# Nutrients in Food

# NUTRIENTS IN FOOD

**ELIZABETH S. HANDS**
*Founder and President, ESHA Research*



LIPPINCOTT WILLIAMS & WILKINS
A **Wolters Kluwer** Company
Philadelphia • Baltimore • New York • London
Buenos Aires • Hong Kong • Sydney • Tokyo

*Editor:* Donna Balado
*Managing Editor:* Matthew Hauber
*Marketing Manager:* Anne Smith
*Project Editor:* Paula C. Williams



351 West Camden Street
Baltimore, Maryland 21201-2436 USA

227 East Washington Square
Philadelphia, PA 19106



The publisher is not responsible (as a matter of product liability, negligence or otherwise) for any injury resulting from any material contained herein. This publication contains information relating to general principles of medical care which should not be construed as specific instructions for individual patients. Manufacturers' product information and package inserts should be reviewed for current information, including contraindications, dosages, and precautions.

*Printed in the United States of America*

**Library of Congress Cataloging-in-Publication Data**

Hands, Elizabeth S.
Nutrients in food / Elizabeth S. Hands.
p. cm.
Includes index.
ISBN 0-683-30705-3
1. Food—Composition—Tables. 2. Food analysis—Tables.
I. Title.
TX551.H274 1999
613.2—dc21
99–17028
CIP

*The publishers have made every effort to trace the copyright holders for borrowed material. If they have inadvertently overlooked any, they will be pleased to make the necessary arrangements at the first opportunity.*

To purchase additional copies of this book, call our customer service department at (800) 638-3030 or fax orders to (301) 824-7390. International customers should call (301) 714-2324.

00 01 02 03
1 2 3 4 5 6 7 8 9 10

To my father, B. Franklin Hunt, and all the other individuals
who inspire curiosity and the love of learning.

# PREFACE

The mission of *Nutrients in Foods* is to provide an excellent reference for those interested in detailed, authoritative information about nutrients in foods, nutrition standards, summary information about each nutrient, and other related information.

*Nutrients in Foods* offers information in an easy-to-read written form, and, in an easy-to-lookup computerized format through CD-ROM lookups. In addition, the reference code for each food can be used in the leading nutrition software packages to build instant nutrition calculations for daily intakes, recipes, or menus. This multi-faceted approach is intended to better assist researchers, dietitians, other health professionals, students, and interested individuals in their work and studies.

We welcome your comments and suggestions about the book and CD-ROM. Your comments will assist us in providing superior products and information to you in the future.

## Your Information Reference—Hard Copy and CD-ROM

This book and CD-ROM offer nutrition standards for the U.S. and Canada, and a means to look up the nutrient content of thousands of elemental, prepared and brand-name foods. The reference code listed for each food item allows menu, recipe, and diet evaluation and planning using the leading nutrition analysis programs: The Food Processor®; Genesis R&D® (ESHA Research, Salem, Oregon); the Nutrition Recipe Analyzer™ (the National Restaurant Association, Chicago, Illinois); and nutrition software for over 80% of college students.

Also provided are information summaries for nutrient factors: 13 vitamins, 11 minerals, and 7 basic food components (proximates): protein, fat, cholesterol, carbohydrate and carbohydrate components, dietary fiber, sugars and other carbohydrates. (VERIFY after final format selection) Supplemental tables of information for many other nutrition components in foods are included also. (See detailed listing in the Contents section.)

## How the Information Is Organized

### Section 1: Introduction

Section 1 includes background and overview information about the nutrient data. Serving sizes of foods (household measure and gram weight) are listed as a reference for the "Nutrients Ranked in Serving Size order" lists for the vitamins and minerals.

### Section 2: Nutrient Standards

Standards for food intake, nutrient intake, ideal weight for height used in the United States and Canada are presented, as well as the Atwater calorie factors for major food groups, sugar, alcohols, and organic acids.

### Section 3: References and Useful Guides

Weight and description of food serving sizes used in the rank order of tables in Sections 5 and 6; conversion factors for weights and measures, food names and synonyms, and abbreviations used in food descriptions are listed here.

### Section 4: Basic Components of Foods

The energy-producing nutrients—proteins, carbohydrates, fats—are discussed in this section, along with water, ash, and alcohol.

### Section 5: Vitamins

Functions, consequences of deficiencies, losses, antagonists, recommended intake, safe upper limits, and other interesting facts are summarized for each vitamin. General food sources are stated and specific food sources are listed in rank order by serving size.

### Section 6: Minerals

Functions, consequences of deficiencies, losses, antagonists, recommended intake, safe upper limits, and other interesting facts are summarized for each mineral. General food sources are stated and specific food sources are listed in rank order by serving size.

### Section 7: Food Nutrient Tables

Use the Contents and the Index to locate food groups and individual foods. Within food groups, foods are listed alphabetically, with two exceptions. Within *Beverages,* Regular beverages are placed before Alcoholic beverages. (Apologies to those who have a different point of view, but we just couldn't bring ourselves to list alcohol at the beginning of a nutrition book.) *Miscellaneous* is at the end, and includes Baking Ingredients (other than flours and sugar), Condiments, and Salsas.

Most food groups are clear, but there are a few tricky areas where a food can be found in more than one food group, or the food group simply may not be obvious. Examples are:

- *Baking Ingredients:* A subcategory of *Miscellaneous.*
- *Cheese & Cheese Substitutes:* Includes dairy and soy products (cheese substitutes, tofu, etc.)
- *Beverages and Beverage Mixes:* Includes fruit flavored drinks, while actual juices are located in their own category—*Fruit, Vegetables & Blended Juices.* Includes beverage mixes and those prepared with milk. Similar products are found in the *Supplements and Formulas* category.
- *Dairy Products and Substitutes:* Includes soy and rice milk as milk substitutes, as well as milks, creams and yogurts from cow milk. Frozen yogurt is listed in Desserts under *Frozen*

*Desserts;* Cheese in *Cheeses and Cheese Substitutes;* and Puddings in Desserts under *Puddings, Custards, & Pie Fillings.*

- *Fats & Oils, Margarines & Shortenings:* Includes butter, margarines, and shortening. Salad dressings and mayonnaise are in a separate group because there are so many non-fat formulas.
- *Fruit, Vegetable & Blended Juices:* Are their own category.
- *Grain Products—Prepared and Baked Goods:* Mostly baked goods, with mixes listed dry and prepared. Sweet rolls, pastries and pie crusts are listed under *Desserts.* Also includes dry and cooked Pasta and Rice, while mixed dishes are in *Meals, Entrees & Dishes.* Seasoning mixes are in *Grains, Flours, Fractions.*
- *Granola Bars, Cereal Bars & Diet Bars* are their own category. Similar products are located in the *Supplements and Formulas* section.
- *Fast Foods:* There are 40 nutrient factors displayed for "generic" fast foods, while brand name items only have the 14-16 "label" nutrients provided by the manufacturer. If you require more accurate and complete data, use the generic data at the beginning of this section.
- *Meals, Entrees, and Dishes:* Includes many mixed dishes, from frozen, dry, and canned forms. Brand Name foods may only include the 14-16 "label" nutrients provided by the manufacturer.
- *Miscellaneous:* Includes baking ingredients, condiments, vinegars, and salsas.
- *Pasta and Rice:* Both cooked and dry forms are subcategories of *Grain Products.* In prepared mixed dishes, they are included in *Meal, Entrées & Dishes.*
- *Salad Dressings, Dips & Mayonnaise.* Dips are included here because of similarities in composition.
- *Salsas & Condiments:* A subcategory of Miscellaneous.
- Soybeans and soy products enjoy multiple status. Versions may be found in *Vegetables & Legumes* (soybeans); *Dairy* (soy milk); *Nuts & Seeds* (soynuts—roasted soybeans); *Cheese* (cheese substitutes—miso, natto, tempeh, tofu); and *Meat Substitutes, Tofu and other Soy/Vegetarian Foods* (soyburgers, etc.)
- *Sauces & Gravies:* Includes tomato sauces for Spaghetti and Pizza and other condiment type sauces.
- *Syrups:* Pancake and Fruit based syrups are listed under *Sweeteners & Sweet Substitutes.* Chocolate and Candy type syrups are listed under *Dessert Toppings.*
- *Vegetables, Legumes & Some Dishes:* Includes dried mature beans and peas (legumes), and some soy products like miso, natto, tempeh and tofu. Although a few vegetable dishes are included here, most are in *Meals, Entrees, & Dishes* and *Snack Foods* (potato chips).

To find a specific food by name, use the Index in the back of the book to locate an exact page number.

### Section 8: Supplementary Tables

This section includes tables for amino acids, alcohol, caffeine, phytosterol, pectin, and theobromine.

## Acknowledgments

Special acknowledgment is given to Elizabeth Braithwaite, R.D., who manages the food/nutrient data at ESHA Research, and Kelly Annotti, lead researcher. These talented individuals are key to the continuing accuracy of the nutrient database and the organization and selection of the foods in this book. Special thanks to Layne Westover, R.D. and Elizabeth Braithwaite for their excellent comments and additions to the narratives.

Finally, a special acknowledgment to all the talented researchers and scientists who use their skills to study the connections between good health and nutrients in foods. The nutrient database herein is a compilation of thousands of their research papers and findings.

# CONTENTS

## SECTION 5 VITAMINS 29



## SECTION 6 MINERALS 53



## SECTION 7 FOOD NUTRIENT TABLES 77

# SECTION 1

# INTRODUCTION

Research for this book began over 18 years ago when we were building an accurate, complete nutrient database for a nutrition analysis software program. At that time, information for nutrients in foods was incomplete and not extensive. So the authors started researching nutrient data sources to create an accurate nutrient database with few missing values.

Hundreds and hundreds of scientific research journals and food composition tables have been reviewed and researched to gather information. Methods and protocols were developed to combine data from multiple sources, reduce missing values, correct errors, and provide quality control to build an enormous repository of information about nutrients in foods. The over 1,200 scientific sources used to compile the ESHA Nutrient database are listed in the CD-ROM that accompanies this book.

The "ESHA" nutrient DataBank now tracks over 165 nutrient factors and is constantly growing and being updated. A selection of those foods and values are part of the leading nutrition software programs[1] and this book. Now, the ESHA Nutrient DataBank is considered a quality standard and is used in major research efforts across the United States and in over 80 other countries.

We are grateful for the many fine researchers, dietitians, and other health professionals throughout the nation who have contributed to the scientific knowledge of nutrition. We also are grateful for those food manufacturers who have contributed information about their products.

## About the Nutrient Data

The most current nutritional data available are presented here, including recently updated values for folate enrichment in foods. These data have been compiled from over 1200 scientific sources of information, including the most recent USDA Data; scientific journal articles; food composition tables from England, Canada, Europe, and Asia; information from other nutrient data banks and publications; unpublished scientific data; and manufacturers' data. These data also reflect information from valuable conversations with researchers throughout the nation, including the professional staff members of the USDA/ARS.

All available sources of nutrient data are considered before data are reported for a food. When multiple values are reported for a nutrient, the numbers are averaged and weighed with consideration for the original number of samples in the separate sources as well as the type of analytical technique applied. When water percentages are available, estimates of nutrient amounts are adjusted for water content. When a reported weight appears inconsistent, kitchen tests are made, and the average weight of the typical product is presented.

Weights for foods are for the edible portion only, unless otherwise specified. For example, the weight of a chicken leg is for the meat only, not the bone. When a serving is 1 ounce, it refers to the measurement, which is often reported as 28 g, 28.4 g, or 28.35 g and not the liquid ounce (fluid oz = fl oz), which is a volume measure that can have varying weight according to the *density* of the item.

## *It Is Important to Know . . .*

Many different nutrient values can be reported for a single food. The values listed here represent average values, and individual food items may vary significantly. Many factors influence nutrients in foods: mineral content of the soil, fertilizer used, genetics of the plant or animal, diet of the animal, method of processing, season of the year, length of storage, method of storage, and cooking method. Other differences can occur in the laboratories: different methods of analysis, variations in moisture content of the samples, and actual conditions in the lab. Manufactured foods may vary because of changes in product formulation, changes in ingredients from a supplier, and changes in package size.

We have attempted to provide the most accurate data available at the time of printing; however, nutrition information is dynamic. There will be changes in nutrient data, new scientific research, and new analytical techniques to measure nutrient content. As a result, nutrient data in this publication should be

[1]The major nutrition programs that contain the ESHA database are *The Food Processor®* and *Genesis R&D®*, published by ESHA Research of Salem, Oregon. Portions of the ESHA Database can be found in the *Nutrition Recipe Analysis*™ (NRA) system from the National Restaurant Association; as well as student versions used by over 80% of all college nutrition students through college text publishers.

viewed and used as a guide—a close approximation of nutrient content of foods. The CD-ROM version will be updated more often; if there is any difference in values, the CD-ROM values should be viewed as the most current resource.

## *Manufactured/Brand Name Food Items—Fewer Nutrients*

The Nutrition Label Education Act (NLEA) standardizes nutritional information on food packaging to assist the public in gaining a better understanding of the foods they are buying. It standardizes serving sizes, eliminates erroneous and misleading health claims, and provides a standardized label format for all food products. The manufacturer is responsible for determining the nutritional content of their product and for accurately presenting the data in terms of the rounding rules laid out by the law for the nutrition facts panel.

Since NLEA was passed, most food manufacturers have been reporting only the 14 or so nutrients required by law. These label data, in addition to being only a subset of nutrients available in foods, are rounded and less accurate for health research. In a time in which the diet-health connection is increasingly known and valued, and diets are comprised of more and more processed foods, this lack of full data development has inadvertently set back health research efforts.

Fortunately, some manufacturers provide the prelabel data, which has not been rounded and is more accurate. Also, some manufacturers are starting to provide information on additional nutrients as they realize how important it is for health research. We use the most accurate manufacturers' data provided.

## *Interpreting the Information*

Keep in mind that nutrient data should be viewed and used only as a guide, a close approximation of nutrient content. Here are some examples:

- Small variations do not signify that one food is nutritionally superior than another food, because it is possible to get small variations between foods that are "mathematical" in nature, not material. Most nutrient data are values derived by averaging multiple test results; values from just one analysis, or just one sample are important, but are not considered as reliable.
- If two samples of the same food contain differing amounts of *moisture,* the dryer item will contain more nutrients by weight. A small change in moisture content of a food item will alter the nutrient content, sometimes significantly.
- Local water supplies contain minerals that are unique to an area, and may affect processed food items that use this water. This information can be obtained from local government agencies.
- Sometimes frozen foods will show a larger amount of a nutrient compared to the same portion of the fresh or cooked from fresh item. This is because freezing breaks down the cell walls of the food, resulting in a denser food when cooked or served.
- Cooking sometimes causes moisture loss. This loss of moisture results in more dry matter and, therefore, a higher nutrient density for some nutrients.
- Nutrient values for recipes and combination foods are derived from average recipes. Obviously, the data will vary for specific recipes. In addition, manufacturers modify their formulations and recipes from time to time, and values will change accordingly.
- Cuts of meat are typically common cuts. What we commonly think of as a breast of chicken is referred to as a half breast in research data. In this document, we use the more common term, one breast of chicken (two per bird).
- Niacin values are for preformed niacin and do not include additional niacin that may form in the body from the conversion of tryptophan.
- Folate values are for total folate in foods, and do not allow for the increased bioavailability of the folic acid added to enrich breads and rice and grain products such as pasta.

# Sources of Data

The sources of data are listed on the CD-ROM accompanying this book. A bibliography for information on basic food components is also listed at the end of Section 6, Minerals and Food Sources.

# SECTION 2

# NUTRITION STANDARDS

The nutrition standards are intended to provide guidance for good health by estimating necessary intake levels of essential nutrients and energy. These values result from the collective scientific judgment of many research scientists who evaluate current research information and relationships between nutrition and disease.

Where information is known, standards allow and provide for: bioavailability; interactions with other nutrients; precursor forms; the larger average size of males if appropriate; variation in individual metabolisms; the availability in the food supply; and any other relevant factors. Keep in mind the following considerations about the values in these recommendations:

- The nutrient values refer to individuals' average nutrient intake over time. The amount taken from day to day can vary substantially without ill effect.
- These amounts are for healthy people. They may not be sufficient for individuals who are already malnourished or have disease states that result in malabsorption syndrome; those who are receiving dialysis treatments; or those who have increased nutrient requirements for other health reasons. A Registered Dietitian or nutrition-knowledgeable health *professional* should be consulted to determine appropriate values.
- The values refer to a standard average size man or woman with a light to moderate activity level, and require adjustment if the individual is significantly different from the norms. If differences are a result of obesity, then a Registered Dietitian should be consulted to determine appropriate values.
- We eat *foods*—not nutrients. Therefore, nutrient standards for food intake patterns are important. Refer to *Dietary Guidelines for Americans* and *The Food Pyramid.*
- Enjoy your food! It should be pleasurable to smell the aroma of food cooking, to consume good flavors and textures, and to enjoy the company of your family and friends while you are eating.

## Dietary Guidelines for Americans

These guidelines[1] are designed to provide advice for healthy Americans about food choices that promote health and prevent disease. To meet these guidelines, select a diet with most of the calories from grain products, vegetables, fruits, lowfat milk products, lean meats, fish, poultry, and dry beans. Choose fewer calories from fats and sweets. These choices refer to diets consumed over several days, not to single meals or foods.

- **Eat a variety of foods daily.**
  No single food can supply all nutrients in the amounts required. Therefore, to obtain the nutrients, energy, and other factors you need for good health, a variety of foods should be consumed. To ensure an adequate intake of nutrients and other substances you need for good health, choose the recommended number of servings from the food groups in the Food Guide Pyramid.
- **Balance the food you eat with physical activity—maintain or reduce your weight.**
  Increase physical activity. Spend more time walking, using stairs, and doing other physical activities. Try to do 30 minutes or more of moderate physical activity every day. Many Americans spend much of their working day at a desk—a low-energy activity. In addition, many spend leisure time being inactive, for example, watching television. To evaluate your body weight, see Table 2.2.

[1]Source: Adapted from Dietary Guidelines for Americans, 4th Edition, US Department of Agriculture, US Department of Health and Human Services, Nutrition and Your Health, Washington, D.C. Government Printing Office, 1995.

- **Consume a diet with plenty of grain products (breads, pasta, cereal, and rice), vegetables, and fruits. Eat cooked dry beans, lentils, and peas more often.**
  These key foods are generally nutrient dense and low in fat. In addition, they give the body a feeling of satiety and fullness because they provide bulk and are rich in complex carbohydrates (fiber and starch).
- **Choose a diet low in fat, saturated fat, and cholesterol.**
  Dietary fats are important for good health. They supply essential fatty acids, promote absorption of the fat-soluble vitamins A, D, E, and K, and provide energy. However, fat also provides twice the number of calories of an equal amount of protein or carbohydrate.

  Because fat also provides a feeling of satiety, too much fat in the diet may crowd out the desire to consume nutrient-rich foods like grains, vegetables, and fruits. Over time, an excess fat intake may lead to obesity. Therefore, it is suggested that no more than 30% of daily calories come from fat. This advice does not apply to children below 5 years of age.
- **Select a diet moderate in sugars.**
  Use less sugar, syrup, and honey; and reduce concentrated sweets like candy, soft drinks, cookies, etc., because they provide many calories and few nutrients. Select fresh fruits or fruits canned in light syrup or their own juices. Read food labels—sucrose, glucose, dextrose, maltose, lactose, fructose, syrups, and honey are all sugars. Eating less sugar also reduces dental caries.
- **Choose a diet moderate in salt and sodium.**
  Learn to enjoy the flavors of unsalted foods; flavor foods with herbs, spices, lemon juice, and vinegar. Reduce salt in cooking and add little or less salt at the table. Limit salty foods like potato chips, pretzels, salted nuts, popcorn, condiments (soy sauce, steak sauce, and garlic salt), some cheeses, pickled foods and cured meats, and some canned vegetables and soups. Read food labels for sodium or salt contents, especially in processed and snack foods; use low-sodium products.
- **If you drink alcoholic beverages, do so in moderation.**
  For individuals who choose to drink, limit all alcoholic beverages (including wine, beer, liquors, etc.) to one or two drinks per day. "One drink" means 12 oz of beer, 3 oz of wine, or 1-1/2 oz of distilled spirits. If you drink, do not drive. Pregnant women should refrain from the use of alcohol.

## Nutrients from Foods or from Supplements

The nutrient standards are established for needed nutrients, *but not all of them.* Researchers are continually learning of factors that are essential to good health and disease prevention, such as phytochemicals, flavonoids, carotenoids, anthocyanins, and many more, primarily from vegetables, fruits, nuts, and grains. Foods, therefore, are our best source for known and unknown vitamins and minerals.

Nutrient supplements cannot provide the "yet to be discovered" nutrients in foods, but they can provide concentrated amounts of known nutrients to compensate for dietary deficiencies. They can also provide concentrated high intake levels, which for some nutrients and individual situations have resulted in excellent health benefits. Although some studies are showing good benefits of concentrated dosages for some forms of supplements, there are also more reports of potential adverse effects of such prolonged concentrated intake. Not enough information is available yet to understand the safety limits or to know if there is long-term potential harm; however, these concerns should not be ignored. Here are some considerations regarding the positive use and misuse of nutrients in supplemental form.

- Nutrients seldom work in isolation from others. Most nutrients require other nutrients to be present to do their job well. A mixed diet provides this needed variety.
- Some food volume is usually necessary for most nutrients to be absorbed into the body, and oil-soluble nutrients require some fat to be absorbed (vitamins A, D, E, K, and the carotenoids). There are exceptions to this. *Some* supplements are even more bioavailable than the forms found in food. For example, the chemical form of folate and some chemical forms of vitamin A retinol are almost fully absorbed if taken without food.
- Supplements can deliver therapeutic levels of nutrients to correct a problem, to enhance health, and to compensate for diet deficiencies.
- Carotenoids are stable in foods and many keep their activity even when cooked. However, if dried or freeze-dried in the presence of air, carotenoids become oxidized and ineffective; retention is better if prepared in a closed-air process. Some supplements contain the dried form of fruits and vegetables. If the preparation was done in a *closed-air* process, nutrient activity may be only partially affected. If they are dried or freeze-dried in the presence of air, they may oxidize and be ineffective. More research is needed on this subject.
- Toxicity from *food intake* of nutrients is not known (with the *extremely* rare exception of vitamin A toxicity from consuming a lot of polar bear liver). However, nutrient load from supplements sometimes confounds and overwhelms the body's mechanisms for absorbing some nutrients into the body, resulting in one of several possible situations:
  —When one nutrient intake dominates excessively over others (as in supplement-size doses) it may block the absorption of the others, resulting in deficiencies in other nutrients even when dietary intake is otherwise adequate.
  —Overload may prevent absorption. The body has mechanisms for refusing additional nutrients when the body has enough, or when the body transport systems are filled up. This means that excess nutrients pass unused out of the body. This is true for most nutrients, but not all. Divided doses over time (similar to meals and snacks throughout the day) are best.
  —Toxicity may occur. If excessive doses are absorbed over an extended period of time, it may overwhelm the body balance. Reports of nutrient toxicity has increased for some supplements.

## The Food Pyramid

The Food Pyramid is another tool for providing dietary guidance. To ensure a good foundation of nutrient factors in foods, the pyramid recommends a daily intake based on different proportions of foods within major food groups. The serving sizes shown in Table 2.1 are averages, and those who eat significantly more or less food should look at the relative proportions, not just the number of servings.

TABLE 2.1 Pyramid Daily Food Servings for Health—Example Portions

| Pyramid Food Group | # of Servings | Serving Size Examples |
|---|---|---|
| Bread, cereal, rice & pasta | 6–11 servings | 1 slice of bread<br>1 oz of ready-to-eat cereal<br>1/2 cup of cooked cereal, rice, or pasta. |
| Vegetable group | 3–5 servings | 1 cup of raw leafy vegetables<br>1/2 cup of other vegetables, cooked, or chopped raw<br>3/4 cup of vegetable juice |
| Fruit group | 2–4 servings | 1 medium apple, banana, orange<br>1/2 cup of chopped, cooked, or canned fruit<br>3/4 cup of fruit juice |
| Meat, Poultry, Fish, Dry Beans, Eggs, Nuts & Soy Products | 2–3 servings; or about 5–7 oz of meat a day | 2–3-1/2 oz of cooked lean meat, poultry, or fish<br>These foods count as 1 oz of lean meat:<br>1/2 cup of cooked dry beans[a]<br>1 egg<br>2 Tbsp peanut butter, 1/3 cup nuts<br>1/2 cup of soy products, tofu, etc. |
| Milk, Yogurt & Cheese Group | 2 servings, or<br>3 servings if pregnant or breast feeding | 1 cup of milk or yogurt<br>1-1/2 oz of natural cheese<br>2 oz of processed cheese |
| Fats & Oils, cream, margarine & butter, salad dressings, sweets, soft drinks, alcohol, most desserts. | Use sparingly | These items consist of *added* fat and sugar that do not naturally occur in the food. No serving sizes are specified. |

[a]Dried beans, peas, and lentils can be counted in either the meat and beans or the vegetable group.

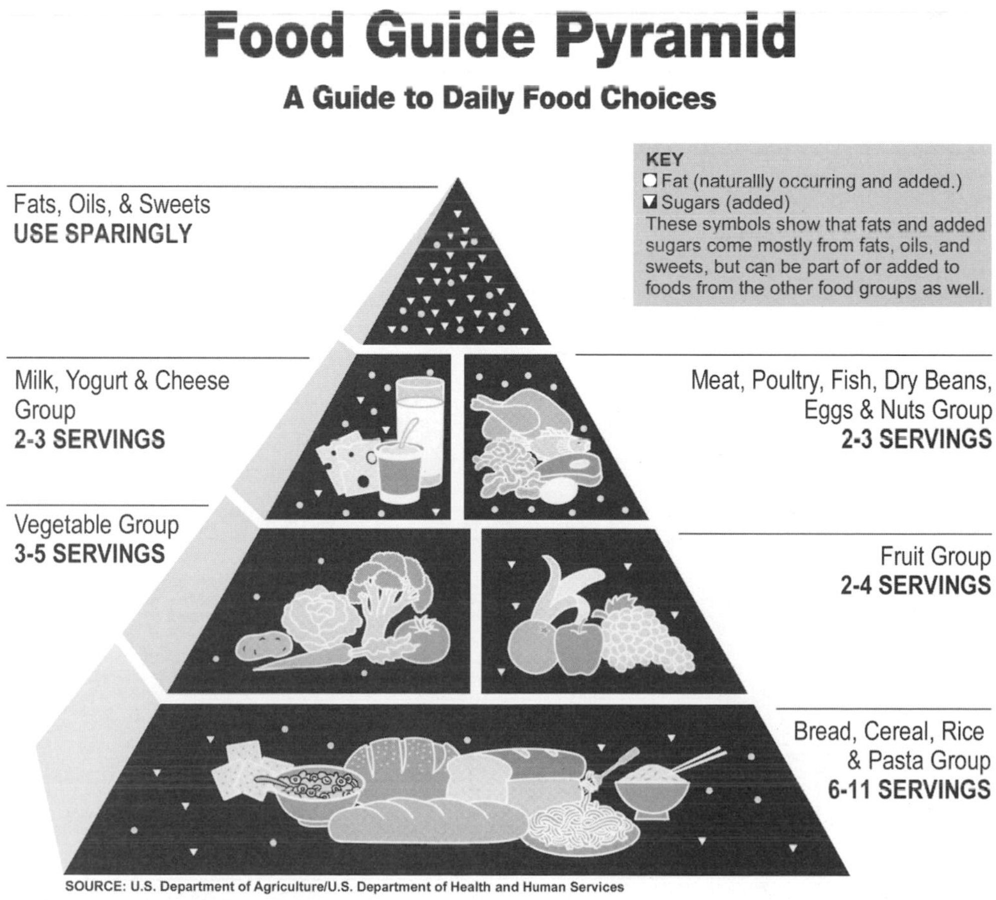

TABLE 2.2 **Evaluate Your Weight for Height**

| Body Mass Index (BMI) Height | 18 | 19 | 20 | 21 | 22 | 23 | 24 | 25 | 26 | 27 | 28 | 29 | 30 | 31 | 32 | 33 | 34 | 35 | 36 | 37 | 38 | 39 | 40 |
|---|---|---|---|---|---|---|---|---|---|---|---|---|---|---|---|---|---|---|---|---|---|---|---|
| | | | | | | | | Body Weight (lb) | | | | | | | | | | | | | | | |
| 4'10" | 86 | 91 | 96 | 100 | 105 | 110 | 115 | 119 | 124 | 129 | 134 | 138 | 143 | 148 | 153 | 158 | 162 | 167 | 172 | 177 | 181 | 186 | 191 |
| 4'11" | 89 | 94 | 99 | 104 | 109 | 114 | 119 | 124 | 128 | 133 | 138 | 143 | 148 | 153 | 158 | 163 | 168 | 173 | 178 | 183 | 188 | 193 | 198 |
| 5'0" | 92 | 97 | 102 | 107 | 112 | 118 | 123 | 128 | 133 | 138 | 143 | 148 | 153 | 158 | 163 | 168 | 174 | 179 | 184 | 189 | 194 | 199 | 204 |
| 5'1" | 95 | 100 | 106 | 111 | 116 | 122 | 127 | 132 | 137 | 143 | 148 | 153 | 158 | 164 | 169 | 174 | 180 | 185 | 190 | 195 | 201 | 206 | 211 |
| 5'2" | 98 | 104 | 109 | 115 | 120 | 126 | 131 | 136 | 142 | 147 | 153 | 158 | 164 | 169 | 175 | 180 | 186 | 191 | 196 | 202 | 207 | 213 | 218 |
| 5'3" | 102 | 107 | 113 | 118 | 124 | 130 | 135 | 141 | 146 | 152 | 158 | 163 | 169 | 175 | 180 | 186 | 191 | 197 | 203 | 208 | 214 | 220 | 225 |
| 5'4" | 105 | 110 | 116 | 122 | 128 | 134 | 140 | 145 | 151 | 157 | 163 | 169 | 174 | 180 | 186 | 192 | 197 | 204 | 209 | 215 | 221 | 227 | 232 |
| 5'5" | 108 | 114 | 120 | 126 | 132 | 138 | 144 | 150 | 156 | 162 | 168 | 174 | 180 | 186 | 192 | 198 | 204 | 210 | 216 | 222 | 228 | 234 | 240 |
| 5'6" | 112 | 118 | 124 | 130 | 136 | 142 | 148 | 155 | 161 | 167 | 173 | 179 | 186 | 192 | 198 | 204 | 210 | 216 | 223 | 229 | 235 | 241 | 247 |
| 5'7" | 115 | 121 | 127 | 134 | 140 | 146 | 153 | 159 | 166 | 172 | 178 | 185 | 191 | 198 | 204 | 211 | 217 | 223 | 230 | 236 | 242 | 249 | 255 |
| 5'8" | 118 | 125 | 131 | 138 | 144 | 151 | 158 | 164 | 171 | 177 | 184 | 190 | 197 | 203 | 210 | 216 | 223 | 230 | 236 | 243 | 249 | 256 | 262 |
| 5'9" | 122 | 128 | 135 | 142 | 149 | 155 | 162 | 169 | 176 | 182 | 189 | 196 | 203 | 209 | 216 | 223 | 230 | 236 | 243 | 250 | 257 | 263 | 270 |
| 5'10" | 126 | 132 | 139 | 146 | 153 | 160 | 167 | 174 | 181 | 188 | 195 | 202 | 209 | 216 | 222 | 229 | 236 | 243 | 250 | 257 | 264 | 271 | 278 |
| 5'11" | 129 | 136 | 143 | 150 | 157 | 165 | 172 | 179 | 186 | 193 | 200 | 208 | 215 | 222 | 229 | 236 | 243 | 250 | 257 | 265 | 272 | 279 | 286 |
| 6'0" | 132 | 140 | 147 | 154 | 162 | 169 | 177 | 184 | 191 | 199 | 206 | 213 | 221 | 228 | 235 | 242 | 250 | 258 | 265 | 272 | 279 | 287 | 294 |
| 6'1" | 136 | 144 | 151 | 159 | 166 | 174 | 182 | 189 | 197 | 204 | 212 | 219 | 227 | 235 | 242 | 250 | 257 | 265 | 272 | 280 | 288 | 295 | 302 |
| 6'2" | 141 | 148 | 155 | 163 | 171 | 179 | 186 | 194 | 202 | 210 | 218 | 225 | 233 | 241 | 249 | 256 | 264 | 272 | 280 | 287 | 295 | 303 | 311 |
| 6'3" | 144 | 152 | 160 | 168 | 176 | 184 | 192 | 200 | 208 | 216 | 224 | 232 | 240 | 248 | 256 | 264 | 272 | 279 | 287 | 295 | 303 | 311 | 319 |
| 6'4" | 148 | 156 | 164 | 172 | 180 | 189 | 197 | 205 | 213 | 221 | 230 | 238 | 246 | 254 | 263 | 271 | 279 | 287 | 295 | 304 | 312 | 320 | 328 |
| 6'5" | 151 | 160 | 168 | 176 | 185 | 193 | 202 | 210 | 218 | 227 | 235 | 244 | 252 | 261 | 269 | 277 | 286 | 294 | 303 | 311 | 319 | 328 | 336 |
| 6'6" | 155 | 164 | 172 | 181 | 190 | 198 | 207 | 216 | 224 | 233 | 241 | 250 | 259 | 267 | 276 | 284 | 293 | 302 | 310 | 319 | 328 | 336 | 345 |
| Underweight (<18.5) | | Healthy Weight (18.5–24.9) | | | | | | Overweight (25–29.9) | | | | | | | | Obese (≥30) | | | | | | | |

Source and Credit: "A Better Way to Check Your Weight" from the Tufts University Health and Nutrition Letter, April 1997, published by Tufts University, New York, NY.

## Your Body Mass Index and Acceptable Weight for Height

Tables 2.2 and 2.3 allow you to determine your body mass index (BMI) without a calculator and to determine your acceptable weight range for your height. The BMI is calculated by dividing weight in kilograms by height in meters squared. To use the table, find your height in the first column then scan across that row to find your weight. If your weight is in the white area (columns 19–25), your weight for height is considered fine. If your weight is in the lightly shaded areas (columns 26–27), you are pushing the edge.

Most researchers generally agree that the larger numbers (columns 28 and greater) are associated with more health risk of being overweight. Please note, however, that some individuals with high BMIs may not be "fat." Body builders, or others with high muscle mass, may score a high BMI because muscle is about twice the weight of fat. *Where* a person carries their fat is also important for health risk. Fat carried around the abdomen (an apple shape) is associated with much more health risk than fat deposited around the hips and thighs (a pear shape).

TABLE 2.3 **Body Mass Index and Grades of Chronic Protein-Energy Malnutrition and Obesity**

| Grade | Body Mass Index |
|---|---|
| Obesity | |
| III | >40 |
| II | 30–40 |
| I | 25–29.9 |
| Normal | ≥18.5–<25 |
| Protein-energy malnutrition | |
| I | 17.0–18.4 |
| II | 16.0–16.9 |
| III | <16 |

(Adapted from James, W. P. T., Ferro-Luzzi, A., Waterlow, J. C.: Eur J Clin Nutr, 42:969–981; and McLaren, D.S.: A fresh look at anthropometric classification schemes in protein-energy malnutrition. In Anthropometric Assessment of Nutritional Status. Edited by J. H. Himes. New York, Wiley-Liss, 1991, pp. 273–286.)

## Dietary Intake Standards for the U.S.—the DRIs[2]

In 1997 and 1998, new recommendations were published for 14 nutrients. The new recommendations are the result of an extensive effort, including input from nutrition experts from both the United States and Canada.

The title for these new standards, the Dietary Reference Intakes (DRIs), will replace the title of Recommended Dietary Allowances (the RDAs) that have served as the Nutrient Standard for more than 50 years. Table 2.4 combines the new recommendations with the remaining 1989 RDAs (9 nutrients).

The RDA term will still be used for those nutrient recommendations that have the widest based assurance of research behind the values, and all recommended amounts are based on the nutrient amounts to maintain a healthy population. Some of the changes and basic considerations are listed as follows:

- Amounts are recommended for healthy individuals and may not be adequate for individuals who are already malnourished; have disease states that result in malabsorption syndrome; are receiving dialysis treatments; or have increased nutrient requirements for other health reasons.
- The nutrient values refer to an average nutrient intake of individuals over time. The amount taken from day to day can vary substantially without ill effect.
- Recommendations for biotin, choline, fluoride, and pantothenic acid have been added. All, except for choline, were previously listed under the 1989 Estimated Safe and Adequate Intake list.
- Folate is now measured in mcg of Folate Equivalents (FE) or Dietary Folate Equivalents (DFE). The equivalency measure was used because flour and breads are now enriched with folate, and the chemical form of folate is more bioavailable than regular food folate.
- Age groups are now called life-stages. The new standards have added a category for those age 70 years and older, and have slightly modified some of the younger age groups.

### *Terms and Definitions*

- RDA is the average intake of essential nutrients that is sufficient to meet the nutrient requirement of nearly all (97–98%) healthy persons in a particular life stage. Within the DRI framework, the RDA is only used as a goal for individuals.
- AI, or Adequate Intake, is the term used when an RDA cannot be determined for a nutrient, and is based on observed or experimentally determined approximations of nutrient intake by a group or groups of healthy people. The AI serves to emphasize the need for more research on requirements of that nutrient. All recommendations for infants are considered Adequate Intakes (AIs), and are the mean, or average, intake for healthy breast-fed infants.
- The UL, or Tolerable Upper Limit, is the highest level of daily nutrient intake that is likely to pose no risks of adverse health effects to almost all individuals in the general population. ULs are useful because of the increased interest and availability of fortified foods and dietary supplements.
- The EAR, or Estimated Average Requirement, is estimated to meet the requirement of half the healthy individuals in a group. It is used to assess the nutrient adequacy of population groups and is a component used to develop RDAs.

## U.S. Estimated Safe and Adequate Daily Intakes

The 1989 Estimated Safe and Adequate Intakes (ESAI) (Table 2.5) are presented as a range of values because there is less scientific information on which to base a single recommended amount. It is recommended that the upper values for these trace elements should not be exceeded habitually because toxic levels may only be several times the usual intakes.

[2]Sources: The 1997 Dietary Reference Intakes: Calcium, Phosphorus, Magnesium, Vitamin D, and Fluoride; A Report of the Standing Committee on the Scientific Evaluation of Dietary Reference Intakes of the Food and Nutrition Board, Institute of Medicine, National Academy of Sciences. Washington, D.C.: National Academy Press, 1997. The 1998 Dietary Reference Intakes: Thiamin, Riboflavin, Niacin, Vitamin B6, Folate, Vitamin B12, Pantothenic Acid, Biotin, and Choline; A Report of the Standing Committee on the Scientific Evaluation of Dietary Reference Intakes of the Food and Nutrition Board, Institute of Medicine, National Academy of Sciences, with the involvement of Health Canada. Washington, D.C.: National Academy Press, 1998.

TABLE 2.4 **U.S. Recommendations for Nutrient Intakes**

| Reference Size | | | | | Recommended Dietary Allowances (RDA) 1989 | | | | | | | | |
|---|---|---|---|---|---|---|---|---|---|---|---|---|---|
| Age | Weight kg | Weight lb | Height cm | Height in | Protein (g) | Vit A (RE) | Vit E (mg aTE) | Vit K (mcg) | Vit C (mg) | Iodine (mcg) | Iron (mg) | Selenium (mcg) | Zinc (mg) |
| **Infants** | | | | | | | | | | | | | |
| 0.0–0.5 | 6 | 13 | 60 | 24 | 13 | 375 | 3 | 5 | 30 | 40 | 6 | 10 | 5 |
| 0.5–1.0 | 9 | 20 | 71 | 28 | 14 | 375 | 4 | 10 | 35 | 50 | 10 | 15 | 5 |
| **Children** | | | | | | | | | | | | | |
| 1–3 | 13 | 29 | 90 | 35 | 16 | 400 | 6 | 15 | 40 | 70 | 10 | 20 | 10 |
| 4–6 | 20 | 44 | 112 | 44 | 24 | 500 | 7 | 20 | 45 | 90 | 10 | 20 | 10 |
| 7–10 | 28 | 62 | 132 | 52 | 28 | 700 | 7 | 30 | 45 | 120 | 10 | 30 | 10 |
| **Males** | | | | | | | | | | | | | |
| 11–14 | 45 | 99 | 157 | 62 | 45 | 1000 | 10 | 45 | 50 | 150 | 12 | 40 | 15 |
| 15–18 | 66 | 145 | 176 | 69 | 59 | 1000 | 10 | 65 | 60 | 150 | 12 | 50 | 15 |
| 19–24 | 72 | 160 | 177 | 70 | 58 | 1000 | 10 | 70 | 60 | 150 | 10 | 70 | 15 |
| 25–50 | 79 | 174 | 176 | 70 | 63 | 1000 | 10 | 80 | 60 | 150 | 10 | 70 | 15 |
| 51 + | 77 | 170 | 173 | 68 | 63 | 1000 | 10 | 80 | 60 | 150 | 10 | 70 | 15 |
| **Females** | | | | | | | | | | | | | |
| 11–14 | 46 | 101 | 157 | 62 | 46 | 800 | 8 | 45 | 50 | 150 | 15 | 45 | 12 |
| 15–18 | 55 | 120 | 163 | 64 | 44 | 800 | 8 | 55 | 60 | 150 | 15 | 50 | 12 |
| 19–24 | 58 | 128 | 164 | 65 | 46 | 800 | 8 | 60 | 60 | 150 | 15 | 55 | 12 |
| 25–50 | 63 | 138 | 163 | 64 | 50 | 800 | 8 | 65 | 60 | 150 | 15 | 55 | 12 |
| 51 + | 65 | 143 | 160 | 63 | 50 | 800 | 8 | 65 | 60 | 150 | 10 | 55 | 12 |
| Pregnant | | | | | | | | | | | | | |
| | | | | | 60 | 800 | 10 | 65 | 70 | 175 | 30 | 65 | 15 |
| Breastfeeding/Lactating | | | | | | | | | | | | | |
| 1st 6 mo. | | | | | 65 | 1300 | 12 | 65 | 95 | 200 | 15 | 75 | 19 |
| 2nd 6 mo. | | | | | 62 | 1200 | 11 | 65 | 90 | 200 | 15 | 75 | 16 |

| Dietary Reference Intakes (DRI) 1997–1998 | | | | | | | | | | | | | | |
|---|---|---|---|---|---|---|---|---|---|---|---|---|---|---|
| Life-Stage Group | Thiamin (mg) | Riboflavin (mg) | Niacin (mg NE) | Vit B6 (mg) | Folate (FE) | Vit B12 (mcg) | Vit D (mcg) | Calcium (mg) | Phosphorus (mg) | Magnesium (mg) | Fluoride (mg) | Pantothenic (mg) | Biotin (mcg) | Choline (mg) |
| **Infants** | | | | | | | | | | | | | | |
| 0.0–0.5 | 0.2 | 0.3 | 2 | 0.1 | 65 | 0.4 | 5 | 210 | 100 | 30 | 0.01 | 1.7 | 5 | 125 |
| 0.5–1.0 | 0.3 | 0.4 | 3 | 0.3 | 80 | 0.5 | 5 | 270 | 275 | 75 | 0.5 | 1.8 | 6 | 150 |
| **Children** | | | | | | | | | | | | | | |
| 1–3 | 0.5 | 0.5 | 6 | 0.5 | 150 | 0.9 | 5 | 500 | 460 | 80 | 0.7 | 2 | 8 | 200 |
| 4–8 | 0.6 | 0.6 | 8 | 0.6 | 200 | 1.2 | 5 | 800 | 500 | 130 | 1.1 | 3 | 12 | 250 |
| **Males** | | | | | | | | | | | | | | |
| 9–13 | 0.9 | 0.9 | 12 | 1.0 | 300 | 1.8 | 5 | 1300 | 1250 | 240 | 2.0 | 4 | 20 | 375 |
| 14–18 | 1.2 | 1.3 | 16 | 1.3 | 400 | 2.4 | 5 | 1300 | 1250 | 410 | 3.2 | 5 | 25 | 550 |
| 19–30 | 1.2 | 1.3 | 16 | 1.3 | 400 | 2.4 | 5 | 1000 | 700 | 400 | 3.8 | 5 | 30 | 550 |
| 31–50 | 1.2 | 1.3 | 16 | 1.3 | 400 | 2.4 | 5 | 1000 | 700 | 420 | 3.8 | 5 | 30 | 550 |
| 51–70 | 1.2 | 1.3 | 16 | 1.7 | 400 | 2.4 | 10 | 1200 | 700 | 420 | 3.8 | 5 | 30 | 550 |
| > 70 | 1.2 | 1.3 | 16 | 1.7 | 400 | 2.4 | 15 | 1200 | 700 | 420 | 3.8 | 5 | 30 | 550 |
| **Females** | | | | | | | | | | | | | | |
| 9–13 | 0.9 | 0.9 | 12 | 1.0 | 300 | 1.8 | 5 | 1300 | 1250 | 240 | 2.0 | 4 | 20 | 375 |
| 14–18 | 1.1 | 1.0 | 14 | 1.2 | 400 | 2.4 | 5 | 1300 | 1250 | 360 | 2.9 | 5 | 25 | 400 |
| 19–30 | 1.1 | 1.1 | 14 | 1.3 | 400 | 2.4 | 5 | 1000 | 700 | 310 | 3.1 | 5 | 30 | 425 |
| 31–50 | 1.1 | 1.1 | 14 | 1.3 | 400 | 2.4 | 5 | 1000 | 700 | 320 | 3.1 | 5 | 30 | 425 |
| 51–70 | 1.1 | 1.1 | 14 | 1.5 | 400 | 2.4 | 10 | 1200 | 700 | 320 | 3.1 | 5 | 30 | 425 |
| >70 | 1.1 | 1.1 | 14 | 1.5 | 400 | 2.4 | 15 | 1200 | 700 | 320 | 3.1 | 5 | 30 | 425 |
| Pregnant | | | | | | | | | | | | | | |
| | 1.4 | 1.4 | 18 | 1.9 | 600 | 2.6 | nc | nc | nc | +40 | nc | 6 | 30 | 450 |
| Breastfeeding/Lactating | | | | | | | | | | | | | | |
| | 1.5 | 1.6 | 17 | 2.0 | 500 | 2.8 | nc | nc | nc | nc | nc | 7 | 35 | 550 |

nc = no change

Table adapted from information from three publications of the National Academy of Sciences, Food and Nutrition Board, National Academy Press: *Recommended Dietary Allowances*, 10th edition, 1989; *Dietary Reference Intakes for Calcium, Phosphorus, Magnesium, Vitamin D, & Fluoride*, 1997; and Dietary Reference Intakes for Folate, Thiamin, Riboflavin, Niacin, Vitamin B6, Vitamin B12, Pantothenic Acid, Biotin and Choline, 1998. Adaptation © copyright

TABLE 2.5 U.S. Estimated Safe and Adequate Daily Intake of Selected Vitamins and Minerals, 1989

| | Age (years) | Biotin[a] (mcg) | Pantothenic[a] (mg) | Fluoride[a] (mg) | Chromium (mcg) | Copper (mg) | Manganese (mg) | Molybdenum (mcg) |
|---|---|---|---|---|---|---|---|---|
| Infants | 0.0–0.5 | 10 | 2 | 0.1–0.5 | 10–40 | 0.4–0.6 | 0.3–0.6 | 15–30 |
| | 0.5–1.0 | 15 | 3 | 0.2–1.0 | 20–60 | 0.6–0.7 | 0.6–1.0 | 20–40 |
| Children | 1–3 | 20 | 3 | 0.5–1.5 | 20–80 | 0.7–1.0 | 1.0–1.5 | 25–50 |
| | 4–6 | 25 | 3–4 | 1.0–2.5 | 30–120 | 1.0–1.5 | 1.5–2.0 | 30–75 |
| | 7–10 | 30 | 4–5 | 1.5–2.5 | 50–200 | 1.0–2.0 | 2.0–3.0 | 50–150 |
| | 11+ | 30–100 | 4–7 | 1.5–2.5 | 50–200 | 1.5–2.5 | 2.0–5.0 | 75–250 |
| Adults | | 30–100 | 4–7 | 1.5–4.0 | 50–200 | 1.5–3.0 | 2.0–5.0 | 75–250 |

Source: Recommended Dietary Allowances, 10th ed. National Academy Press, Washington, D.C., 1989, page 284.
[a]The values for Biotin, Pantothenic Acid, and Fluoride are provided for reference purposes only. The shaded columns identify those nutrient values that have been updated and are now part of the 1998 Daily Reference Intakes.

TABLE 2.6 Estimated Minimum Daily Intakes for Sodium, Chloride, and Potassium

| Reference | | Sodium[a] (mg) | Chloride[a] (mg) | Potassium[a] (mg) |
|---|---|---|---|---|
| Age | Weight (kg) | | | |
| 0–5 mo | 4.5 | 120 | 180 | 500 |
| 6–11 mo | 8.9 | 200 | 300 | 700 |
| 1 yr | 11 | 225 | 350 | 1,000 |
| 2–5 yr | 16 | 300 | 500 | 1,400 |
| 6–9 yr | 25 | 400 | 600 | 1,600 |
| 10–18 yr | 50 | 500 | 750 | 2,000 |
| Over 18 yr | 70 | 500 | 750 | 2,000 |

Source: Adapted from the Recommended Dietary Allowances, 10th ed. National Academy Press, Washington, D.C., 1989, page 243.
[a]Minimums, not optimums.

## Estimated Minimums for Sodium, Chloride, and Potassium

Although *minimums* have been estimated, *optimums* have not. In these minimum values, there is no allowance for large prolonged losses from sweating or any special needs due to ill health. Desirable intakes of potassium, for example, considerably exceed these values and range about 3500 mg for adults. The values in Table 2.6 are suggested minimum intake levels for persons in good health. Read more about these minerals in Section 5.

## Reference Values Used for Food Labels

Nutrition facts panels on food labels use reference values to standardize the label information. The reference daily intakes (RDI) are based on those nutrients with Recommended Dietary Allowances—protein, vitamins, and minerals.

The Daily Reference Values (DRVs) are for other nutrients with more general standards—energy/calories, sodium, and potassium. The sources of energy assume 2000 kcalories a day with 10% from protein, 60% from carbohydrate, 30% from fat, and 10% from saturated fat.

Together the two sets of information (DRVs and RDAs) comprise the Daily Values used on food labels. The mandatory and voluntary components for adults and children over 4 years of age are shown in Table 2.7.

## Recommended Energy Intake

The calorie values shown in Tables 2.8 to 2.10 represent the *average* needs of individuals. Depending on the individual's personal metabolism, these values can vary ±20% within the light-to-moderate activity level. The numbers listed for calories per day are calculated based on FAO equations and then rounded. The Multiples[1] of the Resting Energy Expenditure (REE) are factors that represent average additional caloric needs for persons with light-to-moderate activity, as suggested by the World Health Organization (WHO).

## Diabetic Food Exchanges

Food Exchanges (Table 2.11), also referred to as Diabetic Exchanges, are a popular method for understanding and gaining control over calorie intake from fat and carbohydrates. Although Food Exchanges do not consider vitamin and mineral intake and are not precise, they provide a excellent tool for many individuals.

The exchange system is based on eight groupings of foods. Within each group, foods have similar calorie, protein, carbohydrate, and fat values per serving. In this way, a food from one group can be "exchanged" for another food in that group. This is useful to add variety in meal planning. The following are the eight groupings of foods:

| | |
|---|---|
| Bread/Starch | Fruit |
| Other Carbohydrates | Vegetables |
| Very Lean Meat | Milk (nonfat) |
| Lean Meat | Fat |

Foods that are high in sugar carbohydrates, e.g., cakes, cookies, fat-free ice cream, pies, puddings, etc., are assigned to "Other Carbohydrate" exchanges. (Previous exchange definitions

TABLE 2.7 **Mandatory and Voluntary Reference Value Components for U.S. Food Labels**

| Mandatory Components | | Voluntary Components | |
|---|---|---|---|
| Total Fat | 65 g | Vitamin D | (10 mcg[a]) or 400 IU |
| Saturated Fat | 20 g | | |
| Cholesterol | 300 mg | Vitamin E | (20 α-TE[a]) or 30 IU |
| Sodium | 2,400 mg | | |
| Total Carbohydrate | 300 g | Vitamin K | 80 mcg |
| Dietary Fiber | 25 g | Thiamin | 1.5 mg |
| Vitamin A | (1,000 RE[a]) | Riboflavin | 1.7 mg |
| | or 5,000 IU | Niacin | 20 mg |
| Vitamin C | 60 mg | Vitamin B-6 | 2.0 mg |
| Calcium | 1,000 mg | Folic Acid | 400 mcg |
| Iron | 18 mg | Vitamin B-12 | 6.0 mcg |
| | | Biotin | 300 mcg |
| | | Pantothenic Acid | 10 mg |
| | | Phosphorus | 1,000 mg |
| | | Iodine | 150 mcg |
| | | Magnesium | 400 mcg |
| | | Zinc | 15 mg |
| | | Selenium | 70 mcg |
| | | Copper | 2.0 mg |
| | | Manganese | 2.0 mg |
| | | Chromium | 120 mcg |
| | | Molybdenum | 75 mcg |
| | | Chloride | 3.4 mg |
| | | Potassium | 3,500 mg |
| | | Protein[b] | 50 g |
| | | Stearic Acid[c] | no standard |

Source: From the Code of Federal Regulations, Food and Drugs, Title 21, part 101.9, Nutrition Labeling of Food. The Office of the Federal Register. Washington, D.C.: US Government Printing Office, 1996.

[a]The Federal Code for food labels uses an older standard of measure for these nutrients—IUs (International Units). The other measures (REs, mcgs and α-TE) are the standards of measure used in research, in food composition tables, and for nutrient standards.

[b]Assumes 10% of calories from protein and is different for different lifestages: 60 g for pregnant women, 65 g for nursing mothers, 16 g for children 1–4 years old, and 14 g for infants under 1 year.

[c]Stearic acid is a saturated fat that is *not* considered a health risk. Manufacturers may list the amount of this fat in their food product on the Nutrition Facts Label under saturated fat to indicate the favorable health component.

assigned sweets and desserts to a fruit exchange and/or starch exchange.)

Individual foods within the Bread/Starch, Fruit and Vegetable categories are fairly self-evident because the name of the exchange is similar to a food group. However, some foods may not seem to belong to the exchange group to which they have been assigned. For example:

- Many nonmeat foods appear as meat exchanges because of their meat-like protein and fat levels. Cheese and peanut butter are two common examples.
- Vegetable exchanges do not include all vegetables. For example, because their carbohydrate and protein contents are more similar to bread/starches, vegetables such as lima beans, peas, and corn, are listed as a bread/starch exchange rather than a vegetable.
- Not all starch and bread exchanges are breads. This group also includes starchy vegetables (such as lima beans, peas, and corn), cereals, pasta, and other grain products.
- Alcohol is counted as a fat exchange because of a similar level of per gram calorie content.
- Some food items are not assigned an exchange, because they are considered "free foods." A free food contains less than 20 calories per serving, and there is no stated limit on consumption. A list of "free foods" can be found in the *Exchange Lists for Meal Planning*, published by The American Diabetes Association, Alexandria, VA.

## Sources of Energy/Calories

Protein, carbohydrates, fat, and alcohol are the components of foods that contribute calories to our diet. They do not contribute calories equally, however. Fats contribute over twice the calories per gram as protein or carbohydrates. Organic acids and sugar alcohols contribute calories as well, but on a much smaller scale.

TABLE 2.8 **Recommended Average Energy Intake Per Day for U.S. Individuals with Light to Medium Activity Level Based on Median Reference Heights and Weights and Resting Energy Expenditure**

| | | | | | | | Average Energy Allowance | | |
|---|---|---|---|---|---|---|---|---|---|
| Category | Age (years) | Weight (kg) | Weight (lb) | Height (cm) | Height (in) | Resting Energy Expenditure in kCal/day | Multiples REE | Calories per kg | Calories per Day |
| Infants | 0.0–0.5 | 6 | 13 | 60 | 24 | 320 | | 108 | 650 |
| | 0.5–1.0 | 9 | 20 | 71 | 28 | 500 | | 98 | 850 |
| Children | 1–3 | 13 | 29 | 90 | 35 | 740 | | 102 | 1300 |
| | 4–6 | 20 | 44 | 112 | 44 | 950 | | 90 | 1800 |
| | 7–10 | 28 | 62 | 132 | 52 | 1130 | | 70 | 2000 |
| Males | 11–14 | 45 | 99 | 157 | 62 | 1440 | 1.70 | 55 | 2500 |
| | 15–18 | 66 | 145 | 176 | 69 | 1760 | 1.67 | 45 | 3000 |
| | 19–24 | 72 | 160 | 177 | 70 | 1780 | 1.67 | 40 | 2900 |
| | 25–50 | 79 | 174 | 176 | 70 | 1800 | 1.60 | 37 | 2900 |
| | 51+ | 77 | 170 | 173 | 68 | 1530 | 1.50 | 30 | 2300 |
| Females | 11–14 | 46 | 101 | 157 | 62 | 1310 | 1.67 | 47 | 2200 |
| | 15–18 | 55 | 120 | 163 | 64 | 1370 | 1.60 | 40 | 2200 |
| | 19–24 | 58 | 128 | 164 | 65 | 1350 | 1.60 | 38 | 2200 |
| | 25–50 | 63 | 138 | 163 | 64 | 1380 | 1.55 | 36 | 2200 |
| | 51+ | 65 | 143 | 160 | 63 | 1280 | 1.50 | 30 | 1900 |
| Pregnant | 1st trimester | | | | | | | | +0 |
| | 2nd trimester | | | | | | | | +300 |
| | 3rd trimester | | | | | | | | +300 |
| Lactating/Breastfeeding | | | | | | | | | +500 |

Source: Adapted from the Recommended Dietary Allowances, 10th ed. National Academy Press, Washington, D.C., 1989, page 33.

TABLE 2.9 **Canadian Recommended Nutrient Intakes (RNI)**

| Energy/Proximates | | | | | | Vitamins | | | | | | | | | Minerals | | | | | |
|---|---|---|---|---|---|---|---|---|---|---|---|---|---|---|---|---|---|---|---|---|
| Age | Weight (kg) | Energy kCal | Protein (g) | n-3 PUFA (g) | n-6 PUFA (g) | Thiamin (mg)[a] | Riboflavin (mg)[a] | Niacin (mg NE)[a] | Vit A (RE) | Vit D (mcg) | Vit E (mg) | Vit C[d] (mg) | Folate (mcg) | Vit B-12 (mcg) | Calcium (mg) | Phosphorus (mg) | Magnesium (mg) | Iron (mg) | Iodine (mcg) | Zinc (mg) |
| Infant | | | | | | | | | | | | | | | | | | | | |
| 0–4 mo | 6.0 | 600 | 12[b] | 0.5 | 3 | 0.3 | 0.3 | 4 | 400 | 10 | 3 | 20 | 25 | 0.3 | 250 | 150[b] | 20 | 0.3 | 30[b] | 2 |
| 5–12 mo | 9.0 | 900 | 12[b] | 0.5 | 3 | 0.4 | 0.5 | 7 | 400 | 10 | 3 | 20 | 40 | 0.4 | 400 | 200 | 32 | 7 | 40 | 3 |
| Children | | | | | | | | | | | | | | | | | | | | |
| 1 | 11 | 1100 | 13 | 0.6 | 4 | 0.5 | 0.6 | 8 | 400 | 10 | 3 | 20 | 40 | 0.5 | 500 | 300 | 40 | 6 | 55 | 4 |
| 2–3 | 14 | 1300 | 16 | 0.7 | 4 | 0.6 | 0.7 | 9 | 400 | 5 | 4 | 20 | 50 | 0.6 | 550 | 350 | 50 | 6 | 65 | 4 |
| 4–6 | 18 | 1800 | 19 | 1.0 | 6 | 0.7 | 0.9 | 13 | 500 | 5 | 5 | 25 | 70 | 0.8 | 600 | 400 | 65 | 8 | 85 | 5 |
| Male | | | | | | | | | | | | | | | | | | | | |
| 7–9 | 25 | 2200 | 26 | 1.2 | 7 | 0.9 | 1.1 | 16 | 700 | 2.5 | 7 | 25 | 90 | 1.0 | 700 | 500 | 100 | 8 | 110 | 7 |
| 10–12 | 34 | 2500 | 34 | 1.4 | 8 | 1.0 | 1.3 | 18 | 800 | 2.5 | 8 | 25 | 120 | 1.0 | 900 | 700 | 130 | 8 | 125 | 9 |
| 13–15 | 50 | 2800 | 49 | 1.4 | 9 | 1.1 | 1.4 | 20 | 900 | 5 | 9 | 30 | 175 | 1.0 | 1100 | 900 | 185 | 10 | 160 | 12 |
| 16–18 | 62 | 3200 | 58 | 1.8 | 11 | 1.3 | 1.6 | 23 | 1000 | 5 | 10 | 40 | 220 | 1.0 | 900 | 1000 | 230 | 10 | 160 | 12 |
| 19–24 | 71 | 3000 | 61 | 1.6 | 10 | 1.2 | 1.5 | 22 | 1000 | 2.5 | 10 | 40 | 220 | 1.0 | 800 | 1000 | 240 | 9 | 160 | 12 |
| 25–49 | 74 | 2700 | 64 | 1.5 | 9 | 1.1 | 1.4 | 19 | 1000 | 2.5 | 9 | 40 | 230 | 1.0 | 800 | 1000 | 250 | 9 | 160 | 12 |
| 50–74 | 73 | 2300 | 63 | 1.3 | 8 | 0.9 | 1.0 | 16 | 1000 | 5 | 7 | 40 | 230 | 1.0 | 800 | 1000 | 250 | 9 | 160 | 12 |
| 75+ | 69 | 2000 | 59 | 1.1 | 7 | 0.8 | 1.0 | 14 | 1000 | 5 | 6 | 40 | 215 | 1.0 | 800 | 1000 | 230 | 9 | 160 | 12 |
| Female | | | | | | | | | | | | | | | | | | | | |
| 7–9 | 25 | 1900 | 26 | 1.0 | 6 | 0.8 | 1.0 | 14 | 700 | 2.5 | 6 | 25 | 90 | 1.0 | 700 | 500 | 100 | 8 | 95 | 7 |
| 10–12 | 36 | 2200 | 36 | 1.1 | 7 | 0.9 | 1.1 | 16 | 800 | 5 | 7 | 25 | 130 | 1.0 | 1100 | 800 | 135 | 8 | 110 | 9 |
| 13–15 | 48 | 2200 | 46 | 1.2 | 7 | 0.9 | 1.1 | 16 | 800 | 5 | 7 | 30 | 170 | 1.0 | 1000 | 850 | 180 | 13 | 160 | 9 |
| 16–18 | 53 | 2100 | 47 | 1.2 | 7 | 0.8 | 1.1 | 15 | 800 | 2.5 | 7 | 30 | 190 | 1.0 | 700 | 850 | 200 | 12 | 160 | 9 |
| 19–24 | 58 | 2100 | 50 | 1.2 | 7 | 0.8 | 1.1 | 15 | 800 | 2.5 | 7 | 30 | 180 | 1.0 | 700 | 850 | 200 | 13 | 160 | 9 |
| 25–49 | 59 | 2000 | 51 | 1.1[c] | 7[c] | 0.8 | 1.0 | 14 | 800 | 2.5 | 6 | 30 | 185 | 1.0 | 700 | 850 | 200 | 13 | 160 | 9 |
| 50–74 | 63 | 1800 | 54 | 1.1[c] | 7[c] | 0.8 | 1.0 | 14 | 800 | 5 | 6 | 30 | 195 | 1.0 | 800 | 850 | 210 | 8 | 160 | 9 |
| 75+ | 64 | 1700 | 55 | 1.1[c] | 7[c] | 0.8 | 1.0 | 14 | 800 | 5 | 5 | 30 | 200 | 1.0 | 800 | 850 | 210 | 8 | 160 | 9 |
| Pregnancy—Additional Amounts | | | | | | | | | | | | | | | | | | | | |
| 1st Trimester | | 100 | 5 | 0.05 | 0.3 | 0.1 | 0.1 | 1.0 | 0 | 2.5 | 2 | 0 | 200 | 0.2 | 500 | 200 | 15 | 0 | 25 | 6 |
| 2nd Trimester | | 300 | 20 | 0.16 | 0.9 | 0.1 | 0.3 | 2.0 | 0 | 2.5 | 2 | 10 | 200 | 0.2 | 500 | 200 | 45 | 5 | 25 | 6 |
| 3rd Trimester | | 300 | 24 | 0.16 | 0.9 | 0.1 | 0.3 | 2.0 | 0 | 2.5 | 2 | 10 | 200 | 0.2 | 500 | 200 | 45 | 10 | 25 | 6 |
| Lactation | | 500 | 20 | 0.25 | 1.5 | 0.2 | 0.4 | 3.0 | 400 | 2.5 | 3 | 25 | 100 | 0.2 | 500 | 200 | 65 | 0 | 50 | 6 |

Information Source: Nutrition Recommendations 1990, pages 203–204, Health and Welfare Canada Scientific Review committee with adjustments made after the first printing, and calculations from formula for thiamin, riboflavin, and niacin.

Modifications and table © ESHA Research 1999.

[a]Thiamin, riboflavin, and niacin recommendations are by formula related to protein intake. At age 24 and older, amounts shown are minimums only.

[b]Protein and iodine for infants are assumed to be from breast milk. Infant formula with high phosphorus should contain 37 mg of calcium.

[c]Minimums only.

[d]Smokers should increase vitamin C by 50%.

## *Calculating Total Calories*

To calculate total calories in foods, the general 4-4-9 formula (see Table 2.12) has been used for many years. One would multiply the known weight of carbohydrate and protein by 4, and the known weight of fat by 9, then add the numbers together for the total calories in the food.

It is a good reference formula to calculate an approximate total calories for mixed foods, but it is not exact and usually overstates actual calories. Table 2.12 lists the general formula and the actual range of calories.

Until recently, most reported values for calories were calculated by using the 4-4-9 formula. Manufacturers and labs are now able to use other methods to more accurately report calories in foods, including the Atwater Factors (see Table 2.13) or a modified 4-4-9 formula. The modified 4-4-9 formula subtracts the weight of insoluble fiber from total carbohydrate before applying the 4-4-9 formula.

## *Calories from Organic Acids*

Organic acids contribute a small amount of energy for very few foods. Estimated caloric amounts are listed here for acetic, citric, malic, and lactic acids. For example, the approximately 5 g of acetic acid per 100 ml of vinegar contribute about 17 calories. Oxalic and tartaric acids are not included because they are not metabolized in significant quantities.

| | | |
|---|---|---|
| Acetic acid | = | 3.5 Calories per gram |
| Citric acid | = | 2.4 Calories per gram |
| Lactic acid | = | 3.6 Calories per gram |
| Malic acid | = | 2.4 Calories per gram |

TABLE 2.10 **Canadian Average Energy Requirements Nutrition Recommendations of Canada, 1990**

| Age | Gender | Height (cm) | Weight (kg) | Index BMI[a] | kCal/kg | kCal/day | KCal/cm Height |
|---|---|---|---|---|---|---|---|
| (1st yr) | | | | | | | |
| 0–2 mo | both | 55 | 4.5 | | 120–100[b] | 500 | 9.0 |
| 3–5 mo | both | 63 | 7.0 | | 100–95[b] | 700 | 11.0 |
| 6–8 mo | both | 69 | 8.5 | | 95–97[b] | 800 | 11.5 |
| 9–11 mo | both | 73 | 9.5 | | 97–99[b] | 950 | 12.5 |
| Years | | | | | | | |
| 1 | both | 82 | 11 | | 101 | 1100 | 13.5 |
| 2–3 | both | 95 | 14 | | 94 | 1300 | 13.5 |
| 4–6 | both | 107 | 18 | | 100 | 1800 | 17.0 |
| 7–9 | Male | 126 | 25 | | 88 | 2200 | 17.5 |
| | Female | 125 | 25 | | 76 | 1900 | 15.0 |
| 10–12 | Male | 141 | 34 | | 73 | 2500 | 17.5 |
| | Female | 143 | 36 | | 61 | 2200 | 15.5 |
| 13–15 | Male | 159 | 50 | | 57 | 2800 | 17.5 |
| | Female | 157 | 48 | | 46 | 2200 | 14.0 |
| 16–18 | Male | 172 | 62 | | 51 | 3200 | 18.5 |
| | Female | 160 | 53 | | 40 | 2100 | 13.0 |
| 19–24 | Male | 175 | 71 | 23.18 | 42 | 3000 | 17.1 |
| | Female | 160 | 58 | 22.66 | 36 | 2100 | 13.1 |
| 25–49 | Male | 172 | 74 | 25.01 | 36 | 2700 | 15.7 |
| | Female | 160 | 59 | 23.05 | 32 | 1900 | 11.9 |
| 50–74 | Male | 170 | 73 | 25.26 | 31 | 2300 | 13.6 |
| | Female | 160 | 63 | 25.24 | 29 | 1800 | 11.4 |
| 75+ | Male | 168 | 69 | 24.45 | 29 | 2000 | 11.9 |
| | Female | 155 | 64 | 26.64 | 23 | 1500 | 9.7 |

[a]BMI = Weight (kg) divided by Height in meters$^2$.
Source: Adapted from Nutrition Recommendations 1990, Report of the Health and Welfare Canada Scientific Review Committee, Health and Welfare, Canada, pages 25 and 27.

TABLE 2.11 **Approximate Carbohydrate, Protein, and Fat Per Exchange Category**

| Exchange Category | Carbs (g) | Protein (g) | Fat (g) | Approx. Calories |
|---|---|---|---|---|
| Carbohydrate Group: | | | | |
| Starch | 15 | 3 | 1 or less | 80 |
| Fruit | 15 | — | — | 60 |
| Other Carbohydrates | 15 | varies | varies | varies |
| Vegetables | 5 | 2 | — | 25 |
| Milk[a] | | | | |
| Nonfat/Skim | 12 | 8 | 0–3 | 90 |
| Low-fat (1–2% fat) | 12 | 8 | 5 | 120 |
| Whole | 12 | 8 | 8 | 150 |
| Meat[a] & Meat Substitutes: | | | | |
| Very lean | — | 7 | 0–1 | 35 |
| Lean | — | 7 | 3 | 55 |
| Medium-fat | — | 7 | 5 | 75 |
| High-fat | — | 7 | 8 | 100 |
| Fat Exchange | — | — | 5 | 45 |

[a]Meats and milks can have various levels of fat and can be calculated two different ways: 1) as a "shaded exchange" that already includes some fat; or 2) as a combination of a *lean* meat (or *nonfat* milk) exchange and one or more fat exchanges.

TABLE 2.12 **4-4-9 Formula for Calculating Total Calories**

| Source | Formula | Actual Range |
|---|---|---|
| Protein | 4 kcal/g | 1.82–4.27 kcal/g |
| Carbohydrate | 4 | 1.33–4.16 |
| Fat | 9 | 8.37–9.02 |
| Alcohol | 7 | 6.93 |

TABLE 2.13 **Calories Per Gram of Common Foods—The Atwater Factors**

| Food Item | Protein | Carbs | Fat |
|---|---|---|---|
| Baked beans w/pork+ tomato sauce | 3.5 | 4.00 | 8.80 |
| Baked beans w/tomato sauce | 3.4 | 4.00 | 8.40 |
| Beans & Peas, mature, dry | 3.47 | 4.07 | 8.37 |
| Beans, refried | 3.5 | 4.10 | 8.90 |
| Beef | 4.27 | — | 9.02 |
| Beef, processed meat | 4.27 | 3.68–3.87 | 9.02 |
| Beef tongue | 4.27 | 4.11 | 9.02 |
| Beverages: | | | |
| Carbonated soda | 3.36 | 3.87 | 8.37 |
| Coffee | 3.47 | 4.07 | 8.37 |
| Fruit-flavored drinks | 3.36 | 3.90 | 8.37 |
| Lemonade/Limeade | 3.36 | 3.80 | 8.37 |
| Tea, unsweetened (all) | 2.44 | 3.57–3.80 | 8.37 |
| Beverages, alcoholic*: | | | |
| Beer* | 3.87 | 4.12 | 8.37 |
| Distilled spirits (whiskey/all)* | — | 4.12 | — |
| Wine* | 3.36 | 3.92 | 8.37 |

*Calories from alcohol are at 6.93 calories per gram of alcohol

| Food Item | Protein | Carbs | Fat |
|---|---|---|---|
| Bran (all—corn, rice, wheat, oat) | 1.82 | 2.35 | 8.30–8.37 |
| Breakfast cereals | 1.82–3.82 | 2.80–4.16 | 8.37–8.80 |
| Corn grits | 2.73 | 4.03 | 8.37 |
| Chili w/beans | 3.5 | 4.00 | 8.70 |
| Chocolate/Cocoa | 1.83 | 1.33 | 8.37 |
| Eggs | 4.36 | 3.68 | 9.02 |
| Fish | 4.27 | — | 9.02 |
| Flour: | | | |
| Corn flour | 2.73 | 3.95 | 8.37 |
| Rice flour, brown | 3.41 | 4.12–4.16 | 8.37 |
| Rice flour, white | 3.82 | 4.12 | 8.37 |
| Rye flour, medium | 3.23 | 4.16 | 8.37 |
| Soy flour | 3.47 | 4.07 | 8.37 |
| White wheat flour, all types | 4.05 | 4.12 | 8.37 |
| Whole wheat flour | 3.59 | 3.78 | 8.37 |
| Fruits, raw | 3.36 | 2.48–3.60 | 8.37 |
| Fruits, canned | 3.36 | 3.60–3.78 | 8.37 |
| Grains & Grain products: | | | |
| Barley | 3.55 | 3.95 | 8.37 |
| Bulgar wheat | 3.59 | 3.78 | 8.37 |
| Buckwheat | 3.37 | 3.78 | 8.37 |
| Cornmeal, degermed | 3.47 | 4.16 | 8.37 |
| Couscous, Farina, Semolina | 4.05 | 4.12 | 8.37 |
| Millet | 3.87 | 4.12 | 8.37 |
| Quinoa | 3.47 | 4.07 | 8.37 |
| Sorghum | 0.91 | 4.03 | 8.37 |
| Triticale | 3.32 | 3.82 | 8.37 |
| Wheat | 3.59 | 3.78 | 8.37 |
| Milk, milk products, butter | 4.27 | 3.87 | 8.79 |
| Nuts | 3.47 | 4.07 | 8.37 |
| Pastas & Noodles | | | |
| Cellophane/long rice, dry | 3.47 | 4.07 | 8.37 |
| Chow mein noodles | 3.93 | 4.12 | 8.93 |
| Egg noodles | 3.93 | 4.09 | 8.41 |
| Egg noodles, spinach | 3.88 | 4.08 | 8.41 |
| Soba noodles | 3.37 | 3.78 | 8.37 |
| Somen noodles | 3.91 | 4.12 | 8.37 |
| Macaroni or Spaghetti | | | |
| Regular-semolina, wheat | 3.91 | 4.12 | 8.37 |
| Vegetable | 3.86 | 4.11 | 8.37 |
| Whole wheat | 3.59 | 3.78 | 8.37 |
| Pork & Ham | 4.27 | 3.68–3.87 | 9.02 |
| Poultry & processed meats | 4.27 | 3.87 | 9.02 |
| Rice, brown | 3.41 | 4.12 | 8.37 |
| Rice, white | 3.82 | 4.16 | 8.37 |
| Rice & pasta w/seasonings | 3.87 | 4.14 | 8.37 |
| Shellfish | 4.27 | 4.11 | 9.02 |
| Soybeans, soy products | 3.47 | 4.07 | 8.37 |
| Sugar (beet or cane) | — | 3.87 | — |
| Vegetables: | | | |
| Beans & Peas, green, veg | 3.47 | 4.07 | 8.37 |
| Beans & Peas, dry legumes | 3.47 | 4.07 | 8.37 |
| Mushrooms | 2.62 | 3.48 | 8.37 |
| Potatoes, regular | 2.78 | 3.48 | 8.37 |
| Potatoes, fried | 2.80 | 4.00 | 8.80 |
| Potato salad | 3.60 | 4.00 | 8.90 |
| Tomato sauce | 2.60 | 3.70 | 8.40 |
| Zuccini | 2.00 | 3.70 | 8.40 |
| Other vegetables, avg all | 2.44 | 3.57 | 8.37 |
| Wheat—all: grain, germ, sprouted | 3.59 | 3.78 | 8.37 |
| Wild Rice | 3.55 | 3.95 | 8.37 |

# SECTION 3

# REFERENCES AND USEFUL GUIDES

## Reference for Serving Sizes in Rank Order

Within the discussions for the vitamins and minerals in Sections 5 and 6, there are lists of food sources *in rank order.* To make this listing relevant for actual food consumption, this rank order is by *serving size* (which means different possible weights) and in *ready-to-eat form.* The approximate gram weight for each food serving is listed according to the way they would be consumed—fresh or cooked, and for some foods, both raw and cooked forms.

### Serving Sizes Used in Ranking[1]

*Milk, coffee, tea, juices:* 1 c all liquids (242–250 g); except 1/2 c pineapple juice (125 g), and 3/4 c prune juice (192 g).

*Dairy:* 1 c plain lowfat yogurt (245 g); 1/2 c 2% cottage cheese (113 g); 1 oz cheeses (28 g); 1 c whole milk (244 g); 1 c nonfat milk (245 g); 1/2 c vanilla ice cream (66 g).

*Fruits:* 1/2 avocado (100 g); apple w/peel (138 g); apple without peel (128 g); banana (118 g); 1/2 c blackberries (72 g); 1/2 c blueberries, fresh or frozen (75 g); 1 c cantaloupe cubes (160 g); 1 c fresh sweet cherries (145 g); 1 c grapes (160 g); 1/2 grapefruit—pink/red (123 g), white (118 g); kiwifruit (76 g); 2 T lemon or lime juice (30.5 g); mango (207 g); small orange (96 g); 1 c papaya cubes (140 g); medium peach (98 g); medium pear (166 g); 1/2 c (≈10) prunes (85 g); 1/2 c fresh raspberries (62 g); 1/4 c raisins (36 g); fresh strawberry halves (152 g); 1 c watermelon dices (152 g).

*Eggs:* 1 cooked (48–50 g).

*Grains:* 1/2 c ckd barley (78 g); 1 c ckd oatmeal (234 g); 1/2 c ckd brown rice (98 g); 1/2 c ckd white rice (79 g); 1 c ckd white pasta (all types—spaghetti, macaroni, etc.) (140 g); 1 c ckd whole wheat pasta, all types (140 g); 1 c ckd fresh pasta (150 g).

*Grain products (baked goods):* 2.5 oz plain bagel (71 g); 1 pce white bread (30 g); 1 pce wheat bread (part white/part whole wheat) (25 g); 1 pce whole wheat bread (28 g); 10″ flour tortilla (72 g); 1 corn tortilla (26 g).

*Meats—all types:* beef, chicken, lamb, pork and ham, turkey, seafood, organ meats, and lunchmeat/hot dogs: 3.5 ounces all (100 g)—weight is for edible portion only.

*Nuts and seeds products:* 1/2 c almonds (70–78 g); 1/2 c brazil nuts (70 g); 1/2 c cashews (65 g); 1/2 c chestnuts (72 g); 1/4 c fresh grated coconut (33 g); 1/4 c dried coconut (20 g); 1/2 c filberts (68 g); 1/2 c macadamias (68 g); 1/4 c or 2.5 oz pumpkin seed kernels (57 g); 1/4 c sunflower seed kernels (33 g); 1/2 c peanuts (72 g); 2 T peanut butter (32 g); 1/2 c chopped pecans (60 g); 1/2 c pistachios (64 g); 1/4 c pumpkin seed kernels rstd, 2 oz (57 g); 1 tsp sesame seed kernels (9 g); 1/2 c roasted soybeans (soynuts) (86 g); 1/2 c chopped walnuts (60 g). Weight is for edible portion only.

*Legumes (beans and peas cooked from dry):* 1/2 c baked beans w/pork (126 g); 1/2 c black beans (86 g); 1/2 c ckd black-eyed peas, ckd fr/dry (120 g); 1/2 c ckd lentils (99 g); 1/2 c large lima beans, ckd fr/dry (94 g); 1/2 c ckd kidney beans (89 g); 1/2 c ckd navy beans (131 g); 1/2 c ckd green split peas (98 g); 1/2 c pinto beans (120 g)—1/2 c refried pinto beans (126 g).

*Vegetables:* cooked whole artichoke (120 g); 1/2 c ckd artichoke hearts (84 g); 4 spears ckd asparagus (60 g); 1/2 c ckd mung bean sprouts (62 g); 1/2 c ckd diced beets (85 g); 1/2 c ckd beet greens (72 g); 1/2 c black-eyed peas or cowpeas, ckd fr/frozen (85 g); 1/2 c ckd chopped broccoli (85 g); 1/2 c ckd Brussels sprouts (78 g); 1/2 c raw cabbage (35 g); 1/2 c ckd cabbage (75 g); 7-1/2″ raw carrot (72 g); 1/2 c ckd sliced carrots (76 g); 1/2 c raw cauliflower (50 g); 1/2 c ckd cauliflower (62 g); 1/2 c raw celery (60 g); 7.6″ stalk of celery (40 g); 1/2 c ckd celery (75 g); 1/2 c chayote (80 g); 1/2 c ckd collard greens (90 g); 1/2 c ckd yellow corn (75 g); 1/2 c ckd green beans (65 g); 1/2 c ckd kale (65 g); 1 c chopped lettuce, any kind (56 g); 1/2 c baby lima beans, ckd fr/frozen (90 g); 1/4 c raw mushroom slices (17.5 g); 1/4 c ckd mushrooms (39 g); 1/2 c ckd mustard greens (70 g); 1/2 c okra (92 g); 1/2 c ckd

[1]Source: The Food Finder, ESHA Research, Salem, Oregon, 1999. Printed with permission.

green peas (80 g); 1/2 c ckd green pea pods (80 g); 1/4 c raw chopped sweet pepper (37 g); 1/4 c ckd chopped sweet pepper (≈36 g); baked potato w/skin (122 g); 1/2 c ckd potatoes (±105 g); 1/2 c ckd sweet potatoes (128 g); 1/2 c cnd pumpkin (123 g); 1/4 c raw seaweed (20 g); 1/2 c green soybeans, cooked from fresh (90 g); 1/2 c ckd summer squash (90 g); 1/2 c ckd winter squash (acorn or butternut) (123 g); 1/2 c chopped fresh tomatoes (90 g); 1/2 c cnd tomato sauce (123 g); 1 c raw chopped spinach greens (30 g); 1/2 c ckd spinach (95 g). (Broccoli, Brussels sprouts, carrots, green beans, and collard greens are the average of cooked fr/fresh and fr/frozen.)

*Fats and oils:* 1 T oil (13.5 g); 1 T fat (12.8 g).

*Other:* 1 oz unsweetened chocolate (28.35 g); 2 T honey (43 g); 2 T maple syrup (40 g); 2 T molasses (41 g); 1/2 c tofu (124 g); 1 T oat bran (5.9 g); 1 T wheat bran (3.6 g); 2 T toasted wheat germ (14 g); 2 T brewer's yeast ≈ 1/2 oz (16 g). Tablespoons are a level tablespoon measure.

# Conversion Factors for Nutrients

## *Kilocalories (Calories) to Kilojoules (kJ)*

To convert kcalories to kilojoules, multiply kcals by 4.184. (Calories is the "popular" term for kilocalories.)
To convert kJ to kcals, multiply kJ by 0.239.
1 kilojoule = 0.239 kilocalories.
1 kilocalorie (kcals) = 4.184 kilojoules.

## *Converting International Units (IUs) to Newer Measures*

International Units (IU) are the older unit of measure for vitamins A, D, and E. Current research and nutrition standards, however, report vitamin A in Retinol Equivalents (REs), vitamin D in micrograms (mcg), and vitamin E in alpha-tocopherol equivalents (α-TE), respectively. These new measures account for the different activity levels of the different forms of the vitamin. Because food labels use the older IUs according to the labeling law, conversion measures are provided here.

## *Vitamin A*

Vitamin A comprises several different forms with different activity levels. The conversion factors depend on the source (animal, plant, or dairy) and a few other factors. To convert IUs into mcg of RE, divide IUs from animal/retinol sources by 3.33; divide IUs from plant foods by 10.

1 mcg RE Vitamin A =

| | |
|---|---|
| 10.0 IU | from plant foods (average of carotenoids) |
| 6.0 IU | from beta carotene |
| 12.0 IU | from alpha carotene and cryptoxanthin |
| 3.33 IU | from animal foods and chemicals for fortifying foods |
| 5.0 IU | from mixed foods, a general average—not precise |
| 3.5 IU | from cheese |
| 4.1 IU | from yogurt and milk |

## *Vitamin D*

40 IU vitamin D = 1 mcg of vitamin D. To convert IU of vitamin D to mcg, divide IUs by 40, or multiply by 0.025.

## *Niacin and Niacin Equivalents*

Niacin in food and for food labels are reported in mg of niacin. The standards for recommended intake, however, use mg of niacin equivalents (NEs). This is mg of niacin, plus the amount that can be potentially converted from the amino acid tryptophan. For some foods, this is significant; see the two lists of foods after the discussion on niacin.

1 mg of NE = niacin (mg) + [tryptophan (mg) ÷ 60]

## *Vitamin E*

Vitamin E comprises tocopherols and tocotrienols, and each form has its own activity level. To accurately convert vitamin E values from the older IU measure to mg of alpha-tocopherol equivalents (α-TE), one must know the amounts of *each* vitamin E component, apply the activity factor (listed below) and add the weighted components together. On a general basis only (not precise), IUs can be converted into mg α-TE by dividing by 1.5.

| | | |
|---|---|---|
| 1 mg alpha-tocopherol (natural) | = | 1.0 α-TE (100% activity) or 1.5 IU vit E |
| 1 mg beta-tocopherol | = | 0.5 α-TE (assays range 0.25–0.50) |
| 1 mg gamma-tocopherol | = | 0.1 α-TE (assays range 0.10–0.35) |
| 1 mg delta-tocopherol | = | 0.03 α-TE |
| 1 mg alpha-tocotrienol | = | 0.30 α-TE |
| 1 mg beta-tocotrienol | = | 0.05 α-TE |

| | | |
|---|---|---|
| 1 mg of *natural* vitamin E | = | 1.5 IU of vitamin E (by definition) |
| 1 IU of vitamin E | = | 0.67 mg of *natural* vitamin E or 1.00 mg of *synthetic* vitamin E |
| 1 mg of *synthetic* vitamin E (acetate form) | = | 0.74 α-TE—that is 74% of the activity of natural form |

## *Folate and Folate Equivalents*

Folate has always been measured in micrograms (mcg or μg). However, with the recent folate enrichment of foods in 1998, a new standard of measure was needed. Here's why: The natural folate within foods is about 50% available to the body, and the 1989 RDAs anticipated this with a slightly larger recommended intake to compensate. However, the type of folate used for enriching foods is more available—about 85% is absorbed when taken with food, or 1.7 times more available (85/50 = 1.7). However, when taken in supplement form without food, folate is 100% available to the body.

Therefore, because our food intake is now a combination of different sources and strengths of folate, a new measure for folate has been established—FE (Folate Equivalents) or DFE (Dietary Folate Equivalents). The nutrient standards will use this FE or DFE measure, but it will be some time before food tables can actually report food data this way. The lab assays of food can only report total folate, not the bioavailability of the components.

| | | |
|---|---|---|
| 1 mcg of FE (or DFE) | = | 1.0 mcg of food folate (natural) |
| | = | 0.6 mcg of folic acid with meals (synthetic) |
| | = | 0.5 mcg of folic acid on an empty stomach (synthetic) |
| 1 mcg of synthetic folic acid on an empty stomach | = | 2 mcg FE (or DFE) |
| 1 mcg of synthetic folic acid with meals | = | 1.67 mcg FE (or DFE) |
| 1 mcg of natural food folate | = | 1 mcg FE (or DFE) |

## Conversion Factors for Measures

| Energy Units | | |
|---|---|---|
| 1 kcalorie (kcal/Calorie) | = | 4.2 kilojoules (kJ) |
| 1 kilojoule (kJ) | = | 0.24 kcal |
| 1 g protein | = | 1.82–4.27 kcal/g (average 4) |
| 1 g carbohydrate | = | 1.33–4.16 kcal/g (average 4) |
| 1 g fat | = | 8.37–9.02 kcal/g (average 9) |
| 1 g alcohol | = | 6.93 kcal/g (≈ 7) |

| Length/Height | | |
|---|---|---|
| 1 cm (centimeter) | = | 0.394 in or 0.01 m |
| 1 m (meter) | = | 39.37 in or 100 cm |
| 1 in (inch) | = | 2.54 cm |
| 1 ft (foot) | = | 12 in or 30.48 cm |

| Volume Measures | | |
|---|---|---|
| 1 fl oz | = | 2 T = 1/8 c = 29.6 ml (30 ml) |
| 1/4 cup | = | 2 fl oz = 4 T = 59.1 ml |
| 1/3 cup | = | 5 T + 1 t = 78.9 ml |
| 1/2 cup | = | 8 T = 4 fl oz = 118.3 ml |
| 1 cup (c) | = | 8 fl oz = 16 T = 237 ml |
| 1 t/tsp (teaspoon) | = | 5 ml ≈ 5g |
| 3 teaspoons | = | 1 T = 1/2 fl oz = 15 ml |
| 1 T/Tbsp (Tablespoon) | = | 3 t = 1/2 fl oz = 15 ml |
| 1 ml (milliliter/mL) | = | 1 cc = 0.001 L = 0.034 fl oz |
| 1000 ml | = | 1 L = 34 fl oz |
| 1 L (liter) | = | 1000 ml, 1.06 qt, or 0.85 imperial gal |
| 1 qt (quart) | = | 4 cups = 2 pints = 32 fl oz = 0.95 L |
| 1 gal ( gallon) | = | 4 qt = 3.79 L |

| Weight | | |
|---|---|---|
| 1 g | = | 1000 mg = 1,000,000 mcg = 0.035 oz = 0.001 kg |
| 454 g | = | 1 lb = 0.454 kg |
| 1 mg | = | 1000 mcg or 0.001 g |
| 1 mcg (1 μg) | = | 0.001 mg |
| 1 oz | = | 28.35 g, often rounded to 28 g |
| 16 oz | = | 1 lb = 453.59 g (454 g) = 0.454 kg |
| 1 kg | = | 1000 g or 2.2 lb |
| 1 pound | = | 454 g = 0.454 kg |
| 1 c | = | Varies—see next table for weight of various foods |

**Weight of 1 Level Cup for Example Foods**

| Food Item | | Approximate Weight Per Cup |
|---|---|---|
| Popcorn, popped | = | 8 g |
| Looseleaf lettuce, shredded | = | 56 g |
| Broccoli, chopped, fresh | = | 88 g |
| Apple slices, peeled | = | 110 g |
| Cheddar cheese, shredded | = | 113 g |
| Chopped nuts (most all) | = | 125 g |
| Ice cream, vanilla | = | 132 g |
| Cooked spaghetti noodles | = | 140 g |
| Salted peanuts | = | 144 g |
| Cooked broccoli | = | 156 g |
| Cooked white rice | = | 158 g |
| Creamed cottage cheeses | = | 210–225 g |
| Vegetable oil, all types | ≈ | 218 g |
| Water | = | 237 g |
| Whole milk | = | 244 g |
| Nonfat/Skim milk | = | 245 g |
| Apple juice | = | 248 g |
| Spaghetti sauce | = | 250 g |
| Refried beans | = | 252 g |
| Peanut butter | = | 256 g |

## Food Name Synonyms

| Synonym | Other Name Used in the Food Composition Tables |
|---|---|
| Asparagus beans | Yardlong Beans |
| Aubergine | Eggplant |
| Awa | Milkfish |
| Barbados Cherry | Acerola |
| Beer Salami | Beerwurst |
| Bilberries | Blueberries |
| Bitter gourd | Balsam Apple |
| Black-eyed Peas | Cowpeas |
| Butterbeans | Lima Beans |
| Cabbage, Chinese | Cabbage, Pak Choi |
| Cabbage, Chinese | Cabbage, Pe-Tsai |
| Capsicum | Sweet peppers |
| Celeriac | Celery Root |
| Cervelat | Thuringer Sausage |
| Chick Peas | Garbanzo Beans |
| Chinese Parsley | Coriander |
| Cilantro | Coriander |
| Citronella | Lemon Grass |
| Daikon | Radish, Oriental |
| Dasheen | Taro |
| Dolphinfish | MahiMahi |
| Fava Beans | Broadbeans |
| Flatfish | Flounder Fish/Sole |
| Goa Beans | Winged Beans |
| Goober Peas/Ground Nuts | Peanuts |
| Groundcherries | Gooseberries |
| Hake Fish | Whiting Fish |
| Hazelnuts | Filberts |
| Hot Chocolate | Cocoa drink |

| | |
|---|---|
| Hot Dog | Frankfurter |
| Huckleberries | Blueberries |
| Jicama | Yambean |
| Ladie's Finger | Okra |
| Lichees/Lichis/Litche | Lychees |
| Lily Root | Lotus Root |
| Linseed | Flaxseed |
| Lox | Salmon, Smoked |
| Litchees/Litchis | Lychees |
| Mandarin Oranges | Tangerines |
| Manioc | Cassava |
| Matai | Waterchestnuts |
| Muskmelon | Cantaloupe |
| Natal Plum | Carissa |
| Okra | Gumbo |
| Oysterplant | Salsify |
| Papri Beans | Hyacinth Beans |
| Pawpaw | Papaya |
| Pignolia/Piñon | Pine Nuts |
| Pork Fat | Lard |
| Pork Liver Sausage | Braunschweiger |
| Scallions | Shallots |
| Seaweed | Agar, Dulse, Nori, Kombu |
| Snow Peas | Peas, edible-podded |
| Sole Fish | Flounder/Flatfish |
| Soybean Curd | Tofu |
| Starfruit | Carambola |
| Sugar Snap Peas | Peas, edible, podded |
| Sunchoke | Artichoke, Jerusalem |
| Swedes | Turnips |
| Tahini | Sesame Butter |
| Tallow | Beef Fat |
| White Kidney Beans | Cannellini Beans |
| Yam | Sweet Potato |

## Abbreviations Used in Tables

### Proximates/Basic Components

| | |
|---|---|
| Cals/Cal | calories/kcalories |
| $H_2O$ | water |
| Prot | protein |
| sugr | sugar |
| carbs/CHO | carbohydrate |
| fol | folate/folacin/folic acid |
| fiber/DFib | dietary fiber |
| kcalories/ kcals | kilocalories/calories |
| sat/sfa | saturated fat |
| mono/MUFA | monounsaturated fat |
| poly/PUFA | polyunsaturated fat |
| chol/choles | cholesterol |

### Vitamins

| | |
|---|---|
| bio/biot | Biotin |
| thiamin | vitamin B-1 |
| riboflavin | vitamin B-2 |
| niacin | vitamin B-3 |
| fol | folate/folacin/folic acid |
| cobalamin | vitamin B-12 |
| panto/pant | pantothenic acid |

### Minerals

| | |
|---|---|
| Ca | Calcium |
| Cl | Chloride |
| Cr | Chromium |
| Cu | Copper |
| F | Fluoride |
| Fe | Iron |
| I | Iodine |
| K | Potassium |
| Mg/Mag | Magnesium |
| Mn/Mang | Manganese |
| Mo/Molyb | Molybdenum |
| Na | Sodium |
| P | Phosphorus |
| Se | Selenium |
| Zn | Zinc |
| Chln | Choline |

### Amino Acids/Proteins

| | |
|---|---|
| Arg | Arginine |
| Cys | Cystine |
| His/Hist | Histidine |
| Iso | Isoleucine |
| Leu | Leucine |
| Lys | Lysine |
| Meth/Met | Methionine |
| Phen | Phenylalanine |
| Thr/Thre | Threonine |
| Tyr | Tyrosine |
| Tryp | Tryptophan |
| Val | Valine |

### Abbreviations for Food Descriptions and Measures

| | |
|---|---|
| amt | amount |
| AP | as purchased |
| aTE/αTE/α-TE | alpha tocopherol equivalents (vit E) |
| bld | boiled |
| brld | broiled |
| Cal/cal/kcal | calories/kilocalories |
| cnd | canned |
| cinn | cinnamon |
| choc | chocolate |
| ckd | cooked |
| conc | concentrate |
| crm | cream |
| diam/dia/dm | diameter |
| DFE/FE | dietary folate equivalents |
| enr | enriched |
| EP | edible portion |
| Flv/flav | flavor |
| fl oz | fluid ounce |
| FE/DFE | dietary folate equivalents |
| fort | fortified |
| frzn/fzn | frozen |
| g | grams |
| hpng | heaping |
| hyd/hydr | hydrogenated |
| imit | imitation |
| inst | instant |
| IU | international units |
| jce | juice |
| jr | junior baby food |
| Kcal/cal | kilocalories/calories |
| L | Liter |
| lb | pound |
| marg | margarine |
| mcg/μg | micrograms |
| med | medium |
| mg | milligrams |
| microwv/mc/wv | microwave cooked |
| ml | milliliter |
| NE | niacin equivalents |
| nfdm | nonfat dry milk solids |

| | |
|---|---|
| orig | original |
| oz | ounce |
| pce | piece |
| pkg | package |
| pkt | packet |
| prep/prpd | prepared |
| rd/rnd | round |
| RE | retinol equivalents (vit A) |
| recon | reconstituted |
| rdu/cal | reduced calories |
| ref | reference # to ESHA software |
| refrig | refrigerated |
| reg | regular |
| RTD | ready to drink |
| RTE | ready to eat |
| RTH | ready to heat |
| RTS | ready to serve |
| sce | sauce |
| sep | separable |
| sq | square |
| std | standard |
| str | strained baby food |
| sub | substitute |
| sucr | sucrose |
| T/tbsp | tablespoon |
| t/tsp | teaspoon |
| tr | trace |
| unenr | unenriched |
| van | vanilla |
| vit | vitamin |

# SECTION 4

# BASIC FOOD COMPONENTS

The basic components of foods, often referred to as proximates, are water, protein, carbohydrate, fat, and ash. Ash is simply the residue remaining after complete combustion of a food item and represents approximately 1 to 2% of the total weight of a food. Ash consists of mineral matter and inorganic constituents. Alcohol (ethanol) is also considered a component, if present. The sum of these basic components equals the total weight of a food.

Minerals are usually included within the ash component; vitamins are included within the protein, fat, or carbohydrate components. Energy, as measured in calories, comes only from protein, carbohydrate, fat, or alcohol.

## Water

*Water is essential for nutrient transport. It is a medium for and participant in chemical reactions. Water is necessary for hydrolysis; as a solvent; for acid-base balance; for transport of oxygen and waste; as a lubricant; as a cleanser; and for temperature regulation.*

Water is often ignored because it is considered so ordinary and so abundant, but water is absolutely vital—an essential nutrient—involved in every part and every function of the body. Water is necessary for the proper functioning of the following: digestive, circulatory, and excretory functions; absorption of nutrients; transport of nutrients to every cell; transport of waste products in and out of the cells; and transport of waste products out of the body. Approximately 60% of the adult human body is water. It is a higher percentage in infants and declines with age.

When body water is low, the previously described functions (and more) are impaired, the blood does not flow as well, and the heart has to work harder to do its job. In addition, the kidneys may find it difficult to adequately dilute and flush out metabolic waste and harmful products from the body. Eight 8-oz glasses of water per day is the recommended intake. You can go without food for about 8 weeks; but you can only survive a few days without water.

## Proteins (Amino Acids)

*Protein makes life possible. All enzymes, antibodies, and most hormones are proteins. Proteins provide the transport of nutrients, oxygen, waste, and other factors throughout the body; provide the structure and contracting capability of muscles; provide collagen to the connecting tissue of the body and to the tissues of the skin, hair, and nails.*

Foods supply amino acids, the building blocks for protein. All animal and plant proteins are made from approximately 20 common amino acids, which the body uses to build all the proteins essential for virtually every function in the body. All enzymes are proteins, which are essential in all body processes including digestion of foods, release and regulation of energy in the body, muscle movement, and blood clotting.

All antibodies are proteins, which are essential for maintaining the body's immune system. Many of the body's hormones include amino acids, which are essential for maintaining the basic metabolic rate, regulation of digestion, absorption processes, regulation of blood glucose levels, and the blood clotting response, to name only a few.

Proteins help maintain the quantity and location of fluids in the body and the acid-base balance. They provide transport for compounds moving in and out of cells and throughout the body. The proteins hemoglobin and myoglobin are involved in transporting oxygen from the lungs to the blood, across the cell wall into the cells, and also transporting carbon dioxide back to the lungs. The light-sensing pigments in the eye are also proteins.

Protein provides the framework for the growth and development of bones, teeth, collagen, and all other tissues. The amino acid tyrosine is a precursor to the pigment melanin and for the neurotransmitters norepinephrine and epinephrine. The amino acid tryptophan is a precursor for niacin and the neurotransmitter serotonin.

### *Deficiency*

A deficiency of protein rarely occurs in isolation of deficiencies of other nutrients. Prolonged deficiency of protein results in starvation and wasting; in children, this deficiency causes the failure to grow and thrive and abdominal edema. Abdominal edema occurs when body fluid leaks from the cells and settles into and expands the abdomen. Symptoms also include poor muscles, thin and fragile hair, skin lesions, hormonal imbalances, and more.

High protein diets are not toxic. On the contrary, in countries where protein intake is consistently high, the populations tend to grow slightly larger than those in countries where protein intake is limited.

## Essential Amino Acids

Nine amino acids exist that the body cannot create and must be provided by the food we eat. These are referred to as essential or indispensable amino acids.

If the body is in short supply of an essential amino acid, it will break down other proteins to create what it needs. Distinctions can blur, however, because some amino acids can be precursors for others, and a short supply of one of these precursors may render a nonessential protein essential.

| Essential Amino Acids (Indispensable) | Nonessential Amino Acids (The Body Can Create Them) |
|---|---|
| Histidine | Alanine |
| Isoleucine | Arginine[a] |
| Leucine | Aspartic acid |
| Lysine | Cysteine[a] |
| Methionine | Cystine |
| Phenylalanine | Glutamic acid |
| Threonine | Glutamine |
| Tryptophan | Glycine |
| Valine | Proline |
| | Serine |
| | Tyrosine[a] |

[a]Conditionally essential amino acids.

## Limiting Protein

The body requires more of some essential amino acids than others. If the diet supplies an essential amino acid in quantities *below* what is needed, protein synthesis will be impaired. When this occurs, the amino acid in short supply is called a *limiting* amino acid, because it limits the use of other available amino acids, and thereby limits the amount of protein actually available to the body.

At one time, it was thought that complete proteins had to be consumed in certain proportions for every meal. Now it is known that the body stores amino acids, and in a mixed diet, limitations seldom occur. Only a dietary deficiency well beyond 24 hours may contribute to this *limiting* effect. This limiting effect is not relevant for a meal or a single day or for a diet of mixed and varied foods.

Protein from animal sources, such as meats, eggs, milk, and cheese, provide nearly complete protein; that is, protein that contains all the essential amino acids. Gelatin is an exception, which is an animal protein that lacks tryptophan. Proteins from plant sources, such as vegetables, grains, legumes, nuts and seeds, may be limited in one or more essential amino acid. Eaten together, however, plant foods can offset each other's limiting amino acids and provide the full array needed—the full protein of meat, without the fat. Only a few amino acids are likely to be limited in a mixed diet. Typically they are lysine, tryptophan, threonine, and methionine plus cystine.

The Amino Acid Requirement Pattern of a mixed diet is a calculation best performed with a computer software program containing an extensive database of amino acids. This calculation can rapidly and accurately identify any limiting amino acids in daily or multiday diets.

Table 4.1 shows the estimated daily recommended amino acid pattern for children ages 2 to 5 as established by WHO in 1989. This age group's requirement pattern is usually used for all ages. To interpret this information, read the numbers in the shaded column as follows: for every 339 parts of essential amino acids, 19 parts should be histidine, 28 parts should be isoleucine, 66 parts should be leucine, and so forth.

## Lysine

Some individual amino acids have provided pharmaceutical relief for some clinical conditions. Lysine in supplement form is well known for its ability to relieve herpes infections and cold sores. It doesn't cure them, but it does relieve the symptoms for many individuals.

## Glucosamine

For many individuals, regular intake of supplemental glucosamine sulphate relieves the pain of osteoarthritis without the side effects that occur with other pain relievers. Short-term studies have also shown evidence that glucosamine sulphate may promote cartilage repair and regeneration and revitalize the bone covering at the joints. Larger long-term research is underway to identify the mechanisms at work and to verify the initial study findings.

TABLE 4.1 **Estimated Amino Acid Requirement Pattern—for Protein**

| Amino Acid In mg/g of protein | Infants (3–4 mo) | Children (2–5 yr) | Children (10–12 yr) | Adult | For Comparison Egg | Cow Milk | Beef |
|---|---|---|---|---|---|---|---|
| Histidine | 26 (18–36) | 19 | 19 | 16 | 22 | 27 | 34 |
| Isoleucine | 46 (41–53) | 28 | 28 | 13 | 54 | 47 | 48 |
| Leucine | 93 (83–107) | 66 | 44 | 19 | 86 | | 81 |
| Lysine | 66 (53–76) | 58 | 44 | 16 | 70 | 78 | 89 |
| Methionine and Cystine | 42 (29–60) | 25 | 22 | 17 | 57 | 33 | 40 |
| Phenylalanine and Tyrosine | 72 (68–118) | 63 | 22 | 19 | 93 | 102 | 80 |
| Threonine | 43 (40–45) | 34 | 28 | 9 | 47 | 44 | 46 |
| Tryptophan | 17 (16–17) | 11 | 9 | 5 | 17 | 14 | 12 |
| Valine | 55 (44–77) | 35 | 25 | 13 | 66 | 64 | 50 |
| Total Amino Acids | 460 (408–588) | 339 | 241 | 127 | 512 | 504 | 479 |

Sources: Protein Quality Evaluation. Report of a Joint FAO/WHO Expert Consultation held in Bethesda, MD, USA, December 4–8, 1989. FAO: Rome, Italy, 1990, p. 23. Energy and Protein Requirements: Report of a Joint FAO/WHO/UNU Expert Technical Report Series No. 724.,WHO: Geneva, Switzerland, 1985.

### *Protein Supplements*

If a person wants to build muscles, they need to exercise and lift weights. Despite all the marketing claims (and hopes), protein supplements cannot build muscle mass. Some companies have created products called "predigested" proteins. Although this is an interesting concept, the body's method for absorbing proteins is a process that requires selecting the amino acids it needs the most and then using specific receptor sites to absorb them. The "predigested" protein products on the market can actually cause more harm than good, because the free amino acids from such products may attach and use up the body's receptor sites before the body can select the amino acids it needs. This incorrect absorption can inadvertently set up deficiencies in some amino acids.

### *Calculating Protein in Foods*

The protein content of foods is an estimate based on the quantity of nitrogen present, and in most foods, nitrogen comprises 16% of the total weight of protein. Therefore, the nitrogen content is assayed, and the protein content is calculated by multiplying the nitrogen value by 6.25 for meats and most other foods. Other factors for converting grams of nitrogen to protein are as follows: 5.83 for whole-wheat flour; 5.70 for all purpose (white) flour, pasta and soy; 6.25 for corn; 5.95 for rice; 5.83 for barley, oats, and rye; 5.41 for peanuts and Brazil nuts; 5.18 for almonds; and approximately 5.30 for other nuts.

### *Recommended Protein Intake*

The recommended daily intake of protein (actually, amino acids) can be expressed in different ways:

- As a percentage of calories. Protein is suggested at 10 to 15% of calories.
- As a formula based on body weight. Protein for healthy adults is suggested at 0.8 g protein per kg of body weight per day.
- As a single amount. Protein is suggested at approximately 50 g/day for a healthy adult weighing about 64 kg, or about 141 lb.

## Carbohydrates

***Carbohydrates are a major energy source for the body; they contribute bulk to the diet with fewer calories than fat.***

Carbohydrate is a large family of compounds from plant foods. The two major categories of carbohydrate are *refined carbohydrates* and *complex carbohydrates*. Refined carbohydrates are sugars. Complex carbohydrates (starches and fiber) are long complex chains of sugars bound together. CHO and Carbs are abbreviations used for carbohydrates.

Sugars and starches supply the major source of energy for all the body's cells, including the brain and the blood. The digestive process converts carbohydrate to glucose, the form the body uses for energy. Excess is stored in the liver, or stored elsewhere in the body as fat.

In addition to energy, carbohydrate contributes bulk to the diet and gives feelings of satisfaction (with less than half the calories of fat). Most fiber is not digested by the body, and the undigested bulk assists normal movement of food through the body.

### *The Family of Carbohydrates*

**Simple or Refined Carbohydrates—Sugars:**

Monosaccharides:
- *Glucose*
- *Fructose*
- *Galactose*

Disaccharides:
- *Sucrose = glucose + fructose*
- *Lactose = glucose + galactose*
- *Maltose = glucose + glucose*

**Complex Carbohydrates:**

Starch (polysaccharides)

Dietary Fiber (nonstarch polysaccharides):
- *Insoluble fiber:*
  - Cellulose
  - Hemicellulose
  - Lignin (a noncarbohydrate component of dietary fiber)
- *Soluble fiber:*
  - Pectin
  - Gums
  - Mucilages

**Other Carbohydrates:**
- Organic acids
- Sugar alcohols
- Other substances that do not fit a cateogry

### *Calculating Carbohydrates in Foods*

If you think there is a lab analysis for carbohydrate, you are mistaken. It may be a surprise to learn that carbohydrate in food is not calculated by lab analysis. When 100 g of food is analyzed, the water content and the dry matter—protein, fat, and ash—are determined. The residual weight, or difference, is considered carbohydrate. Because so many foods comprise 80 to 90% water, a small change in the water content can have a significant impact on the dry matter, and therefore, an even larger impact on the amount that is considered carbohydrate. As a result, there may be a wide variety of reported values for a given carbohydrate in a food, and differences may only represent differences in moisture content.

But there is more. Carbohydrate comprises sugars, starches, and insoluble and soluble fiber fractions, for which there *are* analytical techniques. Because the analyses for these food components are usually conducted with separate samples, these values almost always add to an amount that differs from the reported total carbohydrate that is "calculated by difference."

And there is more. Different analytical techniques for fiber can give different results for the same food. Sometimes the data is the result of the method, rather than the actual fiber content. Food mixtures with large amounts of fat or low concentrations of fiber can influence results; some techniques work best for grains, whereas other techniques work better for vegetables and other foods.

### *Available Carbohydrate*

Because only portions of the carbohydrate family are actually available to the body, this term continues to grow in use. In foods, it represents primarily the sugars, starches, and *soluble fiber.* Available carbohydrate can be quickly calculated by subtracting the insoluble fiber value from the total carbohydrate value. This value more accurately represents the carbohydrate value to be used when calculating calories in foods.

## *Recommended Intake*

It is recommended that 50 to 60% of the calories we consume come from carbohydrates—primarily complex carbohydrates.

## *Simple Carbohydrates—The Sugars*

Sugar is a basic contributor of energy for the body, which the body converts into sugars the body can use. In recent years, however, there have been concerns regarding the large quantities of refined sugar added to our diets. However, sugar is not a poison; it is a delicious part of foods. Large amounts of refined sugar can be a concern if sugar-laden foods *displace* the foods that contain more nutrients. If a person has filled themselves with soft drinks, candies, and concentrated sweets, they will not be eating as much of the protein and complex carbohydrate-rich foods the body needs. They will not have room for the foods with more vitamins, minerals, fiber, and other nutrient factors that make us look and feel healthy.

Consuming sugar in the diet will *not* cause diabetes. Although control of blood sugar is central to diabetes, controlling dietary sugar is part of the treatment, not part of the cause.

A definite connection exists between sugar and dental caries (cavities). Foods most likely to contribute to dental caries are those that are sticky or do not clear out of the mouth, such as pastries, jam, caramels, peanut butter, raisins, and other dried fruit. Eating other foods along with sticky foods will reduce this effect. Caries development also depends on exposure time. If a person sips sweet liquids all day, continually exposing their teeth to sugar, this will allow bacteria to produce decay-causing acids. Rinsing the mouth with plain water right after eating can help minimize this problem.

There has been much discussion concerning sugar and hyperactivity in children. Indeed, sugary foods will give children (and adults) more energy for short periods. If high-sugar foods dominate the diet, they will *displace nutrient laden foods* needed for good health and proper growth and the fiber that moderates the body's absorption of sugar.

Many studies have been done on this subject, but they have not consistently proven any connection beyond the factors just listed. It is possible that the effects of sugar produce an elevated response in growing children who have a marginal deficiency in other nutrients.

The three basic monosaccharide sugars are glucose, fructose, and galactose (Table 4.2). When these basic sugars are each bound with another glucose sugar, they are known as disaccharides. Disaccharides are the predominant sugars in foods.

### Monosaccharides—Single Sugars

Glucose, fructose, and galactose are monosaccharides, or single sugars. Glucose is the most prevalent naturally occurring sugar. It is a component of all disaccharide sugars, starches, and glycogen, the major form of storing energy in the body. Dextrose is an older name for glucose.

Fructose is the sweetest tasting of all natural sugars and occurs primarily in fruits, honey, and products using high-fructose corn syrup. An older name for fructose is levulose. Galactose usually only occurs as a part of lactose in milk.

### Disaccharides (Sucrose, Lactose, Maltose)

Sucrose, lactose, and maltose are disaccharides, which is a combination of two sugar molecules, one of which is glucose. Sucrose is table sugar, a combination of glucose and fructose. Lactose, milk sugar, is made up of glucose and galactose. Maltose, usually a breakdown product of starch, is composed of two molecules of glucose.

TABLE 4.2 **Sugar Detail for Sample Foods**

| 100 g of Food Item | Glucose | Fructose | Galactose | Sucrose | Lactose | Maltose | Total Sugar |
|---|---|---|---|---|---|---|---|
| Brown sugar | 5.2 | 0.40 | 0 | 84.3 | 0 | — | 97.3 |
| Corn syrup | 20.6 | 2.2 | 0 | — | 0 | 15 | 51.1 |
| Honey | 31.0 | 38.5 | 0 | 1.5 | 0 | 7.2 | 78.2 |
| Molasses | 11.2 | 12.9 | 0 | 34.7 | 0 | — | 59.9 |
| Raw-turbinado sugar | — | — | — | 95.9 | 0 | — | 95.9 |
| White sugar | — | — | — | 96.8 | 0 | — | 96.8 |
| Apple w/peel | 2.3 | 6.0 | 0 | 2.5 | 0 | 0.1 | 12.0 |
| Banana | 3.9 | 3.7 | 0 | 10.4 | 0 | 0 | 18.5 |
| Blueberries, fresh | 3.5 | 3.6 | 0 | 0.20 | 0 | — | 11.4 |
| Green seedless grapes | 6.0 | 7.1 | 0.5 | 0.32 | 0 | 2.88 | 16.8 |
| Peaches, fresh | 1.1 | 1.3 | 0 | 5.60 | 0 | 0.7 | 8.82 |
| Prunes, dried | 23.1 | 14.0 | 0 | 0.80 | 0 | — | 43.0 |
| Strawberries, fresh | 1.8 | 2.02 | 0 | 0.82 | 0 | 0.081 | 4.72 |
| Watermelon | 1.2 | 2.4 | 0 | 2.71 | 0 | 0.37 | 6.68 |
| Broccoli, ckd fr/frozen | 0.6 | 1.0 | 0 | 0.2 | 0 | 0 | 1.8 |
| Corn, ckd fr/frozen | 0.4 | 0.2 | 0 | 1.2 | 0 | — | 1.8 |
| Peas, ckd fr/frozen | 0.2 | 0.1 | 0 | 4.8 | 0 | 0.2 | 5.8 |
| Baked Potato, no skin | 0.4 | 0.4 | 0 | 0.2 | 0 | — | 1.7 |
| Nonfat Milk | 0 | 0 | 0 | 0 | 4.66 | 0 | 4.66 |
| Lowfat Yogurt | 0 | 0 | 1.72 | 0 | 4.56 | 0 | 7.04 |
| Cheddar Cheese | 0.1 | 0 | 0.8 | 0 | 0.38 | 0 | 1.28 |
| White Pasta | 0.3 | 0.3 | 0 | 0.3 | 0 | 0.4 | 1.3 |
| Whole Wheat Pasta | 0.2 | 0.1 | 0 | 0.1 | 0 | 0.3 | 0.8 |
| White Rice | 0.2 | — | 0 | 0.2 | 0 | 0.1 | 0.5 |

## *Complex Carbohydrates—Starches and Fiber*

### Starches (Polysaccharides)

Starch is a complex carbohydrate that is the major energy source for the body. Starches are long chains of sugar molecules, primarily glucose. Starchy foods are mostly found in grains and cereals, cooked dried beans and peas, and tubers (potatoes, yams, and cassava). As many foods mature, the sweetness declines as the sugar forms into starch. Therefore, sugar/starch data for fruits and vegetables in food composition tables may vary significantly.

### Dietary Fiber

Dietary fiber is a complex carbohydrate primarily composed of the indigestible components of plant cell walls. It consists of long chains of connected sugars called polysaccharides and oligosaccharides and can absorb water and resist digestion into the body. Dietary fiber is of great interest, because a diet high in fiber is connected with better colon health, a reduced incidence of adult onset diabetes, lower blood pressure and cholesterol, and less risk of cardiovascular disease. People who eat a lot of fruits and vegetables have regular elimination of wastes, so there is less constipation and less incidence of diverticulitis.

The average American consumes about 12 g of fiber per day. It is recommended that adults consume about 25 to 30 g per day. Recommendations vary according to body size, and more fiber should be consumed if the diet contains more fat. A general guideline for children suggests that they consume daily grams of dietary fiber equal to their age in years plus 5. For example, a 10-year-old child should consume about 15 grams of fiber per day.

Dietary fiber should not be confused with crude fiber, an obsolete term referring to the residue of an assay method. Foods generally contain more dietary fiber than crude, but unfortunately no consistent relationship exists.

#### *Insoluble Fiber*

Insoluble fiber is resistant to absorption into the body; therefore, it moves food quickly through the digestive system, reducing problems in the digestive tract. It also absorbs water, making stools softer and bulkier. These properties prevent the accumulation of digested food in the intestines, resulting in the normal daily elimination of stool, preventing constipation, hemorrhoids, diverticulosis, and appendicitis.

The rapid passage through the colon may also reduce the possibility of potential carcinogens interacting with the intestinal surface. It used to be thought that insoluble fiber reduced the incidence of colon cancer, but that is not a proven connection.

Insoluble fiber is found primarily in whole grains (especially whole wheat and wheat bran), nuts and seeds, cocoa (yes, chocolate), vegetables, and cooked dried beans and peas (legumes). Most foods contain a mixture of both soluble and insoluble fiber.

#### *Soluble Fiber*

Soluble fiber is associated with reducing blood cholesterol levels. It will bind with certain substances and prevent their absorption either by binding bile acids or by coating the intestines. Some soluble fiber is digestible and may be absorbed into the body.

Soluble fiber is inside and around plant cells and includes pectins, gums, and mucilages that can dissolve in water. Sources are primarily in oat bran, apples, barley, fruits, seaweed, and cooked dried beans and peas (legumes).

## *Other Carbohydrates*

Other carbohydrates include organic acids and any other compounds that are not strictly sugars, starches, or fiber. Organic acids provide sweetness and far fewer calories than sugar. In addition, they appear to not promote dental caries because the bacteria in the mouth cannot metabolize them as quickly as sugar. Organic acids include sorbitol, mannitol, maltitol found in fruits, and xylitol.

Substances other than sugar that can sweeten our foods include artificial sweeteners and sugar alcohols. *Artificial sweeteners* include saccharin, aspartame, and acesulfame-K. These provide a sweet taste, but the body does not absorb them. Other artificial sweeteners include alitame, cyclamate, and sucralose. The FDA has established an Acceptable Daily Intake (ADI) for artificial sweeteners. The ADI for aspartame is 50 mg/kg of body weight per day.

A plant that grows in central South America called stevia has been used as a sweetener for hundreds of years in that region. Stevia is very sweet to the taste and is not metabolized as a sugar. Derivatives are currently being explored in the United States as a potential commercial sweetener. Stevia is already available in health food stores, but has yet to be approved as an additive in foods at this time.

## Lipids/Fats (Fatty Acids and Triglycerides)

***Lipids and fats are basic components of every cell and for many important hormones. They are essential for the body's use of fat-soluble vitamins A, D, E and K; are an important energy source; keep us warm; and protect bones and organs from shock.***

Fats are a good thing. It is *excessive* fat that is *not so good* a thing. Fats offer an important supply of energy, provide a layer of warmth, are a basic component of every cell, and are the basic components for important hormones.

Fat is necessary for absorbing and transporting the important fat-soluble vitamins—vitamin A, the carotenoids, and vitamins D, E, and K. Stores of fat serve as cushions for our bones and organs to protect them from shock. They are an important component of cell structures, particularly in the brain and nervous system; and as a key component in all cell membranes, lipids protect the internal structure of the cell.

Dietary fat carries much of the flavor and aromas of food and the tenderness in meats; it is part of the good mouth feel to our food and the sense of fullness and satiety after a meal.

Lipids are the body's most concentrated source of energy, supplying approximately 9 kcal per gram. A person cannot burn this body fat, however, without burning some muscle. When fat is broken down by the body for energy for movement and muscles, it requires a little bit of glucose to do so, and glucose is released during the breakdown of muscle. Energy for the brain, nervous system, and red blood cells requires glucose exclusively.

The term fats and oils is often used as the umbrella term, but it really is a subset (the major subset) of lipids, and comprises 95% of all lipids in foods. Another term for fats and oils is triglycerides. Phospholipids and sterols comprise the remaining 5% of lipids.

## Lipids—The Family

### Triglycerides (Fats and Oils):

Fatty Acids
- Saturated fats (Sat)
  - *Trans-fatty acids*
- Monounsaturated (Mono)
- Polyunsaturated (PUFA or Poly)
  - *Omega 3 (n-3)*
  - *Omega 6 (n-6)*

Glycerol

### Phospholipids and Sterols

## Saturated Fats

Saturated fats are hard at room temperature. Chemically, this is because the carbon atoms within the fatty acid structure are all bound with hydrogen, and they do not "bend" (Table 4.3). Saturated fats are found in large amounts in the fat of animals: beef, pork, lamb, less in poultry and fish. Plant sources have little saturated fat, with the exception of coconut and palm oils. Large intakes of saturated fat are associated with high risk of heart disease and atherosclerosis. Stearic acid, a saturated fat, does not exhibit this risk association. Conversely, high intakes are also associated with protection against cancer.

It is recommended that saturated fats should comprise approximately 1/3 (or a little less) of total daily fat intake. Assuming 30% of calories from fat, this would equate to 8 to 10% of total calories.

## The Other Saturated Fat—Hydrogenated Fats and Trans-Fatty Acids

Trans-fatty acids are formed during hydrogenation of oils to make them more solid and have a longer shelf-life. Chemically, oils are primarily monounsaturated and polyunsaturated fats in which some of the carbon atoms in the fatty acid structure are not fully saturated with hydrogen atoms. The carbons connect with each other by double bonds and are more flexible. This flexibility makes them liquid and also makes them more reactive to oxygen in the air, thereby becoming rancid.

Food manufacturers can increase the stability of oils by the process of hydrogenation—adding hydrogen to the oil molecules. This transformation results in a large percentage of molecules called trans-fatty acids. These fats are indistinguishable from natural saturated fat and are rare, almost nonexistent, in nature. Very small quantities are made microscopically in the milk of ruminants (cows, sheep).

Trans-fatty acids are not currently listed on nutrition labels, therefore manufacturers list the original polyunsaturated or monounsaturated oils on their products. Current research, however, now confirms the concerns raised by scientists in the past about trans-fatty acids. Studies indicate that trans-fats present the same health risks as saturated fats, and some research has found a link with prostate cancer. More research continues.

Trans-fatty acids in foods are found in margarines, shortening, and *all the baked goods that contain them*—crackers, cookies, snack foods, and other baked and fried items. Partially hydrogenated vegetable oils have a relatively low level of saturation; however, margarines and shortenings can contain 20 to 40% trans-fatty acids. Because health risks have been proven, it is expected that the amounts of trans-fatty acids will be reduced in food products in the future as different processes are created to minimize this outcome.

TABLE 4.3 **Saturated Fats**

| Structure[a] | Name |
|---|---|
| 4:0 | Butyric |
| 6:0 | Caprioc |
| 8:0 | Caprylic |
| 10:0 | Capric |
| 12:0 | Lauric |
| 14:0 | Myristic |
| 15:0 | Pentadecanoic |
| 16:0 | Palmitic |
| 17:0 | Margaric |
| 18:0 | Stearic |
| 20:0 | Arachidic |
| 22:0 | Behenic |
| 24:0 | Lignoceric |

[a]Number of carbons : number of double bonds.

## Monounsaturated Fats (Mono)

Monounsaturated fats (Table 4.4) are primarily found in olive oil, canola oil, and chicken fat. Additional sources are sunflower oil (the over 70% oleic form), almond oil, and hazelnut oil. Their intake is associated with lowered blood cholesterol and healthy cuisine. Olive oil is the main oil in the Mediterranean diet. Studies show that diets rich in mono fats are as effective at lowering cholesterol levels as diets rich in poly fats.

It is recommended that monounsaturated fats should comprise approximately 1/3 (or a little more) of total daily fat intake. Assuming 30% of calories from fat, this would equate to 10 to 12% of total calories.

## Polyunsaturated Fats (PUFA or Poly)

Polyunsaturated fats (Table 4.5) and their hormonelike compounds help regulate blood clot formation, cholesterol and blood lipid concentrations, the immune response, blood pressure, and other body functions.

TABLE 4.4 **Monounsaturated Fats**

| Structure[a] | Name |
|---|---|
| 14:1 | Myristol |
| 15:1 | Pentadecenoic |
| 16:1 | Palmitol |
| 17:1 | Heptadecanoic |
| 18:1 | Oleic |
| 20:1 | Eicosenoic |
| 22:1 | Erucic |
| 24:1 | Nervonic |

[a]Number of carbons : number of double bonds.

When poly fat intake replaces saturated fat in the diet, blood cholesterol levels are lowered. These fats are found primarily in fruits and vegetables and most plant oils, with the highest concentrations in safflower, sunflower (linoleic over 60%), soy, cottonseed, and corn oils.

It is recommended that approximately 1/3 of total daily fat intake should be from polyunsaturated fats. Assuming 30% of calories from fat, this would equate to 10% of total calories. Because poly fats have two or more double bonds, and are more reactive than other fats to oxidation, additional vitamin E in the diet is recommended. A diet very high in polyunsaturated fats is connected with some cancers.

## *Essential Fatty Acids*

Linoleic acid, alpha-linolenic, and arachidonic fatty acids (18:2, 18:3, and 20:4) are considered essential because the body cannot synthesize them. These fatty acids are plentiful in foods, and deficiencies are usually only seen in those persons on parenteral or enteral feeding or infant formula that does not contain these fats.

When essential fatty acids are missing from the diet, symptoms include dry scaly skin, liver abnormalities, poor wound healing, growth failure in infants, and impaired vision and hearing.

## *Omega Fatty Acids (n-3 and n-6)*

As a natural part of fish and fish oils, omega fatty acids (Table 4.6) generate much interest because their intake is associated with a lowered risk of heart disease. Certain omega fatty acids (EPA, eicosatrienoic acid, and arachidonate) are precursors to eicosanoids, which are important in the regulation of widely diverse physiological processes. The n-3s are more potent than n-6s for reducing triglycerides and in lowering cholesterol. A deficiency of n-3 fatty acids can lead to subtle neurologic and visual problems; a deficiency of n-6 fatty acids can lead to skin lesions.

Recently, for easier terminology, the term omega (ω) is being replaced by the letter "n."

TABLE 4.5 **Polyunsaturated Fats**

| Structure[a] | Name |
|---|---|
| 18:2 | Linoleic (n-6) |
| 18:3 | α-Linolenic (n-3) |
| 18:4 | Stearidonic |
| 20:3 | Eicosatrienoic (n-6) |
| 20:4 | Arachidonate (n-6) |
| 20:5 | EPA—Eicosapentanoic acid (n-3) |
| 22:5 | DPA—Docosapentanoic acid |
| 22:6 | DHA —Docosahexaenoic acid (n-3) |

[a]Number of carbons : number of double bonds.

TABLE 4.6 **Omega Fatty Acids**

| | |
|---|---|
| 18:3 Linolenic | 18:2 Linoleic |
| 20:5 EPA | 20:3 Eicosatrienoic acid |
| 22:6 DHA | 20:4 Arachidonate |

The 1990 Report of the Scientific Review Committee Nutrition Recommendations of Canada recommended a ratio between 4 and 6 g of omega-6 fatty acids to 1 g of omega-3 fatty acids. The 1989 Committee on Diet and Health of the Food and Nutrition Board recommended that an RDA be established in the future for these nutrients.

## *Phospholipids and Sterols*

Phospholipids and sterols are part of the structures of all cells. These compounds have the unique ability to dissolve in both water and fat, which helps them move nutrients, hormones, and other substances in and out of the cells and allows them to act as emulsifying agents to help keep fats suspended in the blood and fluids of the body. One phospholipid form (the sphingomyelins) occurs in the myelin sheath of nerve tissues.

Lecithin, a triglyceride containing choline, is the best known of these phospholipids. Choline's importance has been recognized, evidenced by its addition to the list of DRI nutrients in 1998. Other phospholipids include ethanolamine, serine, and inositol.

## *Cholesterol*

All living cells contain cholesterol. It is the starting material for making hormones, including the sex hormones (estrogens, androgens, progesterone, and testosterone) and the adrenal hormones (cortisol and others).

Most of the body's supply of cholesterol is made by the liver. In foods, cholesterol is only found in foods of animal origin. There is no cholesterol in foods of plant origin—fruits, vegetables, nuts, and grains. The cholesterol in meat is fairly evenly distributed between the lean parts and the fat of meats, except for the greater concentrations in organ meats such as the liver and kidney.

## *Blood Levels of Cholesterol and Disease*

In atherosclerosis, blood vessel walls become caked with *deposits* of cholesterol, narrowing the blood flow, and making the vessel walls less flexible. A high blood serum level of cholesterol is an indicator of the problem; a *risk factor,* however, is not the same as the cause.

Recent studies suggest that high blood levels of homocysteine may irritate and damage the cell walls, causing deposits of cholesterol to occur. These high levels of homocysteine, which can be caused by an enzyme deficiency, are *easily corrected by adequate to temporarily higher intakes of vitamin B-6, vitamin B-12, and folate.*

There are several types of blood serum cholesterol. HDL (high-density lipoprotein—the "healthy or good" type) carries cholesterol in the blood back to the liver. LDL (low-density lipoprotein) and VLDL (very-low density) are considered the "bad" cholesterol.

High dietary intake of *saturated fats* is also associated with high blood cholesterol levels and risk of heart disease. Dietary intake of cholesterol may contribute to increased LDL and VLDL levels in *sensitive* persons, but regardless of food intake, the liver is busy making cholesterol all the time anyway.

# SECTION 5

# VITAMINS

| | | | |
|---|---|---|---|
| Vitamin A | Niacin (vitamin B-3) | Pantothenic acid | Vitamin K |
| Carotenoids | Vitamin B-6 | Vitamin C | Biotin |
| Thiamin (vitamin B-1) | Folate | Vitamin D | Choline |
| Riboflavin (vitamin B-2) | Vitamin B-12 | Vitamin E | |

## Vitamin A

*Vitamin A is vital for vision, growth, the immune system, and reproduction. It is essential for the integrity of the mucous membranes throughout the body and necessary for healthy skin, bone, and tooth growth.*

### *The Vitamin A Family*

Vitamin A comprises a large family of fat-soluble compounds—retinols and carotenoids. The carotenoids are precursors of vitamin A and the body converts it into the active vitamin form. The retinols are already active vitamin A.

#### Retinoids (Retinol, Retinal, and Retinoic Acid)

Animal foods and vitamin A-fortified foods supply this form of vitamin A. Natural sources are primarily liver and dairy products, and the chemical form is used to fortify foods like breakfast cereals. It is easily absorbed and excess is stored in the liver and fat tissue. This is the only form that can become toxic if taken in extremely large quantities, such as from supplements.

#### Carotenoids (Beta-Carotene and Other Carotenoids)

The carotenoids are precursors of vitamin A and are found in fruits and vegetables and in a small amount in dairy foods. There are hundreds of carotenoids and approximately 10% of them have some vitamin A activity. The most active vitamin A precursor is beta-carotene. The value of the carotenoids, however, may exceed vitamin A activity. Many have been found to have other antioxidant functions and health-protective activity that researchers are now studying.

Beta-carotene is responsible for the rich, yellow orange red pigment of fruits and vegetables, but carotenoids are plentiful in dark green vegetables in which chlorophyll masks the orange color. An individual cannot consume toxic doses of *this* form of vitamin A because the body can regulate the absorption. Read more about carotenoids at the end of this vitamin A section.

#### Vitamin A Activity

Vitamin A activity is measured in retinol equivalents (RE) because various forms of the vitamin have different activity levels. The list that follows shows the estimated conversion rates from IUs to REs (international units is an older unit of measure).

#### One RE Vitamin A (in mcg) equals:

10.00 IU from plant foods (average estimate for avg. carotenoids)
6.00 IU from beta-carotene (carotenoid with the most A activity)
12.00 IU from alpha-carotene or cryptoxanthin (carotenoids)
3.33 IU from animal foods and the chemical form used to fortify foods
3.50 IU from cheese (a mixture of retinols and carotenoids)
4.10 IU from yogurt and milk (a mixture of retinols and carotenoids)

### *Vitamin A Functions*

Vitamin A was first identified as a plant substance that prevented eye disorders and is therefore best known for its vital role in promoting and maintaining good vision. Interestingly enough, only one-thousandth of the vitamin A in our bodies is found in the eyes; most is in the blood stream and tissues. The vitamin A that is not flowing through our system is stored in the liver.

Vitamin A is essential for healthy skin and epithelial tissue—the inside surfaces of the mucous membranes, the linings of the mouth, throat, lungs, stomach, intestines, urinary tract, and the reproductive tract. It plays an important role in the body's immune reactions and some forms of vitamin A function as important antioxidants.

Vitamin A is important for normal body growth and formation of soft tissue, maintains the stability of the cell membranes, helps manufacture red blood cells, maintains nerve cell sheaths, and helps ensure a normal output of thyroxin from the thyroid gland. In the formative years, it is important for spacing of teeth, tooth enamel, and the formation of bones.

As antioxidants, beta-carotene and other carotenoids protect the body from disease and the actions of unstable and highly reactive molecules called free radicals. Beta-carotene works with vitamins C and E in the body to build a strong immune system.

## *Vitamin A Losses, Antagonists, and Deficiencies*

Vitamin A destroyers include: tannic acid found in black tea; nitrates and benzoate from preserved food; aspirin; barbiturates; artificial lemon flavoring called citral; ferrous sulfate, an iron supplement; and pollutants such as nitrates from high nitrogen fertilizers, nitrogen dioxide, and ozone.

As a fat-soluble vitamin, the body's absorption of vitamin A is substantially reduced in very low-fat diets. Mineral oil (sold as a laxative) and some fat replacers are not readily absorbed by the body and will attach to the vitamin A and carry it unused from the body. General cooking retention is fairly good and ranges from approximately 70 to 90%; however, high temperatures in the presence of oxygen (air) will destroy much more vitamin A.

Deficiencies of other nutrients, such as vitamin E, iron, zinc, and protein, may adversely affect the absorption, transport, storage, and utilization of vitamin A. There is increased risk of deficiency for alcohol abusers, those with celiac disease or other intestinal malabsorption disorders, tobacco users, smokers, and cancer patients. Also, individuals who dine regularly on hamburgers, french fries, soft drinks, snacks, and candies (and eat few fruits or vegetables) may also run a risk of vitamin A deficiency.

## *Vitamin A Recommended Intake*

The 1989 recommended daily allowance (RDA) values for vitamin A are listed next. The lower amount for women is based on their lower average body size. The RDAs are estimates for healthy individuals; therefore, amounts may vary for those persons with certain health or living conditions:

| | | |
|---|---|---|
| Men | 11 years + | 1,000 RE/day |
| Women | 11 years + | 800 RE/day |
| Pregnant | | 800 RE/day |
| Breastfeeding | | 1,300 RE/day |

Prompted by more recent research findings, many health professionals and organizations are currently recommending higher intakes. The University of California Wellness Newsletter recommends daily amounts of the beta-carotene form of Vitamin A, with vitamins C and E:

- 10,000–25,000 IU (≈1,600–4,000 RE) of *beta-carotene*,
- 250–500 mg of vitamin C, and
- 200–800 IU (133–533 mg) of vitamin E

The 1990 Canadian recommendations for vitamin A are 1,000 RE/day for adult men and 800 RE/day for adult women. There is 400 RE/day additional for breastfeeding, but no change for pregnancy.

## *Vitamin A Upper Limits*

No official UL (upper limit) has been established, but adverse effects are only from the retinol form of vitamin A. A person can*not* overdose on vitamin A from plants (the carotenoid or beta-carotene form), because the body controls the amount it absorbs. However, a person may have problems from the *retinoid* form by ingesting large amounts of polar bear liver (where toxic doses were first noticed), or from megadoses in supplements taken over a period of time (approximately 25,000 IU or 7,500 RE per day of the retinol form).

## *Vitamin A Food Sources*

All dark-green vegetables and yellow-orange vegetables and fruits are excellent sources of beta-carotene and carotenoid forms of vitamin A (Table 5.1). Vegetable-based soups are good sources as well. Dark-green leaves are more nutritious than pale leaves. Romaine lettuce has about eight times the beta-carotene (and six times the vitamin C) as iceberg lettuce.

Good sources of the *retinoid* form are fortified breakfast cereals, milk, and cheese; natural sources are liver, fish liver oils, and eggs (the yolk). Poor sources are meats (except liver), nuts and seeds, and unfortified grain products and cereals.

# Carotenoids

***Carotenoids act as antioxidants in the body and may help protect eyes against the effects of aging.***

## *Some Are Vitamin A Precursors*

Beta-carotene, the best known carotenoid (Table 5.2), is the most active Vitamin A precursor and gives fruits and vegetables their deep orange color. (The dark green of chlorophyll in vegetable greens will mask this orange color.) Vitamin A activity is found in lesser amounts in about 10% of the carotenoids, including alpha-carotene and cryptoxanthin.

## *Nonvitamin A Carotenoids*

Of the 600 to 1,000 or more carotenoids identified, 90% are not vitamin A precursors but perform other disease-preventing, health-promoting functions. These carotenoids, along with other phytochemicals, have antioxidant activity beyond vitamin A that we are only beginning to identify and understand. As vitamins C and E work synergistically with the beta-carotene form of Vitamin A, these carotenoids may also work together rather than individually. Preliminary research suggests that carotenoids lutein and zeaxanthin act to protect eyes against age-related macular degeneration. Lycopene may help prevent or delay prostate cancer.

## *Cooking/Processing Retention*

Preliminary research finds that foods cooked and canned with little contact with air have high nutrient retention rates for

TABLE 5.1 Vitamin A Sources in Rank Order by Serving Size

| | Weight (g) | Vit A (RE) |
|---|---|---|
| **1000–10,000 RE/serving:** | | |
| 3.5 oz ckd beef liver | 100 | 10,700 |
| 3.5 oz ckd veal liver | 100 | 5,600 |
| 3.5 oz ckd chicken liver | 100 | 4,900 |
| 1 T cod liver oil | 13.6 | 4,080 |
| 3.5 oz ckd turkey liver | 100 | 3,700 |
| 7.5″ raw carrot | 72 | 2,025–3,800 |
| 1/2 c ckd sliced carrots | 76 | 1,300–1,900 |
| 1/2 c cnd pumpkin | 123 | 2,700 |
| 1/2 c cnd sweet potatoes | 128 | 1,940 |
| 1 small baked sweet potato | 60 | 1,310 |
| **500–999 RE:** | | |
| 1/2 c ckd butternut squash | 123 | 857 |
| 1 mango | 207 | 805 |
| 1/2 c spinach ckd fr/frzn | 95 | 739 |
| 1/2 c chopped raw broccoli *leaves* | 44 | 704 |
| 4 baby fresh carrots | 40 | 600 |
| 1 c cantaloupe cubes | 160 | 561 |
| 1/2 c collard greens, ckd f/frzn | 90 | 502 |
| **250–499 RE:** | | |
| 1/2 c ckd kale | 65 | 481 |
| 3.5 oz ckd beef kidney | 100 | 373 |
| 1/2 c ckd beet greens | 72 | 367 |
| 1 c vegetable tomato juice | 242 | 283 |
| 1/2 c ckd Swiss chard | 88 | 275 |
| 1/2 c collard greens ckd f/fresh | 90 | 260 |
| **150–249 RE:** | | |
| 1/2 c ckd mustard greens | 70 | 212 |
| 1/4 c sweet chopped red peppers | 37 | 212 |
| 1 c raw spinach | 30 | 202 |
| 3.5 oz ckd veal kidney | 100 | 201 |
| 2 fresh apricots | 70 | 183 |
| 3.5 oz steamed clams | 100 | 171 |
| 1/2 c broccoli ckd from frzn | 92 | 174 |
| 3 oz prunes (≈10) | 85 | 169 |
| **100–149 RE:** | | |
| 1/2 c ckd artichoke hearts | 84 | 149 |
| 1 c nonfat milk added w/vit A | 245 | 149 |
| 3.5 oz ckd oysters | 100 | 146 |
| 1 c romaine lettuce | 56 | 146 |
| 1 c tomato juice | 243 | 136 |
| 1/2 c cnd tomato sauce | 123 | 120 |
| 1/2 c broccoli ckd fr/fresh | 78 | 109 |
| 1 T butter or margarine | 14.2 | 109 |
| 1 c looseleaf lettuce | 56 | 106 |
| 1/2 c raw broccoli flowerets | 36 | 106 |
| 1/4 c raw lavar seaweed | 20 | 104 |
| 4 dried apricots halves | 14 | 101 |
| **50–99 RE/serving:** | | |
| 3.5 oz farmed trout | 100 | 86 |
| 1 oz cheddar cheese | 28.4 | 86 |
| 1 cooked egg | 48–50 | 84 |
| 1 oz American cheese | 28.4 | 82 |
| 3.5 oz raw pacific oysters | 100 | 81 |
| 1/2 c vanilla ice cream | 66 | 77 |
| 1 oz Swiss or provolone cheese | 28.4 | 73 |
| 3.5 oz small ckd shrimp | 100 | 66 |
| 1 half avocado | 100 | 61 |
| 1 c watermelon cubes | 152 | 56 |
| 1/2 c chopped raw tomato | 90 | 56 |
| 1/2 c Brussels sprouts ckd f/fresh | 78 | 56 |
| 1/2 c ckd green peas | 80 | 54 |
| 3.5 oz halibut | 100 | 54 |
| 1 medium peach | 98 | 53 |
| 1 c fresh orange juice | 248 | 50 |
| **15–49 RE:** | | |
| 1/2 c ckd okra | 92 | 46 |
| 1/2 c Brussels sprouts, ckd f/fzn | 78 | 46 |
| 4 spears ckd asparagus | 60 | 40 |
| 1 c papaya cubes | 140 | 39 |
| 1 c lowfat yogurt | 245 | 39 |
| 1 pink/red grapefruit half | 123 | 32 |
| 1/2 c ckd green beans | 65 | 27 |
| 3.5 oz ckd dark chicken meat | 100 | 24 |
| 1/2 c 2% fat cottage cheese | 28.4 | 23 |
| 1 whole ckd artichoke | 120 | 22 |
| 1/4 c pumpkin seed kernels, rstd | 57 | 22 |
| 1 c chilled orange juice | 249 | 20 |
| 1 c iceberg lettuce | 56 | 18 |
| 1 T raw chicken fat | 12.8 | 18 |
| 1/2 c ckd broccoli stalks | 85 | 18 |
| 1/2 c pistachios | 64 | 15 |
| 3.5 oz farmed catfish or salmon | 100 | 15 |
| 1/2 c ckd green soybeans | 90 | 14.4 |

Listing includes elemental and enriched foods; does not include additionally fortified products like breakfast cereals.
Source: The Food Finder, ESHA Research, Salem, Oregon, 1999. Printed with permission.

carotenoids. However, they oxidize and lose value when they have been dehydrated or freeze dried in the presence of air. Retention is high if the drying or freeze-drying process is closed to air exposure. Because vitamin A and carotenoids are fat soluble, more is available if cooked in a little oil or butter.

## *Bioavailability*

Preliminary information finds that far more beta-carotene is bioavailable in cooked carrots than in raw. The carotenoid lycopene in cooked and processed tomatoes is more easily absorbed than that in raw tomatoes.

## Carotenoids, Phytochemicals, Flavonoids, and More

Keep a watch for new research findings. Many foods contain compounds with strong antioxidant and health-promoting properties that exceed the vitamins they contain. A good example are berries, which contain many such compounds.

TABLE 5.2 Sources of Carotenoids

| Carotenoid type | Food Sources |
|---|---|
| Alpha-carotene | *Fruits:* Orange juice.<br>*Vegetables:* Carrots, tomatoes, pumpkin. |
| Beta-carotene | *Fruits:* Apricots, cantaloupe, grapefruit, mango, peaches, orange juice, watermelon.<br>*Vegetables:* Carrots, pumpkin, sweet potatoes, winter squash. Broccoli, especially broccoli leaves, greens of all kinds (beet, collards, mustard, fennel, fresh parsley, kale, romaine lettuce, spinach) red peppers, tomatoes and tomato products (juice, sauces, paste). |
| Lutein & Zeaxanthin | *Fruits:* Peaches, orange juice.<br>*Vegetables:* Kale, spinach, broccoli, pumpkin, summer squash, Brussels sprouts, fresh parsley, dark-green leaf lettuce (not iceberg), green peas, leeks, mustard greens, Swiss chard, chicory, tomatoes, okra, carrots. |
| Lycopene | *Fruits:* Pink grapefruit, dried apricots, guava or guava juice, watermelon.<br>*Vegetables:* Red tomatoes, tomato based products (catsup, sauces, juice, paste). |
| Cryptoxanthin | *Fruits:* Oranges, orange juice, nectarines, papayas, peaches, tangerines, mangos. |

# Thiamin (Vitamin B-1)

***Thiamin is essential for helping cells convert carbohydrate into energy and necessary for healthy nerve cell, brain, and heart function.***

## *Thiamin Functions*

Thiamin is essential for making the energy in food available to the body. It works with other "B" vitamins in the many stages of metabolism to convert carbohydrates into a usable form of energy (glucose). In this role, it is pivotal in providing fuel to the brain, heart, nerves, and other body cells. Thiamin also plays an important, but less understood, role in regulating normal nerve transmissions. More thiamin is needed if you are very active and consume a high calorie diet, or if a high percentage of your calories comes from carbohydrates.

## *Thiamin Deficiencies*

Because the brain and nervous system rely on glucose for energy, they are sensitive to a shortfall of this vitamin. Mild deficiencies result in the inability to concentrate, poor coordination, irritability, depression, and muscle weakness. Major deficiencies produce far more severe symptoms: edema, atrophy of leg muscles, peripheral nerve changes, paralysis, and heart failure. The clinical condition of severe, prolonged deficiency, called Beriberi, led to the discovery of this vitamin.

Thiamin is needed to metabolize alcohol, and concurrently, alcohol decreases the absorption of thiamin. Also at risk are those who consume large quantities of unenriched white rice or baked goods made with *un*enriched white flour, or smokers and those with chronic fevers and kidney diseases. Deficiencies may be created with a continual diet of only dry snacks (such as corn chips and pretzels that are not made with enriched flour), or a continual diet of soft drinks and candy (a low-nutrient, high-calorie diet).

The practice of removing the outer hull of rice to produce the white appearance started with affluent members of eastern societies more than 4,000 years ago. The hull that was polished off was rich in thiamin along with other "B" vitamins and several more nutrients.

As "pale" rice replaced whole grain rice and became the staple of the diet, the prevalence of beriberi increased to epidemic proportions. It took a long time for researchers to discover that Beriberi was the result of something NOT in the food, rather than by some bacteria or substance IN the food. It wasn't until the late 19th century that a surgeon in the Japanese navy demonstrated that beriberi could be prevented by adding thiamin-rich foods such as meat and whole grains to the diet.

## *Thiamin Losses*

Thiamin is not heat-stable and, therefore, is one of the vitamins most easily destroyed by cooking or by the milling of grains. Thiamin is a water-soluble vitamin and will dissolve into the cooking liquid. If the liquid is retained and used, there should be fairly complete retention. The Enrichment Act of 1942 required thiamin (and several other nutrients) to be added to flour and cereals to compensate for the loss of nutrients during the milling and processing of grain.

## *Thiamin Recommended Intake*

Because thiamin is essential to the metabolism of energy (calories), the recommended amount of thiamin in the 1989 RDAs was indexed to the calories consumed at 0.5 mg thiamin/1,000 kcal/day with a 1 mg/day minimum. The 1998 RDA/DRI for thiamin converted the amount to a single daily value regardless of caloric intake.

| | | |
|---|---|---|
| Men | 14 years + | 1.2 mg/day |
| Women | 14 years + | 1.1 mg/day |
| Pregnant | | 1.4 mg/day |
| Breastfeeding | | 1.5 mg/day w/ 1.0 mg minimum |

The recommended daily allowance (RDA) values are estimates for healthy individuals. Amounts may increase for individuals who are very athletic and active, and those persons with certain health conditions, such as those being treated with dialysis, individuals with malabsorption syndrome, women carrying more than one fetus, or those who are nursing more than one infant.

The 1990 Canadian RNIs recommended a thiamin intake of 0.40 mg/1,000 cal/day for adults, with a minimum of 0.9 mg/day.

## *Thiamin Upper Limits*

There have been no reported cases of thiamin toxicity from foods; therefore, no official upper limit (UL) was set in the 1998 recommendations. As a water-soluble vitamin, excess amounts are easily excreted in the urine.

TABLE 5.3 Thiamin Sources—Vitamin B-1 in Rank Order by Serving Size

| | Weight (g) | Thiamin (mg) |
|---|---|---|
| **0.5–2.5 mg/serving:** | | |
| 2 T brewers yeast | 16 | 2.3 |
| 3.5 oz ckd roast pork | 100 | 0.9 |
| 3.5 oz ckd ham | 100 | 0.7 |
| 1/2 c brazil nuts | 70 | 0.7 |
| 1/2 c pistachios | 64 | 0.5 |
| 1/2 c chopped pecans | 60 | 0.5 |
| **0.25–0.49 mg:** | | |
| 3.5 oz ckd farmed catfish | 100 | 0.4 |
| 2 oz bagel | 71 | 0.4 |
| 1/2 c soynuts (roasted soybeans) | 86 | 0.4 |
| 1/2 c filberts | 68 | 0.3 |
| 1 c ckd pasta | 140 | 0.3 |
| 1/2 c cashews | 65 | 0.3 |
| 1 c ckd oatmeal | 234 | 0.26 |
| 1 c orange juice | 248 | 0.25 |
| 3.5 oz ckd veal liver | 100 | 0.25 |
| **0.20–0.24 mg:** | | |
| 3.5 oz ckd trout | 100 | 0.24 |
| 1/2 c ckd green soybeans | 90 | 0.23 |
| 1/2 c ckd green peas | 80 | 0.23 |
| 1/2 c chopped walnuts | 60 | 0.23 |
| 1/2 c macadamias | 68 | 0.23 |
| 3.5 oz ckd beef liver | 100 | 0.21 |
| 1/2 c ckd black beans | 86 | 0.21 |
| 1/2 c peanuts | 72 | 0.20 |
| **0.15–0.19 mg:** | | |
| 1/2 c ckd green split peas | 98 | 0.19 |
| 1/2 c ckd navy beans | 131 | 0.19 |
| 1 c ckd whole wheat pasta | 140 | 0.15 |
| 1/2 c lima beans ckd fr/dry | 94 | 0.15 |
| 3.5 oz steamed clams | 100 | 0.15 |
| 1 c grapes | 160 | 0.15 |
| **0.10–0.14 mg:** | | |
| 1/2 c ckd kidney beans | 89 | 0.14 |
| 1 piece white bread | 30 | 0.14 |
| 1 baked potato w/skin | 122 | 0.14 |
| 3.5 oz ckd oysters | 100 | 0.13 |
| 1/2 c ckd white rice | 79 | 0.13 |
| 1/2 c ckd acorn squash | 123 | 0.12 |
| 1 c watermelon | 152 | 0.12 |
| 1 c pink grapefruit juice | 247 | 109 |
| 1 mango | 207 | 0.12 |
| 3.5 oz ckd beef, all kinds | 100 | 0.12 |
| 1 c tomato-vegetable juice | 242 | 0.11 |
| 3.5 oz beef/pork hotdog | 100 | 0.11 |
| 1/4 c pumpkin seed kernels | 57 | 0.11 |
| 5 oz ckd lamb | 100 | 0.11 |
| 1 c lowfat yogurt | 245 | 0.11 |
| 1 avocado half | 100 | 0.11 |
| 1 c tomato juice | 243 | 0.11 |
| 1/2 c cnd pinto beans | 120 | 0.10 |
| 1/2 c almonds | 78 | 0.10 |
| **0.05–0.09 mg:** | | |
| 1/2 c ckd brown rice | 98 | 0.09 |
| 3.5 oz ckd dark chicken meat | 100 | 0.09 |
| 1 c milk | 245 | 0.09 |
| 1/2 c pineapple juice | 125 | 0.09 |
| 1/2 c mashed potatoes | 105 | 0.09 |
| 1/2 c ckd beet greens | 72 | 0.08 |
| 1 whole ckd artichoke | 120 | 0.08 |
| 1/2 c ckd peapods | 80 | 0.08 |
| 3.5 oz ckd light chicken meat | 100 | 0.07 |
| 1/4 c sunflower seeds | 68 | 0.07 |
| 7.5" raw carrot | 72 | 0.07 |
| 1 T oat bran | 6 | 0.07 |
| 3.5 oz ckd dark turkey meat | 100 | 0.06 |

Listing includes elemental and enriched foods; does not include additionally fortified products like breakfast cereals.
Source: The Food Finder, ESHA Research, Salem, Oregon, 1999. Printed with permission.

## *Thiamin Food Sources*

Excellent sources include pork, bacon, and ham, most nuts, fish, enriched grain products (breads, pasta, and fortified breakfast cereals), soy and soy products, cooked dried beans and peas, wheat germ, and various vegetables and fruits (Table 5.3).

# Riboflavin (Vitamin B-2)

***Riboflavin helps cells convert carbohydrates into energy and is essential for cell growth, production of red blood cells, and healthy skin and eyes.***

## *Riboflavin Functions*

Riboflavin is needed to release the body's stored energy for use. It works with the other B vitamins and is essential to the activation and functioning of vitamins B-6, folate, niacin, and vitamin K. As a component of several different enzymes, riboflavin is essential to many steps in the metabolism of carbohydrates, fats, and protein. People who are more active need more riboflavin.

Cell growth cannot occur without riboflavin. It is necessary for building and maintaining body tissue, for making red blood cells, for helping the body protect itself from common skin and eye disorders, and for synthesizing corticosteroids. Riboflavin is a water-soluble, yellow fluorescent compound.

## *Riboflavin Deficiencies*

A riboflavin deficiency most often occurs in combination with a deficiency of other B vitamins. Symptoms include an inflamed mouth with cracks in the corners, scaly, dry facial skin, confusion, and poor wound healing. Rapidly growing tissues such as skin and the mucous membranes lining the eyes, mouth, and tongue are first to be affected.

## *Riboflavin Losses*

Riboflavin is processed out of whole grain when it is milled into flour and out of rice when it is polished. It is restored to white wheat flour and cornmeal through "enrichment"; therefore, products made from enriched flour provide a good source of riboflavin. Enriched white rice contains additional thiamin, folate, niacin, and iron, but not riboflavin.

Riboflavin is water-soluble and fairly heat-stable. Small amounts of riboflavin will leach into cooking water because it is water-soluble, but if the cooking water is used there should be fairly complete retention. Riboflavin is light sensitive, however. Ever wonder why milk is seldom sold in clear glass bottles? Fifty percent of the riboflavin in a clear bottle is destroyed in 2 hours if exposed to direct sunlight, and approximately 20% is destroyed on an overcast day.

## *Riboflavin Recommended Intake*

The 1998 Dietary Reference Intakes for riboflavin are listed next. The lower amount for women is based on average lower body size.

| | | |
|---|---|---|
| Men | 14 years + | 1.3 mg/day |
| Women | 14 years + | 1.1 mg/day |
| Pregnant | | 1.4 mg/day |
| Breastfeeding | | 1.6 mg/day w/1.0 mg min. |

The Canadian 1990 RNIs recommend 0.5 mg of riboflavin/1,000 kcal of daily intake for adults.

## *Riboflavin Upper Limits*

There are no reported cases of riboflavin toxicity; therefore, no official UL has been set. As a water-soluble vitamin, and because of riboflavin's yellow fluorescent color, excess amounts are excreted, resulting in bright yellow urine.

## *Riboflavin Food Sources*

The best riboflavin sources (Table 5.4) are organ meats (liver, kidney, heart), almonds, brewers yeast, soynuts, shellfish (oysters, clams), yogurt and cheeses, milk, meats, poultry (especially the dark meat), eggs, enriched breads, fortified breakfast cereals, spinach, avocados, mangos, bananas, mushrooms, and sweet potatoes.

TABLE 5.4 **Riboflavin Sources—Vitamin B-2 in Rank Order by Serving Size**

| | Weight (g) | Riboflavin (mg) |
|---|---|---|
| **1–5 mg/serving:** | | |
| 3.5 oz ckd beef liver | 100 | 4.14 |
| 3.5 oz ckd beef kidney | 100 | 4.10 |
| 3.5 oz ckd veal liver | 100 | 3.36 |
| 3.5 oz ckd chicken liver | 100 | 1.75 |
| 3.5 oz ckd beef heart | 100 | 1.5 |
| 3.5 oz ckd turkey liver | 100 | 1.4 |
| **0.5–1.0 mg:** | | |
| 1/2 c almonds | 78 | 0.78 |
| 2 T brewer's yeast | 16 | 0.69 |
| 1/2 c soynuts (roasted soybeans) | 86 | 0.65 |
| 3.5 oz ckd mackerel | 100 | 0.54 |
| 1 c lowfat yogurt | 245 | 0.52 |
| 3.5 oz steamed clams | 100 | 0.43 |
| **0.25–0.49 mg:** | | |
| 3.5 oz ckd veal | 100 | 0.36 |
| 1 c nonfat milk | 245 | 0.34 |
| 3.5 oz ckd pork loin | 100 | 0.31 |
| 3.5 oz ckd lean beef steak | 100 | 0.28 |
| 3.5 oz ckd lamb | 100 | 0.28 |
| 3.5 oz ckd herring | 100 | 0.28 |
| 1 cooked egg | 48–50 | 0.26 |
| 3.5 oz ckd oysters | 100 | 0.25 |
| 3.5 oz ckd dark chicken or turkey | 100 | 0.25 |
| **0.15–0.24 mg:** | | |
| 3.5 oz ckd ground beef | 100 | 0.23 |
| 1 c fresh pasta | 150 | 0.23 |
| 2.5 oz plain bagel | 71 | 0.22 |
| 10" flour tortilla | 72 | 0.22 |
| 1/2 c cottage cheese | 28.4 | 0.21 |
| 1/2 c ckd beet greens | 72 | 0.21 |
| 1/4 c pumpkin seed kernels, rstd | 57 | 0.18 |
| 1/2 c spinach ckd, fr/frzn | 95 | 0.16 |
| 3.5 oz raw oysters | 100 | 0.15 |
| **0.10–0.14 mg:** | | |
| 1/2 c ckd green soybeans | 90 | 0.14 |
| 3.5 oz ckd white turkey meat | 100 | 0.14 |
| 3 oz prunes (≈10) | 85 | 0.14 |
| 1 c regular ckd pasta | 140 | 0.14 |
| 3/4 c prune juice | 192 | 0.13 |
| 3.5 oz ckd light chicken meat | 100 | 0.13 |
| 3.5 oz ckd ham | 100 | 0.13 |
| 1 avocado half | 100 | 0.12 |
| 1 medium mango | 207 | 0.12 |
| 1 banana | 118 | 0.12 |
| 1/4 c ckd mushrooms | 39 | 0.12 |
| 2 T wheat germ | 14 | 0.12 |
| 1/2 c cnd sweet potatoes | 128 | 0.12 |
| 1/2 c pistachios | 64 | 0.11 |
| 1 c fresh strawberry halves | 152 | 0.11 |
| 1 oz cheddar cheese | 28.4 | 0.11 |
| 1 piece white bread | 30 | 0.10 |
| 1/2 c tofu | 124 | 0.10 |
| **0.05–0.09 mg** | | |
| 1/2 c black-eyed peas, ckd fr/dry | 120 | 0.09 |
| 1/2 c ckd broccoli | 85 | 0.09 |
| 1/2 c ckd Brussels sprouts | 78 | 0.09 |
| 1/4 c sunflower seeds | 68 | 0.09 |
| 1 whole ckd artichoke | 120 | 0.08 |
| 1/2 c ckd pintos | 120 | 0.08 |
| 1/2 c ckd lentils | 99 | 0.08 |
| 1/2 c ckd navy beans | 131 | 0.07 |
| 1 T oat bran | 6 | 0.07 |
| 1/2 c ckd Swiss chard | 88 | 0.07 |
| 1 c ckd oatmeal | 234 | 0.05 |

Listing includes elemental and enriched foods; does not include additionally fortified products like breakfast cereals.
Source: The Food Finder, ESHA Research, Salem, Oregon, 1999. Printed with permission.

## Niacin (Vitamin B-3, Nicotinic Acid, Nicotinamide, and Niacinamide)

***Niacin is central to the release of energy from foods and helps maintain healthy skin, nerves, and the digestive tract.***

### *Niacin Functions*

Niacin is essential to almost every biochemical link in the metabolism of carbohydrates, proteins, and fats for energy. If there is a shortfall, the energy reactions are blocked. As a result, the amount of niacin needed is generally proportional to the calories eaten. Niacin protects the skin, nervous tissues, and the digestive tract from disorders, aids in calcium mobilization, and is required in DNA repair.

Large doses of niacin have been shown to lower blood cholesterol levels, lower blood triglycerides, and lower the low-density lipoproteins (LDLs), while raising HDLs (the good cholesterol). However, therapeutic use of niacin should be conducted under a doctor's supervision, because at high dosages, niacin is no longer acting as a vitamin—it's a drug. (See upper limits.)

There are several forms of niacin, and niacin reported in food composition tables represents the niacin already available in foods. However, there is also a precursor—the amino acid tryptophan. About 60 mg of tryptophan can be converted to 1 mg of niacin. (The actual equivalency data ranges from 39 to 86 mg, and appears to be influenced by hormones—larger amounts are converted during pregnancy or when contraceptive pills are taken.)

When this additional form of niacin is considered, the combined total is called Niacin Equivalents (NEs), which is the measure the RDAs use. Because tryptophan is also needed as a protein, the body makes the choice of how much is converted into niacin. The conversion requires the coenzyme forms of vitamin B-6 and riboflavin; therefore, niacin status is also dependent on the availability of these nutrients.

### *Niacin Deficiencies*

Deficiencies include symptoms such as fatigue, decreased appetite, indigestion, diarrhea, nervous irritability, and sometimes a swollen, red, sore tongue. A pigmented rash may develop symmetrically in areas of the skin exposed to sunlight. Mental symptoms include irritability, headaches, loss of memory, emotional instability, psychosis, and delirium. Children with a niacin deficiency can be weak and show poor growth.

Symptoms of a severe deficiency include skin and gastrointestinal lesions, inflammation of the mucous membranes, and mental disorders leading to dementia and death. This condition is called pellagra. At the turn of the century, pellagra was a severe problem in the South where the diet of the poor was dependent primarily on refined cornmeal and salt pork (really just fat). The niacin-deficient grain combined with the generally low protein diet led to the development of pellagra. Niacin played a big role in "curing" large numbers of mental patients in the South after the turn of the century—nearly half of the psychiatric cases at that time were cleared up with niacin. Clinical pellagra may also represent the combined deficiency of niacin and riboflavin.

### *Niacin Losses*

When cereal grains are milled into flour, large amounts of niacin are lost. Because of enrichment, however, enriched grain products are a good source of niacin. Niacin in meats is in a different form and appears to be more available. Niacin in cooked mature beans, liver, and in fortified foods is in the free form and is highly available. Studies now show that niacin intake in the United States is generous and typically exceeds the RDAs.

Niacin is fairly stable in food preparation and storage; however, as a water-soluble vitamin, some will dissolve into cooking liquid. If the liquid is retained and consumed, losses are minimized. Prolonged treatment with the drug Isoniazid will reduce the conversion of tryptophan to niacin, but will not interfere with preformed niacin.

### *Niacin Recommended Intake*

The recommendations assume sources of niacin from both preformed niacin *and* the amount that can be converted from tryptophan. The combined measure is called niacin equivalents (NEs) (Table 5.5).

Average diets in the United States supply about 700 mg of tryptophan for adult women and 1,100 mg for adult men. This converts to about 11.7 mg to 18.3 mg of niacin over and above the amount of preformed niacin already in food.

The 1998 RDAs for niacin are for healthy individuals. Additional niacin intake may be required for persons on dialysis, those with malabsorption syndrome, pregnant women bearing multiple fetuses, and women breastfeeding more than one infant. The 1998 Dietary Reference Intakes for niacin were adjusted down from the 1989 recommendations.

| | | |
|---|---|---|
| Men | 14 years + | 16 mg NE/day |
| Women | 14 years + | 14 mg NE/day |
| Pregnant | | 18 mg NE/day |
| Breastfeeding | | 17 mg NE/day |

The 1990 Canadian RNI recommends 7.2 NE per 1,000 kcal of food intake, with a minimum of 14.4 NE/day for age 19 years and older.

### *Niacin Upper Limits*

Adverse affects have been observed at prolonged, very high niacin intakes of the *nicotinic acid* form. Because the first noticed side effect is usually flushing, the intakes can be readily adjusted to a lower amount. Flushing is the result of a release of histamine and can cause reddening of the face, arms, and chest and a burning, tingling, or itching sensation in the hands and feet. Other

TABLE 5.5 **Comparison of Niacin and Niacin Equivalent (NE) for Selected Foods**

| Food Item | mg | mg NE |
|---|---|---|
| 3.5 oz light chicken meat | 13.4 | 19.8 |
| 3.5 oz dark chicken meat | 7.1 | 12.8 |
| 3.5 oz salmon | 8.1 | 12.2 |
| 3.5 oz ground beef | 5.3 | 10.0 |
| 3.5 oz pork/ham | 4.8 | 11.0 |
| 2 T peanut butter | 4.4 | 5.6 |
| 1 c nonfat milk | 0.2 | 2.1 |
| 1/2 c 2% fat cottage cheese | 0.2 | 2.8 |
| 1 c lowfat yogurt | 0.3 | 1.4 |
| 1 c cooked oatmeal | 0.3 | 1.7 |

reported symptoms include nausea, diarrhea, high blood uric acid levels, high blood sugar, and heart arrhythmia. The nicotinamide form does not cause these toxic effects, but it also does not reduce blood lipid levels.

Toxic levels of niacin intake may cause adverse effects for those who have liver dysfunction or a history of liver disease, diabetes, active peptic ulcer disease, gout, cardiac arrhythmia, migraine headaches, alcoholism, or inflammatory bowel disease. However, there are also documented cases in which severe liver dysfunction has occurred in healthy individuals as a result of the prolonged intake of high amounts of niacin.

Upper limits were established with the 1998 Dietary Reference Intakes and do not apply to persons receiving niacin therapy under a doctor's care.

| | |
|---|---|
| 10 mg/day | Ages 1–3 years |
| 15 mg/day | Ages 4–8 years |
| 20 mg/day | Ages 9–13 years |
| 30 mg/day | Ages 14–18 years |
| 35 mg/day | Adults over 19 years and women who are pregnant or breastfeeding. |

## *Niacin Food Sources*

The best niacin sources (Tables 5.6 and 5.7) are organ meats such as liver, fish, poultry, peanuts, nutritional yeast, lamb, veal, pork and ham, polish sausage, peanut butter, beef, enriched breads, fortified breakfast cereals, tofu, enriched pasta, almonds, shrimp, sunflower seeds, soybeans, potatoes, rice, mushrooms, tomato sauces, sweet potatoes, green peas, corn, and lentils.

Other foods are good sources when the availability of the niacin precursor tryptophan is considered. Milk products, legumes, more vegetables, and some fruits also become excellent sources. In rank order, they are cheeses (most of them), tofu, avocados, milk, cooked dried beans, green peas, mangos, corn, yogurt, eggs, cooked collard greens, spinach, broccoli, Brussels sprouts, prune juice, peaches, orange juice, raisins, and strawberries.

TABLE 5.6 **Niacin Sources–Vitamin B-3 in Rank Order by Serving Size**

| | Weight (g) | Niacin (mg) |
|---|---|---|
| **10–17 mg/serving:** | | |
| 3.5 oz ckd veal liver | 100 | 16.9 |
| 3.5 oz ckd beef liver | 100 | 14.4 |
| 1/2 c peanuts | 72 | 10.5 |
| 3.5 oz ckd chicken white meat | 100 | 13.4 |
| 3.5 oz ckd mackerel | 100 | 10.7 |
| **5–10 mg:** | | |
| 3.5 oz ckd trout | 100 | 8.8 |
| 3.5 oz ckd salmon | 100 | 8.0 |
| 3.5 oz ckd veal, ranges 6.4–9.3 | 100 | 7.9 |
| 3.5 oz ckd chicken dark meat | 100 | 7.1 |
| 3.5 oz ckd lamb | 100 | 6.6 |
| 3.5 oz ckd turkey white meat | 100 | 6.2 |
| 2 T brewers yeast | 16 | 6.1 |
| 3.5 oz ckd turkey liver | 100 | 5.9 |
| 3.5 oz ckd ground beef | 100 | 5.3 |
| 3.5 oz beef kidney, ranges 4.6–6.0 | 100 | 5.3 |
| **2.5–4.9 mg:** | | |
| 3.5 oz ckd pork ranges 4.1–5.4 | 100 | 4.8 |
| 3.5 oz ckd chicken dark meat | 100 | 4.5 |
| 2 T peanut butter | 32 | 4.4 |
| 3.5 oz ckd beef heart | 100 | 4.1 |
| 3.5 oz beef steak, ranges 3.6–4.5 | 100 | 4.1 |
| 1/4 c sunflower seeds | 68 | 3.4 |
| 3.5 oz ckd turkey dark meat | 100 | 3.7 |
| 3.5 oz ckd oysters | 100 | 3.6 |
| 2.5 oz plain bagel | 71 | 3.3 |
| 1/2 c almonds | 78 | 2.7 |
| 3.5 oz ckd shrimp | 100 | 2.6 |
| 10″ flour tortilla | 72 | 2.6 |
| **1.5–2.4 mg:** | | |
| 1 c ckd pasta | 140 | 2.3 |
| 1 baked potato w/skin | 122 | 2.0 |
| 1 avocado half | 100 | 1.9 |
| 1/4 c ckd mushrooms | 39 | 1.7 |
| 3 oz prunes (≈10) | 85 | 1.7 |
| 1/2 c ckd barley | 78 | 1.6 |
| **1–1.5 mg:** | | |
| 3/4 c prune juice | 192 | 1.5 |
| 1 medium mango | 207 | 1.5 |
| 1/2 c ckd brown rice | 98 | 1.5 |
| 3.5 oz ckd lunchmeats-average | 100 | 1.5 |
| 1/2 c ckd lentils | 99 | 1.4 |
| 1/2 c macadamias | 68 | 1.4 |
| 1/2 c tomato sauce | 123 | 1.4 |
| 1/2 c cnd sweet potatoes | 128 | 1.2 |
| 1/2 c ckd white rice | 79 | 1.2 |
| 1 piece white bread | 30 | 1.2 |
| 1 ckd whole artichoke | 120 | 1.2 |
| 1/2 c ckd butternut squash | 123 | 1.2 |
| 1/2 c ckd green peas | 80 | 1.2 |
| 1/2 c mashed potatoes | 105 | 1.1 |
| 1/2 c ckd green soybeans | 90 | 1.1 |
| 1/2 c ckd corn | 75 | 1.1 |
| 1 medium peach | 98 | 1.0 |
| 1/2 c pumpkin seed kernels-rstd | 57 | 1.0 |
| 1 c cantaloupe cubes | 160 | 0.9 |
| 1/2 c ckd green split peas | 98 | 0.9 |
| 1/2 c ckd artichoke hearts | 84 | 0.8 |
| 1 T wheat germ | 14 | 0.8 |

Listing includes elemental and enriched foods; does not include additionally fortified products like breakfast cereals.
Source: The Food Finder, ESHA Research, Salem, Oregon, 1999. Printed with permission.

TABLE 5.7 Niacin Equivalents (Niacin + Tryptophan ÷ by 60) in Rank Order by Serving Size

| | Weight (g) | Niacin NE |
|---|---|---|
| **15–20 mg NE/serving:** | | |
| 3.5 oz light chicken meat | 100 | 19.8 |
| 3.5 oz veal liver | 100 | 16.9 |
| 3.5 oz mackerel | 100 | 15.5 |
| **10–14.9 NE:** | | |
| 3.5 oz ckd beef liver | 100 | 14.4 |
| 1/2 c peanuts | 72 | 13.5 |
| 3.5 oz ckd farmed trout | 100 | 13.3 |
| 3.5 oz ckd lamb | 100 | 13.3 |
| 3.5 oz ckd dark chicken meat | 100 | 12.8 |
| 3.5 oz ckd farmed salmon | 100 | 12.2 |
| 3.5 oz ckd halibut | 100 | 12.1 |
| 3.5 oz ckd veal | 100 | 11.8 |
| 3.5 oz ckd lamb | 100 | 11.8 |
| 3.5 oz ckd light turkey meat | 100 | 11.5 |
| 3.5 oz ckd pork and ham | 100 | 10.9 |
| 3.5 oz ckd ground beef | 100 | 10.1 |
| **7.5–9.9 NE:** | | |
| 3.5 oz ckd dark turkey meat | 100 | 9.1 |
| 3.5 oz fish, ranges 6.5 –9.2 | 100 | 8.5 |
| 3.5 oz ckd beef | 100 | 8.7 |
| 1/2 c soynuts (roasted soybeans) | 86 | 8.7 |
| 3.5 oz steamed clams | 100 | 8.1 |
| **5.0–7.4 NE** | | |
| 3.5 oz ckd shrimp | 100 | 7.4 |
| 1/2 c almonds | 78 | 6.9 |
| 2 T brewer's yeast | 16 | 6.1 |
| 3.5 oz beef kidney | 100 | 6.0 |
| 3.5 oz farmed catfish | 100 | 6.0 |
| 3.5 oz turkey liver | 100 | 5.9 |
| 1/4 c pumpkin seed kernels | 57 | 5.7 |
| 2 T peanut butter | 32 | 5.6 |
| 1 oz soy protein Isolate | 28.4 | 5.3 |
| 2.5 oz plain bagel | 71 | 4.7 |
| **2.5–4.9 NE:** | | |
| 3.5 oz veal liver | 100 | 4.6 |
| 3.5 oz chicken liver | 100 | 4.5 |
| 3.5 oz beef heart | 100 | 4.1 |
| 1/2 c cashews | 65 | 3.9 |
| 1/2 c macadamias | 68 | 3.8 |
| 1 10" flour tortilla | 72 | 3.85 |
| 1/2 c ckd green soybeans | 90 | 3.8 |
| 1/2 c brazil nuts | 70 | 3.75 |
| 1/4 c sunflower seed kernels | 68 | 3.4 |
| 1/2 c pistachios | 64 | 3.4 |
| 1/2 c filberts | 68 | 2.85 |
| 1 baked potato with skin | 122 | 2.75 |
| 1/2 c cottage cheese | 113 | 2.75 |
| 1/2 c tofu | 124 | 2.6 |
| 1/2 c navy beans | 131 | 2.6 |
| 1/2 c chopped walnuts | 60 | 2.5 |
| 1/2 c chopped pecans | 60 | 2.5 |
| **2.0–2.4 NE:** | | |
| 1/2 c ckd lentils | 99 | 2.4 |
| 1/2 c ckd split peas | 98 | 2.4 |
| 1 avocado half | 100 | 2.3 |
| 1 c nonfat milk | 245 | 2.1 |
| 1/4 c ckd mushrooms | 39 | 2.1 |
| 1/2 c ckd kidney beans | 89 | 2.0 |
| 1/2 c black-eyed peas, ckd fr/frzn | 85 | 2.0 |
| 1/2 c baby lima beans, ckd fr/frzn | 90 | 2.0 |
| 1 c whole milk | 244 | 2.0 |
| 1/2 c black beans, ckd fr/dry | 86 | 1.9 |
| 1/2 c baked beans, canned | 127 | 1.9 |
| 1 c tomato juice | 243 | 1.8 |
| 1/2 c lima beans, ckd fr/dry | 94 | 1.8 |
| **1.5–1.75 NE:** | | |
| 1 oz Swiss cheese | 28.4 | 1.75 |
| 1 c vegetable-tomato juice | 242 | 1.75 |
| 1/2 c cnd sweet potato | 128 | 1.7 |
| 1 piece bread–avg all | 28 | 1.7 |
| 2T wheat germ | 14 | 1.7 |
| 1 c ckd oatmeal | 234 | 1.7 |
| 3 oz prunes (≈10) | 85 | 1.7 |
| 1/2 c ckd green peas | 80 | 1.6 |
| 1/2 c mashed potatoes | 105 | 1.6 |
| 1/2 c canned tomato sauce | 123 | 1.6 |
| 1 oz provolone cheese | 28.4 | 1.5 |
| 1 oz American cheese | 28.4 | 1.5 |
| 1/2 c ckd corn | 82 | 1.5 |
| 1/2 c cnd pinto beans | 120 | 1.5 |
| 3/4 c prune juice | 192 | 1.5 |
| 1 medium mango | 207 | 1.5 |
| 1/2 c butternut squash | 123 | 1.5 |
| **1.0–1.4 NE:** | | |
| 1 oz cheddar cheese | 28.4 | 1.4 |
| 1 c lowfat yogurt | 245 | 1.4 |
| 1 ckd egg | 48–50 | 1.3 |
| 1 whole ckd artichoke | 120 | 1.2 |
| 1 c cantaloupe cubes | 160 | 1.1 |
| 1/2 c ckd collards | 90 | 1.1 |
| 1 small orange | 96 | 1.1 |
| 1/2 c ckd spinach | 95 | 1.1 |
| 1 oz unsweetened chocolate | 28.4 | 1.0 |
| 1 medium peach | 98 | 1.0 |
| 1/2 c ckd okra | 92 | 1.0 |
| **0.4–0.9 NE:** | | |
| 1/2 c ckd peapods | 80 | 0.9 |
| 1/2 c ckd Brussels sprouts | 78 | 0.9 |
| 1/2 c ckd broccoli | 85 | 0.9 |
| 1/4 c raw mushrooms | 17.5 | 0.9 |
| 1/2 c ckd artichoke hearts | 84 | 0.8 |
| 1/2 c ckd beet greens | 72 | 0.8 |
| 7.5" raw carrot | 72 | 0.8 |
| 1/2 c ckd bean sprouts | 62 | 0.8 |
| 1/2 c blueberries | 75 | 0.8 |
| 1 T wheat bran | 3.6 | 0.7 |
| 1 c papaya cubes | 140 | 0.7 |
| 1 corn tortilla | 26 | 0.6 |
| 1 T oat bran | 5.9 | 0.4 |

Listing includes elemental and enriched foods; does not include additionally fortified products like breakfast cereals.
Source: The Food Finder, ESHA Research, Salem, Oregon, 1999. Printed with permission.

# Vitamin B-6 (Pyridoxal, Pyridoxine, Pyridoxamine, and Their Phosphates)

*Vitamin B-6 is a vital part in more than 100 enzymes and coenzymes involved in amino acid and glycogen metabolism. It is necessary for brain function and formation of red blood cells, helps convert tryptophan to niacin, is involved in the immune function and steroid hormone activity, and reduces risk of atherosclerosis.*

## *Vitamin B-6 Functions*

Vitamin B-6 plays several important roles in the body, especially in the metabolism of amino acids into body proteins. If there is an increase in protein in the diet, the need for B-6 increases to convert extra protein into energy. It also releases energy by converting body stores of glycogen into glucose.

Vitamin B-6 is required for building some amino acids and for converting others to hormones. It is necessary for the synthesis of niacin from tryptophan, the production of red blood cells and white blood cells, and the functioning of nerve tissue. It may also be involved with the metabolism of polyunsaturated fats. B-6 is stored in the liver and muscle tissue.

Vitamin B-6 has been reported as a useful treatment for carpal tunnel syndrome, in which pressure on the nerves of the hands causes weakness and pain. Short-term supplemental doses of vitamin B-6 are also used to treat PMS (premenstrual syndrome), depression, and muscular fatigue.

## *Vitamin B-6 Deficiencies*

A vitamin B-6 deficiency can result in diseases of the skin, tongue and mouth sores, small-cell type anemia, insulin sensitivity, nausea, nervousness, and convulsions. Neurologic symptoms can include weakness, tingling and pain in the hands and arms, depression, headaches, confusion, and seizures.

Deficiencies of vitamin B-6 along with folate and vitamin B-12 can result in elevated blood levels of homocysteine, which are associated with atherosclerosis and heart disease. The body's utilization of vitamin B-6 may be impaired if there is a deficiency of riboflavin. Deficiencies rarely occur alone, however, and are most likely to be seen in people who are deficient in several B-complex vitamins.

## *Vitamin B-6 Losses and Antagonists*

Vitamin B-6 is easily lost. Processed and refined foods often contain less than 50% of that found in the original unprocessed or uncooked form, and exposure to sunlight (ultraviolet light) may reduce vitamin content even more. About 50 to 70% can be lost freezing fruits and vegetables and in processing luncheon meats. Approximately 50 to 90% is lost in milling cereal grains, and it is not added back through enrichment.

In addition to the consumption of alcohol, there are about 40 medicines known to affect the metabolism or bioavailability of vitamin B-6. The drugs INH (isonicotinic acid hydrazide for treating tuberculosis) and hydralazine (for high blood pressure) decrease the absorption of B-6 and promote the destruction and loss from the body. Vitamin B-6 needs are increased if certain drugs are taken, such as penicillamine, isoniazid, and some diuretics.

Vitamin B-6 from meats is more bioavailable than B-6 from plant foods, although plant fiber does not appear to affect absorption. In a mixed diet, approximately 75% is bioavailable.

## *Vitamin B-6 Recommended Intake*

The 1998 Dietary Reference Intakes for vitamin B6 recommendations are listed next. These allowances assume that the reported average protein intakes are approximately 100 g/day for men and 60 g/day for women. These intakes may not be sufficient for those whose habitual protein intake is at or above this amount for extended periods. The previous 1989 RDAs were 2.0 mg/day for adult men; 1.6 mg/day for adult women; 2.2 mg if pregnant; and 2.1 mg if breastfeeding.

| | | |
|---|---|---|
| Men | 14–50 years | 1.3 mg/day |
| | 51 years + | 1.7 mg/day |
| Women | 14–18 years | 1.2 mg/day |
| | 19–50 years | 1.3 mg/day |
| | 51 years + | 1.5 mg/day |
| Pregnant | | 1.9 mg/day |
| Breastfeeding | | 2.0 mg/day |

The 1990 Canadian RNI recommends 15 mcg (0.015 mg) of B-6 *per gram of protein* for adults. For a 50 g intake of protein, this would result in a recommended amount of 750 mcg, or 0.75 mg, of Vitamin B6.

## *Vitamin B-6 Upper Limits*

Vitamin B-6 is a water-soluble vitamin, but unlike other water-soluble vitamins, excesses apparently are not completely excreted from the body. There are no upper limits for dietary vitamin B-6; however, the 1998 RDA/DRIs set upper limits for *supplemental* B-6. When megadoses of vitamin B-6 are taken in "gram" quantities over an extended period, numbness, nerve damage, and other neurologic symptoms occur. Several weeks of intake may not show any toxicity, but more than 2 months may.

Toxicity can result from taking very large doses of supplements or from prescribed doses over extended periods to treat PMS, mental, or other disorders. Toxicity cannot occur with food sources. Reported consequences can vary from permanent nerve damage to reversal of the symptoms when the overdoses are eliminated.

Upper limits were established with the 1998 RDA/DRIs as follows:

| | |
|---|---|
| 30 mg/day | Ages 1–3 |
| 40 mg/day | Ages 4–8 |
| 60 mg/day | Ages 9–13 |
| 80 mg/day | Ages 14–18 |
| 100 mg/day | Ages 19 and older |

## *Vitamin B-6 Food Sources*

Vitamin B-6 is available in a large variety of *unprocessed* foods. The best sources (Table 5.8) are liver, poultry, meats, fish, nuts and seeds (especially filberts and sunflower seeds, peanuts and peanut butter), and fruits (bananas, avocados, mangos, prune juice, grapes).

Other sources include vegetables such as tomato juice and sauces, soybeans, Brussels sprouts, lima beans (the cooked-from-dry legume form), winter squash, brown rice, molasses, and wheat germ. Breakfast cereals fortified with vitamin B-6 are also good sources. Vitamin B-6 is also found in cinnamon and cocoa.

TABLE 5.8 **Vitamin B-6 Sources in Rank Order by Serving Size**

| | Weight (g) | Vit B-6 (mg) |
|---|---|---|
| **0.5–1.5 mg/serving:** | | |
| 3.5 oz ckd beef liver | 100 | 1.43 |
| 3.5 oz ckd veal liver | 100 | 0.9 |
| 2 T brewer's yeast | 16 | 0.8 |
| 1 banana | 118 | 0.7 |
| 3.5 oz ckd salmon | 100 | 0.65 |
| 3.5 oz ckd light chicken meat | 100 | 0.63 |
| 3.5 oz ckd chicken liver | 100 | 0.60 |
| 3.5 oz ckd herring | 100 | 0.52 |
| 3.5 oz ckd turkey liver | 100 | 0.52 |
| 3.5 oz ckd turkey light meat | 100 | 0.50 |
| 3.5 oz ckd beef kidney | 100 | 0.50 |
| **0.35–0.49 mg:** | | |
| 1 baked potato w/skin | 122 | 0.42 |
| 1/2 c baked beans w/pork | 127 | 0.42 |
| 3/4 c prune juice | 192 | 0.42 |
| 1/2 c filberts | 68 | 0.41 |
| 3.5 oz ckd halibut | 100 | 0.40 |
| 3.5 oz ckd shrimp | 100 | 0.40 |
| 3.5 oz ckd beef, roasts/steak | 100 | 0.40 |
| 3.5 oz ckd dark turkey meat | 100 | 0.36 |
| 3.5 oz ckd dark chicken meat | 100 | 0.37 |
| 1/2 c roasted chestnuts | 72 | 0.36 |
| **0.25–0.34 mg:** | | |
| 1 c vegetable-tomato juice | 242 | 0.34 |
| 1/2 c chopped walnuts | 60 | 0.34 |
| 3.5 oz ckd veal | 100 | 0.30 |
| 1/2 c cnd sweet potatoes | 128 | 0.30 |
| 2 T blackstrap molasses | 41 | 0.29 |
| 1 avocado half | 100 | 0.28 |
| 1 mango | 207 | 0.28 |
| 2 T molasses | 41 | 0.28 |
| 1 c tomato juice | 243 | 0.27 |
| 3.5 oz ckd ground beef | 100 | 0.26 |
| 1/4 c sunflower seed kernels | 33 | 0.26 |
| **0.15–0.24 mg:** | | |
| 1/2 c mashed potatoes | 105 | 0.24 |
| 1/2 c Brussels sprouts | 78 | 0.23 |
| 3 oz prunes (≈10) | 85 | 0.22 |
| 1 c watermelon cubes | 152 | 0.22 |
| 3.5 oz ckd beef heart | 100 | 0.21 |
| 1/2 c soynuts (roasted soybeans) | 86 | 0.19 |
| 1/2 c canned tomato sauce | 123 | 0.19 |
| 1 c cantaloupe cubes | 160 | 0.18 |
| 1/2 c peanuts | 72 | 0.18 |
| 1/2 c lentils | 99 | 0.18 |
| 1 c grapes | 160 | 0.18 |
| 1/2 c brazil nuts | 70 | 0.18 |
| 1/2 c cooked carrots | 78 | 0.18 |
| 1/2 c cashews | 65 | 0.18 |
| 1 c grape juice | 253 | 0.16 |
| 1/2 c lima beans ckd fr/dry | 94 | 0.15 |
| 2 T peanut butter | 32 | 0.15 |
| 1/2 c winter squash | 123 | 0.15 |
| **0.10–0.14 mg:** | | |
| 1/2 c ckd brown rice | 98 | 0.14 |
| 1/2 c ckd spinach | 95 | 0.14 |
| 2 T wheat germ | 14 | 0.14 |
| 1/2 c ckd navy beans | 131 | 0.14 |
| 1 c orange juice | 248 | 0.13 |
| 1 whole ckd artichoke | 120 | 0.13 |
| 1 c lowfat yogurt | 245 | 0.12 |
| 1/2 c ckd peapods | 80 | 0.12 |
| 1/2 c ckd broccoli | 85 | 0.11 |
| 1 c ckd whole wheat pasta | 140 | 0.11 |
| 1/2 c cauliflower raw (50 g) or ckd | 62 | 0.11 |
| 7.5" raw carrot | 72 | 0.11 |
| 1/2 c ckd corn | 75 | 0.11 |
| 1/2 c ckd kidney beans | 89 | 0.11 |
| 1/2 c ckd red cabbage | 75 | 0.11 |
| 1 c milk | 245 | 0.10 |
| 1/2 c ckd collard greens | 90 | 0.10 |
| **0.02–0.09 mg:** | | |
| 1/2 c ckd artichoke hearts | 84 | 0.09 |
| 1/2 c pineapple juice | 125 | 0.09 |
| 1/2 c ckd kale | 65 | 0.09 |
| 1/2 c ckd barley | 78 | 0.09 |
| 1/2 c cnd pinto beans | 120 | 0.09 |
| 1 c fresh strawberry halves | 152 | 0.09 |
| 1/2 c cottage cheese | 28.4 | 0.09 |
| 1 c grapefruit juice | 247 | 0.08 |
| 1/2 c ckd white rice | 79 | 0.07 |
| 1 cooked egg | 48–50 | 0.07 |
| 1/2 c ckd black beans | 86 | 0.06 |
| 1 corn tortilla | 26 | 0.06 |
| 1/2 c ckd green soybeans | 90 | 0.05 |
| 1 c ckd oatmeal | 234 | 0.05 |
| 1/4 c pumpkin seed kernels, roasted | 57 | 0.05 |
| 1/2 c ckd split green peas | 80 | 0.05 |
| 1/2 c ckd okra | 92 | 0.04 |
| 1 T wheat bran | 3.6 | 0.05 |
| 1 oz cocoa | 28.4 | 0.03 |
| 1 T cinnamon | 6.8 | 0.02 |

Listing includes elemental and enriched foods; does not include additionally fortified products like breakfast cereals.
Source: The Food Finder, ESHA Research, Salem, Oregon, 1999. Printed with permission.

# Folate (Folacin, Folic Acid, and Pteroylmonoglutamic Acid)

***Folate is important in synthesis of DNA and RNA, new cell formation, protein metabolism, and for normal growth. Adequate intake reduces risk of certain birth defects and heart disease—atherosclerosis.***

## *Folate Functions*

Folate is essential for the formation of DNA and RNA. This function is especially important in tissues that have rapid cell production and turn-over, such as the bone marrow that produces blood cells and the intestinal tract where regeneration of some cells occurs every few days. The health of the intestinal tract, of course, affects the ability to absorb other nutrients.

Folate is also required for the synthesis and breakdown of amino acids. Approximately 1/3 of folate is stored in the liver, and the rest is stored in body tissues.

A deficiency can affect the nervous system and brain function; in the developing fetus, neural tube defects, such as spina-bifida and anencephaly may occur. Therefore, adequate folate intake is essential *before* and during pregnancy for the growth of the fetus. To reduce the risk of neural tube defects for women capable of becoming pregnant, folate fortification of cereal grains and flours began in 1998 in the U.S., and is authorized in Canada as well.

Folate, along with vitamins B-6 and B-12, are protective against heart disease (coronary heart disease and atherosclerosis) by reducing blood homocysteine levels. This mechanism is not completely understood, but it is thought that excessive levels of homocysteine can lead to atherosclerotic lesions and increase the adhesiveness of platelets and affect several factors related to clotting. Higher intakes of folate are also associated with reduced incidence of colon cancer.

Folate is the general term for all forms of this vitamin. The naturally occurring vitamin in food is generally referred to as folate or folacin. The form used in fortification and vitamin supplements is called folic acid (pteroylmonoglutamic acid) and rarely occurs naturally in food.

## Folate Deficiencies

Deficiencies can occur from alcohol abuse, poor food intake, and any condition that requires increased cell production, such as burns, blood loss, skin diseases (measles, chicken pox), and pregnancies, especially those involving multiple births. Some drugs may be antagonistic to folate and will reduce the folate in the body—anticancer drugs, aspirin, antacids, and oral contraceptives.

Those at risk of deficiency include pregnant women and premature infants, due to rapid cell division and growth; the elderly, due to limited intake of high folate foods; alcoholics, because alcohol inhibits folate absorption; and smokers, because smoke inactivates folate in the cells lining the lungs.

Deficiencies of folate, vitamin B-6, and vitamin B-12 can result in elevated blood homocysteine levels, which can promote heart disease and atherosclerosis. Other deficiency symptoms include poor growth, problems in nerve development and function, diarrhea, inflammation of the tongue, mental confusions, and anemia.

## Folate Losses and Bioavailability

It is estimated that 50 to 95% of the original folate in food can be lost in food preparation or food processing. Most natural folate is unstable and easily degraded by heat, oxidation, and sunlight, and as a result, processing can drastically reduce folate content of foods. Normal household preparation can destroy as much as 50% in vegetables, and re-heating destroys even more.

Bioavailability is another matter. Food folate is approximately 50% bioavailable. Synthetic folate used in fortifying food is about 85% available when eaten as part of a meal. When taken as a supplement without any food, folate is almost 100% available. Therefore, folic acid in fortified foods is about 1.7 times more bioavailable than food folate.

Studies have found impaired folate status associated with chronic use of some medications: certain anticonvulsants, methotrexate used to treat a variety of disease conditions, pyrimethamine (malaria), trimethoprim (bacterial infections), trimetrexate and sulfasalazine, and others.

## Folate Recommended Intake

The 1998 Recommended Intakes for folate are measured in mcg of Dietary Folate Equivalents (DFE) or Folate Equivalents (FE). This recognizes the different bioavailability of the folate used to enrich foods, which began in 1998. Unfortunately analytical techniques for food can only measure total folate—no technique can measure bioavailability. So food data for folate will "understate" the actual (FE) available, especially if the person consumes grain products fortified with folate in the United States and Canada.

| | | |
|---|---|---|
| Men | 19 years and over | 400 mcg DFE/day |
| Women | 19 years and over | 400 mcg DFE/day |
| Pregnant | | 600 mcg DFE/day |
| Breastfeeding | | 500 mcg DFE/day |

1990 Canadian RNI recommendations for adults are based on 3.1 mcg/kg of body weight per day. Using the Canadian standard reference weights, the mean daily intake is 205 mcg/day for men and 149 mcg/day for women.

## Folate Upper Limits

No adverse effects have been observed associated with excess folate from foods. However, excessive intakes (from supplements or fortified foods) may obscure and delay the diagnosis of vitamin B-12 deficiency. This can result in risk of progressive unrecognized neurologic damage, in addition to pernicious anemia. Because this has been shown in animal studies, there is a concern that this hazard may be true for humans. This supports caution in the use of folic acid supplements by individuals, especially those who eat no animal foods (vegans) who may be at risk for B-12 deficiency. For these and other reasons, upper limits have been set at the following:

| | |
|---|---|
| Ages 1–3 years | 300 mcg/day |
| Ages 4–8 years | 400 mcg/day |
| Ages 9–13 years | 600 mcg/day |
| Ages 14–18 years | 800 mcg/day |
| Adults 19 years and over | 1000 mcg (1 mg)/day |

## Folate Food Sources

Rich sources of natural folate (Table 5.9) are primarily found in liver, legumes, nuts, many dark-green vegetables, and many fruits, with lesser amounts in fish, eggs, and dairy foods. The enrichment of grains and flour with folate now provide excellent additional sources of folate. Rice, pasta and breads, baked goods, and breakfast cereals made with enriched flour are now excellent sources, and white bread contains twice that of whole wheat bread.

Milk, green tea, and black tea have small amounts but if consumed in large quantities can contribute to the dietary intake of folacin. Except for organ meats, meats are not rich sources.

*Note:* The food data in this publication includes the new levels of folate resulting from fortification of wheat flour, corn meal, rice, and their products—breads, pastas, etc.

TABLE 5.9 Folate Sources in Rank Order by Serving Size

| | Weight (g) | Folate (mcg) |
|---|---|---|
| **300–770 mcg/serving:** | | |
| 3.5 oz ckd chicken liver | 100 | 770 |
| 3.5 oz ckd turkey liver | 100 | 666 |
| 2 T brewer's yeast | 16 | 626 |
| 3.5 oz ckd veal liver | 100 | 320 |
| **100–299 mcg:** | | |
| 3.5 oz ckd beef liver | 100 | 220 |
| 1/2 c lentils | 99 | 179 |
| 1/2 c ckd okra | 92 | 134 |
| 1/2 c ckd black beans | 86 | 128 |
| 1/2 c black-eyed peas, ckd fr/frzn | 85 | 120 |
| 1/2 c ckd kidney beans | 89 | 115 |
| 1/2 c ckd spinach | 95 | 103 |
| 1/2 c ckd green soybeans | 90 | 100 |
| **75–99 mcg:** | | |
| 1 c ckd white pasta | 140 | 98 |
| 3.5 oz ckd beef kidney | 100 | 98 |
| 1/2 c peanuts | 72 | 90 |
| 10″ flour tortilla | 72 | 88 |
| 1/2 c collard greens, ckd fr/fresh | 90 | 88 |
| 4 ckd asparagus spears | 60 | 84 |
| 1/2 c ckd navy beans | 131 | 81 |
| 1/4 c sunflower kernels | 68 | 77 |
| 1 c romaine lettuce | 56 | 76 |
| 1 c fresh orange juice | 248 | 75 |
| **50–74 mcg:** | | |
| 1/2 c cnd pinto beans | 120 | 72 |
| 1/2 c ckd beets | 85 | 68 |
| 1/2 c ckd Brussels sprouts | 78 | 67 |
| 1/2 c collard greens, ckd fr/frzn | 90 | 65 |
| 1/2 c ckd split peas | 98 | 64 |
| 1 half avocado | 100 | 62 |
| 1/2 c black-eyed peas, ckd fr/fzn | 85 | 60 |
| 1 c fresh chopped spinach | 30 | 58 |
| 1/2 c tofu | 124 | 55 |
| 1 c papaya cubes | 140 | 53 |
| 1/2 c ckd chopped broccoli | 85 | 52 |
| 3.5 oz ckd crab | 100 | 51 |
| 1/2 c ckd mustard greens | 70 | 51 |
| 1 c vegetable-tomato juice | 242 | 51 |
| 1/2 c almonds | 78 | 50 |
| 1/2 c roasted chestnuts | 72 | 50 |
| 2 T wheat germ | 14 | 50 |
| **30–49 mcg:** | | |
| 1/2 c ckd white rice | 79 | 48 |
| 1/2 c filberts | 68 | 48 |
| 1/2 c ckd green peas | 80 | 47 |
| 1 c chilled orange juice | 249 | 45 |
| 1/2 c baked beans | 127 | 45 |
| 1/2 c cashews | 65 | 44 |
| 1/2 c ckd artichoke hearts | 84 | 43 |
| 1/2 c chopped walnuts | 60 | 40 |
| 1/2 c pistachios | 64 | 37 |
| 1/4 c raw seaweed | 20 | 36 |
| 1/2 c ckd okra | 92 | 36 |
| 1 banana | 118 | 35 |
| 3.5 oz ckd salmon | 100 | 34 |
| 1/4 c pumpkin seed kernels, rstd | 57 | 33 |
| 1/2 c chopped broccoli *leaves* | 44 | 31 |
| 1 c iceberg lettuce | 56 | 31 |
| 1 corn tortilla | 26 | 30 |
| **25–29 mcg:** | | |
| 1 small orange | 96 | 29 |
| 1 medium mango | 207 | 29 |
| 1 kiwifruit | 76 | 29 |
| 3.5 oz steamed clams | 100 | 30 |
| 1 piece white bread | 30 | 29 |
| 1/2 c cauliflower, raw (50 g) or ckd | 62 | 28 |
| 1 c lowfat yogurt | 245 | 28 |
| 1 c cantaloupe cubes | 160 | 27 |
| 1 c fresh strawberry halves | 152 | 27 |
| 3.5 oz ckd oysters | 100 | 27 |
| 1/2 c ckd peapods | 80 | 26 |
| 1/2 c raw broccoli flowerets | 36 | 25 |
| 1 c grapefruit juice | 247 | 25 |
| 1/2 c ckd corn | 75 | 25 |
| 1/2 c blackberries | 72 | 25 |
| **8–24 mcg:** | | |
| 3.5 oz ckd trout | 100 | 24 |
| 1/2 c chopped pecans | 60 | 23 |
| 1 cooked egg | 48–50 | 20 |
| 1/2 c ckd green beans | 65 | 18 |
| 1/2 c ckd summer squash | 90 | 18 |
| 3.5 oz raw oysters | 100 | 16 |
| 1/2 c red raspberries | 62 | 16 |
| 1/2 c green cabbage, raw (35 g) or ckd | 75 | 15 |
| 1/2 c ckd chopped chayote | 80 | 15 |
| 1/2 c baby lima beans, ckd fr/frzn | 90 | 14 |
| 1/2 c cnd sweet potatoes | 128 | 14 |
| 1 baked potato w/skin | 122 | 13 |
| 1/2 c pineapple juice | 125 | 13 |
| 1 oz cheddar cheese | 28.4 | 12 |
| 1 c milk | 245 | 12 |
| 1 c green tea | 237 | 12 |
| 1 c black tea | 237 | 10 |
| 7.5″ raw carrot | 72 | 10 |
| 1/2 c mashed potatoes | 105 | 8 |

Listing includes elemental and enriched foods; does not include additionally fortified products like breakfast cereals.
Source: The Food Finder, ESHA Research, Salem, Oregon, 1999. Printed with permission.

## Vitamin B-12 (Cobalamin and Cyanocobalamin)

***Vitamin B-12 is necessary for development of red blood cells, maintains normal functioning of the nervous system, is essential for normal functioning of folate, and helps protect against risk factors associated with heart disease and atherosclerosis.***

### *Vitamin B-12 Functions*

Vitamin B-12 is required for several enzymatic reactions to synthesize certain amino acids, and to protect against atherosclerosis by functioning as a coenzyme for converting homocysteine to other forms. It plays an important role in building and maintaining the sheath that protects the nerve fibers. Vitamin B-12 is needed—along with folacin—where new cell growth is required and to help manufacture red blood cells. Because folacin and B-12 work together for cell formation and growth, a deficiency in one can impair the function of the other.

### *Vitamin B-12 Deficiencies*

Deficiencies are more likely from inadequate *absorption* rather than inadequate intake. Although a strict long-term vegetarian diet may induce a deficiency because B-12 is not found in plant foods.

The absorption of vitamin B-12 requires a factor in the stomach called the intrinsic factor. It attaches to B-12 and facilitates the absorption in the intestine. If this intrinsic factor is lacking (such as in pernicious anemia, and often in the elderly), malabsorption of B-12 results.

Deficiencies in B-12 or folacin can cause a form of anemia, and can result in an increasing paralysis of the muscles and nerves due to degeneration of myelin sheath that coats the nerves, spinal cord, and brain. Since the early symptoms are not detectable from a blood test, and early detection is necessary to prevent permanent damage, this type of "sneaky" deficiency damage has earned the name *pernicious anemia.*

Symptoms of deficiency may include those of anemia (skin pallor, diminished energy, shortness of breath, and palpitations) and neurologic defects (tingling and numbness of extremities [worse in the lower limbs], motor disturbances, gait abnormalities, loss of concentration, memory loss, and disorientation).

Because folacin and B-12 work together, folacin intake will clear up the early anemia condition and mask the more serious B-12 deficiency. As a result, over-the-counter preparations of folacin are limited by law to 400 mcg, an amount too low to have this masking effect over vitamin B-12.

Deficiency of vitamin B-12 along with vitamin B-6 and folate can result in elevated blood levels of homocysteine, which can promote coronary heart disease and atherosclerosis. Gastritis, and iron and vitamin B-6 deficiencies will decrease absorption of vitamin B-12.

### *Vitamin B-12 Food Losses*

Vitamin B-12 is generally fairly stable in food; however, there can be small losses in cooking and processing. Up to 10% is lost in milk during pasteurization, another 30% can be destroyed by boiling for several minutes, and about 50% can be lost if boiled for 10 minutes. Canned evaporated milk contains only about 25% of the B-12 of whole fluid milk for example.

### *Vitamin B-12 Recommended Intake*

Because 10 to 30% of older people may not be able to absorb B-12 normally, the committee of scientists for the 1998 RDA/DRIs advises those over 50 years of age to consume foods fortified with B-12 or take a B-12-containing supplement, which is more bioavailable. Individuals who are unable to absorb B-12 (caused by lack of the intrinsic factor) require medical treatment. Strict vegetarians who eat no animal food (vegans) may need supplements.

The 1998 Dietary Reference Intakes for vitamin B-12 recommend amounts that are a little less than the 1989 recommendations.

| | | |
|---|---|---|
| Men | 14 years and over | 2.4 mcg/day |
| Women | 14 years and over | 2.4 mcg/day |
| Pregnant | | 2.6 mcg/day |
| Breastfeeding | | 2.8 mcg/day |

1990 Canadian RNI is 1.0 mcg for adults; 1.2 mcg if pregnant or breastfeeding/lactating.

### *Vitamin B-12 Upper Limits*

There was insufficient evidence of toxic levels to establish upper limits with the 1998 recommendations. No toxic effects have been observed with B-12 intakes of up to 100 mcg daily. When high doses are given orally, the body compensates and smaller percentages of B-12 are actually absorbed.

### *Vitamin B-12 Food Sources*

Vitamin B-12 is found in meats, eggs, and dairy products (Table 5.10). For those who are strict vegetarians (vegans), fortified breakfast cereals and other foods fortified with vitamin B-12 are good sources. There is none in plant foods, although some might be produced by bacteria if a food has fermented. Nutritional yeast and beer, for example, have small amounts.

## Pantothenic Acid

***Pantothenic acid is vital for the synthesis and maintenance of coenzyme A, which is involved in the metabolism of fatty acids and many essential body chemicals. Pantothenic acid is involved in over 100 different steps in the synthesis of fats, neurotransmitters, steroid hormones, and hemoglobin. It is required for production of energy from protein, carbohydrate, and fat.***

### *Pantothenic Acid Functions*

As a constituent of coenzyme A, pantothenic acid plays a central role in the metabolic process for fats, amino acids, and carbohydrates. It plays an important role for synthesizing fatty acids, phospholipids, cholesterol, acetylcholine, vitamin A, vitamin D, and steroid hormones, and for the formation of certain other nerve-regulating substances and hormones.

TABLE 5.10 **Vitamin B-12 Sources in Rank Order by Serving Size**

| | Weight (g) | Vit B-12 (mcg) |
|---|---|---|
| **25–112 mcg:** | | |
| 3.5 oz ckd beef liver | 100 | 112 |
| 3.5 oz steamed clams | 100 | 99 |
| 3.5 oz ckd veal liver | 100 | 64 |
| 3.5 oz ckd beef/veal kidney | 100 | 51 |
| 3.5 oz ckd turkey liver | 100 | 48 |
| 3.5 oz ckd oysters | 100 | 27 |
| **5–24 mcg:** | | |
| 3.5 oz ckd chicken liver | 100 | 19 |
| 3.5 oz raw oysters | 100 | 16 |
| 3.5 oz ckd beef heart | 100 | 14 |
| 3.5 oz ckd herring | 100 | 10 |
| 3.5 oz ckd crab | 100 | 9 |
| 3.5 oz ckd trout | 100 | 5 |
| **1–4 mcg:** | | |
| 3.5 oz ckd pollock | 100 | 3.7 |
| 3.5 oz ckd catfish | 100 | 2.8 |
| 3.5 oz ckd salmon | 100 | 2.8 |
| 3.5 oz ckd beef | 100 | 2.5 |
| 3.5 oz ckd lamb | 100 | 2.4 |
| 3.5 oz fish ranges from 0.6–1.4 | 100 | 2.0 |
| 3.5 oz cnd tuna | 100 | 1.8 |
| 3.5 oz ckd shrimp | 100 | 1.5 |
| 1 c lowfat yogurt | 245 | 1.4 |
| **Less than 1 mcg:** | | |
| 1 c nonfat milk | 245 | 0.93 |
| 1 c whole milk | 244 | 0.87 |
| 1/2 c cottage cheese | 28.4 | 0.80 |
| 1/4 c feta cheese | 28.4 | 0.63 |
| 3.5 oz ckd pork | 100 | 0.60 |
| 1 cooked egg | 48–50 | 0.49 |
| 1 oz Swiss cheese | 28.4 | 0.48 |
| 2 T brewer's yeast varies from 0.12–0.84 | 16 | 0.48 |
| 1 oz provolone | 28.4 | 0.41 |
| 3.5 oz ckd turkey | 100 | 0.37 |
| 3.5 oz ckd light chicken meat | 100 | 0.36 |
| 3.5 oz ckd dark chicken meat | 100 | 0.32 |
| 1 oz cheddar cheese | 28.4 | 0.24 |
| 1 oz American processed cheese | 28.4 | 0.20 |

Listing includes elemental and enriched foods; does not include additionally fortified products like breakfast cereals.
Source: The Food Finder, ESHA Research, Salem, Oregon, 1999. Printed with permission.

## *Pantothenic Acid Deficiencies*

Dietary deficiencies are not known. However, experimentally induced deficiencies can create weakness and fatigue, reduced antibody production, muscle cramps, and reduced adrenal function.

## *Pantothenic Acid Losses*

Fresh, unprocessed foods are best. Milling destroys at least half the pantothenic acid in grains, and it is not replaced by enrichment. It is readily destroyed by heat, and canned and frozen fruits and vegetables show average losses of 50% or more from the fresh or raw form.

## *Pantothenic Acid Recommended Intake*

The 1998 Dietary Reference Intakes for pantothenic acid are based on Adequate Intakes (AIs). There was not sufficient information to establish values for the RDA designation:

| | | |
|---|---|---|
| Men | 14 years and over | 5 mg/day |
| Women | 14 years and over | 5 mg/day |
| Pregnant | | 6 mg/day |
| Breastfeeding | | 7 mg/day |

The 1990 Canadian RNI recommends 5 mg to 7 mg per day for adults.

## *Pantothenic Acid Upper Limits*

With no reported adverse effects, no upper limits have been identified.

## *Pantothenic Acid Food Sources*

Good sources (Table 5.11) include liver, nuts, peanuts and seeds, yogurt, chicken and turkey (especially the dark meat), fish and shellfish, eggs, vegetables (especially mushrooms, tomato juice, potatoes, peas, sweet potatoes), pork, whole grain products, oatmeal, and orange juice.

Pantothenic acid is severely reduced in processed foods. Whole wheat pasta and breads have twice the vitamin of white pasta and breads, for example.

# Vitamin C (Ascorbic Acid)

***Vitamin C is essential for the formation and maintenance of the protein collagen, the base structure of all connective tissue in the body (blood vessel walls, scar tissue, matrix for bones and teeth, etc.). As a major antioxidant, it strengthens resistance to infection and counters the adverse effects of free radicals. It is necessary in the metabolism of proteins, for the synthesis of hormones and neurotransmitters, and enhances the absorption of iron.***

## *Vitamin C Functions*

Vitamin C is a very reactive vitamin. It is convertible into different forms, and as a water-soluble compound is excreted rapidly when excessive amounts are taken. Vitamin C is important in maintaining and forming the protein collagen, an essential part of the connective tissue that binds the body's cells together. Bones and teeth continually need vitamin C to repair connective tissues. It aids in the healing of cuts and burns, which cannot heal without collagen. Vitamin C also helps keep capillaries and other blood vessels strong.

TABLE 5.11 Pantothenic Acid Sources in Rank Order by Serving Size

| | Weight (g) | Panto (mg) |
|---|---|---|
| **1.0–6.0 mg/serving:** | | |
| 3.5 oz ckd turkey liver | 100 | 6.0 |
| 3.5 oz ckd chicken liver | 100 | 5.4 |
| 3.5 oz ckd beef & veal liver | 100 | 5.3 |
| 1/4 c sunflower seeds | 68 | 2.3 |
| 1 c lowfat yogurt | 245 | 1.45 |
| 3.5 oz ckd salmon | 100 | 1.35 |
| 2 T brewer's yeast | 16 | 1.35 |
| 3.5 oz dark chicken & turkey | 100 | 1.3 |
| 3.5 oz light chicken & turkey | 100 | 1.0 |
| 1/2 c chopped pecans | 60 | 1.0 |
| 1/2 c peanuts | 72 | 1.0 |
| 1 avocado half | 100 | 1.0 |
| **0.75–0.90 mg:** | | |
| 3.5 oz ckd western oysters | 100 | 0.9 |
| 3.5 oz ckd bass | 100 | 0.9 |
| 3.5 oz ckd beef heart | 100 | 0.9 |
| 3.5 oz ckd herring | 100 | 0.85 |
| 1/2 c ckd mushrooms | 39 | 0.84 |
| 1 c milk | 245 | 0.8 |
| 1/2 c filberts | 68 | 0.8 |
| 1/2 c cashews | 65 | 0.8 |
| 1/2 c pistachios | 64 | 0.8 |
| 3.5 oz steamed clams | 100 | 0.7 |
| 1 baked potato w/skin | 122 | 0.7 |
| 3.5 oz ckd lamb | 100 | 0.7 |
| 1/2 c ckd peapods | 80 | 0.7 |
| **0.50–0.74 mg:** | | |
| 1/2 c cnd sweet potato | 128 | 0.66 |
| 1 cooked egg | 48–50 | 0.65 |
| 1 c vegetable-tomato juice | 242 | 0.64 |
| 1/2 c ckd lentils | 99 | 0.6 |
| 1 c tomato juice | 243 | 0.6 |
| 1/2 c mashed potatoes | 105 | 0.6 |
| 3.5 oz ckd catfish | 100 | 0.6 |
| 3.5 oz ckd pork | 100 | 0.6 |
| 1 c whole wheat pasta | 140 | 0.6 |
| 1/2 c cooked split peas | 98 | 0.6 |
| 1/2 c cottage cheese | 28.4 | 0.55 |
| 1 c fresh strawberry halves | 152 | 0.54 |
| 3.5 oz raw western oysters | 100 | 0.50 |
| 1/2 c pumpkin | 123 | 0.50 |
| **0.25–0.49 mg:** | | |
| 1 c grapefruit juice | 247 | 0.47 |
| 1 c orange juice | 248 | 0.47 |
| 1 c ckd oatmeal | 234 | 0.47 |
| 1/2 c butternut squash | 123 | 0.44 |
| 1 ckd whole artichoke | 120 | 0.41 |
| 1/2 c soy nuts | 86 | 0.41 |
| 10" flour tortilla | 72 | 0.40 |
| 1/2 c ckd broccoli | 85 | 0.40 |
| 1/2 c lima beans ckd fr/dry | 94 | 0.40 |
| 3 oz (10 prunes) | 85 | 0.39 |
| 3.5 oz ckd beef–ranges 0.28–0.38 | 100 | 0.38 |
| 3.5 oz ckd halibut | 100 | 0.38 |
| 1/2 c chopped walnuts | 60 | 0.38 |
| 1/2 c tomato sauce | 123 | 0.38 |
| 2 T peanut butter | 32 | 0.36 |
| 1 grapefruit half | 118–123 | 0.35 |
| 3.5 oz ckd turkey/chicken hot dog | 100 | 0.35 |
| 1 medium mango | 207 | 0.33 |
| 1 c watermelon cubes | 152 | 0.32 |
| 1 c papaya cubes | 140 | 0.30 |
| 1 banana | 118 | 0.30 |
| 1/2 c ckd rice, avg all | 88 | 0.30 |
| 1 c ckd fresh pasta | 150 | 0.27 |
| 1/2 c ckd corn | 75 | 0.25 |
| **0.10–0.24 mg:** | | |
| 1/2 c baked navy beans | 129 | 0.23 |
| 1/2 c black-eyed peas, ckd fr/dry | 120 | 0.23 |
| 1 kiwifruit | 76 | 0.22 |
| 1/2 c black-eyed peas, ckd fr/frzn | 85 | 0.18 |
| 1 medium peach | 98 | 0.17 |
| 1/2 c ckd red cabbage | 75 | 0.17 |
| 1 c papaya cubes | 140 | 0.15 |
| 1 c ckd white pasta | 140 | 0.15 |
| 1/2 c ckd chopped celery | 75 | 0.15 |
| 1/2 c ckd Swiss chard | 88 | 0.14 |
| 1 piece white bread | 30 | 0.12 |

Listing includes elemental and enriched foods; does not include additionally fortified products like breakfast cereals.
Source: The Food Finder, ESHA Research, Salem, Oregon, 1999. Printed with permission.

As an antioxidant, vitamin C serves as a bodyguard by becoming oxidized to protect other items from a similar fate. As one of the most versatile antioxidants in the body, vitamin C is the major antioxidant substance present in the airway surface of the lungs and is protective to vitamins A, E, folate, and possibly others. It is sometimes added to food products to protect them from oxidation (turning brown) as well as to improve their overall nutritional value. Vitamin C also enhances absorption of iron from foods.

Vitamin C is also involved in the metabolism of several amino acids (proteins) and the precursor hormones epinephrine and norepinephrine. It is needed for the synthesis of thyroxin, which helps regulate metabolism. Extreme stress can increase the need for vitamin C as well.

## *Vitamin C Deficiencies*

A severe deficiency can result in scurvy, which is how the vitamin was eventually discovered and named. The name *ascorbic acid* was derived from the anti-scorbutic (anti-scurvy) factor. Because vitamin C is the major antioxidant present in the airway surface of the lungs, higher intake of vitamin C appears to offer protection for smokers, persons exposed to environmental oxidants (pollution), and adults with symptoms of asthma. Marginal deficiencies are far more likely, but more difficult to identify.

## *Vitamin C Losses and Antagonists*

Vitamin C is more readily destroyed than the other vitamins. It is stable in growing plants, but when they are cut or bruised, an enzyme is activated that destroys the vitamin. Blanching vegetables (heating in water for a few minutes) inactivates the enzyme. This vitamin is also easily destroyed by exposure to air, heat, iron and copper pans, and will leach easily into cooking water. It is most stable in acid fruits (they don't have the destroying enzyme). Refrigerated citrus fruit juices stored in a sealed container with small airspace will retain most of their vitamin C; however, in the presence of air (oxygen), juices will retain less vitamin C. Loss of flavor usually parallels loss of nutrients.

Massive doses of vitamin C may conflict with anticlotting medications, may interfere with some tests used to determine diabetes, and are a problem for persons with iron overload (hemochromatosis) because vitamin C enhances iron intake.

## *Vitamin C Recommended Intake*

We probably don't know all the things vitamin C does for the body, thus the recommended amounts vary all over the scientific map. The 1989 RDA of 60 mg a day for adults was a controversial recommendation at the time, and still is. The RDA recommendations also suggested 100 mg/day for smokers.

| | | |
|---|---|---|
| Men | 15 years and over | 60 mg/day |
| Women | 15 years and over | 60 mg/day |
| Pregnant | | 70 mg/day |
| Breastfeeding 1st 6 mo. | | 95 mg/day |
| Breastfeeding 2nd 6 mo. | | 90 mg/day |

Research findings since the 1989 RDA was established have prompted other recommendations:

- Researchers of the University of California at Berkeley have steadfastly recommended 250 to 500 mg of vitamin C per day in their Wellness Newsletter, along with 10,000 to 25,000 IU (≈1,600 to 4,000 RE) Vitamin A in the form of beta-carotene; and 200 to 800 IU (or 133 to 533 mg of TE) of vitamin E.
- Current Dietary Guidelines and the Food Pyramid suggest 5 to 9 servings of fresh fruits and vegetables a day. This will provide from 200–250+ mg a day of vitamin C.

1990 Canadian RNI recommend 40 mg for adult men, 30 mg for adult women, 40 mg for the last two trimesters of pregnancy, and 55 mg if breastfeeding.

## *Vitamin C Upper Limits*

There is no evidence of harm for persons who take regular supplemental doses of 500 to 1,000 mg of vitamin C per day. On the other hand, proven benefits above 100 mg a day are not obvious. In significant studies regarding vitamin C protection for the common cold, 1,000 mg a day (or 1 g) was no more effective than 50 mg a day.

High levels of vitamin C from supplements may require the body to handle vitamin C differently by limiting absorption and excreting more vitamin C than normal. It is theorized, *but not proven,* that if the person reduces intake suddenly the body may not be able to adjust as quickly. So it is recommended to decrease high doses gradually.

## *Vitamin C Food Sources*

Citrus fruits (oranges, grapefruit, lemons, limes) have been known for their contribution of vitamin C (Table 5.12). Other excellent fruit sources include papaya, strawberries, kiwifruit, cantaloupes, mangos, grapes, avocados, watermelons, and berries. Vegetable sources include red peppers, broccoli, Brussels sprouts, cauliflower, cabbages, dark-green vegetables of all kinds, tomatoes, and potatoes (the fresher they are, the more vitamin C). Dark-green leaves are more nutritious than pale leaves. Romaine lettuce has about six times the vitamin C (and eight times the beta-carotene) as iceberg lettuce.

Poor sources are dairy products, grains and grain products, nuts, meats, cooked dried beans and peas. Many luncheon meats use a form of vitamin C as a preservative, but it is not a form that is bioavailable to our bodies.

# Vitamin D (Calciferol, Ergocalciferol, Cholecalciferol, and Dihydroxy Vitamin D)

***Vitamin D is vital for the proper mineralization of bone and helps maintain proper blood levels of calcium and phosphorus.***

## *Vitamin D Functions*

Vitamin D regulates the efficiency of the small intestine to absorb calcium and phosphorus, and promotes the growth of strong bones. Vitamin D signals the GI tract to absorb more calcium, the bones to release more, and the kidneys to retain more in the body. Thus, vitamin D maintains the blood calcium and phosphorus at needed levels.

This is an unusual nutrient in that it is photosynthesized by the body from the action of sunlight (ultraviolet B radiation) on the skin. Given enough sun, a person will have sufficient vitamin D. Darker skinned people require longer exposure to sunlight than lighter skinned people to make the same amount of vitamin D—approximately 3 hours versus about 30 minutes.

## *Vitamin D Deficiencies*

People who completely avoid sunlight or who do not consume sufficient dietary vitamin D are at risk of deficiency. The body's production of vitamin D is reduced by the application of sunscreen, and it will also vary according to the intensity of the sun, as affected by geographical latitude, time of day, and season. Those who do not want to consider additional time in sunlight should consider vitamin D supplements if their dietary intake is limited. For most persons, the vitamin D that is synthesized during the summer and fall months of sunshine can be stored in the fat for use throughout the winter.

Rickets is the disease that results from inadequate exposure to sunlight or inadequate dietary intake of vitamin D as an infant. It is characterized by bowed legs, narrow rib cages and other deformities. The effects show up when children start to walk. Their legs bow out because their bones are not strong enough to support the weight of their bodies. Unfortunately, rickets still affects many children worldwide. Rickets has also been observed in children with fat malabsorption and vegetarian children who do not consume milk.

With an "indoor lifestyle," many people do not get sufficient exposure to sunlight to create enough vitamin D for their needs, which can result in the adult form of rickets called osteomalacia. Curvature of the spine and bowed legs are only some of the results of bone softening due to vitamin D deficiency.

TABLE 5.12 **Vitamin C Sources in Rank Order by Serving Size**

| | Weight (g) | Vit C (mg) |
|---|---|---|
| **50–124 mg/serving:** | | |
| 1 c fresh orange juice | 248 | 124 |
| 1 c chilled orange juice | 249 | 82 |
| 1 c fresh grapefruit juice | 247 | 94 |
| 1 c papaya cubes | 140 | 86 |
| 1 c fresh strawberry halves | 152 | 86 |
| 1 kiwifruit | 76 | 74 |
| 1 c canned grapefruit juice | 247 | 72 |
| 1/4 c raw red pepper, chopped | 37 | 71 |
| 1 c cantaloupe cubes | 160 | 67.5 |
| 1 c tomato-vegetable juice | 242 | 67 |
| 1/2 c broccoli, ckd fr/fresh | 92 | 62 |
| 1 mango | 207 | 57 |
| 1 small orange | 96 | 51 |
| **25–49 mg:** | | |
| 1/2 c Brussels sprouts, ckd fr/fresh | 78 | 48 |
| 1 pink/red grapefruit half | 123 | 46 |
| 1 c tomato juice | 243 | 44 |
| 1 white grapefruit half | 118 | 41 |
| 1/2 c peapods, ckd fr/fresh | 80 | 38 |
| 1/2 c broccoli, ckd fr/frzn | 92 | 37 |
| 1 c cantaloupe cubes | 160 | 37 |
| 1/2 c Brussels sprouts ckd f/fzn | 78 | 35 |
| 1/4 c raw green pepper, chopped | 37 | 33 |
| 1/2 c ckd cauliflower | 62 | 27 |
| 1/2 c ckd kale | 65 | 27 |
| 1/2 c ckd red cabbage | 75 | 26 |
| 1/4 c ckd red pepper | 37 | 25 |
| **15–24 mg:** | | |
| 1/2 c collard greens, ckd fr/frzn | 90 | 22 |
| 3.5 oz steamed clams | 100 | 22 |
| 1/2 c ckd butternut squash | 123 | 18 |
| 1/2 c ckd beet greens | 72 | 18 |
| 1/2 c peapods, ckd fr/frzn | 80 | 18 |
| 1 c grapes | 160 | 17 |
| 1/2 c fresh chopped tomatoes | 90 | 17 |
| 1/2 c ckd mustard greens | 70 | 17 |
| 1 baked potato w/skin | 122 | 16 |
| 1/2 c tomato sauce | 123 | 16 |
| 1/2 c ckd Swiss chard | 88 | 16 |
| 1/2 c ckd green soybeans | 90 | 15 |
| 1/2 c fresh raspberries | 62 | 15 |
| 1/2 c fresh blackberries | 72 | 15 |
| 1/4 c ckd green pepper | 34 | 15 |
| 1/2 c pineapple juice | 125 | 15 |
| 1 small baked sweet potato | 60 | 15 |
| **10–14 mg:** | | |
| 1 c watermelon cubes | 152 | 14 |
| 2 T fresh lemon juice | 30.5 | 14 |
| 1 c romaine lettuce | 56 | 13 |
| 1/2 c pineapple juice | 125 | 13 |
| 3.5 oz ckd pacific oysters | 100 | 13 |
| 1/2 c collard greens, ckd fr/ fresh | 90 | 12 |
| 1 ckd artichoke | 120 | 12 |
| 1/2 c fresh pineapple | 78 | 12 |
| 1/2 c spinach, ckd fr/frzn | 95 | 12 |
| 1/2 c ckd okra | 92 | 11 |
| 1 banana | 118 | 11 |
| 1 c looseleaf lettuce | 56 | 10 |
| **5.0–9.9 mg:** | | |
| 1/2 c fresh blueberries | 73 | 9.0 |
| 2 T fresh lime juice | 30.5 | 9.0 |
| 1/2 c spinach, ckd fr/fresh | 90 | 8.8 |
| 1/2 c ckd artichoke hearts | 84 | 8.4 |
| 1 half avocado | 100 | 8.0 |
| 3.5 oz raw pacific oysters | 100 | 8.0 |
| 1 medium apple w/peel | 138 | 7.9 |
| 1/2 c green peas, ckd fr/frzn | 80 | 7.9 |
| 3/4 c prune juice | 192 | 7.9 |
| 2 T bottled lemon juice | 30.5 | 7.6 |
| 1/2 c ckd bean sprouts | 62 | 7.1 |
| 2 fresh apricots | 70 | 7.0 |
| 7.5″ raw carrot | 72 | 6.7 |
| 1/2 c cnd sweet potatoes | 128 | 6.7 |
| 1/2 c mashed potatoes | 105 | 6.4 |
| 3.5 oz ckd eastern oysters | 100 | 6.0 |
| 1 medium apple, peeled | 128 | 5.1 |
| 1/2 c canned pumpkin | 123 | 5.1 |
| **2.0–4.9 mg:** | | |
| 3.5 oz raw eastern oysters | 100 | 4.7 |
| 1/2 c green beans, ckd fr/frzn | 68 | 2.8 |
| 3 oz prunes (≈10) | 85 | 2.8 |
| 1 c iceberg lettuce | 56 | 2.1 |
| 2 T bottled lime juice | 30.5 | 2.0 |
| 1 c milk, avg all | 245 | 2.0 |
| 1/2 c frzn blueberries, thawed | 78 | 1.9 |

Listing includes elemental and enriched foods; does not include additionally fortified products like breakfast cereals.
Source: The Food Finder, ESHA Research, Salem, Oregon 1999. Printed with permission.

Other conditions that may create deficiencies include intestinal malabsorption, liver failure, Crohn's disease, and sprue. One study found that as the human skin ages, it may produce less vitamin D from sunlight. In adults over age 65, there was a fourfold decrease in the ability to produce vitamin D. Because vitamin D is fat soluble, low-fat diets may also affect the uptake of this vitamin.

## *Vitamin D Recommended Intake*

The 1998 Dietary Reference Intake (DRI) for Vitamin D is in the form of Adequate Intakes (AIs). Because both sunlight and dietary intake play a role in providing vitamin D, the RDA category is not used. Intake is expressed in international units (IUs) or micrograms (mcg or g). One IU = 0.025 mcg; or one mcg of vitamin D = 40 IU.

| | | |
|---|---|---|
| Men and Women | 19–50 years | 5.0 mcg (200 IU)/day |
| | 51–70 years | 10.0 mcg (400 IU)/day |
| | 71 years and over | 15.0 mcg (600 IU)/day |
| Pregnant or Breastfeeding | | 5.0 mcg (200 IU)/day |

The 1990 Canadian RNI recommends 2.5 mcg per day (100 IU) for adults and 5.0 mcg (200 IU) per day for women who are pregnant or breastfeeding.

## *Vitamin D Upper Limits*

Vitamin D toxicity can occur by consuming supplements only. Toxic effects are potentially severe and can include calcification of soft tissues, reduced kidney function because of calcification, and central nervous system disorders. Toxicity cannot occur when vitamin D is formed from sunlight because the body controls the amount formed. In 1998, upper limits were estimated at the following:

| | |
|---|---|
| 25 mcg (2000 IU)/day | 0–12 months of age |
| 50 mcg (2000 IU)/day | Children and Adults, all ages |
| 50 mcg (2000 IU)/day | Pregnant or Breastfeeding |

## *Vitamin D Food Sources*

Self-synthesis of vitamin D through exposure to sunlight (Table 5.13) is the easiest and safest source for most people because the body regulates the amount it creates. For those who are very sensitive to the sun, foods fortified with vitamin D or the careful use of supplements are alternatives. The very few foods that have vitamin D naturally are fish liver oils, fatty fish, and egg yolks from chickens that have been fed vitamin D.

Some foods have been fortified to provide dietary vitamin D, such as milk, some yogurts, some infant formulas, some margarines, and some fortified cereals. However, three surveys in the last 10 years have found that milk did not contain the vitamin D amounts stated. About 62% of the milks sampled contained less than 80% of the Vitamin D stated on the label, and 14% of the nonfat milk samples had no detectable vitamin D at all.

TABLE 5.13 **Vitamin D Sources in Rank Order by Serving Size**

| | |
|---|---|
| Exposure to sunlight[a] | Exact measure not possible |
| 1 T cod liver oil | 34.0 mcg (1360 IU) |
| 1 T herring oil | 20.0 mcg ( 800 IU) |
| 3.5 oz ckd pacific oysters | 16.0 mcg ( 640 IU) |
| 1 T salmon oil | 13.6 mcg ( 544 IU) |
| 3.5 oz cnd mackerel | 9.0 mcg ( 360 IU) |
| 3.5 oz raw pacific oysters | 8.0 mcg ( 320 IU) |
| 3.5 oz most fish (1.0–3.4) | 2.2 mcg ( 88 IU) |
| 1 c fortified milk (2.4–2.5) | 2.45 mcg ( 100 IU) |
| 1 cooked egg | 0.65 mcg ( 26 IU) |
| 3.5 oz beef, chicken, pork, turkey & organ meats | 0.30 mcg ( 12 IU) |
| 1 T butter | 0.20 mcg ( 8 IU) |
| 3.5 oz beef | 0.18 mcg ( 7 IU) |
| 3.5 oz lamb | 0.13 mcg ( 5 IU) |
| 1 c yogurt | 0.10 mcg ( 4 IU) |
| 1 oz cheddar cheese | 0.09 mcg ( 3.6 IU) |
| 1 oz American cheese | 0.06 mcg ( 2.4 IU) |

[a]Regular sunlight on un-sunblocked skin can provide all you need.

# Vitamin E (Alpha Tocopherol, other Tocopherols, and Tocotrienols)

***Vitamin E, an important antioxidant, provides special protection of polyunsaturated fatty acids (PUFA), vitamin A, and carotenoids. It stabilizes cell membranes, promotes healing of tissues, protects red and white blood cells, and regulates oxidation reactions.***

## *Vitamin E Functions*

Vitamin E acts as an antioxidant to prevent cell-membrane damage. It helps to protect unsaturated fats in the body, especially the polyunsaturated fats (PUFA) from oxidation. It also detoxifies radicals (a good word for destructive substances). Vitamin E aids in the growth of new tissue and the healing of damaged tissue from surgery or burns. It also protects red and white blood cells. In older adults, it improves the immune response. Vitamin E appears to prevent the oxidation of the bad cholesterol (LDL) in the bloodstream. When LDL is oxidized, it is more likely to promote the buildup of fatty plaque in the artery walls (atherosclerosis).

Vitamin E is comprised of eight forms: the alpha, beta, gamma, and delta tocopherols and the alpha, beta, gamma, and delta tocotrienols. The most active form is alpha-tocopherol. Other forms are considered less active, but there is evidence that some forms may work better in the presence of others, a synergy that cannot be quantified in the terms of activity. Alpha and gamma tocopherol together may be more effective than one alone.

## *Measuring Vitamin E Activity*

The total weight of vitamin E present, without regard for activity or the various forms, is simply called *total vitamin E.* The Nutrition Facts labels on food packages use this total value using the older international unit (IU) measure. As a reference, 1 IU of vitamin E is the same as 0.67 mg of vitamin E.

A different measure is used for dietary recommendations - alpha tocopherol equivalents (TEs). Using alpha tocopherol as the standard of 1, the amount of each vitamin E component is weighted according to its activity factor, as listed next. Then all the *weighted* components of E are added together.

| | | |
|---|---|---|
| 1 mg alpha tocopherol | = | 1.00 α-TE |
| 1 mg beta tocopherol | = | 0.50 α-TE (assays range from 0.25–0.50) |
| 1 mg gamma tocopherol | = | 0.10 α-TE (assays range from 0.10–0.35) |
| 1 mg delta tocopherol | = | 0.03 α-TE |
| 1 mg alpha tocotrienol | = | 0.33 α-TE |
| 1 mg beta tocotrienol | = | 0.05 α-TE |

The natural form of vitamin E is D-tocopherol. The synthetic version is a "mirror image" version called L-tocopherol, and has about 74% of the activity of the natural vitamin.

Current research is showing important health factors for the gamma tocopherol form of Vitamin E, aside from the vitamin A activity. Excellent sources of the gamma tocopherol form of vitamin E include palm oil, soybean oil, grapeseed oil, tofu, and several nuts (almonds, cashews, pumpkin seeds, and walnuts).

## *Vitamin E Deficiencies*

Deficiencies are rare and are usually associated with diseases of fat malabsorption such as cystic fibrosis and in individuals consuming very low-fat diets for a prolonged period. When blood concentration of vitamin E is in a severe deficiency state, the red blood cells tend to break open. A prolonged deficiency state can cause neuromuscular dysfunction with loss of muscle coordination and impaired vision. If untreated, the conditions may become permanent.

### Vitamin E Losses

The milling of whole grains into flour takes out a high percentage of vitamin E, and the bleaching of flour eliminates any vitamin E remaining. Vitamin E is fairly stable at regular cooking temperatures, but high frying temperatures will destroy more of the vitamin. A continual diet of processed convenience foods over a long period may contribute to vitamin E deficiency. If a person ingests mineral oil, it will absorb vitamin E and carry it unused out of the body.

### Vitamin E Recommended Intake

The 1989 Dietary Reference Intakes for vitamin E are as follows:

| | | |
|---|---|---|
| Men | 11 years and over | 10 mg TE/day |
| Women | 11 years and over | 8 mg TE/day |
| Pregnant | | 10 mg TE/day |
| Breastfeeding 1st 6 mo. | | 12 mg TE/day |
| Breastfeeding 2nd 6 mo. | | 11 mg TE/day |

Since the 1989 recommendations, research findings have prompted higher recommendations from other health professionals. The University of California at Berkeley Wellness Letter, for example, recommends daily amounts of the following:

- 200 to 800 IU of vitamin E; along with
- 250 to 500 mg of vitamin C; and
- 10,000 to 25,000 IU of the beta-carotene form of vitamin A (≈1,600 to 4,000 RE) per day.

The 1990 Canadian RNI recommends 6 to 10 mg/day for adults, with an additional 2 mg for pregnancy, and an additional 3 mg for lactation.

### Vitamin E Upper Limits

There is not enough information to set upper limits; however, extremely high doses may interfere with blood clotting and enhance the effects of drugs used to oppose blood clotting, such as aspirin, or anticoagulants.

### Vitamin E Food Sources

Vitamin E is predominantly found in vegetable and seed oils, nuts and seeds, green and leafy green vegetables, and some fruits (Table 5.14). Best sources of vitamin E are wheat germ oil, sunflower seeds, filberts, sunflower seed oil, safflower oil, cottonseed oil, peanuts and peanut butter, almonds, turkey liver, cod liver oil, palm oil, soybean oil, corn oil, canola oil, wheat germ, other nuts, and selected fruits and vegetables. Because oils are a major ingredient of margarines and salad dressings, many of these products contain some vitamin E as well.

When taking supplements, any form of vitamin E is worth taking, but if you have a choice it is recommended to take mixed tocopherols. Animal foods are not good sources of vitamin E except for liver.

## Vitamin K (Phylloquinone—the Naturally Occurring Form, Menadione, Menaquinone, Naphthoquinone)

***Vitamin K is necessary for normal blood clotting, including the protein prothrombin.***

### Vitamin K Functions

The K comes from the Danish word for coagulation, spelled koagulation. Vitamin K is part of the synthesis of blood clotting proteins and a protein that regulates blood calcium. To make blood clot, it takes 13 different proteins plus calcium. Vitamin K is essential for the synthesis prothrombin and at least five other clotting factors to produce fibrin, the protein structure of blood clots. Blood clots are needed to prevent the effects of injuries and the normal wear and tear that causes small rips in blood vessels.

This vitamin is also important for the synthesis of other proteins in the bone, plasma, and kidney. Vitamin K is unique in that bacteria in the GI tract can synthesize it. Bacterial production alone is not enough to meet the body's total need, however, so it is important that the body gets adequate of amounts of vitamin K from the diet.

Fat-soluble vitamins are dependent on the presence of other fat-soluble vitamins in order to function. For example, three of the four fat-soluble vitamins (A, D, K) play important roles in bone remodeling: Vitamin K helps in the synthesis of a specific bone protein, and vitamin D regulates the synthesis.

### Vitamin K Deficiency

Vitamin K deficiency is seldom seen except in an unusual combination of circumstances. Prolonged antibiotic drug therapy, especially sulfa drugs, can kill intestinal bacteria that make vitamin K, thereby causing a deficiency. Deficiencies may also occur whenever fat absorption is impaired, such as in diarrhea or when bile production is faulty.

The only major sign of Vitamin K deficiency is that the blood cannot clot, coagulation is lacking, resulting in hemorrhagic disease. However, vitamin K deficiency is not the only cause of hemorrhagic disease, because there are other factors involved with normal blood clotting as well. Because the body can store this vitamin, deficiency is unlikely; the body can rely on its stores when dietary intake is low.

Newborn infants have a sterile digestive tract at birth, and vitamin K in breast milk is minimal; therefore, newborns may be susceptible to vitamin K deficiency, which may be seen as hemorrhages. Most babies born in hospitals are given an injection of vitamin K at birth to protect them from possible deficiencies. Infant formulas are fortified with vitamin K for this reason.

TABLE 5.14 Vitamin E Sources in Rank Order by Serving Size

| | Weight (g) | Vit E (αTE) |
|---|---|---|
| **10.0–26.0 αTE/serving:** | | |
| 1 T wheat germ oil | 13.6 | 26 |
| 1/4 c sunflower seed kernels | 33 | 17 |
| 1/2 c filberts | 68 | 16 |
| **3.0–9.0 αTE:** | | |
| 1 T sunflower oil, linoleic <60% | 13.6 | 7.0 |
| 1 T hazelnut/filbert oil | 13.6 | 6.0 |
| 1/2 c peanuts | 72 | 5.0 |
| 1 T almond oil | 13.6 | 5.0 |
| 1/2 c brazil nuts | 70 | 5.0 |
| 1 T grapeseed oil | 13.6 | 4.4 |
| 1/2 c almonds | 78 | 4.3 |
| 1/2 c pistachios | 64 | 3.3 |
| 2 T peanut butter | 32 | 3.3 |
| 3.5 oz ckd turkey liver | 100 | 3.0 |
| 1 T cod liver oil | 100 | 3.0 |
| **1.5–2.9 αTE:** | | |
| 1 T corn oil | 13.6 | 2.9 |
| 1 T canola oil | 13.6 | 2.9 |
| 1 T salmon oil | 13.6 | 2.6 |
| 2 T wheat germ | 13.6 | 2.6 |
| 3.5 oz cnd *white* tuna in oil | 100 | 2.5 |
| 1 mango | 207 | 2.3 |
| 3.5 oz steamed clams | 100 | 2.0 |
| 1/2 c chopped pecans | 60 | 1.8 |
| 3.5 oz ckd pacific oysters | 100 | 1.8 |
| 1 T peanut oil | 13.6 | 1.7 |
| 3.5 oz ckd chicken liver | 100 | 1.7 |
| 1/2 c tomato sauce | 123 | 1.7 |
| 3.5 oz ckd mackerel | 100 | 1.7 |
| 1 T olive oil | 13.6 | 1.7 |
| 1/2 c ckd Swiss chard | 88 | 1.65 |
| 3.5 oz cnd *white* tuna in water | 100 | 1.6 |
| 1 c papaya cubes | 140 | 1.6 |
| 1/2 c chopped walnuts | 60 | 1.6 |
| **1.0–1.4 αTE:** | | |
| 1/2 c ckd mustard greens | 70 | 1.4 |
| 1 avocado half | 100 | 1.4 |
| 1/2 c pumpkin | 123 | 1.3 |
| 3.5 oz ckd catfish | 100 | 1.3 |
| 3.5 oz ckd herring | 100 | 1.3 |
| 1 T herring oil | 13.6 | 1.3 |
| 3 oz prunes (≈10) | 85 | 1.2 |
| 3.5 oz cnd *light* tuna in oil | 100 | 1.2 |
| 1/2 c pinto beans | 120 | 1.1 |
| 1 c grapes | 160 | 1.1 |
| 3.5 oz ckd carp | 100 | 1.1 |
| 3.5 oz ckd crab | 100 | 1.0 |
| **0.8–0.9 αTE:** | | |
| 1/2 c ckd broccoli | 85 | 0.9 |
| 1/2 c ckd spinach | 95 | 0.9 |
| 3.5 oz ckd farmed salmon | 100 | 0.9 |
| 3.5 oz raw pacific oysters | 100 | 0.9 |
| 1 pear | 166 | 0.8 |
| 3.5 oz ckd eastern oysters | 100 | 0.8 |
| 1 c tomato-vegetable juice | 242 | 0.8 |
| 3.5 oz ckd salmon | 100 | 0.8 |
| 1/2 c frzn blueberries-thawed | 78 | 0.8 |
| **0.50–0.79 αTE:** | | |
| 1/2 c fresh blueberries | 73 | 0.7 |
| 3.5 oz ckd beef heart | 100 | 0.7 |
| 1 medium peach | 98 | 0.7 |
| 3.5 oz raw eastern oysters | 100 | 0.7 |
| 1/2 c ckd Brussels sprouts | 78 | 0.7 |
| 1/2 c ckd okra | 92 | 0.6 |
| 2 fresh apricots | 70 | 0.6 |
| 1/2 c baby lima beans, ckd fr/frzn | 90 | 0.6 |
| 1/4 c pumpkin seed kernels, rstd | 57 | 0.6 |
| 1/2 c ckd kale | 65 | 0.55 |
| 1/2 c ckd collards | 90 | 0.55 |
| 3.5 oz ckd beef liver | 100 | 0.55 |
| 1 cooked egg | 48–50 | 0.5 |
| 3.5 oz cnd *light* tuna in water | 100 | 0.5 |
| 1/2 c fresh blackberries | 72 | 0.5 |
| 1/2 c navy/baked beans | 127 | 0.5 |
| **0.2–0.49 αTE:** | | |
| 1 apple w/peel | 138 | 0.44 |
| 3.5 oz ckd pork | 100 | 0.40 |
| 1/2 c ckd split peas | 98 | 0.40 |
| 1/2 c cnd sweet potatoes | 128 | 0.35 |
| 1 oz chocolate | 28.4 | 0.35 |
| 7.5″ raw carrot | 72 | 0.3 |
| 1 banana | 118 | 0.3 |
| 1/2 c ckd sliced carrots | 76 | 0.3 |
| 1/2 c mashed potatoes | 105 | 0.3 |
| 1 grapefruit half | 118–123 | 0.3 |
| 1/2 c peapods, ckd fr/fresh | 80 | 0.3 |
| 3.5 oz ckd ham | 100 | 0.3 |
| 1 piece whole wheat bread | 28 | 0.3 |
| 1 c romaine lettuce | 56 | 0.3 |
| 1 c looseleaf lettuce | 56 | 0.3 |
| 1/2 c fresh raspberries | 62 | 0.3 |
| 1/2 c brown rice | 98 | 0.26 |
| 1/4 c raisins | 36 | 0.25 |
| 1 c cantaloupe cubes | 160 | 0.24 |
| 1 c ckd oatmeal | 234 | 0.23 |
| 1 whole ckd artichoke | 120 | 0.2 |
| 1 c fresh strawberry halves | 152 | 0.2 |
| 4 dried apricot halves | 14 | 0.2 |
| 1/2 c peapods, ckd fr/frzn | 80 | 0.2 |

Listing includes elemental and enriched foods; does not include additionally fortified products like breakfast cereals.
Source: The Food Finder, ESHA Research, Salem, Oregon, 1999. Printed with permission.

## *Vitamin K Recommended Intake*

The RDAs for vitamin K were established in 1989 as follows:

| | | |
|---|---|---|
| Men | 19–24 years | 70 mcg/day |
| | 25 years and over | 80 mcg/day |
| Women | 19–24 years | 60 mcg/day |
| | 25 years and over | 65 mcg/day |
| Pregnant | | 65 mcg/day |
| Breastfeeding | | 65 mcg/day |

The 1990 Canadian RNI states that there is evidence that a basic need may range from 0.03 to 1.5 mcg/kg of body weight per day. Greatest need may be during the time immediately after birth.

## *Vitamin K Upper Limit*

There is no upper limit for vitamin K at this time. Toxicity is rare, but it may be possible to intake too much of the supplement form. Since vitamin K is fat-soluble and stored in the liver, the body cannot excrete the excess. Excessive doses can result in the clotting and breaking of blood cells. One of the symptoms of toxicity is jaundice.

## *Vitamin K Food Sources*

The best food sources (Table 5.15) are green vegetables (especially Brussels sprouts, kale, broccoli, spinach, and looseleaf lettuce). Other sources include eggs (the egg yolk), milk, strawberries, avocados, tomato sauces, and other vegetables and fruit.

# Biotin

***Biotin is part of a coenzyme needed for metabolizing protein, carbohydrates, and fats into energy. It is needed to synthesize glycogen and certain fats.***

## *Biotin Functions*

Biotin is important to human metabolism as a part of a coenzyme that serves as a carrier of carbon dioxide. It plays crucial roles in synthesizing certain fatty acids and glycogen and in breaking down certain fatty acids and proteins. Biotin is water-soluble, and what the body does not need is excreted in the urine. A small amount is produced by intestinal bacteria.

## *Biotin Deficiencies*

Biotin is widely distributed in foods so deficiencies are rare. Deficiencies can occur with the use of certain anticonvulsants, and for individuals with malabsorption syndrome. Raw egg whites contain a substance (avidin) that binds biotin and prevents absorption. This effect does not occur with cooked egg whites. (Researchers have induced deficiencies in adults and animals by feeding over two dozen raw egg whites daily, which is an extreme amount.)

Deficiency symptoms include thinning of hair, sometimes loss of hair color, nausea, rashes, depression, lethargy, hallucinations and other neurologic symptoms, and sometimes tingling in extremities.

TABLE 5.15 **Vitamin K Sources in Rank Order by Serving Size**

| | Weight (g) | Vit K (mcg) |
|---|---|---|
| **100–460 mcg/serving:** | | |
| 1/2 c ckd Brussels sprouts | 78 | 460 |
| 1/2 c ckd chopped broccoli | 85 | 248 |
| 1/2 c ckd chopped chayote | 80 | 138 |
| 1/2 c raw cauliflower | 50 | 150 |
| 1/2 c ckd Swiss chard | 88 | 123 |
| 1 c raw spinach | 30 | 120 |
| 1 c looseleaf lettuce | 56 | 118 |
| 7.5″ raw carrot | 72 | 104 |
| **20–99 mcg:** | | |
| 1/2 c green beans ckd fr/fresh | 63 | 49 |
| 4 spears ckd asparagus | 60 | 34 |
| 1/2 c green beans ckd fr/frzn | 68 | 32 |
| 1 cooked egg | 48–50 | 24 |
| 1 c fresh strawberry halves | 152 | 23 |
| 1 avocado half | 100 | 20 |
| 1/2 c ckd peapods | 80 | 20 |
| **10–19 mcg:** | | |
| 1 whole artichoke ckd | 120 | 17 |
| 1/2 c ckd artichoke hearts | 84 | 12 |
| **5–9 mcg:** | | |
| 1 c whole milk | 244 | 9.8 |
| 1 c nonfat milk | 245 | 8.6 |
| 1/2 c canned tomato sauce | 123 | 8.6 |
| 1 medium apple with peel | 128 | 6.9 |
| 1 T sunflower oil, 60% + linoleic | 13.6 | 6.9 |
| 1/4 c raw sweet peppers, red or green | 37 | 6.0 |
| 1 c orange juice | 249 | 5.5 |
| 1 c apple juice | 244 | 5.4 |
| 1/2 c fresh tomatoes, chopped | 90 | 5.4 |
| 1 T cottonseed oil | 13.6 | 5.2 |
| 1/2 c cnd sweet potatoes | 128 | 5.1 |
| **1.0–4.9 mcg:** | | |
| 1 medium peach | 98 | 4.9 |
| 1 baked potato w/skin | 122 | 4.9 |
| 2 canned peach halves | 98 | 3.3 |
| 1 T palm oil | 13.6 | 3.0 |
| 1 T wheat bran | 3.6 | 2.9 |
| 2 T wheat germ | 14 | 2.6 |
| 1 T peanut oil | 13.6 | 1.7 |
| 1 T soybean oil | 13.6 | 2.5 |
| 1 T mayonnaise (soybean oil) | 13.8 | 1.6 |
| 1 banana | 118 | 1.2 |
| 3.5 oz ckd white chicken meat | 100 | 1.2 |

Listing includes elemental and enriched foods; does not include additionally fortified products like breakfast cereals.
Source: The Food Finder, ESHA Research, Salem, Oregon, 1999. Printed with permission.

## Biotin Recommended Intake

The 1998 Dietary Reference Intakes for biotin are in the form of Adequate Intakes (AIs). There is insufficient information on which to make recommendations in the RDA category.

| | | |
|---|---|---|
| Men | 19 years and over | 30 mcg/day |
| Women | 19 years and over | 30 mcg/day |
| Pregnant | | 30 mcg/day |
| Breastfeeding | | 35 mcg/day |

## Biotin Upper Limits

There is insufficient data on which to base an upper limit for Biotin. Toxicity has not been reported in patients treated for biotin deficiency with daily doses up to 200 mg orally and up to 20 mg intravenously.

## Biotin Food Sources

Good sources of biotin (Table 5.16) are nuts (peanuts, filberts, almonds, walnuts), liver, egg yolks (or cooked eggs), soybeans, sweet potatoes and fish. Bananas, some green leafy vegetables, milk, cheeses, onions and yeast are also good sources. Many other foods contain biotin, but in small amounts. The uptake of biotin by the body varies in foods; however, people who consume a variety of foods will obtain sufficient biotin in their diet.

# Choline

***Choline is important for the structural integrity of cell membranes, methyl metabolism, lipid-cholesterol transport, and metabolism. It assists neurotransmissions and functions as a precursor of acetylcholine and phospholipids.***

## Choline Functions

Choline is essential to life. Human cells grown in culture have an absolute requirement for choline because when deprived, they die. The demand for choline is also interdependent on the presence of folic acid, vitamin B-12, and methionine (an amino acid). With such close relationships, it is difficult to measure needs for choline without considering the other nutrients. There may also be an interrelationship with vitamin B-6.

Choline accelerates the production and release of acetylcholine and is therefore involved in memory storage, muscle control, and many other functions. As a precursor for the synthesis of phospholipids, it is important for the structure and function of membranes, intracellular messages, export of very low density lipoproteins, and a platelet activating factor. Choline is a precursor for betaine, which is required for kidney function and other body processes.

## Choline Recommended Intake

The 1998 DRIs estimate Adequate Intakes (AIs) of choline, but there is not sufficient data to derive RDAs. The higher amount for men is based on preliminary findings that males may have a higher choline requirement than females.

| | | |
|---|---|---|
| Men | 19 years and over | 550 mg/day |
| Women | 19 years and over | 425 mg/day |
| Pregnant | | 450 mg/day |
| Breastfeeding | | 550 mg/day |

The recommended amounts may be influenced by the availability of methionine, folate, and vitamin B-12 in the diet. After menopause, a woman's needs may increase. There is also some preliminary evidence that transport of choline across the blood-brain barrier may be diminished in the elderly.

## Choline Upper Limits

High doses of choline have been associated with fishy body odor, vomiting, salivation, sweating, and gastrointestinal effects. The fishy body odor results from the excessive production of trimethylamine, a product of metabolism from one form of choline. A form of choline that does *not* contribute to this symptom is the choline form that is part of the phospholipid lecithin.

Persons with renal disease, liver disease, depression, and Parkinson's disease may have adverse effects of high intakes of choline compared with healthy individuals. Upper limits are estimated as follows:

| | |
|---|---|
| 1 g/day | Ages 1–8 years |
| 2 g/day | Ages 9–13 |
| 3 g/day | Ages 14–18 |
| 3.5 g/day | Adults over 19 years |

## Choline Food Sources

Choline is widely distributed in foods. Especially rich sources include milk, liver, cauliflower, iceberg lettuce, and peanuts. Lecithins added during food processing may also contribute added amounts.

Current food data values for choline are incomplete or understated, because older assay techniques did not include all forms of choline.

TABLE 5.16 **Biotin Sources in Rank Order by Serving Size**

| | Weight (g) | Biotin (mcg) |
|---|---|---|
| **10–75 mcg/serving:** | | |
| 1/2 c peanuts | 72 | 73 |
| 1/2 c filberts | 68 | 51 |
| 1/2 c almonds | 78 | 34 |
| 2 T peanut butter | 32 | 32 |
| 1/2 c chopped walnuts | 60 | 11 |
| **5–9 mcg:** | | |
| 1 oz soy protein isolate | 28.4 | 8.5 |
| 1 cooked egg | 48–50 | 8.1 |
| 1/2 c cashew nuts | 65 | 8.9 |
| 1 c lowfat yogurt | 245 | 7.4 |
| 3.5 oz ckd mackerel | 100 | 6.0 |
| 3.5 oz ckd haddock | 100 | 6.0 |
| 1/2 c cnd sweet potatoes | 128 | 5.5 |
| 1/2 c ckd Swiss chard | 88 | 5.3 |
| 3.5 oz ckd salmon | 100 | 5.0 |
| **3.0–4.9 mcg:** | | |
| 1 whole ckd artichoke | 120 | 4.9 |
| 1 c nonfat milk | 245 | 4.9 |
| 1/2 c tomato sauce | 123 | 4.7 |
| 1 c whole milk | 244 | 4.6 |
| 1/2 c macadamia nuts | 67 | 4.0 |
| 1/2 c ckd sliced carrots | 76 | 3.9 |
| 1 avocado half | 100 | 3.6 |
| 1/2 c fresh chopped tomatoes | 90 | 3.6 |
| 7.5″ raw carrot | 72 | 3.6 |
| 1/2 c ckd artichoke hearts | 84 | 3.4 |
| 1/4 c ckd mushrooms | 39 | 3.3 |
| 1 c papaya cubes | 140 | 3.1 |
| 1 banana | 118 | 3.1 |
| 3.5 oz ckd pork | 100 | 3.0 |
| 3.5 oz cnd tuna in oil | 100 | 3.0 |
| **2.0–2.9 mcg:** | | |
| 1/4 c sliced raw mushrooms | 17.5 | 2.8 |
| 1 c pink/red grapefruit juice | 247 | 2.6 |
| 1 c grape juice | 253 | 2.5 |
| 1 c white grapefruit juice | 247 | 2.5 |
| 1 oz camembert cheese | 28.4 | 2.2 |
| 1 T oat bran | 6 | 2.1 |
| 1/4 c ckd onions | 53 | 2.0 |
| 3.5 oz ckd lamb | 100 | 2.0 |
| 3.5 oz cnd tuna in water | 100 | 2.0 |
| 3.5 oz ckd turkey dark meat | 100 | 2.0 |
| 3.5 oz ckd lobster | 100 | 2.0 |
| 1 c apple juice | 244 | 2.0 |
| 1 c orange juice, varies 1.2–2.5 mcg | 249 | 1.9± |
| 1 c cantaloupe cubes | 160 | 1.8 |
| 1 medium apple w/peel | 138 | 1.7 |
| 1 piece whole wheat bread | 28 | 1.7 |
| 1 c fresh strawberry halves | 152 | 1.7 |
| 1 T wheat bran | 3.6 | 1.6 |
| 1/2 c vanilla ice cream | 66 | 1.6 |
| 1 oz brie cheese | 28.4 | 1.6 |
| 1 piece wheat bread | 25 | 1.5 |
| 1 c watermelon cubes | 152 | 1.5 |
| **1.0–1.4 mcg:** | | |
| 1 medium apple, peeled | 128 | 1.4 |
| 1/4 c chopped raw onions | 40 | 1.4 |
| 1 half pink/red grapefruit | 123 | 1.2 |
| 1/2 c strawberries-frzn, thawed | 111 | 1.2 |
| 1 half white grapefruit | 118 | 1.2 |
| 1/2 c fresh raspberries | 62 | 1.2 |
| 1 oz Swiss cheese | 28.4 | 1.1 |
| 1 oz provolone cheese | 28.4 | 1.1 |
| 1 oz monterey jack cheese | 28.4 | 1.1 |
| 1 oz mozzarella cheese | 28.4 | 1.1 |
| 1 c lettuce-average all | 56 | 1.1 |
| 1 small orange | 96 | 1.0 |
| **0.5–0.9 mcg:** | | |
| 1/4 c feta cheese | 28.4 | 0.9 |
| 10″ flour tortilla | 72 | 0.84 |
| 1/2 c ckd cabbage | 75 | 0.8 |
| 1/2 c ckd cauliflower | 62 | 0.8 |
| 1/2 c ckd white rice | 79 | 0.8 |
| 1 oz blue cheese | 28.4 | 0.8 |
| 1/2 c raw cauliflower | 50 | 0.75 |
| 1 oz Swiss processed cheese | 28.4 | 0.7 |
| 1/4 c raisins | 36 | 0.7 |
| 2.5 oz bagel | 71 | 0.7 |
| 1/2 c raw shredded cabbage | 35 | 0.7 |
| 1 oz American cheese | 28.4 | 0.7 |
| 1 c fresh sweet cherries | 145 | 0.6 |
| 1/2 c ckd barley | 78 | 0.6 |
| 1 corn tortilla | 26 | 0.54 |
| 1/2 c ckd green beans | 65 | 0.5 |
| 1 c grapes | 160 | 0.5 |
| **0.03–0.49 mcg:** | | |
| 1 medium pear | 166 | 0.30 |
| 1 piece white bread | 30 | 0.30 |
| 1/2 c fresh blackberries | 72 | 0.30 |
| 1 medium peach | 98 | 0.20 |
| 1/2 c spinach, ckd fr/frzn | 95 | 0.10 |
| 1/2 c ckd celery | 75 | 0.08 |
| 1/2 c raw chopped celery | 60 | 0.06 |
| 1 c raw chopped spinach | 30 | 0.03 |

Listing includes elemental and enriched foods; does not include additionally fortified products like breakfast cereals.
Source: The Food Finder, ESHA Research, Salem, Oregon, 1999. Printed with permission.

# SECTION 6

# MINERALS

| | | | |
|---|---|---|---|
| Calcium | Iodine | Molybdenum | Selenium |
| Chloride | Iron | Phosphorus | Sodium |
| Chromium | Magnesium | Potassium | Zinc |
| Copper | Manganese | | |

## Calcium (Ca)

***Calcium is vital for strong bones and teeth, nerve transmissions, and proper balance of muscle contractions (including the heart muscle). It plays important roles in cells and cell membranes, blood clotting, and other functions.***

### *Calcium Functions*

About 99% of the body's calcium is in the bones and teeth. It provides structure and strength but is also surprisingly dynamic. Calcium deposits are constantly being moved back into the bloodstream and redeposited into the bones, according to the body's needs and the current balance of other nutrients.

The remaining 1% of calcium is vital to the body fluids, and plays important roles in muscle, blood, and other tissues. Calcium is necessary for the transmission of nerve impulses, blood clotting, and for muscle contractions, including the rhythm of the heart muscle. Calcium is also essential for the production and activity of numerous enzymes and hormones that regulate digestion, metabolism of energy and fat, and the production of saliva.

Calcium aids in the transport of nutrients and other substances across cell membranes, helps maintain connective tissue, and is part of the glue that holds body cells together. It is involved in maintaining normal blood pressure and the absorption of vitamin B-12.

Calcium works with magnesium in tooth enamel and is a strong partner with phosphorus in our bone structure. Our bones are composed primarily of calcium phosphate.

Good muscle tone requires a balance between calcium, sodium, potassium, and magnesium. Other nutrients that are essential for, or complimentary to, the proper utilization of calcium include copper, zinc, manganese, fluoride, silicon, and boron. Hormones regulate the comings and goings of calcium between the bones and body fluids.

### *Calcium Absorption and Bioavailability*

Nutrient absorption and bioavailability are difficult to measure because so many different factors can affect the amount of calcium available in the body. First, dietary calcium requires the presence of vitamin D for absorption. Next, absorption increases when accompanied by food, and greater amounts are absorbed when a person is in deficient or marginal calcium status. Less calcium is absorbed if body stores are adequate or if antagonist substances are present.

Greater amounts will be absorbed if the person puts frequent and recurrent stress on the bones (weight-bearing exercises). In one study when the astronauts returned from low-gravity space, their calcium statuses were surprisingly low. This was the first strong indication regarding the importance of weight-bearing exercise for retaining calcium and strong bones. People who do not exercise or are bedridden can rapidly become deficient as the body adjusts to the lower exercise level and the reduced requirement for bone strength.

The absorption of calcium from supplements appears to be greatest when taken with a meal and in relatively small doses—500 mg or less. When large doses are consumed, calcium absorption appears to be substantially lower.

## *Calcium Losses, Antagonists, and Deficiencies*

Symptoms of calcium deficiency include stunted growth in children, fragile bones and bone loss in adults (osteoporosis), and hypertension or high blood pressure.

Many factors contribute to the bone loss associated with osteoporosis, only one of which is the lack of dietary calcium. Other factors include lack of exercise, lack of other needed nutrients, such as sunlight or vitamin D, and diets excessive in protein. Diminished estrogen production in women accelerates bone loss at menopause, and not all this loss can be prevented by increasing calcium intake.

Absorption of calcium is reduced with the intake of drugs such as tetracycline, diuretics, aluminum-containing antacids, or excessive intake of alcohol. Calcium absorption may be slightly reduced if the diet is very high in insoluble fiber, oxalic acid (spinach, rhubarb), or phytic acid (nonyeast leavened breads, some nuts and seeds, grains and soy isolates).

Because vitamin D is necessary for the absorption and use of calcium, a deficiency of sunlight exposure or a deficient intake of vitamin D-fortified foods will reduce the amount of calcium available to the body. Calcium, manganese, magnesium, copper, zinc, and iron compete for absorption into our bodies at the same site in the intestine. Therefore, excessively high intakes of any one mineral may reduce the absorption of the other minerals. High stress levels may also increase calcium needs.

High intakes of caffeine or salt (sodium chloride) have only a modest negative impact on calcium retention. However diets high in protein, at levels twice the RDA amounts, can promote urinary excretion of calcium, and coincidentally, American and Canadian diets are very high in protein. Canada and the United States recommendations are twice the amount of the World Health Organization.

Many countries do not have the prevalence of osteoporosis that we have, even though they may have far lower calcium intakes and do not consume dairy foods. Several possibilities have been theorized: their average body size is smaller; they obtain calcium from larger dietary intake of vegetables; they do not have excessive dietary intake of protein; and their everyday work may include much more physical activity than ours. In addition, with lower calcium intake, their bodies may have increased absorptive capabilities.

## *Calcium Recommended Intake*

The 1998 DRI recommendations for calcium estimate these adequate intakes (AIs) for adults. There is no change for pregnancy or breastfeeding status.

| | | |
|---|---|---|
| Men and Women | 9–18 years | 1,300 mg/day |
| | 19–50 years | 1,000 mg/day |
| | 51 years + | 1,200 mg/day |

Recommended values for over age 51 are based on the fact that calcium absorption is known to decrease with advancing age. The evidence for values at the age 19 to 50 range are less certain and may be an underestimate, according to the DRI committee.

The 1990 Canadian RNIs recommend 800 mg/day of calcium for adult men, 700 mg/day for adult women, and 1,300 mg/day if pregnant or breastfeeding.

## *Calcium Upper Limits*

Excess calcium intake from calcium supplements can cause disturbances to calcium metabolism, and may result in reduced efficiency in the use of calcium. The 1998 DRIs set upper limits (ULs) for calcium intake at 2,500 mg/day for all ages over 1 year. Excesses may cause constipation, may inhibit the absorption of iron, zinc, magnesium and other essential minerals, and may be connected to kidney stone formation.

The incidence of a syndrome called hypercalcemia, which can lead to deposition of calcium in the soft tissues and affect renal function if deposited in the kidneys, is connected to a treatment for peptic ulcers, which includes excessive intake of calcium in the form of treatment for peptic ulcers. As this treatment has changed (systemically absorbed antacids and large quantities of milk used to be prescribed), the incidence of this syndrome has decreased.

## *Calcium Food Sources*

The best sources (Table 6.1) are dairy products—milk, yogurt, and cheeses. Other excellent sources are calcium-set tofu, nuts, canned sardines with the bones, molasses, and dark-green leafy vegetables (beet, collard, and mustard greens; Swiss chard, kale, and spinach). Orange juice enriched with calcium and hard tap water in certain areas are also good sources. Cooked dried beans and peas (legumes), peanuts, broccoli, and lime-processed corn tortillas also provide good amounts. Calcium absorption is relatively high from soybeans even though they contain large amounts of phytic acid.

Calcium supplements are recommended by many health professionals for older adults, especially those at risk of osteoporosis. At this time, it is believed most effective to consume supplements with meals and in doses divided over meals rather than a single large dose.

# Chloride (Cl)

*As a part of stomach acid, chloride is essential for the digestion of food. It helps regulate acid-base balance and is part of the extracellular fluids in the body. Chloride is essential in maintaining fluid and electrolyte balance.*

## *Chloride Functions*

Chloride works with sodium and potassium in our bodies to help maintain the normal balance and distribution of fluids throughout the body, regulate pH (acid-base) balance, maintain normal muscle contraction and relaxation, and maintain normal nerve transmission and function. With sodium, chloride is part of the extracellular fluid, which is the fluid between cells. Chloride occurs in blood plasma, and in more concentrated forms, in cerebrospinal fluid and gastrointestinal secretions.

As a component of hydrochloric acid in our stomach, chloride is essential for digestion of our food. Chlorine gas ($Cl_2$) is a related compound added in tiny amounts to our water supplies. The careful use of this normally poisonous form has resulted in one of our most important and successful public health measures by eliminating water-borne diseases such as typhoid fever in our country.

TABLE 6.1 **Calcium Sources in Rank Order by Serving Size**

| | Weight (g) | Calcium (mg) |
|---|---|---|
| **290–450 mg/serving:** | | |
| 1 c lowfat yogurt | 245 | 448 |
| 3.5 oz atlantic sardines w/bones | 100 | 380 |
| 2 T blackstrap molasses | 41 | 350 |
| 1 c nonfat milk | 245 | 300 |
| 1 c whole milk | 244 | 290 |
| **150–289 mg:** | | |
| 1 oz Swiss cheese | 28.4 | 272 |
| 3.5 oz pacific sardines w/bones | 100 | 240 |
| 1 oz provolone cheese | 28.4 | 214 |
| 1 oz cheddar cheese | 28.4 | 204 |
| 1/2 c almonds | 78 | 183 |
| 1 oz American cheese | 28.4 | 174 |
| 1/2 c cottage cheese | 28.4 | 153 |
| **100–149 mg:** | | |
| 1/2 c ckd spinach | 95 | 140 |
| 1/2 c tofu | 124 | 138 |
| 1/2 c ckd green soybeans | 90 | 130 |
| 1/2 c filberts | 68 | 127 |
| 1/2 c brazil nuts | 70 | 123 |
| 1/2 c soynuts (roasted soybeans) | 86 | 119 |
| 1/2 c ckd collard greens | 90 | 100 |
| **50–99 mg:** | | |
| 1/2 c vanilla ice cream | 66 | 85 |
| 2 T molasses | 41 | 84 |
| 3.5 oz sardines, no skin | 100 | 84 |
| 1/2 c ckd beet greens | 72 | 82 |
| 1/2 c navy/baked beans | 127 | 64 |
| 1 whole ckd artichoke | 120 | 54 |
| 1/2 c cnd pinto beans | 120 | 52 |
| 1/2 c ckd mustard greens | 70 | 51 |
| 1/2 c ckd Swiss chard | 88 | 51 |
| 1/2 c peanuts | 72 | 50 |
| 1/2 c ckd butternut squash | 123 | 50 |
| 1/2 c ckd okra | 92 | 50 |
| **30–49 mg:** | | |
| 1/2 c ckd kale | 65 | 47 |
| 3.5 oz turkey/chicken hot dog | 100 | 44 |
| 3 oz, ≈10 prunes | 85 | 43 |
| 1/2 c ckd broccoli | 85 | 42 |
| 1 small orange | 96 | 38 |
| 1 c looseleaf lettuce | 56 | 38 |
| 1/2 c cnd sweet potato | 128 | 38 |
| 1/2 c ckd artichoke hearts | 84 | 37 |
| 1/2 c ckd peapods | 80 | 35 |
| 1 c papaya cubes | 140 | 34 |
| 2 T brewers yeast | 16 | 34 |
| 1/2 c ckd green beans | 65 | 33 |
| 1/4 c raw seaweed—kelp, nori, kombu, oarweed | 20 | 33 |
| 1/2 c ckd pumpkin | 123 | 32 |
| 1/2 c ckd acorn squash | 123 | 32 |
| 1 piece white bread | 30 | 32 |
| 1/2 c ckd celery | 75 | 31 |
| 1 c raw spinach | 30 | 30 |
| **20–29 mg:** | | |
| 1/2 c ckd red cabbage | 75 | 27 |
| 2 T maple syrup | 40 | 27 |
| 1/2 c mashed potatoes, avg | 105 | 27 |
| 1 c vegetable-tomato juice | 242 | 27 |
| 1 c orange juice | 248 | 26 |
| 1 piece wheat bread | 25 | 26 |
| 1 cooked egg | 48–50 | 25 |
| 1/4 c pumpkin seed kernels, rstd | 57 | 24 |
| 1/2 c lima beans, ckd fr/dry | 94 | 24 |
| 1/2 c black-eyed peas, ckd fr/dry | 120 | 24 |
| 1/2 c ckd Brussels sprouts | 78 | 24 |
| 3/4 c prune juice | 192 | 23 |
| 1/2 c ckd black beans | 86 | 23 |
| 1/2 c fresh blackberries | 72 | 23 |
| 1 c grape juice | 253 | 23 |
| 1/2 c ckd green cabbage | 75 | 23 |
| 1 c fresh sweet cherries | 145 | 22 |
| 1 c tomato juice | 243 | 22 |
| 1 c grapefruit juice | 247 | 22 |
| 1 c fresh strawberry halves | 152 | 21 |
| 1 oz unsweetened chocolate | 28.4 | 21 |
| 1 mango | 207 | 21 |
| 1 kiwifruit | 76 | 20 |
| 2 T white sugar | 25 | 20 |
| 1 c romaine lettuce | 56 | 20 |
| **5–19 mg:** | | |
| 7.5″ raw carrot | 72 | 19 |
| 1/2 c ckd green peas | 80 | 19 |
| 1 c ckd oatmeal | 234 | 18 |
| 1 pear | 166 | 18 |
| 1 c grapes | 160 | 18 |
| 1 c cantaloupe cubes | 160 | 18 |
| 1/2 c cnd tomato sauce | 123 | 17 |
| 1/2 c shredded green cabbage | 35 | 16 |
| 1 c papaya cubes | 140 | 15 |
| 1 grapefruit half | 118–123 | 14 |
| 1/2 c pineapple juice | 125 | 14 |
| 1/2 c ckd green split peas | 98 | 14 |
| 2 T peanut butter | 32 | 13 |
| 1 baked potato w/skin | 122 | 13 |
| 1 avocado half | 100 | 11 |
| 1 medium apple w/peel | 138 | 10 |
| 1/2 c ckd bean sprouts | 62 | 7 |
| 1 banana | 118 | 7 |
| 2 T wheat germ | 14 | 6.4 |

Listing includes elemental and enriched foods; does not include additionally fortified products like breakfast cereals.
Source: The Food Finder, ESHA Research, Salem, Oregon, 1999. Printed with permission.

### *Chloride Deficiencies*

Chloride deficiency doesn't occur under normal circumstances. Loss would tend to parallel losses of sodium; therefore, heavy, persistent sweating, chronic diarrhea, vomiting, and renal disease might cause losses. Deficiency is uncommon as the element is consumed in table salt (sodium chloride).

### *Chloride Recommended Intake*

No RDA has been established. Nutrition requirements of chloride are minimal because the element is easily obtained in a normal diet.

### *Chloride Upper Limits*

The only known dietary condition of too much chloride (measured in blood serum) is water-deficiency dehydration.

### *Chloride Food Sources*

Dietary chloride comes almost entirely from sodium chloride—table salt, and smaller amounts from potassium chloride (salt substitutes), and even smaller amounts from natural chloride in natural waters (not the same form as the chlorine used in water supplies). Dietary sources of chloride are the same as those for sodium, and processed foods are the main source.

## Chromium (Cr)

*Chromium works with insulin to facilitate the uptake of blood sugar (glucose) into the cells and to regulate blood sugar levels. It helps release energy and participates in metabolism of carbohydrate and lipids.*

### *Chromium Functions*

Chromium is required for maintaining normal glucose metabolism, is a cofactor of insulin, and essential for helping the body metabolize carbohydrates and lipids. As a component of Glucose Tolerance Factor (GTF), chromium works with insulin to transport glucose into the cells. GTF also contains niacin, the amino acid glycine, glutamic acid, cysteine, and other compounds. The chromium-insulin combination also stimulates the synthesis of protein.

Scientific studies do not support claims that chromium picolinate promotes weight loss, builds muscle, burns fat, and performs a few other functions. As a result, the FTC stopped marketers from making these statements.

### *Chromium Deficiencies*

In a chromium deficiency, a diabetes-like condition similar to that seen in adult onset diabetes may develop. Research on humans has shown that diets low in chromium (the definition of low is still under research) may inhibit glucose tolerance, may inhibit glucagon response, and impair insulin activity. Diets high in sugar, refined white breads and rice, and processed or convenience foods, may lead to a deficiency of chromium. Higher levels of chromium are excreted in the urine with diets high in simple sugars.

In the United States, blood and tissue levels of chromium decrease as a person ages. In contrast, people in primitive cultures have chromium levels 2 to 3 times higher than most Americans, their chromium status does not decline with age, and cardiovascular and diabetic diseases are infrequent to nonexistent.

Supplementation with chromium appears to improve the symptoms of hypoglycemia, a condition in which blood sugar levels drop to low levels because of excessive levels of insulin (the opposite of diabetes).

### *Chromium Losses and Gains*

Food processing takes a heavy toll on the chromium content of foods. When milled and processed, grains, cereals, and sugar cane lose most of their chromium. Stainless steel cookware may contribute chromium to the foods prepared in them, especially if food mixtures are acidic, like tomato sauces.

### *Chromium Recommended Intake*

The 1989 Estimated Safe and Adequate Dietary Intakes recommend a range of 50 to 200 mcg per day for healthy adults. Research suggests that U.S. adults consume less than the recommended 50 mcg per day.

### *Chromium Upper Limits*

No upper limit has been set for chromium consumed in food; no dietary toxicity has been reported in humans. However, toxic levels can be correlated to exposure to work conditions where there is dust containing the chromate form, which is a completely different form than that consumed in foods. This exposure can lead to bronchial cancer.

### *Chromium Food Sources*

Unprocessed, unrefined foods are the best sources of chromium. Those with high bioavailability include nutritional or brewer's yeast, cheeses, liver, and wheat germ. Other sources include molasses, nuts, whole grain breads and cereals, lean meats, cantaloupe, dark-green lettuces, onions, mushrooms, artichokes, prunes, tomatoes, asparagus, wine, and beer (yes, because beer is brewed with brewer's yeast). Not all foods have been analyzed for chromium, so this list is not complete.

Poor sources of chromium are any refined and processed foods. Studies have found substantial differences in the biological activity of different chromium compounds. The chromic chloride form is not as well absorbed as the naturally occurring form of chromium found in foods, nutritional yeast, or chromium picolinate.

## Copper (Cu)

*Copper is part of many essential enzymes in the body that affect the formation and maintenance of the blood vessels and heart, the nerve sheaths and brain, bones, skin, hair color, connective tissue, and collagen. It is also essential for absorption and use of iron.*

### *Copper Functions*

Copper is essential and plays a key role as part of several enzymes and as a catalyst. It is involved in the production of red blood cells, transportation and absorption of iron, creation and maintenance of the sheath around nerve fibers, formation of bone, synthesis of RNA, development of collagen, and healing of wounds. Copper also plays a role in controlling the oxidation of vitamin C and in the metabolism of fatty acids.

It is interesting to note that copper is more concentrated in the young and growing parts of foods than in the mature forms. This illustrates the importance of copper in the formation and maintenance of the skeleton; the formation of connective tissue and collagen; the development and maintenance of the blood vessels, red blood cells, and the heart; and the structure and function of the nervous system, including the brain.

Copper also strengthens immunity as a component of the antioxidant enzyme superoxide dismutase, helps break down fats in fat tissue, is necessary for normal functioning of insulin, and influences hair and skin color as a part of the pigment melanin. In addition, copper aids in the conversion of protein, carbohydrates, and fat to energy. It also contributes to the synthesis of prostaglandins that regulate a variety of body functions including heartbeat, blood pressure and wound healing.

Approximately 33% of the copper in the body is located in the muscles, about 33% is in the brain and liver, about 15% is in the bones, and the rest is in the heart, kidney, and all other tissues. Blood levels of copper are elevated when there is a niacin deficiency, although the significance of this association is unknown.

### *Copper Deficiencies*

Severe copper deficiency is rare in human beings, although marginal deficiencies might be more common. Copper is stored in the liver, so deficiencies develop slowly. High zinc intake (from supplements) over time can cause a copper deficiency, as can prolonged intake of the medication B-penicillamine. The balance between iron, zinc, and copper is important in the absorption and utilization of all three of these minerals. Excessive intake of one might result in a secondary deficiency of the other.

Deficiencies can occur, however, where there is impaired copper utilization (an extremely rare inherited disease) or if an adult or infant is exclusively fed supplemental feeding over an extended period.

Since copper is necessary for the normal development and maintenance of many tissues, a deficiency may cause a variety of disorders. Data on copper deficiencies in animals indicate the following potential conditions in humans: anemia (copper affects iron absorption), skeletal defects (e.g., scoliosis), impaired nervous system function, reproductive failure, defects in pigmentation and structure of the hair, and decreased arterial elasticity.

### *Copper Recommended Intake*

Because there is uncertainty about the level of copper required, it is not possible to establish an RDA for this element. Therefore, a range of 1.5 to 3.0 mg per day that was estimated as a safe and adequate daily intake for U.S. adults was established in 1989. The 1990 Canadian RNI estimates 2.0 mg per day for adults as an adequate and safe intake.

### *Copper Upper Limits*

Toxicity is rare; therefore, no upper levels have been established at this time. Daily intakes of more than 10 to 20 mg may cause nausea and vomiting in some persons. Wilson's disease (an inherited disorder) is characterized by excessive accumulation of copper in the tissues, liver disease, mental retardation, tremor, and loss of coordination. Treatment includes eating a low-copper diet and taking penicillamine, which binds to copper and increases its excretion.

### *Copper Food Sources*

The best sources of copper (Table 6.2) are liver, oysters and clams, nuts and seeds, peanuts, molasses, beef heart, chocolate, brewer's yeast, and vegetable-tomato juice. Baked potatoes, artichokes, avocados, prunes, and legumes (cooked beans and peas), whole wheat pasta, shrimp, dark turkey/chicken meat, and dark-green leafy vegetables contain good amounts of copper as well.

There are considerably higher levels of both copper and zinc in the peel rather than in the flesh of some fruits. Drinking water can be a good source of copper in locations where copper pipe is used in plumbing or the mineral content of the water is high. Milk and milk products are generally poor sources.

## Fluoride

*Fluoride is essential for strong bones and helps make teeth resistant to decay.*

### *Fluoride Functions*

Fluoride is involved in the formation of bones and teeth and helps teeth to be resistant to decay. Intake is especially critical during the first eight years of childhood. Adequate fluoride intake is estimated to reduce the occurrence of dental caries by 50 to 65%. Where diets are high in fluorine, the crystalline deposits in bones and teeth are larger and more perfectly formed; and bones are more stable and resistant to degeneration and osteoporosis.

Fluoride works with calcium, phosphorus, magnesium, and vitamin D in this task. Fluoride might also aid in wound healing and enhance iron absorption. Recently studies are looking at the possible capability of certain forms of fluoride to strengthen bones in adults.

### *Fluoride Recommended Intake*

The 1998 DRIs established these recommendations for adults as Adequate Intakes (AIs) for fluoride. There is no change for pregnancy or breastfeeding status.

| | | |
|---|---|---|
| Men | 14–18 years | 3.2 mg/day |
| | 19 years + | 3.8 mg/day |
| Women | 14–18 years | 2.9 mg/day |
| | 19 years + | 3.1 mg/day |

TABLE 6.2 Copper Sources in Rank Order by Serving Size

| | Weight (g) | Copper (mg) |
|---|---|---|
| **3.0–10.0 mg/serving:** | | |
| 3.5 oz ckd veal liver | 100 | 9.9 |
| 3.5 oz ckd beef liver | 100 | 4.5 |
| **1.0–2.9 mg:** | | |
| 3.5 oz ckd oysters | 100 | 2.0 |
| 1/2 c cashews | 65 | 1.4 |
| 1/2 c brazil nuts | 70 | 1.2 |
| 3.5 oz ckd Alaska king crab | 100 | 1.2 |
| 3.5 oz ckd raw oysters | 100 | 1.1 |
| 1/2 c filberts | 68 | 1.0 |
| 1/2 c almonds | 78 | 1.0 |
| **0.70–0.99 mg:** | | |
| 1/2 c soynuts (roasted soybeans) | 86 | 0.90 |
| 1/2 c chopped walnuts | 60 | 0.80 |
| 2 T blackstrap molasses | 41 | 0.84 |
| 1/4 c pumpkin seed kernels, rstd | 57 | 0.78 |
| 1/2 c pistachios | 64 | 0.76 |
| 1/2 c peanuts | 72 | 0.75 |
| 3.5 oz ckd beef heart | 100 | 0.74 |
| 1/2 c chopped pecans | 60 | 0.70 |
| **0.50–0.69 mg:** | | |
| 3.5 oz steamed clams | 100 | 0.69 |
| 3.5 oz ckd blue crab | 100 | 0.65 |
| 1 oz unsweetened chocolate | 28.4 | 0.62 |
| 1/4 c sunflower seed kernels | 33 | 0.60 |
| 3.5 oz ckd turkey liver | 100 | 0.56 |
| 2 T brewers yeast | 16 | 0.52 |
| **0.25–0.49 mg:** | | |
| 1 c vegetable-tomato juice | 242 | 0.48 |
| 2 T blackstrap molasses | 41 | 0.42 |
| 1 baked potato w/skin | 122 | 0.38 |
| 3.5 oz ckd chicken liver | 100 | 0.37 |
| 3 oz, ≈10 prunes | 85 | 0.37 |
| 1/2 c roasted chestnuts | 72 | 0.36 |
| 1/2 c cnd sweet potato | 128 | 0.36 |
| 1 whole ckd artichoke | 120 | 0.28 |
| 1/2 c navy/baked beans | 127 | 0.27 |
| 1 avocado half | 100 | 0.27 |
| 1/2 c ckd lentils | 99 | 0.25 |
| **0.15–0.24 mg:** | | |
| 1/2 c tofu | 124 | 0.24 |
| 1/2 c tomato sauce | 123 | 0.24 |
| 1 c ckd whole wheat pasta | 140 | 0.23 |
| 3.5 oz sardines, avg all | 100 | 0.23 |
| 1 tsp spirulina | < 4 | 0.23 |
| 1 mango | 207 | 0.23 |
| 1/2 c baby lima beans, ckd fr/frzn | 90 | 0.22 |
| 1/2 c ckd kidney beans | 89 | 0.21 |
| 1/2 c ckd mushrooms | 39 | 0.20 |
| 3.5 oz ckd shrimp | 100 | 0.20 |
| 1/2 c ckd artichoke hearts | 84 | 0.20 |
| 6″ flour tortilla | 72 | 0.19 |
| 1/2 c ckd black beans | 86 | 0.18 |
| 1/2 c beet greens | 72 | 0.18 |
| 1/2 c lima beans, ckd fr/dry | 94 | 0.18 |
| 1/2 c ckd dried split peas | 98 | 0.18 |
| 1/2 c pinto beans | 120 | 0.17 |
| 2 T peanut butter | 32 | 0.17 |
| 3.5 oz ckd dark turkey meat | 100 | 0.16 |
| 1/4 c coconut dry (20 g) or fresh | 33 | 0.15 |
| **0.10–0.14 mg:** | | |
| 3.5 oz beef roasts/steaks (0.12–0.16) | 100 | 0.15 |
| 1/2 c mashed potatoes | 105 | 0.14 |
| 1/2 c ckd Swiss chard | 88 | 0.14 |
| 1 c ckd regular pasta | 140 | 0.14 |
| 1/2 c black-eyed peas, ckd fr/frzn | 85 | 0.14 |
| 1 c grapes | 160 | 0.14 |
| 1/2 c spinach, ckd fr/frzn | 95 | 0.13 |
| 3/4 c prune juice | 192 | 0.13 |
| 1 c ckd oatmeal | 234 | 0.13 |
| 1/2 c ckd pumpkin | 123 | 0.13 |
| 3.5 oz ckd veal | 100 | 0.12 |
| 3.5 oz ckd lamb | 100 | 0.12 |
| 1 banana | 118 | 0.12 |
| 1 kiwifruit | 76 | 0.12 |
| 2.5 oz plain bagel | 71 | 0.12 |
| 1/4 c raisins | 36 | 0.11 |
| 1/2 c pineapple juice | 125 | 0.11 |
| 1/2 c ckd winter squash | 123 | 0.11 |
| 1/2 c ckd green peas | 80 | 0.11 |
| 1/2 c ckd green soybeans | 90 | 0.11 |
| 1 c orange juice | 248 | 0.10 |
| 1/2 c fresh blackberries | 72 | 0.10 |
| 1/2 c ckd kale | 65 | 0.10 |
| 1/2 c ckd brown rice | 98 | 0.10 |
| **0.075–0.09 mg:** | | |
| 1/2 c ckd summer squash | 90 | 0.09 |
| 1/2 c fresh pineapple | 78 | 0.09 |
| 3.5 oz ckd turkey light meat | 100 | 0.09 |
| 1 c grapefruit juice | 247 | 0.09 |
| 3.5 oz ckd dark chicken | 100 | 0.09 |
| 2 T wheat germ | 14 | 0.09 |
| 3.5 oz ckd ground beef, ranges 0.07–0.09 | 100 | 0.08 |
| 1 piece whole wheat bread | 28 | 0.08 |
| 1/2 c ckd barley | 78 | 0.08 |
| 1/2 c ckd mung bean sprouts | 62 | 0.08 |
| 1 c fresh strawberry halves | 152 | 0.08 |
| 1/2 c ckd sliced carrots | 76 | 0.08 |
| 3.5 oz ckd pork & ham | 100 | 0.08 |
| **0.050–0.075 mg:** | | |
| 3.5 oz ckd fish, ranges 0.04–0.10 | 100 | 0.07 |
| 1/2 c fresh tomatoes | 90 | 0.07 |
| 1 c cantaloupe cubes | 160 | 0.07 |
| 2 fresh apricots | 70 | 0.06 |
| 4 dried apricot halves | 14 | 0.06 |
| 1/2 c ckd Brussels sprouts | 78 | 0.06 |
| 3.5 oz ckd light chicken meat | 100 | 0.05 |
| 1 piece wheat bread | 25 | 0.05 |
| 1/2 c ckd red cabbage | 75 | 0.05 |
| 1/2 c ckd broccoli | 85 | 0.05 |
| 1 c apple juice | 244 | 0.05 |
| 1/2 c ckd white rice | 79 | 0.05 |
| **Less than 0.04 mg:** | | |
| 1 corn tortilla | 26 | 0.04 |
| 1 T wheat bran | 3.6 | 0.04 |
| 7.5″ raw whole carrot | 72 | 0.04 |
| 1 T oat bran | 6 | 0.02 |
| your local water supply | Amounts vary | |

Listing includes elemental and enriched foods; does not include additionally fortified products like breakfast cereals.
Source: The Food Finder, ESHA Research, Salem, Oregon, 1999. Printed with permission.

### Fluoride Upper Limits

Mottling, pitting, and dulling of the teeth has been observed in areas where fluoride is a natural ingredient in the water at levels of 2 ppm to 6 ppm. Intake greater than 8 ppm can cause fluorosis of the bones that produces arthritis-like symptoms. Fatal poisoning can occur if fluoride is greater than 2,500 times the recommended intake. Chronic ingestion of 50 mg/day can occur with some forms of air or environmental pollution, resulting in bone and tooth deformities. The 1998 DRI recommendations set upper limits for fluoride at:

| | |
|---|---|
| 0–6 months | 0.9 mg/day |
| 6–12 months | 0.7 mg/day |
| 1–3 years | 1.3 mg/day |
| 4–8 years | 2.2 mg/day |

### Fluoride Food Sources

The best source of fluoride is fluoridated water, where the fluorine is actually more available than the protein bound fluorine in foods. Topical application of fluoride to the teeth is not as effective in preventing cavities as is ingested fluoride. The fluoride in food is dependent on the content in the soil where it is grown.

An average cup of tea provides about 0.3 mg of fluoride. Tea leaves have the ability to accumulate concentrations of fluoride exceeding 10 mg/100 g of dry weight; however, brewed tea can range from 1 to 6 mg/L. Concentrations of decaffeinated teas usually contain more fluoride than regular tea. There is also fluoride in the meat of marine fish.

## Iodine (I)

***Iodine is an essential part of thyroid hormones that regulate basal metabolic rate, growth, and development and promote protein synthesis.***

### Iodine Functions

Iodine is an important constituent of the thyroid hormones, which are involved in many roles in the body, including growth, reproduction, nerve and muscle function, the synthesis of proteins, the growth of skin and hair, body temperature, making of blood cells, and the use of oxygen in cells. One of these hormones, thyroxin, regulates the metabolic rate, which is an important regulator of body weight.

More than 60% of iodine in the body is found in the thyroid gland. The remaining 40% is distributed throughout the body, particularly in the ovaries, muscles, and blood. In addition to dietary intake, iodine also can be absorbed through the skin.

### Iodine Deficiencies

Iodine deficiency causes an enlargement of the thyroid gland, which leads to a swelling at the neck called goiter. Lack of iodine can also cause sluggishness and weight gain. A deficiency during pregnancy will impair the development of the fetus causing extreme mental and physical retardation. The condition is called cretinism. These conditions used to occur with high incidence in the Central Plains states, where the soil is low in iodine. In 1924, to solve the problem of iodine deficiency, iodine was added to something everyone would eat—salt. Iodized salt has greatly reduced the prevalence of these diseases and conditions in the United States.

### Iodine Recommended Intake

The 1989 RDA is 150 mcg/day for adults, 175 mcg if pregnant, and 200 mcg if breastfeeding. It is thought that the average American gets more than twice this amount in their diet. The 1990 Canadian RNI recommends 160 mcg/day for adults, 185 mcg if pregnant, and 210 mcg if breastfeeding.

### Iodine Upper Limits

There is not enough information to set an official upper limit amount of iodine at this time because the potential chronic toxic effects of dietary iodine are not clear. Prolonged, excessive intakes of iodine are known to depress thyroid function and cause a goiter condition, like that seen in deficiency. However, iodine intakes of up to about 2,000 mcg per day have caused no adverse reactions in healthy adults.

An overactive thyroid is called Graves' disease. This is the result of a disruption in the regulatory mechanisms that control the thyroid hormone function, not the result of over-consumption of iodine.

### Iodine Food Sources

Iodized salt is the most reliable source, as plant sources vary widely with the iodine content of the soil they grow in (Table 6.3). Good sources include seafood; seaweed; plants grown in iodine-rich soil and animals that feed on those plants; dairy products; and breads (dough conditioners contain forms of iodine).

In seashore areas, seafood, water, and even the ocean mist are sources of iodine. Further inland, the iodine content of plant and animal products can vary depending on fertilizing and feeding practices. If the area was a sea in ancient times, the soil will contain iodine. Dairy products contain iodine because it is contained in the feed additives and disinfectants. Many dough stabilizers contain the iodate form of iodine, so a slice of this bread may contain as much as 150 mcg of iodine.

## Iron

***Iron is essential for making oxygen available to every tissue of the body and transporting carbon dioxide out of the body. It is important to a strong immune system, plays a role in enzymes and hormones, and helps convert energy for normal cell activities.***

### Iron Functions

The greatest portion of iron in our bodies—approximately 80%—is contained in the hemoglobin of blood cells. This is what makes our blood red. Hemoglobin carries oxygen from the lungs to all the cells in the body and transfers the oxygen to myoglobin, which also contains iron. Myoglobin accepts, stores, and releases oxygen in the muscles for muscle contraction. Iron is therefore the main determinant of how much oxygen is available to body tissues, including the brain, muscles, heart, and liver. It helps convert substances to energy for normal cell activities.

Iron also plays a role in transporting carbon dioxide from the cells back to the lungs. Iron plays a role in several enzymes and is needed to make certain amino acids, hormones, and neurotransmitters. In addition, it strengthens the immune system, increasing resistance to colds, infections, and disease. Some iron is stored in combination with proteins in the spleen, liver, and bone marrow.

TABLE 6.3 Iodine Sources in Rank Order by Serving Size

| | Weight (g) | Iodine (mcg) |
|---|---|---|
| **100–200 mcg/serving:** | | |
| 1/2 t iodized table salt, all kinds | 2.5–3 | 195 |
| 3.5 oz haddock/cod filet, bkd | 100 | 116 |
| **75–99 mcg:** | | |
| 1 chicken pot pie | 230 | 89 |
| 1 c chocolate milkshake, fast food | 166 | 88 |
| 1 c plain lowfat yogurt (8 oz) | 245 | 84 |
| 1 c chocolate drink, fr/dry + milk | 266 | 82 |
| 1 c evaporated milk, avg all | 256 | 80 |
| 1 c lasagna-home recipe | 245 | 80 |
| 1 c flavored yogurt—vanilla, coffee, lemon | 227 | 79 |
| 1 c hot cocoa-prep w/whole milk | 250 | 75 |
| **50–74 mcg:** | | |
| 3.5 oz fish sticks, ckd fr/frzn | 100 | 63 |
| 1/2 c bread pudding w/raisins | 126 | 63 |
| 1 c 1%-2% chocolate milk | 250 | 63 |
| 1 c 1%-2% lowfat milk | 247 | 59 |
| 1 c buttermilk, skim, cultured | 245 | 59 |
| 1 c spaghetti in tomato sce, cnd | 250 | 57 |
| 1 c chicken noodle casserole-recipe | 250 | 56 |
| 1 piece apple pie (1/8 of 9″ frzn pie) | 125 | 55 |
| 10″ flour tortilla | 72 | 54 |
| 1 c nonfat/skim milk | 245 | 54 |
| 1/2 c mashed potatoes fr/instant | 105 | 54 |
| 1 c whole milk, 3.3% fat | 244 | 53 |
| 1/2 c choc pudding fr/mix | 147 | 52 |
| 1/2 c ckd white rice | 79 | 50 |
| 1/2 c tapioca pudding, recipe | 147 | 50 |
| **35–49 mcg:** | | |
| 1/2 c vanilla pudding | 142 | 48 |
| 1 c lowfat yogurt w/fruit or nuts | 245 | 47 |
| 1 c spaghetti w/meat sce, recipe | 250 | 47 |
| 1 cooked egg, avg | 50 | 46 |
| 1 white roll, ranges 10–46 mcg | 57 | 46 |
| 1 c chili con carne w/beans, cnd | 254 | 45 |
| 1 piece pumpkin pie—1/6 of 8″ fzn pie | 109 | 45 |
| 1 c beef stew | 245 | 44 |
| 1 piece cornbread | 65 | 44 |
| 2 pancakes fr/mix 4″ diam | 76 | 43 |
| 3.5 oz beef/calf liver, pan fried | 100 | 42 |
| 3.5 oz shrimp, breaded, ckd fr/frzn | 100 | 41 |
| 3.5 oz bkd turkey breast | 100 | 40 |
| 3.5 oz meatloaf, homemade | 100 | 38 |
| 1 medium baked potato w/peel | 122 | 38 |
| 1/2 c corn grits, ckd | 128 | 36 |
| 1/2 c navy beans, cooked | 91 | 36 |
| 1 ice cream sandwich, avg | 59 | 35 |
| **25–34 mcg:** | | |
| 1/4 pound hamburger w/condiments–fast food sandwich | 166 | 33 |
| 1/2 c macaroni + cheese fr/mix | 98 | 33 |
| 1/2 c chocolate ice cream | 66 | 31 |
| 3.5 oz breaded onion rings/ckd fr/frzn | 100 | 30 |
| 1 piece yellow cake w/white icing | 64 | 30 |
| 1 danish pastry/sweet roll | 65 | 29 |
| 1 blueberry muffin | 50 | 29 |
| 1/2 c white sauce, med, recipe | 144 | 27 |
| 1 c tomato soup, cnd, prep w/milk | 248 | 27 |
| 1 piece white bread | 30 | 27 |
| 1/2 c vanilla ice cream | 66 | 27 |
| 1/2 c cottage cheese, avg all | 105–112 | 27 |
| 1/2 c cnd red beans | 128 | 27 |
| 1 ckd egg yolk | 17 | 26 |
| 1 c corn flakes cereal | 28 | 26 |
| 1/2 c baby lima beans, ckd fr/frzn | 82 | 25 |
| 1/2 c french fried potatoes, fr/frzn | 86 | 25 |
| **15–24 mcg:** | | |
| 1/2 c egg custard, recipe | 141 | 24 |
| 1/2 c flan w/caramel | 133 | 23 |
| 1/2 c black-eyed peas/cowpeas, ckd from fresh | 85 | 22 |
| 3.5 oz pan fried sausage | 100 | 21 |
| 1 grilled cheese sandwich | 128 | 21 |
| 1 egg bagel, large | 110 | 21 |
| 3.5 oz tuna, cnd in oil | 100 | 20 |
| 1/2 c ice milk or ice cream, vanilla | 66 | 19 |
| 3.5 oz veal cutlet, breaded/fried | 100 | 19 |
| 1/2 c red beans, cooked | 88 | 18.5 |
| 1 piece coffee cake rte/frzn | 63 | 18 |
| 4 saltine crackers | 12 | 18 |
| 1 piece whole wheat bread | 28 | 18 |
| 1/2 c sweet potatoes, candied-recipe | 117 | 18 |
| 1 c crispy rice cereal, rte | 26 | 17 |
| 3.5 oz beef roast or pan fried, avg | 10 | 15–17 |
| 2 chocolate cookies w/crème filling | 22 | 17 |
| 1/2 c gelatin dessert, fr/mix | 135 | 16 |
| 2 T honey | 42 | 16 |
| 1 piece rye bread | 32 | 16 |
| 1 pce choc cake w/choc icing | 64 | 15 |
| **10–14 mcg:** | | |
| 3.5 oz ground beef, pan fried | 100 | 14 |
| 1 buttermilk biscuit, avg fr/mix | 77 | 14 |
| 1 oz Swiss, asiago, provolone, cheshire, caraway, fontina, monterey jack cheese | 28 | 13 |
| 1/2 c macaroni, cooked | 70 | 13 |
| 1/2 c pinto beans, cooked | 86 | 13 |
| 1 medium potato, boiled wo/peel | 135 | 12 |
| 3.5 oz ham, baked | 100 | 12 |
| 1/2 c granola w/raisins | 45 | 12 |
| 1 cake-type doughnut | 28 | 12 |
| 1 c shredded wheat cereal | 43 | 12 |
| 1 oz cheddar/colby cheese, avg | 28 | 11.5 |
| 1 c oat ring cereal (like Cheerios) | 23 | 11 |
| 3.5 oz lamb chop, pan fried | 100 | 11 |
| 1 c raisin bran cereal | 56 | 11 |
| 4 prunes | 34 | 10 |
| 1 oz mozzarella cheese | 28 | 10 |
| 2 T pancake syrup | 40 | 10 |
| **0–9 mcg:** | | |
| 1 piece Swiss processed cheese | 21 | 9 |
| 1/4 c mozzarella processed cheese shredded | 28 | 9 |
| 1 oz corn chips, snack | 28 | 8 |
| 1 piece American processed cheese | 21 | 8 |
| 1 c apple juice, canned | 248 | 7 |
| 1/2 c corn, ckd fr/frzn | 82 | 7 |
| 2 c popcorn, popped in oil | 22 | 6 |
| 1 c grape juice | 253 | 5 |
| 1 oz peanuts, avg, range 2–5 mcg | 28 | 4 |
| 1 c brewed tea | 220 | 4.4 |
| 1 oz cashews, avg | 21 | 3 |
| 1 Tbsp sugar | 12.5 | 2.8 |
| 1 oz potato chips | 28 | 1.4 |
| Most all fruits, vegetables are low in iodine (excluding beans and a few others previously listed) | 0–3 mcg/100g | |

## *Iron Deficiencies*

Iron deficiency anemia can result from inadequate food intake of iron, but it can also be caused indirectly by a deficiency in other nutrients. For example, a deficiency in vitamin B-6, vitamin E, folacin, vitamin B-12, vitamin A, vitamin C, or copper can affect the hemoglobin level in the body and can indirectly create an iron deficiency.

Iron deficiency in children can show up as psychological disturbances before anemia is evident—short attention span, apathy, irritability, hyperactivity, impaired development, and reduced ability to learn. A severe, long-standing deficiency can result in reduced intelligence. In adults, deficiency can result in lowered immunity, anemia, irregular heartbeat, impaired mental skills, fatigue, decreased work capacity, behavior changes, reduced resistance to cold, pale nail beds, and concave nails.

To reduce these deficiency problems, white wheat flour, cornmeal, pastas and breads are enriched with iron to help provide more iron in the diet.

Sometimes a craving for nonfood items (called pica) such as ice, clay, or starch can occur. Such behavior was once thought to relate to iron deficiency because of the potential iron in the object craved (like clay); however, some analyses of the desired dirt did not always confirm this.

## *Iron Bioavailability—Heme and Nonheme*

Iron comes in heme and nonheme forms, which are absorbed by different mechanisms and therefore have different bioavailability. Heme iron is the predominant form in meat and is highly absorbable; nonheme iron, which is more difficult to absorb, is the only form in plant foods and accounts for a smaller portion of iron in meats.

Not all meats are the same, however. The iron in ground beef, beef loin, lamb chops, and cured ham (pork) is about 75 to 79% heme iron. The iron in pork shoulder is 65% heme; beef round is 55% heme; ground turkey or a chicken drumstick is 40% heme. The iron in a chicken thigh is 32% heme; chicken breast is 29% heme; and a pork loin is 22% heme.

Absorption of nonheme iron is increased if consumed with foods containing meat (heme iron) and vitamin C. Foods cooked in iron vessels provide more iron, especially if cooked with acidic type foods like tomato sauces.

Many factors affect nonheme iron absorption. Because of the inhibiting and enhancing factors, absorption may vary up to tenfold, depending on the content of the overall diet. When body stores are high, the body compensates and reduces the absorption of dietary iron; when body stores are low, absorption is increased. Therefore, predicting iron intake by measuring dietary iron may not necessarily predict the iron actually absorbed by the body.

## *Iron Losses*

Coffee and tea consumed an hour before or after a meal or an iron supplement will prevent the absorption of up to 39% of the nonheme form of iron. This effect is caused by the tannic acid and phenols in those beverages (not from the caffeine). Spinach contains iron, but it is not completely available because the oxalic acid in raw spinach will bind some of it and make most of it unavailable to the body.

Iron uptake varies from person to person, and the same person will have a different uptake from day to day. Iron absorption will be reduced in the presence of antacids, phosphate salts, as well as the calcium and phosphate in milk, EDTA in food additives, calcium phosphate, phytates, bran, and high fiber foods. Excess consumption of calcium, copper, or magnesium carbonate will also reduce the absorption of iron. Because iron competes with calcium, manganese, and zinc for absorption in the intestine, an excess intake of any one of these minerals (usually from supplements) might produce a deficiency of the others.

## *Iron Recommended Intake*

The 1989 RDAs for iron for adults are listed next. The RDAs recommend increased levels of iron for women to account for monthly menstrual losses. Additional amounts may be necessary if there is external bleeding from a wound or from internal hemorrhaging; higher iron intake may be needed for those whose diet has little meat or vitamin C.

| | | |
|---|---|---|
| Men | 19 years + | 10 mg/day |
| Women | 19–50 years | 15 mg/day |
| | 51 years + | 15 mg/day |
| Pregnant | | 30 mg/day |
| Breastfeeding | | 15 mg/day |

The 1990 Canadian RNI recommends 9 mg/day for adult men and 13 mg/day for adult women. During pregnancy, 13 mg for the 1st trimester is recommended, 18 mg for 2nd trimester, and 23 mg/day for the 3rd trimester; 13 mg/day if breastfeeding.

## *Iron Upper Limits*

Iron absorption is usually regulated by need, and excesses are merely eliminated from the body. However, iron supplementation may cause iron overload and toxicity. After aspirin, iron pills are the second most common cause of accidental poisoning in children. As few as 6 to 12 tablets of supplemental iron or vitamins containing iron, have caused deaths in children. Apparently the mechanisms that limit iron absorption in adults are not mature and active in children. It is estimated that the lethal dose of ferrous sulfate for a 2-year-old child is about 3 g; for adults it is approximately 200 to 250 mg of iron per kg of body weight.

Iron overload in adults has been seen in individuals who have had many blood transfusions, sickle cell anemia, and fibromyalgia. Full-blown iron overload, however, is seen in individuals with hemochromatosis, a disease in which a hereditary defect allows absorption without regard for need.

In hemochromatosis, large amounts of iron are deposited in the liver, spleen, and other tissues, causing pronounced impairment in function and tissue damage. Symptoms include weakness, arthritis and joint pain, chronic fatigue, headache, weight loss, heart palpitations, and mouth soreness. It is estimated that one in eight persons may carry this gene, and when combined with another gene, will create the disease in their offspring. Individuals with fibromyalgia should be tested for iron overload.

## *Iron Food Sources*

Good sources of iron (Table 6.4) include shellfish (clams and oysters), organ meats (liver, kidney, and heart), pumpkin seed kernels, pistachios, beef, legumes (dried beans and peas), eggs, nuts and seeds, dark chicken/turkey meat, dark molasses, prune juice, breads and pasta (both regular and whole wheat), and green vegetables. Breads and cereals that are fortified with iron are also good sources. If iron supplements are needed, ferrous sulfate and iron chelate are the more bioavailable forms.

TABLE 6.4 Iron Sources in Rank Order by Serving Size

The shaded items indicate that the iron content is more bioavailable. Read discussion about bioavailability.

| | Weight (g) | Iron (mg) |
|---|---|---|
| **10–28 mg/serving:** | | |
| 3.5 oz steamed clams range 15–28 | 100 | 22.0 |
| **5–9 mg:** | | |
| 3.5 oz ckd oysters | 100 | 8.5 |
| 3.5 oz ckd chicken liver | 100 | 8.5 |
| 1/4 c pumpkin seed kernels-rstd | 57 | 8.5 |
| 3.5 oz ckd turkey liver | 100 | 7.8 |
| 3.5 oz ckd beef heart | 100 | 7.5 |
| 3.5 oz ckd beef kidney | 100 | 7.3 |
| 1/2 c tofu | 124 | 6.7 |
| 3.5 oz ckd beef liver | 100 | 6.3 |
| 3.5 oz ckd raw oysters | 100 | 5.4 |
| 3.5 oz ckd veal liver | 100 | 5.2 |
| **2.5–4.9 mg:** | | |
| 1/2 c pistachios | 64 | 4.4 |
| 2 T blackstrap molasses | 41 | 3.6 |
| 3.5 oz ckd beef chuck/loin roast | 100 | 3.5 |
| 3 oz ckd ground beef | 85 | 2.2 |
| 3.5 oz ckd lamb | 100 | 1.8 |
| 1/4 c raw Irish moss seaweed | 20 | 1.8 |
| 1 oz unsweetened chocolate | 28.4 | 1.8 |
| 1/2 c ckd peapods | 80 | 1.75 |
| 1/4 c raisins | 36 | 1.75 |
| 1/2 c cnd pinto beans | 120 | 1.75 |
| **1.50–1.74 mg:** | | |
| 1/4 c sunflower seed kernels | 33 | 1.7 |
| 1/2 c cnd sweet potatoes | 128 | 1.7 |
| 1 c ckd fresh pasta | 150 | 1.7 |
| 1/2 c ckd pumpkin | 123 | 1.7 |
| 1/2 c baked potato with skin | 122 | 1.7 |
| 3.5 oz ckd turkey light meat | 100 | 1.6 |
| 1 c ckd oatmeal | 234 | 1.6 |
| 1/2 c macadamia nuts | 67 | 1.6 |
| 1 ckd whole artichoke | 120 | 1.6 |
| 1 c ckd whole wheat pasta | 140 | 1.5 |
| 1/2 c chopped walnuts | 60 | 1.5 |
| **1.25–1.49 mg:** | | |
| 1/2 c spinach, ckd fr/frzn | 95 | 1.4 |
| 1 c tomato juice | 243 | 1.4 |
| 3.5 oz ckd veal | 100 | 1.3 |
| 3.5 oz ckd canned tuna | 100 | 1.3 |
| 1/2 c ckd split green peas | 80 | 1.3 |
| 1/2 c ckd green peas | 80 | 1.3 |
| 1/2 c chopped pecans | 60 | 1.3 |
| **1.0–1.24 mg:** | | |
| 3.5 oz ckd pork and ham | 100 | 1.2 |
| 1/2 c peanuts | 72 | 1.2 |
| 1/2 c black-eyed peas, ckd fr/dry | 120 | 1.2 |
| 1.8 oz chicken drumstick | 52 | 1.1 |
| 1/2 c ckd artichoke hearts | 84 | 1.1 |
| 1 tsp spirulina | < 4 | 1.1 |
| 1/2 c ckd barley | 78 | 1.0 |
| 1 avocado half | 100 | 1.0 |
| 1 c veg tomato juice | 243 | 1.0 |
| 3.5 oz ckd veal | 100 | 1.0 |
| 1/2 c white rice | 79 | 1.0 |
| 3.5 oz ckd fish, ranges 0.3–1.0 | 100 | 1.0 |
| **0.40–0.99 mg:** | | |
| 1/2 c tomato sauce | 123 | 0.94 |
| 2.2 oz chicken thigh | 85 | 0.90 |
| 1 piece bread, range 0.83–.91 | 28.4 | 0.87 |
| 1 c raw spinach | 30 | 0.80 |
| 1/4 c fresh grated coconut | 33 | 0.79 |
| 1 c looseleaf lettuce | 56 g | 0.78 |
| 1 c apple juice | 244 g | 0.75 |
| 1/2 c ckd Brussels sprouts | 78 | 0.75 |
| 3.5 oz chicken breast | 100 | 0.71 |
| 3.5 oz hot dogs | 100 | 0.70 |
| 1/2 c ckd green beans | 65 | 0.70 |
| 1/2 c ckd winter squash | 123 | 0.70 |
| 1/2 c ckd broccoli | 85 | 0.68 |
| 1/2 c ckd mushrooms | 39 | 0.68 |
| 1/2 c beets | 85 | 0.67 |
| 4 dried apricot halves | 14 | 0.66 |
| 1 c romaine lettuce | 56 | 0.62 |
| 1 c grape juice | 253 | 0.60 |
| 1 c fresh strawberry halves | 152 | 0.60 |
| 1/2 c ckd kale | 65 | 0.59 |
| 1 c sweet cherries | 145 | 0.57 |
| 1/2 c ckd collards | 90 | 0.55 |
| 1 c grapes | 160 | 0.42 |
| 1/2 c ckd sliced carrots | 76 | 0.41 |
| 1/2 c ckd brown rice | 98 | 0.41 |
| 1/2 c fresh blackberries | 72 | 0.41 |
| 1/2 c ckd mung bean sprouts | 62 | 0.40 |

Listing includes elemental and enriched foods; does not include additionally fortified products like breakfast cereals.
Source: The Food Finder, ESHA Research, Salem, Oregon, 1999. Printed with permission.

Keep in mind that iron from plant foods (nonheme) is better absorbed when eaten with vitamin C-rich foods *and* meat or eggs (which contain 40% of its iron in the heme form). For example, only about 2% of the iron in nuts is absorbed if eaten alone. When consumed in a meal with chicken (heme-iron) and a salad (vitamin C), as much as 7 to 10% of the iron in the nuts is absorbed.

## Magnesium

*Magnesium is important for bone mineralization and the building of protein. It is necessary for energy metabolism and normal muscle contraction, critical for nerve impulse transmission, and important for good strong teeth. It is involved with the metabolism of fat and nucleic acids, the membrane transport system, normal blood clotting. Magnesium is a necessary component for over 300 enzymes.*

## *Magnesium Functions*

Approximately 50 to 60% of the body's magnesium works with calcium and phosphorus to make and maintain strong bones. About two-thirds of the magnesium is fixed there; about one-third is exchangeable. In addition to being essential for bone structure, magnesium promotes resistance to tooth decay by holding calcium in tooth enamel.

Magnesium is found throughout the body and has a wide variety of functions. Approximately 40% of magnesium is in the muscles and soft tissues; approximately 1% is in the extracellular fluid. Normal heart and nerve function is dependent on magnesium. This positively charged ion is integral in maintaining electrical potentials across nerve and muscle membranes and transmitting impulses from nerves to muscles. Magnesium helps relax muscles after contraction and is vital to conduction of nerve impulses. Muscle contraction and membrane transport systems require magnesium, potassium, and sodium to work closely together.

More than 300 enzymes are activated by magnesium, including most of the enzymes that use thiamin, riboflavin, vitamin B6, vitamin C, and vitamin E. Because it is so necessary to the function of the B vitamins, magnesium is important for protein metabolism. It is also necessary for the body's use of vitamin D, calcium, sodium, and potassium.

Magnesium works with calcium to facilitate blood clotting and the constriction and relaxation of blood vessels, which are important regulators of blood pressure. Recent studies suggest that an adequate magnesium intake may help discourage osteoporosis. It appears that insufficient magnesium intake can result in insufficient available calcium. Animal studies suggest that low magnesium diets lead to arterial wall degeneration, elevated cholesterol levels, and atherosclerosis. Recent studies have shown that dietary magnesium supplements have improved glucose tolerance and insulin response in elderly noninsulin-dependent diabetics.

## *Magnesium Deficiencies*

Clinical deficiencies are rare, but marginal subclinical deficiencies may be more common. Deficiencies may result from the use of diuretics, alcohol abuse, kidney disease, diabetes, malabsorption syndrome, protein malnutrition, or from excessive vomiting, or prolonged diarrhea. Some of the effects of magnesium deficiency include muscular weakness and spasms, irregular pulse, confusion or nervousness, convulsions, bizarre muscle movements (especially of the eyes and face), hallucinations and difficulty in swallowing. In youth, disturbances in behavior and growth may be a sign of magnesium deficiency.

Stress may increase the need for this mineral. Because magnesium is essential to most of the enzymes that use the B vitamins and vitamins C and E, a deficiency may result in symptoms that mimic the deficiencies of these other vitamins.

## *Magnesium Losses*

As a mineral, magnesium is not lost from food due to heat or light. However, some magnesium is lost in food processing and a small amount leaches into cooking water during food preparation. More than 80% of magnesium in whole grains is lost during milling. This mineral is not added back to foods through "enrichment." The presence of phytate and fiber may decrease absorption.

Magnesium is absorbed much more efficiently from foods than from high doses found in supplements. Excessive calcium supplementation (over 2,600 mg/day) has been reported to decrease magnesium balance.

## *Magnesium Recommended Intake*

The 1998 Daily Reference Intakes (DRIs) Recommended Daily Allowances (RDAs) for adults are:

| | | |
|---|---|---|
| Men | 19–30 years | 400 mg/day |
| | 31 years + | 420 mg/day |
| Women | 19–30 years | 310 mg/day |
| | 31 years + | 320 mg/day |
| Pregnant or Breastfeeding | | + 40 mg/day |

## *Magnesium Upper Limits*

There is no Upper Limit (UL) for magnesium from *food sources*, and toxic effects are not reported for healthy adults. Persons who take laxative preparations containing magnesium salts will experience diarrhea, as intended, but no other ill effects.

However, ULs are established for the *nonfood* sources, or supplemental forms of magnesium, because toxic effects can occur in persons who have impaired kidney function *and* consume excessive intakes of magnesium supplements or drugs containing magnesium. Early symptoms are diarrhea, nausea, vomiting, and low blood pressure; later symptoms include cardiovascular abnormalities. There is no documented evidence of magnesium being harmful to people with normal kidney function.

| | |
|---|---|
| 0–12 months | Not able to establish |
| 1–3 years | 65 mg/day |
| 4–8 years | 110 mg/day |
| 9 + all ages, pregnant or breastfeeding | 350 mg/day |

## *Magnesium Food Sources*

Good sources of magnesium (Table 6.5) include nuts and seeds, peanuts, soybeans, tofu, chocolate, dark-green vegetables (artichokes, lima beans, okra), cooked dried beans and peas, yogurt, whole wheat pasta, brown rice, fish, prunes, brewer's yeast, bananas, crab, baked potatoes, milk, sweet potatoes, chicken, turkey, whole wheat breads, and beef heart and liver. Because milk consumption is high, it supplies about 22% of the magnesium in the American diet. Water in some locations may also be a good source.

# Manganese

***As a cofactor for many enzymes manganese is necessary for many body processes and cell functions. It is a part of blood clotting, urea synthesis, and formation of connective tissue, fats, cholesterol, and bones. It also strengthens immunity as part of some antioxidants.***

## *Manganese Functions*

Manganese is an essential element that acts as a cofactor for many enzymes. In this capacity it is involved with many cell functions and works with many other nutrients. Its functions

TABLE 6.5 Magnesium Sources in Rank Order by Serving Size

| | Weight (g) | Magnesium (mg) |
|---|---|---|
| **200–303 mg/serving:** | | |
| 1/4 c pumpkin seed kernels, rstd | 57 | 303 |
| 1/2 c almonds | 78 | 238 |
| **150–199 mg:** | | |
| 1/2 c soynuts (roasted soybeans) | 86 | 196 |
| 1/2 c filberts | 68 | 192 |
| 1/2 c Brazil nuts | 70 | 166 |
| 1/2 c cashews | 65 | 157 |
| **100–149 mg:** | | |
| 1/2 c tofu | 124 | 128 |
| 1/2 c peanuts | 72 | 125 |
| 1/2 c chopped walnuts | 60 | 101 |
| 1/2 c pistachios | 64 | 101 |
| 2 T molasses | 41 | 100 |
| **50–99 mg:** | | |
| 1/4 c sunflower seeds, range 42–118 mg | 68 | 82 avg |
| 1 oz unsweetened chocolate | 28.4 | 88 |
| 1/2 c ckd green soybeans | 90 | 83 |
| 1/2 c macadamias | 68 | 77 |
| 1/2 c chopped pecans | 60 | 76 |
| 1/2 c ckd Swiss chard | 88 | 75 |
| ckd whole artichoke | 120 | 72 |
| 1/2 c spinach, ckd fr/frzn | 95 | 66 |
| 1/2 c ckd black beans | 86 | 60 |
| 1 c ckd oatmeal | 234 | 56 |
| 1/2 c ckd green soybeans | 90 | 54 |
| 2 T peanut butter | 32 | 51 |
| 1/2 c navy/baked beans | 127 | 52 |
| 1/2 c ckd artichoke hearts | 84 | 50 |
| 1/2 c baby lima beans, ckd fr/frzn | 90 | 50 |
| **35–49 mg:** | | |
| 1/2 c ckd beet greens | 72 | 49 |
| 1/2 c ckd okra | 92 | 46 |
| 2 T wheat germ | 14 | 45 |
| 3.5 oz ckd Alaska king crab | 100 | 43 |
| 1 c lowfat yogurt | 245 | 43 |
| 1/2 c black-eyed peas, ckd fr/frzn | 85 | 43 |
| 1 c ckd whole wheat pasta | 140 | 42 |
| 1/2 c ckd brown rice | 98 | 42 |
| 1/2 c lima beans, ckd fr/dry | 94 | 40 |
| 1/2 c kidney beans | 89 | 40 |
| 1 avocado half | 100 | 39 |
| 3.5 oz ckd oysters | 100 | 39 |
| 3.5 oz ckd fish average all | 100 | 30–40 |
| 3.5 oz, ≈10 prunes | 85 | 38 |
| 3/4 c prune juice | 192 | 36 |
| 2 T brewer's yeast | 16 | 37 |
| 1/2 c ckd lentils | 99 | 36 |
| 1/2 c ckd butternut squash | 123 | 36 |
| 1/2 c ckd dry split peas | 98 | 35 |
| **25–34 mg:** | | |
| 1 banana | 118 | 34 |
| 3.5 oz ckd shrimp | 100 | 34 |
| 1/2 c black-eyed peas, ckd fr/dry | 120 | 34 |
| 3.5 oz ckd blue crab | 100 | 33 |
| 1 baked potato with skin | 122 | 33 |
| 1 c whole milk | 244 | 33 |
| 1/2 c cnd pinto beans | 120 | 32 |
| 1 tsp sesame seeds | 9.4 | 32 |
| 1/2 c cnd sweet potato | 128 | 31 |
| 3.5 oz ckd light chicken meat | 100 | 29 |
| 1/2 c ckd pumpkin | 123 | 28 |
| 1 c skim milk | 245 | 28 |
| 3.5 oz ckd light turkey meat | 100 | 26 |
| 1 c orange juice | 248 | 27 |
| 1 c grapefruit juice | 247 | 27 |
| 3/4 c prune juice | 192 | 27 |
| 1 c tomato juice | 243 | 27 |
| 1 c tomato veg juice | 242 | 27 |
| 3.5 oz ckd beef steak | 100 | 26 |

*continued*

include the formation of connective tissues, fats, cholesterol, bones, blood clotting factors, proteins, and the synthesis of urea. Manganese is found in the bones, liver, kidneys, and body tissues. It is involved in carbohydrate and lipid metabolism as well as brain function.

## *Manganese Deficiencies*

Manganese deficiency in animals alters fat metabolism. Signs of deficiency include impaired fertility, growth retardation, birth abnormalities, abnormalities in brain function, abnormal malformations in bone and cartilage, impaired glucose tolerance, and abnormal lipid metabolism. Deficiencies have not been reported in humans. The body's requirements for this mineral are low, and most plant foods contain an adequate supply. A diet that includes a variety of foods will meet the requirements for manganese.

## *Manganese Recommended Intake*

The estimated safe and adequate dietary intake for manganese is 2.5 to 5.0 mg/day.

## *Manganese Upper Limits*

Manganese toxicity from food intake has not been observed. However, workers exposed to high concentrations of manganese dust or fumes (miners) can have adverse effects to the central nervous system. Dietary toxicity might occur if an individual consumes high dosage supplements for several years, especially if there is diminished function to produce bile. The body appears to regulate excessive manganese by excreting it in bile into the intestinal tract. Therefore, if intakes exceed the body's ability to excrete manganese, toxic levels would result in damage to the nervous system.

## *Manganese Food Sources*

The best sources (Table 6.6) of manganese are wheat germ, nuts and seeds, whole wheat pasta, oatmeal, oysters, dark molasses, brown rice, sweet potatoes, tofu, chocolate, and brewed tea. Generally, fruits and vegetables have somewhat less, but pineapple, tomato juice, grape juice, and others provide good amounts. Dairy products, meat, fish, and poultry are poor sources.

TABLE 6.5 *(Continued)* **Magnesium Sources in Rank Order by Serving Size**

| | Weight (g) | Magnesium (mg) | | Weight (g) | Magnesium (mg) |
|---|---|---|---|---|---|
| 1 c grape juice | 253 | 25 | 1/2 c fresh pineapple | 78 | 18 |
| 1 c dark chicken | 100 | 25 | 1 c cantaloupe cubes | 160 | 17 |
| 3.5 oz ckd dark turkey meat | 100 | 24 | 1/2 c ckd Brussels sprouts | 78 | 18 |
| 3.5 oz ckd beef roast | 100 | 24 | 1/2 c ckd barley | 78 | 17 |
| 3.5 oz ckd veal | 100 | 25 | 1 c watermelon cubes | 152 | 16 |
| 3.5 oz ckd beef heart | 100 | 25 | 1 c fresh strawberry halves | 152 | 16 |
| 1 c ckd regular pasta | 140 | 25 | 1/2 c ckd green beans | 65 | 16 |
| | | | 3.5 oz ckd turkey liver | 100 | 15 |
| **20–24 mg:** | | | **5–14 mg:** | | |
| 1 piece whole wheat bread | 28 | 24 | 1/2 c blackberries | 72 | 14 |
| 1/4 c seaweed (dried agar=4 g), raw Irish moss, kelp, nori, kombu, oarweed | 20 | 24 | 1 c papaya cubes | 140 | 14 |
| 1 c raw spinach | 30 | 24 | 1 T oat bran | 6 | 13 |
| 3.5 oz ckd pork | 100 | 20–25 | 1/4 c raisins | 36 | 12 |
| 1/2 c ckd green peas | 80 | 23 | 1 c brewed coffee | 240 | 12 |
| 3.5 oz ckd beef liver | 100 | 23 | 1 piece wheat bread | 25 | 12 |
| 1 kiwifruit | 76 | 23 | 1/2 c pineapple juice | 125 | 11 |
| 3.5 oz ckd oysters | 100 | 23 | 1/2 c raspberries | 62 | 11 |
| 1 T wheat bran | 3.6 | 23 | 1/2 c fresh pineapple | 78 | 11 |
| 3.5 oz ckd ham | 100 | 22 | 7.5″ whole raw carrot | 72 | 11 |
| 3.5 oz ckd lamb | 100 | 22 | 1 oz Swiss cheese | 28.4 | 10 |
| 1/2 c ckd collard greens | 90 | 21 | 1 pear | 166 | 10 |
| 3.5 oz ckd chicken liver | 100 | 21 | 1 grapefruit half | 118–123 | 10 |
| 1/2 c ckd peapods | 80 | 21 | 1 c grapes | 160 | 9.6 |
| 2.5 oz bagel | 71 | 21 | 1 small orange | 96 | 9.6 |
| 3.5 oz ckd ground beef | 100 | 20 | 1/2 c ckd white rice | 79 | 9.5 |
| 1/2 c ckd beets | 85 | 20 | 1/2 c ckd bean sprouts | 62 | 8.6 |
| | | | 1 oz cheddar cheese | 28.4 | 7.9 |
| **15–19 mg:** | | | 1 oz provolone cheese | 28.4 | 7.8 |
| 1/2 c ckd broccoli | 85 | 19 | 1 apple w/peel | 138 | 6.9 |
| 1/2 c mashed potatoes | 105 | 19 | 1 piece white bread | 30 | 7.2 |
| 10″ flour tortilla | 72 | 19 | 4 halves dried apricots | 14 | 6.6 |
| 1 mango | 207 | 18 | 1 oz American cheese | 28.4 | 6.3 |
| 3.5 oz steamed clams | 100 | 18 | 1 cooked egg | 48–50 | 5.0 |

Listing includes elemental and enriched foods; does not include additionally fortified products like breakfast cereals.
Source: The Food Finder, ESHA Research, Salem, Oregon, 1999. Printed with permission.

# Molybdenum

***As part of several enzymes, molybdenum facilitates many cell functions and processes.***

## *Molybdenum Functions*

All tissues contain small amounts of molybdenum, with the largest amounts found in the liver, kidney, bone, and skin. It is a component of several enzymes, including xanthine oxidase that aids in the formation of uric acid, a normal breakdown product of metabolism. It works with thiamin in the conversion of food to energy, is important in the mobilization of iron from storage, and is necessary for normal growth and development.

## *Molybdenum Deficiencies*

Molybdenum deficiency, uncomplicated by other antagonists or causes, is not reported in humans. Controlled experiments with animals have induced deficiencies with symptoms of stunted growth, loss of appetite, weight loss, impaired reproduction, and shortened life.

## *Molybdenum Recommended Intake*

The 1989 Estimated Safe and Adequate Amounts for molybdenum are 75 to 250 mcg for adults.

## *Molybdenum Food Sources*

Good sources (Table 6.7) are milk, cooked dried beans and peas (legumes), nuts and seeds, yogurt, egg, liver, cottage cheese, milk, coconut, tomatoes, carrots, all meats and fish, celery, cauliflower, onions, and "hard" tap water. Information on food sources is limited because not all foods have been analyzed for molybdenum.

The amount of molybdenum in food varies considerably, depending on the soil content where the plants are grown, and where the animals graze. Plants grown on rich soil can contain

TABLE 6.6 Manganese Sources in Rank Order by Serving Size

| | Weight (g) | Manganese (mg) | | Weight (g) | Manganese (mg) |
|---|---|---|---|---|---|
| **1.5–2.8 mg/serving:** | | | 1 c fresh strawberry halves | 152 | 0.46 |
| 2 T wheat germ | 14 | 2.80 | 1/2 c ckd green soybeans | 90 | 0.45 |
| 1/4 c chopped pecans | 60 | 2.68 | 1/2 c ckd sliced carrots | 76 | 0.44 |
| 1 c ckd whole wheat pasta | 140 | 1.93 | 3.5 oz ckd beef liver | 100 | 0.42 |
| 1/2 c soynuts (roasted soybeans) | 86 | 1.88 | 1 c looseleaf lettuce | 56 | 0.42 |
| 1/2 c chopped walnuts | 60 | 1.74 | 1 T wheat bran | 3.6 | 0.42 |
| 1/4 c pumpkin seed kernels, rstd | 57 | 1.71 | 1 c ckd regular pasta | 140 | 0.40 |
| 1/2 c almonds | 78 | 1.55 | 3.5 oz raw eastern oysters | 100 | 0.40 |
| **1.0–1.49 mg:** | | | **0.30–0.39 mg:** | | |
| 1/2 c filberts | 68 | 1.4 | 1/2 c ckd split green peas | 80 | 0.39 |
| 1 c ckd oatmeal | 234 | 1.4 | 1/2 c ckd black beans | 86 | 0.38 |
| 1/2 c peanuts | 72 | 1.3 | 2.5 oz bagel | 71 | 0.38 |
| 1/2 c cnd sweet potatoes | 128 | 1.27 | 1/2 c ckd white rice | 79 | 0.37 |
| 1/2 c fresh pineapple | 78 | 1.25 | 1 c romaine lettuce | 56 | 0.36 |
| 1/2 c pineapple juice | 125 | 1.2 | 1/2 c black-eyed peas, ckd fr/dry | 120 | 0.34 |
| 3.5 oz ckd pacific oysters | 100 | 1.2 | 10″ flour tortilla | 72 | 0.33 |
| 2 T blackstrap molasses | 41 | 1.1 | 1 T oat bran | 6 | 0.33 |
| 1 c tomato juice | 243 | 1.0 | 1/2 c ckd green peas | 80 | 0.33 |
| | | | 1 whole ckd artichoke | 120 | 0.31 |
| **0.75–0.99 mg:** | | | 3.5 oz ckd chicken liver | 100 | 0.30 |
| 1/2 c blackberries | 72 | 0.93 | | | |
| 1 c grape juice | 253 | 0.91 | **0.20–0.29 mg:** | | |
| 1/2 c spinach, ckd fr/frzn | 95 | 0.90 | 3/4 c prune juice | 192 | 0.29 |
| 1/2 c ckd brown rice | 98 | 0.88 | 1/2 c ckd Swiss chard | 88 | 0.29 |
| 1/2 c roasted chestnuts | 72 | 0.84 | 1 baked potato w/skin | 122 | 0.28 |
| 3.5 oz ckd eastern oysters | 100 | 0.80 | 1/2 c ckd kale | 65 | 0.27 |
| 1/2 c tofu | 124 | 0.75 | 1/2 c spinach, ckd fr/frzn | 95 | 0.27 |
| | | | 3.5 oz ckd turkey liver | 100 | 0.25 |
| **0.50–0.74 mg:** | | | 1/2 c ckd broccoli | 85 | 0.24 |
| 1/4 c sunflower seeds | 68 | 0.73 | 1 half avocado | 100 | 0.23 |
| 1/2 c baby lima beans, ckd fr/frzn | 90 | 0.73 | 1 c apple juice | 244 | 0.22 |
| 1/2 c ckd green soybeans | 90 | 0.70 | 1/2 c ckd Brussels sprouts | 78 | 0.21 |
| 1/2 c black-eyed peas, ckd fr/frzn | 85 | 0.67 | 3.5 oz ckd veal liver | 100 | 0.21 |
| 2 T maple syrup | 40 | 0.66 | 1/2 c ckd green beans | 65 | 0.20 |
| 3.5 oz raw pacific oysters | 100 | 0.64 | 1/2 c ckd barley | 78 | 0.20 |
| 2 T molasses | 41 | 0.63 | | | |
| 1/2 c raspberries | 62 | 0.62 | **0.10–0.19 mg:** | | |
| 1/2 c cashews | 65 | 0.55 | 1/2 c ckd summer squash | 90 | 0.19 |
| 1 oz unsweetened chocolate | 28.4 | 0.54 | 1/2 c ckd mustard greens | 70 | 0.19 |
| 1/2 c brazil nuts | 70 | 0.54 | 3 oz, ≈10 prunes | 85 | 0.19 |
| 1 c brewed tea | 237 | 0.52 | 1 banana | 118 | 0.18 |
| | | | 3.5 oz sardines | 100 | 0.15 |
| **0.40–0.49 mg:** | | | 1/2 c mashed potatoes | 105 | 0.12 |
| 1/4 c coconut, dry (20 g) or fresh | 33 | 0.49 | 1 piece white bread | 30 | 0.12 |
| 1/2 c lima beans, ckd fr/dry | 94 | 0.49 | 1 corn tortilla | 26 | 0.11 |
| 1/2 c navy/baked beans | 127 | 0.48 | 5″ raw carrot | 72 | 0.10 |

Listing includes elemental and enriched foods; does not include additionally fortified products like breakfast cereals.
Source: The Food Finder, ESHA Research, Salem, Oregon, 1999. Printed with permission.

as much as 500 times the amount as those grown on depleted soil. However, this vitamin is in good supply in the average American diet.

# Phosphorus

***Phosphorus is an essential component of bones and teeth, key enzymes, DNA and RNA, and glycogen. It is necessary for growth, maintenance, and repair of all body tissues and is needed for metabolism of carbohydrates, protein and fat, and much more.***

## *Phosphorus Functions*

Phosphorus is an essential component of bones and teeth, and approximately 85% of the body's phosphorus is stored in the bones as calcium phosphate. The remaining phosphorus is active in a variety of essential functions and metabolic processes and is found in every cell of the body.

Phosphorus is fundamental to the growth, maintenance, and repair of all body tissues. Many key enzymes and the B vitamins require phosphorus for the metabolism of carbohydrates, protein, and fat. Phosphorus is a component of glycogen (the stor-

TABLE 6.7 Molybdenum Sources in Rank Order by Serving Size

| | Weight (g) | Molybdenum (mcg) | | Weight (g) | Molybdenum (mcg) |
|---|---|---|---|---|---|
| **50–99 mcg/serving:** | | | 3.5 oz ckd veal liver | 100 | 8.9 |
| 1/2 c ckd navy beans | 131 | 98 | 3.5 oz ckd turkey liver | 100 | 8.9 |
| 1/2 c black-eyed peas, ckd fr/dry | 120 | 90 | 1/2 c ckd green soybeans | 90 | 6.4 |
| 1/2 c ckd lentils | 99 | 74 | 1/2 c cottage cheese | 28.4 | 5.2 |
| 1/2 c ckd dry split peas | 98 | 74 | **2.5–4.9 mcg:** | | |
| 1/2 c large lima beans, ckd fr/dry | 94 | 71 | 1 c milk | 245 | 4.9 |
| 1/2 c ckd kidney beans | 89 | 66 | 1/2 c fresh tomatoes | 90 | 4.5 |
| 1/2 c ckd black beans | 86 | 65 | 7.5″ raw carrot | 72 | 3.6 |
| **25–49 mcg:** | none identified | | 3.5 oz ckd avg, all meats—beef, veal, pork, ham, turkey, fish | 100 | 3.4 |
| **10–24 mcg:** | | | 1 c lettuce | 56 | 3.4 |
| 1/2 c almonds | 78 | 23.1 | 1/2 c raw celery | 60 | 3.0 |
| 1/2 c peanuts | 72 | 21.2 | 1/2 c raw cauliflower | 50 | 2.5 |
| 1/2 c chestnuts | 72 | 21.1 | **<1.0–2.4 mcg:** | | |
| 1/2 c macadamias | 68 | 19.8 | 1/2 c onion , raw (40 g) or ckd | 53 | 2.0 |
| 1/2 c cashews | 65 | 19.1 | 1/4 c raw green pepper | 37 | 1.9 |
| 1/2 c pistachios | 64 | 18.9 | 1/2 c raw cabbage | 35 | 1.75 |
| 1/2 c chopped walnuts | 60 | 17.5 | 1 c raw spinach | 30 | 1.5 |
| 1 c lowfat yogurt | 245 | 11.3 | 1 oz cheese | 28.4 | 1.3 |
| **5.0–9.9 mcg:** | | | 1/4 c sliced mushrooms | 18 | 0.88 |
| 1/2 c coconut, dry (20 g) or fresh | 33 | 9.6 | | | |
| 1 cooked egg | 48–50 | 9.0 | | | |

Listing includes elemental and enriched foods; does not include additionally fortified products like breakfast cereals.
Source: The Food Finder, ESHA Research, Salem, Oregon, 1999. Printed with permission.

age form of energy in the body) and facilitates the absorption of nutrients such as glucose. It is necessary for new cell formation and growth, moving nutrients into and out of cells, and is used in many hormones. Phosphorus is found in all cells as a part of the DNA and RNA genetic code

As a part of phospholipids, phosphorus is a major component of most biological membranes, nucleotides, nucleic acids, and red blood cells. It also helps transport some fats in the bloodstream (plasma lipoproteins). Phospholipids help maintain normal body acid-base balance, transfer energy from metabolic fluids, and activate many catalytic proteins.

## *Phosphorus Deficiencies*

Long-term and excessive use of anticonvulsant medications, calcium carbonate, or antacids containing aluminum hydroxide will reduce the absorption of phosphorus. Phosphorus deficiency symptoms are bone loss, weakness, and loss of appetite. However, phosphorus is so prevalent in foods, near total starvation is required to produce a deficiency.

## *Phosphorus Bioavailability and Phytate*

The body's absorption mechanism for phosphorus appears to vary very little with different levels of phosphorus intake. It continues at the same level even when extremely high doses (through supplements) are ingested. This is in sharp contrast to calcium in which the absorption efficiency decreases when calcium intakes are elevated.

All plant seeds (beans, peas, cereals, nuts) contain a form of phosphate called phytic acid, which is normally not available to the body. However, some foods, and some colonic bacteria, contain the enzyme phytase, which can make this form of phosphorus available. Yeast can also make phytic acid more bioavailable, so yeast-leavened whole grain breads have higher phosphate bioavailability than breakfast cereals, or unleavened breads. As a result, about one half of the phosphate in the phytate form can be absorbed.

## *Phosphorus Recommended Intake*

In the past the calcium-phosphorus ratio was used to determine the recommended amount of phosphorus intake. This ratio has some use under conditions of rapid growth, but is not relevant in adults. The new 1998 recommendations for phosphorus are based on much more scientific evidence of human requirements and absorption patterns and are somewhat lower than past recommendations:

| | |
|---|---|
| Adult men and women | 700 mg/day age 19 years and older |

There is no change for pregnancy or breastfeeding conditions. For professional athletes and military trainees, or for anyone whose level of energy consumption is greater than 6,000 calories a day, the need for phosphorus may exceed the recommendations.

The 1990 Canadian RNI recommends 800 mg/day for adult men and 700 mg/day for adult women; 1,300 mg if pregnant or lactating.

## *Phosphorus Upper Limits*

Excess phosphorus can lower blood calcium, which releases parathyroid hormone, possibly causing mineral loss from bone.

However, dietary intake of phosphorus in the presence of adequate calcium and vitamin D is not likely to be harmful. During pregnancy, absorption for phosphorus rises approximately 15%. Upper limits have been set with the 1998 RDA/DRIs:

| | |
|---|---|
| Infants | No values—not possible to establish |
| 1–8 years | 3.0 g/day (3,000 mg) |
| 9–70 years | 4.0 g/day (4,000 mg) |
| 70 years and older | 3.0 g/day (3,000 mg) |
| Pregnant | 3.5 g/day (3,500 mg) |
| Breastfeeding | 4.0 g/day (3,500 mg) |

### *Phosphorus Food Sources*

Excellent sources (Table 6.8) include nuts and seeds, canned sardines with bones, yogurt, clams, fish, meats, cheese, poultry (chicken/turkey), wheat germ, and whole wheat products. Lesser, but good, amounts are found in a wide variety of vegetables, fruits, and grains.

Milk is a good source of both calcium and phosphorus, and food additives can contribute as much as 30% of dietary phosphorus. Soft drinks contain as much as 500 mg of phosphoric acid per serving and can contribute to excessive phosphorus intake if consumed regularly.

## Potassium

***As the body's principal intracellular electrolyte, potassium maintains fluid volume inside the cells and maintains acid-base balance. It is vital for nerve transmissions and important for normal blood pressure.***

### *Potassium Functions*

Potassium plays a vital role in maintaining fluid and electrolyte balance and cell integrity. It is a positively charged ion found *inside* body cells. When there is significant water loss from the body, sodium is lost and potassium is pulled out of the cells and excreted. Because a potassium deficiency can quickly affect the brain cells, the need for water may not be perceived, resulting in dehydration.

Nerve and muscle cells are especially dependent on potassium to function well. When muscles and nerves are being used, sodium and potassium are exchanged within the cell wall for contraction, and pump the minerals back into their original place in relaxation. Potassium is a key player during nerve transmissions and is important to the maintenance of normal blood pressure. It is also believed that potassium plays a catalytic role in carbohydrate and protein metabolism as well.

### *Potassium Deficiencies and Losses*

A diet *very* low or absent in fruits and vegetables may result in low potassium status, but dietary deficiencies are otherwise uncommon. Excessive losses may result from diabetic acidosis, dehydration, laxative abuse, steroid intake, use of diuretics, prolonged vomiting, or diarrhea. Only minimal amounts of potassium are lost from sweat. Deficiency symptoms include weakness, nausea, listlessness, apprehension, drowsiness, irrational behavior, and anorexia. Severe deficiency may affect the heart muscle and result in irregular heart rhythm that can be fatal.

### *Potassium Recommended Intake*

An adult intake of about 3,500 mg/day would be more in accordance with the government recommendation to eat more fruits and vegetables. This is the amount that may reduce the incidence of hypertension. In relationship to the uses within the body, there should be slightly more potassium than sodium in the diet.

### *Potassium Upper Limits*

Potassium toxicity is not a concern from foods, but can be created from the misuse of supplements, the overuse of potassium salt (marketed as a sodium-free salt), or sudden enteral or parenteral increases of potassium, especially for an infant or a person with heart disease. If large amounts of potassium are ingested, faster than the kidneys can excrete it, or if potassium is injected rapidly into a vein, bypassing the vomiting reflex, it may cause cardiac arrest.

### *Potassium Food Sources*

Potassium is widely distributed in fresh fruits, vegetables, cooked dried beans and peas (legumes), shellfish, nuts and seeds, and molasses (Table 6.9). Fresh foods contain much more potassium than sodium. In contrast, once foods are processed and refined, they usually contain much more sodium than potassium, such as canned vegetables, ready-to-eat cereals, and luncheon meats.

Excellent sources are soynuts, pistachios, prunes, clams, molasses, yogurt, tomato juice, prune juice, baked potatoes, cantaloupe, cooked dried beans, orange juice, bananas, peanuts, artichokes, fish, beef and lamb, brewer's yeast, avocados, and apple juice.

## Selenium

***Selenium is a strong antioxidant that works with and can replace vitamin E activity and protects polyunsaturated fats, red blood cells, and cell membranes. It is needed for synthesis of thyroid hormones.***

### *Selenium Functions*

Selenium is a component of the antioxidant enzyme glutathione peroxidase. This enzyme protects polyunsaturated fatty acids (PUFA), red blood cells, and cell membranes from damage by highly reactive free radicals. Selenium is needed for the synthesis of thyroid hormones and works closely with, and in some cases can replace, the antioxidant activities of vitamin E.

People who consume a selenium-rich diet are less likely to develop certain cancers; this anticancer effect is enhanced by vitamin E. Selenium is involved in the production of prostaglandins, which among other things, regulate the inflammation process in arthritis. Selenium supplementation has been considered as an aid in the treatment of rheumatoid arthritis, but results at this time are inconclusive.

A large selenium study recently found statistical connections between selenium intakes of 200 mcg/day and a lower risk for prostate, colon, and lung cancer rates and deaths. The protective effect occurred very quickly after supplementation was implemented.

TABLE 6.8 Phosphorus Sources in Rank Order by Serving Size

| | Weight (g) | Phosphorus (mg) |
|---|---|---|
| **450–700 mg/serving:** | | |
| 1/4 c pumpkin seed kernels, rstd | 57 | 665 |
| 1/2 c soynuts (roasted soybeans) | 86 | 558 |
| **300–449 mg:** | | |
| 1/2 c almonds | 78 | 429 |
| 3.5 oz sardines w/bones | 100 | 425 |
| 1/2 c brazil nuts | 70 | 420 |
| 1/4 c sunflower seed kernels | 33 | 377 |
| 1 c lowfat yogurt | 245 | 352 |
| 3.5 oz steamed clams | 100 | 338 |
| 1/2 c pistachios | 64 | 322 |
| **250–299 mg:** | | |
| 1/2 c peanuts | 72 | 295 |
| 3.5 oz ckd herring or bluefish | 100 | 292 |
| 3.5 oz ckd halibut | 100 | 285 |
| 2 T brewer's yeast | 16 | 280 |
| 1/2 c cashews | 65 | 277 |
| 3.5 oz ckd salmon or trout | 100 | 252–266 |
| **200–249 mg:** | | |
| 1 c nonfat milk | 245 | 247 |
| 3.5 oz ckd pork | 100 | 230 |
| 1 c whole milk | 244 | 228 |
| 3.5 oz ckd beef, roasts/steak | 100 | 218 |
| 3.5 oz ckd chicken light meat | 100 | 221 |
| 3.5 oz ckd fish, ranges 140–250 | 100 | 195 |
| 3.5 oz ckd veal | 100 | 220 |
| 1 oz American cheese | 28.4 | 211 |
| 1/2 c filberts | 68 | 211 |
| 3.5 oz ckd turkey meat | 100 | 204 |
| **150–199 mg:** | | |
| 1/2 c chopped walnuts | 60 | 190 |
| 3.5 oz ckd chicken dark meat | 100 | 184 |
| 3.5 oz ckd lamb | 100 | 182 |
| 1/2 c ckd lentils | 99 | 178 |
| 1 c ckd oatmeal | 234 | 178 |
| 1/2 c chopped pecans | 60 | 173 |
| 1 oz Swiss cheese | 28.4 | 171 |
| 1/2 c cottage cheese | 28.4 | 170 |
| 1 T wheat germ | 14 | 162 |
| 3.5 oz ckd beef, ground beef | 100 | 155 |
| 1/2 c navy/baked beans | 127 | 155 |
| **100–149 mg:** | | |
| 1 oz cheddar cheese | 28.4 | 145 |
| 1/2 c ckd green soybeans | 90 | 142 |
| 1 oz provolone cheese | 28.4 | 140 |
| 1/2 c canned tuna | 100 | 138 |
| 1/2 c ckd kidney beans | 89 | 126 |
| 1 c ckd whole wheat pasta | 140 | 125 |
| 1/2 c tofu | 124 | 120 |
| 1/2 c ckd black beans | 86 | 120 |
| 1 oz unsweetened chocolate | 28.4 | 118 |
| 1/2 c cnd pinto beans | 120 | 110 |
| 1/2 c large lima beans, ckd fr/dry | 94 | 104 |
| 1/2 c black-eyed peas ckd fr/frzn | 85 | 104 |
| 1 ckd whole artichoke | 120 | 103 |
| 2 T peanut butter | 32 | 101 |
| 1/2 c baby lima beans, ckd fr/frzn | 90 | 101 |
| **50–99 mg:** | | |
| 1 baked potato w/skin | 122 | 98 |
| 1/2 c ckd dry split peas | 98 | 97 |
| 1 c ckd fresh pasta | 150 | 94 |
| 10″ flour tortilla | 72 | 89 |
| 1 cooked egg | 48–50 | 88 |
| 1/2 c black-eyed peas, ckd fr/dry | 120 | 84 |
| 1 corn tortilla | 26 | 82 |
| 1/2 c ckd brown rice | 98 | 81 |
| 1 c ckd white pasta | 140 | 76 |
| 1/2 c ckd artichoke hearts | 84 | 72 |
| 1/2 c ckd green peas | 80 | 72 |
| 2.5 oz plain bagel | 71 | 68 |
| 1/2 c cnd sweet potato | 128 | 67 |
| 1/2 c ckd broccoli | 85 | 51 |
| **20–49 mg:** | | |
| 1/2 c mashed potatoes | 105 | 48 |
| 3/4 c prune juice | 192 | 48 |
| 1/2 c ckd corn | 75 | 47 |
| 1 c tomato juice | 243 | 46 |
| 1/2 c ckd peapods | 80 | 45 |
| 1 T oat bran | 6 | 43 |
| 1/2 c ckd barley | 78 | 42 |
| 1/2 c ckd Brussels sprouts | 78 | 42 |
| 1 c veg tomato juice | 243 | 41 |
| 1/2 c cnd tomato sauce | 123 | 39 |
| 1 piece wheat bread | 25 | 38 |
| 1/4 c raisins | 36 | 35 |
| 1/2 c ckd summer squash | 90 | 35 |
| 1/4 c ckd mushrooms | 39 | 34 |
| 1 c avg orange juice | 248 | 34 |
| 1/2 c ckd white rice | 79 | 34 |
| 1/2 c ckd winter squash | 123 | 33 |
| 1 c grapefruit juice | 247 | 31 |
| 1 c fresh strawberry halves | 152 | 30 |
| 1/2 c ckd Swiss chard | 88 | 29 |
| 1 c cantaloupe cubes | 160 | 28 |
| 1 piece white bread | 30 | 28 |
| 1 c grape juice | 253 | 28 |
| 1 c fresh sweet cherries | 145 | 28 |
| 1 kiwifruit | 76 | 30 |
| 1 mango | 207 | 23 |

Listing includes elemental and enriched foods; does not include additionally fortified products like breakfast cereals.
Source: The Food Finder, ESHA Research, Salem, Oregon, 1999. Printed with permission.

## *Selenium Deficiencies*

Symptoms of selenium deficiency in humans include predisposition to Keshan disease (a form of heart disease). Patients on intravenous feedings (total parenteral nutrition-TPN) that lacked selenium experienced weakness and muscular discomfort. However, because selenium and vitamin E work very closely together, deficiencies are difficult to observe in isolation. Selenium deficiencies, with adequate levels of vitamin E present, have only been demonstrated in animals.

In animals, deficiency during pregnancy can have irreversible effects on the baby's development and growth and can have detrimental effects on the formation of the immune system. In

TABLE 6.9 **Potassium Sources in Rank Order by Serving Size**

| | Weight (g) | Potassium (mg) | | Weight (g) | Potassium (mg) |
|---|---|---|---|---|---|
| **500–1200 mg/serving:** | | | 1/2 c chopped walnuts | 60 | 301 |
| 1/2 c soynuts (roasted soybeans) | 86 | 1176 | 1/2 c filberts | 68 | 300 |
| 2 T blackstrap molasses | 41 | 1022 | | | |
| 1/2 c pistachios | 64 | 700 | **250–299 mg:** | | |
| 1/2 c ckd beet greens | 72 | 654 | 3.5 oz ckd lamb | 100 | 298 |
| 3 oz, ≈10 prunes | 85 | 633 | 1 c apple juice | 244 | 298 |
| 3.5 oz steamed clams | 100 | 628 | 1/2 c ckd artichoke hearts | 84 | 297 |
| 1 avocado half | 100 | 602 | 1 c grapes | 160 | 296 |
| 2 T molasses | 41 | 600 | 1/2 c cnd pinto beans | 120 | 291 |
| | | | 3.5 oz ckd turkey dark meat | 100 | 290 |
| **500–575 mg:** | | | 1 c spinach, ckd fr/frzn | 95 | 283 |
| 1 c lowfat yogurt | 245 | 573 | 1/4 c raisins | 36 | 272 |
| 1/2 c almonds | 78 | 536 | 1/2 c cnd sweet potatoes | 128 | 269 |
| 1 c tomato juice | 243 | 534 | 3.5 oz light chicken meat | 100 | 263 |
| 3/4 c prune juice | 192 | 530 | 3.5 oz ckd turkey light meat | 100 | 262 |
| 1 baked potato w/skin | 122 | 510 | 1/2 c beets | 85 | 259 |
| | | | 1/2 c ckd okra | 92 | 257 |
| **400–500 mg:** | | | 3.5 oz dark chicken meat | 100 | 253 |
| 1 c cantaloupe cubes | 160 | 494 | 1 c fresh strawberry halves | 152 | 252 |
| 1 c orange juice | 248 | 484 | 1/2 c pumpkin | 123 | 252 |
| 1/2 c ckd Swiss chard | 88 | 480 | 1 kiwifruit | 76 | 252 |
| 1/2 c lima beans, ckd fr/dry | 94 | 477 | | | |
| 1 banana | 118 | 467 | **200–249 mg:** | | |
| 1 c veg tomato juice | 243 | 467 | 1/2 c ckd Brussels sprouts | 78 | 249 |
| 1/4 c pumpkin seed kernels, rstd | 57 | 457 | 1/2 c macadamia nuts | 67 | 246 |
| 1/2 c cnd tomato sauce | 123 | 454 | 2 T peanut butter | 32 | 239 |
| 1/2 c peanuts | 72 | 453 | 1 oz unsweetened chocolate | 28.4 | 236 |
| 3.5 oz ckd fish | 100 | 380–450 | 3.5 oz ckd beef heart | 100 | 233 |
| 3.5 oz ckd veal liver | 100 | 438 | 1/2 c chpd pecans | 60 | 233 |
| 1 ckd whole artichoke | 120 | 425 | 7.5″ raw carrot | 72 | 232 |
| 1/2 c chestnuts | 72 | 423 | 1/4 c sunflower seeds | 68 | 217 |
| 1/2 c brazil nuts | 70 | 420 | 1/2 c ckd celery | 75 | 213 |
| 1 c nonfat milk | 245 | 407 | 1/2 c ckd collards | 90 | 213 |
| | | | 1 pear | 166 | 207 |
| **350–399 mg:** | | | 2 fresh apricots | 70 | 207 |
| 3.5 oz sardines-average | 100 | 397 | 1/2 c black-eyed peas, ckd fr/dry | 120 | 206 |
| 1 c grapefruit juice | 247 | 388 | 1/2 c fresh chopped tomatoes | 90 | 200 |
| 1/2 c navy/baked beans | 127 | 384 | | | |
| 1 c whole milk | 244 | 371 | **150–199 mg:** | | |
| 1/2 c baby lima beans, ckd fr/frzn | 90 | 370 | 3.5 oz ckd turkey liver | 100 | 194 |
| 1/2 c ckd lentils | 99 | 365 | 4 dried apricot halves | 14 | 193 |
| 3.5 oz ckd beef liver | 100 | 364 | 1 medium peach | 98 | 193 |
| 1 c papaya cubes | 140 | 360 | 1/2 c ckd peapods | 80 | 183 |
| 1/2 c ckd kidney beans | 89 | 357 | 1 c watermelon cubes | 152 | 176 |
| 1/2 c ckd split peas | 98 | 355 | 1/2 c pineapple juice | 125 | 170 |
| | | | 1/2 c tofu | 124 | 150 |
| **300–349 mg:** | | | | | |
| 3.5 oz ckd veal | 100 | 346 | **75–149 mg:** | | |
| 1/2 c cashews | 65 | 344 | 1/2 c blackberries | 72 | 141 |
| 1 c grape juice | 253 | 334 | 3.5 oz ckd chicken liver | 100 | 140 |
| 1 c sweet cherries, fresh | 145 | 324 | 1/2 c ckd chopped chayote | 80 | 138 |
| 3.5 oz ckd beef, avg | 100 | 323 | 2 T wheat germ | 14 | 134 |
| 1/2 c black-eyed peas, ckd fr/frzn | 85 | 319 | 1 c ckd oatmeal | 234 | 131 |
| 1/2 c black beans | 86 | 305 | 1/4 c coconut, dry (20 g) or fresh | 33 | 110 |
| 1/2 c mashed potato | 105 | 303 | 1/2 c cottage cheese | 28.4 | 109 |
| 2 T brewers yeast | 16 | 302 | 2 T maple syrup | 40 | 81 |

Listing includes elemental and enriched foods; does not include additionally fortified products like breakfast cereals.
Source: The Food Finder, ESHA Research, Salem, Oregon, 1999. Printed with permission.

areas where the soil is selenium-poor, many farm animals are given selenium-fortified feed, and some newborns are given intravenous shots of selenium to compensate.

Selenium deficiency was found to be associated with heart disease in thousands of children and young mothers in China in the 1970s. This sparked researchers to look further into the effects of selenium deficiency. It was later found that the heart disease in China also included the involvement of a virus, but the selenium deficiency was a major part of the diagnosis; when diets contained sufficient amounts of selenium, the disease (Keshan disease) was preventable.

### *Selenium Losses*

Some selenium is lost when foods are processed or refined; some forms are volatile and are lost in cooking steam.

### *Selenium Recommended Intake*

The 1989 RDAs recommend 0.87 mcg/day of selenium per kilogram of body weight. Pregnant women tend to conserve slightly more dietary selenium, but there is no clear understanding of why. Assuming the reference weights for an average adult man and woman, the recommendations are as follows:

| | | |
|---|---|---|
| Men | 19 years + | 70 mcg/day |
| Women | 19 years + | 55 mcg/day |
| Pregnant | | 65 mcg/day |
| Breastfeeding | | 75 mcg/day |

### *Selenium Upper Limits*

Like several other nutrients, intake of selenium in moderate amounts is absolutely necessary; in large doses it can be toxic. Upper limits have not been set, but large daily doses over 750 to 1,000 mcg (0.75 to 1 mg) can cause nausea, vomiting, diarrhea, loss of hair and nails, tenderness and swelling of the fingers, fatigue, irritability, skin lesions, tooth damage, and problems with the nervous system.

There is more potential for toxic doses of selenium from supplements rather than food. Selenium supplements are often taken for their antioxidant activity, without realizing the potential adverse effects of excessive intakes. Doses 2 to 3 times the RDA appear harmless. The organic forms of selenium (selenomethionine and selenocysteine) are better absorbed and less likely to cause toxic symptoms than the inorganic forms of the mineral (sodium selenite and selenate). Organic forms are available in selenium-rich nutritional yeast, whole grain products, and some supplements.

A person consuming 1 mg (1,000 mcg) of sodium selenite daily for over 2 years had thickened fragile nails and a garlic odor. Some selenium compounds smell like garlic, and, interestingly enough, garlic tends to be higher in selenium than other vegetables. One case of selenium toxicity was diagnosed because the patient had garlic breath, but had never eaten garlic.

### *Selenium Food Sources*

Excellent sources of selenium (Table 6.10) are Brazil nuts, oysters and clams, pork and ham, whole grain and regular pasta, chicken and turkey, sunflower seeds, beef and lamb, breads (including bagels, tortillas), oatmeal, soynuts, eggs, nuts and seeds, and lowfat dairy products. Brazil nuts are a variable, but unusually high, source of selenium. Lower selenium levels are found in higher fat meats, sausages, and cream. Fruits and vegetables contain only small amounts.

Selenium is a soil-dependent mineral whose concentrations in foods can vary 200-fold. Because most food supplies are not restricted to just locally grown products, the multiregional supply of foods from many locations compensates for a deficiency in one area. Deficiency is unlikely if a variety of foods are eaten. Grains such as whole wheat, brown rice, and oatmeal are excellent sources if the grain was grown in selenium rich soil.

Meat and poultry are a reliable source of selenium because farm animals have this added to their feed. The FDA approved selenium as a food additive to the feed of most species in 1979 because of its nutritional importance and affect on the growth of certain farm animals. Many plants and animals fail to thrive without sufficient selenium.

## Sodium

***Sodium functions as an electrolyte, maintaining the extracellular fluid balance in the body. This mineral is essential for muscle contractions and nerve transmissions.***

### *Sodium Functions*

Sodium is a major element in regulating fluid balance in the body, and its function is balanced by potassium. When people ingest salt in the diet, thirst assures that the body will restore the appropriate water-to-sodium ratio. Sodium along with chloride make up common table salt. Sodium, potassium, and chloride are electrolytes—salts that dissolve in water.

The movement of fluids in and out of the cells is largely a function of the relative concentration of the electrolytes on either side of the semipermeable cell membrane. The sodium ion is on the outside of the cell and the potassium ion is on the inside. Fairly equal intakes of both minerals are needed to maintain this balance. Only under extreme conditions of heavy, long-term sweating (tri-athletes) would more sodium be needed to replace the sodium lost through sweat. Sodium is also involved with generating nerve impulses, acid-base balance, and the metabolism of carbohydrates and protein.

For years, sodium intake, particularly in the form of table salt, was thought to be the cause of high blood pressure or hypertension. Recent studies, however, have shed new light on this topic and present a significantly different point of view. A large study, called the DASH study, found that a diet high in fruits and vegetables (10 servings per day), low in fat, and with low-fat dairy foods, was very successful in lowering high blood pressure. Sodium intake averaged about 2,800 mg a day in this diet.

It is now known that hypertension is better controlled by weight loss and other factors. People with diabetes, chronic renal disease, those who are black, and those whose parents had hypertension are more likely to be salt sensitive and may be able to slightly lower their blood pressure with some salt restriction.

However, only about 1 in 5 persons is sodium sensitive. Of the people *with high blood pressure,* approximately 50 to 67% are *not* sensitive to sodium intake. And, in a recent study on chronic fatigue syndrome, it was found that many cases were virtually cured with a regimen that included a high salt diet and blood pressure medication.

### *Sodium Recommended Intake*

The Food and Nutrition Board Committee recommends approximately 2,000 to 2,400 mg of sodium/day, with a minimum requirement of 500 mg. The American Heart Association

TABLE 6.10 **Selenium Sources in Rank Order by Serving Size**

| | Weight (g) | Selenium (mcg) |
|---|---|---|
| **100–2100 mcg/serving:** | | |
| 1/2 c brazil nuts–average of range | 70 | 2072 |
| 3.5 oz ckd oysters | 100 | 115 |
| **50–99 mcg:** | | |
| 3.5 oz ckd chicken liver | 100 | 71 |
| 3.5 oz ckd raw oysters | 100 | 70 |
| 3.5 oz steamed clams | 100 | 64 |
| 3.5 oz ckd beef liver | 100 | 57 |
| **25–49 mcg:** | | |
| 3.5 oz sardines, avg | 100 | 46 |
| 3.5 oz ckd pork | 100 | |
| 3.5 oz ckd crab | 100 | 40 |
| 3.5 oz ckd salt water fish, avg | 100 | 40 |
| 1 c whole wheat pasta | 140 | 36 |
| 3.5 oz ckd dark chicken meat | 100 | 35 |
| 3.5 oz ckd light chicken meat | 100 | 32 |
| 1 c regular pasta | 140 | 30 |
| 3.5 oz ckd turkey liver | 100 | 27 |
| 3.5 oz ckd lamb | 100 | 26 |
| 1/4 c sunflower seed kernels | 33 | 26 |
| **15–24 mcg:** | | |
| 2.5 oz plain bagel | 71 | 23 |
| 3.5 oz ckd imitation crab, surimi, processed fish | 100 | 22 |
| 3.5 oz ckd beef heart | 100 | 21 |
| 1 c ckd oatmeal | 234 | 19 |
| 10″ flour tortilla | 72 | 17 |
| 1/2 c soynuts (roasted soybeans) | 86 | 17 |
| 3.5 oz ckd freshwater fish | 100 | 15 |
| **10–14 mcg:** | | |
| 1 cooked egg | 48–50 | 13 |
| 3.5 oz ckd veal | 100 | 13 |
| 1/2 c cottage cheese | 28.4 | 12 |
| 1/2 c tofu | 124 | 11 |
| 1 piece whole wheat bread | 28 | 10 |
| **5.0–9.9 mcg:** | | |
| 1/2 c ckd brown rice | 98 | 9.6 |
| 2 T wheat germ | 14 | 9.2 |
| 1 piece white bread | 30 | 8.6 |
| 1/2 c cnd pinto beans | 120 | 8.5 |
| 1 c lowfat yogurt | 245 | 8.1 |
| 1 cooked egg yolk | 16.6 | 7.5 |
| 1/2 c cashews | 65 | 7.5 |
| 2 T molasses | 41 | 7.3 |
| 1/2 c ckd navy/baked beans | 127 | 6.8 |
| 1/2 c ckd barley | 78 | 6.8 |
| 2 T brewer's yeast | 16 | 6.7 |
| 1/2 c ckd white rice | 79 | 5.9 |
| 1/2 c peanuts | 72 | 5.4 |
| 1 c nonfat milk | 245 | 5.2 |
| **2.5–4.9 mcg:** | | |
| 1 c whole milk | 244 | 4.9 |
| 1/4 c ckd mushrooms | 39 | 4.6 |
| 1/2 c large lima beans, ckd fr/dry | 94 | 4.2 |
| 1 oz corn nuts | 28.4 | 4.2 |
| 1/2 c pistachios | 64 | 4.1 |
| 1 oz American cheese | 28.4 | 4.1 |
| 1/2 c almonds | 78 | 3.8 |
| 1/4 c coconut, dry(20 g) or fresh | 33 | 3.4 |
| 1/4 c pumpkin seed kernels, rstd | 57 | 3.2 |
| 1/2 c chopped pecans | 60 | 3.1 |
| 1/2 c macadamias | 68 | 3.1 |
| 1/2 c ckd lentils | 99 | 2.9 |
| 1/2 c black-eyed peas, ckd fr/frzn | 85 | 2.9 |
| 1 T wheat bran | 3.6 | 2.8 |
| 1/2 c ckd broccoli | 85 | 2.8 |
| 1/2 c chopped walnuts | 60 | 2.7 |
| 1/2 c filberts | 68 | 2.7 |
| 1 T oat bran | 6 | 2.7 |
| **1.0–2.4 mcg:** | | |
| 2 T peanut butter | 32 | 2.4 |
| 1 oz chocolate | 28.4 | 2.1 |
| 3 oz, ≈10 prunes | 85 | 2.0 |
| 1 pear | 166 | 1.7 |
| 1/2 c spinach, ckd fr/frzn | 95 | 1.6 |
| 1/2 c baby lima beans, ckd fr/frzn | 90 | 1.5 |
| 1 grapefruit half | 118–123 | 1.5 |
| 1 corn tortilla | 26 | 1.4 |
| 1 banana | 118 | 1.3 |
| 1/2 c ckd green soybeans | 90 | 1.3 |
| 1/2 c Brussels sprouts | 78 | 1.15 |
| 1/2 c ckd collards | 90 | 1.15 |
| 3/4 c prune juice | 192 | 1.15 |
| 1 c fresh strawberry halves | 152 | 1.1 |
| 1/2 c black beans | 86 | 1.0 |
| 1/2 c cnd sweet potato | 128 | 1.0 |
| **0.24–0.90 mcg:** | | |
| 1 c papaya cubes | 140 | 0.84 |
| 7.5″ fresh carrot | 72 | 0.79 |
| 1/2 c ckd Swiss chard | 88 | 0.79 |
| 1 c cantaloupe cubes | 160 | 0.64 |
| 1/2 c ckd split green peas | 80 | 0.59 |
| 1/2 c mashed potatoes | 105 | 0.53 |
| 1/2 c blueberries | 75 | 0.45 |
| 1/2 c blackberries | 72 | 0.43 |
| 1 avocado half | 100 | 0.40 |
| 1 c brewed coffee | 240 | 0.24 |

Listing includes elemental and enriched foods; does not include additionally fortified products like breakfast cereals.
Source: The Food Finder, ESHA Research, Salem, Oregon, 1999. Printed with permission.

recommends limiting sodium intake to 3 grams daily (3,000 mg); and people who have hypertension (high blood pressure) *and* are salt-sensitive, may benefit from a restriction to 2 grams of sodium per day (2,000 mg).

## *Sodium Upper Limits*

No upper limits of sodium have been set. When there is excess body sodium, thirst causes the consumption of more fluids. The excess fluid and sodium are then excreted in the urine. A high intake of sodium is not a health threat as long as water needs are met and the kidneys are functioning properly. (Read the previous discussion about recent findings on hypertension and that high sodium intake is *not* the cause.)

## *Sodium Food Sources*

Table salt, soy sauce, pickles, sauerkraut, catsup, lunch meats, and other processed foods contain the most sodium. Some local tap waters contain sodium, depending on the location. Despite the title "saltwater" fish, unless canned, smoked, or pickled, they do not have more sodium than freshwater varieties. Salt is sodium chloride and is 39% sodium by weight. Therefore, 5 grams of salt (about a teaspoon) equates to about 2 grams of sodium. In the current American diet, approximately 75% of sodium is found in processed foods.

Most people are unaware of the sodium they consume each day because it is assumed it will taste salty. Processed foods may contain additives for preservation that contain sodium as part of the chemical compound. For instance, there is more sodium in one cup of round puffed oat cereal with honey, or in one plain English muffin, than in 1 oz of oil roasted salted peanuts. People may think that the peanuts have more salt, but this is because the salt is on the surface, the first taste the tongue receives.

# Zinc

***Zinc is necessary for many enzymes, including those associated with energy metabolism. This mineral is needed for the synthesis of proteins and for genetic material, immune reactions, taste, wound healing, the hormone insulin, normal growth of the fetus, the making of sperm, and the transport of vitamin A in the body.***

## *Zinc Functions*

Zinc plays a necessary and versatile role in enzyme production for the body's metabolism of protein, carbohydrate, fat, alcohol, and many other functions. Over 100 enzymes require zinc as a cofactor. Zinc is needed for the synthesis of proteins, stabilizing cell membranes, and for the maintenance of DNA and RNA. It is important for proper functioning of the immune system, for proper storage and release of the hormone insulin, for growth and repair of tissues, for wound healing, and for the ability to taste foods.

The active form of vitamin A and the cell's ability to produce and dispose of carbon dioxide requires zinc. It is important to the production of prostaglandins that regulate many body processes including blood pressure, the heart rate, and the normal functioning of the oil glands of the skin.

Zinc also is involved with the mineralization of bone and may protect the body from heavy-metal (lead) poisoning. Zinc is involved in blood clotting, affects the functions of the thyroid hormone, helps maintain blood cholesterol levels, and influences behavior and learning performance. Children have very high zinc needs because of their rapid growth. It is very important for the development of the fetus, in pregnancy, and in the making of sperm.

Zinc is found throughout the body including the bones, eyes, prostate gland, and testes, with the highest concentrations found in the muscles (over 60%). It is also found in the skin, kidneys, and in the saliva and pancreatic fluids, which assist in the digestion of foods. The rate of absorption is dependent on stored levels in the body. Histidine (an amino acid) and blood albumin (a protein) seem to enhance absorption.

## *Zinc Losses, Deficiencies, and Antagonists*

Overt zinc deficiency is rare in the United States. Marginal status can be found in groups at risk due to poor diet: alcoholics, the elderly, low-income children and families, and vegetarians, particularly female vegans. Symptoms include anemia, slowed growth, birth defects, spontaneous abortion, delayed sexual maturation, sterility, reduced taste perception, slow healing of wounds, poor alcohol tolerance, glucose intolerance, mental disorders, skin and hair problems, loss of appetite, skeletal abnormalities, and poor resistance to infection.

Excessive intakes of iron or copper may interfere with absorption of zinc and produce a zinc deficiency. In turn, excessive intakes of zinc can inhibit copper and iron absorption and result in deficiencies of these minerals. The body uses similar absorption mechanisms for zinc, copper, and iron. When there is an oversupply of one mineral (from a continuous over-consumption from supplements or heavily fortified foods), the dominant mineral may use up all the receptor capabilities and create a deficiency of the other minerals.

Phytate and fiber in plant foods reduce the amount of zinc available for absorption, but in spite of this, whole grain foods still provide more zinc than refined foods (foods with less fiber and phytate). Yeast breads have higher zinc availability because the yeast produces enzymes that destroy phytate.

Zinc absorption can vary from 15 to 40% depending on several factors. The body absorbs small amounts of zinc better than large amounts. More is absorbed if the body is depleted; less is absorbed if the body has sufficient zinc. Zinc from meats is four times more available than that from fibrous foods like cereals, because fiber and phytate bind some of the zinc. For infants, zinc is better absorbed from breast milk than formula.

## *Zinc Recommended Intake*

The 1989 RDAs recommended zinc intakes are listed next. These amounts are for healthy adults, and the amount for men is higher because of their greater average weight than women.

| | | |
|---|---|---|
| Men | 11 years + | 15 mg/day |
| Women | 11 years + | 12 mg/day |
| Pregnant | | 15 mg/day |
| Breastfeeding | | 19 mg/day 1st 6 months |
| | | 16 mg/day over 6 months |

The 1990 Canadian RNI recommend 12 mg/day for adult men, 9 mg/day for adult women, and 15 mg/day if pregnant or breastfeeding (lactating).

## *Zinc Upper Limits*

Zinc in excess may cause problems, but there is insufficient information with which to set an Upper Limit. Doses of 80 to 150 mg of zinc per day may cause a decline of "healthy" HDL cholesterol and affect cholesterol metabolism. Doses of 150 to 300 mg+ a day over time (over 10 times the RDA) can lower levels of white blood cells, and lower blood levels of copper. Such doses are also associated with changed cholesterol metabolism and appear to possibly accelerate development of atherosclerosis. Severe gastrointestinal irritation and vomiting have occurred following an intake of 2 g (2,000 mg) of zinc sulphate.

## *Zinc Food Sources*

Excellent sources (Table 6.11) are oysters, beef, liver, crab, seafood, poultry (especially the dark meat), organ meats, nuts and seeds, whole grain breads and cereals, tofu, legumes, and milk. Vegetables and fruits contain less. Zinc in breast milk is better absorbed than the zinc in formula or cow's milk.

Zinc levels have been shown to vary according to genetic breeding of some plants, soil conditions, and the amount of fertilizer applied. There are considerably higher levels of both zinc and copper in the peel rather than in the flesh of some fruits.

TABLE 6.11 **Zinc Sources in Rank Order by Serving Size**

| | Weight (g) | Zinc (mg) |
|---|---|---|
| **10–40 mg/serving:** | | |
| 3.5 oz ckd oysters | 100 | 39 |
| 3.5 oz raw oysters | 100 | 27 |
| **5–9 mg:** | | |
| 3.5 oz ckd beef pot roast | 100 | 8.5 |
| 3.5 oz ckd veal liver | 100 | 7.8 |
| 3.5 oz ckd Alaska king crab | 100 | 7.6 |
| 3.5 oz ckd ground beef | 100 | 5.5 |
| **2.5– 4.9 mg:** | | |
| 3.5 oz ckd beef steak | 100 | 5.4 |
| 3.5 oz ckd beef liver | 100 | 4.5 |
| 3.5 oz ckd turkey dark meat | 100 | 4.5 |
| 3.5 oz ckd veal | 100 | 4.4 |
| 3.5 oz ckd chicken liver | 100 | 4.3 |
| 1/4 c pumpkin seed kernels-rstd | 57 | 4.2 |
| 3.5 oz ckd blue crab | 100 | 4.2 |
| 3.5 oz ckd beef kidney | 100 | 4.2 |
| 1/2 c soynuts (roasted soybeans) | 86 | 4.1 |
| 3.5 oz ckd lamb | 100 | 4.0 |
| 1/2 c almonds | 78 | 3.9 |
| 1/2 c peanuts | 72 | 3.5 |
| 1/2 c chopped pecans | 60 | 3.6 |
| 1/2 c brazil nuts | 70 | 3.2 |
| 3.5 oz ckd turkey liver | 100 | 3.1 |
| 1/2 c cashews | 65 | 3.1 |
| 3.5 oz ckd dark chicken meat | 100 | 2.9 |
| 3.5 oz steamed clams | 100 | 2.7 |
| **1.5–2.4 mg:** | | |
| 3.5 oz ckd pork | 100 | 2.4 |
| 2 T wheat germ | 14 | 2.4 |
| 1 c lowfat yogurt | 245 | 2.2 |
| 3.5 oz ckd light turkey meat | 100 | 2.1 |
| 1/2 c baked beans w/ham | 127 | 1.8 |
| 1/4 c sunflower seeds | 68 | 1.7 |
| 3.5 oz ckd turkey ham | 100 | 1.7 |
| 2 T maple syrup | 40 | 1.7 |
| 1/2 c chopped walnuts | 60 | 1.6 |
| 1/2 c filberts | 68 | 1.6 |
| 3.5 oz ckd shrimp | 100 | 1.6 |
| **1.0–1.4 mg:** | | |
| 3.5 oz turkey hot dog | 100 | 1.4 |
| 3.5 oz sardines-avg | 100 | 1.4 |
| 3.5 oz ckd light chicken meat | 100 | 1.3 |
| 2 T brewers yeast | 16 | 1.3 |
| 1/2 c ckd lentils | 99 | 1.3 |
| 3.5 oz beef hot dog | 100 | 1.2 |
| 1/2 c black-eyed peas, ckd fr/frzn | 85 | 1.2 |
| 1/2 c macadamia nuts | 68 | 1.2 |
| 1 c ckd oatmeal | 234 | 1.15 |
| 1 c ckd whole wheat pasta | 140 | 1.1 |
| 1 oz Swiss cheese | 28.4 | 1.1 |
| 3.5 oz ckd catfish | 100 | 1.1 |
| 1/2 c tofu | 124 | 1.0 |
| 1/2 c ckd split peas | 98 | 1.0 |
| 1 c nonfat milk | 245 | 1.0 |
| 1 tsp sesame seeds | 9.4 | 1.0 |
| 1/2 c ckd black beans | 86 | 1.0 |
| 1/2 c ckd kidney beans | 89 | 1.0 |
| **0.75–0.90 mg:** | | |
| 1 c whole milk | 244 | 0.9 |
| 1 oz provolone cheese | 28.4 | 0.9 |
| 2 T peanut butter | 32 | 0.9 |
| 1/2 c lima beans, ckd fr/dry | 94 | 0.9 |
| 1 oz cheddar cheese | 28.4 | 0.9 |
| 1/2 c pistachios | 64 | 0.9 |
| 1 oz American cheese | 28.4 | 0.85 |
| 1 c ckd fresh pasta | 150 | 0.84 |
| 1/2 c black-eyed peas, ckd fr/dry | 120 | 0.84 |
| 1/2 c ckd green soybeans | 90 | 0.80 |
| 1/2 c ckd green peas | 80 | 0.75 |
| **0.50–0.74 mg:** | | |
| 1 c ckd regular pasta | 140 | 0.74 |
| 1/2 c spinach, ckd fr/frzn | 95 | 0.67 |
| 1/2 c ckd barley | 78 | 0.64 |
| 2.5 oz bagel | 71 | 0.63 |
| 1/2 c ckd brown rice | 98 | 0.61 |
| 1 ckd whole artichoke | 120 | 0.59 |
| 1 piece whole wheat bread | 28 | 0.54 |
| 1 cooked egg | 48–50 | 0.54 |
| 10″ flour tortilla | 72 | 0.51 |
| 3.5 oz ckd fish, ranges .40 –.60 | 100 | 0.50 |
| **0.35–0.49 mg:** | | |
| 1 c veg tomato juice | 243 | 0.48 |
| 3 oz, ≈10 prunes | 85 | 0.45 |
| 1/2 c ckd okra | 92 | 0.44 |
| 1 avocado half | 100 | 0.42 |
| 1/2 c ckd artichoke hearts | 84 | 0.41 |
| 2 T black molasses | 41 | 0.41 |
| 3/4 c prune juice | 192 | 0.40 |
| 1 baked potato w/skin | 122 | 0.39 |
| 1/4 c raw Irish moss seaweed | 20 | 0.39 |

*(continued)*

TABLE 6.11 *(Continued)* **Zinc Sources in Rank Order by Serving Size**

| | Weight (g) | Zinc (mg) | | Weight (g) | Zinc (mg) |
|---|---|---|---|---|---|
| 1/2 c ckd white rice | 79 | 0.39 | 1/2 c cnd sweet potatoes | 128 | 0.27 |
| 1/2 c ckd beet greens | 72 | 0.36 | 1 T wheat bran | 3.6 | 0.26 |
| 1/2 c ckd summer squash | 90 | 0.35 | 1 piece wheat bread | 25 | 0.26 |
| **0.25–0.34 mg:** | | | 1/4 c raw seaweed—kelp, nori, kombu, oarweed | 20 | 0.26 |
| 1 c tomato juice | 243 | 0.34 | 1 c cantaloupe cubes | 160 | 0.26 |
| 1/2 c ckd peapods | 80 | 0.34 | | | |
| 1/2 c ckd mushrooms | 39 | 0.34 | **0.10–0.24 mg:** | | |
| 1/2 c ckd corn | 75 | 0.33 | 1 corn tortilla | 26 | 0.24 |
| 1/2 c ckd beets | 85 | 0.30 | 1/2 c ckd collards | 90 | 0.23 |
| 1/2 c ckd bean sprouts | 62 | 0.29 | 1 c fresh strawberry halves | 152 | 0.21 |
| 1/2 c ckd broccoli | 85 | 0.29 | 1 pear | 166 | 0.20 |
| 1/2 c ckd Swiss chard | 88 | 0.29 | 1 piece white bread | 30 | 0.19 |
| 1/2 c mashed potatoes | 105 | 0.28 | 1 T oat bran | 6 | 0.18 |
| 1/2 c fresh red raspberries | 62 | 0.28 | 2 fresh apricots | 70 | 0.18 |
| 1/2 c ckd green beans | 65 | 0.28 | 1 c looseleaf lettuce | 56 | 0.16 |
| 1/2 c ckd Brussels sprouts | 78 | 0.27 | 1 c romaine lettuce | 56 | 0.14 |

Listing includes elemental and enriched foods; does not include additionally fortified products like breakfast cereals.
Source: The Food Finder, ESHA Research, Salem, Oregon, 1999. Printed with permission.

## PARTIAL BIBLIOGRAPHY FOR INFORMATION ON BASIC FOOD COMPONENTS, VITAMINS, AND MINERALS

Recommended Dietary Allowances, 10th edition. Subcommittee on the Tenth Edition of the RDAs, Food and Nutrition Board, Commission on Life Sciences, National Research Council. National Academy Press, Washington, DC, 1989.

Dietary Reference Intakes for Calcium, Phosphorus, Magnesium, Vitamin D, and Fluoride. A Report of the Standing Committee on the Scientific Evaluation of Dietary Reference Intakes. Food and Nutrition Board, Institute of Medicine. National Academy Press, Washington, DC, 1997.

Dietary Reference Intakes for Thiamin, Riboflavin, Niacin, Vitamin B6, Folate, Vitamin B12, Pantothenic Acid, Biotin, and Choline. A Report of the Standing Committee on the Scientific Evaluation of Dietary Reference Intakes; and its Panel on Folate, Other B Vitamins, and Choline; and Subcommittee on Upper Reference Levels of Nutrients. Food and Nutrition Board, Institute of Medicine. National Academy Press, Washington, DC, 1998.

McCance and Widdowson's The Composition of Foods, by B. Holland, A.A. Welch, I.D. Unwin, D.H. Buss, A.A. Paul, and D.A.T. Southgate; The Royal Society of Chemistry and Ministry of Agriculture, Fisheries and Food, Cambridge, UK, the 5th revised and extended edition, 1991.

Nutrition Recommendations. The Report of the Scientific Review Committee, National Health and Welfare, Canada, 1990.

Advanced Nutrition and Human Metabolism. Sara M. Hunt and James L Groff. West Publishing Company, St. Paul, MN, 1990.

Understanding Normal and Clinical Nutrition, 5th edition. Eleanor Whitney, Corinne Cataldo, Sharon Rady Rolfes. West/Wadsworth Publishing, International Thomson Publishing Company, 1998.

Genesis® R&D and The Food Processor® User Manuals, special topics sections, E.S. Hands, ESHA Research, Salem, OR, 1996–1998.

Nutrients ranked by serving size: The ESHA nutrient database through The Food Processor® and Genesis® nutrition software programs; and The Food Finder, 3rd and 4th editions, Elizabeth Hands, ESHA Research, Salem, OR, 1995 and 1998. ESHA Research, Salem, Oregon, 1998. Printed with permission.

Sources of nutrient data used to compile the ESHA Food Nutrient database (over 1,200 sources) are listed separately on the CD-ROM that accompanies this publication.

Nutrition and health articles from the University of California Berkeley, Wellness Newsletters: Health Letter Associates, Palm Coast, FL, 1994–1999.

Nutrition and health articles from the Harvard Health Letter, President and Fellows of Harvard College, Palm Coast, FL, 1994–1999.

Nutrition and health articles from the Tufts University Health and Nutrition Letter, Tufts University, New York, NY, 1994–1999.

Nutrition and health articles from Nutrition Action, Center for Science in the Public Interest, Washington, DC, 1994–1999.

Nutrition and health articles from the Mayo Clinic Health Letter, Mayo Foundation, Boulder, CO, 1996–1999.

Discussions with many researchers and scientists in the field.

SECTION 7

# FOOD NUTRIENT TABLES

| Code | Amount | Description | Weight (g) | Calories | % Water | Protein (g) | Carbs (g) | Fiber (g) | Sugar (g) | Other Carbs (g) | Fat (g) | Sat Fat (g) | Mono Fat (g) | Poly Fat (g) | Omega 3 (g) | Omega 6 (g) | Choles (mg) |
|---|---|---|---|---|---|---|---|---|---|---|---|---|---|---|---|---|---|
| | | **BEVERAGE AND BEVERAGE MIXES** | | | | | | | | | | | | | | | |
| | | *CARBONATED DRINKS, 1 1/2 cups, 12 fl oz* | | | | | | | | | | | | | | | |
| 20467 | 1 1/2 cup | Birch Beer, diet, Shasta | 360 | 0 | 100 | 0.0 | 0.0 | 0.0 | 0.0 | 0.0 | 0.0 | 0.0 | 0.0 | 0.0 | 0.00 | 0.00 | 0 |
| | | Black Cherry | | | | | | | | | | | | | | | |
| 20462 | 1 1/2 cup | Diet, Shasta | 360 | 0 | 100 | 0.0 | 0.0 | 0.0 | 0.0 | 0.0 | 0.0 | 0.0 | 0.0 | 0.0 | 0.00 | 0.00 | 0 |
| 20528 | 1 1/2 cup | Minute Maid | 375 | 165 | 88 | 0.0 | 43.5 | 0.0 | 43.5 | 0.0 | 0.0 | 0.0 | 0.0 | 0.0 | 0.00 | 0.00 | 0 |
| 20170 | 1 1/2 cup | Shasta | 360 | 170 | 88 | 0.0 | 41.0 | 0.0 | 41.0 | 0.0 | 0.0 | 0.0 | 0.0 | 0.0 | 0.00 | 0.00 | 0 |
| 20529 | 1 1/2 cup | Blueberry, Minute Maid | 376 | 165 | 88 | 0.0 | 43.6 | 0.0 | 43.6 | 0.0 | 0.0 | 0.0 | 0.0 | 0.0 | 0.00 | 0.00 | 0 |
| 20171 | 1 1/2 cup | Cherry Cola, Shasta | 360 | 160 | 89 | 0.0 | 39.0 | 0.0 | 39.0 | 0.0 | 0.0 | 0.0 | 0.0 | 0.0 | 0.00 | 0.00 | 0 |
| 20481 | 1 1/2 cup | Cherry Cola, diet, Shasta | 360 | 0 | 100 | 0.0 | 0.0 | 0.0 | 0.0 | 0.0 | 0.0 | 0.0 | 0.0 | 0.0 | 0.00 | 0.00 | 0 |
| 20006 | 1 1/2 cup | Club Soda, avg | 355 | 0 | 100 | 0.0 | 0.0 | 0.0 | 0.0 | 0.0 | 0.0 | 0.0 | 0.0 | 0.0 | 0.00 | 0.00 | 0 |
| 20028 | 1 1/2 cup | Cream Soda, avg | 371 | 189 | 87 | 0.0 | 49.3 | 0.0 | 49.3 | 0.0 | 0.0 | 0.0 | 0.0 | 0.0 | 0.00 | 0.00 | 0 |
| 20624 | 1 1/2 cup | Cream Soda, diet, avg | 355 | 0 | 100 | 0.0 | 0.4 | 0.0 | 0.0 | 0.4 | 0.0 | 0.0 | 0.0 | 0.0 | 0.00 | 0.00 | 0 |
| | | Cola | | | | | | | | | | | | | | | |
| 20005 | 1 1/2 cup | Avg | 372 | 153 | 89 | 0.0 | 38.7 | 0.0 | 38.7 | 0.0 | 0.0 | 0.0 | 0.0 | 0.0 | 0.00 | 0.00 | 0 |
| 20030 | 1 1/2 cup | Diet, avg | 355 | 4 | 100 | 0.4 | 0.4 | 0.0 | 0.0 | 0.4 | 0.0 | 0.0 | 0.0 | 0.0 | 0.00 | 0.00 | 0 |
| 20473 | 1 1/2 cup | Diet, caff free, Shasta | 360 | 0 | 100 | 0.0 | 0.0 | 0.0 | 0.0 | 0.0 | 0.0 | 0.0 | 0.0 | 0.0 | 0.00 | 0.00 | 0 |
| | | Coca Cola | | | | | | | | | | | | | | | |
| 20148 | 1 1/2 cup | Classic | 373 | 145 | 91 | 0.0 | 40.5 | 0.0 | 40.5 | 0.0 | 0.0 | 0.0 | 0.0 | 0.0 | 0.00 | 0.00 | 0 |
| 20513 | 1 1/2 cup | Classic, caff free | 373 | 145 | 89 | 0.0 | 40.5 | 0.0 | 40.5 | 0.0 | 0.0 | 0.0 | 0.0 | 0.0 | 0.00 | 0.00 | 0 |
| 20514 | 1 1/2 cup | Classic, diet | 359 | 1 | 100 | 0.0 | 0.1 | 0.0 | 0.1 | 0.0 | 0.0 | 0.0 | 0.0 | 0.0 | 0.00 | 0.00 | 0 |
| 20149 | 1 1/2 cup | Cherry | 375 | 156 | 89 | 0.0 | 42.0 | 0.0 | 42.0 | 0.0 | 0.0 | 0.0 | 0.0 | 0.0 | 0.00 | 0.00 | 0 |
| 20515 | 1 1/2 cup | Cherry, diet | 359 | 1 | 100 | 0.0 | 0.1 | 0.0 | 0.1 | 0.0 | 0.0 | 0.0 | 0.0 | 0.0 | 0.00 | 0.00 | 0 |
| 20433 | 1 1/2 cup | Fruit Flvd Punch, avg | 372 | 170 | 89 | 0.0 | 42.0 | 0.0 | 42.0 | 0.0 | 0.0 | 0.0 | 0.0 | 0.0 | 0.00 | 0.00 | 0 |
| 20008 | 1 1/2 cup | Ginger Ale, avg | 366 | 124 | 91 | 0.0 | 31.8 | 0.0 | 31.8 | 0.0 | 0.0 | 0.0 | 0.0 | 0.0 | 0.00 | 0.00 | 0 |
| 20627 | 1 1/2 cup | Ginger Ale, diet, avg | 355 | 0 | 100 | 0.0 | 0.4 | 0.0 | 0.0 | 0.4 | 0.0 | 0.0 | 0.0 | 0.0 | 0.00 | 0.00 | 0 |
| 20031 | 1 1/2 cup | Grape, avg | 372 | 160 | 89 | 0.0 | 41.7 | 0.0 | 41.7 | 0.0 | 0.0 | 0.0 | 0.0 | 0.0 | 0.00 | 0.00 | 0 |
| 20460 | 1 1/2 cup | Grape, diet, Shasta | 360 | 0 | 100 | 0.0 | 0.0 | 0.0 | 0.0 | 0.0 | 0.0 | 0.0 | 0.0 | 0.0 | 0.00 | 0.00 | 0 |
| 20192 | 1 1/2 cup | Grapefruit, diet, Shasta | 360 | 0 | 100 | 0.0 | 0.0 | 0.0 | 0.0 | 0.0 | 0.0 | 0.0 | 0.0 | 0.0 | 0.00 | 0.00 | 0 |
| | | Lemon-Lime | | | | | | | | | | | | | | | |
| 20032 | 1 1/2 cup | Avg | 368 | 147 | 90 | 0.0 | 38.3 | 0.0 | 37.5 | 0.7 | 0.0 | 0.0 | 0.0 | 0.0 | 0.00 | 0.00 | 0 |
| 20536 | 1 1/2 cup | Diet, Fresca | 359 | 4 | 100 | 0.0 | 0.3 | 0.0 | 0.3 | 0.0 | 0.0 | 0.0 | 0.0 | 0.0 | 0.00 | 0.00 | 0 |
| 20207 | 1 1/2 cup | Diet, 7-Up | 360 | 4 | 100 | 0.4 | 0.4 | 0.0 | | | 0.0 | 0.0 | 0.0 | 0.0 | 0.00 | 0.00 | 0 |
| 20209 | 1 1/2 cup | Diet, 7-Up Gold | 360 | 4 | 99 | 0.0 | 2.0 | | | | 0.0 | 0.0 | 0.0 | 0.0 | 0.00 | 0.00 | 0 |
| 20068 | 1 1/2 cup | Diet, Slice | 360 | 0 | 97 | 0.0 | 1.0 | 0.0 | 0.0 | 1.0 | 0.0 | 0.0 | 0.0 | 0.0 | 0.00 | 0.00 | 0 |
| 20164 | 1 1/2 cup | Diet, Sprite | 359 | 4 | 100 | 0.0 | 0.0 | 0.0 | 0.0 | 0.0 | 0.0 | 0.0 | 0.0 | 0.0 | 0.00 | 0.00 | 0 |
| 20055 | 1 1/2 cup | 7-Up | 360 | 42 | 97 | 0.0 | 10.4 | 0.0 | | | 0.0 | 0.0 | 0.0 | 0.0 | 0.00 | 0.00 | 0 |
| 20208 | 1 1/2 cup | 7-Up Gold | 360 | 156 | 89 | 0.0 | 38.0 | | | | 0.0 | 0.0 | 0.0 | 0.0 | 0.00 | 0.00 | 0 |
| 20408 | 1 1/2 cup | Slice | 360 | 150 | 89 | 0.0 | 40.0 | 0.0 | 39.0 | 1.0 | 0.0 | 0.0 | 0.0 | 0.0 | 0.00 | 0.00 | 0 |
| 20163 | 1 1/2 cup | Sprite | 373 | 144 | 89 | 0.0 | 39.0 | 0.0 | 39.0 | 0.0 | 0.0 | 0.0 | 0.0 | 0.0 | 0.00 | 0.00 | 0 |
| | | Mountain Dew | | | | | | | | | | | | | | | |
| 20407 | 1 1/2 cup | Caff free | 360 | 170 | 87 | 0.0 | 46.0 | 0.0 | 46.0 | 0.0 | 0.0 | 0.0 | 0.0 | 0.0 | 0.00 | 0.00 | 0 |
| 20272 | 1 1/2 cup | Diet | 360 | 0 | 97 | 0.0 | 0.0 | 0.0 | 0.0 | 0.0 | 0.0 | 0.0 | 0.0 | 0.0 | 0.00 | 0.00 | 0 |
| 20273 | 1 1/2 cup | Diet, caff free | 360 | 0 | 97 | 0.0 | 0.0 | 0.0 | 0.0 | 0.0 | 0.0 | 0.0 | 0.0 | 0.0 | 0.00 | 0.00 | 0 |
| 20271 | 1 1/2 cup | Regular | 360 | 170 | 87 | 0.0 | 46.0 | 0.0 | 46.0 | 0.0 | 0.0 | 0.0 | 0.0 | 0.0 | 0.00 | 0.00 | 0 |
| | | Orange | | | | | | | | | | | | | | | |
| 20029 | 1 1/2 cup | Avg | 372 | 179 | 88 | 0.0 | 45.8 | 0.0 | 45.8 | 0.0 | 0.0 | 0.0 | 0.0 | 0.0 | 0.00 | 0.00 | 0 |
| 20527 | 1 1/2 cup | Diet, Minute Maid | 360 | 3 | 100 | 0.0 | 0.0 | 0.0 | 0.0 | 0.0 | 0.0 | 0.0 | 0.0 | 0.0 | 0.00 | 0.00 | 0 |
| 20153 | 1 1/2 cup | Fanta | 377 | 177 | 87 | 0.0 | 48.0 | 0.0 | 48.0 | 0.0 | 0.0 | 0.0 | 0.0 | 0.0 | 0.00 | 0.00 | 0 |
| 20160 | 1 1/2 cup | Minute Maid | 377 | 177 | 87 | 0.0 | 48.1 | 0.0 | 48.1 | 0.0 | 0.0 | 0.0 | 0.0 | 0.0 | 0.00 | 0.00 | 0 |
| 20477 | 1 1/2 cup | Peach, Shasta | 360 | 170 | 88 | 0.0 | 43.0 | 0.0 | 43.0 | 0.0 | 0.0 | 0.0 | 0.0 | 0.0 | 0.00 | 0.00 | 0 |
| | | Pepsi Cola | | | | | | | | | | | | | | | |
| 20268 | 1 1/2 cup | Caff free | 360 | 150 | 86 | 0.0 | 41.0 | 0.0 | 41.0 | 0.0 | 0.0 | 0.0 | 0.0 | 0.0 | 0.00 | 0.00 | 0 |
| 20167 | 1 1/2 cup | Diet | 360 | 0 | 100 | 0.0 | 0.0 | 0.0 | 0.0 | 0.0 | 0.0 | 0.0 | 0.0 | 0.0 | 0.00 | 0.00 | 0 |
| 20269 | 1 1/2 cup | Diet, caff free | 360 | 0 | 100 | 0.0 | 0.0 | 0.0 | 0.0 | 0.0 | 0.0 | 0.0 | 0.0 | 0.0 | 0.00 | 0.00 | 0 |
| 20166 | 1 1/2 cup | Regular | 360 | 150 | 88 | 0.0 | 41.0 | 0.0 | 41.0 | 0.0 | 0.0 | 0.0 | 0.0 | 0.0 | 0.00 | 0.00 | 0 |
| 20270 | 1 1/2 cup | Wild Cherry | 360 | 160 | 86 | 0.0 | 43.0 | 0.0 | 43.0 | 0.0 | 0.0 | 0.0 | 0.0 | 0.0 | 0.00 | 0.00 | 0 |
| 20533 | 1 1/2 cup | Pineapple, Minute Maid | 376 | 164 | 88 | 0.0 | 45.1 | 0.0 | 45.1 | 0.0 | 0.0 | 0.0 | 0.0 | 0.0 | 0.00 | 0.00 | 0 |
| | | Root Beer | | | | | | | | | | | | | | | |
| 20009 | 1 1/2 cup | Avg | 370 | 152 | 89 | 0.0 | 39.2 | 0.0 | 39.2 | 0.0 | 0.0 | 0.0 | 0.0 | 0.0 | 0.00 | 0.00 | 0 |
| 20518 | 1 1/2 cup | Barqs | 376 | 167 | 88 | 0.0 | 45.0 | 0.0 | 45.0 | 0.0 | 0.0 | 0.0 | 0.0 | 0.0 | 0.00 | 0.00 | 0 |
| 20485 | 1 1/2 cup | Diet, avg | 370 | 0 | 100 | 0.0 | 0.4 | 0.0 | | | 0.0 | 0.0 | 0.0 | 0.0 | 0.00 | 0.00 | 0 |
| 20519 | 1 1/2 cup | Diet, Barqs | 359 | 1 | 100 | 0.0 | 0.1 | 0.0 | 0.1 | 0.0 | 0.0 | 0.0 | 0.0 | 0.0 | 0.00 | 0.00 | 0 |
| 20275 | 1 1/2 cup | Diet, Mug | 360 | 0 | 100 | 0.0 | 0.0 | 0.0 | 0.0 | 0.0 | 0.0 | 0.0 | 0.0 | 0.0 | 0.00 | 0.00 | 0 |
| 20409 | 1 1/2 cup | Mug | 360 | 160 | | 0.0 | 43.0 | 0.0 | 43.0 | 0.0 | 0.0 | 0.0 | 0.0 | 0.0 | 0.00 | 0.00 | 0 |

| Code | Description | Vit A (IU) | Vit A (RE) | Retinol (RE) | Carotenoids (RE) | Beta Carotene (mcg) | Thiamin (mg) | Riboflavin(mg) | Niacin (NE) | Vit B6 (mg) | Vit B12 (mcg) | Folate (mcg) | Panto (mg) | Vit C (mg) | Vit D (mg) | Vit E (α TE) | Calcium (mg) | Copper (mg) | Iron (mg) | Magnes (mg) | Mang (mg) | Phos (mg) | Potassium (mg) | Selenium (mcg) | Sodium (mg) | Zinc (mg) |
|---|---|---|---|---|---|---|---|---|---|---|---|---|---|---|---|---|---|---|---|---|---|---|---|---|---|---|
| | **BEVERAGE AND BEVERAGE MIXES** | | | | | | | | | | | | | | | | | | | | | | | | | |
| | *CARBONATED DRINKS, 1 1/2 cups, 12 fl oz* | | | | | | | | | | | | | | | | | | | | | | | | | |
| 20467 | Birch Beer, diet, Shasta | | | | | | | | | | 0.00 | | | | | | | | | | | | | | 55 | |
| | Black Cherry | | | | | | | | | | | | | | | | | | | | | | | | | |
| 20462 | Diet, Shasta | | | | | | | | | | 0.00 | | | | | | | | | | | | | | 45 | |
| 20528 | Minute Maid | 0 | 0 | 0 | 0 | 0 | | | | | | | | 0.0 | | | 0 | | 0.0 | | | 0 | 0 | | 16 | |
| 20170 | Shasta | 0 | 0 | 0 | 0 | 0 | | | | | 0.00 | | | | | | | | | | | | 0 | | 45 | |
| 20529 | Blueberry, Minute Maid | 0 | 0 | 0 | 0 | 0 | | | | | | | | 0.0 | | | 0 | | 0.0 | | | 0 | 0 | | 14 | |
| 20171 | Cherry Cola, Shasta | | | | | | | | | | 0.00 | | | | | | | | | | | 58 | 0 | | 45 | |
| 20481 | Cherry Cola, diet, Shasta | | | | | | | | | | 0.00 | | | | | | | | | | | | | | 45 | |
| 20006 | Club Soda, avg | 0 | 0 | 0 | 0 | 0 | 0.00 | 0.00 | 0.00 | 0.00 | 0.00 | 0.0 | 0.00 | 0.0 | 0.0 | 0.0 | 18 | 0.0 | 0.0 | 4 | 0.0 | 0 | 7 | 0.0 | 75 | 0.35 |
| 20028 | Cream Soda, avg | 0 | 0 | 0 | 0 | 0 | 0.00 | 0.00 | 0.00 | 0.00 | 0.00 | 0.0 | 0.00 | 0.0 | 0.0 | 0.0 | 19 | 0.0 | 0.2 | 4 | 0.0 | 0 | 4 | 0.0 | 45 | 0.26 |
| 20624 | Cream Soda, diet, avg | 0 | 0 | 0 | 0 | 0 | 0.00 | 0.00 | 0.00 | 0.00 | 0.00 | 0.0 | | 0.0 | 0.0 | 0.0 | 14 | 0.1 | 0.1 | 4 | 0.0 | 39 | 7 | | 57 | 0.18 |
| | Cola | | | | | | | | | | | | | | | | | | | | | | | | | |
| 20005 | Avg | 0 | 0 | 0 | 0 | 0 | 0.00 | 0.00 | 0.00 | 0.00 | 0.00 | 0.0 | 0.00 | 0.0 | 0.0 | 0.0 | 11 | 0.0 | 0.1 | 4 | 0.1 | 45 | 4 | 0.4 | 15 | 0.04 |
| 20030 | Diet, avg | 0 | 0 | 0 | 0 | 0 | 0.02 | 0.08 | 0.00 | 0.00 | 0.00 | 0.0 | 0.00 | 0.0 | 0.0 | 0.0 | 14 | 0.0 | 0.1 | 4 | 0.1 | 32 | 0 | 0.4 | 21 | 0.28 |
| 20473 | Diet, caff free, Shasta | | | | | | | | | | 0.00 | | | | | | | | | | | | | | 45 | |
| | Coca Cola | | | | | | | | | | | | | | | | | | | | | | | | | |
| 20148 | Classic | 0 | 0 | 0 | 0 | 0 | 0.00 | 0.00 | 0.00 | 0.00 | 0.00 | 0.0 | 0.00 | 0.0 | 0.0 | 0.0 | 13 | 0.0 | 0.1 | 4 | | 61 | 0 | | 13 | 0.04 |
| 20513 | Classic, caff free | 0 | 0 | 0 | 0 | 0 | | | | | | | | 0.0 | | | 0 | | 0.0 | | | 61 | 0 | | 13 | |
| 20514 | Classic, diet | 0 | 0 | 0 | 0 | 0 | | | | | | | | 0.0 | | | 0 | | 0.0 | | | 27 | 18 | | 6 | |
| 20149 | Cherry | 0 | 0 | 0 | 0 | 0 | 0.00 | 0.00 | 0.00 | 0.00 | 0.00 | 0.0 | | 0.0 | 0.0 | 0.0 | 10 | 0.0 | 0.1 | 3 | | 55 | 0 | | 6 | 0.03 |
| 20515 | Cherry, diet | 0 | 0 | 0 | 0 | 0 | | | | | | | | 0.0 | | | 0 | | 0.0 | | | 27 | 18 | | 6 | |
| 20433 | Fruit Flvd Punch, avg | 0 | 0 | 0 | 0 | 0 | 0.00 | 0.00 | 0.02 | 0.00 | 0.00 | 0.0 | 0.00 | 0.0 | 0.0 | 0.0 | 15 | 0.1 | 0.3 | 4 | 0.0 | 2 | 20 | 0.0 | 48 | 0.27 |
| 20008 | Ginger Ale, avg | 0 | 0 | 0 | 0 | 0 | 0.00 | 0.00 | 0.00 | 0.00 | 0.00 | 0.0 | 0.00 | 0.0 | 0.0 | 0.0 | 11 | 0.1 | 0.7 | 4 | 0.0 | 0 | 4 | 0.4 | 26 | 0.18 |
| 20627 | Ginger Ale, diet, avg | 0 | 0 | 0 | 0 | 0 | 0.00 | 0.00 | 0.00 | 0.00 | 0.00 | 0.0 | | 0.0 | 0.0 | 0.0 | 14 | 0.1 | 0.1 | 4 | | 39 | 7 | | 57 | 0.18 |
| 20031 | Grape, avg | 0 | 0 | 0 | 0 | 0 | 0.00 | 0.00 | 0.00 | 0.00 | 0.00 | 0.0 | 0.00 | 0.0 | 0.0 | 0.0 | 11 | 0.1 | 0.3 | 4 | 0.0 | 0 | 4 | 0.0 | 56 | 0.26 |
| 20460 | Grape, diet, Shasta | | | | | | | | | | 0.00 | | | | | | | | | | | | | | 45 | |
| 20192 | Grapefruit, diet, Shasta | | | | | | | | | | 0.00 | | | | | | | | | | | 0 | 8 | | 55 | |
| | Lemon-Lime | | | | | | | | | | | | | | | | | | | | | | | | | |
| 20032 | Avg | 0 | 0 | 0 | 0 | 0 | 0.00 | 0.00 | 0.06 | 0.00 | 0.00 | 0.0 | 0.00 | 0.0 | 0.0 | 0.0 | 7 | 0.0 | 0.3 | 4 | 0.0 | 0 | 4 | 0.0 | 40 | 0.18 |
| 20536 | Diet, Fresca | 0 | 0 | 0 | 0 | 0 | | | | | | | | 0.0 | | | 0 | | 0.0 | | | | 82 | | 1 | |
| 20207 | Diet, 7-Up | 0 | 0 | 0 | 0 | 0 | 0.00 | 0.00 | | 0.00 | 0.00 | | | 0.0 | | | 7 | | 0.2 | | | | 27 | | 10 | |
| 20209 | Diet, 7-Up Gold | 0 | 0 | 0 | 0 | 0 | | | | | 0.00 | | | | | | | | | | | 68 | | | 70 | |
| 20068 | Diet, Slice | 0 | 0 | 0 | 0 | 0 | | | | | 0.00 | | | 0.0 | | | 0 | | 0.0 | | | 0 | | | 35 | |
| 20164 | Diet, Sprite | 0 | 0 | 0 | 0 | 0 | 0.00 | 0.00 | 0.00 | 0.00 | 0.00 | 0.0 | | 0.0 | 0.0 | 0.0 | 15 | 0.1 | 0.1 | | | 0 | 100 | | 0 | 0.18 |
| 20055 | 7-Up | 0 | 0 | 0 | 0 | 0 | 0.00 | 0.00 | | 0.00 | 0.00 | | | 0.0 | 0.0 | 0.0 | 1 | | 0.1 | | | | 8 | | 3 | |
| 20208 | 7-Up Gold | 0 | 0 | 0 | 0 | 0 | | | | | 0.00 | | | | | | | | | | | 68 | | | 70 | |
| 20408 | Slice | 0 | 0 | 0 | 0 | 0 | | | | | 0.00 | | | 0.0 | | | 0 | | 0.0 | | | 0 | | | 55 | |
| 20163 | Sprite | 0 | 0 | 0 | 0 | 0 | 0.00 | 0.00 | 0.07 | 0.00 | 0.00 | 0.0 | 0.00 | 0.0 | 0.0 | 0.0 | 7 | 0.0 | 0.3 | 3 | 0.0 | 0 | 0 | | 34 | 0.19 |
| | Mountain Dew | | | | | | | | | | | | | | | | | | | | | | | | | |
| 20407 | Caff free | 0 | 0 | 0 | 0 | 0 | | | | | 0.00 | | | 0.0 | | | 0 | | 0.0 | | | 0 | | | 70 | |
| 20272 | Diet | 0 | 0 | 0 | 0 | 0 | | | | | 0.00 | | | 0.0 | | | 0 | | 0.0 | | | 0 | | | 35 | |
| 20273 | Diet, caff free | 0 | 0 | 0 | 0 | 0 | | | | | 0.00 | | | 0.0 | | | 0 | | 0.0 | | | 0 | | | 35 | |
| 20271 | Regular | 0 | 0 | 0 | 0 | 0 | | | | | 0.00 | | | 0.0 | | | 0 | | 0.0 | | | 0 | | | 70 | |
| | Orange | | | | | | | | | | | | | | | | | | | | | | | | | |
| 20029 | Avg | 0 | 0 | 0 | 0 | 0 | 0.00 | 0.00 | 0.00 | 0.00 | 0.00 | 0.0 | 0.00 | 0.0 | 0.0 | 0.0 | 19 | 0.1 | 0.2 | 4 | 0.0 | 4 | 7 | 0.0 | 45 | 0.37 |
| 20527 | Diet, Minute Maid | 0 | 0 | 0 | 0 | 0 | | | | | | | | 0.0 | | | 0 | | 0.0 | | | 0 | 65 | | 0 | |
| 20153 | Fanta | 0 | 0 | 0 | 0 | 0 | 0.00 | 0.00 | 0.08 | 0.00 | 0.00 | 0.0 | 0.00 | 0.0 | 0.0 | 0.0 | 8 | 0.0 | 0.3 | 3 | | 0 | 0 | | 14 | 0.19 |
| 20160 | Minute Maid | 0 | 0 | 0 | 0 | 0 | 0.00 | 0.00 | 0.00 | 0.00 | 0.00 | 0.0 | 0.00 | 0.0 | 0.0 | 0.0 | 8 | 0.0 | 0.3 | 3 | | 0 | 21 | | 0 | 0.19 |
| 20477 | Peach, Shasta | | | | | | | | | | 0.00 | | | | | | | | | | | | | | 45 | |
| | Pepsi Cola | | | | | | | | | | | | | | | | | | | | | | | | | |
| 20268 | Caff free | 0 | 0 | 0 | 0 | 0 | | | | | 0.00 | | | 0.0 | | | 0 | | 0.0 | | | 53 | | | 35 | |
| 20167 | Diet | 0 | 0 | 0 | 0 | 0 | | | | | 0.00 | | | 0.0 | | | 0 | | 0.0 | | | 41 | 8 | | 35 | |
| 20269 | Diet, caff free | 0 | 0 | 0 | 0 | 0 | | | | | 0.00 | | | 0.0 | | | 0 | | 0.0 | | | 41 | | | 35 | |
| 20166 | Regular | 0 | 0 | 0 | 0 | 0 | | | | | 0.00 | | | 0.0 | | | 0 | | 0.0 | | | 53 | | | 35 | |
| 20270 | Wild Cherry | 0 | 0 | 0 | 0 | 0 | | | | | 0.00 | | | 0.0 | | | 0 | | 0.0 | | | 53 | | | 35 | |
| 20533 | Pineapple, Minute Maid | 0 | 0 | 0 | 0 | 0 | | | | | | | | 0.0 | | | 0 | | 0.0 | | | 0 | 0 | | 14 | |
| | Root Beer | | | | | | | | | | | | | | | | | | | | | | | | | |
| 20009 | Avg | 0 | 0 | 0 | 0 | 0 | 0.00 | 0.00 | 0.00 | 0.00 | 0.00 | 0.0 | 0.00 | 0.0 | 0.0 | 0.0 | 19 | 0.0 | 0.2 | 4 | 0.0 | 0 | 4 | 0.4 | 48 | 0.26 |
| 20518 | Barqs | 0 | 0 | 0 | 0 | 0 | | | | | | | | 0.0 | | | 0 | | 0.0 | | | 0 | | | 36 | |
| 20485 | Diet, avg | 0 | 0 | 0 | 0 | 0 | 0.00 | 0.00 | 0.00 | 0.00 | 0.00 | 0.0 | | 0.0 | | 0.0 | 15 | 0.1 | 0.1 | 4 | | 41 | 7 | | 59 | 0.19 |
| 20519 | Diet, Barqs | 0 | 0 | 0 | 0 | 0 | | | | | | | | 0.0 | | | 0 | | 0.0 | | | 0 | | | 36 | |
| 20275 | Diet, Mug | 0 | 0 | 0 | 0 | 0 | | | | | 0.00 | | | 0.0 | | | 0 | | 0.0 | | | 0 | | | 65 | |
| 20409 | Mug | 0 | 0 | 0 | 0 | 0 | | | | | 0.00 | | | 0.0 | | | 0 | | 0.0 | | | 0 | | | 65 | |

| Code | Amount | Description | Weight (g) | Calories | % Water | Protein (g) | Carbs (g) | Fiber (g) | Sugar (g) | Other Carbs (g) | Fat (g) | Sat Fat (g) | Mono Fat (g) | Poly Fat (g) | Omega 3 (g) | Omega 6 (g) | Choles (mg) | Vit A (IU) | Vit A (RE) | Retinol (RE) | Carotenoids (RE) | Beta Carotene (mcg) | Thiamin (mg) | Riboflavin (mg) | Niacin (NE) | Vit B6 (mg) | Vit B12 (mcg) | Folate (mcg) | Panto (mg) | Vit C (mg) | Vit D (mg) | Vit E (α TE) | Calcium (mg) | Copper (mg) | Iron (mg) | Magnes (mg) | Mang (mg) | Phos (mg) | Potassium (mg) | Selenium (mcg) | Sodium (mg) | Zinc (mg) |
|---|---|---|---|---|---|---|---|---|---|---|---|---|---|---|---|---|---|---|---|---|---|---|---|---|---|---|---|---|---|---|---|---|---|---|---|---|---|---|---|---|---|---|
| | | | **Basic Components** | | | | | | | | | **Additional Fats** | | | | | | **Vit A & Components** | | | | | **Vitamins** | | | | | | | | | | **Minerals** | | | | | | | | | |
| 20169 | 1 1/2 ea | Royal Crown Cola | 537 | 260 | 84 | 0.0 | 64.8 | | | | 0.0 | 0.0 | 0.0 | 0.0 | 0.00 | 0.00 | 0 | | | | | | | | | | 0.00 | | | | | | | | | | | | 90 | | 2 | |
| 20173 | 1 1/2 ea | Royal Crown Cola, Diet Rite | 537 | 2 | 100 | 0.0 | 0.3 | | | | 0.0 | 0.0 | 0.0 | 0.0 | 0.00 | 0.00 | 0 | | | | | | | | | | 0.00 | | | | | | | | | | | | 90 | | 15 | |
| 20534 | 1 1/2 cup | Strawberry, Minute Maid | 377 | 183 | 87 | 0.0 | 49.5 | 0.0 | 49.5 | 0.0 | 0.0 | 0.0 | 0.0 | 0.0 | 0.00 | 0.00 | 0 | 0 | 0 | 0 | 0 | 0 | | | | | | | | 0.0 | | | 0 | | 0.0 | | | 0 | 0 | | 14 | |
| 20165 | 1 1/2 cup | Tab | 359 | 1 | 100 | 0.0 | 0.4 | 0.0 | 0.0 | 0.4 | 0.0 | 0.0 | 0.0 | 0.0 | 0.00 | 0.00 | 0 | 0 | 0 | 0 | 0 | 0 | 0.00 | 0.00 | | 0.00 | 0.00 | 0.0 | | 0.0 | 0.0 | 0.0 | 12 | | 0.1 | | | 45 | 18 | | 6 | |
| | | *COFFEE AND SUBSTITUTES* | | | | | | | | | | | | | | | | | | | | | | | | | | | | | | | | | | | | | | | | |
| 20012 | 1 cup | Brewed Coffee, avg | 237 | 5 | 99 | 0.2 | 0.9 | 0.0 | 0.0 | 0.9 | 0.0 | 0.0 | 0.0 | 0.0 | 0.00 | 0.00 | 0 | 0 | 0 | 0 | 0 | 0 | 0.00 | 0.00 | 0.53 | 0.00 | 0.00 | 0.2 | 0.00 | 0.0 | 0.0 | 0.0 | 5 | 0.0 | 0.1 | 12 | 0.1 | 2 | 128 | 0.2 | 5 | 0.05 |
| 20065 | 1 cup | Brewed Coffee, decaf, avg | 240 | 5 | 99 | 0.2 | 1.0 | 0.0 | 1.0 | 0.0 | 0.0 | 0.0 | 0.0 | 0.0 | 0.00 | 0.00 | 0 | 0 | 0 | 0 | 0 | 0 | 0.00 | 0.00 | 0.53 | 0.00 | 0.00 | 0.2 | 0.00 | 0.0 | 0.0 | 0.0 | 5 | 0.0 | 0.1 | 12 | 0.0 | 2 | 130 | | 5 | 0.05 |
| | | Cappuccino | | | | | | | | | | | | | | | | | | | | | | | | | | | | | | | | | | | | | | | | |
| 20252 | 1 cup | Cinnamon, Maxwell House | 257 | 90 | 92 | 2.0 | 16.0 | 0.0 | 16.0 | 0.0 | 1.5 | 0.0 | | | | | 0 | 0 | 0 | 0 | 0 | 0 | | | | | 0.00 | | | 0.0 | | | 60 | | 0.0 | | | | 150 | | 70 | |
| 20248 | 1 cup | Iced, Maxwell House | 236 | 130 | | 2.0 | 24.0 | 0.0 | 21.0 | 3.0 | 2.5 | 1.5 | | | | | 5 | 0 | 0 | 0 | 0 | 0 | | | | | 0.00 | | | 0.0 | | | 100 | | 0.0 | | | | 280 | | 120 | |
| 20232 | 1 cup | Italian, General Foods | 249 | 50 | 95 | 0.5 | 10.0 | 0.0 | 8.0 | 2.0 | 1.5 | 0.5 | | | | | 0 | 0 | 0 | 0 | 0 | 0 | | | | | 0.00 | | | 0.0 | | | 0 | | 0.0 | | | | 85 | | 50 | |
| 20258 | 1 cup | Mocha, decaf, Maxwell House | 259 | 100 | 92 | 2.0 | 17.0 | 0.0 | 16.0 | 1.0 | 2.5 | 1.0 | | | | | 0 | 0 | 0 | 0 | 0 | 0 | | | | | 0.00 | | | 0.0 | | | 60 | | 0.0 | | | | 150 | | 70 | |
| 20256 | 1 cup | Mocha, Maxwell House | 259 | 100 | 92 | 2.0 | 17.0 | 0.0 | 16.0 | 1.0 | 2.5 | 1.0 | | | | | 0 | 0 | 0 | 0 | 0 | 0 | | | | | 0.00 | | | 0.0 | | | 80 | | 0.0 | | | | 160 | | 70 | |
| 20235 | 1 cup | Orange, General Foods | 252 | 70 | 94 | 0.5 | 11.0 | 0.0 | 9.0 | 2.0 | 2.0 | 0.5 | | | | | 0 | 0 | 0 | 0 | 0 | 0 | | | | | 0.00 | | | 0.0 | | | 0 | | 0.0 | | | | 140 | | 100 | |
| 20244 | 1 cup | Orange, sugar free, General Foods | 243 | 30 | 98 | 0.5 | 3.0 | 0.0 | 0.0 | 3.0 | 1.5 | 0.5 | | | | | 0 | 0 | 0 | 0 | 0 | 0 | | | | | 0.00 | | | 0.0 | | | 0 | | 0.0 | | | | 110 | | 75 | |
| 20044 | 1 cup | Plain, w/sugar, avg | 256 | 82 | 93 | 0.5 | 14.3 | 0.0 | 9.5 | 4.9 | 2.8 | 2.4 | 0.2 | 0.1 | 0.00 | 0.05 | 0 | 0 | 0 | 0 | 0 | 0 | 0.02 | 0.01 | 0.43 | 0.00 | 0.00 | 0.0 | 0.01 | 0.0 | 0.0 | | 10 | 0.0 | 0.2 | 13 | 0.0 | 36 | 159 | 0.5 | 138 | 0.10 |
| 20254 | 1 cup | Plain, Maxwell House | 258 | 90 | 92 | 1.0 | 18.0 | 0.0 | 17.0 | 1.0 | 1.0 | 0.0 | | | | | 0 | 0 | 0 | 0 | 0 | 0 | | | | | 0.00 | | | 0.0 | | | 40 | | 0.0 | | | | 180 | | 65 | |
| 20262 | 1 cup | Vanilla, decaf, Maxwell House | 258 | 90 | 92 | 1.0 | 19.0 | 0.0 | 18.0 | 1.0 | 1.0 | 0.0 | | | | | 0 | 0 | 0 | 0 | 0 | 0 | | | | | 0.00 | | | 0.0 | | | 60 | | 0.0 | | | | 90 | | 65 | |
| 20260 | 1 cup | Vanilla, Maxwell House | 258 | 90 | 92 | 1.0 | 19.0 | 0.0 | 18.0 | 1.0 | 1.0 | 0.0 | | | | | 0 | 0 | 0 | 0 | 0 | 0 | | | | | 0.00 | | | 0.0 | | | 60 | | 0.0 | | | | 105 | | 65 | |
| 20439 | 1 cup | Espresso, brewed, avg | 237 | 21 | 98 | 0.0 | 3.6 | 0.0 | 0.0 | 3.6 | 0.4 | 0.2 | 0.0 | 0.2 | 0.00 | 0.21 | 0 | 0 | 0 | 0 | 0 | 0 | 0.00 | 0.42 | 12.35 | 0.00 | 0.00 | 2.4 | 0.07 | 0.5 | 0.0 | 0.0 | 5 | 0.1 | 0.3 | 190 | 0.1 | 17 | 273 | 0.0 | 33 | 0.12 |
| 20064 | 1 cup | Espresso, brewed, decaf, avg | 240 | 5 | 99 | 0.2 | 1.0 | 0.0 | 1.0 | 0.0 | 0.0 | 0.0 | 0.0 | 0.0 | 0.00 | 0.00 | 0 | 0 | 0 | 0 | 0 | 0 | 0.00 | 0.00 | 0.53 | 0.00 | 0.00 | 0.2 | 0.00 | 0.0 | 0.0 | 0.0 | 5 | 0.0 | 0.1 | 12 | 0.0 | 2 | 130 | | 5 | 0.05 |
| 20593 | 1 1/2 cup | Frappuccino, Tall, Starbucks | 344 | 290 | | 8.0 | 59.0 | 1.0 | 3.1 | 54.9 | 2.0 | 1.0 | | | | | 15 | 1250 | 250 | | | | 0.38 | 0.43 | 5.00 | 0.50 | 1.50 | 100.0 | 2.50 | 15.0 | 2.5 | | | | | | | | 270 | | 230 | |
| | | Instant Coffee | | | | | | | | | | | | | | | | | | | | | | | | | | | | | | | | | | | | | | | | |
| 20013 | 1 tsp | Powdered, avg | 2 | 5 | 3 | 0.2 | 0.8 | 0.0 | 0.5 | 0.3 | 0.0 | 0.0 | 0.0 | 0.0 | 0.00 | 0.00 | 0 | 0 | 0 | 0 | 0 | 0 | 0.00 | 0.00 | 0.56 | 0.00 | 0.00 | 0.0 | 0.00 | 0.0 | 0.0 | 0.0 | 3 | 0.0 | 0.1 | 7 | 0.0 | 6 | 71 | 0.3 | 1 | 0.01 |
| 20090 | 1 tsp | Powdered, decaf, avg | 2 | 4 | 3 | 0.2 | 0.9 | 0.0 | 0.5 | 0.3 | 0.0 | 0.0 | 0.0 | 0.0 | 0.00 | 0.00 | 0 | 0 | 0 | 0 | 0 | 0 | 0.00 | 0.03 | 0.56 | 0.00 | 0.00 | 0.0 | 0.00 | 0.0 | 0.0 | 0.0 | 3 | 0.0 | 0.1 | 6 | 0.0 | 6 | 70 | 0.2 | 0 | 0.00 |
| 20089 | 1 cup | Pre-lightened, prep, avg | 180 | 27 | 97 | 0.3 | 2.9 | 0.0 | 2.7 | 0.2 | 1.6 | 1.5 | 0.0 | 0.0 | | | 0 | 9 | 1 | 0 | 1 | | 0.00 | 0.01 | 0.28 | 0.00 | 0.00 | 0.0 | 0.00 | 0.0 | 0.0 | | 5 | 0.0 | 0.1 | 5 | 0.0 | 22 | 72 | | 14 | 0.08 |
| 20023 | 1 cup | Prep f/pwd, avg | 238 | 5 | 99 | 0.2 | 1.0 | 0.0 | 0.6 | 0.4 | 0.0 | 0.0 | 0.0 | 0.0 | 0.00 | 0.00 | 0 | 0 | 0 | 0 | 0 | 0 | 0.00 | 0.00 | 0.67 | 0.00 | 0.00 | 0.0 | 0.00 | 0.0 | 0.0 | 0.0 | 7 | 0.0 | 0.1 | 10 | 0.0 | 7 | 86 | 0.2 | 7 | 0.07 |
| 20091 | 1 cup | Prep f/pwd, decaf, avg | 179 | 4 | 99 | 0.2 | 0.7 | 0.0 | 0.4 | 0.3 | 0.0 | 0.0 | 0.0 | 0.0 | 0.00 | 0.00 | 0 | 0 | 0 | 0 | 0 | 0 | 0.00 | 0.03 | 0.50 | 0.00 | 0.00 | 0.0 | 0.00 | 0.0 | 0.0 | 0.0 | 5 | 0.0 | 0.1 | 7 | 0.0 | 5 | 63 | 0.2 | 5 | 0.05 |
| 20087 | 1 cup | Pre-swtnd w/sugar, prep, avg | 180 | 29 | 96 | 0.1 | 7.0 | 0.0 | 6.8 | 0.2 | 0.0 | 0.0 | 0.0 | 0.0 | | | 0 | 0 | 0 | 0 | 0 | 0 | 0.00 | 0.00 | 0.28 | 0.00 | 0.00 | 0.0 | 0.00 | 0.0 | 0.0 | 0.0 | 5 | 0.0 | 0.1 | 5 | 0.0 | 4 | 36 | | 5 | 0.06 |
| 20088 | 1 cup | Pre-swtnd w/sugar & pre-lightnd, prep, avg | 180 | 50 | 93 | 0.3 | 9.2 | 0.0 | 9.0 | 0.2 | 1.5 | 1.4 | 0.0 | 0.0 | | | 0 | 9 | 1 | 0 | 1 | | 0.00 | 0.01 | 0.27 | 0.00 | 0.00 | 0.0 | 0.00 | 0.0 | 0.0 | | 5 | 0.0 | 0.1 | 5 | 0.0 | 22 | 70 | | 13 | 0.08 |
| 20092 | 2 tsp | With Chicory, pwd, avg | 4 | 14 | 4 | 0.4 | 3.0 | 0.0 | 1.8 | 1.2 | 0.0 | 0.0 | 0.0 | 0.0 | 0.00 | 0.00 | 0 | 0 | 0 | 0 | 0 | 0 | 0.00 | 0.01 | 0.87 | 0.00 | 0.00 | 0.0 | 0.00 | 0.0 | 0.0 | 0.0 | 4 | 0.0 | 0.2 | 9 | 0.0 | 11 | 136 | 0.4 | 11 | 0.01 |
| 20093 | 1 cup | With Chicory, prep f/pwd, avg | 179 | 7 | 99 | 0.2 | 1.3 | 0.0 | 0.8 | 0.5 | 0.0 | 0.0 | 0.0 | 0.0 | 0.00 | 0.00 | 0 | 0 | 0 | 0 | 0 | 0 | 0.00 | 0.01 | 0.39 | 0.00 | 0.00 | 0.0 | 0.00 | 0.0 | 0.0 | 0.0 | 5 | 0.0 | 0.1 | 5 | 0.0 | 5 | 61 | 0.2 | 11 | 0.05 |
| | | Instant Flavored Coffee | | | | | | | | | | | | | | | | | | | | | | | | | | | | | | | | | | | | | | | | |
| 20224 | 1 cup | Amaretto, prep, General Foods | 249 | 60 | 95 | 0.5 | 8.0 | 0.0 | 5.0 | 3.0 | 3.0 | 0.5 | | | | | 0 | 0 | 0 | 0 | 0 | 0 | | | | | 0.00 | | | 0.0 | | | 0 | | 0.0 | | | | 150 | | 105 | |
| 20225 | 1 cup | Francais, prep, General Foods | 249 | 60 | 95 | 0.5 | 7.0 | 0.0 | 5.0 | 2.0 | 3.5 | 1.0 | | | | | 0 | 0 | 0 | 0 | 0 | 0 | | | | | 0.00 | | | 0.0 | | | 0 | | 0.0 | | | | 270 | | 25 | |
| 20096 | 2 tsp | French, w/sugar, dry pwd, avg | 12 | 60 | 2 | 0.5 | 6.9 | 0.0 | 4.5 | 2.4 | 3.6 | 3.1 | 0.2 | 0.1 | 0.00 | 0.06 | 0 | 0 | 0 | 0 | 0 | 0 | 0.00 | 0.00 | 0.70 | 0.00 | 0.00 | 0.0 | 0.00 | 0.0 | 0.0 | 0.0 | 4 | 0.0 | 0.1 | 6 | 0.0 | 42 | 142 | 0.3 | 25 | 0.01 |
| 20108 | 1 cup | French, w/sugar, prep f/pwd, avg | 252 | 76 | 94 | 0.8 | 8.8 | 0.0 | 5.3 | 3.5 | 4.5 | 3.9 | 0.3 | 0.1 | 0.00 | 0.08 | 0 | 0 | 0 | 0 | 0 | 0 | 0.00 | 0.00 | 0.90 | 0.00 | 0.00 | 0.0 | 0.00 | 0.0 | 0.0 | 0.0 | 10 | 0.0 | 0.0 | 3 | 0.0 | 55 | 181 | 0.5 | 40 | 0.05 |
| 20228 | 1 cup | French Vanilla, prep, General Foods | 250 | 60 | 95 | 0.5 | 10.0 | 0.0 | 8.0 | 2.0 | 2.5 | 0.5 | | | | | 0 | 0 | 0 | 0 | 0 | 0 | | | | | 0.00 | | | 0.0 | | | 0 | | 0.0 | | | | 75 | | 55 | |
| 20243 | 1 cup | French Vanilla, sugar free, prep, General Foods | 243 | 35 | 97 | 0.5 | 4.0 | 0.0 | 0.0 | 4.0 | 2.0 | 0.5 | | | | | 0 | 0 | 0 | 0 | 0 | 0 | | | | | 0.00 | | | 0.0 | | | 0 | | 0.0 | | | | 70 | | 55 | |
| 20230 | 1 cup | Hazelnut Belgian, prep, General Foods | 252 | 70 | 94 | 0.5 | 12.0 | 0.0 | 9.0 | 3.0 | 2.0 | 0.5 | | | | | 0 | 0 | 0 | 0 | 0 | 0 | | | | | 0.00 | | | 0.0 | | | 0 | | 0.0 | | | | 130 | | 65 | |
| 20234 | 1 cup | Kahlua, prep, General Foods | 249 | 60 | 95 | 0.5 | 10.0 | 0.0 | 7.0 | 3.0 | 2.0 | 0.5 | | | | | 0 | 0 | 0 | 0 | 0 | 0 | | | | | 0.00 | | | 0.0 | | | 0 | | 0.0 | | | | 80 | | 55 | |
| 20094 | 2 tsp | Mocha, w/sugar, dry pwd, avg | 12 | 53 | 2 | 0.5 | 8.8 | 0.1 | 5.4 | 3.2 | 2.0 | 1.7 | 0.1 | 0.0 | 0.00 | 0.04 | 0 | 0 | 0 | 0 | 0 | 0 | 0.00 | 0.00 | 0.27 | 0.00 | 0.00 | 0.0 | 0.01 | 0.0 | 0.0 | 0.0 | 4 | 0.1 | 0.2 | 8 | 0.1 | 30 | 124 | 0.3 | 32 | 0.12 |
| 20109 | 1 cup | Mocha, w/sugar, prep f/pwd, avg | 250 | 68 | 94 | 0.8 | 11.3 | 0.3 | 7.5 | 3.5 | 2.5 | 2.1 | 0.1 | 0.0 | 0.00 | 0.04 | 0 | 0 | 0 | 0 | 0 | 0 | 0.01 | 0.01 | 0.34 | 0.00 | 0.00 | 0.0 | 0.01 | 0.0 | 0.0 | | 10 | 0.1 | 0.3 | 12 | 0.1 | 38 | 158 | 0.3 | 48 | 0.20 |
| 20236 | 1 cup | Suisse Mocha, prep, General Foods | 249 | 60 | 95 | 0.5 | 8.0 | 0.0 | 6.0 | 2.0 | 2.5 | 0.5 | | | | | 0 | 0 | 0 | 0 | 0 | 0 | | | | | 0.00 | | | 0.0 | | | 0 | | 0.0 | | | | 140 | | 50 | |
| 20238 | 1 cup | Suisse Mocha, decaf, prep, General Foods | 249 | 60 | 95 | 0.5 | 8.0 | 0.0 | 6.0 | 2.0 | 3.0 | 0.5 | | | | | 0 | 0 | 0 | 0 | 0 | 0 | | | | | 0.00 | | | 0.0 | | | 0 | | 0.0 | | | | 130 | | 40 | |
| 20247 | 1 cup | Suisse Mocha, decaf, sugar free, General Foods | 243 | 30 | 97 | 0.5 | 4.0 | 0.0 | 0.0 | 4.0 | 1.5 | 0.5 | | | | | 0 | 0 | 0 | 0 | 0 | 0 | | | | | 0.00 | | | 0.0 | | | 0 | | 0.0 | | | | 115 | | 75 | |
| 20245 | 1 cup | Suisse Mocha, sugar free, prep, General Foods | 243 | 30 | 97 | 0.5 | 4.0 | 0.0 | 0.0 | 4.0 | 2.0 | 0.5 | | | | | 0 | 0 | 0 | 0 | 0 | 0 | | | | | 0.00 | | | 0.0 | | | 0 | | 0.0 | | | | 105 | | 30 | |
| 20043 | 1 cup | Swiss mocha, prep, avg | 188 | 51 | 94 | 0.5 | 8.4 | 0.1 | 4.9 | 3.4 | 1.9 | 1.6 | 0.1 | 0.0 | | | 0 | 0 | 0 | 0 | 0 | 0 | 0.00 | 0.00 | 0.26 | 0.00 | 0.00 | 0.0 | 0.01 | 0.0 | 0.0 | 0.0 | 8 | 0.1 | 0.3 | 9 | 0.1 | 28 | 118 | | 36 | 0.16 |
| 20226 | 1 cup | Vienna, prep, General Foods | 252 | 70 | 94 | 0.5 | 11.0 | 0.0 | 10.0 | 1.0 | 2.5 | 0.5 | | | | | 0 | 0 | 0 | 0 | 0 | 0 | | | | | 0.00 | | | 0.0 | | | 0 | | 0.0 | | | | 130 | | 110 | |
| 20241 | 1 cup | Vienna, sugar free, prep, General Foods | 243 | 30 | 98 | 0.5 | 3.0 | 0.0 | 0.0 | 3.0 | 1.5 | 0.5 | | | | | 0 | 0 | 0 | 0 | 0 | 0 | | | | | 0.00 | | | 0.0 | | | 0 | | 0.0 | | | | 110 | | 75 | |
| 20240 | 1 cup | Viennese Chocolate, prep, Gen Foods | 249 | 60 | 95 | 0.5 | 10.0 | 0.0 | 9.0 | 1.0 | 2.0 | 0.5 | | | | | 0 | 0 | 0 | 0 | 0 | 0 | | | | | 0.00 | | | 0.0 | | | 0 | | 0.0 | | | | 75 | | 30 | |
| | | Substitutes for coffee | | | | | | | | | | | | | | | | | | | | | | | | | | | | | | | | | | | | | | | | |
| 20097 | 1 tsp | Cereal Grain, pwd, avg | 2 | 7 | 5 | 0.1 | 1.6 | 0.2 | | | 0.1 | 0.0 | 0.0 | 0.0 | 0.00 | 0.03 | 0 | 0 | 0 | 0 | 0 | 0 | 0.01 | 0.00 | 0.34 | 0.02 | 0.00 | 0.5 | 0.02 | 0.0 | 0.0 | | 1 | 0.0 | 0.1 | 5 | 0.0 | 12 | 37 | 0.3 | 1 | 0.01 |
| 20048 | 1 cup | Cereal Grain, prep f/pwd, avg | 240 | 12 | 99 | 0.2 | 2.4 | 0.0 | | | 0.0 | 0.0 | 0.0 | 0.0 | 0.00 | 0.00 | 0 | 0 | 0 | 0 | 0 | 0 | 0.02 | 0.00 | 0.52 | 0.03 | 0.00 | 0.7 | 0.02 | 0.0 | 0.0 | 0.0 | 7 | 0.0 | 0.1 | 10 | 0.0 | 17 | 58 | 0.5 | 10 | 0.07 |
| 20128 | 1 cup | Coffee Substitute w/milk, avg | 247 | 161 | 87 | 8.2 | 13.8 | 0.2 | | | 8.2 | 5.1 | 2.4 | 0.4 | 0.13 | 0.23 | 32 | 306 | 77 | | | | 0.03 | 0.40 | 0.72 | 0.10 | 0.86 | 12.1 | 0.77 | 2.2 | 2.3 | | 294 | 0.0 | 0.3 | 40 | 0.0 | 245 | 425 | 13.6 | 121 | 0.94 |
| 20313 | 1 tsp | Instant, coffee flvd, dry pwd, Postum | 3 | 10 | | 0.0 | 3.0 | 0.0 | 0.0 | 3.0 | 0.0 | 0.0 | 0.0 | 0.0 | 0.00 | 0.00 | 0 | 0 | 0 | 0 | 0 | 0 | | | | | 0.00 | | | 0.0 | | | 0 | | 0.0 | | | | 110 | | 0 | |
| 20312 | 1 tsp | Instant, dry pwd, Postum | 3 | 10 | 0 | 3.0 | 0.0 | 0.0 | 0.0 | 0.0 | 0.0 | 0.0 | 0.0 | 0.0 | 0.00 | 0.00 | 0 | 0 | 0 | 0 | 0 | 0 | | | | | 0.00 | | | 0.0 | | | 0 | | 0.0 | | | | 110 | | 0 | |
| | | *DAIRY MIXED DRINKS AND MIXES* | | | | | | | | | | | | | | | | | | | | | | | | | | | | | | | | | | | | | | | | |
| 43 | 1 Tbs | Carob Beverage, dry mix, avg | 12 | 45 | 3 | 0.2 | 11.2 | 1.0 | | | 0.0 | 0.0 | 0.0 | 0.0 | 0.00 | 0.01 | 0 | 0 | 0 | 0 | 0 | 0 | 0.00 | 0.00 | 0.09 | 0.01 | 0.00 | 0.0 | 0.00 | 0.0 | 0.0 | 0.0 | 4 | 0.0 | 0.6 | 1 | 0.0 | 1 | 12 | 0.2 | 12 | 0.01 |
| 44 | 1 cup | Carob Beverage, prep f/mix, avg | 256 | 195 | 84 | 8.2 | 22.5 | 1.0 | | | 8.2 | 5.1 | 2.4 | 0.3 | 0.12 | 0.19 | 33 | 307 | 77 | 72 | 5 | | 0.09 | 0.39 | 0.30 | 0.12 | 0.87 | 12.3 | 0.77 | 2.3 | 2.3 | | 292 | 0.0 | 0.7 | 33 | 0.0 | 228 | 369 | 5.1 | 133 | 0.92 |
| | | Chocolate Drinks & Mixes | | | | | | | | | | | | | | | | | | | | | | | | | | | | | | | | | | | | | | | | |
| 14 | 1 Tbs | Mix, avg | 26 | 91 | 1 | 0.9 | 23.5 | 1.5 | 21.3 | 0.6 | 0.8 | 0.5 | 0.3 | 0.0 | 0.00 | 0.02 | 0 | 5 | 0.5 | 0 | 0.5 | | 0.01 | 0.04 | 0.13 | 0.00 | 0.00 | 1.5 | 0.01 | 0.2 | 0.0 | | 10 | 0.2 | 0.8 | 25 | 0.2 | 33 | 154 | 0.7 | 55 | 0.40 |
| 74 | 1 ea | Mix, sugar free, avg, dry env | 21 | 63 | 13 | 5.3 | 10.5 | 0.3 | 9.9 | 0.3 | 0.5 | 0.4 | 0.1 | 0.0 | 0.00 | 0.01 | 2 | 242 | 72 | | | | 0.02 | 0.41 | 0.26 | 0.02 | 0.50 | 8.8 | 0.45 | 0.3 | | | 185 | 0.2 | 1.6 | 44 | 0.2 | 179 | 470 | 3.2 | 164 | 0.76 |
| 39 | 1 cup | Prep w/milk, avg | 266 | 226 | 81 | 8.8 | 30.9 | 1.3 | 29.5 | 0.0 | 8.3 | 5.5 | 2.6 | 0.3 | 0.12 | 0.20 | 32 | 311 | 77 | 72 | 5 | | 0.10 | 0.43 | 0.32 | 0.10 | 0.88 | 12.2 | 0.77 | 2.4 | 4.0 | | 301 | 0.2 | 0.8 | 53 | 0.2 | 255 | 497 | 5.3 | 165 | 1.28 |
| 151 | 1 cup | Prep w/water, sugar free, avg | 272 | 84 | 91 | 7.1 | 14.1 | 0.5 | 12.8 | 0.8 | 0.8 | 0.5 | 0.1 | 0.0 | 0.00 | 0.02 | 3 | 326 | 98 | | | | 0.03 | 0.55 | 0.36 | 0.03 | 0.68 | 12.0 | 0.61 | 0.3 | 0.0 | | 256 | 0.2 | 2.2 | 63 | 0.2 | 242 | 639 | 4.4 | 228 | 1.09 |

| Code | Amount | Description | Basic Components | | | | | | | | | Additional Fats | | | | | | Vit A & Components | | | | | Vitamins | | | | | | | | | | Minerals | | | | | | | | | |
|---|---|---|---|---|---|---|---|---|---|---|---|---|---|---|---|---|---|---|---|---|---|---|---|---|---|---|---|---|---|---|---|---|---|---|---|---|---|---|---|---|---|---|
| | | | Weight (g) | Calories | % Water | Protein (g) | Carbs (g) | Fiber (g) | Sugar (g) | Other Carbs (g) | Fat (g) | Sat Fat (g) | Mono Fat (g) | Poly Fat (g) | Omega 3 (g) | Omega 6 (g) | Choles (mg) | Vit A (IU) | Vit A (RE) | Retinol (RE) | Carotenoids (RE) | Beta Carotene (mcg) | Thiamin (mg) | Riboflavin (mg) | Niacin (NE) | Vit B6 (mg) | Vit B12 (mcg) | Folate (mcg) | Panto (mg) | Vit C (mg) | Vit D (mg) | Vit E (α TE) | Calcium (mg) | Copper (mg) | Iron (mg) | Magnes (mg) | Mang (mg) | Phos (mg) | Potassium (mg) | Selenium (mcg) | Sodium (mg) | Zinc (mg) |
| 37 | 1 Tbs | Chocolate Malt, dry mix, avg | 5 | 18 | 2 | 0.2 | 4.2 | 0.0 | 2.0 | 2.1 | 0.2 | 0.1 | 0.0 | 0.0 | 0.00 | 0.01 | 0 | 655 | 196 | | | | 0.15 | 0.21 | 2.55 | 0.22 | 0.01 | 4.7 | 0.03 | 7.5 | 1.1 | | 22 | 0.0 | 0.9 | 5 | 0.0 | 20 | 60 | 0.4 | 30 | 0.05 |
| 38 | 1 cup | Chocolate Malt, prep f/mix, avg | 265 | 225 | 81 | 9.0 | 29.2 | 0.3 | 17.2 | 11.7 | 8.7 | 5.5 | 2.6 | 0.4 | 0.13 | 0.24 | 34 | 3058 | 901 | | | | 0.73 | 1.26 | 10.89 | 1.02 | 0.87 | 31.8 | 0.91 | 33.9 | 10.6 | | 384 | 0.2 | 3.8 | 53 | 0.1 | 313 | 620 | 6.4 | 244 | 1.17 |
| | | Chocolate Milk | | | | | | | | | | | | | | | | | | | | | | | | | | | | | | | | | | | | | | | | |
| 86 | 1 cup | Prep w/lowfat milk & syrup, avg | 250 | 180 | 82 | 7.8 | 30.2 | 0.6 | 27.9 | 1.7 | 4.5 | 2.8 | 1.3 | 0.2 | | | 15 | 454 | 124 | 119 | 5 | | 0.09 | 0.38 | 0.30 | 0.09 | 0.79 | 12.4 | | 2.1 | | | 268 | 0.2 | 0.8 | 52 | | 250 | 410 | 4.8 | 140 | 1.09 |
| 87 | 1 cup | Prep w/nonfat milk & syrup, avg | 250 | 150 | 84 | 8.0 | 30.3 | 0.6 | 27.9 | 1.7 | 0.7 | 0.4 | 0.2 | 0.0 | | | 5 | 452 | 133 | 132 | 1 | | 0.08 | 0.32 | 0.30 | 0.09 | 0.82 | 12.6 | | 2.2 | | | 272 | 0.2 | 0.8 | 48 | | 262 | 432 | 4.8 | 142 | 1.11 |
| 70 | 1 cup | Prep w/whole milk & syrup, avg | 263 | 197 | 84 | 8.4 | 23.7 | 0.3 | 21.8 | 1.6 | 8.4 | 5.2 | 2.4 | 0.3 | 0.11 | 0.20 | 34 | 1126 | 321 | | | | 0.09 | 0.55 | 6.52 | 0.11 | 0.87 | 12.1 | 0.77 | 2.4 | 3.9 | | 292 | 0.0 | 2.7 | 32 | 0.0 | 229 | 460 | 5.0 | 147 | 0.92 |
| | | Cocoa | | | | | | | | | | | | | | | | | | | | | | | | | | | | | | | | | | | | | | | | |
| 48 | 1 cup | Hot, prep w/water, avg | 275 | 138 | 86 | 4.1 | 30.0 | 3.3 | 26.7 | 0.0 | 1.7 | 0.9 | 0.5 | 0.0 | 0.00 | 0.04 | 3 | 6 | 0.5 | 0 | 0.5 | | 0.04 | 0.21 | 0.22 | 0.04 | 0.50 | 0.0 | 0.34 | 0.6 | 0.0 | | 129 | 0.1 | 0.5 | 33 | 0.1 | 118 | 270 | 1.1 | 198 | 0.61 |
| 77 | 1 cup | Hot, prep w/water, low cal, avg | 256 | 64 | 92 | 5.1 | 11.3 | 0.5 | 10.9 | 0.0 | 0.5 | 0.3 | 0.2 | 0.0 | 0.00 | 0.02 | 3 | 320 | 72 | | | | 0.05 | 0.28 | 0.22 | 0.06 | 0.38 | 3.1 | 0.76 | 0.0 | 2.3 | | 292 | 0.2 | 1.0 | 44 | 0.1 | 325 | 540 | 3.6 | 138 | 0.74 |
| 21 | 1 cup | Hot, prep w/whole milk, avg | 250 | 192 | 81 | 9.8 | 29.5 | 2.0 | 21.9 | 5.6 | 5.8 | 3.6 | 1.7 | 0.2 | 0.07 | 0.14 | 20 | 515 | 138 | 125 | 12 | | 0.10 | 0.44 | 0.38 | 0.12 | 0.93 | 15.0 | 0.82 | 2.5 | 2.4 | | 315 | 0.3 | 1.1 | 70 | 0.3 | 292 | 500 | 6.8 | 128 | 1.47 |
| 61 | 1 ea | Hot Mix, dry pkt, avg | 31 | 119 | 2 | 1.9 | 23.9 | 0.9 | 22.9 | 0.0 | 3.0 | 1.8 | 1.0 | 0.1 | 0.00 | 0.08 | 1 | 497 | 149 | | | | 0.15 | 0.17 | 1.99 | 0.04 | 0.41 | 0.0 | 0.28 | 6.0 | 2.2 | | 100 | 0.1 | 1.8 | 22 | 0.1 | 110 | 401 | 0.5 | 200 | 0.22 |
| 75 | 1 ea | Hot Mix, low cal, dry pkt, avg | 19 | 61 | 3 | 4.8 | 10.8 | 0.5 | 8.9 | 1.4 | 0.6 | 0.3 | 0.2 | 0.0 | 0.00 | 0.02 | 2 | 304 | 68 | | | | 0.05 | 0.27 | 0.21 | 0.06 | 0.37 | 2.8 | 0.73 | 0.0 | 0.0 | | 274 | 0.1 | 0.9 | 40 | 0.1 | 310 | 513 | 3.5 | 124 | 0.65 |
| 166 | 1 ea | Hot Mix, w/marsh, dry pkt, Carnation | 28 | 112 | 2 | 1.3 | 24.2 | 0.5 | 20.9 | 2.8 | 1.0 | 0.4 | 0.3 | 0.4 | 0.02 | 0.33 | 2 | 0 | 0 | 0 | 0 | 0 | 0.03 | 0.12 | 0.10 | 0.03 | 0.12 | 1.1 | 0.28 | 0.0 | 2.0 | | 41 | 0.1 | 0.2 | 16 | 0.1 | 58 | 142 | | 96 | 0.20 |
| 172 | 1 ea | Hot Mix, Rich Chocolate, dry pkt, Carnation | 28 | 112 | 2 | 1.3 | 24.2 | 0.7 | 20.8 | 2.8 | 1.1 | 0.3 | 0.3 | 0.3 | 0.01 | 0.25 | 2 | 0 | 0 | 0 | 0 | 0 | 0.03 | 0.12 | 0.16 | 0.03 | 0.10 | 2.0 | 0.25 | 0.0 | 2.0 | | 40 | 0.2 | 0.3 | 27 | 0.2 | 71 | 194 | | 102 | 0.36 |
| 83 | 1 cup | Prep w/2% milk, avg | 250 | 185 | 82 | 8.3 | 29.7 | 1.2 | | | 5.0 | 3.1 | 1.5 | 0.2 | | | 18 | 474 | 131 | 127 | 5 | | 0.09 | 0.41 | 0.30 | 0.10 | 0.83 | 12.9 | | 2.3 | | | 288 | 0.2 | 0.8 | 52 | | 245 | 475 | | 158 | 1.22 |
| 84 | 1 cup | Prep w/nonfat milk, avg | 250 | 152 | 83 | 8.5 | 29.8 | 1.2 | | | 1.1 | 0.6 | 0.3 | 0.0 | | | 5 | 472 | 140 | 140 | 0 | | 0.09 | 0.35 | 0.31 | 0.09 | 0.87 | 13.1 | | 2.4 | | | 290 | 0.2 | 0.7 | 48 | | 258 | 502 | | 162 | 1.24 |
| 73 | 1 cup | Prep w/water, avg | 279 | 159 | 85 | 2.5 | 32.1 | 1.1 | 31.0 | 0.0 | 3.9 | 2.4 | 1.3 | 0.1 | 0.01 | 0.11 | 0 | 670 | 201 | | | | 0.20 | 0.23 | 2.68 | 0.05 | 0.56 | 0.0 | 0.37 | 8.1 | 2.6 | | 139 | 0.1 | 2.4 | 31 | 0.1 | 148 | 541 | 0.6 | 276 | 0.36 |
| 227 | 1 cup | Prep w/whole milk, avg | 250 | 212 | 81 | 8.2 | 29.3 | 1.2 | | | 8.3 | 5.1 | 2.4 | 0.3 | | | 30 | 293 | 72 | 65 | 7 | | 0.09 | 0.40 | 0.30 | 0.10 | 0.82 | 12.6 | | 2.3 | | | 282 | 0.2 | 0.8 | 50 | | 240 | 470 | | 155 | 1.19 |
| | | Eggnog | | | | | | | | | | | | | | | | | | | | | | | | | | | | | | | | | | | | | | | | |
| 17 | 1 cup | Avg | 254 | 343 | 74 | 9.7 | 34.3 | 0.0 | 34.3 | 0.0 | 19.0 | 11.3 | 5.7 | 0.9 | 0.26 | 0.59 | 150 | 894 | 203 | 185 | 18 | | 0.09 | 0.48 | 0.27 | 0.13 | 1.14 | 2.3 | 1.06 | 3.8 | 1.1 | | 330 | 0.0 | 0.5 | 46 | 0.0 | 277 | 419 | 10.7 | 137 | 1.17 |
| 45 | 1 Tbs | Mix, avg | 14 | 55 | 0 | 0.1 | 13.6 | 0.4 | | | 0.1 | 0.0 | 0.1 | 0.0 | 0.00 | 0.02 | 3 | 5 | 1.4 | | | | 0.00 | 0.00 | 0.02 | 0.00 | 0.01 | 0.3 | 0.86 | 0.0 | | | 0 | 0.0 | 0.1 | 0 | 0.0 | 1 | 1 | 0.0 | 22 | 0.01 |
| 98 | 1 cup | Mix, prep w/2% milk, avg | 254 | 188 | 85 | 12.1 | 16.6 | 0.0 | 16.4 | 0.2 | 8.1 | 3.7 | 2.7 | 0.7 | | | 193 | 686 | 197 | 193 | 4 | | 0.11 | 0.55 | 0.21 | 0.15 | 1.17 | 30.1 | 1.18 | 1.9 | 0.5 | | 269 | 0.0 | 0.7 | 33 | 0.0 | 269 | 366 | | 155 | 1.26 |
| | | Instant Breakfast | | | | | | | | | | | | | | | | | | | | | | | | | | | | | | | | | | | | | | | | |
| 24 | 1 ea | Mix, avg, dry env | 37 | 131 | 7 | 7.4 | 24.5 | 0.1 | 24.3 | 0.0 | 0.5 | 0.3 | 0.1 | 0.0 | | | 4 | 1844 | 554 | 554 | 0 | | 0.31 | 0.07 | 5.27 | 0.42 | 0.63 | 105.5 | 2.00 | 28.5 | 0.1 | | 105 | 0.5 | 4.7 | 84 | | 158 | 350 | 2.8 | 142 | 3.16 |
| 101 | 1 cup | Prep w/1% milk, avg | 281 | 233 | 79 | 15.4 | 36.2 | 0.2 | 36.0 | 0.0 | 3.1 | 2.0 | 0.9 | 0.1 | 0.04 | 0.06 | 14 | 2344 | 698 | 695 | 3 | | 0.41 | 0.48 | 5.47 | 0.53 | 1.53 | 117.9 | 2.79 | 30.8 | 2.5 | | 406 | 0.6 | 4.9 | 118 | 0.0 | 393 | 731 | 9.2 | 266 | 4.12 |
| 26 | 1 cup | Prep w/2% milk, avg | 281 | 252 | 78 | 15.5 | 36.2 | 0.2 | 36.0 | 0.0 | 5.2 | 3.3 | 1.5 | 0.2 | 0.07 | 0.10 | 23 | 2344 | 693 | 688 | 5 | | 0.41 | 0.48 | 5.46 | 0.53 | 1.52 | 117.9 | 2.78 | 30.8 | 2.5 | | 401 | 0.5 | 4.9 | 118 | 0.0 | 390 | 726 | 9.2 | 264 | 4.12 |
| 27 | 1 cup | Prep w/nonfat milk, avg | 282 | 216 | 80 | 15.7 | 36.4 | 0.2 | 36.3 | 0.0 | 1.0 | 0.7 | 0.3 | 0.0 | 0.00 | 0.01 | 9 | 2343 | 703 | 703 | 0 | | 0.40 | 0.42 | 5.47 | 0.52 | 1.56 | 118.2 | 2.81 | 30.9 | 2.5 | | 407 | 0.6 | 4.8 | 112 | 0.0 | 406 | 755 | 9.4 | 268 | 4.14 |
| 25 | 1 cup | Prep w/whole milk, avg | 281 | 280 | 77 | 15.4 | 35.9 | 0.2 | 35.7 | 0.0 | 8.7 | 5.4 | 2.5 | 0.3 | 0.12 | 0.18 | 38 | 2151 | 630 | 623 | 7 | | 0.41 | 0.47 | 5.46 | 0.52 | 1.50 | 117.7 | 2.77 | 30.7 | 2.5 | 0.1 | 396 | 0.6 | 4.9 | 117 | 0.0 | 385 | 719 | 5.8 | 262 | 4.09 |
| 51 | 1 cup | Kefir, avg | 117 | 75 | 88 | 3.9 | 5.6 | 0.0 | 5.6 | 0.0 | 4.1 | | | | | | | | | | | | | | | | | | | | | | | | 0.2 | 16 | | 105 | 187 | | 54 | |
| 175 | 1 Tbs | Malted Milk, dry pwd, Kraft | 7 | 30 | 2 | 1.0 | 5.0 | 0.0 | 3.3 | 1.7 | 0.7 | 0.3 | | | | | 2 | 0 | 0 | 0 | 0 | 0 | | | | | | | | 0.0 | | | 13 | | 0.0 | | | | 47 | | 28 | |
| 176 | 1 cup | Malted Milk, dry pwd, prep w/2% milk, Kraft | 264 | 210 | 81 | 11.0 | 27.0 | 0.0 | 22.0 | 5.0 | 7.0 | 4.0 | | | | | 25 | 500 | 122 | | | | | | | | | | | 2.4 | | | 35 | | 0.0 | | | | 510 | | 205 | |
| | | Milk Shakes | | | | | | | | | | | | | | | | | | | | | | | | | | | | | | | | | | | | | | | | |
| 197 | 1 cup | Chocolate, avg | 227 | 270 | 72 | 6.9 | 48.1 | 0.7 | 30.6 | 16.8 | 6.1 | 3.8 | 1.8 | 0.2 | 0.09 | 0.14 | 23 | 195 | 48 | 34 | 14 | | 0.11 | 0.50 | 0.28 | 0.06 | 0.72 | 11.1 | 0.82 | 0.0 | 2.3 | | 300 | 0.1 | 0.7 | 36 | 0.1 | 286 | 508 | 4.3 | 252 | 1.09 |
| 62405 | 1 cup | Strawberry, Menu Magic | 260 | 400 | 66 | 12.0 | 62.7 | 0.0 | 34.0 | 28.7 | 12.0 | 2.0 | | | | | 5 | 1333 | 267 | | | | 0.40 | 0.45 | 5.33 | 0.53 | 1.60 | 106.7 | 2.67 | 16.0 | 2.7 | | 400 | 0.5 | 4.8 | 161 | | 268 | 468 | | 268 | 4.00 |
| 199 | 1 cup | Vanilla, avg | 227 | 254 | 74 | 8.8 | 40.4 | 0.0 | 30.6 | 9.8 | 6.9 | 4.3 | 2.0 | 0.3 | 0.10 | 0.15 | 27 | 259 | 64 | 45 | 18 | | 0.07 | 0.44 | 0.33 | 0.10 | 1.18 | 15.0 | 0.84 | 0.0 | 2.3 | | 331 | 0.1 | 0.2 | 27 | 0.0 | 261 | 415 | 5.2 | 216 | 0.89 |
| 40 | 1 Tbs | Strawberry Milk, dry mix, avg | 26 | 101 | 0 | 0.0 | 25.8 | 0.1 | 24.8 | 0.9 | 0.1 | 0.0 | 0.0 | 0.0 | 0.00 | 0.03 | 0 | 0 | 0 | 0 | 0 | 0 | 0.00 | 0.03 | 0.02 | 0.00 | 0.00 | 0.0 | 0.00 | 0.1 | 0.0 | 0.0 | 0 | 0.0 | 0.1 | 0 | 0.0 | 0 | 1 | 0.0 | 10 | 0.00 |
| 41 | 1 cup | Strawberry Milk, prep f/mix, avg | 266 | 234 | 81 | 8.0 | 32.7 | 0.0 | 31.5 | 1.2 | 8.2 | 5.1 | 2.4 | 0.3 | 0.12 | 0.18 | 32 | 309 | 74 | | | | 0.09 | 0.42 | 0.22 | 0.10 | 0.88 | 12.2 | 0.77 | 2.4 | 2.7 | | 293 | 0.0 | 0.2 | 32 | 0.0 | 229 | 370 | 4.8 | 128 | 0.93 |
| 93 | 1 cup | Vanilla Milk, low cal, prep f/mix, avg | 276 | 105 | 90 | 7.5 | 16.9 | 0.5 | | | 0.8 | 0.7 | 0.1 | 0.0 | | | 6 | 368 | 90 | 78 | 13 | | 0.04 | 0.11 | 0.40 | 0.04 | 0.76 | 13.4 | | 0.4 | | | 287 | 0.3 | 2.5 | 66 | | 47 | 704 | | 257 | 1.22 |
| | | *JUICE AND FRUIT FLAVORED DRINKS* | | | | | | | | | | | | | | | | | | | | | | | | | | | | | | | | | | | | | | | | |
| | | Capri Sun All Natural Juice Drinks | | | | | | | | | | | | | | | | | | | | | | | | | | | | | | | | | | | | | | | | |
| 20609 | 1 ea | Fruit Punch, 9.5 fl oz pkg | 210 | 100 | 88 | 0.0 | 26.0 | 0.0 | 26.0 | 0.0 | 0.0 | 0.0 | 0.0 | 0.0 | 0.00 | 0.00 | 0 | 0 | 0 | 0 | 0 | 0 | | | | | 0.00 | | | 0.0 | | | 0 | | 0.0 | | | | 25 | | 20 | |
| 20610 | 1 ea | Grape, 9.5 fl oz pkg | 211 | 110 | 87 | 0.0 | 28.0 | 0.0 | 28.0 | 0.0 | 0.0 | 0.0 | 0.0 | 0.0 | 0.00 | 0.00 | 0 | 0 | 0 | 0 | 0 | 0 | | | | | 0.00 | | | 0.0 | | | 0 | | 0.0 | | | | 15 | | 20 | |
| 20611 | 1 ea | Maui Punch, 9.5 fl oz pkg | 211 | 110 | 87 | 0.0 | 28.0 | 0.0 | 28.0 | 0.0 | 0.0 | 0.0 | 0.0 | 0.0 | 0.00 | 0.00 | 0 | 0 | 0 | 0 | 0 | 0 | | | | | 0.00 | | | 0.0 | | | 0 | | 0.0 | | | | 35 | | 20 | |
| 20612 | 1 ea | Mountain Cooler, 9.5 fl oz pkg | 210 | 100 | 88 | 0.0 | 26.0 | 0.0 | 26.0 | 0.0 | 0.0 | 0.0 | 0.0 | 0.0 | 0.00 | 0.00 | 0 | 0 | 0 | 0 | 0 | 0 | | | | | 0.00 | | | 0.0 | | | 0 | | 0.0 | | | | 20 | | 20 | |
| 20280 | 1 ea | Orange, 9.5 fl oz pkg | 211 | 100 | 88 | 0.0 | 26.0 | 0.0 | 26.0 | 0.0 | 0.0 | 0.0 | 0.0 | 0.0 | 0.00 | 0.00 | 0 | 0 | 0 | 0 | 0 | 0 | | | | | 0.00 | | | 0.0 | | | 0 | | 0.0 | | | | 110 | | 25 | |
| 20613 | 1 ea | Pacific Cooler, 9.5 fl oz pkg | 211 | 110 | 87 | 0.0 | 29.0 | 0.0 | 29.0 | 0.0 | 0.0 | 0.0 | 0.0 | 0.0 | 0.00 | 0.00 | 0 | 0 | 0 | 0 | 0 | 0 | | | | | 0.00 | | | 0.0 | | | 0 | | 0.0 | | | | 25 | | 20 | |
| 20614 | 1 ea | Red Berry, 9.5 fl oz pkg | 211 | 100 | 87 | 0.0 | 28.0 | 0.0 | 28.0 | 0.0 | 0.0 | 0.0 | 0.0 | 0.0 | 0.00 | 0.00 | 0 | 0 | 0 | 0 | 0 | 0 | | | | | 0.00 | | | 0.0 | | | 0 | | 0.0 | | | | 25 | | 20 | |
| 20615 | 1 ea | Safari Punch, 9.5 fl oz pkg | 210 | 100 | 88 | 0.0 | 25.0 | 0.0 | 25.0 | 0.0 | 0.0 | 0.0 | 0.0 | 0.0 | 0.00 | 0.00 | 0 | 0 | 0 | 0 | 0 | 0 | | | | | 0.00 | | | 0.0 | | | 0 | | 0.0 | | | | 25 | | 20 | |
| 20616 | 1 ea | Strawberry Cooler, 9.5 fl oz pkg | 210 | 100 | 88 | 0.0 | 26.0 | 0.0 | 26.0 | 0.0 | 0.0 | 0.0 | 0.0 | 0.0 | 0.00 | 0.00 | 0 | 0 | 0 | 0 | 0 | 0 | | | | | 0.00 | | | 0.0 | | | 0 | | 0.0 | | | | 10 | | 20 | |
| 20617 | 1 ea | Surfer Cooler, 9.5 fl oz pkg | 210 | 100 | 87 | 0.0 | 27.0 | 0.0 | 27.0 | 0.0 | 0.0 | 0.0 | 0.0 | 0.0 | 0.00 | 0.00 | 0 | 0 | 0 | 0 | 0 | 0 | | | | | 0.00 | | | 0.0 | | | 0 | | 0.0 | | | | 30 | | 20 | |
| 20618 | 1 ea | Wild Cherry, 9.5 fl oz pkg | 212 | 110 | 86 | 0.0 | 30.0 | 0.0 | 30.0 | 0.0 | 0.0 | 0.0 | 0.0 | 0.0 | 0.00 | 0.00 | 0 | 0 | 0 | 0 | 0 | 0 | | | | | 0.00 | | | 0.0 | | | 0 | | 0.0 | | | | 25 | | 20 | |
| 20619 | 1 ea | Yo Yogi Berry, 9.5 fl oz pkg | 210 | 100 | 87 | 0.0 | 27.0 | 0.0 | 27.0 | 0.0 | 0.0 | 0.0 | 0.0 | 0.0 | 0.00 | 0.00 | 0 | 0 | 0 | 0 | 0 | 0 | | | | | 0.00 | | | 0.0 | | | 0 | | 0.0 | | | | 20 | | 20 | |
| 20098 | 1/8 cup | Citrus Drink, conc, avg | 35 | 57 | 57 | 0.4 | 14.1 | 0.0 | | | 0.0 | 0.0 | 0.0 | 0.0 | 0.00 | 0.00 | 0 | 51 | 5 | 0 | 5 | | 0.02 | 0.01 | 0.22 | 0.03 | 0.00 | 2.5 | 0.16 | 33.4 | 0.0 | 0.0 | 9 | 0.0 | 1.4 | 7 | 0.1 | 13 | 138 | 0.0 | 1 | 0.04 |
| 20052 | 1 cup | Citrus Drink, prep f/conc, avg | 248 | 114 | 88 | 0.7 | 28.5 | 0.0 | 28.4 | 0.1 | 0.0 | 0.0 | 0.0 | 0.0 | 0.00 | 0.00 | 0 | 104 | 10 | 0 | 10 | | 0.03 | 0.03 | 0.45 | 0.06 | 0.00 | 5.0 | 0.33 | 67.2 | 0.0 | 0.0 | 22 | 0.1 | 2.8 | 15 | 0.2 | 25 | 278 | 0.0 | 7 | 0.12 |
| 20123 | 1 cup | Citrus Juice, calcium fort, avg | 240 | 113 | 88 | 0.8 | 27.7 | 0.1 | 27.5 | 0.0 | 0.2 | 0.0 | 0.0 | 0.0 | 0.01 | 0.04 | 0 | 13 | 1.4 | 0 | 1.4 | | 0.06 | 0.03 | 0.31 | 0.06 | 0.00 | 5.2 | | 79.8 | 0.0 | | 317 | 0.1 | 0.2 | 17 | | 22 | 197 | | 5 | 0.10 |
| 20563 | 1 cup | Cranberry Apple Cocktail, Minute Maid | 252 | 167 | 83 | 0.0 | 42.1 | 0.0 | 40.1 | 2.0 | 0.0 | 0.0 | 0.0 | 0.0 | 0.00 | 0.00 | | 0 | 0 | 0 | 0 | 0 | | | | | | | | 0.0 | | | 0 | | 0.0 | | | | 35 | | 26 | |
| 20566 | 1 cup | Cranberry Apple Raspberry Blend, Minute Maid | 252 | 123 | 87 | 0.0 | 33.1 | 0.0 | 31.1 | 2.0 | 0.0 | 0.0 | 0.0 | 0.0 | 0.00 | 0.00 | | 0 | 0 | 0 | 0 | 0 | | | | | | | | 0.0 | | | 0 | | 0.0 | | | | 47 | | 24 | |
| | | Crystal Light | | | | | | | | | | | | | | | | | | | | | | | | | | | | | | | | | | | | | | | | |
| 20215 | 1/2 tsp | Citrus Blend, low cal, dry mix | 1 | 4 | 2 | 0.0 | 0.0 | 0.0 | 0.0 | 0.0 | 0.0 | 0.0 | 0.0 | 0.0 | 0.00 | 0.00 | 0 | 0 | 0 | 0 | 0 | 0 | | | | | 0.00 | | | 4.3 | | | 0 | | 0.0 | | | | 32 | | 0 | |
| 20314 | 1 cup | Citrus Blend, low cal, prep f/dry mix | 238 | 5 | 100 | 0.0 | 0.0 | 0.0 | 0.0 | 0.0 | 0.0 | 0.0 | 0.0 | 0.0 | 0.00 | 0.00 | 0 | 0 | 0 | 0 | 0 | 0 | | | | | 0.00 | | | 6.0 | | | 0 | | 0.0 | | | | 45 | | 0 | |
| 20348 | 1/2 tsp | Cranberry Breeze, low cal, dry mix | 1 | 4 | 2 | 0.0 | 0.0 | 0.0 | 0.0 | 0.0 | 0.0 | 0.0 | 0.0 | 0.0 | 0.00 | 0.00 | 0 | 0 | 0 | 0 | 0 | 0 | | | | | 0.00 | | | 4.3 | | | 0 | | 0.0 | | | | 7 | | 0 | |
| 20380 | 1 cup | Cranberry Breeze, low cal, prep f/dry mix | 239 | 5 | 100 | 0.0 | 0.0 | 0.0 | 0.0 | 0.0 | 0.0 | 0.0 | 0.0 | 0.0 | 0.00 | 0.00 | 0 | 0 | 0 | 0 | 0 | 0 | | | | | 0.00 | | | 6.0 | | | 0 | | 0.0 | | | | 10 | | 0 | |
| 20214 | 1/2 tsp | Fruit Punch, low cal, dry mix | 1 | 4 | 2 | 0.0 | 0.0 | 0.0 | 0.0 | 0.0 | 0.0 | 0.0 | 0.0 | 0.0 | 0.00 | 0.00 | 0 | 0 | 0 | 0 | 0 | 0 | | | | | 0.00 | | | 5.0 | | | 0 | | | | | | 37 | | 0 | |
| 20317 | 1 cup | Fruit Punch, low cal, prep f/dry mix | 238 | 5 | 100 | 0.0 | 0.0 | 0.0 | 0.0 | 0.0 | 0.0 | 0.0 | 0.0 | 0.0 | 0.00 | 0.00 | 0 | 0 | 0 | 0 | 0 | 0 | | | | | 0.00 | | | 6.0 | | | 0 | | 0.0 | | | | 45 | | 0 | |
| 20213 | 1/2 tsp | Lemonade, low cal, dry mix | 2 | 5 | 2 | 0.0 | 0.0 | 0.0 | 0.0 | 0.0 | 0.0 | 0.0 | 0.0 | 0.0 | 0.00 | 0.00 | 0 | 0 | 0 | 0 | 0 | 0 | | | | | 0.00 | | | 6.0 | | | 0 | | 0.0 | | | | 60 | | 0 | |
| 20357 | 1 cup | Lemonade, low cal, prep f/dry mix | 239 | 5 | 100 | 0.0 | 0.0 | 0.0 | 0.0 | 0.0 | 0.0 | 0.0 | 0.0 | 0.0 | 0.00 | 0.00 | 0 | 0 | 0 | 0 | 0 | 0 | | | | | 0.00 | | | 6.0 | | | 0 | | 0.0 | | | | 60 | | 0 | |
| 20210 | 1/2 tsp | Lemon Lime, low cal, dry mix | 2 | 6 | 2 | 0.0 | 0.0 | 0.0 | 0.0 | 0.0 | 0.0 | 0.0 | 0.0 | 0.0 | 0.00 | 0.00 | 0 | 0 | 0 | 0 | 0 | 0 | | | | | 0.00 | | | 7.1 | | | 0 | | 0.0 | | | | 6 | | 0 | |
| 20316 | 1 cup | Lemon Lime, low cal, prep f/dry mix | 239 | 5 | 100 | 0.0 | 0.0 | 0.0 | 0.0 | 0.0 | 0.0 | 0.0 | 0.0 | 0.0 | 0.00 | 0.00 | 0 | 0 | 0 | 0 | 0 | 0 | | | | | 0.00 | | | 6.0 | | | 0 | | 0.0 | | | | 5 | | 0 | |
| 20351 | 1/2 tsp | Pink Grapefruit, low cal, dry mix | 2 | 6 | 2 | 0.0 | 0.0 | 0.0 | 0.0 | 0.0 | 0.0 | 0.0 | 0.0 | 0.0 | 0.00 | 0.00 | 0 | 0 | 0 | 0 | 0 | 0 | | | | | 0.00 | | | 7.1 | | | 0 | | 0.0 | | | | 59 | | 0 | |
| 20383 | 1 cup | Pink Grapefruit, low cal, prep f/dry mix | 239 | 5 | 100 | 0.0 | 0.0 | 0.0 | 0.0 | 0.0 | 0.0 | 0.0 | 0.0 | 0.0 | 0.00 | 0.00 | 0 | 0 | 0 | 0 | 0 | 0 | | | | | 0.00 | | | 6.0 | | | 0 | | 0.0 | | | | 50 | | 0 | |

| Code | Amount | Description | Basic Components | | | | | | | | | Additional Fats | | | | | | Vit A & Components | | | | | Vitamins | | | | | | | | | | Minerals | | | | | | | | | |
|---|---|---|---|---|---|---|---|---|---|---|---|---|---|---|---|---|---|---|---|---|---|---|---|---|---|---|---|---|---|---|---|---|---|---|---|---|---|---|---|---|---|---|
| | | | Weight (g) | Calories | % Water | Protein (g) | Carbs (g) | Fiber (g) | Sugar (g) | Other Carbs (g) | Fat (g) | Sat Fat (g) | Mono Fat (g) | Poly Fat (g) | Omega 3 (g) | Omega 6 (g) | Choles (mg) | Vit A (IU) | Vit A (RE) | Retinol (RE) | Carotenoids (RE) | Beta Carotene (mcg) | Thiamin (mg) | Riboflavin (mg) | Niacin (NE) | Vit B6 (mg) | Vit B12 (mcg) | Folate (mcg) | Panto (mg) | Vit C (mg) | Vit D (mg) | Vit E (α TE) | Calcium (mg) | Copper (mg) | Iron (mg) | Magnes (mg) | Mang (mg) | Phos (mg) | Potassium (mg) | Selenium (mcg) | Sodium (mg) | Zinc (mg) |
| 20352 | 1/2 tsp | Raspberry Ice, low cal, dry mix | 1 | 0 | 1 | 0.0 | 0.0 | 0.0 | 0.0 | 0.0 | 0.0 | 0.0 | 0.0 | 0.0 | 0.00 | 0.00 | 0 | 0 | 0 | 0 | 0 | 0 | | | | | 0.00 | | | 6.0 | | | 0 | | 0.0 | | | | 0 | | 0 | |
| 20384 | 1 cup | Raspberry Ice, low cal, prep f/dry mix | 238 | 5 | 100 | 0.0 | 0.0 | 0.0 | 0.0 | 0.0 | 0.0 | 0.0 | 0.0 | 0.0 | 0.00 | 0.00 | 0 | 0 | 0 | 0 | 0 | 0 | | | | | 0.00 | | | 6.0 | | | 0 | | 0.0 | | | | 0 | | 0 | |
| 20564 | 1 cup | Five Alive, Minute Maid | 251 | 123 | 87 | 0.0 | 31.0 | 0.0 | 29.0 | 2.0 | 0.0 | 0.0 | 0.0 | 0.0 | 0.00 | 0.00 | | 0 | 0 | 0 | 0 | 0 | | | | | | | | 5.0 | | | 0 | | 0.0 | | | | 184 | | 26 | |
| 20081 | 1 cup | Fruit Drink, low cal, avg | 240 | 43 | 95 | 0.0 | 11.3 | 0.0 | | | 0.0 | 0.0 | 0.0 | 0.0 | 0.00 | 0.00 | 0 | 29 | 2.4 | 0 | 2.4 | | 0.02 | 0.05 | 0.05 | 0.00 | 0.00 | 4.8 | | 77.5 | 0.0 | 0.0 | 17 | 0.1 | 0.6 | 5 | | 5 | 50 | | 50 | 0.26 |
| | | Fruit Flavored Beverage | | | | | | | | | | | | | | | | | | | | | | | | | | | | | | | | | | | | | | | | |
| 20061 | 1 Tbs | Low Sugar, pwd, avg | 12 | 44 | 0 | 0.0 | 11.0 | 0.0 | 11.0 | 0.0 | 0.0 | 0.0 | 0.0 | 0.0 | 0.00 | 0.00 | 0 | 0 | 0 | 0 | 0 | 0 | 0.00 | 0.00 | 0.00 | 0.00 | 0.00 | 0.0 | | 0.0 | 0.0 | 0.0 | 0 | 0.0 | 0.0 | 0 | 0.0 | 20 | 18 | | 81 | 0.00 |
| 20124 | 1 cup | Low Sugar, prep f/pwd, avg | 240 | 2 | 99 | 0.1 | 0.1 | 0.0 | 0.0 | 0.1 | 0.0 | 0.0 | 0.0 | 0.0 | 0.00 | 0.00 | 0 | 0 | 0 | 0 | 0 | 0 | 0.00 | 0.00 | 0.00 | 0.00 | 0.00 | 0.0 | | 6.0 | 0.0 | 0.0 | 38 | 0.0 | 0.0 | 2 | | 14 | 46 | | 7 | 0.07 |
| | | Fruitopia Drink | | | | | | | | | | | | | | | | | | | | | | | | | | | | | | | | | | | | | | | | |
| 20547 | 1 cup | Fruit Integration | 251 | 125 | 88 | 0.0 | 31.0 | 0.0 | 30.0 | 1.0 | 0.0 | 0.0 | 0.0 | 0.0 | 0.00 | 0.00 | 0 | 0 | 0 | 0 | 0 | 0 | | | | | | | | 0.0 | | | 0 | | 0.0 | | | | 35 | | 26 | |
| 20567 | 1 cup | Fruit Integration + calcium | 251 | 111 | 88 | 0.0 | 29.0 | 0.0 | 29.0 | 0.0 | 0.0 | 0.0 | 0.0 | 0.0 | 0.00 | 0.00 | 0 | 0 | 0 | 0 | 0 | 0 | | | | | | | | 0.0 | | | 116 | | 0.0 | | | | 35 | | 22 | |
| 20552 | 1 cup | Grape Beyond | 251 | 127 | 87 | 0.0 | 32.0 | 0.0 | 31.0 | 1.0 | 0.0 | 0.0 | 0.0 | 0.0 | 0.00 | 0.00 | 0 | 0 | 0 | 0 | 0 | 0 | | | | | | | | 0.0 | | | 0 | | 0.0 | | | | 54 | | 26 | |
| 20556 | 1 cup | Grape Beyond + calcium | 251 | 113 | 88 | 0.0 | 30.0 | 0.0 | 30.0 | 0.0 | 0.0 | 0.0 | 0.0 | 0.0 | 0.00 | 0.00 | 0 | 0 | 0 | 0 | 0 | 0 | | | | | | | | 0.0 | | | 119 | | 0.0 | | | | 41 | | 21 | |
| 20548 | 1 cup | Pink Lemonade Euphoria | 250 | 117 | 88 | 0.0 | 29.0 | 0.0 | 28.0 | 1.0 | 0.0 | 0.0 | 0.0 | 0.0 | 0.00 | 0.00 | 0 | 0 | 0 | 0 | 0 | 0 | | | | | | | | 0.0 | | | 0 | | 0.0 | | | | 28 | | 26 | |
| 20549 | 1 cup | Raspberry Psychic Lemonade | 251 | 121 | 88 | 0.0 | 29.0 | 0.0 | 29.0 | 0.0 | 0.0 | 0.0 | 0.0 | 0.0 | 0.00 | 0.00 | 0 | 0 | 0 | 0 | 0 | 0 | | | | | | | | 0.0 | | | 0 | | 0.0 | | | | 25 | | 26 | |
| 20550 | 1 cup | Strawberry Passion Awareness | 251 | 124 | 88 | 0.0 | 31.0 | 0.0 | 30.0 | 1.0 | 0.0 | 0.0 | 0.0 | 0.0 | 0.00 | 0.00 | 0 | 0 | 0 | 0 | 0 | 0 | | | | | | | | 0.0 | | | 0 | | 0.0 | | | | 40 | | 30 | |
| 20554 | 1 cup | Strawberry Passion Awareness + calcium | 251 | 115 | 88 | 0.0 | 30.0 | 0.0 | 30.0 | 0.0 | 0.0 | 0.0 | 0.0 | 0.0 | 0.00 | 0.00 | 0 | 0 | 0 | 0 | 0 | 0 | | | | | | | | 0.0 | | | 111 | | 0.0 | | | | 40 | | 22 | |
| 20551 | 1 cup | Tangerine Wavelength | 250 | 119 | 88 | 0.0 | 30.0 | 0.0 | 29.0 | 1.0 | 0.0 | 0.0 | 0.0 | 0.0 | 0.00 | 0.00 | 0 | 0 | 0 | 0 | 0 | 0 | | | | | | | | 0.0 | | | 0 | | 0.0 | | | | 47 | | 24 | |
| 20555 | 1 cup | Tangerine Wavelength + calcium | 250 | 110 | 88 | 0.0 | 29.0 | 0.0 | 28.0 | 1.0 | 0.0 | 0.0 | 0.0 | 0.0 | 0.00 | 0.00 | 0 | 0 | 0 | 0 | 0 | 0 | | | | | | | | 0.0 | | | 112 | | 0.0 | | | | 47 | | 21 | |
| 20553 | 1 cup | Tropical Consideration | 251 | 75 | 92 | 0.0 | 19.0 | 0.0 | 18.0 | 1.0 | 0.0 | 0.0 | 0.0 | 0.0 | 0.00 | 0.00 | 0 | 0 | 0 | 0 | 0 | 0 | | | | | | | | 0.0 | | | 0 | | 0.0 | | | | 39 | | 24 | |
| | | Fruit Punch | | | | | | | | | | | | | | | | | | | | | | | | | | | | | | | | | | | | | | | | |
| 20024 | 1 cup | Canned, avg | 248 | 117 | 88 | 0.0 | 29.5 | 0.2 | | | 0.0 | 0.0 | 0.0 | 0.0 | 0.00 | 0.00 | 0 | 35 | 3.5 | 0 | 3.5 | | 0.05 | 0.06 | 0.05 | 0.00 | 0.00 | 3.2 | 0.03 | 73.4 | | 0.0 | 20 | 0.1 | 0.5 | 5 | 0.5 | 2 | 62 | 0.0 | 55 | 0.30 |
| 20034 | 1/8 cup | Concentrate, avg | 35 | 57 | 58 | 0.1 | 14.5 | 0.1 | 12.7 | 1.7 | 0.0 | 0.0 | 0.0 | 0.0 | 0.00 | 0.00 | 0 | 14 | 1.4 | 0 | 1.4 | | 0.01 | 0.02 | 0.03 | 0.01 | 0.00 | 1.2 | 0.01 | 54.6 | 0.0 | 0.0 | 3 | 0.0 | 0.1 | 2 | 0.1 | 1 | 15 | 0.0 | 3 | 0.02 |
| 20130 | 2 Tbs | Dry mix, avg | 25 | 96 | 1 | 0.0 | 24.4 | 0.0 | 24.4 | 0.0 | 0.0 | 0.0 | 0.0 | 0.0 | 0.00 | 0.00 | 0 | 1.2 | 0.2 | 0 | 0.2 | | 0.00 | 0.01 | 0.00 | 0.00 | 0.00 | 0.2 | 0.00 | 30.5 | 0.0 | 0.0 | 36 | 0.0 | 0.1 | 0 | 0.0 | 52 | 1 | 0.2 | 10 | 0.03 |
| 20531 | 1 cup | Minute Maid | 250 | 119 | 87 | 0.0 | 32.0 | 0.0 | 32.0 | 0.0 | 0.0 | 0.0 | 0.0 | 0.0 | 0.00 | 0.00 | 0 | 0 | 0 | 0 | 0 | 0 | | | | | | | | 0.0 | | | 0 | | 0.0 | | | 0 | 45 | | 5 | |
| 20565 | 1 cup | Minute Maid, w/10% juice | 250 | 125 | 87 | 0.0 | 31.0 | 0.0 | 30.0 | 1.0 | 0.0 | 0.0 | 0.0 | 0.0 | 0.00 | 0.00 | 0 | 0 | 0 | 0 | 0 | 0 | | | | | | | | 0.0 | | | 0 | | 0.0 | | | | 36 | | 26 | |
| 20035 | 1 cup | Prep f/conc, avg | 247 | 114 | 88 | 0.0 | 28.9 | 0.2 | 25.2 | 3.5 | 0.0 | 0.0 | 0.0 | 0.0 | 0.00 | 0.00 | 0 | 27 | 2.5 | 0 | 2.5 | | 0.02 | 0.03 | 0.05 | 0.01 | 0.00 | 2.2 | 0.02 | 108.4 | 0.0 | 0.0 | 10 | 0.1 | 0.2 | 5 | 0.3 | 2 | 32 | 0.0 | 10 | 0.10 |
| 20016 | 1 cup | Prep f/dry mix, avg | 262 | 97 | 90 | 0.0 | 24.9 | 0.0 | 24.9 | 0.0 | 0.0 | 0.0 | 0.0 | 0.0 | 0.00 | 0.00 | 0 | 0 | 0 | 0 | 0 | 0 | 0.00 | 0.01 | 0.00 | 0.00 | 0.00 | 0.3 | 0.00 | 30.9 | 0.0 | 0.0 | 42 | 0.0 | 0.1 | 3 | 0.0 | 52 | 3 | 0.3 | 37 | 0.08 |
| 20413 | 1 1/2 cup | Slice | 360 | 190 | 86 | 0.0 | 48.0 | 0.0 | 48.0 | 0.0 | 0.0 | 0.0 | 0.0 | 0.0 | 0.00 | 0.00 | 0 | 0 | 0 | 0 | 0 | 0 | | | | | 0.00 | | | 0.0 | | | 0 | | 0.0 | | | 0 | | | 55 | |
| | | Grape Juice Drink | | | | | | | | | | | | | | | | | | | | | | | | | | | | | | | | | | | | | | | | |
| 20026 | 1 cup | Avg | 250 | 125 | 87 | 0.3 | 32.3 | 0.3 | 32.0 | 0.0 | 0.0 | 0.0 | 0.0 | 0.0 | 0.00 | 0.00 | 0 | 5 | 0.5 | 0 | 0.5 | | 0.02 | 0.02 | 0.25 | 0.05 | 0.00 | 2.0 | 0.03 | 40.0 | 0.0 | 0.0 | 8 | 0.0 | 0.3 | 10 | 0.3 | 10 | 88 | 0.0 | 2 | 0.07 |
| 20562 | 1 cup | Concord Punch, Minute Maid | 251 | 127 | 87 | 0.0 | 32.0 | 0.0 | 31.0 | 1.0 | 0.0 | 0.0 | 0.0 | 0.0 | 0.00 | 0.00 | 0 | 0 | 0 | 0 | 0 | 0 | | | | | | | | 0.0 | | | 0 | | 0.0 | | | | 54 | | 26 | |
| 20082 | 1 cup | Low Calorie, avg | 240 | 43 | 95 | 0.0 | 11.3 | 0.0 | | | 0.0 | 0.0 | 0.0 | 0.0 | 0.00 | 0.00 | 0 | 29 | 2.4 | 0 | 2.4 | | 0.02 | 0.05 | 0.05 | 0.00 | 0.00 | 4.8 | | 77.5 | 0.0 | 0.0 | 17 | 0.1 | 0.6 | 5 | | 5 | 50 | | 50 | 0.26 |
| 20450 | 1 1/2 cup | Shasta | 354 | 170 | 88 | 0.0 | 41.9 | 0.0 | 41.9 | 0.0 | 0.0 | 0.0 | 0.0 | 0.0 | 0.00 | 0.00 | 0 | | | | | | | | | | 0.00 | | | 59.9 | | | | | | | | | | | 45 | |
| | | Hi-C Fruit Drink, w/10% Juice | | | | | | | | | | | | | | | | | | | | | | | | | | | | | | | | | | | | | | | | |
| 20573 | 1 ea | Blue Cooler, 8.45 fl oz box | 251 | 130 | 87 | 0.0 | 33.1 | 0.0 | 32.1 | 1.0 | 0.0 | 0.0 | 0.0 | 0.0 | 0.00 | 0.00 | 0 | 0 | 0 | 0 | 0 | 0 | | | | | | | | 100.2 | | | | | | | | | | | 30 | |
| 20576 | 1 cup | Boppin Berry | 236 | 107 | 87 | 0.0 | 28.5 | 0.0 | 27.6 | 0.9 | 0.0 | 0.0 | 0.0 | 0.0 | 0.00 | 0.00 | 0 | 0 | 0 | 0 | 0 | 0 | | | | | | | | 89.1 | | | | | | | | | | | 134 | |
| 20577 | 1 cup | Ectocooler | 236 | 107 | 87 | 0.0 | 28.5 | 0.0 | 27.6 | 0.9 | 0.0 | 0.0 | 0.0 | 0.0 | 0.00 | 0.00 | 0 | 0 | 0 | 0 | 0 | 0 | | | | | | | | 89.1 | | | | | | | | | | | 134 | |
| 20579 | 1 cup | Fruit Punch | 236 | 98 | 89 | 0.0 | 25.9 | 0.0 | 25.9 | 0.0 | 0.0 | 0.0 | 0.0 | 0.0 | 0.00 | 0.00 | 0 | 0 | 0 | 0 | 0 | 0 | | | | | | | | 89.4 | | | | | | | | | | | 134 | |
| 20580 | 1 cup | Grape | 236 | 98 | 89 | 0.0 | 25.9 | 0.0 | 25.9 | 0.0 | 0.0 | 0.0 | 0.0 | 0.0 | 0.00 | 0.00 | 0 | 0 | 0 | 0 | 0 | 0 | | | | | | | | 89.2 | | | | | | | | | | | 134 | |
| 20157 | 1 ea | Orange, 8.45 fl oz box | 250 | 120 | 86 | 0.0 | 33.9 | 0.0 | 32.9 | 1.0 | 0.0 | 0.0 | 0.0 | 0.0 | 0.00 | 0.00 | 0 | 0 | 0 | 0 | 0 | 0 | | | | | 0.00 | | | 99.7 | | | | | | | | | | | 30 | |
| 20571 | 1 ea | Tropical Punch, 8.45 fl oz box | 250 | 120 | 87 | 0.0 | 32.0 | 0.0 | 31.0 | 1.0 | 0.0 | 0.0 | 0.0 | 0.0 | 0.00 | 0.00 | | 0 | 0 | 0 | 0 | 0 | | | | | | | | 100.0 | | | | | | | | | | | 30 | |
| 20574 | 1 ea | Watermelon Rapids, 8.45 fl oz box | 251 | 130 | 87 | 0.0 | 33.1 | 0.0 | 32.1 | 1.0 | 0.0 | 0.0 | 0.0 | 0.0 | 0.00 | 0.00 | 0 | 0 | 0 | 0 | 0 | 0 | | | | | | | | 100.2 | | | | | | | | | | | 30 | |
| | | Kool-Aid | | | | | | | | | | | | | | | | | | | | | | | | | | | | | | | | | | | | | | | | |
| 20629 | 1 ea | Cherry, Bursts, 6.75 fl oz | 210 | 100 | 88 | 0.0 | 25.0 | 0.0 | 25.0 | 0.0 | 0.0 | 0.0 | 0.0 | 0.0 | 0.00 | 0.00 | 0 | 0 | 0 | 0 | 0 | 0 | | | | | 0.00 | | | 0.0 | | | 0 | | 0.0 | | | | 15 | | 35 | |
| 20330 | 1 ea | Cherry, sugar free, dry pkt | 10 | 42 | 2 | 0.0 | 0.0 | 0.0 | 0.0 | 0.0 | 0.0 | 0.0 | 0.0 | 0.0 | 0.00 | 0.00 | 0 | 0 | 0 | 0 | 0 | 0 | | | | | 0.00 | | | 50.0 | | | 0 | | 0.0 | | | | 0 | | 42 | |
| 20398 | 1 cup | Cherry, sugar free, prep f/dry mix | 237 | 5 | 100 | 0.0 | 0.0 | 0.0 | 0.0 | 0.0 | 0.0 | 0.0 | 0.0 | 0.0 | 0.00 | 0.00 | 0 | 0 | 0 | 0 | 0 | 0 | | | | | 0.00 | | | 6.0 | | | 0 | | 0.0 | | | | 0 | | 5 | |
| 20318 | 1 ea | Cherry, sugar swtnd, dry pkt | 136 | 480 | 5 | 0.0 | 128.0 | 0.0 | 128.0 | 0.0 | 0.0 | 0.0 | 0.0 | 0.0 | 0.00 | 0.00 | 0 | 0 | 0 | 0 | 0 | 0 | | | | | 0.00 | | | 48.0 | | | 0 | | 0.0 | | | | 0 | | 0 | |
| 20385 | 1 cup | Cherry, sugar swtnd, prep f/dry mix | 254 | 60 | 94 | 0.0 | 16.0 | 0.0 | 16.0 | 0.0 | 0.0 | 0.0 | 0.0 | 0.0 | 0.00 | 0.00 | 0 | 0 | 0 | 0 | 0 | 0 | | | | | 0.00 | | | 6.0 | | | 0 | | 0.0 | | | | 0 | | 0 | |
| 20630 | 1 ea | Grape, Bursts, 6.75 fl oz | 210 | 100 | 88 | 0.0 | 25.0 | 0.0 | 25.0 | 0.0 | 0.0 | 0.0 | 0.0 | 0.0 | 0.00 | 0.00 | 0 | 0 | 0 | 0 | 0 | 0 | | | | | 0.00 | | | 0.0 | | | 0 | | 0.0 | | | | 15 | | 30 | |
| 20322 | 1 ea | Orange, sugar swtnd, dry pkt | 136 | 480 | 5 | 0.0 | 128.0 | 0.0 | 128.0 | 0.0 | 0.0 | 0.0 | 0.0 | 0.0 | 0.00 | 0.00 | 0 | 0 | 0 | 0 | 0 | 0 | | | | | 0.00 | | | 48.0 | | | 0 | | 0.0 | | | | 0 | | 40 | |
| 20390 | 1 cup | Orange, sugar swtnd, prep f/dry mix | 254 | 60 | 94 | 0.0 | 16.0 | 0.0 | 16.0 | 0.0 | 0.0 | 0.0 | 0.0 | 0.0 | 0.00 | 0.00 | 0 | 0 | 0 | 0 | 0 | 0 | | | | | 0.00 | | | 6.0 | | | 0 | | 0.0 | | | | 0 | | 5 | |
| 20323 | 1 ea | Raspberry, sugar swtnd, dry pkt | 136 | 480 | 0 | 0.0 | 136.0 | 0.0 | 136.0 | 0.0 | 0.0 | 0.0 | 0.0 | 0.0 | 0.00 | 0.00 | 0 | 0 | 0 | 0 | 0 | 0 | | | | | 0.00 | | | 48.0 | | | 0 | | 0.0 | | | | 0 | | 0 | |
| 20391 | 1 cup | Raspberry, sugar swtnd, prep f/dry mix | 254 | 60 | 93 | 0.0 | 17.0 | 0.0 | 17.0 | 0.0 | 0.0 | 0.0 | 0.0 | 0.0 | 0.00 | 0.00 | 0 | 0 | 0 | 0 | 0 | 0 | | | | | 0.00 | | | 6.0 | | | 0 | | 0.0 | | | | 0 | | 0 | |
| | | Lemonade | | | | | | | | | | | | | | | | | | | | | | | | | | | | | | | | | | | | | | | | |
| 20001 | 1/8 cup | Concentrate, avg | 36 | 65 | 52 | 0.1 | 17.0 | 0.1 | 14.9 | 1.9 | 0.1 | 0.0 | 0.0 | 0.0 | 0.01 | 0.02 | 0 | 34 | 3.5 | 0 | 3.6 | | 0.01 | 0.03 | 0.03 | 0.01 | 0.00 | 3.6 | 0.02 | 6.4 | 0.0 | 0.0 | 3 | 0.0 | 0.3 | 2 | 0.0 | 3 | 24 | 0.1 | 1 | 0.03 |
| 20582 | 1 cup | Fresh, Sun Orchard | 264 | 110 | 89 | 0.0 | 28.0 | 0.0 | 24.0 | 4.0 | 0.0 | 0.0 | 0.0 | 0.0 | 0.00 | 0.00 | 0 | 0 | 0 | 0 | 0 | 0 | | | | | | | | 24.0 | | | 0 | | 0.4 | | | | 290 | | | |
| 20583 | 1 cup | Fresh strawberry, Sun Orchard | 264 | 100 | 90 | 0.0 | 25.0 | 0.0 | 24.0 | 1.0 | 0.0 | 0.0 | 0.0 | 0.0 | 0.00 | 0.00 | 0 | 0 | 0 | 0 | 0 | 0 | | | | | | | | 18.0 | | | 0 | | 0.4 | | | | | | 0 | |
| 20047 | 1 cup | Low Calorie, prep f/dry mix, Country Time | 237 | 5 | 99 | 0.0 | 1.2 | 0.0 | 1.2 | 0.0 | 0.0 | 0.0 | 0.0 | 0.0 | 0.00 | 0.00 | 0 | 0 | 0 | 0 | 0 | 0 | 0.00 | 0.00 | 0.00 | 0.00 | 0.00 | 0.2 | 0.00 | 5.9 | 0.0 | 0.0 | 50 | 0.0 | 0.1 | 2 | 0.0 | 24 | 0 | 0.2 | 7 | 0.07 |
| 20116 | 1/8 cup | Pink, conc, avg | 36 | 65 | 52 | 0.1 | 17.0 | 0.1 | 15.0 | 1.8 | 0.1 | 0.0 | 0.0 | 0.0 | 0.01 | 0.02 | 0 | 3 | 0.4 | 0 | 0.4 | | 0.01 | 0.03 | 0.03 | 0.01 | 0.00 | 3.6 | 0.02 | 6.4 | 0.0 | 0.0 | 3 | 0.0 | 0.3 | 2 | 0.0 | 3 | 24 | 0.0 | 1 | 0.03 |
| 20117 | 1 cup | Pink, prep f/conc, avg | 247 | 99 | 89 | 0.2 | 25.9 | 0.0 | 22.7 | 3.3 | 0.0 | 0.0 | 0.0 | 0.0 | 0.00 | 0.00 | 0 | 5 | 0.5 | 0 | 0.5 | | 0.01 | 0.05 | 0.04 | 0.01 | 0.00 | 5.4 | 0.03 | 9.6 | 0.0 | 0.0 | 7 | 0.0 | 0.4 | 5 | 0.0 | 5 | 37 | 0.0 | 7 | 0.10 |
| 20000 | 1 cup | Prep f/conc, avg | 248 | 99 | 89 | 0.2 | 26.0 | 0.2 | 22.8 | 3.0 | 0.0 | 0.0 | 0.0 | 0.0 | 0.00 | 0.00 | 0 | 52 | 5 | 0 | 5 | | 0.01 | 0.05 | 0.04 | 0.01 | 0.00 | 5.5 | 0.03 | 9.7 | 0.0 | 0.0 | 7 | 0.0 | 0.4 | 5 | 0.0 | 5 | 37 | 0.2 | 7 | 0.10 |
| 20083 | 1 cup | Prep, low cal, avg | 240 | 43 | 95 | 0.0 | 11.3 | 0.2 | | | 0.0 | 0.0 | 0.0 | 0.0 | 0.00 | 0.00 | 0 | 29 | 2 | 0 | 2 | | 0.02 | 0.02 | 0.05 | 0.00 | 0.00 | 7.2 | | 16.1 | 0.0 | 0.0 | 7 | 0.1 | 0.4 | 5 | | 2 | 38 | | 7 | 0.07 |
| 20451 | 1 1/2 cup | Shasta | 354 | 170 | 88 | 0.0 | 41.9 | 0.0 | 41.9 | 0.0 | 0.0 | 0.0 | 0.0 | 0.0 | 0.00 | 0.00 | 0 | | | | | | | | | | 0.00 | | | 59.9 | | | | | | | | | | | 45 | |
| 20346 | 1/2 tsp | Sugar Free, dry mix, Country Time | 2 | 5 | 2 | 0.0 | 0.0 | 0.0 | 0.0 | 0.0 | 0.0 | 0.0 | 0.0 | 0.0 | 0.00 | 0.00 | 0 | 0 | 0 | 0 | 0 | 0 | | | | | 0.00 | | | 6.3 | | | 0 | | 0.0 | | | | 42 | | 0 | |
| 20378 | 1 cup | Sugar Free, prep f/ mix, Country Time | 239 | 5 | 100 | 0.0 | 0.0 | 0.0 | 0.0 | 0.0 | 0.0 | 0.0 | 0.0 | 0.0 | 0.00 | 0.00 | 0 | 0 | 0 | 0 | 0 | 0 | | | | | 0.00 | | | 6.0 | | | 0 | | 0.0 | | | | 40 | | 0 | |
| 20343 | 1 ea | Sugar Sweetened, dry pkt, County Time | 18 | 70 | 5 | 0.0 | 17.0 | 0.0 | 17.0 | 0.0 | 0.0 | 0.0 | 0.0 | 0.0 | 0.00 | 0.00 | 0 | 0 | 0 | 0 | 0 | 0 | | | | | 0.00 | | | 6.0 | | | 0 | | 0.0 | | | | 5 | | 15 | |
| 20375 | 1 cup | Sugar Sweetened, prep f/mix, County Time | 255 | 70 | 93 | 0.0 | 17.0 | 0.0 | 17.0 | 0.0 | 0.0 | 0.0 | 0.0 | 0.0 | 0.00 | 0.00 | 0 | 0 | 0 | 0 | 0 | 0 | | | | | 0.00 | | | 6.0 | | | 0 | | 0.0 | | | | 5 | | 15 | |
| 20447 | 1 1/2 cup | Lemon-Lime drink, Shasta | 360 | 90 | 94 | 0.0 | 23.0 | 0.0 | 23.0 | 0.0 | 0.0 | 0.0 | 0.0 | 0.0 | 0.00 | 0.00 | 0 | | | | | | | | | | 0.00 | | | | | | | | | | | | 35 | | 145 | |
| 20003 | 1/8 cup | Limeade, conc, avg | 36 | 67 | 50 | 0.1 | 17.8 | 0.1 | 14.2 | 3.5 | 0.0 | 0.0 | 0.0 | 0.0 | 0.00 | 0.01 | 0 | 0 | 0 | 0 | 0 | 0 | 0.00 | 0.00 | 0.04 | 0.00 | 0.00 | 1.4 | 0.03 | 4.3 | 0.0 | 0.0 | 2 | 0.0 | 0.0 | 1 | 0.0 | 2 | 21 | 0.0 | 0 | 0.01 |
| 20002 | 1 cup | Limeade, prep f/conc, avg | 247 | 101 | 89 | 0.0 | 27.2 | 0.2 | 21.6 | 5.4 | 0.0 | 0.0 | 0.0 | 0.0 | 0.00 | 0.00 | 0 | 0 | 0 | 0 | 0 | 0 | 0.00 | 0.00 | 0.05 | 0.00 | 0.00 | 2.5 | 0.05 | 6.7 | 0.0 | 0.0 | 7 | 0.0 | 0.1 | 2 | 0.0 | 2 | 32 | 0.0 | 5 | 0.05 |

| Code | Amount | Description | Weight (g) | Calories | % Water | Protein (g) | Carbs (g) | Fiber (g) | Sugar (g) | Other Carbs (g) | Fat (g) | Sat Fat (g) | Mono Fat (g) | Poly Fat (g) | Omega 3 (g) | Omega 6 (g) | Choles (mg) |
|---|---|---|---|---|---|---|---|---|---|---|---|---|---|---|---|---|---|
| | | | Basic Components | | | | | | | | | Additional Fats | | | | | |
| 20538 | 1 cup | Nestea Cool Drink | 248 | 82 | 91 | 0.0 | 22.0 | 0.0 | 22.0 | 0.0 | 0.0 | 0.0 | 0.0 | 0.0 | 0.00 | 0.00 | 0 |
| 20539 | 1 cup | Nestea Cool Drink, diet | 240 | 1 | 100 | 0.0 | 0.1 | 0.0 | 0.1 | 0.0 | 0.0 | 0.0 | 0.0 | 0.0 | 0.00 | 0.00 | 0 |
| | | Orange drinks and mixes | | | | | | | | | | | | | | | |
| 20070 | 1 cup | Cnd, avg | 248 | 126 | 87 | 0.0 | 32.0 | 0.2 | 31.7 | 0.0 | 0.0 | 0.0 | 0.0 | 0.0 | 0.00 | 0.00 | 0 |
| 20110 | 1/8 cup | Conc, avg | 35 | 60 | 55 | 0.0 | 15.0 | 0.1 | 14.9 | 0.0 | 0.2 | 0.0 | 0.1 | 0.1 | 0.00 | 0.06 | 0 |
| 20107 | 3 tsp | Dry Mix, avg | 24 | 88 | 0 | 0.0 | 22.0 | 0.1 | 23.7 | 0.0 | 0.0 | 0.0 | 0.0 | 0.0 | 0.00 | 0.00 | 0 |
| 20340 | 2 Tbs | Dry Mix, Tang | 26 | 100 | 7 | 0.0 | 24.0 | 0.0 | 24.0 | 0.0 | 0.0 | 0.0 | 0.0 | 0.0 | 0.00 | 0.00 | 0 |
| 20341 | 2 Tbs | Dry Mix, sugar free, Tang | 15 | 30 | | 0.0 | 6.0 | 0.0 | 0.0 | 6.0 | 0.0 | 0.0 | 0.0 | 0.0 | 0.00 | 0.00 | 0 |
| 20004 | 1 cup | Prep f/dry mix, avg | 248 | 114 | 88 | 0.0 | 29.3 | 0.0 | 26.8 | 2.5 | 0.0 | 0.0 | 0.0 | 0.0 | 0.00 | 0.00 | 0 |
| 20445 | 1 1/2 cup | Shasta | 360 | 90 | 94 | 0.0 | 23.0 | 0.0 | 23.0 | 0.0 | 0.0 | 0.0 | 0.0 | 0.0 | 0.00 | 0.00 | 0 |
| 20058 | 1 cup | Orange Apricot, juice drink, cnd, avg | 250 | 128 | 87 | 0.8 | 31.8 | 0.3 | 31.8 | 0.0 | 0.3 | 0.0 | 0.1 | 0.1 | 0.01 | 0.05 | 0 |
| 20448 | 1 1/2 cup | Pineapple Drink, Shasta | 354 | 170 | 88 | 0.0 | 40.9 | 0.0 | 40.9 | 0.0 | 0.0 | 0.0 | 0.0 | 0.0 | 0.00 | 0.00 | 0 |
| 20059 | 1 cup | Pineapple Grapefruit, juice drink, cnd, avg | 250 | 118 | 88 | 0.5 | 29.0 | 0.3 | 29.0 | 0.0 | 0.3 | 0.0 | 0.0 | 0.1 | 0.03 | 0.04 | 0 |
| 20025 | 1 cup | Pineapple Orange Drink, cnd, avg | 250 | 125 | 87 | 3.3 | 29.5 | 0.3 | 29.3 | 0.0 | 0.0 | 0.0 | 0.0 | 0.0 | 0.00 | 0.00 | 0 |
| | | Sport Drinks | | | | | | | | | | | | | | | |
| 20421 | 1 cup | Fruit Punch, avg | 240 | 53 | 94 | 0.0 | 14.7 | 0.0 | 14.7 | 0.0 | 0.0 | 0.0 | 0.0 | 0.0 | 0.00 | 0.00 | 0 |
| 20557 | 1 cup | Fruit Punch, Powerade | 247 | 72 | 92 | 0.0 | 19.0 | 0.0 | 15.0 | 4.0 | 0.0 | 0.0 | 0.0 | 0.0 | 0.00 | 0.00 | 0 |
| 20424 | 1 cup | Grape, avg | 240 | 53 | 94 | 0.0 | 13.3 | 0.0 | 13.3 | 0.0 | 0.0 | 0.0 | 0.0 | 0.0 | 0.00 | 0.00 | 0 |
| 20558 | 1 cup | Grape, Powerade | 247 | 73 | 92 | 0.0 | 19.0 | 0.0 | 15.0 | 4.0 | 0.0 | 0.0 | 0.0 | 0.0 | 0.00 | 0.00 | 0 |
| 20422 | 1 cup | Lemon Lime, avg | 240 | 47 | 94 | 0.0 | 13.3 | 0.0 | 12.7 | 0.7 | 0.0 | 0.0 | 0.0 | 0.0 | 0.00 | 0.00 | 0 |
| 20559 | 1 cup | Lemon Lime, Powerade | 247 | 72 | 92 | 0.0 | 19.0 | 0.0 | 15.0 | 4.0 | 0.0 | 0.0 | 0.0 | 0.0 | 0.00 | 0.00 | 0 |
| 20560 | 1 cup | Mountain Blast, Powerade | 247 | 73 | 92 | 0.0 | 19.0 | 0.0 | 15.0 | 4.0 | 0.0 | 0.0 | 0.0 | 0.0 | 0.00 | 0.00 | 0 |
| 20423 | 1 cup | Orange, avg | 240 | 47 | 94 | 0.0 | 13.3 | 0.0 | 12.7 | 0.7 | 0.0 | 0.0 | 0.0 | 0.0 | 0.00 | 0.00 | 0 |
| 20561 | 1 cup | Orange, Powerade | 247 | 72 | 92 | 0.0 | 19.0 | 0.0 | 15.0 | 4.0 | 0.0 | 0.0 | 0.0 | 0.0 | 0.00 | 0.00 | 0 |
| 20589 | 1 cup | Sugar Cane Beverage, avg | 240 | 163 | 81 | 0.0 | 42.4 | 0.0 | | | 0.0 | 0.0 | 0.0 | 0.0 | 0.00 | 0.00 | 0 |
| 20142 | 1 cup | Thirst Quencher Drink, avg | 241 | 60 | 94 | 0.0 | 15.2 | 0.0 | | | 0.0 | 0.0 | 0.0 | 0.0 | 0.00 | 0.00 | 0 |
| | | *TEAS* | | | | | | | | | | | | | | | |
| | | Brewed Tea & Tea Bags/Leaves | | | | | | | | | | | | | | | |
| 20014 | 1 cup | Brewed Tea, black, avg | 237 | 2 | 100 | 0.0 | 0.7 | 0.0 | 0.0 | 0.7 | 0.0 | 0.0 | 0.0 | 0.0 | 0.00 | 0.00 | 0 |
| 20118 | 1 cup | Brewed Tea, chamomile, avg | 237 | 2 | 100 | 0.0 | 0.5 | 0.0 | 0.0 | 0.5 | 0.0 | 0.0 | 0.0 | 0.0 | 0.00 | 0.00 | 0 |
| 20036 | 1 cup | Brewed Tea, herbal, avg | 237 | 2 | 100 | 0.0 | 0.5 | 0.0 | 0.0 | 0.5 | 0.0 | 0.0 | 0.0 | 0.0 | 0.00 | 0.00 | 0 |
| 20493 | 1 cup | Brewed Tea, rice, avg | 245 | 100 | 89 | 0.3 | 25.4 | 0.2 | | | 0.0 | 0.0 | 0.0 | 0.0 | | | 0 |
| 20496 | 1 ea | Tea Bag, dry, decaf, Lipton | 2 | 0 | | 0.0 | 0.0 | 0.0 | 0.0 | 0.0 | 0.0 | 0.0 | 0.0 | 0.0 | 0.00 | 0.00 | 0 |
| 20495 | 1 ea | Tea Bag, dry, Lipton | 2 | 0 | | 0.0 | 0.0 | 0.0 | 0.0 | 0.0 | 0.0 | 0.0 | 0.0 | 0.0 | 0.00 | 0.00 | 0 |
| 20482 | 1 oz | Tea Leaves, Chinese, green, dry , avg | 28 | 84 | 8 | 7.9 | 12.3 | | | | 1.3 | | | | | | |
| 20483 | 1 oz | Tea Leaves, Indian, dry, avg | 28 | 30 | 9 | 5.5 | 0.8 | | | | 0.6 | | | | | | |
| | | Frozen Tea | | | | | | | | | | | | | | | |
| 20498 | 1/2 cup | Ginger Mango, Botanica | 88 | 104 | | 0.3 | 25.0 | 0.0 | 15.0 | 10.0 | 0.0 | 0.0 | 0.0 | 0.0 | 0.00 | 0.00 | 0 |
| 20499 | 1/2 cup | Lemon Ginseng, Botanica | 88 | 104 | | 0.3 | 25.0 | 0.0 | 15.0 | 10.0 | 0.0 | 0.0 | 0.0 | 0.0 | 0.00 | 0.00 | 0 |
| 20500 | 1/2 cup | Peach, Botanica | 88 | 103 | | 0.3 | 25.0 | 0.0 | 15.0 | 10.0 | 0.0 | 0.0 | 0.0 | 0.0 | 0.00 | 0.00 | 0 |
| 20501 | 1/2 cup | Wildberry, Botanica | 88 | 103 | | 0.3 | 25.0 | 0.0 | 15.0 | 10.0 | 0.0 | 0.0 | 0.0 | 0.0 | 0.00 | 0.00 | 0 |
| | | Instant Iced Tea | | | | | | | | | | | | | | | |
| 20349 | 1 tsp | Decaf, dry mix, Crystal Light | 2 | 10 | 4 | 0.0 | 0.0 | 0.0 | 0.0 | 0.0 | 0.0 | 0.0 | 0.0 | 0.0 | 0.00 | 0.00 | 0 |
| 20381 | 1 cup | Decaf, prep, Crystal Light | 238 | 5 | 100 | 0.0 | 0.0 | 0.0 | 0.0 | 0.0 | 0.0 | 0.0 | 0.0 | 0.0 | 0.00 | 0.00 | 0 |
| 20039 | 1 tsp | Lemon, diet, dry mix, avg | 1 | 3 | 4 | 0.0 | 0.8 | 0.0 | 0.0 | 0.8 | 0.0 | 0.0 | 0.0 | 0.0 | 0.00 | 0.00 | 0 |
| 20040 | 1 cup | Lemon, diet, prep, avg | 237 | 5 | 99 | 0.0 | 1.2 | 0.0 | 0.0 | 1.2 | 0.0 | 0.0 | 0.0 | 0.0 | 0.00 | 0.00 | 0 |
| 20120 | 1 cup | Lemon, w/sugar, vit C, prep, avg | 182 | 701 | 0 | 1.1 | 177.6 | 0.0 | 177.6 | 0.0 | 0.5 | 0.1 | 0.0 | 0.2 | 0.11 | 0.05 | 0 |
| 20350 | 1 tsp | Low Calorie, dry mix, Crystal Light | 2 | 9 | 4 | 0.0 | 0.0 | 0.0 | 0.0 | 0.0 | 0.0 | 0.0 | 0.0 | 0.0 | 0.00 | 0.00 | 0 |
| 20382 | 1 cup | Low Calorie, prep, Crystal Light | 238 | 5 | 100 | 0.0 | 0.0 | 0.0 | 0.0 | 0.0 | 0.0 | 0.0 | 0.0 | 0.0 | 0.00 | 0.00 | 0 |
| 20342 | 1 ea | With Sugar, dry, Country Time, 1/8 cap | 18 | 70 | 5 | 0.0 | 17.0 | 0.0 | 17.0 | 0.0 | 0.0 | 0.0 | 0.0 | 0.0 | 0.00 | 0.00 | 0 |
| 20374 | 1 cup | With Sugar, prep, Country Time | 255 | 70 | 93 | 0.0 | 17.0 | 0.0 | 17.0 | 0.0 | 0.0 | 0.0 | 0.0 | 0.0 | 0.00 | 0.00 | 0 |
| | | Ready to Serve | | | | | | | | | | | | | | | |
| 20541 | 1 cup | Earl Grey, Nestea | 246 | 68 | 93 | 0.0 | 18.0 | 0.0 | 18.0 | 0.0 | 0.0 | 0.0 | 0.0 | 0.0 | 0.00 | 0.00 | |
| 20543 | 1 cup | Extra Sweet w/ Lemon, Nestea | 249 | 100 | 89 | 0.0 | 27.0 | 0.0 | 27.0 | 0.0 | 0.0 | 0.0 | 0.0 | 0.0 | 0.00 | 0.00 | |
| 20540 | 1 cup | Lemon, diet, Nestea | 240 | 2 | 99 | 0.0 | 1.2 | 0.0 | 1.2 | 0.0 | 0.0 | 0.0 | 0.0 | 0.0 | 0.00 | 0.00 | |
| 20542 | 1 cup | Lemon, swtnd, Nestea | 247 | 80 | 91 | 0.0 | 22.0 | | 0.0 | 22.0 | 0.0 | 0.0 | 0.0 | 0.0 | 0.00 | 0.00 | |
| | | *WATER* | | | | | | | | | | | | | | | |
| 20041 | 1 cup | Ice cubes, avg | 237 | 0 | 100 | 0.0 | 0.0 | 0.0 | 0.0 | 0.0 | 0.0 | 0.0 | 0.0 | 0.0 | 0.00 | 0.00 | 0 |
| 20050 | 1 cup | Perrier | 237 | 0 | 100 | 0.0 | 0.0 | 0.0 | 0.0 | 0.0 | 0.0 | 0.0 | 0.0 | 0.0 | 0.00 | 0.00 | 0 |
| 20051 | 1 cup | Poland Springs | 237 | 0 | 100 | 0.0 | 0.0 | 0.0 | 0.0 | 0.0 | 0.0 | 0.0 | 0.0 | 0.0 | 0.00 | 0.00 | 0 |
| 90073 | 1 cup | Pure, bottled, avg | 237 | 0 | 100 | 0.0 | 0.0 | 0.0 | 0.0 | 0.0 | 0.0 | 0.0 | 0.0 | 0.0 | 0.00 | 0.00 | 0 |
| 20444 | 1 cup | Shasta A' Sante | 237 | 0 | 100 | 0.0 | 0.0 | 0.0 | 0.0 | 0.0 | 0.0 | 0.0 | 0.0 | 0.0 | 0.00 | 0.00 | 0 |
| 20041 | 1 cup | Tap, avg | 237 | 0 | 100 | 0.0 | 0.0 | 0.0 | 0.0 | 0.0 | 0.0 | 0.0 | 0.0 | 0.0 | 0.00 | 0.00 | 0 |
| 20010 | 1 1/2 cup | Tonic/Quinine, 12 fl oz, avg | 366 | 124 | 91 | 0.0 | 32.2 | 0.0 | 32.2 | 0.0 | 0.0 | 0.0 | 0.0 | 0.0 | 0.00 | 0.00 | 0 |
| 20633 | 1 1/2 cup | Tonic/Quinine, diet, 12 fl oz, avg | 355 | 0 | 100 | 0.0 | 0.4 | 0.0 | 0.4 | 0.0 | 0.0 | 0.0 | 0.0 | 0.0 | 0.00 | 0.00 | 0 |
| | | **BEVERAGES, ALCOHOLIC** | | | | | | | | | | | | | | | |
| 22757 | 1 ea | Ale, Miller Reserve Amber, 12 fl oz | 356 | 158 | 96 | 2.1 | 12.2 | | | | 0.0 | 0.0 | 0.0 | 0.0 | 0.00 | 0.00 | 0 |
| | | Beer, 12 fl oz | | | | | | | | | | | | | | | |
| 22738 | 1 ea | Avg | 356 | 146 | 92 | 1.1 | 13.2 | 0.7 | 12.5 | 0.0 | 0.0 | 0.0 | 0.0 | 0.0 | 0.00 | 0.00 | 0 |
| 22742 | 1 ea | Avg, light | 354 | 99 | 95 | 0.7 | 4.6 | 0.0 | 4.6 | 0.0 | 0.0 | 0.0 | 0.0 | 0.0 | 0.00 | 0.00 | 0 |

| Code | Vit A (IU) | Vit A (RE) | Retinol (RE) | Carotenoids (RE) | Beta Carotene (mcg) | Thiamin (mg) | Riboflavin (mg) | Niacin (NE) | Vit B6 (mg) | Vit B12 (mcg) | Folate (mcg) | Panto (mg) | Vit C (mg) | Vit D (mg) | Vit E (α TE) | Calcium (mg) | Copper (mg) | Iron (mg) | Magnes (mg) | Mang (mg) | Phos (mg) | Potassium (mg) | Selenium (mcg) | Sodium (mg) | Zinc (mg) |
|---|---|---|---|---|---|---|---|---|---|---|---|---|---|---|---|---|---|---|---|---|---|---|---|---|---|
| | Vit A & Components | | | | | Vitamins | | | | | | | | | | Minerals | | | | | | | | | |
| 20538 | 0 | 0 | 0 | 0 | 0 | | | | | | | | 0.0 | | | 0 | | 0.0 | | | 73 | 38 | | 33 | |
| 20539 | 0 | 0 | 0 | 0 | 0 | | | | | | | | 0.0 | | | 0 | | 0.0 | | | 69 | 26 | | 27 | |
| 20070 | 45 | 5 | 0 | 5 | | 0.01 | 0.01 | 0.08 | 0.02 | 0.00 | 5.5 | 0.04 | 84.6 | 0.0 | 0.0 | 15 | 0.0 | 0.7 | 5 | 0.0 | 2 | 45 | 0.0 | 40 | 0.22 |
| 20110 | 0 | 0 | 0 | 0 | 0 | 0.15 | 0.05 | 0.00 | 0.00 | 0.00 | 28.0 | 0.01 | 85.0 | 0.0 | 0.0 | 38 | 0.0 | 0.1 | 1 | 0.0 | 27 | 152 | 0.0 | 8 | 0.02 |
| 20107 | 480 | 144 | 144 | 0 | 0 | 0.00 | 0.16 | 1.92 | 0.19 | 0.00 | 0.0 | 0.00 | 57.6 | 0.0 | 0.0 | 89 | 0.0 | 0.0 | 0 | 0.0 | 41 | 46 | 0.1 | 2 | 0.01 |
| 20340 | 500 | 100 | | | | | 0.15 | 2.00 | 0.20 | 0.00 | 40.0 | | 60.0 | | | 80 | | 0.0 | | | | 50 | | 0 | |
| 20341 | 3000 | 600 | | | | | 0.90 | 12.00 | 1.20 | 0.00 | 240.0 | | 360.0 | | | 0 | | 0.0 | | | | 390 | | 0 | |
| 20004 | 1835 | 551 | 0 | 551 | | 0.00 | 0.04 | 0.00 | 0.00 | 0.00 | 142.8 | 0.00 | 121.0 | 0.0 | 0.0 | 62 | 0.0 | 0.2 | 2 | 0.0 | 37 | 50 | 0.2 | 12 | 0.10 |
| 20445 | | | | | | | | | | 0.00 | | | | | | | | | | | | 35 | | 145 | |
| 20058 | 1450 | 145 | 0 | 145 | | 0.05 | 0.02 | 0.50 | 0.07 | 0.00 | 14.5 | 0.19 | 50.0 | 0.0 | 0.0 | 12 | 0.1 | 0.3 | 10 | 0.0 | 20 | 200 | 0.0 | 5 | 0.13 |
| 20448 | | | | | | | | | | 0.00 | | | 59.9 | | | | | | | | | | | 45 | |
| 20059 | 88 | 10 | 0 | 10 | | 0.07 | 0.04 | 0.67 | 0.10 | 0.00 | 26.3 | 0.13 | 115.0 | 0.0 | 0.0 | 18 | 0.1 | 0.8 | 15 | 1.0 | 15 | 152 | 0.0 | 35 | 0.15 |
| 20025 | 1328 | 133 | 0 | 133 | | 0.07 | 0.05 | 0.52 | 0.12 | 0.00 | 27.3 | 0.14 | 56.3 | 0.0 | 0.0 | 12 | 0.1 | 0.7 | 15 | 0.9 | 10 | 115 | 0.0 | 8 | 0.15 |
| 20421 | 0 | 0 | 0 | 0 | 0 | | | | | 0.00 | | | 0.0 | | | 0 | | 0.0 | | | 7 | 37 | | 37 | |
| 20557 | 0 | 0 | 0 | 0 | 0 | | | | | | | | 0.0 | | | 0 | | 0.0 | | | | 32 | | 28 | |
| 20424 | 0 | 0 | 0 | 0 | 0 | | | | | 0.00 | | | 0.0 | | | 0 | | 0.0 | | | 0 | 37 | | 37 | |
| 20558 | 0 | 0 | 0 | 0 | 0 | | | | | | | | 0.0 | | | 0 | | 0.0 | | | | 32 | | 28 | |
| 20422 | 0 | 0 | 0 | 0 | 0 | | | | | 0.00 | | | 0.0 | | | 0 | | 0.0 | | | 25 | 37 | | 37 | |
| 20559 | 0 | 0 | 0 | 0 | 0 | | | | | | | | 0.0 | | | 0 | | 0.0 | | | | 32 | | 28 | |
| 20560 | 0 | 0 | 0 | 0 | 0 | | | | | | | | | | | 0 | | 0.0 | | | | 32 | | 28 | |
| 20423 | 0 | 0 | 0 | 0 | 0 | | | | | 0.00 | | | 0.0 | | | 0 | | 0.0 | | | 23 | 37 | | 37 | |
| 20561 | 0 | 0 | 0 | 0 | 0 | | | | | | | | 0.0 | | | 0 | | 0.0 | | | | 32 | | 28 | |
| 20589 | 0 | 0 | 0 | 0 | 0 | 0.08 | 0.04 | 0.06 | 0.00 | 0.00 | 0.0 | | 0.0 | | 0.0 | 12 | 0.0 | 2.3 | 7 | | 5 | 38 | | 41 | 0.17 |
| 20142 | 0 | 0 | 0 | 0 | 0 | 0.01 | 0.00 | 0.00 | 0.00 | 0.00 | 0.0 | 0.00 | 0.0 | 0.0 | 0.0 | 0 | 0.0 | 0.1 | 2 | 0.0 | 22 | 27 | 0.7 | 96 | 0.05 |
| 20014 | 0 | 0 | 0 | 0 | 0 | 0.00 | 0.03 | 0.00 | 0.00 | 0.00 | 12.3 | 0.03 | 0.0 | 0.0 | 0.0 | 0 | 0.0 | 0.0 | 7 | 0.5 | 2 | 88 | 0.0 | 7 | 0.05 |
| 20118 | 47 | 5 | 0 | 5 | | 0.02 | 0.01 | 0.00 | 0.00 | 0.00 | 1.4 | 0.03 | 0.0 | 0.0 | | 5 | 0.0 | 0.2 | 2 | 0.1 | 0 | 21 | 0.0 | 2 | 0.09 |
| 20036 | 0 | 0 | 0 | 0 | 0 | 0.02 | 0.01 | 0.00 | 0.00 | 0.00 | 1.4 | 0.03 | 0.0 | 0.0 | 0.0 | 5 | 0.0 | 0.2 | 2 | 0.1 | 0 | 21 | 0.0 | 2 | 0.09 |
| 20493 | 1 | 0.1 | 0 | 0.1 | | 0.01 | 0.01 | 0.14 | 0.01 | 0.00 | 0.4 | | 0.1 | | | 12 | 0.0 | 0.3 | 2 | | 5 | 7 | | 7 | 0.12 |
| 20496 | 0 | 0 | 0 | 0 | 0 | | | | | 0.00 | | | 0.0 | | | 0 | | 0.0 | | | | | | 0 | |
| 20495 | 0 | 0 | 0 | 0 | 0 | | | | | 0.00 | | | 0.0 | | | 0 | | 0.0 | | | | | | 0 | |
| 20482 | | | | | | 0.11 | 0.35 | 1.29 | | 0.00 | | | 64.4 | | | 69 | | 5.3 | | | | | | 17 | |
| 20483 | 0 | 0 | 0 | 0 | 0 | 0.04 | 0.34 | 2.10 | | 0.00 | | | | | | 120 | 0.4 | 4.3 | 70 | | | 605 | | 13 | 0.84 |
| 20498 | | | | | | | | | | | | | | | | | | | | | | | | 63 | |
| 20499 | | | | | | | | | | | | | | | | | | | | | | | | 107 | |
| 20500 | | | | | | | | | | | | | | | | | | | | | | | | 72 | |
| 20501 | | | | | | | | | | | | | | | | | | | | | | | | 67 | |
| 20349 | 0 | 0 | 0 | 0 | 0 | | | | | 0.00 | | | 12.0 | | | 0 | | 0.0 | | | | 40 | | 0 | |
| 20381 | 0 | 0 | 0 | 0 | 0 | | | | | 0.00 | | | 6.0 | | | 0 | | 0.0 | | | | 20 | | 0 | |
| 20039 | 0 | 0 | 0 | 0 | 0 | 0.00 | 0.01 | 0.04 | 0.00 | 0.00 | 2.9 | 0.01 | 0.0 | 0.0 | 0.0 | 0 | 0.0 | 0.1 | 1 | 0.3 | 1 | 25 | 0.0 | 10 | 0.01 |
| 20040 | 0 | 0 | 0 | 0 | 0 | 0.00 | 0.01 | 0.06 | 0.00 | 0.00 | 4.5 | 0.02 | 0.0 | 0.0 | 0.0 | 5 | 0.0 | 0.1 | 5 | 0.5 | 2 | 40 | 0.0 | 24 | 0.07 |
| 20120 | 0 | 0 | 0 | 0 | 0 | 0.00 | 0.36 | 0.74 | 0.04 | 0.00 | 77.3 | 0.20 | 182.0 | 0.0 | 0.0 | 5 | 0.0 | 0.3 | 20 | 5.4 | 25 | 395 | 1.3 | 9 | 0.18 |
| 20350 | 0 | 0 | 0 | 0 | 0 | | | | | 0.00 | | | 10.9 | | | 0 | | 0.0 | | | | 36 | | 0 | |
| 20382 | 0 | 0 | 0 | 0 | 0 | | | | | 0.00 | | | 6.0 | | | 0 | | 0.0 | | | | 20 | | 0 | |
| 20342 | 0 | 0 | 0 | 0 | 0 | | | | | 0.00 | | | 6.0 | | | 0 | | 0.0 | | | | 10 | | 0 | |
| 20374 | 0 | 0 | 0 | 0 | 0 | | | | | 0.00 | | | 6.0 | | | 0 | | 0.0 | | | | 10 | | 0 | |
| 20541 | 0 | 0 | 0 | 0 | 0 | | | | | | | | 0.0 | | | 0 | | 0.0 | | | 34 | 35 | | 2 | |
| 20543 | 0 | 0 | 0 | 0 | 0 | | | | | | | | 0.0 | | | 0 | | 0.0 | | | 0 | 18 | | | |
| 20540 | 0 | 0 | 0 | 0 | 0 | | | | | | | | 0.0 | | | 0 | | 0.0 | | | 0 | 64 | | | |
| 20542 | 0 | 0 | 0 | 0 | 0 | | | | | | | | 0.0 | | | 0 | | 0.0 | | | 0 | 64 | | | |
| 20041 | 0 | 0 | 0 | 0 | 0 | 0.00 | 0.00 | 0.00 | 0.00 | 0.00 | 0.0 | 0.00 | 0.0 | 0.0 | 0.0 | 5 | 0.0 | 0.0 | 2 | 0.0 | 0 | 0 | 0.0 | 7 | 0.07 |
| 20050 | 0 | 0 | 0 | 0 | 0 | 0.00 | 0.00 | 0.00 | 0.00 | 0.00 | 0.0 | 0.00 | 0.0 | 0.0 | 0.0 | 33 | 0.0 | 0.0 | 0 | 0.0 | 0 | 0 | 0.0 | 2 | 0.00 |
| 20051 | 0 | 0 | 0 | 0 | 0 | 0.00 | 0.00 | 0.00 | 0.00 | 0.00 | 0.0 | 0.00 | 0.0 | 0.0 | 0.0 | 2 | 0.0 | 0.0 | 2 | 0.0 | 0 | 0 | 0.0 | 2 | 0.00 |
| 90073 | 0 | 0 | 0 | 0 | 0 | 0.00 | 0.00 | 0.00 | 0.00 | 0.00 | 0.0 | 0.00 | 0.0 | 0.0 | 0.0 | 0 | 0.0 | 0.0 | 0 | 0.0 | 0 | 0 | 0.0 | 0 | 0.00 |
| 20444 | | | | | | | | | | 0.00 | | | | | | | | | | | | | | 0 | |
| 20041 | 0 | 0 | 0 | 0 | 0 | 0.00 | 0.00 | 0.00 | 0.00 | 0.00 | 0.0 | 0.00 | 0.0 | 0.0 | 0.0 | 5 | 0.0 | 0.0 | 2 | 0.0 | 0 | 0 | 0.0 | 7 | 0.07 |
| 20010 | 0 | 0 | 0 | 0 | 0 | 0.00 | 0.00 | 0.00 | 0.00 | 0.00 | 0.0 | 0.00 | 0.0 | 0.0 | 0.0 | 4 | 0.0 | 0.0 | 0 | 0.0 | 0 | 0 | 0.0 | 15 | 0.37 |
| 20633 | 0 | 0 | 0 | 0 | 0 | 0.00 | 0.00 | 0.00 | 0.00 | 0.00 | 0.0 | | 0.0 | 0.0 | 0.0 | 14 | 0.1 | 0.1 | 4 | | 39 | 7 | | 57 | 0.18 |
| 22757 | | | | | | | | | | 0.00 | | | | | | | | | | | | | | 6 | |
| 22738 | 0 | 0 | 0 | 0 | 0 | 0.02 | 0.09 | 1.61 | 0.18 | 0.07 | 21.4 | 0.21 | 0.0 | 0.0 | 0.0 | 18 | 0.0 | 0.1 | 21 | 0.0 | 43 | 89 | 4.3 | 18 | 0.07 |
| 22742 | 0 | 0 | 0 | 0 | 0 | 0.03 | 0.11 | 1.39 | 0.12 | 0.04 | 14.5 | 0.13 | 0.0 | 0.0 | 0.0 | 18 | 0.1 | 0.1 | 18 | 0.1 | 42 | 64 | 4.2 | 11 | 0.11 |

| Code | Amount | Description | Basic Components | | | | | | | | | Additional Fats | | | | | | |
|---|---|---|---|---|---|---|---|---|---|---|---|---|---|---|---|---|---|---|
| | | | Weight (g) | Calories | % Water | Protein (g) | Carbs (g) | Fiber (g) | Sugar (g) | Other Carbs (g) | Fat (g) | Sat Fat (g) | Mono Fat (g) | Poly Fat (g) | Omega 3 (g) | Omega 6 (g) | Choles (mg) |
| 22824 | 1 ea | Bud Dry | 356 | 130 | 97 | 1.1 | 7.8 | | | | 0.0 | 0.0 | 0.0 | 0.0 | 0.00 | 0.00 | 0 |
| 22822 | 1 ea | Bud Light | 356 | 110 | 98 | 1.2 | 6.6 | | | | 0.0 | 0.0 | 0.0 | 0.0 | 0.00 | 0.00 | 0 |
| 22737 | 1 ea | Budweiser | 357 | 145 | 93 | 1.3 | 10.6 | | | | 0.0 | 0.0 | 0.0 | 0.0 | 0.00 | 0.00 | 0 |
| 22606 | 1 ea | Coors Cutter, nonalcoholic | 356 | 82 | 95 | 0.7 | 15.1 | 0.0 | 10.5 | 4.6 | 0.0 | 0.0 | 0.0 | 0.0 | 0.00 | 0.00 | 0 |
| 22739 | 1 ea | Coors Premium | 360 | 141 | 92 | 1.0 | 11.6 | | | | 0.0 | 0.0 | 0.0 | 0.0 | 0.00 | 0.00 | |
| 22632 | 1 ea | Icehouse | 355 | 132 | | 1.2 | 8.7 | | | | 0.0 | 0.0 | 0.0 | 0.0 | 0.00 | 0.00 | 0 |
| 22610 | 1 ea | Lowenbrau Dark | 355 | 158 | 95 | 1.4 | 14.3 | | | | 0.0 | 0.0 | 0.0 | 0.0 | 0.00 | 0.00 | 0 |
| 22743 | 1 ea | Lowenbrau Malt Liquor | 356 | 167 | | 0.4 | 11.8 | | | | 0.0 | 0.0 | 0.0 | 0.0 | 0.00 | 0.00 | 0 |
| 22744 | 1 ea | Lowenbrau Special | 356 | 158 | 95 | 1.4 | 14.3 | | | | 0.0 | 0.0 | 0.0 | 0.0 | 0.00 | 0.00 | 0 |
| 22745 | 1 ea | Magnum | 356 | 155 | 97 | 1.1 | 9.0 | | | | 0.0 | 0.0 | 0.0 | 0.0 | 0.00 | 0.00 | 0 |
| 22747 | 1 ea | Meister Brau | 356 | 130 | 97 | 0.9 | 11.1 | | | | 0.0 | 0.0 | 0.0 | 0.0 | 0.00 | 0.00 | 0 |
| 22748 | 1 ea | Meister Brau, light | 356 | 102 | 98 | 0.8 | 4.5 | | | | 0.0 | 0.0 | 0.0 | 0.0 | 0.00 | 0.00 | 0 |
| 22749 | 1 ea | Miller Genuine Draft | 356 | 143 | 96 | 1.0 | 13.1 | | | | 0.0 | 0.0 | 0.0 | 0.0 | 0.00 | 0.00 | 0 |
| 22750 | 1 ea | Miller Genuine Draft, light | 356 | 98 | 99 | 0.8 | 3.5 | | | | 0.0 | 0.0 | 0.0 | 0.0 | 0.00 | 0.00 | 0 |
| 22751 | 1 ea | Miller High Life | 356 | 143 | 96 | 1.0 | 13.1 | | | | 0.0 | 0.0 | 0.0 | 0.0 | 0.00 | 0.00 | 0 |
| 22753 | 1 ea | Miller High Life, light | 356 | 98 | 99 | 0.8 | 3.5 | | | | 0.0 | 0.0 | 0.0 | 0.0 | 0.00 | 0.00 | 0 |
| 22752 | 1 ea | Miller High Life Ice | 356 | 142 | 97 | 1.0 | 9.2 | | | | 0.0 | 0.0 | 0.0 | 0.0 | 0.00 | 0.00 | 0 |
| 22754 | 1 ea | Miller Lite | 356 | 96 | 99 | 0.9 | 3.2 | | | | 0.0 | 0.0 | 0.0 | 0.0 | 0.00 | 0.00 | 0 |
| 22755 | 1 ea | Miller Lite Ice 5.0 | 356 | 113 | 98 | 0.9 | 4.0 | | | | 0.0 | 0.0 | 0.0 | 0.0 | 0.00 | 0.00 | 0 |
| 22758 | 1 ea | Miller Reserve Lager | 356 | 142 | 97 | 2.2 | 8.6 | | | | 0.0 | 0.0 | 0.0 | 0.0 | 0.00 | 0.00 | 0 |
| 22759 | 1 ea | Miller Reserve Velvet Stout | 356 | 157 | 96 | 1.9 | 13.2 | | | | 0.0 | 0.0 | 0.0 | 0.0 | 0.00 | 0.00 | 0 |
| 22760 | 1 ea | Milwaukee's Best | 356 | 133 | 96 | 0.9 | 11.4 | | | | 0.0 | 0.0 | 0.0 | 0.0 | 0.00 | 0.00 | 0 |
| 22761 | 1 ea | Milwaukee's Best Ice | 356 | 135 | 98 | 0.9 | 6.9 | | | | 0.0 | 0.0 | 0.0 | 0.0 | 0.00 | 0.00 | 0 |
| 22762 | 1 ea | Milwaukee's Best, light | 356 | 98 | 99 | 0.8 | 3.5 | | | | 0.0 | 0.0 | 0.0 | 0.0 | 0.00 | 0.00 | 0 |
| 22691 | 1 ea | Near Beer, nonalcoholic | 356 | 32 | 98 | 1.1 | 5.0 | 0.0 | | | 0.0 | 0.0 | 0.0 | 0.0 | 0.00 | 0.00 | 0 |
| 22826 | 1 ea | O'Doul's, nonalcoholic | 361 | 70 | 96 | 0.7 | 15.0 | | | | 0.0 | 0.0 | 0.0 | 0.0 | 0.00 | 0.00 | 0 |
| 22764 | 1 ea | Red Dog | 356 | 147 | 96 | 0.7 | 14.1 | | | | 0.0 | 0.0 | 0.0 | 0.0 | 0.00 | 0.00 | 0 |
| 20608 | 1 ea | Sharp's, non alcoholic | 356 | 58 | 96 | 0.4 | 12.1 | | | | 0.0 | 0.0 | 0.0 | 0.0 | 0.00 | 0.00 | 0 |
| | | Distilled Spirits, 80 Proof, avg, 1.5 fl oz | | | | | | | | | | | | | | | |
| 22696 | 1 ea | Bourbon | 42 | 97 | 67 | 0.0 | 0.0 | 0.0 | 0.0 | 0.0 | 0.0 | 0.0 | 0.0 | 0.0 | 0.00 | 0.00 | 0 |
| 22692 | 1 ea | Brandy | 42 | 97 | 67 | 0.0 | 0.0 | 0.0 | 0.0 | 0.0 | 0.0 | 0.0 | 0.0 | 0.0 | 0.00 | 0.00 | 0 |
| 22693 | 1 ea | Gin | 42 | 97 | 67 | 0.0 | 0.0 | 0.0 | 0.0 | 0.0 | 0.0 | 0.0 | 0.0 | 0.0 | 0.00 | 0.00 | 0 |
| 22729 | 1 ea | Rum | 42 | 97 | 67 | 0.0 | 0.0 | 0.0 | 0.0 | 0.0 | 0.0 | 0.0 | 0.0 | 0.0 | 0.00 | 0.00 | 0 |
| 22731 | 1 ea | Vodka | 42 | 97 | 67 | 0.0 | 0.0 | 0.0 | 0.0 | 0.0 | 0.0 | 0.0 | 0.0 | 0.0 | 0.00 | 0.00 | 0 |
| 22694 | 1 ea | Tequila | 42 | 97 | 67 | 0.0 | 0.0 | 0.0 | 0.0 | 0.0 | 0.0 | 0.0 | 0.0 | 0.0 | 0.00 | 0.00 | 0 |
| 22695 | 1 ea | Whiskey | 42 | 97 | 67 | 0.0 | 0.0 | 0.0 | 0.0 | 0.0 | 0.0 | 0.0 | 0.0 | 0.0 | 0.00 | 0.00 | 0 |
| | | Liqueur or Cordial, avg, 1.5 fl oz | | | | | | | | | | | | | | | |
| 22547 | 1 ea | Amaretto | 30 | 106 | 30 | 0.0 | 13.3 | 0.0 | 12.1 | 1.2 | 0.1 | 0.0 | 0.0 | 0.0 | | | 0 |
| 22548 | 1 ea | Anisette | 30 | 106 | 30 | 0.0 | 13.3 | 0.0 | 12.1 | 1.2 | 0.1 | 0.0 | 0.0 | 0.0 | | | 0 |
| 22597 | 1 ea | Cherry Brandy | 48 | 122 | 48 | | 15.6 | | 15.6 | 0.0 | 0.0 | 0.0 | 0.0 | 0.0 | 0.00 | 0.00 | |
| 22734 | 1 ea | Coffee Liqueur | 52 | 175 | 31 | 0.1 | 24.3 | 0.0 | 20.3 | 4.1 | 0.2 | 0.1 | 0.0 | 0.1 | 0.00 | 0.05 | 0 |
| 22736 | 1 ea | Coffee Liqueur, w/cream | 47 | 154 | 46 | 1.3 | 9.8 | 0.0 | 9.8 | 0.0 | 7.4 | 4.5 | 2.1 | 0.3 | 0.11 | 0.21 | 7 |
| 22732 | 1 ea | Crème De Menthe | 50 | 186 | 28 | 0.0 | 20.8 | 0.0 | 20.8 | 0.0 | 0.2 | 0.0 | 0.0 | 0.1 | 0.05 | 0.03 | 0 |
| 22549 | 1 ea | Drambuie | 30 | 106 | 30 | 0.0 | 13.3 | 0.0 | 12.1 | 1.2 | 0.1 | 0.0 | 0.0 | 0.0 | | | 0 |
| 22550 | 1 ea | Grenadine | 30 | 106 | 30 | 0.0 | 13.3 | 0.0 | 12.1 | 1.2 | 0.1 | 0.0 | 0.0 | 0.0 | | | 0 |
| 22551 | 1 ea | Kahlua | 30 | 106 | 30 | 0.0 | 13.3 | 0.0 | 12.1 | 1.2 | 0.1 | 0.0 | 0.0 | 0.0 | | | 0 |
| 20606 | 1 ea | Lime Liqueur | 57 | 64 | 70 | 0.1 | 17.0 | 0.0 | 17.0 | 0.0 | 0.0 | 0.0 | 0.0 | 0.0 | 0.00 | 0.00 | 0 |
| 22552 | 1 ea | Sloe Gin | 30 | 106 | 30 | 0.0 | 13.3 | 0.0 | 12.1 | 1.2 | 0.1 | 0.0 | 0.0 | 0.0 | | | 0 |
| 22553 | 1 ea | Tia Maria | 30 | 106 | 30 | 0.0 | 13.3 | 0.0 | 12.1 | 1.2 | 0.1 | 0.0 | 0.0 | 0.0 | | | 0 |
| 22554 | 1 ea | Triple Sec | 30 | 106 | 30 | 0.0 | 13.3 | 0.0 | 12.1 | 1.2 | 0.1 | 0.0 | 0.0 | 0.0 | | | 0 |
| | | Mixed Drinks, avg | | | | | | | | | | | | | | | |
| 22555 | 1 ea | Bacardi Cocktail | 63 | 117 | 68 | 0.0 | 6.1 | 0.0 | 5.9 | 0.2 | 0.0 | 0.0 | 0.0 | 0.0 | | | 0 |
| 22563 | 1 ea | Black Russian | 90 | 243 | 53 | 0.0 | 15.8 | 0.0 | 13.2 | 2.6 | 0.1 | 0.0 | 0.0 | 0.0 | | | 0 |
| 22795 | 1 ea | Bloody Mary | 238 | 186 | 86 | 1.2 | 7.9 | 0.7 | 6.4 | 0.8 | 0.2 | 0.0 | 0.0 | 0.1 | 0.00 | 0.06 | 0 |
| 22796 | 1 ea | Bourbon & Soda | 232 | 209 | 87 | 0.0 | 0.0 | 0.0 | 0.0 | 0.0 | 0.0 | 0.0 | 0.0 | 0.0 | 0.00 | 0.00 | 0 |
| 22802 | 1 ea | Coffee Royale | 211 | 207 | 86 | 0.7 | 5.1 | 0.0 | 5.1 | 0.0 | 10.5 | 6.5 | 3.0 | 0.4 | | | 38 |
| 22797 | 1 ea | Coquito, P.R., coconut & rum | 263 | 623 | 58 | 12.4 | 45.3 | 0.9 | | | 23.8 | 16.3 | 4.8 | 1.0 | | | 189 |
| 22546 | 1 ea | Daiquiri | 288 | 187 | 83 | 0.2 | 47.5 | 0.9 | 46.6 | 0.0 | 0.2 | 0.0 | 0.0 | 0.0 | | | 0 |
| 22682 | 1 ea | Gibson | 213 | 475 | 68 | 0.1 | 0.6 | 0.0 | | | 0.0 | 0.0 | 0.0 | 0.0 | 0.00 | 0.00 | 0 |
| 22572 | 1 ea | Gin Fizz | 225 | 140 | 90 | 0.1 | 5.4 | 0.0 | 5.3 | 0.0 | 0.0 | 0.0 | 0.0 | 0.0 | | | 0 |
| 22800 | 1 ea | Gin & Tonic | 240 | 182 | 86 | 0.0 | 16.8 | 0.0 | 16.8 | 0.0 | 0.0 | 0.0 | 0.0 | 0.0 | 0.00 | 0.00 | 0 |
| 22559 | 1 ea | Harvey Wallbanger | 213 | 183 | 83 | 1.2 | 18.5 | 0.3 | 18.1 | 0.0 | 0.1 | 0.0 | 0.0 | 0.0 | | | 0 |
| 22556 | 1 ea | High Ball | 160 | 104 | 90 | 0.0 | 0.0 | 0.0 | 0.0 | 0.0 | 0.0 | 0.0 | 0.0 | 0.0 | 0.00 | 0.00 | 0 |
| 22808 | 1 ea | Hot Buttered Rum | 211 | 266 | 82 | 0.2 | 3.8 | 0.0 | | | 10.0 | 6.3 | 2.8 | 0.4 | | | 25 |
| 22801 | 1 ea | Irish Coffee | 211 | 207 | 86 | 0.7 | 5.1 | 0.0 | 5.1 | 0.0 | 10.5 | 6.5 | 3.0 | 0.4 | | | 38 |

| Code | Description | Vit A & Components | | | | | Vitamins | | | | | | | | | | Minerals | | | | | | | | | |
|---|---|---|---|---|---|---|---|---|---|---|---|---|---|---|---|---|---|---|---|---|---|---|---|---|---|---|
| | | Vit A (IU) | Vit A (RE) | Retinol (RE) | Carotenoids (RE) | Beta Carotene (mcg) | Thiamin (mg) | Riboflavin (mg) | Niacin (NE) | Vit B6 (mg) | Vit B12 (mcg) | Folate (mcg) | Panto (mg) | Vit C (mg) | Vit D (mg) | Vit E (α TE) | Calcium (mg) | Copper (mg) | Iron (mg) | Magnes (mg) | Mang (mg) | Phos (mg) | Potassium (mg) | Selenium (mcg) | Sodium (mg) | Zinc (mg) |
| 22824 | Bud Dry | | | | | | | 0.07 | 2.14 | 17.80 | 0.00 | | 14.24 | 0.0 | | | 11 | | | 17 | | 151 | 102 | | 9 | 0.00 |
| 22822 | Bud Light | | | | | | | 0.07 | 1.63 | 0.18 | 0.00 | | 0.18 | 0.0 | | | 11 | | | 17 | | 139 | 90 | | 9 | |
| 22737 | Budweiser | | | | | | 0.01 | 0.14 | 1.40 | 0.16 | 0.00 | | 0.41 | 0.0 | | | 16 | 0.0 | 0.0 | 22 | 0.0 | 147 | 111 | | 9 | 0.01 |
| 22606 | Coors Cutter, nonalcoholic | | | | | | 0.04 | 0.07 | 1.25 | | 0.00 | | | | | | 17 | | | | | | 42 | | 9 | |
| 22739 | Coors Premium | | | | | | 0.04 | 0.09 | 1.40 | | 0.00 | | | | | | 12 | | | | | | 83 | | 15 | |
| 22632 | Icehouse | | | | | | | | | | 0.00 | | | | | | | | | | | | | | 8 | |
| 22610 | Lowenbrau Dark | | | | | | | | | | 0.00 | | | | | | | | | | | | | | 7 | |
| 22743 | Lowenbrau Malt Liquor | | | | | | | | | | 0.00 | | | | | | | | | | | | | | 5 | |
| 22744 | Lowenbrau Special | | | | | | | | | | 0.00 | | | | | | | | | | | | | | 7 | |
| 22745 | Magnum | | | | | | | | | | 0.00 | | | | | | | | | | | | | | 6 | |
| 22747 | Meister Brau | | | | | | | | | | 0.00 | | | | | | | | | | | | | | 3 | |
| 22748 | Meister Brau, light | | | | | | | | | | 0.00 | | | | | | | | | | | | | | 3 | |
| 22749 | Miller Genuine Draft | | | | | | | | | | 0.00 | | | | | | | | | | | | | | 7 | |
| 22750 | Miller Genuine Draft, light | | | | | | | | | | 0.00 | | | | | | | | | | | | | | 6 | |
| 22751 | Miller High Life | | | | | | | | | | 0.00 | | | | | | | | | | | | | | 7 | |
| 22753 | Miller High Life, light | | | | | | | | | | 0.00 | | | | | | | | | | | | | | 6 | |
| 22752 | Miller High Life Ice | | | | | | | | | | 0.00 | | | | | | | | | | | | | | 5 | |
| 22754 | Miller Lite | | | | | | | | | | 0.00 | | | | | | | | | | | | | | 6 | |
| 22755 | Miller Lite Ice 5.0 | | | | | | | | | | 0.00 | | | | | | | | | | | | | | 7 | |
| 22758 | Miller Reserve Lager | | | | | | | | | | 0.00 | | | | | | | | | | | | | | 6 | |
| 22759 | Miller Reserve Velvet Stout | | | | | | | | | | 0.00 | | | | | | | | | | | | | | 6 | |
| 22760 | Milwaukee's Best | | | | | | | | | | 0.00 | | | | | | | | | | | | | | 6 | |
| 22761 | Milwaukee's Best Ice | | | | | | | | | | 0.00 | | | | | | | | | | | | | | 5 | |
| 22762 | Milwaukee's Best, light | | | | | | | | | | 0.00 | | | | | | | | | | | | | | 6 | |
| 22691 | Near Beer, nonalcoholic | 0 | 0 | 0 | 0 | 0 | 0.02 | 0.09 | 1.61 | 0.18 | 0.07 | 21.4 | | 0.0 | | 0.0 | 25 | 0.0 | 0.0 | 32 | | 110 | 89 | | 18 | 0.04 |
| 22826 | O'Doul's, nonalcoholic | | | | | | | 0.10 | 2.59 | | 0.00 | | 0.29 | 0.0 | | | 17 | | | 24 | | 165 | 139 | | 9 | 0.00 |
| 22764 | Red Dog | | | | | | | | | | 0.00 | | | | | | | | | | | | | | 4 | |
| 20608 | Sharp's, non alcoholic | | | | | | | | | | 0.00 | | | | | | | | | | | | | | 3 | |
| | Distilled Spirits, 80 Proof, avg, 1.5 fl oz | | | | | | | | | | | | | | | | | | | | | | | | | |
| 22696 | Bourbon | 0 | 0 | 0 | 0 | 0 | 0.00 | 0.00 | 0.01 | 0.00 | 0.00 | 0.0 | 0.00 | 0.0 | 0.0 | 0.0 | 0 | 0.0 | 0.0 | 0 | 0.0 | 2 | 1 | 0.0 | 0 | 0.02 |
| 22692 | Brandy | 0 | 0 | 0 | 0 | 0 | 0.00 | 0.00 | 0.01 | 0.00 | 0.00 | 0.0 | 0.00 | 0.0 | 0.0 | 0.0 | 0 | 0.0 | 0.0 | 0 | 0.0 | 2 | 1 | 0.0 | 0 | 0.02 |
| 22693 | Gin | 0 | 0 | 0 | 0 | 0 | 0.00 | 0.00 | 0.01 | 0.00 | 0.00 | 0.0 | 0.00 | 0.0 | 0.0 | 0.0 | 0 | 0.0 | 0.0 | 0 | 0.0 | 2 | 1 | 0.0 | 0 | 0.02 |
| 22729 | Rum | 0 | 0 | 0 | 0 | 0 | 0.00 | 0.00 | 0.00 | 0.00 | 0.00 | 0.0 | 0.00 | 0.0 | 0.0 | 0.0 | 0 | 0.0 | 0.1 | 0 | 0.0 | 2 | 1 | 0.0 | 0 | 0.03 |
| 22731 | Vodka | 0 | 0 | 0 | 0 | 0 | 0.00 | 0.00 | 0.00 | 0.00 | 0.00 | 0.0 | 0.00 | 0.0 | 0.0 | 0.0 | 0 | 0.0 | 0.0 | 0 | 0.0 | 2 | 0 | 0.0 | 0 | 0.00 |
| 22694 | Tequila | 0 | 0 | 0 | 0 | 0 | 0.00 | 0.00 | 0.01 | 0.00 | 0.00 | 0.0 | 0.00 | 0.0 | 0.0 | 0.0 | 0 | 0.0 | 0.0 | 0 | 0.0 | 2 | 1 | 0.0 | 0 | 0.02 |
| 22695 | Whiskey | 0 | 0 | 0 | 0 | 0 | 0.00 | 0.00 | 0.01 | 0.00 | 0.00 | 0.0 | 0.00 | 0.0 | 0.0 | 0.0 | 0 | 0.0 | 0.0 | 0 | 0.0 | 2 | 1 | 0.0 | 0 | 0.02 |
| | Liqueur or Cordial, avg, 1.5 fl oz | | | | | | | | | | | | | | | | | | | | | | | | | |
| 22547 | Amaretto | 0 | 0 | 0 | 0 | 0 | 0.00 | 0.00 | 0.02 | 0.00 | 0.00 | 0.0 | 0.00 | 0.0 | 0.0 | 0.0 | 0 | 0.0 | 0.0 | 1 | 0.0 | 1 | 5 | | 2 | 0.01 |
| 22548 | Anisette | 0 | 0 | 0 | 0 | 0 | 0.00 | 0.00 | 0.02 | 0.00 | 0.00 | 0.0 | 0.00 | 0.0 | 0.0 | 0.0 | 0 | 0.0 | 0.0 | 1 | 0.0 | 1 | 5 | | 2 | 0.01 |
| 22597 | Cherry Brandy | | | | | | | | | | 0.00 | | | 0.0 | | | 0 | | 0.0 | | | | 7 | | 1 | |
| 22734 | Coffee Liqueur | 0 | 0 | 0 | 0 | 0 | 0.00 | 0.01 | 0.07 | 0.00 | 0.00 | 0.0 | 0.00 | 0.0 | 0.0 | 0.0 | 1 | 0.0 | 0.0 | 2 | 0.0 | 3 | 16 | 0.2 | 4 | 0.02 |
| 22736 | Coffee Liqueur, w/cream | 82 | 20 | 19 | 1 | | 0.00 | 0.03 | 0.04 | 0.01 | 0.06 | 0.0 | 0.04 | 0.0 | 0.0 | | 8 | 0.0 | 0.1 | 1 | 0.0 | 23 | 15 | 0.1 | 43 | 0.08 |
| 22732 | Crème De Menthe | 0 | 0 | 0 | 0 | 0 | 0.00 | 0.00 | 0.00 | 0.00 | 0.00 | 0.0 | 0.00 | 0.0 | 0.0 | 0.0 | 0 | 0.0 | 0.0 | 0 | 0.0 | 0 | 0 | 0.2 | 2 | 0.02 |
| 22549 | Drambuie | 0 | 0 | 0 | 0 | 0 | 0.00 | 0.00 | 0.02 | 0.00 | 0.00 | 0.0 | 0.00 | 0.0 | 0.0 | 0.0 | 0 | 0.0 | 0.0 | 1 | 0.0 | 1 | 5 | | 2 | 0.01 |
| 22550 | Grenadine | 0 | 0 | 0 | 0 | 0 | 0.00 | 0.00 | 0.02 | 0.00 | 0.00 | 0.0 | 0.00 | 0.0 | 0.0 | 0.0 | 0 | 0.0 | 0.0 | 1 | 0.0 | 1 | 5 | | 2 | 0.01 |
| 22551 | Kahlua | 0 | 0 | 0 | 0 | 0 | 0.00 | 0.00 | 0.02 | 0.00 | 0.00 | 0.0 | 0.00 | 0.0 | 0.0 | 0.0 | 0 | 0.0 | 0.0 | 1 | 0.0 | 1 | 5 | | 2 | 0.01 |
| 20606 | Lime Liqueur | 6 | 0.6 | 0 | 0.6 | 3 | 0.01 | | | | 0.00 | | | 0.6 | | | 5 | | 0.2 | | | | 28 | 0.1 | 5 | |
| 22552 | Sloe Gin | 0 | 0 | 0 | 0 | 0 | 0.00 | 0.00 | 0.02 | 0.00 | 0.00 | 0.0 | 0.00 | 0.0 | 0.0 | 0.0 | 0 | 0.0 | 0.0 | 1 | 0.0 | 1 | 5 | | 2 | 0.01 |
| 22553 | Tia Maria | 0 | 0 | 0 | 0 | 0 | 0.00 | 0.00 | 0.02 | 0.00 | 0.00 | 0.0 | 0.00 | 0.0 | 0.0 | 0.0 | 0 | 0.0 | 0.0 | 1 | 0.0 | 1 | 5 | | 2 | 0.01 |
| 22554 | Triple Sec | 0 | 0 | 0 | 0 | 0 | 0.00 | 0.00 | 0.02 | 0.00 | 0.00 | 0.0 | 0.00 | 0.0 | 0.0 | 0.0 | 0 | 0.0 | 0.0 | 1 | 0.0 | 1 | 5 | | 2 | 0.01 |
| | Mixed Drinks, avg | | | | | | | | | | | | | | | | | | | | | | | | | |
| 22555 | Bacardi Cocktail | 2 | 0.3 | 0 | 0.3 | | 0.01 | 0.00 | 0.03 | 0.01 | 0.00 | 1.2 | 0.01 | 1.0 | 0.0 | | 3 | 0.0 | 0.1 | 2 | 0.0 | 4 | 15 | | 13 | 0.03 |
| 22563 | Black Russian | 0 | 0 | 0 | 0 | 0 | 0.00 | 0.01 | 0.06 | 0.00 | 0.00 | 0.0 | 0.00 | 0.0 | 0.0 | 0.0 | 0 | 0.0 | 0.0 | 1 | 0.0 | 4 | 11 | | 4 | 0.03 |
| 22795 | Bloody Mary | 816 | 81 | | | | 0.08 | 0.05 | 1.03 | 0.17 | 0.00 | 31.7 | 0.39 | 32.8 | 0.0 | | 17 | 0.2 | 0.9 | 19 | 0.1 | 33 | 347 | 1.1 | 533 | 0.21 |
| 22796 | Bourbon & Soda | 0 | 0 | 0 | 0 | 0 | 0.01 | 0.00 | 0.04 | 0.00 | 0.00 | 0.0 | 0.00 | 0.0 | 0.0 | 0.0 | 7 | 0.0 | 0.0 | 2 | 0.0 | 5 | 5 | 0.0 | 32 | 0.19 |
| 22802 | Coffee Royale | 415 | 119 | 116 | 3 | | 0.01 | 0.03 | 0.32 | 0.01 | 0.05 | 1.2 | 0.07 | 0.2 | 0.4 | | 21 | 0.0 | 0.1 | 8 | 0.0 | 21 | 97 | | 15 | 0.11 |
| 22797 | Coquito, P.R., coconut & rum | 596 | 155 | 148 | 7 | | 0.12 | 0.55 | 0.58 | 0.12 | 0.76 | 35.8 | | 4.1 | | | 373 | 0.1 | 1.4 | 47 | | 397 | 558 | | 163 | 1.78 |
| 22546 | Daiquiri | 14 | 1 | 0 | 1 | | 0.03 | 0.02 | 0.00 | 0.00 | 0.00 | 0.0 | | 6.0 | 0.0 | 0.0 | 9 | 0.0 | 0.3 | 3 | | 14 | 63 | | 233 | 0.22 |
| 22682 | Gibson | 0 | 0 | 0 | 0 | 0 | 0.01 | 0.01 | 0.06 | 0.01 | 0.00 | 0.5 | | 0.0 | | 0.0 | 4 | 0.0 | 0.2 | 4 | | 13 | 43 | | 4 | 0.10 |
| 22572 | Gin Fizz | 2 | 0.3 | 0 | 0.3 | | 0.01 | 0.00 | 0.03 | 0.01 | 0.00 | 1.7 | 0.01 | 4.1 | 0.0 | | 9 | 0.0 | 0.0 | 2 | 0.0 | 2 | 20 | | 38 | 0.17 |
| 22800 | Gin & Tonic | 2 | 0.2 | | | | 0.00 | 0.00 | 0.03 | 0.00 | 0.00 | 1.2 | 0.01 | 1.0 | 0.0 | 0.0 | 5 | 0.0 | 0.0 | 2 | 0.0 | 2 | 12 | | 10 | 0.19 |
| 22559 | Harvey Wallbanger | 133 | 14 | 0 | 14 | | 0.14 | 0.03 | 0.35 | 0.08 | 0.00 | 74.8 | 0.26 | 66.5 | 0.0 | | 15 | 0.1 | 0.2 | 17 | 0.0 | 30 | 326 | | 2 | 0.10 |
| 22556 | High Ball | 0 | 0 | 0 | 0 | 0 | 0.00 | 0.00 | 0.00 | 0.00 | 0.00 | 0.0 | | 0.0 | 0.0 | 0.0 | 6 | 0.0 | 0.0 | 2 | | 2 | 3 | | 26 | 0.13 |
| 22808 | Hot Buttered Rum | 365 | 90 | 80 | 10 | | 0.01 | 0.01 | 0.03 | 0.00 | 0.01 | 0.9 | | 0.0 | | | 6 | 0.0 | 0.1 | 4 | | 8 | 8 | | 6 | 0.09 |
| 22801 | Irish Coffee | 415 | 119 | 116 | 3 | | 0.01 | 0.03 | 0.32 | 0.01 | 0.05 | 1.2 | 0.07 | 0.2 | 0.4 | | 21 | 0.0 | 0.1 | 8 | 0.0 | 21 | 97 | | 15 | 0.11 |

| Code | Amount | Description | Basic Components | | | | | | | | | Additional Fats | | | | | | Vit A & Components | | | | | Vitamins | | | | | | | | | | Minerals | | | | | | | | | |
|---|---|---|---|---|---|---|---|---|---|---|---|---|---|---|---|---|---|---|---|---|---|---|---|---|---|---|---|---|---|---|---|---|---|---|---|---|---|---|---|---|---|---|
| | | | Weight (g) | Calories | % Water | Protein (g) | Carbs (g) | Fiber (g) | Sugar (g) | Other Carbs (g) | Fat (g) | Sat Fat (g) | Mono Fat (g) | Poly Fat (g) | Omega 3 (g) | Omega 6 (g) | Choles (mg) | Vit A (IU) | Vit A (RE) | Retinol (RE) | Carotenoids (RE) | Beta Carotene (mcg) | Thiamin (mg) | Riboflavin (mg) | Niacin (NE) | Vit B6 (mg) | Vit B12 (mcg) | Folate (mcg) | Panto (mg) | Vit C (mg) | Vit D (mg) | Vit E (α TE) | Calcium (mg) | Copper (mg) | Iron (mg) | Magnes (mg) | Mang (mg) | Phos (mg) | Potassium (mg) | Selenium (mcg) | Sodium (mg) | Zinc (mg) |
| 22566 | 1 ea | Mai Tai | 126 | 305 | 54 | 0.1 | 29.4 | 0.0 | 28.1 | 1.3 | 0.1 | 0.0 | 0.0 | 0.0 | | | 0 | 2.5 | 0.3 | 0 | 0.3 | | 0.01 | 0.01 | 0.06 | 0.01 | 0.00 | 1.2 | 0.02 | 1.0 | 0.0 | | 4 | 0.0 | 0.1 | 3 | 0.0 | 5 | 24 | | 11 | 0.07 |
| 22804 | 1 ea | Manhattan | 228 | 511 | 66 | 0.2 | 7.3 | 0.0 | 7.3 | 0.0 | 0.0 | 0.0 | 0.0 | 0.0 | 0.00 | 0.00 | 0 | 0 | 0 | 0 | 0 | 0 | 0.03 | 0.01 | 0.21 | 0.00 | 0.00 | 0.2 | 0.02 | 0.0 | 0.0 | 0.0 | 5 | 0.1 | 0.2 | 5 | 0.1 | 16 | 59 | 0.0 | 7 | 0.11 |
| 22557 | 1 ea | Margarita | 77 | 168 | 61 | 0.0 | 10.5 | 0.0 | 9.8 | 0.7 | 0.1 | 0.0 | 0.0 | 0.0 | | | 0 | 2.5 | 0.3 | 0 | 0.3 | | 0.01 | 0.00 | 0.04 | 0.00 | 0.00 | 1.2 | 0.01 | 1.0 | 0.0 | | 2 | 0.0 | 0.1 | 2 | 0.0 | 4 | 15 | | 276 | 0.03 |
| 22805 | 1 ea | Martini | 226 | 504 | 68 | 0.0 | 0.7 | 0.0 | 0.7 | 0.0 | 0.0 | 0.0 | 0.0 | 0.0 | 0.00 | 0.00 | 0 | 0 | 0 | 0 | 0 | 0 | 0.00 | 0.01 | 0.03 | 0.01 | 0.00 | 0.5 | 0.01 | 0.0 | 0.0 | 0.0 | 5 | 0.0 | 0.2 | 5 | 0.1 | 7 | 41 | 0.0 | 7 | 0.05 |
| 22803 | 1 ea | Mexican Eggnog, rompope | 243 | 406 | 69 | 9.4 | 37.2 | 0.0 | 37.2 | 0.0 | 13.3 | 5.6 | 4.6 | 1.3 | | | 367 | 712 | 204 | 198 | 5 | | 0.09 | 0.39 | 0.13 | 0.15 | 1.09 | 35.9 | 1.22 | 1.2 | 2.2 | | 211 | 0.0 | 1.1 | 22 | 0.1 | 272 | 248 | | 85 | 1.43 |
| 22558 | 1 ea | Mint Julep | 65 | 157 | 62 | 0.0 | 4.1 | 0.0 | 4.0 | 0.1 | 0.0 | 0.0 | 0.0 | 0.0 | 0.00 | 0.00 | 0 | 0 | 0 | 0 | 0 | 0 | 0.00 | 0.00 | 0.01 | 0.00 | 0.00 | 0.0 | 0.00 | 0.0 | 0.0 | 0.0 | 0 | 0.0 | 0.0 | 0 | 0.0 | 3 | 1 | | 1 | 0.03 |
| 22568 | 1 ea | Long Island Iced Tea | 125 | 119 | 83 | 0.1 | 8.9 | 0.0 | 8.8 | 0.0 | 0.0 | 0.0 | 0.0 | 0.0 | | | 0 | 2 | 0.2 | 0 | 0.2 | | 0.01 | 0.00 | 0.03 | 0.01 | 0.00 | 1.3 | 0.01 | 3.2 | 0.0 | | 4 | 0.0 | 0.1 | 1 | 0.0 | 11 | 15 | | 6 | 0.03 |
| 22805 | 1 ea | Pina Colada | 251 | 560 | 68 | 0.0 | 0.8 | 0.0 | 0.8 | 0.0 | 0.0 | 0.0 | 0.0 | 0.0 | 0.00 | 0.00 | 0 | 0 | 0 | 0 | 0 | 0 | 0.00 | 0.01 | 0.04 | 0.01 | 0.00 | 0.5 | 0.02 | 0.0 | 0.0 | 0.0 | 5 | 0.0 | 0.2 | 5 | 0.1 | 8 | 45 | 0.0 | 8 | 0.05 |
| 22809 | 1 ea | Screwdriver | 243 | 199 | 84 | 1.2 | 20.9 | 0.5 | 20.4 | 0.0 | 0.1 | 0.0 | 0.0 | 0.0 | 0.01 | 0.02 | 0 | 153 | 15 | | | | 0.16 | 0.04 | 0.39 | 0.09 | 0.00 | 85.3 | 0.31 | 75.8 | 0.0 | | 17 | 0.1 | 0.2 | 19 | 0.0 | 34 | 372 | 0.3 | 2 | 0.10 |
| 22565 | 1 ea | Singapore Sling | 225 | 227 | 83 | 0.1 | 12.0 | 0.0 | 11.9 | 0.0 | 0.1 | 0.0 | 0.0 | 0.0 | | | 0 | 2 | 0.2 | 0 | 0.2 | | 0.01 | 0.00 | 0.04 | 0.01 | 0.00 | 1.5 | 0.01 | 3.8 | 0.0 | | 9 | 0.0 | 0.1 | 2 | 0.0 | 4 | 20 | | 32 | 0.17 |
| 22560 | 1 ea | Slo-Screw | 213 | 183 | 83 | 1.2 | 18.5 | 0.3 | 18.1 | 0.0 | 0.1 | 0.0 | 0.0 | 0.0 | | | 0 | 133 | 14 | 0 | 14 | | 0.14 | 0.03 | 0.35 | 0.08 | 0.00 | 74.8 | 0.26 | 66.5 | 0.0 | | 15 | 0.1 | 0.2 | 17 | 0.0 | 30 | 326 | | 2 | 0.10 |
| 22562 | 1 ea | Sloe Gin Fizz | 222 | 122 | 91 | 0.1 | 3.0 | 0.0 | 2.9 | 0.0 | 0.0 | 0.0 | 0.0 | 0.0 | | | 0 | 2 | 0.2 | 0 | 0.2 | | 0.01 | 0.00 | 0.04 | 0.01 | 0.00 | 1.5 | | 3.8 | 0.0 | | 9 | 0.0 | 0.1 | 2 | 0.0 | 2 | 20 | | 38 | 0.19 |
| 22810 | 1 ea | Tequila Sunrise | 250 | 275 | 80 | 0.8 | 21.5 | 0.5 | 21.0 | 0.0 | 0.3 | 0.0 | 0.0 | 0.1 | 0.01 | 0.04 | 0 | 243 | 25 | | | | 0.09 | 0.04 | 0.47 | 0.13 | 0.00 | 26.5 | 0.22 | 48.3 | 0.0 | | 15 | 0.1 | 0.7 | 18 | 0.0 | 25 | 260 | 0.3 | 10 | 0.15 |
| 22812 | 1 ea | Tom Collins | 237 | 130 | 91 | 0.0 | 3.1 | 0.0 | 3.0 | 0.0 | 0.0 | 0.0 | 0.0 | 0.0 | 0.00 | 0.01 | 0 | 2 | 0.2 | | | | 0.01 | 0.00 | 0.03 | 0.01 | 0.00 | 1.7 | 0.01 | 4.0 | 0.0 | 0.0 | 9 | 0.0 | 0.0 | 2 | 0.0 | 2 | 19 | | 40 | 0.19 |
| 22564 | 1 ea | White Russian | 100 | 256 | 56 | 0.3 | 16.2 | 0.0 | 13.6 | 2.6 | 1.3 | 0.8 | 0.3 | 0.1 | | | 4 | 44 | 11 | 10 | 1 | | 0.01 | 0.02 | 0.06 | 0.00 | 0.03 | 0.3 | 0.03 | 0.1 | 0.0 | | 11 | 0.0 | 0.1 | 2 | 0.0 | 14 | 24 | | 7 | 0.08 |
| 22813 | 1 ea | Whiskey Sour | 243 | 362 | 73 | 0.0 | 31.8 | 0.0 | 31.8 | 0.0 | 0.0 | 0.0 | 0.0 | 0.0 | 0.00 | 0.00 | 0 | 32 | 2 | 0 | 2 | | 0.03 | 0.01 | 0.05 | 0.00 | 0.00 | 0.0 | 0.02 | 3.9 | 0.0 | 0.0 | 2 | 0.0 | 0.2 | 2 | 0.0 | 15 | 12 | 0.2 | 49 | 0.15 |
| | | Wine, 6 fl oz, avg | | | | | | | | | | | | | | | | | | | | | | | | | | | | | | | | | | | | | | | | |
| 22769 | 1 ea | All table types | 177 | 124 | 89 | 0.4 | 2.5 | 0.0 | 2.3 | 0.2 | 0.0 | 0.0 | 0.0 | 0.0 | 0.00 | 0.00 | 0 | 0 | 0 | 0 | 0 | 0 | 0.01 | 0.03 | 0.13 | 0.04 | 0.02 | 1.9 | 0.05 | 0.0 | 0.0 | 0.0 | 14 | 0.0 | 0.7 | 18 | 0.3 | 25 | 158 | 0.4 | 14 | 0.12 |
| 22780 | 1 ea | Chinese wine | 177 | 124 | 89 | 0.4 | 2.5 | 0.0 | | | 0.0 | 0.0 | 0.0 | 0.0 | 0.00 | 0.00 | 0 | 0 | 0 | 0 | 0 | 0 | 0.01 | 0.03 | 0.13 | 0.04 | 0.02 | 1.9 | | 0.0 | | 0.0 | 14 | 0.0 | 0.7 | 18 | | 25 | 158 | | 14 | 0.12 |
| 22778 | 1 ea | Japanese Mirin wine | 178 | 402 | 54 | 0.9 | 56.1 | 0.0 | 56.1 | 0.0 | 0.0 | 0.0 | 0.0 | 0.0 | 0.00 | 0.00 | | 0 | 0 | 0 | 0 | 0 | 0.00 | 0.00 | 0.00 | | 0.00 | | | 0.0 | | | 14 | | 0.2 | | | 12 | | | | |
| 22779 | 1 ea | Japanese Plum wine | 178 | 274 | 70 | 0.2 | 31.3 | 0.0 | 31.3 | 0.0 | 0.4 | | | | | | | 0 | 0 | 0 | 0 | 0 | 0.00 | 0.00 | 0.00 | | 0.00 | | | 0.0 | | | 2 | | 0.5 | | | 5 | | | | |
| 22782 | 1 ea | Japanese Rice wine | 177 | 237 | 78 | 0.9 | 8.9 | 0.0 | | | 0.0 | 0.0 | 0.0 | 0.0 | 0.00 | 0.00 | 0 | 0 | 0 | 0 | 0 | 0 | 0.00 | 0.00 | 0.00 | 0.00 | 0.00 | 0.0 | | 0.0 | | 0.0 | 9 | 0.0 | 0.2 | 11 | | 11 | 44 | | 4 | 0.04 |
| 22794 | 1 ea | Japanese Sake/Saki wine | 178 | 239 | 78 | 0.9 | 8.9 | 0.0 | 8.9 | 0.0 | 0.0 | 0.0 | 0.0 | 0.0 | 0.00 | 0.00 | | 0 | 0 | 0 | 0 | 0 | 0.00 | 0.00 | 0.00 | | 0.00 | | | 0.0 | | | 0 | | 0.2 | | | 11 | | | | |
| 22790 | 1 ea | Red wine | 177 | 127 | 88 | 0.4 | 3.0 | 0.0 | | | 0.0 | 0.0 | 0.0 | 0.0 | 0.00 | 0.00 | 0 | 0 | 0 | 0 | 0 | 0 | 0.01 | 0.05 | 0.14 | 0.06 | 0.02 | 3.5 | 0.06 | 0.0 | 0.0 | 0.0 | 14 | 0.0 | 0.8 | 23 | 1.1 | 25 | 198 | 0.4 | 9 | 0.16 |
| 22792 | 1 ea | Red Burgundy wine | 176 | 123 | 89 | 0.4 | 2.5 | 0.0 | 2.5 | 0.0 | 0.0 | 0.0 | 0.0 | 0.0 | 0.00 | 0.00 | 0 | 0 | 0 | 0 | 0 | 0 | 0.01 | 0.03 | 0.13 | 0.04 | 0.02 | 1.9 | 0.00 | 0.0 | 0.0 | 0.0 | 14 | 0.0 | 0.7 | 18 | 0.2 | 25 | 157 | 0.0 | 14 | 0.12 |
| 22793 | 1 ea | Red Claret wine | 176 | 123 | 89 | 0.4 | 2.5 | 0.0 | 2.5 | 0.0 | 0.0 | 0.0 | 0.0 | 0.0 | 0.00 | 0.00 | 0 | 0 | 0 | 0 | 0 | 0 | 0.01 | 0.03 | 0.13 | 0.04 | 0.02 | 1.9 | 0.00 | 0.0 | 0.0 | 0.0 | 14 | 0.0 | 0.7 | 18 | 0.2 | 25 | 157 | 0.0 | 14 | 0.12 |
| 22771 | 1 ea | Red Rose' wine | 177 | 126 | 89 | 0.4 | 2.5 | 0.0 | | | 0.0 | 0.0 | 0.0 | 0.0 | 0.00 | 0.00 | 0 | 0 | 0 | 0 | 0 | 0 | 0.01 | 0.03 | 0.13 | 0.04 | 0.02 | 1.9 | 0.05 | 0.0 | 0.0 | 0.0 | 14 | 0.1 | 0.7 | 18 | 0.2 | 27 | 175 | 0.4 | 9 | 0.11 |
| 22791 | 1 ea | Red Sherry wine, dry | 176 | 123 | 89 | 0.4 | 2.5 | 0.0 | 2.5 | 0.0 | 0.0 | 0.0 | 0.0 | 0.0 | 0.00 | 0.00 | 0 | 0 | 0 | 0 | 0 | 0 | 0.01 | 0.03 | 0.13 | 0.04 | 0.02 | 1.9 | 0.00 | 0.0 | 0.0 | 0.0 | 14 | 0.0 | 0.7 | 18 | 0.2 | 25 | 157 | 0.0 | 14 | 0.12 |
| 22770 | 1 ea | Sangria wine | 177 | 145 | 83 | 0.2 | 20.2 | 0.0 | | | 0.0 | 0.0 | 0.0 | 0.0 | | | 0 | 20 | 2 | 0 | 2 | | 0.01 | 0.01 | 0.08 | 0.02 | 0.00 | 3.9 | | 6.7 | | | 7 | 0.0 | 0.2 | 5 | | 9 | 62 | | 12 | 0.10 |
| 22768 | 1 ea | White wine, medium | 177 | 120 | 90 | 0.2 | 1.4 | 0.0 | | | 0.0 | 0.0 | 0.0 | 0.0 | 0.00 | 0.00 | 0 | 0 | 0 | 0 | 0 | 0 | 0.01 | 0.01 | 0.12 | 0.02 | 0.00 | 0.4 | 0.04 | 0.0 | 0.0 | 0.0 | 16 | 0.0 | 0.6 | 18 | 0.8 | 25 | 142 | 0.4 | 9 | 0.12 |
| 27765 | 1 ea | Wine Cooler, 12 fl oz | 340 | 231 | 90 | 0.3 | 2.7 | 0.0 | | | 0.0 | 0.0 | 0.0 | 0.0 | 0.00 | 0.00 | 0 | 0 | 0 | 0 | 0 | 0 | 0.01 | 0.02 | 0.23 | 0.05 | 0.00 | 0.7 | 0.07 | 0.0 | 0.0 | 0.0 | 31 | 0.1 | 1.1 | 34 | 1.6 | 48 | 272 | 0.7 | 17 | 0.24 |
| 22766 | 1 ea | Wine Spritzer, 12 fl oz | 340 | 143 | 93 | 0.4 | 2.8 | 0.0 | | | 0.0 | 0.0 | 0.0 | 0.0 | 0.00 | 0.00 | 0 | 0 | 0 | 0 | 0 | 0 | 0.01 | 0.03 | 0.15 | 0.05 | 0.02 | 2.2 | | 0.0 | | 0.0 | 24 | 0.0 | 0.8 | 20 | | 27 | 184 | | 44 | 0.28 |
| | | Cooking Wine | | | | | | | | | | | | | | | | | | | | | | | | | | | | | | | | | | | | | | | | |
| 22603 | 2 Tbs | Burgundy | 30 | 19 | 95 | 0.3 | 1.0 | | | 1.0 | 0.3 | 0.0 | 0.0 | 0.0 | | | 0 | 9 | 2 | | | | 0.00 | 0.00 | 0.06 | | 0.00 | | | 0.9 | | | 1 | | 0.1 | | | | 7 | | 229 | |
| 22605 | 2 Tbs | Chablis | 30 | 17 | 97 | 0.3 | 0.4 | | | 0.4 | 0.3 | 0.0 | 0.0 | 0.0 | | | 0 | 9 | 2 | | | | 0.00 | 0.00 | 0.00 | | 0.00 | | | 0.9 | | | 1 | | 0.1 | | | | 6 | | 189 | |
| 22608 | 2 Tbs | Red, Fleischmann's | 30 | 20 | 88 | 0.0 | 0.2 | 0.0 | 0.2 | 0.0 | 0.0 | 0.0 | 0.0 | 0.0 | 0.00 | 0.00 | | 0.3 | 0.06 | | | | 0.15 | 0.15 | 0.15 | | 0.00 | | | 0.2 | | | 2 | | 0.2 | | | 5 | 24 | | 180 | |
| 27074 | 2 Tbs | Sauterne, Regina | 30 | 20 | 88 | 0.0 | 3.0 | 0.0 | 0.0 | 3.0 | 0.0 | 0.0 | 0.0 | 0.0 | 0.00 | 0.00 | 0 | | | | | | | | | | 0.00 | | | | | | | | | | | | 25 | | 361 | |
| 22607 | 2 Tbs | Sherry, Fleischmann's | 30 | 29 | 84 | 0.0 | 0.2 | 0.0 | 0.2 | 0.0 | 0.0 | 0.0 | 0.0 | 0.0 | 0.00 | 0.00 | | 0.3 | 0.06 | | | | 0.15 | 0.15 | 0.15 | | 0.00 | | | 0.2 | | | 2 | | 0.2 | | | 4 | 18 | | 180 | |
| | | Dessert Wine, 6 fl oz | | | | | | | | | | | | | | | | | | | | | | | | | | | | | | | | | | | | | | | | |
| 22785 | 1 ea | Dry dessert wine | 177 | 223 | 80 | 0.4 | 7.3 | 0.0 | 7.3 | 0.0 | 0.0 | 0.0 | 0.0 | 0.0 | 0.00 | 0.00 | 0 | 0 | 0 | 0 | 0 | 0 | 0.03 | 0.03 | 0.38 | 0.00 | 0.00 | 0.7 | 0.06 | 0.0 | 0.0 | 0.0 | 14 | 0.1 | 0.4 | 16 | 0.2 | 16 | 163 | 0.7 | 16 | 0.12 |
| 22789 | 1 ea | Madeira dessert wine | 177 | 271 | 72 | 0.4 | 20.9 | 0.0 | 20.9 | 0.0 | 0.0 | 0.0 | 0.0 | 0.0 | 0.00 | 0.00 | 0 | 0 | 0 | 0 | 0 | 0 | 0.03 | 0.03 | 0.38 | 0.00 | 0.00 | 0.7 | 0.06 | 0.0 | 0.0 | 0.0 | 14 | 0.1 | 0.4 | 16 | 0.2 | 16 | 163 | 0.9 | 16 | 0.12 |
| 22787 | 1 ea | Marsala dessert wine | 177 | 271 | 72 | 0.4 | 20.9 | 0.0 | 20.9 | 0.0 | 0.0 | 0.0 | 0.0 | 0.0 | 0.00 | 0.00 | 0 | 0 | 0 | 0 | 0 | 0 | 0.03 | 0.03 | 0.38 | 0.00 | 0.00 | 0.7 | 0.06 | 0.0 | 0.0 | 0.0 | 14 | 0.1 | 0.4 | 16 | 0.2 | 16 | 163 | 0.9 | 16 | 0.12 |
| 22788 | 1 ea | Port dessert wine | 177 | 271 | 72 | 0.4 | 20.9 | 0.0 | 20.9 | 0.0 | 0.0 | 0.0 | 0.0 | 0.0 | 0.00 | 0.00 | 0 | 0 | 0 | 0 | 0 | 0 | 0.03 | 0.03 | 0.38 | 0.00 | 0.00 | 0.7 | 0.06 | 0.0 | 0.0 | 0.0 | 14 | 0.1 | 0.4 | 16 | 0.2 | 16 | 163 | 0.9 | 16 | 0.12 |
| 22786 | 1 ea | Sweet dessert wine | 177 | 271 | 72 | 0.4 | 20.9 | 0.0 | 20.9 | 0.0 | 0.0 | 0.0 | 0.0 | 0.0 | 0.00 | 0.00 | 0 | 0 | 0 | 0 | 0 | 0 | 0.03 | 0.03 | 0.38 | 0.00 | 0.00 | 0.7 | 0.06 | 0.0 | 0.0 | 0.0 | 14 | 0.1 | 0.4 | 16 | 0.2 | 16 | 163 | 0.9 | 16 | 0.12 |
| 22784 | 1 ea | Sweet vermouth dessert wine | 180 | 275 | 72 | 0.4 | 21.2 | 0.0 | 21.2 | 0.0 | 0.0 | 0.0 | 0.0 | 0.0 | 0.00 | 0.00 | 0 | 0 | 0 | 0 | 0 | 0 | 0.03 | 0.03 | 0.38 | 0.00 | 0.00 | 0.7 | 0.06 | 0.0 | 0.0 | 0.0 | 14 | 0.1 | 0.4 | 16 | 0.2 | 16 | 166 | 0.4 | 16 | 0.13 |
| | | **CANDIES AND CONFECTIONS, GUM** | | | | | | | | | | | | | | | | | | | | | | | | | | | | | | | | | | | | | | | | |
| | | Baking Chocolate and Coating | | | | | | | | | | | | | | | | | | | | | | | | | | | | | | | | | | | | | | | | |
| 23439 | 1 ea | Bittersweet Bar, Hersheys | 28 | 157 | 1 | 1.9 | 16.0 | 2.2 | 12.7 | 1.2 | 9.4 | 5.8 | 0.8 | 0.1 | | | 1 | 2 | 0.4 | | | | | | | | | | | 0.0 | | | 1 | | 0.1 | | | | 107 | | 1 | |
| 23208 | 1 oz | Bittersweet Coating, Blue Ribbon | 28 | 134 | 1 | 2.0 | 14.6 | 0.3 | | | 10.4 | 5.9 | | | | | 0 | 10 | 1 | 0 | 1 | | 0.01 | 0.03 | 0.25 | | | | | 0.0 | | | 13 | | 1.1 | | | 64 | 137 | | 8 | |
| 23044 | 1 ea | Bittersweet Square, avg | 28 | 134 | 2 | 2.2 | 13.1 | 0.9 | 0.5 | 11.7 | 11.1 | 6.2 | 4.1 | 0.2 | 0.00 | 0.22 | 0 | 11 | 3 | 0 | 3 | | 0.01 | 0.05 | 0.28 | 0.01 | 0.00 | 3.4 | 0.05 | 0.0 | 0.0 | | 16 | 0.2 | 1.4 | 28 | | 80 | 172 | 0.6 | 1 | 1.11 |
| 23329 | 2 pce | German's Sweet Bar, Baker's | 13 | 60 | 2 | 1.0 | 8.0 | 0.5 | 8.0 | | 3.5 | 2.0 | | | | | 0 | 0 | 0 | 0 | 0 | 0 | | | | | | | | 0.0 | | | 0 | | 0.4 | | | | 50 | | 0 | |
| 23418 | 1 ea | Mexican Squares, avg | 20 | 85 | 2 | 0.7 | 15.5 | 0.8 | 0.7 | 14.0 | 3.1 | 1.7 | 1.0 | 0.2 | 0.01 | 0.22 | 0 | 4 | 0.4 | | | | 0.01 | 0.02 | 0.37 | 0.01 | 0.00 | 0.4 | 0.04 | 0.0 | 0.0 | | 7 | 0.1 | 0.4 | 19 | 0.1 | 28 | 79 | 0.4 | 1 | 0.25 |
| 23209 | 1 oz | Milk Chocolate Coating, avg | 28 | 143 | 1 | 1.1 | 18.2 | 0.1 | | | 7.8 | 4.8 | | | | | 3 | 34 | 9 | | | | 0.01 | 0.06 | 0.06 | | | | | 0.3 | | | 34 | | 0.2 | | | 36 | 67 | | 19 | |
| 23401 | 1 pce | Semi-Sweet Bar, Baker's | 28 | 130 | | 2.0 | 17.0 | 2.0 | 13.0 | 2.0 | 9.0 | 5.0 | | | | | 0 | 0 | 0 | 0 | 0 | 0 | | | | | | | | 0.0 | | | 0 | | 1.4 | | | | 140 | | 0 | |
| 23440 | 1 ea | Semi-Sweet Bar, Hersheys's | 28 | 149 | 1 | 1.4 | 18.0 | 1.4 | 14.7 | 1.9 | 8.0 | 5.0 | 2.7 | 0.3 | | | 2 | | | | | | | | | | | | | | | | 8 | | 0.7 | | | | 94 | | 5 | |
| 23180 | 1 oz | Semi-Sweet Bar, Nestle | 28 | 140 | 1 | 1.6 | 18.0 | 4.0 | 14.0 | 0.0 | 8.1 | 5.0 | | | | | 0 | 0 | 0 | 0 | 0 | 0 | 0.02 | 0.00 | 0.20 | | | | | 0.0 | | | 0 | | 0.7 | | | | 108 | 1.1 | 0 | |
| 23200 | 1/2 cup | Semi-Sweet Chocolate, w/butter, avg | 85 | 405 | 1 | 3.6 | 53.9 | 5.0 | | | 25.2 | 14.9 | 8.4 | 0.8 | 0.16 | 0.64 | 15 | 51 | 5 | | | | 0.05 | 0.08 | 0.36 | 0.04 | 0.00 | 2.6 | 0.09 | 0.0 | | | 27 | 0.6 | 2.7 | 98 | 0.7 | 112 | 310 | 2.7 | 9 | 1.38 |
| 23441 | 1 ea | Unsweetened Bar, Hershey's | 28 | 178 | 2 | 4.0 | 8.1 | 4.4 | 0.1 | 3.6 | 14.4 | 8.8 | 5.1 | 0.4 | | | 0 | | | | | | | | | | | | | | | | 25 | | 1.7 | | | | 262 | | 5 | |
| 23178 | 1 oz | Unsweetened, ChocoBake, pre-mltd | 28 | 160 | 4 | 0.0 | 10.0 | 6.0 | 0.0 | 4.0 | 16.0 | 10.1 | | | | | 0 | 0 | 0 | 0 | 0 | 0 | 0.04 | 0.04 | 0.36 | | | | | 0.0 | | | 0 | | 1.4 | | | | | 1.1 | 0 | |
| 23010 | 1 ea | Unsweetened Square, avg | 28 | 146 | 1 | 2.9 | 7.9 | 4.3 | 0.2 | 3.4 | 15.5 | 9.1 | 5.2 | 0.5 | 0.00 | 0.49 | 0 | 27 | 3 | 0 | 3 | | 0.02 | 0.05 | 0.31 | 0.03 | 0.00 | 2.0 | 0.06 | 0.0 | 0.0 | | 21 | 0.6 | 1.8 | 87 | 0.5 | 117 | 233 | 2.1 | 4 | 1.12 |
| 23011 | 1/2 cup | Unsweetened Square, grated, avg | 66 | 345 | 1 | 6.8 | 18.7 | 10.2 | 0.4 | 8.1 | 36.5 | 21.5 | 12.2 | 1.2 | 0.00 | 1.16 | 0 | 65 | 6 | 0 | 6 | | 0.05 | 0.11 | 0.73 | 0.06 | 0.00 | 4.6 | 0.13 | 0.0 | 0.0 | | 49 | 1.4 | 4.2 | 205 | 1.3 | 275 | 550 | 5.0 | 9 | 2.65 |
| 23179 | 1 oz | Unsweetened Bar, Nestle | 28 | 160 | 0 | 4.0 | 9.0 | 6.0 | 0.0 | 3.0 | 14.0 | 3.9 | 5.2 | 0.7 | 0.03 | 0.67 | 0 | 0 | 0 | 0 | 0 | 0 | 0.03 | 0.04 | 0.38 | | | | | 0.0 | | | 0 | | 0.0 | | | | 236 | 1.1 | 0 | |
| 23072 | 1 oz | Unsweetened White, Nestle Toll House | 28 | 160 | | 2.0 | 16.0 | 0.0 | 16.0 | 0.0 | 10.1 | 5.9 | | | | | 6 | 0 | 0 | 0 | 0 | 0 | | | | | | | | 0.0 | | | 80 | | 0.0 | | | | | | 30 | |
| | | Baking Chips & Morsels | | | | | | | | | | | | | | | | | | | | | | | | | | | | | | | | | | | | | | | | |
| 23119 | 1/2 cup | Butterscotch Chips, avg | 85 | 458 | 1 | 1.9 | 57.0 | 0.0 | 57.9 | 2.5 | 24.7 | 20.5 | 1.9 | 0.4 | 0.01 | 0.36 | 0 | 0 | 0 | 0 | 0 | 0 | 0.07 | 0.00 | 0.06 | 0.01 | 0.09 | 0.9 | 0.13 | 0.1 | | | 29 | 0.0 | 0.1 | 4 | 0.0 | 27 | 159 | 1.1 | 76 | 0.10 |
| 23475 | 1/2 cup | Butterscotch Chips, Bakeshoppe | 120 | 649 | 1 | 4.6 | 77.3 | 0.5 | 73.9 | 2.9 | 35.8 | 31.8 | 3.4 | 0.5 | | | 7 | | | | | | | | | | | | | | | | 162 | | 0.0 | | | | 258 | | 94 | |
| 23184 | 1/2 cup | Butterscotch Morsels, Toll House | 86 | 491 | 1 | 0.0 | 61.4 | 0.0 | 61.4 | 0.0 | 24.9 | 24.9 | 0.0 | 0.0 | 0.00 | 0.00 | 0 | 0 | 0 | 0 | 0 | 0 | 0.06 | 0.09 | 0.05 | | | | | 0.0 | | | 0 | | 0.0 | | | | 159 | | 92 | |
| 23243 | 1/2 cup | Carob Chips, avg | 85 | 459 | 2 | 6.9 | 47.9 | 3.2 | | | 26.7 | 24.7 | 0.4 | 0.3 | 0.03 | 0.22 | 3 | 20 | 7 | | | | 0.09 | 0.15 | 0.88 | 0.11 | 0.85 | 23.8 | 0.64 | 0.4 | | | 258 | 0.2 | 1.1 | 31 | 0.1 | 107 | 538 | 4.4 | 91 | 3.00 |
| 23246 | 30 pce | Carob Chips, unswtnd, avg | 6 | 28 | | 0.9 | 3.3 | 0.0 | 2.1 | 1.2 | 1.3 | 1.2 | | | | | 1 | 4 | 1 | | | | | | | | | | | 0.3 | | | 38 | | 0.1 | | | | | | 26 | |
| 23245 | 30 pce | Carob Vegan Malted Chips, avg | 14 | 68 | 3 | 0.4 | 10.0 | 0.0 | 4.3 | 5.7 | 3.1 | 2.8 | | | | | 0 | 0.3 | 0.06 | | | | | | | | | | | 0.0 | | | 10 | | 0.4 | | | | | | 4 | |

| Code | Amount | Description | Basic Components | | | | | | | | | Additional Fats | | | | | |
|---|---|---|---|---|---|---|---|---|---|---|---|---|---|---|---|---|---|
| | | | Weight (g) | Calories | % Water | Protein (g) | Carbs (g) | Fiber (g) | Sugar (g) | Other Carbs (g) | Fat (g) | Sat Fat (g) | Mono Fat (g) | Poly Fat (g) | Omega 3 (g) | Omega 6 (g) | Choles (mg) |
| 23207 | 1/2 cup | Chocolate Bittersweet Chips, Ambrosia | 86 | 404 | 1 | 4.3 | 57.6 | 0.8 | | | 22.4 | 12.9 | | | | | 0 |
| 23378 | 2 Tbs | Crunch Pieces, choc&crspd rice, Nestle | 24 | 125 | 1 | 1.4 | 15.6 | 0.5 | 13.4 | 1.6 | 6.3 | 3.6 | 2.[illegible] | 0.2 | 0.00 | 0.20 | 3 |
| 23423 | 1 Tbs | Milk Chocolate, M&M's mini bits | 14 | 70 | 2 | 0.7 | 9.4 | 0.4 | 8.6 | 0.4 | 3.3 | 2.0 | 1.[illegible] | 0.1 | 0.00 | 0.10 | 2 |
| 23382 | 1 oz | Milk Chocolate Chips, Bakers | 28 | 140 | | 2.0 | 18.0 | 0.0 | 16.0 | 2.0 | 8.0 | 4.0 | | | | | 0 |
| 23474 | 1/2 cup | Milk Chocolate Chips, Bakeshoppe | 120 | 647 | 2 | 8.8 | 72.1 | 0.7 | 64.5 | 7.0 | 35.9 | 21.1 | 6.[illegible] | 0.[illegible] | | | 25 |
| 23444 | 10 ea | Milk Chocolate Kisses, mini, Hershey's | 14 | 76 | 2 | 1.0 | 8.1 | 0.3 | 7.1 | 0.7 | 4.4 | 2.8 | 1.5 | 0.[illegible] | | | 3 |
| 23181 | 1/2 cup | Milk Chocolate Morsel Chips, Toll House | 86 | 430 | 3 | 0.0 | 55.3 | 0.0 | 49.1 | 6.1 | 27.5 | 15.5 | | | | | 18 |
| 23476 | 1/2 cup | Peanut Butter Chips, Reese's | 120 | 629 | 3 | 24.8 | 55.9 | 4.9 | 45.8 | 5.2 | 34.0 | 28.7 | 3.5 | 1.7 | | | 2 |
| 23012 | 1/2 cup | Semi-Sweet Chocolate Chips, avg | 84 | 402 | 1 | 3.5 | 53.0 | 5.0 | 47.8 | 0.3 | 25.2 | 15.0 | 8.[illegible] | 0.8 | 0.05 | 0.76 | 0 |
| 23328 | 1 oz | Semi-Sweet Chocolate flvd Chips, Bakers | 28 | 140 | 5 | 0.0 | 20.0 | 1.0 | 18.0 | 1.0 | 6.0 | 6.0 | | | | | 0 |
| 23313 | 1 oz | Semi-Sweet Real Chocolate Chips, Bakers | 28 | 120 | 1 | 2.0 | 18.0 | 1.0 | 16.0 | 1.0 | 7.0 | 4.0 | | | | | 0 |
| 23473 | 1/2 cup | Semi-Sweet Chocolate Chips, Bakeshoppe | 120 | 635 | 1 | 5.6 | 78.9 | 1.[illegible] | 66.1 | 11.7 | 32.6 | 18.8 | 3.[illegible] | 0.4 | | | 7 |
| 23421 | 1 Tbs | Semi-Sweet Chocolate Mini Bits, M&M's | 14 | 73 | 1 | 0.6 | 9.2 | 0.9 | 7.4 | 0.9 | 3.7 | 2.2 | 1.[illegible] | 0.1 | 0.00 | 0.12 | 0 |
| 23182 | 1/2 cup | Semi-Sweet Chocolate Morsels, Toll House | 86 | 430 | 5 | 0.0 | 55.3 | 0.2 | 43.0 | 12.0 | 24.9 | 12.0 | | | | | 0 |
| 23183 | 1/2 cup | Semi-Sweet Chocolate Mini Morsels, Toll House | 86 | 430 | 5 | 0.0 | 55.3 | 0.2 | 43.0 | 12.0 | 24.9 | 12.0 | 8.[illegible] | 1.1 | | | 0 |
| 23121 | 1/2 cup | White Chips, avg | 85 | 458 | 1 | 5.0 | 50.4 | 0.0 | 51.0 | 3.3 | 27.3 | 16.5 | 7.[illegible] | 0.9 | 0.09 | 0.77 | 18 |
| 23477 | 1/2 cup | Vanilla Chips, Hershey's | 120 | 637 | 2 | 9.3 | 73.4 | 0.0 | 72.1 | 1.2 | 34.0 | 20.6 | 1.[illegible] | 0.4 | | | 5 |
| | | Candy and Candy Bars | | | | | | | | | | | | | | | |
| 23049 | 1 ea | Almond Joy, 1.73 oz bar | 49 | 229 | 10 | 2.1 | 28.6 | 2.4 | 22.3 | 3.9 | 13.1 | 8.5 | 3.[illegible] | 0.7 | 0.04 | 0.63 | 2 |
| 23405 | 1 ea | Almond Joy, fun size, .7 oz bar | 20 | 93 | 10 | 0.8 | 11.7 | 1.0 | 9.1 | 1.6 | 5.4 | 3.5 | 1.[illegible] | 0.3 | 0.02 | 0.23 | [illegible] |
| 23085 | 1 pce | Almond Roca candy | 11 | 48 | 5 | 0.8 | 7.3 | 0.3 | 6.7 | 0.4 | 2.0 | 1.1 | 0.[illegible] | 0.2 | | | [illegible] |
| 23077 | 1 ea | Alpine, white chocolate & almonds, 1.23 oz bar | 35 | 193 | 1 | 3.4 | 17.7 | 1.5 | | | 12.9 | 7.0 | 5.[illegible] | 0.9 | 0.06 | 0.85 | 4 |
| 23110 | 1 ea | Baby Ruth , 2.12 oz bar | 60 | 289 | 5 | 4.5 | 39.1 | 1.7 | 31.2 | 6.2 | 12.7 | 7.1 | 3.[illegible] | 1.9 | 0.00 | 1.90 | 2 |
| 23269 | 1 ea | Baby Ruth, fun size, .5 oz bar | 14 | 67 | 5 | 1.0 | 9.1 | 0.4 | 7.3 | 1.4 | 3.0 | 1.7 | 0.5 | 0.4 | 0.00 | 0.44 | [illegible] |
| 23111 | 1 ea | Bar None, 1.52 oz bar | 43 | 224 | 4 | 3.5 | 22.4 | 1.4 | | | 14.6 | 9.4 | 3.[illegible] | 1.0 | 0.01 | 0.94 | [illegible] |
| 23112 | 5 pce | Bit-O-Honey Chews | 40 | 155 | 7 | 1.1 | 32.4 | | | | 3.2 | | | | | | 0 |
| 23254 | 1 ea | Buncha Crunch, 1.4 oz bar | 40 | 202 | 3 | 2.0 | 26.3 | 0.8 | 20.2 | 5.3 | 10.0 | 5.2 | | | | | 5 |
| 23115 | 5 pce | Butterscotch candy, avg | 30 | 119 | 1 | 0.0 | 28.6 | 0.0 | 28.6 | 0.0 | 1.1 | 0.3 | 0.2 | 0.0 | 0.01 | 0.01 | 3 |
| 23225 | 1 pce | Breath Savers mints, asstd flvrs | 2 | 10 | | 0.0 | 0.0 | 0.0 | 0.0 | 0.0 | 0.0 | 0.0 | 0.0 | 0.0 | 0.00 | 0.00 | 0 |
| 23309 | 5 pce | Butter Mints, Kraft | 11 | 44 | | 0.0 | 10.3 | 0.0 | 10.3 | 0.0 | 0.0 | 0.0 | 0.0 | 0.0 | 0.00 | 0.00 | 0 |
| 23116 | 1 ea | Caramello, 1.6 oz bar | 45 | 213 | 7 | 2.7 | 28.5 | 0.7 | 21.6 | 6.2 | 9.8 | 6.3 | 3.2 | 0.3 | | | 12 |
| 23435 | 2 Tbs | Caramel Dip, Marie's | 35 | 150 | 15 | 0.5 | 24.0 | 1.0 | 18.0 | 5.0 | 5.0 | 4.0 | | | | | 5 |
| 23015 | 5 pce | Caramels, avg | 50 | 191 | 8 | 2.3 | 38.5 | 0.6 | 32.8 | 5.2 | 4.1 | 3.3 | 0.4 | 0.1 | 0.01 | 0.08 | 4 |
| 23117 | 5 ea | Caramels, chocolate flvd roll, avg | 25 | 90 | 7 | 0.5 | 21.8 | 0.2 | 18.8 | 2.9 | 0.6 | 0.1 | 0.3 | 0.2 | 0.01 | 0.18 | 0 |
| 23308 | 5 pce | Caramels, Kraft | 41 | 170 | 8 | 2.0 | 32.0 | 0.0 | 27.0 | 5.0 | 3.0 | 1.0 | | | | | 2 |
| 23118 | 1 ea | Carob, avg, 3.1 oz. bar | 87 | 470 | 2 | 7.1 | 49.0 | 3.3 | | | 27.3 | 25.[illegible] | 0.4 | 0.3 | 0.03 | 0.23 | 3 |
| 23020 | 1/2 cup | Chocolate Coated Almonds, avg | 82 | 466 | 2 | 10.1 | 32.5 | 6.9 | 22.1 | 3.4 | 36.4 | 6.1 | 23.9 | 6.5 | | 4.51 | 1 |
| 23113 | 1 ea | Chocolate Covered Banana, w/nuts, avg | 145 | 336 | 51 | 6.8 | 43.2 | 4.6 | | | 18.3 | 7.0 | 7.5 | 3.1 | | | 0 |
| 23023 | 5 ea | Chocolate Covered Fondant/Mints, avg | 55 | 201 | 8 | 1.2 | 44.1 | 0.8 | 42.9 | 0.4 | 5.1 | 3.0 | 1.7 | 0.2 | 0.00 | 0.17 | 0 |
| 23122 | 1 ea | Chunky, 1.4 oz. bar | 40 | 198 | 3 | 3.6 | 22.8 | 1.9 | 20.2 | 0.7 | 11.7 | 9.3 | 0.1 | 1.8 | 0.05 | 1.71 | 4 |
| 23098 | 1 ea | Crisped Rice Almond bar, 1 oz, avg | 28 | 128 | 7 | 2.0 | 18.1 | 1.0 | 8.7 | 8.4 | 5.7 | 1.[illegible] | 2.1 | 2.2 | 0.09 | 2.08 | 0 |
| 23099 | 1 ea | Crisped Rice Chocolate Chip bar, 1 oz, avg | 28 | 113 | 7 | 1.4 | 20.4 | 0.6 | 10.1 | 9.7 | 3.8 | 1.5 | 1.1 | 1.0 | 0.05 | 0.97 | 0 |
| 23133 | 1 ea | Crunch, milk chocolate bar, 1.4 oz | 40 | 209 | 1 | 2.4 | 26.1 | 1.0 | 22.4 | 2.5 | 10.5 | 6.[illegible] | 3.4 | 0.3 | 0.00 | 0.34 | 5 |
| 23134 | 1 ea | Crunch, milk chocolate mini bar, .35 oz | 10 | 52 | 1 | 0.6 | 6.5 | 0.3 | 5.6 | 0.7 | 2.6 | 1.5 | 0.9 | 0.1 | 0.00 | 0.09 | 1 |
| 23311 | 1 oz | Dark Chocolate Coffee Beans, avg | 28 | 111 | 1 | 0.8 | 13.8 | 1.2 | 11.5 | 1.1 | 7.2 | 4.3 | 2.4 | 0.2 | | | 1 |
| 23079 | 5 ea | Dietetic Chocolate Cvrd Candy, avg | 80 | 439 | 4 | 10.1 | 34.6 | 5.6 | | | 31.5 | 25.[illegible] | 3.6 | 0.5 | | | 3 |
| 23074 | 5 pce | Dietetić, hard candies, low calorie, avg | 15 | 56 | 1 | 0.0 | 14.0 | 0.0 | 0.0 | 14.0 | 0.0 | 0.0 | 0.0 | 0.0 | 0.00 | 0.00 | 0 |
| 23053 | 1 pce | Divinity Candy, w/o nuts, recipe, avg | 11 | 38 | 9 | 0.1 | 9.8 | 0.0 | 9.7 | 0.1 | 0.0 | 0.0 | 0.0 | 0.0 | 0.00 | 0.00 | 0 |
| 23125 | 1 ea | 5TH Avenue, 2 oz bar | 57 | 280 | 2 | 5.1 | 37.7 | 1.3 | 25.7 | 10.7 | 12.1 | 4.5 | 5.7 | [illegible].9 | 0.0[illegible] | 1.92 | 3 |
| 23024 | 1 pce | Candy Corn, recipe, avg | 16 | 57 | 7 | 0.0 | 14.8 | 0.0 | 14.3 | 0.5 | 0.0 | 0.0 | 0.0 | 0.0 | 0.00 | 0.00 | 0 |
| 23078 | 1 pce | Candy Corn, chocolate cvrd, avg | 14 | 51 | 8 | 0.3 | 11.2 | 0.2 | | | 1.3 | 0.8 | 0.4 | 0.0 | | | 0 |
| 23369 | 1 oz | Fruit By The Foot, asstd flvrs | 28 | 104 | 13 | 0.2 | 22.4 | 0.4 | 12.9 | 9.[illegible] | 1.7 | 0.7 | 0.9 | 0.0 | 0.00 | 0.00 | 0 |
| 23404 | 1 ea | Fruit Leather, avg, .74 oz | 21 | 73 | 11 | 0.2 | 17.7 | 0.8 | 9.0 | 7.9 | 0.6 | 0.1 | 0.3 | 0.[illegible] | 0.02 | 0.09 | 0 |
| 23364 | 1 ea | Fruit Roll-Ups, asstd flvrs, .5 oz | 14 | 53 | 10 | 0.1 | 11.8 | 0.3 | 5.2 | 6.3 | 0.7 | 0.3 | 0.3 | 0.0 | 0.00 | 0.00 | 0 |
| 23025 | 1 pce | Fudge, chocolate, recipe, avg | 17 | 65 | 10 | 0.3 | 13.5 | 0.1 | 12.9 | 0.5 | 1.4 | 0.9 | 0.4 | 0.[illegible] | 0.01 | 0.04 | 2 |
| 23026 | 1 pce | Fudge, chocolate w/nuts, recipe, avg | 19 | 81 | 7 | 0.6 | 13.8 | 0.2 | 12.7 | 0.9 | 3.1 | 1.1 | 0.8 | 1.0 | 0.18 | 0.84 | 3 |
| 23126 | 1 pce | Fudge chocolate marshmallow, recipe, avg | 20 | 84 | 8 | 0.5 | 14.3 | 0.0 | 13.9 | 0.5 | 3.4 | 2.0 | 1.0 | 0.1 | 0.02 | 0.09 | 5 |
| 23127 | 1 pce | Fudge chocolate marsh w/nuts recipe, avg | 22 | 96 | 7 | 0.7 | 15.1 | 0.4 | 14.4 | 0.4 | 4.3 | 2.1 | 1.3 | 0.7 | 0.13 | 0.57 | 5 |
| 23128 | 1 pce | Fudge, peanut butter, recipe, avg | 16 | 59 | 11 | 0.6 | 12.5 | 0.1 | 12.2 | 0.2 | 1.0 | 0.2 | 0.5 | 0.3 | 0.00 | 0.26 | 1 |
| 23124 | 1 pce | Fudge, penuche w/brn sugar & nuts, avg | 14 | 55 | 8 | 0.4 | 10.9 | 0.1 | | | 1.4 | 0.2 | 0.3 | 0.8 | 0.14 | 0.62 | 1 |
| 23027 | 1 pce | Fudge, vanilla, recipe, avg | 16 | 59 | 11 | 0.2 | 13.2 | 0.0 | 13.2 | 0.0 | 0.9 | 0.5 | 0.2 | 0.[illegible] | 0.01 | 0.02 | 3 |
| 23028 | 1 pce | Fudge, vanilla w/nuts, recipe, avg | 15 | 62 | 8 | 0.4 | 11.3 | 0.1 | 11.0 | 0.2 | 2.0 | 0.6 | 0.5 | 0.[illegible] | 0.15 | 0.68 | 2 |
| 23307 | 1 pce | Fudgies candy, Kraft | 8 | 35 | 8 | 0.2 | 6.2 | 0.0 | 5.3 | 1.0 | 1.0 | 0.5 | | | | | 0 |
| 23129 | 1 ea | Golden Almond Chocolate, 3 oz bar | 85 | 488 | 2 | 10.5 | 38.8 | 4.1 | 32.1 | 2.6 | 32.4 | 13.9 | 15.0 | 3.3 | | | 13 |
| 23130 | 1 ea | Golden Almond Solitaires, 2.75 oz pkg | 78 | 444 | 2 | 9.4 | 36.6 | 3.4 | 28.9 | 4.2 | 28.9 | 11.9 | 13.8 | 3.3 | 0.09 | 3.16 | 10 |
| 23131 | 1 ea | Golden III Chocolate, 3.2 oz bar | 91 | 471 | 3 | 5.9 | 50.8 | 5.2 | 44.0 | 1.5 | 30.0 | | | | | | 17 |
| 23257 | 1/2 cup | Goobers, milk chocolate cvrd peanuts | 82 | 421 | 2 | 11.2 | 39.9 | 5.0 | 27.3 | 7.6 | 27.5 | 10.0 | 12.1 | 4.2 | 0.05 | 4.12 | 7 |
| 23029 | 5 pce | Gumdrops candy, avg | 18 | 69 | 1 | 0.0 | 17.8 | 0.0 | 15.7 | 2.1 | 0.0 | 0.0 | 0.0 | 0.0 | 0.00 | 0.00 | 0 |
| 23030 | 5 pce | Gummy Bears | 11 | 42 | 1 | 0.0 | 10.9 | 0.0 | 9.6 | 1.3 | 0.0 | 0.0 | 0.0 | 0.0 | 0.00 | 0.00 | 0 |
| 23410 | 5 pce | Gummy Dinosaurs | 32 | 124 | 1 | 0.0 | 31.6 | 0.0 | 27.9 | 3.7 | 0.0 | 0.0 | 0.0 | 0.0 | 0.00 | 0.00 | 0 |

| Code | Vit A & Components | | | | | Vitamins | | | | | | | | | | Minerals | | | | | | | | | |
|---|---|---|---|---|---|---|---|---|---|---|---|---|---|---|---|---|---|---|---|---|---|---|---|---|---|
| | Vit A (IU) | Vit A (RE) | Retinol (RE) | Carotenoids (RE) | Beta Carotene (mcg) | Thiamin (mg) | Riboflavin (mg) | Niacin (NE) | Vit B6 (mg) | Vit B12 (mcg) | Folate (mcg) | Panto (mg) | Vit C (mg) | Vit D (mg) | Vit E (α TE) | Calcium (mg) | Copper (mg) | Iron (mg) | Magnes (mg) | Mang (mg) | Phos (mg) | Potassium (mg) | Selenium (mcg) | Sodium (mg) | Zinc (mg) |
| 23207 | 18 | 2 | 0 | 2 | | 0.02 | 0.07 | 0.43 | | | | | 0.0 | | | 23 | | 1.7 | | | 112 | 249 | | 22 | |
| 23378 | 17 | 5 | | | | 0.08 | 0.13 | 0.95 | 0.10 | 0.09 | 19.0 | 0.10 | 0.1 | 0.0 | | 41 | 0.1 | 0.1 | 14 | 0.1 | 48 | 83 | | 32 | 0.34 |
| 23423 | 31 | 6 | | | | 0.01 | 0.03 | 0.03 | 0.00 | 0.04 | 0.7 | 0.05 | 0.1 | 0.0 | | 16 | 0.0 | 0.2 | 6 | 0.0 | 23 | 41 | | 10 | 0.15 |
| 23382 | 0 | 0 | 0 | 0 | 0 | | | | | | | | 0.0 | | | 40 | | 0.0 | | | | 100 | | 20 | |
| 23474 | 277 | 55 | | | | | | | | | | | 1.0 | | | 211 | | 1.8 | | | | 492 | | 83 | |
| 23444 | | | | | | | | | | | | | | | | 29 | | 0.2 | | | | 54 | | 11 | |
| 23181 | 0 | 0 | 0 | 0 | 0 | 0.07 | 0.15 | 0.21 | | | | | 0.0 | | | 0 | | 0.0 | | | | 249 | | 0 | |
| 23476 | | | | | | | | | | | | | | | | 151 | | 1.4 | | | | 697 | | 259 | |
| 23012 | 18 | 2 | 0 | 2 | | 0.05 | 0.08 | 0.36 | 0.03 | 0.00 | 2.5 | 0.09 | 0.0 | 1.9 | | 27 | 0.6 | 2.6 | 97 | 0.7 | 111 | 307 | 2.6 | 9 | 1.36 |
| 23328 | 0 | 0 | 0 | 0 | 0 | | | | | | | | 0.0 | | | 0 | | 0.7 | | | | 140 | | 20 | |
| 23313 | 0 | 0 | 0 | 0 | 0 | | | | | | | | 0.0 | | | 0 | | 0.7 | | | | 120 | | 0 | |
| 23473 | 100 | 20 | | | | | | | | | | | 0.0 | | | 35 | | 3.0 | | | | 368 | | 2 | |
| 23421 | 10 | 1 | | | | 0.01 | 0.01 | 0.06 | 0.01 | 0.00 | 3.9 | 0.01 | 0.0 | 0.0 | | 5 | 0.1 | 0.4 | 15 | 0.1 | 17 | 47 | | 0 | 0.21 |
| 23182 | 0 | 0 | 0 | 0 | 0 | 0.06 | | 0.37 | | | | | 0.0 | | | 0 | | 0.0 | | | 136 | 274 | | 0 | |
| 23183 | 0 | 0 | 0 | 0 | 0 | 0.06 | | 0.37 | | | | | 0.0 | | | 0 | | 0.0 | | | 136 | 274 | | 0 | |
| 23121 | 30 | 3 | 0 | 3 | | 0.05 | 0.24 | 0.63 | 0.05 | 0.52 | 14.5 | 0.52 | 0.4 | 0.0 | | 169 | 0.1 | 0.2 | 10 | 0.0 | 150 | 243 | 4.5 | 77 | 0.63 |
| 23477 | 9 | 2 | | | | | | | | | | | 1.7 | | | 323 | | 0.1 | | | | 461 | | 258 | |
| 23049 | 6 | 2 | | | | 0.01 | 0.07 | 0.23 | 0.03 | 0.06 | | 0.12 | 0.1 | 0.0 | | 30 | 0.1 | 0.7 | 32 | 0.3 | 69 | 121 | | 72 | 0.39 |
| 23405 | 3 | 1 | | | | 0.01 | 0.03 | 0.09 | 0.01 | 0.02 | | 0.05 | 0.0 | 0.0 | | 12 | 0.1 | 0.3 | 13 | 0.1 | 28 | 49 | | 29 | 0.16 |
| 23085 | 8 | 2 | 2 | 0 | | 0.01 | 0.02 | 0.16 | 0.01 | 0.01 | 3.2 | | 0.0 | | | 16 | 0.0 | 0.1 | 5 | | 19 | 34 | | 20 | 0.11 |
| 23077 | 29 | 9 | 8 | 1 | | 0.03 | 0.15 | 0.28 | 0.03 | 0.30 | 4.5 | 0.22 | 0.1 | | | 81 | 0.0 | 0.2 | 13 | 0.0 | 82 | 146 | | 26 | 0.40 |
| 23110 | 0 | 0 | 0 | 0 | 0 | 0.06 | 0.06 | 1.67 | 0.04 | 0.03 | 18.6 | 0.20 | 0.0 | 0.0 | | 25 | 0.3 | 0.1 | 48 | 0.5 | 91 | 238 | 2.0 | 136 | 0.78 |
| 23269 | 0 | 0 | 0 | 0 | 0 | 0.01 | 0.01 | 0.39 | 0.01 | 0.01 | 4.3 | 0.05 | 0.0 | 0.0 | | 6 | 0.1 | 0.0 | 11 | 0.1 | 21 | 55 | 0.5 | 32 | 0.18 |
| 23111 | 57 | 10 | | | | 0.03 | 0.12 | 0.68 | 0.03 | 0.18 | 12.0 | 0.24 | 0.0 | | | 62 | 0.1 | 0.5 | 31 | 0.2 | 86 | 168 | | 45 | 0.53 |
| 23112 | 0 | 0 | 0 | 0 | 0 | 0.00 | 0.10 | 0.02 | 0.01 | 0.00 | 1.6 | 0.07 | 0.0 | | | 22 | 0.0 | 0.1 | 8 | 0.0 | 26 | 50 | | 104 | 0.14 |
| 23254 | 0 | 0 | 0 | 0 | 0 | | | | | | | | 0.0 | | | 40 | | 0.0 | | | | | | 96 | |
| 23115 | 42 | 10 | | | | 0.00 | 0.01 | 0.00 | 0.00 | 0.00 | 0.0 | 0.00 | 0.0 | 0.0 | 0.0 | 1 | 0.0 | 0.0 | 0 | 0.0 | 1 | 1 | 0.2 | 110 | 0.01 |
| 23225 | | | | | | | | | | | | | | | | | | | | | | 0 | | 0 | |
| 23309 | 0 | 0 | 0 | 0 | 0 | | | | | | | | 0.0 | | | 0 | | 0.0 | | | | 0 | | 18 | |
| 23116 | 148 | 35 | | | | 0.02 | 0.18 | 0.52 | 0.02 | 0.28 | | 0.22 | 0.2 | 0.0 | | 83 | 0.1 | 0.3 | 19 | 0.1 | 72 | 153 | | 52 | 0.43 |
| 23435 | 0 | 0 | 0 | 0 | 0 | | | | | | | | 0.0 | | | 20 | | 0.0 | | | | | | 75 | |
| 23015 | 16 | 4 | | | | 0.00 | 0.09 | 0.13 | 0.02 | 0.00 | 2.5 | 0.30 | 0.3 | 0.5 | | 69 | 0.0 | 0.1 | 8 | 0.0 | 57 | 107 | 0.9 | 122 | 0.22 |
| 23117 | 2 | 1 | | | | 0.00 | 0.02 | 0.02 | 0.00 | 0.01 | 0.3 | 0.04 | 0.0 | 0.0 | | 6 | 0.1 | 0.1 | 8 | 0.0 | 10 | 26 | 0.4 | 20 | 0.13 |
| 23308 | 0 | 0 | 0 | 0 | 0 | | | | | | | | 0.0 | | | 80 | | 0.0 | | | | 120 | | 110 | |
| 23118 | 21 | 7 | | | | 0.09 | 0.15 | 0.90 | 0.11 | 0.87 | 24.4 | 0.65 | 0.4 | | | 264 | 0.2 | 1.1 | 31 | 0.1 | 110 | 551 | 4.5 | 93 | 3.07 |
| 23020 | 0 | 0 | 0 | 0 | 0 | 0.10 | 0.43 | 1.39 | 0.06 | 0.00 | 63.6 | 0.33 | 0.0 | 0.7 | | 166 | 0.7 | 2.3 | 181 | | 280 | 447 | 2.3 | 48 | 2.09 |
| 23113 | 36 | 9 | 0 | 9 | | 0.10 | 0.19 | 3.28 | 0.63 | 0.00 | 42.3 | | 9.0 | | | 29 | 0.5 | 1.4 | 93 | | 154 | 596 | | 6 | 1.76 |
| 23023 | 11 | 1 | 0 | 1 | | 0.01 | 0.03 | 0.32 | 0.00 | 0.00 | 1.1 | 0.01 | 0.0 | 0.0 | | 9 | 0.2 | 0.9 | 35 | 0.2 | 52 | 92 | 0.7 | 14 | 0.25 |
| 23122 | 25 | 4 | | | | 0.03 | 0.16 | 0.76 | 0.05 | 0.15 | 8.3 | 0.20 | 0.1 | 0.0 | | 57 | 0.2 | 0.5 | 29 | 0.2 | 83 | 214 | | 21 | 0.74 |
| 23098 | 741 | 74 | 0 | 74 | | 0.37 | 0.42 | 4.93 | 0.49 | 0.00 | 0.0 | 0.16 | 3.2 | | | 21 | 0.1 | 1.8 | 20 | 0.4 | 47 | 64 | | 66 | 1.48 |
| 23099 | 494 | 49 | | | | 0.15 | 0.17 | 1.97 | 0.20 | 0.00 | 39.2 | 0.00 | 0.0 | 0.0 | | 6 | 0.1 | 1.8 | 13 | 0.3 | 38 | 47 | 2.7 | 78 | 0.24 |
| 23133 | 28 | 8 | | | | 0.14 | 0.22 | 1.58 | 0.16 | 0.15 | 31.6 | 0.17 | 0.1 | 0.0 | | 68 | 0.1 | 0.2 | 23 | 0.2 | 81 | 138 | | 53 | 0.57 |
| 23134 | 7 | 2 | | | | 0.03 | 0.06 | 0.40 | 0.04 | 0.04 | 7.9 | 0.04 | 0.0 | 0.0 | | 17 | 0.0 | 0.1 | 6 | 0.0 | 20 | 34 | | 13 | 0.14 |
| 23311 | 19 | 2 | | | | 0.00 | 0.00 | 0.00 | 0.00 | 0.00 | 0.0 | | 0.0 | | | 6 | 0.0 | 0.5 | 0 | | 0 | 63 | | 1 | 0.00 |
| 23079 | 6 | 16 | 16 | 0 | | 0.16 | 0.38 | 1.81 | 0.14 | 0.58 | 50.4 | | 1.1 | | | 242 | 0.7 | 1.2 | 103 | | 266 | 485 | | 87 | 1.98 |
| 23074 | 0 | 0 | 0 | 0 | 0 | 0.00 | 0.00 | 0.00 | 0.00 | 0.00 | 0.0 | 0.00 | 0.0 | 0.0 | 0.0 | 0 | 0.0 | 0.0 | 0 | 0.0 | 0 | 0 | 0.0 | 0 | 0.00 |
| 23053 | 0 | 0 | | | | 0.00 | 0.01 | 0.00 | 0.00 | 0.00 | 0.0 | 0.00 | 0.0 | 0.0 | | 0 | 0.0 | 0.0 | 0 | 0.0 | 0 | 2 | 0.7 | 5 | 0.00 |
| 23125 | 32 | 9 | | | | 0.08 | 0.07 | 1.97 | 0.05 | 0.07 | 21.7 | 0.28 | 0.1 | 0.0 | | 42 | 0.2 | 0.7 | 36 | 0.4 | 88 | 169 | 2.1 | 54 | 0.70 |
| 23024 | 0.3 | 0.05 | | | | 0.00 | 0.00 | 0.00 | 0.00 | 0.00 | 0.0 | 0.00 | 0.0 | 0.0 | 0.0 | 0 | 0.0 | 0.0 | 0 | 0.0 | 0 | 3 | 0.1 | 6 | 0.01 |
| 23078 | 3 | 0.3 | 0 | 0.3 | | 0.00 | 0.01 | 0.08 | 0.00 | 0.00 | 0.1 | | 0.0 | | | 2 | 0.1 | 0.2 | 9 | | 13 | 24 | | 4 | 0.06 |
| 23369 | | | | | | 0.00 | 0.00 | 0.00 | | | | | | | | 6 | | 0.1 | | | | 45 | | 55 | |
| 23404 | 24 | 2.5 | 0 | 2.5 | | 0.01 | 0.00 | 0.02 | 0.06 | 0.00 | 1.7 | 0.07 | 1.3 | 0.0 | | 7 | 0.0 | 0.2 | 4 | 0.0 | 7 | 62 | 0.6 | 13 | 0.04 |
| 23364 | | | | | | 0.00 | 0.00 | 0.00 | | | | | 24.5 | | | 4 | | 0.1 | | | | 19 | | 40 | |
| 23025 | 32 | 3 | 3 | 0 | | 0.00 | 0.01 | 0.02 | 0.00 | 0.01 | 0.3 | 0.02 | 0.0 | 0.0 | | 7 | 0.0 | 0.1 | 4 | 0.0 | 10 | 18 | 0.3 | 11 | 0.07 |
| 23026 | 38 | 9 | 9 | 0 | | 0.01 | 0.02 | 0.04 | 0.02 | 0.01 | 1.9 | 0.03 | 0.1 | 0.0 | | 9 | 0.1 | 0.1 | 9 | 0.1 | 18 | 30 | 0.4 | 11 | 0.14 |
| 23126 | 56 | 15 | 15 | 0 | | 0.00 | 0.02 | 0.03 | 0.00 | 0.01 | 0.4 | 0.02 | 0.0 | 0.0 | | 9 | 0.0 | 0.2 | 7 | 0.0 | 13 | 28 | | 21 | 0.11 |
| 23127 | 57 | 15 | 15 | 0 | | 0.01 | 0.02 | 0.05 | 0.01 | 0.01 | 1.5 | 0.03 | 0.1 | 0.0 | | 11 | 0.1 | 0.2 | 10 | 0.1 | 18 | 37 | 0.4 | 21 | 0.16 |
| 23128 | 7 | 2 | [illegible] | 0.03 | | 0.00 | 0.01 | 0.24 | 0.01 | 0.01 | 1.8 | 0.03 | 0.0 | 0.0 | | 7 | 0.0 | 0.0 | 4 | 0.0 | 10 | 21 | | 12 | 0.07 |
| 23124 | 11 | 2 | [illegible] | 0.05 | | 0.01 | 0.01 | 0.03 | 0.01 | 0.00 | 1.5 | 0.04 | 0.1 | 0.0 | | 16 | 0.1 | 0.3 | 7 | 0.1 | 12 | 52 | | 14 | 0.09 |
| 23027 | 33 | 3 | 3 | 0.1 | | 0.00 | 0.01 | 0.00 | 0.00 | 0.01 | 0.2 | 0.02 | 0.0 | 0.0 | | 6 | 0.0 | 0.0 | 1 | 0.0 | 5 | 8 | 0.2 | 11 | 0.02 |
| 23028 | 30 | [illegible] | [illegible] | 0.1 | | 0.01 | 0.01 | 0.03 | 0.01 | 0.01 | 1.5 | 0.03 | 0.1 | 0.0 | | 7 | 0.0 | 0.1 | 4 | 0.1 | 11 | 17 | 0.3 | 9 | 0.08 |
| 23307 | 0 | 0 | [illegible] | 0 | 0 | | | | | | | | 0.0 | | | 4 | | 0.1 | | | | 27 | | 13 | |
| 23129 | 125 | 3 | | | | 0.05 | 0.45 | 0.90 | 0.04 | 0.37 | | 0.32 | 0.2 | 0.0 | | 190 | 0.3 | 1.5 | 94 | 0.7 | 230 | 400 | | 57 | 1.45 |
| 23130 | 39 | [illegible] | | | | 0.05 | 0.39 | 0.84 | 0.04 | 0.37 | | 0.30 | 0.2 | | | 147 | 0.3 | 1.8 | 92 | 0.6 | 234 | 393 | | 44 | 1.44 |
| 23131 | 32 | 2[illegible] | | | | 0.06 | 0.25 | 0.15 | 0.10 | 0.41 | 10.9 | 0.53 | 0.8 | | | 275 | 0.3 | 0.5 | 61 | 0.4 | 200 | 413 | | 79 | 1.00 |
| 23257 | 0 | [illegible] | | 0 | 0 | 0.10 | 0.17 | 4.26 | 0.17 | 0.24 | 6.6 | 0.47 | 0.0 | 0.0 | | 104 | 0.7 | 1.1 | 98 | 0.7 | 243 | 412 | | 34 | 1.80 |
| 23029 | 0 | [illegible] | | 0 | 0 | 0.00 | 0.00 | 0.00 | 0.00 | 0.00 | 0.0 | 0.00 | 0.0 | 0.0 | 0.0 | 1 | 0.0 | 0.1 | 0 | 0.0 | 0 | 1 | 0.1 | 8 | 0.00 |
| 23030 | 0 | [illegible] | | 0 | 0 | 0.00 | 0.00 | 0.00 | 0.00 | 0.00 | 0.0 | 0.00 | 0.0 | 0.0 | 0.0 | 0 | 0.0 | 0.0 | 0 | 0.0 | 0 | 1 | 0.1 | 5 | 0.00 |
| 23410 | 0 | [illegible] | | 0 | 0 | 0.00 | 0.00 | 0.00 | 0.00 | 0.00 | 0.0 | 0.00 | 0.0 | 0.0 | 0.0 | 1 | 0.0 | 0.1 | 0 | 0.0 | 0 | 2 | 0.2 | 14 | 0.00 |

| Code | Amount | Description | Weight (g) | Calories | % Water | Protein (g) | Carbs (g) | Fiber (g) | Sugar (g) | Other Carbs (g) | Fat (g) | Sat Fat (g) | Mono Fat (g) | Poly Fat (g) | Omega 3 (g) | Omega 6 (g) | Choles (mg) |
|---|---|---|---|---|---|---|---|---|---|---|---|---|---|---|---|---|---|
| | | | Basic Components | | | | | | | | | Additional Fats | | | | | |
| 23411 | 5 pce | Gummy Fish | 25 | 96 | 1 | 0.0 | 24.7 | 0.0 | 21.8 | 2.9 | 0.0 | 0.0 | 0.0 | 0.0 | 0.00 | 0.00 | 0 |
| 23412 | 5 pce | Gummy Worms | 37 | 143 | 1 | 0.0 | 36.6 | 0.0 | 32.3 | 4.3 | 0.0 | 0.0 | 0.0 | 0.0 | 0.00 | 0.00 | 0 |
| 23031 | 1 pce | Hard Candy, all flvrs, avg | 6 | 24 | 1 | 0.0 | 5.9 | 0.0 | 3.8 | 2.1 | 0.0 | 0.0 | 0.0 | 0.0 | 0.00 | 0.00 | 0 |
| 23033 | 10 pce | Jellybeans, avg | 11 | 40 | 6 | 0.0 | 10.2 | 0.0 | | | 0.1 | 0.0 | 0.0 | 0.0 | 0.00 | 0.01 | 0 |
| 23413 | 5 pce | Jelly Ring candy, avg | 50 | 193 | 1 | 0.0 | 49.5 | 0.0 | 43.7 | 5.8 | 0.0 | 0.0 | 0.0 | 0.0 | 0.00 | 0.00 | 0 |
| 23034 | 7 ea | Jordan Almonds, sugar ctd, avg | 28 | 128 | 2 | 2.2 | 19.7 | 1.3 | 10.4 | 8.0 | 5.2 | 0.4 | 3.6 | 1.1 | | | 0 |
| 23060 | 1 ea | Kit Kat, 1.48 oz bar | 42 | 216 | 2 | 3.0 | 26.9 | 0.8 | 17.9 | 8.2 | 10.7 | 6.8 | 3.1 | 0.3 | 0.04 | 0.30 | 3 |
| 23016 | 1 ea | Kisses, milk chocolate, 1.6 oz pkg, Hershey's | 44 | 226 | 1 | 3.0 | 26.0 | 1.5 | 23.0 | 1.5 | 13.5 | 8.1 | 4.4 | 0.5 | 0.04 | 0.42 | 10 |
| 23063 | 6 pce | Kisses, milk chocolate, 1 oz, Hershey's | 28 | 144 | 1 | 1.9 | 16.6 | 0.8 | 14.1 | 1.8 | 8.6 | 5.1 | 2.8 | 0.3 | | | 6 |
| 23061 | 1 ea | Krackel, chocolate & crisped rice bar, 1.45 oz | 41 | 218 | 2 | 2.7 | 25.3 | 0.9 | 20.7 | 3.6 | 11.8 | 7.4 | 3.9 | 0.4 | 0.00 | 0.37 | 8 |
| 23087 | 1 oz | Licorice, avg | 28 | 103 | 6 | 0.0 | 26.1 | 0.0 | 26.0 | 0.0 | 0.1 | 0.1 | 0.0 | 0.0 | 0.00 | 0.00 | 0 |
| 23032 | 1 ea | Lollipop, avg | 6 | 24 | 1 | 0.0 | 5.9 | 0.0 | 3.8 | 2.1 | 0.0 | 0.0 | 0.0 | 0.0 | 0.00 | 0.00 | 0 |
| 23427 | 1 ea | M&M's, mini milk chocolate, 5 oz pkg | 142 | 707 | 2 | 6.8 | 95.3 | 3.8 | 91.9 | 0.0 | 33.1 | 20.6 | 10.8 | 1.0 | 0.00 | 0.99 | 21 |
| 23479 | 1 ea | M&M's, peanut, 25 pces, 1.74 oz pkg | 49 | 253 | 2 | 4.6 | 29.6 | 1.7 | 24.9 | 3.1 | 12.8 | 5.0 | 5.4 | 2.1 | 0.00 | 0.39 | 4 |
| 23480 | 1 ea | M&M's, plain, 69 pces, 1.69 oz pkg | 48 | 236 | 2 | 2.1 | 34.2 | 1.2 | 30.6 | 2.4 | 10.1 | 6.3 | 3.3 | 0.3 | 0.00 | 0.30 | 7 |
| 23037 | 1 ea | Mars Almond bar, 1.76 oz | 50 | 234 | 4 | 4.1 | 31.4 | 1.0 | 26.0 | 4.3 | 11.5 | 3.6 | 5.3 | 2.0 | 0.13 | 1.85 | 8 |
| 4711 | 100 g | Marzipan | 100 | 410 | 10 | 7.4 | 60.0 | 4.8 | 54.1 | 1.1 | 18.1 | | | | | | 0 |
| 23192 | 1 ea | Milk Chocolate candy bar, 1.45 oz, Nestle | 41 | 219 | 1 | 4.0 | 22.9 | 2.0 | 20.9 | 0.0 | 13.1 | 7.0 | 5.0 | 0.5 | | | 10 |
| 23058 | 1 ea | Milk Chocolate candy bar w/crsp rice, 1.4 oz, avg | 40 | 198 | 2 | 2.5 | 25.4 | 1.2 | 22.0 | 2.1 | 10.6 | 6.4 | 3.5 | 0.3 | 0.02 | 0.29 | 8 |
| 23019 | 1 ea | Milk Chocolate candy bar w/peanuts, 1 oz, avg | 28 | 155 | 1 | 4.5 | 10.8 | 1.6 | 7.3 | 1.9 | 11.5 | 3.4 | 5.1 | 2.5 | 0.00 | 2.53 | 3 |
| 23242 | 100 g | Milk Chocolate Coffee Beans, avg | 100 | 529 | 1 | 7.1 | 67.0 | | | | 24.7 | | | | | | |
| 23022 | 1/2 cup | Milk Chocolate Cvrd Raisins, avg | 95 | 370 | 11 | 3.9 | 64.9 | 4.0 | 59.1 | 1.8 | 14.1 | 8.4 | 4.5 | 0.5 | 0.05 | 0.43 | 3 |
| 23419 | 5 pce | Milk Chocolate Coated Peanuts, 5 pces | 20 | 104 | 2 | 2.6 | 9.9 | 0.9 | 7.1 | 1.9 | 6.7 | 2.9 | 2.6 | 0.9 | 0.01 | 0.86 | 2 |
| 23193 | 1 pce | Milk Chocolate After 8 Mint, Nestle | 8 | 29 | 6 | 0.2 | 6.1 | 0.2 | 5.6 | 0.4 | 1.1 | 0.7 | 0.4 | 0.0 | 0.00 | 0.04 | 0 |
| 23018 | 1 ea | Milk chocolate w/almonds, 1.45 oz bar, avg | 41 | 216 | 2 | 3.7 | 21.8 | 2.5 | 18.0 | 1.3 | 14.1 | 7.0 | 5.5 | 0.9 | 0.05 | 0.89 | 8 |
| 23038 | 1 ea | Milky Way bar, 2.12 oz | 60 | 254 | 6 | 2.7 | 43.0 | 1.0 | 36.4 | 5.6 | 9.7 | 4.7 | 3.6 | 0.4 | 0.02 | 0.34 | 8 |
| 23039 | 1 ea | Milky Way bar, fun size, .63 oz | 18 | 76 | 6 | 0.8 | 12.9 | 0.3 | 10.9 | 1.7 | 2.9 | 1.4 | 1.1 | 0.1 | 0.01 | 0.10 | 3 |
| 23035 | 1 ea | Mounds, 1.87 oz bar | 53 | 253 | 11 | 2.0 | 31.2 | 3.1 | 14.8 | 13.3 | 13.3 | 10.8 | 2.3 | 0.3 | 0.00 | 0.26 | 1 |
| 23062 | 1 ea | Mr. Goodbar, 1.73 oz bar | 49 | 267 | 1 | 5.2 | 25.3 | 1.7 | 22.1 | 1.5 | 17.1 | 7.3 | 5.7 | 2.4 | 0.00 | 2.35 | 4 |
| 23153 | 1 ea | Nibs Cherry candy, 1 oz pkg | 28 | 105 | 1 | 0.8 | 25.9 | 0.0 | 25.9 | 0.0 | 0.6 | | | | | | 0 |
| 23196 | 5 pce | Nips Caramel candy | 36 | 154 | 2 | 0.0 | 30.9 | 0.0 | 30.9 | 0.0 | 4.0 | 4.0 | | | | | 0 |
| 23194 | 5 pce | Nips Chocolate Parfait candy | 36 | 154 | 3 | 1.3 | 28.3 | 0.0 | 25.7 | 2.6 | 5.0 | 5.0 | | | | | 0 |
| 23191 | 5 pce | Nips Coffee candy | 25 | 107 | 2 | 0.0 | 21.4 | 0.0 | 21.4 | 0.0 | 2.8 | 1.8 | | | | | 0 |
| 23189 | 1 oz | Nips Licorice candy | 28 | 120 | 2 | 0.0 | 24.0 | 0.0 | 24.0 | 0.0 | 3.1 | 3.1 | | | | | 0 |
| 23190 | 1 oz | Nips Peanut Butter Parfait candy | 28 | 120 | 2 | 2.0 | 22.0 | 0.0 | 22.0 | 0.0 | 3.9 | 3.9 | 0.0 | 0.0 | 0.00 | 0.00 | 0 |
| 23135 | 1 ea | Oh Henry, 2 oz bar | 57 | 246 | 6 | 6.2 | 36.9 | 2.0 | 33.6 | 1.3 | 9.6 | 3.8 | 3.8 | 1.6 | 0.00 | 1.55 | 5 |
| 23137 | 1 ea | Peanut Bar, 1.4 oz, avg | 40 | 209 | 2 | 6.2 | 19.0 | 2.3 | 16.9 | 1.6 | 13.5 | 1.9 | 6.7 | 4.3 | 0.00 | 4.24 | 0 |
| 23284 | 5 pce | Peanut Brittle, 1.3 oz, Kraft | 38 | 170 | 2 | 3.0 | 29.0 | 1.0 | 21.0 | 7.0 | 5.0 | 1.0 | | | | | 0 |
| 23081 | 1/2 cup | Peanut Brittle, recipe, avg | 74 | 335 | 2 | 5.6 | 51.3 | 1.5 | 48.3 | 1.5 | 14.1 | 3.7 | 6.3 | 3.5 | 0.05 | 3.41 | 10 |
| 23120 | 1/2 cup | Peanut Butter candy, avg | 84 | 417 | 6 | 15.4 | 37.7 | 7.1 | 24.4 | 6.3 | 25.0 | 11.0 | 8.1 | 4.5 | 0.00 | 4.49 | 0 |
| 23080 | 1 ea | Planters Peanut bar, 1.4 oz | 40 | 209 | 2 | 6.2 | 19.0 | 1.3 | 13.2 | 4.5 | 13.5 | 1.7 | 6.7 | 4.3 | | | 3 |
| 23138 | 1 pce | Praline Candy, recipe, avg | 39 | 177 | 10 | 1.1 | 24.2 | 1.1 | 22.7 | 0.5 | 9.5 | 0.7 | 5.9 | 2.4 | 0.10 | 2.25 | 0 |
| 23214 | 1 ea | Raisinets, milk choc cvrd raisins, 1.59 oz pkg | 45 | 185 | 6 | 2.1 | 32.0 | 2.3 | 27.5 | 2.2 | 7.2 | 3.3 | 2.7 | 0.9 | 0.05 | 0.80 | 2 |
| 23424 | 5 ea | Reese's Peanut Butter Cups, mini, 1.2 oz | 35 | 189 | 2 | 3.6 | 19.1 | 1.1 | 16.3 | 1.6 | 11.0 | 3.9 | 4.6 | 2.0 | 0.00 | 1.96 | 2 |
| 23043 | 1 ea | Reese's Peanut Butter Cups, 1.76 oz pkg | 50 | 270 | 2 | 5.2 | 27.3 | 1.6 | 23.4 | 2.3 | 15.6 | 5.6 | 6.6 | 2.8 | 0.00 | 2.80 | 2 |
| 23436 | 1 ea | Reese's Pieces candy, 1.6 oz pkg | 46 | 226 | 3 | 6.3 | 28.2 | 1.3 | 24.3 | 2.6 | 9.7 | 8.3 | 1.0 | 0.5 | 0.03 | 0.43 | 1 |
| 23426 | 1 ea | Rolo Caramels, milk chocolate, 1.87 oz pkg | 53 | 218 | 20 | 2.6 | 28.4 | 0.4 | 25.5 | 2.4 | 10.6 | 6.5 | 3.3 | 0.3 | 0.01 | 0.31 | 10 |
| 23142 | 20 pce | Sesame Crunch candy, avg | 35 | 181 | 2 | 4.1 | 17.6 | 2.8 | 12.3 | 2.6 | 11.7 | 1.6 | 4.4 | 5.1 | 0.09 | 5.01 | 0 |
| 23485 | 1 ea | Skittles, bite size candy, 2.17 oz pkg | 62 | 251 | 4 | 0.1 | 56.2 | 0.0 | 47.1 | 9.1 | 2.7 | 0.5 | 1.8 | 0.1 | 0.00 | 0.01 | 0 |
| 23036 | 1 ea | Skor English Toffee, 1.38 oz bar | 39 | 217 | 3 | 1.8 | 22.5 | 0.6 | 20.9 | 1.1 | 13.3 | 8.5 | 4.3 | 0.5 | | | 20 |
| 23040 | 1 ea | Snickers, 2 oz. bar | 57 | 273 | 5 | 4.6 | 33.7 | 1.4 | 28.1 | 4.2 | 14.0 | 5.1 | 6.0 | 2.8 | 0.01 | 0.17 | 7 |
| 23041 | 1 ea | Snickers, fun size, .5 oz. bar | 15 | 72 | 5 | 1.2 | 8.9 | 0.4 | 7.4 | 1.1 | 3.7 | 1.3 | 1.6 | 0.7 | 0.00 | 0.04 | 2 |
| 23057 | 1 ea | Special Dark Chocolate, 1.45 oz bar, Hershey's | 41 | 226 | 1 | 2.0 | 24.8 | 2.0 | 19.1 | 3.6 | 13.3 | 8.3 | 4.6 | 0.4 | 0.01 | 0.40 | 0 |
| 23414 | 5 pce | Spice drop candy, avg | 120 | 463 | 1 | 0.0 | 118.7 | 0.0 | 104.8 | 13.9 | 0.0 | 0.0 | 0.0 | 0.0 | 0.00 | 0.00 | 0 |
| 23415 | 5 pce | Spice Stick candy, avg | 48 | 185 | 1 | 0.0 | 47.5 | 0.0 | 41.9 | 5.6 | 0.0 | 0.0 | 0.0 | 0.0 | 0.00 | 0.00 | 0 |
| 23144 | 5 pce | Starburst Fruit Chews candy | 25 | 99 | 7 | 0.1 | 21.1 | 0.0 | 16.7 | 4.4 | 2.1 | 0.3 | 0.9 | 0.8 | 0.05 | 0.73 | 0 |
| 23145 | 1 ea | Sweet Chocolate bar, 1.45 oz, avg | 41 | 207 | 0 | 1.6 | 24.4 | 2.3 | 19.3 | 2.9 | 14.0 | 8.2 | 4.6 | 0.4 | 0.01 | 0.39 | 0 |
| 23146 | 1 ea | Symphony Milk Chocolate bar, 1.4 oz | 40 | 221 | 1 | 2.9 | 23.2 | 0.8 | 20.0 | 2.4 | 13.1 | | | | | | 9 |
| 23147 | 1 pce | Taffy candy, homemade, avg | 15 | 56 | 5 | 0.0 | 13.7 | 0.0 | | | 0.5 | 0.3 | 0.1 | 0.0 | 0.01 | 0.01 | 1 |
| 23136 | 1 ea | 100 Grand bar, 1.5 oz | 43 | 200 | 5 | 2.1 | 30.4 | 0.6 | 27.3 | 2.5 | 7.8 | 4.8 | 2.5 | 0.3 | 0.00 | 0.25 | 8 |
| 23375 | 1 ea | 100 Grand mini bar, .74 oz | 21 | 98 | 5 | 1.0 | 14.8 | 0.3 | 13.3 | 1.2 | 3.8 | 2.4 | 1.2 | 0.1 | 0.00 | 0.12 | 4 |
| 23075 | 1 ea | 3 Musketeers bar, 2.12 oz | 60 | 250 | 6 | 1.9 | 46.1 | 1.0 | 39.7 | 5.4 | 7.7 | 3.9 | 2.6 | 0.3 | 0.05 | 0.22 | 7 |
| 23076 | 1 ea | 3 Musketeers, fun size bar, .58 oz | 16 | 67 | 6 | 0.5 | 12.3 | 0.3 | 10.6 | 1.4 | 2.1 | 1.0 | 0.7 | 0.1 | 0.01 | 0.06 | 2 |
| 23173 | 1 pce | Toffee candy, homemade, avg | 12 | 65 | 1 | 0.1 | 7.7 | 0.0 | 7.7 | 0.0 | 3.9 | 2.4 | 1.1 | 0.1 | 0.06 | 0.09 | 13 |
| 23148 | 1 pce | Truffles candy, homemade, avg | 12 | 59 | 14 | 0.7 | 5.4 | 0.3 | 4.8 | 0.3 | 4.1 | 2.1 | 1.8 | 0.2 | 0.01 | 0.18 | 6 |
| 23123 | 1 pce | Turtles, choc, caramel & pecans candy, Nestle | 17 | 82 | 6 | 1.1 | 9.9 | 0.4 | 6.6 | 2.8 | 4.7 | 1.8 | 1.9 | 0.8 | 0.04 | 0.75 | 4 |
| 23149 | 1 ea | Twix Caramel Cookie bar, 2 oz pkg | 57 | 284 | 4 | 2.6 | 37.4 | 0.6 | 27.4 | 9.4 | 13.9 | 5.1 | 7.6 | 0.5 | 0.05 | 0.43 | 3 |
| 23150 | 1 ea | Twix Peanut Butter Cookie bar, 1.9 oz pkg | 54 | 286 | 2 | 5.5 | 28.5 | 1.8 | 19.1 | 7.6 | 17.4 | 6.2 | 8.0 | 2.3 | 0.16 | 2.11 | 3 |
| 23448 | 1 ea | Twizzlers Cherry Bits Licorice, 1.38 oz pkg | 39 | 135 | | 1.1 | 30.6 | 0.5 | 16.9 | 13.2 | 1.0 | 0.2 | | | | | 0 |
| 23154 | 1 ea | Twizzlers Strawberry Bits Licorice, 2.5 oz pkg | 71 | 237 | 17 | 2.4 | 55.0 | 1.0 | 26.1 | 27.8 | 1.1 | 0.3 | | | | | 0 |

| Code | Vit A (IU) | Vit A (RE) | Retinol (RE) | Carotenoids (RE) | Beta Carotene (mcg) | Thiamin (mg) | Riboflavin (mg) | Niacin (NE) | Vit B6 (mg) | Vit B12 (mcg) | Folate (mcg) | Panto (mg) | Vit C (mg) | Vit D (mg) | Vit E (α TE) |
|---|---|---|---|---|---|---|---|---|---|---|---|---|---|---|---|
| | Vit A & Components | | | | | Vitamins | | | | | | | | | |
| 23411 | 0 | 0 | 0 | 0 | 0 | 0.00 | 0.00 | 0.00 | 0.00 | 0.00 | 0.0 | 0.00 | 0.0 | 0.0 | 0.0 |
| 23412 | 0 | 0 | 0 | 0 | 0 | 0.00 | 0.00 | 0.00 | 0.00 | 0.00 | 0.0 | 0.00 | 0.0 | 0.0 | 0.0 |
| 23031 | 0 | 0 | 0 | 0 | 0 | 0.00 | 0.00 | 0.00 | 0.00 | 0.00 | 0.0 | 0.00 | 0.0 | 0.0 | 0.0 |
| 23033 | 0 | 0 | 0 | 0 | 0 | 0.00 | 0.00 | 0.00 | 0.00 | 0.00 | 0.0 | 0.00 | 0.0 | 0.0 | 0.0 |
| 23413 | 0 | 0 | 0 | 0 | 0 | 0.00 | 0.00 | 0.00 | 0.00 | 0.00 | 0.0 | 0.00 | 0.0 | 0.0 | 0.0 |
| 23034 | 0 | 0 | 0 | 0 | 0 | 0.01 | 0.08 | 0.28 | 0.02 | 0.00 | 16.0 | 0.09 | 0.0 | 0.0 | |
| 23060 | 68 | 20 | 0 | 12 | | 0.07 | 0.23 | 1.07 | 0.05 | 0.07 | 59.6 | 0.45 | 0.3 | 0.0 | |
| 23016 | 81 | 24 | 0 | 24 | | 0.03 | 0.13 | 0.14 | 0.02 | 0.17 | 3.5 | 0.19 | 0.2 | 1.8 | |
| 23063 | 52 | 13 | 11 | 3 | | 0.02 | 0.08 | 0.09 | 0.01 | 0.11 | 2.0 | 0.20 | 0.1 | | |
| 23061 | 20 | 5 | | | | 0.02 | 0.12 | 0.18 | 0.01 | 0.24 | | 0.23 | 0.2 | 1.7 | |
| 23087 | 0 | 0 | 0 | 0 | 0 | 0.00 | 0.00 | 0.00 | 0.00 | 0.00 | 0.0 | | 0.0 | | 0.0 |
| 23032 | 0 | 0 | 0 | 0 | 0 | 0.00 | 0.00 | 0.00 | 0.00 | 0.00 | 0.0 | 0.00 | 0.0 | 0.0 | 0.0 |
| 23427 | 318 | 64 | | | | 0.09 | 0.33 | 0.35 | 0.05 | 0.41 | 7.1 | 0.46 | 0.9 | 2.9 | |
| 23479 | 46 | 12 | | | | 0.05 | 0.08 | 1.84 | 0.04 | 0.09 | 17.1 | 0.27 | 0.2 | 0.0 | |
| 23480 | 97 | 25 | | | | 0.03 | 0.10 | 0.11 | 0.01 | 0.13 | 2.9 | 0.14 | 0.2 | 0.0 | |
| 23037 | 94 | 25 | 22 | 1 | | 0.02 | 0.16 | 0.47 | 0.03 | 0.18 | 9.5 | 0.20 | 0.3 | 0.0 | |
| 4711 | 0 | 0 | 0 | 0 | 0 | | 0.15 | | | 0.00 | | | 0.0 | | |
| 23192 | 0 | 0 | 0 | 0 | 0 | 0.03 | 0.14 | 0.11 | | | | | 0.0 | | |
| 23058 | 23 | 4 | 3 | 1 | | 0.02 | 0.12 | 0.19 | 0.02 | 0.14 | 3.6 | 0.24 | 0.1 | 0.0 | |
| 23019 | 23 | 6 | 5 | 1 | | 0.08 | 0.05 | 2.12 | 0.04 | 0.05 | 23.2 | 0.27 | 0.0 | 0.5 | |
| 23242 | | | | | | | | | | | | | | | |
| 23022 | 36 | 7 | 5 | 2 | | 0.08 | 0.15 | 0.38 | 0.08 | 0.17 | 4.8 | 0.21 | 0.2 | 2.3 | |
| 23419 | 0 | 0 | 0 | 0 | 0 | 0.02 | 0.03 | 0.85 | 0.04 | 0.05 | 1.6 | 0.11 | 0.0 | 0.5 | |
| 23193 | 1.6 | 0.16 | | | | 0.00 | 0.00 | 0.02 | 0.00 | 0.00 | 0.1 | 0.00 | 0.0 | 0.0 | |
| 23018 | 30 | 6 | | | | 0.02 | 0.18 | 0.30 | 0.02 | 0.14 | 4.9 | 0.18 | 0.1 | 0.7 | |
| 23038 | 65 | 19 | | | | 0.02 | 0.13 | 0.21 | 0.03 | 0.19 | 6.0 | 0.18 | 0.6 | 0.0 | |
| 23039 | 19 | 6 | | | | 0.01 | 0.04 | 0.06 | 0.01 | 0.06 | 1.8 | 0.05 | 0.2 | 0.0 | |
| 23035 | 3 | 0.5 | | | | 0.02 | 0.03 | 0.15 | 0.05 | 0.00 | 1.6 | 0.13 | 0.2 | 0.0 | |
| 23062 | 70 | 18 | | | | 0.08 | 0.12 | 1.62 | 0.04 | 0.15 | 19.1 | 0.32 | 0.1 | 1.4 | |
| 23153 | 6 | 0.6 | | | | 0.01 | 0.01 | 0.03 | 0.00 | 0.00 | 0.0 | 0.00 | 0.0 | 0.0 | |
| 23196 | 0 | 0 | 0 | 0 | 0 | | | | | | | | 0.0 | | |
| 23194 | 0 | 0 | 0 | 0 | 0 | | | | | | | | 0.0 | | |
| 23191 | 0 | 0 | 0 | 0 | 0 | | | | | | | | 0.0 | | |
| 23189 | 0 | 0 | 0 | 0 | 0 | | | | | | | | 0.0 | | |
| 23190 | 0 | 0 | 0 | 0 | 0 | | | | | | | | 0.0 | | |
| 23135 | 27 | 5 | | | | 0.01 | 0.09 | 1.60 | 0.04 | 0.12 | 17.1 | 0.27 | 0.1 | 0.0 | |
| 23137 | 0 | 0 | 0 | 0 | 0 | 0.04 | 0.06 | 3.17 | 0.06 | 0.00 | 31.2 | 0.35 | 0.0 | 0.0 | |
| 23284 | 0 | 0 | 0 | 0 | 0 | | | | | | | | 0.0 | | |
| 23081 | 141 | 35 | | | | 0.14 | 0.04 | 2.59 | 0.08 | 0.01 | 51.8 | 0.39 | 0.0 | 0.0 | |
| 23120 | 17 | 2 | | | | 0.04 | 0.17 | 6.89 | 0.19 | 0.05 | 80.6 | 0.96 | 0.1 | 0.0 | |
| 23080 | 203 | 20 | 15 | 6 | | 0.04 | 0.06 | 3.17 | 0.04 | 0.01 | 24.0 | | 0.0 | | |
| 23138 | 18 | 2 | | | | 0.12 | 0.02 | 0.13 | 0.03 | 0.00 | 5.5 | 0.25 | 0.3 | | |
| 23214 | 17 | 4 | | | | 0.04 | 0.10 | 0.18 | 0.05 | 0.09 | 2.3 | 0.13 | 0.1 | 1.1 | |
| 23424 | 26 | 7 | | | | 0.09 | 0.06 | 1.62 | 0.05 | 0.05 | 19.3 | 0.30 | 0.1 | 0.0 | |
| 23043 | 37 | 10 | | | | 0.12 | 0.09 | 2.31 | 0.07 | 0.08 | 27.5 | 0.43 | 0.1 | 0.0 | |
| 23436 | 1 | 0.1 | | | | 0.04 | 0.07 | 1.31 | 0.03 | 0.10 | 12.9 | 0.22 | 0.2 | 0.0 | |
| 23426 | 77 | 20 | | | | 0.03 | 0.12 | 0.11 | 0.02 | 0.15 | 2.6 | 0.17 | 0.2 | 1.1 | |
| 23142 | 0.4 | 0.04 | | | | 0.19 | 0.06 | 1.29 | 0.19 | 0.00 | 22.8 | 0.01 | 0.0 | 0.0 | |
| 23485 | 0 | 0 | 0 | 0 | 0 | 0.00 | 0.01 | 0.01 | 0.00 | 0.00 | 0.0 | 0.00 | 41.5 | 0.0 | |
| 23036 | 109 | 27 | 27 | 0.4 | | 0.01 | 0.13 | 0.04 | 0.01 | 0.11 | | 0.12 | 0.1 | 0.0 | |
| 23040 | 87 | 22 | | | | 0.06 | 0.09 | 2.39 | 0.05 | 0.09 | 22.8 | 0.32 | 0.3 | 0.0 | |
| 23041 | 23 | 6 | | | | 0.01 | 0.02 | 0.63 | 0.01 | 0.02 | 6.0 | 0.08 | 0.1 | 0.0 | |
| 23057 | 14 | 2 | | | | 0.01 | 0.03 | 0.16 | 0.01 | 0.00 | 0.8 | 0.03 | 0.0 | 0.0 | |
| 23414 | 0 | 0 | 0 | 0 | 0 | 0.00 | 0.00 | 0.00 | 0.00 | 0.00 | 0.0 | 0.01 | 0.0 | 0.0 | 0.0 |
| 23415 | 0 | 0 | 0 | 0 | 0 | 0.00 | 0.00 | 0.00 | 0.00 | 0.00 | 0.0 | 0.00 | 0.0 | 0.0 | 0.0 |
| 23144 | 0 | 0 | 0 | 0 | 0 | 0.00 | 0.00 | 0.00 | 0.00 | 0.00 | 0.0 | 0.01 | 13.2 | 0.0 | |
| 23145 | 8 | 1 | | | | 0.01 | 0.10 | 0.27 | 0.02 | 0.00 | 1.2 | 0.03 | 0.0 | | |
| 23146 | 28 | 5 | | | | 0.04 | 0.15 | 0.13 | 0.02 | 0.16 | | 0.17 | 0.2 | 0.0 | |
| 23147 | 20 | 5 | | | | 0.00 | 0.00 | 0.00 | 0.00 | 0.00 | 0.0 | 0.00 | 0.0 | | |
| 23136 | 35 | 10 | | | | 0.12 | 0.19 | 1.42 | 0.14 | 0.11 | 30.1 | 0.12 | 0.2 | 0.0 | |
| 23375 | 17 | 5 | | | | 0.06 | 0.09 | 0.69 | 0.07 | 0.05 | 14.7 | 0.06 | 0.1 | 0.0 | |
| 23075 | 48 | 14 | | | | 0.02 | 0.08 | 0.14 | 0.01 | 0.10 | 0.0 | 0.14 | 0.2 | 0.6 | |
| 23076 | 13 | 4 | | | | 0.01 | 0.02 | 0.04 | 0.00 | 0.03 | 0.0 | 0.04 | 0.1 | 0.2 | |
| 23173 | 152 | 38 | | | | 0.00 | 0.01 | 0.00 | 0.00 | 0.01 | 0.2 | 0.02 | 0.0 | 0.0 | |
| 23148 | 62 | 17 | | | | 0.01 | 0.03 | 0.03 | 0.00 | 0.04 | 0.1 | 0.05 | 0.0 | | |
| 23123 | 28 | 6 | | | | 0.03 | 0.04 | 0.06 | 0.01 | 0.07 | 1.7 | 0.09 | 0.1 | 0.3 | |
| 23149 | 54 | 14 | 0 | 14 | | 0.09 | 0.13 | 0.68 | 0.02 | 0.10 | 13.7 | 0.16 | 0.2 | 0.0 | |
| 23150 | 39 | 10 | 0 | 10 | | 0.05 | 0.08 | 2.18 | 0.08 | 0.07 | 13.5 | 0.26 | 0.3 | 0.0 | |
| 23448 | | | | | | | | | | | | | | | |
| 23154 | 0 | 0 | 0 | 0 | 0 | 0.01 | 0.03 | 0.07 | 0.01 | 0.00 | | 0.00 | 0.0 | 0.0 | |

| Code | Calcium (mg) | Copper (mg) | Iron (mg) | Magnes (mg) | Mang (mg) | Phos (mg) | Potassium (mg) | Selenium (mcg) | Sodium (mg) | Zinc (mg) |
|---|---|---|---|---|---|---|---|---|---|---|
| | Minerals | | | | | | | | | |
| 23411 | 1 | 0.0 | 0.1 | 0 | 0.0 | 0 | 1 | 0.2 | 11 | 0.00 |
| 23412 | 1 | 0.0 | 0.1 | 0 | 0.0 | 0 | 2 | 0.2 | 16 | 0.00 |
| 23031 | 0 | 0.0 | 0.0 | 0 | 0.0 | 0 | 0 | 0.0 | 2 | 0.00 |
| 23033 | 0 | 0.0 | 0.1 | 0 | 0.0 | 0 | 4 | 0.1 | 3 | 0.01 |
| 23413 | 2 | 0.0 | 0.2 | 0 | 0.0 | 0 | 2 | 0.3 | 22 | 0.00 |
| 23034 | 28 | 0.1 | 0.5 | 45 | | 46 | 71 | 0.7 | 6 | 0.52 |
| 23060 | 69 | 0.1 | 0.4 | 16 | 0.1 | 100 | 122 | 2.0 | 31 | 0.52 |
| 23016 | 84 | 0.2 | 0.6 | 26 | 0.1 | 95 | 169 | 1.7 | 36 | 0.61 |
| 23063 | 53 | 0.1 | 0.4 | 17 | 0.1 | 60 | 108 | 1.1 | 23 | 0.39 |
| 23061 | 72 | 0.2 | 0.4 | 23 | 0.1 | 91 | 140 | | 57 | 0.50 |
| 23087 | 1 | 0.0 | 0.3 | 1 | | 1 | 10 | | 7 | 0.01 |
| 23032 | 0 | 0.0 | 0.0 | 0 | 0.0 | 0 | 0 | 0.0 | 2 | 0.00 |
| 23427 | 165 | 0.4 | 1.7 | 65 | 0.3 | 236 | 416 | | 97 | 1.51 |
| 23479 | 49 | 0.3 | 0.6 | 36 | 0.3 | 112 | 170 | 1.9 | 24 | 1.13 |
| 23480 | 50 | 0.1 | 0.5 | 20 | 0.1 | 72 | 128 | 1.4 | 29 | 0.46 |
| 23037 | 84 | 0.1 | 0.6 | 36 | 0.2 | 117 | 162 | 0.8 | 85 | 0.56 |
| 4711 | 110 | | 1.4 | 59 | | | 120 | | 12 | 1.40 |
| 23192 | 80 | | 0.0 | 18 | | 76 | 159 | | 30 | |
| 23058 | 68 | 0.1 | 0.3 | 20 | 0.1 | 77 | 137 | 2.2 | 58 | 0.45 |
| 23019 | 33 | 0.2 | 0.5 | 35 | 0.4 | 82 | 150 | 1.6 | 11 | 0.68 |
| 23242 | | | | | | | | | | |
| 23022 | 82 | 0.3 | 1.6 | 43 | 0.3 | 136 | 488 | 2.2 | 34 | 0.77 |
| 23419 | 21 | 0.1 | 0.3 | 19 | 0.2 | 42 | 100 | 1.0 | 8 | 0.39 |
| 23193 | 2 | 0.0 | 0.1 | 4 | 0.0 | 5 | 13 | | 1 | 0.05 |
| 23018 | 92 | 0.2 | 0.7 | 37 | 0.3 | 108 | 182 | 1.6 | 30 | 0.55 |
| 23038 | 78 | 0.1 | 0.5 | 20 | 0.1 | 86 | 145 | 3.4 | 144 | 0.43 |
| 23039 | 23 | 0.0 | 0.1 | 6 | 0.0 | 26 | 43 | 1.0 | 43 | 0.13 |
| 23035 | 8 | 0.2 | 1.1 | 30 | 0.5 | 48 | 131 | 3.3 | 79 | 0.52 |
| 23062 | 53 | 0.2 | 0.6 | 42 | 0.3 | 122 | 219 | 2.3 | 73 | 0.89 |
| 23153 | 18 | 0.3 | 0.2 | 2 | 0.0 | 87 | 18 | | 66 | 0.04 |
| 23196 | 0 | | 0.0 | | | | 62 | | 103 | 0.10 |
| 23194 | 0 | | 0.0 | 14 | | | 93 | | 90 | 0.24 |
| 23191 | 0 | | 0.0 | | | | 60 | | 80 | |
| 23189 | 0 | | 0.0 | 3 | | | 54 | | 80 | 0.08 |
| 23190 | 0 | | 0.0 | 8 | | | 69 | | 80 | 0.06 |
| 23135 | 62 | 0.2 | 0.3 | 35 | 0.3 | 94 | 185 | 2.0 | 135 | 0.69 |
| 23137 | 31 | 0.3 | 0.4 | 46 | 0.5 | 129 | 163 | 2.0 | 62 | 1.65 |
| 23284 | 0 | | 0.0 | | | | 75 | | 310 | |
| 23081 | 22 | 0.3 | 1.0 | 37 | 0.4 | 82 | 154 | 2.0 | 334 | 0.72 |
| 23120 | 92 | 0.3 | 1.4 | 92 | 1.2 | 260 | 424 | 2.3 | 210 | 1.68 |
| 23080 | 31 | 0.1 | 0.4 | 30 | | 61 | 163 | | 96 | 0.55 |
| 23138 | 12 | 0.2 | 0.5 | 20 | 0.7 | 43 | 82 | | 24 | 0.79 |
| 23214 | 49 | 0.2 | 0.5 | 20 | 0.1 | 65 | 231 | | 16 | 0.36 |
| 23424 | 27 | 0.2 | 0.4 | 31 | 0.3 | 71 | 123 | 1.6 | 111 | 0.64 |
| 23043 | 39 | 0.3 | 0.6 | 44 | 0.4 | 102 | 176 | 2.3 | 158 | 0.92 |
| 23436 | 38 | 0.1 | 0.4 | 20 | 0.2 | 61 | 106 | 0.8 | 68 | 0.35 |
| 23426 | 81 | 0.1 | 0.3 | 21 | 0.1 | 79 | 131 | 2.1 | 93 | 0.49 |
| 23142 | 229 | 0.3 | 1.5 | 88 | 0.6 | 148 | 113 | 1.4 | 58 | 1.32 |
| 23485 | 0 | 0.0 | 0.0 | 1 | 0.0 | 1 | 3 | 0.4 | 10 | 0.02 |
| 23036 | 51 | 0.1 | 0.2 | 13 | 0.1 | 58 | 93 | | 108 | 0.30 |
| 23040 | 54 | 0.3 | 0.4 | 41 | 0.4 | 127 | 185 | 2.6 | 152 | 1.34 |
| 23041 | 14 | 0.1 | 0.1 | 11 | 0.1 | 33 | 49 | 0.7 | 40 | 0.35 |
| 23057 | 11 | 0.3 | 1.0 | 46 | 0.3 | 61 | 123 | 1.2 | 3 | 0.59 |
| 23414 | 4 | 0.0 | 0.5 | 1 | 0.0 | 1 | 6 | 0.7 | 53 | 0.00 |
| 23415 | 1 | 0.0 | 0.2 | 0 | 0.0 | 0 | 2 | 0.3 | 21 | 0.00 |
| 23144 | 1 | 0.0 | 0.0 | 0 | 0.0 | 2 | 0 | 0.2 | 14 | 0.00 |
| 23145 | 10 | 0.2 | 1.1 | 46 | 0.2 | 60 | 119 | 1.1 | 7 | 0.62 |
| 23146 | 86 | 0.1 | 0.5 | 22 | 0.1 | 100 | 154 | | 37 | 0.45 |
| 23147 | 0 | 0.0 | 0.0 | 0 | 0.0 | 0 | 1 | | 13 | 0.00 |
| 23136 | 49 | 0.1 | 0.1 | 16 | 0.1 | 58 | 97 | 1.0 | 89 | 0.42 |
| 23375 | 24 | 0.1 | 0.1 | 8 | 0.1 | 28 | 47 | 0.5 | 43 | 0.21 |
| 23075 | 50 | 0.1 | 0.4 | 17 | 0.1 | 55 | 80 | 1.5 | 116 | 0.33 |
| 23076 | 13 | 0.0 | 0.1 | 5 | 0.0 | 15 | 21 | 0.4 | 31 | 0.09 |
| 23173 | 4 | 0.0 | 0.0 | 0 | 0.0 | 4 | 6 | | 22 | 0.02 |
| 23148 | 19 | 0.0 | 0.1 | 6 | 0.0 | 21 | 37 | | 9 | 0.13 |
| 23123 | 27 | 0.1 | 0.2 | 9 | 0.1 | 33 | 52 | | 16 | 0.24 |
| 23149 | 51 | 0.1 | 0.5 | 18 | 0.2 | 68 | 115 | 1.1 | 110 | 0.44 |
| 23150 | 42 | 0.2 | 0.5 | 40 | 0.5 | 103 | 192 | 5.6 | 147 | 0.76 |
| 23448 | 2 | | 0.1 | | | | | | 83 | |
| 23154 | 5 | 0.6 | 0.2 | 4 | 0.1 | 220 | 45 | | 175 | 0.11 |

| Code | Amount | Description | Weight (g) | Calories | % Water | Protein (g) | Carbs (g) | Fiber (g) | Sugar (g) | Other Carbs (g) | Fat (g) | Sat Fat (g) | Mono Fat (g) | Poly Fat (g) | Omega 3 (g) | Omega 6 (g) | Choles (mg) |
|---|---|---|---|---|---|---|---|---|---|---|---|---|---|---|---|---|---|
| | | | Basic Components | | | | | | | | | Additional Fats | | | | | |
| 23151 | 1 ea | Whatchamacallit, 1.69 oz bar | 48 | 214 | 10 | 4.3 | 28.9 | 1.0 | 21.2 | 6.7 | 9.3 | 4.5 | 2.8 | 1.5 | 0.09 | 1.42 | 5 |
| 23084 | 10 ea | Whoppers, malted milk balls | 29 | 144 | 2 | 1.8 | 18.4 | 0.8 | 14.6 | 3.0 | 7.7 | 4.6 | 2.5 | 0.2 | | | 5 |
| 23408 | 100 g | Yogurt Coated candy, avg | 100 | 521 | 2 | 5.9 | 63.7 | 0.[illegible] | | | 27.0 | 24.1 | 0.5 | 0.5 | 0.03 | 0.49 | 1 |
| 23089 | 1/2 cup | Yogurt Covered Raisins, avg | 96 | 382 | 9 | 4.3 | 68.8 | 3.[illegible] | | | 12.5 | 7.2 | 3.9 | 0.4 | | | 9 |
| 23088 | 1/2 cup | Yogurt Covered Peanuts, avg | 85 | 387 | 4 | 7.5 | 32.0 | 3.6 | | | 26.1 | 5.0 | 12.8 | 7.0 | | | 3 |
| 23152 | 1 ea | York Peppermint Patty, 1.48 oz pkg | 42 | 165 | 10 | 0.9 | 33.6 | 0.[illegible] | 26.6 | 6.2 | 3.0 | 1.8 | 1.0 | 0.1 | | | 0 |
| | | Gum | | | | | | | | | | | | | | | |
| 23082 | 1 pce | Average | 3 | 10 | 3 | 0.0 | 2.9 | 0.0 | 2.9 | 0.0 | 0.0 | 0.0 | 0.0 | 0.0 | 0.00 | 0.00 | 0 |
| 23083 | 1 pce | Sugarless, avg | 4 | 11 | 4 | 0.0 | 3.8 | 0.0 | 0.0 | 3.8 | 0.0 | 0.0 | 0.0 | 0.0 | 0.00 | 0.00 | 0 |
| 25128 | 1 pce | Assorted flvrs, Beechnut | 3 | 10 | | 0.0 | 3.0 | 1.0 | 2.0 | 0.0 | 0.0 | 0.0 | 0.0 | 0.0 | 0.00 | 0.00 | 0 |
| | | Marshmallows | | | | | | | | | | | | | | | |
| 23064 | 2 Tbs | Crème, Kraft | 12 | 40 | 16 | 0.0 | 10.0 | 0.0 | 8.0 | 2.0 | 0.0 | 0.0 | 0.0 | 0.0 | 0.00 | 0.00 | 0 |
| 23302 | 5 pce | Funmallows, Kraft | 40 | 138 | 16 | 0.0 | 32.5 | 0.0 | 25.0 | 7.5 | 0.0 | 0.0 | 0.0 | 0.0 | 0.00 | 0.00 | 0 |
| 23304 | 5 pce | Jet puffed, Kraft | 34 | 110 | 16 | 1.0 | 27.0 | 0.0 | 20.0 | 7.0 | 0.0 | 0.0 | 0.0 | 0.0 | 0.00 | 0.00 | 0 |
| 23008 | 1 cup | Miniature, avg | 46 | 146 | 16 | 0.8 | 37.4 | 0.0 | 25.8 | 11.6 | 0.1 | 0.0 | 0.0 | 0.0 | 0.00 | 0.02 | 0 |
| 23305 | 1 cup | Miniature, Kraft | 60 | 200 | 16 | 2.0 | 50.0 | 0.0 | 34.0 | 16.0 | 0.0 | 0.0 | 0.0 | 0.0 | 0.00 | 0.00 | 0 |
| 23303 | 1 cup | Miniature Funmallows, Kraft | 60 | 200 | 16 | 2.0 | 50.0 | 0.0 | 36.0 | 14.0 | 0.0 | 0.0 | 0.0 | 0.0 | 0.00 | 0.00 | 0 |
| 23306 | 1 cup | Teddy Bear, Kraft | 60 | 200 | 16 | 2.0 | 46.0 | 0.0 | 32.0 | 14.0 | 0.0 | 0.0 | 0.0 | 0.0 | 0.00 | 0.00 | 0 |
| | | **CEREALS, BREAKFAST TYPE** | | | | | | | | | | | | | | | |
| | | *CEREALS, COOKED AND DRY* | | | | | | | | | | | | | | | |
| | | Arrowhead Mills | | | | | | | | | | | | | | | |
| 40441 | 1/4 cup | Bear Mush, dry | 45 | 160 | 9 | 5.0 | 33.0 | 2.0 | 0.0 | 31.0 | 1.0 | 0.0 | | | | | 0 |
| 40440 | 1/4 cup | Bits O Barley, dry | 34 | 103 | 9 | 3.7 | 25.9 | 4.4 | 0.7 | 20.7 | 0.7 | 0.0 | | | | | 0 |
| 40439 | 1/4 cup | Bulgur Wheat, dry | 43 | 150 | 9 | 5.0 | 33.0 | 4.0 | 0.0 | 29.0 | 0.5 | 0.0 | | | | | 0 |
| 40438 | 1/4 cup | Cracked Wheat, dry | 41 | 140 | 10 | 5.0 | 29.0 | 6.0 | 0.0 | 23.0 | 0.5 | 0.0 | | | | | 0 |
| 40437 | 1/4 cup | Oat Bran, dry | 29 | 112 | 7 | 5.9 | 17.1 | 5.2 | 0.0 | 11.9 | 1.9 | 0.0 | | | | | 0 |
| 40444 | 1/4 cup | Rice & Shine, dry | 42 | 150 | 6 | 3.0 | 32.0 | 2.0 | 0.0 | 30.0 | 1.0 | 0.0 | | | | | 0 |
| 40443 | 1/4 cup | Seven Grain, dry | 30 | 105 | 10 | 4.5 | 18.8 | 3.3 | 0.0 | 15.0 | 1.1 | 0.0 | | | | | 0 |
| 40442 | 1/4 cup | Seven Grain Wheat Free, dry | 35 | 120 | 10 | 4.0 | 25.0 | 2.0 | 0.0 | 23.0 | 1.5 | 0.0 | | | | | 0 |
| 40445 | 1/4 cup | Steel Cut Oats, dry | 43 | 170 | 9 | 6.0 | 29.0 | 5.0 | 0.0 | 24.0 | 3.0 | 0.5 | | | | | 0 |
| | | Corn Grits | | | | | | | | | | | | | | | |
| 40093 | 1 cup | Enriched, white, ckd, avg | 242 | 145 | 85 | 3.4 | 31.5 | 0.5 | 0.1 | 30.9 | 0.5 | 0.1 | 0.1 | 0.2 | 0.00 | 0.19 | 0 |
| 40150 | 1/4 cup | Enriched, white, dry, avg | 39 | 145 | 10 | 3.4 | 31.0 | 0.6 | 0.1 | 30.3 | 0.5 | 0.1 | 0.1 | 0.2 | 0.00 | 0.19 | 0 |
| 38007 | 1 cup | Enriched, yellow, ckd, avg | 242 | 145 | 85 | 3.4 | 31.5 | 0.5 | 0.1 | 30.9 | 0.5 | 0.1 | 0.1 | 0.2 | 0.00 | 0.19 | 0 |
| 38006 | 1/4 cup | Enriched, yellow, dry, avg | 39 | 145 | 10 | 3.4 | 31.0 | 0.6 | 0.0 | 30.4 | 0.5 | 0.1 | 0.1 | 0.2 | 0.00 | 0.19 | 0 |
| 38349 | 1/4 cup | Hominy, Quick, yellow, dry, Albers | 40 | 140 | 10 | 3.0 | 31.0 | 1.0 | 0.0 | 30.0 | 0.4 | 0.0 | | | 0.00 | 0.00 | 0 |
| 38349 | 1/4 cup | Hominy, white, dry, Albers | 40 | 140 | 10 | 3.0 | 31.0 | 1.0 | 0.0 | 30.0 | 0.4 | 0.0 | | | 0.00 | 0.00 | 0 |
| 40363 | 1 ea | Instant Butter flvr, dry pkt, Quaker | 28 | 101 | 9 | 2.3 | 20.9 | 1.3 | 0.2 | 19.4 | 1.4 | 0.3 | 0.3 | 0.3 | 0.01 | 0.24 | 0 |
| 40376 | 1 ea | Instant Butter flvr, prep f/dry pkt, Quaker | 147 | 101 | 82 | 2.3 | 20.9 | 1.3 | 0.1 | 19.5 | 1.4 | 0.3 | 0.3 | 0.3 | 0.01 | 0.24 | 0 |
| 40152 | 1 ea | Instant Cheese flvr, dry pkt, Quaker | 28 | 102 | 8 | 2.3 | 20.5 | 1.2 | 0.6 | 18.8 | 1.6 | 0.5 | 0.4 | 0.2 | 0.01 | 0.19 | 1 |
| 40233 | 1 cup | Instant Cheese flvr, prep, Quaker | 178 | 125 | 82 | 2.8 | 24.9 | 1.4 | 0.1 | 23.4 | 2.0 | 0.6 | 0.5 | 0.3 | 0.02 | 0.23 | 0 |
| 40153 | 1 ea | Instant Imit Bacon, dry pkt, Quaker | 28 | 98 | 7 | 2.8 | 21.7 | 1.5 | 0.1 | 20.1 | 0.5 | 0.[illegible] | 0.1 | 0.2 | 0.00 | 0.11 | 0 |
| 40243 | 1 ea | Instant Imit Bacon, prep f/dry pkt, Quaker | 141 | 94 | 82 | 2.7 | 20.9 | 1.4 | 0.1 | 19.4 | 0.5 | 0.[illegible] | 0.1 | 0.2 | 0.00 | 0.11 | 0 |
| 40154 | 1 ea | Instant Imit Ham Bits, dry pkt, Quaker | 28 | 95 | 7 | 2.8 | 21.1 | 1.4 | 0.1 | 19.5 | 0.5 | 0.[illegible] | 0.1 | 0.1 | 0.00 | 0.11 | 0 |
| 40234 | 1 cup | Instant Ham Bits prep, Quaker | 176 | 114 | 82 | 3.3 | 25.2 | 1.6 | 0.1 | 23.5 | 0.6 | 0.1 | 0.2 | 0.1 | 0.00 | 0.14 | 0 |
| 40094 | 1 cup | Unenriched, white, ckd, avg | 242 | 145 | 85 | 3.4 | 31.5 | 0.5 | 0.1 | 30.3 | 0.5 | 0.1 | 0.1 | 0.2 | 0.00 | 0.19 | 0 |
| 40173 | 1/4 cup | Unenriched, white, dry, avg | 39 | 145 | 10 | 3.4 | 31.0 | 0.6 | 0.0 | 30.4 | 0.5 | 0.1 | 0.1 | 0.2 | 0.00 | 0.19 | 0 |
| 40081 | 1 cup | Unenriched, yellow, ckd, avg | 242 | 145 | 85 | 3.4 | 31.5 | 0.5 | 0.1 | 30.3 | 0.5 | 0.1 | 0.1 | 0.2 | 0.00 | 0.19 | 0 |
| 40174 | 1/4 cup | Unenriched, yellow, dry, avg | 39 | 145 | 10 | 3.4 | 31.0 | 0.6 | 0.0 | 30.4 | 0.5 | 0.1 | 0.1 | 0.2 | 0.00 | 0.19 | 0 |
| 40078 | 1 cup | Cream of Rice, ckd, avg | 244 | 127 | 88 | 2.2 | 27.8 | 0.2 | 0.2 | 27.3 | 0.2 | 0.1 | 0.1 | 0.1 | 0.01 | 0.05 | 0 |
| 40155 | 1/4 cup | Cream of Rice, dry, avg | 43 | 159 | 10 | 2.7 | 35.4 | 0.3 | 0.3 | 34.8 | 0.2 | 0.1 | 0.1 | 0.1 | 0.01 | 0.05 | 0 |
| | | Cream of Wheat | | | | | | | | | | | | | | | |
| 40162 | 1 ea | Apple, Banana & Maple, dry pkt, avg | 35 | 131 | 8 | 2.4 | 28.6 | 0.9 | 0.1 | 27.6 | 0.4 | 0.1 | 0.1 | 0.2 | 0.02 | 0.19 | 0 |
| 40163 | 1 ea | Apple, Banana & Maple, prep f/dry pkt, avg | 150 | 132 | 78 | 2.4 | 28.9 | 0.5 | 0.2 | 28.3 | 0.5 | 0.1 | 0.0 | 0.1 | 0.01 | 0.10 | 0 |
| 40157 | 1 cup | Cooked, avg | 251 | 133 | 87 | 3.8 | 27.6 | 1.8 | 0.3 | 25.6 | 0.5 | 0.1 | 0.1 | 0.3 | 0.03 | 0.25 | 0 |
| 40156 | 1/4 cup | Dry, avg | 43 | 159 | 11 | 4.5 | 32.9 | 1.6 | 0.1 | 31.[illegible] | 0.6 | 0.1 | 0.1 | 0.4 | 0.04 | 0.32 | 0 |
| 40159 | 1/4 cup | Instant, dry, avg | 44 | 161 | 10 | 4.7 | 33.2 | 1.4 | 0.1 | 31.7 | 0.6 | 0.1 | 0.1 | 0.3 | 0.04 | 0.30 | 0 |
| 40160 | 1 cup | Prep f/instant, avg | 241 | 154 | 84 | 4.3 | 31.6 | 2.9 | 0.2 | 28.4 | 0.5 | 0.1 | 0.1 | 0.3 | 0.03 | 0.24 | 0 |
| 40158 | 1/4 cup | Quick, dry, avg | 44 | 159 | 10 | 4.5 | 33.0 | 1.2 | 0.1 | 31.6 | 0.6 | 0.1 | 0.1 | 0.3 | 0.03 | 0.28 | 0 |
| 40079 | 1 cup | Quick, prep, avg | 239 | 129 | 87 | 3.6 | 26.8 | 1.2 | 0.2 | 25.3 | 0.5 | 0.1 | 0.1 | 0.3 | 0.03 | 0.23 | 0 |
| | | Fantastic Foods Cereal in a Cup | | | | | | | | | | | | | | | |
| 40498 | 1 ea | Apple Cinnamon Oatmeal, dry pkg | 47 | 170 | 4 | 6.0 | 37.0 | 4.0 | 12.0 | 21.0 | 2.0 | 0.0 | | | 0.00 | 0.00 | 0 |
| 40499 | 1 ea | Banana Nut Barley, dry pkg | 46 | 170 | 1 | 4.0 | 39.0 | 6.0 | 12.0 | 21.0 | 2.5 | 0.0 | | | 0.00 | 0.00 | 0 |
| 40500 | 1 ea | Cranberry Orange Oatmeal, dry pkg | 49 | 180 | 6 | 6.0 | 38.0 | 4.0 | 13.0 | 21.0 | 2.0 | 0.0 | | | 0.00 | 0.00 | 0 |
| 40501 | 1 ea | Maple Raisin 3 Grain, dry pkg | 52 | 180 | 7 | 5.0 | 42.0 | 5.0 | 16.0 | 21.0 | 1.0 | 0.0 | | | 0.00 | 0.00 | 0 |

| Code | Vit A (IU) | Vit A (RE) | Retinol (RE) | Carotenoids (RE) | Beta Carotene (mcg) | Thiamin (mg) | Riboflavin (mg) | Niacin (NE) | Vit B6 (mg) | Vit B12 (mcg) | Folate (mcg) | Panto (mg) | Vit C (mg) | Vit D (mg) | Vit E (α TE) | Calcium (mg) | Copper (mg) | Iron (mg) | Magnes (mg) | Mang (mg) | Phos (mg) | Potassium (mg) | Selenium (mcg) | Sodium (mg) | Zinc (mg) |
|---|---|---|---|---|---|---|---|---|---|---|---|---|---|---|---|---|---|---|---|---|---|---|---|---|---|
| | Vit A & Components | | | | | Vitamins | | | | | | | | | | Minerals | | | | | | | | | |
| 23151 | 34 | 9 | | | | 0.22 | 0.29 | 3.52 | 0.27 | 0.16 | 4.8 | 0.27 | 0.1 | 0.0 | | 55 | 0.1 | 0.3 | 29 | 0.4 | 87 | 148 | 1.1 | 99 | 0.62 |
| 23084 | 17 | 3 | 2.3 | 0.6 | | 0.02 | 0.08 | 0.13 | 0.02 | 0.11 | 2.6 | 0.17 | 0.1 | | | 50 | 0.1 | 0.2 | 14 | 0.1 | 56 | 99 | | 42 | 0.32 |
| 23408 | 35 | 1 | | | | 0.06 | 0.28 | 0.75 | 0.06 | 0.75 | 17.0 | 0.61 | 0.5 | | | 199 | 0.1 | 0.2 | 12 | 0.0 | 176 | 286 | 3.7 | 90 | 0.74 |
| 23089 | 90 | 26 | 25 | 1 | | 0.11 | 0.16 | 0.52 | 0.16 | 0.30 | 7.9 | | 2.0 | | | 110 | 0.2 | 1.2 | 20 | | 131 | 541 | | 42 | 0.50 |
| 23088 | 82 | 21 | 18 | 3 | | 0.09 | 0.06 | 4.73 | 0.09 | 0.34 | 96.1 | | 1.8 | | | 33 | 0.7 | 0.9 | 50 | | 126 | 214 | | 29 | 1.71 |
| 23152 | 2 | 0.2 | | | | 0.01 | 0.04 | 0.36 | 0.00 | 0.01 | | 0.02 | 0.0 | 0.0 | | 6 | 0.2 | 0.4 | 26 | 0.2 | 40 | 54 | | 10 | 0.32 |
| 23082 | 0 | 0 | 0 | 0 | 0 | 0.00 | 0.00 | 0.00 | 0.00 | 0.00 | 0.0 | 0.00 | 0.0 | 0.0 | 0.0 | 0 | 0.0 | 0.0 | 0 | 0.0 | 0 | 0 | 0.0 | 0 | 0.00 |
| 23083 | 0 | 0 | 0 | 0 | 0 | 0.00 | 0.00 | 0.00 | 0.00 | 0.00 | 0.0 | | 0.0 | | 0.0 | 1 | 0.0 | 0.0 | 0 | | 0 | 0 | | 0 | 0.00 |
| 25128 | | | | | | | | | | | | | | | | | | | | | | 0 | | 0 | |
| 23064 | 0 | 0 | 0 | 0 | 0 | | | | | | | | 0.0 | | 0.0 | 0 | | 0.0 | | | | 0 | | 10 | |
| 23302 | 0 | 0 | 0 | 0 | 0 | | | | | | | | 0.0 | | | 0 | | 0.0 | | | | 0 | | 25 | |
| 23304 | 0 | 0 | 0 | 0 | 0 | | | | | | | | 0.0 | | | 0 | | 0.0 | | | | 0 | | 40 | |
| 23008 | 0.5 | 0.05 | 0 | 0.05 | | 0.00 | 0.00 | 0.04 | 0.00 | 0.00 | 0.5 | 0.00 | 0.0 | 0.0 | 0.0 | 1 | 0.0 | 0.1 | 1 | 0.0 | 4 | 2 | 0.9 | 22 | 0.02 |
| 23305 | 0 | 0 | 0 | 0 | 0 | | | | | | | | 0.0 | | | 0 | | 0.0 | | | | 0 | | 60 | |
| 23303 | 0 | 0 | 0 | 0 | 0 | | | | | | | | 0.0 | | | 0 | | 0.0 | | | | 0 | | 40 | |
| 23306 | 0 | 0 | 0 | 0 | 0 | | | | | | | | 0.0 | | | 0 | | 0.0 | | | | 100 | | 50 | |
| 40441 | 0 | 0 | 0 | 0 | 0 | 0.09 | 0.03 | 1.20 | | | | | 0.0 | | | 150 | | 0.7 | | | | 40 | | 0 | |
| 40440 | 0 | 0 | 0 | 0 | 0 | 0.00 | 0.03 | 0.89 | | | | | 0.0 | | | 0 | | 1.1 | | | | 170 | | 0 | |
| 40439 | 0 | 0 | 0 | 0 | 0 | 0.09 | 0.07 | 2.00 | | | | | 0.0 | | | 0 | | 3.6 | | | | 100 | | 0 | |
| 40438 | 0 | 0 | 0 | 0 | 0 | 0.22 | 0.03 | 1.60 | | | | | 0.0 | | | 20 | | 1.4 | | | | 150 | | 0 | |
| 40437 | 0 | 0 | 0 | 0 | 0 | 0.04 | 0.08 | 0.30 | | | | | 0.0 | | | 30 | | 2.7 | | | | 208 | | 0 | |
| 40444 | 0 | 0 | 0 | 0 | 0 | 0.15 | | 2.00 | | | | | 0.0 | | | 0 | | 0.7 | | | | 90 | | 0 | |
| 40443 | 0 | 0 | 0 | 0 | 0 | 0.04 | 0.13 | 1.50 | | | | | 0.0 | | | 30 | | 1.1 | | | | 30 | | 0 | |
| 40442 | 0 | 0 | 0 | 0 | 0 | 0.15 | 0.03 | 0.80 | | | | | 0.0 | | | 20 | | 1.1 | | | | 100 | | 0 | |
| 40445 | 0 | 0 | 0 | 0 | 0 | 0.22 | 0.07 | 0.40 | | | | | 0.0 | | | 20 | | 1.8 | | | | 150 | | 0 | |
| 40093 | 0 | 0 | 0 | 0 | 0 | 0.24 | 0.15 | 1.96 | 0.06 | 0.00 | 75.0 | 0.15 | 0.0 | 0.0 | 0.0 | 0 | 0.0 | 1.5 | 10 | 0.0 | 29 | 53 | 7.5 | 0 | 0.17 |
| 40150 | 0 | 0 | 0 | 0 | 0 | 0.25 | 0.15 | 1.93 | 0.06 | 0.00 | 72.9 | 0.19 | 0.0 | 0.0 | 0.0 | 1 | 0.0 | 1.5 | 11 | 0.0 | 28 | 53 | 6.6 | 0 | 0.16 |
| 38007 | 145 | 5 | 0 | 15 | | 0.24 | 0.15 | 1.96 | 0.06 | 0.00 | 75.0 | 0.15 | 0.0 | 0.0 | 0.0 | 0 | 0.0 | 1.5 | 10 | 0.0 | 29 | 53 | 7.5 | 0 | 0.17 |
| 38006 | 172 | 7 | 0 | 17 | | 0.25 | 0.15 | 1.93 | 0.06 | 0.00 | 72.9 | 0.19 | 0.0 | 0.0 | 0.0 | 1 | 0.0 | 1.5 | 11 | 0.0 | 28 | 53 | 6.6 | 0 | 0.16 |
| 38349 | 0 | 0 | 0 | 0 | 0 | 0.15 | 0.10 | 1.20 | | | | | 0.0 | | | 0 | | 1.1 | | | | | | 0 | |
| 38349 | 0 | 0 | 0 | 0 | 0 | 0.15 | 0.10 | 1.20 | | | | | 0.0 | | | 0 | | 1.1 | | | | | | 0 | |
| 40363 | 54 | 5 | 0 | 5 | 32 | 0.13 | 0.20 | 2.37 | 0.03 | 0.00 | 47.0 | 0.11 | 0.0 | 0.0 | | 2 | 0.0 | 8.1 | 8 | 0.0 | 25 | 54 | 4.5 | 323 | 0.11 |
| 40376 | 54 | 5 | 0 | 5 | 32 | 0.15 | 0.08 | 1.40 | 0.03 | 0.00 | 47.0 | 0.11 | 0.0 | 0.0 | | 4 | 0.0 | 8.3 | 9 | 0.0 | 25 | 54 | | 328 | 0.15 |
| 40152 | 3.6 | 1.1 | | | | 0.17 | 0.18 | 2.20 | 0.04 | 0.06 | 43.7 | 0.11 | 0.0 | 0.0 | | 13 | 0.0 | 8.1 | 10 | 0.1 | 39 | 48 | 4.5 | 522 | 0.21 |
| 40233 | 3.6 | 1.8 | | | | 0.17 | 0.10 | 1.58 | 0.06 | 0.07 | 53.4 | 0.14 | 0.0 | 0.0 | | 18 | 0.0 | 9.9 | 48 | 0.1 | 30 | 57 | 5.3 | 639 | 0.30 |
| 40153 | 0 | 0 | 0 | 0 | 0 | 0.13 | 0.20 | 2.35 | 0.06 | 0.00 | 46.8 | 0.11 | 0.0 | 0.0 | | 11 | 0.0 | 8.1 | 10 | 0.0 | 39 | 71 | 4.5 | 341 | 0.26 |
| 40243 | 0 | 0 | 0 | 0 | 0 | 0.15 | 0.09 | 1.38 | 0.06 | 0.00 | 45.1 | 0.11 | 0.0 | 0.0 | | 13 | 0.0 | 8.0 | 10 | 0.0 | 38 | 68 | | 331 | 0.28 |
| 40154 | 0 | 0 | 0 | 0 | 0 | 0.17 | 0.20 | 2.34 | 0.06 | 0.06 | 46.5 | 0.11 | 0.0 | 0.0 | | 15 | 0.1 | 8.1 | 14 | 0.1 | 37 | 50 | 4.5 | 493 | 0.24 |
| 40234 | 0 | 0 | 0 | 0 | 0 | 0.19 | 0.11 | 0.11 | 0.08 | 0.07 | 56.3 | 0.13 | 0.0 | 0.0 | | 21 | 0.1 | 9.9 | 18 | 0.1 | 39 | 72 | | 637 | 0.32 |
| 40094 | 0 | 0 | 0 | 0 | 0 | 0.05 | 0.02 | 0.48 | 0.06 | 0.00 | 2.4 | 0.15 | 0.0 | 0.0 | | 0 | 0.0 | 0.5 | 10 | 0.0 | 29 | 53 | 7.5 | 0 | 0.17 |
| 40173 | 0 | 0 | 0 | 0 | 0 | 0.05 | 0.02 | 0.47 | 0.06 | 0.00 | 1.9 | 0.19 | 0.0 | 0.0 | | 1 | 0.0 | 0.4 | 11 | 0.0 | 28 | 53 | 6.6 | 0 | 0.16 |
| 40081 | 145 | 15 | 0 | 15 | | 0.05 | 0.02 | 0.48 | 0.06 | 0.00 | 2.4 | 0.15 | 0.0 | 0.0 | | 0 | 0.0 | 0.5 | 10 | 0.0 | 29 | 53 | 7.5 | 0 | 0.17 |
| 40174 | 172 | 17 | 0 | 17 | | 0.05 | 0.02 | 0.47 | 0.06 | 0.00 | 1.9 | 0.19 | 0.0 | 0.0 | | 1 | 0.0 | 0.4 | 11 | 0.0 | 28 | 53 | 6.6 | 0 | 0.16 |
| 40078 | 0 | 0 | 0 | 0 | 0 | 0.00 | 0.00 | 0.98 | 0.07 | 0.00 | 7.3 | 0.19 | 0.0 | 0.0 | | 7 | 0.1 | 0.5 | 7 | 0.4 | 41 | 49 | 7.3 | 2 | 0.39 |
| 40155 | 0 | 0 | 0 | 0 | 0 | 0.09 | 0.04 | 1.29 | 0.08 | 0.00 | 12.5 | 0.24 | 0.0 | 0.0 | | 10 | 0.1 | 0.6 | 10 | 0.4 | 53 | 61 | 8.2 | 3 | 0.48 |
| 40162 | 1236 | 124 | 0 | 124 | 742 | 0.38 | 0.24 | 4.93 | 0.49 | 0.00 | 98.7 | 0.12 | 0.0 | 0.0 | | 40 | 0.1 | 8.0 | 9 | 0.2 | 20 | 54 | 7.0 | 238 | 0.23 |
| 40163 | 1251 | 125 | 0 | 125 | 750 | 0.45 | 0.30 | 4.95 | 0.45 | 0.00 | 100.5 | 0.12 | 0.0 | 0.0 | | 40 | 0.1 | 8.1 | 9 | 0.1 | 20 | 56 | 17.1 | 242 | 0.23 |
| 40157 | 0 | 0 | 0 | 0 | 0 | 0.25 | 0.00 | 1.51 | 0.04 | 0.00 | 45.2 | 0.19 | 0.0 | 0.0 | | 50 | 0.1 | 10.3 | 10 | 0.2 | 43 | 43 | 32.1 | 3 | 0.33 |
| 40156 | 0 | 0 | 0 | 0 | 0 | 0.22 | 0.09 | 1.81 | 0.05 | 0.00 | 52.0 | 0.22 | 0.0 | 0.0 | | 61 | 0.1 | 12.3 | 12 | 0.3 | 49 | 52 | 8.6 | 3 | 0.38 |
| 40159 | 0 | 0 | 0 | 0 | 0 | 0.22 | 0.09 | 1.85 | 0.04 | 0.00 | 157.1 | 0.21 | 0.0 | 0.0 | | 62 | 0.1 | 12.6 | 15 | 0.3 | 45 | 51 | 8.8 | 7 | 0.43 |
| 40160 | 0 | 0 | 0 | 0 | 0 | 0.24 | 0.00 | 1.69 | 0.03 | 0.00 | 149.4 | 0.17 | 0.0 | 0.0 | | 60 | 0.1 | 12.1 | 14 | 0.2 | 43 | 48 | 27.5 | 7 | 0.41 |
| 40158 | 0 | 0 | 0 | 0 | 0 | 0.22 | 0.09 | 1.85 | 0.04 | 0.00 | 53.2 | 0.21 | 0.0 | 0.0 | | 62 | 0.1 | 12.6 | 15 | 0.3 | 124 | 57 | 8.8 | 172 | 0.43 |
| 40079 | 0 | 0 | 0 | 0 | 0 | 0.24 | 0.00 | 1.43 | 0.03 | 0.00 | 107.6 | 0.17 | 0.0 | 0.0 | | 50 | 0.1 | 10.3 | 12 | 0.2 | 100 | 45 | 30.6 | 139 | 0.33 |
| 40498 | 0 | 0 | 0 | 0 | 0 | | | | | | | | 0.0 | | | 20 | | 1.8 | | | | | | 240 | |
| 40499 | 0 | 0 | 0 | 0 | 0 | | | | | | | | 0.0 | | | 0 | | 1.1 | | | | | | 240 | |
| 40500 | 0 | 0 | 0 | 0 | 0 | | | | | | | | 6.0 | | | 20 | | 1.4 | | | | | | 210 | |
| 40501 | 0 | 0 | 0 | 0 | 0 | | | | | | | | 0.0 | | | 20 | | 1.4 | | | | | | 240 | |

| Code | Amount | Description | Basic Components | | | | | | | | | Additional Fats | | | | | | Vit A & Components | | | | | Vitamins | | | | | | | | | | Minerals | | | | | | | | | |
|---|---|---|---|---|---|---|---|---|---|---|---|---|---|---|---|---|---|---|---|---|---|---|---|---|---|---|---|---|---|---|---|---|---|---|---|---|---|---|---|---|---|---|
| | | | Weight (g) | Calories | % Water | Protein (g) | Carbs (g) | Fiber (g) | Sugar (g) | Other Carbs (g) | Fat (g) | Sat Fat (g) | Mono Fat (g) | Poly Fat (g) | Omega 3 (g) | Omega 6 (g) | Choles (mg) | Vit A (IU) | Vit A (RE) | Retinol (RE) | Carotenoids (RE) | Beta Carotene (mcg) | Thiamin (mg) | Riboflavin(mg) | Niacin (NE) | Vit B6 (mg) | Vit B12 (mcg) | Folate (mcg) | Panto (mg) | Vit C (mg) | Vit D (mg) | Vit E (α TE) | Calcium (mg) | Copper (mg) | Iron (mg) | Magnes (mg) | Mang (mg) | Phos (mg) | Potassium (mg) | Selenium (mcg) | Sodium (mg) | Zinc (mg) |
| 40502 | 1 ea | Mellow Mango w/Oat Bran, dry pkg | 50 | 180 | 5 | 6.0 | 39.0 | 5.0 | 13.0 | 21.0 | 2.5 | 0.0 | | | 0.00 | 0.00 | 0 | 750 | 150 | | | | | | | | | | | 4.8 | | | 20 | | 1.8 | | | | | | 140 | |
| 40503 | 1 ea | Peachberry Wheat & Oat, dry pkg | 50 | 190 | 2 | 5.0 | 42.0 | 5.0 | 14.0 | 23.0 | 1.5 | 0.0 | | | 0.00 | 0.00 | 0 | 200 | 40 | | | | | | | | | | | 4.8 | | | 20 | | 1.8 | | | | | | 260 | |
| 40504 | 1 ea | Strawberry Banana 3 Grain, dry pkg | 48 | 180 | 2 | 5.0 | 40.0 | 4.0 | 12.0 | 24.0 | 1.5 | 0.0 | | | 0.00 | 0.00 | 0 | 0 | 0 | 0 | 0 | 0 | | | | | | | | 4.8 | | | 40 | | 1.1 | | | | | | 220 | |
| 40505 | 1 ea | Wheat N' Berries, dry pkg | 49 | 170 | 6 | 5.0 | 40.0 | 5.0 | 12.0 | 23.0 | 1.0 | 0.0 | | | 0.00 | 0.00 | 0 | 0 | 0 | 0 | 0 | 0 | | | | | | | | 4.8 | | | 0 | | 1.4 | | | | | | 230 | |
| | | Farina | | | | | | | | | | | | | | | | | | | | | | | | | | | | | | | | | | | | | | | | |
| 40006 | 1 cup | Enriched, ckd, avg | 233 | 116 | 88 | 3.3 | 24.7 | 3.3 | 0.2 | 21.2 | 0.2 | 0.0 | 0.0 | 0.1 | 0.00 | 0.07 | 0 | 0 | 0 | 0 | 0 | 0 | 0.19 | 0.12 | 1.28 | 0.02 | 0.00 | 53.6 | 0.13 | 0.0 | 0.0 | | 5 | 0.0 | 1.2 | 5 | 0.2 | 28 | 30 | 21.2 | 0 | 0.16 |
| 40370 | 1/4 cup | Enriched, dry, Quaker | 44 | 154 | 12 | 4.8 | 33.5 | 1.3 | 0.1 | 32.1 | 0.4 | 0.1 | 0.0 | 0.2 | 0.01 | 0.06 | 0 | 0 | 0 | 0 | 0 | 0 | 0.19 | 0.11 | 1.55 | 0.02 | 0.00 | 67.8 | 0.19 | 0.0 | 0.0 | | 5 | 0.1 | 13.2 | 7 | 0.1 | 37 | 43 | | 1 | 0.27 |
| 38496 | 1 cup | Enriched, prep, Quaker | 233 | 119 | 87 | 3.6 | 26.3 | 0.9 | 0.2 | 25.2 | 0.2 | 0.0 | 0.1 | 0.0 | 0.00 | 0.04 | 0 | 0 | 0 | 0 | 0 | 0 | 0.16 | 0.11 | 1.81 | 0.02 | 0.00 | 53.6 | 0.12 | 0.0 | 0.0 | | 9 | 0.0 | 11.0 | 7 | 0.1 | 30 | 33 | | 7 | 0.23 |
| 40077 | 1 cup | Unenriched, ckd, avg | 233 | 116 | 88 | 3.3 | 24.7 | 3.3 | 0.2 | 21.2 | 0.2 | 0.0 | 0.0 | 0.1 | 0.00 | 0.07 | 0 | 0 | 0 | 0 | 0 | 0 | 0.02 | 0.02 | 0.23 | 0.02 | 0.00 | 4.7 | 0.13 | 0.0 | 0.0 | | 5 | 0.0 | 0.0 | 5 | 0.2 | 28 | 30 | 21.2 | 0 | 0.16 |
| 40183 | 1/4 cup | Unenriched, dry, avg | 44 | 162 | 10 | 4.7 | 34.3 | 0.8 | 0.1 | 33.4 | 0.2 | 0.0 | 0.0 | 0.1 | 0.01 | 0.09 | 0 | 0 | 0 | 0 | 0 | 0 | 0.03 | 0.04 | 0.31 | 0.03 | 0.00 | 10.6 | 0.18 | 0.0 | 0.0 | | 6 | 0.0 | 0.7 | 6 | 0.3 | 39 | 41 | 10.3 | 1 | 0.23 |
| | | Malt-o-Meal | | | | | | | | | | | | | | | | | | | | | | | | | | | | | | | | | | | | | | | | |
| 40188 | 1 cup | Chocolate, ckd w/salt, avg | 240 | 122 | 88 | 3.6 | 25.9 | 1.0 | 1.0 | 24.0 | 0.2 | 0.0 | 0.1 | 0.0 | 0.00 | 0.04 | 0 | 0 | 0 | 0 | 0 | 0 | 0.48 | 0.24 | 5.76 | 0.02 | 0.00 | 4.8 | 0.14 | 0.0 | 0.0 | | 5 | 0.0 | 9.6 | 5 | 0.2 | 24 | 31 | | 324 | 0.17 |
| 40187 | 1/4 cup | Chocolate, dry, avg | 41 | 151 | 10 | 4.3 | 31.9 | 1.7 | 1.2 | 29.0 | 0.4 | 0.1 | 0.1 | 0.0 | 0.00 | 0.04 | 0 | 0 | 0 | 0 | 0 | 0 | 0.53 | 0.37 | 7.22 | 0.02 | 0.00 | 9.8 | 0.17 | 0.0 | 0.0 | | 6 | 0.0 | 11.7 | 5 | 0.3 | 29 | 39 | | 4 | 0.22 |
| 40014 | 1 cup | Plain, ckd, avg | 240 | 122 | 88 | 3.6 | 25.7 | 1.0 | 1.0 | 23.8 | 0.2 | 0.1 | 0.1 | 0.0 | 0.00 | 0.04 | 0 | 0 | 0 | 0 | 0 | 0 | 0.48 | 0.24 | 5.76 | 0.02 | 0.00 | 4.8 | 0.14 | 0.0 | 0.0 | | 5 | 0.0 | 9.6 | 5 | 0.2 | 24 | 31 | 8.0 | 2 | 0.17 |
| 40165 | 1/4 cup | Plain, dry, avg | 41 | 151 | 10 | 4.3 | 31.9 | 1.7 | 0.7 | 29.4 | 0.4 | 0.1 | 0.1 | 0.0 | 0.00 | 0.04 | 0 | 0 | 0 | 0 | 0 | 0 | 0.53 | 0.37 | 7.22 | 0.02 | 0.00 | 9.8 | 0.17 | 0.0 | 0.0 | | 6 | 0.0 | 11.7 | 5 | 0.3 | 29 | 39 | 9.6 | 3 | 0.22 |
| 40235 | 1 cup | Maltex, wheat cereal, ckd, avg | 249 | 179 | 81 | 5.7 | 39.6 | 3.0 | 0.2 | 36.4 | 1.0 | 0.2 | 0.1 | 0.4 | 0.02 | 0.39 | 0 | 0 | 0 | 0 | 0 | 0 | 0.25 | 0.10 | 2.39 | 0.08 | 0.00 | 22.4 | 0.23 | 0.0 | 0.0 | | 17 | 0.3 | 1.8 | 57 | 0.4 | 179 | 266 | | 10 | 1.87 |
| 40164 | 1/4 cup | Maltex, wheat cereal, dry, avg | 38 | 134 | 8 | 4.3 | 29.4 | 1.6 | 0.2 | 27.6 | 0.8 | 0.1 | 0.1 | 0.3 | 0.01 | 0.29 | 0 | 0 | 0 | 0 | 0 | 0 | 0.20 | 0.08 | 1.77 | 0.06 | 0.00 | 21.7 | 0.26 | 0.0 | 0.0 | | 14 | 0.2 | 1.3 | 42 | 0.3 | 133 | 198 | 26.9 | 6 | 1.38 |
| 40015 | 1 cup | Maypo, ckd, avg | 240 | 170 | 83 | 5.8 | 31.9 | 5.8 | 7.2 | 19.0 | 2.4 | 0.4 | 0.7 | 0.9 | 0.01 | 0.84 | 0 | 2338 | 703 | 703 | 0 | 0 | 0.72 | 0.72 | 9.36 | 0.96 | 2.88 | 9.6 | 0.34 | 28.8 | 0.0 | | 125 | 0.2 | 8.4 | 50 | 1.7 | 247 | 211 | 18.5 | 10 | 1.49 |
| 40166 | 1/4 cup | Maypo, dry, avg | 24 | 92 | 6 | 3.2 | 17.3 | 2.6 | 3.9 | 10.8 | 1.3 | 0.2 | 0.4 | 0.5 | 0.00 | 0.46 | 0 | 1270 | 381 | 381 | 0 | 0 | 0.38 | 0.43 | 5.09 | 0.50 | 1.51 | 6.5 | 0.18 | 15.4 | 0.0 | | 68 | 0.1 | 4.6 | 28 | 0.9 | 135 | 115 | 10.0 | 5 | 0.80 |
| 40138 | 1 cup | Multi-Grain Cereal, ckd, avg | 246 | 199 | 78 | 6.8 | 40.0 | 3.9 | 1.0 | 35.1 | 2.2 | 0.4 | 0.9 | 0.6 | | | 0 | 1147 | 115 | 0 | 115 | | 0.39 | 0.46 | 4.39 | 0.46 | 0.00 | 17.1 | | 0.0 | 0.0 | | 69 | 0.1 | 5.4 | 66 | | 182 | 138 | | 760 | 0.90 |
| | | Oatmeal | | | | | | | | | | | | | | | | | | | | | | | | | | | | | | | | | | | | | | | | |
| 90076 | 1 ea | Apple Cinnamon, dry pkt, Quaker | 35 | 128 | 6 | 3.3 | 26.9 | 2.6 | 7.5 | 16.9 | 1.5 | 0.3 | 0.5 | 0.6 | 0.02 | 0.51 | 0 | 1050 | 315 | | | | 0.31 | 0.36 | 4.20 | 0.42 | 0.00 | 84.0 | 0.15 | 0.3 | 0.0 | | 106 | 0.1 | 4.0 | 30 | 0.9 | 116 | 108 | 7.9 | 121 | 0.69 |
| 40073 | 1 ea | Apple Cinnamon, prep f/dry pkt, Quaker | 149 | 125 | 79 | 3.2 | 26.2 | 2.5 | 7.3 | 16.4 | 1.4 | 0.3 | 0.5 | 0.6 | 0.02 | 0.49 | 0 | 1019 | 305 | | | | 0.30 | 0.35 | 4.08 | 0.41 | 0.00 | 93.9 | 0.15 | 0.3 | 0.0 | | 104 | 0.1 | 3.9 | 30 | 0.9 | 113 | 106 | 7.6 | 121 | 0.70 |
| 90077 | 1 ea | Brown Sugar & Raisins, dry pkt, Quaker | 42 | 156 | 8 | 4.8 | 30.0 | 3.2 | 12.5 | 14.3 | 1.8 | 0.3 | 0.6 | 0.7 | 0.04 | 0.71 | 0 | 1577 | 474 | | | | 0.55 | 0.63 | 8.02 | 0.75 | 0.00 | 153.3 | 0.45 | 0.4 | 0.0 | 0.2 | 171 | 0.3 | 7.5 | 56 | 1.6 | 203 | 233 | 9.0 | 244 | 1.33 |
| 38317 | 1 ea | Brown Sugar & Raisins, prep f/dry pkt, Quaker | 195 | 158 | 80 | 4.9 | 30.4 | 5.5 | 12.5 | 12.5 | 2.0 | 0.4 | 0.6 | 0.8 | 0.04 | 0.75 | 0 | 1599 | 480 | | | | 0.57 | 0.64 | 8.13 | 0.76 | 0.00 | 156.0 | 0.45 | 0.0 | 0.0 | 0.2 | 174 | 0.3 | 7.6 | 57 | 1.6 | 207 | 236 | 15.8 | 248 | 1.35 |
| 40365 | 1 ea | Cinnamagic, dry pkt, Quaker | 40 | 144 | 8 | 3.8 | 29.6 | 3.0 | 13.9 | 12.7 | 2.0 | 0.4 | 0.7 | 0.6 | 0.04 | 0.53 | 0 | 1275 | 383 | | | | 0.36 | 0.23 | 3.85 | 0.42 | 0.00 | 103.2 | 0.18 | 0.1 | 0.0 | | 178 | 0.1 | 6.3 | 37 | 1.2 | 130 | 118 | | 165 | 0.85 |
| 40385 | 1 ea | Cinnamagic, prep f/dry pkt Quaker | 159 | 145 | 77 | 3.8 | 29.7 | 3.0 | | | 2.0 | 0.4 | 0.7 | 0.6 | 0.04 | 0.54 | 0 | 1278 | 385 | | | | 0.36 | 0.23 | 3.86 | 0.43 | 0.00 | 103.3 | 0.18 | 0.2 | 0.0 | | 181 | 0.1 | 6.3 | 38 | 1.2 | 130 | 118 | | 169 | 0.89 |
| 40446 | 1 ea | Cinn Raisin Almond, dry pkt, Arrowhead Mills | 35 | 130 | 10 | 5.0 | 24.0 | 2.0 | 4.0 | 18.0 | 2.0 | 0.0 | | | | | 0 | 0 | 0 | 0 | 0 | 0 | 0.12 | 0.03 | 0.40 | | | | | 0.0 | | | 0 | | 1.1 | | | | 120 | | 0 | |
| 90079 | 1 ea | Cinnamon Spice, dry pkt, Quaker | 46 | 172 | 6 | 3.9 | 35.8 | 3.0 | 15.4 | 17.4 | 2.1 | 0.4 | 0.8 | 0.6 | 0.03 | 0.58 | 0 | 1144 | 344 | | | | 0.41 | 0.26 | 4.24 | 0.54 | 0.08 | 124.2 | 0.20 | 0.0 | 0.0 | | 190 | 0.1 | 9.8 | 40 | 1.3 | 144 | 116 | 10.0 | 288 | 0.91 |
| 40074 | 1 ea | Cinnamon Spice, prep f/dry pkt, Quaker | 161 | 177 | 73 | 4.8 | 35.1 | 2.6 | 15.5 | 17.1 | 1.9 | 0.4 | 0.6 | 0.7 | 0.01 | 0.65 | 0 | 1578 | 473 | | | | 0.56 | 0.34 | 5.65 | 0.77 | 0.00 | 152.9 | 0.38 | 0.0 | 0.0 | | 172 | 0.1 | 6.6 | 52 | 1.5 | 145 | 105 | 10.0 | 280 | 0.97 |
| 40000 | 1 cup | Cooked, avg | 234 | 145 | 85 | 6.1 | 25.3 | 4.0 | 0.9 | 20.4 | 2.3 | 0.4 | 0.7 | 0.9 | 0.05 | 0.82 | 0 | 37 | 5 | 0 | 5 | | 0.26 | 0.05 | 0.30 | 0.05 | 0.00 | 9.4 | 0.47 | 0.0 | 0.0 | | 19 | 0.1 | 1.6 | 56 | 1.4 | 178 | 131 | 19.0 | 2 | 1.15 |
| 40366 | 1 ea | Fruit & Cream Variety, dry pkt, Quaker | 35 | 135 | 6 | 2.9 | 26.3 | 2.2 | 10.8 | 13.3 | 2.5 | 0.5 | 0.8 | 0.6 | 0.03 | 0.52 | 0 | 1050 | 315 | | | | 0.31 | 0.36 | 4.20 | 0.42 | 0.01 | 84.0 | 0.13 | 0.1 | 0.0 | | 106 | 0.1 | 4.0 | 28 | 0.8 | 105 | 97 | | 169 | 0.61 |
| 40367 | 1 ea | Fruit & Cream Variety, prep f/dry pkt, Quaker | 154 | 182 | 71 | 3.9 | 35.6 | 2.9 | 14.6 | 18.0 | 3.4 | 0.7 | 1.0 | 0.8 | 0.05 | 0.71 | 0 | 1418 | 427 | | | | 0.42 | 0.48 | 5.67 | 0.57 | 0.02 | 114.0 | 0.18 | 0.2 | 0.0 | | 145 | 0.1 | 5.4 | 38 | 1.1 | 142 | 131 | | 231 | 0.86 |
| 40436 | 1 ea | Instant, dry pkt, General Mills | 35 | 110 | 11 | 4.0 | 19.0 | 2.0 | 1.0 | 16.0 | 2.0 | 0.0 | | | | | 0 | 0 | 0 | 0 | 0 | 0 | 0.09 | 0.10 | | | | | | 0.0 | | | 0 | | 0.7 | | | | 70 | | 0 | |
| 40447 | 1 ea | Maple Apple Spice, dry pkt, Arrowhead Mills | 35 | 130 | 10 | 4.0 | 25.0 | 2.0 | 6.0 | 17.0 | 2.0 | 0.0 | | | | | 0 | 0 | 0 | 0 | 0 | 0 | 0.09 | 0.03 | | | | | | 0.0 | | | 0 | | 0.7 | | | | 95 | | 40 | |
| 40167 | 1 ea | Maple & Brown Sugar, dry pkt, Quaker | 42 | 156 | 6 | 4.2 | 32.0 | 2.6 | 13.9 | 15.4 | 1.8 | 0.4 | 0.6 | 0.8 | 0.04 | 0.70 | 0 | 1026 | 308 | | | | 0.30 | 0.35 | 4.10 | 0.41 | 0.00 | 81.9 | 0.34 | 0.0 | 0.0 | | 105 | 0.1 | 3.9 | 39 | 1.2 | 135 | 114 | 9.1 | 234 | 0.88 |
| 40075 | 1 ea | Maple & Brown Sugar, prep f/dry pkt, Quaker | 155 | 153 | 75 | 4.2 | 31.5 | 2.6 | 13.8 | 15.0 | 1.8 | 0.4 | 0.6 | 0.7 | 0.04 | 0.69 | 0 | 1007 | 302 | | | | 0.30 | 0.34 | 4.03 | 0.40 | 0.00 | 80.6 | 0.34 | 0.0 | 0.0 | | 105 | 0.1 | 3.9 | 39 | 1.2 | 132 | 112 | | 234 | 0.90 |
| 40347 | 1/4 cup | Multigrain, dry, Quaker | 20 | 67 | 11 | 2.3 | 14.7 | 2.4 | 0.0 | 12.3 | 0.5 | 0.1 | 0.1 | 0.3 | 0.02 | 0.19 | 0 | 1.4 | 0.2 | | | | 0.06 | 0.03 | 0.71 | 0.05 | 0.00 | 5.2 | 0.10 | 0.0 | 0.0 | | 7 | 0.1 | 0.6 | 23 | 0.5 | 69 | 82 | 8.3 | 1 | 0.64 |
| 38499 | 1 cup | Multigrain, prep, Quaker | 234 | 143 | 84 | 4.9 | 31.6 | 5.1 | 0.0 | 26.4 | 1.1 | 0.2 | 0.2 | 0.5 | 0.04 | 0.41 | 0 | 2 | 0.2 | 0 | 0.2 | | 0.12 | 0.06 | 1.54 | 0.10 | 0.00 | 11.7 | 0.22 | 0.0 | 0.0 | | 19 | 0.2 | 1.3 | 51 | 1.1 | 150 | 175 | | 7 | 1.43 |
| 40140 | 1/4 cup | Quick, dry, General Mills | 20 | 72 | 14 | 2.8 | 13.0 | 1.8 | 0.0 | 11.2 | 1.4 | 0.3 | 0.5 | 0.6 | | | 0 | | | | | | 0.11 | 0.03 | 0.12 | | | | | | | | 10 | | 0.9 | | | | 68 | 6.8 | 0 | |
| 40364 | 1 ea | Power Rangers Fruit Punch flvr, dry pkt | 40 | 149 | 6 | 3.5 | 30.6 | 2.6 | | | 2.0 | 0.4 | 0.8 | 0.6 | 0.02 | 0.54 | 0 | 1273 | 382 | | | | 0.35 | 0.22 | 3.83 | 0.42 | 0.00 | 108.0 | 0.16 | 0.0 | | | 176 | 0.1 | 6.2 | 35 | 1.1 | 121 | 99 | | 165 | 0.80 |
| 40373 | 1 ea | Power Rangers Fruit Punch flvr, prep f/dry pkt | 159 | 149 | 76 | 3.6 | 30.7 | 2.5 | | | 2.1 | 0.4 | 0.8 | 0.6 | 0.02 | 0.54 | 0 | 1277 | 383 | | | | 0.35 | 0.22 | 3.85 | 0.42 | 0.00 | 108.1 | 0.16 | 0.0 | 0.0 | | 178 | 0.1 | 6.2 | 37 | 1.1 | 121 | 99 | | 169 | 0.83 |
| 40432 | 1 ea | Raisin, Dates & Walnuts, dry pkt, Quaker | 37 | 135 | 8 | 3.3 | 27.3 | 2.4 | 12.0 | 12.8 | 2.0 | 0.3 | 0.6 | 0.8 | 0.07 | 0.69 | 0 | 1050 | 315 | | | | 0.31 | 0.36 | 4.22 | 0.42 | 0.00 | 84.0 | 0.16 | 0.2 | 0.0 | | 107 | 0.1 | 4.0 | 33 | 1.0 | 109 | 130 | 7.8 | 237 | 0.72 |
| 40375 | 1 ea | Raisin, Dates & Walnuts, prep f/dry pkt, Quaker | 156 | 181 | 71 | 4.4 | 36.7 | 3.3 | 16.1 | 17.3 | 2.7 | 0.5 | 0.9 | 1.0 | 0.09 | 0.93 | 0 | 1412 | 424 | | | | 0.42 | 0.48 | 5.65 | 0.57 | 0.00 | 112.3 | 0.22 | 0.3 | 0.0 | | 145 | 0.1 | 5.4 | 45 | 1.3 | 147 | 175 | | 323 | 1.00 |
| 90080 | 1 ea | Raisin Spice, dry pkt, Quaker | 42 | 152 | 8 | 4.4 | 31.3 | 2.7 | 14.5 | 14.1 | 1.8 | 0.3 | 0.7 | 0.6 | 0.03 | 0.53 | 0 | 1139 | 342 | | | | 0.35 | 0.21 | 3.60 | 0.48 | 0.04 | 108.4 | 0.21 | 0.2 | 0.0 | | 168 | 0.1 | 5.6 | 39 | 1.2 | 126 | 156 | 8.8 | 244 | 0.89 |
| 40076 | 1 ea | Raisin Spice, prep f/dry pkt, Quaker | 158 | 161 | 75 | 4.3 | 31.9 | 2.2 | 14.9 | 14.9 | 1.7 | 0.3 | 0.6 | 0.6 | 0.01 | 0.58 | 0 | 1468 | 441 | | | | 0.51 | 0.36 | 5.48 | 0.75 | 0.00 | 150.1 | 0.37 | 0.0 | 0.0 | | 166 | 0.1 | 6.6 | 36 | 0.9 | 133 | 150 | 9.0 | 226 | 0.71 |
| 40141 | 1/4 cup | Regular, dry, General Mills | 20 | 73 | 12 | 3.0 | 13.2 | 1.8 | 0.0 | 11.4 | 1.4 | 0.2 | 0.4 | 0.3 | | | 0 | | | | | | 0.08 | 0.03 | 0.19 | | | | | | | | 11 | | 0.9 | | | | 76 | 6.8 | 1 | |
| 38008 | 1/4 cup | Rolled Oats, dry, avg | 20 | 77 | 9 | 3.2 | 13.4 | 2.1 | 0.4 | 10.9 | 1.3 | 0.2 | 0.4 | 0.5 | 0.02 | 0.44 | 0 | 20 | 2 | 0 | 2 | | 0.15 | 0.03 | 0.16 | 0.02 | 0.00 | 6.4 | 0.25 | 0.0 | 0.0 | | 10 | 0.1 | 0.8 | 30 | 0.7 | 95 | 70 | 6.8 | 1 | 0.61 |
| 38417 | 1/4 cup | Rolled Oats, flakes, Arrowhead Mills | 26 | 99 | 9 | 3.8 | 17.6 | 3.1 | 0.8 | 13.8 | 1.9 | 0.4 | | | | | 0 | 0 | 0 | 0 | 0 | 0 | 0.17 | 0.03 | 0.31 | | | | | 0.0 | | | 0 | | 1.1 | | | | 92 | | 0 | |
| 40088 | 1 cup | Ralston Cereal, ckd | 253 | 134 | 86 | 5.6 | 28.3 | 6.1 | 0.3 | 22.0 | 0.8 | 0.1 | 0.1 | 0.4 | 0.03 | 0.34 | 0 | 0 | 0 | 0 | 0 | 0 | 0.20 | 0.18 | 2.05 | 0.11 | 0.11 | 17.7 | 0.33 | 0.0 | 0.0 | | 13 | 0.2 | 1.6 | 58 | 2.0 | 147 | 154 | | 5 | 1.42 |
| 40168 | 1/4 cup | Ralston Cereal, dry | 30 | 102 | 10 | 4.2 | 21.6 | 4.0 | 0.1 | 17.5 | 0.6 | 0.1 | 0.1 | 0.3 | 0.02 | 0.26 | 0 | 0 | 0 | 0 | 0 | 0 | 0.16 | 0.14 | 1.57 | 0.09 | 0.08 | 18.0 | 0.22 | 0.0 | 0.0 | | 11 | 0.2 | 1.3 | 46 | 1.5 | 113 | 118 | 21.2 | 3 | 1.08 |
| | | Roman Meal | | | | | | | | | | | | | | | | | | | | | | | | | | | | | | | | | | | | | | | | |
| 40016 | 1 cup | Cooked, avg | 241 | 147 | 83 | 6.5 | 33.0 | 8.2 | 0.5 | 24.3 | 1.0 | 0.1 | 0.1 | 0.4 | 0.03 | 0.38 | 0 | 0 | 0 | 0 | 0 | 0 | 0.24 | 0.12 | 3.08 | 0.11 | 0.00 | 24.1 | 0.37 | 0.0 | 0.0 | | 29 | 0.3 | 2.1 | 108 | 2.3 | 214 | 301 | 9.3 | 2 | 1.78 |
| 40083 | 1/4 cup | Dry, avg | 24 | 77 | 9 | 3.5 | 17.3 | 4.3 | 0.2 | 12.7 | 0.5 | 0.1 | 0.1 | 0.2 | 0.02 | 0.22 | 0 | 0 | 0 | 0 | 0 | 0 | 0.12 | 0.06 | 1.61 | 0.06 | 0.00 | 16.8 | 0.19 | 0.0 | 0.0 | | 16 | 0.2 | 1.1 | 57 | 1.2 | 113 | 158 | 10.6 | 1 | 0.93 |
| 40172 | 1 cup | W/oats, ckd, avg | 240 | 170 | 82 | 7.2 | 34.1 | 7.0 | 0.7 | 26.4 | 1.9 | 0.2 | | | | | 0 | 22 | 2 | 0 | 2 | | 0.31 | 0.22 | 3.26 | 0.38 | 0.00 | 24.0 | 0.25 | 0.0 | 0.0 | | 26 | 0.1 | 1.4 | 74 | 1.4 | 235 | 257 | | 10 | 1.94 |
| 40171 | 1/4 cup | W/oats, dry, avg | 25 | 85 | 11 | 3.6 | 17.1 | 3.5 | 0.3 | 13.3 | 1.0 | 0.1 | | | | | 0 | 11 | 1 | 0 | 1 | | 0.16 | 0.11 | 1.63 | 0.19 | 0.00 | 17.5 | 0.13 | 0.0 | 0.0 | | 14 | 0.1 | 0.7 | 38 | 0.7 | 118 | 128 | 14.6 | 5 | 0.98 |
| 40080 | 1 cup | Wheatena, whole wheat cereal, ckd | 243 | 136 | 85 | 4.9 | 28.7 | 6.6 | 1.0 | 21.1 | 1.2 | 0.2 | 0.2 | 0.6 | 0.05 | 0.57 | 0 | 0 | 0 | 0 | 0 | 0 | 0.02 | 0.05 | 1.34 | 0.05 | 0.00 | 17.0 | 0.10 | 0.0 | 0.0 | | 10 | 0.1 | 1.4 | 49 | 2.0 | 146 | 187 | 27.0 | 5 | 1.68 |
| 40169 | 1/4 cup | Wheatena, whole wheat cereal, dry | 35 | 125 | 6 | 4.6 | 26.5 | 4.5 | 0.0 | 22.0 | 1.0 | 0.2 | 0.1 | 0.5 | 0.04 | 0.47 | 0 | 0 | 0 | 0 | 0 | 0 | 0.02 | 0.05 | 1.23 | 0.04 | 0.00 | 20.6 | 0.09 | 0.0 | 0.0 | | 10 | 0.1 | 1.2 | 45 | 1.8 | 134 | 172 | 24.7 | 5 | 1.54 |
| 40002 | 1 cup | Whole Wheat Natural Cereal, ckd, avg | 240 | 149 | 84 | 4.8 | 32.9 | 3.8 | 1.0 | 28.1 | 1.0 | 0.1 | 0.1 | 0.5 | 0.04 | 0.45 | 0 | 0 | 0 | 0 | 0 | 0 | 0.17 | 0.12 | 2.14 | 0.18 | 0.00 | 26.4 | 0.40 | 0.0 | 0.0 | | 17 | 0.2 | 1.5 | 53 | 1.4 | 166 | 170 | 26.6 | 0 | 1.15 |
| 40001 | 1/4 cup | Whole Wheat Natural Cereal, dry, avg | 21 | 72 | 10 | 2.4 | 15.8 | 2.0 | 0.2 | 13.6 | 0.4 | 0.1 | 0.1 | 0.2 | 0.02 | 0.20 | 0 | 0 | 0 | 0 | 0 | 0 | 0.08 | 0.06 | 1.03 | 0.08 | 0.00 | 16.4 | 0.19 | 0.0 | 0.0 | | 8 | 0.1 | 0.7 | 26 | 0.7 | 80 | 82 | 14.8 | 0 | 0.56 |
| | | *CEREALS, READY TO EAT* | | | | | | | | | | | | | | | | | | | | | | | | | | | | | | | | | | | | | | | | |
| 40344 | 1 cup | Almond Crunch w/Raisins, Healthy Choice | 58 | 209 | 6 | 5.0 | 45.6 | 4.9 | 16.3 | 24.4 | 2.7 | 0.4 | 1.3 | 0.8 | 0.03 | 0.42 | 0 | 500 | 50 | 0 | 50 | | 0.52 | 0.58 | 7.02 | 0.70 | 2.09 | 116.0 | 3.48 | 0.0 | 2.0 | | 28 | 0.2 | 6.3 | 52 | 1.3 | 137 | 209 | 4.8 | 227 | 1.51 |
| 40480 | 1 cup | Almond Delight, Ralston Purina | 38 | 149 | 2 | 2.8 | 31.2 | 2.0 | | | 2.2 | | | | | | | 0 | 0 | 0 | 0 | 0 | 0.52 | | 6.79 | 0.68 | 2.04 | 135.7 | | 20.4 | 0.0 | | 33 | | 2.4 | | | | | | 270 | 2.04 |
| 40322 | 1 cup | Almond Delight Honey, Ralston Purina | 51 | 210 | 3 | 5.0 | 41.0 | 4.0 | 12.0 | 25.0 | 3.0 | 0.0 | | | | | 0 | 0 | 0 | 0 | 0 | 0 | 0.38 | | 5.00 | 0.50 | 1.50 | 100.0 | 0.20 | 6.0 | | | 20 | 0.2 | 1.8 | 40 | | 100 | | | 410 | 1.50 |
| 40258 | 1 cup | Alpha Bits, Post | 28 | 110 | 1 | 2.2 | 24.2 | 1.2 | 10.6 | 12.4 | 0.6 | 0.1 | 0.2 | 0.2 | 0.00 | 0.23 | 0 | 1235 | 371 | 371 | 0 | 0 | 0.36 | 0.42 | 4.93 | 0.50 | 1.48 | 98.8 | 0.14 | 0.0 | 1.0 | | 8 | 0.1 | 2.7 | 17 | 0.5 | 51 | 54 | 10.0 | 178 | 1.48 |

| Code | Amount | Description | Basic Components | | | | | | | | | Additional Fats | | | | | | Vit A & Components | | | | | Vitamins | | | | | | | | | | Minerals | | | | | | | | | |
|---|---|---|---|---|---|---|---|---|---|---|---|---|---|---|---|---|---|---|---|---|---|---|---|---|---|---|---|---|---|---|---|---|---|---|---|---|---|---|---|---|---|---|
| | | | Weight (g) | Calories | % Water | Protein (g) | Carbs (g) | Fiber (g) | Sugar (g) | Other Carbs (g) | Fat (g) | Sat Fat (g) | Mono Fat (g) | Poly Fat (g) | Omega 3 (g) | Omega 6 (g) | Choles (mg) | Vit A (IU) | Vit A (RE) | Retinol (RE) | Carotenoids (RE) | Beta Carotene (mcg) | Thiamin (mg) | Riboflavin (mg) | Niacin (NE) | Vit B6 (mg) | Vit B12 (mcg) | Folate (mcg) | Panto (mg) | Vit C (mg) | Vit D (mg) | Vit E (α TE) | Calcium (mg) | Copper (mg) | Iron (mg) | Magnes (mg) | Mang (mg) | Phos (mg) | Potassium (mg) | Selenium (mcg) | Sodium (mg) | Zinc (mg) |
| 40280 | 1 cup | Alpha Bits w/Marshmallows, Post | 29 | 120 | 1 | 2.0 | 25.0 | 1.0 | 14.0 | 10.0 | 1.0 | 0.0 | | | | | 0 | 1250 | 375 | 375 | 0 | 0 | 0.38 | 0.43 | 5.00 | 0.50 | 1.50 | 100.0 | | 0.0 | 1.0 | | 0 | 0.0 | 2.7 | 16 | | 60 | 45 | | 160 | 1.50 |
| 40456 | 1 cup | Amaranth Flakes, Arrowhead Mills | 34 | 130 | 4 | 4.0 | 25.0 | 3.0 | 3.0 | 19.0 | 2.0 | 0.0 | | | | | 0 | 0 | 0 | 0 | 0 | 0 | 0.09 | 0.00 | | | | | | 0.0 | | | 0 | | 1.4 | | | | 210 | | 0 | |
| 40228 | 1 cup | Apple Cinnamon O's, fat free, Health Valley | 86 | 303 | 11 | 9.1 | 63.7 | 9.1 | | | 0.0 | 0.0 | 0.0 | 0.0 | 0.00 | 0.00 | 0 | 1517 | 455 | 455 | 0 | 0 | 0.46 | 0.10 | 3.64 | | | | | | | | 61 | | 3.3 | | | | 243 | | 46 | |
| 40097 | 1 cup | Apple Cinnamon Squares, Kellogg's | 73 | 242 | 10 | 5.3 | 58.5 | 6.3 | 15.5 | 36.7 | 1.3 | 0.3 | 0.4 | 0.7 | 0.03 | 0.62 | 0 | 0 | 0 | 0 | 0 | 0 | 0.51 | 0.58 | 6.64 | 0.66 | 1.97 | 146.0 | 0.47 | 0.0 | 0.0 | | 28 | 0.1 | 21.5 | 64 | 2.3 | 204 | 220 | 3.0 | 26 | 1.97 |
| 40098 | 1 cup | Apple Jacks, Kellogg's | 33 | 127 | 3 | 1.6 | 29.5 | 0.6 | 15.9 | 13.0 | 0.4 | 0.1 | 0.1 | 0.2 | 0.01 | 0.18 | 0 | 825 | 248 | 248 | 0 | 0 | 0.43 | 0.46 | 5.51 | 0.56 | 0.00 | 116.5 | 0.09 | 16.5 | 1.0 | | 4 | 0.1 | 5.0 | 10 | 0.1 | 33 | 35 | 2.4 | 148 | 4.13 |
| 40099 | 1 cup | Apple Raisin Crisp, Kellogg's | 53 | 178 | 5 | 3.3 | 45.0 | 4.2 | 15.0 | 25.8 | 0.5 | 0.1 | 0.2 | 0.2 | 0.02 | 0.19 | 0 | 750 | 225 | 225 | 0 | 0 | 0.37 | 0.42 | 4.98 | 0.48 | 1.48 | 106.0 | 0.36 | 0.0 | 1.0 | | 14 | 0.1 | 1.8 | 10 | 0.7 | 83 | 82 | 4.8 | 360 | 1.48 |
| 40278 | 1 cup | Banana Nut Crunch, Post | 59 | 250 | 7 | 5.0 | 43.0 | 4.0 | 11.0 | 28.0 | 6.0 | 1.0 | | | | | 0 | 1250 | 375 | 375 | 0 | 0 | 0.38 | 0.43 | 5.00 | 0.50 | 1.50 | 100.0 | | 0.0 | 1.0 | | 20 | 0.3 | 1.8 | 40 | | | 190 | | 200 | 1.50 |
| 40394 | 1 cup | Basic 4, General Mills | 55 | 201 | 7 | 4.2 | 42.0 | 3.4 | 12.5 | 26.1 | 2.8 | 0.4 | 1.0 | 1.1 | 0.07 | 0.44 | 0 | 1250 | 375 | 375 | 0 | 0 | 0.37 | 0.42 | 5.00 | 0.50 | 0.00 | 99.6 | 0.29 | 15.0 | 1.8 | | 310 | 0.2 | 4.5 | 40 | 0.9 | 232 | 162 | 9.4 | 323 | 3.75 |
| 40279 | 1 cup | Blueberry Morning, Post | 46 | 186 | 7 | 3.2 | 36.3 | 1.6 | 11.3 | 23.4 | 2.8 | 0.4 | | | | | 0 | 1009 | 303 | 303 | 0 | 0 | 0.30 | 0.34 | 4.04 | 0.40 | 1.21 | 80.7 | | 0.0 | 0.8 | | 0 | 0.1 | 1.5 | 19 | | 65 | 85 | | 202 | 0.73 |
| 40100 | 1 cup | Blueberry Squares, Kellogg's | 72 | 238 | 10 | 5.5 | 57.3 | 6.3 | 14.8 | 36.2 | 1.3 | 0.3 | 0.3 | 0.7 | 0.03 | 0.54 | 0 | 0 | 0 | 0 | 0 | 0 | 0.50 | 0.58 | 6.70 | 0.65 | 2.02 | 144.0 | 0.44 | 0.0 | 2.4 | | 25 | 0.1 | 21.6 | 67 | 1.7 | 212 | 240 | 3.0 | 27 | 2.02 |
| 40411 | 1 cup | Body Buddies, General Mills | 30 | 115 | 2 | 1.5 | 25.8 | 0.9 | 5.6 | 19.4 | 0.9 | 0.2 | 0.3 | 0.0 | 0.00 | 0.02 | 0 | 750 | 225 | 225 | 0 | 0 | 0.38 | 0.43 | 5.01 | 0.50 | 1.50 | 99.9 | 1.00 | 15.0 | 1.0 | | 50 | 0.3 | 8.1 | 7 | 0.0 | 50 | 26 | 6.0 | 288 | 3.75 |
| 40405 | 1 cup | Boo Berry, General Mills | 30 | 116 | 2 | 1.0 | 27.3 | 0.4 | 14.9 | 12.0 | 0.5 | 0.1 | 0.2 | 0.0 | 0.00 | 0.03 | 0 | 0 | 0 | 0 | 0 | 0 | 0.38 | 0.43 | 5.01 | 0.50 | 0.00 | 99.9 | 0.03 | 15.0 | 1.0 | | 20 | 0.0 | 4.5 | 3 | 0.0 | 31 | 18 | 2.0 | 214 | 3.75 |
| | | Bran Cereals | | | | | | | | | | | | | | | | | | | | | | | | | | | | | | | | | | | | | | | | |
| 40281 | 1 cup | 100% Bran Flakes, Nabisco | 66 | 178 | 3 | 8.3 | 48.1 | 19.5 | 15.8 | 12.7 | 3.3 | 0.6 | 0.6 | 1.9 | 0.13 | 1.75 | 0 | 0 | 0 | 0 | 0 | 0 | 1.58 | 1.78 | 20.92 | 2.11 | 6.27 | 46.9 | 1.27 | 62.7 | 0.0 | | 46 | 1.0 | 8.1 | 312 | 6.0 | 801 | 652 | 5.3 | 457 | 5.74 |
| 40170 | 1 cup | 40% Bran Flakes, Ralston Purina | 37 | 120 | 2 | 4.3 | 29.5 | 5.2 | 6.5 | 17.8 | 0.5 | 0.1 | 0.3 | 0.1 | 0.00 | 0.07 | 0 | 1631 | 490 | 490 | 0 | 0 | 0.48 | 0.56 | 6.51 | 0.67 | 1.96 | 130.6 | 0.51 | 19.6 | 1.2 | | 17 | 0.3 | 5.9 | 89 | 1.7 | 206 | 216 | | 344 | 1.54 |
| 40095 | 1 cup | All-Bran, Kellogg's | 62 | 164 | 3 | 7.6 | 47.1 | 20.0 | 11.8 | 15.3 | 1.9 | 0.4 | 0.4 | 1.1 | 0.08 | 1.03 | 0 | 1550 | 466 | 466 | 0 | 0 | 0.81 | 0.87 | 10.35 | 1.05 | 3.10 | 186.0 | 1.07 | 31.0 | 2.0 | | 219 | 0.7 | 9.3 | 266 | 5.7 | 608 | 706 | 5.8 | 126 | 7.75 |
| 40096 | 1 cup | All-Bran w/extra fiber, Kellogg's | 52 | 92 | 4 | 6.4 | 39.3 | 26.6 | 0.8 | 11.9 | 1.6 | 0.3 | 0.3 | 1.0 | 0.07 | 0.94 | 0 | 1500 | 450 | 450 | 0 | 0 | 0.73 | 0.83 | 9.98 | 0.99 | 3.02 | 208.0 | 0.83 | 30.0 | 2.0 | | 200 | 0.5 | 9.0 | 207 | 3.8 | 498 | 520 | 4.9 | 220 | 7.49 |
| 40029 | 1 cup | Bran Buds, Kellogg's | 91 | 251 | 3 | 8.6 | 72.7 | 36.3 | 24.4 | 12.0 | 2.2 | 0.4 | 0.5 | 1.4 | 0.10 | 1.26 | 0 | 2275 | 683 | 683 | 0 | 0 | 1.18 | 1.27 | 15.20 | 1.55 | 0.00 | 273.0 | 1.36 | 45.5 | 3.0 | | 61 | 0.6 | 13.7 | 253 | 7.5 | 504 | 818 | 26.3 | 606 | 19.57 |
| 40259 | 1 cup | Bran Flakes, Post | 47 | 152 | 3 | 5.3 | 37.3 | 9.2 | 5.7 | 22.4 | 0.8 | 0.1 | 0.1 | 0.4 | 0.03 | 0.34 | 0 | 2072 | 622 | 622 | 0 | 0 | 0.61 | 0.70 | 8.27 | 0.85 | 2.49 | 165.9 | 0.65 | 0.0 | 1.7 | | 21 | 0.3 | 13.4 | 102 | 2.3 | 296 | 251 | 4.7 | 431 | 2.49 |
| 40274 | 1 cup | Bran'nola Original, Post | 106 | 400 | 3 | 8.0 | 86.0 | 10.0 | 30.0 | 46.0 | 6.0 | 1.0 | | | | | 0 | 2500 | 751 | 751 | 0 | 0 | 0.75 | 0.85 | 10.00 | 1.00 | 3.00 | 200.0 | | 0.0 | 2.0 | | 0 | 0.3 | 9.0 | 120 | | 300 | 400 | | 480 | 3.00 |
| 40275 | 1 cup | Bran'nola with raisins, Post | 110 | 400 | 3 | 8.0 | 88.0 | 10.0 | 36.0 | 42.0 | 6.0 | 1.0 | | | | | 0 | 2500 | 751 | 751 | 0 | 0 | 0.75 | 0.85 | 10.00 | 1.00 | 3.00 | 200.0 | | 0.0 | 2.0 | | 0 | 0.3 | 9.0 | 80 | | 200 | 440 | | 440 | 3.00 |
| | | Cap'n Crunch | | | | | | | | | | | | | | | | | | | | | | | | | | | | | | | | | | | | | | | | |
| 40476 | 1 cup | Choco, Quaker | 43 | 178 | 1 | 2.3 | 36.5 | | | | 2.6 | | | | | | | 0 | 0 | 0 | 0 | 0 | 0.57 | 0.40 | 7.68 | 0.77 | 1.54 | 153.6 | 3.07 | | | | 8 | 0.1 | 6.9 | 12 | 0.0 | 31 | 69 | | 264 | 3.07 |
| 40032 | 1 cup | Original, Quaker | 37 | 147 | 2 | 1.9 | 31.6 | 1.2 | 14.6 | 15.8 | 1.9 | 0.5 | 0.4 | 0.3 | 0.01 | 0.23 | 0 | 49 | 5 | 0 | 5 | | 0.51 | 0.58 | 6.85 | 0.68 | 0.00 | 137.3 | 0.13 | 0.0 | 0.0 | | 7 | 0.1 | 6.2 | 13 | 0.3 | 39 | 47 | 7.4 | 286 | 5.14 |
| 40034 | 1 cup | Peanut Butter, Quaker | 35 | 146 | 2 | 2.5 | 27.9 | 1.0 | 12.6 | 14.3 | 3.0 | 0.7 | 1.1 | 0.7 | 0.01 | 0.62 | 0 | 48 | 5 | 0 | 5 | | 0.49 | 0.55 | 6.47 | 0.65 | 0.00 | 129.8 | 0.16 | 0.0 | 0.0 | | 3 | 0.1 | 5.8 | 24 | 0.3 | 67 | 80 | 7.0 | 264 | 4.86 |
| 40033 | 1 cup | Crunchberries, Quaker | 35 | 140 | 2 | 1.7 | 30.0 | 0.8 | 13.9 | 15.3 | 1.7 | 0.5 | 0.3 | 0.3 | 0.01 | 0.22 | 0 | 44 | 6 | | | | 0.50 | 0.57 | 6.72 | 0.67 | 0.01 | 134.8 | 0.13 | 0.0 | 0.0 | | 9 | 0.0 | 6.1 | 13 | 0.2 | 40 | 49 | 7.0 | 256 | 5.39 |
| | | Cheerios | | | | | | | | | | | | | | | | | | | | | | | | | | | | | | | | | | | | | | | | |
| 40295 | 1 cup | Apple Cinnamon, General Mills | 40 | 157 | 3 | 2.5 | 33.4 | 2.1 | 17.5 | 13.8 | 2.2 | 0.4 | 0.9 | 0.3 | 0.02 | 0.26 | 0 | 1000 | 300 | 300 | 0 | 0 | 0.50 | 0.57 | 6.68 | 0.67 | 0.00 | 133.2 | 0.21 | 20.0 | 0.0 | | 47 | 0.1 | 6.0 | 27 | 0.6 | 87 | 80 | 15.0 | 200 | 5.00 |
| 40399 | 1 cup | Frosted, General Mills | 30 | 115 | 2 | 2.0 | 25.5 | 1.5 | 13.7 | 10.3 | 1.0 | 0.2 | 0.4 | 0.4 | 0.01 | 0.35 | 0 | 750 | 225 | 225 | 0 | 0 | 0.38 | 0.43 | 5.01 | 0.50 | 0.00 | 99.9 | 0.15 | 15.0 | 0.0 | | 32 | 0.1 | 4.5 | 18 | 0.4 | 66 | 58 | 11.3 | 192 | 3.75 |
| 40051 | 1 cup | Honey Nut, General Mills | 33 | 126 | 2 | 3.1 | 26.7 | 1.7 | 12.6 | 12.4 | 1.4 | 0.3 | 0.5 | 0.2 | 0.01 | 0.13 | 0 | 825 | 248 | 248 | 0 | 0 | 0.41 | 0.47 | 5.51 | 0.55 | 0.00 | 109.9 | 0.16 | 16.5 | 1.2 | | 22 | 0.1 | 5.0 | 32 | 0.8 | 113 | 94 | 7.8 | 285 | 4.13 |
| 40301 | 1 cup | Multigrain, General Mills | 30 | 112 | 3 | 2.6 | 24.5 | 1.9 | 6.3 | 16.3 | 1.1 | 0.2 | 0.3 | 0.2 | 0.01 | 0.14 | 0 | 750 | 225 | 225 | 0 | 0 | 0.38 | 0.43 | 5.01 | 0.50 | 0.00 | 99.9 | 0.20 | 15.0 | 0.0 | | 57 | 0.1 | 8.1 | 30 | 0.6 | 114 | 97 | | 254 | 3.75 |
| 40297 | 1 cup | Original, General Mills | 23 | 84 | 3 | 2.4 | 17.5 | 2.0 | 1.1 | 14.4 | 1.4 | 0.3 | 0.5 | 0.2 | 0.01 | 0.16 | 0 | 958 | 238 | 288 | 0 | 0 | 0.29 | 0.33 | 3.84 | 0.33 | 0.00 | 76.6 | 0.02 | 11.5 | 0.8 | | 42 | 0.1 | 6.2 | 25 | 0.1 | 87 | 68 | 8.6 | 218 | 2.88 |
| | | Chex Cereals | | | | | | | | | | | | | | | | | | | | | | | | | | | | | | | | | | | | | | | | |
| 40323 | 1 cup | Bran, Ralston Purina | 49 | 156 | 2 | 5.0 | 39.1 | 7.9 | 8.9 | 22.2 | 1.4 | 0.2 | 0.3 | 0.7 | 0.04 | 0.63 | 0 | 107 | 11 | 0 | 11 | | 0.64 | 0.26 | 8.62 | 0.83 | 2.60 | 173.0 | 0.50 | 26.0 | 0.0 | | 29 | 0.4 | 14.0 | 69 | 2.5 | 173 | 216 | 4.4 | 345 | 6.47 |
| 40325 | 1 cup | Corn, Ralston Purina | 28 | 110 | 2 | 2.0 | 24.6 | 0.5 | 2.9 | 21.2 | 0.1 | 0.0 | 0.0 | 0.0 | 0.00 | 0.05 | 0 | 141 | 14 | 0 | 14 | | 0.36 | 0.07 | 4.93 | 0.50 | 1.48 | 98.8 | 0.05 | 14.8 | 0.0 | | 3 | 0.0 | 8.0 | 4 | 0.0 | 11 | 23 | 1.0 | 306 | 0.10 |
| 40327 | 1 cup | Crispy Mini Grahams, Ralston Purina | 52 | 210 | 4 | 3.0 | 45.0 | 1.0 | 17.0 | 27.0 | 1.5 | 0.0 | | | | | 0 | 0 | 0 | 0 | 0 | 0 | 0.38 | | 5.00 | 0.50 | 1.50 | 100.0 | | 6.0 | | | 0 | | 16.2 | 16 | | 60 | 80 | | 340 | 5.25 |
| 40481 | 1 cup | Crispy Oatmeal Raisin, Ralston Purina | 29 | 107 | 7 | 2.3 | 23.7 | 1.3 | | | 0.4 | | | | | | | | | | | | 0.29 | 0.24 | 3.82 | 0.38 | 1.14 | 76.3 | 0.06 | 3.1 | | | 9 | 0.1 | | 21 | | 65 | 8 | | 128 | 2.86 |
| 40326 | 1 cup | Double, Ralston Purina | 24 | 96 | 6 | 0.8 | 21.6 | 0.0 | 6.4 | 15.2 | 0.0 | 0.0 | 0.0 | 0.0 | 0.00 | 0.00 | 0 | 0 | 0 | 0 | 0 | 0 | 0.30 | | 4.00 | 0.40 | 1.20 | 80.0 | | 4.8 | | | 0 | | 7.2 | | | | 48 | | 134 | |
| 40333 | 1 cup | Rice, Ralston Purina | 33 | 130 | 3 | 1.7 | 29.4 | 0.6 | 2.6 | 26.2 | 0.1 | 0.0 | 0.0 | 0.0 | 0.01 | 0.03 | 0 | 20 | 2 | 0 | 2 | | 0.43 | 0.01 | 5.81 | 0.59 | 1.75 | 116.5 | 0.12 | 17.5 | 0.0 | | 5 | 0.1 | 9.4 | 8 | 0.3 | 32 | 38 | 1.3 | 276 | 0.46 |
| 40335 | 1 cup | Wheat, Ralston Purina | 46 | 169 | 2 | 4.6 | 37.8 | 4.1 | 4.6 | 29.1 | 1.1 | 0.2 | 0.1 | 0.5 | 0.02 | 0.45 | 0 | 0 | 0 | 0 | 0 | 0 | 0.60 | 0.17 | 8.10 | 0.83 | 2.44 | 162.4 | 0.21 | 24.4 | 0.0 | | 18 | 0.3 | 13.2 | 58 | 1.3 | 182 | 173 | 2.3 | 308 | 1.23 |
| 40207 | 1 cup | Cinnamon Mini Buns, Kellogg's | 40 | 154 | 2 | 2.0 | 35.5 | 0.9 | 16.0 | 18.6 | 0.8 | 0.2 | 0.2 | 0.4 | 0.01 | 0.35 | 0 | 1000 | 300 | 300 | 0 | 0 | 0.52 | 0.56 | 6.68 | 0.68 | 0.00 | 120.0 | 0.13 | 20.0 | 1.3 | | 5 | 0.0 | 6.0 | 15 | 0.2 | 32 | 49 | 4.8 | 277 | 5.00 |
| 40358 | 1 cup | Cinnamon Oatmeal Squares, Quaker | 60 | 232 | 2 | 7.6 | 47.2 | 4.6 | 9.7 | 32.9 | 2.5 | 0.5 | 0.9 | 1.1 | 0.05 | 1.03 | 0 | 548 | 165 | 165 | 0 | 0 | 0.41 | 0.46 | 5.48 | 0.55 | 0.00 | 109.3 | 0.43 | 6.6 | 0.0 | | 41 | 0.2 | 14.6 | 70 | 1.9 | 182 | 250 | 10.4 | 266 | 4.11 |
| 40126 | 1 cup | Cinnamon Toast Crunch, General Mills | 40 | 166 | 2 | 2.2 | 31.8 | 2.0 | 14.2 | 15.6 | 4.0 | 0.7 | 1.2 | 0.7 | 0.27 | 0.43 | 0 | 1000 | 300 | 300 | 0 | 0 | 0.50 | 0.57 | 6.68 | 0.67 | 0.00 | 133.2 | 0.31 | 20.0 | 1.3 | | 56 | 0.1 | 6.0 | 18 | 1.1 | 99 | 59 | 1.7 | 280 | 5.00 |
| 40378 | 1 cup | Clusters, General Mills | 55 | 213 | 3 | 5.4 | 43.4 | 4.2 | 14.5 | 24.6 | 3.5 | 0.4 | 1.8 | 0.4 | 0.02 | 0.35 | 0 | 0 | 0 | 0 | 0 | 0 | 0.37 | 0.42 | 5.01 | 0.50 | 0.00 | 100.1 | 0.63 | 9.0 | 1.8 | | 72 | 0.2 | 4.5 | 52 | 2.7 | 153 | 171 | 5.9 | 239 | 1.04 |
| 40102 | 1 cup | Cocoa Krispies, Kellogg's | 41 | 159 | 2 | 2.0 | 36.0 | 0.5 | 17.3 | 18.2 | 1.1 | 0.3 | 0.1 | 0.2 | 0.01 | 0.15 | 0 | 992 | 298 | 298 | 0 | 0 | 0.49 | 0.57 | 6.60 | 0.66 | 0.00 | 123.0 | 0.37 | 19.8 | 1.3 | | 5 | 0.1 | 2.4 | 15 | 1.0 | 39 | 80 | 5.7 | 278 | 1.97 |
| 40257 | 1 cup | Cocoa Pebbles, Post | 32 | 131 | 2 | 1.5 | 27.5 | 0.5 | 14.7 | 12.3 | 1.7 | 1.1 | 0.4 | 0.1 | 0.01 | 0.13 | 0 | 1411 | 424 | 424 | 0 | 0 | 0.42 | 0.48 | 5.63 | 0.58 | 1.70 | 113.0 | 0.09 | 0.0 | 1.1 | | 5 | 0.1 | 2.0 | 13 | 0.3 | 25 | 53 | | 180 | 1.70 |
| 40425 | 1 cup | Cocoa Puffs, General Mills | 30 | 119 | 2 | 1.1 | 26.7 | 0.2 | 13.8 | 12.8 | 0.9 | 0.2 | 0.3 | 0.0 | 0.00 | 0.04 | 0 | 0 | 0 | 0 | 0 | 0 | 0.33 | 0.43 | 5.01 | 0.50 | 0.00 | 99.9 | 0.03 | 15.0 | 0.0 | | 33 | 0.0 | 4.5 | 7 | 0.0 | 43 | 52 | 2.0 | 181 | 3.75 |
| 40324 | 1 cup | Cookie Crisp, Ralston Purina | 30 | 120 | 2 | 1.5 | 26.3 | 0.4 | 13.7 | 12.1 | 1.1 | 0.6 | 0.2 | 0.2 | 0.01 | 0.15 | 0 | 0 | 0 | 0 | 0 | 0 | 0.39 | 0.27 | 5.28 | 0.54 | 1.59 | 105.9 | 0.06 | 0.0 | 0.8 | | 6 | 0.1 | 4.8 | 8 | 0.2 | 24 | 29 | 2.2 | 207 | 3.18 |
| 40036 | 1 cup | Corn Bran, Quaker | 36 | 120 | 3 | 2.5 | 30.3 | 6.4 | 7.7 | 16.2 | 1.2 | 0.3 | 0.3 | 0.4 | 0.01 | 0.33 | 0 | 50 | 5 | 0 | 5 | | 0.10 | 0.57 | 6.66 | 0.67 | 0.00 | 133.6 | 0.14 | 0.0 | 0.0 | | 27 | 0.1 | 10.1 | 19 | 0.5 | 48 | 75 | 4.3 | 338 | 5.00 |
| | | Corn Flakes | | | | | | | | | | | | | | | | | | | | | | | | | | | | | | | | | | | | | | | | |
| 40424 | 1 cup | Country, General Mills | 30 | 114 | 3 | 1.8 | 26.0 | 0.5 | 2.5 | 23.0 | 0.5 | 0.2 | 0.1 | 0.0 | 0.00 | 0.03 | 0 | 750 | 225 | 225 | 0 | 0 | 0.38 | 0.43 | 5.01 | 0.50 | 0.00 | 99.9 | 0.07 | 15.0 | 1.0 | | 53 | 0.0 | 8.1 | 7 | 0.0 | 39 | 41 | 1.5 | 284 | 3.75 |
| 40298 | 1 cup | Frosted, General Mills | 41 | 161 | 2 | 1.6 | 36.9 | 0.4 | 14.3 | 22.1 | 0.5 | 0.1 | | | | | 0 | 1708 | 513 | 513 | 0 | 0 | 0.51 | 0.58 | 6.83 | 0.68 | | 0.1 | | 20.5 | 1.4 | | 1 | 0.1 | 6.2 | | | | 39 | | 257 | |
| 40492 | 1 cup | Honey Crunch, Kellogg's | 40 | 147 | 3 | 2.7 | 34.7 | 1.3 | 13.3 | 20.0 | 1.3 | 0.0 | | | | | 0 | 1000 | 300 | 300 | 0 | 0 | 0.50 | 0.57 | 6.67 | 0.67 | | 133.3 | | 20.0 | 1.3 | | 0 | | 6.0 | | | | 47 | | 360 | |
| 40195 | 1 cup | Kellogg's | 28 | 102 | 3 | 1.8 | 24.2 | 0.8 | 1.9 | 21.5 | 0.2 | 0.1 | 0.0 | 0.1 | 0.00 | 0.10 | 0 | 700 | 210 | 210 | 0 | 0 | 0.36 | 0.39 | 4.68 | 0.48 | 0.00 | 98.8 | 0.09 | 14.0 | 1.0 | | 1 | 0.0 | 8.7 | 3 | 0.1 | 11 | 25 | 1.4 | 298 | 0.17 |
| 40145 | 1 cup | Low sodium, avg | 25 | 100 | 3 | 1.9 | 22.2 | 0.3 | 1.7 | 20.2 | 0.1 | 0.0 | 0.0 | 0.0 | 0.00 | 0.03 | 0 | 95 | 9.5 | 0 | 9.5 | | 0.00 | 0.05 | 0.10 | 0.02 | 0.00 | 1.8 | 0.03 | 0.0 | | | 11 | 0.0 | 0.6 | 3 | 0.0 | 12 | 18 | 1.3 | 2 | 0.07 |
| 40103 | 1 cup | Common Sense, Kellogg's | 40 | 145 | 3 | 5.2 | 31.0 | 5.3 | 8.4 | 17.2 | 1.6 | 0.5 | 0.8 | 0.3 | 0.01 | 0.31 | 0 | 1000 | 300 | 300 | 0 | 0 | 0.52 | 0.56 | 6.68 | 0.68 | 2.00 | 120.0 | 0.42 | 0.0 | 1.3 | | 20 | 0.1 | 11.2 | 64 | 1.6 | 204 | 160 | 6.8 | 360 | 5.00 |
| 40206 | 1 cup | Corn Pops, Kellogg's | 31 | 118 | 3 | 1.1 | 28.4 | 0.4 | 13.1 | 14.9 | 0.2 | 0.1 | 0.1 | 0.0 | 0.00 | 0.03 | 0 | 775 | 233 | 233 | 0 | 0 | 0.40 | 0.43 | 5.18 | 0.53 | 0.00 | 109.4 | 0.09 | 15.5 | 1.0 | | 2 | 0.0 | 1.9 | 2 | 0.1 | 7 | 23 | 2.0 | 123 | 1.55 |
| 40402 | 1 cup | Count Chocula, General Mills | 30 | 117 | 2 | 1.4 | 26.4 | 0.5 | 12.5 | 13.5 | 0.9 | 0.2 | 0.3 | 0.0 | 0.00 | 0.03 | 0 | 0 | 0 | 0 | 0 | 0 | 0.38 | 0.43 | 5.01 | 0.50 | 0.00 | 99.9 | 0.03 | 15.0 | 1.0 | | 29 | 0.1 | 4.5 | 9 | 0.0 | 41 | 63 | 2.0 | 209 | 3.75 |
| 40205 | 1 cup | Cracklin' Oat Bran, Kellogg's | 65 | 266 | 4 | 5.5 | 47.4 | 7.7 | 21.4 | 18.3 | 8.3 | 3.5 | 3.8 | 0.9 | 0.04 | 0.82 | 0 | 995 | 299 | 299 | 0 | 0 | 0.50 | 0.56 | 6.63 | 0.66 | 0.00 | 180.7 | 0.49 | 19.9 | 1.3 | | 29 | 0.2 | 2.4 | 90 | 2.0 | 220 | 301 | 14.3 | 231 | 1.95 |
| 40104 | 1 cup | Crispix, Kellogg's | 29 | 108 | 3 | 2.1 | 25.0 | 0.6 | 3.0 | 21.4 | 0.3 | 0.1 | 0.1 | 0.1 | 0.00 | 0.11 | 0 | 750 | 225 | 225 | 0 | 0 | 0.38 | 0.44 | 4.99 | 0.49 | 0.00 | 87.0 | 0.27 | 15.0 | 1.0 | | 3 | 0.1 | 1.8 | 7 | 0.5 | 27 | 35 | 3.2 | 240 | 1.51 |
| 40487 | 1 cup | Crisp Rice, Krusteaz, Continental Mills | 32 | 130 | 2 | 3.0 | 27.0 | 0.0 | 3.0 | 24.0 | 0.0 | 0.0 | 0.0 | 0.0 | 0.00 | 0.00 | 0 | 1250 | 375 | 375 | 0 | 0 | | | | | | | | 15.0 | | | 0 | | 8.1 | | | | 40 | | 260 | |
| 40318 | 1 cup | Crisp Brn Rice, honey swtnd, fat free, Health Valley | 37 | 110 | 16 | 1.0 | 30.0 | 1.0 | 5.0 | 24.0 | 0.0 | 0.0 | 0.0 | 0.0 | 0.00 | 0.00 | 0 | 0 | 0 | 0 | 0 | 0 | | | | | | | | 0.0 | | | 0 | | 0.0 | | | | | | 0 | |
| 40453 | 1 cup | Crispy Puffs, Arrowhead Mills | 20 | 80 | 4 | 2.0 | 16.0 | 1.0 | 3.0 | 12.0 | 1.0 | 0.0 | | | | | 0 | 0 | 0 | 0 | 0 | 0 | | | 0.40 | | | | | 0.0 | | | 0 | | 0.4 | | | | 50 | | 0 | |
| 40017 | 1 cup | Crispy Rice, avg | 28 | 111 | 2 | 1.8 | 24.8 | 0.3 | 2.5 | 22.0 | 0.1 | 0.0 | 0.0 | 0.0 | 0.01 | 0.02 | 0 | 1235 | 371 | 371 | 0 | 0 | 0.52 | 0.59 | 6.92 | 0.69 | 0.08 | 138.3 | 0.11 | 14.8 | 1.0 | | 5 | 0.1 | 0.7 | 12 | 0.4 | 31 | 27 | 4.3 | 206 | 0.46 |
| 40240 | 1 cup | Crispy Rice, low sod, avg+D935 | 28 | 113 | 3 | 1.5 | 25.5 | 0.4 | 2.5 | 22.6 | 0.1 | 0.0 | 0.0 | 0.0 | 0.00 | 0.01 | 0 | 0 | 0 | 0 | 0 | 0 | 0.00 | 0.05 | 0.38 | 0.04 | 0.00 | 3.1 | 0.15 | 0.0 | 0.0 | | 19 | 0.1 | 0.9 | 11 | 0.3 | 29 | 22 | 4.3 | 3 | 0.42 |
| 40040 | 1 cup | Crispy Wheat 'N Raisins, General Mills | 43 | 150 | 7 | 3.5 | 34.7 | 2.7 | 17.2 | 14.7 | 0.6 | 0.1 | 0.1 | 0.1 | 0.01 | 0.12 | 0 | 977 | 293 | 293 | 0 | 0 | 0.29 | 0.33 | 3.91 | 0.39 | 0.00 | 77.8 | 0.28 | 0.0 | 0.0 | | 54 | 0.1 | 3.5 | 33 | 1.1 | 110 | 180 | 3.0 | 223 | 0.85 |
| 40362 | 1 cup | Crispy Whole Grain w/Raisins, low fat, Quaker | 100 | 389 | 4 | 8.3 | 80.7 | 6.0 | | | 5.3 | 1.5 | 2.5 | 1.1 | 0.06 | 0.38 | 1 | 18 | 2 | 0 | 2 | | 0.29 | 0.11 | 1.82 | 0.14 | 0.00 | 23.0 | 0.45 | 0.7 | | | 60 | 0.3 | 2.6 | 79 | 2.0 | 237 | 338 | 17.3 | 258 | 1.84 |
| 40475 | 1 cup | Crunchy Nut Ohs, Quaker | 28 | 129 | 1 | 1.7 | 21.2 | 0.8 | | | 4.2 | 2.4 | 0.5 | 0.3 | | | | 0 | 0 | 0 | 0 | 0 | 0.61 | 0.41 | 8.12 | 0.71 | 1.89 | 208.0 | 3.47 | 0.0 | | | 10 | 0.1 | 5.7 | 14 | 0.3 | 40 | 45 | | 135 | 2.97 |
| 40030 | 1 cup | C.W. Post, Post | 97 | 421 | 2 | 9.1 | 72.7 | 7.2 | 22.3 | 43.2 | 12.8 | 1.7 | 6.0 | 4.7 | 0.12 | 4.52 | 0 | 4277 | 1284 | 1284 | 0 | 0 | 1.26 | 1.46 | 17.07 | 1.75 | 5.14 | 342.4 | 0.79 | 0.0 | 3.4 | | 47 | 0.4 | 15.4 | 67 | | 224 | 198 | 11.0 | 167 | 1.64 |
| 40031 | 1 cup | C.W. Post w/raisins, Post | 103 | 446 | 4 | 9.0 | 74.0 | 13.6 | 24.7 | 35.6 | 14.7 | 11.0 | 1.7 | 1.4 | 0.06 | 1.32 | 0 | 4541 | 1364 | 1364 | 0 | 0 | 1.34 | 1.54 | 18.13 | 1.85 | 5.46 | 363.6 | 0.77 | 0.0 | 3.6 | | 50 | 0.4 | 16.4 | 74 | | 232 | 261 | 11.6 | 161 | 1.64 |

| Code | Amount | Description | Basic Components | | | | | | | | | Additional Fats | | | | | | Vit A & Components | | | | | Vitamins | | | | | | | | | | Minerals | | | | | | | | | |
|---|---|---|---|---|---|---|---|---|---|---|---|---|---|---|---|---|---|---|---|---|---|---|---|---|---|---|---|---|---|---|---|---|---|---|---|---|---|---|---|---|---|---|
| | | | Weight (g) | Calories | % Water | Protein (g) | Carbs (g) | Fiber (g) | Sugar (g) | Other Carbs (g) | Fat (g) | Sat Fat (g) | Mono Fat (g) | Poly Fat (g) | Omega 3 (g) | Omega 6 (g) | Choles (mg) | Vit A (IU) | Vit A (RE) | Retinol (RE) | Carotenoids (RE) | Beta Carotene (mcg) | Thiamin (mg) | Riboflavin (mg) | Niacin (NE) | Vit B6 (mg) | Vit B12 (mcg) | Folate (mcg) | Panto (mg) | Vit C (mg) | Vit D (mg) | Vit E (α TE) | Calcium (mg) | Copper (mg) | Iron (mg) | Magnes (mg) | Mang (mg) | Phos (mg) | Potassium (mg) | Selenium (mcg) | Sodium (mg) | Zinc (mg) |
| 40208 | 1 cup | Double Dip Crunch, Kellogg's | 39 | 149 | 3 | 1.3 | 35.5 | 0.6 | 14.8 | 20.1 | 0.2 | 0.0 | 0.0 | 0.2 | 0.00 | 0.08 | 0 | 1009 | 303 | 303 | 0 | 0 | 0.51 | 0.58 | 6.71 | 0.66 | 0.00 | 117.0 | 0.05 | 20.2 | 1.3 | | 3 | 0.0 | 2.4 | 7 | 0.0 | 25 | 28 | 1.8 | 229 | 2.03 |
| 40119 | 1 cup | 4-Grain Plus Flax, Arrowhead Mills | 180 | 600 | 18 | 24.0 | 112.0 | 24.0 | 0.0 | 88.0 | 8.0 | 0.0 | | | | | 0 | 0 | 0 | 0 | 0 | 0 | 0.48 | 0.14 | 3.20 | | 0.00 | | | 0.0 | | | 80 | | 7.2 | | | 576 | 760 | | 0 | |
| 40130 | 1 cup | Fiber One, General Mills | 60 | 123 | 4 | 5.6 | 48.0 | 28.5 | 1.1 | 18.4 | 1.7 | 0.3 | 0.3 | 0.1 | 0.01 | 0.11 | 0 | 0 | 0 | 0 | 0 | 0 | 0.75 | 0.85 | 10.02 | 1.00 | 0.00 | 199.8 | 0.67 | 18.0 | 0.0 | | 117 | 0.4 | 9.0 | 136 | 3.3 | 337 | 434 | 5.4 | 285 | 2.48 |
| 40400 | 1 cup | Frankenberry, General Mills | 30 | 117 | 2 | 1.0 | 27.3 | 0.2 | 14.6 | 12.5 | 0.5 | 0.1 | 0.2 | 0.0 | 0.00 | 0.03 | 0 | 0 | 0 | 0 | 0 | 0 | 0.38 | 0.43 | 5.01 | 0.50 | 0.00 | 99.9 | 0.04 | 15.0 | 1.0 | | 25 | 0.0 | 4.5 | 3 | 0.0 | 28 | 16 | 5.9 | 209 | 3.75 |
| 40218 | 1 cup | Froot Loops, Kellogg's | 32 | 125 | 2 | 1.6 | 28.2 | 0.6 | 15.0 | 12.6 | 0.9 | 0.4 | 0.2 | 0.3 | 0.01 | 0.27 | 0 | 750 | 225 | 225 | 0 | 0 | 0.42 | 0.45 | 5.34 | 0.54 | 0.00 | 96.0 | 0.09 | 15.0 | 1.0 | | 4 | 0.0 | 4.5 | 9 | 0.1 | 22 | 34 | 2.3 | 150 | 4.00 |
| 40198 | 1 cup | Frosted Bran, Kellogg's | 60 | 203 | 3 | 4.7 | 50.8 | 6.7 | 18.9 | 25.2 | 0.7 | 0.1 | 0.2 | 0.4 | 0.01 | 0.35 | 0 | 1451 | 436 | 436 | 0 | 0 | 0.72 | 0.84 | 9.66 | 0.96 | 2.88 | 180.0 | 0.32 | 29.0 | 0.6 | | 19 | 0.2 | 8.7 | 76 | 1.2 | 185 | 244 | 5.6 | 413 | 7.26 |
| 40217 | 1 cup | Frosted Flakes, Kellogg's | 41 | 158 | 3 | 1.6 | 37.4 | 0.8 | 17.2 | 19.4 | 0.2 | 0.1 | 0.0 | 0.1 | 0.00 | 0.08 | 0 | 992 | 298 | 298 | 0 | 0 | 0.49 | 0.57 | 6.60 | 0.66 | 0.00 | 123.0 | 0.14 | 19.8 | 1.3 | | 1 | 0.0 | 5.9 | 4 | 0.1 | 11 | 27 | 1.8 | 264 | 0.20 |
| 40043 | 1 cup | Frosted Mini-Wheats, Kellogg's | 51 | 173 | 5 | 4.8 | 42.1 | 5.5 | 10.0 | 26.6 | 0.8 | 0.2 | 0.1 | 0.6 | 0.03 | 0.51 | 0 | 0 | 0 | 0 | 0 | 0 | 0.36 | 0.41 | 5.00 | 0.46 | 1.48 | 102.0 | 0.38 | 0.0 | 0.0 | | 18 | 0.2 | 14.3 | 52 | 1.4 | 148 | 170 | 2.1 | 2 | 1.48 |
| 40146 | 1 cup | Frosted Rice Krinkles, avg | 45 | 173 | 2 | 2.2 | 41.0 | 0.3 | 17.5 | 23.2 | 0.1 | 0.0 | 0.0 | 0.0 | 0.00 | 0.02 | 0 | 1984 | 596 | 596 | 0 | 0 | 0.58 | 0.67 | 7.92 | 0.81 | 2.38 | 158.8 | 0.20 | 0.0 | | | 6 | 0.1 | 2.8 | 12 | 0.5 | 31 | 23 | 6.9 | 283 | 2.38 |
| 40282 | 1 cup | Frosted Wheat Bites, Nabisco | 52 | 190 | 5 | 4.0 | 44.0 | 5.0 | 12.0 | 27.0 | 1.0 | 0.0 | | | 0.00 | 0.00 | 0 | 0 | 0 | 0 | 0 | 0 | 0.38 | 0.43 | 5.00 | 0.50 | 1.50 | 100.0 | | 0.0 | 0.0 | | 20 | 0.2 | 1.8 | 40 | | 150 | 170 | | 10 | 1.50 |
| | | Fruit & Fibre Cereal, Post | | | | | | | | | | | | | | | | | | | | | | | | | | | | | | | | | | | | | | | | |
| 40493 | 1 cup | W/dates, raisins & nuts, Post | 57 | 193 | 9 | 4.8 | 43.3 | 7.6 | 15.4 | 20.3 | 3.0 | 0.4 | 1.3 | 1.0 | | | 0 | 2415 | 725 | 725 | 0 | | 0.75 | 0.86 | 10.05 | 1.00 | 3.02 | 201.2 | 0.00 | 0.0 | 2.5 | | 30 | 0.3 | 10.1 | 81 | | 221 | 335 | 7.0 | 270 | 3.02 |
| 40262 | 1 cup | W/dates, raisins & walnuts, Post | 60 | 210 | 11 | 4.0 | 46.0 | 6.0 | 18.0 | 22.0 | 3.0 | 0.5 | | | | | 0 | 1500 | 450 | 450 | 0 | 0 | 0.45 | 0.51 | 6.00 | 0.60 | 1.80 | 120.0 | | 0.0 | 1.5 | | 20 | 0.3 | 6.3 | 80 | | 150 | 260 | | 260 | 1.50 |
| 40256 | 1 cup | W/peaches, raisins & almonds, Post | 60 | 210 | 9 | 4.0 | 46.0 | 6.0 | 15.0 | 25.0 | 3.0 | 0.5 | | | | | 0 | 1500 | 450 | 450 | 0 | 0 | 0.45 | 0.51 | 6.00 | 0.60 | 1.80 | 120.0 | | 0.0 | 1.5 | | 20 | 0.3 | 6.0 | 80 | | 200 | 280 | | 270 | 1.50 |
| | | Fruit Wheats Cereal, Nabisco | | | | | | | | | | | | | | | | | | | | | | | | | | | | | | | | | | | | | | | | |
| 40283 | 1 cup | Blueberry | 68 | 227 | 8 | 5.3 | 54.7 | 5.3 | 13.3 | 36.0 | 1.3 | 0.0 | | | 0.00 | 0.00 | 0 | 1000 | 300 | 340 | 0 | 0 | 0.50 | 0.57 | 6.67 | 0.67 | 2.00 | 133.3 | | 0.0 | 1.3 | | 27 | 0.2 | 2.4 | 53 | | 133 | 227 | | 20 | 2.00 |
| 40284 | 1 cup | Raspberry | 65 | 212 | 8 | 5.3 | 53.1 | 5.3 | 13.3 | 34.5 | 0.7 | 0.0 | | | 0.00 | 0.00 | 0 | 995 | 298 | 298 | 0 | 0 | 0.50 | 0.56 | 6.63 | 0.66 | 1.99 | 132.7 | | 0.0 | 1.3 | | 27 | 0.2 | 2.4 | 53 | | 133 | 212 | | 20 | 1.99 |
| 40285 | 1 cup | Strawberry | 68 | 227 | 10 | 5.3 | 54.7 | 5.3 | 16.0 | 33.3 | 0.7 | 0.0 | | | 0.00 | 0.00 | 0 | 1000 | 300 | 300 | 0 | 0 | 0.50 | 0.57 | 6.67 | 0.67 | 2.00 | 133.3 | | 0.0 | 1.3 | | 27 | 0.2 | 2.4 | 53 | | 333 | 213 | | 20 | 2.00 |
| 40490 | 1 cup | Fruit Whirls, Krusteaz | 40 | 160 | 5 | 4.0 | 32.0 | 1.3 | 14.7 | 16.0 | 1.3 | 0.0 | | | 0.00 | 0.00 | 0 | 1667 | 501 | 501 | 0 | 0 | | | | | | | | 80.0 | | | 0 | | 6.0 | | | | 87 | | 373 | |
| 40106 | 1 cup | Fruity Marshmallow Krispies, Kellogg's | 37 | 140 | 3 | 1.7 | 33.4 | 0.4 | 17.4 | 15.7 | 0.1 | 0.0 | 0.0 | 0.1 | 0.03 | 0.04 | 0 | 991 | 298 | 298 | 0 | 0 | 0.48 | 0.56 | 6.62 | 0.67 | 0.00 | 148.0 | 0.18 | 19.8 | 1.3 | 0.0 | 2 | 0.1 | 2.4 | 8 | 0.2 | 24 | 22 | 5.1 | 221 | 0.33 |
| 40266 | 1 cup | Fruity Pebbles, Post | 32 | 130 | 3 | 1.3 | 27.6 | 0.4 | 13.6 | 13.6 | 1.7 | 1.4 | 0.1 | 0.1 | 0.01 | 0.06 | 0 | 1411 | 424 | 424 | 0 | 0 | 0.42 | 0.48 | 5.63 | 0.58 | 1.70 | 113.0 | 0.10 | 0.0 | 1.1 | | 4 | 0.0 | 2.0 | 9 | 0.3 | 19 | 24 | | 178 | 1.70 |
| 40299 | 1 cup | Golden Grahams, General Mills | 39 | 150 | 3 | 2.1 | 33.4 | 1.2 | 13.8 | 18.3 | 1.4 | 0.2 | 0.4 | 0.2 | 0.01 | 0.19 | 0 | 975 | 293 | 293 | 0 | 0 | 0.49 | 0.55 | 6.51 | 0.65 | 0.00 | 129.9 | 0.11 | 19.5 | 1.4 | | 19 | 0.1 | 5.8 | 12 | 0.3 | 47 | 69 | 2.2 | 357 | 4.88 |
| 40506 | 1 cup | Graham Crackos, avg | 37 | 134 | 3 | 2.8 | 32.0 | 2.3 | | | 0.2 | 0.0 | 0.1 | 0.1 | | | 0 | 1631 | 490 | 490 | 0 | 0 | 0.48 | 0.56 | 6.51 | 0.67 | 0.00 | 130.6 | 0.24 | 19.6 | | | 17 | 0.1 | 2.3 | 31 | 1.0 | 81 | 134 | | 242 | 1.96 |
| | | Granola Cereals | | | | | | | | | | | | | | | | | | | | | | | | | | | | | | | | | | | | | | | | |
| 40064 | 1 cup | Apple Cinnamon, 100% Nat, Quaker | 104 | 477 | 2 | 11.0 | 69.8 | 6.9 | 21.8 | 41.1 | 19.6 | 15.5 | 1.8 | 1.3 | 0.06 | 1.28 | 0 | 57 | 6 | 0 | 6 | | 0.33 | 0.57 | 1.87 | 0.11 | 0.30 | 16.6 | 1.09 | 1.0 | 0.0 | | 157 | 0.4 | 2.9 | 72 | 1.9 | 350 | 514 | 18.0 | 52 | 2.00 |
| 40309 | 1 cup | Cinnamon & Raisin, Nature Valley | 73 | 312 | 5 | 6.5 | 51.0 | 3.8 | 18.0 | 29.3 | 10.2 | 1.3 | 6.3 | 2.4 | 0.08 | 1.59 | 0 | 0 | 0 | 0 | 0 | 0 | 0.24 | 0.06 | 0.74 | 0.11 | 0.00 | 11.0 | 0.55 | 0.0 | 0.0 | | 57 | 0.2 | 1.7 | 73 | 1.6 | 212 | 250 | 12.6 | 117 | 1.21 |
| 40312 | 1 cup | Fruit, Nature Valley, General Mills | 83 | 320 | 4 | 6.9 | 66.1 | 5.1 | 28.6 | 32.3 | 4.5 | 0.5 | 2.1 | 0.8 | 0.04 | 0.79 | 0 | 0 | 0 | 0 | 0 | 0 | 0.14 | 0.07 | 1.43 | 0.09 | 0.00 | 10.8 | 0.62 | 0.0 | 0.0 | | 60 | 0.2 | 2.1 | 28 | 1.7 | 272 | 244 | 14.4 | 310 | 1.32 |
| 40310 | 1 cup | Fruit N' Nut, Nature Valley, General Mills | 83 | 382 | 5 | 8.9 | 51.7 | 5.1 | 18.8 | 27.8 | 16.8 | 2.9 | 10.7 | 3.1 | 0.10 | 2.13 | 0 | 0 | 0 | 0 | 0 | 0 | 0.29 | 0.14 | 0.97 | 0.10 | 0.00 | 14.9 | 0.65 | 0.0 | 0.0 | | 69 | 0.3 | 2.6 | 84 | 1.8 | 236 | 292 | 14.4 | 116 | 1.64 |
| 40276 | 1 cup | Hearty, C.W. Post | 92 | 422 | 2 | 7.5 | 67.9 | 6.0 | 22.6 | 39.2 | 13.6 | 1.5 | | | | | 0 | 1885 | 566 | 566 | 0 | 0 | 0.57 | 0.64 | 7.54 | 0.75 | 2.26 | 150.8 | | 0.0 | 1.5 | | 30 | 0.3 | 6.8 | 60 | | 226 | 173 | | 226 | 1.36 |
| 40137 | 1 cup | Lowfat, avg | 94 | 362 | 3 | 9.0 | 75.3 | 6.0 | 27.1 | 42.2 | 6.0 | 0.0 | | | | | 0 | 2259 | 452 | | | | 1.13 | 1.28 | 15.04 | 1.50 | 4.52 | 301.7 | | | 3.0 | | | 0.2 | 5.4 | 72 | | 241 | 286 | 18.8 | 180 | 11.28 |
| 40048 | 1 cup | Lowfat, oat & wheat germ, homemade, avg | 122 | 570 | 5 | 17.9 | 64.7 | 12.8 | 33.4 | 18.4 | 30.0 | 5.8 | 9.6 | 12.9 | 0.68 | 12.02 | 0 | 45 | 5 | 0 | 5 | | 0.90 | 0.34 | 2.50 | 0.39 | 0.00 | 104.9 | 0.74 | 1.7 | 0.0 | | 99 | 0.7 | 5.1 | 217 | | 564 | 656 | 24.8 | 29 | 4.95 |
| 38361 | 1 cup | Lowfat, Kellogg's | 98 | 380 | 4 | 8.2 | 78.7 | 5.8 | 24.0 | 48.9 | 5.8 | 0.9 | 1.2 | 3.7 | 0.15 | 2.60 | 0 | 1500 | 451 | 451 | 0 | 0 | 0.78 | 0.88 | 10.00 | 0.98 | 3.04 | 196.0 | 0.00 | 2.9 | 2.0 | | 40 | 0.2 | 3.6 | 83 | 2.7 | 240 | 245 | 17.0 | 240 | 7.55 |
| 40008 | 1 cup | Lowfat, NatureValley, General Mills | 113 | 510 | 4 | 12.0 | 74.5 | 7.2 | 23.1 | 44.2 | 19.9 | 2.6 | 13.3 | 3.8 | 0.13 | 2.61 | 0 | 0 | 0 | 0 | 0 | 0 | 0.35 | 0.12 | 1.25 | 0.16 | 0.00 | 17.0 | 0.94 | 0.0 | 0.0 | | 85 | 0.3 | 3.5 | 107 | 2.7 | 329 | 375 | 19.5 | 183 | 2.27 |
| 40311 | 1 cup | Lowfat, Toasted Oat, 100% natural | 80 | 361 | 4 | 8.0 | 52.8 | 4.8 | 16.0 | 32.0 | 14.1 | 1.8 | | | | | 0 | | | | | | 0.22 | | 0.58 | | | | | | | | 58 | 0.2 | 2.1 | 58 | | 218 | 266 | | 130 | 1.28 |
| 40197 | 1 cup | Lowfat, w/raisins, Kelloggs | 90 | 330 | 5 | 7.4 | 71.5 | 5.4 | 26.3 | 39.8 | 4.5 | 1.5 | 1.1 | 1.9 | 0.10 | 1.76 | 0 | 1125 | 338 | 338 | 0 | 0 | 0.54 | 0.63 | 7.47 | 0.72 | 2.25 | 180.0 | 0.00 | 2.7 | 1.5 | | 40 | 0.2 | 3.1 | 75 | | 208 | 255 | 15.6 | 202 | 5.67 |
| 40063 | 1 cup | Lowfat, 100%Natural Oats & Honey, Quaker | 104 | 462 | 2 | 10.9 | 71.3 | 7.8 | 25.2 | 38.4 | 17.2 | 7.5 | 7.5 | 2.2 | 0.14 | 2.02 | 1 | 7 | 1 | | | | 0.36 | 0.17 | 1.84 | 0.19 | 0.11 | 26.0 | 0.78 | 0.3 | 0.0 | | 100 | 0.7 | 3.1 | 109 | 3.0 | 322 | 457 | 18.0 | 28 | 2.50 |
| 40360 | 1 cup | Lowfat, 100% Natural w/raisins, Quaker | 102 | 437 | 4 | 9.7 | 71.7 | 7.3 | 25.0 | 39.4 | 14.6 | 6.4 | 6.3 | 1.6 | 0.10 | 1.48 | 1 | 7 | 1 | | | | 0.29 | 0.17 | 1.54 | 0.15 | 0.10 | 23.5 | 0.56 | 0.6 | 0.0 | | 78 | 0.6 | 3.3 | 96 | 2.4 | 300 | 427 | 17.6 | 22 | 2.16 |
| 40065 | 1 cup | Lowfat, 100% Natural Raisin & Dates, Quaker | 110 | 496 | 4 | 11.7 | 72.4 | 7.3 | 19.4 | 45.8 | 20.4 | 13.6 | 3.7 | 1.7 | 0.07 | 1.64 | 0 | 61 | 7 | 0 | 7 | | 0.31 | 0.65 | 2.09 | 0.17 | 0.15 | 45.1 | 0.94 | 0.0 | 0.0 | | 160 | 0.5 | 3.1 | 124 | 1.8 | 348 | 538 | 18.8 | 47 | 2.11 |
| 40315 | 1 cup | O's fat free, Almond, Health Valley | 41 | 159 | 4 | 4.0 | 34.4 | 4.0 | 4.0 | 26.5 | 0.0 | 0.0 | 0.0 | 0.0 | 0.00 | 0.00 | 0 | 132 | 40 | 0 | 40 | | | | | | | | | 0.0 | | | 0 | | 1.4 | | | | | | 13 | |
| 40314 | 1 cup | O's fat free, Apple Cinn, Health Valley | 41 | 159 | 4 | 4.0 | 34.4 | 4.0 | 4.0 | 26.5 | 0.0 | 0.0 | 0.0 | 0.0 | 0.00 | 0.00 | 0 | 132 | 40 | 0 | 40 | | | | | | | | | 0.0 | | | 0 | | 1.4 | | | | | | 13 | |
| 40313 | 1 cup | O's fat free, Honey Crunch, Health Valley | 41 | 159 | 4 | 4.0 | 34.4 | 4.0 | 4.0 | 26.5 | 0.0 | 0.0 | 0.0 | 0.0 | 0.00 | 0.00 | 0 | 132 | 40 | 0 | 40 | | | | | | | | | 0.0 | | | 0 | | 1.4 | | | | | | 13 | |
| 40277 | 1 cup | Grape Nuts, Post | 109 | 389 | 3 | 13.4 | 89.4 | 10.9 | 9.9 | 68.6 | 0.4 | 0.1 | 0.1 | 0.2 | 0.01 | 0.19 | 0 | 4806 | 1443 | 1443 | 0 | 0 | 1.42 | 1.63 | 19.18 | 1.96 | 5.78 | 384.8 | 1.04 | 0.0 | 3.8 | | 11 | 0.4 | 31.2 | 73 | 2.6 | 274 | 364 | 10.5 | 758 | 2.40 |
| 40265 | 1 cup | Grape Nuts Flakes, Post | 39 | 144 | 3 | 4.4 | 31.6 | 3.9 | 4.8 | 22.9 | 1.1 | 0.6 | 0.1 | 0.2 | 0.01 | 0.22 | 0 | 1720 | 516 | 516 | 0 | 0 | 0.51 | 0.58 | 6.86 | 0.70 | 2.07 | 137.7 | 0.40 | 0.0 | 1.4 | | 16 | 0.2 | 11.2 | 43 | 1.0 | 116 | 136 | 3.5 | 220 | 0.78 |
| 40290 | 1 cup | Great Grains, Crunchy, Post | 80 | 332 | 7 | 7.5 | 57.4 | 6.0 | 12.1 | 39.2 | 9.1 | 1.5 | | | | | 0 | 1887 | 566 | 566 | 0 | 0 | 0.57 | 0.64 | 7.55 | 0.75 | 2.26 | 150.9 | | 0.0 | 1.5 | | 30 | 0.3 | 4.1 | 60 | | 226 | 181 | | 226 | 1.81 |
| 40291 | 1 cup | Great Grains, Raisins, Dates & Pecans, Post | 82 | 319 | 10 | 6.1 | 59.2 | 6.1 | 19.7 | 33.4 | 7.6 | 0.8 | | | | | 0 | 2278 | 683 | 683 | 0 | 0 | 0.68 | 0.77 | 9.11 | 0.91 | 2.73 | 182.2 | | 0.0 | 2.3 | | 30 | 0.3 | 5.5 | 61 | | 228 | 228 | | 228 | 1.82 |
| 40478 | 1 cup | Halfsies, Quaker | 32 | 129 | 1 | 2.1 | 27.4 | | | | 1.3 | | | | | | | | | | | | 0.42 | 0.30 | 5.71 | 0.57 | 1.14 | 114.3 | 2.29 | | | | 14 | 0.1 | 9.3 | 9 | 0.0 | 33 | 42 | | 278 | 2.29 |
| | | Heartland Cereal | | | | | | | | | | | | | | | | | | | | | | | | | | | | | | | | | | | | | | | | |
| 40236 | 1 cup | Natural, avg | 115 | 499 | 4 | 11.6 | 78.5 | 7.0 | | | 17.7 | 4.5 | 4.8 | 7.1 | 0.32 | 6.70 | 0 | 64 | 7 | 0 | 7 | | 0.36 | 0.16 | 1.61 | 0.19 | 0.00 | 64.4 | 0.96 | 1.1 | | | 75 | 0.3 | 4.3 | 147 | | 416 | 385 | 19.9 | 293 | 3.04 |
| 40237 | 1 cup | Natural, w/coconut, avg | 105 | 463 | 3 | 10.9 | 71.3 | 7.5 | | | 17.1 | 6.2 | 4.0 | 5.7 | 0.26 | 5.38 | 0 | 57 | 6 | 0 | 6 | | 0.35 | 0.15 | 1.78 | 0.16 | 0.00 | 56.7 | 0.84 | 1.0 | | | 66 | 0.5 | 5.4 | 138 | | 380 | 384 | 18.2 | 213 | 2.74 |
| 40238 | 1 cup | Natural, w/raisins | 110 | 468 | 5 | 10.7 | 75.9 | 6.1 | | | 15.6 | 4.0 | 4.2 | 6.2 | 0.29 | 5.90 | 0 | 63 | 7 | 0 | 7 | | 0.32 | 0.14 | 1.54 | 0.20 | 0.00 | 44.0 | 0.91 | 1.1 | | | 66 | 0.5 | 4.0 | 141 | | 376 | 415 | 19.0 | 226 | 2.83 |
| 40129 | 1 cup | Heartwise, avg | 39 | 113 | 4 | 3.9 | 31.2 | 8.6 | | | 0.9 | 0.2 | 0.3 | 0.4 | | | 0 | 1032 | 310 | 310 | 0 | | 0.51 | 0.58 | 7.02 | 0.69 | 1.95 | 136.5 | | 0.0 | 0.0 | | 30 | 0.1 | 6.2 | 55 | | 154 | 265 | | 168 | 2.06 |
| 40052 | 1 cup | Honey Bran, avg | 35 | 119 | 2 | 3.1 | 28.6 | 3.9 | | | 0.7 | 0.3 | 0.1 | 0.3 | 0.02 | 0.24 | 0 | 1543 | 463 | 463 | 0 | 0 | 0.45 | 0.52 | 6.16 | 0.63 | 1.86 | 23.4 | 0.20 | 18.5 | 0.0 | | 16 | 0.2 | 5.6 | 46 | 1.3 | 132 | 150 | 2.5 | 202 | 0.90 |
| 40084 | 1 cup | Honey Bucwheat Crisp, avg | 38 | 147 | 5 | 4.0 | 30.8 | 3.4 | 11.2 | 16.2 | 1.3 | 0.2 | 0.3 | 0.6 | | | 0 | 3015 | 913 | 913 | 0 | | 0.90 | 1.03 | 12.06 | 1.88 | 3.62 | 11.4 | | 36.2 | 0.0 | | 54 | 0.1 | 10.9 | 43 | | 107 | 142 | 3.2 | 361 | 0.68 |
| 40292 | 1 cup | Honey Bunches of Oats, Post | 41 | 172 | 2 | 4.0 | 31.7 | 1.3 | 7.9 | 22.5 | 4.0 | 0.7 | | | | | 0 | 1653 | 496 | 496 | 0 | 0 | 0.50 | 0.56 | 6.61 | 0.66 | 1.98 | 132.3 | | 0.0 | 1.3 | | 0 | 0.1 | 3.6 | 32 | | 79 | 86 | | 238 | 0.40 |
| 40293 | 1 cup | Honey Bunches of Oats w/Almonds, Post | 41 | 172 | 2 | 4.0 | 31.7 | 1.3 | 7.9 | 22.5 | 4.0 | 0.7 | | | | | 0 | 1653 | 496 | 496 | 0 | 0 | 0.50 | 0.56 | 6.61 | 0.66 | 1.98 | 132.3 | | 0.0 | 1.3 | | 0 | 0.1 | 3.6 | 32 | | 79 | 86 | | 238 | 0.40 |
| | | Honey Cluster Flakes | | | | | | | | | | | | | | | | | | | | | | | | | | | | | | | | | | | | | | | | |
| 40319 | 1 cup | Almond, fat free, Health Valley | 41 | 172 | 4 | 4.0 | 34.4 | 5.3 | 5.3 | 23.8 | 0.0 | 0.0 | 0.0 | 0.0 | 0.00 | 0.00 | 0 | 132 | 40 | 40 | 0 | 0 | | | | | | | | 1.6 | | | 0 | | 0.5 | | | | | | 26 | |
| 40320 | 1 cup | Apple Cinn, fat free, Health Valley | 41 | 172 | 4 | 4.0 | 34.4 | 5.3 | 5.3 | 23.8 | 0.0 | 0.0 | 0.0 | 0.0 | 0.00 | 0.00 | 0 | 132 | 40 | 40 | 0 | 0 | | | | | | | | 1.6 | | | 0 | | 0.5 | | | | | | 26 | |
| 40321 | 1 cup | Honey Crunch, fat free, Health Valley | 41 | 172 | 4 | 4.0 | 34.4 | 5.3 | 5.3 | 23.8 | 0.0 | 0.0 | 0.0 | 0.0 | 0.00 | 0.00 | 0 | 132 | 40 | 40 | 0 | 0 | | | | | | | | 1.6 | | | 0 | | 0.5 | | | | | | 26 | |
| 40264 | 1 cup | Honey Comb, Post | 22 | 86 | 1 | 1.3 | 19.6 | 0.6 | 8.5 | 10.5 | 0.4 | 0.2 | 0.1 | 0.1 | 0.00 | 0.11 | 0 | 970 | 291 | 291 | 0 | 0 | 0.29 | 0.33 | 3.87 | 0.40 | 1.17 | 77.7 | 0.09 | 0.0 | 0.8 | | 4 | 0.0 | 2.1 | 7 | 0.1 | 22 | 25 | 2.6 | 124 | 1.17 |
| 40427 | 1 cup | Honey Graham OH!S, Quaker | 36 | 149 | 2 | 1.8 | 30.3 | 0.9 | 14.7 | 14.7 | 2.5 | 0.7 | 1.4 | 0.4 | 0.02 | 0.34 | 0 | 1338 | 402 | 402 | 0 | 0 | 0.50 | 0.57 | 6.70 | 0.67 | 0.00 | 133.9 | 0.11 | 16.1 | 0.0 | | 17 | 0.1 | 6.0 | 17 | 0.2 | 56 | 60 | 3.1 | 237 | 5.00 |
| 40361 | 1 cup | Honey Nut Toasted Oatmeal, Quaker | 49 | 191 | 2 | 4.9 | 39.0 | 3.3 | 13.0 | 22.6 | 2.7 | 0.5 | 1.2 | 0.7 | 0.04 | 0.69 | 0 | 500 | 150 | 150 | 0 | 0 | 0.37 | 0.42 | 5.00 | 0.50 | 0.01 | 100.0 | 0.33 | 6.0 | 0.0 | | 27 | 0.2 | 4.5 | 53 | 1.4 | 166 | 185 | 8.5 | 166 | 3.92 |
| 40491 | 1 cup | Honey Nut Toasted Oats, Krusteaz | 40 | 160 | 3 | 4.0 | 30.7 | 1.3 | 13.3 | 16.0 | 2.7 | 0.0 | | | 0.00 | 0.00 | 0 | 1667 | 501 | 501 | 0 | 0 | | | | | | | | 20.0 | | | 133 | | 6.0 | | | | 80 | | 293 | |
| 40068 | 1 cup | Honey Smacks, Kellogg's | 36 | 137 | 3 | 2.3 | 31.5 | 1.3 | 19.6 | 10.7 | 0.7 | 0.4 | 0.1 | 0.3 | 0.01 | 0.23 | 0 | 1000 | 300 | 300 | 0 | 0 | 0.50 | 0.58 | 6.66 | 0.68 | 0.00 | 133.2 | 0.13 | 20.2 | 1.3 | | 4 | 0.1 | 2.4 | 21 | 0.5 | 53 | 56 | 17.5 | 68 | 0.47 |
| | | Just Right Cereal, Kellogg's | | | | | | | | | | | | | | | | | | | | | | | | | | | | | | | | | | | | | | | | |
| 40108 | 1 cup | Crunchy Nuggets | 56 | 208 | 3 | 4.3 | 46.9 | 2.9 | 11.9 | 32.1 | 1.5 | 0.1 | 0.3 | 1.1 | 0.04 | 0.98 | 0 | 1273 | 382 | 382 | 0 | 0 | 0.39 | 0.45 | 5.10 | 0.50 | 1.51 | 104.2 | 0.00 | 0.0 | 1.0 | | 15 | 0.1 | 16.5 | 35 | 1.2 | 108 | 123 | 2.9 | 344 | 0.90 |
| 40109 | 1 cup | Fruit & Nut | 60 | 210 | 7 | 4.5 | 48.3 | 3.0 | 15.0 | 30.3 | 1.7 | 0.3 | 0.8 | 0.6 | 0.02 | 0.51 | 0 | 1250 | 376 | 376 | 0 | 0 | 0.36 | 0.42 | 4.98 | 0.48 | 1.50 | 120.0 | 0.00 | 0.0 | 1.0 | | 0 | 0.1 | 16.2 | 36 | | 119 | 170 | 3.1 | 290 | 1.14 |
| 40134 | 1 cup | Regular | 43 | 152 | 2 | 4.6 | 36.4 | 3.1 | 10.7 | 22.7 | 0.9 | 0.2 | 0.2 | 0.4 | | | 0 | 1137 | 341 | 341 | 0 | | 2.27 | 2.58 | 30.34 | 3.03 | 9.10 | 606.7 | | 0.0 | | | 11 | 0.1 | 27.3 | 29 | | 94 | 98 | | 288 | 22.75 |
| 40410 | 1 cup | Kaboom, General Mills | 24 | 94 | 3 | 2.1 | 19.4 | 1.2 | 5.9 | 12.3 | 0.9 | 0.2 | 0.3 | 0.1 | 0.00 | 0.09 | 0 | 600 | 180 | 180 | 0 | 0 | 0.30 | 0.34 | 4.01 | 0.40 | 0.00 | 79.9 | 0.14 | 12.0 | 0.0 | | 40 | 0.0 | 6.5 | 15 | 0.4 | 70 | 48 | 4.8 | 220 | 3.00 |
| 40452 | 1 cup | Kamut Flakes, Arrowhead Mills | 32 | 120 | 3 | 4.0 | 25.0 | 3.0 | 2.0 | 20.0 | 1.0 | 0.0 | | | | | 0 | 0 | 0 | 0 | 0 | 0 | 0.06 | 0.00 | 0.40 | | | | | 0.0 | | | 0 | | 1.4 | | | | 190 | | 65 | |

| Code | Amount | Description | Basic Components | | | | | | | | | Additional Fats | | | | | | V t A & Components | | | | | Vitamins | | | | | | | | | | Minerals | | | | | | | | | |
|---|---|---|---|---|---|---|---|---|---|---|---|---|---|---|---|---|---|---|---|---|---|---|---|---|---|---|---|---|---|---|---|---|---|---|---|---|---|---|---|---|---|---|
| | | | Weight (g) | Calories | % Water | Protein (g) | Carbs (g) | Fiber (g) | Sugar (g) | Other Carbs (g) | Fat (g) | Sat Fat (g) | Mono Fat (g) | Poly Fat (g) | Omega 3 (g) | Omega 6 (g) | Choles (mg) | Vit A (IU) | Vit A (RE) | Retinol (RE) | Carotenoids (RE) | Beta Carotene (mcg) | Thiamin (mg) | Riboflavin (mg) | Niacin (NE) | Vit B6 (mg) | Vit B12 (mcg) | Folate (mcg) | Panto (mg) | Vit C (mg) | Vit D (mg) | Vit E (α TE) | Calcium (mg) | Copper (mg) | Iron (mg) | Magnes (mg) | Mang (mg) | Phos (mg) | Potassium (mg) | Selenium (mcg) | Sodium (mg) | Zinc (mg) |
| 40054 | 1 cup | King Vitaman, Quaker | 21 | 81 | 2 | 1.5 | 17.7 | 0.8 | 4.4 | 12.4 | 0.7 | 0.2 | 0.3 | 0.2 | 0.01 | 0.22 | 0 | 707 | 212 | 212 | 0 | 0 | 0.26 | 0.30 | 3.53 | 0.35 | 1.06 | 70.8 | 0.10 | 8.4 | 3.0 | | 3 | 0.1 | 5.9 | 18 | 0.2 | 54 | 58 | 4.2 | 176 | 2.65 |
| 40010 | 1 cup | Kix , General Mills | 19 | 72 | 2 | 1.2 | 16.4 | 0.5 | 2.1 | 13.8 | 0.4 | 0.1 | 0.1 | 0.0 | 0.00 | 0.02 | 0 | 792 | 238 | 238 | 0 | 0 | 0.24 | 0.27 | 3.17 | 0.32 | 0.00 | 63.3 | 0.08 | 9.5 | 0.7 | | 28 | 0.0 | 5.1 | 6 | 0.2 | 27 | 26 | 3.8 | 167 | 2.38 |
| 40296 | 1 cup | Kix, Berry Berry, General Mills | 40 | 160 | 2 | 1.7 | 34.8 | 0.2 | 12.0 | 22.6 | 1.5 | 0.3 | 0.6 | 0.1 | 0.00 | 0.08 | 0 | 1000 | 300 | 300 | 0 | 0 | 0.50 | 0.57 | 6.68 | 0.67 | 0.00 | 133.2 | 0.11 | 20.0 | 0.0 | | 88 | 0.0 | 6.0 | 8 | 0.2 | 50 | 32 | 8.0 | 246 | 5.00 |
| | | Life Cereal, Quaker | | | | | | | | | | | | | | | | | | | | | | | | | | | | | | | | | | | | | | | | |
| 40426 | 1 cup | Cinnamon Oat | 50 | 190 | 4 | 4.4 | 40.4 | 3.0 | 15.6 | 21.8 | 1.7 | 0.3 | 0.6 | 0.8 | 0.03 | 0.71 | 0 | 16 | 1.5 | 0 | 1.5 | | 0.63 | 0.71 | 8.40 | 0.83 | 0.00 | 167.5 | 0.28 | 0.1 | 0.0 | | 134 | 0.1 | 7.6 | 42 | 1.6 | 181 | 113 | 11.8 | 220 | 6.30 |
| 40011 | 1 cup | Regular | 44 | 167 | 4 | 4.3 | 34.6 | 2.8 | 9.3 | 22.5 | 1.8 | 0.3 | 0.6 | 0.8 | 0.03 | 0.72 | 0 | 16 | 1.6 | 0 | 1.5 | | 0.55 | 0.62 | 7.35 | 0.73 | 0.00 | 147.0 | 0.29 | 0.0 | 0.0 | | 134 | 0.1 | 12.3 | 43 | 1.3 | 187 | 109 | 10.4 | 240 | 5.50 |
| 40479 | 1 cup | With Raisins | 43 | 161 | 10 | 8.4 | 25.8 | 0.9 | | | 2.8 | | | | | | | | | | | | 0.57 | 0.64 | 7.68 | 0.06 | 0.00 | 27.6 | 0.00 | | | | 92 | 0.3 | 12.4 | 69 | 1.5 | 154 | 356 | | 247 | 1.54 |
| 40300 | 1 cup | Lucky Charms, General Mills | 32 | 124 | 2 | 2.3 | 26.8 | 1.3 | 13.9 | 11.7 | 1.2 | 0.2 | 0.4 | 0.2 | 0.01 | 0.15 | 0 | 800 | 240 | 240 | 0 | 0 | 0.40 | 0.45 | 5.34 | 0.53 | 0.00 | 106.6 | 0.23 | 16.0 | 1.1 | | 35 | 0.0 | 4.8 | 21 | 0.7 | 81 | 58 | 6.3 | 217 | 4.00 |
| 40451 | 1 cup | Maple Corns, Arrowhead Mills | 53 | 190 | 3 | 5.0 | 43.0 | 6.0 | 11.0 | 26.0 | 3.0 | 0.5 | | | | | 0 | 0 | 0 | 0 | 0 | 0 | 0.15 | 0.03 | 0.80 | | | | | 0.0 | | | 20 | | 1.1 | | | | 105 | | 140 | |
| 40056 | 1 cup | Most Cereal, avg | 52 | 175 | 5 | 7.4 | 39.6 | 7.3 | | | 0.6 | 0.1 | 0.2 | 0.3 | | | 0 | 9171 | 2754 | 2754 | 0 | | 2.76 | 3.13 | 36.66 | 3.69 | 11.02 | 733.7 | 0.70 | 110.2 | 0.0 | | 79 | 0.3 | 33.0 | 103 | 3.6 | 361 | 340 | | 276 | 2.76 |
| | | Mueslix Cereal | | | | | | | | | | | | | | | | | | | | | | | | | | | | | | | | | | | | | | | | |
| 40417 | 1 cup | Apple & Almond Crunch, Kelloggs | 71 | 272 | 4 | 7.0 | 52.8 | 6.0 | 12.0 | 34.7 | 6.4 | 1.3 | 3.3 | 1.3 | 0.07 | 1.28 | 0 | 1005 | 302 | 302 | 0 | 0 | 0.50 | 0.57 | 6.67 | 0.64 | 1.63 | 142.0 | 2.70 | 0.0 | 3.4 | | 43 | 0.1 | 6.0 | 81 | 1.7 | 226 | 270 | 12.3 | 349 | 4.05 |
| 40328 | 1 cup | Blueberry Pecan, Ralston Purina | 54 | 200 | 10 | 5.0 | 41.0 | 4.0 | 14.0 | 23.0 | 2.5 | 1.5 | | | | | 0 | 1500 | 450 | 450 | 0 | 0 | 0.45 | 0.51 | 6.00 | 0.60 | 1.80 | 120.0 | | 0.0 | 1.0 | | 0 | | 4.5 | | | | | | 170 | 1.50 |
| 40124 | 1 cup | Five Grain, avg | 82 | 279 | 5 | 7.4 | 63.1 | 7.4 | 21.7 | 34.0 | 3.3 | 0.5 | 1.0 | 1.2 | | | 0 | 2488 | 747 | 747 | 0 | | 0.75 | 0.84 | 9.84 | 0.99 | 3.28 | 196.8 | | 0.8 | 0.0 | | 38 | 0.1 | 8.9 | 82 | | 215 | 369 | | 107 | 7.46 |
| 40329 | 1 cup | Cranberry Walnut, Ralston Purina | 72 | 267 | 11 | 6.7 | 53.3 | 5.3 | 18.7 | 29.3 | 4.0 | | | | | | 0 | 2000 | 600 | 600 | 0 | 0 | 0.60 | 0.68 | 8.00 | 0.80 | 2.40 | 160.0 | | 0.0 | 0.0 | | 0 | | 6.0 | | | | | | 240 | 2.00 |
| 40330 | 1 cup | Peach Pecan, Ralston Purina | 71 | 268 | 11 | 6.7 | 52.2 | 5.4 | 16.1 | 30.8 | 4.0 | 0.0 | | | | | 0 | 2009 | 603 | 603 | 0 | 0 | 0.60 | 0.68 | 8.04 | 0.80 | 2.41 | 160.8 | | 0.0 | 1.3 | | 0 | | 6.0 | | | | | | 228 | 2.01 |
| 40332 | 1 cup | Raspberry Almond, Ralston Purina | 77 | 292 | 10 | 6.6 | 58.4 | 5.3 | 18.6 | 34.5 | 4.0 | 0.0 | | | | | 0 | 2323 | 698 | 698 | 0 | 0 | 0.70 | 0.79 | 9.29 | 0.93 | 2.79 | 185.9 | | 0.0 | 1.3 | | 0 | | 6.0 | | | | | | 226 | 1.99 |
| 40418 | 1 cup | Raisin & Almond Crunch w/Dates, Kelloggs | 82 | 298 | 10 | 6.6 | 60.4 | 5.6 | 2.5 | 52.3 | 4.8 | 0.6 | 2.9 | 1.3 | 0.06 | 1.21 | 0 | 298 | 39 | 39 | 0 | 0 | 0.57 | 0.66 | 7.46 | 0.00 | 2.21 | 164.0 | 3.69 | 0.0 | 0.3 | | 30 | 0.2 | 6.7 | 70 | 1.8 | 198 | 343 | 14.2 | 239 | 5.58 |
| 40331 | 1 cup | Strawberry Pecan, Ralston Purina | 54 | 210 | 8 | 5.0 | 42.0 | 3.0 | 14.0 | 25.0 | 2.5 | 0.0 | | | | | 0 | 1500 | 450 | 450 | 0 | 0 | 0.45 | 0.51 | 6.00 | 0.60 | 1.80 | 120.0 | | 0.0 | 1.0 | | 0 | | 4.5 | | | | | | 170 | 1.50 |
| 40450 | 1 cup | Multi-grain Flakes, Arrowhead Mills | 35 | 140 | 4 | 3.0 | 29.0 | 3.0 | 3.0 | 23.0 | 1.5 | 0.0 | | | | | 0 | 0 | 0 | 0 | 0 | 0 | 0.09 | 0.03 | 0.80 | | | | | 0.0 | | | 20 | | 1.1 | | | | 110 | | 130 | |
| 40350 | 1 cup | Multi-grain Flakes, Healthy Choice, Kelloggs | 41 | 142 | 3 | 3.5 | 34.5 | 3.5 | 8.5 | 22.1 | 0.5 | 0.0 | 0.2 | 0.2 | 0.01 | 0.23 | 0 | 683 | 205 | 205 | 0 | 0 | 0.74 | 0.82 | 9.55 | 0.94 | 2.87 | 123.0 | 4.80 | 0.0 | 2.6 | | 12 | 0.1 | 8.6 | 40 | 1.2 | 118 | 137 | 4.2 | 238 | 2.05 |
| 40449 | 1 cup | Nature O's, Arrowhead Mills | 32 | 130 | 3 | 5.0 | 24.0 | 3.0 | 1.0 | 20.0 | 2.0 | 0.5 | | | | | 0 | 0 | 0 | 0 | 0 | 0 | 0.09 | 0.07 | 0.80 | | | | | 0.0 | | | 0 | | 1.1 | | | | 120 | | 5 | |
| 40112 | 1 cup | Nut & Honey Crunch, Kelloggs | 37 | 150 | 2 | 2.7 | 30.9 | 0.5 | 12.0 | 18.4 | 1.7 | 0.3 | 0.8 | 0.5 | 0.02 | 0.54 | 0 | 505 | 152 | 152 | 0 | 0 | 0.26 | 0.30 | 3.37 | 0.33 | 0.00 | 74.0 | 0.00 | 10.1 | 0.7 | | 4 | 0.0 | 3.0 | 3 | 0.1 | 24 | 40 | 2.7 | 249 | 0.26 |
| 40115 | 1 cup | Nutri-grain Almond & Raisin, Kelloggs | 39 | 143 | 6 | 3.1 | 30.3 | 3.1 | 5.6 | 21.6 | 2.2 | 0.1 | 1.0 | 1. | 0.03 | 1.10 | 0 | 0 | 0 | 0 | 0 | 0 | 0.27 | 0.31 | 3.55 | 0.35 | 1.05 | 78.0 | 0.00 | 0.0 | 0.0 | | 119 | 0.0 | 1.0 | 9 | 0.9 | 133 | 139 | 4.0 | 138 | 2.65 |
| 40213 | 1 cup | Nutri-grain Wheat, Kelloggs | 40 | 134 | 4 | 4.0 | 32.0 | 5.0 | 0.5 | 26.5 | 1.3 | 0.1 | 0.3 | 0.3 | 0.00 | 0.91 | 0 | 0 | 0 | 0 | 0 | 0 | 0.52 | 0.56 | 6.68 | 0.68 | 2.00 | 120.0 | 0.00 | 20.0 | 0.0 | | 13 | 0.1 | 1.3 | 32 | 0.9 | 144 | 146 | 4.2 | 294 | 5.00 |
| 40434 | 1 cup | Oat Bran, Quaker | 46 | 172 | 4 | 6.9 | 33.4 | 4.3 | 7.3 | 21.3 | 2.4 | 0.4 | 0.8 | 1.0 | 0.04 | 0.91 | 0 | 419 | 126 | 126 | 0 | 0 | 0.31 | 0.35 | 4.19 | 0.42 | 0.00 | 83.7 | 0.39 | 5.0 | 0.0 | | 24 | 0.1 | 12.9 | 80 | 1.8 | 247 | 207 | 14.0 | 166 | 3.14 |
| 40448 | 1 cup | Oat Bran Flakes, Arrowhead Mills | 34 | 110 | 4 | 6.0 | 22.0 | 4.0 | 8.0 | 10.0 | 2.0 | 1.0 | | | | | 0 | 0 | 0 | 0 | 0 | 0 | 0.22 | 0.10 | 3.00 | | | | | 0.0 | | | 0 | | 1.8 | | | | 120 | | 60 | |
| 40041 | 1 cup | Oat Flakes, Post | 48 | 180 | 3 | 7.9 | 36.1 | 1.4 | 10.6 | 24.1 | 1.0 | 0.2 | 0.3 | 0.1 | 0.01 | 0.34 | 0 | 2116 | 636 | 636 | 0 | 0 | 0.62 | 0.72 | 8.45 | 0.86 | 2.54 | 169.4 | 0.49 | 0.0 | 1.7 | | 68 | 0.3 | 13.7 | 58 | 1.4 | 176 | 228 | 6.8 | 220 | 2.54 |
| 40348 | 1 cup | Oatmeal Crisp w/Almonds, General Mills | 55 | 219 | 2 | 5.8 | 42.0 | 4.3 | 15.5 | 22.1 | 4.6 | 0.5 | 2.4 | 1. | 0.05 | 1.05 | 0 | 0 | 0 | 0 | 0 | 0 | 0.37 | 0.42 | 5.00 | 0.50 | 0.00 | 99.6 | 0.35 | 9.0 | | | 36 | 0.2 | 4.5 | 57 | 1.1 | 144 | 185 | 9.5 | 250 | 3.75 |
| 40342 | 1 cup | Oatmeal Crisp w/Apples, General Mills | 55 | 205 | 2 | 4.3 | 46.2 | 4.5 | 19.4 | 22.4 | 1.8 | 0.4 | 0.6 | 0. | 0.01 | 0.19 | 0 | 0 | 0 | 0 | 0 | 0 | 0.37 | 0.42 | 5.00 | 0.50 | 0.00 | 99.6 | 0.42 | 9.0 | 0.0 | | 23 | 0.1 | 4.5 | 45 | 1.1 | 122 | 160 | 9.5 | 282 | 3.75 |
| 40302 | 1 cup | Oatmeal Raisin Crisp, General Mills | 55 | 204 | 6 | 4.4 | 43.7 | 3.5 | 18.9 | 21.3 | 2.4 | 0.4 | 1.2 | 0. | 0.02 | 0.35 | 0 | 750 | 226 | 226 | 0 | 0 | 0.37 | 0.42 | 5.01 | 0.50 | 0.00 | 100.1 | 0.34 | 0.0 | 1.0 | | 38 | 0.2 | 4.5 | 45 | 0.0 | 117 | 212 | 9.5 | 224 | 3.75 |
| 40430 | 1 cup | Oatmeal Squares, Quaker | 56 | 216 | 2 | 7.3 | 43.3 | 4.3 | 9.0 | 30.1 | 2.6 | 0.5 | 0.8 | 1. | 0.04 | 0.97 | 0 | 563 | 169 | 169 | 0 | 0 | 0.42 | 0.48 | 5.66 | 0.56 | 0.00 | 112.6 | 0.44 | 6.8 | 0.0 | | 36 | 0.2 | 15.7 | 70 | 2.0 | 186 | 228 | 9.7 | 253 | 4.22 |
| 40474 | 1 cup | Popeye Sweet Crunch, Quaker | 28 | 115 | 3 | 1.3 | 23.4 | 0.7 | | | 1.8 | 1.0 | 0.2 | 0. | | | | 0 | 0 | 0 | 0 | 0 | 0.48 | 0.67 | 4.84 | 0.70 | 2.61 | 2.8 | 0.03 | 0.0 | | | 4 | | 5.7 | 21 | | 32 | 37 | | 209 | 0.08 |
| 40216 | 1 cup | Product 19, Kellogg's | 30 | 110 | 3 | 2.7 | 25.0 | 1.0 | 3.5 | 20.5 | 0.4 | 0.0 | 0.2 | 0. | 0.01 | 0.19 | 0 | 750 | 225 | 225 | 0 | 0 | 1.50 | 1.71 | 20.01 | 2.01 | 6.00 | 390.0 | 9.99 | 60.0 | 1.0 | | 3 | 0.0 | 18.0 | 12 | 0.3 | 33 | 41 | 3.6 | 216 | 15.00 |
| 40462 | 1 cup | Puffed Corn, Arrowhead Mills | 22 | 80 | 4 | 3.0 | 16.0 | 1.0 | 0.0 | 15.0 | 0.0 | 0.0 | 0.0 | 0. | 0.00 | 0.00 | 0 | 0 | 0 | 0 | 0 | 0 | 0.00 | 0.00 | 0.00 | | | | | 0.0 | | | 0 | | 1.1 | | | | 70 | | 0 | |
| 40316 | 1 cup | Puffed Corn, Honey Swtnd, fat free, Health Valley | 23 | 80 | 3 | 2.0 | 20.0 | 2.0 | 3.0 | 15.0 | 0.0 | 0.0 | 0.0 | 0. | 0.00 | 0.00 | 0 | 0 | 0 | 0 | 0 | 0 | | | | | | | | 0.0 | | | 0 | | 0.4 | | | | | | 0 | |
| 40461 | 1 cup | Puffed Kamut, Arrowhead Mills | 16 | 50 | 4 | 2.0 | 11.0 | 2.0 | 0.0 | 9.0 | 0.0 | 0.0 | 0.0 | 0. | 0.00 | 0.00 | 0 | 0 | 0 | 0 | 0 | 0 | 0.03 | | 0.40 | | | | | 0.0 | | | 0 | | 0.4 | | | | 70 | | 0 | |
| 40460 | 1 cup | Puffed Millet, Arrowhead Mills | 25 | 90 | 4 | 3.0 | 19.0 | 1.0 | 0.0 | 18.0 | 0.5 | 0.0 | | | | | 0 | 0 | 0 | 0 | 0 | 0 | 0.00 | 0.00 | 0.80 | | | | | 0.0 | | | 0 | | 0.7 | | | | 70 | | 0 | |
| 40018 | 1 cup | Puffed rice, Quaker | 14 | 54 | 4 | 1.0 | 12.3 | 0.2 | 0.0 | 12.1 | 0.1 | 0.0 | 0.0 | 0. | 0.01 | 0.04 | 0 | 0 | 0 | 0 | 0 | 0 | 0.06 | 0.01 | 0.88 | 0.00 | 0.00 | 1.4 | 0.05 | 0.0 | 0.0 | | 1 | 0.1 | 0.4 | 4 | 0.1 | 17 | 16 | 1.5 | 1 | 0.15 |
| 40023 | 1 cup | Puffed Wheat, Quaker | 12 | 44 | 4 | 2.0 | 9.2 | 1.1 | 0.2 | 7.9 | 0.3 | 0.0 | 0.0 | 0. | 0.01 | 0.12 | 0 | 1.3 | 0.1 | 0 | 0.1 | | 0.05 | 0.03 | 1.43 | 0.02 | 0.05 | 4.1 | 0.06 | 0.0 | 0.0 | | 3 | 0.1 | 0.6 | 16 | 0.2 | 40 | 44 | 14.8 | 1 | 0.37 |
| 40066 | 1 cup | Quisp, Quaker | 30 | 121 | 3 | 1.5 | 25.5 | 0.8 | 12.8 | 12.0 | 1.7 | 0.5 | 0.4 | 0. | 0.01 | 0.20 | 0 | 37 | 4 | 0 | 4 | | 0.42 | 0.48 | 5.67 | 0.56 | 0.00 | 113.1 | 0.10 | 0.0 | 0.0 | | 6 | 0.1 | 5.1 | 15 | 0.2 | 47 | 40 | 6.0 | 216 | 4.26 |
| | | Raisin Bran Cereal | | | | | | | | | | | | | | | | | | | | | | | | | | | | | | | | | | | | | | | | |
| 40209 | 1 cup | Kellogg's | 61 | 186 | 8 | 5.6 | 47.1 | 8.2 | 18.3 | 20.6 | 1.5 | 0.0 | 0.2 | 0. | 0.03 | 0.36 | 0 | 332 | 250 | 250 | 0 | 0 | 0.43 | 0.49 | 5.55 | 0.55 | 1.65 | 122.0 | 0.40 | 0.0 | 1.0 | | 35 | 0.2 | 5.0 | 89 | 1.9 | 214 | 437 | 4.3 | 354 | 4.15 |
| 40393 | 1 cup | Nut Bran, Kelloggs | 55 | 209 | 4 | 5.2 | 41.5 | 5.1 | 16.0 | 20.4 | 4.4 | 0.7 | 1.9 | 0. | 0.03 | 0.43 | 0 | 0 | 0 | 0 | 0 | 0 | 0.37 | 0.42 | 5.00 | 0.50 | 0.00 | 99.6 | 0.34 | 0.0 | 0.0 | | 74 | 0.2 | 4.5 | 54 | 1.3 | 163 | 218 | 3.9 | 246 | 1.11 |
| 40260 | 1 cup | Post | 56 | 172 | 9 | 5.2 | 42.3 | 7.9 | 14.9 | 19.5 | 1.1 | 0.2 | 0.1 | 0. | 0.04 | 0.47 | 0 | 2469 | 741 | 741 | 0 | 0 | 0.73 | 0.84 | 9.86 | 1.01 | 2.97 | 197.7 | 0.41 | 0.0 | 2.1 | | 26 | 0.3 | 8.9 | 95 | 2.1 | 235 | 345 | 4.0 | 365 | 2.97 |
| 40117 | 1 cup | Raisin Squares, Kelloggs | 71 | 241 | 10 | 5.7 | 55.4 | 6.7 | 15.1 | 33.7 | 2.0 | 0.2 | 0.1 | 0. | 0.05 | 0.59 | 0 | 0 | 0 | 0 | 0 | 0 | 0.50 | 0.57 | 6.67 | 0.64 | 1.99 | 142.0 | 0.00 | 0.0 | 0.0 | | 24 | 0.1 | 21.7 | 62 | 1.6 | 206 | 335 | 2.9 | 4 | 1.99 |
| 40343 | 1 cup | Reese's Peanut Butter Puffs, General Mills | 40 | 172 | 2 | 3.4 | 30.6 | 0.5 | 15.5 | 14.5 | 4.3 | 0.8 | 1.9 | 0. | 0.02 | 0.78 | 0 | 1000 | 300 | 300 | 0 | 0 | 0.50 | 0.57 | 6.68 | 0.67 | 0.00 | 133.2 | 0.19 | 20.0 | 0.0 | | 28 | 0.1 | 6.0 | 21 | 0.4 | 58 | 82 | 2.6 | 236 | 5.00 |
| 40338 | 1 cup | Rice, w/other grains & raisins, avg | 46 | 155 | 6 | 2.6 | 39.3 | 2.6 | 12.2 | 24.4 | 0.1 | 0.0 | 0.0 | 0. | 0.01 | 0.04 | 0 | 1558 | 468 | 468 | 0 | 0 | 0.46 | 0.55 | 6.26 | 0.64 | 1.89 | 124.7 | 0.34 | 0.5 | | | 10 | 0.1 | 5.6 | 20 | | 50 | 144 | | 350 | 4.69 |
| 40303 | 1 cup | Rice Crunchins, General Mills | 21 | 84 | 4 | 1.7 | 17.9 | 0.2 | 1.3 | 16.4 | 0.3 | 0. | | | | | 0 | 875 | 263 | 263 | 0 | 0 | 0.26 | 0.30 | 3.50 | 0.35 | | 0.1 | | 10.5 | 0.7 | | 5 | 0.1 | 5.7 | 6 | | 28 | 24 | | 192 | 0.21 |
| | | Rice Krispies | | | | | | | | | | | | | | | | | | | | | | | | | | | | | | | | | | | | | | | | |
| 40340 | 1 cup | Apple Cinnamon, Kelloggs | 39 | 145 | 3 | 2.0 | 34.7 | 0.6 | 14.8 | 19.3 | 0.2 | 0. | 0.0 | 0. | 0.02 | 0.07 | 0 | 1009 | 303 | 303 | 0 | 0 | 0.51 | 0.58 | 6.71 | 0.66 | 0.00 | 117.0 | 0.36 | 20.2 | 1.3 | | 3 | 0.0 | 2.4 | 10 | 1.0 | 32 | 40 | 6.0 | 290 | 0.43 |
| 40105 | 1 cup | Frosted, Kelloggs | 35 | 132 | 2 | 1.6 | 31.6 | 0.4 | 12.9 | 18.3 | 0.2 | 0. | 0.1 | 0. | 0.01 | 0.06 | 0 | 1010 | 303 | 303 | 0 | 0 | 0.49 | 0.56 | 6.72 | 0.66 | 0.00 | 140.0 | 0.24 | 20.2 | 1.3 | | 2 | 0.0 | 2.4 | 8 | 0.3 | 28 | 27 | 5.4 | 256 | 0.42 |
| 40210 | 1 cup | Kelloggs | 26 | 98 | 3 | 1.6 | 22.5 | 0.3 | 2.4 | 19.3 | 0.3 | 0. | 0.1 | 0. | 0.02 | 0.09 | 0 | 650 | 195 | 195 | 0 | 0 | 0.34 | 0.36 | 4.34 | 0.44 | 0.00 | 91.8 | 0.25 | 13.0 | 0.8 | | 3 | 0.1 | 1.6 | 12 | 0.3 | 34 | 33 | 4.0 | 279 | 0.47 |
| 40420 | 1 cup | Treats Cereal, Kelloggs | 40 | 160 | 4 | 1.5 | 34.2 | 0.4 | 11.5 | 22.3 | 2.1 | 0.5 | 1.3 | 0. | 0.03 | 0.29 | 0 | 1000 | 300 | 300 | 0 | 0 | 0.52 | 0.56 | 6.68 | 0.68 | 2.00 | 120.0 | 0.00 | 20.0 | 1.3 | | 2 | 0.0 | 2.4 | 8 | 0.2 | 27 | 25 | 4.8 | 253 | 0.40 |
| | | Shredded Wheat | | | | | | | | | | | | | | | | | | | | | | | | | | | | | | | | | | | | | | | | |
| 40062 | 1 ea | Large biscuit, 1.7 oz, avg | 47 | 169 | 4 | 5.1 | 38.2 | 4.6 | 0.2 | 33.4 | 0.8 | 0. | 0.1 | 0. | 0.03 | 0.38 | 0 | 0 | 0 | 0 | 0 | 0 | 0.13 | 0.13 | 2.15 | 0.12 | 0.00 | 23.5 | 0.38 | 0.0 | 0.0 | | 19 | 0.2 | 1.5 | 80 | 1.4 | 171 | 154 | 2.8 | 1 | 1.18 |
| 40288 | 1 cup | N' Bran, Nabisco | 47 | 159 | 5 | 5.6 | 37.4 | 6.4 | 0.8 | 30.3 | 0.8 | 0.0 | | | 0.00 | 0.00 | 0 | 0 | 0 | 0 | 0 | 0 | 0.12 | 0.03 | 3.19 | 0.13 | 0.00 | 19.1 | | 0.0 | 0.0 | | 16 | 0.2 | 2.2 | 64 | | 199 | 199 | | 0 | 1.79 |
| 40022 | 1 cup | Small biscuit, avg | 43 | 154 | 5 | 4.7 | 34.6 | 4.2 | 0.2 | 30.2 | 0.7 | 0.1 | 0.1 | 0. | 0.03 | 0.35 | 0 | 0 | 0 | 0 | 0 | 0 | 0.11 | 0.12 | 2.26 | 0.11 | 0.00 | 21.5 | 0.36 | 0.0 | 0.0 | | 16 | 0.3 | 1.8 | 57 | 1.3 | 152 | 155 | 2.5 | 4 | 1.42 |
| 40287 | 1 cup | Spoon size, Nabisco | 49 | 170 | 5 | 5.0 | 41.0 | 5.0 | 0.0 | 36.0 | 0.5 | 0.0 | | | 0.00 | 0.00 | 0 | 0 | 0 | 0 | 0 | 0 | 0.12 | 0.03 | 3.00 | 0.16 | 0.00 | 16.0 | | 0.0 | 0.0 | | 20 | 0.2 | 1.4 | 60 | | 200 | 200 | | 0 | 1.20 |
| 40396 | 1 cup | S'Mores Grahams, General Mills | 40 | 156 | 3 | 2.2 | 34.1 | 1.1 | 16.6 | 16.4 | 1.6 | 0.2 | 0.5 | 0.2 | 0.01 | 0.19 | 0 | 1000 | 300 | 300 | 0 | 0 | 0.50 | 0.57 | 6.68 | 0.67 | 0.00 | 133.2 | 0.13 | 20.0 | 1.3 | | 19 | 0.1 | 6.0 | 14 | 0.4 | 54 | 64 | 6.0 | 283 | 5.00 |
| 40211 | 1 cup | Special K, Kelloggs | 31 | 115 | 3 | 6.4 | 22.4 | 1.0 | 3.0 | 18.5 | 0.3 | 0.0 | 0.0 | 0.2 | 0.01 | 0.13 | 0 | 750 | 225 | 225 | 0 | 0 | 0.53 | 0.59 | 7.01 | 0.71 | 0.00 | 93.0 | 0.00 | 15.0 | 1.0 | | 5 | 0.0 | 8.7 | 18 | 0.9 | 51 | 55 | 17.0 | 250 | 3.75 |
| 40457 | 1 cup | Spelt Flakes, Arrowhead Mills | 30 | 100 | 3 | 5.0 | 22.0 | 3.0 | 2.0 | 17.0 | 1.0 | 0.0 | | | | | 0 | 0 | 0 | 0 | 0 | 0 | 0.09 | 0.03 | 0.80 | | | | | 0.0 | | | 0 | | 1.1 | | | | 140 | | 60 | |
| 40118 | 1 cup | Strawberry Squares, Kelloggs | 67 | 228 | 9 | 5.4 | 52.9 | 6.2 | 11.7 | 35.1 | 1.6 | 0.3 | 0.3 | 1.0 | 0.06 | 0.75 | 0 | 0 | 0 | 0 | 0 | 0 | 0.54 | 0.60 | 6.70 | 0.67 | 2.01 | 134.0 | 0.00 | 0.0 | 0.0 | | 27 | 0.2 | 21.7 | 80 | 1.6 | 206 | 228 | 2.7 | 20 | 2.01 |
| 40149 | 1 cup | Sugar Frosted Flakes, Ralston | 38 | 149 | 2 | 2.0 | 34.2 | 0.8 | 15.0 | 18.4 | 0.5 | 0.3 | 0.1 | 0.1 | 0.00 | 0.09 | 0 | 1675 | 503 | 503 | 0 | 0 | 0.49 | 0.57 | 6.69 | 0.68 | 2.01 | 2.7 | 0.01 | 20.1 | | | 4 | 0.0 | 0.9 | 3 | 0.0 | 9 | 24 | 1.7 | 247 | 0.82 |
| 40339 | 1 cup | Sugar Sparkled Flakes, avg | 38 | 146 | 2 | 2.0 | 34.6 | 0.5 | 15.0 | 19.1 | 0.1 | 0.0 | 0.0 | 0.0 | 0.00 | 0.03 | 0 | 1675 | 503 | 503 | 0 | 0 | 0.49 | 0.57 | 6.69 | 0.68 | 2.01 | 134.1 | 0.01 | 0.0 | | | 5 | 0.1 | 0.5 | 4 | 0.0 | 10 | 85 | 1.7 | 215 | 0.07 |
| 40349 | 1 cup | Sun Crunchers, General Mills | 55 | 216 | 3 | 4.9 | 43.7 | 2.2 | 16.5 | 25.0 | 3.2 | 0.3 | 2.0 | 0.3 | 0.01 | 0.32 | 0 | 750 | 225 | 225 | 0 | 0 | 0.37 | 0.42 | 5.00 | 0.50 | 0.00 | 99.6 | 0.45 | 15.0 | | | 85 | 0.2 | 4.5 | 43 | 1.0 | 172 | 130 | 5.6 | 380 | 0.80 |
| | | Sunflakes | | | | | | | | | | | | | | | | | | | | | | | | | | | | | | | | | | | | | | | | |
| 40482 | 1 cup | Corn & Rice, Ralston Purina | 36 | 141 | | 1.8 | 30.9 | 1.3 | | | 1.2 | | | | | | | | | | | | 0.49 | 0.17 | 6.43 | 0.64 | 1.93 | 128.6 | 0.44 | 19.3 | | | 12 | | 2.3 | 15 | | 32 | 40 | | 305 | 0.24 |
| 40334 | 1 cup | Ralston Purina | 36 | 147 | 3 | 2.7 | 30.7 | 1.3 | 0.0 | 29.3 | 1.3 | 0.0 | | | | | 0 | 1333 | 400 | 400 | 0 | 0 | 0.40 | | 5.33 | 0.53 | 1.60 | 106.7 | | 16.0 | 10.7 | | 0 | | 1.9 | | | | | | 280 | |
| 40483 | 1 cup | Wheat & Rice, Ralston Purina | 36 | 174 | | 3.0 | 30.9 | | | | 4.4 | | | | | | | | | | | | 0.49 | | 6.43 | 0.64 | 1.93 | 128.6 | 0.62 | 19.3 | | | | | 2.3 | | | | 90 | | 234 | |

| Code | Amount | Description | Weight (g) | Calories | % Water | Protein (g) | Carbs (g) | Fiber (g) | Sugar (g) | Other Carbs (g) | Fat (g) | Sat Fat (g) | Mono Fat (g) | Poly Fat (g) | Omega 3 (g) | Omega 6 (g) | Choles (mg) | Vit A (IU) | Vit A (RE) | Retinol (RE) | Carotenoids (RE) | Beta Carotene (mcg) |
|---|---|---|---|---|---|---|---|---|---|---|---|---|---|---|---|---|---|---|---|---|---|---|
| | | **Basic Components** | | | | | | | | | | **Additional Fats** | | | | | | **Vit A & Components** | | | | |
| 40261 | 1 cup | Super Golden Crisp, Post | 33 | 123 | 2 | 2.3 | 29.8 | 0.5 | 17.4 | 11.9 | 0.3 | 0.1 | 0.1 | 0.1 | 0.01 | 0.11 | 0 | 1455 | 437 | 437 | 0 | 0 |
| 40070 | 1 cup | Tasteeos, avg | 24 | 94 | 2 | 3.1 | 19.0 | 2.5 | 0.7 | 15.8 | 0.7 | 0.2 | 0.2 | 0.2 | 0.01 | 0.17 | 0 | 1058 | 318 | 318 | 0 | 0 |
| 40289 | 1 cup | Team Flakes, Nabisco | 46 | 178 | 3 | 3.2 | 39.5 | 0.8 | 8.1 | 30.7 | 0.0 | 0.0 | 0.0 | 0.0 | 0.00 | 0.00 | 0 | 1009 | 303 | 303 | 0 | 0 |
| 40071 | 1 cup | Team Rice, Nabisco | 42 | 164 | 4 | 2.8 | 36.0 | 0.5 | 7.5 | 28.0 | 0.8 | 0.1 | 0.2 | 0.3 | 0.02 | 0.30 | 0 | 1852 | 556 | 556 | 0 | 0 |
| 40351 | 1 cup | Temptations, French Vanilla Almond, Kelloggs | 35 | 139 | 3 | 2.5 | 28.8 | 0.9 | 10.2 | 17.7 | 1.9 | 1.2 | 0.4 | 0.3 | 0.02 | 0.26 | 0 | 1010 | 303 | 303 | 0 | 0 |
| 40352 | 1 cup | Temptations, Honey Roasted Pecan, Kelloggs | 43 | 175 | 3 | 2.6 | 35.0 | 1.0 | 13.8 | 20.2 | 3.2 | 0.7 | 1.7 | 0.8 | 0.04 | 0.68 | 0 | 1112 | 334 | 334 | 0 | 0 |
| 40346 | 1 cup | Toasted Brown Sugar Squares, Healthy Choice | 54 | 186 | 5 | 5.1 | 44.2 | 5.0 | 9.0 | 30.1 | 1.0 | 0.2 | 0.2 | 0.4 | 0.02 | 0.40 | 0 | 500 | 50 | 0 | 50 | |
| 40485 | 1 cup | Toasted Oats, Krusteaz | 29 | 120 | 3 | 3.0 | 23.0 | 2.0 | 2.0 | 19.0 | 2.0 | 0.0 | | | 0.00 | 0.00 | 0 | 1250 | 375 | 375 | 0 | 0 |
| 40484 | 1 cup | Toasted Oats Apple Cinnamon, Krusteaz | 40 | 173 | 3 | 2.7 | 33.3 | 1.3 | 13.3 | 18.7 | 2.7 | 0.0 | | | 0.00 | 0.00 | 0 | 1667 | 501 | 501 | 0 | 0 |
| 40263 | 1 cup | Toasties, Post | 24 | 93 | 3 | 2.0 | 20.6 | 0.8 | 1.6 | 18.1 | 0.0 | 0.0 | 0.0 | 0.0 | 0.00 | 0.02 | 0 | 1058 | 318 | 318 | 0 | 0 |
| 40435 | 1 cup | Total, General Mills | 40 | 149 | 3 | 2.4 | 34.2 | 1.0 | 4.0 | 29.2 | 0.6 | 0.2 | 0.1 | 0.0 | 0.00 | 0.03 | 0 | 1667 | 500 | 500 | 0 | 0 |
| 40021 | 1 cup | Total Wheat w/calcium, General Mills | 40 | 140 | 3 | 4.0 | 31.8 | 3.5 | 5.6 | 22.7 | 0.9 | 0.2 | 0.2 | 0.1 | 0.01 | 0.10 | 0 | 1667 | 500 | 500 | 0 | 0 |
| 40305 | 1 cup | Triples, General Mills | 30 | 116 | 3 | 2.4 | 25.0 | 0.8 | 6.1 | 18.0 | 1.0 | 0.3 | 0.3 | 0.0 | 0.00 | 0.03 | 0 | 1250 | 375 | 375 | 0 | 0 |
| 40306 | 1 cup | Trix, General Mills | 28 | 114 | 2 | 0.9 | 24.3 | 0.7 | 12.2 | 11.5 | 1.6 | 0.4 | 0.8 | 0.3 | 0.02 | 0.26 | 0 | 700 | 210 | 210 | 0 | 0 |
| 40128 | 1 cup | Uncle Sam's High Fiber, U.S. Mills | 55 | 213 | 6 | 8.4 | 39.7 | 14.5 | | | 2.3 | 0.2 | 0.5 | 1.5 | | | 0 | 0 | 0 | 0 | 0 | 0 |
| 40307 | 1 cup | Wheaties, General Mills | 29 | 106 | 3 | 3.1 | 23.0 | 2.0 | 2.9 | 18.1 | 0.9 | 0.2 | 0.2 | 0.1 | 0.01 | 0.13 | 0 | 725 | 218 | 218 | 0 | 0 |
| 40308 | 1 cup | Wheaties, Honey Frosted, General Mills | 40 | 146 | 3 | 2.3 | 35.2 | 2.0 | 12.6 | 20.6 | 0.4 | 0.1 | 0.1 | 0.0 | 0.00 | 0.04 | 0 | 1000 | 300 | 300 | 0 | 0 |
| | | **CHEESE AND CHEESE SUBSTITUTES** | | | | | | | | | | | | | | | | | | | | |
| | | *NATURAL CHEESES* | | | | | | | | | | | | | | | | | | | | |
| | | Asiago | | | | | | | | | | | | | | | | | | | | |
| 1027 | 1/4 cup | Avg | 27 | 102 | 37 | 7.7 | 0.9 | 0.0 | 0.9 | 0.0 | 7.4 | 4.8 | 2.0 | 0.3 | 0.10 | 0.17 | 25 | 228 | 68 | 66 | 2 | |
| 1231 | 1 oz | Aged, Stella Foods | 28 | 110 | | 9.0 | 0.5 | 0.0 | 0.5 | 0.0 | 8.0 | 5.0 | | | | | 25 | 300 | 60 | | | |
| 1233 | 1 oz | Mellow, Stella Foods | 28 | 100 | | 7.0 | 2.0 | 0.0 | 0.0 | 2.0 | 7.0 | 4.5 | | | | | 25 | 500 | 100 | | | |
| 1234 | 1 oz | Mild, Stella Foods | 28 | 110 | | 7.0 | 0.5 | 0.0 | 0.5 | 0.0 | 9.0 | 5.0 | | | | | 20 | 300 | 60 | | | |
| 1232 | 1/4 cup | Shred, Stella Foods | 28 | 120 | | 8.0 | 0.0 | 0.0 | 0.0 | 0.0 | 8.0 | 6.0 | | | | | 20 | 400 | 80 | | | |
| 1613 | 1 oz | Auribella, Belgioioso | 28 | 108 | 36 | 7.0 | 0.6 | 0.0 | 0.6 | 0.0 | 9.0 | 5.0 | | | | | 28 | 250 | 71 | | | |
| 1542 | 1 oz | Bakers Franklin County Cheese | 28 | 27 | | 5.6 | 0.8 | | 0.5 | | 0.1 | 0.1 | | | | | 2 | 4 | 1 | | | |
| 1003 | 1/4 cup | Blue, avg | 34 | 120 | 42 | 7.3 | 0.8 | 0.0 | 0.8 | 0.0 | 9.8 | 6.4 | 2.6 | 0.3 | 0.09 | 0.18 | 26 | 245 | 78 | 67 | 10 | |
| 1004 | 1/4 cup | Brie, avg | 36 | 120 | 48 | 7.5 | 0.2 | 0.0 | 0.2 | 0.0 | 10.0 | 6.3 | 2.9 | 0.3 | 0.11 | 0.18 | 36 | 240 | 66 | 58 | 7 | |
| 1037 | 1/4 cup | Brick, avg | 28 | 104 | 41 | 6.5 | 0.8 | 0.0 | 0.8 | 0.0 | 8.3 | 5.3 | 2.4 | 0.2 | 0.08 | 0.14 | 26 | 303 | 85 | 81 | 4 | |
| 1109 | 1/4 cup | Brick, w/salami, avg | 28 | 101 | 43 | 6.2 | 0.8 | 0.0 | 0.8 | 0.0 | 8.0 | 5.0 | 2.4 | 0.3 | 0.09 | 0.17 | 25 | 273 | 76 | 73 | 3 | |
| 1006 | 1/4 cup | Camembert, avg | 62 | 186 | 52 | 12.3 | 0.3 | 0.0 | 0.3 | 0.0 | 15.1 | 9.5 | 4.4 | 0.4 | 0.17 | 0.28 | 45 | 572 | 156 | 126 | 30 | |
| 1593 | 1 oz | Caraway, avg | 28 | 110 | 39 | 7.0 | 0.0 | 0.0 | 0.0 | 0.0 | 9.0 | 5.0 | 3.0 | 0.5 | | | 30 | | | | | |
| | | Cheddar | | | | | | | | | | | | | | | | | | | | |
| 1008 | 1/4 cup | Avg | 28 | 113 | 37 | 7.0 | 0.4 | 0.0 | 0.4 | 0.0 | 9.3 | 5.9 | 2.6 | 0.3 | 0.10 | 0.16 | 29 | 297 | 78 | 70 | 8 | |
| 1601 | 1 oz | Cabot | 28 | 109 | 35 | 6.9 | 1.0 | 0.0 | 0.0 | 1.0 | 8.9 | 4.9 | | | | | 30 | 296 | 85 | | | |
| 1486 | 1/4 cup | Fat Free, fancy, Healthy Choice | 30 | 45 | 57 | 9.0 | 2.0 | 0.0 | 0.0 | 2.0 | 0.0 | 0.0 | 0.0 | 0.0 | 0.00 | 0.00 | 5 | 200 | 57 | | | |
| 1224 | 1/4 cup | Fat Free, Lifetime | 31 | 44 | 64 | 8.9 | 1.1 | 0.0 | 1.1 | 0.0 | 0.0 | 0.0 | 0.0 | 0.0 | 0.00 | 0.00 | 6 | 332 | 95 | | | |
| 1285 | 1/4 cup | Fat Free, sharp, Healthy Choice | 29 | 45 | | 10.0 | 1.0 | 0.0 | 0.0 | 1.0 | 0.0 | 0.0 | 0.0 | 0.0 | 0.00 | 0.00 | 2 | 400 | 114 | | | |
| 1202 | 1 pce | Fat Free, sharp, Weight Watchers | 11 | 15 | 65 | 2.6 | 1.0 | 0.0 | 0.5 | 0.5 | 0.0 | 0.0 | 0.0 | 0.0 | 0.00 | 0.00 | 0 | 103 | 30 | | | |
| 1485 | 1/4 cup | Fat Free, shreds, Healthy Choice | 30 | 45 | 57 | 9.0 | 2.0 | 0.0 | 0.0 | 2.0 | 0.0 | 0.0 | 0.0 | 0.0 | 0.00 | 0.00 | 5 | 200 | 57 | | | |
| 1604 | 1 oz | Five Peppercorn, Cabot | 28 | 109 | 35 | 6.9 | 1.0 | 0.0 | 0.0 | 1.0 | 8.9 | 4.9 | | | | | 30 | 296 | 85 | | | |
| 1603 | 1 oz | Garlic & Dill, Cabot | 28 | 109 | 35 | 6.9 | 1.0 | 0.0 | 0.0 | 1.0 | 8.9 | 4.9 | | | | | 30 | 296 | 85 | | | |
| 1089 | 1/4 cup | Low Fat, low sod, avg | 28 | 48 | 65 | 6.8 | 0.5 | 0.0 | 0.5 | 0.0 | 2.0 | 1.2 | 0.6 | 0.1 | 0.02 | 0.04 | 6 | 65 | 17 | 16 | 1 | |
| 1451 | 1/4 cup | Low Sod, avg | 28 | 111 | 39 | 6.8 | 0.5 | 0.0 | 0.0 | 0.5 | 9.1 | 5.8 | 2.6 | 0.3 | 0.11 | 0.17 | 28 | 293 | 81 | | | |
| 1210 | 1/4 cup | Low Sod, mild, Weight Watchers | 31 | 87 | 49 | 8.7 | 1.1 | 0.0 | 0.0 | 1.1 | 5.5 | 3.3 | | | | | 16 | 328 | 94 | | | |
| 1423 | 1/4 cup | Reduced Fat, Alpine Lace | 31 | 89 | 48 | 10.0 | 1.1 | 0.0 | 0.0 | 1.1 | 5.0 | 3.3 | | | | | 17 | 332 | 95 | | | |
| 1517 | 1 ea | Reduced Fat 50%, slice, Cabot | 28 | 69 | 52 | 7.9 | 1.0 | 0.0 | 0.0 | 1.0 | 4.0 | 3.0 | | | | | 15 | 296 | 85 | | | |
| 1598 | 1 oz | Reduced Fat 50%, Jalapeno, Cabot | 28 | 69 | 51 | 7.9 | 1.0 | 0.0 | 0.0 | 1.0 | 4.4 | 3.0 | | | | | 15 | 296 | 85 | | | |
| 1516 | 1/4 cup | Reduced Fat 50%, Shredded, Cabot | 28 | 70 | 50 | 8.0 | 1.0 | 0.0 | 0.0 | 1.0 | 4.5 | 3.0 | | | | | 15 | 300 | 86 | | | |
| 1600 | 1 oz | Sun Dried Tomato Basil, Cabot | 28 | 109 | 35 | 6.9 | 1.0 | 0.0 | 0.0 | 1.0 | 8.9 | 4.9 | | | | | 30 | 296 | 85 | | | |
| 1602 | 1 oz | Toasted Onion & Chive, Cabot | 28 | 110 | 35 | 7.0 | 1.0 | 0.0 | 0.0 | 1.0 | 9.0 | 5.0 | | | | | 30 | 300 | 86 | | | |
| 1010 | 1/4 cup | Colby, avg | 28 | 110 | 38 | 6.7 | 0.7 | 0.0 | 0.7 | 0.0 | 9.0 | 5.7 | 2.6 | 0.3 | 0.08 | 0.19 | 27 | 290 | 77 | 72 | 5 | |
| 1430 | 1/4 cup | Colby, red fat, Alpine Lace | 31 | 89 | 47 | 10.0 | 1.1 | 0.0 | 0.0 | 1.1 | 5.5 | 3.3 | | | | | 17 | 332 | 95 | | | |
| | | Cottage Cheese | | | | | | | | | | | | | | | | | | | | |
| 1502 | 1/2 cup | Fat Free, Darigold | 115 | 80 | 83 | 13.0 | 6.0 | 0.0 | 5.0 | 1.0 | 0.0 | 0.0 | 0.0 | 0.0 | 0.00 | 0.00 | 5 | | | | | |
| 1501 | 1/2 cup | Fat Free, dry curd, Darigold | 75 | 60 | 79 | 13.5 | 1.5 | 0.0 | 0.0 | 1.5 | 0.0 | 0.0 | 0.0 | 0.0 | 0.00 | 0.00 | 0 | | | | | |
| 1047 | 1/2 cup | 1% Fat, avg | 113 | 81 | 82 | 14.0 | 3.1 | 0.0 | 3.1 | 0.0 | 1.2 | 0.7 | 0.3 | 0.0 | 0.01 | 0.02 | 5 | 42 | 13 | 12 | 1 | |
| 1012 | 1/2 cup | 1% Fat, small curd, avg | 105 | 108 | 79 | 13.1 | 2.8 | 0.0 | 0.6 | 2.2 | 4.7 | 3.0 | 1.4 | 0.1 | 0.04 | 0.10 | 16 | 171 | 50 | 48 | 2 | |
| 1013 | 1/2 cup | 1% Fat, large curd, avg | 112 | 115 | 79 | 14.0 | 3.0 | 0.0 | 0.7 | 2.3 | 5.1 | 3.2 | 1.4 | 0.2 | 0.04 | 0.11 | 17 | 183 | 54 | 52 | 2 | |
| 1099 | 1/2 cup | 1% Fat, low sod, avg | 112 | 81 | 84 | 13.9 | 3.0 | 0.0 | 3.0 | 0.0 | 1.1 | 0.7 | 0.3 | 0.0 | 0.01 | 0.02 | 4 | 41 | 12 | 12 | 0 | |
| 1622 | 1/2 cup | 1.5% Fat, w/fruit, Knudsen | 113 | 120 | | 11.0 | 15.0 | 0.0 | 13.0 | 2.0 | 2.0 | 1.5 | | | | | 10 | 0 | 0 | 0 | 0 | 0 |
| 1049 | 1/2 cup | 2% Fat, creamed w/fruit, avg | 113 | 140 | 72 | 11.2 | 15.0 | 0.0 | 15.0 | 0.0 | 3.8 | 2.4 | 1.1 | 0.1 | 0.03 | 0.08 | 12 | 139 | 41 | 40 | 1 | |
| 1354 | 1/2 cup | 4% Fat, large curd, Breakstone's | 120 | 120 | 79 | 14.0 | 4.0 | 0.0 | 3.0 | 1.0 | 5.0 | 3.5 | | | | | 25 | 200 | 57 | | | |
| 1355 | 1/2 cup | 4% Fat, small curd, Breakstone's | 120 | 120 | 79 | 14.0 | 4.0 | 0.0 | 3.0 | 1.0 | 5.0 | 3.5 | | | | | 25 | 200 | 57 | | | |

| Code | Thiamin (mg) | Riboflavin (mg) | Niacin (NE) | Vit B6 (mg) | Vit B12 (mcg) | Folate (mcg) | Panto (mg) | Vit C (mg) | Vit D (mg) | Vit E (α TE) | Calcium (mg) | Copper (mg) | Iron (mg) | Magnes (mg) | Mang (mg) | Phos (mg) | Potassium (mg) | Selenium (mcg) | Sodium (mg) | Zinc (mg) |
|---|---|---|---|---|---|---|---|---|---|---|---|---|---|---|---|---|---|---|---|---|
| | **Vitamins** | | | | | | | | | | **Minerals** | | | | | | | | | |
| 40261 | 0.43 | 0.50 | 5.81 | 0.59 | 1.75 | 116.5 | 0.12 | 0.0 | 1.2 | | 7 | 0.1 | 2.1 | 20 | 0.3 | 44 | 48 | 16.0 | 51 | 1.75 |
| 40070 | 0.31 | 0.36 | 4.22 | 0.43 | 1.27 | 84.7 | 0.12 | 12.7 | 0.0 | | 11 | 0.1 | 6.9 | 26 | | 96 | 71 | 9.0 | 183 | 0.69 |
| 40289 | 0.30 | 0.34 | 4.04 | 0.40 | 1.21 | 0.0 | | 12.1 | 0.0 | | 0 | 0.1 | 6.5 | 19 | | 65 | 65 | | 291 | 0.73 |
| 40071 | 0.55 | 0.63 | 7.39 | 0.76 | 2.23 | 6.7 | 0.31 | 22.3 | 0.0 | | 6 | 0.2 | 12.0 | 12 | 0.5 | 65 | 71 | 6.0 | 260 | 0.58 |
| 40351 | 0.49 | 0.56 | 6.72 | 0.66 | 0.00 | 140.0 | 0.00 | 20.2 | 1.3 | | 13 | 0.0 | 6.1 | 8 | 0.2 | 24 | 48 | 5.1 | 241 | 0.24 |
| 40352 | 0.56 | 0.64 | 7.40 | 0.73 | 0.00 | 129.0 | 0.00 | 22.2 | 1.5 | | 1 | 0.0 | 6.7 | 4 | 0.2 | 11 | 41 | 2.2 | 356 | 0.17 |
| 40346 | 0.54 | 0.59 | 7.02 | 0.70 | 2.11 | 108.0 | 3.51 | 0.0 | 2.0 | | 18 | 0.1 | 6.3 | 58 | 1.6 | 191 | 210 | 6.6 | 2 | 1.51 |
| 40485 | | | | | | | | 15.0 | | | 100 | | 8.1 | | | | 65 | | 210 | |
| 40484 | | | | | | | | 20.0 | | | 80 | | 6.0 | | | | 73 | | 200 | |
| 40263 | 0.31 | 0.36 | 4.22 | 0.43 | 1.27 | 84.7 | 0.03 | 0.0 | 0.8 | | 1 | 0.0 | 0.6 | 4 | 0.0 | 11 | 28 | 1.2 | 252 | 0.07 |
| 40435 | 2.00 | 2.27 | 26.80 | 2.67 | 10.84 | 533.2 | 15.72 | 80.0 | 1.3 | | 316 | 0.0 | 24.0 | 10 | 0.0 | 146 | 45 | 2.0 | 270 | 20.00 |
| 40021 | 2.00 | 2.27 | 26.80 | 2.67 | 10.24 | 533.2 | 14.60 | 80.0 | 0.3 | | 344 | 0.2 | 24.0 | 43 | 1.3 | 281 | 129 | 1.9 | 265 | 20.00 |
| 40305 | 0.38 | 0.43 | 5.01 | 0.50 | 0.00 | 99.9 | 0.20 | 15.0 | 1.0 | | 41 | 0.5 | 8.1 | 7 | 0.4 | 35 | 31 | 1.3 | 191 | 3.75 |
| 40306 | 0.35 | 0.40 | 4.68 | 0.47 | 0.00 | 93.2 | 0.04 | 14.0 | 1.0 | | 30 | 0.1 | 4.2 | 3 | 0.0 | 24 | 17 | 5.6 | 184 | 3.50 |
| 40128 | 1.31 | 1.39 | 11.55 | 0.07 | 0.00 | 42.9 | | 0.0 | | | 39 | 0.3 | 2.0 | 67 | | 208 | 259 | | 125 | 1.46 |
| 40307 | 0.36 | 0.41 | 4.84 | 0.48 | 0.00 | 96.6 | 0.23 | 14.5 | 1.0 | | 53 | 0.1 | 7.8 | 31 | 0.9 | 92 | 101 | 1.4 | 215 | 0.68 |
| 40308 | 0.50 | 0.57 | 6.68 | 0.67 | 0.00 | 133.2 | 0.14 | 20.0 | 0.0 | | 10 | 0.0 | 6.0 | 14 | 0.4 | 72 | 74 | 1.9 | 281 | 5.00 |
| 1027 | 0.01 | 0.10 | 0.02 | 0.02 | 0.45 | 1.7 | 0.12 | 0.0 | 0.3 | | 259 | 0.0 | 0.0 | 10 | 0.0 | 163 | 30 | 3.4 | 70 | 1.05 |
| 1231 | | | | | | | | 0.0 | | | 250 | | | | | | | | 310 | |
| 1233 | | | | | | | | 0.0 | | | 250 | | 0.0 | | | | | | 0 | |
| 1234 | | | | | | | | 0.0 | | | 200 | | 0.0 | | | | | | 330 | |
| 1232 | | | | | | | | 0.0 | | | 240 | | 0.0 | | | | | | 320 | |
| 1613 | | | | | | | | 0.0 | | | 200 | | 0.2 | | | | | | 265 | |
| 1542 | | | | | | | | 0.0 | | | 24 | | | | | | | | 25 | |
| 1003 | 0.01 | 0.13 | 0.35 | 0.06 | 0.41 | 12.4 | 0.59 | 0.0 | 0.1 | | 180 | 0.0 | 0.1 | 8 | 0.0 | 132 | 87 | 4.9 | 474 | 0.90 |
| 1004 | 0.03 | 0.19 | 0.14 | 0.08 | 0.59 | 23.4 | 0.25 | 0.0 | 0.1 | | 66 | 0.0 | 0.2 | 7 | 0.0 | 68 | 55 | 5.2 | 226 | 0.86 |
| 1037 | 0.00 | 0.10 | 0.03 | 0.02 | 0.35 | 5.7 | 0.08 | 0.0 | 0.1 | | 189 | 0.0 | 0.1 | 7 | 0.0 | 126 | 38 | 4.1 | 157 | 0.73 |
| 1109 | 0.01 | 0.10 | 0.13 | 0.02 | 0.42 | 5.2 | 0.10 | 0.3 | 0.1 | | 170 | 0.0 | 0.2 | 6 | 0.0 | 117 | 40 | 3.1 | 171 | 0.72 |
| 1006 | 0.02 | 0.30 | 0.39 | 0.14 | 0.81 | 38.6 | 0.84 | 0.0 | 0.2 | | 241 | 0.0 | 0.2 | 12 | 0.0 | 215 | 116 | 9.0 | 522 | 1.48 |
| 1593 | | | | | | | | | | | 200 | | 0.0 | | | | 20 | | 170 | |
| 1008 | 0.01 | 0.11 | 0.02 | 0.02 | 0.23 | 5.1 | 0.12 | 0.0 | 0.1 | | 202 | 0.0 | 0.2 | 8 | 0.0 | 143 | 27 | 3.9 | 174 | 0.87 |
| 1601 | | | | | | | | 0.0 | | | 198 | | 0.0 | | | | | | 178 | |
| 1486 | 0.00 | 0.07 | 0.00 | | | | | 0.0 | | | 250 | | 0.0 | | | | | | 200 | |
| 1224 | | | | | | | | | | | 443 | | | | | | | | 244 | |
| 1285 | | 0.14 | | | 0.24 | | | 0.0 | | | 250 | | 0.0 | 8 | | 150 | 20 | | 220 | 1.20 |
| 1202 | | | | | | | | 0.0 | | | 52 | | 0.0 | | | | 34 | | 160 | |
| 1485 | 0.00 | 0.07 | 0.00 | | | | | 0.0 | | | 250 | | 0.0 | | | | | | 200 | |
| 1604 | | | | | | | | 0.0 | | | 198 | | 0.0 | | | | | | 178 | |
| 1603 | | | | | | | | 0.0 | | | 198 | | 0.0 | | | | | | 178 | |
| 1089 | 0.01 | 0.01 | 0.03 | 0.02 | 0.23 | 5.0 | 0.06 | 0.0 | 0.0 | | 197 | 0.0 | 0.2 | 8 | 0.0 | 136 | 31 | 3.1 | 6 | 0.87 |
| 1451 | 0.01 | 0.11 | 0.02 | 0.02 | 0.23 | 5.0 | 0.09 | 0.0 | 0.0 | | 197 | 0.0 | 0.2 | 8 | 0.0 | 136 | 31 | 4.1 | 6 | 0.87 |
| 1210 | | | | | | | | 0.0 | | | 219 | | 0.0 | | | | 46 | | 77 | |
| 1423 | | | | | | | | 1.3 | | | 277 | | 0.4 | | | | | | 105 | |
| 1517 | | | | | | | | 0.0 | | | 198 | | 0.0 | | | | | | 168 | |
| 1598 | | | | | | | | 0.0 | | | 198 | | 0.0 | | | | | | 168 | |
| 1516 | | | | | | | | 0.0 | | | 200 | | 0.0 | | | | | | 170 | |
| 1600 | | | | | | | | 0.0 | | | 198 | | 0.0 | | | | | | 178 | |
| 1602 | | | | | | | | 0.0 | | | 200 | | 0.0 | | | | | | 180 | |
| 1010 | 0.00 | 0.11 | 0.03 | 0.02 | 0.23 | 5.1 | 0.06 | 0.0 | 0.1 | | 192 | 0.0 | 0.2 | 7 | 0.0 | 128 | 36 | 4.1 | 169 | 0.86 |
| 1430 | | | | | | | | 1.3 | | | 387 | | 0.4 | | | | | | 127 | |
| 1502 | | | | | | | | 0.0 | | | 120 | | 0.0 | | 0.0 | | 190 | | 500 | |
| 1501 | | | | | | | | 0.0 | | | 22 | | 0.0 | | 0.0 | | 45 | | 795 | |
| 1047 | 0.02 | 0.19 | 0.14 | 0.08 | 0.72 | 14.0 | 0.24 | 0.0 | 0.0 | | 69 | 0.0 | 0.2 | 6 | 0.0 | 151 | 97 | 10.2 | 459 | 0.43 |
| 1012 | 0.02 | 0.17 | 0.13 | 0.07 | 0.65 | 12.8 | 0.22 | 0.0 | 0.0 | | 63 | 0.0 | 0.1 | 5 | 0.0 | 139 | 88 | 9.4 | 425 | 0.39 |
| 1013 | 0.02 | 0.18 | 0.14 | 0.08 | 0.70 | 13.7 | 0.24 | 0.0 | 0.0 | | 67 | 0.0 | 0.2 | 6 | 0.0 | 148 | 94 | 10.1 | 454 | 0.41 |
| 1099 | 0.02 | 0.18 | 0.15 | 0.08 | 0.71 | 13.4 | 0.22 | 0.0 | 0.0 | | 68 | 0.0 | 0.2 | 6 | 0.0 | 150 | 96 | 6.7 | 15 | 0.43 |
| 1622 | 0.03 | 0.25 | | | 0.48 | | | 0.0 | | | 40 | | 0.0 | | | 100 | 100 | | 300 | |
| 1049 | 0.02 | 0.15 | 0.11 | 0.06 | 0.56 | 11.0 | 0.19 | 0.0 | 0.0 | | 54 | 0.0 | 0.1 | 5 | 0.0 | 119 | 76 | 8.0 | 458 | 0.33 |
| 1354 | 0.03 | 0.17 | | | 0.48 | | | 0.0 | | | 100 | | 0.0 | | | 150 | 105 | | 400 | |
| 1355 | 0.03 | 0.17 | | | 0.48 | | | 0.0 | | | 100 | | 0.0 | | | 150 | 105 | | 400 | |

| Code | Amount | Description | Basic Components | | | | | | | | | Additional Fats | | | | | | Vit A & Components | | | | | Vitamins | | | | | | | | | | Minerals | | | | | | | | | |
|---|---|---|---|---|---|---|---|---|---|---|---|---|---|---|---|---|---|---|---|---|---|---|---|---|---|---|---|---|---|---|---|---|---|---|---|---|---|---|---|---|---|---|
| | | | Weight (g) | Calories | % Water | Protein (g) | Carbs (g) | Fiber (g) | Sugar (g) | Other Carbs (g) | Fat (g) | Sat Fat (g) | Mono Fat (g) | Poly Fat (g) | Omega 3 (g) | Omega 6 (g) | Choles (mg) | Vit A (IU) | Vit A (RE) | Retinol (RE) | Carotenoids (RE) | Beta Carotene (mcg) | Thiamin (mg) | Riboflavin (mg) | Niacin (NE) | Vit B6 (mg) | Vit B12 (mcg) | Folate (mcg) | Panto (mg) | Vit C (mg) | Vit D (mg) | Vit E (α TE) | Calcium (mg) | Copper (mg) | Iron (mg) | Magnes (mg) | Mang (mg) | Phos (mg) | Potassium (mg) | Selenium (mcg) | Sodium (mg) | Zinc (mg) |
| 1506 | 1/2 cup | 4% Fat, Chive, Darigold | 114 | 115 | 78 | 13.0 | 5.0 | 0.0 | 4.0 | 1.0 | 5.0 | 3.0 | 1.5 | 0.0 | 0.00 | 0.00 | 25 | | | | | | | | | | | | | | | | 90 | | 0.0 | | | | 160 | | 450 | |
| 1507 | 1/2 cup | 4% Fat, Pineapple, Darigold | 126 | 140 | 75 | 12.0 | 14.0 | 0.0 | 12.0 | 2.0 | 4.0 | 2.5 | 1.0 | 0.0 | 0.00 | 0.00 | 20 | | | | | | | | | | | | | | | | 165 | | 0.0 | | | | 160 | | 420 | |
| 1046 | 1 oz | Chesire Cheese, avg | 28 | 108 | 38 | 6.6 | 1.3 | 0.0 | 1.3 | 0.0 | 8.6 | 5.5 | 2.4 | 0.2 | 0.09 | 0.15 | 29 | 276 | 69 | 62 | 7 | | 0.01 | 0.08 | 0.02 | 0.02 | 0.23 | 5.1 | 0.12 | 0.0 | 0.1 | | 180 | 0.0 | 0.1 | 6 | 0.0 | 130 | 27 | 4.1 | 136 | 0.78 |
| 1045 | 1 oz | Caraway Cheese, avg | 28 | 105 | 39 | 7.1 | 0.9 | 0.0 | 0.8 | 0.0 | 8.2 | 5.2 | 2.3 | 0.2 | 0.09 | 0.14 | 26 | 335 | 81 | 77 | 4 | | 0.01 | 0.13 | 0.05 | 0.02 | 0.08 | 5.1 | 0.05 | 0.0 | 0.1 | | 188 | 0.0 | 0.2 | 6 | 0.0 | 137 | 26 | 4.1 | 193 | 0.82 |
| | | Cream Cheese | | | | | | | | | | | | | | | | | | | | | | | | | | | | | | | | | | | | | | | | |
| 1015 | 1 Tbs | Avg | 14 | 49 | 54 | 1.1 | 0.4 | 0.0 | 0.2 | 0.1 | 4.9 | 3.1 | 1.4 | 0.2 | 0.07 | 0.11 | 15 | 200 | 53 | 49 | 5 | | 0.00 | 0.03 | 0.01 | 0.01 | 0.06 | 1.8 | 0.04 | 0.0 | 0.0 | | 11 | 0.0 | 0.2 | 1 | 0.0 | 15 | 17 | 0.3 | 41 | 0.08 |
| 1452 | 1 Tbs | Fat Free, avg | 14 | 13 | 76 | 2.0 | 0.8 | 0.0 | 0.0 | 0.8 | 0.2 | 0.1 | 0.0 | 0.0 | 0.00 | 0.01 | 1 | 130 | 39 | | | | 0.01 | 0.02 | 0.02 | 0.01 | 0.08 | 5.2 | 0.03 | 0.0 | 0.0 | | 26 | 0.0 | 0.0 | 2 | 0.0 | 61 | 23 | 0.7 | 76 | 0.12 |
| 1217 | 1 ea | Fat Free, Garden Vegetable, slice, Lifetime | 28 | 40 | 64 | 8.0 | 1.0 | 0.0 | 1.0 | 0.0 | 0.0 | 0.0 | 0.0 | 0.0 | 0.00 | 0.00 | 5 | 300 | 60 | | | | | | | | | | | | | | 400 | | | | | | | | 220 | |
| 1484 | 1 Tbs | Fat Free, Herb & Garlic, Healthy Choice | 15 | 12 | 76 | 2.0 | 1.0 | 0.5 | | | 0.0 | 0.0 | 0.0 | 0.0 | 0.00 | 0.00 | 2 | 50 | 14 | | | | 0.00 | 0.02 | 0.00 | | | | | 0.0 | | | 10 | | 0.0 | | | | | | 100 | |
| 1218 | 1 ea | Fat Free, Onion & Chives, slice, Lifetime | 28 | 40 | 64 | 8.0 | 1.0 | 0.0 | 1.0 | 0.0 | 0.0 | 0.0 | 0.0 | 0.0 | 0.00 | 0.00 | 5 | 300 | 86 | | | | | | | | | | | | | | 400 | | | | | | | | 220 | |
| 1188 | 1 Tbs | Fat Free, Philadelphia | 16 | 14 | 78 | 2.3 | 1.1 | 0.0 | 0.6 | 0.6 | 0.0 | 0.0 | 0.0 | 0.0 | 0.00 | 0.00 | 1 | 286 | 82 | | | | | 0.04 | | | 0.07 | | | 0.0 | | | 46 | | 0.0 | 0 | | 57 | 29 | | 77 | 0.17 |
| 1115 | 1 Tbs | Fat Free, Soft, Philadelphia | 16 | 15 | 78 | 2.4 | 1.0 | 0.0 | 0.5 | 0.5 | 0.0 | 0.0 | 0.0 | 0.0 | 0.00 | 0.00 | 1 | 242 | 69 | | | | | 0.16 | | | 0.06 | | | 0.0 | | | 48 | | 0.0 | 0 | | 73 | 32 | | 78 | 0.15 |
| 1483 | 1 Tbs | Fat Free, Strawberry, Healthy Choice | 15 | 18 | 69 | 2.0 | 2.5 | 0.5 | 0.0 | 2.0 | 0.0 | 0.0 | 0.0 | 0.0 | 0.00 | 0.00 | 2 | 200 | 57 | | | | 0.00 | 0.02 | 0.00 | | | | | 0.0 | | | 10 | | 0.0 | | | | | | 100 | |
| 1098 | 1 Tbs | Light, avg | 15 | 35 | 64 | 1.7 | 1.1 | 0.0 | 1.1 | 0.0 | 2.6 | 1.7 | 0.9 | 0.1 | 0.04 | 0.06 | 8 | 108 | 33 | 31 | 2 | | 0.00 | 0.04 | 0.02 | 0.01 | 0.09 | 2.7 | 0.06 | 0.0 | 0.0 | | 17 | 0.0 | 0.3 | 1 | 0.0 | 22 | 25 | 0.5 | 44 | 0.11 |
| 1171 | 1 Tbs | Light, Garlic, Bongrain | 16 | 34 | | 1.7 | 1.1 | | | | 2.8 | | | | | | 8 | | | | | | | | | | | | | | | | 11 | | | | | | | | 73 | |
| 1173 | 1 Tbs | Light, Herbs & Garlic, Bongrain | 16 | 34 | | 1.7 | 1.1 | | | | 2.8 | | | | | | 8 | | | | | | | | | | | | | | | | 11 | | | | | | 28 | | 73 | |
| 1352 | 1 Tbs | Light, Soft, Philadelphia | 16 | 35 | 68 | 1.5 | 1.0 | 0.0 | 1.0 | 0.0 | 2.5 | 1.5 | | | | | 8 | 200 | 57 | | | | | 0.02 | | | 0.00 | | | 0.0 | | | 20 | | 0.0 | 0 | | 20 | 28 | | 75 | 0.00 |
| 1170 | 1 Tbs | Light, Vegetables, Bongrain | 16 | 34 | | 0.6 | 2.8 | | | | 3.5 | | | | | | | | | | | | | | | | | | | | | | 11 | | | | | | 28 | | 68 | |
| 1275 | 1 Tbs | Light, Weight Watchers | 15 | 21 | 76 | 1.6 | 0.5 | 0.0 | 0.5 | 0.0 | 1.3 | 0.8 | | | | | 5 | 212 | 60 | | | | | | | | | | | 0.0 | | | 11 | | 0.0 | | | | 23 | | 56 | |
| 1343 | 1 Tbs | Soft, Chives & Onions, Philadelphia | 16 | 57 | 54 | 1.0 | 1.0 | 0.0 | 0.3 | 0.3 | 5.2 | 3.6 | | | | | 15 | 206 | 59 | | | | | 0.04 | | | 0.00 | | | 0.0 | | | 10 | | 0.0 | 0 | | 10 | 26 | | 57 | 0.00 |
| 1344 | 1 Tbs | Soft, Herb & Garlic, Philadelphia | 16 | 57 | 57 | 0.5 | 1.0 | 0.0 | 0.3 | 0.3 | 5.2 | 3.6 | | | | | 15 | 206 | 59 | | | | | 0.04 | | | 0.00 | | | 0.0 | | | 21 | | 0.0 | 0 | | 21 | 36 | | 93 | 0.00 |
| 1345 | 1 Tbs | Soft, Olive & Pimento, Philadelphia | 16 | 52 | 57 | 1.0 | 1.0 | 0.0 | 0.3 | 0.3 | 4.6 | 3.1 | | | | | 15 | 206 | 59 | | | | | 0.02 | | | 0.00 | | | 0.0 | | | 10 | | 0.0 | 0 | | 10 | 23 | | 88 | 0.00 |
| 1346 | 1 Tbs | Soft, w/Pineapple, Philadelphia | 16 | 50 | 52 | 1.0 | 2.0 | 0.0 | 1.5 | 0.5 | 4.5 | 3.0 | | | | | 15 | 150 | 43 | | | | | 0.02 | | | 0.00 | | | 0.0 | | | 10 | | 0.0 | 0 | | 10 | 22 | | 50 | 0.00 |
| 1347 | 1 Tbs | Soft, w/Smkd Salmon, Philadelphia | 16 | 52 | 60 | 1.0 | 0.5 | 0.0 | 0.3 | 0.3 | 4.6 | 3.1 | | | | | 15 | 103 | 29 | | | | | 0.02 | | | 0.00 | | | 0.0 | | | 10 | | 0.0 | 0 | | 10 | 23 | | 103 | 0.00 |
| 1348 | 1 Tbs | Soft, w/Strawberries, Philadelphia | 16 | 50 | 52 | 0.5 | 2.5 | 0.0 | 1.5 | 1.0 | 4.5 | 3.0 | | | | | 15 | 150 | 43 | | | | | 0.02 | | | | | | 0.0 | | | 10 | | 0.0 | 0 | | 10 | 30 | | 32 | 0.00 |
| 1341 | 1 oz | W/Chives, Philadelphia | 28 | 90 | 58 | 2.0 | 0.5 | 0.0 | 0.5 | 0.0 | 9.0 | 6.0 | | | | | 30 | 300 | 85 | | | | | 0.03 | | | 0.00 | | | 0.0 | | | 0 | | 0.0 | 0 | | 20 | 25 | | 150 | 0.00 |
| 1342 | 1 oz | W/Pimentos, Philadelphia | 28 | 90 | 58 | 2.0 | 0.5 | 0.0 | 0.5 | 0.0 | 9.0 | 6.0 | | | | | 30 | 300 | 85 | | | | | 0.03 | | | 0.00 | | | 0.0 | | | 0 | | 0.0 | 0 | | 20 | 30 | | 150 | 0.00 |
| 1453 | 1 Tbs | Whipped, avg | 10 | 35 | 54 | 0.8 | 0.3 | 0.0 | 0.2 | 0.1 | 3.5 | 2.2 | 1.0 | 0.1 | 0.05 | 0.08 | 11 | 143 | 38 | 35 | 3 | | 0.00 | 0.02 | 0.01 | 0.00 | 0.04 | 1.3 | 0.03 | 0.0 | 0.0 | | 8 | 0.0 | 0.1 | 1 | 0.0 | 10 | 12 | 0.2 | 30 | 0.05 |
| 1350 | 1 Tbs | Whipped, w/Smkd Salmon, Philadelphia | 10 | 33 | 56 | 0.7 | 0.7 | 0.0 | 0.3 | 0.3 | 3.0 | 2.0 | | | | | 10 | 133 | 38 | | | | | 0.01 | | | 0.00 | | | 0.0 | | | 7 | | 0.0 | 0 | | 7 | 17 | | 67 | 0.00 |
| 1050 | 1/4 cup | Edam, avg | 33 | 118 | 42 | 8.3 | 0.5 | 0.0 | 0.5 | 0.0 | 9.2 | 5.8 | 2.7 | 0.2 | 0.08 | 0.14 | 29 | 302 | 84 | 74 | 10 | | 0.01 | 0.13 | 0.03 | 0.03 | 0.51 | 5.3 | 0.09 | 0.0 | 0.3 | | 241 | 0.0 | 0.1 | 10 | 0.0 | 177 | 62 | 4.8 | 318 | 1.24 |
| 1283 | 1 oz | Farmers, avg | 28 | 100 | 45 | 6.0 | 0.5 | 0.0 | 0.0 | 0.5 | 8.0 | 6.0 | | | | | 25 | 300 | 85 | | | | | 0.07 | | | 0.48 | | | 0.0 | | | 200 | | 0.0 | 8 | | 150 | 25 | | 190 | 0.90 |
| 1016 | 1/4 cup | Feta Cheese, avg | 38 | 100 | 55 | 5.4 | 1.6 | 0.0 | 1.6 | 0.0 | 8.1 | 5.7 | 1.8 | 0.2 | 0.10 | 0.12 | 34 | 170 | 49 | 47 | 2 | | 0.06 | 0.32 | 0.38 | 0.16 | 0.64 | 12.2 | 0.37 | 0.0 | 0.2 | | 187 | 0.0 | 0.2 | 7 | 0.0 | 128 | 24 | 5.7 | 424 | 1.09 |
| 1052 | 1/4 cup | Fontina Cheese, avg | 27 | 105 | 38 | 6.9 | 0.4 | 0.0 | 0.4 | 0.0 | 8.4 | 5.2 | 2.3 | 0.4 | 0.21 | 0.23 | 31 | 317 | 79 | 70 | 9 | | 0.01 | 0.06 | 0.04 | 0.02 | 0.45 | 1.5 | 0.12 | 0.0 | 0.1 | | 149 | 0.0 | 0.1 | 4 | 0.0 | 93 | 17 | 3.9 | 216 | 0.95 |
| 1151 | 1/4 cup | Fresco, avg | 62 | 90 | 73 | 7.4 | 3.4 | 0.0 | | | 5.2 | 3.2 | 1.5 | 0.2 | | | 20 | 232 | 71 | 68 | 6 | | 0.01 | 0.12 | 0.05 | 0.01 | 0.19 | 8.5 | | 0.0 | | | 177 | 0.0 | 0.3 | 10 | | 119 | 82 | | 81 | 0.87 |
| 1132 | 1 oz | Gjetost, avg | 28 | 130 | 13 | 2.7 | 12.0 | 0.0 | 12.0 | 0.0 | 8.3 | 5.4 | 2.2 | 0.3 | 0.12 | 0.14 | 26 | 312 | 77 | 68 | 8 | | 0.09 | 0.39 | 0.23 | 0.08 | 0.68 | 1.3 | 0.94 | 0.0 | 0.1 | | 112 | 0.0 | 0.1 | 20 | 0.0 | 124 | 395 | 4.1 | 168 | 0.32 |
| | | Goat Cheese | | | | | | | | | | | | | | | | | | | | | | | | | | | | | | | | | | | | | | | | |
| 1078 | 1 oz | Hard, avg | 28 | 127 | 29 | 8.5 | 0.6 | 0.0 | 0.6 | 0.0 | 10.0 | 6.9 | 2.3 | 0.2 | 0.00 | 0.24 | 29 | 445 | 134 | | | | 0.04 | 0.33 | 0.67 | 0.02 | 0.03 | 1.1 | 0.11 | 0.0 | 0.1 | | 251 | 0.2 | 0.5 | 15 | 0.1 | 204 | 13 | 1.5 | 97 | 0.45 |
| 1079 | 1 oz | Semi-soft, avg | 28 | 102 | 46 | 6.0 | 0.7 | 0.0 | 0.7 | 0.0 | 8.3 | 5.8 | 1.9 | 0.2 | 0.00 | 0.20 | 22 | 374 | 112 | | | | 0.02 | 0.19 | 0.32 | 0.02 | 0.06 | 0.6 | 0.05 | 0.0 | 0.1 | | 83 | 0.2 | 0.5 | 8 | 0.0 | 105 | 44 | 1.1 | 144 | 0.18 |
| 1080 | 1/4 cup | Soft, avg | 62 | 166 | 61 | 11.5 | 0.6 | 0.0 | 0.6 | 0.0 | 13.1 | 9.1 | 3.0 | 0.3 | 0.00 | 0.31 | 29 | 534 | 175 | | | | 0.04 | 0.24 | 0.27 | 0.16 | 0.12 | 7.4 | 0.42 | 0.0 | 0.1 | | 87 | 0.5 | 1.2 | 10 | 0.1 | 159 | 16 | 1.7 | 223 | 0.57 |
| 1241 | 1/4 cup | Gorganzola, crumbled, avg | 28 | 100 | 40 | 6.0 | 0.5 | 0.0 | 0.5 | 0.0 | 9.0 | 6.0 | | | | | 25 | 300 | 60 | | | | | | | | | | | 0.0 | | | 150 | | 0.0 | | | | | | 390 | |
| 1054 | 1/4 cup | Gouda, avg | 33 | 117 | 42 | 8.2 | 0.7 | 0.0 | 0.7 | 0.0 | 9.0 | 5.8 | 2.6 | 0.2 | 0.13 | 0.09 | 38 | 213 | 57 | 52 | 5 | | 0.01 | 0.11 | 0.02 | 0.03 | 0.51 | 6.9 | 0.11 | 0.0 | 0.1 | | 231 | 0.0 | 0.1 | 10 | 0.0 | 180 | 40 | 4.8 | 270 | 1.29 |
| 1074 | 1/4 cup | Gruyere, avg | 27 | 112 | 33 | 8.0 | 0.1 | 0.0 | 0.1 | 0.0 | 8.7 | 5.1 | 2.7 | 0.5 | 0.12 | 0.35 | 30 | 329 | 81 | 72 | 9 | | 0.02 | 0.08 | 0.03 | 0.02 | 0.43 | 2.8 | 0.15 | 0.0 | 0.1 | | 273 | 0.0 | 0.0 | 10 | 0.0 | 163 | 22 | 3.9 | 91 | 1.05 |
| 1284 | 1 oz | Havarti, Kraft | 28 | 120 | | 6.0 | 0.0 | 0.0 | 0.0 | 0.0 | 11.0 | 7.0 | | | | | 35 | 300 | 86 | | | | | 0.10 | | | 0.12 | | | 0.0 | | | 150 | | 0.0 | 0 | | 100 | 10 | | 240 | 0.90 |
| 1243 | 1 oz | Kasseri, Stella Foods | 28 | 110 | | 7.0 | 0.5 | 0.0 | 0.5 | 0.0 | 9.0 | 5.0 | | | | | 25 | 300 | 60 | | | | | | | | | | | 0.0 | | | 200 | | 0.0 | | | | | | 290 | |
| 1055 | 1/4 cup | Limburger, avg | 34 | 111 | 48 | 6.8 | 0.2 | 0.0 | 0.2 | 0.0 | 9.3 | 5.7 | 2.9 | 0.2 | 0.05 | 0.12 | 31 | 436 | 107 | 102 | 5 | | 0.03 | 0.17 | 0.05 | 0.03 | 0.35 | 19.6 | 0.40 | 0.0 | 0.1 | | 169 | 0.0 | 0.0 | 7 | 0.0 | 134 | 44 | 4.9 | 272 | 0.71 |
| | | Lorraine Cheese | | | | | | | | | | | | | | | | | | | | | | | | | | | | | | | | | | | | | | | | |
| 1244 | 1 oz | Stella Foods | 28 | 110 | | 7.0 | 0.5 | 0.0 | 0.5 | 0.0 | 9.0 | 5.0 | | | | | 30 | 300 | 60 | | | | | | | | | | | 0.0 | | | 200 | | 0.0 | | | | | | 30 | |
| 1247 | 1 oz | Smoked, Stella Foods | 28 | 110 | | 7.0 | 0.5 | 0.0 | 0.5 | 0.0 | 9.0 | 5.0 | | | | | 25 | 300 | 60 | | | | | | | | | | | 0.0 | | | 200 | | 0.0 | | | | | | 30 | |
| 1245 | 1 oz | W/Chives & Onion, Stella Foods | 28 | 110 | | 7.0 | 0.5 | 0.0 | 0.5 | 0.0 | 9.0 | 5.0 | | | | | 25 | 300 | 60 | | | | | | | | | | | 0.0 | | | 200 | | 0.0 | | | | | | 30 | |
| 1246 | 1 oz | W/Jalapeno Pepper, Stella Foods | 28 | 100 | | 6.0 | 0.5 | 0.0 | 0.5 | 0.0 | 8.0 | 5.0 | | | | | 25 | 300 | 60 | | | | | | | | | | | 0.0 | | | 200 | | 0.0 | | | | | | 30 | |
| 1615 | 1 oz | Mascarpone, Belgioioso | 28 | 124 | 41 | 2.0 | 0.6 | 0.0 | 0.6 | 0.0 | 13.0 | 7.0 | | | | | 36 | 350 | 100 | | | | | | | | | | | 0.0 | | | 30 | | 0.0 | | | | | | 16 | |
| | | Mexican Cheese | | | | | | | | | | | | | | | | | | | | | | | | | | | | | | | | | | | | | | | | |
| 1146 | 1/4 cup | Anejo, aged, avg | 33 | 123 | 38 | 7.1 | 1.5 | 0.0 | | | 9.9 | 6.3 | 2.9 | 0.2 | | | 32 | 241 | 73 | 73 | 0 | | 0.01 | 0.07 | 0.01 | 0.02 | 0.46 | 0.0 | | 0.0 | | | 224 | 0.0 | 0.2 | 9 | | 147 | 29 | | 381 | 0.97 |
| 1443 | 1/4 cup | Asadero, aged, avg | 33 | 117 | 42 | 7.5 | 0.9 | 0.0 | | | 9.3 | 5.9 | 2.7 | 0.3 | 0.11 | 0.17 | 35 | 74 | 21 | | | | 0.01 | 0.07 | 0.06 | 0.02 | 0.33 | 2.6 | 0.08 | 0.0 | | | 218 | 0.0 | 0.2 | 9 | 0.0 | 146 | 28 | 4.8 | 216 | 1.00 |
| 1146 | 1/4 cup | Chihuahua, aged, avg | 28 | 104 | 38 | 6.0 | 1.3 | 0.0 | | | 8.4 | 5.3 | 2.4 | 0.2 | | | 27 | 204 | 62 | 62 | 0 | | 0.01 | 0.06 | 0.01 | 0.01 | 0.39 | 0.0 | | 0.0 | | | 190 | 0.0 | 0.1 | 8 | | 124 | 24 | | 323 | 0.82 |
| 1228 | 1/4 cup | Queso, fat free, mild, Lifetime | 31 | 44 | 64 | 8.9 | 1.1 | 0.0 | 1.1 | 0.0 | 0.0 | 0.0 | 0.0 | 0.0 | 0.00 | 0.00 | 6 | 332 | 95 | | | | | | | | | | | | | | 443 | | | | | | | | 244 | |
| 1489 | 1/4 cup | Shreds, fat free, Healthy Choice | 30 | 45 | 57 | 9.0 | 2.0 | 0.0 | 0.0 | 2.0 | 0.0 | 0.0 | 0.0 | 0.0 | 0.00 | 0.00 | 5 | 200 | 57 | | | | 0.00 | 0.07 | 0.00 | | | | | 0.0 | | | 250 | | 0.0 | | | | | | 200 | |
| | | Monterey Jack | | | | | | | | | | | | | | | | | | | | | | | | | | | | | | | | | | | | | | | | |
| 1017 | 1/4 cup | Avg | 28 | 104 | 41 | 6.9 | 0.2 | 0.0 | 0.2 | 0.0 | 8.5 | 5.3 | 2.5 | 0.3 | 0.07 | 0.18 | 25 | 266 | 71 | 62 | 9 | | 0.00 | 0.11 | 0.03 | 0.02 | 0.23 | 5.1 | 0.06 | 0.0 | 0.1 | | 209 | 0.0 | 0.2 | 8 | 0.0 | 124 | 23 | 4.1 | 150 | 0.84 |
| 1216 | 1 ea | Fat Free, Jalapeno, slice, Lifeline | 28 | 40 | 64 | 8.0 | 1.0 | 0.0 | 1.0 | 0.0 | 0.0 | 0.0 | 0.0 | 0.0 | 0.00 | 0.00 | 5 | 300 | 60 | | | | | | | | | | | | | | 400 | | | | | | | | 220 | |
| 1223 | 1/4 cup | Fat Free, Lifeline | 31 | 44 | 64 | 8.9 | 1.1 | 0.0 | 1.1 | 0.0 | 0.0 | 0.0 | 0.0 | 0.0 | 0.00 | 0.00 | 6 | 332 | 95 | | | | | | | | | | | | | | 443 | | | | | | | | 244 | |
| 1595 | 1 oz | Pepper, Cabot | 28 | 109 | 35 | 6.9 | 1.0 | 0.0 | 0.0 | 1.0 | 8.9 | 4.9 | | | | | 30 | 296 | 85 | | | | | | | | | | | 0.0 | | | 198 | | 0.0 | | | | | | 168 | |
| 1426 | 1/4 cup | Reduced Fat, Alpine Lace | 31 | 77 | 47 | 8.9 | 1.1 | 0.0 | 0.0 | 1.1 | 5.0 | 3.3 | | | | | 17 | 332 | 95 | | | | | | | | | | | 1.3 | | | 221 | | 0.4 | | | | | | 188 | |
| 1586 | 1 oz | Reduced Fat, red sod, Darigold | 28 | 80 | 50 | 8.0 | 0.0 | 0.0 | 0.0 | 0.0 | 5.0 | | | | | | 5 | | | | | | | | | | | | | 0.0 | | | 260 | | 0.0 | | 0.0 | | | | 120 | |
| 1325 | 1 oz | Reduced Fat, w/Jalapeno Pepper, Kraft | 28 | 110 | 38 | 7.0 | 0.5 | 0.0 | 0.0 | 0.5 | 9.0 | 6.0 | | | | | 30 | 400 | 80 | | | | | 0.10 | | | 0.24 | | | 0.0 | | | 200 | | 0.0 | 0 | | 100 | 15 | | 190 | 0.90 |
| 1512 | 1/4 cup | Shredded, Cabot | 28 | 110 | 35 | 7.0 | 1.0 | 0.0 | 0.0 | 1.0 | 9.0 | 5.0 | | | | | 30 | 300 | 86 | | | | | | | | | | | 0.0 | | | 200 | | 0.0 | | | | | | 170 | |
| | | Mozzarella | | | | | | | | | | | | | | | | | | | | | | | | | | | | | | | | | | | | | | | | |
| 1226 | 1/4 cup | Fat Free, Lifeline | 31 | 44 | 64 | 8.9 | 1.1 | 0.0 | 1.1 | 0.0 | 0.0 | 0.0 | 0.0 | 0.0 | 0.00 | 0.00 | 6 | 332 | 95 | | | | | | | | | | | | | | 443 | | | | | | | | 244 | |
| 1478 | 1/4 cup | Fat Free, Shreds, ConAgra | 30 | 45 | 57 | 9.0 | 2.0 | 0.0 | 0.0 | 2.0 | 0.0 | 0.0 | 0.0 | 0.0 | 0.00 | 0.00 | 5 | 200 | 57 | | | | 0.00 | 0.07 | 0.00 | | | | | 0.0 | | | 250 | | 0.0 | | | | | | 200 | |
| 1476 | 1 ea | Fat Free, String Cheese Stick, ConAgra | 30 | 36 | 65 | 5.7 | 2.9 | 0.0 | 0.0 | 2.9 | 0.0 | 0.0 | 0.0 | 0.0 | 0.00 | 0.00 | 7 | 423 | 122 | | | | 0.00 | 0.14 | 0.00 | | | | | 0.0 | | | 214 | | 0.0 | | | | | | 286 | |

| Code | Amount | Description | Basic Components | | | | | | | | | Additional Fats | | | | | | Vit A & Components | | | | | Vitamins | | | | | | | | | | Minerals | | | | | | | | | |
|---|---|---|---|---|---|---|---|---|---|---|---|---|---|---|---|---|---|---|---|---|---|---|---|---|---|---|---|---|---|---|---|---|---|---|---|---|---|---|---|---|---|---|
| | | | Weight (g) | Calories | % Water | Protein (g) | Carbs (g) | Fiber (g) | Sugar (g) | Other Carbs (g) | Fat (g) | Sat Fat (g) | Mono Fat (g) | Poly Fat (g) | Omega 3 (g) | Omega 6 (g) | Choles (mg) | Vit A (IU) | Vit A (RE) | Retinol (RE) | Carotenoids (RE) | Beta Carotene (mcg) | Thiamin (mg) | Riboflavin(mg) | Niacin (NE) | Vit B6 (mg) | Vit B12 (mcg) | Folate (mcg) | Panto (mg) | Vit C (mg) | Vit D (mg) | Vit E (α TE) | Calcium (mg) | Copper (mg) | Iron (mg) | Magnes (mg) | Mang (mg) | Phos (mg) | Potassium (mg) | Selenium (mcg) | Sodium (mg) | Zinc (mg) |
| 1100 | 1/4 cup | Low Sodium Mozzarella, Lifeline | 28 | 78 | 50 | 7.7 | 0.9 | 0.0 | 0.9 | 0.0 | 4.8 | 3.0 | 1.4 | 0.1 | 0.04 | 0.10 | 15 | 176 | 54 | 51 | 3 | | 0.01 | 0.10 | 0.03 | 0.02 | 0.26 | 2.8 | 0.03 | 0.0 | 0.0 | | 205 | 0.0 | 0.1 | 7 | 0.0 | 147 | 27 | 3.1 | 4 | 0.88 |
| 1058 | 1/4 cup | Part Skim, avg | 28 | 71 | 54 | 6.8 | 0.8 | 0.0 | 0.8 | 0.0 | 4.5 | 2.8 | 1.3 | 0.1 | 0.04 | 0.09 | 16 | 164 | 50 | 38 | 11 | | 0.01 | 0.08 | 0.03 | 0.02 | 0.23 | 2.5 | 0.02 | 0.0 | 0.0 | | 181 | 0.0 | 0.1 | 6 | 0.0 | 130 | 24 | 4.0 | 130 | 0.77 |
| 1556 | 1 oz | Part Skim, red fat, avg | 28 | 78 | 49 | 7.7 | 0.9 | 0.0 | | | 4.8 | 3.0 | 1.4 | 0.1 | | | 15 | 176 | 54 | 51 | 3 | | 0.01 | 0.10 | 0.03 | 0.02 | 0.26 | 2.8 | | 0.0 | | | 205 | 0.0 | 0.1 | 7 | | 147 | 27 | | 148 | 0.88 |
| 1294 | 1/4 cup | Part Skim, shredded, Kraft | 30 | 90 | | 8.0 | 0.5 | 0.0 | 0.5 | 0.0 | 6.0 | 4.0 | | | | | 20 | 200 | 57 | | | | | 0.07 | | | 0.36 | | | 0.0 | | | 250 | | 0.0 | 0 | | 150 | 20 | | 210 | 1.20 |
| 1292 | 1 ea | Part Skim, string cheese stick, Kraft | 28 | 80 | | 7.0 | 0.5 | 0.0 | 0.0 | 0.5 | 6.0 | 3.5 | | | | | 20 | 200 | 57 | | | | | 0.07 | | | 0.48 | | | 0.0 | | | 150 | | 0.0 | 0 | | 100 | 20 | | 240 | 1.20 |
| 1056 | 1/4 cup | Whole Milk, avg | 28 | 79 | 54 | 5.4 | 0.6 | 0.0 | 0.1 | 0.5 | 6.0 | 3.7 | 1.8 | 0.2 | 0.10 | 0.11 | 22 | 222 | 67 | 55 | 13 | | 0.00 | 0.07 | 0.02 | 0.02 | 0.18 | 2.0 | 0.02 | 0.0 | 0.0 | | 145 | 0.0 | 0.1 | 5 | 0.0 | 104 | 19 | 4.1 | 104 | 0.62 |
| 1021 | 1/4 cup | Muenster, avg | 29 | 107 | 42 | 6.8 | 0.3 | 0.0 | 0.3 | 0.0 | 8.7 | 5.5 | 2.5 | 0.2 | 0.07 | 0.12 | 28 | 325 | 92 | 88 | 4 | | 0.00 | 0.09 | 0.03 | 0.02 | 0.43 | 3.5 | 0.06 | 0.0 | 0.1 | | 208 | 0.0 | 0.1 | 8 | 0.0 | 136 | 39 | 4.2 | 182 | 0.81 |
| 1102 | 1/4 cup | Muenster, low sod, avg | 33 | 121 | 43 | 7.7 | 0.4 | 0.0 | 0.4 | 0.0 | 9.9 | 6.3 | 2.9 | 0.2 | 0.08 | 0.14 | 32 | 370 | 104 | 100 | 4 | | 0.00 | 0.11 | 0.03 | 0.02 | 0.49 | 4.0 | 0.06 | 0.0 | 0.1 | | 237 | 0.0 | 0.1 | 9 | 0.0 | 154 | 44 | 2.3 | 6 | 0.93 |
| | | Neufchatel | | | | | | | | | | | | | | | | | | | | | | | | | | | | | | | | | | | | | | | | |
| 1060 | 1/4 cup | Avg | 58 | 151 | 62 | 5.8 | 1.7 | 0.0 | 1.7 | 0.0 | 13.6 | 8.6 | 3.9 | 0.4 | 0.12 | 0.26 | 44 | 658 | 174 | 149 | 25 | | 0.01 | 0.11 | 0.07 | 0.02 | 0.15 | 6.6 | 0.33 | 0.0 | 0.1 | | 43 | 0.0 | 0.2 | 5 | 0.0 | 79 | 66 | 1.7 | 231 | 0.30 |
| 1389 | 1 Tbs | Classic Ranch, Spreadery | 15 | 40 | 62 | 1.5 | 0.5 | 0.0 | 0.3 | 0.3 | 3.5 | 2.5 | | | | | 10 | 100 | 29 | | | | | 0.02 | | | 0.00 | | | 0.0 | | | 10 | | 0.0 | 0 | | 10 | 18 | | 105 | 0.00 |
| 1390 | 1 Tbs | Garden Vegetables, Spreadery | 15 | 35 | 62 | 1.5 | 1.0 | 0.0 | 0.5 | 0.5 | 3.0 | 2.0 | | | | | 10 | 200 | 57 | | | | | 0.02 | | | 0.00 | | | 0.0 | | | 10 | | 0.0 | 0 | | 10 | 22 | | 115 | 0.00 |
| 1391 | 1 Tbs | Garlic & Herb, Spreadery | 15 | 40 | 62 | 1.5 | 0.5 | 0.0 | 0.3 | 0.3 | 3.5 | 2.5 | | | | | 10 | 100 | 29 | | | | | 0.02 | | | 0.00 | | | 10.0 | | | 10 | | 0.0 | 0 | | 10 | 18 | | 90 | 0.00 |
| | | Parmesan | | | | | | | | | | | | | | | | | | | | | | | | | | | | | | | | | | | | | | | | |
| 1422 | 1/4 cup | Fat Free, Alpine Lace | 31 | 44 | 54 | 8.9 | 2.2 | 0.0 | 1.1 | 1.1 | 0.0 | 0.0 | 0.0 | 0.0 | 0.00 | 0.00 | 6 | 332 | 95 | | | | | | | | | | | 1.3 | | | 221 | | 0.4 | | | | | | 387 | |
| 1208 | 1 Tbs | Fat Free, grated, Weight Watchers | 6 | 14 | 33 | 1.9 | 1.9 | 0.0 | 1.0 | 1.0 | 0.0 | 0.0 | 0.0 | 0.0 | 0.00 | 0.00 | 5 | 0 | 0 | 0 | 0 | 0 | | | | | | | | 0.0 | | | 38 | | 0.0 | | | | 29 | | 43 | |
| 1075 | 1 Tbs | Grated, avg | 6 | 27 | 18 | 2.5 | 0.2 | 0.0 | 0.2 | 0.0 | 1.8 | 1.1 | 0.5 | 0.0 | 0.02 | 0.02 | 5 | 42 | 10 | 9 | 1 | | 0.00 | 0.02 | 0.02 | 0.01 | 0.08 | 0.5 | 0.03 | 0.0 | 0.0 | | 82 | 0.0 | 0.1 | 3 | 0.0 | 48 | 6 | 1.6 | 112 | 0.19 |
| 1061 | 1 ea | Hard, cube, avg | 10 | 39 | 29 | 3.6 | 0.3 | 0.0 | 0.3 | 0.0 | 2.6 | 1.6 | 0.8 | 0.1 | 0.03 | 0.03 | 7 | 60 | 15 | 14 | 1 | | 0.00 | 0.03 | 0.03 | 0.01 | 0.12 | 0.7 | 0.05 | 0.0 | 0.1 | | 118 | 0.0 | 0.1 | 4 | 0.0 | 69 | 9 | 2.3 | 160 | 0.28 |
| 1103 | 1 Tbs | Low Sod, avg | 6 | 27 | 22 | 2.5 | 0.2 | 0.0 | 0.2 | 0.0 | 1.8 | 1.2 | 0.5 | 0.0 | 0.02 | 0.02 | 5 | 42 | 11 | 9 | 2 | | 0.00 | 0.02 | 0.02 | 0.01 | 0.08 | 0.5 | 0.03 | 0.0 | 0.0 | | 83 | 0.0 | 0.1 | 3 | 0.0 | 48 | 6 | 1.4 | 4 | 0.19 |
| 1112 | 1 Tbs | Shredded, avg | 5 | 21 | 25 | 1.9 | 0.2 | 0.0 | 0.2 | 0.0 | 1.4 | 0.9 | 0.4 | 0.0 | 0.02 | 0.01 | 4 | 32 | 9 | 8 | 1 | | 0.00 | 0.02 | 0.01 | 0.01 | 0.07 | 0.4 | 0.03 | 0.0 | 0.0 | | 63 | 0.0 | 0.0 | 3 | 0.0 | 37 | 5 | 1.2 | 85 | 0.16 |
| 1062 | 1/4 cup | Port Du Salut, avg | 28 | 99 | 46 | 6.7 | 0.2 | 0.0 | 0.2 | 0.0 | 7.9 | 4.7 | 2.6 | 0.2 | 0.10 | 0.11 | 34 | 373 | 104 | 96 | 8 | | 0.00 | 0.07 | 0.02 | 0.01 | 0.42 | 5.1 | 0.06 | 0.0 | 0.1 | | 182 | 0.0 | 0.1 | 7 | 0.0 | 101 | 38 | 4.1 | 150 | 0.73 |
| | | Provolone | | | | | | | | | | | | | | | | | | | | | | | | | | | | | | | | | | | | | | | | |
| 1023 | 1/4 cup | Avg | 33 | 116 | 41 | 8.4 | 0.7 | 0.0 | 0.7 | 0.0 | 8.8 | 5.6 | 2.4 | 0.3 | 0.09 | 0.16 | 23 | 269 | 87 | 85 | 2 | | 0.01 | 0.11 | 0.05 | 0.02 | 0.48 | 3.4 | 0.16 | 0.0 | 0.1 | | 249 | 0.0 | 0.2 | 9 | 0.0 | 164 | 46 | 4.8 | 289 | 1.07 |
| 1255 | 1 oz | Aged, Stella Foods | 28 | 100 | 40 | 7.0 | 0.5 | 0.0 | 0.5 | 0.0 | 8.0 | 4.5 | | | | | 20 | 200 | 40 | | | | | | | | | | | 0.0 | | | 200 | | 0.0 | | | | | | 290 | |
| 1256 | 1 oz | Lite, Stella Foods | 28 | 70 | 52 | 8.0 | 0.5 | 0.0 | 0.5 | 0.0 | 3.5 | 2.0 | | | | | 20 | 200 | 40 | | | | | | | | | | | 0.0 | | | 250 | | 0.0 | | | | | | 120 | |
| 1257 | 1 oz | Mellow, Stella Foods | 28 | 100 | 44 | 7.0 | 0.5 | 0.0 | 0.0 | 0.5 | 7.0 | 4.0 | | | | | 20 | | | | | | | | | | | | | | | | | | | | | | | | 290 | |
| 1258 | 1 oz | Mild, Stella Foods | 28 | 100 | 44 | 7.0 | 0.5 | 0.0 | 0.0 | 0.5 | 7.0 | 4.0 | | | | | 20 | 200 | 40 | | | | | | | | | | | 0.0 | | | 200 | | 0.0 | | | | | | 290 | |
| 1424 | 1/4 cup | Reduced Fat, Alpine Lace | 31 | 77 | 45 | 10.0 | 1.1 | 0.0 | 0.0 | 1.1 | 5.5 | 3.3 | | | | | 17 | 332 | 95 | | | | | | | | | | | 1.3 | | | 387 | | 0.4 | | | | | | 133 | |
| 1328 | 1 oz | With Smoke flvr, Kraft | 28 | 100 | 44 | 7.0 | 0.5 | 0.0 | 0.5 | 0.0 | 7.0 | 5.0 | | | | | 25 | 300 | 86 | | | | | 0.07 | | | 0.48 | | | 0.0 | | | 200 | | 0.0 | 0 | | 150 | 25 | | 240 | 0.90 |
| 1024 | 1/4 cup | Ricotta, part skim, avg | 62 | 86 | 74 | 7.1 | 3.2 | 0.0 | 0.9 | 2.3 | 4.9 | 3.1 | 1.4 | 0.2 | 0.04 | 0.12 | 19 | 268 | 70 | 65 | 5 | | 0.01 | 0.11 | 0.05 | 0.01 | 0.18 | 8.1 | 0.15 | 0.0 | 0.0 | | 169 | 0.0 | 0.3 | 9 | 0.0 | 113 | 78 | 10.4 | 78 | 0.83 |
| 1064 | 1/4 cup | Ricotta, whole milk, avg | 62 | 108 | 72 | 7.0 | 1.9 | 0.0 | 0.9 | 1.0 | 8.1 | 5.1 | 2.3 | 0.2 | 0.07 | 0.17 | 32 | 304 | 83 | 77 | 6 | | 0.01 | 0.12 | 0.06 | 0.03 | 0.21 | 7.6 | 0.13 | 0.0 | 0.1 | | 128 | 0.0 | 0.2 | 7 | 0.0 | 98 | 65 | 9.0 | 52 | 0.72 |
| | | Romano | | | | | | | | | | | | | | | | | | | | | | | | | | | | | | | | | | | | | | | | |
| 1066 | 1 Tbs | Avg | 6 | 23 | 31 | 1.9 | 0.2 | 0.0 | 0.2 | 0.0 | 1.6 | 1.0 | 0.5 | 0.0 | 0.02 | 0.02 | 6 | 34 | 9 | 8 | 1 | | 0.00 | 0.02 | 0.00 | 0.01 | 0.07 | 0.4 | 0.03 | 0.0 | 0.0 | | 64 | 0.0 | 0.0 | 2 | 0.0 | 46 | 5 | 0.9 | 72 | 0.15 |
| 1266 | 1 Tbs | Grated, Di Giorno | 8 | 40 | 23 | 3.2 | 0.0 | 0.0 | 0.0 | 0.0 | 2.4 | 1.6 | | | | | 8 | 0 | 0 | 0 | 0 | 0 | | 0.00 | | | 0.00 | | | 0.0 | | | 96 | | 0.0 | 0 | | 64 | 0 | | 144 | 0.00 |
| 1262 | 1 oz | Shredded, Di Giorno | 28 | 110 | 31 | 8.0 | 0.5 | 0.0 | 0.5 | 0.0 | 8.0 | 5.0 | | | | | 30 | 200 | 40 | | | | | | | | | | | 0.0 | | | 300 | | 0.0 | | | | | | 390 | |
| 1026 | 1 Tbs | Roquefort, avg | 8 | 30 | 39 | 1.7 | 0.2 | 0.0 | 0.2 | 0.0 | 2.4 | 1.5 | 0.7 | 0.1 | 0.06 | 0.05 | 7 | 84 | 24 | 23 | 1 | | 0.00 | 0.05 | 0.06 | 0.01 | 0.05 | 3.9 | 0.14 | 0.0 | 0.0 | | 53 | 0.0 | 0.0 | 2 | 0.0 | 31 | 7 | 1.2 | 145 | 0.17 |
| | | Swiss | | | | | | | | | | | | | | | | | | | | | | | | | | | | | | | | | | | | | | | | |
| 1027 | 1/4 cup | Avg | 27 | 102 | 37 | 7.7 | 0.9 | 0.0 | 0.9 | 0.0 | 7.4 | 4.8 | 2.0 | 0.3 | 0.10 | 0.17 | 25 | 228 | 68 | 66 | 2 | | 0.01 | 0.10 | 0.02 | 0.02 | 0.45 | 1.7 | 0.12 | 0.0 | 0.3 | | 259 | 0.0 | 0.0 | 10 | 0.0 | 163 | 30 | 3.4 | 70 | 1.05 |
| 1225 | 1/4 cup | Fat Free, Lifetime | 31 | 44 | 64 | 8.9 | 1.1 | 0.0 | 1.1 | 0.0 | 0.0 | 0.0 | 0.0 | 0.0 | 0.00 | 0.00 | 6 | 332 | 95 | | | | | | | | | | | | | | 443 | | | | | | | | 244 | |
| 1093 | 1/4 cup | Lowfat, avg | 33 | 59 | 60 | 9.4 | 1.1 | 0.0 | 1.1 | 0.0 | 1.7 | 1.1 | 0.5 | 0.0 | 0.02 | 0.02 | 12 | 89 | 21 | 19 | 3 | | 0.01 | 0.12 | 0.03 | 0.03 | 0.55 | 2.0 | 0.13 | 0.0 | 0.0 | | 317 | 0.0 | 0.1 | 12 | 0.0 | 200 | 37 | 4.5 | 86 | 1.29 |
| 1104 | 1/4 cup | Low Sod, avg | 33 | 124 | 38 | 9.4 | 1.1 | 0.0 | 1.1 | 0.0 | 9.0 | 5.9 | 2.4 | 0.3 | 0.12 | 0.20 | 30 | 279 | 83 | 81 | 3 | | 0.01 | 0.12 | 0.03 | 0.03 | 0.55 | 2.0 | 0.13 | 0.0 | 0.1 | | 317 | 0.0 | 0.1 | 12 | 0.0 | 200 | 37 | 4.5 | 5 | 1.29 |
| 1428 | 1/4 cup | Reduced Fat, Alpine Lace | 31 | 100 | 43 | 8.9 | 1.1 | 0.0 | 0.0 | 1.1 | 6.6 | 4.4 | | | | | 22 | 332 | 95 | | | | | | | | | | | 1.3 | | | 277 | | 0.4 | | | | | | 39 | |
| 1067 | 1/4 cup | Tilsit, whole milk, avg | 28 | 95 | 43 | 6.8 | 0.5 | 0.0 | 0.5 | 0.0 | 7.3 | 4.7 | 2.0 | 0.2 | 0.09 | 0.11 | 29 | 293 | 81 | 74 | 7 | | 0.02 | 0.10 | 0.06 | 0.02 | 0.59 | 5.6 | 0.10 | 0.0 | 0.1 | | 196 | 0.0 | 0.1 | 4 | 0.0 | 140 | 18 | 4.1 | 211 | 0.98 |
| 1085 | 1 oz | Yogurt Cheese, avg | 28 | 21 | 76 | 2.2 | 2.9 | 0.0 | | | 0.1 | 0.0 | 0.0 | 0.0 | | | 1 | 2 | 0.6 | | | | 0.01 | 0.06 | 0.03 | 0.01 | 0.17 | 3.4 | | 0.3 | | | 56 | 0.0 | 0.0 | 5 | | 44 | 71 | | 21 | 0.27 |
| | | *PROCESSED CHEESE AND CHEESE SUBSTITUTES* | | | | | | | | | | | | | | | | | | | | | | | | | | | | | | | | | | | | | | | | |
| | | American Process Cheese & Cheese Food | | | | | | | | | | | | | | | | | | | | | | | | | | | | | | | | | | | | | | | | |
| 1425 | 1/4 cup | Alpine Lace | 31 | 89 | 46 | 6.6 | 2.2 | 0.0 | 0.0 | 2.2 | 6.6 | 4.4 | | | | | 22 | 332 | 95 | | | | | | | | | | | 1.3 | | | 277 | | 0.4 | | | | | | 221 | |
| 1393 | 1/4 cup | Cheez Whiz | 66 | 180 | 52 | 10.0 | 4.0 | 0.0 | 4.0 | 0.0 | 14.0 | 10.0 | | | | | 40 | 600 | 171 | | | | | 0.20 | | | 0.48 | | | 0.0 | | | 300 | | 0.0 | 0 | | 600 | 150 | | 1120 | 1.20 |
| 1001 | 1 oz | Cold Pack, avg | 28 | 93 | 43 | 5.5 | 2.3 | 0.0 | 2.3 | 0.0 | 6.9 | 4.3 | 2.0 | 0.2 | 0.07 | 0.13 | 18 | 197 | 57 | 53 | 3 | | 0.01 | 0.12 | 0.02 | 0.04 | 0.36 | 1.5 | 0.27 | 0.0 | 0.2 | | 139 | 0.0 | 0.2 | 8 | 0.0 | 112 | 102 | 4.5 | 270 | 0.84 |
| 1363 | 1 pce | Deluxe, slice, Kraft | 28 | 110 | 43 | 5.0 | 0.5 | 0.0 | 0.0 | 0.5 | 9.0 | 6.0 | | | | | 25 | 300 | 86 | | | | | 0.10 | | | 0.12 | | | 0.0 | | | 150 | | 0.0 | 0 | | 200 | 25 | | 460 | 0.60 |
| 1314 | 1 oz | Deluxe, 25% less fat, Kraft | 28 | 93 | | 5.3 | 1.3 | 0.0 | 1.3 | 0.0 | 6.7 | 4.0 | | | | | 20 | 267 | 76 | | | | | 0.14 | | | 0.16 | | | 0.0 | | | 267 | | 0.0 | 0 | | 200 | 53 | | 467 | 0.80 |
| 1427 | 1/4 cup | Fat Free, Alpine Lace | 31 | 44 | 56 | 8.9 | 2.2 | 0.0 | 1.1 | 1.1 | 0.0 | 0.0 | 0.0 | 0.0 | 0.00 | 0.00 | 6 | 332 | 95 | | | | | | | | | | | 1.3 | | | 221 | | 0.4 | | | | | | 310 | |
| 1409 | 1 oz | Fat Free, Lunch Wagon | 28 | 88 | 51 | 4.4 | 0.7 | 0.0 | 0.0 | 0.7 | 7.4 | 1.5 | | | | | 0 | 295 | 84 | | | | | 0.05 | | | 0.18 | | | 0.0 | | | 221 | | 0.0 | 0 | | 221 | 15 | | 309 | 0.44 |
| 1480 | 1 pce | Fat Free, slice, Con Agra | 19 | 25 | 62 | 4.0 | 2.0 | 0.0 | 0.0 | 2.0 | 0.0 | 0.0 | 0.0 | 0.0 | 0.00 | 0.00 | 5 | 300 | 86 | | | | 0.01 | 0.05 | 0.00 | | | | | 0.0 | | | 150 | | 0.0 | | | | | | 180 | |
| 1387 | 1 pce | Fat Free, slice, Harvest Moon | 19 | 50 | 52 | 4.0 | 1.0 | 0.0 | 1.0 | 0.0 | 3.0 | 2.0 | | | | | 10 | 100 | 29 | | | | | 0.07 | | | 0.24 | | | 0.0 | | | 150 | | 0.0 | 0 | | 100 | 45 | | 280 | 0.30 |
| 1204 | 1 pce | Fat Free, slice, Weight Watchers | 11 | 15 | 65 | 2.6 | 1.0 | 0.0 | 0.5 | 0.5 | 0.0 | 0.0 | 0.0 | 0.0 | 0.00 | 0.00 | 0 | 103 | 30 | | | | | | | | | | | 0.0 | | | 52 | | 0.0 | | | | 34 | | 160 | |
| 1406 | 1 oz | Golden Image | 28 | 93 | 43 | 6.7 | 1.3 | 0.0 | 0.7 | 0.7 | 6.7 | 2.0 | | | | | 7 | 533 | 152 | | | | | 0.09 | | | 0.32 | | | 0.0 | | | 200 | | 0.0 | 0 | | 133 | 53 | | 360 | 0.80 |
| 1380 | 1/4 cup | Grated, Kraft | 20 | 100 | 24 | 4.0 | 4.0 | 0.0 | 4.0 | 0.0 | 6.0 | 4.0 | | | | | 8 | 0 | 0 | 0 | 0 | 0 | | 0.14 | | | 0.48 | | | 0.0 | | | 160 | | 0.0 | 0 | | 240 | 200 | | 540 | 0.00 |
| 1189 | 1/4 cup | Light, Cheez Whiz | 70 | 160 | 54 | 12.0 | 12.0 | 0.0 | 6.0 | 6.0 | 6.0 | 4.0 | | | | | 30 | 800 | 229 | | | | | 0.27 | | | 0.24 | | | 0.0 | | | 300 | | 0.0 | 16 | | 700 | 220 | | 1080 | 1.20 |
| 1580 | 1 oz | Light, Land O' Lakes | 28 | 70 | 57 | 7.0 | 1.0 | 0.0 | 1.0 | 0.0 | 4.0 | 3.0 | | | | | 20 | 500 | 143 | | | | | | | | | | | 0.0 | | | 200 | | 0.0 | | | | | | 360 | |
| 1229 | 1 oz | Light,Velveeta | 28 | 60 | 57 | 6.0 | 3.0 | 0.0 | 3.0 | 0.0 | 3.0 | 2.0 | | | | | 10 | 300 | 86 | | | | | 0.14 | | | 0.36 | | | 0.0 | | | 150 | | 0.0 | 8 | | 250 | 75 | | 420 | 0.60 |
| 1096 | 1/4 cup | Lowfat, avg | 28 | 50 | 59 | 7.1 | 1.0 | 0.0 | 1.0 | 0.0 | 2.0 | 1.2 | 0.6 | 0.1 | 0.02 | 0.04 | 10 | 76 | 18 | 16 | 2 | | 0.01 | 0.11 | 0.02 | 0.02 | 0.22 | 2.5 | 0.11 | 0.0 | 0.0 | | 192 | 0.0 | 0.1 | 7 | 0.0 | 232 | 50 | 2.7 | 400 | 0.93 |
| 1207 | 1 pce | Low Sod, slice, Weight Watchers | 11 | 15 | 62 | 2.6 | 1.0 | 0.0 | 1.0 | 0.0 | 0.0 | 0.0 | 0.0 | 0.0 | 0.00 | 0.00 | 3 | 103 | 30 | | | | | | | | | | | 0.0 | | | 103 | | 0.0 | | | | 145 | | 57 | |
| 1289 | 1 pce | Sharp Cheddar flvr, fat free, slice, Kraft | 21 | 30 | | 5.0 | 3.0 | 0.0 | 2.0 | 1.0 | 0.0 | 0.0 | 0.0 | 0.0 | 0.00 | 0.00 | 2 | 300 | 86 | | | | | 0.10 | | | 0.24 | | | 0.0 | | | 150 | | 0.0 | 0 | | 200 | 55 | | 290 | 0.60 |
| 1367 | 1/4 cup | Shredded, avg | 27 | 110 | 37 | 6.0 | 0.5 | 0.0 | 0.0 | 0.5 | 9.0 | 6.0 | | | | | 30 | 400 | 114 | | | | | 0.10 | | | 0.12 | | | 0.0 | | | 150 | | 0.0 | 0 | | 200 | 15 | | 440 | 0.90 |

| Code | Amount | Description | Weight (g) | Calories | % Water | Protein (g) | Carbs (g) | Fiber (g) | Sugar (g) | Other Carbs (g) | Fat (g) | Sat Fat (g) | Mono Fat (g) | Poly Fat (g) | Omega 3 (g) | Omega 6 (g) | Choles (mg) | Vit A (IU) | Vit A (RE) | Retinol (RE) | Carotenoids (RE) | Beta Carotene (mcg) | Thiamin (mg) | Riboflavin (mg) | Niacin (NE) | Vit B6 (mg) | Vit B12 (mcg) | Folate (mcg) | Panto (mg) | Vit C (mg) | Vit D (mg) | Vit E (α TE) | Calcium (mg) | Copper (mg) | Iron (mg) | Magnes (mg) | Mang (mg) | Phos (mg) | Potassium (mg) | Selenium (mcg) | Sodium (mg) | Zinc (mg) |
|---|---|---|---|---|---|---|---|---|---|---|---|---|---|---|---|---|---|---|---|---|---|---|---|---|---|---|---|---|---|---|---|---|---|---|---|---|---|---|---|---|---|---|
| | | **Basic Components / Additional Fats / Vit A & Components / Vitamins / Minerals** | | | | | | | | | | | | | | | | | | | | | | | | | | | | | | | | | | | | | | | | |
| 1383 | 1/4 cup | Shredded, Velveeta | 36 | 130 | 40 | 8.0 | 3.0 | 0.0 | 3.0 | 0.0 | 9.0 | 6.0 | | | | | 30 | 750 | 214 | | | | | 0.17 | | | 0.48 | | | 0.0 | | | 200 | | 0.0 | 8 | | 150 | 100 | | 500 | 0.90 |
| 1287 | 1 pce | Singles, fat free, slice, Kraft | 21 | 30 | | 5.0 | 3.0 | 0.0 | 2.0 | 1.0 | 0.0 | 0.0 | 0.0 | 0.0 | 0.00 | 0.00 | 2 | 86 | 24 | | | | | 0.10 | | | 0.24 | | | 0.0 | | | 150 | | 0.0 | 0 | | 200 | 60 | | 320 | 0.60 |
| 1373 | 1 pce | Singles, slice, Kraft | 21 | 70 | 43 | 4.0 | 2.0 | 0.0 | 1.0 | 1.0 | 5.0 | 3.5 | | | | | 15 | 300 | 86 | | | | | 0.10 | | | 0.12 | | | 0.0 | | | 100 | | 0.0 | 0 | | 100 | 50 | | 290 | 0.30 |
| 1315 | 1 oz | Singles,1/3 less fat, Kraft | 28 | 67 | | 6.7 | 2.7 | 0.0 | 1.3 | 1.3 | 4.0 | 2.7 | | | | | 13 | 400 | 114 | | | | | 0.09 | | | 0.32 | | | 0.0 | | | 200 | | 0.0 | 0 | | 133 | 73 | | 440 | 0.80 |
| 1072 | 1 pce | Slice, avg | 21 | 69 | 43 | 4.1 | 1.5 | 0.0 | 1.5 | 0.0 | 5.2 | 3.2 | 1.5 | 0.2 | 0.05 | 0.10 | 13 | 132 | 46 | 43 | 3 | | 0.01 | 0.09 | 0.03 | 0.03 | 0.24 | 1.5 | 0.12 | 0.0 | 0.1 | | 121 | 0.0 | 0.2 | 7 | 0.0 | 96 | 59 | 3.4 | 250 | 0.63 |
| 1368 | 1 pce | Slice, Harvest Moon | 19 | 70 | 42 | 4.0 | 0.0 | 0.0 | 0.0 | 0.0 | 6.0 | 4.0 | | | | | 20 | 200 | 57 | | | | | 0.07 | | | 0.12 | | | 0.0 | | | 100 | | 0.0 | 0 | | 150 | 15 | | 320 | 0.60 |
| 1288 | 1 pce | White, fat free, slice, Kraft | 21 | 30 | | 5.0 | 3.0 | 0.0 | 2.0 | 1.0 | 0.0 | 0.0 | 0.0 | 0.0 | 0.00 | 0.00 | 2 | 200 | 57 | | | | | 0.10 | | | 0.12 | | | 0.0 | | | 150 | | 0.0 | 0 | | 200 | 60 | | 320 | 0.60 |
| 1203 | 1 pce | White, fat free, slice, Weight Watchers | 11 | 15 | 65 | 2.6 | 1.0 | 0.0 | 0.5 | 0.5 | 0.0 | 0.0 | 0.0 | 0.0 | 0.00 | 0.00 | 0 | 103 | 30 | | | | | | | | | | | 0.0 | | | 52 | | 0.0 | | | | 34 | | 160 | |
| 1206 | 1 pce | White, low sod, slice, Weight Watchers | 5 | 7 | 66 | 1.2 | 0.5 | 0.0 | 0.2 | 0.2 | 0.0 | 0.0 | 0.0 | 0.0 | 0.00 | 0.00 | 1 | 47 | 13 | | | | | | | | | | | 0.0 | | | 47 | | 0.0 | | | | 66 | | 26 | |
| 1364 | 1 pce | White, slice, Kraft | 28 | 110 | 39 | 6.0 | 0.5 | 0.0 | 0.0 | 0.5 | 9.0 | 6.0 | | | | | 25 | 300 | 86 | | | | | 0.10 | | | 0.24 | | | 0.0 | | | 150 | | 0.0 | 0 | | 200 | 25 | | 460 | 0.60 |
| | | American Cheese Sauces | | | | | | | | | | | | | | | | | | | | | | | | | | | | | | | | | | | | | | | | |
| 1386 | 1 Tbs | Cheese Whiz, Squeezable | 16 | 48 | 55 | 1.0 | 1.9 | 0.0 | 0.5 | 1.5 | 3.9 | 1.9 | | | | | 7 | 48 | 14 | | | | | 0.02 | | | 0.00 | | | 0.0 | | | 19 | | 0.0 | 0 | | 97 | 15 | | 228 | 0.00 |
| 1397 | 1 Tbs | Cheese Whiz, Zap-a-pack | 16 | 44 | 52 | 1.5 | 1.5 | 0.0 | 1.5 | 0.0 | 3.9 | 2.4 | | | | | 10 | 145 | 42 | | | | | 0.07 | | | 0.06 | | | 0.0 | | | 48 | | 0.0 | 4 | | 145 | 53 | | 281 | 0.15 |
| 1440 | 1 Tbs | Fondue, avg | 14 | 32 | 62 | 2.0 | 0.5 | 0.0 | | | 1.9 | 1.2 | 0.5 | 0.1 | 0.02 | 0.04 | 6 | 58 | 16 | | | | 0.03 | 0.03 | 0.03 | 0.01 | 0.12 | 1.1 | 0.03 | 0.0 | | | 67 | 0.0 | 0.1 | 3 | 0.0 | 43 | 15 | 1.3 | 18 | 0.27 |
| 1441 | 1 Tbs | Prep f/Recipe, avg | 15 | 30 | 67 | 1.5 | 0.8 | 0.0 | | | 2.2 | 1.2 | 0.7 | 0.2 | 0.03 | 0.18 | 6 | 91 | 24 | 21 | 3 | | 0.01 | 0.04 | 0.03 | 0.01 | 0.05 | 1.5 | 0.03 | 0.1 | | | 47 | 0.0 | 0.1 | 3 | 0.0 | 34 | 21 | 1.0 | 74 | 0.19 |
| | | American Cheese Spreads | | | | | | | | | | | | | | | | | | | | | | | | | | | | | | | | | | | | | | | | |
| 1002 | 1 Tbs | Avg | 15 | 44 | 48 | 2.5 | 1.3 | 0.0 | 1.3 | 0.0 | 3.2 | 2.0 | 0.9 | 0.1 | 0.03 | 0.06 | 8 | 118 | 29 | 27 | 2 | | 0.01 | 0.06 | 0.02 | 0.02 | 0.06 | 1.1 | 0.10 | 0.0 | 0.0 | | 84 | 0.0 | 0.0 | 4 | 0.0 | 107 | 36 | 1.7 | 202 | 0.39 |
| 1625 | 1 oz | Cheddar Base, low fat, avg | 28 | 50 | 62 | 7.1 | 1.0 | 0.0 | 1.0 | 0.0 | 2.0 | 1.2 | 0.6 | 0.1 | 0.02 | 0.04 | 10 | 76 | 18 | 16 | 2 | | 0.01 | 0.11 | 0.02 | 0.02 | 0.22 | 2.5 | 0.11 | 0.0 | 0.0 | | 192 | 0.0 | 0.1 | 7 | 0.0 | 232 | 50 | 2.7 | 2 | 0.93 |
| 1398 | 1 oz | Harvest Moon | 28 | 88 | 47 | 4.4 | 2.9 | 0.0 | 1.5 | 1.5 | 5.9 | 3.7 | | | | | 22 | 147 | 42 | | | | | 0.10 | | | 0.18 | | | 0.0 | | | 118 | | 0.0 | 0 | | 118 | 81 | | 398 | 0.44 |
| 1272 | 1 oz | Velveeta | 28 | 80 | 46 | 5.0 | 3.0 | 0.0 | 2.0 | 1.0 | 6.0 | 4.0 | | | | | 20 | 300 | 86 | | | | | 0.14 | | | 0.24 | | | 0.0 | | | 150 | | 0.0 | 8 | | 250 | 80 | | 420 | 0.60 |
| 1411 | 1/4 cup | Blue Cheese, Roka Brand Spread | 64 | 160 | 57 | 6.0 | 4.0 | 0.0 | 2.0 | 2.0 | 14.0 | 9.0 | | | | | 40 | 600 | 171 | | | | | 0.14 | | | 0.24 | | | 0.0 | | | 80 | | 0.0 | 0 | | 80 | 120 | | 680 | 0.00 |
| | | Cheddar Cheese / Process Cheese / Cheese Food | | | | | | | | | | | | | | | | | | | | | | | | | | | | | | | | | | | | | | | | |
| 1371 | 1 Tbs | Extra Sharp, cold pack, Cracker Barrel | 16 | 52 | 44 | 2.6 | 1.5 | 0.0 | 1.5 | 0.0 | 4.1 | 0.8 | | | | | 13 | 155 | 44 | | | | | 0.09 | | | 0.19 | | | 0.0 | | | 77 | | 0.0 | 4 | | 52 | 59 | | 150 | 0.31 |
| 1369 | 1 oz | Old English | 28 | 100 | 39 | 6.0 | 0.5 | 0.0 | 0.0 | 0.5 | 9.0 | 6.0 | | | | | 25 | 400 | 114 | | | | | 0.10 | | | 0.24 | | | 0.0 | | | 150 | | 0.0 | 0 | | 200 | 20 | | 440 | 0.90 |
| 1372 | 1 Tbs | Sharp Cheddar, cold pack, Cracker Barrel | 16 | 52 | 41 | 2.6 | 2.1 | 0.0 | 1.5 | 0.5 | 4.1 | 2.6 | | | | | 13 | 155 | 44 | | | | | 0.09 | | | 0.19 | | | 0.0 | | | 77 | | 0.0 | 4 | | 52 | 67 | | 150 | 0.31 |
| 1577 | 1 oz | Sharp Cheddar, Land O' Lakes | 28 | 110 | 37 | 6.0 | 1.0 | 0.0 | 0.0 | 1.0 | 9.0 | 6.0 | | | | | 30 | 500 | 167 | | | | | | | | | | | 0.0 | | | 150 | | 0.0 | | | | | | 380 | |
| 1377 | 1 pce | Sharp Cheddar Singles, Kraft | 21 | 70 | 46 | 4.0 | 0.5 | 0.0 | 0.0 | 0.5 | 6.0 | 4.0 | | | | | 20 | 300 | 86 | | | | | 0.07 | | | 0.12 | | | 0.0 | | | 100 | | 0.0 | 0 | | 100 | 25 | | 300 | 0.30 |
| 1317 | 1 oz | Sharp Cheddar Singles, 1/3 less fat, Kraft | 28 | 67 | | 6.7 | 2.7 | 0.0 | 1.3 | 1.3 | 4.0 | 2.7 | | | | | 13 | 400 | 114 | | | | | 0.09 | | | 0.32 | | | 0.0 | | | 200 | | 0.0 | 0 | | 133 | 80 | | 400 | 0.80 |
| 1408 | 1/4 cup | Shredded, Harvest Moon | 36 | 120 | 46 | 6.0 | 3.0 | 0.0 | 2.0 | 1.0 | 9.0 | 2.0 | | | | | 0 | 750 | 214 | | | | | 0.07 | | | 0.12 | | | 0.0 | | | 250 | | 0.0 | 8 | | 250 | 65 | | 480 | 0.60 |
| | | Cheddar Cheese Spreads | | | | | | | | | | | | | | | | | | | | | | | | | | | | | | | | | | | | | | | | |
| 1400 | 1 Tbs | Old English Sharp Cheddar, Kraft | 16 | 45 | 52 | 2.5 | 0.3 | 0.0 | 0.0 | 0.3 | 4.0 | 2.5 | | | | | 12 | 250 | 71 | | | | | 0.03 | | | 0.06 | | | 0.0 | | | 75 | | 0.0 | 0 | | 150 | 8 | | 260 | 0.30 |
| 1401 | 1 Tbs | Squeez-A-Snak Sharp Cheddar, Kraft | 16 | 45 | 52 | 2.5 | 0.3 | 0.0 | 0.0 | 0.3 | 4.0 | 2.5 | | | | | 12 | 150 | 43 | | | | | 0.03 | | | 0.12 | | | 0.0 | | | 75 | | 0.0 | 0 | | 125 | 8 | | 220 | 0.45 |
| 1193 | 1 Tbs | Spreadery Medium Cheddar | 16 | 41 | 57 | 2.6 | 1.5 | 0.0 | 1.0 | 0.5 | 2.3 | 1.5 | | | | | 8 | 52 | 15 | | | | | 0.09 | | | 0.25 | | | 0.0 | | | 77 | | 0.0 | 4 | | 77 | 88 | | 150 | 0.31 |
| 1388 | 1 Tbs | Spreadery Sharp Cheddar | 16 | 41 | 55 | 2.6 | 1.5 | 0.0 | 1.0 | 0.5 | 2.3 | 1.5 | | | | | 8 | 52 | 15 | | | | | 0.09 | | | 0.19 | | | 0.0 | | | 77 | | 0.0 | 4 | | 77 | 88 | | 150 | 0.31 |
| 1190 | 1 Tbs | Spreadery White Cheddar | 16 | 41 | 57 | 2.6 | 1.5 | 0.0 | 1.0 | 0.5 | 2.3 | 1.5 | | | | | 8 | 52 | 15 | | | | | 0.09 | | | 0.19 | | | 0.0 | | | 77 | | 0.0 | 4 | | 77 | 88 | | 150 | 0.31 |
| 1184 | 1 Tbs | Wine flavored, Wispride Lite | 16 | 45 | | 2.3 | 2.3 | | | | 2.8 | 1.1 | | | | | 8 | | | | | | | | | | | | | | | | 85 | | | | | | | | 113 | |
| 1399 | 1 Tbs | Limburger, Mohawk Valley, spread, Kraft | 16 | 40 | 60 | 2.0 | 0.0 | 0.0 | 0.0 | 0.0 | 3.5 | 2.3 | | | | | 10 | 150 | 43 | | | | | 0.02 | | | 0.00 | | | 0.0 | | | 75 | | 0.0 | 0 | | 125 | 8 | | 250 | 0.30 |
| 1376 | 1 pce | Monterey Jack, Singles, slice, Kraft | 21 | 70 | 42 | 4.0 | 2.0 | 0.0 | 0.5 | 1.5 | 5.0 | 3.5 | | | | | 15 | 100 | 29 | | | | | 0.10 | | | 0.24 | | | 0.0 | | | 100 | | 0.0 | 0 | | 100 | 55 | | 290 | 0.30 |
| | | Mozzarella Process Cheese | | | | | | | | | | | | | | | | | | | | | | | | | | | | | | | | | | | | | | | | |
| 1092 | 1/4 cup | Avg | 28 | 50 | 61 | 4.5 | 3.4 | 0.0 | 3.4 | 0.0 | 2.0 | 1.3 | 0.6 | 0.1 | | | 5 | 86 | 22 | 20 | 2 | | 0.01 | 0.11 | 0.05 | 0.04 | 0.13 | 1.1 | 0.02 | 0.0 | 0.0 | | 160 | 0.0 | 0.0 | 8 | 0.0 | 204 | 65 | 3.4 | 321 | 0.73 |
| 1559 | 1 Tbs | E-Z Melt , imit, Whitehall Specialties | 6 | 20 | 48 | 0.8 | 0.4 | 0.0 | 0.0 | 0.4 | 1.6 | 0.2 | | | | | 0 | 20 | 4 | | | | | | | | | | | 0.0 | | | 0 | | 0.0 | | | | | | 74 | |
| 1421 | 1/4 cup | Fat Free, Alpine Lace | 31 | 44 | 54 | 8.7 | 2.2 | 0.0 | 1.1 | 1.1 | 0.0 | 0.0 | 0.0 | 0.0 | 0.00 | 0.00 | 5 | 328 | 94 | | | | | | | | | | | 1.3 | | | 219 | | 0.4 | | | | | | 306 | |
| 1321 | 1/4 cup | Low Moist, part skim, Harvest Moon | 36 | 110 | | 8.0 | 1.0 | 0.0 | 0.0 | 1.0 | 8.0 | 1.5 | | | | | 0 | 0 | 0 | 0 | 0 | 0 | | 0.00 | | | 0.24 | | | 0.0 | | | 300 | | 0.0 | 8 | | 250 | 0 | | 430 | 0.90 |
| | | Swiss Process Cheese and Cheese Food | | | | | | | | | | | | | | | | | | | | | | | | | | | | | | | | | | | | | | | | |
| 1458 | 1 pce | Avg, slice | 21 | 70 | 42 | 5.2 | 0.4 | 0.0 | 0.4 | 0.0 | 5.3 | 3.4 | 1.5 | 0.1 | 0.06 | 0.07 | 18 | 170 | 48 | 47 | 1 | | 0.00 | 0.06 | 0.01 | 0.01 | 0.26 | 1.2 | 0.05 | 0.0 | 0.0 | | 162 | 0.0 | 0.1 | 6 | 0.0 | 160 | 45 | 3.3 | 288 | 0.76 |
| 1097 | 1/4 cup | Lowfat, avg | 35 | 59 | 59 | 9.1 | 1.5 | 0.0 | 1.5 | 0.0 | 1.8 | 1.1 | 0.5 | 0.0 | 0.02 | 0.02 | 12 | 95 | 23 | 20 | 3 | | 0.01 | 0.14 | 0.03 | 0.03 | 0.27 | 3.1 | 0.11 | 0.0 | 0.0 | | 239 | 0.0 | 0.2 | 8 | 0.0 | 289 | 63 | 4.3 | 500 | 1.16 |
| 1330 | 1 oz | Baby, Kraft | 28 | 110 | 37 | 7.0 | 0.0 | 0.0 | 0.0 | 0.0 | 9.0 | 6.0 | | | | | 25 | 300 | 85 | | | | | 0.10 | | | 0.36 | | | 0.0 | | | 200 | | 0.0 | 0 | | 150 | 15 | | 110 | 0.90 |
| 1624 | 1 pce | Nonfat, Deluxe, slice, Kraft | 28 | 40 | | 6.7 | 4.0 | 0.0 | 2.7 | 1.3 | 0.0 | 0.0 | 0.0 | 0.0 | 0.00 | 0.00 | 3 | 400 | 114 | | | | | 0.14 | | | 0.32 | | | 0.0 | | | 200 | | 0.0 | 0 | | 267 | 80 | | 387 | 0.80 |
| 1378 | 1 pce | Singles, slice, Kraft | 21 | 70 | 48 | 4.0 | 1.0 | 0.0 | 1.0 | 0.0 | 5.0 | 3.5 | | | | | 15 | 200 | 57 | | | | | 0.07 | | | 0.36 | | | 0.0 | | | 150 | | 0.0 | 0 | | 100 | 50 | | 320 | 0.30 |
| 1318 | 1 pce | Singles, 1/3 less fat, slice, Kraft | 28 | 67 | | 6.7 | 2.7 | 0.0 | 1.3 | 1.3 | 3.3 | 2.0 | | | | | 13 | 267 | 75 | | | | | 0.09 | | | 0.32 | | | 0.0 | | | 200 | | 0.0 | 0 | | 133 | 80 | | 360 | 0.80 |
| | | Cheese Mixtures | | | | | | | | | | | | | | | | | | | | | | | | | | | | | | | | | | | | | | | | |
| 1410 | 1 Tbs | Bacon flvd Spread, Kraft | 16 | 45 | 52 | 2.5 | 0.3 | 0.0 | 0.0 | 0.3 | 4.0 | 2.5 | | | | | 12 | 250 | 71 | | | | | 0.03 | | | 0.06 | | | 0.0 | | | 75 | | 0.0 | 0 | | 150 | 10 | | 285 | 0.15 |
| 1566 | 1 oz | Cheddarella, Land O' Lakes | 28 | 100 | 42 | 7.0 | 0.0 | 0.0 | 0.0 | 0.0 | 8.0 | 5.0 | | | | | 25 | 300 | 85 | | | | | | | | | | | 0.0 | | | 200 | | 0.0 | | | | | | 200 | |
| 1282 | 1 oz | Colby & Monterey Jack, Kraft | 28 | 110 | 39 | 7.0 | 0.0 | 0.0 | 0.0 | 0.0 | 9.0 | 6.0 | | | | | 30 | 300 | 85 | | | | | 0.10 | | | 0.24 | | | 0.0 | | | 200 | | 0.0 | 0 | | 150 | 15 | | 190 | 0.90 |
| 1333 | 1/4 cup | Colby & Monterey Jack, shredded, Kraft | 30 | 120 | 38 | 7.0 | 0.5 | 0.0 | 0.0 | 0.5 | 10.0 | 6.0 | | | | | 30 | 300 | 85 | | | | | 0.10 | | | 0.24 | | | 0.0 | | | 200 | | 0.0 | 8 | | 150 | 20 | | 200 | 0.90 |
| 1518 | 1/4 cup | Fancy Blend, shredded, Cabot | 28 | 100 | 42 | 7.0 | 1.0 | 0.0 | 0.0 | 1.0 | 7.0 | 4.0 | | | | | 20 | 300 | 85 | | | | | | | | | | | 0.0 | | | 200 | | 0.0 | | | | | | 180 | |
| 1381 | 1 oz | Garlic flvd Cheese Food, Kraft | 28 | 90 | 44 | 5.0 | 2.0 | 0.0 | 2.0 | 0.0 | 7.0 | 5.0 | | | | | 20 | 300 | 85 | | | | | 0.10 | | | 0.36 | | | 0.0 | | | 150 | | 0.0 | 8 | | 250 | 75 | | 370 | 0.60 |
| 1338 | 1 Tbs | Italian Blend, grated, Kraft | 9 | 38 | | 4.5 | 0.0 | 0.0 | 0.0 | 0.0 | 2.3 | 1.5 | | | | | 3 | 0 | 0 | 0 | 0 | 0 | | 0.00 | | | 0.36 | | | 0.0 | | | 120 | | 0.0 | 0 | | 90 | 0 | | 142 | 0.45 |
| 1299 | 1 Tbs | Italian, lowfat, grated, Kraft | 9 | 38 | | 3.0 | 1.5 | 0.0 | 0.0 | 1.5 | 1.5 | 0.8 | | | | | 3 | 0 | 0 | 0 | 0 | 0 | | 0.00 | | | 0.18 | | | 0.0 | | | 120 | | 0.0 | 0 | | 60 | 0 | | 172 | 0.45 |
| 1242 | 1 oz | Italian, Sharp, Stella Foods | 28 | 100 | | 8.0 | 0.5 | 0.0 | 0.5 | 0.0 | 7.0 | 4.5 | | | | | 30 | 300 | 60 | | | | | | | | | | | 0.0 | | | 200 | | 0.0 | | | | | | 330 | |
| 1402 | 1 oz | Velveeta Italiana Spread, Kraft | 28 | 80 | 50 | 5.0 | 2.0 | 0.0 | 2.0 | 0.0 | 6.0 | 4.0 | | | | | 20 | 200 | 57 | | | | | 0.14 | | | 0.36 | | | 0.0 | | | 100 | | 0.0 | 0 | | 200 | 75 | | 430 | 0.30 |
| | | Jalapeno Flavored Cheese | | | | | | | | | | | | | | | | | | | | | | | | | | | | | | | | | | | | | | | | |
| 1384 | 1/4 cup | Hot Mexican Cheese Food w/Jalepeno, Velveeta | 36 | 130 | 40 | 8.0 | 3.0 | 0.0 | 2.0 | 1.0 | 9.0 | 6.0 | | | | | 30 | 750 | 214 | | | | | 0.14 | | | 0.48 | | | 0.0 | | | 200 | | 0.0 | 8 | | 150 | 100 | | 540 | 0.90 |
| 1385 | 1/4 cup | Mild Mexican Cheese Food w/ Jalepeno, Velveeta | 36 | 130 | 40 | 8.0 | 3.0 | 0.0 | 2.0 | 1.0 | 9.0 | 6.0 | | | | | 30 | 750 | 214 | | | | | 0.14 | | | 0.48 | | | 0.0 | | | 200 | | 0.0 | 8 | | 150 | 95 | | 520 | 0.90 |
| 1327 | 1 oz | Nacho Blend w/peppers, Kraft | 28 | 110 | 41 | 7.0 | 0.0 | 0.0 | 0.0 | 0.0 | 9.0 | 6.0 | | | | | 30 | 300 | 60 | | | | | 0.10 | | | 0.24 | | | 0.0 | | | 200 | | 0.0 | 0 | | 150 | 15 | | 250 | 1.20 |
| 1382 | 1 oz | Past Proc Cheese Food w/Jalapenos, Kraft | 28 | 90 | 46 | 5.0 | 2.0 | 0.0 | 2.0 | 0.0 | 7.0 | 5.0 | | | | | 20 | 300 | 85 | | | | | 0.10 | | | 0.24 | | | 0.0 | | | 150 | | 0.0 | 0 | | 200 | 80 | | 370 | 0.30 |
| 1375 | 1 pce | Mexican Past Proc Cheese Food Singles, Kraft | 21 | 70 | 42 | 4.0 | 2.0 | 0.0 | 1.0 | 1.0 | 5.0 | 3.5 | | | | | 15 | 300 | 85 | | | | | 0.10 | | | 0.24 | | | 0.0 | | | 100 | | 0.0 | 0 | | 100 | 55 | | 330 | 0.30 |
| | | Pimento Flavored Cheese | | | | | | | | | | | | | | | | | | | | | | | | | | | | | | | | | | | | | | | | |
| 1365 | 1 pce | Deluxe, slice, Kraft | 28 | 100 | 42 | 6.0 | 0.5 | 0.0 | 0.0 | 0.5 | 8.0 | 6.0 | | | | | 25 | 300 | 85 | | | | | 0.10 | | | 0.24 | | | 0.0 | | | 150 | | 0.0 | 0 | | 200 | 25 | | 430 | 0.60 |
| 1200 | 1 Tbs | Olive & Pimiento Spread, Kraft | 16 | 35 | 62 | 1.0 | 1.5 | 0.0 | 1.0 | 0.5 | 3.0 | 2.0 | | | | | 10 | 150 | 43 | | | | | 0.02 | | | 0.00 | | | 0.0 | | | 10 | | 0.0 | 0 | | 10 | 25 | | 110 | 0.00 |

| Code | Amount | Description | Weight (g) | Calories | % Water | Protein (g) | Carbs (g) | Fiber (g) | Sugar (g) | Other Carbs (g) | Fat (g) | Sat Fat (g) | Mono Fat (g) | Poly Fat (g) | Omega 3 (g) | Omega 6 (g) | Choles (mg) |
|---|---|---|---|---|---|---|---|---|---|---|---|---|---|---|---|---|---|
| 1379 | 1 pce | Singles, slice, Kraft | 21 | 70 | 42 | 4.0 | 2.0 | 0.0 | 0.5 | 1.5 | 5.0 | 3.5 | | | | | 15 |
| 1069 | 1/4 cup | Spread, avg | 28 | 105 | 39 | 6.2 | 0.5 | 0.0 | 0.5 | 0.0 | 8.7 | 5.5 | 2.5 | 0.3 | 0.11 | 0.17 | 26 |
| 1199 | 1 Tbs | Spread, Kraft | 16 | 40 | 62 | 1.0 | 1.5 | 0.0 | 1.0 | 0.5 | 3.0 | 2.0 | | | | | 10 |
| 1392 | 1 Tbs | Spreadery Snack Spread | 16 | 52 | 46 | 2.1 | 1.5 | 0.0 | 1.0 | 0.5 | 4.1 | 2.6 | | | | | 10 |
| 1196 | 1 Tbs | Pineapple Cheese Spread, Kraft | 15 | 33 | 62 | 0.9 | 1.9 | 0.0 | 1.9 | 0.0 | 2.3 | 1.6 | | | | | 7 |
| | | Pizza Cheese | | | | | | | | | | | | | | | |
| 1336 | 1/4 cup | Cheddar & Monterey Jack, shredded, Kraft | 26 | 100 | 40 | 6.0 | 0.5 | 0.0 | 0.0 | 0.5 | 8.0 | 6.0 | | | | | 25 |
| 1334 | 1/4 cup | Four Cheese, Pizza Style, shredded, Kraft | 27 | 90 | | 7.0 | 0.5 | 0.0 | 0.0 | 0.5 | 7.0 | 4.5 | | | | | 20 |
| 1296 | 1/4 cup | Mozzarella, shredded, Kraft | 26 | 90 | | 6.0 | 0.5 | 0.0 | 0.5 | 0.0 | 7.0 | 5.0 | | | | | 20 |
| 1322 | 1/4 cup | Mozzarella & Cheddar, low moist, shredded, Kraft | 27 | 100 | | 6.0 | 0.5 | 0.0 | 0.0 | 0.5 | 8.0 | 5.0 | | | | | 25 |
| 1337 | 1/4 cup | Mozzarella & Provolone, w/smoke flvr, Kraft | 27 | 90 | 46 | 6.0 | 0.5 | 0.0 | 0.5 | 0.0 | 7.0 | 4.5 | | | | | 20 |
| 1395 | 1 Tbs | Salsa flvd Cheese Whiz, mild, Kraft | 16 | 44 | 52 | 2.4 | 1.0 | 0.0 | 0.5 | 0.5 | 3.4 | 2.4 | | | | | 12 |
| 1394 | 1 Tbs | Salsa flvd Cheese Whiz, hot, Kraft | 16 | 44 | 52 | 2.4 | 1.0 | 0.0 | 0.5 | 0.5 | 3.4 | 2.4 | | | | | 12 |
| | | Substitutes | | | | | | | | | | | | | | | |
| 70525 | 1 pce | Better Than Cheese Tofutti, slice, Life Lite | 57 | 180 | 51 | 2.0 | 16.0 | | | | 10.0 | 4.0 | 0.0 | 6.0 | | | 0 |
| 70526 | 1 Tbs | Better Than Cream Cheese Tofutti, Life Lite | 14 | 39 | 65 | 0.5 | 0.5 | | | | 3.9 | 1.5 | 1.5 | 1.0 | | | 0 |
| 7656 | 1 oz | Cheddar Style Veg Cheese, White Almond | 28 | 54 | 58 | 6.9 | 3.0 | 1.0 | 2.0 | 0.0 | 1.0 | 0.0 | 1.0 | 0.0 | 0.00 | 0.00 | 0 |
| 7655 | 1 oz | Garlic & Herb Veg Cheese, White Almond | 28 | 54 | 58 | 6.9 | 3.0 | 1.0 | 2.0 | 0.0 | 1.0 | 0.0 | 1.0 | 0.0 | 0.00 | 0.00 | 0 |
| 7657 | 1 oz | Jalapeno Jack Style Veg Cheese, White Almond | 28 | 57 | 52 | 7.5 | 3.4 | 1.4 | 0.1 | 1.9 | 1.5 | 0.2 | 1.0 | 0.4 | | | 0 |
| 7654 | 1 oz | Mozzarella Style Veg Cheese, White Almond | 28 | 54 | 55 | 6.9 | 2.9 | 1.2 | 2.0 | | 1.6 | 0.2 | 1.0 | 0.0 | 0.00 | 0.00 | 0 |
| | | **DAIRY PRODUCTS AND SUBSTITUTES** | | | | | | | | | | | | | | | |
| | | *CREAMS AND SUBSTITUTES* | | | | | | | | | | | | | | | |
| | | Cream | | | | | | | | | | | | | | | |
| 500 | 1 Tbs | Half & half, avg | 15 | 20 | 81 | 0.4 | 0.6 | 0.0 | | | 1.7 | 1.1 | 0.5 | 0.1 | 0.03 | 0.04 | 6 |
| 501 | 1 Tbs | Light, avg | 15 | 29 | 74 | 0.4 | 0.5 | 0.0 | | | 2.9 | 1.8 | 0.8 | 0.1 | 0.04 | 0.07 | 10 |
| 527 | 1 Tbs | Medium, 25% fat, avg | 15 | 37 | 68 | 0.4 | 0.5 | 0.0 | | | 3.8 | 2.3 | 1.1 | 0.1 | 0.05 | 0.08 | 13 |
| 587 | 1 Tbs | Whipping, heavy, avg | 15 | 52 | 58 | 0.3 | 0.4 | 0.0 | 0.4 | 0.0 | 5.6 | 3.5 | 1.6 | 0.2 | 0.08 | 0.13 | 21 |
| 503 | 1 Tbs | Whipping, heavy, whipped, avg | 15 | 52 | 58 | 0.3 | 0.4 | 0.0 | 0.4 | 0.0 | 5.6 | 3.5 | 1.6 | 0.2 | 0.08 | 0.13 | 21 |
| 586 | 1 Tbs | Whipping, light, avg | 15 | 44 | 64 | 0.3 | 0.4 | 0.0 | | | 4.6 | 2.9 | 1.4 | 0.1 | 0.04 | 0.09 | 17 |
| 515 | 1 Tbs | Whipping, light, whipped, avg | 15 | 20 | 80 | 0.4 | 0.6 | 0.0 | | | 1.8 | 1.1 | 0.5 | 0.1 | 0.03 | 0.04 | 6 |
| | | Creamers | | | | | | | | | | | | | | | |
| 545 | 1 Tbs | Coffee Rich, light, Rich's | 14 | 12 | | 0.5 | 1.0 | | | | 0.5 | 0.0 | | | | | |
| 548 | 1 Tbs | Coffee Rich, Rich's | 14 | 24 | | 0.5 | 1.9 | | | | 1.9 | 0.0 | | | | | |
| 534 | 1 Tbs | Coffee whitener, avg | 15 | 20 | 77 | 0.2 | 1.7 | 0.0 | | | 1.5 | 0.3 | 1.1 | 0.0 | 0.00 | 0.00 | 0 |
| 541 | 1 Tbs | Lite, Coffee Mate | 9 | 45 | | 0.0 | 6.0 | 0.0 | 0.0 | 6.0 | 1.5 | 0.0 | | | | | 0 |
| 539 | 1 Tbs | Non-Dairy, Coffee Mate | 6 | 30 | | 0.0 | 3.0 | 0.0 | 0.0 | 3.0 | 1.5 | 1.5 | 0.0 | 0.0 | 0.00 | 0.00 | 0 |
| 540 | 1 Tbs | Non Dairy, Cremora | 6 | 30 | | 0.0 | 3.0 | | | | 1.5 | 1.5 | | | | | |
| 544 | 1 Tbs | Non Dairy, light, Rich's | 14 | 10 | | 0.5 | 0.5 | | | | 0.5 | 0.0 | | | | | |
| 542 | 1 Tbs | Non Dairy, lite, Cremora | 6 | 24 | | 1.5 | 6.0 | | | | 1.5 | 0.0 | | | 0.00 | 0.00 | |
| 517 | 1 Tbs | Non Dairy, Mocha Mix | 14 | 19 | 79 | 0.0 | 1.2 | 0.0 | | | 1.6 | 0.3 | 0.0 | 0.7 | | | 0 |
| 547 | 1 Tbs | Non Dairy, Rich's | 14 | 19 | | 0.5 | 1.0 | | | | 1.9 | 0.0 | | | | | |
| 506 | 1 Tbs | Powder, avg | 6 | 33 | 2 | 0.3 | 3.3 | 0.0 | 3.3 | 0.0 | 2.1 | 1.9 | 0.1 | 0.0 | 0.00 | 0.00 | 0 |
| 546 | 1 ea | Powder, dry pkt, Coffee Mate | 3 | 15 | | 0.0 | 2.0 | 0.0 | 0.0 | 2.0 | 1.0 | 1.0 | | | | | 0 |
| | | Dessert Toppings | | | | | | | | | | | | | | | |
| 513 | 2 Tbs | Dry Mix, avg | 3 | 17 | 1 | 0.1 | 1.6 | 0.0 | 1.6 | 0.0 | 1.2 | 1.1 | 0.0 | 0.0 | 0.00 | 0.01 | 0 |
| 508 | 2 Tbs | Frozen, semi solid, avg | 9 | 29 | 50 | 0.1 | 2.1 | 0.0 | 2.1 | 0.0 | 2.3 | 2.0 | 0.1 | 0.0 | 0.02 | 0.03 | 0 |
| 509 | 2 Tbs | Prep w/milk, avg | 10 | 19 | 67 | 0.4 | 1.6 | 0.0 | 1.6 | 0.0 | 1.2 | 1.1 | 0.1 | 0.0 | 0.00 | 0.02 | 1 |
| 514 | 2 Tbs | Pressurized, avg | 9 | 24 | 60 | 0.1 | 1.4 | 0.0 | 1.4 | 0.0 | 2.0 | 1.7 | 0.2 | 0.0 | 0.00 | 0.02 | 0 |
| 559 | 2 Tbs | Real Cream Topping, D-Zerta | 7 | 20 | | 0.0 | 1.0 | 0.0 | 1.0 | 0.0 | 1.5 | 1.0 | | | | | 5 |
| 526 | 2 Tbs | Whipped Cream Substitute, non dairy, prep, avg | 10 | 5 | 82 | 0.2 | 1.1 | 0.0 | 1.1 | 0.0 | 0.6 | 0.6 | 0.0 | 0.0 | | | 0 |
| 510 | 2 Tbs | Whipped Cream Topping, pressurized, avg | 8 | 21 | 61 | 0.3 | 1.0 | 0.0 | 1.0 | 0.0 | 1.8 | 1.1 | 0.5 | 0.1 | 0.03 | 0.04 | 6 |
| 569 | 2 Tbs | Whipped Topping, dry mix, Dream Whip | 2 | 12 | | 0.0 | 1.6 | 0.0 | 1.6 | 0.0 | 0.4 | 0.4 | 0.0 | 0.0 | 0.00 | 0.00 | 0 |
| 560 | 2 Tbs | Whipped Topping, D-Zerta | 7 | 20 | | 0.0 | 1.0 | 0.0 | 1.0 | 0.0 | 1.5 | 1.0 | | | | | 0 |
| 566 | 2 Tbs | Whipped Topping, extra creamy, Cool Whip | 9 | 30 | 55 | 0.0 | 2.0 | 0.0 | 2.0 | 0.0 | 2.0 | 2.0 | 0.0 | 0.0 | 0.00 | 0.00 | 0 |
| 565 | 2 Tbs | Whipped Topping, lite, Cool Whip | 8 | 20 | 62 | 0.0 | 2.0 | 0.0 | 1.0 | 1.0 | 1.0 | 1.0 | 0.0 | 0.0 | 0.00 | 0.00 | 0 |
| 564 | 2 Tbs | Whipped Topping, non dairy, Cool Whip | 8 | 25 | 56 | 0.0 | 2.0 | 0.0 | 1.0 | 1.0 | 1.5 | 1.5 | 0.0 | 0.0 | 0.00 | 0.00 | 0 |
| 70563 | 2 Tbs | Whipped Topping, non dairy, Mrs Smiths | 10 | 29 | 58 | 0.0 | 2.1 | | | | 2.1 | | | | | | 0 |
| 582 | 2 Tbs | Whipped Topping, prep w/milk & vanilla, Dream Whip | 10 | 20 | 69 | 0.0 | 2.0 | 0.0 | 2.0 | 0.0 | 1.0 | 1.0 | 0.0 | 0.0 | 0.00 | 0.00 | 0 |
| 568 | 2 Tbs | Whipped Topping, red cal, D-Zerta | 10 | 50 | | 0.0 | 5.0 | 0.0 | 0.0 | 5.0 | 5.0 | 2.5 | | | | | 0 |
| | | Sour Cream | | | | | | | | | | | | | | | |
| 504 | 2 Tbs | Avg | 29 | 62 | 71 | 0.9 | 1.2 | 0.0 | | | 6.1 | 3.8 | 1.8 | 0.2 | 0.09 | 0.14 | 13 |
| 555 | 2 Tbs | Breakstone's | 30 | 60 | 76 | 1.0 | 1.0 | 0.0 | 1.0 | 0.0 | 5.0 | 4.0 | | | | | 25 |
| 550 | 2 Tbs | Fat free, Breakstone's | 32 | 35 | | 2.0 | 6.0 | 0.0 | 2.0 | 4.0 | 0.0 | 0.0 | 0.0 | 0.0 | 0.00 | 0.00 | 2 |
| 515 | 2 Tbs | Half & Half, avg | 30 | 41 | 80 | 0.9 | 1.3 | 0.0 | | | 3.6 | 2.2 | 1.0 | 0.1 | 0.05 | 0.08 | 11 |
| 554 | 2 Tbs | Half & Half, Breakstone's | 31 | 45 | 78 | 1.0 | 2.0 | 0.0 | 2.0 | 0.0 | 3.5 | 2.5 | | | | | 15 |

| Code | Description | Vit A (IU) | Vit A (RE) | Retinol (RE) | Carotenoids (RE) | Beta Carotene (mcg) | Thiamin (mg) | Riboflavin (mg) | Niacin (NE) | Vit B6 (mg) | Vit B12 (mcg) | Folate (mcg) | Panto (mg) | Vit C (mg) | Vit D (mg) | Vit E (α TE) |
|---|---|---|---|---|---|---|---|---|---|---|---|---|---|---|---|---|
| 1379 | Singles, slice, Kraft | 300 | 86 | | | | | 0.07 | | | 0.24 | | | 0.0 | | |
| 1069 | Spread, avg | 353 | 90 | 76 | 14 | | 0.01 | 0.10 | 0.02 | 0.02 | 0.19 | 2.2 | 0.14 | 0.6 | 0.1 | |
| 1199 | Spread, Kraft | 150 | 43 | | | | | 0.03 | | | 0.00 | | | 0.0 | | |
| 1392 | Spreadery Snack Spread | 103 | 29 | | | | | 0.04 | | | 0.00 | | | 0.0 | | |
| 1196 | Pineapple Cheese Spread, Kraft | 94 | 27 | | | | | 0.02 | | | 0.00 | | | 0.0 | | |
| | Pizza Cheese | | | | | | | | | | | | | | | |
| 1336 | Cheddar & Monterey Jack, shredded, Kraft | 400 | 114 | | | | | 0.10 | | | 0.24 | | | 0.0 | | |
| 1334 | Four Cheese, Pizza Style, shredded, Kraft | 200 | 57 | | | | | 0.10 | | | 0.48 | | | 0.0 | | |
| 1296 | Mozzarella, shredded, Kraft | 300 | 86 | | | | | 0.07 | | | 0.36 | | | 0.0 | | |
| 1322 | Mozzarella & Cheddar, low moist, shredded, Kraft | 300 | 86 | | | | | 0.07 | | | 0.36 | | | 0.0 | | |
| 1337 | Mozzarella & Provolone, w/smoke flvr, Kraft | 200 | 57 | | | | | 0.07 | | | 0.48 | | | 0.0 | | |
| 1395 | Salsa flvd Cheese Whiz, mild, Kraft | 145 | 42 | | | | | 0.03 | | | 0.06 | | | 0.0 | | |
| 1394 | Salsa flvd Cheese Whiz, hot, Kraft | 145 | 42 | | | | | 0.03 | | | 0.06 | | | 0.0 | | |
| | Substitutes | | | | | | | | | | | | | | | |
| 70525 | Better Than Cheese Tofutti, slice, Life Lite | | | | | | | | | | | | | | | |
| 70526 | Better Than Cream Cheese Tofutti, Life Lite | | | | | | | | | | | | | | | |
| 7656 | Cheddar Style Veg Cheese, White Almond | 44 | 9 | | | | | | | | | | | 0.2 | | |
| 7655 | Garlic & Herb Veg Cheese, White Almond | 44 | 9 | | | | | | | | | | | 0.2 | | |
| 7657 | Jalapeno Jack Style Veg Cheese, White Almond | 1400 | 280 | | | | | | | | | | | 0.2 | | |
| 7654 | Mozzarella Style Veg Cheese, White Almond | 44 | 9 | | | | | | | | | | | 0.2 | | |
| | **DAIRY PRODUCTS AND SUBSTITUTES** | | | | | | | | | | | | | | | |
| | *CREAMS AND SUBSTITUTES* | | | | | | | | | | | | | | | |
| | Cream | | | | | | | | | | | | | | | |
| 500 | Half & half, avg | 65 | 16 | 15 | 0.6 | | 0.01 | 0.02 | 0.01 | 0.01 | 0.05 | 0.4 | 0.04 | 0.1 | 0.1 | |
| 501 | Light, avg | 95 | 27 | 26 | 1.6 | | 0.00 | 0.02 | 0.01 | 0.00 | 0.03 | 0.3 | 0.04 | 0.1 | 0.1 | |
| 527 | Medium, 25% fat, avg | 141 | 35 | 32 | 2.4 | | 0.00 | 0.02 | 0.01 | 0.00 | 0.03 | 0.3 | 0.04 | 0.1 | 0.1 | |
| 587 | Whipping, heavy, avg | 221 | 63 | 61 | 2 | | 0.00 | 0.02 | 0.01 | 0.00 | 0.03 | 0.6 | 0.04 | 0.1 | 0.2 | |
| 503 | Whipping, heavy, whipped, avg | 221 | 63 | 61 | 2 | | 0.00 | 0.02 | 0.01 | 0.00 | 0.03 | 0.6 | 0.04 | 0.1 | 0.2 | |
| 586 | Whipping, light, avg | 169 | 44 | 41 | 3 | | 0.00 | 0.02 | 0.01 | 0.00 | 0.03 | 0.6 | 0.04 | 0.1 | 0.0 | |
| 515 | Whipping, light, whipped, avg | 68 | 17 | 15 | 2 | | 0.01 | 0.02 | 0.01 | 0.00 | 0.05 | 1.6 | 0.05 | 0.1 | 0.0 | |
| | Creamers | | | | | | | | | | | | | | | |
| 545 | Coffee Rich, light, Rich's | | | | | | | | | | | | | | | |
| 548 | Coffee Rich, Rich's | | | | | | | | | | | | | | | |
| 534 | Coffee whitener, avg | 13 | 1.3 | | | | 0.00 | 0.00 | 0.00 | 0.00 | 0.00 | 0.0 | 0.00 | 0.0 | | |
| 541 | Lite, Coffee Mate | 0 | 0 | 0 | 0 | 0 | | | | | | | | 0.0 | | |
| 539 | Non-Dairy, Coffee Mate | 0 | 0 | 0 | 0 | 0 | | | | | | | | 0.0 | | |
| 540 | Non Dairy, Cremora | | | | | | | | | | | | | | | |
| 544 | Non Dairy, light, Rich's | | | | | | | | | | | | | | | |
| 542 | Non Dairy, lite, Cremora | | | | | | | | | | | | | | | |
| 517 | Non Dairy, Mocha Mix | | | | | | | | | | | | | | | |
| 547 | Non Dairy, Rich's | | | | | | | | | | | | | | | |
| 506 | Powder, avg | 12 | 1 | 0 | 1 | | 0.00 | 0.01 | 0.00 | 0.00 | 0.00 | 0.0 | 0.00 | 0.0 | 0.0 | |
| 546 | Powder, dry pkt, Coffee Mate | 0 | 0 | 0 | 0 | 0 | | | | | | | | 0.0 | | |
| | Dessert Toppings | | | | | | | | | | | | | | | |
| 513 | Dry Mix, avg | 32 | 3 | | | | 0.00 | 0.00 | 0.00 | 0.00 | 0.00 | 0.0 | 0.00 | 0.0 | 0.0 | |
| 508 | Frozen, semi solid, avg | 77 | 8 | 0 | 8 | | 0.00 | 0.00 | 0.00 | 0.00 | 0.00 | 0.0 | 0.00 | 0.0 | 0.0 | |
| 509 | Prep w/milk, avg | 36 | 5 | 2 | 3 | | 0.00 | 0.01 | 0.01 | 0.00 | 0.03 | 0.4 | 0.02 | 0.1 | 0.1 | |
| 514 | Pressurized, avg | 43 | 4 | | | | 0.00 | 0.00 | 0.00 | 0.00 | 0.00 | 0.0 | 0.00 | 0.0 | 0.0 | |
| 559 | Real Cream Topping, D-Zerta | 0 | 0 | 0 | 0 | 0 | | | | | | | | 0.0 | | |
| 526 | Whipped Cream Substitute, non dairy, prep, avg | 0 | 0 | 0 | 0 | 0 | 0.00 | 0.00 | 0.00 | 0.00 | 0.00 | 0.0 | 0.00 | 0.0 | 0.0 | |
| 510 | Whipped Cream Topping, pressurized, avg | 67 | 17 | 15 | 2 | | 0.00 | 0.01 | 0.01 | 0.00 | 0.02 | 0.2 | 0.02 | 0.0 | 0.0 | |
| 569 | Whipped Topping, dry mix, Dream Whip | 0 | 0 | 0 | 0 | 0 | | | | | | | | 0.0 | | |
| 560 | Whipped Topping, D-Zerta | 0 | 0 | 0 | 0 | 0 | | | | | | | | 0.0 | | |
| 566 | Whipped Topping, extra creamy, Cool Whip | 0 | 0 | 0 | 0 | 0 | | | | | | | | 0.0 | | |
| 565 | Whipped Topping, lite, Cool Whip | 0 | 0 | 0 | 0 | 0 | | | | | | | | 0.0 | | |
| 564 | Whipped Topping, non dairy, Cool Whip | 0 | 0 | 0 | 0 | 0 | | | | | | | | 0.0 | | |
| 70563 | Whipped Topping, non dairy, Mrs Smiths | 0 | 0 | 0 | 0 | 0 | 0.00 | 0.00 | 0.00 | | | | | 0.0 | | |
| 582 | Whipped Topping, prep w/milk & vanilla, Dream Whip | 0 | 0 | 0 | 0 | 0 | | | | | | | | 0.0 | | |
| 568 | Whipped Topping, red cal, D-Zerta | 0 | 0 | 0 | 0 | 0 | | | | | | | | 0.0 | | |
| | Sour Cream | | | | | | | | | | | | | | | |
| 504 | Avg | 229 | 57 | 51 | 6 | | 0.01 | 0.04 | 0.02 | 0.00 | 0.09 | 3.1 | 0.10 | 0.2 | 0.0 | |
| 555 | Breakstone's | 200 | 49 | | | | 0.00 | 0.03 | | | 0.00 | | | 0.0 | | |
| 550 | Fat free, Breakstone's | 200 | 49 | | | | 0.00 | 0.07 | | | 0.12 | | | 0.0 | | |
| 515 | Half & Half, avg | 136 | 34 | 30 | 4 | | 0.01 | 0.04 | 0.02 | 0.00 | 0.09 | 3.2 | 0.11 | 0.3 | 0.0 | |
| 554 | Half & Half, Breakstone's | 100 | 24 | | | | 0.00 | 0.07 | | | 0.12 | | | 0.0 | | |

| Code | Description | Calcium (mg) | Copper (mg) | Iron (mg) | Magnes (mg) | Mang (mg) | Phos (mg) | Potassium (mg) | Selenium (mcg) | Sodium (mg) | Zinc (mg) |
|---|---|---|---|---|---|---|---|---|---|---|---|
| 1379 | Singles, slice, Kraft | 100 | | 0.0 | 0 | | 100 | 55 | | 290 | 0.30 |
| 1069 | Spread, avg | 172 | 0.0 | 0.1 | 6 | 0.0 | 208 | 45 | 4.1 | 400 | 0.83 |
| 1199 | Spread, Kraft | 10 | | 0.0 | 0 | | 10 | 30 | | 85 | 0.00 |
| 1392 | Spreadery Snack Spread | 52 | | 0.0 | 0 | | 77 | 21 | | 165 | 0.15 |
| 1196 | Pineapple Cheese Spread, Kraft | 9 | | 0.0 | 0 | | 9 | 26 | | 56 | 0.00 |
| | Pizza Cheese | | | | | | | | | | |
| 1336 | Cheddar & Monterey Jack, shredded, Kraft | 150 | | 0.0 | 0 | | 100 | 25 | | 180 | 0.90 |
| 1334 | Four Cheese, Pizza Style, shredded, Kraft | 200 | | 0.0 | 8 | | 150 | 20 | | 230 | 1.20 |
| 1296 | Mozzarella, shredded, Kraft | 150 | | 0.0 | 0 | | 100 | 25 | | 170 | 0.90 |
| 1322 | Mozzarella & Cheddar, low moist, shredded, Kraft | 150 | | 0.0 | 0 | | 100 | 25 | | 190 | 0.90 |
| 1337 | Mozzarella & Provolone, w/smoke flvr, Kraft | 150 | | 0.0 | 0 | | 100 | 20 | | 210 | 0.90 |
| 1395 | Salsa flvd Cheese Whiz, mild, Kraft | 73 | | 0.0 | 0 | | 291 | 29 | | 257 | 0.29 |
| 1394 | Salsa flvd Cheese Whiz, hot, Kraft | 73 | | 0.0 | 0 | | 145 | 32 | | 262 | 0.29 |
| | Substitutes | | | | | | | | | | |
| 70525 | Better Than Cheese Tofutti, slice, Life Lite | | | | | | 35 | 80 | | 110 | |
| 70526 | Better Than Cream Cheese Tofutti, Life Lite | | | | | | | | | 99 | |
| 7656 | Cheddar Style Veg Cheese, White Almond | 138 | | 0.4 | | | | | | 217 | |
| 7655 | Garlic & Herb Veg Cheese, White Almond | 138 | | 0.4 | | | | | | 217 | |
| 7657 | Jalapeno Jack Style Veg Cheese, White Almond | 279 | | 0.2 | | | | | | 321 | |
| 7654 | Mozzarella Style Veg Cheese, White Almond | 137 | | 0.4 | | | | | | 504 | |
| | **DAIRY PRODUCTS AND SUBSTITUTES** | | | | | | | | | | |
| | *CREAMS AND SUBSTITUTES* | | | | | | | | | | |
| | Cream | | | | | | | | | | |
| 500 | Half & half, avg | 16 | 0.0 | 0.0 | 2 | 0.0 | 14 | 20 | 0.3 | 6 | 0.08 |
| 501 | Light, avg | 14 | 0.0 | 0.0 | 1 | 0.0 | 12 | 18 | 0.1 | 6 | 0.04 |
| 527 | Medium, 25% fat, avg | 14 | 0.0 | 0.0 | 1 | 0.0 | 11 | 17 | | 6 | 0.04 |
| 587 | Whipping, heavy, avg | 10 | 0.0 | 0.0 | 1 | 0.0 | 9 | 11 | 0.1 | 6 | 0.03 |
| 503 | Whipping, heavy, whipped, avg | 10 | 0.0 | 0.0 | 1 | 0.0 | 9 | 11 | 0.1 | 6 | 0.03 |
| 586 | Whipping, light, avg | 10 | 0.0 | 0.0 | 1 | 0.0 | 9 | 15 | 0.1 | 5 | 0.04 |
| 515 | Whipping, light, whipped, avg | 16 | 0.0 | 0.0 | 2 | 0.0 | 14 | 19 | 0.3 | 6 | 0.08 |
| | Creamers | | | | | | | | | | |
| 545 | Coffee Rich, light, Rich's | | | | | | | 14 | | 5 | |
| 548 | Coffee Rich, Rich's | | | | | | | 5 | | 10 | |
| 534 | Coffee whitener, avg | 1 | 0.0 | 0.0 | 0 | 0.0 | 10 | 29 | 0.2 | 12 | 0.00 |
| 541 | Lite, Coffee Mate | 0 | | 0.0 | | | | | | 0 | |
| 539 | Non-Dairy, Coffee Mate | 0 | | 0.0 | | | | | | 0 | |
| 540 | Non Dairy, Cremora | | | | | | | 45 | | 15 | |
| 544 | Non Dairy, light, Rich's | | | | | | | 19 | | 5 | |
| 542 | Non Dairy, lite, Cremora | | | | | | | 45 | | 6 | |
| 517 | Non Dairy, Mocha Mix | 1 | | | 0 | | 8 | 20 | 0.1 | 7 | |
| 547 | Non Dairy, Rich's | | | | | | | 19 | | 5 | |
| 506 | Powder, avg | 1 | 0.0 | 0.1 | 0 | 0.0 | 25 | 49 | 0.0 | 11 | 0.03 |
| 546 | Powder, dry pkt, Coffee Mate | 0 | | 0.0 | | | | | | 0 | |
| | Dessert Toppings | | | | | | | | | | |
| 513 | Dry Mix, avg | 1 | 0.0 | 0.0 | 0 | 0.0 | 2 | 5 | 0.0 | 4 | 0.00 |
| 508 | Frozen, semi solid, avg | 1 | 0.0 | 0.0 | 0 | 0.0 | 1 | 2 | 0.2 | 2 | 0.00 |
| 509 | Prep w/milk, avg | 9 | 0.0 | 0.0 | 1 | 0.0 | 9 | 15 | 0.5 | 7 | 0.03 |
| 514 | Pressurized, avg | 0 | 0.0 | 0.0 | 0 | 0.0 | 2 | 2 | 0.1 | 6 | 0.00 |
| 559 | Real Cream Topping, D-Zerta | 0 | | 0.0 | | | | 5 | | 0 | |
| 526 | Whipped Cream Substitute, non dairy, prep, avg | 0 | 0.0 | 0.0 | 0 | 0.0 | 3 | 3 | | 11 | 0.00 |
| 510 | Whipped Cream Topping, pressurized, avg | 8 | 0.0 | 0.0 | 1 | 0.0 | 7 | 12 | 0.1 | 10 | 0.03 |
| 569 | Whipped Topping, dry mix, Dream Whip | 0 | | 0.0 | | | | 0 | | 0 | |
| 560 | Whipped Topping, D-Zerta | 0 | | 0.0 | | | | 0 | | 0 | |
| 566 | Whipped Topping, extra creamy, Cool Whip | 0 | | 0.0 | | | | 5 | | 5 | |
| 565 | Whipped Topping, lite, Cool Whip | 0 | | 0.0 | | | | 5 | | 0 | |
| 564 | Whipped Topping, non dairy, Cool Whip | 0 | | 0.0 | | | | 0 | | 0 | |
| 70563 | Whipped Topping, non dairy, Mrs Smiths | 0 | | 0.0 | | | | 0 | | 0 | |
| 582 | Whipped Topping, prep w/milk & vanilla, Dream Whip | 0 | | 0.0 | | | | 15 | | 10 | |
| 568 | Whipped Topping, red cal, D-Zerta | 0 | | 0.0 | | | | 50 | | 50 | |
| | Sour Cream | | | | | | | | | | |
| 504 | Avg | 34 | 0.0 | 0.0 | 3 | 0.0 | 25 | 42 | 0.6 | 15 | 0.08 |
| 555 | Breakstone's | 20 | | 0.0 | | | 20 | 45 | | 15 | |
| 550 | Fat free, Breakstone's | 40 | | 0.0 | | | 40 | 70 | | 25 | |
| 515 | Half & Half, avg | 31 | 0.0 | 0.0 | 3 | 0.0 | 29 | 39 | 0.6 | 12 | 0.15 |
| 554 | Half & Half, Breakstone's | 40 | | 0.0 | | | 20 | 65 | | 20 | |

| Code | Amount | Description | Weight (g) | Calories | % Water | Protein (g) | Carbs (g) | Fiber (g) | Sugar (g) | Other Carbs (g) | Fat (g) | Sat Fat (g) | Mono Fat (g) | Poly Fat (g) | Omega 3 (g) | Omega 6 (g) | Choles (mg) | Vit A (IU) | Vit A (RE) | Retinol (RE) | Carotenoids (RE) | Beta Carotene (mcg) | Thiamin (mg) | Riboflavin (mg) | Niacin (NE) | Vit B6 (mg) | Vit B12 (mcg) | Folate (mcg) | Panto (mg) | Vit C (mg) | Vit D (mg) | Vit E (α TE) | Calcium (mg) | Copper (mg) | Iron (mg) | Magnes (mg) | Mang (mg) | Phos (mg) | Potassium (mg) | Selenium (mcg) | Sodium (mg) | Zinc (mg) |
|---|---|---|---|---|---|---|---|---|---|---|---|---|---|---|---|---|---|---|---|---|---|---|---|---|---|---|---|---|---|---|---|---|---|---|---|---|---|---|---|---|---|---|
| | | | Basic Components | | | | | | | | | Additional Fats | | | | | | Vit A & Components | | | | | Vitamins | | | | | | | | | | Minerals | | | | | | | | | |
| 505 | 2 Tbs | Imitation, avg | 29 | 60 | 71 | 0.7 | 1.9 | 0.0 | 1.9 | 0.0 | 5.7 | 5.2 | 0.2 | 0.0 | 0.00 | 0.02 | 0 | 0 | 0 | 0 | 0 | 0 | 0.00 | 0.00 | 0.00 | 0.00 | 0.00 | 0.0 | 0.00 | 0.0 | 0.0 | | 1 | 0.0 | 0.1 | 2 | 0.0 | 13 | 47 | 0.7 | 30 | 0.34 |
| 553 | 2 Tbs | Light, Knudsen | 31 | 40 | | 2.0 | 2.0 | 0.0 | 2.0 | 0.0 | 2.5 | 2.0 | | | | | 10 | 200 | 49 | | | | 0.00 | 0.07 | | | 0.12 | | | 0.0 | | | 40 | | 0.0 | | | 40 | 70 | | 20 | |
| | | *MILKS AND NON-DAIRY MILKS* | | | | | | | | | | | | | | | | | | | | | | | | | | | | | | | | | | | | | | | | |
| | | Cow Milk | | | | | | | | | | | | | | | | | | | | | | | | | | | | | | | | | | | | | | | | |
| 32 | 1/3 cup | Buttermilk, dried, avg | 40 | 155 | 3 | 13.7 | 19.6 | 0.0 | 19.6 | 0.0 | 2.3 | 1.4 | 0.7 | 0.1 | 0.03 | 0.25 | 23 | 87 | 22 | 19 | 2 | | 0.16 | 0.63 | 0.35 | 0.14 | 1.53 | 19.0 | 1.27 | 2.3 | 2.0 | | 474 | 0.0 | 0.1 | 44 | 0.0 | 373 | 637 | 8.1 | 207 | 1.61 |
| 217 | 1 cup | Buttermilk, low fat 1%, avg | 245 | 110 | 89 | 9.0 | 13.0 | 0.0 | 12.0 | 1.0 | 2.5 | 1.5 | 0.5 | 0.0 | 0.00 | 0.00 | 15 | | | | | | | | | | | | | | | | 270 | | 0.0 | | 0.0 | | 400 | | 260 | |
| 58 | 1 cup | Buttermilk, reconstd f/dry, avg | 245 | 93 | 90 | 8.8 | 11.8 | 0.0 | 11.8 | 0.0 | 1.4 | 0.9 | 0.4 | 0.1 | 0.02 | 0.03 | 17 | 53 | 13 | 12 | 1 | | 0.10 | 0.38 | 0.21 | 0.08 | 0.92 | 11.5 | 0.74 | 1.4 | 0.1 | | 292 | 0.0 | 0.1 | 29 | 0.0 | 225 | 385 | 2.5 | 132 | 1.04 |
| 7 | 1 cup | Buttermilk, skim, cultured, avg | 245 | 98 | 90 | 8.1 | 11.7 | 0.0 | 11.7 | 0.0 | 2.2 | 1.3 | 0.6 | 0.1 | 0.03 | 0.05 | 10 | 81 | 20 | 17 | 2 | | 0.08 | 0.38 | 0.14 | 0.08 | 0.54 | 12.3 | 0.67 | 2.4 | 0.1 | | 284 | 0.0 | 0.1 | 27 | 0.0 | 218 | 370 | 4.9 | 257 | 1.03 |
| 11 | 1/4 cup | Condensed milk, sweet, cnd, avg | 76 | 244 | 27 | 6.0 | 41.3 | 0.0 | 41.3 | 0.0 | 6.6 | 4.2 | 1.8 | 0.3 | 0.09 | 0.16 | 25 | 249 | 62 | 55 | 6 | | 0.07 | 0.32 | 0.16 | 0.04 | 0.34 | 8.5 | 0.57 | 2.0 | 0.1 | | 216 | 0.0 | 0.1 | 20 | 0.0 | 192 | 282 | 11.2 | 97 | 0.71 |
| 188 | 1/4 cup | Condensed milk, sweet, fat free, Borden | 78 | 217 | 29 | 6.9 | 47.0 | | 47.3 | | 0.2 | | | | | | 5 | 0.6 | 0.1 | | | | 0.09 | 0.33 | 0.16 | | | | | 0.8 | | | 218 | | 0.0 | 20 | | 181 | 288 | | 82 | 0.69 |
| 187 | 1/4 cup | Condensed milk, sweet, low fat, Borden | 78 | 234 | 28 | 6.1 | 45.5 | | 49.8 | | 3.0 | 1.9 | 0.6 | 0.1 | | | 12 | 200 | 49 | | | | 0.05 | 0.30 | 0.13 | | | | | 0.8 | | | 214 | | 0.1 | 18 | | 170 | 282 | | 78 | 0.73 |
| 224 | 1 cup | Eggnog, Darigold | 254 | 360 | 77 | 6.0 | 44.0 | 0.0 | 32.0 | 12.0 | 18.0 | 10.0 | 5.0 | 1.0 | | | 140 | | | | | | | | | | | | | | | | 180 | | 1.0 | | | | 340 | | 210 | |
| 213 | 1 cup | Eggnog, low fat, Darigold | 254 | 240 | 77 | 10.0 | 44.0 | 0.0 | 38.0 | 6.0 | 2.0 | | | | | | 90 | 686 | 197 | | | | | | | | | | | | | | 300 | | 1.0 | | | | 460 | | 160 | |
| 80 | 1 cup | Evaporated, 2% fat, avg | 252 | 232 | 78 | 18.7 | 28.1 | 0.0 | 28.1 | 0.0 | 4.9 | 3.1 | 1.4 | 0.2 | 0.07 | 0.11 | 20 | 1138 | 331 | 328 | 3 | | 0.11 | 0.77 | 0.43 | 0.14 | 0.59 | 21.3 | 1.76 | 3.1 | | | 716 | 0.0 | 0.7 | 68 | 0.0 | 484 | 822 | 3.0 | 285 | 2.23 |
| 10 | 1 cup | Evaporated, skim milk, cnd, avg | 256 | 200 | 79 | 19.3 | 29.2 | 0.0 | 29.2 | 0.0 | 0.5 | 0.3 | 0.2 | 0.0 | 0.01 | 0.01 | 10 | 1004 | 300 | 300 | 0 | 0 | 0.12 | 0.79 | 0.45 | 0.14 | 0.61 | 22.0 | 1.89 | 3.2 | 5.1 | | 742 | 0.0 | 0.7 | 69 | 0.0 | 499 | 850 | 6.4 | 294 | 2.30 |
| 15 | 1 cup | Evaporated, whole milk, cnd, avg | 252 | 338 | 74 | 17.2 | 25.2 | 0.0 | 25.2 | 0.0 | 19.1 | 11.6 | 5.9 | 0.6 | 0.20 | 0.42 | 73 | 612 | 136 | 117 | 19 | | 0.12 | 0.80 | 0.49 | 0.13 | 0.41 | 19.9 | 1.61 | 4.7 | 2.5 | | 658 | 0.0 | 0.5 | 60 | 0.0 | 512 | 764 | 5.8 | 267 | 1.94 |
| 196 | 1 cup | Filled Milk, fluid w/blend of hydro veg oil, avg | 244 | 154 | 88 | 8.1 | 11.6 | 0.0 | | | 8.4 | 1.9 | 4.3 | 1.8 | 0.07 | 1.75 | 5 | 17 | 5 | | | | 0.07 | 0.30 | 0.21 | 0.10 | 0.83 | 11.7 | 0.73 | 2.2 | | | 312 | 0.0 | 0.1 | 32 | 0.0 | 237 | 339 | 4.9 | 139 | 0.88 |
| 4 | 1 cup | Lowfat milk, 1%, acidophilus w/added vit A, avg | 244 | 102 | 90 | 8.0 | 11.7 | 0.0 | 11.7 | 0.0 | 2.6 | 1.6 | 0.7 | 0.1 | 0.04 | 0.05 | 10 | 500 | 144 | 134 | 10 | | 0.10 | 0.41 | 0.21 | 0.10 | 0.90 | 12.4 | 0.79 | 2.4 | 2.4 | 0.1 | 300 | 0.0 | 0.1 | 34 | 0.0 | 234 | 381 | 5.4 | 122 | 0.95 |
| 53 | 1 cup | Lowfat milk, 1%, avg | 247 | 104 | 90 | 8.5 | 11.8 | 0.0 | 11.8 | 0.0 | 2.6 | 1.7 | 0.6 | 0.1 | 0.01 | 0.07 | 10 | 506 | 146 | 143 | 3 | | 0.10 | 0.41 | 0.21 | 0.11 | 0.91 | 12.6 | 0.74 | 2.4 | 2.5 | | 551 | 0.0 | 0.1 | 35 | 0.0 | 237 | 385 | 4.9 | 124 | 0.96 |
| 19 | 1 cup | Lowfat milk, 1%, chocolate, avg | 250 | 158 | 84 | 8.1 | 26.0 | 1.3 | 22.1 | 2.6 | 2.5 | 1.5 | 0.8 | 0.1 | 0.03 | 0.05 | 8 | 500 | 147 | 146 | 1 | | 0.09 | 0.41 | 0.32 | 0.10 | 0.86 | 12.0 | 0.75 | 2.3 | 2.5 | | 288 | 0.2 | 0.6 | 32 | 0.2 | 258 | 425 | 4.8 | 152 | 1.02 |
| 54 | 1 cup | Lowfat milk, 1%, low lactose, avg | 246 | 103 | 90 | 8.5 | 11.8 | 0.0 | 11.8 | 0.0 | 2.6 | 1.6 | 0.8 | 0.1 | 0.04 | 0.05 | 10 | 504 | 145 | 143 | 2 | | 0.10 | 0.41 | 0.21 | 0.11 | 0.91 | 12.5 | 0.74 | 2.4 | 2.5 | | 303 | 0.0 | 0.1 | 34 | 0.0 | 236 | 384 | 4.9 | 123 | 0.96 |
| 55 | 1 cup | Lowfat milk, 1%, low lactose, fort w/calc, avg | 247 | 104 | 90 | 8.5 | 11.8 | 0.0 | 11.8 | 0.0 | 2.6 | 1.6 | 0.8 | 0.1 | 0.04 | 0.05 | 10 | 506 | 146 | 143 | 3 | | 0.10 | 0.41 | 0.21 | 0.11 | 0.91 | 12.6 | 0.74 | 2.4 | 2.5 | | 551 | 0.0 | 0.1 | 35 | | 237 | 385 | 4.9 | 124 | 0.96 |
| 64 | 1 cup | Lowfat milk, 1%, protein fort w/added vit A, avg | 246 | 118 | 89 | 9.7 | 13.6 | 0.0 | 13.6 | 0.0 | 2.9 | 1.8 | 0.8 | 0.1 | 0.04 | 0.05 | 10 | 499 | 145 | 135 | 10 | | 0.11 | 0.47 | 0.25 | 0.12 | 1.05 | 14.5 | 0.92 | 2.8 | 2.5 | | 349 | 0.0 | 0.1 | 39 | 0.0 | 273 | 443 | 6.2 | 143 | 1.11 |
| 79 | 1 cup | Lowfat milk, 1%, reconstd f/dry, avg | 245 | 83 | 91 | 8.0 | 11.9 | 0.0 | 11.9 | 0.0 | 0.4 | 0.3 | 0.1 | 0.0 | 0.00 | 0.01 | 5 | 549 | 164 | 163 | 0.5 | | 0.09 | 0.40 | 0.20 | 0.08 | 0.91 | 11.3 | 0.74 | 1.3 | 2.5 | | 284 | 0.0 | 0.1 | 29 | 0.0 | 223 | 387 | 6.1 | 132 | 1.07 |
| 2 | 1 cup | Lowfat milk, 2%, acidophilus w/added vit A, avg | 244 | 122 | 89 | 8.1 | 11.7 | 0.0 | 11.7 | 0.0 | 4.7 | 2.9 | 1.4 | 0.2 | 0.07 | 0.10 | 20 | 500 | 139 | 129 | 10 | | 0.10 | 0.40 | 0.21 | 0.10 | 0.89 | 12.4 | 0.78 | 2.3 | 2.4 | 0.1 | 298 | 0.0 | 0.1 | 34 | 0.0 | 232 | 376 | 5.4 | 122 | 0.95 |
| 18 | 1 cup | Lowfat milk, 2%, chocolate, avg | 250 | 180 | 84 | 8.0 | 26.0 | 1.3 | 22.1 | 2.6 | 5.0 | 3.1 | 1.5 | 0.2 | 0.06 | 0.12 | 18 | 500 | 143 | 138 | 5 | | 0.09 | 0.41 | 0.31 | 0.10 | 0.85 | 12.0 | 0.75 | 2.3 | 2.5 | | 285 | 0.2 | 0.6 | 32 | 0.2 | 255 | 422 | 4.8 | 150 | 1.02 |
| 63 | 1 cup | Lowfat milk, 2%, protein fort w/added vit A, avg | 246 | 138 | 88 | 9.7 | 13.5 | 0.0 | 13.5 | 0.0 | 4.9 | 3.0 | 1.4 | 0.2 | 0.07 | 0.11 | 20 | 499 | 140 | 130 | 10 | | 0.11 | 0.48 | 0.25 | 0.13 | 1.05 | 14.8 | 0.92 | 2.8 | 2.5 | 0.1 | 352 | 0.0 | 0.1 | 39 | 0.0 | 276 | 448 | 6.4 | 145 | 1.11 |
| 132 | 1 cup | Nonfat/Skim milk, avg | 245 | 86 | 91 | 8.4 | 11.9 | 0.0 | 11.9 | 0.0 | 0.4 | 0.3 | 0.1 | 0.0 | 0.00 | 0.01 | 5 | 17 | 2.5 | | | | 0.09 | 0.34 | 0.22 | 0.10 | 0.93 | 12.3 | 0.81 | 2.4 | 2.5 | | 301 | 0.0 | 0.1 | 27 | 0.0 | 247 | 407 | 5.1 | 127 | 0.98 |
| 210 | 1 cup | Nonfat/Skim milk, acidoph w/add vit A & D, avg | 245 | 100 | 89 | 10.0 | 15.0 | 0.0 | 14.0 | 1.0 | 0.0 | 0.0 | 0.0 | 0.0 | 0.00 | 0.00 | 5 | 500 | 150 | | | | | | | | | | | | 2.5 | | 300 | | 0.0 | | 0.0 | | 460 | | 150 | |
| 59 | 1 cup | Nonfat/Skim milk, chocolate, avg | 250 | 145 | 85 | 9.0 | 26.7 | 1.5 | 22.8 | 2.4 | 1.2 | 0.7 | 0.4 | 0.0 | 0.01 | 0.03 | 5 | 475 | 142 | 142 | 0.1 | | 0.09 | 0.34 | 0.28 | 0.10 | 0.88 | 13.6 | 0.75 | 2.3 | 2.5 | | 292 | 0.2 | 0.7 | 45 | 0.2 | 265 | 485 | 4.8 | 120 | 1.20 |
| 131 | 1/3 cup | Nonfat/Skim milk, dry pwd, avg | 23 | 81 | 5 | 8.2 | 11.9 | 0.0 | 11.9 | 0.0 | 0.0 | 0.0 | 0.0 | 0.0 | 0.00 | 0.00 | 0 | 2 | 0.5 | | | | 0.04 | 0.38 | 0.15 | 0.07 | 0.92 | 11.4 | 0.76 | 1.5 | | | 64 | 0.0 | 0.1 | 14 | 0.0 | 233 | 156 | 6.3 | 524 | 0.93 |
| 69 | 1/3 cup | Nonfat/Skim milk, instant, dry, avg | 23 | 82 | 4 | 8.1 | 12.0 | 0.0 | 12.0 | 0.0 | 0.2 | 0.1 | 0.0 | 0.0 | 0.00 | 0.00 | 4 | 6 | 1 | | | | 0.09 | 0.40 | 0.20 | 0.08 | 0.92 | 11.5 | 0.74 | 1.3 | 2.5 | | 283 | 0.0 | 0.1 | 27 | 0.0 | 227 | 392 | 6.3 | 126 | 1.01 |
| 57 | 1 cup | Nonfat/Skim milk, instant, reconstd, avg | 245 | 81 | 91 | 8.4 | 11.9 | 0.0 | 11.9 | 0.0 | 0.2 | 0.1 | 0.1 | 0.0 | 0.00 | 0.00 | 5 | 539 | 152 | 161 | 0.3 | | 0.09 | 0.40 | 0.20 | 0.08 | 0.91 | 11.3 | 0.79 | 1.3 | 2.5 | | 284 | 0.0 | 0.1 | 29 | 0.0 | 223 | 387 | 6.4 | 132 | 1.07 |
| 56 | 1 cup | Nonfat/Skim milk, low lactose, avg | 245 | 86 | 91 | 8.8 | 11.9 | 0.0 | 11.9 | 0.0 | 0.4 | 0.3 | 0.1 | 0.0 | 0.00 | 0.01 | 5 | 500 | 149 | 149 | 0 | | 0.09 | 0.34 | 0.22 | 0.10 | 0.93 | 12.7 | 0.74 | 2.4 | 2.5 | | 301 | 0.0 | 0.1 | 27 | 0.0 | 247 | 407 | 5.1 | 127 | 0.98 |
| 65 | 1 cup | Nonfat/Skim milk, protein fort w/added vit A, avg | 246 | 101 | 89 | 9.7 | 13.7 | 0.0 | 13.7 | 0.0 | 0.6 | 0.4 | 0.2 | 0.0 | 0.01 | 0.01 | 5 | 499 | 150 | 140 | 10 | | 0.11 | 0.48 | 0.25 | 0.12 | 1.05 | 14.8 | 0.92 | 2.8 | 2.5 | 0.0 | 352 | 0.0 | 0.1 | 39 | 0.0 | 276 | 448 | 5.9 | 145 | 1.11 |
| 20 | 1 cup | Whole milk, chocolate, avg | 250 | 208 | 82 | 7.9 | 25.8 | 2.0 | 22.1 | 1.6 | 8.5 | 5.3 | 2.5 | 0.3 | 0.12 | 0.20 | 30 | 303 | 73 | 65 | 8 | | 0.09 | 0.41 | 0.31 | 0.10 | 0.83 | 11.8 | 0.74 | 2.3 | 2.5 | | 280 | 0.2 | 0.6 | 32 | 0.2 | 252 | 418 | 4.8 | 150 | 1.02 |
| 66 | 1/3 cup | Whole milk, dry pwd, avg | 43 | 213 | 2 | 11.3 | 16.5 | 0.0 | 16.5 | 0.0 | 11.5 | 7.2 | 3.4 | 0.3 | 0.09 | 0.20 | 42 | 396 | 120 | | | | 0.12 | 0.52 | 0.28 | 0.13 | 1.40 | 15.9 | 0.98 | 3.7 | 3.6 | | 392 | 0.0 | 0.2 | 36 | 0.0 | 334 | 571 | 7.0 | 160 | 1.44 |
| 52 | 1 cup | Whole milk, low sod, avg | 244 | 149 | 88 | 7.6 | 10.9 | 0.0 | 10.9 | 0.0 | 8.4 | 5.2 | 2.4 | 0.3 | 0.12 | 0.19 | 34 | 317 | 78 | 73 | 5 | | 0.05 | 0.26 | 0.10 | 0.03 | 0.88 | 12.2 | 0.74 | 2.3 | 2.4 | 0.1 | 246 | 0.0 | 0.1 | 12 | 0.0 | 210 | 617 | 4.9 | 5 | 0.93 |
| 78 | 1 cup | Whole milk, reconstd f/dry pwd, avg | 244 | 149 | 88 | 7.9 | 11.5 | 0.0 | 11.5 | 0.0 | 8.0 | 5.0 | 2.4 | 0.2 | 0.06 | 0.14 | 29 | 277 | 34 | 81 | 2.0 | | 0.09 | 0.36 | 0.19 | 0.09 | 0.98 | 11.1 | 0.66 | 2.6 | 2.4 | | 278 | 0.0 | 0.2 | 27 | 0.0 | 232 | 400 | 3.0 | 117 | 1.07 |
| 1 | 1 cup | Whole milk, 3.3% fat, avg | 244 | 149 | 88 | 8.0 | 11.4 | 0.0 | 11.4 | 0.0 | 8.1 | 5.1 | 2.4 | 0.3 | 0.12 | 0.18 | 34 | 307 | 76 | 71 | 5 | | 0.09 | 0.40 | 0.20 | 0.10 | 0.87 | 12.2 | 0.77 | 2.3 | 2.4 | 0.1 | 290 | 0.0 | 0.1 | 32 | 0.0 | 227 | 371 | 4.9 | 120 | 0.93 |
| 62 | 1 cup | Whole milk, 3.7% fat, avg | 244 | 156 | 88 | 8.0 | 11.3 | 0.0 | 11.3 | 0.0 | 8.9 | 5.5 | 2.6 | 0.3 | 0.13 | 0.20 | 34 | 337 | 83 | 78 | 5 | | 0.09 | 0.39 | 0.20 | 0.10 | 0.87 | 12.2 | 0.76 | 3.6 | 2.4 | | 290 | 0.0 | 0.1 | 32 | 0.0 | 227 | 368 | 4.9 | 120 | 0.93 |
| 23 | 1 cup | Goat milk, avg | 244 | 168 | 87 | 8.7 | 10.9 | 0.0 | 10.9 | 0.0 | 10.1 | 6.5 | 2.7 | 0.4 | 0.10 | 0.27 | 27 | 451 | 137 | 137 | 0 | | 0.12 | 0.34 | 0.68 | 0.11 | 0.16 | 1.5 | 0.76 | 3.1 | 0.7 | | 327 | 0.1 | 0.1 | 34 | 0.0 | 271 | 498 | 3.4 | 122 | 0.73 |
| 22 | 1 cup | Human breast milk, avg | 246 | 172 | 88 | 2.5 | 16.9 | 0.0 | 16.9 | 0.0 | 10.8 | 4.9 | 4.1 | 1.2 | 0.13 | 0.98 | 34 | 593 | 167 | 148 | 10 | | 0.03 | 0.09 | 0.44 | 0.03 | 0.11 | 12.8 | 0.55 | 12.3 | 0.2 | 2.2 | 79 | 0.1 | 0.1 | 7 | 0.1 | 34 | 125 | 4.4 | 42 | 0.42 |
| 150 | 1 cup | Indian buffalo milk, avg | 244 | 237 | 83 | 9.2 | 12.6 | 0.0 | 12.6 | 0.0 | 16.8 | 11.2 | 4.4 | 0.4 | 0.19 | 0.17 | 46 | 434 | 129 | | | | 0.13 | 0.33 | 0.22 | 0.06 | 0.89 | 13.7 | 0.47 | 5.5 | | | 412 | 0.1 | 0.3 | 76 | 0.0 | 285 | 434 | | 127 | 0.54 |
| | | Non Dairy Milks | | | | | | | | | | | | | | | | | | | | | | | | | | | | | | | | | | | | | | | | |
| 38404 | 1 cup | Oatmeal beverage (Puerto Rican), avg | 245 | 105 | 89 | 0.7 | 26.0 | 0.5 | | | 0.3 | 0.1 | 0.1 | 0.1 | | | 0 | 5 | 0.5 | 0.5 | 0 | | 0.03 | 0.01 | 0.04 | 0.00 | 0.00 | 1.5 | | 0.0 | | | 7 | 0.0 | 0.2 | 10 | | 22 | 17 | | 7 | 0.21 |
| 38362 | 1 cup | Rice beverage, Mexican, avg | 245 | 100 | 89 | 0.3 | 25.4 | 0.2 | | | 0.0 | 0.0 | 0.0 | 0.0 | | | 0 | 1 | 0.1 | 0 | 0.1 | | 0.01 | 0.01 | 0.14 | 0.01 | 0.00 | 0.4 | | 0.1 | | | 12 | 0.0 | 0.3 | 2 | | 5 | 7 | | 7 | 0.12 |
| 20440 | 1 cup | Rice Dream beverage, cnd, Imagine Foods | 245 | 120 | 89 | 0.4 | 24.7 | 0.0 | 12.3 | 12.5 | 2.0 | 0.2 | 1.3 | 0.3 | 0.00 | 0.31 | 0 | 5 | 0 | 0 | 0 | | 0.08 | 0.01 | 1.91 | 0.04 | 0.00 | 90.7 | 0.14 | 1.2 | 0.0 | | 20 | 0.1 | 0.2 | 10 | 0.1 | 34 | 69 | | 86 | 0.25 |
| 42 | 1 cup | Sheep milk, avg | 245 | 265 | 81 | 14.7 | 13.1 | 0.0 | 13.1 | 0.0 | 17.1 | 11.3 | 4.2 | 0.8 | 0.31 | 0.44 | 66 | 350 | 103 | 93 | 10 | | 0.16 | 0.87 | 1.02 | 0.15 | 1.74 | 17.1 | 1.00 | 10.2 | 0.4 | | 473 | 0.1 | 0.2 | 44 | 0.0 | 387 | 336 | 4.2 | 108 | 1.32 |
| 143 | 1 Tbs | Whey, acid, dried, avg | 3 | 10 | 4 | 0.4 | 2.2 | 0.0 | 2.2 | 0.0 | 0.0 | 0.0 | 0.0 | 0.0 | 0.00 | 0.02 | 0 | 2 | 0.3 | 0.1 | 0.1 | | 0.02 | 0.06 | 0.03 | 0.02 | 0.07 | 1.0 | 0.17 | 0.0 | 0.0 | | 62 | 0.0 | 0.0 | 6 | 0.0 | 40 | 69 | 0.8 | 29 | 0.19 |
| 144 | 1 cup | Whey, acid, fluid, avg | 246 | 59 | 93 | 1.9 | 12.6 | 0.0 | 12.6 | 0.0 | 0.2 | 0.1 | 0.1 | 0.0 | 0.00 | 0.01 | 0 | 17 | 2 | | | | 0.10 | 0.34 | 0.19 | 0.10 | 0.44 | 5.4 | 0.94 | 0.1 | 0.0 | | 253 | 0.0 | 0.2 | 25 | 0.0 | 192 | 352 | 4.4 | 118 | 1.06 |
| 145 | 1 Tbs | Whey, sweet, dried, avg | 8 | 28 | 3 | 1.0 | 6.0 | 0.0 | 6.0 | 0.0 | 0.1 | 0.1 | 0.0 | 0.0 | 0.00 | 0.02 | 0 | 3.5 | 0.8 | 0.6 | 0.2 | | 0.04 | 0.18 | 0.10 | 0.05 | 0.19 | 0.9 | 0.45 | 0.1 | 0.0 | | 64 | 0.0 | 0.1 | 14 | 0.0 | 75 | 166 | 2.2 | 86 | 0.16 |
| 146 | 1 cup | Whey, sweet, fluid, avg | 246 | 66 | 93 | 2.1 | 12.6 | 0.0 | 12.6 | 0.0 | 0.9 | 0.5 | 0.2 | 0.0 | 0.01 | 0.02 | 5 | 39 | 10 | | | | 0.03 | 0.39 | 0.18 | 0.08 | 0.68 | 2.0 | 0.94 | 0.2 | 0.0 | | 116 | 0.0 | 0.1 | 20 | 0.0 | 113 | 396 | 4.7 | 133 | 0.32 |
| | | *YOGURTS* | | | | | | | | | | | | | | | | | | | | | | | | | | | | | | | | | | | | | | | | |
| 2468 | 1 ea | Apricot Mango, lowfat, 8 oz, Darigold | 227 | 250 | 74 | 10.0 | 46.0 | 0.0 | 40.0 | 6.0 | 2.5 | 1.5 | | | | | 15 | 300 | [illegible] | | | | | | | | | | | 2.4 | | | 250 | | 0.0 | | | | | | 150 | |
| 2508 | 1 ea | Banana Berry, lowfat, 4.4 oz, Light n' Lively | 125 | 130 | | 5.0 | 24.0 | 0.0 | 21.0 | 3.0 | 1.0 | 1.0 | | | | | 10 | 0 | 0 | 0 | 0 | 0 | 0.03 | 0.17 | | | 0.48 | | | 0.0 | | | 150 | | 0.0 | | | 150 | 230 | | 65 | |
| 2504 | 1 ea | Berry Blue, lowfat, 4.4 oz, Light n' Lively | 125 | 150 | | 5.0 | 30.0 | 0.0 | 26.0 | 4.0 | 1.0 | 0.5 | | | | | 10 | 0 | 0 | 0 | 0 | 0 | 0.00 | 0.17 | | | 0.48 | | | 0.0 | | | 150 | | 0.0 | | | 150 | 270 | | 65 | |
| 2513 | 1 ea | Black Cherry, nonfat, 6 oz, Knudsen | 170 | 70 | | 7.0 | 12.0 | 0.0 | 9.0 | 3.0 | 0.0 | 0.0 | 0.0 | 0.0 | 0.00 | 0.00 | 5 | 0 | 0 | 0 | 0 | 0 | 0.03 | 0.25 | | | 0.60 | | | 0.0 | | | 200 | | 0.0 | | | 150 | 270 | | 85 | |
| | | Blueberry Yogurt | | | | | | | | | | | | | | | | | | | | | | | | | | | | | | | | | | | | | | | | |
| 2495 | 1 ea | Lowfat, 4.4 oz, Light n' Lively | 125 | 140 | | 5.0 | 27.0 | 0.0 | 24.0 | 3.0 | 1.0 | 0.5 | | | | | 10 | 0 | 0 | 0 | 0 | 0 | 0.00 | 0.17 | | | 0.48 | | | 0.0 | | | 15 | | 0.0 | | | 150 | 220 | | 65 | |
| 2472 | 1 ea | Lowfat, 8 oz, Darigold | 227 | 240 | 74 | 10.0 | 45.0 | 0.0 | 40.0 | 5.0 | 2.5 | 1.5 | | | | | 15 | 100 | 24 | | | | | | | | | | | 1.2 | | | 250 | | 0.0 | | | | | | 150 | |
| 2551 | 1 ea | N' Crème, nonfat, 8 oz, Weight Watchers | 227 | 90 | 89 | 8.0 | 14.0 | 3.0 | 9.0 | 2.0 | 0.0 | 0.0 | 0.0 | 0.0 | 0.00 | 0.00 | 5 | 0 | 0 | 0 | 0 | 0 | | | | | | | | 0.0 | | | 250 | | | | | | 240 | | 140 | |
| 2514 | 1 ea | Nonfat, 6 oz, Knudsen | 170 | 70 | | 7.0 | 12.0 | 0.0 | 8.0 | 4.0 | 0.0 | 0.0 | 0.0 | 0.0 | 0.00 | 0.00 | 5 | 0 | 0 | 0 | 0 | 0 | 0.03 | 0.25 | | | 0.60 | | | 0.0 | | | 200 | | 0.0 | | | 150 | 280 | | 80 | |
| 2538 | 1 ea | Nonfat, 4.4 oz, Light n' Lively | 125 | 50 | | 5.0 | 8.0 | 0.0 | 6.0 | 2.0 | 0.0 | 0.0 | 0.0 | 0.0 | 0.00 | 0.00 | 2 | 0 | 0 | 0 | 0 | 0 | 0.00 | 0.17 | | | 0.48 | | | 0.0 | | | 150 | | 0.0 | | | 100 | 200 | | 60 | |
| 2474 | 1 ea | Boysenberry, lowfat, 8 oz, Darigold | 227 | 240 | 74 | 10.0 | 45.0 | 0.0 | 39.0 | 6.0 | 2.5 | 1.5 | | | | | 15 | 100 | 24 | | | | | | | | | | | 1.2 | | | 250 | | 0.4 | | | | | | 170 | |

| Code | Amount | Description | Weight (g) | Calories | % Water | Protein (g) | Carbs (g) | Fiber (g) | Sugar (g) | Other Carbs (g) | Fat (g) | Sat Fat (g) | Mono Fat (g) | Poly Fat (g) | Omega 3 (g) | Omega 6 (g) | Choles (mg) |
|---|---|---|---|---|---|---|---|---|---|---|---|---|---|---|---|---|---|
| | | | Basic Components | | | | | | | | | Additional Fats | | | | | |
| 2568 | 1 ea | Breakfast, whole milk, 6 oz, Yoplait | 170 | 230 | | 8.0 | 41.0 | 0.2 | | | 4.0 | 2.6 | 1.1 | 0.1 | | | 10 |
| 2476 | 1 ea | Caffe Latte, lowfat, 8 oz, Darigold | 227 | 240 | 74 | 10.0 | 46.0 | 0.0 | 40.0 | 6.0 | 2.5 | 1.5 | | | | | 15 |
| 2552 | 1 ea | Cappuccino, nonfat, D17328 oz, Weight Watchers | 227 | 90 | 89 | 8.0 | 14.0 | 0.0 | 7.0 | 7.0 | 0.0 | 0.0 | 0.0 | 0.0 | 0.00 | 0.00 | 5 |
| 2553 | 1 ea | Cherry Jubilee, nonfat, 8 oz, Weight Watchers | 227 | 90 | 89 | 8.0 | 14.0 | 0.0 | 8.0 | 6.0 | 0.0 | 0.0 | 0.0 | 0.0 | 0.00 | 0.00 | 5 |
| 2471 | 1 ea | Cherry, lowfat, 8 oz, Darigold | 227 | 240 | 75 | 10.0 | 44.0 | 0.0 | 39.0 | 5.0 | 2.5 | 1.5 | | | | | 15 |
| 2563 | 1 ea | Chocolate, whole milk, 8 oz, avg | 245 | 247 | 77 | 11.9 | 33.1 | 0.0 | 29.3 | 3.9 | 7.8 | 4.9 | 2.2 | 0.3 | | | 25 |
| | | Coffee Yogurt | | | | | | | | | | | | | | | |
| 2579 | 1 ea | Lowfat, 8 oz, avg | 245 | 208 | 79 | 12.1 | 33.8 | 0.0 | 33.8 | 0.0 | 3.1 | 2.0 | 0.8 | 0.1 | 0.02 | 0.06 | 12 |
| 2574 | 1 ea | Nonfat, 8 oz, avg | 227 | 207 | 76 | 11.6 | 39.7 | 0.0 | 39.6 | 0.1 | 0.4 | 0.2 | 0.1 | 0.0 | 0.00 | 0.01 | 5 |
| 2575 | 1 ea | Whole milk, 8 oz, avg | 227 | 229 | 77 | 11.0 | 30.7 | 0.0 | 30.7 | 0.0 | 7.2 | 4.5 | 2.0 | 0.2 | 0.07 | 0.17 | 23 |
| 2554 | 1 ea | Cranberry Raspberry, nonfat,8 oz, Weight Watchers | 227 | 90 | 89 | 8.0 | 14.0 | 0.0 | 7.0 | 7.0 | 0.0 | 0.0 | 0.0 | 0.0 | 0.00 | 0.00 | 5 |
| | | Custard Yogurt | | | | | | | | | | | | | | | |
| 2572 | 1 ea | Berry, whole milk, 6 oz, Yoplait | 170 | 180 | | 7.0 | 30.0 | | | | 4.0 | | | | | | 15 |
| 2573 | 1 ea | Vanilla, whole milk, 6 oz, Yoplait | 170 | 180 | | 7.0 | 30.0 | | | | 4.0 | | | | | | 15 |
| 2569 | 1 ea | Whole milk, 6 oz, Yoplait | 170 | 190 | | 7.0 | 32.0 | 0.0 | | | 4.0 | 2.6 | 1.1 | 0.1 | | | 15 |
| | | Fruit Yogurt | | | | | | | | | | | | | | | |
| 2493 | 1 ea | Lowfat, 8 oz, avg | 245 | 250 | 74 | 10.7 | 46.8 | 0.0 | 46.5 | 0.2 | 2.6 | 1.7 | 0.7 | 0.1 | 0.02 | 0.05 | 10 |
| 2102 | 1 ea | Lowfat, w/nuts, 8 oz, avg | 227 | 268 | 72 | 10.1 | 43.2 | 0.4 | 42.3 | 0.5 | 6.9 | 1.9 | 3.4 | 1.2 | | | 9 |
| 2511 | 1 ea | Nonfat, 8 oz, avg | 241 | 123 | 86 | 11.6 | 19.4 | 1.3 | 18.1 | 0.0 | 0.4 | 0.2 | 0.1 | 0.0 | 0.01 | 0.03 | 2 |
| 2570 | 1 ea | Whole milk, 6 oz, Yoplait | 170 | 190 | | 8.0 | 32.0 | 0.2 | | | 3.0 | 1.9 | 0.8 | 0.1 | | | 10 |
| 2467 | 1 ea | Keylime Pie, lowfat, 8 oz, Darigold | 227 | 240 | 75 | 10.0 | 44.0 | 0.0 | 40.0 | 4.0 | 2.5 | 1.5 | | | | | 15 |
| | | Lemon Yogurt | | | | | | | | | | | | | | | |
| 2578 | 1 ea | Lowfat, 8 oz, avg | 245 | 208 | 79 | 12.1 | 33.8 | 0.0 | 33.8 | 0.0 | 3.1 | 2.0 | 0.8 | 0.1 | 0.02 | 0.06 | 12 |
| 2097 | 1 ea | Nonfat, 8 oz, avg | 227 | 207 | 76 | 11.6 | 39.7 | 0.0 | 39.6 | 0.1 | 0.4 | 0.2 | 0.1 | 0.0 | 0.00 | 0.01 | 5 |
| 2515 | 1 ea | Nonfat, 6 oz, Knudsen | 170 | 70 | | 7.0 | 11.0 | 0.5 | 8.0 | 2.5 | 0.0 | 0.0 | 0.0 | 0.0 | 0.00 | 0.00 | 5 |
| 2555 | 1 ea | Nonfat, 8 oz, Weight Watchers | 227 | 90 | 89 | 8.0 | 14.0 | 1.0 | 7.0 | 6.0 | 0.0 | 0.0 | 0.0 | 0.0 | 0.00 | 0.00 | 5 |
| 2576 | 1 ea | Whole milk, 8 oz, avg | 227 | 229 | 77 | 11.0 | 30.7 | 0.0 | 30.7 | 0.0 | 7.2 | 4.5 | 2.0 | 0.2 | 0.07 | 0.17 | 23 |
| 2492 | 1 ea | Maple, lowfat, 8 oz, avg | 245 | 208 | 79 | 12.1 | 33.8 | 0.0 | 33.8 | 0.0 | 3.1 | 2.0 | 0.8 | 0.1 | 0.02 | 0.06 | 12 |
| 2521 | 1 ea | Mixed Berry, nonfat, 6 oz, Knudsen | 170 | 170 | | 8.0 | 33.0 | 0.0 | 29.0 | 4.0 | 0.0 | 0.0 | 0.0 | 0.0 | 0.00 | 0.00 | 5 |
| | | Peach Yogurt | | | | | | | | | | | | | | | |
| 2477 | 1 ea | Lowfat, 8 oz, Darigold | 227 | 240 | 74 | 10.0 | 45.0 | 0.0 | 40.0 | 5.0 | 2.5 | 1.5 | | | | | 15 |
| 2496 | 1 ea | Lowfat, 4.4 oz, Light n' Lively | 125 | 140 | | 5.0 | 27.0 | 0.0 | 24.0 | 3.0 | 1.0 | 0.5 | | | | | 10 |
| 2516 | 1 ea | Nonfat, 6 oz, Knudsen | 170 | 70 | | 7.0 | 11.0 | 0.5 | 9.0 | 1.5 | 0.0 | 0.0 | 0.0 | 0.0 | 0.00 | 0.00 | 5 |
| 2540 | 1 ea | Nonfat, 4.4 oz, Light n' Lively | 125 | 50 | | 5.0 | 9.0 | 0.0 | 6.0 | 3.0 | 0.0 | 0.0 | 0.0 | 0.0 | 0.00 | 0.00 | 2 |
| 2556 | 1 ea | Nonfat, 8 oz, Weight Watchers | 227 | 90 | 89 | 8.0 | 14.0 | 0.0 | 7.0 | 7.0 | 0.0 | 0.0 | 0.0 | 0.0 | 0.00 | 0.00 | 5 |
| 2497 | 1 ea | Pineapple, lowfat, 4.4 oz, Light n' Lively | 125 | 140 | | 5.0 | 27.0 | 0.0 | 24.0 | 3.0 | 1.0 | 0.5 | | | | | 5 |
| 2517 | 1 ea | Pineapple, nonfat, 6 oz, Knudsen | 170 | 70 | | 7.0 | 11.0 | 0.0 | 8.0 | 3.0 | 0.0 | 0.0 | 0.0 | 0.0 | 0.00 | 0.00 | 5 |
| | | Plain Yogurt | | | | | | | | | | | | | | | |
| 2494 | 1 ea | Lowfat, 8 oz, avg | 245 | 154 | 85 | 12.9 | 17.2 | 0.0 | 17.2 | 0.0 | 3.8 | 2.5 | 1.0 | 0.1 | 0.03 | 0.08 | 15 |
| 2510 | 1 ea | Nonfat, 8 oz, avg | 245 | 137 | 85 | 14.0 | 18.8 | 0.0 | 18.8 | 0.0 | 0.4 | 0.3 | 0.1 | 0.0 | 0.00 | 0.01 | 5 |
| 2557 | 1 ea | Nonfat, 8 oz, Weight Watchers | 227 | 90 | 89 | 8.0 | 14.0 | 0.0 | 8.0 | 6.0 | 0.0 | 0.0 | 0.0 | 0.0 | 0.00 | 0.00 | 5 |
| 2565 | 1 ea | Whole milk, 8 oz, avg | 245 | 149 | 88 | 8.5 | 11.4 | 0.0 | 11.4 | 0.0 | 8.0 | 5.1 | 2.2 | 0.2 | 0.07 | 0.16 | 32 |
| 2571 | 1 ea | Whole milk, 6 oz, Yoplait | 170 | 120 | | 10.0 | 14.0 | 0.0 | | | 3.0 | 1.9 | 0.8 | 0.1 | | | 20 |
| | | Raspberry Yogurt | | | | | | | | | | | | | | | |
| 2469 | 1 ea | Lowfat, 8 oz, Darigold | 227 | 240 | 75 | 10.0 | 44.0 | 0.0 | 39.0 | 5.0 | 2.5 | 1.5 | | | | | 15 |
| 2558 | 1 ea | N' Crème, nonfat, 8 oz, Weight Watchers | 227 | 90 | 89 | 8.0 | 14.0 | 0.0 | 7.0 | 7.0 | 0.0 | 0.0 | 0.0 | 0.0 | 0.00 | 0.00 | 5 |
| 2498 | 1 ea | Red, lowfat, 4.4 oz, Light n' Lively | 125 | 130 | | 5.0 | 24.0 | 0.0 | 21.0 | 3.0 | 1.0 | 1.0 | | | | | 10 |
| 2523 | 1 ea | Red, nonfat, 6 oz, Knudsen | 170 | 160 | | 8.0 | 31.0 | 0.0 | 28.0 | 3.0 | 0.0 | 0.0 | 0.0 | 0.0 | 0.00 | 0.00 | 5 |
| 2536 | 1 ea | Red, nonfat, 4.4 oz, Light n' Lively | 125 | 50 | | 5.0 | 8.0 | 0.0 | 6.0 | 2.0 | 0.0 | 0.0 | 0.0 | 0.0 | 0.00 | 0.00 | 2 |
| | | Strawberry Yogurt | | | | | | | | | | | | | | | |
| 2470 | 1 ea | Lowfat, 8 oz, Darigold | 227 | 240 | 74 | 10.0 | 45.0 | 0.0 | 39.0 | 6.0 | 2.5 | 1.5 | | | | | 15 |
| 2499 | 1 ea | Lowfat, 4.4 oz, Light n' Lively | 125 | 140 | | 5.0 | 26.0 | 0.0 | 24.0 | 2.0 | 1.0 | 1.0 | | | | | 10 |
| 2527 | 1 ea | Nonfat, 6 oz, Knudsen | 170 | 70 | 89 | 7.0 | 11.0 | 0.0 | 8.0 | 3.0 | 0.0 | 0.0 | 0.0 | 0.0 | 0.00 | 0.00 | 5 |
| 2539 | 1 ea | Nonfat, 4.4 oz, Light n' Lively | 125 | 50 | | 5.0 | 8.0 | 0.0 | 6.0 | 2.0 | 0.0 | 0.0 | 0.0 | 0.0 | 0.00 | 0.00 | 2 |
| 2560 | 1 ea | Nonfat, 8 oz, Weight Watchers | 227 | 90 | 89 | 8.0 | 14.0 | 2.0 | 7.0 | 5.0 | 0.0 | 0.0 | 0.0 | 0.0 | 0.00 | 0.00 | 5 |
| | | Strawberry Banana Yogurt | | | | | | | | | | | | | | | |
| 2503 | 1 ea | Lowfat, 4.4 oz, Light n' Lively | 125 | 140 | | 5.0 | 28.0 | 0.0 | 25.0 | 3.0 | 1.0 | 0.5 | | | | | 10 |
| 2520 | 1 ea | Nonfat, 6 oz, Knudsen | 170 | 70 | | 7.0 | 11.0 | 0.0 | 8.0 | 3.0 | 0.0 | 0.0 | 0.0 | 0.0 | 0.00 | 0.00 | 5 |
| 2544 | 1 ea | Nonfat, 4.4 oz, Light n' Lively | 125 | 50 | | 5.0 | 8.0 | 0.0 | 6.0 | 2.0 | 0.0 | 0.0 | 0.0 | 0.0 | 0.00 | 0.00 | 2 |
| 2559 | 1 ea | Nonfat, 8 oz, Weight Watchers | 227 | 90 | 89 | 8.0 | 14.0 | 2.0 | 7.0 | 5.0 | 0.0 | 0.0 | 0.0 | 0.0 | 0.00 | 0.00 | 5 |
| 2478 | 1 ea | Strawberry Kiwi, lowfat, 8 oz, Darigold | 227 | 240 | 74 | 10.0 | 45.0 | 0.0 | 40.0 | 5.0 | 2.5 | 1.5 | | | | | 15 |
| 2506 | 1 ea | Tropical Punch, lowfat, 4.4 oz, Light n' Lively | 125 | 140 | | 5.0 | 27.0 | 0.0 | 24.0 | 3.0 | 1.0 | 0.5 | | | | | 10 |
| | | Vanilla Yogurt | | | | | | | | | | | | | | | |
| 2577 | 1 ea | Lowfat, 8 oz, avg | 245 | 208 | 79 | 12.1 | 33.8 | 0.0 | 33.8 | 0.0 | 3.1 | 2.0 | 0.8 | 0.1 | 0.02 | 0.06 | 12 |
| 2473 | 1 ea | Lowfat, 8 oz, Darigold | 227 | 240 | 74 | 10.0 | 45.0 | 0.0 | 41.0 | 4.0 | 2.5 | 1.5 | | | | | 15 |

| Code | Vit A (IU) | Vit A (RE) | Retinol (RE) | Carotenoids (RE) | Beta Carotene (mcg) | Thiamin (mg) | Riboflavin (mg) | Niacin (NE) | Vit B6 (mg) | Vit B12 (mcg) | Folate (mcg) | Panto (mg) | Vit C (mg) | Vit D (mg) | Vit E (α TE) | Calcium (mg) | Copper (mg) | Iron (mg) | Magnes (mg) | Mang (mg) | Phos (mg) | Potassium (mg) | Selenium (mcg) | Sodium (mg) | Zinc (mg) |
|---|---|---|---|---|---|---|---|---|---|---|---|---|---|---|---|---|---|---|---|---|---|---|---|---|---|
| | Vit A & Components | | | | | Vitamins | | | | | | | | | | Minerals | | | | | | | | | |
| 2568 | 85 | 21 | | | | 0.09 | 0.34 | | 0.06 | | | | 0.3 | | | 510 | | 0.5 | | | 400 | 370 | | 90 | |
| 2476 | 100 | 24 | | | | | | | | | | | 1.2 | | | 250 | | 0.0 | | | | | | 150 | |
| 2552 | 0 | 0 | 0 | 0 | 0 | | | | | | | | 0.0 | | | 250 | | 0.0 | | | | 260 | | 140 | |
| 2553 | 0 | 0 | 0 | 0 | 0 | | | | | | | | 0.0 | | | 250 | | 0.0 | | | | 280 | | 140 | |
| 2471 | 100 | 24 | | | | | | | | | | | 1.2 | | | 250 | | 0.0 | | | | | | 150 | |
| 2563 | 310 | 76 | 68 | 7 | | 0.10 | 0.48 | 0.26 | 0.11 | 1.27 | 25.2 | 1.23 | 1.8 | 0.1 | | 412 | 0.0 | 0.2 | 39 | 0.0 | 323 | 527 | 3.4 | 159 | 1.99 |
| 2579 | 132 | 32 | 29 | 2 | | 0.10 | 0.49 | 0.26 | 0.11 | 1.29 | 25.7 | 1.35 | 1.8 | 0.1 | | 419 | 0.0 | 0.2 | 39 | 0.0 | 331 | 537 | 12.0 | 162 | 2.03 |
| 2574 | 14 | 4 | 4 | 0 | | 0.10 | 0.48 | 0.25 | 0.11 | 1.24 | 24.7 | 1.13 | 1.8 | 0.1 | | 404 | 0.0 | 0.2 | 39 | 0.1 | 318 | 518 | 4.8 | 154 | 1.97 |
| 2575 | 287 | 70 | 63 | 7 | | 0.09 | 0.45 | 0.24 | 0.10 | 1.17 | 23.4 | 1.13 | 1.7 | 0.1 | | 381 | 0.0 | 0.2 | 36 | 0.0 | 300 | 488 | 4.5 | 148 | 1.85 |
| 2554 | 0 | 0 | 0 | 0 | 0 | | | | | | | | 0.0 | | | 250 | | 0.0 | | | | | | 140 | |
| 2572 | 85 | 21 | | | | 0.05 | 0.31 | | | 0.36 | | | | | | 200 | | | | | 150 | 310 | | 95 | |
| 2573 | 100 | 24 | | | | 0.05 | 0.26 | | | 0.36 | | | | | | 250 | | | | | 200 | 290 | | 110 | 0.60 |
| 2569 | 100 | 24 | | | | 0.05 | 0.26 | | 0.07 | 0.36 | | | 1.0 | | | 200 | | 0.3 | | | 150 | 290 | | 95 | 0.60 |
| 2493 | 113 | 27 | 25 | 2 | | 0.09 | 0.44 | 0.23 | 0.10 | 1.14 | 22.8 | 1.20 | 1.6 | 0.1 | | 372 | 0.2 | 0.2 | 37 | 0.2 | 292 | 478 | 7.6 | 142 | 1.81 |
| 2102 | 110 | 25 | 22 | 3 | | 0.14 | 0.40 | 0.27 | 0.10 | 1.03 | 23.1 | 1.13 | 1.6 | 0.1 | | 336 | 0.1 | 0.3 | 41 | 0.1 | 281 | 454 | 4.5 | 129 | 1.99 |
| 2511 | 40 | 6 | 4 | 2 | | 0.10 | 0.45 | 0.50 | 0.11 | 1.11 | 32.2 | 1.18 | 26.4 | 0.1 | | 369 | 0.1 | 0.6 | 41 | 0.1 | 292 | 549 | 4.8 | 140 | 1.83 |
| 2570 | 85 | 21 | | | | 0.09 | 0.34 | | 0.07 | 0.36 | | | 0.3 | | | 250 | | 0.2 | | | 200 | 350 | | 105 | 0.60 |
| 2467 | 100 | 24 | | | | | | | | | | | 2.4 | | | 250 | | 0.0 | | | | | | 150 | |
| 2578 | 132 | 32 | 29 | 2 | | 0.10 | 0.49 | 0.26 | 0.11 | 1.29 | 25.7 | 1.35 | 1.8 | 0.1 | | 419 | 0.0 | 0.2 | 39 | 0.0 | 331 | 537 | 12.0 | 162 | 2.03 |
| 2097 | 14 | 4 | 4 | 0 | | 0.10 | 0.48 | 0.25 | 0.11 | 1.24 | 24.7 | 1.13 | 1.8 | 0.1 | | 404 | 0.0 | 0.2 | 39 | 0.1 | 318 | 518 | 4.8 | 154 | 1.97 |
| 2515 | 0 | 0 | 0 | 0 | 0 | 0.03 | 0.25 | | | 0.60 | | | 0.0 | | | 200 | | 0.0 | | | 150 | 270 | | 100 | |
| 2555 | 0 | 0 | 0 | 0 | 0 | | | | | | | | 0.0 | | | 250 | | 0.0 | | | | 305 | | 140 | |
| 2576 | 287 | 70 | 63 | 7 | | 0.09 | 0.45 | 0.24 | 0.10 | 1.17 | 23.4 | 1.13 | 1.7 | 0.1 | | 381 | 0.0 | 0.2 | 36 | 0.0 | 300 | 488 | 4.5 | 148 | 1.85 |
| 2492 | 132 | 32 | 29 | 2 | | 0.10 | 0.49 | 0.26 | 0.11 | 1.29 | 25.7 | 1.35 | 1.8 | 0.1 | | 419 | 0.0 | 0.2 | 39 | 0.0 | 331 | 537 | 12.0 | 162 | 2.03 |
| 2521 | 0 | 0 | 0 | 0 | 0 | 0.03 | 0.25 | | | 0.90 | | | 0.0 | | | 250 | | 0.0 | | | 200 | 370 | | 105 | |
| 2477 | 200 | 49 | | | | | | | | | | | 1.2 | | | 250 | | 0.0 | | | | | | 150 | |
| 2496 | 0 | 0 | 0 | 0 | 0 | 0.00 | 0.17 | | | 0.48 | | | 3.6 | | | 150 | | 0.0 | | | 150 | 230 | | 65 | |
| 2516 | 0 | 0 | 0 | 0 | 0 | 0.03 | 0.25 | | | 0.60 | | | 0.0 | | | 200 | | 0.0 | | | 150 | 270 | | 80 | |
| 2540 | 0 | 0 | 0 | 0 | 0 | 0.00 | 0.17 | | | 0.48 | | | 0.0 | | | 150 | | 0.0 | | | | 100 | | 60 | |
| 2556 | 0 | 0 | 0 | 0 | 0 | | | | | | | | 0.0 | | | 250 | | 0.0 | | | | | | 140 | |
| 2497 | 0 | 0 | 0 | 0 | 0 | 0.03 | 0.17 | | | 0.48 | | | 3.6 | | | 150 | | 0.0 | | | 150 | 250 | | 60 | |
| 2517 | 0 | 0 | 0 | 0 | 0 | 0.03 | 0.25 | | | 0.60 | | | 0.0 | | | 200 | | 0.0 | | | 150 | 270 | | 80 | |
| 2494 | 162 | 39 | 37 | 2 | | 0.11 | 0.52 | 0.28 | 0.12 | 1.38 | 27.4 | 1.45 | 2.0 | 0.1 | | 448 | 0.0 | 0.2 | 44 | 0.0 | 353 | 573 | 8.1 | 172 | 2.18 |
| 2510 | 17 | 5 | 5 | 0.1 | | 0.12 | 0.57 | 0.30 | 0.13 | 1.50 | 29.9 | 1.57 | 2.1 | 0.1 | | 488 | 0.0 | 0.2 | 47 | 0.0 | 385 | 625 | 8.8 | 186 | 2.38 |
| 2557 | 0 | 0 | 0 | 0 | 0 | | | | | | | | 0.0 | | | 300 | | 0.0 | | | | 320 | | 150 | |
| 2565 | 301 | 74 | 66 | 7 | | 0.07 | 0.35 | 0.18 | 0.08 | 0.91 | 18.1 | 0.95 | 1.3 | 0.1 | | 296 | 0.0 | 0.1 | 29 | 0.0 | 233 | 380 | 5.4 | 113 | 1.45 |
| 2571 | 100 | 27 | | | | 0.09 | 0.43 | | 0.08 | 0.36 | | | 1.4 | | | 300 | | 0.1 | | | 250 | 370 | | 120 | 0.60 |
| 2469 | 100 | 24 | | | | | | | | | | | 2.4 | | | 250 | | 0.0 | | | | | | 150 | |
| 2558 | 0 | 0 | 0 | 0 | 0 | | | | | | | | 0.0 | | | 250 | | 0.0 | | | | 210 | | 140 | |
| 2498 | 0 | 0 | 0 | 0 | 0 | 0.03 | 0.17 | | | 0.48 | | | 0.0 | | | 200 | | 0.0 | | | 150 | 230 | | 65 | |
| 2523 | 0 | 0 | 0 | 0 | 0 | 0.03 | 0.25 | | | 0.90 | | | 0.0 | | | 250 | | 0.0 | | | 200 | 360 | | 105 | |
| 2536 | 0 | 0 | 0 | 0 | 0 | 0.00 | 0.17 | | | 0.48 | | | 0.0 | | | 150 | | 0.0 | | | 100 | 220 | | 60 | |
| 2470 | 100 | 24 | | | | | | | | | | | 4.8 | | | 250 | | 0.4 | | | | | | 150 | |
| 2499 | 0 | 0 | 0 | 0 | 0 | 0.03 | 0.17 | | | 0.48 | | | 0.0 | | | 150 | | 0.0 | | | 150 | 230 | | 65 | |
| 2527 | 0 | 0 | 0 | 0 | 0 | 0.03 | 0.25 | | 0.09 | 0.60 | | | 0.0 | | | 200 | | 0.0 | | | 150 | 290 | | 85 | |
| 2539 | 0 | 0 | 0 | 0 | 0 | 0.00 | 0.17 | | | 0.48 | | | 0.0 | | | 150 | | 0.0 | | | 100 | 210 | | 60 | |
| 2560 | 0 | 0 | 0 | 0 | 0 | | | | | | | | 0.0 | | | 250 | | 0.0 | | | | 290 | | 140 | |
| 2503 | 0 | 0 | 0 | 0 | 0 | 0.03 | 0.17 | | | 0.48 | | | 2.4 | | | 150 | | 0.0 | | | 150 | 230 | | 60 | |
| 2520 | 0 | 0 | 0 | 0 | 0 | 0.03 | 0.25 | | | 0.60 | | | 0.0 | | | 200 | | 0.0 | | | 150 | 270 | | 85 | |
| 2544 | 0 | 0 | 0 | 0 | 0 | 0.00 | 0.17 | | | 0.48 | | | 0.0 | | | 150 | | 0.0 | | | 100 | 210 | | 60 | |
| 2559 | 0 | 0 | 0 | 0 | 0 | | | | | | | | 0.0 | | | 250 | | 0.0 | | | | 305 | | 140 | |
| 2478 | 100 | 24 | | | | | | | | | | | 4.8 | | | 250 | | 0.0 | | | | | | 150 | |
| 2506 | 0 | 0 | 0 | 0 | 0 | 0.00 | 0.17 | | | 0.48 | | | 0.0 | | | 150 | | 0.0 | | | 150 | 220 | | 65 | |
| 2577 | 132 | 32 | 29 | 3 | | 0.10 | 0.49 | 0.26 | 0.11 | 1.29 | 25.7 | 1.35 | 1.8 | 0.1 | | 419 | 0.0 | 0.2 | 39 | 0.0 | 331 | 537 | 12.0 | 162 | 2.03 |
| 2473 | 100 | 24 | | | | | | | | | | | 1.2 | | | 250 | | 0.4 | | | | | | 150 | |

| Code | Amount | Description | Basic Components | | | | | | | | | Additional Fats | | | | | | Vit A & Components | | | | | | Vitamins | | | | | | | | | | Minerals | | | | | | | | | |
|---|---|---|---|---|---|---|---|---|---|---|---|---|---|---|---|---|---|---|---|---|---|---|---|---|---|---|---|---|---|---|---|---|---|---|---|---|---|---|---|---|---|---|
| | | | Weight (g) | Calories | % Water | Protein (g) | Carbs (g) | Fiber (g) | Sugar (g) | Other Carbs (g) | Fat (g) | Sat Fat (g) | Mono Fat (g) | Poly Fat (g) | Omega 3 (g) | Omega 6 (g) | Choles (mg) | Vit A (IU) | Vit A (RE) | Retinol (RE) | Carotenoids (RE) | Beta Carotene (mcg) | Thiamin (mg) | Riboflavin (mg) | Niacin (NE) | Vit B6 (mg) | Vit B12 (mcg) | Folate (mcg) | Panto (mg) | Vit C (mg) | Vit D (mg) | Vit E (α TE) | Calcium (mg) | Copper (mg) | Iron (mg) | Magnes (mg) | Mang (mg) | Phos (mg) | Potassium (mg) | Selenium (mcg) | Sodium (mg) | Zinc (mg) |
| 2098 | 1 ea | Nonfat, 8 oz, avg | 227 | 207 | 76 | 11.6 | 39.7 | 0.0 | 39.6 | 0.1 | 0.4 | 0.2 | 0.1 | 0.0 | 0.00 | 0.01 | 5 | 14 | 4 | 4 | 0 | | 0.10 | 0.48 | 0.25 | 0.11 | 1.24 | 24.7 | 1.13 | 1.8 | 0.1 | | 404 | 0.0 | 0.2 | 39 | 0.1 | 318 | 518 | 4.8 | 154 | 1.97 |
| 2526 | 1 ea | Nonfat, 6 oz, Knudsen | 170 | 70 | 89 | 7.0 | 11.0 | 0.0 | 8.0 | 3.0 | 0.0 | 0.0 | 0.0 | 0.0 | 0.00 | 0.00 | 5 | 0 | 0 | 0 | 0 | 0 | 0.03 | 0.25 | | 0.09 | 0.60 | | | 0.0 | | | 200 | | 0.0 | | | 150 | 270 | | 80 | |
| 2562 | 1 ea | Nonfat, 8 oz, Weight Watchers | 227 | 90 | 89 | 8.0 | 14.0 | 0.0 | 7.0 | 7.0 | 0.0 | 0.0 | 0.0 | 0.0 | 0.00 | 0.00 | 5 | 0 | 0 | 0 | 0 | 0 | | | | | | | | 0.0 | | | 250 | | 0.0 | | | | 260 | | 140 | |
| 2564 | 1 ea | Whole milk, 8 oz, avg | 227 | 229 | 77 | 11.0 | 30.7 | 0.0 | 30.7 | 0.0 | 7.2 | 4.5 | 2.0 | 0.2 | 0.07 | 0.17 | 23 | 287 | 70 | 63 | 7 | | 0.09 | 0.45 | 0.24 | 0.10 | 1.17 | 23.4 | 1.13 | 1.7 | 0.1 | | 381 | 0.0 | 0.2 | 36 | 0.0 | 300 | 488 | 4.5 | 148 | 1.85 |
| 2475 | 1 ea | White Choc Raspberry, lowfat, 8 oz, Darigold | 227 | 240 | 74 | 10.0 | 45.0 | 0.0 | 41.0 | 4.0 | 2.5 | 1.5 | | | | | 15 | 100 | 24 | | | | | | | | | | | 2.4 | | | 250 | | 0.0 | | | | | | 150 | |
| 2502 | 1 ea | Wild Berry, lowfat, 4.4 oz, Light n' Lively | 125 | 140 | | 5.0 | 27.0 | 0.0 | 24.0 | 3.0 | 1.0 | 0.5 | | | | | 10 | 0 | 0 | 0 | 0 | 0 | 0.00 | 0.17 | | | 0.48 | | | 0.0 | | | 150 | | 0.0 | | | 150 | 220 | | 65 | |
| | | **DESSERTS** | | | | | | | | | | | | | | | | | | | | | | | | | | | | | | | | | | | | | | | | |
| | | *BROWNIES AND BARS* | | | | | | | | | | | | | | | | | | | | | | | | | | | | | | | | | | | | | | | | |
| | | Bars | | | | | | | | | | | | | | | | | | | | | | | | | | | | | | | | | | | | | | | | |
| 47494 | 1 ea | Fudge Nut, Gold Medal | 69 | 321 | | 4.0 | 49.1 | 1.0 | 31.1 | 17.0 | 13.0 | 3.0 | 4.0 | 2.0 | | | 15 | 0 | 0 | 0 | 0 | 0 | 0.12 | 0.10 | 1.20 | | | | | | | | 20 | | 1.4 | | | | 110 | | 181 | |
| 47587 | 1 ea | Lemon, Gold Medal | 57 | 249 | | 3.0 | 45.8 | 0.5 | 29.8 | 15.4 | 6.0 | 1.5 | 2.5 | 1.5 | | | 50 | 99 | 20 | | | | 0.09 | 0.03 | 0.80 | | | | | 0.0 | | | 0 | | 0.7 | | | | 35 | | 149 | |
| | | Brownies | | | | | | | | | | | | | | | | | | | | | | | | | | | | | | | | | | | | | | | | |
| 47151 | 1 ea | A La Mode, Weight Watchers | 91 | 95 | 75 | 3.0 | 17.5 | 2.0 | 12.0 | 3.5 | 2.0 | 0.5 | 1.0 | 1.5 | | | 2 | 0 | 0 | 0 | 0 | 0 | 0.03 | 0.01 | 0.10 | 0.01 | | | | 0.0 | | | 40 | | 0.5 | | | | 115 | | 80 | |
| 49092 | 1 ea | Bar w/Caramel Top, fat free, Health Valley | 38 | 110 | 22 | 3.0 | 26.0 | 4.0 | 17.0 | 5.0 | 0.0 | 0.0 | 0.0 | 0.0 | 0.00 | 0.00 | 0 | 100 | 20 | | | | | | | | | | | 0.0 | | | 0 | | 1.1 | | | | | | 30 | |
| 47075 | 1 ea | Butterscotch, avg | 34 | 149 | 11 | 1.6 | 21.7 | 0.3 | 15.8 | 5.6 | 6.6 | 1.2 | 2.6 | 2.3 | | | 18 | 291 | 76 | 70 | 6 | | 0.05 | 0.06 | 0.41 | 0.02 | 0.04 | 3.9 | 0.07 | 0.1 | 0.1 | | 24 | 0.1 | 0.7 | 10 | 0.1 | 26 | 80 | | 96 | 0.17 |
| 47320 | 1 ea | Chocolate Frosted, Weight Watchers | 35 | 99 | 25 | 2.0 | 21.7 | 3.0 | 17.8 | 1.0 | 2.5 | 1.0 | | | | | 0 | 0 | 0 | 0 | 0 | 0 | | | | | | | | 0.0 | | | 79 | | 0.7 | | | | 128 | | 133 | |
| 47368 | 1 ea | Double Fudge Parfait, Weight Watchers | 75 | 95 | | 3.0 | 19.5 | 1.0 | 10.0 | 8.5 | 1.2 | 1.0 | | | | | 2 | 0 | 0 | 0 | 0 | 0 | | | | | | | | 0.0 | | | 100 | | 0.5 | | | | 110 | | 85 | |
| 47577 | 1 ea | Fudge Walnut, Tasty Kake | 85 | 370 | | 5.0 | 52.0 | 1.0 | 37.0 | 14.0 | 17.0 | 4.0 | | | | | 80 | 100 | 20 | | | | | | | | | | | 0.0 | | | 20 | | 1.1 | | | | | | 150 | |
| 47589 | 1 ea | Gold Medal | 42 | 188 | | 2.0 | 31.6 | 1.0 | 22.7 | 7.9 | 4.9 | 2.0 | 2.0 | 1.5 | | | 15 | 0 | 0 | 0 | 0 | 0 | 0.09 | 0.10 | 0.00 | | | | | 0.0 | | | 0 | | 1.1 | | | | 148 | | 124 | |
| 47030 | 1 ea | Low Calorie, low sod, avg | 22 | 84 | 13 | 0.8 | 15.7 | 0.8 | 9.5 | 5.4 | 2.4 | 1.1 | 1.0 | 0.2 | 0.01 | 0.17 | 0 | 0 | 0 | 0 | 0 | 0 | 0.02 | 0.03 | 0.22 | 0.00 | 0.00 | 7.5 | 0.01 | 0.0 | 0.0 | | 3 | 0.0 | 0.3 | 1 | 0.1 | 11 | 69 | 0.6 | 21 | 0.03 |
| 47683 | 1 oz | Low Calorie, low sod, dry mix, avg | 28 | 119 | 4 | 0.8 | 22.5 | 1.2 | 15.0 | 6.4 | 3.5 | 0.6 | 1.5 | 1.3 | 0.09 | 1.19 | 0 | 0 | 0 | 0 | 0 | 0 | 0.04 | 0.03 | 0.35 | 0.00 | 0.00 | 13.4 | 0.03 | 0.0 | 0.0 | | 3 | 0.0 | 0.4 | 1 | 0.1 | 16 | 94 | 0.6 | 23 | 0.04 |
| 47323 | 1 ea | Peanut Butter Fudge, Weight Watchers | 35 | 110 | 24 | 2.0 | 21.1 | 3.0 | 16.1 | 2.0 | 2.5 | 0.5 | | | | | 0 | 0 | 0 | 0 | 0 | 0 | | | | | | | | 0.0 | | | 20 | | 1.1 | | | | 100 | | 141 | |
| 47669 | 1 ea | With Icing, fzn, avg | 25 | 104 | 12 | 1.2 | 15.2 | 0.9 | | | 5.2 | 1.7 | 2.6 | 1.8 | | 0.57 | 10 | 55 | 17 | 14 | 2 | | 0.03 | 0.03 | 0.17 | 0.01 | 0.05 | 2.0 | 0.11 | 0.1 | | | 10 | 0.1 | 0.4 | 10 | | 31 | 45 | 2.9 | 50 | 0.33 |
| 47000 | 1 ea | With Nuts, avg | 61 | 247 | 14 | 2.9 | 39.0 | 1.3 | 27.5 | 10.2 | 9.9 | 2.6 | 5.5 | 1.4 | 0.10 | 1.23 | 10 | 42 | 4 | | | | 0.16 | 0.13 | 1.05 | 0.02 | 0.04 | 12.8 | 0.33 | 0.0 | 0.1 | | 18 | 0.1 | 1.4 | 19 | 0.1 | 62 | 91 | 3.8 | 190 | 0.44 |
| 47028 | 1 ea | Without Nuts, avg | 33 | 140 | 13 | 1.4 | 20.4 | 0.9 | 14.2 | 5.2 | 6.6 | 1.3 | 2.0 | 2.8 | 0.28 | 2.56 | 9 | 15 | 4 | 4 | 0.2 | | 0.04 | 0.05 | 0.45 | 0.01 | 0.02 | 2.6 | 0.05 | 0.0 | 0.0 | | 6 | 0.1 | 0.6 | 11 | 0.2 | 26 | 61 | | 83 | 0.19 |
| 47027 | 1 oz | Without Nuts, dry mix, avg | 28 | 122 | 3 | 1.1 | 21.4 | 0.9 | 15.0 | 5.6 | 4.2 | 0.7 | 1.4 | 1.8 | 0.22 | 1.55 | 0 | 3 | 0.3 | | | | 0.05 | 0.05 | 0.53 | 0.02 | 0.00 | 9.8 | 0.04 | 0.1 | 0.0 | | 5 | 0.1 | 0.6 | 11 | 0.1 | 23 | 61 | 0.7 | 85 | 0.18 |
| 47019 | 1 ea | With Walnuts, prep f/rec, avg | 24 | 112 | 13 | 1.5 | 12.0 | 0.5 | 8.4 | 3.1 | 7.0 | 1.8 | 2.6 | 2.3 | 0.23 | 2.03 | 18 | 184 | 48 | 44 | 4 | | 0.03 | 0.05 | 0.24 | 0.02 | 0.04 | 7.0 | 0.08 | 0.1 | 0.0 | | 14 | 0.1 | 0.4 | 13 | 0.1 | 32 | 42 | 2.8 | 82 | 0.23 |
| | | *CAKES* | | | | | | | | | | | | | | | | | | | | | | | | | | | | | | | | | | | | | | | | |
| | | Angel Food cake | | | | | | | | | | | | | | | | | | | | | | | | | | | | | | | | | | | | | | | | |
| 46049 | 1 oz | Dry mix, avg | 28 | 104 | 3 | 2.5 | 23.8 | 0.1 | 19.3 | 4.5 | 0.1 | 0.0 | 0.0 | 0.1 | 0.00 | 0.05 | 0 | 0 | 0 | 0 | 0 | 0 | 0.05 | 0.09 | 0.08 | 0.00 | 0.01 | 10.9 | 0.07 | 0.0 | 0.0 | | 34 | 0.0 | 0.1 | 3 | 0.0 | 94 | 55 | 3.5 | 206 | 0.04 |
| 46004 | 1 pce | Prep, avg | 28 | 72 | 33 | 1.7 | 16.2 | 0.4 | 12.8 | 2.9 | 0.2 | 0.0 | 0.0 | 0.1 | 0.01 | 0.10 | 0 | 0 | 0 | 0 | 0 | 0 | 0.03 | 0.14 | 0.25 | 0.01 | 0.02 | 9.8 | 0.06 | 0.0 | 0.0 | | 39 | 0.0 | 0.1 | 3 | 0.0 | 9 | 26 | 2.0 | 210 | 0.02 |
| 46050 | 1 pce | Prep f/mix, avg | 50 | 128 | 33 | 3.0 | 29.4 | 0.1 | 23.7 | 5.5 | 0.2 | 0.0 | 0.0 | 0.1 | 0.00 | 0.06 | 0 | 0 | 0 | 0 | 0 | 0 | 0.05 | 0.10 | 0.09 | 0.00 | 0.01 | 15.0 | 0.05 | 0.0 | 0.0 | | 42 | 0.0 | 0.1 | 4 | 0.0 | 116 | 68 | 7.7 | 254 | 0.06 |
| 46051 | 1 pce | Prep f/rec, avg | 53 | 142 | 32 | 4.0 | 31.5 | 0.2 | 25.5 | 5.8 | 0.1 | 0.0 | 0.0 | 0.0 | 0.00 | 0.03 | 0 | 0 | 0 | 0 | 0 | 0 | 0.05 | 0.17 | 0.44 | 0.00 | 0.05 | 2.1 | 0.05 | 0.0 | 0.0 | | 3 | 0.0 | 0.4 | 5 | 0.1 | 13 | 116 | | 96 | 0.07 |
| 46102 | 1 pce | Applesauce cake, w/icing, avg | 108 | 399 | 19 | 2.9 | 69.8 | 1.5 | 55.4 | 12.9 | 13.3 | 3.2 | 5.7 | 3.6 | | | 21 | 188 | 49 | 45 | 4 | | 0.12 | 0.12 | 1.00 | 0.05 | 0.05 | 5.3 | 0.11 | 0.9 | 0.1 | | 21 | 0.1 | 1.3 | 10 | 0.2 | 45 | 137 | | 293 | 0.24 |
| 46098 | 1 pce | Applesauce cake, w/o icing, avg | 87 | 313 | 22 | 3.0 | 52.0 | 1.7 | 36.7 | 13.6 | 11.4 | 2.9 | 4.9 | 2.9 | | | 23 | 38 | 11 | 10 | 0.4 | | 0.14 | 0.13 | 1.10 | 0.06 | 0.04 | 5.6 | 0.09 | 0.9 | 0.1 | | 17 | 0.1 | 1.4 | 10 | 0.3 | 46 | 145 | | 285 | 0.25 |
| | | Banana cake | | | | | | | | | | | | | | | | | | | | | | | | | | | | | | | | | | | | | | | | |
| 46243 | 1 pce | Crunch, fat free, Entenmann's, | 53 | 140 | | 2.0 | 33.0 | 2.0 | 20.0 | 11.0 | 0.0 | 0.0 | 0.0 | 0.0 | 0.00 | 0.00 | 0 | 0 | 0 | 0 | 0 | 0 | | | | | | | | 0.0 | | | 40 | | 0.0 | | | | 115 | | 150 | |
| 46294 | 1 oz | Dry Mix, Pillsbury | 28 | 117 | 4 | 1.0 | 22.7 | 0.3 | 13.5 | 8.9 | 2.5 | 0.8 | | | | | 0 | 0 | 0 | 0 | 0 | 0 | | | | | | | | 0.0 | | | 23 | | 0.6 | | | | | | 169 | |
| 46244 | 1 pce | Loaf, fat free, Entenmann's | 57 | 150 | | 2.0 | 34.0 | 1.0 | 20.0 | 13.0 | 0.0 | 0.0 | 0.0 | 0.0 | 0.00 | 0.00 | 0 | 0 | 0 | 0 | 0 | 0 | | | | | | | | 0.0 | | | 20 | | 0.0 | | | | 140 | | 190 | |
| 46104 | 1 pce | With Icing, avg | 108 | 309 | 34 | 3.5 | 58.5 | 1.1 | | | 7.6 | 1.6 | 3.2 | 2.3 | | | 30 | 419 | 135 | 94 | 10 | | 0.13 | 0.17 | 1.10 | 0.25 | 0.08 | 12.5 | 0.22 | 3.5 | 0.1 | | 27 | 0.1 | 1.0 | 17 | 0.1 | 49 | 198 | | 292 | 0.29 |
| 46103 | 1 pce | Without Icing, avg | 87 | 245 | 37 | 3.1 | 43.3 | 1.1 | | | 7.3 | 1.6 | 3.1 | 2.2 | | | 30 | 401 | 130 | 90 | 10 | | 0.12 | 0.15 | 1.05 | 0.24 | 0.07 | 12.0 | 0.17 | 3.4 | 0.1 | | 26 | 0.1 | 1.0 | 17 | 0.1 | 45 | 185 | | 257 | 0.27 |
| 42327 | 1 pce | Black Forest cake, avg | 80 | 280 | 34 | 3.0 | 32.5 | 5.6 | 24.0 | 2.9 | 15.4 | | | | | | 46 | 426 | 36 | 80 | 16 | | 0.02 | 0.14 | | | | | | 0.0 | | | 46 | | 2.1 | 19 | | | 130 | | 224 | 0.48 |
| 46245 | 1 pce | Blueberry cake, Crunch, fat free, Entenmann's | 57 | 140 | | 2.0 | 32.0 | 2.0 | 18.0 | 12.0 | 0.0 | 0.0 | 0.0 | 0.0 | 0.00 | 0.00 | 0 | 100 | 20 | | | | | | | | | | | 0.0 | | | 40 | | 0.0 | | | | 75 | | 200 | |
| 46002 | 1 pce | Boston Cream Pie cake, coml prep, avg | 92 | 232 | 45 | 2.2 | 39.5 | 1.3 | 24.7 | 13.5 | 7.8 | 2.3 | 4.2 | 0.9 | 0.05 | 0.87 | 34 | 74 | 21 | 20 | 1 | | 0.38 | 0.25 | 0.18 | 0.02 | 0.15 | 13.8 | 0.28 | 0.2 | 0.6 | | 21 | 0.0 | 0.3 | 6 | 0.0 | 45 | 36 | 3.8 | 132 | 0.15 |
| 46052 | 1 pce | Boston Cream Pie cake, prep f/rec, avg | 93 | 293 | 34 | 4.3 | 43.0 | 0.8 | 27.1 | 15.0 | 12.3 | 3.9 | 5.0 | 2.6 | 0.17 | 2.43 | 43 | 180 | 51 | 49 | 2 | | 0.13 | 0.18 | 1.02 | 0.03 | 0.15 | 8.4 | 0.26 | 0.2 | 0.4 | | 93 | 0.1 | 1.2 | 16 | 0.2 | 91 | 95 | | 309 | 0.44 |
| 46260 | 1 pce | Butter cake, Entenmann's | 57 | 220 | 22 | 3.0 | 31.0 | 0.0 | 18.0 | 13.0 | 10.0 | 6.0 | | | | | 80 | 400 | 30 | | | | | | | | | | | 0.0 | | | 20 | | 0.0 | | | | 45 | | 290 | |
| 46223 | 1 pce | Caramel cake, avg | 63 | 243 | 23 | 2.8 | 33.8 | | | | 10.9 | 2.9 | 5.3 | 2.2 | 0.00 | 2.18 | 49 | 113 | 23 | | | | 0.09 | 0.11 | 0.76 | | | | | 0.1 | | | 49 | | 1.4 | | | 67 | 43 | | 192 | |
| | | Carrot cake | | | | | | | | | | | | | | | | | | | | | | | | | | | | | | | | | | | | | | | | |
| 46262 | 1 pce | Entenmann's | 71 | 290 | 23 | 3.0 | 35.0 | 0.5 | 26.0 | 8.5 | 16.0 | 3.5 | | | | | 35 | 1750 | 350 | | | | | | | | | | | 0.0 | | | 20 | | 0.4 | | | | 105 | | 240 | |
| 46246 | 1 pce | Fat free, Entenmann's | 71 | 170 | | 3.0 | 40.0 | 1.0 | 27.0 | 12.0 | 0.0 | 0.0 | 0.0 | 0.0 | 0.00 | 0.00 | 0 | 2250 | 450 | | | | | | | | | | | 0.0 | | | 40 | | 0.7 | | | | 150 | | 230 | |
| 46053 | 1 oz | Pudding Type, dry mix, avg | 28 | 116 | 4 | 1.4 | 22.2 | 0.7 | 14.2 | 7.3 | 2.7 | 0.4 | 1.1 | 1.0 | 0.07 | 0.96 | 0 | 540 | 117 | 14 | 103 | | 0.07 | 0.05 | 0.62 | 0.02 | 0.01 | 18.8 | 0.08 | 0.3 | 0.0 | | 48 | 0.0 | 0.5 | 2 | 0.1 | 69 | 47 | 4.2 | 159 | 0.06 |
| 46010 | 1 pce | With Cream Cheese Frosting, prep f/rec, avg | 111 | 484 | 21 | 5.1 | 52.4 | 1.3 | 37.4 | 13.7 | 29.3 | 5.4 | 7.2 | 15.1 | 1.94 | 13.12 | 60 | 3827 | 426 | 53 | 373 | | 0.15 | 0.17 | 1.12 | 0.08 | 0.11 | 13.3 | 0.25 | 1.2 | 0.2 | | 28 | 0.2 | 1.4 | 20 | 0.4 | 79 | 124 | 9.8 | 273 | 0.54 |
| 46054 | 1 pce | Without Frosting, prep f/mix, avg | 70 | 239 | 31 | 3.6 | 32.7 | 1.4 | 20.9 | 10.4 | 11.0 | 1.8 | 3.4 | 5.0 | 0.51 | 4.52 | 51 | 790 | 173 | 21 | 152 | | 0.09 | 0.12 | 0.83 | 0.06 | 0.81 | 8.4 | 0.19 | 1.7 | 0.1 | | 77 | 0.0 | 0.9 | 5 | 0.2 | 122 | 84 | 2.1 | 249 | 0.22 |
| | | Cheesecake | | | | | | | | | | | | | | | | | | | | | | | | | | | | | | | | | | | | | | | | |
| 46233 | 1 pce | Almond Amaretto, Weight Watchers | 85 | 170 | 56 | 8.0 | 24.0 | 3.0 | 13.0 | 8.0 | 5.0 | 2.5 | | | | | 5 | 200 | 40 | | | | | | | | | | | 0.0 | | | 80 | | 0.4 | | | | 105 | | 160 | |
| 46230 | 1 pce | Brownie, Weight Watchers | 99 | 200 | 51 | 9.0 | 32.9 | 4.0 | 12.0 | 17.0 | 6.0 | 2.0 | | | | | 5 | 0 | 0 | 0 | 0 | 0 | | | | | | | | 0.0 | | | 80 | | 1.1 | | | | 185 | | 219 | |
| 46391 | 1 oz | Cherry, no bake mix, Jell-o | 28 | 85 | 29 | 1.5 | 16.6 | 0.2 | 10.3 | 6.1 | 1.5 | 0.7 | | | | | 0 | 0 | 0 | 0 | 0 | 0 | | | | | | | | 0.0 | | | 29 | | 0.3 | | | | 74 | | 111 | |
| 46469 | 1 pce | Cherry, prep f/no bake mix, Jell-o | 126 | 330 | 45 | 5.0 | 51.0 | 1.0 | 33.0 | 17.0 | 12.0 | 4.0 | | | | | 5 | 400 | 30 | | | | | | | | | | | 0.0 | | | 150 | | 0.7 | | | | 280 | | 390 | |
| 46452 | 1 pce | Lemon, fat free, fzn, Krusteaz | 130 | 229 | 55 | 10.8 | 46.8 | 1.7 | 33.8 | 11.3 | 0.2 | 0.0 | 0.0 | 0.0 | | | 1 | 144 | 29 | | | | | | | | | | | 0.0 | | | 77 | | 0.9 | | | | 138 | | 415 | |
| 46195 | 1 oz | Plain, dry mix, General Mills | 28 | 109 | 8 | 3.9 | 19.9 | 0.0 | 16.8 | 3.1 | 1.4 | 0.6 | 0.7 | 0.0 | | | 3 | | | | | | 0.02 | 0.18 | 0.04 | | | | | | | | 157 | | 0.1 | | | | 207 | | 276 | |
| 46411 | 1 pce | Plain, prep f/mix, General Mills | 31 | 71 | 45 | 3.0 | 12.1 | 0.0 | 10.1 | 2.0 | 1.5 | 0.5 | 0.0 | 0.0 | 0.00 | 0.00 | 2 | 0 | 0 | 0 | 0 | 0 | 0.00 | 0.10 | 0.00 | | | | | 0.0 | | | 101 | | 0.0 | | | | 141 | | 162 | |
| 46453 | 1 pce | Strawberry, fat free, fzn, Krusteaz | 130 | 234 | 55 | 10.7 | 46.8 | 1.6 | 33.8 | 11.4 | 0.2 | 0.1 | 0.1 | 0.1 | | | 0 | 246 | 49 | | | | | | | | | | | 0.0 | | | 82 | | 0.7 | | | | 144 | | 400 | |
| 2181 | 1 ea | Strawberry, Weight Watchers | 111 | 180 | 62 | 7.0 | 28.0 | 2.0 | 9.0 | 17.0 | 5.0 | 2.0 | 1.0 | 2.0 | | | 15 | 200 | 40 | | | | 0.06 | 0.07 | 1.60 | | | | | 2.4 | | | 80 | | 0.4 | | | | 115 | | 230 | |
| 46234 | 1 pce | Triple Chocolate, Weight Watchers | 89 | 199 | 52 | 7.0 | 31.9 | 1.0 | 19.9 | 11.0 | 5.0 | 2.5 | | | | | 10 | 0 | 0 | 0 | 0 | 0 | | | | | | | | 0.0 | | | 80 | | 1.1 | | | | 169 | | 199 | |
| 46183 | 1 oz | Cherry cake, dry mix, Gold Medal | 28 | 119 | 7 | 1.7 | 20.7 | 0.2 | 12.0 | 8.5 | 3.4 | 1.2 | 1.1 | 1.2 | | | 7 | | | | | | 0.09 | 0.06 | 0.52 | | | | | | | | 6 | | 0.5 | | | | 24 | | 219 | |
| 46404 | 1 pce | Cherry cake, prep f/mix, Gold Medal | 44 | 198 | 14 | 2.0 | 25.7 | 0.0 | 14.8 | 10.9 | 9.9 | 2.5 | 3.0 | 3.0 | | | 25 | 0 | 0 | 0 | 0 | 0 | 0.09 | 0.07 | 0.40 | | | | | 0.0 | | | 0 | | 0.4 | | | | 35 | | 277 | |
| | | Chocolate cake | | | | | | | | | | | | | | | | | | | | | | | | | | | | | | | | | | | | | | | | |
| 46252 | 1 pce | Chip, fat free, Entenmann's | 53 | 130 | | 3.0 | 31.0 | 1.0 | 19.0 | 11.0 | 0.0 | 0.0 | 0.0 | 0.0 | 0.00 | 0.00 | 0 | 100 | 20 | | | | | | | | | | | 0.0 | | | 0 | | 0.7 | | | | 100 | | 220 | |
| 46013 | 1 pce | Commercial, w/frosting, avg | 64 | 235 | 23 | 2.6 | 34.9 | 1.8 | 31.2 | 1.9 | 10.5 | 3.1 | 5.6 | 1.2 | 0.06 | 1.12 | 27 | 54 | 16 | | | | 0.02 | 0.09 | 0.37 | 0.03 | 0.09 | 10.9 | 0.13 | 0.1 | 0.2 | 0.0 | 28 | 0.2 | 1.4 | 22 | 0.2 | 78 | 128 | 2.1 | 214 | 0.44 |
| 46247 | 1 pce | Crunch, fat free, Entenmann's | 50 | 130 | | 2.0 | 32.0 | 2.0 | 20.0 | 10.0 | 0.0 | 0.0 | 0.0 | 0.0 | 0.00 | 0.00 | 0 | 0 | 0 | 0 | 0 | 0 | | | | | | | | 0.0 | | | 0 | | 1.1 | | | | 200 | | 170 | |

| Code | Amount | Description | Weight (g) | Calories | % Water | Protein (g) | Carbs (g) | Fiber (g) | Sugar (g) | Other Carbs (g) | Fat (g) | Sat Fat (g) | Mono Fat (g) | Poly Fat (g) | Omega 3 (g) | Omega 6 (g) | Choles (mg) | Vit A (IU) | Vit A (RE) | Retinol (RE) | Carotenoids (RE) | Beta Carotene (mcg) |
|---|---|---|---|---|---|---|---|---|---|---|---|---|---|---|---|---|---|---|---|---|---|---|
| | | **Basic Components** | | | | | | | | | | **Additional Fats** | | | | | | **Vit A & Components** | | | | |
| 46387 | 1 pce | Devil's Food, Gold Medal | 44 | 208 | 14 | 3.0 | 24.7 | 0.0 | 15.8 | 8.9 | 9.9 | 3.0 | 3.0 | 3.5 | | | 25 | 0 | 0 | 0 | 0 | 0 |
| 46058 | 1 oz | Dry Mix, avg | 28 | 120 | 3 | 1.7 | 20.4 | 0.7 | 14.1 | 5.6 | 4.4 | 0.9 | 1.8 | 1.4 | 0.10 | 1.31 | 0 | 1 | 0.1 | 0 | 0.1 | |
| 46232 | 1 pce | Double Fudge, Weight Watchers | 78 | 190 | 42 | 4.0 | 36.0 | 2.0 | 22.0 | 12.0 | 4.5 | 1.0 | | | | | 0 | 0 | 0 | 0 | 0 | 0 |
| 46265 | 1 pce | Fudge, Entenmann's | 85 | 310 | 23 | 3.0 | 47.0 | 2.0 | 35.0 | 10.0 | 14.0 | 5.0 | | | | | 45 | 0 | 0 | 0 | 0 | 0 |
| 46250 | 1 pce | Fudge Iced, fat free, Entenmann's | 85 | 210 | | 3.0 | 51.0 | 2.0 | 38.0 | 11.0 | 0.0 | 0.0 | 0.0 | 0.0 | 0.00 | 0.00 | 0 | 0 | 0 | 0 | 0 | 0 |
| 46066 | 1 pce | German, w/icing, avg | 11 | 40 | 27 | 0.4 | 5.5 | 0.2 | 4.1 | 1.2 | 2.0 | 0.5 | 0.9 | 0.5 | 0.05 | 0.49 | 5 | 8 | 2 | 2 | 0.1 | |
| 46368 | 1 pce | Juniors, Tastykake | 94 | 360 | | 4.0 | 57.0 | 2.0 | 35.0 | 20.0 | 13.0 | 2.5 | | | | | 70 | 100 | 20 | | | |
| 46248 | 1 pce | Loaf, fat free, Entenmann's | 53 | 130 | | 3.0 | 30.0 | 1.0 | 18.0 | 11.0 | 0.0 | 0.0 | 0.0 | 0.0 | 0.00 | 0.00 | 0 | 0 | 0 | 0 | 0 | 0 |
| 46061 | 1 pce | Low sod, w/fructose, avg | 38 | 116 | 24 | 1.4 | 23.0 | 0.6 | | | 2.9 | 1.4 | 1.2 | 0.2 | 0.01 | 0.20 | 0 | 0.4 | 0 | | | |
| 46407 | 1 pce | Milk, Gold Medal | 44 | 198 | 11 | 3.0 | 25.7 | 0.0 | 14.8 | 10.9 | 9.9 | 2.5 | 3.0 | 3.0 | | | 25 | 0 | 0 | 0 | 0 | 0 |
| 46257 | 1 pce | Mocha Iced, Entenmann's | 85 | 200 | | 3.0 | 46.0 | 1.0 | 32.0 | 13.0 | 0.0 | 0.0 | 0.0 | 0.0 | 0.00 | 0.00 | 0 | 0 | 0 | 0 | 0 | 0 |
| 46059 | 1 pce | Prep f/mix, avg | 65 | 198 | 32 | 3.6 | 31.8 | 1.4 | 22.1 | 8.3 | 7,6 | 1.8 | 3.1 | 2.3 | 0.16 | 2.14 | 35 | 54 | 16 | 15 | 1 | |
| 46117 | 1 pce | With Cream Cheese Icing, avg | 103 | 355 | 26 | 3.7 | 57.2 | 1.0 | 44.5 | 11.7 | 14.2 | 3.7 | 6.5 | 3.2 | 0.19 | 2.99 | 35 | 200 | 60 | | | |
| 46120 | 1 pce | With Fluffy White Icing, avg | 91 | 262 | 33 | 4.0 | 48.1 | 1.0 | 38.3 | 8.9 | 7.6 | 1.7 | 3.1 | 2.3 | 0.16 | 2.14 | 35 | 54 | 16 | | | |
| 46118 | 1 pce | With Vanilla Icing, avg | 103 | 358 | 25 | 3.7 | 58.2 | 1.0 | 47.7 | 9.6 | 14.0 | 3.6 | 6.4 | 3.2 | 0.19 | 2.97 | 35 | 337 | 102 | | | |
| | | Coffee cake | | | | | | | | | | | | | | | | | | | | |
| 46261 | 1 pce | Banana Crunch, Entenmann's | 57 | 220 | 23 | 2.0 | 32.0 | 0.5 | 18.0 | 13.5 | 9.0 | 2.0 | | | | | 40 | 100 | 20 | | | |
| 46092 | 1 pce | Cheese, avg | 76 | 258 | 32 | 5.3 | 33.7 | 0.8 | | | 11.6 | 4.1 | 5.4 | 1.3 | 0.10 | 1.15 | 65 | 218 | 66 | 66 | 0 | |
| 46492 | 1 oz | Cinnamon, w/crumb top, dry mix, avg | 28 | 122 | 3 | 1.3 | 21.8 | 0.5 | 13.6 | 7.6 | 3.4 | 0.8 | 1.3 | 1.2 | 0.05 | 0.81 | 0 | 6 | 0.6 | 0.5 | 0.04 | |
| 46093 | 1 pce | Cinnamon, w/crumb top, prep f/mix, avg | 63 | 263 | 22 | 4.3 | 29.4 | 1.3 | 18.5 | 9.7 | 14.7 | 3.7 | 8.2 | 2.0 | 0.10 | 1.86 | 20 | 70 | 21 | 21 | 0 | 0 |
| 46249 | 1 pce | Cinnamon Apple, fat free, Entenmann's | 54 | 130 | | 2.0 | 29.0 | 2.0 | 16.0 | 11.0 | 0.0 | 0.0 | 0.0 | 0.0 | 0.00 | 0.00 | 0 | 0 | 0 | 0 | 0 | 0 |
| 46096 | 1 pce | Crème Filled, w/chocolate frosting, avg | 90 | 298 | 29 | 4.5 | 48.4 | 1.8 | | | 9.7 | 2.5 | 5.1 | 1.3 | 0.07 | 1.25 | 62 | 111 | 33 | 33 | 0 | 0 |
| 46259 | 1 pce | French Crumb, Entenmann's | 50 | 210 | | 3.0 | 29.0 | 0.0 | 15.0 | 14.0 | 10.0 | 6.0 | | | | | 60 | 300 | 60 | | | |
| 46097 | 1 pce | Fruit, avg | 50 | 156 | 32 | 2.6 | 25.8 | 1.3 | 20.5 | 4.0 | 5.1 | 1.3 | 2.8 | 0.7 | 0.04 | 0.69 | 4 | 70 | 10 | 9 | 0.7 | |
| 46360 | 1 pce | Koffee Kake Cup Cake, Tastykake | 28 | 118 | | 1.5 | 17.2 | 0.0 | 9.8 | 7.4 | 4.4 | 1.0 | | | | | 17 | 0 | 0 | 0 | 0 | 0 |
| 46206 | 1 pce | Plain, avg | 63 | 263 | 22 | 4.3 | 29.4 | 1.3 | 18.5 | 9.7 | 14.7 | 3.7 | 8.2 | 2.0 | 0.10 | 1.86 | 20 | 70 | 21 | 19 | 2 | |
| 46005 | 1 pce | Plain, prep f/mix, avg | 56 | 178 | 30 | 3.1 | 29.6 | 0.7 | 18.5 | 10.3 | 5.4 | 1.0 | 2.2 | 1.8 | 0.12 | 1.65 | 27 | 78 | 22 | 21 | 2 | |
| 46095 | 1 pce | Plain, prep f/rec, avg | 60 | 240 | 21 | 3.9 | 30.2 | 0.9 | 18.9 | 10.4 | 12.1 | 2.2 | 4.6 | 4.7 | 0.47 | 4.18 | 36 | 383 | 99 | 92 | 7 | |
| 46277 | 1 pce | Coconut Layer, Pepperidge Farm | 80 | 300 | 27 | 2.0 | 41.0 | 1.0 | 22.0 | 18.0 | 14.0 | 4.0 | | | | | 40 | 0 | 0 | 0 | 0 | 0 |
| 46369 | 1 pce | Coconut, Juniors, Tastykake | 94 | 320 | | 4.0 | 59.0 | 1.0 | 36.0 | 22.0 | 8.0 | 4.0 | | | | | 65 | 100 | 20 | | | |
| 46205 | 1 pce | Fruit cake, avg | 43 | 139 | 25 | 1.2 | 26.5 | 1.6 | | | 3.9 | 0.5 | 1.8 | 1.4 | 0.14 | 1.27 | 2 | 9 | 2 | | | |
| 46063 | 1 pce | Fruit cake, prep f/rec, avg | 84 | 302 | 19 | 3.0 | 54.4 | 3.1 | 38.1 | 13.3 | 9.7 | 1.2 | 4.0 | 3.8 | 0.36 | 3.48 | 24 | 60 | 13 | 12 | 1 | |
| 45562 | 1 pce | Funnel cake, avg | 90 | 284 | 41 | 7.3 | 29.1 | 0.9 | | | 15.3 | 3.9 | 4.5 | 5.9 | | | 67 | 169 | 46 | 44 | 2 | |
| | | Gingerbread cake | | | | | | | | | | | | | | | | | | | | |
| 46067 | 1 oz | Dry Mix, avg | 28 | 122 | 4 | 1.2 | 20.9 | 0.5 | 10.5 | 9.9 | 3.9 | 1.0 | 2.2 | 0.5 | 0.03 | 0.47 | 0 | 1 | 0.1 | 0 | 0.1 | |
| 46006 | 1 pce | Prep f/Mix, avg | 67 | 207 | 33 | 2.7 | 34.0 | 0.8 | 16.1 | 17.1 | 6.8 | 1.8 | 3.8 | 0.9 | 0.04 | 0.85 | 23 | 37 | 11 | 11 | 0.07 | |
| 46000 | 1 pce | Prep f/Recipe, avg | 74 | 263 | 28 | 2.9 | 36.4 | 0.6 | 18.2 | 17.6 | 12.1 | 3.0 | 5.3 | 3.1 | 0.19 | 2.93 | 24 | 36 | 10 | 10 | 0.07 | |
| 46108 | 1 pce | Graham Cracker cake, avg | 45 | 156 | 28 | 2.7 | 21.9 | 0.4 | 15.9 | 5.6 | 6.9 | 1.7 | 3.0 | 1.8 | | | 34 | 304 | 80 | 75 | 5 | |
| 46109 | 1 pce | Ice Cream cake, chocolate, avg | 34 | 102 | 39 | 1.4 | 13.6 | 0.3 | 9.2 | 4.1 | 5.0 | 2.2 | 1.8 | 0.7 | | | 16 | 76 | 21 | 20 | 2 | |
| | | Lemon cake | | | | | | | | | | | | | | | | | | | | |
| 46187 | 1 oz | Dry Mix, Gold Medal | 28 | 119 | 7 | 1.7 | 20.7 | 0.2 | 12.3 | 8.2 | 3.4 | 1.2 | 1.1 | 0.2 | | | 7 | | | | | |
| 46281 | 1 pce | Mousse, Pepperidge Farm | 69 | 250 | 30 | 2.0 | 34.0 | 1.0 | 21.0 | 12.0 | 12.0 | 4.0 | | | | | 40 | 0 | 0 | 0 | 0 | 0 |
| 46406 | 1 pce | Prep f/Mix, Gold Medal | 44 | 198 | 14 | 2.0 | 25.7 | 0.0 | 15.8 | 9.9 | 9.9 | 2.5 | 3.0 | 3.0 | | | 25 | 0 | 0 | 0 | 0 | 0 |
| 46111 | 1 pce | With Icing, avg | 109 | 388 | 21 | 2.8 | 70.3 | 0.5 | 67.1 | 2.6 | 11.3 | 2.6 | 5.2 | 2.7 | | | 34 | 298 | 79 | 74 | 5 | |
| | | Marble cake | | | | | | | | | | | | | | | | | | | | |
| 46256 | 1 pce | Fat Free, Entenmann's | 50 | 130 | | 2.0 | 29.0 | 1.0 | 18.0 | 10.0 | 0.0 | 0.0 | 0.0 | 0.0 | 0.00 | 0.00 | 0 | 0 | 0 | 0 | 0 | 0 |
| 46119 | 1 pce | Prep w/Chocolate Icing, avg | 111 | 404 | 25 | 3.5 | 58.5 | 0.9 | 52.3 | 5.3 | 19.1 | 4.4 | 7.4 | 6.2 | 0.54 | 5.68 | 53 | 329 | 99 | | | |
| 46068 | 1 oz | Pudding Type, dry mix, avg | 28 | 116 | 3 | 1.0 | 22.2 | 0.8 | 19.3 | 2.1 | 3.3 | 0.7 | 1.3 | 1.1 | 0.07 | 0.98 | 0 | 0.6 | 0.06 | 0 | 0.06 | |
| 46069 | 1 pce | Pudding Type, prep f/mix, avg | 73 | 253 | 30 | 3.1 | 34.5 | 1.3 | 29.9 | 3.3 | 12.4 | 2.3 | 4.0 | 5.4 | 0.54 | 4.87 | 53 | 80 | 24 | 22.6 | 1.5 | |
| 46112 | 1 pce | Oatmeal cake, w/icing, avg | 110 | 410 | 19 | 3.0 | 70.5 | 1.5 | 66.4 | 2.5 | 14.0 | 3.4 | 6.1 | 3.8 | | | 20 | 219 | 57 | 53 | 4 | |
| 46113 | 1 pce | Peanut Butter cake, w/icing, avg | 109 | 409 | 20 | 6.1 | 61.9 | 1.3 | 44.7 | 15.9 | 16.3 | 5.8 | 6.3 | 3.2 | | | 56 | 479 | 124 | 114 | 10 | |
| 46070 | 1 pce | Pineapple cake, upside down, prep f/rec, avg | 115 | 367 | 32 | 4.0 | 58.1 | 0.9 | 39.3 | 17.8 | 13.9 | 3.4 | 6.0 | 3.8 | 0.21 | 3.56 | 25 | 291 | 75 | 70 | 5 | |
| 46282 | 1 pce | Pineapple cake, Cream, w/coconut, Pepp Farm | 76 | 240 | 33 | 2.0 | 38.0 | 1.0 | 24.0 | 13.0 | 10.0 | 3.0 | | | | | 30 | 0 | 0 | 0 | 0 | 0 |
| 46106 | 1 pce | Plum Pudding cake, avg | 42 | 131 | 35 | 1.7 | 19.2 | 0.9 | 13.4 | 4.9 | 5.7 | 3.0 | 1.9 | 0.3 | | | 16 | 30 | 8 | 7.6 | 0.4 | |
| 46114 | 1 pce | Poppy Seed cake, w/icing, avg | 90 | 354 | 24 | 6.5 | 43.2 | 1.1 | 22.7 | 19.4 | 17.5 | 6.5 | 4.6 | 5.3 | | | 79 | 371 | 94 | 87 | 7 | |
| | | Pound cake | | | | | | | | | | | | | | | | | | | | |
| 46493 | 1 oz | Dry Mix, Gold Medal | 28 | 138 | | 1.7 | 18.8 | 0.0 | 12.6 | 6.2 | 6.4 | 1.8 | 3.1 | 0.4 | | | 16 | | | | | |
| 46495 | 1 pce | Fat Free, avg | 80 | 226 | 31 | 4.3 | 48.8 | 0.9 | 28.3 | 19.6 | 1.0 | 0.2 | 0.1 | 0.3 | 0.02 | 0.32 | 0 | 77 | 23 | | | |
| 46073 | 1 pce | Prep w/Butter, avg | 54 | 206 | 23 | 3.2 | 28.4 | 0.4 | 16.6 | 11.4 | 9.0 | 5.2 | 2.7 | 0.5 | 0.13 | 0.36 | 62 | 372 | 96 | 87 | 9 | |
| 46074 | 1 pce | Prep wMmarg, avg | 54 | 206 | 23 | 3.2 | 28.5 | 0.4 | 16.7 | 11.4 | 9.0 | 2.0 | 3.8 | 2.6 | 0.12 | 2.50 | 41 | 396 | 104 | 95 | 9 | |
| 46395 | 1 pce | Prep f/Mix, Gold Medal | 22 | 112 | | 1.0 | 14.3 | 0.0 | 10.2 | 4.1 | 5.1 | 1.5 | 2.5 | 0.0 | 0.00 | 0.00 | 15 | 0 | 0 | 0 | 0 | 0 |
| 46270 | 1 pce | Raisin cake, Entenmann's | 57 | 220 | | 3.0 | 32.0 | 0.5 | 21.0 | 10.5 | 9.0 | 2.0 | | | | | 50 | 0 | 0 | 0 | 0 | 0 |
| 46258 | 1 pce | Raisin cake, fat free, Entenmann's | 53 | 140 | | 2.0 | 33.0 | 1.0 | 21.0 | 11.0 | 0.0 | 0.0 | 0.0 | 0.0 | 0.00 | 0.00 | 0 | 100 | 20 | | | |
| | | Snack cake | | | | | | | | | | | | | | | | | | | | |
| 46365 | 1 ea | Butter Cream, mini, Tastykake | 14 | 55 | | 0.5 | 9.0 | 0.5 | 6.0 | 2.5 | 2.0 | 0.5 | | | | | 2 | 0 | 0 | 0 | 0 | 0 |
| 46372 | 1 ea | Butterscotch Iced, Tastykake | 28 | 103 | | 1.0 | 19.6 | 0.5 | 12.3 | 6.9 | 2.5 | 0.7 | | | | | 25 | 49 | 10 | | | |
| 46357 | 1 ea | Chocolate, cup cake, Tastykake | 30 | 110 | | 1.5 | 19.5 | 1.0 | 12.0 | 6.5 | 3.0 | 0.8 | | | | | 5 | 0 | 0 | 0 | 0 | 0 |
| 46364 | 1 ea | Chocolate, mini, Tastykake | 14 | 55 | | 0.5 | 9.0 | 0.5 | 6.0 | 2.5 | 2.0 | 0.5 | | | | | 2 | 0 | 0 | 0 | 0 | 0 |
| 46383 | 1 ea | Chocolate, Tastykake | 19 | 90 | | 1.0 | 11.7 | 0.7 | 7.3 | 3.7 | 4.3 | 2.7 | | | | | 2 | 0 | 0 | 0 | 0 | 0 |
| 46362 | 1 ea | Chocolate Cream filled, Tastykake | 32 | 100 | | 1.5 | 21.0 | 1.0 | 10.0 | 10.0 | 1.5 | 0.5 | | | | | 0 | 0 | 0 | 0 | 0 | 0 |

| Code | Thiamin (mg) | Riboflavin (mg) | Niacin (NE) | Vit B6 (mg) | Vit B12 (mcg) | Folate (mcg) | Panto (mg) | Vit C (mg) | Vit D (mg) | Vit E (α TE) | Calcium (mg) | Copper (mg) | Iron (mg) | Magnes (mg) | Mang (mg) | Phos (mg) | Potassium (mg) | Selenium (mcg) | Sodium (mg) | Zinc (mg) |
|---|---|---|---|---|---|---|---|---|---|---|---|---|---|---|---|---|---|---|---|---|
| | **Vitamins** | | | | | | | | | | **Minerals** | | | | | | | | | |
| 46387 | 0.09 | 0.10 | 0.40 | | | | | 0.0 | | | 20 | | 1.1 | | | | 168 | | 267 | |
| 46058 | 0.05 | 0.04 | 0.45 | 0.01 | 0.00 | 15.1 | 0.04 | 0.0 | 0.0 | | 42 | 0.1 | 1.3 | 13 | 0.1 | 76 | 92 | 3.5 | 231 | 0.22 |
| 46232 | | | | | | | | 0.0 | | | 80 | | 1.4 | | | | 200 | | 200 | |
| 46265 | | | | | | | | 0.0 | | | 40 | | 2.7 | | | | 350 | | 260 | |
| 46250 | | | | | | | | 0.0 | | | 20 | | 1.4 | | | | 210 | | 270 | |
| 46066 | 0.01 | 0.01 | 0.11 | 0.00 | 0.01 | 0.4 | 0.01 | 0.0 | 0.1 | | 5 | 0.0 | 0.1 | 2 | 0.0 | 17 | 15 | | 37 | 0.05 |
| 46368 | | | | | | | | 0.0 | | | 40 | | 1.8 | | | | | | 270 | |
| 46248 | | | | | | | | 0.0 | | | 0 | | | | | | 210 | | 250 | |
| 46061 | 0.05 | 0.07 | 0.52 | 0.01 | 0.01 | 2.3 | 0.04 | 0.0 | 0.1 | | 11 | 0.3 | 0.8 | 14 | 0.2 | 102 | 82 | | 130 | 0.25 |
| 46407 | 0.09 | 0.07 | 0.40 | | | | | 0.0 | | | 20 | | 1.1 | | | | 104 | | 257 | |
| 46257 | | | | | | | | 0.0 | | | 20 | | 0.7 | | | | 46 | | 270 | |
| 46059 | 0.06 | 0.10 | 0.63 | 0.02 | 0.06 | 7.1 | 0.14 | 0.0 | 0.2 | | 70 | 0.2 | 2.1 | 21 | 0.3 | 132 | 153 | | 370 | 0.45 |
| 46117 | 0.06 | 0.10 | 0.64 | 0.02 | 0.06 | 7.2 | 0.14 | 0.0 | | | 71 | 0.2 | 2.1 | 22 | 0.0 | 133 | 167 | | 460 | 0.45 |
| 46120 | 0.06 | 0.11 | 0.80 | 0.02 | 0.07 | 7.7 | 0.15 | 0.0 | | | 71 | 0.2 | 2.1 | 22 | 0.0 | 133 | 173 | | 410 | 0.45 |
| 46118 | 0.06 | 0.10 | 0.64 | 0.02 | 0.06 | 7.2 | 0.14 | 0.0 | 0.0 | | 71 | 0.2 | 2.1 | 22 | 0.0 | 147 | 168 | | 404 | 0.45 |
| 46261 | | | | | | | | 0.0 | | | 0 | | 0.0 | | | | 70 | | 280 | |
| 46092 | 0.08 | 0.09 | 0.52 | 0.04 | 0.26 | 29.6 | 0.30 | 0.1 | | | 45 | 0.0 | 0.5 | 11 | 0.1 | 77 | 220 | 10.1 | 258 | 0.45 |
| 46492 | 0.08 | 0.04 | 0.70 | 0.01 | 0.00 | 20.2 | 0.04 | 0.1 | 0.3 | | 41 | 0.1 | 0.5 | 5 | 0.1 | 72 | 24 | 4.5 | 167 | 0.10 |
| 46093 | 0.13 | 0.14 | 1.06 | 0.02 | 0.11 | 38.4 | 0.41 | 0.2 | 0.1 | | 34 | 0.1 | 1.2 | 14 | 0.3 | 68 | 77 | 10.8 | 221 | 0.51 |
| 46249 | | | | | | | | 0.0 | | | 20 | | 0.4 | | | | 75 | | 110 | |
| 46096 | 0.07 | 0.07 | 0.76 | 0.04 | 0.18 | 36.9 | 0.35 | 0.1 | | | 34 | 0.1 | 0.5 | 13 | 0.2 | 67 | 70 | 13.0 | 291 | 0.40 |
| 46259 | | | | | | | | 0.0 | | | 20 | | 0.0 | | | | 50 | | 240 | |
| 46097 | 0.02 | 0.09 | 1.28 | 0.02 | 0.01 | 23.5 | 0.33 | 0.4 | | | 22 | 0.0 | 1.2 | 8 | 0.1 | 59 | 45 | 8.3 | 192 | 0.32 |
| 46360 | | | | | | | | 0.0 | | | 10 | | 0.4 | | | | | | 74 | |
| 46206 | 0.09 | 0.06 | 0.55 | 0.02 | 0.11 | 20.2 | 0.41 | 0.2 | 0.1 | | 34 | 0.1 | 0.5 | 14 | 0.3 | 68 | 77 | 10.8 | 221 | 0.51 |
| 46005 | 0.09 | 0.10 | 0.85 | 0.03 | 0.08 | 38.1 | 0.15 | 0.1 | 0.4 | | 76 | 0.1 | 0.8 | 10 | 0.2 | 120 | 63 | 9.4 | 236 | 0.25 |
| 46095 | 0.11 | 0.12 | 0.67 | 0.05 | 0.09 | 9.0 | 0.24 | 0.2 | 0.1 | | 67 | 0.2 | 1.3 | 24 | 0.4 | 83 | 143 | 10.3 | 233 | 0.49 |
| 46277 | 0.03 | 0.07 | 0.00 | | | | | 0.0 | | | | | 0.7 | | | | | | 200 | |
| 46369 | | | | | | | | 0.0 | | | 40 | | 1.4 | | | | | | 260 | |
| 46205 | 0.02 | 0.04 | 0.34 | 0.02 | 0.00 | 8.2 | 0.10 | 0.2 | | | 14 | 0.0 | 0.9 | 7 | 0.1 | 22 | 66 | 0.9 | 116 | 0.12 |
| 46063 | 0.14 | 0.10 | 0.89 | 0.09 | 0.04 | 8.4 | 0.29 | 3.8 | 0.1 | | 55 | 0.2 | 1.6 | 29 | 0.5 | 66 | 260 | | 121 | 0.59 |
| 45562 | 0.24 | 0.32 | 1.86 | 0.05 | 0.24 | 13.5 | | 0.4 | | | 115 | 0.1 | 1.8 | 18 | | 128 | 153 | | 236 | 0.64 |
| 46067 | 0.10 | 0.07 | 0.71 | 0.01 | 0.00 | 17.1 | 0.07 | 0.1 | 0.0 | | 26 | 0.1 | 1.3 | 6 | 0.2 | 63 | 95 | | 184 | 0.10 |
| 46006 | 0.13 | 0.12 | 1.05 | 0.03 | 0.05 | 6.7 | 0.15 | 0.1 | 0.0 | | 46 | 0.1 | 2.2 | 11 | 0.2 | 113 | 161 | 3.1 | 307 | 0.27 |
| 46000 | 0.14 | 0.12 | 1.29 | 0.14 | 0.04 | 24.4 | 0.28 | 0.1 | 0.1 | | 53 | 0.1 | 2.1 | 52 | 0.5 | 40 | 325 | 12.1 | 242 | 0.29 |
| 46108 | 0.04 | 0.14 | 0.56 | 0.02 | 0.09 | 5.2 | 0.14 | 0.1 | 0.2 | | 44 | 0.0 | 0.7 | 8 | 0.1 | 52 | 78 | | 175 | 0.25 |
| 46109 | 0.04 | 0.07 | 0.30 | 0.01 | 0.08 | 2.3 | 0.10 | 0.1 | 0.1 | | 43 | 0.1 | 0.5 | 9 | 0.0 | 38 | 57 | | 69 | 0.24 |
| 46187 | 0.09 | 0.06 | 0.53 | | | | | | | | 13 | | 0.5 | | | | 24 | | 203 | |
| 46281 | 0.00 | 0.00 | 0.00 | | | | | 0.0 | | | 0 | | 0.0 | | | | | | 100 | |
| 46406 | 0.09 | 0.07 | 0.40 | | | | | 0.0 | | | 0 | | 0.4 | | | | 35 | | 257 | |
| 46111 | 0.09 | 0.12 | 0.81 | 0.02 | 0.07 | 6.0 | 0.22 | 1.4 | 0.1 | | 70 | 0.1 | 0.9 | 5 | 0.1 | 136 | 55 | | 249 | 0.22 |
| 46256 | | | | | | | | 0.0 | | | 0 | | 0.4 | | | | 120 | | 190 | |
| 46119 | 0.07 | 0.12 | 0.66 | 0.03 | 0.10 | 7.3 | 0.21 | 0.0 | | | 43 | 0.1 | 1.4 | 17 | 0.1 | 172 | 143 | | 311 | 0.41 |
| 46068 | 0.05 | 0.04 | 0.43 | 0.01 | 0.00 | 10.1 | 0.03 | 0.0 | 0.0 | | 21 | 0.0 | 0.5 | 5 | 0.0 | 77 | 34 | 0.7 | 145 | 0.10 |
| 46069 | 0.07 | 0.11 | 0.61 | 0.03 | 0.10 | 7.3 | 0.19 | 0.0 | 0.2 | | 40 | 0.1 | 0.9 | 9 | 0.2 | 142 | 69 | | 242 | 0.30 |
| 46112 | 0.15 | 0.11 | 1.10 | 0.05 | 0.05 | 5.0 | | 0.5 | | | 21 | 0.1 | 1.8 | 13 | | 56 | 134 | | 256 | 0.32 |
| 46113 | 0.12 | 0.16 | 2.34 | 0.08 | 0.13 | 13.3 | | 0.1 | | | 134 | 0.2 | 1.6 | 29 | | 111 | 216 | | 542 | 0.65 |
| 46070 | 0.18 | 0.18 | 1.37 | 0.04 | 0.09 | 29.9 | 0.23 | 1.4 | 0.2 | | 138 | 0.1 | 1.7 | 15 | 0.4 | 94 | 129 | 10.8 | 367 | 0.36 |
| 46282 | 0.00 | 0.03 | 0.00 | | | | | 0.0 | | | 0 | | 0.7 | | | | | | 120 | |
| 46106 | 0.04 | 0.06 | 0.40 | 0.08 | 0.05 | 3.4 | 0.13 | 0.4 | 0.1 | | 40 | 0.1 | 0.8 | 23 | 0.2 | 35 | 196 | | 56 | 0.16 |
| 46114 | 0.25 | 0.29 | 1.66 | 0.05 | 0.18 | 16.4 | 0.27 | 0.5 | 0.7 | | 107 | 0.1 | 1.7 | 20 | 0.3 | 122 | 138 | | 251 | 0.74 |
| 46493 | 0.06 | 0.09 | 0.57 | | | | | 0.0 | | | 13 | | 0.4 | | | | 23 | | 107 | |
| 46495 | 0.10 | 0.24 | 0.55 | 0.01 | 0.00 | 28.8 | 0.28 | 0.0 | 0.0 | | 34 | 0.0 | 1.6 | 8 | 0.1 | 117 | 88 | 4.2 | 273 | 0.25 |
| 46073 | 0.11 | 0.14 | 0.85 | 0.02 | 0.10 | 7.0 | 0.19 | 0.1 | 0.3 | | 39 | 0.0 | 0.9 | 6 | 0.1 | 52 | 47 | | 161 | 0.26 |
| 46074 | 0.11 | 0.14 | 0.85 | 0.02 | 0.10 | 6.5 | 0.19 | 0.1 | 0.2 | | 39 | 0.0 | 0.9 | 6 | 0.1 | 52 | 49 | | 172 | 0.26 |
| 46395 | 0.03 | 0.07 | 0.41 | | | | | 0.0 | | | 0 | | 0.0 | | | | 20 | | 87 | |
| 46270 | | | | | | | | 0.0 | | | 20 | | 0.4 | | | | 105 | | 200 | |
| 46258 | | | | | | | | 0.0 | | | 20 | | 0.0 | | | | 120 | | 150 | |
| 46365 | | | | | | | | 0.0 | | | 0 | | 0.4 | | | | | | 60 | |
| 46372 | | | | | | | | 0.0 | | | 10 | | 0.4 | | | | | | 84 | |
| 46357 | | | | | | | | 0.0 | | | 10 | | 0.9 | | | | | | 135 | |
| 46364 | | | | | | | | 0.0 | | | 0 | | 0.4 | | | | | | 58 | |
| 46383 | | | | | | | | 0.0 | | | 7 | | 0.4 | | | | | | 40 | |
| 46362 | | | | | | | | 0.0 | | | 10 | | 0.7 | | | | | | 115 | |

| Code | Amount | Description | Weight (g) | Calories | % Water | Protein (g) | Carbs (g) | Fiber (g) | Sugar (g) | Other Carbs (g) | Fat (g) | Sat Fat (g) | Mono Fat (g) | Poly Fat (g) | Omega 3 (g) | Omega 6 (g) | Choles (mg) | Vit A (IU) | Vit A (RE) | Retinol (RE) | Carotenoids (RE) | Beta Carotene (mcg) |
|---|---|---|---|---|---|---|---|---|---|---|---|---|---|---|---|---|---|---|---|---|---|---|
| | | **Basic Components** | | | | | | | | | **Additional Fats** | | | | | | | **Vit A & Components** | | | | |
| 46379 | 1 ea | Chocolate Creamies, Tastykake | 43 | 180 | | 2.0 | 26.0 | 0.0 | 17.0 | 9.0 | 7.0 | 2.0 | | | | | 15 | 0 | 0 | 0 | 0 | 0 |
| 46011 | 1 ea | Chocolate Creme Filled, w/icing, avg | 50 | 188 | 20 | 1.7 | 30.1 | 0.4 | 17.0 | 12.8 | 7.3 | 1.4 | 2.8 | 2.6 | 0.26 | 2.35 | [illegible] | 9 | 1.5 | 1.9 | 0.6 | |
| 46358 | 1 ea | Chocolate Crème, cup cake, Tastykake | 32 | 125 | | 1.5 | 20.5 | 1.0 | 13.0 | 6.5 | 4.0 | 1.0 | | | | | 5 | 0 | 0 | 0 | 0 | 0 |
| 46240 | 1 ea | Chocolate Finger, Pet Inc | 42 | 143 | | 2.0 | 23.2 | 1.0 | 14.3 | 7.9 | 4.9 | 2.0 | | | | | 10 | 0 | 0 | 0 | 0 | 0 |
| 46426 | 1 ea | Chocolate w/Frosting, low fat, avg | 43 | 131 | 23 | 1.8 | 28.9 | 1.8 | 14.6 | 12.4 | 1.6 | 0.5 | 0.8 | 0.2 | 0.01 | 0.20 | 0 | 0 | 0 | 0 | 0 | 0 |
| 46105 | 1 ea | Chocolate w/Fruit & Cream, avg | 43 | 146 | 27 | 1.9 | 24.1 | 0.4 | 22.5 | 1.2 | 4.8 | 1.4 | 2.2 | 0.8 | | | 23 | 46 | 11 | 10 | 1 | |
| 46385 | 1 ea | Coconut, Tastykake | 19 | 87 | | 1.0 | 11.3 | 0.7 | 7.7 | 3.0 | 4.3 | 3.3 | | | | | [illegible] | 33 | 7 | | | |
| 46366 | 1 ea | Crème Filled, Tastykake | 13 | 55 | | 0.5 | 8.0 | 0.0 | 4.5 | 3.5 | 2.0 | 0.5 | | | | | [illegible] | 0 | 0 | 0 | 0 | 0 |
| 46373 | 1 ea | Jelly Filled, Tastykake | 28 | 93 | | 1.0 | 18.7 | 0.5 | 11.3 | 6.9 | 1.5 | 0.2 | | | | | 22 | 49 | 10 | | | |
| 46361 | 1 ea | Kreme Kup, Tastykake | 25 | 95 | | 1.0 | 15.5 | 0.5 | 9.5 | 5.5 | 3.0 | 0.8 | | | | | 5 | 0 | 0 | 0 | 0 | 0 |
| 46384 | 1 ea | Peanut Butter, Tastykake | 19 | 90 | | 1.5 | 10.5 | 0.5 | 7.5 | 2.5 | 5.0 | 2.0 | | | | | [illegible] | 0 | 0 | 0 | 0 | 0 |
| 46239 | 1 ea | Raspberry Finger, Pet Inc | 42 | 138 | | 2.0 | 24.2 | 1.0 | 14.3 | 8.9 | 4.0 | 2.0 | | | | | [illegible] | 0 | 0 | 0 | 0 | 0 |
| 46008 | 1 ea | Sponge, avg | 42 | 153 | 20 | 1.3 | 26.8 | 0.2 | 25.2 | 1.5 | 4.8 | 1.1 | 1.7 | 1.4 | 0.16 | 1.22 | [illegible] | 7 | 2 | 2 | 0.2 | |
| 46381 | 1 ea | Sprinkled Creamies, Tastykake | 38 | 150 | | 1.0 | 25.0 | 0.0 | 14.0 | 11.0 | 6.0 | 0.5 | | | | | 25 | 0 | 0 | 0 | 0 | 0 |
| 46363 | 1 ea | Vanilla Cream filled, Tastykake | 32 | 105 | | 1.5 | 20.5 | 0.5 | 10.0 | 10.0 | 2.0 | 0.8 | | | | | 0 | 0 | 0 | 0 | 0 | 0 |
| 46380 | 1 ea | Vanilla Creamies, Tastykake | 43 | 190 | | 1.0 | 26.0 | 0.0 | 18.0 | 8.0 | 8.0 | 1.5 | | | | | 30 | 0 | 0 | 0 | 0 | 0 |
| 46238 | 1 ea | Vanilla Finger, Pet Inc | 42 | 143 | | 2.0 | 23.2 | 1.0 | 14.3 | 7.9 | 4.9 | 2.0 | | | | | 5 | 0 | 0 | 0 | 0 | 0 |
| 46382 | 1 ea | Witchy Good Treat, Tastykake | 38 | 150 | | 2.0 | 24.0 | 1.0 | 14.0 | 9.0 | 6.0 | 1.0 | | | | | 30 | 0 | 0 | 0 | 0 | 0 |
| | | Spice cake | | | | | | | | | | | | | | | | | | | | |
| 46242 | 1 pce | Apple, fat free, Entenmann's | 50 | 130 | | 2.0 | 30.0 | 2.0 | 19.0 | 9.0 | 0.0 | 0.0 | 0.0 | 0.0 | 0.00 | 0.00 | 0 | 100 | 20 | | | |
| 46185 | 1 oz | Dry Mix, Gold Medal | 28 | 119 | | 1.7 | 20.7 | 0.2 | 12.3 | 8.2 | 3.4 | 1.2 | 1.1 | 0.2 | | | [illegible] | | | | | |
| 46396 | 1 pce | Prep f/Mix, Gold Medal | 44 | 198 | | 2.0 | 25.7 | 0.0 | 15.8 | 9.9 | 9.9 | 4.2 | 4.1 | 0.6 | | | 25 | 0 | 0 | 0 | 0 | 0 |
| 46116 | 1 pce | Prep w/Icing, avg | 109 | 374 | 24 | 4.3 | 65.2 | 1.0 | 62.1 | 2.1 | 11.3 | 3.8 | 5.1 | 1.4 | | | 4[illegible] | 144 | 40 | 38 | 2 | |
| | | Sponge cake | | | | | | | | | | | | | | | | | | | | |
| 46115 | 1 pce | Chocolate, w/o icing, avg | 66 | 195 | 30 | 5.4 | 35.8 | 1.0 | 27.0 | 7.8 | 4.1 | 1.4 | 1.5 | 0.5 | | | [illegible] | 211 | 63 | 63 | 0.1 | |
| 46001 | 1 pce | Coml Prep, avg | 38 | 110 | 30 | 2.1 | 23.2 | 0.2 | 16.5 | 6.5 | 1.0 | 0.3 | 0.4 | 0.2 | 0.01 | 0.15 | 39 | 59 | 17 | 16 | 2 | |
| 46078 | 1 pce | Prep f/Recipe, avg | 63 | 187 | 29 | 4.6 | 36.4 | 0.4 | 25.8 | 10.1 | 2.7 | 0.8 | 1.0 | 0.4 | 0.02 | 0.39 | 107 | 163 | 49 | 44 | 5 | |
| | | Strawberry cake | | | | | | | | | | | | | | | | | | | | |
| 46283 | 1 pce | Cream, w/coconut, Pepperidge Farm | 76 | 230 | 34 | 2.0 | 38.0 | 1.0 | 23.0 | 14.0 | 9.0 | 3.0 | | | | | 30 | 0 | 0 | 0 | 0 | 0 |
| 46280 | 1 pce | Layer | 90 | 310 | 26 | 2.0 | 47.0 | 1.0 | 22.0 | 24.0 | 13.0 | 4.0 | | | | | 65 | 0 | 0 | 0 | 0 | 0 |
| 46496 | 1 pce | Shortcake, Ala Mode, Weight Watchers | 92 | 90 | | 2.0 | 19.5 | 0.5 | 5.5 | 13.5 | 0.8 | 0.3 | | | | | [illegible] | 100 | 20 | | | |
| | | White cake | | | | | | | | | | | | | | | | | | | | |
| 46082 | 1 pce | Avg | 62 | 190 | 31 | 2.5 | 34.3 | 0.4 | 32.3 | 1.6 | 4.8 | 0.7 | 2.0 | 1.8 | 0.12 | 1.67 | 0 | 0.6 | 0.06 | | | |
| 46184 | 1 oz | Dry Mix, Gold Medal | 28 | 120 | | 1.7 | 20.7 | 0.3 | 12.3 | 8.1 | 3.4 | 1.2 | 1.2 | 0.2 | | | 0 | | | | | |
| 46084 | 1 pce | Low Sod, avg | 38 | 118 | 26 | 1.3 | 23.3 | 0.2 | 19.8 | 3.3 | 2.5 | 0.4 | 1.0 | 0.9 | 0.06 | 0.87 | 0 | 0 | 0 | 0 | 0 | 0 |
| 46400 | 1 pce | Prep f/Mix, Gold Medal | 44 | 198 | | 2.0 | 25.7 | 0.0 | 15.8 | 9.9 | 9.9 | 2.5 | 3.0 | 3.0 | | | 15 | 0 | 0 | 0 | 0 | 0 |
| 46007 | 1 pce | With Choc Icing, prep f/rec, avg | 100 | 364 | 20 | 2.5 | 64.1 | 1.1 | 60.9 | 2.1 | 11.5 | 5.2 | 3.6 | 1.8 | 0.19 | 1.55 | 1[illegible] | 234 | 58 | 52 | 6 | |
| 46003 | 1 pce | With Coconut Icing, prep f/rec, avg | 112 | 399 | 21 | 4.9 | 70.8 | 1.1 | 52.5 | 17.1 | 11.5 | 4.4 | 4.1 | 2.4 | 0.15 | 2.27 | [illegible] | 43 | 12 | 11 | 1 | |
| 46017 | 1 pce | With White Frosting, prep f/rec, avg | 71 | 266 | 20 | 2.3 | 44.7 | 0.7 | 33.9 | 10.2 | 9.6 | 4.3 | 3.8 | 1.0 | 0.09 | 0.84 | 6 | 78 | 23 | 21 | 2 | |
| 46085 | 1 pce | Without Frosting, prep f/rec, avg | 74 | 264 | 23 | 4.0 | 42.3 | 0.6 | 26.5 | 15.2 | 9.2 | 2.4 | 3.9 | 2.3 | 0.15 | 2.13 | [illegible] | 41 | 12 | 11 | 1 | |
| 46276 | 1 pce | Vanilla cake, Pepperidge Farm | 80 | 290 | 29 | 2.0 | 41.0 | 0.5 | 23.0 | 17.5 | 13.0 | 2.5 | | | | | 45 | 0 | 0 | 0 | 0 | 0 |
| | | Yellow cake | | | | | | | | | | | | | | | | | | | | |
| 46089 | 1 oz | Dry Mix, avg | 28 | 121 | 4 | 1.2 | 21.9 | 0.3 | 20.6 | 1.0 | 3.2 | 0.5 | 1.4 | 1.2 | 0.08 | 1.14 | [illegible] | 0.3 | 0.03 | 0 | 0.03 | |
| 46421 | 1 pce | Layer, Pepperidge Farm | 80 | 290 | | 3.0 | 40.0 | 23.0 | 36.0 | | 14.0 | 3.0 | | | | | 50 | 0 | 0 | 0 | 0 | 0 |
| 46429 | 1 pce | Light, avg | 69 | 181 | 37 | 3.0 | 36.8 | 0.6 | 21.7 | 14.6 | 2.4 | 1.1 | 0.9 | 0.2 | 0.00 | 0.15 | 0 | 5.5 | .4 | | | |
| 46090 | 1 pce | Prep f/Mix, avg | 63 | 202 | 30 | 3.0 | 34.3 | 0.5 | 21.1 | 12.7 | 5.9 | 1.0 | 2.5 | 2.0 | 0.14 | 1.83 | 3[illegible] | 54 | 16 | 16 | 0.1 | |
| 46088 | 1 pce | PuddingTtype, avg | 73 | 257 | 30 | 3.3 | 35.1 | 0.3 | 30.5 | 4.3 | 11.6 | 2.4 | 4.3 | 4.3 | 0.45 | 3.80 | 53 | 80 | 24 | 24 | 0.2 | |
| 46012 | 1 pce | With Chocolate Frosting, avg | 64 | 243 | 22 | 2.4 | 35.5 | 1.2 | 24.2 | 10.1 | 11.1 | 3.0 | 6.1 | 1.4 | 0.07 | 1.23 | 35 | 70 | 21 | 21 | 0 | |
| 46015 | 1 pce | With Vanilla Frosting, avg | 64 | 239 | 22 | 2.2 | 37.6 | 0.2 | 28.5 | 8.9 | 9.3 | 1.5 | 3.9 | 3.3 | 0.23 | 3.05 | 35 | 40 | 12 | 12 | 0.1 | |
| 46091 | 1 pce | Without Frosting, prep f/recipe, avg | 80 | 289 | 25 | 4.2 | 42.4 | 0.6 | 26.1 | 15.8 | 11.7 | 3.1 | 5.0 | 2.9 | 0.18 | 2.63 | 43 | 111 | 32 | 32 | 0.3 | |
| | | *COOKIES* | | | | | | | | | | | | | | | | | | | | |
| 47073 | 1 ea | Almond cookie, avg | 10 | 52 | 6 | 0.9 | 5.1 | 0.2 | 2.3 | 2.6 | 3.2 | 0.5 | 1.6 | 0.9 | | | 5 | 109 | 28 | 26 | 2 | |
| 47504 | 1 ea | Almond cookie, Crescent, Archway | 12 | 52 | | 0.5 | 8.9 | 0.3 | 3.1 | 5.5 | 1.8 | 0.3 | | | | | [illegible] | 0 | 0 | 0 | 0 | 0 |
| | | Animal cookie | | | | | | | | | | | | | | | | | | | | |
| 47026 | 1 ea | Avg | 1 | 4 | 4 | 0.1 | 0.7 | 0.0 | 0.4 | 0.3 | 0.1 | 0.0 | 0.1 | 0.0 | 0.00 | 0.02 | 0 | 0 | 0 | 0 | 0 | 0 |
| 47175 | 1 ea | Barnum's | 3 | 13 | | 0.2 | 2.3 | | | | 0.4 | 0.1 | | | | | | | | | | |
| 47176 | 1 ea | Bugs Bunny Graham Crackers | 3 | 13 | | 0.2 | 2.3 | | | | 0.4 | 0.1 | | | | | | | | | | |
| 47201 | 1 ea | Little Debbie's, 1.5 oz pkg | 43 | 182 | | 3.0 | 33.3 | | | | 6.1 | 3.0 | | | | | | | | | | |
| | | Apple cookies | | | | | | | | | | | | | | | | | | | | |
| 49089 | 1 ea | Bakes, fat free, Health Valley | 27 | 70 | 26 | 2.0 | 18.0 | 2.0 | 11.0 | 5.0 | 0.0 | 0.0 | 0.0 | 0.0 | 0.00 | 0.00 | 0 | 100 | 20 | | | |
| 47590 | 1 ea | Cinnamon Bar, Tastykake | 43 | 180 | 7 | 2.0 | 29.0 | 1.0 | 15.0 | 13.0 | 7.0 | 1.5 | | | | | 0 | 0 | 0 | 0 | 0 | 0 |
| 47318 | 1 ea | Filled, fat free, Health Valley | 33 | 70 | 38 | 2.0 | 18.0 | 2.0 | 9.0 | 7.0 | 0.0 | 0.0 | 0.0 | 0.0 | 0.00 | 0.00 | 0 | 500 | 100 | | | |
| 47514 | 1 ea | Filled Oatmeal, Archway | 28 | 111 | 15 | 1.3 | 18.4 | 0.6 | 8.9 | 8.8 | 3.6 | 0.8 | 1.4 | 0.3 | | | 3 | 4 | 0.8 | | | |
| 47287 | 1 ea | Fruit Bar, fat free, Health Valley | 42 | 140 | 8 | 3.0 | 35.0 | 3.0 | 13.0 | 19.0 | 0.0 | 0.0 | 0.0 | 0.0 | 0.00 | 0.00 | 0 | 500 | 100 | | | |
| 47302 | 1 ea | Fruit Filled Center, fat free, Health Valley | 33 | 70 | 38 | 2.0 | 18.0 | 2.0 | 9.0 | 7.0 | 0.0 | 0.0 | 0.0 | 0.0 | 0.00 | 0.00 | 0 | 500 | 100 | | | |
| 47515 | 1 ea | N' Raisin, Archway | 30 | 128 | 11 | 1.6 | 19.7 | 0.9 | 10.7 | 8.2 | 4.8 | 1.1 | 1.9 | 0.5 | | | 6 | 10 | 2 | | | |
| 47152 | 1 ea | Newtons, fat free, Nabisco | 23 | 73 | | 0.8 | 16.2 | | | | 0.0 | 0.0 | 0.0 | 0.0 | 0.00 | 0.00 | | | | | | |
| 47249 | 1 ea | Raisin Bar, Weight Watchers | 21 | 69 | | 1.0 | 13.8 | 2.0 | 4.0 | 7.9 | 2.0 | 0.5 | | | | | 0 | 0 | 0 | 0 | 0 | 0 |
| 47312 | 1 ea | Raisin, fat free, Health Valley | 25 | 80 | 14 | 2.0 | 19.0 | 3.0 | 9.0 | 7.0 | 0.0 | 0.0 | 0.0 | 0.0 | 0.00 | 0.00 | 0 | 100 | 20 | | | |
| 47307 | 1 ea | Spice, fat free, Health Valley | 11 | 33 | 16 | 0.7 | 8.0 | 1.0 | 3.7 | 3.3 | 0.0 | 0.0 | 0.0 | 0.0 | 0.00 | 0.00 | 0 | 167 | 33 | | | |

| Code | Thiamin (mg) | Riboflavin (mg) | Niacin (NE) | Vit B6 (mg) | Vit B12 (mcg) | Folate (mcg) | Panto (mg) | Vit C (mg) | Vit D (mg) | Vit E (α TE) | Calcium (mg) | Copper (mg) | Iron (mg) | Magnes (mg) | Mang (mg) | Phos (mg) | Potassium (mg) | Selenium (mcg) | Sodium (mg) | Zinc (mg) |
|---|---|---|---|---|---|---|---|---|---|---|---|---|---|---|---|---|---|---|---|---|
| | **Vitamins** | | | | | | | | | | **Minerals** | | | | | | | | | |
| 46379 | | | | | | | | 0.0 | | | 20 | | 0.7 | | | | | | 120 | |
| 46011 | 0.11 | 0.15 | 1.22 | 0.01 | 0.03 | 14.5 | 0.11 | 0.0 | 0.0 | | 36 | 0.1 | 1.7 | 20 | 0.2 | 46 | 61 | 1.4 | 212 | 0.25 |
| 46358 | | | | | | | | 0.0 | | | 10 | | 0.9 | | | | | | 135 | |
| 46240 | | | | | | | | 0.0 | | | 30 | | 0.7 | | | | | | 212 | |
| 46426 | 0.02 | 0.06 | 0.31 | 0.00 | 0.00 | 6.5 | 0.10 | 0.0 | 0.0 | | 15 | 0.1 | 0.7 | 11 | 0.1 | 79 | 96 | 2.4 | 178 | 0.24 |
| 46105 | 0.06 | 0.09 | 0.55 | 0.01 | 0.05 | 4.6 | 0.17 | 0.4 | 0.1 | | 46 | 0.0 | 0.6 | 4 | 0.1 | 92 | 34 | | 132 | 0.14 |
| 46385 | | | | | | | | 0.0 | | | 7 | | 0.6 | | | | | | 37 | |
| 46366 | | | | | | | | 0.0 | | | 0 | | 0.2 | | | | | | 32 | |
| 46373 | | | | | | | | 0.0 | | | 10 | | 0.4 | | | | | | 84 | |
| 46361 | | | | | | | | 0.0 | | | 10 | | 0.7 | | | | | | 125 | |
| 46384 | | | | | | | | 0.0 | | | 10 | | 0.4 | | | | | | 40 | |
| 46239 | | | | | | | | 0.0 | | | 30 | | 0.5 | | | | | | 178 | |
| 46008 | 0.06 | 0.06 | 0.51 | 0.01 | 0.05 | 12.2 | 0.12 | 0.0 | 0.0 | | 19 | 0.0 | 0.5 | 3 | 0.1 | 79 | 37 | 1.3 | 153 | 0.12 |
| 46381 | | | | | | | | 0.0 | | | 20 | | 0.7 | | | | | | 115 | |
| 46363 | | | | | | | | 0.0 | | | 10 | | 0.5 | | | | | | 115 | |
| 46380 | | | | | | | | 0.0 | | | 20 | | 0.7 | | | | | | 125 | |
| 46238 | | | | | | | | 0.0 | | | 30 | | 0.7 | | | | | | 212 | |
| 46382 | | | | | | | | 0.0 | | | 20 | | 0.7 | | | | | | 110 | |
| 46242 | | | | | | | | 0.0 | | | 0 | | 0.0 | | | | 65 | | 140 | |
| 46185 | 0.09 | 0.06 | 0.53 | | | | | | | | 16 | | 0.6 | | | | 25 | | 214 | |
| 46396 | 0.09 | 0.07 | 0.40 | | | | | 0.0 | | | 20 | | 0.7 | | | | 35 | | 277 | |
| 46116 | 0.13 | 0.19 | 1.09 | 0.04 | 0.11 | 8.7 | 0.17 | 0.1 | 0.2 | | 77 | 0.1 | 1.6 | 14 | 0.1 | 201 | 150 | | 270 | 0.37 |
| 46115 | 0.09 | 0.21 | 0.66 | 0.05 | 0.26 | 14.3 | 0.33 | 0.9 | 0.4 | | 22 | 0.1 | 1.6 | 20 | 0.2 | 89 | 98 | | 115 | 0.62 |
| 46001 | 0.09 | 0.10 | 0.73 | 0.02 | 0.09 | 14.8 | 0.18 | 0.0 | 0.2 | | 27 | 0.0 | 1.0 | 4 | 0.1 | 52 | 38 | 3.5 | 93 | 0.19 |
| 46078 | 0.10 | 0.19 | 0.76 | 0.04 | 0.23 | 24.6 | 0.34 | 0.0 | 0.3 | | 26 | 0.0 | 1.0 | 6 | 0.1 | 63 | 89 | 11.7 | 144 | 0.37 |
| 46283 | 0.00 | 0.03 | 0.00 | | | | | 0.0 | | | 0 | | 1.1 | | | | | | 115 | |
| 46280 | 0.00 | 0.07 | 0.00 | | | | | 0.0 | | | 0 | | 0.7 | | | | | | 150 | |
| 46496 | | | | | | | | 2.4 | | | 40 | | 0.0 | | | | 65 | | 80 | |
| 46082 | 0.08 | 0.10 | 0.43 | 0.01 | 0.06 | 3.1 | 0.08 | 0.1 | 0.2 | | 86 | 0.0 | 0.6 | 6 | 0.1 | 149 | 59 | | 301 | 0.21 |
| 46184 | 0.09 | 0.06 | 0.54 | | | | | | | | 14 | | 0.5 | | | | 26 | | 199 | |
| 46084 | 0.07 | 0.07 | 0.63 | 0.00 | 0.01 | 1.9 | 0.04 | 0.0 | 0.0 | | 8 | 0.0 | 0.6 | 3 | 0.1 | 87 | 50 | | 83 | 0.09 |
| 46400 | 0.09 | 0.07 | 0.40 | | | | | | | | 0 | | 0.4 | | | | 35 | | 257 | |
| 46007 | 0.07 | 0.09 | 0.40 | 0.01 | 0.06 | 3.0 | 0.08 | 0.1 | 0.1 | | 78 | 0.0 | 0.7 | 5 | 0.0 | 132 | 72 | 0.3 | 308 | 0.20 |
| 46003 | 0.14 | 0.21 | 1.19 | 0.03 | 0.07 | 24.6 | 0.19 | 0.1 | 0.0 | | 101 | 0.1 | 1.3 | 13 | 0.3 | 78 | 111 | 12.0 | 318 | 0.37 |
| 46017 | 0.07 | 0.09 | 0.64 | 0.01 | 0.04 | 4.0 | 0.21 | 0.1 | 0.1 | | 34 | 0.0 | 0.6 | 4 | 0.1 | 46 | 41 | 2.3 | 166 | 0.11 |
| 46085 | 0.14 | 0.18 | 1.13 | 0.02 | 0.06 | 23.7 | 0.14 | 0.1 | 0.2 | | 96 | 0.0 | 1.1 | 9 | 0.1 | 69 | 70 | 9.6 | 242 | 0.24 |
| 46276 | 0.00 | 0.07 | 0.00 | | | | | 0.0 | | | 20 | | 0.4 | | | | | | 190 | |
| 46089 | 0.05 | 0.06 | 0.50 | 0.02 | 0.03 | 18.5 | 0.10 | 0.1 | 0.0 | | 38 | 0.0 | 0.4 | 3 | 0.1 | 87 | 23 | 0.8 | 184 | 0.08 |
| 46421 | 0.00 | 0.07 | 0.40 | | | | | 0.0 | | | 40 | | 1.1 | | | | | | 230 | |
| 46429 | 0.06 | 0.12 | 0.62 | 0.01 | 0.06 | 2.1 | 0.10 | 0.0 | 0.1 | | 69 | 0.0 | 0.6 | 6 | 0.1 | 143 | 41 | | 279 | 0.15 |
| 46090 | 0.07 | 0.12 | 0.71 | 0.04 | 0.12 | 5.7 | 0.20 | 0.1 | 0.2 | | 64 | 0.0 | 0.8 | 6 | 0.1 | 151 | 46 | | 299 | 0.21 |
| 46088 | 0.11 | 0.13 | 1.03 | 0.02 | 0.12 | 7.3 | 0.14 | 0.0 | 0.2 | | 57 | 0.0 | 0.9 | 5 | 0.1 | 133 | 42 | | 317 | 0.26 |
| 46012 | 0.08 | 0.10 | 0.80 | 0.02 | 0.11 | 14.1 | 0.18 | 0.0 | 0.3 | | 24 | 0.1 | 1.3 | 19 | 0.2 | 103 | 114 | 2.2 | 216 | 0.40 |
| 46015 | 0.06 | 0.04 | 0.32 | 0.02 | 0.10 | 17.3 | 0.22 | 0.0 | 0.2 | | 40 | 0.0 | 0.7 | 4 | 0.1 | 92 | 34 | 3.5 | 220 | 0.16 |
| 46091 | 0.15 | 0.19 | 1.17 | 0.03 | 0.13 | 27.2 | 0.25 | 0.2 | 0.4 | | 117 | 0.0 | 1.3 | 10 | 0.2 | 94 | 73 | 11.0 | 274 | 0.36 |
| 47073 | 0.03 | 0.04 | 0.24 | 0.01 | 0.01 | 2.0 | 0.03 | 0.0 | 0.0 | | 7 | 0.0 | 0.2 | 7 | 0.1 | 17 | 21 | | 25 | 0.10 |
| 47504 | | | | | | | | 0.0 | | | 0 | | 0.4 | | | | | | 39 | |
| 47026 | 0.00 | 0.00 | 0.03 | 0.00 | 0.00 | 0.8 | 0.00 | 0.0 | 0.0 | | 0 | 0.0 | 0.0 | 0 | 0.0 | 1 | 1 | 0.1 | 4 | 0.01 |
| 47175 | | | | | | | | | | | | | | | | | | | 15 | |
| 47176 | | | | | | | | | | | | | | | | | | | 15 | |
| 47201 | | | | | | | | | | | | | | | | | | | 167 | |
| 49089 | | | | | | | | 2.4 | | | 0 | | 0.7 | | | | | | 30 | |
| 47590 | | | | | | | | 0.0 | | | 0 | | 0.4 | | | | | | 160 | |
| 47318 | | | | | | | | 1.2 | | | 20 | | 0.4 | | | | | | 20 | |
| 47514 | 0.07 | 0.04 | 0.49 | | | 14.9 | | 0.0 | | | 8 | | 0.9 | | | | 52 | | 116 | |
| 47287 | | | | | | | | 0.0 | | | 0 | | 1.8 | | | | | | 0 | |
| 47302 | | | | | | | | 1.2 | | | 20 | | 0.4 | | | | | | 20 | |
| 47515 | 0.08 | 0.04 | 0.42 | | | | | 0.0 | | | 9 | | 0.7 | | | | 66 | | 140 | |
| 47152 | | | | | | | | | | | | | | | | | | | 40 | |
| 47249 | | | | | | | | 0.0 | | | 0 | | 0.0 | | | | 49 | | 59 | |
| 47312 | | | | | | | | 1.2 | | | 20 | | 1.1 | | | | | | 35 | |
| 47307 | | | | | | | | 0.8 | | | 0 | | 0.2 | | | | | | 17 | |

| Code | Amount | Description | Basic Components | | | | | | | | | Additional Fats | | | | | | Vit A & Components | | | | | Vitamins | | | | | | | | | | Minerals | | | | | | | | | |
|---|---|---|---|---|---|---|---|---|---|---|---|---|---|---|---|---|---|---|---|---|---|---|---|---|---|---|---|---|---|---|---|---|---|---|---|---|---|---|---|---|---|---|
| | | | Weight (g) | Calories | % Water | Protein (g) | Carbs (g) | Fiber (g) | Sugar (g) | Other Carbs (g) | Fat (g) | Sat Fat (g) | Mono Fat (g) | Poly Fat (g) | Omega 3 (g) | Omega 6 (g) | Choles (mg) | Vit A (IU) | Vit A (RE) | Retinol (RE) | Carotenoids (RE) | Beta Carotene (mcg) | Thiamin (mg) | Riboflavin (mg) | Niacin (NE) | Vit B6 (mg) | Vit B12 (mcg) | Folate (mcg) | Panto (mg) | Vit C (mg) | Vit D (mg) | Vit E (α TE) | Calcium (mg) | Copper (mg) | Iron (mg) | Magnes (mg) | Mang (mg) | Phos (mg) | Potassium (mg) | Selenium (mcg) | Sodium (mg) | Zinc (mg) |
| 47074 | 1 ea | Applesauce cookie, avg | 18 | 67 | 18 | 0.9 | 11.3 | 0.6 | 7.5 | 3.3 | 2.2 | 0.4 | 0.9 | 0.7 | | | 4 | 108 | 27 | 25 | 2 | | 0.04 | 0.03 | 0.19 | 0.01 | 0.01 | 1.5 | 0.04 | 0.2 | 0.0 | | 11 | 0.0 | 0.3 | 6 | 0.1 | 22 | 38 | | 54 | 0.12 |
| | | Apricot cookies | | | | | | | | | | | | | | | | | | | | | | | | | | | | | | | | | | | | | | | | |
| 47289 | 1 ea | Bar, fat free, Health Valley | 42 | 140 | 8 | 3.0 | 35.0 | 4.0 | 12.0 | 19.0 | 0.0 | 0.0 | 0.0 | 0.0 | 0.00 | 0.00 | 0 | 500 | 100 | | | | | | | | | | | 0.0 | | | 0 | | 3.6 | | | | 0 | | 5 | |
| 47311 | 1 ea | Delight, fat free, Health Valley | 11 | 33 | 20 | 0.7 | 8.0 | 1.0 | 3.7 | 3.3 | 0.0 | 0.0 | 0.0 | 0.0 | 0.00 | 0.00 | 0 | 167 | 33 | | | | | | | | | | | 0.8 | | | 0 | | 0.2 | | | | | | 17 | |
| 47516 | 1 ea | Filled, Archway | 28 | 112 | 15 | 1.4 | 18.1 | 0.4 | 9.1 | 8.7 | 3.9 | 1.5 | 1.2 | 0.2 | | | 8 | 15 | 3 | | | | 0.07 | 0.06 | 0.55 | | | | | 0.0 | | | 6 | | 0.6 | | | | 35 | | 90 | |
| 47319 | 1 ea | Filled, fat free, Health Valley | 33 | 70 | 38 | 2.0 | 18.0 | 2.0 | 9.0 | 7.0 | 0.0 | 0.0 | 0.0 | 0.0 | 0.00 | 0.00 | 0 | 500 | 100 | | | | | | | | | | | 1.2 | | | 20 | | 0.4 | | | | | | 20 | |
| | | Biscotti cookies | | | | | | | | | | | | | | | | | | | | | | | | | | | | | | | | | | | | | | | | |
| 47455 | 1 ea | Almond, Pepperidge Farm | 23 | 110 | 11 | 2.0 | 14.0 | 1.0 | 6.0 | 7.0 | 4.0 | 2.0 | | | | | 10 | 0 | 0 | 0 | 0 | 0 | 0.09 | 0.07 | 0.80 | | | | | 0.0 | | | 0 | | 1.1 | | | | | | 70 | |
| 47454 | 1 ea | Cranberry Pistachio, Pepperidge Farm | 19 | 90 | 3 | 2.0 | 13.0 | 0.5 | 7.0 | 5.5 | 3.0 | 1.0 | 1.5 | 0.5 | | | 5 | 0 | 0 | 0 | 0 | 0 | 0.09 | 0.03 | 0.80 | | | | | 0.0 | | | 0 | | 0.7 | | | | | | 65 | |
| 47451 | 1 ea | Dark Chocolate, Pepperidge Farm | 12 | 53 | 2 | 0.5 | 9.1 | 0.0 | 4.3 | 4.8 | 1.9 | 1.0 | 0.7 | 0.2 | | | 0 | 0 | 0 | 0 | 0 | 0 | 0.00 | 0.00 | 0.00 | | | | | 0.0 | | | 0 | | | | | | | | 24 | |
| 47604 | 1 ea | LaScala Anise, Pepperidge Farm | 19 | 90 | | 2.0 | 14.0 | 0.0 | 6.0 | 8.0 | 3.0 | 1.0 | 1.0 | 1.0 | | | 5 | 0 | 0 | 0 | 0 | 0 | 0.09 | 0.07 | 0.80 | | | | | 0.0 | | | 0 | | 0.7 | | | | | | 75 | |
| | | Biscuit cookies | | | | | | | | | | | | | | | | | | | | | | | | | | | | | | | | | | | | | | | | |
| 47452 | 1 ea | Blanc-Esprit, Pepperidge Farm | 17 | 80 | 7 | 1.0 | 10.0 | 0.0 | 3.0 | 7.0 | 4.5 | 2.5 | 1.5 | 0.5 | | | 10 | 0 | 0 | 0 | 0 | 0 | 0.00 | 0.00 | 0.00 | | | | | 0.0 | | | 0 | | 0.0 | | | | | | 50 | |
| 47602 | 1 ea | Choc A L' Orange, Pepperidge Farm | 16 | 77 | | 1.0 | 11.9 | 0.0 | 5.7 | 6.2 | 3.1 | 1.1 | 1.3 | 0.7 | | | 1 | 0 | 0 | 0 | 0 | 0 | 0.00 | 0.00 | 0.00 | | | | | 0.0 | | | 0 | | 0.2 | | | | | | 10 | |
| 47447 | 1 ea | Noir Dark Choc Esprit, Pepperidge Farm | 17 | 90 | 4 | 1.0 | 10.0 | 0.0 | 3.0 | 7.0 | 5.0 | 3.5 | | | | | 10 | 0 | 0 | 0 | 0 | 0 | 0.00 | 0.00 | 0.00 | | | | | 0.0 | | | 0 | | 0.0 | | | | | | 50 | |
| | | Blueberry cookies | | | | | | | | | | | | | | | | | | | | | | | | | | | | | | | | | | | | | | | | |
| 47300 | 1 ea | Apple Bakes, Health Valley, fat free | 38 | 110 | 25 | 2.0 | 26.0 | 3.0 | 13.0 | 10.0 | 0.0 | 0.0 | 0.0 | 0.0 | 0.00 | 0.00 | 0 | 500 | 100 | | | | | | | | | | | 1.2 | | | 20 | | 0.7 | | | | | | 25 | |
| 47517 | 1 ea | Filled, Archway | 28 | 110 | | 1.0 | 19.0 | 0.5 | 14.0 | 4.5 | 4.0 | 1.5 | | | | | 5 | 0 | 0 | 0 | 0 | 0 | | | | | | | | 0.0 | | | 0 | | 0.7 | | | | | | 115 | |
| 62417 | 1 ea | Menu Magic | 49 | 200 | 15 | 6.0 | 27.0 | 1.0 | 16.0 | 10.0 | 8.0 | 0.0 | | | | | 4 | 0 | 0 | 0 | 0 | 0 | | | | | | | | 0.0 | | | 20 | | 1.1 | | | 90 | 90 | | 280 | |
| 47495 | 1 oz | Mrs Rich's Family Recipe | 28 | 145 | 0 | 1.5 | 18.4 | 0.4 | 8.9 | 9.1 | 7.3 | 3.1 | 2.4 | 0.4 | | | 15 | 148 | 30 | | | | 0.06 | 0.05 | 0.57 | 0.00 | 0.00 | 3.3 | 0.01 | 0.1 | 0.0 | 0.0 | 15 | 0.0 | 0.5 | 3 | | 30 | 17 | | 147 | 0.10 |
| 47005 | 1 ea | Butter cookie, avg | 5 | 23 | 5 | 0.3 | 3.4 | 0.0 | 1.6 | 1.8 | 0.9 | 0.6 | 0.3 | 0.0 | 0.01 | 0.04 | 6 | 34 | 8 | | | | 0.02 | 0.02 | 0.16 | 0.00 | 0.02 | 2.0 | 0.02 | 0.0 | 0.0 | | 1 | 0.0 | 0.1 | 1 | 0.0 | 5 | 6 | 0.4 | 18 | 0.02 |
| 47337 | 1 ea | Butter cookie, Chessman, Pepperidge Farm | 9 | 42 | | 0.7 | 6.2 | 0.2 | 1.7 | 4.3 | 1.7 | 1.0 | 0.5 | 0.0 | 0.00 | 0.00 | 7 | 0 | 0 | 0 | 0 | 0 | 0.02 | 0.01 | 0.14 | | | | | 0.0 | | | 0 | | 0.1 | | | | | | 28 | |
| 47076 | 1 ea | Carob cookie, avg | 13 | 51 | 5 | 1.2 | 8.5 | 0.8 | | | 2.2 | 0.4 | 1.0 | 0.7 | | | 8 | 12 | 3.6 | 3.5 | 0.05 | | 0.02 | 0.05 | 0.26 | 0.03 | 0.04 | 3.0 | 0.08 | 0.1 | 0.1 | | 35 | 0.0 | 0.3 | 8 | 0.1 | 29 | 70 | | 40 | 0.19 |
| 47518 | 1 ea | Carrot cookie, Cake, Archway | 28 | 120 | 11 | 1.1 | 18.0 | 0.5 | 10.6 | 6.8 | 5.0 | 1.5 | 1.6 | 0.6 | | | 4 | 251 | 50 | | | | 0.06 | 0.04 | 0.41 | | | | | 0.0 | | | 11 | | 0.7 | | | | 63 | | 176 | |
| | | Cherry cookies | | | | | | | | | | | | | | | | | | | | | | | | | | | | | | | | | | | | | | | | |
| 47475 | 1 ea | Cobbler, Pepperidge Farm | 16 | 70 | 7 | 1.0 | 11.0 | 0.0 | 5.0 | 6.0 | 2.5 | 1.0 | | | | | 5 | 0 | 0 | 0 | 0 | 0 | 0.03 | 0.00 | 0.00 | | | | | 0.0 | | | 0 | | 0.0 | | | | | | 45 | |
| 47519 | 1 ea | Filled, Archway | 28 | 113 | 15 | 1.4 | 18.1 | 0.4 | 8.8 | 8.9 | 3.9 | 1.5 | 1.2 | 0.2 | | | 8 | 24 | 5 | | | | 0.07 | 0.06 | 0.53 | | | | | 0.0 | | | 7 | | 0.6 | | | | 34 | | 92 | |
| 47506 | 1 ea | Nougat, Archway | 9 | 48 | | 0.3 | 5.8 | 0.0 | 3.9 | 1.9 | 2.9 | 0.5 | | | | | 0 | 0 | 0 | 0 | 0 | 0 | | | | | | | | 0.0 | | | 0 | | 0.1 | | | | | | 13 | |
| | | Cinnamon cookies | | | | | | | | | | | | | | | | | | | | | | | | | | | | | | | | | | | | | | | | |
| 47502 | 1 ea | Honey Heart, fat free, Archway | 10 | 35 | 11 | 0.5 | 8.2 | 0.1 | 4.3 | 3.8 | 0.1 | 0.0 | 0.0 | 0.0 | | | 0 | 0.06 | 0.01 | | | | 0.03 | 0.02 | 0.26 | | | 7.9 | | 0.0 | | | 2 | | 0.3 | | | | 7 | | 41 | |
| 47525 | 1 ea | Snap, Archway | 6 | 30 | | 0.2 | 4.0 | 0.0 | 1.6 | 2.4 | 1.4 | 0.3 | | | | | 1 | 0 | 0 | 0 | 0 | 0 | | | | | | | | 0.0 | | | 0 | | 0.1 | | | | | | 24 | |
| 47670 | 1 ea | Teddy Graham, Nabisco | 1 | 5 | | 0.1 | 0.8 | 0.0 | 0.3 | 0.5 | 0.1 | 0.0 | 0.1 | 0.0 | 0.00 | 0.00 | 0 | | | | | | | | | | | | | | | | | | 0.0 | | | | 1 | | 5 | |
| | | Chocolate cookies | | | | | | | | | | | | | | | | | | | | | | | | | | | | | | | | | | | | | | | | |
| 47671 | 1 ea | Aquarium, Pepperidge Farm | 2 | 9 | 2 | 0.1 | 1.5 | 0.1 | 0.5 | 0.8 | 0.3 | 0.1 | | | | | 1 | 0 | 0 | 0 | 0 | 0 | 0.01 | 0.00 | 0.05 | | | | | 0.0 | | | 0 | | 0.1 | | | | | | 6 | |
| 49088 | 1 ea | Caramel, Health Valley | 16 | 34 | 41 | 1.0 | 8.2 | 1.5 | 4.8 | 1.9 | 0.0 | 0.0 | 0.0 | 0.0 | 0.00 | 0.00 | 0 | 48 | 10 | | | | | | | | | | | 0.0 | | | 0 | | 0.5 | | | | | | 10 | |
| 47472 | 1 ea | Milano, Pepperidge Farm | 11 | 58 | 1 | 0.6 | 6.8 | 0.3 | 3.6 | 2.9 | 3.2 | 1.1 | | | | | 3 | 0 | 0 | 0 | 0 | 0 | 0.03 | 0.02 | 0.26 | | | | | 0.0 | | | 0 | | 0.3 | | | | | | 26 | |
| 47598 | 1 ea | Milk Chocolate Bordeaux, Pepperidge Farm | 11 | 55 | 4 | 0.7 | 6.5 | 0.0 | 2.8 | 3.8 | 3.1 | 1.2 | | | | | 0 | 0 | 0 | 0 | 0 | 0 | 0.02 | 0.01 | 0.14 | | | | | 0.0 | | | 0 | | 0.4 | | | | | | 33 | |
| 47478 | 1 ea | Milk Chocolate Toffee, Pepperidge Farm | 26 | 130 | 6 | 1.0 | 16.0 | 1.0 | 9.0 | 6.0 | 7.0 | 2.5 | | | | | 20 | 0 | 0 | 0 | 0 | 0 | 0.06 | 0.03 | 0.40 | | | | | 0.0 | | | 0 | | 0.4 | | | | | | 110 | |
| 47431 | 1 ea | Rocky Road, Archway | 28 | 128 | 9 | 1.6 | 17.5 | 0.7 | 9.3 | 7.5 | 5.9 | 1.5 | 2.0 | 1.2 | | | 11 | 22 | 4 | | | | 0.06 | 0.06 | 0.51 | | | | | 0.0 | | | 6 | | 0.7 | | | | 55 | | 71 | |
| 47248 | 1 ea | Weight Watchers | 7 | 28 | 12 | 0.4 | 4.6 | 0.7 | 1.4 | 2.5 | 1.1 | 0.4 | | | | | 0 | | | | | | | | | | | | | | | | | | 0.3 | | | | 18 | | 25 | |
| | | Chocolate Chip cookies | | | | | | | | | | | | | | | | | | | | | | | | | | | | | | | | | | | | | | | | |
| 47520 | 1 ea | Archway | 9 | 43 | | 0.3 | 5.7 | 0.0 | 3.0 | 2.7 | 2.3 | 0.7 | | | | | 3 | 0 | 0 | 0 | 0 | 0 | | | | | | | | 0.0 | | | 0 | | 0.2 | | | | | | 23 | |
| 47036 | 1 ea | Baked f/refrig dough, avg | 12 | 59 | 3 | 0.6 | 8.2 | 0.2 | 5.4 | 2.6 | 2.7 | 0.9 | 1.4 | 0.3 | 0.01 | 0.26 | 3 | 7 | 2 | 1.9 | 0.2 | | 0.02 | 0.02 | 0.24 | 0.00 | 0.01 | 0.8 | 0.02 | 0.0 | 0.1 | | 3 | 0.0 | 0.3 | 3 | 0.1 | 9 | 24 | 0.7 | 28 | 0.07 |
| 47644 | 1 ea | Big, Grandma's | 39 | 190 | 6 | 2.0 | 25.0 | 1.0 | 11.0 | 13.0 | 9.0 | 2.5 | | | | | 5 | | | | | | | | | | | | | | | | | | | | | | | | 130 | |
| 47356 | 1 ea | Chesapeake w/nuts, Pepperidge Farm | 26 | 140 | | 2.0 | 15.0 | 0.5 | 7.0 | 7.5 | 8.0 | 1.5 | 4.5 | 1.0 | | | 10 | 0 | 0 | 0 | 0 | 0 | 0.06 | 0.03 | 0.40 | | | | | 0.0 | | | 0 | | 0.7 | | | | | | 100 | |
| 47170 | 1 ea | Chips Ahoy | 11 | 55 | | 0.7 | 7.2 | 0.3 | 3.4 | 3.4 | 2.8 | 0.9 | 0.9 | 0.0 | 0.00 | 0.00 | 0 | | | | | | | | | | | | | | | | | | 0.4 | | | | 19 | | 38 | |
| 47575 | 1 ea | Chocolate, Tastykake | 39 | 175 | 7 | 2.0 | 27.0 | 1.0 | 14.5 | 11.5 | 6.5 | 2.0 | | | | | 2 | 0 | 0 | 0 | 0 | 0 | | | | | | | | 0.0 | | | 10 | | 1.4 | | | | | | 80 | |
| 47342 | 1 ea | Chocolate Walnut, Pepperidge Farm | 26 | 130 | | 2.0 | 16.0 | 1.0 | 9.0 | 6.0 | 6.0 | 2.0 | 3.0 | 1.0 | | | 5 | 0 | 0 | 0 | 0 | 0 | 0.12 | 0.07 | 0.40 | | | | | 0.0 | | | 0 | | 0.7 | | | | | | 45 | |
| 47022 | 1 ea | Diet, avg | 5 | 25 | 4 | 0.2 | 3.1 | 0.2 | | | 1.3 | 0.4 | 0.5 | 0.4 | | | 1 | 1.6 | 0.5 | 0.5 | 0 | | 0.01 | 0.01 | 0.07 | 0.00 | 0.01 | 0.5 | | 0.0 | | | 2 | 0.0 | 0.1 | 1 | | 3 | 4 | 0.3 | 1 | 0.04 |
| 47298 | 1 ea | Double Fudge, Health Valley | 11 | 33 | 15 | 1.0 | 8.0 | 1.3 | 2.3 | 4.3 | 0.0 | 0.0 | 0.0 | 0.0 | 0.00 | 0.00 | 0 | 167 | 33 | | | | | | | | | | | 0.0 | | | 0 | | 0.4 | | | | | | 7 | |
| 47672 | 1 oz | Dry Mix, avg | 28 | 139 | 3 | 1.3 | 18.5 | 0.4 | 12.7 | 5.4 | 7.1 | 2.3 | 3.7 | 0.7 | 0.04 | 0.70 | 0 | 1 | 0.2 | | | | 0.05 | 0.06 | 0.56 | 0.00 | 0.00 | 14.3 | 0.05 | 0.0 | 0.0 | | 12 | 0.1 | 0.6 | 10 | 0.1 | 22 | 58 | 0.7 | 81 | 0.17 |
| 47370 | 1 ea | Entenmann's | 10 | 47 | 5 | 0.3 | 6.7 | 0.2 | 3.7 | 2.8 | 2.3 | 0.7 | | | | | 3 | 0 | 0 | 0 | 0 | 0 | | | | | | | | 0.0 | | | 0 | | 0.0 | | | | 15 | | 30 | |
| 47645 | 1 ea | Fudge, avg | 39 | 170 | 9 | 2.0 | 27.0 | 1.0 | 11.0 | 15.0 | 6.0 | 2.0 | | | | | 5 | | | | | | | | | | | | | | | | | | | | | | | | 160 | |
| 47125 | 1 ea | Health Valley | 11 | 33 | 16 | 1.0 | 8.0 | 1.3 | 2.3 | 4.3 | 0.0 | 0.0 | 0.0 | 0.0 | 0.00 | 0.00 | 0 | 167 | 33 | | | | | | | | | | | 0.0 | | | 0 | | 0.4 | | | | | | 7 | |
| 47522 | 1 ea | Iced Box, Archway | 28 | 136 | 6 | 1.3 | 18.0 | 0.3 | 9.8 | 7.9 | 6.6 | 2.0 | 2.5 | 0.3 | | | 9 | 14 | 2.7 | | | | 0.07 | 0.06 | 0.54 | | | | | 0.0 | | | 6 | | 0.7 | | | | 32 | | 69 | |
| 47032 | 1 ea | Low Fat, avg | 10 | 45 | 4 | 0.6 | 7.3 | 0.4 | 4.8 | 2.2 | 1.5 | 0.4 | 0.6 | 0.5 | 0.03 | 0.43 | 0 | 0 | 0 | | | | 0.03 | 0.03 | 0.28 | 0.03 | 0.00 | 7.0 | 0.03 | 0.0 | 0.0 | | 2 | 0.0 | 0.3 | 3 | 0.0 | 8 | 12 | 0.6 | 38 | 0.07 |
| 47341 | 1 ea | Milk Choc w/Macadamia Nuts, Pepp Farm | 26 | 130 | | 1.0 | 16.0 | 1.0 | 9.0 | 6.0 | 6.0 | 2.5 | 3.0 | 0.0 | 0.00 | 0.00 | 10 | 0 | 0 | 0 | 0 | 0 | 0.09 | 0.07 | 0.80 | | | | | 0.0 | | | 0 | | 0.7 | | | | | | 55 | |
| 47566 | 1 ea | Mini, Archway | 2 | 10 | | 0.1 | 1.3 | 0.0 | 0.6 | 0.7 | 0.5 | 0.1 | | | | | 0 | 0 | 0 | 0 | 0 | 0 | | | | | | | | 0.0 | | | 0 | | 0.1 | | | | | | 6 | |
| 47358 | 1 ea | Nantucket, Pepperidge Farm | 26 | 130 | | 1.0 | 16.0 | 0.5 | 8.0 | 7.5 | 7.0 | 3.0 | 3.5 | 0.5 | | | 10 | 0 | 0 | 0 | 0 | 0 | 0.06 | 0.00 | 0.00 | | | | | 0.0 | | | 0 | | 0.4 | | | | | | 75 | |
| 47033 | 1 ea | No Sodium, w/fructose, avg | 7 | 32 | 5 | 0.3 | 5.1 | 0.1 | 3.4 | 1.7 | 1.2 | 0.3 | 0.5 | 0.4 | 0.02 | 0.33 | 0 | 0 | 0 | | | | 0.03 | 0.01 | 0.20 | 0.00 | 0.00 | 3.2 | 0.01 | 0.0 | 0.0 | | 3 | 0.0 | 0.2 | 1 | 0.0 | 8 | 14 | 0.2 | 1 | 0.03 |
| 47369 | 1 ea | Oatmeal, avg | 12 | 40 | | 0.5 | 9.5 | 0.5 | 6.0 | 3.0 | 0.0 | 0.0 | 0.0 | 0.0 | 0.00 | 0.00 | 0 | 0 | 0 | 0 | 0 | 0 | | | | | | | | 0.0 | | | 0 | | 0.2 | | | | 40 | | 55 | |
| 47265 | 1 ea | Old Fashioned, Health Valley | 11 | 33 | 16 | 1.0 | 8.0 | 1.3 | 2.3 | 4.3 | 0.0 | 0.0 | 0.0 | 0.0 | 0.00 | 0.00 | 0 | 167 | 33 | | | | | | | | | | | 0.0 | | | 0 | | 0.4 | | | | | | 7 | |
| 47650 | 1 ea | Peanut Butter, avg | 39 | 190 | 4 | 4.0 | 23.0 | 1.0 | 13.0 | 9.0 | 10.0 | 3.0 | | | | | 5 | | | | | | | | | | | | | | | | | | | | | | | | 170 | |
| 47035 | 1 ea | Prep f/Mix, avg | 16 | 79 | 4 | 0.9 | 10.3 | 0.2 | 6.8 | 3.3 | 4.1 | 1.3 | 2.1 | 0.4 | 0.02 | 0.40 | 7 | 10 | 3 | 2.8 | 0.2 | | 0.02 | 0.04 | 0.28 | 0.00 | 0.01 | 1.3 | 0.03 | 0.0 | 0.0 | | 8 | 0.0 | 0.3 | 6 | 0.1 | 15 | 34 | 1.0 | 47 | 0.11 |
| 47037 | 1 ea | Prep f/Recipe, avg | 16 | 78 | 6 | 0.9 | 9.3 | 0.4 | 6.2 | 2.7 | 4.5 | 2.3 | 1.3 | 0.7 | 0.14 | 0.59 | 11 | 95 | 24 | 21 | 3 | | 0.03 | 0.03 | 0.22 | 0.01 | 0.01 | 5.3 | 0.04 | 0.0 | 0.1 | | 6 | 0.1 | 0.4 | 9 | 0.1 | 16 | 35 | 1.8 | 55 | 0.15 |
| 47013 | 1 ea | Refrig Dough, avg | 16 | 71 | 13 | 0.7 | 9.8 | 0.2 | 6.4 | 3.1 | 3.3 | 1.1 | 1.7 | 0.3 | 0.02 | 0.33 | 4 | 9 | 2.7 | 2.5 | 0.2 | | 0.03 | 0.03 | 0.32 | 0.01 | 0.01 | 9.1 | 0.05 | 0.0 | 0.1 | | 4 | 0.0 | 0.4 | 4 | 0.1 | 11 | 29 | 0.8 | 33 | 0.08 |
| 47470 | 1 ea | Sausalito, Pepperidge Farm | 23 | 120 | 3 | 1.0 | 14.0 | 0.0 | 8.0 | 6.0 | 7.0 | 2.5 | | | | | 5 | 0 | 0 | 0 | 0 | 0 | 0.00 | 0.00 | 0.00 | | | | | 0.0 | | | 0 | | 0.0 | | | | | | 65 | |
| 47166 | 1 ea | Snackwell's | 14 | 60 | 4 | 0.8 | 10.6 | 0.3 | 4.7 | 5.6 | 1.8 | 0.7 | 0.9 | 0.1 | | | 0 | 2 | 0.4 | | | | 0.03 | 0.04 | 0.41 | 0.01 | 0.00 | | | 0.0 | | | 3 | 0.0 | 0.4 | 5 | | 25 | 19 | | 84 | 0.11 |
| 47001 | 1 ea | Soft, avg | 15 | 69 | 12 | 0.5 | 8.9 | 0.5 | | | 3.6 | 1.1 | 2.0 | 0.5 | 0.02 | 0.38 | 0 | 0.5 | 0.1 | | | | 0.02 | 0.03 | 0.24 | 0.02 | 0.00 | 5.9 | 0.04 | 0.0 | 0.1 | | 2 | 0.0 | 0.4 | 5 | 0.1 | 8 | 14 | 0.8 | 49 | 0.07 |
| 47574 | 1 ea | Soft & Chewy, Tastykake | 39 | 175 | 7 | 2.0 | 26.0 | 1.0 | 11.5 | 13.5 | 7.0 | 2.0 | | | | | 8 | 0 | 0 | 0 | 0 | 0 | | | | | | | | 0.0 | | | 10 | | 0.9 | | | | | | 130 | |

| Code | Amount | Description | Basic Components | | | | | | | | | Additional Fats | | | | | | Vit A & Components | | | | | Vitamins | | | | | | | | | | Minerals | | | | | | | | | |
|---|---|---|---|---|---|---|---|---|---|---|---|---|---|---|---|---|---|---|---|---|---|---|---|---|---|---|---|---|---|---|---|---|---|---|---|---|---|---|---|---|---|---|
| | | | Weight (g) | Calories | % Water | Protein (g) | Carbs (g) | Fiber (g) | Sugar (g) | Other Carbs (g) | Fat (g) | Sat Fat (g) | Mono Fat (g) | Poly Fat (g) | Omega 3 (g) | Omega 6 (g) | Choles (mg) | Vit A (IU) | Vit A (RE) | Retinol (RE) | Carotenoids (RE) | Beta Carotene (mcg) | Thiamin (mg) | Riboflavin (mg) | Niacin (NE) | Vit B6 (mg) | Vit B12 (mcg) | Folate (mcg) | Panto (mg) | Vit C (mg) | Vit D (mg) | Vit E (α TE) | Calcium (mg) | Copper (mg) | Iron (mg) | Magnes (mg) | Mang (mg) | Phos (mg) | Potassium (mg) | Selenium (mcg) | Sodium (mg) | Zinc (mg) |
| 47340 | 1 ea | Soft Chunk, Pepperidge Farm | 26 | 130 | | 1.0 | 16.0 | 2.0 | 9.0 | 5.0 | 6.0 | 2.5 | 2.5 | 0.0 | 0.00 | 0.00 | 10 | 0 | 0 | 0 | 0 | 0 | 0.09 | 0.07 | 0.80 | | | | | 0.0 | | | 0 | | 0.7 | | | | | | 35 | |
| 47245 | 1 ea | Weight Watchers | 15 | 70 | | 1.0 | 11.0 | 0.5 | 7.5 | 3.0 | 2.5 | 1.0 | | | | | 0 | 0 | 0 | 0 | 0 | 0 | | | | | | | | 0.0 | | | 10 | | 0.4 | | | | 22 | | 45 | |
| 47524 | 1 ea | With Toffee, Fun Chip, Archway | 29 | 136 | 8 | 1.3 | 18.6 | 0.5 | 9.4 | 8.6 | 6.3 | 1.8 | 2.4 | 0.5 | | | 6 | 21 | 4 | | | | 0.07 | 0.05 | 0.59 | | | | | 0.0 | | | 4 | | 0.6 | | | | 21 | | 128 | |
| | | Chocolate Fudge cookie | | | | | | | | | | | | | | | | | | | | | | | | | | | | | | | | | | | | | | | | |
| 47044 | 1 ea | Avg | 21 | 73 | 12 | 1.0 | 16.4 | 0.6 | | | 0.8 | 0.2 | 0.4 | 0.1 | 0.00 | 0.10 | 0 | 0.4 | 0.1 | | | | 0.05 | 0.04 | 0.25 | 0.01 | 0.02 | 9.0 | 0.05 | 0.0 | | | 7 | 0.1 | 0.5 | 7 | 0.1 | 17 | 29 | 0.8 | 40 | 0.12 |
| 47572 | 1 ea | Bar, Tastykake | 43 | 190 | 7 | 2.0 | 29.0 | 1.0 | 15.0 | 13.0 | 7.0 | 2.0 | | | | | 5 | 0 | 0 | 0 | 0 | 0 | | | | | | | | 0.0 | | | 0 | | 1.1 | | | | | | 100 | |
| 47674 | 1 ea | Bar Swirl, Pillsbury | 33 | 149 | 3 | 1.2 | 25.1 | 0.6 | 16.4 | 8.1 | 5.0 | 1.1 | | | | | 0 | 0 | 0 | 0 | 0 | 0 | | | | | | | | 0.0 | | | 9 | | 0.7 | | | | | | 107 | |
| 47647 | 1 ea | Big Nutty Fudge, Grandma's | 40 | 190 | 9 | 3.0 | 25.0 | 1.0 | 14.0 | 10.0 | 8.0 | 1.5 | | | | | 5 | | | | | | | | | | | | | | | | | | | | | | | | 150 | |
| 47213 | 1 ea | Brownie, fat free, Entenmann's | 12 | 40 | 9 | 0.5 | 10.0 | 0.5 | 6.0 | 3.5 | 0.0 | 0.0 | 0.0 | 0.0 | 0.00 | 0.00 | 0 | 0 | 0 | 0 | 0 | 0 | | | | | | | | 0.0 | | | 0 | | 0.4 | | | | 62 | | 45 | |
| 47324 | 1 ea | Double Fudge, Snackwells | 16 | 53 | 14 | 0.8 | 11.9 | 0.3 | 6.4 | 5.2 | 0.2 | 0.1 | 0.1 | 0.0 | | | 0 | 0.19 | 0.04 | | | | 0.02 | 0.02 | 0.26 | 0.00 | 0.00 | | | 0.0 | | | 3 | 0.0 | 0.3 | 5 | | 11 | 26 | | 71 | 0.08 |
| 47153 | 1 ea | Devils Food, Snackwells | 23 | 79 | 19 | 1.1 | 18.1 | 0.3 | 13.1 | 4.7 | 0.2 | 0.0 | 0.2 | 0.0 | 0.00 | 0.00 | 0 | 1 | 0.1 | | | | 0.02 | 0.03 | 0.35 | 0.01 | 0.02 | | | 0.0 | | | 7 | 0.0 | 0.3 | 5 | | 17 | 24 | | 39 | 0.11 |
| 47536 | 1 ea | Nut Bar, Archway | 28 | 110 | | 2.0 | 17.0 | 0.5 | 8.0 | 8.5 | 4.5 | 1.0 | | | | | 2 | 0 | 0 | 0 | 0 | 0 | | | | | | | | 0.0 | | | 0 | | 0.7 | | | | | | 120 | |
| | | Chocolate Sandwich cookies | | | | | | | | | | | | | | | | | | | | | | | | | | | | | | | | | | | | | | | | |
| 47262 | 1 ea | Cameo Cream, Nabisco | 14 | 65 | | 0.5 | 10.5 | 0.3 | 5.0 | 5.3 | 2.5 | 0.5 | 1.0 | 0.0 | 0.00 | 0.00 | 0 | | | | | | | | | | | | | | | | | | 0.4 | | | | 15 | | 52 | |
| 47468 | 1 ea | Deluxe Bar Oreo, Pillsbury | 30 | 128 | 8 | 1.0 | 22.0 | 0.5 | 13.7 | 7.8 | 4.0 | 1.0 | | | | | 0 | 1 | 0.2 | | | | | | | | | | | 0.1 | | | 8 | | 0.7 | | | | | | 125 | |
| 47267 | 1 ea | Fudge, fat free, Health Valley | 16 | 34 | 41 | 1.0 | 8.2 | 1.5 | 4.8 | 1.9 | 0.0 | 0.0 | 0.0 | 0.0 | 0.00 | 0.00 | 0 | 242 | 48 | | | | | | | | | | | 0.0 | | | 0 | | 0.5 | | | | | | 10 | |
| 47039 | 1 ea | Low Sod, w/fructose, avg | 10 | 46 | 4 | 0.5 | 6.8 | 0.4 | 3.9 | 2.4 | 2.2 | 0.4 | 0.9 | 0.8 | 0.05 | 0.74 | 0 | 0.3 | 0.06 | | | | 0.05 | 0.03 | 0.40 | 0.00 | 0.00 | 6.2 | 0.04 | 0.0 | 0.0 | | 10 | 0.0 | 0.5 | 3 | 0.0 | 20 | 30 | 0.4 | 24 | 0.06 |
| 47180 | 1 ea | Oreo, Nabisco | 11 | 53 | | 0.7 | 7.7 | 0.3 | 4.3 | 3.0 | 2.3 | 0.5 | 1.0 | 0.2 | | | 0 | | | | | | | | | | | | | | | | | | 0.2 | | | | 20 | | 73 | |
| 47244 | 1 ea | Smart Snackers | 15 | 70 | | 1.0 | 11.5 | 0.5 | 8.0 | 3.0 | 1.8 | 0.5 | | | | | 0 | 0 | 0 | 0 | 0 | 0 | | | | | | | | 0.0 | | | 0 | | 0.5 | | | | 28 | | 80 | |
| 47164 | 1 ea | Snackwells | 11 | 45 | 4 | 0.6 | 8.7 | 0.3 | 4.7 | 3.6 | 1.0 | 0.3 | 0.3 | 0.1 | | | 0 | 0.3 | 0.06 | | | | 0.01 | 0.02 | 0.25 | 0.00 | 0.00 | | | 0.0 | | | 6 | 0.0 | 0.3 | 5 | | 22 | 18 | | 84 | 0.08 |
| 47038 | 1 ea | With Chocolate Icing, avg | 17 | 82 | 2 | 0.6 | 11.2 | 0.9 | | | 4.5 | 1.3 | 2.5 | 0.5 | 0.02 | 0.49 | 0 | 0.5 | 0.1 | | | | 0.02 | 0.03 | 0.23 | 0.01 | 0.01 | 3.1 | 0.03 | 0.0 | | | 6 | 0.1 | 0.5 | 7 | 0.1 | 15 | 41 | 0.5 | 55 | 0.10 |
| 47040 | 1 ea | With Extra Crème, avg | 13 | 65 | 2 | 0.5 | 8.9 | 0.3 | | | 3.3 | 0.5 | 1.4 | 1.2 | 0.08 | 1.13 | 0 | 0 | 0 | 0 | 0 | 0 | 0.01 | 0.02 | 0.20 | 0.00 | 0.00 | 5.6 | 0.03 | 0.0 | | | 3 | 0.0 | 0.4 | 4 | 0.0 | 12 | 16 | 0.3 | 64 | 0.08 |
| 47181 | 1 ea | Chocolate Snap cookie, Nabisco | 4 | 17 | | 0.3 | 2.8 | | | | 0.6 | 0.3 | | | | | | | | | | | | | | | | | | | | | | | | | | | | | 23 | |
| 47041 | 1 ea | Chocolate Wafer cookie, avg | 6 | 26 | 4 | 0.4 | 4.3 | 0.2 | | | 0.9 | 0.3 | 0.3 | 0.2 | 0.02 | 0.23 | 0 | 0.8 | 0.2 | | | | 0.01 | 0.02 | 0.17 | 0.00 | 0.01 | 3.0 | 0.02 | 0.0 | 0.0 | | 2 | 0.0 | 0.2 | 3 | 0.0 | 8 | 13 | 0.3 | 35 | 0.07 |
| 47185 | 1 ea | Chocolate Wafer cookie, Nabisco | 6 | 26 | | 0.4 | 4.5 | 0.2 | 2.1 | 2.3 | 0.8 | 0.3 | 0.3 | 0.1 | | | 0 | | | | | | | | | | | | | | | | | | 0.2 | | | | 15 | | 43 | |
| 49014 | 1 ea | Cone, sugar, rolled type, avg | 10 | 40 | 3 | 0.8 | 8.4 | 0.2 | 0.5 | 7.7 | 0.4 | 0.1 | 0.1 | 0.1 | 0.01 | 0.14 | 0 | 0 | 0 | 0 | 0 | 0 | 0.05 | 0.04 | 0.51 | 0.01 | 0.00 | 8.3 | 0.04 | 0.0 | 0.0 | | 4 | 0.0 | 0.4 | 3 | 0.1 | 10 | 15 | 0.5 | 32 | 0.08 |
| 49111 | 1 ea | Cone, wafer type, cake cone, avg | 29 | 121 | 5 | 2.3 | 22.9 | 0.9 | 0.2 | 21.8 | 2.0 | 0.4 | 0.5 | 0.9 | 0.05 | 0.89 | 0 | 0 | 0 | 0 | 0 | 0 | 0.07 | 0.10 | 1.28 | 0.01 | 0.00 | 29.6 | 0.14 | 0.0 | 0.0 | | 7 | 0.1 | 1.0 | 8 | 0.2 | 28 | 32 | 1.4 | 41 | 0.19 |
| 47154 | 1 ea | Cranberry cookie, Newtons, fat free, Nabisco | 21 | 63 | | 0.7 | 14.4 | | | | 0.0 | 0.0 | 0.0 | 0.0 | 0.00 | 0.00 | | | | | | | | | | | | | | | | | | | | | | | | | 70 | |
| 47190 | 1 ea | Cranberry/Orange Fruit cookie, fat free, Pepp Farm | 14 | 44 | | 1.0 | 9.9 | | | | 0.0 | 0.0 | 0.0 | 0.0 | 0.00 | 0.00 | | | | | | | | | | | | | | | | | | | | | | | | | 74 | |
| | | Date cookies | | | | | | | | | | | | | | | | | | | | | | | | | | | | | | | | | | | | | | | | |
| 49090 | 1 ea | Bakes, fat free, Health Valley | 27 | 70 | 26 | 2.0 | 18.0 | 2.0 | 11.0 | 5.0 | 0.0 | 0.0 | 0.0 | 0.0 | 0.00 | 0.00 | 0 | 100 | 20 | | | | | | | | | | | 2.4 | | | 0 | | 0.7 | | | | | | 30 | |
| 47309 | 1 ea | Delight, fat free, Health Valley | 11 | 33 | 16 | 0.7 | 8.0 | 1.0 | 3.7 | 3.3 | 0.0 | 0.0 | 0.0 | 0.0 | 0.00 | 0.00 | 0 | 167 | 33 | | | | | | | | | | | 0.8 | | | 0 | | 0.2 | | | | | | 17 | |
| 47288 | 1 ea | Fruit Bar, fat free, Health Valley | 42 | 140 | 10 | 3.0 | 34.0 | 3.0 | 12.0 | 19.0 | 0.0 | 0.0 | 0.0 | 0.0 | 0.00 | 0.00 | 0 | 500 | 100 | | | | | | | | | | | 0.0 | | | 0 | | 0.7 | | | | | | 5 | |
| 47530 | 1 ea | Oatmeal Filled, Archway | 28 | 111 | 14 | 1.5 | 18.6 | 0.8 | 9.7 | 8.2 | 3.5 | 0.8 | 1.3 | 0.3 | | | 4 | 7 | .4 | | | | 0.07 | 0.05 | 0.50 | | | | | 0.0 | | | 10 | | 0.6 | | | | 59 | | 110 | |
| | | Fig cookies | | | | | | | | | | | | | | | | | | | | | | | | | | | | | | | | | | | | | | | | |
| 47012 | 1 ea | Avg | 16 | 56 | 16 | 0.6 | 11.3 | 0.7 | 6.7 | 3.9 | 1.2 | 0.2 | 0.5 | 0.4 | 0.03 | 0.41 | 0 | 5 | 0.6 | | | | 0.03 | 0.03 | 0.30 | 0.01 | 0.01 | 4.3 | 0.06 | 0.0 | 0.0 | | 10 | 0.0 | 0.5 | 4 | 0.1 | 10 | 33 | 0.5 | 56 | 0.06 |
| 47194 | 1 ea | Bar, Sunshine | 14 | 54 | | 0.5 | 9.9 | | | | 1.2 | 0.2 | | | | | | | | | | | | | | | | | | | | | | | | | | | | | 30 | |
| 47204 | 1 ea | Figaroo's, 1.5 oz pkg, Little Debbie | 43 | 151 | | 1.5 | 31.8 | | | | 3.0 | 1.5 | | | | | | | | | | | | | | | | | | | | | | | | | | | | | 98 | |
| 47161 | 1 ea | Newton, Nabisco | 16 | 60 | | 1.0 | 10.0 | 1.0 | 7.0 | 2.0 | 1.5 | 0.5 | 0.5 | 0.0 | 0.00 | 0.00 | 0 | | | | | | | | | | | | | | | | | | 0.4 | | | | 40 | | 60 | |
| 47242 | 1 ea | Smart Snackers | 20 | 71 | 14 | 1.0 | 16.2 | 0.0 | 9.1 | 7.1 | 0.0 | 0.0 | 0.0 | 0.0 | 0.00 | 0.00 | 0 | 0 | 0 | 0 | 0 | 0 | | | | | | | | 0.0 | | | 20 | | 0.4 | | | | 51 | | 51 | |
| 47043 | 1 ea | Fortune cookie, avg | 8 | 30 | 8 | 0.3 | 6.7 | 0.1 | 3.2 | 3.4 | 0.2 | 0.1 | 0.1 | 0.0 | 0.00 | 0.04 | 0 | 0.2 | 0.08 | 0.08 | 0 | | 0.01 | 0.01 | 0.15 | 0.00 | 0.00 | 4.4 | 0.02 | 0.0 | 0.0 | | 1 | 0.0 | 0.1 | 1 | 0.0 | 3 | 3 | 0.2 | 22 | 0.01 |
| 47367 | 1 ea | Fortune cookie, La Choy | 8 | 30 | 6 | 0.4 | 7.0 | 0.2 | 3.0 | 3.8 | 0.1 | 0.0 | | | | | 0 | | | | | | | | | | | | | 0.0 | | | 1 | | 0.0 | | | | | | 3 | |
| | | Fruit cookies | | | | | | | | | | | | | | | | | | | | | | | | | | | | | | | | | | | | | | | | |
| 47020 | 1 ea | Avg, whole wheat fruit & nut | 14 | 60 | 13 | 1.1 | 7.8 | 0.7 | | | 3.1 | 0.5 | 1.1 | 1.4 | | | 7 | 97 | 25 | 23 | 2 | | 0.02 | 0.02 | 0.23 | 0.03 | 0.02 | 2.8 | 0.06 | 0.1 | 0.0 | | 9 | 0.1 | 0.3 | 10 | 0.2 | 24 | 56 | | 29 | 0.18 |
| 47376 | 1 ea | Bar, fat free, Archway | 28 | 90 | | 2.0 | 21.0 | 0.0 | 11.0 | 10.0 | 0.0 | 0.0 | 0.0 | 0.0 | 0.00 | 0.00 | 0 | 0 | 0 | 0 | 0 | 0 | | | | | | | | 0.0 | | | 0 | | 0.4 | | | | | | 95 | |
| 47507 | 1 ea | Cake, Archway | 11 | 48 | | 0.7 | 6.9 | 0.7 | 4.1 | 2.1 | 2.4 | 0.5 | | | | | 0 | 0 | 0 | 0 | 0 | 0 | | | | | | | | 0.0 | | | 7 | | 0.2 | | | | | | 34 | |
| 47308 | 1 ea | Hawaiian, fat free, Health Valley | 11 | 33 | 16 | 0.7 | 8.0 | 1.0 | 3.7 | 3.3 | 0.0 | 0.0 | 0.0 | 0.0 | 0.00 | 0.00 | 0 | 167 | 33 | | | | | | | | | | | 0.8 | | | 0 | | 0.2 | | | | | | 17 | |
| 47535 | 1 ea | Honey Bar, Archway | 28 | 112 | 14 | 1.3 | 18.9 | 0.5 | 10.0 | 8.3 | 3.5 | 0.8 | 1.3 | 0.3 | | | 6 | 12 | 2 | | | | 0.08 | 0.06 | 0.60 | | | | | 0.0 | | | 7 | | 0.7 | | | | 48 | | 115 | |
| 47119 | 1 ea | Tropical, fat free, Health Valley | 33 | 70 | 38 | 2.0 | 18.0 | 2.0 | 9.0 | 7.0 | 0.0 | 0.0 | 0.0 | 0.0 | 0.00 | 0.00 | 0 | 500 | 100 | | | | | | | | | | | 1.2 | | | 20 | | 0.4 | | | | | | 20 | |
| 47509 | 1 ea | Gingerbread cookie, Archway, Iced | 11 | 51 | 5 | 0.4 | 7.8 | 0.1 | 4.2 | 3.5 | 2.1 | 0.6 | 0.7 | 0.2 | | | 0 | 0.04 | 0.01 | | | | 0.02 | 0.03 | 0.27 | | | 7.5 | | 0.0 | | | 2 | | 0.0 | | | | 7 | | 39 | |
| | | Gingersnap cookies | | | | | | | | | | | | | | | | | | | | | | | | | | | | | | | | | | | | | | | | |
| 47045 | 1 ea | Avg | 7 | 29 | 5 | 0.4 | 5.4 | 0.2 | 2.5 | 2.8 | 0.7 | 0.2 | 0.4 | 0.1 | 0.01 | 0.09 | 0 | 0.14 | 0.03 | | | | 0.01 | 0.02 | 0.23 | 0.01 | 0.00 | 5.0 | 0.03 | 0.0 | 0.0 | | 5 | 0.0 | 0.4 | 3 | 0.1 | 6 | 24 | 0.4 | 46 | 0.04 |
| 47610 | 1 ea | Archway | 6 | 27 | 5 | 0.2 | 4.3 | 0.1 | 2.1 | 2.1 | 1.0 | 0.3 | 0.4 | 0.1 | | | 0 | 0.03 | 0.01 | | | | 0.02 | 0.01 | 0.16 | | | 4.4 | | 0.0 | | | 1 | | 0.2 | | | | 4 | | 22 | |
| 47163 | 1 ea | Old Fashioned, Nabisco | 7 | 30 | | 0.3 | 5.5 | 0.1 | 2.5 | 2.9 | 0.6 | 0.1 | 0.3 | 0.0 | 0.00 | 0.00 | 0 | | | | | | | | | | | | | | | | 5 | | 0.4 | | | | 32 | | 42 | |
| | | Goldfish cookies | | | | | | | | | | | | | | | | | | | | | | | | | | | | | | | | | | | | | | | | |
| 47684 | 1 ea | Chocolate, Pepperidge Farm | 2 | 9 | 3 | 0.1 | 1.4 | 0.1 | 0.5 | 0.8 | 0.3 | 0.1 | 0.2 | 0.0 | | | [illegible] | 0 | 0 | 0 | 0 | 0 | 0.00 | 0.01 | 0.06 | | | | | 0.0 | | | | | 0.1 | | | | | | 6 | |
| 47677 | 1 ea | Chocolate Chunk, Pepperidge Farm | 2 | 10 | | 0.1 | 1.4 | 0.1 | 0.4 | 0.9 | 0.5 | 0.2 | | | | | [illegible] | 0 | 0 | 0 | 0 | 0 | 0.01 | 0.00 | 0.05 | | | | | 0.0 | | | | | 0.0 | | | | | | 3 | |
| 47678 | 1 ea | Cinnamon Graham, Pepperidge Farm | 1 | 5 | 2 | 0.1 | 0.7 | 0.1 | 0.2 | 0.4 | 0.2 | 0.1 | | | | | 0 | 0 | 0 | 0 | 0 | 0 | 0.00 | 0.00 | 0.03 | | | | | 0.0 | | | 0 | | 0.0 | | | | | | 5 | |
| 47675 | 1 ea | Graham, Pepperidge Farm | 2 | 10 | 1 | 0.1 | 1.3 | 0.1 | 0.5 | 0.7 | 0.5 | 0.2 | | | | | [illegible] | 0 | 0 | 0 | 0 | 0 | 0.01 | 0.00 | 0.05 | | | | | 0.0 | | | | | 0.0 | | | | | | 10 | |
| 47685 | 1 ea | Vanilla, Pepperidge Farm | 2 | 10 | | 0.1 | 1.4 | 0.1 | 0.4 | 1.0 | 0.5 | 0.2 | | | | | [illegible] | 0 | 0 | 0 | 0 | 0 | 0.01 | 0.00 | 0.06 | | | | | 0.0 | | | | | 0.1 | | | | | | 4 | |
| 47077 | 1 ea | Granola cookies, avg | 13 | 60 | 3 | 1.1 | 8.7 | 0.6 | | | 2.2 | 1.9 | 0.1 | 0.0 | | | 0 | 1.3 | 0.1 | 0 | 0.1 | | 0.08 | 0.03 | 0.23 | 0.05 | 0.00 | 10.5 | | 0.1 | | | 9 | 0.0 | 0.4 | 13 | | 46 | 47 | | 43 | 0.21 |
| 47343 | 1 ea | Hazelnut cookies, old fash, avg | 11 | 55 | | 0.7 | 7.2 | 0.2 | 2.1 | 5.0 | 2.8 | 0.7 | 1.5 | 0.3 | | | 0 | 0 | 0 | 0 | 0 | 0 | 0.03 | 0.01 | 0.14 | | | | | 0.0 | | | 0 | | 0.2 | | | | | | 46 | |
| 47009 | 1 ea | Ladyfinger cookie, w/lemon juice, avg | 11 | 40 | 20 | 1.2 | 6.6 | 0.1 | 4.4 | 2.1 | 1.0 | 0.4 | 0.5 | 0.2 | 0.01 | 0.16 | 40 | 61 | 18 | 18 | 0 | | 0.03 | 0.05 | 0.23 | 0.01 | 0.08 | 8.5 | 0.12 | 0.4 | 0.1 | | 5 | 0.0 | 0.4 | 1 | 0.0 | 19 | 12 | 2.3 | 16 | 0.13 |
| | | Lemon cookies | | | | | | | | | | | | | | | | | | | | | | | | | | | | | | | | | | | | | | | | |
| 47078 | 1 ea | Bar, avg | 16 | 69 | 12 | 0.8 | 10.0 | 0.1 | 6.9 | 3.0 | 3.0 | 0.6 | 1.3 | 0.9 | | | 12 | 158 | 41 | 38 | 3 | | 0.03 | 0.04 | 0.22 | 0.01 | 0.03 | 1.9 | 0.03 | 0.6 | 0.0 | | 6 | 0.0 | 0.2 | 1 | 0.0 | 11 | 11 | | 39 | 0.06 |
| 47585 | 1 ea | Cheesecake Bar, Pillsbury | 32 | 170 | 4 | 1.1 | 20.0 | 0.2 | 12.7 | 7.1 | 9.5 | 3.2 | | | | | [illegible] | 64 | 13 | | | | | | | | | | | 0.1 | | | 17 | | 0.5 | | | | | | 47 | |
| 47533 | 1 ea | Frosty, Archway | 28 | 120 | 12 | 1.2 | 18.1 | 0.2 | 9.3 | 8.6 | 4.8 | 1.6 | 1.6 | 0.3 | | | 0 | 0.2 | 0.04 | | | | 0.07 | 0.06 | 0.55 | | | 16.6 | | 0.0 | | | 12 | | 0.5 | | | | 26 | | 102 | |
| 47346 | 1 ea | Nut Crunch, Pepperidge Farm | 10 | 55 | | 0.6 | 5.8 | 0.6 | 2.3 | 2.9 | 2.9 | 0.6 | 1.5 | 0.5 | | | 5 | 0 | 0 | 0 | 0 | 0 | 0.02 | 0.01 | 0.13 | | | | | 0.0 | | | 0 | | 0.1 | | | | | | 19 | |
| 47497 | 1 ea | Snaps, Archway | 6 | 29 | 5 | 0.3 | 3.9 | 0.1 | 1.7 | 2.1 | 1.4 | 0.3 | 0.5 | 0.1 | | | [illegible] | 2 | 0.4 | | | | 0.02 | 0.01 | 0.14 | | | 4.5 | | 0.0 | | | 2 | | 0.1 | | | | 5 | | 23 | |
| 47477 | 1 ea | Macadamia Nut cookie, w/White Choc, Pepp Farm | 26 | 130 | 2 | 2.0 | 16.0 | 1.0 | 7.0 | 8.0 | 7.0 | 3.0 | | | | | 15 | 0 | 0 | 0 | 0 | 0 | 0.09 | 0.03 | 0.80 | | | | | 0.0 | | | 20 | | 0.4 | | | | | | 110 | |

| Code | Amount | Description | Basic Components | | | | | | | | | Additional Fats | | | | | | Vit A & Components | | | | | Vitamins | | | | | | | | | | Minerals | | | | | | | | | |
|---|---|---|---|---|---|---|---|---|---|---|---|---|---|---|---|---|---|---|---|---|---|---|---|---|---|---|---|---|---|---|---|---|---|---|---|---|---|---|---|---|---|---|
| | | | Weight (g) | Calories | % Water | Protein (g) | Carbs (g) | Fiber (g) | Sugar (g) | Other Carbs (g) | Fat (g) | Sat Fat (g) | Mono Fat (g) | Poly Fat (g) | Omega 3 (g) | Omega 6 (g) | Choles (mg) | Vit A (IU) | Vit A (RE) | Retinol (RE) | Carotenoids (RE) | Beta Carotene (mcg) | Thiamin (mg) | Riboflavin (mg) | Niacin (NE) | Vit B6 (mg) | Vit B12 (mcg) | Folate (mcg) | Panto (mg) | Vit C (mg) | Vit D (mg) | Vit E (α TE) | Calcium (mg) | Copper (mg) | Iron (mg) | Magnes (mg) | Mang (mg) | Phos (mg) | Potassium (mg) | Selenium (mcg) | Sodium (mg) | Zinc (mg) |
| 47042 | 1 ea | Macaroon Coconut cookie, avg | 24 | 97 | 11 | 0.9 | 17.3 | 0.4 | 16.2 | 0.7 | 3.0 | 2.7 | 0.1 | 0.0 | 0.00 | 0.03 | 0 | 0 | 0 | 0 | 0 | 0 | 0.00 | 0.03 | 0.03 | 0.02 | 0.01 | 1.0 | 0.06 | 0.0 | 0.0 | | 2 | 0.0 | 0.2 | 5 | 0.2 | 10 | 37 | 2.5 | 59 | 0.17 |
| 47526 | 1 ea | Macaroon Coconut cookie, Archway | 23 | 111 | 11 | 0.9 | 12.9 | 0.5 | 9.9 | 2.4 | 6.4 | 5.7 | 0.4 | 0.1 | | | 0 | 0 | 0 | 0 | 0 | 0 | 0.01 | 0.01 | 0.07 | | | 1.2 | | 0.0 | | | 4 | | 0.4 | | | | 60 | | 40 | |
| 47046 | 1 ea | Marshmallow cookie, w/choc coating, avg | 13 | 55 | 10 | 0.5 | 8.8 | 0.3 | 6.9 | 1.6 | 2.2 | 0.6 | 1.2 | 0.3 | 0.01 | 0.24 | 0 | 0.6 | 0.1 | | | | 0.01 | 0.03 | 0.10 | 0.01 | 0.02 | 2.5 | 0.06 | 0.0 | 0.0 | | 6 | 0.0 | 0.3 | 5 | 0.0 | 13 | 24 | 0.6 | 22 | 0.08 |
| 47197 | 1 ea | Marshmallow cookie, Mallopuffs, Sunshine | 19 | 70 | | 1.3 | 12.0 | | | | 2.0 | 1.7 | | | | | | | | | | | | | | | | | | | | | | | | | | | | | 37 | |
| | | Molasses cookies | | | | | | | | | | | | | | | | | | | | | | | | | | | | | | | | | | | | | | | | |
| 47109 | 1 ea | Avg | 15 | 65 | 6 | 0.8 | 11.1 | 0.1 | 5.6 | 5.3 | 1.9 | 0.5 | 1.1 | 0.3 | 0.01 | 0.25 | 0 | 0 | 0 | 0 | 0 | 0 | 0.05 | 0.04 | 0.45 | 0.02 | 0.00 | 11.1 | 0.06 | 0.0 | 0.0 | | 11 | 0.1 | 1.0 | 8 | 0.2 | 14 | 52 | 0.8 | 69 | 0.07 |
| 47646 | 1 ea | Big, Grandma's | 39 | 160 | 9 | 2.0 | 29.0 | 1.0 | 12.0 | 16.0 | 4.0 | 1.0 | | | | | 5 | | | | | | | | | | | | | | | | | | | | | | | | 260 | |
| 47528 | 1 ea | Dark, Archway | 28 | 115 | 8 | 1.2 | 20.1 | 0.3 | 10.2 | 9.6 | 3.4 | 0.8 | 1.3 | 0.2 | | | 0 | | | | | | 0.08 | 0.06 | 0.75 | | | 19.2 | | 0.0 | | | 13 | | 1.2 | | | | 95 | | 154 | |
| 47537 | 1 ea | Iced, Archway | 28 | 114 | 11 | 1.0 | 19.5 | 0.3 | 10.0 | 9.2 | 3.6 | 1.1 | 1.1 | 0.5 | | | 0 | 0.08 | 0.02 | | | | 0.08 | 0.06 | 0.74 | | | | | 0.0 | | | 7 | | 1.2 | | | | 21 | | 130 | |
| 47546 | 1 ea | Old Fashioned, Archway | 28 | 113 | 10 | 1.3 | 19.9 | 0.3 | 10.6 | 8.9 | 3.2 | 0.8 | 1.2 | 0.2 | | | 9 | 13 | 3 | | | | 0.08 | 0.07 | 0.74 | | | | | 0.0 | | | 10 | | 1.3 | | | | 32 | | 148 | |
| 47558 | 1 ea | Soft Drop, Archway | 28 | 110 | | 1.0 | 18.0 | 0.5 | 6.0 | 11.5 | 3.5 | 1.0 | | | | | 2 | 0 | 0 | 0 | 0 | 0 | | | | | | | | 0.0 | | | 0 | | 2.7 | | | | | | 160 | |
| | | Oatmeal cookies | | | | | | | | | | | | | | | | | | | | | | | | | | | | | | | | | | | | | | | | |
| 47047 | 1 ea | Avg | 18 | 81 | 6 | 1.1 | 12.4 | 0.5 | 6.7 | 5.1 | 3.3 | 0.8 | 1.8 | 0.5 | 0.02 | 0.43 | 0 | 3 | 0.4 | 0.4 | 0 | | 0.05 | 0.04 | 0.40 | 0.01 | 0.00 | 8.1 | 0.07 | 0.1 | 0.0 | | 7 | 0.0 | 0.5 | 6 | 0.2 | 25 | 26 | 1.8 | 69 | 0.14 |
| 47541 | 1 ea | Archway | 27 | 115 | 10 | 1.6 | 18.0 | 0.8 | 8.7 | 8.6 | 4.1 | 0.9 | 1.5 | 0.4 | | | 4 | 7 | 1.5 | | | | 0.08 | 0.05 | 0.50 | | | | | 0.0 | | | 8 | | 0.6 | | | | 50 | | 93 | |
| 47681 | 1 oz | Dry Mix, avg | 28 | 129 | 5 | 1.8 | 18.8 | 0.8 | 10.3 | 7.8 | 5.4 | 1.3 | 3.0 | 0.8 | 0.04 | 0.74 | 0 | 8 | 0.6 | | | | 0.04 | 0.04 | 0.36 | 0.01 | 0.00 | 14.0 | 0.13 | 0.0 | 0.0 | | 7 | 0.1 | 0.6 | 13 | 0.3 | 46 | 51 | 3.0 | 132 | 0.22 |
| 47612 | 1 oz | Fat Free, avg | 28 | 91 | 12 | 1.7 | 22.0 | 2.0 | | | 0.4 | 0.1 | 0.1 | 0.2 | 0.01 | 0.17 | 0 | 0 | 0 | 0 | 0 | 0 | 0.04 | 0.07 | 0.33 | 0.02 | 0.00 | 10.1 | 0.10 | 0.0 | | | 11 | 0.1 | 0.6 | 10 | 0.2 | 29 | 59 | 2.2 | 83 | 0.18 |
| 47256 | 1 ea | Homestyle, Nabisco | 13 | 60 | | 0.5 | 9.0 | 0.5 | 3.5 | 5.0 | 2.5 | 0.5 | 1.0 | 0.0 | 0.00 | 0.00 | 0 | | | | | | | | | | | | | | | | | | 0.2 | | | | 15 | | 60 | |
| 47539 | 1 ea | Iced, Archway | 28 | 123 | 10 | 1.5 | 18.5 | 0.6 | 9.8 | 8.0 | 4.9 | 1.5 | 1.5 | 0.7 | | | 3 | 5 | 1 | | | | 0.07 | 0.04 | 0.44 | | | | | 0.0 | | | 8 | | 0.5 | | | | 46 | | 93 | |
| 47465 | 1 ea | Irish, Pepperidge Farm | 9 | 42 | 1 | 0.6 | 6.1 | 0.6 | 2.3 | 3.2 | 1.9 | 0.5 | | | | | 1 | 0 | 0 | 0 | 0 | 0 | 0.02 | 0.01 | 0.13 | | | | | 0.0 | | | 0 | | 0.1 | | | | | | 22 | |
| 47567 | 1 ea | Mini, Archway | 2 | 10 | | 0.1 | 1.3 | 0.1 | 0.5 | 0.7 | 0.5 | 0.1 | | | | | 0 | 0 | 0 | 0 | 0 | 0 | | | | | | | | 0.0 | | | 0 | | 0.0 | | | | | | 9 | |
| 47051 | 1 ea | Prep f/Dry Mix, avg | 16 | 74 | 6 | 1.2 | 10.4 | 0.6 | 5.7 | 4.1 | 3.1 | 0.8 | 1.7 | 0.4 | 0.02 | 0.42 | 7 | 13 | 3.4 | 3.3 | 0.03 | | 0.04 | 0.03 | 0.18 | 0.01 | 0.01 | 1.8 | 0.06 | 0.0 | 0.0 | | 5 | 0.0 | 0.4 | 8 | 0.2 | 28 | 30 | 1.6 | 75 | 0.14 |
| 47048 | 1 ea | Soft Type, avg | 15 | 61 | 11 | 0.9 | 9.9 | 0.4 | 5.4 | 4.1 | 2.2 | 0.5 | 1.2 | 0.3 | 0.02 | 0.31 | 1 | 5 | 1 | 0.7 | 0.01 | | 0.03 | 0.03 | 0.27 | 0.01 | 0.00 | 5.1 | 0.07 | 0.0 | 0.0 | | 14 | 0.1 | 0.4 | 5 | 0.1 | 31 | 20 | 1.6 | 52 | 0.07 |
| 47200 | 1 ea | Soft & Chewy, Tastykake | 39 | 175 | 7 | 2.0 | 26.0 | 1.0 | 11.5 | 13.5 | 7.0 | 1.3 | | | | | 5 | 0 | 0 | 0 | 0 | 0 | | | | | | | | 0.0 | | | 10 | | 0.9 | | | | | | 145 | |
| | | Oatmeal Raisin cookies | | | | | | | | | | | | | | | | | | | | | | | | | | | | | | | | | | | | | | | | |
| 47496 | 1 ea | Archway | 28 | 110 | | 2.0 | 19.0 | 0.5 | 13.0 | 5.5 | 4.0 | 1.0 | | | | | 2 | 0 | 0 | 0 | 0 | 0 | | | | | | | | 0.0 | | | 0 | | 1.1 | | | | | | 115 | |
| 47573 | 1 ea | Bar, Tastykake | 43 | 190 | 7 | 3.0 | 28.0 | 1.0 | 13.0 | 14.0 | 7.0 | 1.5 | | | | | 15 | 0 | 0 | 0 | 0 | 0 | | | | | | | | 0.0 | | | 20 | | 1.1 | | | | | | 180 | |
| 47543 | 1 ea | Bran, Archway | 28 | 115 | 11 | 1.6 | 18.8 | 0.9 | 10.0 | 7.9 | 3.8 | 0.9 | 1.4 | 0.3 | | | 3 | 7 | 1.4 | | | | 0.08 | 0.04 | 0.48 | | | | | 0.0 | | | 9 | | 0.6 | | | | 65 | | 106 | |
| 47023 | 1 ea | Dietetic, avg | 11 | 48 | 10 | 0.7 | 7.0 | 0.3 | | | 2.0 | 0.5 | 0.9 | 0.5 | | | 0 | 0.11 | 0.02 | | | | 0.03 | 0.01 | 0.11 | 0.00 | 0.01 | 1.3 | 0.02 | 0.0 | | | 2 | 0.0 | 0.2 | 3 | 0.1 | 15 | 18 | 1.1 | 0 | 0.10 |
| 47500 | 1 ea | Fat Free, Archway | 28 | 96 | 13 | 1.3 | 22.0 | 0.9 | 12.5 | 8.7 | 0.4 | 0.1 | 0.2 | 0.2 | | | 0 | 0.6 | 0.1 | | | | 0.07 | 0.04 | 0.46 | | | 13.2 | | 0.0 | | | 11 | | 0.9 | | | | 79 | | 149 | |
| 47212 | 1 ea | Fat Free, Entenmann's | 12 | 40 | 18 | 0.5 | 9.0 | 0.3 | 5.5 | 3.3 | 0.0 | 0.0 | 0.0 | 0.0 | 0.00 | 0.00 | 0 | 0 | 0 | 0 | 0 | 0 | | | | | | | | 0.0 | | | 0 | | 0.0 | | | | 30 | | 60 | |
| 47306 | 1 ea | Fat Free, Health Valley | 11 | 33 | 16 | 0.7 | 8.0 | 1.0 | 3.7 | 3.3 | 0.0 | 0.0 | 0.0 | 0.0 | 0.00 | 0.00 | 0 | 167 | 33 | | | | | | | | | | | 0.8 | | | 0 | | 0.2 | | | | | | 17 | |
| 47003 | 1 ea | Prep f/Recipe, avg | 15 | 65 | 6 | 1.0 | 10.3 | 0.5 | 6.1 | 3.7 | 2.4 | 0.5 | 1.0 | 0.8 | 0.03 | 0.72 | 5 | 96 | 25 | 23 | 2 | | 0.04 | 0.02 | 0.19 | 0.01 | 0.01 | 4.5 | 0.05 | 0.1 | 0.0 | | 15 | 0.0 | 0.4 | 6 | 0.1 | 24 | 36 | 2.3 | 81 | 0.13 |
| 47162 | 1 ea | Snackwells | 28 | 115 | 7 | 1.7 | 21.0 | 0.9 | 10.4 | 9.7 | 2.7 | 0.3 | 0.8 | 0.6 | | | 0 | 7 | 1.4 | | | | 0.05 | 0.06 | 0.65 | 0.03 | 0.01 | 0.0 | | 0.2 | | | 21 | 0.0 | 0.7 | 10 | | 74 | 80 | | 140 | 0.19 |
| 47240 | 1 ea | Weight Watchers | 15 | 60 | 13 | 1.0 | 11.0 | 0.5 | 6.5 | 4.0 | 1.0 | 0.0 | | | 0.00 | 0.00 | 0 | 0 | 0 | 0 | 0 | 0 | | | | | | | | 0.0 | | | 0 | | 0.2 | | | | 40 | | 45 | |
| 47049 | 1 ea | Without sodium, w/fructose, avg | 7 | 31 | 6 | 0.3 | 4.9 | 0.2 | 2.9 | 1.8 | 1.3 | 0.2 | 0.5 | 0.5 | 0.03 | 0.44 | 0 | 0.6 | 0.07 | 0.06 | 0.01 | | 0.03 | 0.01 | 0.23 | 0.00 | 0.00 | 3.6 | 0.02 | 0.0 | 0.0 | | 4 | 0.0 | 0.3 | 1 | 0.0 | 9 | 12 | 0.3 | 1 | 0.03 |
| 47564 | 1 ea | Orange Frosty cookie, Archway | 28 | 122 | 11 | 1.3 | 18.2 | 0.2 | 9.5 | 8.4 | 4.9 | 1.5 | 1.6 | 0.6 | | | 0 | 0.2 | 0.04 | | | | 0.07 | 0.06 | 0.52 | | | 16.5 | | 0.0 | | | 12 | | 0.5 | | | | 26 | | 101 | |
| | | Peanut Butter cookie | | | | | | | | | | | | | | | | | | | | | | | | | | | | | | | | | | | | | | | | |
| 49102 | 1 ea | Avg | 15 | 72 | 6 | 1.4 | 8.8 | 0.3 | 4.8 | 3.8 | 3.5 | 0.7 | 1.9 | 0.8 | 0.01 | 0.82 | 0 | 1 | 0.4 | 0.3 | 0.1 | | 0.03 | 0.03 | 0.64 | 0.01 | 0.01 | 9.3 | 0.09 | 0.0 | 0.0 | | 5 | 0.0 | 0.4 | 7 | 0.0 | 13 | 25 | 0.9 | 62 | 0.08 |
| 47549 | 1 ea | Archway | 28 | 134 | 6 | 2.5 | 16.4 | 0.8 | 9.1 | 6.5 | 6.8 | 1.5 | 2.9 | 1.2 | | | 10 | 17 | 3 | | | | 0.07 | 0.06 | 1.22 | | | | | 0.0 | | | 10 | | 0.8 | | | | 59 | | 113 | |
| 47571 | 1 ea | Bar, Tastykake | 43 | 240 | | 2.0 | 18.0 | 0.5 | 17.0 | 0.5 | 11.0 | 3.0 | | | | | 5 | 0 | 0 | 0 | 0 | 0 | | | | | | | | 0.0 | | | 0 | | 0.7 | | | | | | 110 | |
| 47649 | 1 ea | Big, Grandma's | 39 | 190 | 9 | 4.0 | 22.0 | 1.0 | 10.0 | 11.0 | 9.0 | 2.0 | | | | | 5 | | | | | | | | | | | | | | | | | | | | | | | | 180 | |
| 47010 | 1 ea | Prep f/Recipe, avg | 20 | 95 | 6 | 1.8 | 11.8 | 0.4 | 6.5 | 4.9 | 4.8 | 0.9 | 2.2 | 1.4 | 0.04 | 1.40 | 6 | 120 | 31 | 29 | 2 | | 0.04 | 0.04 | 0.70 | 0.02 | 0.02 | 11.0 | 0.07 | 0.0 | 0.0 | | 8 | 0.0 | 0.4 | 8 | 0.1 | 23 | 46 | 3.0 | 104 | 0.16 |
| 47058 | 1 ea | Prep f/Refrig dough | 12 | 60 | 4 | 1.1 | 6.9 | 0.1 | 3.8 | 2.9 | 3.3 | 0.8 | 1.8 | 0.6 | 0.02 | 0.57 | 4 | 6 | 2 | 2 | 0.1 | | 0.02 | 0.02 | 0.49 | 0.01 | 0.01 | 1.1 | 0.04 | 0.0 | 0.0 | | 13 | 0.0 | 0.2 | 5 | 0.1 | 32 | 41 | 0.6 | 52 | 0.09 |
| 47057 | 1 ea | Refrig Dough, avg | 16 | 73 | 13 | 1.3 | 8.3 | 0.2 | 4.6 | 3.5 | 4.0 | 0.9 | 2.1 | 0.8 | 0.02 | 0.75 | 4 | 8 | 2 | 2 | 0.2 | | 0.03 | 0.03 | 0.66 | 0.02 | 0.01 | 9.1 | 0.06 | 0.0 | 0.0 | | 16 | 0.0 | 0.3 | 6 | 0.1 | 39 | 49 | 0.8 | 64 | 0.11 |
| 47056 | 1 ea | Soft Type, avg | 15 | 69 | 12 | 0.8 | 8.7 | 0.3 | 4.8 | 3.6 | 3.7 | 0.9 | 2.1 | 0.5 | 0.01 | 0.46 | 0 | 0 | 0 | 0 | 0 | 0 | 0.04 | 0.02 | 0.32 | 0.00 | 0.00 | 10.1 | 0.05 | 0.0 | 0.0 | | 2 | 0.0 | 0.1 | 5 | 0.1 | 13 | 16 | 0.7 | 50 | 0.08 |
| | | Peanut Butter Sandwich cookies | | | | | | | | | | | | | | | | | | | | | | | | | | | | | | | | | | | | | | | | |
| 47059 | 1 ea | Avg | 14 | 67 | 3 | 1.2 | 9.2 | 0.3 | 4.4 | 4.6 | 3.0 | 0.7 | 1.6 | 0.5 | 0.01 | 0.52 | 0 | 0.6 | 0.1 | | | | 0.05 | 0.04 | 0.52 | 0.02 | 0.03 | 6.2 | 0.13 | 0.0 | 0.0 | | 7 | 0.0 | 0.4 | 7 | 0.1 | 26 | 27 | 1.1 | 52 | 0.15 |
| 47060 | 1 ea | Low Sod, w/fructose, avg | 10 | 54 | 4 | 1.0 | 5.1 | 0.2 | 3.1 | 1.8 | 3.4 | 0.5 | 1.5 | 1.2 | 0.05 | 1.14 | 0 | 0 | 0 | 0 | 0 | 0 | 0.03 | 0.01 | 0.53 | 0.01 | 0.00 | 5.4 | 0.05 | 0.0 | 0.0 | | 4 | 0.0 | 0.3 | 5 | 0.1 | 15 | 29 | 0.3 | 41 | 0.10 |
| 47252 | 1 ea | Nutter Butter | 14 | 65 | | 1.5 | 9.5 | 0.5 | 4.0 | 5.0 | 3.0 | 0.5 | 1.3 | 0.5 | | | 1 | | | | | | | | | | | | | | | | | | 0.4 | | | | 28 | | 55 | |
| | | Pecan cookies | | | | | | | | | | | | | | | | | | | | | | | | | | | | | | | | | | | | | | | | |
| 47338 | 1 ea | Caramel, soft bkd, Pepperidge Farm | 26 | 130 | | 2.0 | 16.0 | 0.5 | 8.0 | 7.5 | 7.0 | 1.5 | 4.0 | 0.5 | | | 20 | 0 | 0 | 0 | 0 | 0 | 0.06 | 0.03 | 0.80 | | | | | 0.0 | | | 20 | | 0.4 | | | | | | | |
| 47551 | 1 ea | Ice Box, Archway | 28 | 140 | 6 | 1.3 | 17.4 | 0.3 | 8.0 | 9.0 | 7.3 | 1.6 | 3.0 | 0.6 | | | 7 | 11 | 2 | | | | 0.08 | 0.06 | 0.66 | | | 20.1 | | 0.0 | | | 5 | | 0.6 | | | | 19 | | 88 | |
| 47553 | 1 ea | Pecan Crunch, Archway | 5 | 25 | | 0.3 | 3.0 | 0.0 | 1.3 | 1.7 | 1.3 | 0.3 | | | | | 2 | 0 | 0 | 0 | 0 | 0 | | | | | | | | 0.0 | | | 0 | | 0.1 | | | | | | 20 | |
| 47062 | 1 ea | Shortbread, avg | 14 | 76 | 3 | 0.7 | 8.2 | 0.3 | 7.0 | 0.9 | 4.6 | 1.1 | 2.6 | 0.6 | 0.03 | 0.55 | 5 | 0.42 | 0.14 | 0.12 | 0.02 | | 0.04 | 0.03 | 0.35 | 0.00 | 0.00 | 8.8 | 0.05 | 0.0 | 0.0 | | 4 | 0.0 | 0.3 | 3 | 0.1 | 12 | 10 | 0.4 | 39 | 0.08 |
| 47351 | 1 ea | Shortbread, Old Fash, Pepperidge Farm | 13 | 70 | | 0.5 | 7.0 | 0.5 | 2.0 | 4.5 | 4.5 | 1.3 | 2.5 | 0.5 | | | 1 | 0 | 0 | 0 | 0 | 0 | 0.03 | 0.02 | 0.20 | | | | | 0.0 | | | 0 | | 0.2 | | | | | | 42 | |
| 47569 | 1 ea | Pineapple cookie, Filled, Archway | 26 | 100 | | 1.0 | 16.0 | 1.0 | 8.0 | 7.0 | 4.0 | 1.0 | | | | | 5 | 0 | 0 | 0 | 0 | 0 | | | | | | | | 0.0 | | | 0 | | 0.7 | | | | | | 75 | |
| | | Raisin cookies | | | | | | | | | | | | | | | | | | | | | | | | | | | | | | | | | | | | | | | | |
| 48091 | 1 ea | Bakes, fat free, Health Valley | 27 | 63 | 52 | 0.5 | 9.4 | 0.3 | 3.9 | 5.3 | 2.7 | 0.5 | 1.1 | 1.0 | 0.06 | 0.89 | 0 | 38 | 9 | 6 | 3 | | 0.00 | 0.01 | 0.08 | 0.01 | 0.00 | 5.9 | 0.04 | 0.7 | 0.0 | | 2 | 0.0 | 0.1 | 1 | 0.0 | 6 | 14 | 0.4 | 88 | 0.04 |
| 47290 | 1 ea | Fruit Bar, Health Valley | 42 | 140 | 8 | 2.0 | 35.0 | 3.0 | 17.0 | 15.0 | 0.0 | 0.0 | 0.0 | 0.0 | 0.00 | 0.00 | 0 | 500 | 100 | | | | | | | | | | | 0.0 | | | 0 | | 3.6 | | | | | | 5 | |
| 47196 | 1 ea | Fruit Biscuits, Sunshine | 29 | 123 | | 2.0 | 23.5 | | | | 2.6 | 0.5 | | | | | | | | | | | | | | | | | | | | | | | | | | | | | 74 | |
| 47310 | 1 ea | Jumbo, Health Valley | 25 | 80 | 16 | 2.0 | 19.0 | 3.0 | 9.0 | 7.0 | 0.0 | 0.0 | 0.0 | 0.0 | 0.00 | 0.00 | 0 | 100 | 20 | | | | | | | | | | | 1.2 | | | 20 | | 1.1 | | | | | | 35 | |
| 47061 | 1 ea | Soft Type, avg | 15 | 60 | 13 | 0.6 | 10.2 | 0.2 | 5.0 | 5.1 | 2.0 | 0.5 | 1.1 | 0.3 | 0.01 | 0.25 | 0 | 1 | 0 | | | | 0.03 | 0.03 | 0.30 | 0.01 | 0.00 | 6.6 | 0.04 | 0.1 | 0.0 | | 7 | 0.1 | 0.3 | 3 | 0.0 | 12 | 21 | 0.4 | 51 | 0.05 |
| | | Raspberry cookies | | | | | | | | | | | | | | | | | | | | | | | | | | | | | | | | | | | | | | | | |
| 47301 | 1 ea | Bakes, fat free, Health Valley | 38 | 110 | 25 | 2.0 | 26.0 | 3.0 | 13.0 | 10.0 | 0.0 | 0.0 | 0.0 | 0.0 | 0.00 | 0.00 | 0 | 500 | 100 | | | | | | | | | | | 1.2 | | | 20 | | 0.7 | | | | | | 25 | |
| 47600 | 1 ea | Chantilly Hazelnut, Pepperidge Farm | 17 | 80 | 7 | 0.5 | 12.0 | 0.5 | 7.0 | 4.5 | 3.0 | 0.5 | | | | | 5 | 0 | 0 | 0 | 0 | 0 | 0.03 | 0.00 | 0.00 | | | | | 0.0 | | | 0 | | 0.4 | | | | | | 50 | |
| 47555 | 1 ea | Filled, Archway | 28 | 113 | 14 | 1.4 | 18.3 | 0.4 | 9.2 | 8.7 | 3.9 | 1.5 | 1.2 | 0.2 | | | 8 | 12 | 2 | | | | 0.09 | 0.06 | 0.54 | | | | | 0.0 | | | 7 | | 0.6 | | | | 35 | | 94 | |
| 47121 | 1 ea | Fruit Center, fat free, Health Valley | 25 | 70 | 18 | 2.0 | 18.0 | 2.0 | 9.0 | 7.0 | 0.0 | 0.0 | 0.0 | 0.0 | 0.00 | 0.00 | 0 | 500 | 100 | | | | | | | | | | | 1.2 | | | 20 | | 0.4 | | | | | | 20 | |
| 47130 | 1 ea | Jumbo, fat free, Health Valley | 25 | 80 | 14 | 2.0 | 19.0 | 3.0 | 9.0 | 7.0 | 0.0 | 0.0 | 0.0 | 0.0 | 0.00 | 0.00 | 0 | 100 | 20 | | | | | | | | | | | 1.2 | | | 20 | | 1.1 | | | | | | 35 | |
| 62418 | 1 ea | Menu Magic | 49 | 200 | 15 | 6.1 | 27.0 | 1.0 | 16.0 | 10.0 | 8.0 | 0.0 | | | | | 4 | 0 | 0 | 0 | 0 | 0 | | | | | | | | 0.0 | | | 20 | | 1.1 | | | 90 | 90 | | 280 | |
| 47613 | 1 ea | Oatmeal, fat free, Archway | 28 | 98 | 11 | 1.3 | 22.5 | 0.9 | 12.9 | 8.7 | 0.4 | 0.1 | 0.2 | 0.2 | | | 0 | 0.8 | 0.2 | | | | 0.08 | 0.04 | 0.46 | | | 13.2 | | 0.0 | | | 11 | | 0.9 | | | | 81 | | 150 | |

| Code | Amount | Description | Weight (g) | Calories | % Water | Protein (g) | Carbs (g) | Fiber (g) | Sugar (g) | Other Carbs (g) | Fat (g) | Sat Fat (g) | Mono Fat (g) | Poly Fat (g) | Omega 3 (g) | Omega 6 (g) | Choles (mg) |
|---|---|---|---|---|---|---|---|---|---|---|---|---|---|---|---|---|---|
| | | **Basic Components** | | | | | | | | | | **Additional Fats** | | | | | |
| 47241 | 1 ea | Smart Snackers | 20 | 71 | 14 | 1.0 | 16.2 | 0.0 | 7.1 | 9.1 | 0.0 | 0.0 | 0.0 | 0.0 | 0.00 | 0.00 | 0 |
| | | Shortbread cookies | | | | | | | | | | | | | | | |
| 47665 | 1 ea | Avg | 15 | 75 | 3 | 1.1 | 9.8 | 0.3 | | | 3.5 | 0.9 | 1.9 | 0.4 | | | 5 |
| 47603 | 1 ea | Highland, Pepperidge Farm | 14 | 73 | | 13.0 | 2.6 | 1.0 | | | 3.6 | 2.6 | | | | | 9 |
| 47254 | 1 ea | Lorna Doone | 7 | 34 | | 0.5 | 4.6 | 0.0 | 1.4 | 3.1 | 1.7 | 0.4 | 0.6 | 0.1 | | | 1 |
| 47348 | 1 ea | Old Fashioned, Pepperidge Farm | 13 | 70 | | 1.0 | 8.0 | 0.3 | 2.5 | 5.3 | 3.5 | 1.3 | 1.8 | 0.3 | | | 5 |
| 47011 | 1 ea | Snickerdoodle cookie, avg | 20 | 81 | 18 | 0.9 | 11.8 | 0.4 | 6.4 | 5.0 | 3.5 | 2.1 | 1.0 | 0.2 | 0.05 | 0.10 | 9 |
| | | Strawberry cookies | | | | | | | | | | | | | | | |
| 47299 | 1 ea | Bakes, fat free, Health Valley | 38 | 110 | 25 | 2.0 | 26.0 | 3.0 | 13.0 | 10.0 | 0.0 | 0.0 | 0.0 | 0.0 | 0.00 | 0.00 | 0 |
| 47560 | 1 ea | Fruit Filled, Archway | 28 | 113 | 15 | 1.4 | 18.1 | 0.4 | 8.9 | 8.8 | 3.9 | 1.5 | 1.2 | 0.2 | | | 8 |
| 90089 | 1 ea | Fruit Filled, Pepperidge Farm | 11 | 48 | | 0.7 | 7.6 | 0.2 | 6.9 | 0.5 | 1.7 | 0.7 | 0.9 | 0.0 | 0.00 | 0.00 | 3 |
| | | Sugar cookies | | | | | | | | | | | | | | | |
| 47064 | 1 ea | Avg | 15 | 72 | 5 | 0.8 | 10.2 | 0.1 | 4.4 | 5.7 | 3.2 | 0.8 | 1.8 | 0.4 | 0.02 | 0.38 | 8 |
| 47561 | 1 ea | Archway | 28 | 120 | | 2.0 | 20.0 | 0.0 | 11.0 | 9.0 | 4.0 | 1.0 | | | | | 2 |
| 47263 | 1 ea | Biscos Wafers, Nabisco | 4 | 20 | | 0.1 | 3.0 | 0.1 | 1.9 | 1.1 | 0.9 | 0.2 | 0.4 | 0.0 | 0.00 | 0.00 | 0 |
| 47069 | 1 ea | Creme filled wafer, avg | 9 | 46 | 1 | 0.4 | 6.3 | 0.1 | 3.0 | 3.3 | 2.2 | 0.3 | 0.9 | 0.8 | 0.06 | 0.77 | 0 |
| 47347 | 1 ea | Old Fashioned, Pepperidge Farm | 10 | 47 | | 0.7 | 6.7 | 0.2 | 3.3 | 3.2 | 2.0 | 0.5 | 1.2 | 0.2 | | | 5 |
| 47004 | 1 ea | Prep f/Refrig Dough, avg | 12 | 58 | 5 | 0.6 | 7.9 | 0.1 | 3.4 | 4.4 | 2.8 | 0.7 | 1.6 | 0.3 | 0.02 | 0.33 | 4 |
| 47066 | 1 ea | Refrig Dough, avg | 16 | 70 | 14 | 0.7 | 9.4 | 0.1 | 4.0 | 5.3 | 3.3 | 0.8 | 1.9 | 0.4 | 0.02 | 0.40 | 5 |
| 47559 | 1 ea | Soft, Archway | 28 | 115 | 10 | 1.4 | 19.3 | 0.3 | 8.8 | 10.2 | 3.6 | 0.9 | 1.3 | 0.2 | | | 6 |
| 47070 | 1 ea | Without Sodium, w/fructose, avg | 4 | 20 | 4 | 0.1 | 2.6 | 0.1 | 1.2 | 1.4 | 1.0 | 0.2 | 0.4 | 0.4 | 0.03 | 0.36 | 0 |
| | | Vanilla Sandwich cookies | | | | | | | | | | | | | | | |
| 47071 | 1 ea | Avg | 10 | 48 | 2 | 0.5 | 7.2 | 0.2 | 4.0 | 3.1 | 2.0 | 0.3 | 0.8 | 0.8 | 0.05 | 0.70 | 0 |
| 47024 | 1 ea | Dietetic, avg | 11 | 50 | 13 | 0.5 | 6.1 | 0.1 | | | 2.7 | 0.7 | 1.2 | 0.7 | | | 0 |
| 47239 | 1 ea | Smart Snackers | 15 | 70 | 2 | 0.5 | 12.5 | 0.5 | 5.0 | 7.0 | 1.5 | 0.5 | | | | | 0 |
| 47160 | 1 ea | Snackwell's | 13 | 55 | 4 | 0.6 | 10.5 | 0.3 | 5.0 | 5.3 | 1.2 | 0.3 | 0.4 | 0.1 | | | 0 |
| | | Vanilla Wafer cookies | | | | | | | | | | | | | | | |
| 47008 | 1 ea | Avg | 4 | 18 | 5 | 0.2 | 2.9 | 0.1 | 1.7 | 1.2 | 0.6 | 0.2 | 0.3 | 0.2 | 0.01 | 0.15 | 2 |
| 47562 | 1 ea | Archway | 6 | 26 | | 0.4 | 4.4 | 0.0 | 3.0 | 1.4 | 0.8 | 0.2 | | | | | 1 |
| 49065 | 1 ea | Keebler | 4 | 20 | | 0.2 | 2.6 | 0.1 | 1.2 | 1.4 | 0.9 | 0.2 | | | | | 0 |
| 47171 | 1 ea | Nilla Wafers, Nabisco | 4 | 18 | | 0.1 | 3.0 | 0.1 | 1.5 | 1.4 | 0.6 | 0.1 | 0.2 | 0.0 | 0.00 | 0.00 | 0 |
| | | Variety Cookie Assortments | | | | | | | | | | | | | | | |
| 47505 | 1 ea | Bells & Stars cookie, Archway | 10 | 52 | | 0.3 | 6.6 | 0.2 | 2.4 | 4.0 | 2.4 | 0.5 | | | | | 2 |
| 47464 | 1 ea | Cafe Favorites cookie, Pepperidge Farm | 7 | 36 | 2 | 0.3 | 4.7 | 0.1 | 2.3 | 2.2 | 1.8 | 0.6 | | | | | 3 |
| 47463 | 1 ea | Dessert Favorites cookie, Pepperidge Farm | 11 | 57 | 1 | 0.7 | 7.0 | 0.3 | 3.7 | 3.0 | 3.0 | 1.0 | | | | | 2 |
| 47473 | 1 ea | Distinctive Collection cookie, Pepperidge Farm | 11 | 55 | 2 | 0.7 | 7.2 | 0.3 | 3.1 | 3.3 | 2.8 | 1.0 | | | | | 3 |
| 47508 | 1 ea | Holiday Pack cookie, Archway | 10 | 50 | | 0.3 | 6.3 | 0.2 | 3.0 | 3.2 | 2.7 | 0.5 | | | | | 1 |
| 47576 | 1 ea | Holiday Tub cookie, Tastykake | 8 | 40 | | 0.5 | 5.5 | 0.3 | 2.3 | 3.0 | 2.0 | 0.4 | | | | | 0 |
| 47448 | 1 ea | Madallion Au Beurre Biscuit, Pepperidge Farm | 8 | 4 | 2 | 0.5 | 6.1 | 0.1 | 2.7 | 3.3 | 1.2 | 0.7 | 0.2 | 0.2 | | | 4 |
| 47609 | 1 ea | Party Favorites cookie, Pepperidge Farm | 11 | 58 | | 0.7 | 7.2 | 0.3 | 3.4 | 3.4 | 2.8 | 1.0 | | | | | 3 |
| 47503 | 1 ea | Select Assortment cookie, Archway | 8 | 40 | | 0.5 | 5.5 | 0.3 | 2.3 | 3.0 | 1.8 | 0.5 | 0.5 | 0.3 | | | 0 |
| 47449 | 1 ea | Selection De Choix Biscuits, Pepperidge Farm | 6 | 31 | 5 | 0.2 | 3.9 | 0.0 | 1.7 | 2.3 | 1.4 | 0.8 | 0.6 | 0.0 | 0.00 | 0.00 | 0 |
| 47513 | 1 ea | Wedding Cake cookies, Archway | 10 | 53 | | 0.3 | 6.7 | 0.0 | 3.0 | 3.7 | 2.7 | 0.5 | | | | | 0 |
| | | *DOUGHNUTS* | | | | | | | | | | | | | | | |
| | | Cake doughnuts | | | | | | | | | | | | | | | |
| 45630 | 1 ea | Buttermilk, glazed, Entenmann's | 64 | 270 | 18 | 3.0 | 36.0 | 0.0 | 22.0 | 14.0 | 13.0 | 3.0 | | | | | 10 |
| 45518 | 1 ea | Chocolate, glazed or sugared, avg | 42 | 175 | 16 | 1.9 | 24.1 | 0.9 | 13.5 | 9.7 | 8.4 | 2.2 | 4.7 | 1.0 | 0.05 | 0.99 | 24 |
| 45524 | 1 ea | Chocolate, iced, avg | 43 | 204 | 14 | 2.2 | 20.6 | 0.9 | 6.4 | 13.4 | 13.3 | 3.5 | 7.5 | 1.6 | 0.08 | 1.54 | 26 |
| 45730 | 1 ea | Chocolate, hole, Dunkin Donut | 19 | 60 | 39 | 0.7 | 7.3 | 0.3 | 4.3 | 2.7 | 3.3 | 0.7 | | | | | 0 |
| 45777 | 1 ea | Churros, avg | 26 | 115 | 22 | 0.7 | 11.9 | 0.2 | 6.5 | 5.3 | 7.4 | 1.4 | 3.0 | 2.5 | | | 2 |
| 45657 | 1 ea | Cinnamon, Tastykake | 48 | 210 | 18 | 3.0 | 24.0 | 1.0 | 11.0 | 12.0 | 12.0 | 2.0 | | | | | 15 |
| 45636 | 1 ea | Cinnamon Sugar, glazed, Entenmann's | 67 | 310 | 18 | 3.0 | 32.0 | 0.5 | 17.0 | 14.5 | 19.0 | 4.0 | | | | | 20 |
| 45509 | 1 ea | Cream Puff, custard filled, avg | 90 | 232 | 54 | 6.0 | 20.6 | 0.4 | 12.2 | 8.0 | 13.9 | 3.3 | 5.9 | 3.7 | 0.17 | 3.57 | 121 |
| 45527 | 1 ea | Cruller, french glazed, avg | 41 | 169 | 18 | 1.3 | 24.4 | 0.5 | 13.9 | 10.0 | 7.5 | 1.9 | 4.3 | 0.9 | 0.05 | 0.39 | 5 |
| 45735 | 1 ea | Cruller, glazed, avg | 86 | 340 | 22 | 3.0 | 49.0 | 2.0 | 25.0 | 22.0 | 14.0 | 3.0 | | | | | 0 |
| 45627 | 1 ea | Crumb Topped, Entenmann's | 60 | 260 | 15 | 3.0 | 34.0 | 0.5 | 19.0 | 14.5 | 13.0 | 3.0 | | | | | 15 |
| 45628 | 1 ea | Devil's Food Crumb, Entenmann's | 60 | 250 | 18 | 3.0 | 33.0 | 1.0 | 19.0 | 13.0 | 12.0 | 3.5 | | | | | 15 |
| 45629 | 1 ea | Frosted Mini, Entenmann's | 26 | 135 | 12 | 1.0 | 11.5 | 0.5 | 6.5 | 4.5 | 10.0 | 3.0 | | | | | 5 |
| 45656 | 1 ea | Frosted, Rich, Mini, Tastykake | 14 | 66 | 12 | 0.8 | 7.2 | 0.5 | 3.8 | 3.0 | 3.8 | 1.8 | | | | | 3 |
| 45655 | 1 ea | Frosted, Rich, Tastykake | 57 | 270 | | 3.0 | 30.0 | 2.0 | 16.0 | 12.0 | 16.0 | 5.0 | | | | | 5 |
| 45525 | 1 ea | Glazed or Sugared, avg | 45 | 192 | 20 | 2.3 | 22.9 | 0.7 | 7.5 | 14.7 | 10.3 | 2.7 | 5.7 | 1.3 | 0.07 | 1.24 | 14 |
| 45653 | 1 ea | Honey Wheat, Tastykake | 57 | 230 | | 2.0 | 33.0 | 1.0 | 19.0 | 13.0 | 10.0 | 2.0 | | | | | 5 |
| 45660 | 1 ea | Honey Wheat, Mini, Tastykake | 12 | 47 | | 0.5 | 6.6 | 0.2 | 3.7 | 2.7 | 2.2 | 0.4 | | | | | 3 |
| 45654 | 1 ea | Orange Glazed, Tastykake | 57 | 220 | | 2.0 | 33.0 | 1.0 | 19.0 | 13.0 | 9.0 | 1.5 | | | | | 5 |
| 45505 | 1 ea | Plain, avg | 47 | 198 | 21 | 2.3 | 23.4 | 0.7 | 7.3 | 15.3 | 10.8 | 1.7 | 4.4 | 3.7 | 0.25 | 3.44 | 17 |
| 45658 | 1 ea | Plain, Tastykake | 41 | 180 | | 3.0 | 19.0 | 1.0 | 7.0 | 11.0 | 11.0 | 2.0 | | | | | 15 |
| 45728 | 1 ea | Sugar Powdered, hole, Dunkin Donut | 14 | 58 | 23 | 0.7 | 6.8 | 0.2 | 2.9 | 3.6 | 3.1 | 0.6 | | | | | 0 |
| 45669 | 1 ea | Sugar Powdered, Mini, Tastykake | 12 | 49 | | 0.7 | 6.8 | 0.2 | 3.2 | 3.4 | 2.0 | 0.4 | | | | | 4 |
| 45659 | 1 ea | Sugar Powdered, Tastykake | 48 | 210 | | 3.0 | 24.0 | 1.0 | 12.0 | 11.0 | 11.0 | 2.0 | | | | | 15 |
| 45729 | 1 ea | Coconut, hole, Dunkin Donut | 17 | 70 | 22 | 0.7 | 8.7 | 0.3 | 4.3 | 4.0 | 3.7 | 1.0 | | | | | 0 |

| Code | Vit A (IU) | Vit A (RE) | Retinol (RE) | Carotenoids (RE) | Beta Carotene (mcg) | Thiamin (mg) | Riboflavin (mg) | Niacin (NE) | Vit B6 (mg) | Vit B12 (mcg) | Folate (mcg) | Panto (mg) | Vit C (mg) | Vit D (mg) | Vit E (α TE) |
|---|---|---|---|---|---|---|---|---|---|---|---|---|---|---|---|
| | **Vit A & Components** | | | | | **Vitamins** | | | | | | | | | |
| 47241 | 0 | 0 | 0 | 0 | 0 | | | | | | | | 0.0 | | |
| 47665 | 12 | 4 | 4 | 0 | | 0.07 | 0.04 | 0.47 | 0.00 | 0.01 | 1.4 | 0.05 | 0.0 | 0.0 | |
| 47603 | 0 | 0 | 0 | 0 | 0 | 0.00 | 0.00 | 0.00 | | | | | 0.0 | | |
| 47254 | | | | | | | | | | | | | | | |
| 47348 | 0 | 0 | 0 | 0 | 0 | 0.03 | 0.02 | 0.40 | | | | | 0.0 | | |
| 47011 | 129 | 32 | 28 | 4 | | 0.05 | 0.04 | 0.41 | 0.01 | 0.01 | 2.0 | 0.04 | 0.1 | 0.1 | 0.1 |
| 47299 | 500 | 100 | | | | | | | | | | | 1.2 | | |
| 47560 | 12 | 2 | | | | 0.07 | 0.06 | 0.54 | | | | | 0.0 | | |
| 90089 | 0 | 0 | 0 | 0 | 0 | 0.02 | 0.00 | 0.00 | | | | | 0.0 | | |
| 47064 | 14 | 4 | 3.9 | 0.1 | | 0.03 | 0.03 | 0.40 | 0.01 | 0.03 | 6.8 | 0.04 | 0.0 | 0.0 | |
| 47561 | 0 | 0 | 0 | 0 | 0 | | | | | | | | 0.0 | | |
| 47263 | | | | | | | | | | | | | | | |
| 47069 | 0 | 0 | 0 | 0 | 0 | 0.01 | 0.02 | 0.22 | 0.00 | 0.00 | 3.9 | 0.02 | 0.0 | 0.0 | |
| 47347 | 0 | 0 | 0 | 0 | 0 | 0.04 | 0.02 | 0.40 | | | | | 0.0 | | |
| 47004 | 4 | 1.3 | .2 | 0.05 | | 0.02 | 0.01 | 0.29 | 0.00 | 0.01 | 6.4 | 0.02 | 0.0 | 0.0 | |
| 47066 | 6 | 2 | 2 | 0.07 | | 0.03 | 0.02 | 0.39 | 0.00 | 0.00 | 12.0 | 0.04 | 0.0 | 0.0 | |
| 47559 | 9 | 2 | | | | 0.09 | 0.06 | 0.69 | | | | | 0.0 | | |
| 47070 | 0 | 0 | 0 | 0 | 0 | 0.01 | 0.00 | 0.06 | 0.00 | 0.00 | 1.7 | 0.00 | 0.0 | 0.0 | |
| 47071 | 0 | 0 | 0 | 0 | 0 | 0.03 | 0.02 | 0.27 | 0.00 | 0.00 | 5.9 | 0.04 | 0.0 | 0.0 | |
| 47024 | 0.1 | 0.02 | | | | 0.02 | 0.02 | 0.14 | 0.00 | 0.00 | 0.7 | | 0.0 | | |
| 47239 | 0 | 0 | 0 | 0 | 0 | | | | | | | | 0.0 | | |
| 47160 | 0.4 | 0.08 | | | | 0.02 | 0.03 | 0.34 | 0.01 | 0.01 | | | 0.0 | | |
| 47008 | 1 | 0.3 | 0.3 | 0 | 0 | 0.01 | 0.01 | 0.12 | 0.00 | 0.01 | 2.0 | 0.02 | 0.0 | 0.0 | |
| 47562 | 0 | 0 | 0 | 0 | 0 | | | | | | | | 0.0 | | |
| 49065 | 0 | 0 | 0 | 0 | 0 | | | | | | | | 0.0 | | |
| 47171 | | | | | | | | | | | | | | | |
| 47505 | 0 | 0 | 0 | 0 | 0 | | | | | | | | 0.0 | | |
| 47464 | 0 | 0 | 0 | 0 | 0 | 0.02 | 0.01 | 0.21 | | | | | | | |
| 47463 | 0 | 0 | 0 | 0 | 0 | 0.03 | 0.01 | 0.27 | | | | | 0.0 | | |
| 47473 | 0 | 0 | 0 | 0 | 0 | 0.02 | 0.01 | 0.28 | | | | | 0.0 | | |
| 47508 | 0 | 0 | 0 | 0 | 0 | | | | | | | | 0.0 | | |
| 47576 | 0 | 0 | 0 | 0 | 0 | | | | | | | | 0.0 | | |
| 47448 | 0 | 0 | 0 | 0 | 0 | 0.00 | 0.00 | 0.00 | | | | | 0.0 | | |
| 47609 | 0 | 0 | 0 | 0 | 0 | 0.03 | 0.01 | 0.28 | | | | | 0.0 | | |
| 47503 | 0 | 0 | 0 | 0 | 0 | | | | | | | | 0.0 | | |
| 47449 | 0 | 0 | 0 | 0 | 0 | 0.00 | 0.00 | 0.00 | | | | | 0.0 | | |
| 47513 | 0 | 0 | 0 | 0 | 0 | | | | | | | | 0.0 | | |
| 45630 | 0 | 0 | 0 | 0 | 0 | | | | | | | | 0.0 | | |
| 45518 | 16 | 5 | 4.4 | 0.3 | | 0.02 | 0.03 | 0.20 | 0.01 | 0.04 | 16.0 | 0.14 | 0.0 | 0.0 | |
| 45524 | 15 | 5 | 4.4 | 0.3 | | 0.05 | 0.05 | 0.56 | 0.02 | 0.10 | 12.5 | 0.18 | 0.1 | 0.0 | |
| 45730 | 0 | 0 | 0 | 0 | 0 | | | | | | | | 0.0 | | |
| 45777 | 24 | 6 | 5.3 | 0.7 | | 0.04 | 0.03 | 0.37 | 0.00 | 0.00 | 1.2 | | 0.0 | | |
| 45657 | 0 | 0 | 0 | 0 | 0 | | | | | | | | 0.0 | | |
| 45636 | 0 | 0 | 0 | 0 | 0 | | | | | | | | 0.0 | | |
| 45509 | 671 | 179 | 170 | 9 | | 0.11 | 0.25 | 0.75 | 0.06 | 0.32 | 25.2 | 0.47 | 0.3 | 0.4 | |
| 45527 | 7 | 12 | 1.2 | 0.06 | | 0.07 | 0.09 | 0.87 | 0.01 | 0.02 | 14.3 | 0.09 | 0.0 | 0.0 | |
| 45735 | 0 | 0 | 0 | 0 | 0 | | | | | | | | 0.0 | | |
| 45627 | 0 | 0 | 0 | 0 | 0 | | | | | | | | 0.0 | | |
| 45628 | 0 | 0 | 0 | 0 | 0 | | | | | | | | 0.0 | | |
| 45629 | 0 | 0 | 0 | 0 | 0 | | | | | | | | 0.0 | | |
| 45656 | 0 | 0 | 0 | 0 | 0 | | | | | | | | 0.0 | | |
| 45655 | 0 | 0 | 0 | 0 | 0 | | | | | | | | 0.0 | | |
| 45525 | 5 | 1.4 | 1.3 | 0.07 | | 0.10 | 0.09 | 0.68 | 0.01 | 0.11 | 20.7 | 0.20 | 0.0 | 0.0 | |
| 45653 | 0 | 0 | 0 | 0 | 0 | | | | | | | | 0.0 | | |
| 45660 | 0 | 0 | 0 | 0 | 0 | | | | | | | | 0.0 | | |
| 45654 | 0 | 0 | 0 | 0 | 0 | | | | | | | | 0.0 | | |
| 45505 | 27 | 3 | 2.6 | 0.4 | | 0.10 | 0.11 | 0.87 | 0.03 | 0.13 | 22.1 | 0.13 | 0.1 | 0.0 | |
| 45658 | 0 | 0 | 0 | 0 | 0 | | | | | | | | 0.0 | | |
| 45728 | 0 | 0 | 0 | 0 | 0 | | | | | | | | 0.3 | | |
| 45669 | 0 | 0 | 0 | 0 | 0 | | | | | | | | 0.0 | | |
| 45659 | 0 | 0 | 0 | 0 | 0 | | | | | | | | 0.0 | | |
| 45729 | 0 | 0 | 0 | 0 | 0 | | | | | | | | 0.0 | | |

| Code | Calcium (mg) | Copper (mg) | Iron (mg) | Magnes (mg) | Mang (mg) | Phos (mg) | Potassium (mg) | Selenium (mcg) | Sodium (mg) | Zinc (mg) |
|---|---|---|---|---|---|---|---|---|---|---|
| | **Minerals** | | | | | | | | | |
| 47241 | 0 | | 0.0 | | | | 15 | | 45 | |
| 47665 | 11 | 0.0 | 0.5 | 3 | 0.1 | 23 | 10 | | 9 | 0.07 |
| 47603 | 0 | | 0.0 | | | | | | 0 | |
| 47254 | | | 0.3 | | | | 6 | | 31 | |
| 47348 | 0 | | 0.2 | | | | | | 52 | |
| 47011 | 8 | 0.0 | 0.5 | 2 | 0.1 | 10 | 24 | 2.7 | 74 | 0.07 |
| 47299 | 20 | | 0.7 | | | | | | 25 | |
| 47560 | 7 | | 0.6 | | | | 38 | | 94 | |
| 90089 | 0 | | 0.1 | | | | | | 36 | |
| 47064 | 3 | 0.0 | 0.3 | 2 | 0.0 | 12 | 9 | 0.3 | 54 | 0.06 |
| 47561 | 0 | | 0.7 | | | | | | 190 | |
| 47263 | | | | | | | 1 | | 6 | |
| 47069 | 2 | 0.0 | 0.2 | 1 | 0.0 | 5 | 5 | 0.2 | 13 | 0.03 |
| 47347 | 0 | | 0.2 | | | | | | 30 | |
| 47004 | 11 | 0.0 | 0.2 | 1 | 0.0 | 22 | 20 | 0.4 | 56 | 0.03 |
| 47066 | 13 | 0.0 | 0.3 | 1 | 0.0 | 27 | 24 | 0.5 | 68 | 0.04 |
| 47559 | 9 | | 0.6 | | | | 23 | | 189 | |
| 47070 | 2 | 0.0 | 0.1 | 0 | 0.0 | 1 | 2 | 0.3 | 0 | 0.01 |
| 47071 | 3 | 0.0 | 0.2 | 1 | 0.0 | 8 | 9 | 0.3 | 35 | 0.04 |
| 47024 | 4 | 0.0 | 0.1 | 3 | | 7 | 11 | | 1 | 0.08 |
| 47239 | 0 | | 0.4 | | | | 5 | | 40 | |
| 47160 | 9 | 0.0 | 0.3 | 2 | | 18 | 14 | | 48 | 0.08 |
| 47008 | 2 | 0.0 | 0.1 | 1 | 0.0 | 4 | 4 | 0.5 | 12 | 0.01 |
| 47562 | 0 | | 0.2 | | | | | | 26 | |
| 49065 | 2 | | 0.1 | | | | | | 15 | |
| 47171 | 2 | | 0.1 | | | | 4 | | 12 | |
| 47505 | 0 | | 0.2 | | | | | | 34 | |
| 47464 | 0 | | 0.1 | | | | | | 22 | |
| 47463 | 0 | | 0.2 | | | | | | 30 | |
| 47473 | 0 | | 0.2 | | | | | | 28 | |
| 47508 | 0 | | 0.2 | | | | | | 32 | |
| 47576 | 0 | | 0.1 | | | | | | 18 | |
| 47448 | 0 | | 0.1 | | | | | | 25 | |
| 47609 | 0 | | 0.2 | | | | | | 31 | |
| 47503 | 0 | | 0.2 | | | | | | 29 | |
| 47449 | 0 | | 0.1 | | | | | | 12 | |
| 47513 | 0 | | 0.2 | | | | | | 15 | |
| 45630 | 80 | | 1.1 | | | | 85 | | 280 | |
| 45518 | 89 | 0.1 | 1.0 | 14 | 0.2 | 68 | 45 | 1.7 | 143 | 0.24 |
| 45524 | 15 | 0.1 | 1.1 | 17 | 0.2 | 87 | 84 | 2.5 | 184 | 0.26 |
| 45730 | 0 | | 0.4 | | | | | | 80 | |
| 45777 | 2 | 0.0 | 0.3 | 2 | | 8 | 8 | | 37 | 0.05 |
| 45657 | 20 | | 0.7 | | | | | | 240 | |
| 45636 | 20 | | 0.4 | | | | 90 | | 300 | |
| 45509 | 59 | 0.0 | 1.1 | 11 | 0.1 | 98 | 103 | 13.9 | 307 | 0.54 |
| 45527 | 11 | 0.0 | 1.0 | 5 | 0.1 | 50 | 32 | 0.9 | 141 | 0.11 |
| 45735 | 20 | | 0.7 | | | | | | 320 | |
| 45627 | 40 | | 0.4 | | | | 60 | | 230 | |
| 45628 | 40 | | 0.7 | | | | 120 | | 240 | |
| 45629 | 0 | | 0.4 | | | | 50 | | 90 | |
| 45656 | 3 | | 0.0 | | | | | | 61 | |
| 45655 | 20 | | 1.4 | | | | | | 180 | |
| 45525 | 27 | 0.0 | 0.5 | 8 | 0.2 | 53 | 46 | 4.3 | 181 | 0.20 |
| 45653 | 20 | | 0.7 | | | | | | 180 | |
| 45660 | 3 | | 0.2 | | | | | | 51 | |
| 45654 | 20 | | 0.7 | | | | | | 200 | |
| 45505 | 21 | 0.0 | 0.9 | 9 | 0.2 | 126 | 60 | 4.4 | 257 | 0.26 |
| 45658 | 20 | | 0.7 | | | | | | 210 | |
| 45728 | 0 | | 0.2 | | | | | | 70 | |
| 45669 | 3 | | 0.1 | | | | | | 59 | |
| 45659 | 20 | | 0.7 | | | | | | 210 | |
| 45729 | 0 | | 0.2 | | | | | | 73 | |

| Code | Amount | Description | Basic Components | | | | | | | | | Additional Fats | | | | | |
|---|---|---|---|---|---|---|---|---|---|---|---|---|---|---|---|---|---|
| | | | Weight (g) | Calories | % Water | Protein (g) | Carbs (g) | Fiber (g) | Sugar (g) | Other Carbs (g) | Fat (g) | Sat Fat (g) | Mono Fat (g) | Poly Fat (g) | Omega 3 (g) | Omega 6 (g) | Choles (mg) |
| | | Raised/Yeast doughnuts | | | | | | | | | | | | | | | |
| 45561 | 1 ea | Carob-coated, w/o egg, avg | 78 | 285 | 27 | 5.3 | 32.5 | 5.3 | | | 17.5 | 2.6 | 6.4 | 7.4 | | | 0 |
| 45508 | 1 ea | Chocolate eclair, avg | 112 | 293 | 52 | 7.2 | 27.1 | 0.7 | 16.4 | 10.1 | 17.6 | 4.6 | 7.3 | 4.4 | 0.21 | 4.21 | 142 |
| 45626 | 1 ea | Chocolate Éclair, Entenmann's | 102 | 250 | 44 | 3.0 | 44.0 | 0.0 | 28.0 | 16.0 | 9.0 | 2.0 | | | | | 70 |
| 49043 | 1 ea | Chocolate Éclair, Weight Watchers | 60 | 151 | 45 | 3.0 | 24.2 | 2.0 | 14.1 | 8.1 | 5.0 | 1.5 | | | | | 0 |
| 45517 | 1 ea | Chocolate w/choc frosting, avg | 71 | 273 | 27 | 4.1 | 30.3 | 2.5 | 17.3 | 10.6 | 16.2 | 7.5 | 6.5 | 1.2 | | | 22 |
| 45563 | 1 ea | Creme filled, avg | 85 | 307 | 38 | 5.4 | 25.5 | 0.7 | 15.0 | 9.8 | 20.8 | 4.6 | 10.3 | 2.6 | 0.14 | 2.48 | 20 |
| 45519 | 1 ea | Custard filled, w/icing, avg | 70 | 260 | 28 | 3.2 | 33.6 | 1.0 | 20.3 | 12.3 | 12.9 | 5.9 | 5.3 | 0.9 | | | 20 |
| 45506 | 1 ea | Glazed, avg | 60 | 242 | 25 | 3.8 | 26.6 | 0.7 | 13.8 | 12.1 | 13.7 | 3.5 | 7.7 | 1.7 | 0.09 | 1.65 | 4 |
| 49109 | 1 ea | Glazed, donut hole, avg | 13 | 52 | 25 | 0.8 | 5.8 | 0.2 | 3.0 | 2.6 | 3.0 | 0.8 | 1.7 | 0.4 | 0.02 | 0.36 | 1 |
| 45731 | 1 ea | Glazed, Dunkin Donuts | 15 | 52 | 22 | 0.8 | 9.0 | 0.3 | 5.0 | 3.8 | 1.8 | 0.4 | | | | | 0 |
| 45507 | 1 ea | Jelly filled, avg | 85 | 289 | 36 | 5.0 | 33.2 | 0.7 | 18.7 | 13.7 | 15.9 | 4.1 | 8.7 | 2.0 | 0.11 | 1.91 | 22 |
| | | *FROZEN DESSERTS* | | | | | | | | | | | | | | | |
| | | Ice Cream | | | | | | | | | | | | | | | |
| 2333 | 1/2 cup | Butter Pecan, Ben & Jerry's | 110 | 310 | 54 | 5.0 | 20.0 | 1.0 | 20.0 | | 25.0 | 11.0 | | | | | 85 |
| 70314 | 1/2 cup | Butter Pecan, Haagan-Dazs | 106 | 288 | 50 | 5.0 | 28.9 | | | | 16.9 | 9.0 | 5.0 | 3.0 | | | 109 |
| 70653 | 1/2 cup | Cappucino Commotion, Haagan-Dazs | 106 | 338 | | 5.0 | 28.9 | | | | 21.9 | | | | | | 100 |
| 70656 | 1/2 cup | Carrot Cake Passion, Haagan-Dazs | 106 | 308 | | 6.0 | 25.9 | | | | 20.9 | | | | | | |
| 2188 | 1/2 cup | Cherry Choc Chip, lowfat, Healthy Choice | 71 | 110 | 65 | 3.0 | 19.0 | 0.5 | 18.5 | 0.0 | 2.0 | 1.5 | | | | | 2 |
| 2050 | 1/2 cup | Chocolate, avg | 66 | 143 | 56 | 2.5 | 18.6 | 0.8 | 17.9 | 0.0 | 7.3 | 4.5 | 2.1 | 0.3 | 0.10 | 0.17 | 22 |
| 2051 | 1/2 cup | Chocolate, soft serve, avg | 86 | 176 | 58 | 3.2 | 24.0 | 0.7 | 22.9 | 0.3 | 8.3 | 5.2 | 2.4 | 0.3 | 0.11 | 0.19 | 22 |
| 2483 | 1/2 cup | Chocolate, Breyers | 70 | 161 | 54 | 3.0 | 20.2 | 0.5 | 19.4 | 0.2 | 8.1 | 5.0 | 2.0 | 0.0 | 0.00 | 0.00 | 20 |
| 70312 | 1/2 cup | Chocolate, Haagan-Dazs | 106 | 269 | 55 | 5.0 | 23.9 | | | | 16.9 | 8.0 | 8.5 | 0.5 | | | 120 |
| 70313 | 1/2 cup | Chocolate Chip, Haagan-Dazs | 106 | 288 | 50 | 5.0 | 27.9 | | | | 19.9 | 10.0 | 9.5 | 0.5 | | | 105 |
| 2216 | 1/2 cup | Chocolate Chip Cookie Dough, Ben & Jerry's | 106 | 270 | | 4.0 | 30.0 | 0.0 | 25.0 | 5.0 | 17.0 | 9.0 | | | | | 80 |
| 70648 | 1/2 cup | Chocolate Fudge, Haagan-Dazs | 106 | 299 | | 5.0 | 27.9 | | | | 14.9 | 9.0 | 5.5 | 0.5 | | | 100 |
| 2334 | 1/2 cup | Chocolate Fudge Brownie, Ben & Jerry's | 106 | 250 | 51 | 4.0 | 33.0 | 2.0 | 30.0 | 1.0 | 14.0 | 8.0 | | | | | 45 |
| 2341 | 1/2 cup | Chocolate Fudge Swirl, Ben & Jerry's | 109 | 260 | 50 | 5.0 | 33.0 | 3.0 | 29.0 | 1.0 | 15.0 | 9.0 | | | | | 55 |
| 2206 | 1/2 cup | Chocolate Mint Cookie, Ben & Jerry's | 107 | 260 | | 4.0 | 27.0 | 1.0 | 23.0 | 3.0 | 17.0 | 10.0 | | | | | 80 |
| 70650 | 1/2 cup | Chocolate Peanut Butter, Haagan-Dazs | 106 | 329 | | 7.0 | 24.9 | | | | 18.9 | | | | | | |
| 2255 | 1/2 cup | Chocolate Tornado, light, Weight Watchers | 113 | 149 | 69 | 4.0 | 25.9 | 1.0 | 21.9 | 3.0 | 3.5 | 1.5 | | | | | 5 |
| 2343 | 1/2 cup | Chubby Hubby, Ben & Jerry's | 114 | 350 | 45 | 8.0 | 31.0 | 2.0 | 26.0 | 3.0 | 23.0 | 11.0 | | | | | 75 |
| 2202 | 1/2 cup | Chunky Monkey, Ben & Jerry's | 106 | 280 | | 4.0 | 29.0 | 1.0 | 28.0 | 0.0 | 19.0 | 10.0 | | | | | 70 |
| 2332 | 1/2 cup | Coffee, Aztec Harvest, Ben & Jerry's | 108 | 230 | 57 | 4.0 | 22.0 | 0.0 | 21.0 | 1.0 | 16.0 | 10.0 | | | | | 90 |
| 70307 | 1/2 cup | Coffee, Haagan-Dazs | 106 | 269 | 56 | 5.0 | 22.9 | | | | 16.9 | 8.0 | 8.5 | 0.5 | | | 120 |
| 2204 | 1/2 cup | Coffee Toffee Crunch, Ben & Jerry's | 106 | 280 | | 4.0 | 28.0 | 0.0 | 28.0 | 0.0 | 19.0 | 10.0 | | | | | 80 |
| 2203 | 1/2 cup | Coconut Almond Fudge Chip, Ben & Jerry's | 109 | 320 | | 6.0 | 24.0 | 2.0 | 21.0 | 1.0 | 25.0 | 14.0 | | | | | 75 |
| 2251 | 1/2 cup | Cookie Dough Craze, light, Weight Watchers | 113 | 140 | 72 | 3.0 | 23.9 | 1.0 | 20.9 | 2.0 | 3.5 | 2.0 | | | | | 5 |
| 70657 | 1/2 cup | Cookie Dough Dynamo, Haagan-Dazs | 106 | 299 | | 4.0 | 30.9 | | | | 17.9 | 7.0 | 8.9 | 2.0 | | | 100 |
| 70659 | 1/2 cup | Cookies & Cream, Haagan-Dazs | 106 | 279 | | 5.0 | 25.9 | | | | 17.9 | | | | | | 109 |
| 2105 | 1/2 cup | Cookies & Cream, lowfat, Healthy Choice | 71 | 120 | 62 | 3.0 | 21.0 | 0.5 | 19.0 | 1.5 | 2.0 | 1.5 | 0.5 | 0.0 | 0.00 | 0.00 | 2 |
| 2184 | 1/2 cup | Fudge Brownie, lowfat, Healthy Choice | 71 | 120 | 60 | 3.0 | 22.0 | 2.0 | 15.0 | 5.0 | 2.0 | 1.0 | 0.3 | 0.7 | | | 2 |
| 70651 | 1/2 cup | Macadamia Brittle, Haagan-Dazs | 106 | 279 | | 4.0 | 24.9 | | | | 17.9 | | | | | | |
| 2185 | 1/2 cup | Mint Choc Chip, lowfat, Healthy Choice | 71 | 120 | 62 | 3.0 | 21.0 | 0.5 | 20.0 | 0.5 | 2.0 | 1.0 | 1.0 | 0.0 | 0.00 | 0.00 | 2 |
| 2218 | 1/2 cup | NY Super Fudge Chunk, Ben & Jerry's | 106 | 290 | | 5.0 | 28.0 | 2.0 | 25.0 | 1.0 | 20.0 | 11.0 | | | | | 50 |
| 70654 | 1/2 cup | Peanut Butter Burst, Haagan-Dazs | 106 | 338 | | 6.0 | 28.9 | | | | 21.9 | 9.0 | 10.9 | 2.0 | | | 94 |
| 2207 | 1/2 cup | Peanut Butter Cup, Ben & Jerry's | 116 | 340 | | 8.0 | 30.0 | 2.0 | 27.0 | 1.0 | 26.0 | 12.0 | | | | | 75 |
| 2107 | 1/2 cup | Praline & Caramel, lowfat, Healthy Choice | 71 | 130 | 56 | 3.0 | 25.0 | 0.5 | 24.0 | 0.5 | 2.0 | 0.5 | 0.1 | 1.4 | | | 2 |
| 2253 | 1/2 cup | Praline Crunch, light, Weight Watchers | 113 | 140 | 71 | 3.0 | 24.9 | 0.0 | 20.9 | 4.0 | 3.0 | 1.5 | | | | | 5 |
| 2254 | 1/2 cup | Rocky Road, light, Weight Watchers | 113 | 140 | 72 | 4.0 | 22.9 | 1.0 | 16.9 | 5.0 | 3.0 | 1.5 | | | | | 5 |
| 2123 | 1/2 cup | Rocky Road, lowfat, Healthy Choice | 71 | 140 | 53 | 3.0 | 28.0 | 2.0 | 19.0 | 7.0 | 1.5 | 1.0 | 0.5 | 0.0 | 0.00 | 0.00 | 2 |
| 70310 | 1/2 cup | Rum Raisin, Haagan-Dazs | 106 | 249 | 58 | 4.0 | 20.9 | | | | 16.9 | 8.0 | 8.5 | 0.5 | | | 109 |
| 2063 | 1/2 cup | Strawberry, avg | 66 | 127 | 60 | 2.1 | 18.2 | 0.2 | 18.1 | 0.0 | 5.5 | 3.4 | 1.6 | 0.2 | | | 19 |
| 2018 | 1/2 cup | Strawberry, Breyers | 70 | 131 | 64 | 2.0 | 16.1 | 0.1 | 16.0 | 0.1 | 6.0 | 4.0 | 2.0 | 0.0 | 0.00 | 0.00 | 20 |
| 2335 | 1/2 cup | Strawberry, fat free, Ben & Jerry's | 95 | 140 | 61 | 3.0 | 31.0 | 0.0 | 25.0 | 6.0 | 0.0 | 0.0 | 0.0 | 0.0 | 0.00 | 0.00 | 0 |
| 70306 | 1/2 cup | Strawberry, Haagan-Dazs | 106 | 249 | 58 | 4.0 | 22.9 | | | | 14.9 | 8.0 | 6.5 | 0.5 | | | 94 |
| 70658 | 1/2 cup | Toffee Crunch, Haagan-Dazs | 106 | 299 | | 4.0 | 26.9 | | | | 18.9 | 9.0 | 8.4 | 1.6 | | | 144 |
| 70652 | 1/2 cup | Triple Brownie Overload, Haagan-Dazs | 106 | 329 | | 5.0 | 27.9 | | | | 21.9 | | | | | | |
| 2330 | 1/2 cup | Triple Chocolate Chunk, lowfat, Healthy Choice | 71 | 110 | 62 | 3.0 | 21.0 | 1.0 | 18.0 | 2.0 | 2.0 | 1.0 | | | | | 2 |
| 2004 | 1/2 cup | Vanilla, avg | 66 | 133 | 61 | 2.3 | 15.6 | 0.0 | 11.6 | 4.0 | 7.3 | 4.5 | 2.1 | 0.3 | 0.11 | 0.17 | 29 |
| 2008 | 1/2 cup | Vanilla, french, soft serve, avg | 86 | 185 | 60 | 3.5 | 19.1 | 0.0 | 18.9 | 0.2 | 11.2 | 6.4 | 3.0 | 0.4 | 0.15 | 0.24 | 78 |
| 2006 | 1/2 cup | Vanilla, rich, 16% fat, avg | 74 | 178 | 57 | 2.6 | 16.6 | 0.0 | 13.0 | 3.6 | 12.0 | 7.4 | 3.4 | 0.4 | 0.17 | 0.27 | 45 |
| 2220 | 1/2 cup | Vanilla, Ben & Jerry's | 108 | 230 | | 4.0 | 21.0 | 0.0 | 21.0 | 0.0 | 17.0 | 10.0 | | | | | 95 |
| 2019 | 1/2 cup | Vanilla, Breyers | 70 | 151 | 62 | 3.0 | 15.1 | 0.1 | 15.0 | 0.1 | 8.1 | 5.0 | 2.0 | 0.3 | 0.12 | 0.18 | 25 |
| 2466 | 1/2 cup | Vanilla, fat free, no added sugar, Darigold | 73 | 80 | 70 | 4.0 | 17.3 | 0.0 | 5.3 | 11.9 | 0.0 | 0.0 | 0.0 | 0.0 | 0.00 | 0.00 | 0 |
| 70311 | 1/2 cup | Vanilla, Haagan-Dazs | 106 | 259 | 56 | 5.0 | 22.9 | | | | 16.9 | 8.0 | 8.5 | 0.5 | | | 120 |
| 2252 | 1/2 cup | Vanilla, light, Weight Watchers | 113 | 120 | 75 | 4.0 | 19.9 | 1.0 | 15.9 | 3.0 | 2.5 | 1.5 | | | | | 5 |
| 2110 | 1/2 cup | Vanilla, lowfat, Healthy Choice | 71 | 100 | 66 | 3.0 | 18.0 | 1.0 | 17.0 | 0.0 | 2.0 | 0.5 | 1.5 | 0.0 | 0.00 | 0.00 | 5 |
| 2339 | 1/2 cup | Vanilla Bean, Ben & Jerry's | 107 | 230 | 58 | 4.0 | 21.0 | 0.0 | 21.0 | 0.0 | 17.0 | 10.0 | | | | | 95 |
| 2338 | 1/2 cup | Vanilla Caramel Fudge Swirl, Ben & Jerry's | 116 | 280 | 52 | 4.0 | 33.0 | 1.0 | 30.0 | 2.0 | 17.0 | 10.0 | | | | | 95 |

| Code | Vit A & Components | | | | | Vitamins | | | | | | | | | | Minerals | | | | | | | | | |
|---|---|---|---|---|---|---|---|---|---|---|---|---|---|---|---|---|---|---|---|---|---|---|---|---|---|
| | Vit A (IU) | Vit A (RE) | Retinol (RE) | Carotenoids (RE) | Beta Carotene (mcg) | Thiamin (mg) | Riboflavin (mg) | Niacin (NE) | Vit B6 (mg) | Vit B12 (mcg) | Folate (mcg) | Panto (mg) | Vit C (mg) | Vit D (mg) | Vit E (α TE) | Calcium (mg) | Copper (mg) | Iron (mg) | Magnes (mg) | Mang (mg) | Phos (mg) | Potassium (mg) | Selenium (mcg) | Sodium (mg) | Zinc (mg) |
| 45561 | 2 | 0.2 | 0 | 0.2 | | 0.14 | 0.13 | 2.29 | 0.16 | 0.00 | 29.6 | | 0.0 | | | 77 | 0.2 | 1.6 | 56 | | 146 | 218 | | 74 | 1.13 |
| 45508 | 804 | 214 | 203 | 11 | | 0.13 | 0.30 | 0.89 | 0.07 | 0.38 | 31.4 | 0.55 | 0.3 | 0.4 | | 71 | 0.1 | 1.3 | 17 | 0.1 | 120 | 131 | 17.5 | 377 | 0.68 |
| 45626 | 100 | 20 | | | | | | | | | | | 0.0 | | | 100 | | 0.4 | | | | 105 | | 220 | |
| 49043 | 0 | 0 | 0 | 0 | 0 | | | | | | | | 0.0 | | | 40 | | 0.0 | | | | 66 | | 151 | |
| 45517 | 40 | 10 | 9 | 1 | | 0.12 | 0.14 | 1.05 | 0.04 | 0.18 | 14.7 | | 0.0 | | | 31 | 0.2 | 1.6 | 35 | | 74 | 110 | 13.6 | 129 | 0.88 |
| 45563 | 55 | 16 | 15 | 1 | | 0.29 | 0.13 | 1.90 | 0.06 | 0.12 | 54.4 | 0.56 | 0.0 | 0.0 | | 21 | 0.1 | 1.6 | 17 | 0.2 | 65 | 68 | 9.2 | 263 | 0.68 |
| 45519 | 13 | 3.7 | 3.3 | 0.3 | | 0.11 | 0.12 | 0.91 | 0.04 | 0.17 | 12.7 | | 0.1 | | | 27 | 0.1 | 1.0 | 13 | | 43 | 50 | | 125 | 0.58 |
| 45506 | 8 | 2.4 | 2.3 | 0.1 | | 0.22 | 0.13 | 1.71 | 0.03 | 0.05 | 25.8 | 0.28 | 0.1 | 0.1 | | 26 | 0.1 | 1.2 | 13 | 0.2 | 56 | 65 | 11.9 | 205 | 0.46 |
| 49109 | 2 | 0.5 | 0.5 | 0.03 | | 0.05 | 0.03 | 0.37 | 0.01 | 0.01 | 5.6 | 0.06 | 0.0 | 0.0 | | 6 | 0.0 | 0.3 | 3 | 0.0 | 12 | 14 | 2.6 | 44 | 0.10 |
| 45731 | 0 | 0 | 0 | 0 | 0 | | | | | | | | 0.0 | | | 0 | | 0.2 | | | | | | 42 | |
| 45507 | 46 | 14 | 13 | 1 | | 0.27 | 0.12 | 1.82 | 0.09 | 0.19 | 52.7 | 0.74 | 0.0 | 0.0 | | 21 | 0.1 | 1.5 | 17 | 0.2 | 72 | 67 | 10.6 | 249 | 0.64 |
| 2333 | 750 | 150 | | | | | 0.22 | | | | | | 0.0 | | | 100 | | 1.1 | | | | | | 125 | |
| 70314 | 353 | 106 | | | | 0.06 | 0.28 | 0.42 | | | | | 0.0 | | | 106 | | 0.4 | | | 106 | 179 | | 100 | |
| 70653 | 353 | 106 | | | | | 0.18 | 0.85 | | | | | | | | 106 | | 0.8 | | | 106 | 189 | | 85 | |
| 70656 | 706 | 212 | | | | | 0.18 | 0.42 | | | | | | | | | | 1.9 | | | 106 | 170 | | 90 | |
| 2188 | 200 | 40 | | | | | | | | | | | 0.0 | | | 10 | | 0.0 | | | 141 | 211 | | 55 | |
| 2050 | 275 | 79 | 73 | 6 | | 0.03 | 0.13 | 0.15 | 0.04 | 0.19 | 10.6 | 0.37 | 0.5 | 0.3 | | 72 | 0.1 | 0.6 | 19 | 0.1 | 71 | 164 | 1.7 | 50 | 0.38 |
| 2051 | 297 | 85 | 65 | 8 | | 0.03 | 0.13 | 0.11 | 0.03 | 0.32 | 4.7 | 0.43 | 0.5 | 0.1 | 0.3 | 102 | 0.1 | 0.3 | 19 | 0.0 | 91 | 191 | 1.3 | 44 | 0.47 |
| 2483 | 140 | 40 | 36 | 4 | | | 0.10 | | | 0.04 | | | | | | 48 | | | | | 32 | 151 | 1.2 | 30 | |
| 70312 | 353 | 101 | | | | | 0.18 | 0.85 | | | | | 0.0 | | | 106 | | 0.4 | | | 106 | 238 | | 50 | |
| 70313 | 353 | 101 | | | | | 0.18 | 0.85 | | | | | 0.0 | | | 85 | | 1.9 | | | 106 | 249 | | 40 | |
| 2216 | 750 | 79 | | | | | | | | | | | 1.2 | | | 100 | | 1.1 | | | | | | 95 | |
| 70648 | 71 | 20 | | | | | 0.14 | | | | | | | | | 106 | | 1.1 | | | 159 | 238 | | 100 | |
| 2334 | 500 | 143 | | | | | | | | | | | 0.0 | | | 100 | | 1.4 | | | | | | 90 | |
| 2341 | 500 | 143 | | | | | | | | | | | 1.2 | | | 100 | | 1.4 | | | | | | 55 | |
| 2206 | 750 | 215 | | | | | | | | | | | 0.0 | | | 100 | | 0.7 | | | | | | 120 | |
| 70650 | 71 | 20 | | | | 0.10 | 0.14 | 2.12 | | | | | | | | 106 | | 1.1 | | | 212 | 299 | | 90 | |
| 2255 | 100 | 29 | | | | | | | | | | | 0.0 | | | 199 | | 1.1 | | | | 199 | | 80 | |
| 2343 | 750 | 215 | | | | | | | | | | | 1.2 | | | 100 | | 0.7 | | | | | | 160 | |
| 2202 | 500 | 143 | | | | | | | | | | | 1.2 | | | 100 | | 1.1 | | | | | | 50 | |
| 2332 | 750 | 215 | | | | | | | | | | | 0.0 | | | 100 | | 0.4 | | | | | | 55 | |
| 70307 | 353 | 101 | | | | 0.03 | 0.28 | 0.85 | | | | | | | | 106 | | 0.4 | | | 106 | 189 | | 55 | |
| 2204 | 750 | 215 | | | | | | | | | | | 0.0 | | | 100 | | 0.4 | | | | | | 120 | |
| 2203 | 500 | 143 | | | | | | | | | | | 0.0 | | | 150 | | 1.4 | | | | | | 85 | |
| 2251 | 0 | 0 | 0 | 0 | 0 | | | | | | | | 0.0 | | | 199 | | 0.4 | | | | 149 | | 85 | |
| 70657 | 282 | 80 | | | | | 0.18 | 0.42 | | | | | | | | 85 | | | | | 85 | 135 | | 109 | |
| 70659 | 529 | 151 | | | | 0.03 | 0.18 | 0.42 | | | | | | | | 159 | | 1.1 | | | 106 | 170 | | 140 | |
| 2105 | 300 | 85 | | | | 0.03 | 0.15 | | | | | | 2.4 | | | 100 | | | | | 141 | 254 | | 90 | |
| 2184 | 200 | 57 | | | | | | | | | | | 0.0 | | | 80 | | 0.0 | | | 113 | 268 | | 55 | |
| 70651 | 71 | 20 | | | | | 0.18 | | | | | | | | | 106 | | 0.4 | | | 106 | 159 | | 59 | |
| 2185 | 200 | 57 | | | | | | | | | | | 0.0 | | | 100 | | 0.0 | | | 141 | 239 | | 50 | |
| 2218 | 500 | 143 | | | | | | | | | | | 0.0 | | | 100 | | 1.4 | | | | | | 55 | |
| 70654 | 282 | 81 | | | | 0.13 | 0.27 | 2.12 | | | | | | | | 85 | | 0.4 | | | 106 | 179 | | 129 | |
| 2207 | 500 | 41 | | | | | | | | | | | 0.0 | | | 150 | | 0.7 | | | | | | 140 | |
| 2107 | 200 | 57 | | | | 0.03 | 0.15 | | | | | | 0.0 | | | 100 | | 0.0 | | | 141 | 225 | | 70 | |
| 2253 | 100 | 29 | | | | | | | | | | | 0.0 | | | 199 | | 1.4 | | | | 100 | | 105 | |
| 2254 | 100 | 29 | | | | | | | | | | | 0.0 | | | 199 | | 0.7 | | | | 179 | | 75 | |
| 2123 | 200 | 58 | | | | 0.03 | 0.15 | | | | | | 0.0 | | | 100 | | 0.0 | | | 9 | 168 | | 60 | |
| 70310 | 353 | 101 | | | | 0.03 | 0.18 | 0.42 | | | | | | | | 85 | | 0.4 | | | 106 | 170 | | 45 | |
| 2063 | 211 | 60 | 46 | 6 | | 0.03 | 0.17 | 0.11 | 0.03 | 0.20 | 7.9 | 0.48 | 5.1 | 0.1 | 0.0 | 79 | 0.0 | 0.1 | 9 | 0.1 | 66 | 124 | 1.6 | 40 | 0.22 |
| 2018 | 140 | 40 | 36 | 4 | | 0.03 | 0.14 | | | 0.08 | | | | | | 64 | | | | | 48 | 126 | 1.2 | 41 | |
| 2335 | 100 | 28 | | | | | | | | | | | 6.0 | | | 100 | | 0.4 | | | | | | 65 | |
| 70306 | 353 | 101 | | | | 0.03 | 0.18 | 0.42 | | | | | | | | 106 | | 0.7 | | | 106 | 159 | | 40 | |
| 70658 | 71 | 21 | | | | 0.03 | 0.18 | | | | | | | | | 159 | | | | | 106 | 179 | | 109 | |
| 70652 | 529 | 151 | | | | | 0.18 | 0.42 | | | | | | | | 85 | | 0.8 | | | 159 | 229 | | 74 | |
| 2330 | 40 | 12 | | | | | | | | | | | 0.0 | | | 100 | | 0.4 | | | | | | 60 | |
| 2004 | 270 | 77 | 69 | 9 | | 0.03 | 0.16 | 0.08 | 0.03 | 0.26 | 3.3 | 0.38 | 0.4 | 0.1 | 0.0 | 84 | 0.0 | 0.1 | 9 | 0.0 | 69 | 131 | 1.7 | 53 | 0.46 |
| 2008 | 464 | 135 | 118 | 15 | | 0.04 | 0.16 | 0.08 | 0.04 | 0.43 | 7.7 | 0.44 | 0.7 | 0.2 | | 113 | 0.0 | 0.2 | 10 | 0.0 | 100 | 152 | 2.6 | 52 | 0.45 |
| 2006 | 476 | 138 | 121 | 15 | | 0.03 | 0.12 | 0.06 | 0.03 | 0.27 | 3.7 | 0.27 | 0.5 | 0.1 | 0.0 | 87 | 0.0 | 0.0 | 8 | 0.0 | 70 | 118 | 1.9 | 41 | 0.30 |
| 2220 | 750 | 218 | | | | | | | | | | | 0.0 | | 0.0 | 150 | | 0.4 | | | | | | 55 | |
| 2019 | 210 | 61 | 52 | 8 | | 0.03 | 0.15 | | | 0.12 | | | | | | 80 | | 0.1 | | | 80 | 141 | 1.2 | 50 | |
| 2466 | 265 | 76 | | | | | | | | | | | 0.0 | | | 106 | | 0.5 | | | | | | 66 | |
| 70311 | 353 | 101 | | | | 0.03 | 0.18 | 0.85 | | | | | 0.0 | | | 106 | | 0.0 | | | 106 | 149 | | 55 | |
| 2252 | 100 | 29 | | | | | | | | | | | 0.0 | | | 199 | | 0.0 | | | | 169 | | 65 | |
| 2110 | 300 | 86 | | | | 0.05 | 0.23 | | | | | | 2.4 | | | 100 | | | | | 141 | 254 | | 50 | |
| 2339 | 750 | 215 | | | | | | | | | | | 0.0 | | | 150 | | 0.4 | | | | | | 55 | |
| 2338 | 750 | 215 | | | | | | | | | | | 1.2 | | | 100 | | 0.4 | | | | | | 75 | |

| Code | Amount | Description | Basic Components | | | | | | | | | Additional Fats | | | | | | Vit A & Components | | | | | Vitamins | | | | | | | | | | Minerals | | | | | | | | | |
|---|---|---|---|---|---|---|---|---|---|---|---|---|---|---|---|---|---|---|---|---|---|---|---|---|---|---|---|---|---|---|---|---|---|---|---|---|---|---|---|---|---|---|
| | | | Weight (g) | Calories | % Water | Protein (g) | Carbs (g) | Fiber (g) | Sugar (g) | Other Carbs (g) | Fat (g) | Sat Fat (g) | Mono Fat (g) | Poly Fat (g) | Omega 3 (g) | Omega 6 (g) | Choles (mg) | Vit A (IU) | Vit A (RE) | Retinol (RE) | Carotenoids (RE) | Beta Carotene (mcg) | Thiamin (mg) | Riboflavin (mg) | Niacin (NE) | Vit B6 (mg) | Vit B12 (mcg) | Folate (mcg) | Panto (mg) | Vit C (mg) | Vit D (mg) | Vit E (α TE) | Calcium (mg) | Copper (mg) | Iron (mg) | Magnes (mg) | Mang (mg) | Phos (mg) | Potassium (mg) | Selenium (mcg) | Sodium (mg) | Zinc (mg) |
| 70649 | 1/2 cup | Vanilla Fudge, Haagan-Dazs | 106 | 269 | | 5.0 | 25.9 | | | | 16.9 | | | | | | | 529 | 148 | | | | | 0.18 | | | | | | | | | 159 | | 0.4 | | | 106 | 199 | | 100 | |
| 2336 | 1/2 cup | Vanilla Fudge Swirl, fat free, Ben & Jerry's | 89 | 150 | 59 | 3.0 | 32.0 | 0.0 | 24.0 | 8.0 | 0.0 | 0.0 | 0.0 | 0.0 | 0.00 | 0.00 | 5 | 100 | 28 | | | | | | | | | | | 0.0 | | | 100 | | 0.4 | | | | | | 80 | |
| 70316 | 1/2 cup | Vanilla Honey, Haagan-Dazs | 106 | 249 | 58 | 5.0 | 21.9 | | | | 15.9 | 8.0 | 7.5 | 0.5 | | | 135 | 353 | 101 | | | | 0.03 | 0.28 | 0.42 | | | | | 0.0 | | | 106 | | 0.0 | | | 106 | 159 | | 55 | |
| 70315 | 1/2 cup | Vanilla Swiss Almond, Haagan-Dazs | 106 | 288 | 53 | 5.0 | 23.9 | | | | 18.9 | 10.0 | 8.0 | 1.0 | | | 109 | 353 | 101 | | | | 0.03 | 0.28 | 1.27 | | | | | 0.0 | | | 106 | | 0.4 | | | 106 | 170 | | 55 | |
| 2208 | 1/2 cup | Wavy Gravy, Ben & Jerry's | 116 | 330 | | 6.0 | 29.0 | 2.0 | 26.0 | 1.0 | 24.0 | 10.0 | | | | | 80 | 500 | 148 | | | | | | | | | | | 1.2 | | | 150 | | 1.1 | | | | | | 95 | |
| 2337 | 1/2 cup | White Russian, Ben & Jerry's | 107 | 220 | 58 | 3.0 | 21.0 | 0.0 | 20.0 | 1.0 | 16.0 | 9.0 | | | | | 85 | 750 | 215 | | | | | | | | | | | 0.0 | | | 100 | | 0.4 | | | | | | 45 | |
| | | Ice Cream Bars | | | | | | | | | | | | | | | | | | | | | | | | | | | | | | | | | | | | | | | | |
| 70684 | 1 ea | Caramel Almond Crunch, Haagan-Dazs | 60 | 242 | | 3.0 | 17.1 | | | | 18.2 | 7.1 | 9.1 | 2.0 | | | 40 | 120 | 35 | | | | | 0.04 | | | | | | | | | 48 | | 0.2 | | | 36 | 141 | | 65 | |
| 2384 | 100 g | Caramel Cone Explosion, Extraas, Haagan-Dazs | 100 | 378 | 34 | 4.5 | 34.2 | 0.9 | 28.6 | 4.7 | 25.2 | 14.8 | | | | | 67 | 379 | 75 | | | | | | | | | | | 0.6 | | | 112 | | 0.8 | | | | | | 167 | |
| 2055 | 1 ea | Chocolate, avg | 101 | 339 | 37 | 3.2 | 36.0 | 2.1 | 31.8 | 2.1 | 23.0 | 13.8 | 7.1 | 0.7 | | | 37 | 393 | 95 | 84 | 11 | | 0.03 | 0.21 | 0.30 | 0.04 | 0.23 | 2.4 | | 0.3 | 0.1 | | 74 | 0.2 | 1.1 | 63 | | 139 | 261 | | 56 | 1.08 |
| 2086 | 1 ea | Chocolate, cake cvrd, avg | 59 | 162 | 39 | 2.7 | 26.4 | 0.8 | 22.4 | 3.2 | 6.0 | 2.6 | 1.9 | 0.8 | | | 30 | 113 | 38 | 31 | 2 | | 0.06 | 0.12 | 0.48 | 0.07 | 0.12 | 4.9 | | 0.1 | 0.1 | | 51 | 0.1 | 0.8 | 17 | | 64 | 80 | | 151 | 0.42 |
| 2085 | 1 ea | Chocolate, caramel cvrd, avg | 54 | 171 | 43 | 2.4 | 16.7 | 0.3 | 13.5 | 2.9 | 10.9 | 6.4 | 2.6 | 0.8 | | | 1 | 105 | 25 | 21 | 4 | | 0.02 | 0.10 | 0.52 | 0.12 | 0.21 | 5.9 | | 0.4 | 0.1 | | 136 | 0.1 | 0.4 | 16 | | 62 | 129 | | 50 | 0.34 |
| 2084 | 1 ea | Chocolate, choc cvrd, avg | 68 | 205 | 48 | 2.0 | 17.4 | 0.2 | 17.1 | 0.2 | 15.2 | 11.6 | 2.3 | 0.4 | | | 24 | 220 | 68 | 57 | 6 | | 0.02 | 0.13 | 0.08 | 0.03 | 0.21 | 2.9 | | 0.3 | 0.1 | | 69 | 0.0 | 0.2 | 11 | | 62 | 126 | | 43 | 0.42 |
| 70639 | 1 ea | Chocolate Dark Chocolate, Haagan-Dazs | 112 | 380 | | 5.0 | 38.0 | | | | 27.0 | 15.0 | 11.5 | 0.5 | | | 85 | 373 | 112 | 112 | 0 | | | 0.11 | | | | | | | | | 112 | | 2.0 | | | 112 | 240 | | 60 | |
| 2257 | 1 ea | Chocolate Mousse, Weight Watchers | 41 | 35 | | 2.0 | 9.0 | 2.0 | 4.5 | 2.5 | 0.5 | 0.3 | | | | | 2 | 150 | 30 | | | | | | | | | | | 0.0 | | | 75 | | 0.4 | | | | 105 | | 40 | |
| 70682 | 1 ea | Chocolate Peanut Butter Crunch, Haagan-Dazs | 63 | 283 | | 6.0 | 16.1 | | | | 21.1 | 7.0 | 11.0 | 3.0 | | | 35 | 84 | 25 | | | | | 0.02 | 1.26 | | | | | | | | 50 | | 0.5 | | | 50 | 191 | | 55 | |
| 2026 | 1 ea | Chocolate, pudding pop, avg | 47 | 72 | 65 | 1.9 | 11.9 | 0.2 | 9.5 | 2.3 | 2.2 | 2.1 | 0.0 | 0.0 | | | 1 | 52 | 15 | 16 | 0 | | 0.02 | 0.08 | 0.06 | 0.01 | 0.25 | 1.4 | 0.16 | 0.2 | 0.0 | | 66 | 0.0 | 0.2 | 10 | 0.0 | 53 | 105 | | 78 | 0.17 |
| 70302 | 1 ea | Chocolate w/Dark Ctng, Haagan-Dazs | 112 | 390 | 41 | 5.0 | 32.0 | | | | 27.0 | | | | | | 85 | 0 | 0 | 0 | 0 | 0 | 0.00 | 0.26 | 0.40 | | | | | | | | 80 | | 0.7 | | | 150 | 270 | | 60 | |
| 70643 | 1 ea | Coffee Almond Crunch, Haagan-Dazs | 106 | 358 | | 5.0 | 27.9 | | | | 25.9 | 14.9 | 7.9 | 3.0 | | | 100 | 529 | 159 | 159 | 0 | | | 0.18 | | | | | | | | | 159 | | 0.4 | | | 106 | 209 | | 89 | |
| 2089 | 1 ea | Cookie Sandwich, avg | 59 | 143 | 48 | 2.6 | 21.8 | 0.6 | 16.1 | 5.1 | 5.6 | 3.3 | 1.7 | 0.4 | | | 20 | 184 | 58 | 48 | 5 | | 0.03 | 0.12 | 0.18 | 0.03 | 0.18 | 4.8 | | 0.3 | 0.1 | | 60 | 0.1 | 0.3 | 12 | | 64 | 122 | 1.9 | 37 | 0.43 |
| 2385 | 100 g | Cookie Dough Dynamo, Extraas, Haagan-Dazs | 100 | 374 | 35 | 4.5 | 33.9 | 1.3 | 27.5 | 5.1 | 24.6 | 14.0 | | | | | 57 | 366 | 73 | | | | | | | | | | | 0.5 | | | 110 | | 0.8 | | | | | | 123 | |
| 2028 | 1 ea | Creamsicle, avg | 66 | 92 | 67 | 1.6 | 17.7 | 0.0 | 17.4 | 0.3 | 2.0 | 1.3 | 0.6 | 0.1 | | | 7 | 85 | 22 | 20 | 2 | | 0.02 | 0.10 | 0.05 | 0.03 | 0.24 | 4.4 | 0.09 | 0.9 | 0.1 | | 62 | 0.0 | 0.1 | 7 | | 48 | 102 | 1.2 | 42 | 0.38 |
| 2029 | 1 ea | Drumstick, avg | 60 | 157 | 48 | 3.4 | 17.9 | 0.7 | 13.8 | 3.5 | 8.8 | 4.3 | 3.1 | 1.0 | | | 20 | 193 | 55 | 49 | 6 | | 0.04 | 0.14 | 0.89 | 0.04 | 0.18 | 7.5 | 0.28 | 0.3 | 0.1 | | 71 | 0.1 | 0.4 | 21 | | 86 | 151 | 4.0 | 48 | 0.72 |
| 2325 | 1 ea | Freezer Bar, asstd flvrs, Haagan-Dazs | 28 | 16 | | 0.0 | 4.6 | 0.0 | 4.6 | 0.0 | 0.0 | 0.0 | 0.0 | 0.0 | 0.00 | 0.00 | 0 | 0 | 0 | 0 | 0 | 0 | | | | | | | | 0.0 | | | 0 | | 0.0 | | | | 0 | | 7 | |
| 2323 | 1 ea | Freezer Bar, asstd flvrs, sugar free, Haagan-Dazs | 28 | 7 | | 0.0 | 1.6 | 0.0 | 0.0 | 1.6 | 0.0 | 0.0 | 0.0 | 0.0 | 0.00 | 0.00 | 0 | 0 | 0 | 0 | 0 | 0 | | | | | | | | 0.0 | | | 0 | | 0.0 | | | | 0 | | 15 | |
| 70685 | 1 ea | Fudge Bar, Haagan-Dazs | 80 | 210 | | 4.0 | 19.0 | | | | 14.0 | 7.0 | 6.5 | 0.5 | | | 75 | 266 | 80 | | | | | 0.05 | | | | | | | | | 80 | | 0.6 | | | 80 | 160 | | 50 | |
| 2030 | 1 ea | Fudgesicle, avg | 73 | 91 | 68 | 3.8 | 18.6 | 0.1 | 14.5 | 3.9 | 0.2 | 0.1 | 0.1 | 0.0 | | | 1 | 8 | 2 | 2 | 0 | | 0.03 | 0.18 | 0.07 | 0.05 | 0.62 | 1.5 | 0.37 | 0.4 | 0.1 | | 129 | 0.0 | 0.1 | 14 | | 99 | 173 | | 55 | 0.34 |
| 2386 | 100 g | Iced Cappuccino, Extraas, Haagan-Dazs | 100 | 345 | 43 | 4.7 | 25.2 | 0.8 | 24.0 | 0.4 | 24.9 | 14.6 | | | | | 85 | 444 | 89 | | | | | | | | | | | 0.6 | | | 137 | | 0.6 | | | | | | 74 | |
| 70686 | 1 ea | Orange & Cream, Haagan-Dazs | 70 | 130 | | 2.0 | 18.0 | | | | 6.0 | 3.0 | | | | | 40 | 140 | 42 | | | | | 0.02 | | | | | | 4.2 | | | 42 | | 0.5 | | | 14 | 60 | | 25 | |
| 70644 | 1 ea | Peanut Butter & Chocolate Chip, Haag Daz | 108 | 399 | | 7.1 | 29.6 | | | | 28.6 | 7.1 | 17.4 | 4.1 | | | | 216 | 65 | 65 | 0 | | | 0.15 | | | | | | | | | 108 | | 0.8 | | | 108 | 245 | | 143 | |
| 2087 | 1 ea | Sandwich, avg | 59 | 143 | 48 | 2.6 | 21.8 | 0.6 | 14.8 | 6.4 | 5.6 | 3.3 | 1.7 | 0.4 | | | 20 | 184 | 58 | 48 | 5 | | 0.03 | 0.12 | 0.18 | 0.03 | 0.18 | 4.8 | | 0.3 | 0.1 | | 60 | 0.1 | 0.3 | 12 | | 64 | 122 | 1.9 | 37 | 0.43 |
| 2387 | 100 g | Triple Brownie Overload, Extraas, Haagan-Dazs | 100 | 374 | 39 | 5.4 | 27.7 | 1.4 | 24.6 | 1.7 | 27.0 | 13.8 | | | | | 93 | 466 | 98 | | | | | | | | | | | 0.4 | | | 111 | | 1.3 | | | | | | 111 | |
| 70642 | 1 ea | Vanilla & Almonds, Haagan-Dazs | 106 | 368 | | 6.0 | 25.9 | | | | 26.9 | 13.9 | 9.9 | 3.0 | | | 89 | 529 | 159 | 159 | 0 | | | 0.18 | | | | | | | | | 159 | | 0.4 | | | 106 | 219 | | 85 | |
| 70638 | 1 ea | Vanilla Caramel Brittle, Haagan-Dazs | 108 | 372 | | 5.0 | 32.2 | | | | 25.1 | 14.1 | 8.0 | 3.0 | | | 85 | 360 | 108 | 108 | 0 | | | 0.18 | 0.43 | | | | | | | | 162 | | 0.4 | | | 108 | 201 | | 171 | |
| 70683 | 1 ea | Vanilla Crisp Crunch, Haagan-Dazs | 59 | 221 | | 3.0 | 16.1 | | | | 16.1 | 6.0 | 8.0 | 2.0 | | | 40 | 118 | 35 | | | | | 0.04 | | | | | | | | | 47 | | 0.2 | | | 24 | 126 | | 55 | |
| 70640 | 1 ea | Vanilla Dark Chocolate, Haagan-Dazs | 112 | 380 | | 5.0 | 38.0 | | | | 27.0 | 15.0 | 11.5 | 0.5 | | | 90 | 373 | 112 | 112 | 0 | | | 0.15 | | | | | | | | | 112 | | 1.6 | | | 112 | 250 | | 65 | |
| 70641 | 1 ea | Vanilla Milk Chocolate, Haagan-Dazs | 100 | 330 | | 5.0 | 25.0 | | | | 24.0 | 14.0 | 7.0 | 3.0 | | | 90 | 333 | 100 | 100 | 0 | | | 0.14 | | | | | | | | | 150 | | 0.4 | | | 100 | 200 | | 75 | |
| 2027 | 1 ea | Vanilla pudding pop, avg | 47 | 75 | 64 | 1.9 | 12.6 | 0.0 | 10.4 | 2.2 | 2.1 | 2.1 | 0.0 | 0.0 | | | 1 | 81 | 24 | 24 | 0 | | 0.02 | 0.09 | 0.02 | 0.02 | 0.17 | 2.3 | 0.18 | 0.1 | 0.0 | | 61 | 0.0 | 0.0 | 5 | 0.0 | 47 | 65 | | 50 | 0.16 |
| 2258 | 1 ea | Vanilla Sandwich, Weight Watchers | 68 | 160 | 43 | 4.0 | 30.0 | 1.0 | 14.0 | 15.0 | 3.5 | 2.0 | | | | | 5 | 0 | 0 | 0 | 0 | 0 | | | | | | | | 0.0 | | | 100 | | 0.7 | | | | 110 | | 180 | |
| 70304 | 1 ea | Vanilla w/Dark Chocolate Ctng, Haagan-Dazs | 112 | 390 | 41 | 5.0 | 32.0 | | | | 27.0 | | | | | | 85 | 0 | 0 | 0 | 0 | 0 | 0.03 | 0.17 | 0.80 | | | | | | | | 80 | | 1.1 | | | 150 | 230 | | 65 | |
| 70305 | 1 ea | Vanilla w/Milk Choc Almond Ctng, Haagan-Dazs | 105 | 370 | 42 | 5.0 | 27.0 | | | | 27.0 | | | | | | 85 | 0 | 0 | 0 | 0 | 0 | 0.00 | 0.14 | 0.80 | | | | | 1.2 | | | 100 | | 0.7 | | | 150 | 190 | | 55 | |
| 70303 | 1 ea | Vanilla w/Milk Chocolate Ctng, Haagan-Dazs | 100 | 360 | 41 | 4.0 | 26.0 | | | | 27.0 | | | | | | 85 | 0 | 0 | 0 | 0 | 0 | 0.00 | 0.10 | 0.40 | | | | | | | | 100 | | 1.1 | | | 100 | 180 | | 55 | |
| | | Ice Cream Cones | | | | | | | | | | | | | | | | | | | | | | | | | | | | | | | | | | | | | | | | |
| 2113 | 1 ea | Chocolate, avg | 78 | 171 | 54 | 3.3 | 24.7 | 0.6 | 19.1 | 4.9 | 7.2 | 4.4 | 2.1 | 0.3 | | | 18 | 250 | 62 | 55 | 7 | | 0.04 | 0.14 | 0.34 | 0.03 | 0.27 | 4.4 | 0.43 | 0.4 | 0.2 | | 96 | 0.1 | 0.4 | 16 | 0.1 | 89 | 175 | 2.2 | 51 | 0.44 |
| 2092 | 1 ea | Chocolate Dipped, avg | 78 | 185 | 52 | 3.1 | 24.0 | 0.4 | 19.0 | 4.5 | 9.3 | 5.7 | 2.8 | 0.4 | | | 29 | 271 | 77 | 70 | 7 | | 0.04 | 0.19 | 0.33 | 0.04 | 0.26 | 3.9 | 0.43 | 0.4 | 0.1 | | 95 | 0.1 | 0.4 | 18 | 0.0 | 89 | 168 | | 66 | 0.60 |
| 2090 | 1 ea | Chocolate Dipped, w/nuts, avg | 78 | 214 | 47 | 4.4 | 22.8 | 1.3 | 17.2 | 4.3 | 12.9 | 5.5 | 5.4 | 1.3 | | | 26 | 244 | 69 | 63 | 7 | | 0.05 | 0.25 | 0.57 | 0.04 | 0.23 | 8.6 | | 0.4 | 0.1 | | 104 | 0.2 | 0.6 | 40 | | 123 | 206 | | 60 | 0.92 |
| 2093 | 1 ea | Vanilla, avg | 78 | 167 | 57 | 3.1 | 21.7 | 0.1 | 17.3 | 4.3 | 8.1 | 4.9 | 2.3 | 0.4 | | | 32 | 294 | 84 | 76 | 8 | | 0.04 | 0.20 | 0.33 | 0.04 | 0.28 | 4.1 | 0.43 | 0.4 | 0.1 | 0.0 | 101 | 0.0 | 0.2 | 11 | 0.0 | 87 | 158 | | 72 | 0.53 |
| 2480 | 1 ea | Vanilla, w/ nuts, avg | 78 | 202 | 51 | 4.5 | 20.6 | 1.0 | | | 12.1 | 4.8 | 5.2 | 1.4 | | | 28 | 262 | 75 | 68 | 7 | | 0.05 | 0.26 | 0.59 | 0.04 | 0.25 | 9.1 | | 0.4 | | | 111 | 0.1 | 0.5 | 36 | | 125 | 199 | | 65 | 0.89 |
| | | Ice Milk | | | | | | | | | | | | | | | | | | | | | | | | | | | | | | | | | | | | | | | | |
| 2057 | 1/2 cup | Chocolate, avg | 66 | 95 | 66 | 2.8 | 17.1 | 0.3 | 16.5 | 0.2 | 2.1 | 1.3 | 0.6 | 0.1 | | | 6 | 72 | 13 | 16 | 2 | | 0.03 | 0.12 | 0.09 | 0.03 | 0.30 | 4.1 | 0.26 | 0.5 | 0.0 | | 95 | 0.0 | 0.2 | 13 | | 79 | 156 | 1.0 | 41 | 0.38 |
| 2058 | 1/2 cup | Strawberry, avg | 68 | 122 | 61 | 3.1 | 18.7 | 0.0 | 18.4 | 0.3 | 4.1 | 2.5 | 0.8 | 0.2 | 0.06 | 0.10 | 16 | 112 | 27 | 24 | 3 | | 0.05 | 0.20 | 0.07 | 0.05 | 0.51 | 2.0 | | 0.5 | 0.0 | | 109 | 0.0 | 0.1 | 11 | | 80 | 162 | 1.0 | 63 | 0.34 |
| 2009 | 1/2 cup | Vanilla, avg | 66 | 92 | 68 | 2.5 | 15.0 | 0.0 | 14.9 | 0.1 | 2.8 | 1.7 | 0.8 | 0.1 | 0.04 | 0.07 | 9 | 109 | 31 | 28 | 3 | | 0.04 | 0.17 | 0.06 | 0.04 | 0.44 | 4.0 | 0.33 | 0.5 | 0.0 | 0.0 | 92 | 0.0 | 0.1 | 10 | 0.0 | 72 | 139 | 1.8 | 56 | 0.29 |
| 2423 | 1/2 cup | Vanilla, ice milk, light, Breyers | 70 | 84 | 74 | 2.1 | 12.6 | | | | 2.8 | 1.4 | 0.7 | 0.0 | 0.00 | 0.00 | 7 | 70 | 20 | | | | 0.02 | 0.11 | | | 0.08 | | | | | | 56 | | | | | 56 | 112 | | 42 | |
| 23204 | 1 ea | Ice Pops, w/added vit C, avg | 52 | 37 | 80 | 0.0 | 9.8 | 0.0 | 6.3 | 3.5 | 0.0 | 0.0 | 0.0 | 0.0 | 0.00 | 0.00 | 0 | 0 | 0 | 0 | 0 | 0 | 0.00 | 0.00 | 0.00 | 0.00 | 0.00 | 0.0 | 0.00 | 5.6 | 0.0 | 0.0 | 0 | 0.0 | 0.0 | 1 | 0.0 | 0 | 2 | 0.0 | 6 | 0.01 |
| | | Ices | | | | | | | | | | | | | | | | | | | | | | | | | | | | | | | | | | | | | | | | |
| 23430 | 1/2 cup | Italian, avg | 116 | 61 | 86 | 0.0 | 15.7 | 0.0 | | | 0.0 | 0.0 | 0.0 | 0.0 | 0.00 | 0.00 | 0 | 194 | 19 | 0 | 19 | | 0.01 | 0.01 | 0.83 | 0.00 | 0.00 | 5.8 | 0.01 | 0.6 | 0.0 | 0.0 | 1 | 0.0 | 0.1 | 0 | 0.0 | 0 | 7 | 0.1 | 5 | 0.03 |
| 23159 | 1/2 cup | Lime, avg | 99 | 127 | 67 | 0.4 | 32.3 | 0.0 | 32.3 | 0.0 | 0.0 | 0.0 | 0.0 | 0.0 | 0.00 | 0.00 | 0 | 0 | 0 | 0 | 0 | 0 | 0.00 | 0.00 | 0.01 | 0.00 | 0.00 | 0.0 | 0.00 | 1.0 | 0.0 | 0.0 | 2 | 0.0 | 0.2 | 1 | 0.0 | 1 | 3 | 0.1 | 22 | 0.02 |
| 23432 | 1/2 cup | Pineapple-coconut, avg | 99 | 112 | 73 | 0.0 | 23.7 | 0.7 | | | 2.6 | 2.3 | 0.1 | 0.0 | | | 0 | 0 | 0 | 0 | 0 | 0 | 0.01 | 0.00 | 0.03 | 0.02 | 0.00 | 1.0 | 0.04 | 13.1 | 0.0 | 0.0 | 0 | 0.0 | 3.5 | 5 | 0.2 | 9 | 17 | 0.9 | 35 | 0.11 |
| 23051 | 1/2 cup | Snow cones/slushy, avg | 96 | 75 | 67 | 0.4 | 31.3 | 0.0 | 31.3 | 0.0 | 0.0 | 0.0 | 0.0 | 0.0 | 0.00 | 0.00 | 0 | 0 | 0 | 0 | 0 | 0 | 0.00 | 0.00 | 0.01 | 0.00 | 0.00 | 0.0 | 0.00 | 1.0 | 0.0 | 0.0 | 2 | 0.0 | 0.2 | 1 | | 1 | 3 | 0.0 | 21 | 0.02 |
| | | Juice Bars | | | | | | | | | | | | | | | | | | | | | | | | | | | | | | | | | | | | | | | | |
| 23174 | 1 ea | Avg | 77 | 63 | 78 | 0.9 | 15.6 | 0.0 | | | 0.1 | 0.0 | 0.0 | 0.0 | 0.01 | 0.02 | 0 | 22 | 2 | 0 | 2 | | 0.01 | 0.01 | 0.12 | 0.02 | 0.00 | 4.6 | 0.03 | 7.3 | 0.0 | 0.0 | 4 | 0.0 | 0.1 | 3 | 0.1 | 5 | 41 | 0.2 | 3 | 0.04 |
| 23160 | 1 ea | Sugar free, aspartame swtnd, avg | 51 | 12 | 93 | 0.3 | 3.2 | 0.0 | 0.0 | 3.2 | 0.1 | 0.0 | | | | | 0 | 0.5 | 0.05 | 0 | 0.05 | 0 | 0.00 | 0.00 | 0.08 | 0.00 | 0.00 | 0.0 | 0.00 | 0.0 | 0.0 | 0.0 | 1 | 0.0 | 0.1 | 1 | 0.0 | 0 | 13 | 0.1 | 3 | 0.02 |
| 23094 | 1 ea | With Cream, avg | 65 | 86 | 67 | 1.0 | 19.3 | 0.1 | 8.8 | 10.4 | 1.3 | 0.8 | 0.4 | 0.0 | | | 5 | 83 | 3 | 0 | 8 | | 0.01 | 0.06 | 0.12 | 0.03 | 0.05 | 3.3 | | 7.5 | | | 29 | 0.0 | 0.1 | 2 | | 5 | 64 | | 19 | 0.05 |
| | | Sherbet/Sorbet | | | | | | | | | | | | | | | | | | | | | | | | | | | | | | | | | | | | | | | | |
| 2066 | 1/2 cup | Citrus, avg | 100 | 92 | 76 | 0.5 | 23.1 | 0.1 | 23.1 | 0.0 | 0.0 | 0.0 | 0.0 | 0.0 | 0.00 | 0.00 | 0 | 272 | 27 | 0 | 27 | | 0.01 | 0.03 | 0.16 | 0.02 | 0.00 | 22.0 | 0.02 | 25.7 | 0.0 | | 9 | 0.0 | 0.5 | 8 | 0.0 | 13 | 100 | 0.6 | 8 | 0.02 |
| 23275 | 1/2 cup | Lemon, sugar free, Diamond Crystal | 43 | 22 | 88 | 0.0 | 5.0 | 0.0 | | | 0.0 | 0.0 | 0.0 | 0.0 | 0.00 | 0.00 | 0 | 0 | 0 | 0 | 0 | 0 | 0.00 | 0.00 | 0.00 | | | | | 35.8 | | | 0 | | 0.0 | | | | 7 | | 22 | |
| 2065 | 1/2 cup | Non citrus, avg | 100 | 70 | 82 | 1.2 | 16.7 | 0.0 | 16.7 | 0.0 | 0.1 | 0.0 | 0.0 | 0.0 | 0.00 | 0.00 | 0 | 0 | 0 | 0 | 0 | 0 | 0.00 | 0.00 | 0.00 | 0.00 | 0.00 | 0.0 | 0.00 | 0.0 | 0.0 | 0.0 | 2 | 0.0 | 0.0 | 1 | 0.0 | 0 | 2 | 0.6 | 46 | 0.03 |
| 2011 | 1/2 cup | Orange, avg | 99 | 137 | 66 | 1.1 | 30.1 | 0.0 | 24.1 | 6.0 | 2.0 | 1.1 | 0.5 | 0.1 | 0.03 | 0.05 | 6 | 75 | 11 | 11 | 3 | | 0.02 | 0.08 | 0.06 | 0.02 | 0.19 | 4.9 | 0.18 | 3.1 | 0.0 | | 53 | 0.0 | 0.1 | 8 | 0.0 | 40 | 95 | 1.3 | 46 | 0.48 |
| 70308 | 1/2 cup | Orange/Vanilla, Haagen-Daz | 106 | 199 | 59 | 3.0 | 29.9 | | | | 8.0 | 4.0 | | | | | 59 | 282 | 85 | | | | 0.03 | 0.11 | 0.85 | | | | | 6.4 | | | 64 | | 0.0 | | | 64 | 114 | | 30 | |
| 70309 | 1/2 cup | Raspberry/Vanilla, Haagen-Daz | 106 | 179 | 64 | 3.0 | 25.9 | | | | 7.0 | 4.0 | | | | | 59 | 424 | 85 | | | | | 0.14 | 0.42 | | | | | | | | 64 | | 0.0 | | | 64 | 114 | | 30 | |

| Code | Amount | Description | Basic Components | | | | | | | | | Additional Fats | | | | | |
|---|---|---|---|---|---|---|---|---|---|---|---|---|---|---|---|---|---|
| | | | Weight (g) | Calories | % Water | Protein (g) | Carbs (g) | Fiber (g) | Sugar (g) | Other Carbs (g) | Fat (g) | Sat Fat (g) | Mono Fat (g) | Poly Fat (g) | Omega 3 (g) | Omega 6 (g) | Choles (mg) |
| 23276 | 1/2 cup | Strawberry, sugar free, Diamond Crystal | 43 | 22 | 88 | 0.0 | 5.0 | 0.0 | | | 0.0 | 0.0 | 0.0 | 0.0 | 0.00 | 0.00 | 0 |
| | | Sundaes | | | | | | | | | | | | | | | |
| 2377 | 1 ea | Chocolate, small, avg | 170 | 290 | 62 | 6.0 | 51.0 | 0.0 | 44.0 | 7.0 | 7.0 | 4.5 | | | | | 25 |
| 2256 | 1 ea | Chocolate Chip Cookie Dough, Weight Watchers | 154 | 180 | | 3.0 | 34.0 | 2.0 | 21.0 | 11.0 | 4.0 | 1.5 | | | | | 5 |
| 2069 | 1 ea | Chocolate w/whippd cream, small, avg | 165 | 417 | 52 | 5.7 | 46.4 | 0.5 | 38.4 | 7.5 | 25.4 | 14.7 | 7.3 | 1.9 | | | 81 |
| 70729 | 1 ea | Praline Toffee Crunch Parfait, Weight Watchers | 145 | 191 | | 5.0 | 40.1 | 2.0 | 20.1 | 18.0 | 3.0 | 2.0 | | | | | 5 |
| | | Tofutti | | | | | | | | | | | | | | | |
| 70518 | 1/2 cup | Cappuccino Love Drop, Life Lite | 75 | 230 | | 3.0 | 26.0 | | | | 12.0 | 3.0 | 3.5 | 5.5 | | | 0 |
| 70520 | 1/2 cup | Chocolate, lite, soft serve, Life Lite | 75 | 90 | 69 | 2.0 | 20.0 | | | | 0.9 | | | | | | 0 |
| 70422 | 1/2 cup | Chocolate Love Drop, Life Lite | 75 | 230 | 44 | 3.0 | 26.0 | | | | 13.0 | 5.0 | 4.0 | 4.0 | | | 0 |
| 70418 | 1/2 cup | Chocolate Supreme, Life Lite | 75 | 210 | 52 | 3.0 | 20.0 | | | | 13.0 | 3.0 | 4.0 | 6.0 | | | 0 |
| 70521 | 1/2 cup | Regular, soft serve, Life Lite | 75 | 158 | 63 | 1.0 | 20.0 | | | | 8.0 | 1.5 | 2.5 | 4.0 | | | 0 |
| 70416 | 1/2 cup | Vanilla, Life Lite | 75 | 200 | | 2.0 | 21.0 | | | | 11.0 | 1.5 | 3.0 | 6.5 | | | 0 |
| 70419 | 1/2 cup | Wildberry, Life Lite | 75 | 210 | 52 | 2.0 | 22.0 | | | | 12.0 | 3.0 | 3.0 | 6.0 | | | 0 |
| | | Yogurt, Frozen | | | | | | | | | | | | | | | |
| 70348 | 1/2 cup | All Flavors, nonfat, Dannon | 86 | 94 | 69 | 3.4 | 21.9 | 0.0 | | | 0.0 | 0.0 | 0.0 | 0.0 | | | 0 |
| 2295 | 1/2 cup | Black Cherry, lowfat, Breyers | 114 | 131 | | 4.0 | 25.1 | 0.0 | 23.6 | 1.5 | 1.3 | 0.8 | | | | | 8 |
| 2296 | 1/2 cup | Blueberry, lowfat, Breyers | 114 | 126 | | 4.0 | 24.1 | 0.0 | 24.1 | 0.0 | 1.3 | 0.8 | | | | | 8 |
| 2461 | 1/2 cup | Blueberry, nonfat, Darigold | 75 | 100 | 65 | 4.0 | 22.0 | 1.0 | 17.0 | 4.0 | 0.0 | 0.0 | 0.0 | 0.0 | 0.00 | 0.00 | 0 |
| 2462 | 1/2 cup | Boysnbry Cheesecake, nonfat, Darigold | 75 | 120 | 61 | 4.0 | 25.0 | 0.0 | 21.0 | 4.0 | 0.0 | 0.0 | 0.0 | 0.0 | 0.00 | 0.00 | 5 |
| 2346 | 1/2 cup | Cappucino, fat free, Ben & Jerry's | 93 | 140 | 61 | 3.0 | 32.0 | 0.0 | 23.0 | 9.0 | 0.0 | 0.0 | 0.0 | 0.0 | 0.00 | 0.00 | 0 |
| 2212 | 1/2 cup | Cherry Garcia, Ben & Jerry's | 106 | 170 | | 4.0 | 31.0 | 0.0 | 30.0 | 1.0 | 3.0 | 2.0 | | | | | 10 |
| 2045 | 1 ea | Chocolate, cone, avg | 78 | 157 | 57 | 3.7 | 21.5 | 1.1 | 13.6 | 6.8 | 7.3 | 3.9 | 2.5 | 0.5 | | | 2 |
| 2039 | 1/2 cup | Chocolate, fat free, avg | 96 | 104 | 70 | 5.4 | 21.2 | 1.5 | 16.1 | 3.6 | 0.8 | 0.5 | 0.3 | 0.0 | | | 1 |
| 2071 | 1/2 cup | Chocolate, lowfat, avg | 96 | 109 | 70 | 5.0 | 20.7 | 1.5 | 17.4 | 1.9 | 1.9 | 1.2 | 0.6 | 0.1 | | | 5 |
| 2344 | 1/2 cup | Chocolate Fudge Brownie, Ben & Jerry's | 106 | 190 | 57 | 6.0 | 36.0 | 1.0 | 34.0 | 1.0 | 3.0 | 1.5 | | | | | 5 |
| 2463 | 1/2 cup | Chocolate Marshmallow, nonfat, Darigold | 75 | 130 | 58 | 4.0 | 27.0 | 1.0 | 20.0 | 6.0 | 0.0 | 0.0 | 0.0 | 0.0 | 0.00 | 0.00 | 5 |
| 2303 | 1/2 cup | Coffee, lowfat, Breyers | 114 | 110 | | 5.0 | 19.1 | 0.0 | 18.6 | 0.5 | 1.5 | 1.0 | | | | | 10 |
| 2213 | 1/2 cup | Coffee Almond Fudge, Ben & Jerry's | 106 | 200 | | 6.0 | 30.0 | 1.0 | 29.0 | 0.0 | 7.0 | 2.0 | | | | | 15 |
| 2464 | 1/2 cup | Cookies 'N Cream, nonfat, Darigold | 75 | 120 | 62 | 4.0 | 24.0 | 0.0 | 17.0 | 7.0 | 0.0 | 0.0 | 0.0 | 0.0 | 0.00 | 0.00 | 5 |
| 2214 | 1/2 cup | English Toffee Crnch, Ben & Jerry's | 106 | 190 | | 4.0 | 32.0 | 0.0 | 32.0 | 0.0 | 6.0 | 2.5 | | | | | 10 |
| 70345 | 1/2 cup | Fruit, Dannon | 86 | 103 | 72 | 3.5 | 17.9 | | | | 2.0 | | | | | | 7 |
| 2304 | 1/2 cup | Lemon, lowfat, Breyers | 114 | 110 | | 5.0 | 19.1 | 0.0 | 18.6 | 0.5 | 1.5 | 1.0 | | | | | 10 |
| 2297 | 1/2 cup | Mixed Berry, lowfat, Breyers | 114 | 126 | | 4.0 | 24.1 | 0.0 | 23.1 | 1.0 | 1.3 | 0.8 | | | | | 8 |
| 2465 | 1/2 cup | Mocha Fudge, nonfat, Darigold | 75 | 120 | 57 | 6.0 | 26.0 | 0.0 | 17.0 | 9.0 | 0.0 | 0.0 | 0.0 | 0.0 | 0.00 | 0.00 | 5 |
| 70628 | 1/2 cup | Orange Tango, Haagan-Dazs | 101 | 132 | | 4.1 | 26.5 | | | | 2.0 | 1.0 | 1.0 | 0.0 | 0.00 | 0.00 | 20 |
| 2298 | 1/2 cup | Peach, lowfat, Breyers | 114 | 126 | | 4.0 | 24.1 | 0.0 | 23.6 | 0.5 | 1.3 | 0.8 | | | | | 8 |
| 2458 | 1/2 cup | Peach, nonfat, Darigold | 75 | 100 | 65 | 4.0 | 22.0 | 0.0 | 17.0 | 5.0 | 0.0 | 0.0 | 0.0 | 0.0 | 0.00 | 0.00 | 0 |
| 2388 | 100 g | Pina Colada, Haagan-Dazs | 100 | 139 | 67 | 3.5 | 26.9 | 0.4 | 22.1 | 4.4 | 1.8 | 1.0 | | | | | 25 |
| 2299 | 1/2 cup | Pineapple, lowfat, Breyers | 114 | 126 | | 4.0 | 24.6 | 0.0 | 24.1 | 0.5 | 1.3 | 0.8 | | | | | 8 |
| 2305 | 1/2 cup | Plain, lowfat, Breyers | 114 | 65 | | 5.5 | 7.5 | 0.0 | 7.5 | 0.0 | 1.5 | 1.0 | | | | | 10 |
| 70630 | 1/2 cup | Praline Pandemonium, Haagan-Dazs | 101 | 240 | | 6.9 | 32.5 | | | | 8.9 | 3.9 | 3.9 | 1.0 | | | 44 |
| 2459 | 1/2 cup | Raspberry, nonfat, Darigold | 75 | 110 | 61 | 4.0 | 25.0 | 1.0 | 20.0 | 4.0 | 0.0 | 0.0 | 0.0 | 0.0 | 0.00 | 0.00 | 0 |
| 2300 | 1/2 cup | Red Raspberry, lowfat, Breyers | 114 | 126 | | | 24.1 | 1.0 | 23.1 | 0.0 | 1.3 | 0.8 | | | | | 8 |
| 2044 | 1 ea | Sandwich, avg | 85 | 180 | 52 | 3.9 | 32.0 | 0.4 | 21.0 | 10.7 | 4.4 | 2.3 | 1.3 | 0.4 | | | 2 |
| 2301 | 1/2 cup | Strawberry, lowfat, Breyers | 114 | 126 | | 4.0 | 23.6 | 0.0 | 23.1 | 0.5 | 1.3 | 0.8 | | | | | 8 |
| 2302 | 1/2 cup | Strawberry Banana, lowfat, Breyers | 114 | 126 | | 4.5 | 25.1 | 0.3 | 22.1 | 2.8 | 1.3 | 0.8 | | | | | 8 |
| 70631 | 1/2 cup | Strawberry Cheescake, Haagan-Dazs | 101 | 208 | | 6.9 | 30.8 | | | | 6.9 | 3.0 | 3.5 | 0.5 | | | 49 |
| 2047 | 1 ea | Vanilla, cone, avg | 78 | 143 | 60 | 3.4 | 21.5 | 0.5 | 14.4 | 6.6 | 5.3 | 2.6 | 1.8 | 0.4 | | | 2 |
| 2079 | 1/2 cup | Vanilla, fat free, avg | 96 | 95 | 74 | 4.8 | 18.9 | 0.0 | 18.8 | 0.0 | 0.2 | 0.1 | 0.0 | 0.0 | | | 2 |
| 2075 | 1/2 cup | Vanilla, lowfat, avg | 96 | 101 | 74 | 4.4 | 18.3 | 0.0 | 18.3 | 0.0 | 1.3 | 0.8 | 0.4 | 0.0 | | | 5 |
| 2306 | 1/2 cup | Vanilla, lowfat, Breyers | 114 | 110 | | 5.0 | 19.1 | 0.0 | 19.1 | 0.0 | 1.5 | 1.0 | | | | | 10 |
| 70636 | 1/2 cup | Vanilla Almond Crunch, Haagan-Dazs | 98 | 201 | | 8.0 | 29.1 | | | | 6.0 | 2.0 | 4.0 | 0.0 | 0.00 | 0.00 | 50 |
| | | Yogurt, Frozen Bar | | | | | | | | | | | | | | | |
| 2083 | 1 ea | Carob Coated, avg | 41 | 100 | 51 | 2.5 | 12.2 | 0.6 | 9.7 | 2.0 | 4.8 | 1.9 | 2.2 | 0.4 | | | 1 |
| 70678 | 1 ea | Cherry Chocolate Fudge, Haagan-Dazs | 74 | 232 | | 5.0 | 28.2 | | | | 12.1 | 7.0 | 4.0 | 1.0 | | | 36 |
| 2043 | 1 ea | Chocolate Coated, avg | 41 | 109 | 51 | 1.3 | 11.8 | 0.1 | 10.1 | 1.6 | 6.7 | 5.4 | 0.8 | 0.2 | | | 1 |
| 70666 | 1 ea | Coffee Chocolate Crunch, Haagan-Dazs | 72 | 209 | | 5.0 | 23.8 | | | | 10.9 | 2.0 | 3.0 | 6.0 | | | 20 |
| 70668 | 1 ea | Peach, Haagan-Dazs | 72 | 100 | | 2.0 | 19.0 | | | | 1.0 | 0.0 | 0.5 | 0.5 | | | 15 |
| 70680 | 1 ea | Pina Colada, Haagan-Dazs | 70 | 100 | | 2.0 | 21.0 | | | | 1.0 | 0.5 | | | | | 15 |
| 70667 | 1 ea | Raspberry, Haagan-Dazs | 72 | 100 | | 3.0 | 19.0 | | | | 1.0 | 0.0 | 0.5 | 0.5 | | | 15 |
| 70681 | 1 ea | Strawberry Daiquiri, Haagan-Dazs | 70 | 100 | | 2.0 | 20.0 | | | | 1.0 | 0.5 | | | | | 20 |
| 70679 | 1 ea | Tropical Orange Passion, Haagan-Dazs | 70 | 100 | | 2.0 | 21.0 | | | | 1.0 | 0.5 | | | | | 20 |
| 70665 | 1 ea | Vanilla Chocolate Crunch, Haagan-Dazs | 72 | 209 | | 5.0 | 22.8 | | | | 10.9 | 2.0 | 3.0 | 6.0 | | | 24 |
| | | *FRUIT DESSERTS* | | | | | | | | | | | | | | | |
| 49018 | 1 ea | Blintz, fruit filled, avg | 70 | 125 | 62 | 3.9 | 17.4 | 0.4 | | | 4.5 | 1.4 | 1.8 | 1.0 | | | 50 |
| 49005 | 1/2 cup | Brown Betty, apple, avg | 103 | 175 | 62 | 2.4 | 30.6 | 2.5 | 16.1 | 12.1 | 5.3 | 2.8 | 1.5 | 0.6 | 0.11 | 0.50 | 11 |
| | | Cobbler | | | | | | | | | | | | | | | |
| 49003 | 1 pce | Apple, avg | 104 | 199 | 57 | 1.9 | 35.0 | 2.1 | 23.2 | 9.7 | 6.4 | 1.2 | 2.8 | 2.0 | 0.15 | 1.83 | 1 |
| 49062 | 1 pce | Apple, Marie Calender's | 125 | 350 | 47 | 2.0 | 45.0 | 2.0 | 26.0 | 17.0 | 18.0 | 4.0 | | | | | 0 |

| Code | Vit A & Components | | | | | Vitamins | | | | | | | | | | Minerals | | | | | | | | | |
|---|---|---|---|---|---|---|---|---|---|---|---|---|---|---|---|---|---|---|---|---|---|---|---|---|---|
| | Vit A (IU) | Vit A (RE) | Retinol (RE) | Carotenoids (RE) | Beta Carotene (mcg) | Thiamin (mg) | Riboflavin (mg) | Niacin (NE) | Vit B6 (mg) | Vit B12 (mcg) | Folate (mcg) | Panto (mg) | Vit C (mg) | Vit D (mg) | Vit E (α TE) | Calcium (mg) | Copper (mg) | Iron (mg) | Magnes (mg) | Mang (mg) | Phos (mg) | Potassium (mg) | Selenium (mcg) | Sodium (mg) | Zinc (mg) |
| 23276 | 0 | 0 | 0 | 0 | 0 | 0.00 | 0.00 | 0.00 | | | | | 35.8 | | | 0 | | 0.0 | | | | 7 | | 22 | |
| 2377 | 500 | 100 | | | | | | | | | | | 0.0 | | | 200 | | 1.1 | | | | | | 150 | |
| 2256 | 0 | 0 | 0 | 0 | 0 | | | | | | | | 0.0 | | | 80 | | 0.7 | | | | 170 | | 120 | |
| 2069 | 776 | 212 | 194 | 18 | | 0.06 | 0.35 | 0.20 | 0.07 | 0.55 | 7.4 | | 1.0 | | | 181 | 0.1 | 0.6 | 35 | | 185 | 302 | 0.5 | 137 | 1.04 |
| 70729 | 0 | 0 | 0 | 0 | 0 | | | | | | | | 0.0 | | | 201 | | 0.0 | | | | 191 | | 140 | |
| 70518 | | | | | | | | | | | | | | | | | | | | | 45 | 85 | | 120 | |
| 70520 | | | | | | | | | | | | | | | | | | | | | 35 | 50 | | 80 | |
| 70422 | | | | | | | | | | | | | | | | | | | | | 65 | 80 | | 100 | |
| 70418 | | | | | | | | | | | | | | | | | | | | | | 40 | | 130 | |
| 70521 | | | | | | | | | | | | | | | | | | | | | 25 | 25 | | 85 | |
| 70416 | | | | | | | | | | | | | | | | | | | | | | 30 | | 90 | |
| 70419 | | | | | | | | | | | | | | | | | | | | | | 10 | | 100 | |
| 70348 | 13 | 4 | | | | 0.04 | 0.20 | | 0.07 | 0.40 | | | 1.0 | | | 127 | | 0.1 | | | | | | 53 | |
| 2295 | 0 | 0 | 0 | 0 | 0 | 0.03 | 0.17 | | | 0.45 | | | 0.0 | | | 151 | | 0.0 | | | 126 | 216 | | 55 | |
| 2296 | 0 | 0 | 0 | 0 | 0 | 0.02 | 0.17 | | | 0.45 | | | 0.0 | | | 151 | | 0.0 | | | 126 | 196 | | 55 | |
| 2461 | 0 | 0 | 0 | 0 | 0 | | | | | | | | 1.2 | | | 100 | | 0.5 | | | | 190 | | 75 | |
| 2462 | 0 | 0 | 0 | 0 | 0 | | | | | | | | 0.0 | | | 100 | | 0.5 | | | | 190 | | 80 | |
| 2346 | 100 | 20 | | | | | | | | | | | 0.0 | | | 100 | | 0.0 | | | | | | 85 | |
| 2212 | 200 | 40 | | | | | | | | | | | 1.2 | | | 150 | | 0.4 | | | | | | 70 | |
| 2045 | 173 | 42 | 35 | 6 | | 0.05 | 0.17 | 0.34 | 0.08 | 0.20 | 6.1 | 0.19 | 0.5 | | | 115 | 0.1 | 0.6 | 29 | | 119 | 193 | | 70 | 0.54 |
| 2039 | 7 | 1.7 | 1.6 | 0.1 | | 0.04 | 0.21 | 0.22 | 0.05 | 0.48 | 11.2 | 0.48 | 0.7 | 0.0 | | 162 | 0.2 | 0.9 | 38 | 0.1 | 159 | 325 | 2.5 | 61 | 1.08 |
| 2071 | 53 | 13 | 11 | 2 | | 0.04 | 0.19 | 0.21 | 0.04 | 0.44 | 10.4 | 0.24 | 0.6 | | | 149 | 0.2 | 0.8 | 37 | | 150 | 309 | | 57 | 1.02 |
| 2344 | 200 | 40 | | | | | | | | | | | 1.2 | | | 150 | | 1.1 | | | | | | 115 | |
| 2463 | 0 | 0 | 0 | 0 | 0 | | | | | | | | 0.0 | | | 100 | | 0.5 | | | | 190 | | 90 | |
| 2303 | 50 | 12 | | | | 0.03 | 0.21 | | | 0.60 | | | 0.0 | | | 176 | | 0.0 | | | 151 | 236 | | 68 | |
| 2213 | 300 | 60 | | | | | | | | | | | 1.2 | | | 150 | | 0.7 | | | | | | 85 | |
| 2464 | 0 | 0 | 0 | 0 | 0 | | | | | | | | 0.0 | | | 100 | | 0.5 | | | | 190 | | 100 | |
| 2214 | 300 | 60 | | | | | | | | | | | 0.0 | | | 150 | | 0.4 | | | | | | 110 | |
| 70345 | 56 | 17 | | | | 0.04 | 0.20 | | | 0.38 | | | | | | 126 | | | | | | | | 52 | |
| 2304 | 50 | 12 | | | | 0.03 | 0.21 | | | 0.60 | | | 0.0 | | | 176 | | 0.0 | | | 151 | 236 | | 70 | |
| 2297 | 0 | 0 | 0 | 0 | 0 | 0.02 | 0.17 | | | 0.45 | | | 0.0 | | | 151 | | 0.0 | | | 126 | 201 | | 55 | |
| 2465 | 0 | 0 | 0 | 0 | 0 | | | | | | | | 0.0 | | | 100 | | 0.5 | | | | 190 | | 85 | |
| 70628 | 0 | 0 | 0 | 0 | 0 | | 0.07 | | | | | | 6.1 | | | 81 | | | | | 61 | 107 | | 30 | |
| 2298 | 0 | 0 | 0 | 0 | 0 | 0.02 | 0.17 | | | 0.45 | | | 0.0 | | | 151 | | 0.0 | | | 126 | 206 | | 55 | |
| 2458 | 0 | 0 | 0 | 0 | 0 | | | | | | | | 2.4 | | | 100 | | 0.5 | | | | 190 | | 75 | |
| 2388 | 103 | 21 | | | | | | | | | | | 7.6 | | | 99 | | 0.3 | | | | | | 27 | |
| 2299 | 0 | 0 | 0 | 0 | 0 | 0.03 | 0.17 | | | 0.45 | | | 0.0 | | | 151 | | 0.0 | | | 126 | 201 | | 55 | |
| 2305 | 50 | 12 | | | | 0.03 | 0.21 | | | 0.60 | | | 0.0 | | | 201 | | 0.0 | | | 151 | 261 | | 75 | |
| 70630 | 67 | 20 | 20 | 0 | | 0.03 | 0.14 | | | | | | 1.2 | | | 151 | | 0.4 | | | 151 | 178 | | 113 | |
| 2459 | 0 | 0 | 0 | 0 | 0 | | | | | | | | 1.2 | | | 100 | | 0.5 | | | | 190 | | 70 | |
| 2300 | 0 | 0 | 0 | 0 | 0 | 0.02 | 0.17 | | | 0.45 | | | 0.0 | | | 15 | | 0.0 | | | 126 | 211 | | 55 | |
| 2044 | 138 | 37 | 34 | 3 | | 0.04 | 0.15 | 0.35 | 0.06 | 0.19 | 7.3 | 0.19 | 0.5 | | | 95 | 0.0 | 0.4 | 12 | | 98 | 151 | | 57 | 0.37 |
| 2301 | 0 | 0 | 0 | 0 | 0 | 0.02 | 0.17 | | | 0.45 | | | 0.6 | | | 151 | | 0.0 | | | 126 | 206 | | 55 | |
| 2302 | 0 | 0 | 0 | 0 | 0 | 0.02 | 0.17 | | | 0.45 | | | 0.6 | | | 151 | | 0.0 | | | 126 | 216 | | 58 | |
| 70631 | 67 | 20 | | | | 0.03 | 0.17 | | | | | | 2.4 | | | 151 | | 0.4 | | | 151 | 148 | | 99 | |
| 2047 | 179 | 44 | 37 | 6 | | 0.05 | 0.17 | 0.32 | 0.08 | 0.21 | 6.1 | 0.19 | 0.6 | | | 119 | 0.0 | 0.4 | 16 | | 107 | 167 | | 73 | 0.39 |
| 2079 | 6 | 2 | 2 | 0 | | 0.04 | 0.20 | 0.10 | 0.04 | 0.51 | 10.2 | 0.24 | 0.7 | | | 166 | 0.0 | 0.1 | 16 | | 131 | 213 | | 64 | 0.81 |
| 2075 | 55 | 13 | 12 | 2 | | 0.04 | 0.18 | 0.10 | 0.04 | 0.47 | 9.4 | 0.24 | 0.7 | | | 153 | 0.0 | 0.1 | 14 | | 120 | 196 | | 59 | 0.75 |
| 2306 | 50 | 12 | | | | 0.03 | 0.21 | | | 0.60 | | | 0.0 | | | 176 | | 0.0 | | | 151 | 241 | | 68 | |
| 70636 | 65 | 20 | 20 | 0 | | | 0.13 | | | | | | | | | 196 | | 0.4 | | | 147 | 151 | | 66 | |
| 2083 | 72 | 19 | 17 | 2 | | 0.01 | 0.13 | 0.20 | 0.04 | 0.18 | 4.8 | 0.10 | 0.4 | | | 88 | 0.0 | 0.2 | 9 | | 67 | 150 | | 41 | 0.26 |
| 70678 | 49 | 15 | | | | | 0.05 | | | | | | | | | 111 | | 0.5 | | | 59 | 171 | | 50 | |
| 2043 | 68 | 18 | 17 | 2 | | 0.01 | 0.07 | 0.10 | 0.03 | 0.09 | 2.0 | 0.09 | 0.3 | | | 46 | 0.0 | 0.1 | 6 | | 43 | 75 | | 28 | 0.15 |
| 70666 | | | | | | | 0.07 | | | | | | | | | 108 | | 0.3 | | | 72 | 168 | | 71 | |
| 70668 | | | | | | | 0.02 | | | | | | 4.3 | | | 43 | | | | | 29 | 80 | | 20 | |
| 70680 | | | | | | 0.02 | 0.02 | | | | | | 4.2 | | | 42 | | | | | 28 | 110 | | 25 | |
| 70667 | | | | | | | 0.05 | | | | | | 3.5 | | | 43 | | | | | 43 | 80 | | 20 | |
| 70681 | | | | | | | 0.02 | | | | | | 4.2 | | | 28 | | | | | 28 | 65 | | 20 | |
| 70679 | | | | | | | 0.02 | | | | | | 2.5 | | | 42 | | | | | 28 | 75 | | 30 | |
| 70665 | | | | | | | 0.07 | | | | | | | | | 72 | | 0.3 | | | 58 | 129 | | 45 | |
| 49018 | 390 | 78 | 59 | 19 | | 0.05 | 0.13 | 0.34 | 0.04 | 0.20 | 7.7 | | 0.5 | | | 33 | 0.0 | 0.8 | 6 | | 55 | 75 | | 151 | 0.27 |
| 49005 | 179 | 41 | 34 | 7 | | 0.15 | 0.09 | 1.26 | 0.05 | 0.01 | 5.0 | 0.08 | 0.2 | 0.1 | 0.1 | 46 | 0.1 | 1.3 | 10 | 0.3 | 33 | 98 | 7.1 | 196 | 0.26 |
| 49003 | 270 | 76 | 67 | 8 | | 0.10 | 0.09 | 0.74 | 0.04 | 0.04 | 3.3 | 0.11 | 0.3 | 0.1 | 0.8 | 21 | 0.0 | 0.8 | 6 | 0.2 | 30 | 106 | 4.9 | 288 | 0.16 |
| 49062 | 20 | 4 | | | | | | | | | | | 42.0 | | | 0 | | 1.4 | | | | | | 170 | |

| Code | Amount | Description | Basic Components | | | | | | | | | Additional Fats | | | | | | V t A & Components | | | | | Vitamins | | | | | | | | | | Minerals | | | | | | | | | |
|---|---|---|---|---|---|---|---|---|---|---|---|---|---|---|---|---|---|---|---|---|---|---|---|---|---|---|---|---|---|---|---|---|---|---|---|---|---|---|---|---|---|---|
| | | | Weight (g) | Calories | % Water | Protein (g) | Carbs (g) | Fiber (g) | Sugar (g) | Other Carbs (g) | Fat (g) | Sat Fat (g) | Mono Fat (g) | Poly Fat (g) | Omega 3 (g) | Omega 6 (g) | Choles (mg) | Vit A (IU) | Vit A (RE) | Retinol (RE) | Carotenoids (RE) | Beta Carotene (mcg) | Thiamin (mg) | Riboflavin (mg) | Niacin (NE) | Vit B6 (mg) | Vit B12 (mcg) | Folate (mcg) | Panto (mg) | Vit C (mg) | Vit D (mg) | Vit E (α TE) | Calcium (mg) | Copper (mg) | Iron (mg) | Magnes (mg) | Mang (mg) | Phos (mg) | Potassium (mg) | Selenium (mcg) | Sodium (mg) | Zinc (mg) |
| 70725 | 1 pce | Apple Crumb Cobbler, Pet-Ritz | 123 | 280 | 50 | 2.0 | 49.0 | 0.0 | 29.0 | 20.0 | 9.0 | 4.0 | 3.0 | 1.0 | | | 5 | 0 | 0 | 0 | 0 | 0 | | | | | | | | 3.6 | | | 0 | | 0.0 | | | | | | 270 | |
| 49019 | 1/2 cup | Berry, avg | 108 | 252 | 47 | 2.8 | 45.9 | 1.9 | | | 6.9 | 1.9 | 2.9 | 1.8 | | | 2 | 64 | 9 | 4 | 5 | | 0.15 | 0.14 | 1.21 | 0.03 | 0.03 | 6.1 | | 6.2 | | | 70 | 0.1 | 1.0 | 10 | | 52 | 94 | | 173 | 0.26 |
| 49064 | 1 pce | Berry, Marie Calender's | 125 | 390 | 49 | 3.0 | 41.0 | 1.0 | 29.0 | 11.0 | 19.0 | 5.0 | | | | | 0 | 0 | 0 | 0 | 0 | 0 | | | | | | | | 3.6 | | | 20 | | 1.8 | | | | | | 170 | |
| 70720 | 1 pce | Blackberry, Pet-Ritz | 123 | 260 | 58 | 2.0 | 38.0 | 1.0 | 22.0 | 15.0 | 11.0 | 4.0 | 4.0 | 1.5 | | | 5 | 0 | 0 | 0 | 0 | 0 | | | | | | | | 0.0 | | | 0 | | 0.7 | | | | | | 230 | |
| 70726 | 1 pce | Blackberry Crumb, Pet-Ritz | 123 | 260 | 53 | 3.0 | 45.0 | 1.0 | 25.0 | 19.0 | 8.0 | 3.0 | 3.0 | 1.0 | | | 5 | 0 | 0 | 0 | 0 | 0 | | | | | | | | 2.4 | | | 0 | | 0.7 | | | | | | 170 | |
| 70721 | 1 pce | Blueberry, Pet-Ritz | 123 | 280 | 53 | 4.0 | 42.0 | 0.0 | 21.0 | 21.0 | 11.0 | 5.0 | 4.0 | 1.5 | | | 5 | 0 | 0 | 0 | 0 | 0 | | | | | | | | 0.0 | | | 0 | | 0.4 | | | | | | 240 | |
| 49020 | 1/2 cup | Cherry, avg | 108 | 214 | 55 | 2.4 | 38.9 | 1.0 | | | 5.9 | 1.6 | 2.5 | 1.5 | | | 1 | 452 | 53 | 12 | 41 | | 0.10 | 0.11 | 0.89 | 0.04 | 0.02 | 5.9 | | 1.1 | | | 58 | 0.1 | 1.7 | 9 | | 43 | 97 | | 176 | 0.20 |
| 70727 | 1 pce | Cherry Crumb, Pet-Ritz | 123 | 280 | 49 | 2.0 | 54.0 | 0.0 | 30.0 | 24.0 | 6.0 | 2.5 | 2.5 | 1.0 | | | 5 | 0 | 0 | 0 | 0 | 0 | | | | | | | | 0.0 | | | 0 | | 0.4 | | | | | | 330 | |
| 49008 | 1 pce | Peach, avg | 130 | 204 | 64 | 2.3 | 36.4 | 1.7 | 25.4 | 9.3 | 6.2 | 1.2 | 2.8 | 1.9 | 0.14 | 1.80 | 1 | 562 | 105 | 67 | 38 | | 0.09 | 0.09 | 1.19 | 0.03 | 0.04 | 5.8 | 0.12 | 3.1 | 0.1 | 0.8 | 24 | 0.1 | 0.9 | 10 | 0.2 | 40 | 159 | 4.9 | 291 | 0.23 |
| 49063 | 1 pce | Peach, Marie Calender's | 125 | 370 | 45 | 3.0 | 47.0 | 0.0 | 24.0 | 23.0 | 18.0 | 3.0 | | | | | 0 | 0 | 0 | 0 | 0 | 0 | | | | | | | | 3.6 | | | 0 | | 1.1 | | | | | | 170 | |
| 70728 | 1 pce | Peach Crumb, Pet-Ritz | 123 | 230 | 61 | 2.0 | 38.0 | 1.0 | 24.0 | 13.0 | 7.0 | 3.0 | 3.0 | 1.0 | | | 5 | 0 | 0 | 0 | 0 | 0 | | | | | | | | 6.0 | | | 0 | | 0.0 | | | | | | 170 | |
| 49021 | 1/2 cup | Plum, avg | 108 | 222 | 53 | 2.4 | 42.0 | 1.5 | | | 5.5 | 1.4 | 2.5 | 1.4 | | | 1 | 188 | 21 | 3 | 18 | | 0.12 | 0.15 | 1.09 | 0.06 | 0.02 | 3.8 | | 4.8 | | | 53 | 0.1 | 0.8 | 10 | | 42 | 145 | | 129 | 0.22 |
| 49022 | 1/2 cup | Rhubarb, avg | 108 | 273 | 43 | 2.6 | 50.7 | 1.4 | | | 7.3 | 1.8 | 3.1 | 2.0 | | | 1 | 186 | 41 | 34 | 7 | | 0.12 | 0.11 | 1.05 | 0.02 | 0.02 | 5.4 | | 3.1 | | | 92 | 0.1 | 0.9 | 12 | | 44 | 177 | | 203 | 0.22 |
| 70724 | 1 pce | Strawberry, Pet-Ritz | 123 | 260 | 57 | 2.0 | 41.0 | 1.0 | 23.0 | 17.0 | 9.0 | 3.0 | 4.0 | 1.0 | | | 5 | 0 | 0 | 0 | 0 | 0 | | | | | | | | 6.0 | | | 0 | | 0.7 | | | | | | 330 | |
| | | Crisps | | | | | | | | | | | | | | | | | | | | | | | | | | | | | | | | | | | | | | | | |
| 49036 | 1 pce | Apple, avg | 78 | 127 | 62 | 1.4 | 25.2 | 1.3 | | | 2.8 | 0.6 | 1.2 | 0.9 | 0.05 | 0.86 | 0 | 107 | 24 | | | | 0.07 | 0.06 | 0.60 | 0.03 | 0.00 | 3.9 | 0.07 | 1.8 | | | 22 | 0.0 | 0.6 | 5 | 0.1 | 19 | 76 | | 142 | 0.12 |
| 49135 | 1 pce | Apricot, avg | 139 | 160 | 74 | 1.5 | 27.9 | 1.7 | 21.0 | 5.3 | 5.4 | 0.9 | 2.5 | 1.7 | 0.12 | 1.62 | 0 | 2132 | 256 | 59 | 197 | | 0.07 | 0.06 | 0.79 | 0.07 | 0.01 | 3.7 | 0.14 | 6.5 | 0.0 | 0.7 | 27 | 0.1 | 0.9 | 16 | 0.2 | 34 | 231 | 3.2 | 70 | 0.20 |
| 49023 | 1/2 cup | Berry, avg | 123 | 354 | 39 | 2.6 | 56.1 | 1.2 | | | 14.2 | 3.1 | 6.6 | 3.6 | | | 0 | 882 | 152 | 96 | 55 | | 0.13 | 0.14 | 1.10 | 0.04 | 0.01 | 8.1 | | 1.3 | | | 79 | 0.1 | 1.9 | 10 | | 141 | 112 | | 296 | 0.17 |
| 49009 | 1 pce | Peach, avg | 139 | 155 | 75 | 1.5 | 27.1 | 2.0 | 20.2 | 5.0 | 5.3 | 0.9 | 2.5 | 1.7 | 0.12 | 1.62 | 0 | 648 | 108 | 59 | 43 | | 0.06 | 0.05 | 1.06 | 0.03 | 0.01 | 5.7 | 0.10 | 5.0 | 0.0 | 0.7 | 20 | 0.1 | 0.9 | 13 | 0.2 | 31 | 189 | 2.9 | 70 | 0.20 |
| 49024 | 1/2 cup | Rhubarb, avg | 123 | 257 | 53 | 1.4 | 48.0 | 2.1 | | | 7.9 | 1.5 | 3.4 | 2.5 | | | 0 | 466 | 110 | 95 | 15 | | 0.08 | 0.07 | 0.71 | 0.03 | 0.01 | 6.7 | | 3.0 | | | 148 | 0.1 | 0.9 | 17 | | 22 | 145 | | 97 | 0.16 |
| | | Dumplings | | | | | | | | | | | | | | | | | | | | | | | | | | | | | | | | | | | | | | | | |
| 49006 | 1 ea | Apple, avg | 151 | 357 | 52 | 2.2 | 53.2 | 2.5 | 38.2 | 12.5 | 16.2 | 3.6 | 8.2 | 3.4 | 0.10 | 3.34 | 0 | 343 | 93 | 82 | 12 | | 0.10 | 0.07 | 0.77 | 0.07 | 0.01 | 6.2 | 0.14 | 5.0 | 0.1 | 1.5 | 50 | 0.2 | 1.3 | 16 | 0.2 | 38 | 212 | 4.9 | 302 | 0.20 |
| 45651 | 1 ea | Apple, Puff Pastry, Pepperidge Farm | 85 | 290 | 29 | 3.0 | 44.0 | 3.0 | 6.0 | 35.0 | 11.0 | 2.5 | | | | | 0 | 0 | 0 | 0 | 0 | 0 | 0.22 | 0.14 | 2.00 | | | | | 2.4 | | | 40 | | 1.1 | | | | | | 160 | |
| 49048 | 1 ea | Cherry, Pepperidge Farm | 85 | 280 | 30 | 3.0 | 47.0 | 2.0 | 13.0 | 32.0 | 9.0 | 2.0 | 6.0 | 0.5 | | | 0 | 0 | 0 | 0 | 0 | 0 | 0.22 | 0.17 | 2.00 | | | | | 4.8 | | | 0 | | 0.7 | | | | | | 280 | |
| 49047 | 1 ea | Peach, Pepperidge Farm | 85 | 300 | 24 | 3.0 | 47.0 | 6.0 | 8.0 | 33.0 | 11.0 | 2.5 | 7.0 | 1.0 | | | 0 | 300 | 60 | | | | 0.22 | 0.17 | 2.00 | | | | | 30.0 | | | 0 | | 1.1 | | | | | | 150 | |
| 45520 | 1 ea | Plain, avg | 32 | 42 | 70 | 1.1 | 6.9 | 0.2 | | | 1.1 | 0.4 | 0.4 | 0.2 | | | 1 | 9 | 2 | 2 | 0 | | 0.06 | 0.05 | 0.45 | 0.01 | 0.02 | 1.9 | | 0.1 | | | 33 | 0.0 | 0.4 | 3 | | 22 | 21 | | 105 | 0.09 |
| | | Fritters | | | | | | | | | | | | | | | | | | | | | | | | | | | | | | | | | | | | | | | | |
| 45515 | 1 ea | Apple, avg | 24 | 87 | 37 | 1.4 | 7.8 | 0.3 | 3.6 | 3.9 | 5.7 | 1.5 | 2.4 | 1.4 | | | 21 | 43 | 12 | 11 | 1 | | 0.04 | 0.06 | 0.30 | 0.02 | 0.06 | 2.9 | | 0.3 | | | 12 | 0.0 | 0.3 | 3 | | 22 | 33 | | 10 | 0.12 |
| 70161 | 1 ea | Apple, Mrs Paul's | 62 | 129 | 55 | 1.5 | 17.9 | 1.0 | 7.4 | 9.4 | 5.5 | 1.7 | | | | | 2 | 7 | 1.5 | | | | 0.06 | 0.04 | 0.60 | | | | | 3.0 | | | 20 | | 0.5 | | | | 22 | | 283 | |
| 45547 | 1 ea | Banana, avg | 34 | 116 | 39 | 1.8 | 11.4 | 0.4 | | | 7.3 | 1.9 | 3.1 | 1.8 | | | 25 | 90 | 23 | 21 | 2 | | 0.05 | 0.09 | 0.43 | 0.10 | 0.07 | 5.0 | | 1.1 | | | 16 | 0.0 | 0.4 | 8 | | 29 | 86 | | 19 | 0.17 |
| 45546 | 1 ea | Berry, avg | 34 | 111 | 44 | 1.8 | 9.9 | 0.6 | | | 7.3 | 1.9 | 3.1 | 1.8 | | | 25 | 93 | 23 | 21 | 2 | | 0.05 | 0.08 | 0.41 | 0.02 | 0.07 | 4.0 | | 1.6 | | | 16 | 0.0 | 0.4 | 4 | | 28 | 41 | | 20 | 0.16 |
| 49046 | 1 ea | Fruit Squares, Apple, Pepperidge Farm | 71 | 210 | 41 | 2.0 | 27.0 | 2.0 | 20.0 | 5.0 | 10.0 | 4.5 | 3.0 | 1.0 | | | 0 | 0 | 0 | 0 | 0 | 0 | 0.03 | 0.00 | 0.00 | | | | | 1.2 | | | 20 | | 0.4 | | | | | | 210 | |
| 45666 | 1 ea | Pastry Pockets, Cherry, Tastykake | 92 | 370 | | 3.0 | 45.0 | 2.0 | 23.0 | 20.0 | 20.0 | 5.0 | | | | | 5 | 0 | 0 | 0 | 0 | 0 | | | | | | | | 0.0 | | | 100 | | 0.0 | | | | | | 190 | |
| 70529 | 1 pce | Streusel, Apple, Mrs. Smith's | 167 | 420 | 48 | 3.0 | 67.0 | | | | 16.0 | | | | | | 5 | 150 | 25 | | | | 0.01 | 0.05 | 0.30 | | | | | 0.0 | | | 21 | | 0.7 | | | | 85 | | 365 | |
| | | Strudels | | | | | | | | | | | | | | | | | | | | | | | | | | | | | | | | | | | | | | | | |
| 49015 | 1 pce | Apple, avg | 71 | 195 | 44 | 2.3 | 29.2 | 1.6 | | | 8.0 | 1.4 | 2.3 | 3.8 | 0.22 | 3.55 | 4 | 21 | 6 | | | | 0.03 | 0.02 | 0.23 | 0.03 | 0.16 | 9.9 | 0.19 | 1.2 | | | 11 | 0.0 | 0.3 | 6 | 0.1 | 23 | 106 | 4.3 | 191 | 0.13 |
| 49057 | 1 pce | Apple, Entenmann's | 110 | 310 | 44 | 3.0 | 44.0 | 2.0 | 19.0 | 23.0 | 14.0 | 3.5 | | | | | 0 | 0 | 0 | 0 | 0 | 0 | | | | | | | | 0.0 | | | 0 | | 0.4 | | | | 75 | | 230 | |
| 49025 | 1 pce | Berry, avg | 64 | 159 | 44 | 2.2 | 29.4 | 1.4 | | | 4.0 | 0.8 | 1.7 | 1.2 | | | 12 | 223 | 53 | 46 | 7 | | 0.09 | 0.09 | 0.83 | 0.02 | 0.03 | 5.7 | | 4.6 | | | 15 | 0.1 | 0.8 | 6 | | 26 | 55 | | 102 | 0.18 |
| 49027 | 1 pce | Cheese, avg | 64 | 195 | 38 | 6.5 | 24.1 | 0.4 | | | 8.2 | 3.9 | 2.7 | 1.1 | | | 42 | 351 | 95 | 88 | 7 | | 0.08 | 0.16 | 0.69 | 0.03 | 0.12 | 8.5 | | 0.4 | | | 90 | 0.0 | 0.8 | 8 | | 86 | 64 | | 116 | 0.60 |
| 49026 | 1 pce | Cherry, avg | 64 | 179 | 39 | 2.7 | 29.3 | 1.1 | | | 6.3 | 0.9 | 2.0 | 2.9 | | | 9 | 552 | 79 | 36 | 43 | | 0.09 | 0.08 | 0.77 | 0.05 | 0.02 | 7.9 | | 3.0 | | | 19 | 0.1 | 0.8 | 15 | | 40 | 100 | | 88 | 0.28 |
| 49028 | 1 pce | Peach, avg | 64 | 124 | 55 | 1.8 | 23.3 | 1.2 | | | 2.9 | 0.6 | 1.3 | 0.9 | | | 8 | 360 | 59 | 34 | 25 | | 0.06 | 0.07 | 0.95 | 0.02 | 0.02 | 4.2 | | 2.9 | | | 12 | 0.1 | 0.6 | 6 | | 22 | 102 | | 76 | 0.17 |
| | | Tarts | | | | | | | | | | | | | | | | | | | | | | | | | | | | | | | | | | | | | | | | |
| 45748 | 1 ea | Apple, Dunkin Donuts | 98 | 290 | 38 | 5.0 | 45.0 | 1.0 | 17.0 | 27.0 | 10.0 | 3.0 | | | | | 0 | 0 | 0 | 0 | 0 | 0 | | | | | | | | 2.4 | | | 0 | | 0.7 | | | | | | 330 | |
| 45745 | 1 ea | Blueberry, Dunkin Donuts | 98 | 300 | 35 | 5.0 | 48.0 | 2.0 | 24.0 | 22.0 | 10.0 | 3.0 | | | | | 0 | 0 | 0 | 0 | 0 | 0 | | | | | | | | 2.4 | | | 0 | | 0.7 | | | | | | 320 | |
| 45746 | 1 ea | Lemon, Dunkin Donuts | 98 | 280 | 39 | 5.0 | 43.0 | 1.0 | 15.0 | 27.0 | 11.0 | 3.0 | | | | | 0 | 0 | 0 | 0 | 0 | 0 | | | | | | | | 2.4 | | | 0 | | 0.7 | | | | | | 340 | |
| 45747 | 1 ea | Raspberry, Dunkin Donuts | 98 | 310 | 32 | 5.0 | 51.0 | 2.0 | 23.0 | 26.0 | 10.0 | 3.0 | | | | | 0 | 0 | 0 | 0 | 0 | 0 | | | | | | | | 2.4 | | | 0 | | 0.7 | | | | | | 350 | |
| 45744 | 1 ea | Strawberry, Dunkin Donuts | 98 | 310 | 32 | 5.0 | 51.0 | 1.0 | 24.0 | 26.0 | 10.0 | 3.0 | | | | | 0 | 0 | 0 | 0 | 0 | 0 | | | | | | | | 4.8 | | | 0 | | 0.7 | | | | | | 340 | |
| | | Turnovers | | | | | | | | | | | | | | | | | | | | | | | | | | | | | | | | | | | | | | | | |
| 45550 | 1 ea | Apple, avg | 82 | 289 | 33 | 2.9 | 36.2 | 1.2 | | | 15.0 | 3.7 | 6.6 | 4.0 | | | 0 | 22 | 4 | 3 | 1 | | 0.17 | 0.13 | 1.51 | 0.02 | 0.00 | 4.8 | | 0.7 | | | 6 | 0.1 | 1.3 | 7 | | 33 | 56 | | 262 | 0.21 |
| 45749 | 1 ea | Apple, Dunkin Donuts | 109 | 350 | 36 | 5.0 | 49.0 | 2.0 | 21.0 | 26.0 | 15.0 | 4.0 | | | | | 0 | 0 | 0 | 0 | 0 | 0 | | | | | | | | 2.4 | | | 0 | | 0.7 | | | | | | 340 | |
| 45640 | 1 ea | Apple, Mini, Pepperidge Farm | 40 | 140 | 35 | 2.0 | 15.0 | 1.0 | 10.0 | 4.0 | 8.0 | 2.0 | | | | | 0 | 0 | 0 | 0 | 0 | 0 | 0.12 | 0.07 | 1.20 | | | | | 0.0 | | | | | 0.7 | | | | | | 80 | |
| 45611 | 1 ea | Apple, Pepperidge Farm | 89 | 330 | 25 | 4.0 | 48.0 | 6.0 | 5.0 | 37.0 | 14.0 | 3.0 | 9.0 | 1.0 | | | 0 | 0 | 0 | 0 | 0 | 0 | 0.22 | 0.17 | 2.00 | | | | | 0.0 | | | 40 | | 1.4 | | | | | | 180 | |
| 45643 | 1 ea | Apple, w/vanilla icing, Pepperidge Farm | 96 | 380 | 24 | 4.0 | 53.0 | 2.0 | 10.0 | 41.0 | 14.0 | 3.0 | | | | | 0 | 0 | 0 | 0 | 0 | 0 | 0.22 | 0.17 | 2.00 | | | | | 40.0 | | | | | 1.4 | | | | | | 190 | |
| 45773 | 1 ea | Berry, avg | 78 | 277 | 32 | 3.0 | 35.6 | 1.4 | | | 13.9 | 3.4 | 6.1 | 3.7 | | | 0 | 23 | 2 | 0 | 2 | | 0.18 | 0.13 | 1.51 | 0.02 | 0.00 | 5.9 | | 3.2 | | | 6 | 0.1 | 1.3 | 8 | | 32 | 55 | | 229 | 0.23 |
| 45750 | 1 ea | Blueberry, Dunkin Donuts | 109 | 370 | 31 | 5.0 | 54.0 | 2.0 | 31.0 | 21.0 | 15.0 | 4.0 | | | | | 0 | 0 | 0 | 0 | 0 | 0 | | | | | | | | 2.4 | | | 0 | | 0.7 | | | | | | 330 | |
| 45609 | 1 ea | Blueberry, Pepperidge Farm | 89 | 340 | 26 | 4.0 | 45.0 | 6.0 | 5.0 | 34.0 | 16.0 | 3.0 | 10.0 | 1.5 | | | 0 | 0 | 0 | 0 | 0 | 0 | 0.22 | 0.17 | 2.00 | | | | | 6.0 | | | 20 | | 1.4 | | | | | | 200 | |
| 45774 | 1 ea | Cherry, avg | 78 | 238 | 41 | 2.5 | 31.2 | 0.9 | | | 11.7 | 2.9 | 5.1 | 3.1 | | | 0 | 244 | 27 | 5 | 23 | | 0.14 | 0.11 | 1.21 | 0.02 | 0.00 | 5.5 | | 0.6 | | | 8 | 0.1 | 1.6 | 7 | | 28 | 58 | | 212 | 0.18 |
| 45608 | 1 ea | Cherry, Pepperidge Farm | 89 | 320 | 28 | 4.0 | 46.0 | 6.0 | 6.0 | 34.0 | 13.0 | 3.0 | 8.0 | 1.0 | | | 0 | 0 | 0 | 0 | 0 | 0 | 0.30 | 0.17 | 2.00 | | | | | 4.8 | | | 0 | | 1.4 | | | | | | 190 | |
| 45555 | 1 ea | Guava, avg | 78 | 239 | 42 | 2.5 | 29.2 | 2.7 | | | 12.9 | 3.2 | 5.6 | 3.5 | | | 0 | 278 | 36 | 12 | 24 | | 0.15 | 0.11 | 1.53 | 0.06 | 0.01 | 6.7 | | 49.3 | | | 14 | 0.1 | 1.1 | 9 | | 34 | 124 | | 105 | 0.25 |
| 45775 | 1 ea | Lemon, avg | 78 | 238 | 42 | 2.7 | 28.8 | 0.6 | | | 12.5 | 3.1 | 5.4 | 3.2 | | | 47 | 115 | 32 | 32 | 1 | | 0.13 | 0.12 | 1.08 | 0.02 | 0.09 | 8.0 | | 1.4 | | | 9 | 0.0 | 1.1 | 5 | | 41 | 31 | | 228 | 0.27 |
| 45752 | 1 ea | Lemon, Dunkin Donuts | 109 | 350 | 37 | 5.0 | 48.0 | 2.0 | 21.0 | 25.0 | 15.0 | 4.0 | | | | | 0 | 0 | 0 | 0 | 0 | 0 | | | | | | | | 2.4 | | | 0 | | 0.7 | | | | | | 360 | |
| 45776 | 1 ea | Peach, avg | 78 | 261 | 36 | 2.9 | 32.9 | 1.3 | | | 13.4 | 3.3 | 5.9 | 3.5 | | | 0 | 139 | 14 | 0 | 14 | | 0.16 | 0.13 | 1.67 | 0.02 | 0.00 | 4.9 | | 1.6 | | | 6 | 0.1 | 1.2 | 8 | | 32 | 89 | | 218 | 0.23 |
| 45589 | 1 ea | Peach, Pepperidge Farm | 89 | 340 | 25 | 4.0 | 47.0 | 6.0 | 5.0 | 36.0 | 15.0 | 3.0 | 9.0 | 1.0 | | | 0 | 300 | 50 | | | | 0.30 | 0.17 | 2.00 | | | | | 36.0 | | | 0 | | 1.4 | | | | | | 180 | |
| 45556 | 1 ea | Pumpkin, avg | 78 | 198 | 53 | 4.3 | 20.2 | 1.3 | | | 11.3 | 3.5 | 4.7 | 2.5 | | | 34 | 6205 | 635 | 23 | 612 | | 0.12 | 0.19 | 1.01 | 0.04 | 0.07 | 9.5 | | 1.2 | | | 72 | 0.1 | 1.3 | 16 | | 83 | 153 | | 103 | 0.41 |
| 45753 | 1 ea | Raspberry, Dunkin Donuts | 109 | 380 | 28 | 5.0 | 57.0 | 2.0 | 29.0 | 26.0 | 15.0 | 4.0 | | | | | 0 | 0 | 0 | 0 | 0 | 0 | | | | | | | | 3.6 | | | 0 | | 0.7 | | | | | | 370 | |

| Code | Amount | Description | Basic Components | | | | | | | | | Additional Fats | | | | | | Vit A & Components | | | | | Vitamins | | | | | | | | | | Minerals | | | | | | | | | |
|---|---|---|---|---|---|---|---|---|---|---|---|---|---|---|---|---|---|---|---|---|---|---|---|---|---|---|---|---|---|---|---|---|---|---|---|---|---|---|---|---|---|---|
| | | | Weight (g) | Calories | % Water | Protein (g) | Carbs (g) | Fiber (g) | Sugar (g) | Other Carbs (g) | Fat (g) | Sat Fat (g) | Mono Fat (g) | Poly Fat (g) | Omega 3 (g) | Omega 6 (g) | Choles (mg) | Vit A (IU) | Vit A (RE) | Retinol (RE) | Carotenoids (RE) | Beta Carotene (mcg) | Thiamin (mg) | Riboflavin (mg) | Niacin (NE) | Vit B6 (mg) | Vit B12 (mcg) | Folate (mcg) | Panto (mg) | Vit C (mg) | Vit D (mg) | Vit E (α TE) | Calcium (mg) | Copper (mg) | Iron (mg) | Magnes (mg) | Mang (mg) | Phos (mg) | Potassium (mg) | Selenium (mcg) | Sodium (mg) | Zinc (mg) |
| 45610 | 1 ea | Raspberry, Pepperidge Farm | 89 | 330 | | 4.0 | 47.0 | 6.0 | 6.0 | 35.0 | 14.0 | 3.0 | 9.0 | 1.0 | | | 0 | 0 | 0 | 0 | 0 | 0 | 0.30 | 0.17 | 2.00 | | | | | 36.0 | | | 0 | | 1.4 | | | | | | 190 | |
| 45751 | 1 ea | Strawberry, Dunkin Donuts | 109 | 380 | 28 | 5.0 | 57.0 | 2.0 | 30.0 | 25.0 | 15.0 | 4.0 | | | | | 0 | 0 | 0 | 0 | 0 | 0 | | | | | | | | 4.8 | | | 0 | | 0.7 | | | | | | 360 | |
| | | *GELATIN DESSERTS* | | | | | | | | | | | | | | | | | | | | | | | | | | | | | | | | | | | | | | | | |
| | | Gelatins | | | | | | | | | | | | | | | | | | | | | | | | | | | | | | | | | | | | | | | | |
| 23155 | 2 1/2 g | Dry Mix, per 1/2 c svg, avg | 2 | 8 | 1 | 0.2 | 1.8 | 0.0 | 1.8 | 0.0 | 0.0 | 0.0 | 0.0 | 0.0 | 0.00 | 0.00 | 0 | 0 | 0 | 0 | 0 | 0 | 0.00 | 0.00 | 0.00 | 0.00 | 0.00 | 0.1 | 0.00 | 0.0 | 0.0 | 0.0 | 0 | 0.0 | 0.0 | 0 | 0.0 | 3 | 0 | 0.1 | 5 | 0.00 |
| 23331 | 2 1/2 g | Dry Mix, per 1/2 c svg, asstd flvrs, Jell-o | 2 | 7 | 4 | 0.2 | 1.7 | 0.0 | 1.7 | 0.0 | 0.0 | 0.0 | 0.0 | 0.0 | 0.00 | 0.00 | 0 | 0 | 0 | 0 | 0 | 0 | | | | | | | | 0.0 | | | 0 | | 0.0 | | | | 0 | | 5 | |
| 23351 | 2 1/2 g | Dry Mix, per 1/2 c svg, 1-2-3, Kraft | 2 | 8 | 4 | 0.1 | 1.7 | 0.0 | 1.4 | 0.3 | 0.1 | | | | | | 0 | 0 | 0 | 0 | 0 | 0 | | | | | | | | | | | | | | | | | | | | |
| 23157 | 1 ea | Dry Mix, sugar free, env, avg | 10 | 35 | 7 | 5.5 | 3.3 | 0.0 | 0.0 | 3.3 | 0.0 | 0.0 | 0.0 | 0.0 | 0.00 | 0.00 | 0 | 0 | 0 | 0 | 0 | 0 | 0.00 | 0.01 | 0.00 | 0.00 | 0.00 | 1.4 | 0.01 | 0.0 | 0.0 | 0.0 | 0 | 0.1 | 0.0 | 0 | 0.0 | 129 | 1 | 2.5 | 217 | 0.01 |
| 23330 | 2 1/2 g | Dry Mix, per 1/2 c svg, sugar free, D-Zerta | 2 | 8 | 15 | 1.6 | 0.0 | 0.0 | 0.0 | 0.0 | 0.0 | 0.0 | 0.0 | 0.0 | 0.00 | 0.00 | 0 | 0 | 0 | 0 | 0 | 0 | | | | | | | | 0.0 | | | 0 | | 0.0 | | | | 36 | | 4 | |
| 23354 | 2 1/2 g | Dry Mix, per 1/2 c svg, sugar free, Kraft | 2 | 8 | 55 | 0.8 | 0.0 | 0.0 | 0.0 | 0.0 | 0.0 | 0.0 | 0.0 | 0.0 | 0.00 | 0.00 | 0 | 0 | 0 | 0 | 0 | 0 | | | | | | | | 0.0 | | | 0 | | 0.0 | | | | 0 | | 48 | |
| 23009 | 1 ea | Dry Mix, unswtnd, env, avg | 7 | 23 | 13 | 6.0 | 0.0 | 0.0 | 0.0 | 0.0 | 0.0 | 0.0 | 0.0 | 0.0 | 0.00 | 0.00 | 0 | 0 | 0 | 0 | 0 | 0 | 0.00 | 0.02 | 0.01 | 0.00 | 0.00 | 2.1 | 0.01 | 0.0 | 0.0 | 0.0 | 4 | 0.2 | 0.1 | 2 | 0.0 | 3 | 1 | 2.8 | 14 | 0.01 |
| 23228 | 1/2 cup | Prep, Fruit flavor, Orville Kent | 120 | 70 | | 2.0 | 15.0 | 2.0 | 16.0 | | 0.0 | 0.0 | 0.0 | 0.0 | 0.00 | 0.00 | 0 | 100 | 20 | | | | | | | | | | | 1.2 | | | 0 | | 0.0 | | | | | | 75 | |
| 23093 | 1/2 cup | Prep, sugar free, avg | 117 | 8 | 98 | 1.3 | 0.8 | 0.0 | 0.0 | 0.8 | 0.0 | 0.0 | 0.0 | 0.0 | 0.00 | 0.00 | 0 | 0 | 0 | 0 | 0 | 0 | 0.00 | 0.00 | 0.00 | 0.00 | 0.00 | 0.0 | 0.00 | 0.0 | 0.0 | 0.0 | 2 | 0.0 | 0.0 | 1 | 0.0 | 32 | 0 | 0.6 | 56 | 0.04 |
| 23274 | 1/2 cup | Prep, sugar free, assorted flvrs, Diamond Crystal | 124 | 5 | 98 | 2.0 | 0.0 | 0.0 | 0.0 | 0.0 | 0.0 | 0.0 | 0.0 | 0.0 | 0.00 | 0.00 | 0 | 0 | 0 | 0 | 0 | 0 | 0.00 | 0.00 | 0.00 | 0.00 | 0.00 | 0.0 | 0.00 | 0.0 | | | 0 | 0.0 | 0.0 | 0 | 0.0 | 0 | 25 | | 0 | 0.00 |
| 23379 | 1/2 cup | Prep, sugar free, assorted flvrs, Menu Magic | 120 | 10 | 99 | 1.0 | 0.5 | 0.0 | 0.0 | 0.5 | 0.0 | 0.0 | 0.0 | 0.0 | 0.00 | 0.00 | 0 | 0 | 0 | 0 | 0 | 0 | | | | | | | | 0.0 | | | 0 | | 0.0 | | | | 0 | | 20 | |
| 23156 | 1/2 cup | Prep, w/added fruit, avg | 106 | 73 | 82 | 1.2 | 17.9 | 0.6 | 17.0 | 0.3 | 0.2 | 0.1 | 0.0 | 0.1 | 0.01 | 0.04 | 0 | 30 | 3 | | | | 0.03 | 0.03 | 0.16 | 0.13 | 0.00 | 4.2 | 0.05 | 3.9 | 0.0 | | 5 | 0.1 | 0.1 | 7 | 0.0 | 22 | 110 | | 30 | 0.05 |
| 23314 | 1 ea | Gelatin Snack, asstd flvrs, Jell-o | 99 | 80 | 80 | 1.0 | 18.0 | 0.0 | 18.0 | 0.0 | 0.0 | 0.0 | 0.0 | 0.0 | 0.00 | 0.00 | 0 | 0 | 0 | 0 | 0 | 0 | | | | | | | | 0.0 | | | 0 | | 0.0 | | | | 0 | | 45 | |
| 23321 | 1 ea | Gelatin Snack, sugar free, Jell-o | 92 | 10 | 98 | 1.0 | 0.0 | 0.0 | 0.0 | 0.0 | 0.0 | 0.0 | 0.0 | 0.0 | 0.00 | 0.00 | 0 | 0 | 0 | 0 | 0 | 0 | | | | | | | | 0.0 | | | 0 | | 0.0 | | | | 0 | | 50 | |
| | | Gelatin Parfaits | | | | | | | | | | | | | | | | | | | | | | | | | | | | | | | | | | | | | | | | |
| 62416 | 1/2 cup | Orange, Menu Magic | 125 | 280 | 55 | 8.0 | 36.0 | 1.0 | 32.0 | 3.0 | 11.0 | 3.0 | | | | | 10 | 1000 | 200 | | | | 0.30 | 0.34 | 4.00 | 0.40 | 1.20 | 80.0 | 2.00 | 12.0 | 2.0 | | 150 | 0.4 | 3.6 | 60 | | 150 | 200 | | 160 | 3.00 |
| 23236 | 1/2 cup | Lime, Orville Kent | 110 | 120 | | 3.0 | 21.0 | 0.0 | 20.0 | 1.0 | 3.0 | 3.0 | | | | | 0 | 0 | 0 | 0 | 0 | 0 | | | | | | | | 9.0 | | | 0 | | 0.0 | | | | | | 105 | |
| 23231 | 1/2 cup | Strawberry, Orville Kent | 110 | 130 | | 3.0 | 22.0 | 1.0 | 20.0 | 1.0 | 3.0 | 3.0 | | | | | 0 | 100 | 20 | | | | | | | | | | | 1.2 | | | 0 | | 0.0 | | | | | | 105 | |
| | | Mousse | | | | | | | | | | | | | | | | | | | | | | | | | | | | | | | | | | | | | | | | |
| 2667 | 1/2 cup | Chocolate, avg | 202 | 446 | 62 | 8.7 | 33.1 | 1.2 | | | 32.9 | 18.5 | 10.3 | 1.7 | 0.34 | 1.35 | 299 | 1133 | 323 | | | | 0.08 | 0.41 | 0.27 | 0.13 | 0.93 | 32.3 | 1.17 | 1.2 | | | 202 | 0.1 | 1.3 | 44 | 0.1 | 259 | 297 | | 87 | 1.43 |
| 2704 | 1 ea | Chocolate, Weight Watchers, svg | 78 | 190 | 44 | 6.0 | 33.0 | 3.0 | 6.0 | 24.0 | 4.0 | 1.5 | | | | | 5 | 0 | 0 | 0 | 0 | 0 | | | | | | | | 0.0 | | | 60 | | 1.8 | | | | 320 | | 150 | |
| 2706 | 1 ea | Chocolate Caramel, Weight Watchers, svg | 78 | 200 | 44 | 5.0 | 34.0 | 2.0 | 16.0 | 16.0 | 4.0 | 1.0 | | | | | 5 | 0 | 0 | 0 | 0 | 0 | | | | | | | | 1.2 | | | 80 | | 1.1 | | | | 190 | | 120 | |
| | | *PASTRIES AND SWEET ROLLS* | | | | | | | | | | | | | | | | | | | | | | | | | | | | | | | | | | | | | | | | |
| 45687 | 1 pce | Baklava, including Kadayif, avg | 78 | 333 | 25 | 5.1 | 29.1 | 1.6 | | | 22.8 | 9.3 | 8.5 | 3.8 | | | 35 | 512 | 124 | 108 | 15 | | 0.17 | 0.13 | 1.31 | 0.05 | 0.02 | 9.2 | | 1.4 | | | 34 | 0.2 | 1.7 | 34 | | 88 | 139 | | 291 | 0.51 |
| | | Buns | | | | | | | | | | | | | | | | | | | | | | | | | | | | | | | | | | | | | | | | |
| 42460 | 1 ea | Apple, fat free, Entenmann's | 66 | 150 | | 3.0 | 33.0 | 1.0 | 17.0 | 15.0 | 0.0 | 0.0 | 0.0 | 0.0 | 0.00 | 0.00 | 0 | 0 | 0 | 0 | 0 | 0 | | | | | | | | 0.0 | | | 20 | | 0.0 | | | | 80 | | 140 | |
| 42461 | 1 ea | Blueberry Cheese, fat free, Entenmann's | 66 | 140 | | 4.0 | 31.0 | 1.0 | 18.0 | 12.0 | 0.0 | 0.0 | 0.0 | 0.0 | 0.00 | 0.00 | 0 | 0 | 0 | 0 | 0 | 0 | | | | | | | | 0.0 | | | 20 | | 0.0 | | | | 65 | | 150 | |
| 42465 | 1 ea | Cinnamon, Entenmann's | 61 | 220 | 25 | 4.0 | 31.0 | 0.5 | 18.0 | 12.5 | 10.0 | 6.0 | | | | | 55 | 300 | 60 | | | | | | | | | | | 0.0 | | | 60 | | 0.7 | | | | 85 | | 190 | |
| 42462 | 1 ea | Cinnamon Raisin, fat free, Entenmann's | 61 | 160 | | 3.0 | 36.0 | 1.0 | 20.0 | 15.0 | 0.0 | 0.0 | 0.0 | 0.0 | 0.00 | 0.00 | 0 | 0 | 0 | 0 | 0 | 0 | | | | | | | | 0.0 | | | 40 | | 0.4 | | | | 95 | | 125 | |
| 42466 | 1 pce | Filbert Ring, Entenmann's | 61 | 270 | 20 | 4.0 | 27.0 | 1.0 | 11.0 | 15.0 | 17.0 | 3.0 | | | | | 30 | 300 | 60 | | | | | | | | | | | 0.0 | | | 40 | | 0.7 | | | | 90 | | 190 | |
| 45661 | 1 ea | Glazed Honey, Tastykake | 92 | 350 | | 5.0 | 47.0 | 0.0 | 22.0 | 25.0 | 17.0 | 4.0 | | | | | 10 | 0 | 0 | 0 | 0 | 0 | | | | | | | | 0.0 | | | 100 | | 1.8 | | | | | | 210 | |
| 45662 | 1 ea | Iced Honey, Tastykake | 92 | 350 | | 5.0 | 47.0 | 0.0 | 22.0 | 25.0 | 17.0 | 4.0 | | | | | 10 | 0 | 0 | 0 | 0 | 0 | | | | | | | | 0.0 | | | 100 | | 1.8 | | | | | | 210 | |
| 45663 | 1 ea | Pecan Twirls, Tastykake | 28 | 108 | | 1.5 | 15.7 | 0.5 | 7.4 | 7.9 | 4.4 | 0.5 | | | | | 0 | 0 | 0 | 0 | 0 | 0 | | | | | | | | 0.0 | | | 10 | | 0.7 | | | | | | 98 | |
| 42463 | 1 ea | Pineapple Cheese, fat free, Entenmann's | 66 | 140 | | 4.0 | 30.0 | 0.5 | 18.0 | 11.5 | 0.0 | 0.0 | 0.0 | 0.0 | 0.00 | 0.00 | 0 | 0 | 0 | 0 | 0 | 0 | | | | | | | | 0.0 | | | 20 | | 0.0 | | | | 70 | | 150 | |
| 42464 | 1 ea | Raspberry Cheese, fat free, Entenmann's | 66 | 160 | | 4.0 | 36.0 | 1.0 | 22.0 | 13.0 | 0.0 | 0.0 | 0.0 | 0.0 | 0.00 | 0.00 | 0 | 0 | 0 | 0 | 0 | 0 | | | | | | | | 0.0 | | | 20 | | 0.0 | | | | 65 | | 135 | |
| 45668 | 1 ea | Whirley Twirls, Tastykake | 28 | 128 | | 1.0 | 17.7 | 0.5 | 9.8 | 7.4 | 6.9 | 3.4 | | | | | 5 | 0 | 0 | 0 | 0 | 0 | | | | | | | | 0.0 | | | 10 | | 0.4 | | | | | | 103 | |
| | | Croissants | | | | | | | | | | | | | | | | | | | | | | | | | | | | | | | | | | | | | | | | |
| 45690 | 1 ea | Almond, Dunkin Donuts | 78 | 360 | 15 | 6.0 | 38.0 | 2.0 | 9.0 | 27.0 | 21.0 | 5.0 | | | | | 10 | 0 | 0 | 0 | 0 | 0 | | | | | | | | 0.0 | | | 60 | | 1.8 | | | | | | 300 | |
| 45522 | 1 ea | Apple, avg | 57 | 145 | 46 | 4.2 | 21.1 | 1.4 | | | 5.0 | 2.8 | 1.4 | 0.4 | 0.06 | 0.30 | 18 | 217 | 56 | | | | 0.13 | 0.09 | 0.91 | 0.02 | 0.11 | 32.5 | 0.34 | 0.3 | | | 17 | 0.0 | 0.6 | 7 | 0.1 | 33 | 51 | 10.8 | 156 | 0.59 |
| 42015 | 1 ea | Butter, avg | 57 | 231 | 23 | 4.7 | 26.1 | 1.5 | 1.8 | 22.8 | 12.0 | 6.7 | 3.2 | 0.6 | 0.17 | 0.45 | 38 | 424 | 106 | 96 | 10 | | 0.22 | 0.14 | 1.25 | 0.03 | 0.09 | 35.3 | 0.49 | 0.1 | 0.1 | | 21 | 0.0 | 1.2 | 9 | 0.2 | 60 | 67 | 12.9 | 424 | 0.43 |
| 45523 | 1 ea | Cheese, avg | 57 | 236 | 21 | 5.2 | 26.8 | 1.5 | | | 11.9 | 6.0 | 3.7 | 1.4 | 0.18 | 1.18 | 32 | 459 | 112 | | | | 0.30 | 0.19 | 1.23 | 0.04 | 0.18 | 42.2 | 0.48 | 0.1 | | | 30 | 0.1 | 1.2 | 14 | 0.2 | 74 | 75 | 15.3 | 316 | 0.54 |
| 45691 | 1 ea | Cheese, Dunkin Donuts | 70 | 240 | 29 | 6.0 | 28.0 | 0.0 | 4.0 | 24.0 | 15.0 | 3.0 | | | | | 5 | 0 | 0 | 0 | 0 | 0 | | | | | | | | 0.0 | | | 20 | | 1.8 | | | | | | 260 | |
| 45545 | 1 ea | Chocolate, avg | 56 | 233 | 22 | 5.2 | 23.4 | 1.6 | | | 14.0 | 8.2 | 4.2 | 0.7 | | | 56 | 419 | 105 | 94 | 11 | | 0.19 | 0.21 | 1.97 | 0.05 | 0.10 | 19.4 | | 0.1 | | | 31 | 0.2 | 1.7 | 27 | | 82 | 113 | | 257 | 0.61 |
| 45689 | 1 ea | Chocolate, Dunkin Donuts | 72 | 370 | 5 | 5.0 | 40.0 | 1.0 | 15.0 | 24.0 | 23.0 | 8.0 | | | | | 10 | 0 | 0 | 0 | 0 | 0 | | | | | | | | 0.0 | | | 40 | | 2.7 | | | | | | 260 | |
| 45688 | 1 ea | Plain, Dunkin Donuts | 60 | 270 | 18 | 4.0 | 27.0 | 0.0 | 3.0 | 24.0 | 17.0 | 4.0 | | | | | 5 | 0 | 0 | 0 | 0 | 0 | | | | | | | | 0.0 | | | 20 | | 1.8 | | | | | | 260 | |
| | | Danish Pastries | | | | | | | | | | | | | | | | | | | | | | | | | | | | | | | | | | | | | | | | |
| 42371 | 1 ea | Apple, Pepperidge Farm | 64 | 210 | 33 | 4.0 | 29.0 | 2.0 | 15.0 | 12.0 | 9.0 | 2.5 | 4.5 | 1.0 | | | 15 | 0 | 0 | 0 | 0 | 0 | 0.22 | 0.10 | 2.00 | | | | | 0.0 | | | 40 | | 1.1 | | | | | | 190 | |
| 45620 | 1 pce | Black Forest, fat free, Entenmann's | 54 | 130 | | 3.0 | 32.0 | 2.0 | 18.0 | 12.0 | 0.0 | 0.0 | 0.0 | 0.0 | 0.00 | 0.00 | 0 | 100 | 20 | | | | | | | | | | | 0.0 | | | 40 | | 0.7 | | | | 100 | | 115 | |
| 45572 | 1 ea | Cheese, avg | 71 | 266 | 31 | 5.7 | 26.4 | 0.7 | 20.0 | 5.8 | 15.5 | 4.8 | 8.0 | 1.8 | 0.12 | 1.71 | 11 | 104 | 32 | | | | 0.13 | 0.18 | 1.42 | 0.03 | 0.12 | 42.6 | 0.22 | 0.1 | 0.0 | | 25 | 0.1 | 1.1 | 11 | 0.2 | 77 | 70 | 13.4 | 319 | 0.50 |
| 42372 | 1 ea | Cheese, Pepperidge Farm | 65 | 230 | 33 | 6.0 | 25.0 | 1.0 | 8.0 | 16.0 | 11.0 | 3.5 | 5.0 | 1.0 | | | 55 | 0 | 0 | 0 | 0 | 0 | 0.22 | 0.14 | 1.60 | | | | | 0.0 | | | 60 | | 1.4 | | | | | | 230 | |
| 45571 | 1 ea | Cinnamon, avg | 65 | 262 | 24 | 4.5 | 29.0 | 0.8 | 18.3 | 9.9 | 14.6 | 3.7 | 8.1 | 1.9 | 0.10 | 1.80 | 14 | 8 | 2 | | | | 0.20 | 0.17 | 1.87 | 0.02 | 0.06 | 40.3 | 0.26 | 0.1 | 0.0 | | 46 | 0.1 | 1.3 | 12 | 0.2 | 70 | 81 | 11.0 | 241 | 0.47 |
| 45569 | 1 ea | Fruit, avg | 71 | 263 | 27 | 3.8 | 33.9 | 1.3 | 20.0 | 12.6 | 13.1 | 3.5 | 7.1 | 1.7 | 0.10 | 1.57 | 81 | 53 | 16 | | | | 0.19 | 0.16 | 1.41 | 0.03 | 0.06 | 23.4 | 0.45 | 2.8 | 0.0 | | 33 | 0.0 | 1.3 | 11 | 0.2 | 63 | 59 | 10.5 | 251 | 0.38 |
| 45573 | 1 ea | Nut, avg | 65 | 279 | 20 | 4.6 | 29.7 | 1.3 | 18.2 | 10.2 | 16.4 | 3.8 | 8.9 | 2.8 | 0.22 | 2.54 | 30 | 34 | 9 | | | | 0.14 | 0.16 | 1.49 | 0.07 | 0.14 | 53.9 | 0.46 | 1.1 | 0.0 | | 61 | 0.1 | 1.2 | 21 | 0.5 | 71 | 62 | 9.2 | 236 | 0.57 |
| 45633 | 1 pce | Pecan, Entenmann's | 53 | 230 | | 3.0 | 23.0 | 1.0 | 11.0 | 11.0 | 15.0 | 3.0 | | | | | 25 | 200 | 40 | | | | | | | | | | | 0.0 | | | 40 | | 0.7 | | | | 95 | | 160 | |
| 45639 | 1 pce | Walnut, Entenmann's | 53 | 230 | | 4.0 | 23.0 | 1.0 | 11.0 | 11.0 | 14.0 | 3.0 | | | | | 25 | 200 | 40 | | | | | | | | | | | 0.0 | | | 40 | | 0.7 | | | | 100 | | 160 | |
| 45590 | 1 ea | Fruit burritos, apple or cherry, avg | 155 | 484 | 36 | 5.2 | 73.3 | | | | 20.0 | 9.6 | 7.2 | 2.2 | 0.00 | 2.22 | 8 | 849 | 78 | 67 | 11 | | 0.36 | 0.37 | 3.89 | 0.16 | 1.07 | 51.1 | 1.98 | 1.5 | | | 33 | 0.2 | 2.2 | 15 | 0.3 | 31 | 219 | 14.4 | 443 | 0.84 |
| 49041 | 7 pce | Nacho chips w/cinnamon & sugar, avg | 109 | 592 | 1 | 7.2 | 63.4 | 3.3 | | | 36.0 | 18.2 | 11.9 | 4.1 | 0.00 | 4.13 | 39 | 108 | 11 | 0 | 11 | | 0.19 | 0.45 | 3.92 | 0.17 | 1.72 | 7.6 | 1.90 | 8.0 | | | 85 | 0.2 | 2.9 | 20 | 0.5 | 33 | 78 | 6.6 | 439 | 0.59 |
| 45652 | 1 oz | Pastry Pocket, Apple, Rich's | 28 | 87 | 39 | 1.4 | 11.4 | 0.3 | 4.2 | 6.9 | 4.0 | 1.0 | 1.0 | 0.8 | | | 8 | 140 | 28 | | | | 0.07 | 0.05 | 0.50 | 0.01 | 0.01 | 3.1 | 0.03 | 0.1 | 0.0 | 0.0 | 12 | 0.0 | 0.4 | 3 | | 29 | 27 | | 158 | 0.10 |
| 45665 | 1 ea | Pastry Pocket, Cheese, Tastykake | 96 | 410 | | 4.0 | 38.0 | 2.0 | 22.0 | 14.0 | 27.0 | 8.0 | | | | | 10 | 0 | 0 | 0 | 0 | 0 | | | | | | | | 0.0 | | | 100 | | 1.4 | | | | | | 210 | |
| | | Pastry Twists | | | | | | | | | | | | | | | | | | | | | | | | | | | | | | | | | | | | | | | | |
| 45619 | 1 pce | Apricot, fat free, Entenmann's | 53 | 150 | | 3.0 | 34.0 | 0.5 | 20.0 | 13.5 | 0.0 | 0.0 | 0.0 | 0.0 | 0.00 | 0.00 | 0 | 0 | 0 | 0 | 0 | 0 | | | | | | | | 0.0 | | | 40 | | 2.0 | | | | 70 | | 110 | |

|Code|Amount|Description|Basic Components|||||||||Additional Fats||||||V t A & Components|||||Vitamins||||||||||Minerals||||||||||
|---|---|---|---|---|---|---|---|---|---|---|---|---|---|---|---|---|---|---|---|---|---|---|---|---|---|---|---|---|---|---|---|---|---|---|---|---|---|---|---|---|---|---|
|||||Weight (g)|Calories|% Water|Protein (g)|Carbs (g)|Fiber (g)|Sugar (g)|Other Carbs (g)|Fat (g)|Sat Fat (g)|Mono Fat (g)|Poly Fat (g)|Omega 3 (g)|Omega 6 (g)|Choles (mg)|Vit A (IU)|Vit A (RE)|Retinol (RE)|Carotenoids (RE)|Beta Carotene (mcg)|Thiamin (mg)|Riboflavin (mg)|Niacin (NE)|Vit B6 (mg)|Vit B12 (mcg)|Folate (mcg)|Panto (mg)|Vit C (mg)|Vit D (mg)|Vit E (α TE)|Calcium (mg)|Copper (mg)|Iron (mg)|Magnes (mg)|Mang (mg)|Phos (mg)|Potassium (mg)|Selenium (mcg)|Sodium (mg)|Zinc (mg)|
|45621|1 pce|Cinnamon Apple, fat free, Entenmann's|53|150||3.0|35.0|0.5|21.0|13.5|0.0|0.0|0.0|0.0|0.00|0.00|0|0|0|0|0|0||||||||0.0|||20||0.0||||55||110||
|45622|1 pce|Lemon, fat free, Entenmann's|53|130||3.0|31.0|1.0|16.0|14.0|0.0|0.0|0.0|0.0|0.00|0.00|0|0|0|0|0|0||||||||0.0|||40||0.0||||70||140||
|45634|1 pce|Raspberry, Entenmann's|53|220|19|3.0|28.0|0.5|15.0|12.5|11.0|3.0|||||20|200|40|||||||||||0.0|||40||0.4||||60||170||
|45624|1 pce|Raspberry, fat free, Entenmann's|53|140||3.0|33.0|2.0|19.0|12.0|0.0|0.0|0.0|0.0|0.00|0.00|0|0|0|0|0|0||||||||0.0|||40||0.4||||70||125||
|||Puff Pastries|||||||||||||||||||||||||||||||||||||||||
|45625|1 ea|Apple, Entenmann's|85|260||2.0|36.0|1.0|19.0|16.0|12.0|3.0|||||0|0|0|0|0|0||||||||0.0|||0||0.0||||60||220||
|45642|1 ea|Dark Chocolate Clouds, Pepperidge Farm|60|288|18|3.0|26.3|2.0|9.4|14.9|18.8|7.4|||||12|0|0|0|0|0|0.00|0.00|0.00|||||0.0|||0||1.8||||||188||
|45650|1 ea|Milk Chocolate Clouds, Pepperidge Farm|60|288|17|3.0|26.8|1.5|12.4|12.9|18.8|7.4|||||27|0|0|0|0|0|0.00|0.00|0.00|||||0.0|||30||1.8||||||198||
|||Sweet Rolls|||||||||||||||||||||||||||||||||||||||||
|42549|1 ea|Apple Cinnamon w/icing, Pillsbury|41|139|27|1.8|21.4|0.7|9.4|11.4|5.2|1.3|||||0|1|0.2|||||||||||0.0|||10||0.8||||||309||
|42164|1 ea|Cheese, avg|66|238|29|4.7|28.8|0.8|12.5|15.5|12.1|4.0|6.0|1.3|0.10|1.24|50|168|51||||0.10|0.09|0.55|0.05|0.20|28.4|0.27|0.1|0.0||78|0.1|0.5|13|0.1|65|90|7.9|236|0.42|
|42166|1 ea|Cinnamon, prep f/refrig dough, w/frosting, avg|30|109|23|1.6|16.8|0.6|7.3|8.9|4.0|1.0|2.2|0.5|0.03|0.50|0|1|0.1||||0.12|0.07|1.09|0.01|0.02|1.8|0.08|0.1|0.1||10|0.0|0.8|4|0.1|104|19||250|0.10|
|42165|1 ea|Cinnamon, refrig dough, w/frosting, avg|30|100|29|1.5|15.5|0.6|6.7|8.2|3.7|0.9|2.1|0.5|0.02|0.45|0|1|0.1||||0.14|0.07|1.11|0.01|0.01|15.0|0.08|0.1|0.1||9|0.0|0.7|3|0.1|96|17|4.9|230|0.09|
|42033|1 ea|Cinnamon Raisin, avg|60|223|25|3.7|30.5|1.4|13.4|15.7|9.8|1.8|2.9|4.5|0.26|4.22|40|129|38|34|4||0.19|0.16|1.43|0.06|0.08|31.2|0.24|1.2|0.8||43|0.1|1.0|10|0.2|46|67|10.2|230|0.35|
|42167|1 ea|Cinnamon Raisin nut, avg|57|196|27|3.8|29.6|1.1|12.9|15.6|7.3|1.4|2.7|2.8|0.30|2.55|13|233|60|54|7||0.16|0.16|1.33|0.05|0.06|17.7|0.19|0.3|0.2||36|0.1|1.5|16|0.3|63|123||185|0.38|
|42365|1 ea|Cinnamon, Pepperidge Farm|64|250|22|4.0|33.0|2.0|15.0|16.0|12.0|2.5|6.0|1.0|||15|0|0|0|0|0|0.22|0.10|1.60|||||0.0|||40||1.4||||||220||
|42094|1 ea|Cinnamon, w/crumb tppng, mex pan dulce, avg|79|291|21|4.5|48.1|1.1|22.1|24.8|9.1|2.0|3.9|2.7|||26|333|88|81|5||0.23|0.21|1.98|0.04|0.06|22.4||0.1|||13|0.1|1.8|9||55|57||140|0.35|
|42362|1 ea|Cinnamon Glazed, Weight Watchers|60|202|24|4.0|33.3|1.0|10.1|22.2|5.0|1.5|||||5|0|0|0|0|0||||||||0.0|||40||0.7||||76||202||
|42399|1 oz|Cinnamon Raisin Swirl Crisps, Pepp Farm|28|228||3.5|33.3|5.3|1.8|26.3|8.8|0.9|6.1|0.0|0.00|0.00|0|0|0|0|0|0|0.26|0.18|2.10|||||0.0|||0||1.9||||||175||
|42263|1 pce|Cinnamon Raisin w/icing, Pillsbury|49|169|28|2.2|25.5|0.6|11.4|13.5|6.5|1.5|||||0|1|0.1|||||||||||0.0|||12||0.9||||||310||
|42264|1 pce|Cinnamon w/Icing, Pillsbury|41|139|28|1.9|21.1|0.5|8.7|12.0|5.2|1.3|||||0|1|0.1|||||||||||0.0|||10||0.8||||||327||
|42187|1 ea|Plain, avg|55|174|32|4.7|27.1|0.7|11.8|14.6|5.0|1.3|2.6|0.7|||18|39|12|12|0||0.20|0.18|1.22|0.06|0.00|17.1|0.17|0.0|0.2||58|0.0|1.2|10|0.2|59|68||214|0.26|
|||Toaster Pastries|||||||||||||||||||||||||||||||||||||||||
|45763|1 ea|Apple Cinnamon w/frosting, lowfat, Pop Tart|52|190|12|2.0|40.0|1.0|20.0|19.0|3.0|0.5|||||0|500|150||||0.15|0.17|2.00|0.20||40.0||0.0|||0||1.8|||20|||210||
|45593|1 ea|Apple Cinnamon w/frosting, Pop Tart|52|210|12|2.0|38.0|1.0|17.0|20.0|5.0|1.0|||||0|500|150||||0.15|0.17|2.00|0.20||40.0||0.0|||0||1.8|||20|||170|0.30|
|45764|1 ea|Blueberry, lowfat, Pop Tart|52|190|12|2.0|40.0|1.0|19.0|20.0|3.0|0.5|||||0|500|100||||0.15|0.17|2.00|0.20||40.0||0.0|||0||1.8|||20|||220||
|45592|1 ea|Blueberry, Pop Tart|52|210|12|2.0|36.0|1.0|16.0|19.0|7.0|1.0|||||0|500|150||||0.15|0.17|2.00|0.20||40.0||0.0|||0|0.1|1.8|8||40|||210|0.60|
|45598|1 ea|Blueberry, w/frosting, Pop Tart|52|200|12|2.0|37.0|1.0|16.0|20.0|5.0|1.0|||||0|500|150||||0.15|0.17|2.00|0.20||40.0||0.0|||0|0.1|1.8|8||40|||210|0.60|
|45683|1 ea|Brown Sugar Cinnamon, avg|50|206|11|2.5|34.0|0.5|15.4|18.2|7.1|1.8|4.0|0.9|0.05|0.85|0|493|112|95|17||0.19|0.29|2.29|0.21|0.11|14.5|0.13|0.1|0.0||17|0.1|2.0|12|0.2|66|57|6.3|212|0.31|
|45765|1 ea|Cherry, lowfat, Pop Tart|52|190|12|2.0|40.0|1.0|19.0|20.0|3.0|0.5|||||0|500|100||||0.15|0.17|2.00|0.20||40.0||0.0|||0||1.8|||20|||220||
|45595|1 ea|Cherry, Pop Tart|52|200|12|2.0|37.0|1.0|16.0|20.0|5.0|1.0|||||0|500|150||||0.15|0.17|2.00|0.20||40.0||0.0|||0|0.1|1.8|8||40|||220|0.60|
|45600|1 ea|Cherry, w/frosting, Pop Tart|52|200|12|2.0|37.0|1.0|19.0|17.0|5.0|1.0|||||0|500|150||||0.15|0.17|2.00|0.20||40.0||0.0|||0|0.1|1.8|0||40|||220|0.90|
|45601|1 ea|Chocolate Fudge w/frosting, Pop Tart|52|200|12|3.0|37.0|1.0|20.0|16.0|5.0|1.0|||||0|500|150||||0.15|0.17|2.00|0.20||40.0||0.0|||0|0.1|1.8|16||40|||200|1.20|
|45596|1 ea|Chocolate Graham, Pop Tart|52|210|12|3.0|36.0|1.0|18.0|17.0|6.0|1.5|||||0|500|150||||0.15|0.17|2.00|0.20||40.0||0.0|||0|0.0|1.8|8||40|||230|0.60|
|45761|1 ea|S'Mores, w/frosting, Pop Tart|52|200|14|3.0|36.0|1.0|19.0|16.0|5.0|1.5|||||0|500|150||||0.15|0.17|2.00|0.20||40.0||0.0|||0|0.0|1.8|8||40|||200||
|45679|1 ea|Strawberry, w/frosting, lowfat, Pop Tart|52|263|7|2.7|28.3|0.8|17.2|10.3|16.2|3.5|7.6|4.0|0.16|3.85|[illegible]|436|114|01|13||0.08|0.11|1.11|0.00|0.01|27.6|0.14|0.0|0.0||16|0.2|1.6|21|0.3|55|87|2.2|349|0.43|
|45762|1 ea|Wild Berry, w/frost, Pop Tart|52|202|12|1.9|37.6|1.0|20.2|16.4|4.8|1.4|||||0|481|144||||0.14|0.16|1.93|0.19||38.5||0.0|||0||1.7|||19|||164||
|||Toaster Strudels|||||||||||||||||||||||||||||||||||||||||
|70295|1 ea|Apple Spice, Pillsbury|54|179|32|2.6|26.4|0.5|10.0|15.8|7.0|1.5|||||6|9|2||||||||||||||6||0.9||||||191||
|70291|1 ea|Blueberry, Pillsbury|54|178|32|2.6|26.2|0.5|9.9|15.8|7.0|1.6|||||6|9|2||||||||||||||6||0.9||||||199||
|70296|1 ea|Cherry, Pillsbury|54|178|32|2.6|26.4|0.5|11.2|14.6|6.9|1.6|||||6|9|2|||||||||||0.0|||6||0.9||||||200||
|70292|1 ea|Cinnamon, Pillsbury|54|183|32|2.6|25.9|0.8|10.1|15.1|7.7|1.7|||||6|9|2||||||||||||||6||0.9||||||196||
|45646|1 ea|Cream Cheese, Pillsbury|54|194|31|3.3|23.1|0.5|7.9|14.7|9.9|3.5|||||0|132|26|||||||||||0.0|||15||1.0||||||228||
|45647|1 ea|Cream Cheese w/Blueberries, Pillsbury|54|188|32|3.0|24.3|0.5|8.6|15.2|8.8|2.8|||||12|85|17|||||||||||0.0|||12||1.0||||||217||
|||*PASTRY, PIE AND DESSERT CRUSTS*|||||||||||||||||||||||||||||||||||||||||
|45530|1 ea|Cookie Crust, chocolate, bkd, whl, avg|219|1130|6|11.4|121.5|3.4|72.9|45.3|69.4|15.0|32.9|17.2|0.68|16.55|[illegible]|1875|[illegible]|436|53||0.34|0.46|4.77|0.00|0.04|0.0|0.62|0.0|0.0||68|0.8|6.7|90|1.2|234|374||1502|1.82|
|45676|1 pce|Cookie Crust, plain, bkd, avg|22|119|7|0.8|11.3|0.3|||8.1|1.7|3.5|2.4|0.11|2.29|9|248|54|57|7||0.04|0.05|0.48|0.01|0.02|1.5|0.07|0.0|0.0||9|0.0|0.4|2|0.0|17|18||116|0.05|
|45500|1 pce|Graham Cracker Crust, bkd, avg|30|148|4|1.3|19.6|0.5|14.3|4.9|7.5|1.6|3.4|2.1|0.09|1.93|0|236|51|54|7||0.03|0.05|0.64|0.01|0.01|7.2|0.07|0.0|0.0||6|0.0|0.7|5|0.1|20|26|1.8|171|0.14|
|70710|1 pce|Graham Cracker Crust, fzn, PET-Ritz,|21|110|3|1.0|13.0|0.0|5.0|8.0|6.0|1.5|||||0|0|0|0|0|0||||||||0.0|||0||0.7||||||120||
|45521|1 ea|Pastry Crust, cream puff shell, 3 1/2 ", avg|66|239|40|5.9|15.0|0.5|0.7|13.9|17.1|3.7|7.3|4.9|0.22|4.65|129|764|203||||0.14|0.24|1.04|0.05|0.26|31.7|0.41|0.0|0.0||24|0.0|1.3|8|0.1|79|64|15.8|368|0.48|
|45528|1 ea|Pastry Crust, phyllo dough, avg|19|57|33|1.3|10.0|0.4|0.2|9.4|1.1|0.3|0.6|0.2|0.02|0.16|0|0|0|0|0|0|0.10|0.06|0.77|0.01|0.00|14.1|0.06|0.0|0.0||2|0.0|0.6|3|0.1|14|14|4.4|92|0.09|
|49044|1 ea|Puff Pastry, dough sheet, Pepperidge Farm|41|200|8|3.0|23.0|3.0|0.0|20.0|11.0|2.5|6.0|1.0|||0|0|0|0|0|0|0.12|0.07|1.20|||||0.0|||0||1.1||||||135||
|49045|1 ea|Patty Sheet, Pepperidge Farm|47|230|13|3.0|23.0|2.0|0.5|20.5|14.0|3.0|9.0|1.0|||0|0|0|0|0|0|0.15|0.10|1.20|||||0.0|||0||0.7||||||135||
|||Pie Crusts|||||||||||||||||||||||||||||||||||||||||
|45617|1 pce|Frozen, 6", Pet|23|110|20|2.0|9.0|0.0|0.0|9.0|7.0|1.5|2.5|0.0|0.00|0.00|0|0|0|0|0|0||||||||0.0|||0||0.7||||||105||
|45614|1 pce|Frozen, 9", Pet|18|90|20|1.0|7.0|0.0|0.0|7.0|6.0|1.5|2.0|0.0|0.00|0.00|0|0|0|0|0|0||||||||0.0|||0||0.4||||||80||
|45615|1 pce|Frozen, 9", deep dish, Pet|20|100|13|2.0|8.0|0.0|0.0|8.0|7.0|1.5|2.5|0.0|0.00|0.00|0|0|0|0|0|0||||||||0.0|||0||0.7||||||95||
|45616|1 pce|Frozen, 10", deep dish, Pet|26|130||2.0|10.0|0.0|0.0|10.0|8.0|2.0|3.0|0.0|0.00|0.00|0|0|0|0|0|0||||||||0.0|||0||0.7||||||120||
|49114|1 pce|Prep f/Mix, avg|20|100|11|1.3|10.1|0.4|0.2|9.5|6.1|1.5|3.5|0.8|0.04|0.73|0|0|0|0|0|0|0.06|0.04|0.47|0.01|0.00|2.4|0.03|0.0|0.0||12|0.0|0.4|3|0.1|17|12|3.0|146|0.08|
|45503|1 ea|Prep f/Mix, whl, avg|160|802|11|10.7|80.6|2.8|1.8|76.0|48.6|12.3|27.7|6.2|0.31|5.84|0|0|0|0|0|0|0.48|0.30|3.79|0.09|0.00|19.2|0.27|0.0|0.0||96|0.1|3.4|24|0.5|134|99|24.0|1166|0.62|
|49115|1 pce|Prep f/Recipe, avg|23|121|10|1.5|10.9|0.4|0.2|10.3|8.0|2.0|3.5|2.1|0.13|1.97|0|0|0|0|0|0|0.09|0.06|0.76|0.01|0.00|15.4|0.04|0.0|0.0||2|0.0|0.7|3|0.1|15|15|4.9|125|0.10|
|45501|1 ea|Prep f/Recipe, whl, avg|180|949|10|11.5|85.5|3.0|1.9|80.6|62.3|15.5|27.4|16.4|1.00|15.41|0|0|0|0|0|0|0.70|0.50|5.96|0.04|0.00|120.6|0.32|0.0|0.0||18|0.2|5.2|25|0.8|121|121|38.0|976|0.79|
|45540|1 ea|Popover Crust, prep f/mix, whl, avg|33|67|55|2.6|10.4|0.3|||1.5|0.4|0.6|0.2|0.01|0.22|37|54|17|16|1||0.05|0.06|0.45|0.02|0.08|5.6|0.14|0.0|||9|0.0|0.6|5|0.1|30|25||143|0.21|
|70712|1 ea|Tart Crust, 3", Pet-Ritz|28|140|20|2.0|11.0|0.0|0.0|11.0|9.0|2.0|3.0|0.5|||0|0|0|0|0|0||||||||0.0|||0||0.7||||||130||
|70711|1 pce|Tart Crust, 6", Pet-Ritz|23|110|20|2.0|9.0|0.0|0.0|9.0|7.0|1.5|2.5|0.0|0.00|0.00|0|0|0|0|0|0||||||||0.0|||0||0.7||||||105||
|||*PIES*|||||||||||||||||||||||||||||||||||||||||
|||Apple Pie|||||||||||||||||||||||||||||||||||||||||
|48061|1 pce|1/8 of 9" pie, avg|125|296|52|2.4|42.5|2.0|21.9|18.6|13.8|4.8|5.5|2.8|0.15|2.59|0|155|38|34|4||0.17|0.20|1.40|0.05|0.01|5.0|0.15|4.0|0.0||14|0.1|1.5|9|0.2|30|81|1.3|332|0.20|
|70537|1 pce|Dutch, Mrs Smith's|163|420|45|5.0|72.0||||13.0||||||[illegible]|246|41||||0.06|0.06|0.20|||||2.0|||23||0.6||||115||420||
|48166|1 pce|Fat Free, Entenmann's|130|270||2.0|65.0|2.0|38.0|25.0|0.0|0.0|0.0|0.0|0.00|0.00|0|0|0|0|0|0||||||||0.0|||0||0.7||||100||330||

| Code | Amount | | Description | Basic Components: Weight (g) | Calories | % Water | Protein (g) | Carbs (g) | Fiber (g) | Sugar (g) | Other Carbs (g) | Fat (g) | Additional Fats: Sat Fat (g) | Mono Fat (g) | Poly Fat (g) | Omega 3 (g) | Omega 6 (g) | Choles (mg) | Vit A & Components: Vit A (IU) | Vit A (RE) | Retinol (RE) | Carotenoids (RE) | Beta Carotene (mcg) | Vitamins: Thiamin (mg) | Riboflavin (mg) | Niacin (NE) | Vit B6 (mg) | Vit B12 (mcg) | Folate (mcg) | Panto (mg) | Vit C (mg) | Vit D (mg) | Vit E (α TE) | Minerals: Calcium (mg) | Copper (mg) | Iron (mg) | Magnes (mg) | Mang (mg) | Phos (mg) | Potassium (mg) | Selenium (mcg) | Sodium (mg) | Zinc (mg) |
|---|---|---|---|---|---|---|---|---|---|---|---|---|---|---|---|---|---|---|---|---|---|---|---|---|---|---|---|---|---|---|---|---|---|---|---|---|---|---|---|---|---|---|---|
| 48013 | 1 | ea | Fried apple pie, avg | 85 | 266 | 40 | 2.4 | 33.1 | 1.5 | 10.2 | 21.4 | 14.4 | 6.5 | 5.8 | 1.2 | 0.12 | 1.04 | 13 | 149 | 33 | 29 | 4 | | 0.10 | 0.08 | 0.98 | 0.03 | 0.08 | 4.3 | 0.15 | 1.1 | 0.0 | 0.4 | 13 | 0.0 | 0.9 | 8 | 0.2 | 37 | 51 | 1.1 | 325 | 0.17 |
| 48076 | 1 | pce | Frozen apple pie, bkd, 1/8 of 9" pie, avg | 125 | 296 | 52 | 2.4 | 42.5 | 2.0 | 21.9 | 18.6 | 13.8 | 4.8 | 5.5 | 2.8 | 0.15 | 2.59 | 0 | 155 | 38 | 34 | 4 | | 0.04 | 0.03 | 0.33 | 0.05 | 0.01 | 27.5 | 0.15 | 4.0 | 0.0 | | 14 | 0.1 | 0.6 | 9 | 0.2 | 30 | 81 | 1.3 | 332 | 0.20 |
| 70528 | 1 | pce | Natural Juice, 1/7 pie, Mrs Smith's | 149 | 420 | 48 | 3.0 | 52.0 | 2.4 | | | 22.0 | 5.7 | 9.6 | 6.1 | | | 5 | 138 | 23 | | | | 0.01 | 0.06 | 0.30 | 0.08 | | | | 0.0 | | | 13 | | 1.4 | | | | 60 | | 370 | |
| 70531 | 1 | pce | Old Fashioned, 1/8 pie, Mrs Smith's | 177 | 530 | 43 | 4.0 | 69.0 | | | | 27.0 | | | | | | 3 | 123 | 21 | | | | 0.05 | 0.07 | 0.20 | | | | | 0.0 | | | 21 | | 0.4 | | | | 120 | | 670 | |
| 48089 | 1 | pce | Prep f/Recipe, 1/8 of 9" pie, avg | 155 | 411 | 47 | 3.7 | 57.5 | 2.2 | 23.7 | 31.6 | 19.4 | 4.7 | 8.4 | 5.2 | 0.32 | 4.85 | 0 | 90 | 19 | 17 | 2 | | 0.23 | 0.17 | 1.91 | 0.05 | 0.00 | 37.2 | 0.14 | 2.6 | 0.0 | | 11 | 0.1 | 1.7 | 11 | 0.3 | 43 | 122 | 12.1 | 327 | 0.29 |
| 70532 | 1 | pce | Raisin, Mrs Smith's | 177 | 560 | 40 | 4.0 | 74.0 | | | | 28.0 | | | | | | 2 | 159 | 27 | | | | 0.04 | 0.18 | 0.20 | | | | | 2.0 | | | 16 | | 0.7 | | | | 215 | | 705 | |
| 48150 | 1 | pce | Sugar Free, 1/9 of 9"pie, Plush Pippin | 126 | 370 | | 2.0 | 43.0 | 2.0 | 6.0 | 35.0 | 22.0 | 4.0 | 7.0 | 0.5 | | | 0 | | | | | | | | | | | | | 2.4 | | | | | | | | | 80 | | 230 | |
| 48105 | 1 | pce | With Sour Cream, 1/8 of 9" pie, avg | 159 | 356 | 53 | 2.8 | 55.5 | 2.6 | | | 14.7 | 5.1 | 5.7 | 3.0 | | | 8 | 185 | 40 | 32 | 7 | | 0.15 | 0.13 | 1.18 | 0.06 | 0.02 | 5.6 | | 3.4 | | | 49 | 0.1 | 1.5 | 16 | | 49 | 235 | | 231 | 0.28 |
| | | | Banana Cream Pie | | | | | | | | | | | | | | | | | | | | | | | | | | | | | | | | | | | | | | | | |
| 48090 | 1 | pce | Prep f/Mix, 1/8 of 9" pie, avg | 92 | 231 | 51 | 3.1 | 29.1 | 0.6 | | | 11.9 | 6.3 | 4.2 | 0.7 | 0.15 | 0.55 | 27 | 375 | 92 | 84 | 8 | | 0.09 | 0.13 | 0.65 | 0.03 | 0.19 | 19.3 | 0.24 | 0.5 | | | 67 | 0.0 | 0.4 | 11 | 0.1 | 154 | 104 | 4.5 | 267 | 0.30 |
| 48069 | 1 | pce | Prep f/Recipe, 1/8 of 9" pie, avg | 144 | 387 | 48 | 6.3 | 47.4 | 1.0 | | | 19.6 | 5.4 | 8.2 | 4.7 | 0.30 | 4.44 | 73 | 376 | 101 | 92 | 9 | | 0.20 | 0.30 | 1.51 | 0.19 | 0.36 | 38.9 | 0.56 | 2.3 | | | 108 | 0.1 | 1.5 | 23 | 0.2 | 132 | 238 | 13.1 | 346 | 0.69 |
| 70553 | 1 | pce | Thaw n Serve, Mrs Smith's | 85 | 240 | 47 | 2.0 | 31.0 | | | | 12.0 | | | | | | 5 | 43 | 9 | | | | 0.04 | 0.14 | 0.60 | | | | | 0.0 | | | 39 | | 0.7 | | | | 70 | | 180 | |
| | | | Blackberry Pie | | | | | | | | | | | | | | | | | | | | | | | | | | | | | | | | | | | | | | | | |
| 48088 | 1 | pce | Avg, 1/8 pie | 150 | 400 | 47 | 3.8 | 55.9 | 4.5 | 22.5 | 28.9 | 18.7 | 4.5 | 8.1 | 5.1 | | | 0 | 213 | 39 | 26 | 12 | | 0.21 | 0.17 | 1.92 | 0.05 | 0.00 | 20.7 | | 13.3 | 0.0 | | 28 | 0.1 | 1.9 | 21 | | 51 | 165 | 1.7 | 292 | 0.43 |
| 70543 | 1 | pce | RTB, 1/8 pie, Mrs Smith's | 163 | 400 | 49 | 4.0 | 62.0 | | | | 16.0 | | | | | | 1 | 114 | 19 | | | | 0.07 | 0.16 | 0.10 | | | | | 2.0 | | | 23 | | 1.8 | | | | 175 | | 470 | |
| 48085 | 1 | pce | Single Crust, avg | 137 | 344 | 48 | 2.4 | 53.7 | 3.8 | | | 14.2 | 3.4 | 6.2 | 3.9 | | | 0 | 172 | 40 | 33 | 6 | | 0.14 | 0.11 | 1.12 | 0.06 | 0.00 | 4.7 | | 10.0 | 0.0 | | 10 | 0.1 | 1.1 | 8 | | 30 | 77 | 1.4 | 248 | 0.25 |
| 48114 | 1 | pce | Black Bottom Pie, 1/8 of 9" pie, avg | 99 | 277 | 48 | 4.9 | 28.2 | 0.7 | | | 16.6 | 7.6 | 5.9 | 2.0 | | | 92 | 626 | 172 | 163 | 9 | | 0.05 | 0.18 | 0.32 | 0.05 | 0.23 | 8.4 | | 0.3 | | | 74 | 0.1 | 0.9 | 27 | | 95 | 173 | | 156 | 0.63 |
| | | | Blueberry Pie | | | | | | | | | | | | | | | | | | | | | | | | | | | | | | | | | | | | | | | | |
| 48091 | 1 | pce | Prep f/Frozen, avg | 125 | 290 | 52 | 2.3 | 43.6 | 1.3 | 17.9 | 24.5 | 12.5 | 2.1 | 5.3 | 4.4 | 0.30 | 4.10 | 0 | 175 | 43 | 30 | 13 | | 0.01 | 0.04 | 0.38 | 0.05 | 0.01 | 27.5 | 0.17 | 3.4 | 0.0 | | 10 | 0.1 | 0.4 | 6 | 0.2 | 29 | 62 | 1.8 | 406 | 0.20 |
| 48092 | 1 | pce | Prep f/Recipe, avg | 147 | 360 | 51 | 4.0 | 49.2 | 2.1 | 20.1 | 27.0 | 17.5 | 4.3 | 7.5 | 4.5 | 0.28 | 4.25 | 0 | 62 | 6 | 4 | 2 | | 0.22 | 0.19 | 1.75 | 0.05 | 0.00 | 33.8 | 0.18 | 1.0 | 0.0 | | 10 | 0.1 | 1.8 | 12 | 0.4 | 44 | 74 | 10.9 | 272 | 0.29 |
| 70551 | 1 | pce | Thaw n Serve, Mrs Smith's | 128 | 290 | 55 | 2.0 | 45.0 | | | | 11.0 | | | | | | 0 | 107 | 22 | | | | 0.04 | 0.06 | 0.10 | | | | | 1.0 | | | 11 | | 0.4 | | | | 75 | | 310 | |
| 70557 | 1 | pce | Boston Cream, Thaw n Serve, 1/8 of 9" pie, Mrs Smith's | 106 | 240 | 48 | 3.0 | 48.0 | 0.8 | | | 4.0 | 1.5 | 1.7 | 0.8 | | | 4 | 35 | 7 | | | | 0.02 | 0.12 | 0.30 | 0.05 | | | | 1.0 | | | 43 | | 0.5 | | | | 105 | | 240 | |
| 48093 | 1 | pce | Butterscotch, prep f/rec, 1/8 of 9" pie, avg | 127 | 354 | 46 | 6.0 | 42.3 | 0.9 | | | 18.2 | 5.1 | 7.6 | 4.4 | 0.27 | 4.08 | 77 | 382 | 107 | 103 | 4 | | 0.18 | 0.27 | 1.26 | 0.07 | 0.38 | 14.0 | 0.54 | 0.6 | | | 128 | 0.1 | 1.6 | 22 | 0.2 | 135 | 221 | | 335 | 0.69 |
| | | | Cheesecake | | | | | | | | | | | | | | | | | | | | | | | | | | | | | | | | | | | | | | | | |
| 49004 | 1 | pce | Avg | 80 | 257 | 46 | 4.4 | 20.4 | 0.3 | 17.9 | 2.2 | 18.0 | 7.9 | 6.9 | 1.3 | 0.18 | 1.10 | 44 | 438 | 117 | | | | 0.02 | 0.15 | 0.16 | 0.04 | 0.14 | 14.4 | 0.46 | 0.3 | | | 41 | 0.0 | 0.5 | 9 | 0.1 | 74 | 72 | 4.2 | 166 | 0.41 |
| 49000 | 1 | pce | Cherry & Cream Cheese Torte, avg | 161 | 448 | 45 | 7.2 | 58.6 | 1.3 | 51.0 | 6.2 | 21.6 | 9.8 | 7.7 | 3.0 | 0.29 | 2.68 | 42 | 1092 | 249 | 209 | 40 | | 0.09 | 0.31 | 0.98 | 0.07 | 0.31 | 14.9 | 0.53 | 4.2 | 0.1 | 0.0 | 158 | 0.1 | 1.7 | 23 | 0.2 | 166 | 273 | 3.9 | 341 | 0.76 |
| 49017 | 1 | pce | Chocolate, avg | 128 | 502 | 29 | 8.3 | 48.5 | 1.9 | 36.9 | 9.8 | 32.3 | 15.5 | 11.0 | 3.9 | | | 118 | 1246 | 347 | 326 | 20 | | 0.16 | 0.29 | 1.29 | 0.05 | 0.23 | 14.0 | | 0.1 | | | 72 | 0.2 | 2.2 | 37 | | 143 | 188 | | 403 | 0.92 |
| 49001 | 1 | pce | Prep f/No Bake Mix, avg | 99 | 271 | 44 | 5.4 | 35.1 | 1.9 | 26.7 | 6.6 | 12.6 | 6.6 | 4.5 | 0.8 | 0.16 | 0.64 | 29 | 362 | 98 | 92 | 6 | | 0.12 | 0.26 | 0.49 | 0.05 | 0.31 | 29.7 | 0.61 | 0.5 | 0.6 | | 170 | 0.0 | 0.5 | 19 | 0.1 | 232 | 209 | 4.7 | 376 | 0.46 |
| 49011 | 1 | pce | With Cherry Topping, avg | 142 | 408 | 49 | 7.1 | 37.6 | 0.6 | 33.0 | 4.0 | 26.3 | 14.5 | 8.3 | 2.2 | 0.37 | 1.81 | 121 | 1275 | 342 | | | | 0.04 | 0.23 | 0.51 | 0.06 | 0.24 | 14.2 | 0.22 | 1.0 | | | 61 | 0.1 | 1.7 | 10 | 0.1 | 101 | 132 | | 288 | 0.57 |
| | | | Cherry Pie | | | | | | | | | | | | | | | | | | | | | | | | | | | | | | | | | | | | | | | | |
| 48113 | 1 | pce | Chiffon, w/liqueur, 1/8 of 9" pie, avg | 99 | 331 | 38 | 4.8 | 33.2 | 0.4 | | | 17.7 | 6.2 | 7.2 | 3.2 | | | 98 | 747 | 205 | 194 | 11 | | 0.07 | 0.17 | 0.52 | 0.04 | 0.24 | 11.2 | | 0.1 | | | 33 | 0.1 | 0.9 | 11 | | 69 | 64 | | 476 | 0.43 |
| 48167 | 1 | pce | Fat Free, Entenmann's | 130 | 270 | | 3.0 | 64.0 | 1.0 | 40.0 | 23.0 | 0.0 | 0.0 | 0.0 | 0.0 | 0.00 | 0.00 | 0 | 400 | 80 | | | | | | | | | | | 2.4 | | | 0 | | 0.7 | | | | 150 | | 310 | |
| 49119 | 1 | ea | Fried, avg | 85 | 266 | 40 | 2.4 | 33.1 | 1.5 | 10.2 | 21.4 | 14.4 | 6.5 | 5.8 | 1.2 | 0.12 | 1.04 | 13 | 149 | 33 | 29 | 4 | | 0.10 | 0.08 | 0.98 | 0.03 | 0.08 | 4.3 | 0.15 | 1.1 | 0.0 | 0.4 | 13 | 0.0 | 0.9 | 8 | 0.2 | 37 | 51 | 1.1 | 325 | 0.17 |
| 70530 | 1 | pce | Natural Juice, 1/7 pie, Mrs Smith's | 149 | 410 | 46 | 4.0 | 59.0 | | | | 18.0 | | | | | | 10 | 84 | 14 | | | | 0.06 | 0.06 | 0.60 | | | | | 0.0 | | | 15 | | 1.1 | | | | 140 | | 380 | |
| 48077 | 1 | pce | Prep f/Frozen, 1/8 of 9" pie, avg | 125 | 325 | 46 | 2.5 | 49.8 | 1.0 | 30.3 | 18.5 | 13.8 | 3.2 | 7.3 | 2.6 | 0.17 | 2.40 | 0 | 351 | 68 | 65 | 2 | | 0.03 | 0.04 | 0.25 | 0.05 | 0.01 | 27.5 | 0.40 | 1.1 | 0.0 | | 15 | 0.0 | 0.6 | 10 | 0.2 | 36 | 101 | 1.5 | 308 | 0.23 |
| 48094 | 1 | pce | Prep f/Recipe, 1/8 pie, avg | 180 | 486 | 46 | 5.0 | 69.3 | 2.7 | 30.2 | 36.4 | 22.0 | 5.4 | 9.6 | 5.8 | 0.36 | 5.49 | 0 | 736 | 86 | 83 | 3 | | 0.27 | 0.22 | 2.30 | 0.06 | 0.00 | 48.6 | 0.22 | 1.8 | 0.0 | | 18 | 0.1 | 3.3 | 16 | 0.4 | 54 | 139 | 14.0 | 344 | 0.36 |
| 70550 | 1 | pce | Thaw n Serve, Mrs Smith's | 128 | 300 | 51 | 3.0 | 50.0 | | | | 10.0 | | | | | | 0 | 360 | 72 | | | | 0.05 | 0.07 | 0.10 | | | | | 1.0 | | | 12 | | 0.4 | | | | 140 | | 305 | |
| | | | Chocolate Pie | | | | | | | | | | | | | | | | | | | | | | | | | | | | | | | | | | | | | | | | |
| 48112 | 1 | pce | Chiffon, 1/8 of 9 " pie, avg | 99 | 321 | 36 | 6.1 | 40.3 | 1.3 | | | 16.0 | 5.1 | 6.6 | 3.3 | | | 107 | 241 | 68 | 66 | 2 | | 0.12 | 0.21 | 0.91 | 0.04 | 0.20 | 12.4 | | 0.0 | | | 21 | 0.2 | 1.5 | 23 | | 86 | 93 | | 185 | 0.62 |
| 48096 | 1 | pce | Cream, RTS, 1/8 of 8" pie, avg | 113 | 344 | 44 | 2.9 | 38.0 | 2.3 | 28.7 | 7.0 | 21.9 | 5.6 | 12.5 | 2.7 | 0.14 | 2.58 | 6 | 0 | 0 | 0 | 0 | 0 | 0.04 | 0.12 | 0.77 | 0.02 | 0.01 | 14.7 | 0.44 | 0.0 | 1.1 | | 41 | 0.1 | 1.2 | 24 | 0.2 | 77 | 144 | 8.5 | 154 | 0.26 |
| 48071 | 1 | pce | Cream, prep f/rec, 1/8 of 9", avg | 142 | 400 | 47 | 6.8 | 44.3 | 2.8 | | | 22.9 | 7.4 | 9.4 | 4.8 | 0.29 | 4.53 | 75 | 375 | 104 | 99 | 5 | | 0.20 | 0.29 | 1.45 | 0.07 | 0.37 | 14.2 | 0.53 | 0.7 | | | 115 | 0.2 | 1.8 | 37 | 0.3 | 156 | 209 | | 348 | 0.91 |
| 70554 | 1 | pce | Cream, Thaw n Serve, Mrs Smith's | 85 | 270 | 41 | 2.0 | 35.0 | 2.9 | | | 13.0 | 4.7 | 5.1 | 2.5 | | | 5 | 65 | 13 | | | | 0.01 | 0.06 | 0.90 | 0.03 | | | | 0.0 | | | 23 | | 0.6 | | | | 115 | | 235 | |
| 48157 | 1 | pce | Cream, Weight Watchers | 78 | 170 | 47 | 6.0 | 31.0 | 2.0 | 20.0 | 9.0 | 4.0 | 1.0 | | | | | 5 | 0 | 0 | 0 | 0 | 0 | | | | | | | | 0.0 | | | 80 | | 0.7 | | | | 200 | | 125 | |
| 48119 | 1 | pce | Meringue, 1/8 of 9" pie, avg | 114 | 287 | 48 | 5.5 | 38.2 | | | | 13.7 | 5.1 | 6.0 | 1.8 | 0.00 | 1.82 | 64 | 217 | 58 | | | | 0.08 | 0.18 | 0.80 | | | | | 0.0 | | | 79 | | 1.3 | | | 112 | 158 | | 292 | |
| 70560 | 1 | pce | Pecan, 1/8 pie, Mrs Smith's | 145 | 570 | 19 | 6.0 | 92.0 | | | | 20.0 | | | | | | 5 | 48 | 10 | | | | 0.07 | 0.14 | 0.10 | | | | | 1.0 | | | 29 | | 1.6 | | | | 155 | | 410 | |
| | | | Coconut Pie | | | | | | | | | | | | | | | | | | | | | | | | | | | | | | | | | | | | | | | | |
| 48099 | 1 | pce | Cream, prep f/rec, 1/8 of 9" pie, avg | 133 | 396 | 44 | 6.4 | 45.5 | 0.7 | | | 21.3 | 7.6 | 8.0 | 4.5 | 0.28 | 4.24 | 77 | 379 | 105 | 101 | 4 | | 0.18 | 0.28 | 1.33 | 0.08 | 0.37 | 14.6 | 0.57 | 0.7 | | | 113 | 0.1 | 1.5 | 21 | 0.4 | 140 | 184 | | 356 | 0.81 |
| 48072 | 1 | pce | Cream, RTS, 1/6 of 7" pie, avg | 64 | 191 | 43 | 1.3 | 23.8 | 0.8 | | | 10.6 | 4.5 | 4.6 | 1.0 | 0.05 | 0.94 | 0 | 58 | 12 | | | | 0.03 | 0.05 | 0.13 | 0.04 | 0.08 | 4.5 | 0.15 | 0.0 | | | 19 | 0.0 | 0.5 | 13 | 0.3 | 54 | 42 | 3.4 | 163 | 0.30 |
| 70555 | 1 | pce | Cream, Thaw n Serve, Mrs Smith's | 85 | 270 | 42 | 2.0 | 33.0 | | | | 14.0 | | | | | | 5 | 40 | 8 | | | | 0.04 | 0.07 | 0.20 | | | | | 0.0 | | | 25 | | 0.7 | | | | 55 | | 220 | |
| 48084 | 1 | pce | Custard, avg | 104 | 270 | 49 | 6.1 | 31.4 | 1.9 | 18.7 | 10.8 | 13.7 | 6.1 | 5.7 | 1.2 | 0.08 | 1.13 | 36 | 114 | 28 | 27 | 1 | | 0.09 | 0.15 | 0.42 | 0.01 | 0.09 | 13.5 | 0.25 | 0.6 | 0.9 | | 84 | 0.1 | 0.8 | 19 | 0.2 | 127 | 182 | 6.7 | 348 | 0.71 |
| 48168 | 1 | pce | Custard, Entenmann's | 125 | 340 | 50 | 7.0 | 35.0 | 1.0 | 21.0 | 13.0 | 19.0 | 8.0 | | | | | 135 | 300 | 60 | | | | | | | | | | | 0.0 | | | 80 | | 0.7 | | | | 190 | | 310 | |
| 70546 | 1 | pce | Custard, RTB, 1/8 pie, Mrs Smith's | 156 | 330 | 59 | 9.0 | 40.0 | | | | 15.0 | | | | | | 50 | 102 | 17 | | | | 0.03 | 0.32 | 0.70 | | | | | 0.0 | | | 123 | | 1.3 | | | | 270 | | 550 | |
| 48084 | 1 | ea | Custard, RTS, whl, avg | 624 | 1622 | 49 | 36.8 | 188.4 | 11.2 | 112.3 | 64.9 | 82.4 | 36.5 | 34.3 | 7.3 | 0.49 | 6.80 | 218 | 686 | 168 | 160 | 8 | | 0.55 | 0.92 | 2.51 | 0.07 | 0.56 | 81.1 | 1.49 | 3.7 | 5.5 | | 505 | 0.4 | 5.0 | 112 | 1.3 | 761 | 1092 | 39.9 | 2090 | 4.24 |
| | | | Egg Custard Pie | | | | | | | | | | | | | | | | | | | | | | | | | | | | | | | | | | | | | | | | |
| 48100 | 1 | pce | Prep f/Recipe, 1/8 of 9" pie, avg | 127 | 262 | 58 | 6.5 | 34.0 | 2.0 | | | 11.3 | 3.5 | 4.6 | 2.4 | 0.17 | 2.24 | 88 | 281 | 81 | 77 | 4 | | 0.12 | 0.29 | 0.84 | 0.06 | 0.30 | 12.7 | 0.51 | 0.5 | | | 107 | 0.0 | 1.0 | 17 | 0.1 | 124 | 159 | | 257 | 0.62 |
| 70547 | 1 | pce | RTB, 1/8 pie, Mrs Smith's | 156 | 300 | 59 | 9.0 | 45.0 | | | | 9.0 | | | | | | 65 | 50 | 15 | | | | 0.06 | 0.42 | 0.00 | | | | | 0.0 | | | 156 | | 0.8 | | | | 240 | | 490 | |
| 48081 | 1 | pce | RTS, 1/6 of 8" pie, avg | 105 | 220 | 61 | 5.8 | 21.8 | 1.7 | 10.5 | 9.7 | 12.2 | 2.5 | 5.0 | 3.9 | 0.27 | 3.63 | 35 | 244 | 70 | 67 | 3 | | 0.04 | 0.22 | 0.31 | 0.05 | 0.45 | 21.0 | 0.70 | 0.6 | 1.0 | | 84 | 0.0 | 0.6 | 12 | 0.1 | 118 | 111 | 7.5 | 252 | 0.55 |
| 49118 | 1 | ea | Fruit pie, fried, avg | 128 | 404 | 38 | 3.8 | 54.5 | 3.3 | 15.4 | 35.8 | 20.6 | 3.1 | 9.5 | 6.9 | 0.73 | 6.16 | 0 | 35 | 4 | 4 | 0.1 | | 0.18 | 0.14 | 1.83 | 0.04 | 0.10 | 23.0 | 0.14 | 1.7 | 0.0 | | 28 | 0.1 | 1.6 | 13 | 0.3 | 55 | 83 | 3.1 | 479 | 0.29 |
| | | | Lemon Pie | | | | | | | | | | | | | | | | | | | | | | | | | | | | | | | | | | | | | | | | |
| 48121 | 1 | pce | Chiffon, 1/8 of 9 " pie, avg | 81 | 254 | 36 | 5.7 | 35.5 | | | | 10.2 | 2.7 | 4.9 | 1.8 | 0.00 | 1.81 | 137 | 138 | 35 | | | | 0.08 | 0.13 | 0.65 | | | | | 2.4 | | | 19 | | 1.2 | | | 67 | 66 | | 211 | |
| 48170 | 1 | pce | Entenmann's | 123 | 340 | 46 | 3.0 | 45.0 | 0.5 | 25.0 | 19.5 | 17.0 | 4.5 | | | | | 45 | 100 | 20 | | | | | | | | | | | 0.0 | | | 0 | | 0.4 | | | | 65 | | 420 | |
| 49120 | 1 | ea | Fried, avg | 85 | 266 | 40 | 2.4 | 33.1 | 1.5 | 10.2 | 21.4 | 14.4 | 6.5 | 5.8 | 1.2 | 0.12 | 1.04 | 13 | 149 | 33 | 29 | 4 | | 0.10 | 0.08 | 0.98 | 0.03 | 0.08 | 4.3 | 0.15 | 1.1 | 0.0 | 0.4 | 13 | 0.0 | 0.9 | 8 | 0.2 | 37 | 51 | 1.1 | 325 | 0.17 |
| 48101 | 1 | pce | Meringue, prep f/rec, 1/8 of 9" pie, avg | 127 | 362 | 43 | 4.8 | 49.7 | 1.5 | 33.4 | 14.7 | 16.4 | 4.1 | 7.1 | 4.2 | 0.24 | 3.99 | 67 | 203 | 56 | 53 | 3 | | 0.15 | 0.20 | 1.20 | 0.03 | 0.15 | 31.8 | 0.27 | 4.2 | 0.3 | | 15 | 0.1 | 1.3 | 8 | 0.2 | 53 | 83 | 14.7 | 307 | 0.36 |
| 48082 | 1 | pce | Meringue, rts, 1/6 of 8" pie, avg | 113 | 303 | 42 | 1.7 | 53.3 | 1.4 | 33.0 | 19.0 | 9.8 | 2.0 | 3.0 | 4.1 | 0.24 | 3.88 | 51 | 198 | 59 | 56 | 3 | | 0.07 | 0.24 | 0.73 | 0.03 | 0.19 | 14.7 | 0.90 | 3.6 | 0.2 | | 63 | 0.0 | 0.7 | 17 | 0.1 | 119 | 101 | 3.4 | 165 | 0.55 |
| 48155 | 1 | pce | Meringue, 1/10 pie, Plush Pippin | 119 | 250 | | 2.0 | 41.0 | 0.5 | 28.0 | 12.5 | 9.0 | 2.0 | 3.0 | 0.0 | 0.00 | 0.00 | 35 | | | | | | | | | | | | | | | | | | 0.7 | | | | 25 | | 180 | |
| 48140 | 1 | pce | 1/3 pie, Banquet | 132 | 360 | 49 | 3.0 | 43.0 | 2.0 | 31.0 | 10.0 | 20.0 | 5.0 | | | | | 2 | 0 | 0 | 0 | 0 | 0 | | 0.03 | | | | | | 0.0 | | | 40 | | 0.4 | | | | | | 240 | |
| 70556 | 1 | pce | Thaw n Serve, 1/8 pie, Mrs Smith's | 85 | 245 | 46 | 2.0 | 32.0 | | | | 12.0 | | | | | | 5 | 88 | 18 | | | | 0.03 | 0.07 | 0.70 | | | | | 0.0 | | | 16 | | 0.6 | | | | 60 | | 185 | |
| | | | Mince Pie | | | | | | | | | | | | | | | | | | | | | | | | | | | | | | | | | | | | | | | | |
| 48146 | 1 | pce | 1/5 pie, Banquet | 113 | 309 | 44 | 3.0 | 45.8 | 2.0 | 25.9 | 17.9 | 13.0 | 6.0 | | | | | 10 | 0 | 0 | 0 | 0 | 0 | 0.03 | 0.03 | 0.30 | | | | | 0.0 | | | 20 | | 0.4 | | | | | | 428 | |
| 48083 | 1 | pce | Prep f/rec, 1/8 of 9", avg | 165 | 477 | 37 | 4.3 | 79.2 | 4.3 | 56.6 | 18.3 | 17.8 | 4.4 | 7.7 | 4.7 | 0.30 | 4.39 | 0 | 36 | 3.3 | 2.9 | 0.4 | | 0.25 | 0.17 | 1.96 | 0.11 | 0.00 | 38.0 | 0.17 | 9.7 | 0.0 | | 36 | 0.2 | 2.5 | 23 | 0.4 | 69 | 335 | 10.9 | 419 | 0.36 |

| Code | Amount | Description | Basic Components | | | | | | | | | Additional Fats | | | | | | Vit A & Components | | | | | Vitamins | | | | | | | | | | Minerals | | | | | | | | | |
|---|---|---|---|---|---|---|---|---|---|---|---|---|---|---|---|---|---|---|---|---|---|---|---|---|---|---|---|---|---|---|---|---|---|---|---|---|---|---|---|---|---|---|
| | | | Weight (g) | Calories | % Water | Protein (g) | Carbs (g) | Fiber (g) | Sugar (g) | Other Carbs (g) | Fat (g) | Sat Fat (g) | Mono Fat (g) | Poly Fat (g) | Omega 3 (g) | Omega 6 (g) | Choles (mg) | Vit A (IU) | Vit A (RE) | Retinol (RE) | Carotenoids (RE) | Beta Carotene (mcg) | Thiamin (mg) | Riboflavin (mg) | Niacin (NE) | Vit B6 (mg) | Vit B12 (mcg) | Folate (mcg) | Panto (mg) | Vit C (mg) | Vit D (mg) | Vit E (α TE) | Calcium (mg) | Copper (mg) | Iron (mg) | Magnes (mg) | Mang (mg) | Phos (mg) | Potassium (mg) | Selenium (mcg) | Sodium (mg) | Zinc (mg) |
| 70544 | 1 pce | RTB, 1/8 pie, Mrs Smith's | 163 | 470 | 41 | 4.0 | 72.0 | 4.7 | | | 19.0 | 4.7 | 8.2 | 5.2 | | | 2 | 66 | 11 | | | | 0.00 | 0.08 | 0.20 | 0.17 | | | | 2.0 | | | 39 | | 1.4 | | | | 240 | | 590 | |
| | | Peach Pie | | | | | | | | | | | | | | | | | | | | | | | | | | | | | | | | | | | | | | | | |
| 48073 | 1 pce | Baked f/Frozen, 1/6 of 8" pie, avg | 117 | 261 | 54 | 2.2 | 38.5 | 1.0 | | | 11.7 | 1.8 | 5.0 | 4.4 | 0.30 | 4.08 | 0 | 123 | 26 | 19 | 7 | | 0.07 | 0.04 | 0.23 | 0.03 | 0.00 | 28.1 | 0.13 | 1.1 | 0.0 | | 9 | 0.1 | 0.6 | 7 | 0.2 | 26 | 146 | 1.5 | 316 | 0.11 |
| 48087 | 1 pce | Prep f/Recipe, 1/8 of 9 " pie, avg | 139 | 375 | 45 | 3.2 | 55.4 | 2.0 | 34.7 | 18.8 | 16.3 | 3.9 | 7.0 | 4.7 | 0.26 | 4.42 | 0 | 310 | 48 | 24 | 24 | | 0.18 | 0.15 | 1.91 | 0.02 | 0.00 | 7.2 | 0.18 | 73.7 | 0.0 | 0.2 | 7 | 0.1 | 1.5 | 10 | 0.2 | 38 | 131 | 0.1 | 253 | 0.23 |
| 70552 | 1 pce | Thaw n Serve, 1/8 pie, Mrs Smith's | 128 | 300 | 54 | 3.0 | 44.0 | | | | 12.0 | | | | | | 0 | 275 | 55 | | | | 0.03 | 0.03 | 0.40 | | | | | 2.0 | | | 9 | | 0.4 | | | | 140 | | 285 | |
| 48106 | 1 pce | Peanut Butter pie, 1/8 of 9" pie, avg | 144 | 441 | 39 | 11.7 | 53.0 | 1.9 | | | 21.0 | 5.8 | 9.0 | 5.0 | | | 65 | 183 | 50 | 47 | 2 | | 0.25 | 0.35 | 3.96 | 0.13 | 0.33 | 26.9 | | 0.6 | | | 112 | 0.2 | 2.0 | 46 | | 187 | 294 | | 415 | 1.10 |
| 70718 | 1 pce | Peanut Butter Pie, Chocolate, fzn, Pet-Ritz | 99 | 300 | | 3.0 | 37.0 | 2.0 | 15.0 | 20.0 | 15.0 | 8.0 | | | | | 5 | 0 | 0 | 0 | 0 | 0 | | | | | | | | 0.0 | | | 20 | | 1.1 | | | | | | 180 | |
| | | Pecan Pie | | | | | | | | | | | | | | | | | | | | | | | | | | | | | | | | | | | | | | | | |
| 48058 | 1 ea | Individual size, avg | 85 | 366 | 17 | 4.2 | 45.2 | 1.5 | | | 20.3 | 3.4 | 10.7 | 5.1 | | | 33 | 75 | 19 | 17 | 2 | | 0.23 | 0.15 | 1.12 | 0.05 | 0.07 | 11.2 | | 0.2 | | | 19 | 0.2 | 1.4 | 26 | | 82 | 104 | | 210 | 1.05 |
| 48102 | 1 pce | Prep f/Recipe, 1/8 of 9" pie, avg | 122 | 503 | 20 | 6.0 | 63.7 | 6.1 | 57.6 | 0.0 | 27.1 | 4.9 | 13.7 | 7.0 | 0.34 | 6.62 | 105 | 410 | 109 | 101 | 8 | | 0.23 | 0.22 | 1.03 | 0.07 | 0.21 | 31.7 | 0.58 | 0.2 | 0.3 | | 39 | 0.3 | 1.8 | 32 | 0.9 | 115 | 162 | 14.6 | 320 | 1.24 |
| 48086 | 1 pce | RTS, 1/6 of 8" pie, avg | 113 | 452 | 19 | 4.5 | 64.6 | 4.0 | 46.9 | 13.8 | 20.9 | 4.0 | 12.1 | 3.6 | 0.16 | 3.42 | 35 | 198 | 53 | 50 | 4 | | 0.10 | 0.14 | 0.28 | 0.02 | 0.11 | 30.5 | 0.48 | 1.2 | 0.3 | | 19 | 0.2 | 1.2 | 20 | 0.9 | 87 | 84 | 5.7 | 479 | 0.64 |
| | | Pineapple Pie | | | | | | | | | | | | | | | | | | | | | | | | | | | | | | | | | | | | | | | | |
| 48123 | 1 pce | 1/8 of 9" pie, avg | 118 | 299 | 48 | 2.6 | 45.0 | | | | 12.6 | 3.1 | 6.3 | 2.8 | 0.00 | 2.83 | 0 | 24 | 6 | | | | 0.14 | 0.11 | 0.83 | | | | | 1.2 | | | 15 | | 1.4 | | | 25 | 85 | | 320 | |
| 48125 | 1 pce | Chiffon, avg | 81 | 233 | 41 | 5.3 | 31.7 | | | | 9.8 | 2.6 | 4.7 | 1.8 | 0.00 | 1.77 | 123 | 284 | 71 | | | | 0.09 | 0.12 | 0.65 | | | | | 0.8 | | | 19 | | 1.2 | | | 62 | 79 | | 207 | |
| 48127 | 1 pce | Custard, avg | 114 | 251 | 54 | 4.6 | 36.6 | | | | 9.9 | 3.0 | 4.6 | 1.7 | 0.00 | 1.74 | 63 | 205 | 51 | | | | 0.09 | 0.15 | 0.68 | | | | | 1.1 | | | 57 | | 0.9 | | | 74 | 111 | | 212 | |
| | | Pumpkin Pie | | | | | | | | | | | | | | | | | | | | | | | | | | | | | | | | | | | | | | | | |
| 48103 | 1 pce | Prep f/rec, 1/8 of 9" pie, avg | 155 | 316 | 58 | 7.0 | 40.9 | 4.2 | 29.3 | 7.4 | 14.4 | 4.9 | 5.7 | 2.8 | 0.20 | 2.60 | 65 | 11833 | 1212 | 98 | 1114 | | 0.14 | 0.31 | 1.21 | 0.07 | 0.14 | 32.5 | 0.69 | 2.6 | 0.7 | | 146 | 0.1 | 2.0 | 29 | 0.3 | 152 | 288 | 11.0 | 349 | 0.71 |
| 48075 | 1 pce | RTS, 1/6 of 8" pie, avg | 109 | 229 | 58 | 4.3 | 29.8 | 2.9 | 17.1 | 9.7 | 10.4 | 2.0 | 4.4 | 3.4 | 0.20 | 3.22 | 22 | 3743 | 405 | 33 | 373 | | 0.06 | 0.17 | 0.20 | 0.06 | 0.28 | 21.8 | 0.55 | 1.1 | 0.5 | | 65 | 0.1 | 0.9 | 16 | 0.3 | 77 | 168 | 2.8 | 307 | 0.49 |
| 70545 | 1 pce | RTB, 1/8 pie, Mrs Smith's | 163 | 310 | 61 | 6.0 | 46.0 | | | | 11.0 | | | | | | 30 | 924 | 154 | | | | 0.06 | 0.26 | 0.00 | | | | | 0.0 | | | 97 | | 0.8 | | | | 210 | | 495 | |
| 48129 | 1 pce | Raisin Pie, 1/8 of 9" pie, avg | 118 | 319 | 42 | 3.1 | 50.7 | | | | 12.6 | 3.1 | 6.3 | 2.8 | 0.00 | 2.83 | 0 | 6 | 1.5 | | | | 0.13 | 0.11 | 1.30 | | | | | 1.2 | | | 21 | | 1.9 | | | 47 | 227 | | 336 | |
| 70542 | 1 pce | Raspberry Pie, RTB, 1/8 pie, Mrs Smith's | 163 | 390 | 51 | 4.0 | 61.0 | | | | 15.0 | | | | | | 2 | 180 | 30 | | | | 0.06 | 0.07 | 0.20 | | | | | 5.0 | | | 23 | | 0.6 | | | | 120 | | 460 | |
| 48131 | 1 pce | Rhubarb Pie, 1/8 of 9" pie, avg | 118 | 299 | 47 | 2.9 | 45.1 | | | | 12.6 | 3.1 | 6.3 | 2.8 | 0.00 | 2.83 | 0 | 59 | 15 | | | | 0.13 | 0.13 | 1.30 | | | | | 3.5 | | | 76 | | 1.7 | | | 31 | 188 | | 319 | |
| 48115 | 1 pce | Shoo Fly Pie, 1/8 of 9" pie, avg | 114 | 397 | 24 | 4.4 | 67.4 | 0.9 | | | 12.7 | 3.2 | 5.4 | 3.2 | | | 36 | 55 | 17 | 16 | 0.03 | | 0.22 | 0.19 | 2.01 | 0.22 | 0.07 | 9.3 | | 0.0 | | | 89 | 0.3 | 3.5 | 83 | | 65 | 541 | | 207 | 0.46 |
| 48107 | 1 pce | Sour Cream & Raisin Pie, 1/8 of 9" pie, avg | 144 | 518 | 35 | 7.6 | 51.3 | 2.5 | | | 32.8 | 12.7 | 12.3 | 5.8 | | | 73 | 682 | 174 | 158 | 15 | | 0.26 | 0.31 | 1.94 | 0.11 | 0.20 | 16.3 | | 1.2 | | | 95 | 0.2 | 2.3 | 27 | | 137 | 346 | | 354 | 0.61 |
| 48108 | 1 pce | Squash Pie, 1/8 of 9" pie, avg | 154 | 296 | 61 | 6.4 | 39.5 | 2.1 | | | 13.0 | 4.1 | 5.2 | 2.8 | | | 69 | 2165 | 246 | 44 | 202 | | 0.16 | 0.26 | 1.19 | 0.10 | 0.24 | 15.0 | | 3.0 | | | 89 | 0.1 | 1.3 | 22 | | 108 | 242 | | 240 | 0.58 |
| | | Strawberry Pie | | | | | | | | | | | | | | | | | | | | | | | | | | | | | | | | | | | | | | | | |
| 48133 | 1 pce | 1/8 of 9" pie, avg | 93 | 184 | 58 | 1.8 | 28.7 | | | | 7.3 | 1.8 | 3.7 | 1.6 | 0.00 | 1.65 | 0 | 37 | 9 | | | | 0.07 | 0.08 | 0.93 | | | | | 23.3 | | | 15 | | 1.1 | | | 23 | 112 | | 180 | |
| 48011 | 1 pce | Chiffon, 1/8 of 9" pie, avg | 139 | 330 | 54 | 4.2 | 41.1 | 1.5 | 27.0 | 12.6 | 17.4 | 7.9 | 7.2 | 1.4 | 0.21 | 1.18 | 35 | 405 | 111 | 05 | 6 | | 0.09 | 0.11 | 0.92 | 0.04 | 0.04 | 15.4 | 0.18 | 26.6 | 0.3 | 0.1 | 44 | 0.1 | 1.1 | 13 | 0.3 | 47 | 131 | 5.2 | 203 | 0.25 |
| 48109 | 1 pce | Cream, 1/8 of 9" pie, avg | 144 | 291 | 61 | 2.1 | 37.2 | 1.9 | | | 15.5 | 7.1 | 5.4 | 2.2 | | | 33 | 365 | 102 | 97 | 5 | | 0.10 | 0.12 | 0.81 | 0.05 | 0.04 | 13.7 | | 33.8 | | | 26 | 0.1 | 0.8 | 10 | | 40 | 130 | | 120 | 0.24 |
| 70541 | 1 pce | Rhubarb, RTB, 1/8 pie, Mrs Smith's | 163 | 410 | 51 | 3.0 | 60.0 | | | | 17.0 | | | | | | | 66 | 11 | | | | 0.05 | 0.05 | 0.20 | | | | | 2.0 | | | 42 | | 0.7 | | | | 190 | | 490 | |
| 48110 | 1 pce | Sweet Potato pie, 1/8 of 9" pie, avg | 154 | 319 | 61 | 6.4 | 35.4 | 1.8 | | | 17.1 | 5.2 | 7.1 | 3.9 | | | 66 | 7620 | 791 | 44 | 747 | | 0.15 | 0.32 | 1.27 | 0.16 | 0.24 | 15.7 | | 7.6 | | | 99 | 0.1 | 1.3 | 18 | | 117 | 222 | | 197 | 0.65 |
| 48116 | 1 pce | Tofu Pie, w/fruit, 1/8 of 9" pie, avg | 144 | 304 | 59 | 7.6 | 32.2 | 1.9 | | | 17.9 | 3.6 | 7.2 | 6.0 | | | 30 | 778 | 193 | 73 | 20 | | 0.07 | 0.18 | 0.60 | 0.07 | 0.09 | 17.2 | | 14.4 | | | 95 | 0.2 | 4.1 | 76 | | 109 | 209 | | 285 | 0.80 |
| 48104 | 1 pce | Vanilla Pie, cream, prep f/rec, 1/8 of 9" pie, avg | 126 | 350 | 47 | 6.0 | 41.1 | 0.8 | | | 18.1 | 5.1 | 7.6 | 4.3 | 0.27 | 4.07 | 78 | 386 | 107 | 02 | 5 | | 0.18 | 0.27 | 1.24 | 0.06 | 0.38 | 32.8 | 0.52 | 0.6 | | | 113 | 0.0 | 1.3 | 16 | 0.2 | 131 | 159 | 12.0 | 328 | 0.67 |
| 70717 | 1 pce | Vanilla Pie, Cream Fudge, fzn, Pet-Ritz | 99 | 300 | 41 | 3.0 | 40.0 | 1.0 | 16.0 | 23.0 | 15.0 | 9.0 | | | | | 5 | 0 | 0 | 0 | 0 | 0 | | | | | | | | 0.0 | | | 20 | | 1.1 | | | | | | 190 | |
| | | *PUDDINGS, CUSTARDS AND PIE FILLINGS* | | | | | | | | | | | | | | | | | | | | | | | | | | | | | | | | | | | | | | | | |
| | | Custard | | | | | | | | | | | | | | | | | | | | | | | | | | | | | | | | | | | | | | | | |
| 2621 | 1 oz | Dry Mix, avg | 28 | 115 | 2 | 1.9 | 23.2 | 0.0 | 23.2 | 0.0 | 1.8 | 0.6 | 0.7 | 0.2 | 0.01 | 0.22 | 70 | 61 | 18 | | | | 0.04 | 0.12 | 0.16 | 0.09 | 0.45 | 8.7 | 0.92 | 0.2 | 0.0 | | 64 | 0.0 | 0.5 | 22 | 0.0 | 141 | 261 | 6.0 | 136 | 0.39 |
| 2795 | 1 oz | Dry Mix, Jell-o | 28 | 107 | 2 | 1.3 | 25.3 | 0.0 | 22.7 | 2.7 | 0.0 | 0.0 | 0.0 | 0.0 | 0.00 | 0.00 | 0 | 0 | 0 | 0 | 0 | 0 | | | | | | | | 0.0 | | | 53 | | 0.0 | | | | 147 | | 173 | |
| 2600 | 1/2 cup | Egg, prep f/rec, avg | 141 | 148 | 79 | 7.2 | 15.1 | 0.0 | 15.1 | 0.0 | 6.6 | 3.3 | 2.1 | 0.5 | 0.08 | 0.42 | 123 | 313 | 35 | 80 | 4 | | 0.05 | 0.32 | 0.12 | 0.07 | 0.44 | 14.1 | 0.67 | 0.7 | 1.5 | | 158 | 0.0 | 0.4 | 20 | 0.0 | 159 | 216 | 9.6 | 109 | 0.75 |
| 2796 | 1/2 cup | Prep f/Mix, Jell-o | 133 | 160 | 75 | 5.0 | 25.0 | 0.0 | 23.0 | 2.0 | 2.5 | 1.5 | | | | | 10 | 200 | 40 | | | | | | | | | | | 0.0 | | | 200 | | 0.0 | | | | 300 | | 190 | |
| | | Flan | | | | | | | | | | | | | | | | | | | | | | | | | | | | | | | | | | | | | | | | |
| 2623 | 1 oz | Caramel, dry mix, avg | 28 | 97 | 8 | 0.0 | 25.6 | 0.0 | 25.6 | 0.0 | 0.0 | 0.0 | 0.0 | 0.0 | 0.00 | 0.00 | 0 | 0 | 0 | 0 | 0 | 0 | 0.00 | 0.00 | 0.00 | 0.00 | 0.00 | 0.0 | 0.00 | 0.0 | 0.0 | 0.0 | 7 | 0.0 | 0.0 | 0 | 0.0 | 0 | 43 | 6.0 | 121 | 0.01 |
| 62238 | 1/2 cup | Caramel, prep f/mix, red cal, Menu Magic | 139 | 81 | 86 | 6.0 | 13.0 | 0.0 | 9.0 | 4.0 | 0.0 | 0.0 | 0.0 | 0.0 | 0.00 | 0.00 | 15 | 556 | 111 | | | | 0.03 | 0.25 | | | | | | 1.2 | | | 200 | | 0.0 | 17 | | 150 | 291 | | 150 | |
| 2624 | 1/2 cup | Caramel, prep w/2% milk, avg | 133 | 136 | 75 | 4.0 | 25.5 | 0.1 | 25.5 | 0.0 | 2.4 | 1.5 | 0.7 | 0.1 | 0.04 | 0.05 | 9 | 249 | 53 | 61 | 2 | | 0.04 | 0.20 | 0.11 | 0.05 | 0.36 | 5.3 | 0.39 | 0.9 | 0.0 | | 153 | 0.0 | 0.1 | 17 | 0.0 | 116 | 194 | 6.8 | 67 | 0.48 |
| 2625 | 1/2 cup | Caramel, prep w/whl milk, avg | 133 | 150 | 74 | 4.0 | 25.4 | 0.1 | 25.4 | 0.0 | 4.1 | 2.5 | 1.2 | 0.2 | 0.07 | 0.09 | 16 | 153 | 35 | 25 | 10 | | 0.04 | 0.20 | 0.10 | 0.05 | 0.35 | 5.3 | 0.38 | 0.9 | 0.0 | | 150 | 0.0 | 0.1 | 16 | 0.0 | 114 | 192 | 6.5 | 65 | 0.47 |
| | | Pie Filling | | | | | | | | | | | | | | | | | | | | | | | | | | | | | | | | | | | | | | | | |
| 48171 | 1 cup | Apple, Libby's | 255 | 240 | 76 | 0.0 | 60.0 | 0.0 | 48.0 | 12.0 | 0.0 | 0.0 | 0.0 | 0.0 | 0.00 | 0.00 | 0 | 0 | 0 | 0 | 0 | 0 | | | | | | | | 0.0 | | | 0 | | 0.0 | | | | | | 31 | |
| 48019 | 1 cup | Blueberry, avg | 262 | 272 | 73 | 1.6 | 67.9 | 3.7 | 57.1 | 7.1 | 0.8 | 0.1 | 0.1 | 0.3 | | | 0 | 157 | 16 | 0 | 16 | | 0.08 | 0.13 | 0.29 | 0.08 | 0.00 | 5.2 | | 2.6 | 0.0 | | 13 | 0.1 | 1.0 | 10 | | 26 | 97 | | 68 | 0.18 |
| 48016 | 1 cup | Cherry, cnd, avg | 264 | 304 | 70 | 1.3 | 77.4 | 1.6 | 63.4 | 12.4 | 0.5 | 0.1 | 0.2 | 0.2 | 0.08 | 0.08 | 0 | 541 | 55 | 8 | 48 | | 0.07 | 0.04 | 0.37 | 0.10 | 0.00 | 10.6 | 0.17 | 9.5 | 0.0 | | 29 | 0.2 | 0.6 | 18 | 0.1 | 40 | 277 | 1.1 | 24 | 0.13 |
| 48018 | 1 cup | Cherry, low cal, avg | 264 | 211 | 79 | 1.6 | 51.2 | 1.6 | 42.8 | 6.9 | 2.1 | 0.4 | 1.0 | 0.7 | | | 0 | 541 | 53 | 0 | 53 | | 0.03 | 0.08 | 0.37 | 0.08 | 0.00 | 10.6 | | 4.2 | | | 24 | 0.2 | 0.6 | 13 | | 21 | 201 | | 24 | 0.16 |
| 48044 | 1 cup | Pumpkin pie, cnd, avg | 270 | 281 | 72 | 2.9 | 71.3 | 22.4 | | | 0.4 | 0.2 | 0.0 | 0.0 | 0.01 | 0.01 | 0 | 22405 | 2241 | | | | 0.04 | 0.32 | 1.01 | 0.43 | 0.00 | 94.5 | 3.08 | 9.4 | | | 100 | 0.2 | 2.9 | 43 | 1.1 | 122 | 373 | 3.0 | 562 | 0.73 |
| 48068 | 1 cup | Peach, R&H Right Choice | 265 | 292 | 70 | 1.3 | 74.2 | 1.3 | 53.0 | 19.9 | 0.3 | | | | | | 0 | 12868 | 2574 | | | | 0.03 | 0.05 | 0.98 | | | | | 6.8 | | | 40 | | 3.4 | | | 27 | 239 | | 305 | |
| | | Pudding | | | | | | | | | | | | | | | | | | | | | | | | | | | | | | | | | | | | | | | | |
| 2630 | 1 oz | Banana, dry mix, avg | 28 | 105 | 4 | 0.0 | 26.0 | 0.1 | 20.3 | 5.6 | 0.1 | 0.0 | 0.0 | 0.0 | 0.00 | 0.04 | 0 | 0 | 0 | 0 | 0 | 0 | 0.00 | 0.00 | 0.00 | 0.00 | 0.00 | 0.0 | 0.00 | 0.0 | 0.0 | | 6 | 0.0 | 0.0 | 2 | 0.0 | 1 | 5 | 0.3 | 221 | 0.03 |
| 2627 | 1 oz | Banana, dry mix, inst, avg | 28 | 103 | 3 | 0.0 | 26.0 | 0.3 | 20.2 | 5.8 | 0.2 | 0.0 | 0.0 | 0.1 | 0.01 | 0.09 | 0 | 0 | 0 | 0 | 0 | 0 | 0.00 | 0.00 | 0.00 | 0.00 | 0.00 | 0.0 | 0.00 | 0.0 | 0.0 | | 2 | 0.0 | 0.0 | 1 | 0.0 | 225 | 4 | 0.2 | 420 | 0.01 |
| 2758 | 1 oz | Banana, dry mix, no sugar/fat, Jell-o | 28 | 88 | 7 | 0.0 | 21.0 | 0.3 | 0.0 | 21.0 | 0.0 | 0.0 | 0.0 | 0.0 | 0.00 | 0.00 | 0 | 0 | 0 | 0 | 0 | 0 | | | | | | | | 0.0 | | | 0 | | 0.0 | | | | 0 | | 1190 | |
| 2628 | 1/2 cup | Banana, prep f/mix, inst, w/2% milk, avg | 147 | 153 | 74 | 4.1 | 29.1 | 0.3 | 22.8 | 6.3 | 2.5 | 1.5 | 0.7 | 0.2 | 0.04 | 0.13 | 9 | 250 | 56 | | | | 0.05 | 0.20 | 0.11 | 0.05 | 0.44 | 5.9 | 0.39 | 1.2 | 1.3 | | 150 | 0.0 | 0.1 | 18 | 0.0 | 318 | 193 | 2.6 | 435 | 0.49 |
| 2631 | 1/2 cup | Banana, prep f/mix, w/2% milk, avg | 140 | 143 | 76 | 4.1 | 25.5 | 0.3 | 19.9 | 5.6 | 2.4 | 1.5 | 0.7 | 0.1 | 0.04 | 0.08 | 10 | 252 | 70 | | | | 0.04 | 0.20 | 0.11 | 0.05 | 0.36 | 5.6 | 0.39 | 1.0 | 1.2 | | 154 | 0.0 | 0.1 | 18 | 0.0 | 118 | 193 | 2.7 | 232 | 0.50 |
| 2787 | 1/2 cup | Banana, prep f/mix, no sugar/fat, Jell-o | 125 | 70 | 86 | 4.0 | 12.0 | 0.3 | 6.0 | 6.0 | 0.0 | 0.0 | 0.0 | 0.0 | 0.00 | 0.00 | 0 | 200 | 40 | | | | | | | | | | | 0.0 | | | 150 | | 0.0 | | | | 210 | | 410 | |
| 2632 | 1 ea | Banana, RTE, 5 oz pkg, avg | 142 | 180 | 72 | 3.4 | 30.1 | 0.1 | 23.4 | 6.5 | 5.1 | 0.3 | 2.2 | 1.9 | 0.13 | 1.76 | 0 | 141 | 43 | 40 | 3 | | 0.03 | 0.21 | 0.23 | 0.03 | 0.26 | 2.8 | 0.23 | 0.7 | 0.0 | | 121 | 0.0 | 0.2 | 11 | 0.0 | 98 | 156 | 2.0 | 278 | 0.40 |
| 2617 | 1/2 cup | Bread w/Raisins, avg | 126 | 212 | 63 | 6.6 | 31.0 | 1.3 | 21.9 | 7.8 | 7.4 | 2.3 | 2.7 | 1.2 | 0.09 | 1.10 | 83 | 304 | 32 | 81 | 1 | | 0.11 | 0.28 | 0.79 | 0.09 | 0.33 | 16.4 | 0.53 | 1.0 | 1.0 | | 144 | 0.1 | 1.4 | 24 | 0.2 | 137 | 282 | 11.0 | 231 | 0.66 |
| 2742 | 1 oz | Butter Pecan, dry mix, Jell-o | 28 | 112 | 4 | 0.0 | 25.8 | 0.0 | 20.2 | 5.6 | 0.6 | 0.0 | | | | | 0 | 0 | 0 | 0 | 0 | 0 | | | | | | | | 0.0 | | | 0 | | 0.0 | | | | 11 | | 332 | |
| 2750 | 1 oz | Butterscotch, dry mix, Jell-o | 28 | 97 | 4 | 0.0 | 25.8 | 0.0 | 20.5 | 5.4 | 0.0 | 0.0 | 0.0 | 0.0 | 0.00 | 0.00 | 0 | 0 | 0 | 0 | 0 | 0 | | | | | | | | 0.0 | | | 0 | | 0.0 | | | | 0 | | 140 | |
| 2753 | 1 oz | Butterscotch, dry mix, no sugar/fat, Jell-o | 28 | 88 | 7 | 0.0 | 21.0 | 0.0 | 0.0 | 21.0 | 0.0 | 0.0 | 0.0 | 0.0 | 0.00 | 0.00 | 0 | 0 | 0 | 0 | 0 | 0 | | | | | | | | 0.0 | | | 0 | | 0.0 | | | | 0 | | 1130 | |
| 2770 | 1/2 cup | Butterscotch, prep f/mix, Jell-o | 150 | 150 | 75 | 4.0 | 29.0 | 0.0 | 24.0 | 5.0 | 2.5 | 1.5 | | | | | 10 | 200 | 40 | | | | | | | | | | | 0.0 | | | 150 | | 0.0 | | | | 190 | | 450 | |
| 2788 | 1/2 cup | Butterscotch, prep f/mix, no sugar/fat, Jell-o | 125 | 70 | 86 | 4.0 | 12.0 | 0.0 | 6.0 | 6.0 | 0.0 | 0.0 | 0.0 | 0.0 | 0.00 | 0.00 | 0 | 200 | 40 | | | | | | | | | | | 0.0 | | | 150 | | 0.0 | | | | 210 | | 400 | |
| 2635 | 1 oz | Chocolate, mix, avg | 28 | 101 | 4 | 0.7 | 24.9 | 0.5 | 18.8 | 5.7 | 0.6 | 0.3 | 0.2 | 0.0 | 0.00 | 0.02 | 0 | 4 | 0.3 | | | | 0.00 | 0.06 | 0.05 | 0.01 | 0.01 | 0.6 | 0.01 | 0.0 | 0.0 | | 15 | 0.1 | 0.5 | 15 | 0.1 | 25 | 59 | 0.5 | 39 | 0.20 |
| 2754 | 1 oz | Chocolate, mix, no sugar/fat, Jell-o | 28 | 89 | 7 | 2.5 | 20.4 | 1.3 | 0.0 | 19.1 | 0.0 | 0.0 | 0.0 | 0.0 | 0.00 | 0.00 | 0 | 0 | 0 | 0 | 0 | 0 | | | | | | | | 0.0 | | | 0 | | 1.8 | | | | 305 | | 840 | |
| 2634 | 1/2 cup | Chocolate, prep f/mix w/2% milk, avg | 147 | 150 | 75 | 4.6 | 27.8 | 0.6 | 21.0 | 6.2 | 2.8 | 1.5 | 0.9 | 0.2 | 0.04 | 0.15 | 9 | 253 | 56 | | | | 0.05 | 0.21 | 0.14 | 0.06 | 0.46 | 5.9 | 0.40 | 1.3 | 1.3 | | 153 | 0.1 | 0.4 | 26 | 0.1 | 353 | 247 | 2.5 | 417 | 0.62 |
| 2605 | 1/2 cup | Chocolate, prep f/mix, w/whl milk, avg | 147 | 163 | 74 | 4.6 | 27.6 | 1.5 | 22.1 | 4.1 | 4.6 | 2.7 | 1.4 | 0.3 | 0.07 | 0.19 | 16 | 157 | 31 | 28 | 3 | | 0.05 | 0.21 | 0.14 | 0.06 | 0.44 | 5.9 | 0.40 | 1.3 | 1.3 | | 150 | 0.1 | 0.4 | 26 | 0.1 | 351 | 244 | 2.5 | 417 | 0.62 |

| Code | Amount | Description | Basic Components | | | | | | | | | Additional Fats | | | | | | Vit A & Components | | | | | Vitamins | | | | | | | | | | Minerals | | | | | | | | | |
|---|---|---|---|---|---|---|---|---|---|---|---|---|---|---|---|---|---|---|---|---|---|---|---|---|---|---|---|---|---|---|---|---|---|---|---|---|---|---|---|---|---|---|
| | | | Weight (g) | Calories | % Water | Protein (g) | Carbs (g) | Fiber (g) | Sugar (g) | Other Carbs (g) | Fat (g) | Sat Fat (g) | Mono Fat (g) | Poly Fat (g) | Omega 3 (g) | Omega 6 (g) | Choles (mg) | Vit A (IU) | Vit A (RE) | Retinol (RE) | Carotenoids (RE) | Beta Carotene (mcg) | Thiamin (mg) | Riboflavin (mg) | Niacin (NE) | Vit B6 (mg) | Vit B12 (mcg) | Folate (mcg) | Panto (mg) | Vit C (mg) | Vit D (mg) | Vit E (α TE) | Calcium (mg) | Copper (mg) | Iron (mg) | Magnes (mg) | Mang (mg) | Phos (mg) | Potassium (mg) | Selenium (mcg) | Sodium (mg) | Zinc (mg) |
| 2793 | 1/2 cup | Chocolate pudding, prep f/mix, no sugar/fat, Jell-o | 125 | 90 | 83 | 5.0 | 12.0 | 1.0 | 6.0 | 5.0 | 2.5 | 1.5 | | | | | 10 | 200 | 40 | | | | | | | | | | | 0.0 | | | 150 | | 1.1 | | | | 330 | | 170 | |
| 2637 | 1/2 cup | Chocolate, prep f/rec, w/2% milk, avg | 157 | 206 | 68 | 4.9 | 40.5 | 1.4 | 21.7 | 17.4 | 3.9 | 2.0 | 1.3 | 0.4 | 0.05 | 0.36 | 9 | 290 | 79 | | | | 0.05 | 0.22 | 0.20 | 0.05 | 0.36 | 6.3 | 0.41 | 0.9 | 1.6 | | 155 | 0.2 | 0.7 | 39 | 0.2 | 149 | 256 | | 138 | 0.79 |
| 2601 | 1/2 cup | Chocolate, prep f/rec, w/whl milk, avg | 157 | 221 | 67 | 4.9 | 40.3 | 1.3 | 31.1 | 8.0 | 5.7 | 3.1 | 1.8 | 0.5 | 0.08 | 0.39 | 17 | 193 | 49 | 46 | 3 | | 0.05 | 0.22 | 0.20 | 0.05 | 0.35 | 6.3 | 0.40 | 0.9 | 1.4 | | 152 | 0.2 | 0.7 | 38 | 0.2 | 148 | 253 | 2.4 | 137 | 0.77 |
| 2610 | 1 ea | Chocolate, RTE, cnd, avg | 142 | 189 | 69 | 3.8 | 32.4 | 1.4 | 26.0 | 5.0 | 5.7 | 1.0 | 2.4 | 2.0 | 0.14 | 1.89 | 4 | 51 | 16 | 14 | 1 | | 0.04 | 0.22 | 0.49 | 0.04 | 0.00 | 4.3 | 0.20 | 2.6 | 1.2 | | 128 | 0.2 | 0.7 | 30 | 0.1 | 114 | 256 | 2.1 | 183 | 0.60 |
| 2618 | 1 ea | Chocolate, RTE, low cal, cnd, avg | 142 | 99 | 83 | 5.0 | 14.4 | 0.1 | 6.5 | 7.8 | 2.9 | 1.7 | 0.8 | 0.1 | 0.04 | 0.07 | 10 | 271 | 75 | 72 | 3 | | 0.04 | 0.23 | 0.16 | 0.05 | 0.26 | 5.4 | 0.14 | 0.8 | 1.1 | | 166 | 0.1 | 0.5 | 31 | 0.1 | 239 | 351 | 2.4 | 271 | 0.62 |
| 2658 | 1 oz | Chocolate, rennin, dry mix, avg | 28 | 102 | 1 | 0.7 | 25.6 | 1.4 | 19.3 | 4.9 | 0.9 | 0.5 | 0.3 | 0.0 | 0.00 | 0.03 | 0 | 1 | 0.2 | | | | 0.00 | 0.02 | 0.09 | 0.01 | 0.00 | 1.7 | 0.01 | 0.0 | 0.0 | | 46 | 0.2 | 0.7 | 23 | 0.2 | 36 | 120 | 0.8 | 20 | 0.44 |
| 2659 | 1/2 cup | Chocolate, rennin, prep f/mix, w/2%milk, avg | 136 | 110 | 80 | 4.4 | 18.4 | 0.7 | 13.6 | 4.1 | 2.9 | 1.7 | 0.8 | 0.1 | 0.04 | 0.07 | 10 | 252 | 60 | | | | 0.05 | 0.21 | 0.15 | 0.06 | 0.45 | 6.8 | 0.40 | 1.2 | 1.2 | | 171 | 0.1 | 0.4 | 27 | 0.1 | 133 | 248 | 3.1 | 71 | 0.69 |
| 2660 | 1/2 cup | Chocolate, rennin, prep f/mix, w/whl milk, avg | 136 | 125 | 79 | 4.4 | 18.1 | 0.7 | 13.6 | 3.8 | 4.5 | 2.8 | 1.3 | 0.2 | 0.07 | 0.11 | 16 | 155 | 33 | | | | 0.05 | 0.21 | 0.14 | 0.06 | 0.44 | 6.8 | 0.39 | 1.1 | 1.2 | | 169 | 0.1 | 0.4 | 27 | 0.1 | 132 | 243 | 3.1 | 69 | 0.68 |
| 2723 | 1 ea | Chocolate Caramel, RTE, cnd, Jell-o | 113 | 160 | 67 | 3.0 | 27.0 | 0.0 | 22.0 | 5.0 | 5.0 | 2.0 | | | | | 0 | 100 | 20 | | | | | | | | | | | 0.0 | | | 100 | | 1.1 | | | | 210 | | 180 | |
| 2638 | 1 oz | Coconut Cream, dry mix, avg | 28 | 108 | 2 | 0.3 | 25.0 | 0.2 | 17.9 | 6.9 | 1.1 | 0.6 | 0.3 | 0.2 | 0.01 | 0.20 | 0 | 0 | 0 | 0 | 0 | 0 | 0.00 | 0.00 | 0.02 | 0.01 | 0.00 | 0.3 | 0.03 | 0.0 | 0.0 | | 2 | 0.0 | 0.2 | 4 | 0.0 | 202 | 6 | 0.6 | 338 | 0.08 |
| 2743 | 1 oz | Coconut Cream, dry mix, Jell-o | 28 | 112 | 4 | 0.0 | 23.5 | 0.6 | 17.9 | 5.0 | 2.2 | 2.2 | | | | | 0 | 0 | 0 | 0 | 0 | 0 | | | | | | | | 0.0 | | | 0 | | 0.0 | | | | 28 | | 291 | |
| 2639 | 1/2 cup | Coconut Cream, prep f/mix, w/2%milk, avg | 147 | 157 | 74 | 4.3 | 28.2 | 0.1 | 25.0 | 3.1 | 3.4 | 2.0 | 0.9 | 0.3 | 0.04 | 0.24 | 9 | 250 | 69 | 63 | 6 | | 0.05 | 0.20 | 0.13 | 0.06 | 0.44 | 5.9 | 0.40 | 1.2 | 1.3 | | 150 | 0.0 | 0.2 | 21 | 0.0 | 295 | 194 | 2.9 | 362 | 0.49 |
| 2615 | 1/2 cup | Coconut Cream, prep f/mix w/whl mlk, avg | 147 | 172 | 73 | 4.3 | 28.1 | 0.1 | 23.4 | 4.5 | 5.1 | 3.1 | 1.4 | 0.4 | 0.07 | 0.28 | 16 | 154 | 37 | 34 | 3 | | 0.05 | 0.20 | 0.12 | 0.05 | 0.44 | 5.9 | 0.39 | 1.2 | 1.5 | | 147 | 0.0 | 0.2 | 21 | 0.0 | 294 | 190 | 2.9 | 362 | 0.49 |
| 2804 | 1/2 cup | Coconut Cream, prep f/mix, Jell-o | 150 | 160 | 75 | 4.0 | 27.0 | 1.0 | 22.0 | 4.0 | 4.5 | 3.5 | | | | | 10 | 200 | 40 | | | | | | | | | | | 0.0 | | | 150 | | 0.0 | | | | 220 | | 320 | |
| 2643 | 1 oz | Lemon, dry mix, avg | 28 | 106 | 1 | 0.0 | 26.7 | 0.0 | 21.3 | 5.4 | 0.2 | 0.0 | 0.1 | 0.1 | 0.01 | 0.06 | 0 | 0 | 0 | 0 | 0 | 0 | 0.00 | 0.00 | 0.00 | 0.00 | 0.00 | 0.0 | 0.00 | 0.0 | 0.0 | | 1 | 0.0 | 0.0 | 0 | 0.0 | 211 | 2 | 0.2 | 373 | 0.01 |
| 2644 | 1/2 cup | Lemon, prep f/mix, w/2% milk, avg | 147 | 154 | 74 | 4.1 | 29.7 | 0.0 | 24.9 | 4.8 | 2.5 | 1.5 | 0.7 | 0.1 | 0.04 | 0.11 | 9 | 250 | 69 | 59 | 10 | | 0.05 | 0.20 | 0.11 | 0.05 | 0.44 | 5.9 | 0.39 | 1.2 | 1.3 | | 148 | 0.0 | 0.1 | 16 | 0.0 | 304 | 190 | 2.6 | 394 | 0.49 |
| 2616 | 1/2 cup | Lemon, prep f/mix, w/whl milk, avg | 147 | 169 | 73 | 4.0 | 29.5 | 0.0 | 24.9 | 4.7 | 4.3 | 2.6 | 1.2 | 0.2 | 0.07 | 0.15 | 16 | 154 | 38 | 37 | 1 | | 0.05 | 0.20 | 0.10 | 0.05 | 0.44 | 5.9 | 0.39 | 1.2 | 1.3 | | 146 | 0.0 | 0.1 | 16 | 0.0 | 301 | 187 | 2.6 | 392 | 0.47 |
| 2647 | 1 ea | Lemon, RTE, cnd, avg | 142 | 177 | 72 | 0.1 | 35.5 | 0.1 | | | 4.3 | 0.6 | 1.8 | 1.6 | 0.11 | 1.51 | 0 | 0 | 0 | 0 | 0 | 0 | 0.00 | 0.01 | 0.00 | 0.00 | 0.00 | 0.0 | 0.01 | 0.1 | 0.0 | | 3 | 0.0 | 0.1 | 1 | 0.0 | 7 | 1 | 2.6 | 199 | 0.04 |
| 2747 | 1 oz | Pistachio, dry mix, Jell-o | 28 | 112 | 4 | 0.0 | 25.8 | 0.0 | 20.2 | 5.6 | 0.6 | 0.0 | | | | | 0 | 0 | 0 | 0 | 0 | 0 | | | | | | | | 0.0 | | | 0 | | 0.0 | | | | 11 | | 392 | |
| 2756 | 1 oz | Pistachio, dry mix, no sugar/fat, Jell-o | 28 | 105 | 7 | 0.0 | 21.0 | 0.0 | 0.0 | 21.0 | 0.0 | 0.0 | 0.0 | 0.0 | 0.00 | 0.00 | 0 | 0 | 0 | 0 | 0 | 0 | | | | | | | | 0.0 | | | 0 | | 0.0 | | | | 18 | | 1120 | |
| 2776 | 1/2 cup | Pistachio, prep f/mix, Jell-o | 150 | 160 | 75 | 4.0 | 29.0 | 0.0 | 24.0 | 5.0 | 3.0 | 1.5 | | | | | 10 | 200 | 40 | | | | | | | | | | | 0.0 | | | 150 | | 0.0 | | | | 200 | | 410 | |
| 2791 | 1/2 cup | Pistachio, prep f/mix, no sugar/fat, Jell-o | 125 | 70 | 86 | 4.0 | 12.0 | 0.0 | 6.0 | 6.0 | 0.0 | 0.0 | 0.0 | 0.0 | 0.00 | 0.00 | 0 | 200 | 40 | | | | | | | | | | | 0.0 | | | 150 | | 0.0 | | | | 210 | | 380 | |
| 2692 | 1 pce | Plum, RTE, cnd, avg | 42 | 116 | 32 | 2.1 | 20.7 | 1.1 | 14.6 | 5.0 | 3.0 | | | | | | 9 | 17 | 2 | 0 | 2 | | | | | | | | | | | | 21 | | 0.4 | 8 | | | 90 | | 145 | 0.21 |
| 2690 | 1/2 cup | Plum/Christmas, prep f/rec, avg | 132 | 384 | 30 | 6.1 | 65.3 | 1.7 | 45.3 | 18.3 | 12.8 | 6.1 | 5.1 | 0.8 | | | 65 | 165 | 33 | 28 | 5 | 28 | 0.11 | 0.11 | | 0.11 | | 10.6 | | 0.0 | | | 104 | | 2.0 | | | | 462 | 9.2 | 264 | 0.66 |
| 2705 | 1 ea | Praline Pecan Mousse, svg, Weight Watchers | 77 | 170 | 49 | 4.0 | 31.1 | 0.0 | 22.0 | 9.0 | 3.5 | 1.0 | | | | | 0 | 0 | 0 | 0 | 0 | 0 | | | | | | | | 1.2 | | | 80 | | 1.8 | | | | 150 | | 140 | |
| 2648 | 1 oz | Rice, dry mix, avg | 28 | 105 | 5 | 0.8 | 25.5 | 0.2 | 16.7 | 8.6 | 0.0 | 0.0 | 0.0 | 0.0 | | | 0 | 0 | 0 | 0 | 0 | 0 | 0.07 | 0.00 | 0.56 | 0.00 | 0.00 | 0.3 | 0.03 | 0.0 | 0.0 | | 4 | 0.0 | 0.5 | 2 | 0.1 | 11 | 1 | 0.1 | 102 | 0.09 |
| 2649 | 1/2 cup | Rice, prep f/mix, w/whl milk, avg | 144 | 161 | 73 | 4.8 | 30.2 | 0.1 | 17.7 | 12.4 | 2.3 | 1.5 | 0.6 | 0.1 | 0.03 | 0.06 | 9 | 249 | 52 | 49 | 3 | | 0.11 | 0.20 | 0.64 | 0.05 | 0.36 | 5.8 | 0.42 | 1.0 | 1.2 | | 151 | 0.0 | 0.5 | 19 | 0.1 | 127 | 190 | 2.7 | 158 | 0.56 |
| 2650 | 1/2 cup | Rice, prep f/rec, avg | 152 | 217 | 66 | 5.5 | 40.1 | 0.8 | 25.5 | 13.8 | 4.3 | 2.6 | 1.2 | 0.2 | 0.08 | 0.14 | 17 | 154 | 38 | 36 | 2 | | 0.12 | 0.21 | 0.82 | 0.09 | 0.24 | 6.1 | 0.50 | 0.9 | 1.5 | | 155 | 0.1 | 1.0 | 24 | 0.2 | 143 | 269 | | 85 | 0.68 |
| 2651 | 1 ea | Rice, RTE, cnd, avg | 142 | 231 | 68 | 2.8 | 31.2 | 0.1 | 18.3 | 12.8 | 10.6 | 1.7 | 4.6 | 4.0 | 0.27 | 3.68 | 1 | 162 | 50 | 47 | 3 | | 0.03 | 0.10 | 0.23 | 0.04 | 0.30 | 4.3 | 0.33 | 0.7 | 0.0 | | 74 | 0.0 | 0.4 | 11 | 0.2 | 97 | 85 | 3.1 | 121 | 0.70 |
| 2652 | 1 oz | Tapioca, dry mix, avg | 92 | 339 | 4 | 0.1 | 86.8 | 0.2 | 59.8 | 26.8 | 0.1 | 0.0 | 0.0 | 0.0 | | | 0 | 0 | 0 | 0 | 0 | 0 | 0.00 | 0.01 | 0.00 | 0.00 | 0.00 | 0.0 | 0.01 | 0.0 | 0.0 | 0.0 | 4 | 0.0 | 0.1 | 2 | 0.0 | 4 | 5 | 0.8 | 439 | 0.07 |
| 2730 | 1 tsp | Tapioca, dry mix, Minute, Kraft | 4 | 13 | 16 | 0.0 | 3.3 | 0.0 | 0.0 | 3.3 | 0.0 | 0.0 | 0.0 | 0.0 | 0.00 | 0.00 | 0 | 0 | 0 | 0 | 0 | 0 | | | | | | | | 0.0 | | | 0 | | 0.0 | | | | 0 | | 0 | |
| 2708 | 1/2 cup | Tapioca, Pearl, Orval Kent | 120 | 150 | | 4.0 | 25.0 | 2.0 | 19.0 | 4.0 | 4.0 | 2.0 | | | | | 35 | 100 | 20 | | | | | | | | | | | 1.2 | | | 150 | | 0.4 | | | | | | 95 | |
| 2653 | 1/2 cup | Tapioca, prep f/mix, w/2% milk, avg | 141 | 147 | 75 | 4.1 | 27.8 | 0.0 | 21.7 | 6.1 | 2.4 | 1.5 | 0.7 | 0.1 | 0.04 | 0.05 | 8 | 251 | 69 | 65 | 4 | | 0.04 | 0.20 | 0.11 | 0.05 | 0.35 | 5.6 | 0.39 | 1.0 | 1.2 | | 149 | 0.0 | 0.1 | 17 | 0.0 | 117 | 189 | 2.8 | 172 | 0.49 |
| 2603 | 1/2 cup | Tapioca, prep f/rec, w/whl milk, avg | 152 | 190 | 73 | 7.2 | 25.8 | 0.0 | 23.2 | 2.7 | 6.5 | 3.3 | 2.1 | 0.5 | 0.09 | 0.41 | 125 | 315 | 87 | 81 | 5 | | 0.05 | 0.32 | 0.12 | 0.08 | 0.56 | 13.7 | 0.67 | 0.9 | 1.5 | | 158 | 0.0 | 0.5 | 20 | 0.0 | 160 | 216 | 1.7 | 289 | 0.74 |
| 2611 | 1 ea | Tapioca, RTE, cnd, avg | 142 | 169 | 74 | 2.8 | 27.5 | 0.1 | 25.1 | 2.3 | 5.3 | 0.9 | 2.2 | 1.9 | 0.14 | 1.79 | 1 | 0 | 0 | 0 | 0 | 0 | 0.03 | 0.14 | 0.44 | 0.03 | 0.31 | 4.3 | 0.28 | 1.0 | 1.4 | | 119 | 0.0 | 0.3 | 11 | 0.0 | 112 | 138 | 2.0 | 226 | 0.38 |
| 2656 | 1 oz | Vanilla, dry mix, avg | 28 | 103 | 4 | 0.1 | 26.2 | 0.1 | 20.4 | 5.7 | 0.1 | 0.0 | 0.0 | 0.0 | 0.00 | 0.04 | 0 | 0 | 0 | 0 | 0 | 0 | 0.00 | 0.00 | 0.00 | 0.00 | 0.00 | 0.0 | 0.00 | 0.0 | 0.0 | | 4 | 0.0 | 0.0 | 0 | 0.0 | 1 | 6 | 0.3 | 211 | 0.01 |
| 2757 | 1 oz | Vanilla, dry mix, no sugar/fat, Jell-o | 28 | 88 | 7 | 0.0 | 21.0 | 0.0 | 0.0 | 21.0 | 0.0 | 0.0 | 0.0 | 0.0 | 0.00 | 0.00 | 0 | 0 | 0 | 0 | 0 | 0 | | | | | | | | 0.0 | | | 0 | | 0.0 | | | | 0 | | 1155 | |
| 2655 | 1/2 cup | Vanilla, prep f/mix, w/2% milk, avg | 142 | 148 | 74 | 4.0 | 28.1 | 0.0 | 15.1 | 13.1 | 2.4 | 1.4 | 0.7 | 0.1 | 0.04 | 0.10 | 9 | 241 | 64 | 60 | 4 | | 0.05 | 0.20 | 0.11 | 0.05 | 0.43 | 5.7 | 0.38 | 1.1 | 1.2 | | 146 | 0.0 | 0.1 | 17 | 0.0 | 283 | 185 | 2.6 | 406 | 0.47 |
| 2608 | 1/2 cup | Vanilla, prep f/mix, w/whl milk, avg | 142 | 162 | 74 | 3.8 | 28.0 | 0.0 | 23.7 | 4.2 | 4.1 | 2.5 | 1.2 | 0.2 | 0.07 | 0.14 | 16 | 149 | 36 | 31 | 5 | | 0.05 | 0.19 | 0.11 | 0.05 | 0.43 | 5.7 | 0.37 | 1.1 | 1.2 | | 143 | 0.0 | 0.1 | 17 | 0.0 | 280 | 182 | 2.3 | 406 | 0.47 |
| 2792 | 1/2 cup | Vanilla, prep f/mix, no sugar/fat, Jell-o | 125 | 70 | 86 | 4.0 | 12.0 | 0.0 | 6.0 | 6.0 | 0.0 | 0.0 | 0.0 | 0.0 | 0.00 | 0.00 | 0 | 200 | 40 | | | | | | | | | | | 0.0 | | | 150 | | 0.0 | | | | 210 | | 400 | |
| 2602 | 1/2 cup | Vanilla, prep f/rec, w/whl milk, avg | 123 | 130 | 77 | 4.1 | 19.6 | 0.0 | 15.6 | 3.9 | 4.1 | 2.5 | 1.2 | 0.2 | 0.06 | 0.10 | 16 | 154 | 37 | 34 | 3 | | 0.03 | 0.20 | 0.10 | 0.04 | 0.23 | 4.9 | 0.38 | 0.7 | 1.1 | | 145 | 0.0 | 0.1 | 16 | 0.0 | 114 | 185 | 1.4 | 113 | 0.47 |
| 2612 | 1 ea | Vanilla, RTS, cnd, avg | 142 | 185 | 71 | 3.3 | 31.1 | 0.1 | 26.7 | 4.3 | 5.1 | 0.8 | 2.2 | 1.9 | 0.13 | 1.76 | 10 | 30 | 9 | 7 | 1 | | 0.03 | 0.20 | 0.36 | 0.02 | 0.14 | 0.0 | 0.25 | 0.0 | 1.2 | | 125 | 0.0 | 0.2 | 11 | 0.0 | 97 | 160 | 2.0 | 192 | 0.35 |
| 2766 | 1 Tbs | Vanilla, rennin, dry mix, avg | 11 | 42 | 0 | 0.0 | 10.9 | 0.0 | | | 0.0 | 0.0 | 0.0 | 0.0 | 0.00 | 0.00 | 0 | 0 | 0 | 0 | 0 | 0 | 0.00 | 0.00 | 0.00 | 0.00 | 0.00 | 0.0 | 0.00 | 0.0 | 0.0 | | 13 | 0.0 | 0.0 | 0 | 0.0 | 10 | 0 | 0.1 | 1 | 0.00 |
| 2662 | 1/2 cup | Vanilla, rennin, prep f/mix, w/2%milk, avg | 133 | 101 | 82 | 4.1 | 16.4 | 0.0 | | | 2.4 | 1.5 | 0.7 | 0.1 | 0.04 | 0.05 | 9 | 251 | 69 | | | | 0.05 | 0.20 | 0.11 | 0.05 | 0.44 | 6.7 | 0.39 | 1.2 | 1.1 | | 161 | 0.0 | 0.1 | 17 | 0.0 | 126 | 189 | 2.8 | 61 | 0.48 |
| 2663 | 1/2 cup | Vanilla, rennin, prep f/mix, w/whl milk, avg | 133 | 116 | 81 | 4.0 | 16.2 | 0.0 | | | 4.1 | 2.5 | 1.2 | 0.2 | 0.07 | 0.09 | 17 | 154 | 33 | | | | 0.05 | 0.20 | 0.10 | 0.05 | 0.44 | 6.7 | 0.38 | 1.2 | 1.1 | | 158 | 0.0 | 0.1 | 16 | 0.0 | 124 | 186 | 2.8 | 61 | 0.47 |
| 2664 | 1/2 cup | Vanilla, rennin, prep f/rec, avg | 137 | 112 | 82 | 4.0 | 15.3 | 0.0 | | | 4.1 | 2.5 | 1.2 | 0.2 | 0.07 | 0.10 | 16 | 153 | 37 | | | | 0.05 | 0.20 | 0.10 | 0.05 | 0.44 | 5.5 | 0.38 | 1.1 | 1.2 | | 151 | 0.0 | 0.1 | 16 | 0.0 | 115 | 185 | | 96 | 0.48 |
| 2726 | 1 ea | Vanilla/Chocolate, RTE, Jell-o | 113 | 160 | 67 | 3.0 | 26.0 | 0.0 | 21.0 | 5.0 | 5.0 | 2.0 | | | | | 0 | 100 | 20 | | | | | | | | | | | 0.0 | | | 100 | | 0.4 | | | | 180 | | 180 | |
| 2728 | 1 ea | Vanilla/Chocolate, RTE, fat free, Jell-o | 113 | 100 | 76 | 3.0 | 23.0 | 0.0 | 17.0 | 6.0 | 0.0 | 0.0 | 0.0 | 0.0 | 0.00 | 0.00 | 0 | 100 | 20 | | | | | | | | | | | 0.0 | | | 80 | | 0.4 | | | | 180 | | 210 | |
| | | **DESSERT TOPPINGS** | | | | | | | | | | | | | | | | | | | | | | | | | | | | | | | | | | | | | | | | |
| | | *FROSTINGS* | | | | | | | | | | | | | | | | | | | | | | | | | | | | | | | | | | | | | | | | |
| 46324 | 2 Tbs | Candy, creamy, RTE, Pillsbury | 34 | 150 | 14 | 0.1 | 21.6 | 0.0 | 19.6 | 2.0 | 7.0 | 2.0 | | | | | 2 | 22 | 4 | | | | | | | | | | | 0.0 | | | 2 | | 0.0 | | | | | | 92 | |
| 46318 | 2 Tbs | Caramel Pecan, RTE, Pillsbury | 35 | 149 | 21 | 0.2 | 19.1 | 0.3 | 15.9 | 2.9 | 8.0 | 1.9 | | | | | 0 | 0 | 0 | 0 | 0 | 0 | | | | | | | | 0.1 | | | 2 | | 0.1 | | | | | | 67 | |
| | | Chocolate Frosting | | | | | | | | | | | | | | | | | | | | | | | | | | | | | | | | | | | | | | | | |
| 46033 | 1 oz | Creamy, dry mix, avg | 28 | 109 | 1 | 0.4 | 25.8 | 0.7 | 24.2 | 0.9 | 1.5 | 0.3 | 0.6 | 0.4 | | | 0 | 0 | 0 | 0 | 0 | 0 | 0.00 | 0.01 | 0.04 | 0.02 | 0.00 | 0.8 | 0.01 | 0.0 | 0.0 | | 3 | 0.1 | 0.3 | 11 | 0.1 | 17 | 50 | 0.4 | 21 | 0.23 |
| 46325 | 2 Tbs | Dark, RTE, Pillsbury | 34 | 134 | 20 | 0.5 | 20.0 | 0.3 | 16.9 | 2.8 | 5.8 | 1.6 | | | | | 0 | 0.3 | 0.1 | | | | | | | | | | | 0.0 | | | 4 | | 0.7 | | | | | | 44 | |
| 23385 | 2 Tbs | Fudge, Amaretto, RTE, fat free, fruit swtnd, Wax Orchards | 30 | 90 | 18 | 1.0 | 21.0 | 3.0 | 18.0 | 0.0 | 0.5 | 0.0 | | | | | 0 | 0 | 0 | 0 | 0 | 0 | | | | | | | | 0.0 | | | 60 | | 1.8 | | | | | | 40 | |
| 23386 | 2 Tbs | Fudge, Orange, RTE, fat free, fruit swtnd, Wax Orchards | 30 | 90 | 18 | 1.0 | 21.0 | 3.0 | 18.0 | 0.0 | 0.5 | 0.0 | | | | | 0 | 0 | 0 | 0 | 0 | 0 | | | | | | | | 0.0 | | | 60 | | 1.8 | | | | | | 40 | |
| 23387 | 2 Tbs | Fudge, Pepprmint, RTE, fat free, fruit swtnd, Wax Orchard | 30 | 90 | 18 | 1.0 | 21.0 | 3.0 | 18.0 | 0.0 | 0.5 | 0.0 | | | | | 0 | 0 | 0 | 0 | 0 | 0 | | | | | | | | 0.0 | | | 60 | | 1.8 | | | | | | 40 | |
| 23383 | 2 Tbs | Fudge, RTE, fat free, fruit swtnd, Wax Orchard | 30 | 90 | 18 | 1.0 | 21.0 | 3.0 | 18.0 | 0.0 | 0.5 | 0.0 | | | | | 0 | 0 | 0 | 0 | 0 | 0 | | | | | | | | 0.0 | | | 60 | | 1.8 | | | | | | 40 | |
| 46168 | 2 Tbs | Fudge, RTE, Pillsbury | 34 | 135 | 20 | 0.4 | 20.5 | 0.2 | 17.7 | 2.5 | 5.8 | 1.6 | | | | | 0 | 0.3 | 0.03 | | | | | | | | | | | 0.0 | | | 4 | | 0.6 | | | | | | 76 | |
| 46335 | 2 Tbs | Fudge, RTE, red fat, Pillsbury | 37 | 135 | 18 | 0.4 | 25.9 | 0.3 | 23.4 | 2.1 | 3.4 | 1.0 | | | | | 0 | 0.4 | 0.04 | | | | | | | | | | | 0.0 | | | 3 | | 0.6 | | | | | | 85 | |
| 46157 | 2 Tbs | Funfetti, RTE, Pillsbury | 32 | 128 | 19 | 0.3 | 19.9 | 0.2 | 17.5 | 2.2 | 5.3 | 1.5 | | | | | 0 | 0.3 | 0.03 | | | | | | | | | | | 0.0 | | | 3 | | 0.5 | | | | | | 69 | |
| 46334 | 2 Tbs | Oreo, RTE, Pillsbury | 34 | 144 | 14 | 0.1 | 23.1 | 0.1 | 20.5 | 2.5 | 5.7 | 1.5 | | | | | 0 | 0 | 0 | 0 | 0 | 0 | | | | | | | | 0.0 | | | 1 | | 0.1 | | | | | | 74 | |
| 46034 | 2 Tbs | Prep f/Mix, w/butter, avg | 34 | 130 | 13 | 0.4 | 24.3 | 0.6 | 22.9 | 0.9 | 4.5 | 1.9 | 0.9 | 0.1 | 0.04 | 0.07 | 8 | 116 | 20 | | | | 0.00 | 0.01 | 0.04 | 0.02 | 0.00 | 0.0 | 0.01 | 0.0 | 0.0 | | 4 | 0.1 | 0.3 | 10 | 0.1 | 17 | 49 | 0.4 | 51 | 0.22 |
| 46035 | 2 Tbs | Prep f/Mix, w/marg, avg | 34 | 130 | 13 | 0.4 | 24.4 | 0.6 | 22.9 | 0.9 | 4.4 | 0.6 | 1.4 | 1.0 | 0.04 | 0.92 | 0 | 125 | 23 | | | | 0.00 | 0.01 | 0.04 | 0.02 | 0.00 | 0.0 | 0.01 | 0.0 | 0.0 | | 4 | 0.1 | 0.3 | 10 | 0.1 | 17 | 49 | 0.4 | 56 | 0.22 |
| 46032 | 2 Tbs | Prep f/Recipe, avg | 34 | 136 | 8 | 0.4 | 26.4 | 0.6 | 24.8 | 1.0 | 3.9 | 2.4 | 1.1 | 0.1 | 0.05 | 0.09 | 10 | 138 | 34 | | | | 0.00 | 0.01 | 0.04 | 0.00 | 0.01 | 0.7 | 0.02 | 0.0 | 0.0 | | 6 | 0.1 | 0.3 | 9 | 0.1 | 16 | 31 | | 65 | 0.13 |
| 46037 | 2 Tbs | RTE, avg | 29 | 115 | 17 | 0.3 | 18.3 | 0.2 | 16.7 | 1.4 | 5.1 | 1.6 | 2.6 | 0.6 | 0.01 | 0.61 | 0 | 190 | 57 | | | | 0.00 | 0.00 | 0.03 | 0.00 | 0.00 | 0.0 | 0.01 | 0.0 | 0.0 | | 2 | 0.1 | 0.4 | 6 | 0.1 | 23 | 57 | 0.2 | 53 | 0.08 |
| | | Coconut Frosting | | | | | | | | | | | | | | | | | | | | | | | | | | | | | | | | | | | | | | | | |
| 46169 | 2 Tbs | Almond, RTE, Pillsbury | 35 | 156 | 21 | 0.7 | 17.4 | 0.9 | 14.0 | 2.5 | 9.3 | 3.8 | | | | | 0 | 0 | 0 | 0 | 0 | 0 | | | | | | | | 0.1 | | | 9 | | 0.3 | | | | | | 60 | |
| 46038 | 2 Tbs | Nut, RTE, avg | 29 | 119 | 21 | 0.4 | 15.3 | 0.4 | 11.6 | 3.3 | 7.0 | 2.0 | 3.5 | 1.0 | 0.05 | 0.94 | 0 | 0 | 0 | 0 | 0 | 0 | 0.01 | 0.01 | 0.06 | 0.02 | 0.00 | 1.7 | 0.08 | 0.1 | 0.0 | | 4 | 0.0 | 0.2 | 6 | 0.2 | 18 | 54 | 0.9 | 57 | 0.12 |

| Code | Amount | Description | Basic Components | | | | | | | | | Additional Fats | | | | | | Vit A & Components | | | | | Vitamins | | | | | | | | | | Minerals | | | | | | | | | |
|---|---|---|---|---|---|---|---|---|---|---|---|---|---|---|---|---|---|---|---|---|---|---|---|---|---|---|---|---|---|---|---|---|---|---|---|---|---|---|---|---|---|---|
| | | | Weight (g) | Calories | % Water | Protein (g) | Carbs (g) | Fiber (g) | Sugar (g) | Other Carbs (g) | Fat (g) | Sat Fat (g) | Mono Fat (g) | Poly Fat (g) | Omega 3 (g) | Omega 6 (g) | Choles (mg) | Vit A (IU) | Vit A (RE) | Retinol (RE) | Carotenoids (RE) | Beta Carotene (mcg) | Thiamin (mg) | Riboflavin (mg) | Niacin (NE) | Vit B6 (mg) | Vit B12 (mcg) | Folate (mcg) | Panto (mg) | Vit C (mg) | Vit D (mg) | Vit E (α TE) | Calcium (mg) | Copper (mg) | Iron (mg) | Magnes (mg) | Mang (mg) | Phos (mg) | Potassium (mg) | Selenium (mcg) | Sodium (mg) | Zinc (mg) |
| 46200 | 1 oz | Pecan, dry mix, General Mills | 28 | 143 | 4 | 0.6 | 18.5 | 0.9 | 13.2 | 4.4 | 7.8 | 3.1 | 2.9 | 0.7 | | | 0 | | | | | | 0.03 | 0.02 | 0.05 | | | | | | | | 10 | | 0.2 | | | | 45 | | 71 | |
| 46413 | 1 oz | Pecan, prep f/mix, General Mills | 28 | 142 | 4 | 0.0 | 19.0 | 0.8 | 12.7 | 5.5 | 7.9 | 3.2 | 3.2 | 0.0 | 0.00 | 0.00 | 0 | 0 | 0 | 0 | 0 | 0 | 0.00 | 0.00 | 0.00 | | | | | 0.0 | | | 0 | | 0.0 | | | | 47 | | 71 | |
| 46170 | 2 Tbs | Pecan, RTE, Pillsbury | 35 | 160 | 20 | 0.5 | 17.1 | 1.0 | 13.7 | 2.4 | 9.9 | 4.1 | | | | | 0 | 0 | 0 | 0 | 0 | 0 | | | | | | | | 0.1 | | | 3 | | 0.2 | | | | | | 60 | |
| 46211 | 1 ea | RTE, can, avg | 462 | 1903 | 21 | 6.9 | 243.9 | 6.5 | 231.0 | 6.5 | 110.9 | 32.5 | 56.4 | 15.8 | 0.74 | 15.01 | 0 | 0 | 0 | 0 | 0 | 0 | 0.16 | 0.09 | 0.98 | 0.25 | 0.00 | 27.7 | 1.23 | 1.4 | 0.0 | | 60 | 0.6 | 2.5 | 88 | 3.9 | 217 | 859 | 14.3 | 901 | 1.89 |
| | | Cream Cheese Frosting | | | | | | | | | | | | | | | | | | | | | | | | | | | | | | | | | | | | | | | | |
| 46415 | 1 oz | Prep f/Mix, General Mills | 28 | 129 | 2 | 0.0 | 22.7 | 0.0 | 17.8 | 4.9 | 4.9 | 2.4 | 2.4 | 0.0 | 0.00 | 0.00 | 0 | 0 | 0 | 0 | 0 | 0 | 0.00 | 0.00 | 0.00 | | | | | 0.0 | | | 0 | | 0.0 | | | | 8 | | 0 | |
| 46212 | 1 ea | RTE, can, avg | 462 | 1908 | 15 | 0.5 | 308.2 | 0.0 | 272.6 | 35.6 | 79.9 | 23.3 | 41.7 | 10.9 | 0.42 | 10.39 | 0 | 5 | 1 | | | | 0.00 | 0.03 | 0.05 | 0.00 | 0.00 | 0.0 | 0.01 | 0.0 | | | 14 | 0.1 | 0.7 | 9 | 0.1 | 14 | 162 | 2.8 | 180 | 0.00 |
| 46171 | 2 Tbs | RTE, Pillsbury | 35 | 147 | 15 | 0.0 | 23.8 | 0.0 | 21.7 | 2.0 | 5.7 | 1.5 | | | | | 0 | 0 | 0 | 0 | 0 | 0 | | | | | | | | 0.0 | | | 1 | | 0.0 | | | | | | 70 | |
| 46330 | 2 Tbs | Lemon Crème, RTE, Pillsbury | 35 | 146 | 15 | 0.0 | 23.4 | 0.0 | 21.1 | 2.3 | 5.8 | 1.6 | | | | | 0 | 0 | 0 | 0 | 0 | 0 | | | | | | | | 0.0 | | | 0 | | 0.1 | | | | | | 76 | |
| 23380 | 2 Tbs | Peanut Butter Fudge, RTE, fruit swtnd, Wax Orchard | 30 | 110 | 22 | 1.0 | 18.0 | 2.0 | 16.0 | 0.0 | 3.0 | 0.0 | | | | | 0 | 0 | 0 | 0 | 0 | 0 | | | | | | | | 0.0 | | | 60 | | 1.8 | | | | | | 40 | |
| 46042 | 1 ea | Sour Cream, RTE, can, avg | 462 | 1903 | 14 | 0.5 | 312.3 | 0.5 | 303.1 | 8.8 | 79.5 | 23.1 | 41.5 | 10.8 | 0.42 | 10.35 | 0 | 1853 | 564 | | | | 0.05 | 0.09 | 3.09 | 0.02 | 0.05 | 4.6 | 0.18 | 0.0 | 0.0 | | 9 | 0.0 | 0.3 | 9 | 0.2 | 18 | 896 | 2.8 | 942 | 0.05 |
| 46336 | 2 Tbs | Strawberry Crème, RTE, Pillsbury | 35 | 146 | 15 | 0.0 | 23.6 | 0.0 | 21.2 | 2.3 | 5.7 | 1.5 | | | | | 0 | 0 | 0 | 0 | 0 | 0 | | | | | | | | 0.0 | | | 0 | | 0.1 | | | | | | 75 | |
| | | Vanilla Frosting | | | | | | | | | | | | | | | | | | | | | | | | | | | | | | | | | | | | | | | | |
| 46043 | 1 ea | Dry Mix pkg, avg | 411 | 1685 | 1 | 1.2 | 385.5 | 0.4 | 374.0 | 11.1 | 20.1 | | | | | | 0 | 0 | 0 | 0 | 0 | 0 | 0.00 | 0.01 | 0.00 | 0.00 | 0.00 | 0.0 | 0.03 | 0.0 | 0.0 | | 12 | 0.1 | 0.0 | 8 | 0.0 | 16 | 29 | 3.3 | 53 | 0.04 |
| 46329 | 2 Tbs | Funfetti, RTE, Pillsbury | 37 | 155 | 15 | 0.0 | 25.2 | 0.0 | 22.8 | 2.4 | 6.0 | 1.6 | | | | | 0 | 0 | 0 | 0 | 0 | 0 | | | | | | | | 0.0 | | | 0 | | 0.0 | | | | | | 74 | |
| 46328 | 2 Tbs | Pink, Funfetti, RTE, Pillsbury | 35 | 146 | 15 | 0.0 | 23.8 | 0.0 | 21.5 | 2.3 | 5.6 | 1.5 | | | | | 0 | 0 | 0 | 0 | 0 | 0 | | | | | | | | 0.0 | | | 0 | | 0.0 | | | | | | 69 | |
| 46044 | 2 Tbs | Prep f/mix, w/butter, avg | 40 | 169 | 12 | 0.1 | 28.3 | 0.0 | 27.5 | 0.8 | 6.7 | 2.9 | 2.2 | 1.3 | 0.12 | 1.13 | 10 | 185 | 38 | | | | 0.01 | 0.01 | 0.14 | 0.00 | 0.00 | 0.0 | 0.02 | 0.0 | 0.0 | | 4 | 0.0 | 0.1 | 1 | 0.0 | 11 | 8 | 0.3 | 84 | 0.05 |
| 46045 | 2 Tbs | Prep f/recipe, w/butter, avg | 40 | 137 | 17 | 0.2 | 31.2 | 0.0 | 30.3 | 1.0 | 1.6 | 1.0 | 0.5 | 0.1 | 0.02 | 0.04 | 5 | 61 | 15 | | | | 0.00 | 0.01 | 0.01 | 0.00 | 0.03 | 0.4 | 0.02 | 0.1 | 0.0 | | 9 | 0.0 | 0.0 | 1 | 0.0 | 7 | 12 | | 26 | 0.04 |
| 46046 | 2 Tbs | Prep f/recipe, w/marg, avg | 40 | 162 | 9 | 0.2 | 31.6 | 0.0 | 30.7 | 1.0 | 4.3 | 0.9 | 1.9 | 1.3 | 0.06 | 1.25 | 0 | 176 | 45 | | | | 0.00 | 0.01 | 0.00 | 0.00 | 0.02 | 0.4 | 0.01 | 0.0 | 0.0 | | 5 | 0.0 | 0.0 | 1 | 0.0 | 4 | 7 | | 82 | 0.02 |
| 46009 | 2 Tbs | RTE, avg | 31 | 130 | 13 | 0.0 | 21.5 | 0.0 | 19.7 | 1.7 | 5.2 | 1.5 | 2.7 | 0.7 | 0.03 | 0.63 | 0 | 231 | 70 | 64 | 6 | | 0.00 | 0.00 | 0.00 | 0.00 | 0.00 | 0.0 | 0.00 | 0.0 | 0.0 | | 1 | 0.0 | 0.0 | 0 | 0.0 | 12 | 11 | 0.2 | 28 | 0.00 |
| 46193 | 1 oz | RTE, General Mills | 28 | 119 | 14 | 0.0 | 20.2 | 0.0 | 18.8 | 1.4 | 4.2 | 1.1 | 1.9 | 0.3 | | | 0 | 158 | 16 | 0 | 16 | | | | | | | | | | | | | | | | | | 10 | | 31 | |
| 46332 | 2 Tbs | RTE, Lovin Lites | 38 | 144 | 15 | 0.0 | 28.9 | 0.2 | 24.9 | 3.9 | 3.1 | 0.8 | | | | | 0 | 0 | 0 | 0 | 0 | 0 | | | | | | | | 0.0 | | | 1 | | 0.0 | | | | | | 69 | |
| 46326 | 2 Tbs | RTE, Pillsbury | 38 | 158 | 15 | 0.0 | 25.3 | 0.0 | 22.9 | 2.5 | 6.2 | 1.7 | | | | | 0 | 0 | 0 | 0 | 0 | 0 | | | | | | | | 0.0 | | | 0 | | 0.1 | | | | | | 78 | |
| | | White Frosting | | | | | | | | | | | | | | | | | | | | | | | | | | | | | | | | | | | | | | | | |
| 46047 | 1 ea | Dry Mix pkg, avg | 207 | 768 | 2 | 4.8 | 196.4 | 0.0 | 195.2 | 1.2 | 0.0 | 0.0 | 0.0 | 0.0 | 0.00 | 0.00 | 0 | 0 | 0 | 0 | 0 | 0 | 0.00 | 0.12 | 2.07 | 0.00 | 0.02 | 6.2 | 0.11 | 0.0 | 0.0 | 0.0 | 8 | 0.1 | 0.2 | 6 | 0.0 | 14 | 242 | 8.5 | 484 | 0.02 |
| 46048 | 2 Tbs | Prep f/Mix, avg | 40 | 98 | 35 | 0.6 | 25.0 | 0.0 | 24.9 | 0.2 | 0.0 | 0.0 | 0.0 | 0.0 | 0.00 | 0.00 | 0 | 0 | 0 | 0 | 0 | 0 | 0.00 | 0.01 | 0.26 | 0.00 | 0.00 | 0.8 | 0.01 | 0.0 | 0.0 | 0.0 | 2 | 0.0 | 0.0 | 1 | 0.0 | 2 | 31 | 1.0 | 62 | 0.01 |
| 46041 | 2 Tbs | Prep f/Recipe, avg | 40 | 127 | 17 | 0.7 | 32.2 | 0.0 | 32.0 | 0.2 | 0.0 | 0.0 | 0.0 | 0.0 | 0.00 | 0.00 | 0 | 0.4 | 0.04 | | | | 0.00 | 0.03 | 0.01 | 0.00 | 0.01 | 0.0 | 0.01 | 0.0 | 0.0 | 0.0 | 1 | 0.0 | 0.0 | 1 | 0.0 | 1 | 26 | | 68 | 0.01 |
| 46474 | 2 Tbs | RTE, Pillsbury | 31 | 127 | | 0.2 | 20.5 | | | | 5.0 | | | | | | | | | | | | | | | | | | | | | | | | | | | | | | 55 | |
| | | *GLAZES* | | | | | | | | | | | | | | | | | | | | | | | | | | | | | | | | | | | | | | | | |
| 23248 | 2 Tbs | Banana, Marie's | 30 | 40 | 70 | 0.0 | 9.0 | 0.0 | 9.0 | 0.0 | 0.0 | 0.0 | 0.0 | 0.0 | 0.00 | 0.00 | 0 | 0 | 0 | 0 | 0 | 0 | | | | | | | | 0.0 | | | 0 | | 0.0 | | | | | | 30 | |
| 23249 | 2 Tbs | Blueberry, Marie's | 30 | 40 | 66 | 0.0 | 10.0 | 0.0 | 8.0 | 2.0 | 0.0 | 0.0 | 0.0 | 0.0 | 0.00 | 0.00 | 10 | 0 | 0 | 0 | 0 | 0 | | | | | | | | 0.0 | | | 0 | | 0.0 | | | | | | 30 | |
| 46337 | 2 Tbs | Chocolate Fudge, RTE, Pillsbury | 35 | 140 | 20 | 0.4 | 21.5 | 0.8 | 18.2 | 2.5 | 5.8 | 1.6 | | | | | 0 | 0.4 | 0.1 | | | | | | | | | | | 0.0 | | | 3 | | 0.6 | | | | | | 61 | |
| 46204 | 1 oz | Cinnamon Raisin Biscuit, dry mix, General Mills | 28 | 117 | 1 | 0.0 | 26.3 | 0.0 | 23.5 | 2.8 | 1.3 | 0.4 | 0.8 | 0.1 | | | 0 | 0 | 0 | 0 | 0 | 0 | 0.00 | 0.00 | 0.00 | | | | | 0.0 | | | | | 0.0 | | | | 1 | | 28 | |
| 46401 | 2 Tbs | Cinnamon Raisin Biscuit, prep f/mix, General Mills | 24 | 101 | | 0.0 | 22.2 | 0.0 | 20.2 | 2.0 | 1.0 | 0.0 | 0.0 | 0.0 | 0.00 | 0.00 | 0 | 0 | 0 | 0 | 0 | 0 | 0.00 | 0.00 | 0.00 | | | | | 0.0 | | | 0 | | 0.0 | | | | 0 | | 20 | |
| 23250 | 2 Tbs | Peach, Marie's | 30 | 40 | 66 | 0.0 | 10.0 | 0.0 | 8.0 | 2.0 | 0.0 | 0.0 | 0.0 | 0.0 | 0.00 | 0.00 | 10 | 0 | 0 | 0 | 0 | 0 | | | | | | | | 0.0 | | | 0 | | 0.0 | | | | | | 50 | |
| 46040 | 2 Tbs | Prep f/Recipe, avg | 40 | 144 | 18 | 0.2 | 29.4 | 0.0 | 28.5 | 0.9 | 3.2 | 0.7 | 1.3 | 0.9 | 0.04 | 0.88 | [illegible] | 127 | 32 | | | | 0.00 | 0.01 | 0.01 | 0.00 | 0.03 | 0.4 | 0.02 | 0.1 | 0.0 | | 9 | 0.0 | 0.0 | 1 | 0.0 | 7 | 12 | 0.3 | 38 | 0.03 |
| 23251 | 2 Tbs | Strawberry, Marie's | 30 | 40 | 70 | 0.0 | 9.0 | 0.0 | 9.0 | 0.0 | 0.0 | 0.0 | 0.0 | 0.0 | 0.00 | 0.00 | 0 | 0 | 0 | 0 | 0 | 0 | | | | | | | | 0.0 | | | 0 | | 0.0 | | | | | | 30 | |
| 46338 | 2 Tbs | Vanilla w/Fudge, RTE, Pillsbury | 37 | 153 | 16 | 0.0 | 24.7 | 0.0 | 22.0 | 2.7 | 6.0 | 1.6 | | | | | 0 | 0 | 0 | 0 | 0 | 0 | | | | | | | | 0.0 | | | 0 | | 0.1 | | | | | | 76 | |
| | | *SPRINKLES* | | | | | | | | | | | | | | | | | | | | | | | | | | | | | | | | | | | | | | | | |
| 23268 | 2 Tbs | Buncha Crunch, topping, Nestle | 20 | 103 | 2 | 1.1 | 13.2 | 0.3 | 9.9 | 3.0 | 5.1 | 2.4 | 1.9 | 0.5 | 0.00 | 0.53 | 3 | 18 | 5 | | | | 0.12 | 0.15 | 1.65 | 0.14 | 0.06 | 29.8 | 0.11 | 0.1 | 0.0 | | 26 | 0.1 | 0.1 | 14 | 0.2 | 42 | 70 | | 46 | 0.34 |
| 23267 | 1 Tbs | Butterfinger, candy topping, Nestle | 25 | 120 | 2 | 3.1 | 16.4 | 0.6 | 12.4 | 3.4 | 4.7 | 2.6 | 1.4 | 0.7 | 0.00 | 0.70 | 0 | 0 | 0 | 0 | 0 | 0 | 0.02 | 0.02 | 0.63 | 0.02 | 0.00 | 6.8 | 0.07 | 0.0 | 0.0 | | 7 | 0.1 | 0.2 | 20 | 0.2 | 33 | 95 | 0.8 | 50 | 0.29 |
| 23252 | 2 Tbs | Mini Morsels, topping, Nestle | 21 | 100 | 0 | 1.0 | 13.4 | 2.0 | 12.0 | | 6.0 | 3.5 | | | | | 0 | 0 | 0 | 0 | 0 | 0 | | | | | | | | 0.0 | | | 0 | | 0.4 | | | | | | 0 | |
| 23187 | 2 Tbs | Rainbow Morsel, topping, Nestle | 28 | 136 | 1 | 1.2 | 20.7 | 1.5 | 17.1 | 2.1 | 5.4 | 3.2 | 1.8 | 0.2 | 0.00 | 0.17 | [illegible] | 1.4 | 0.3 | | | | 0.01 | 0.02 | 0.08 | 0.01 | 0.00 | 0.6 | 0.02 | 0.2 | 0.0 | | 9 | 0.1 | 0.5 | 21 | 0.1 | 25 | 67 | | 1 | 0.30 |
| 23186 | 1 oz | Sno Caps, sweet choc topping, Nestle | 28 | 129 | 2 | 0.9 | 20.6 | 1.3 | 16.3 | 3.0 | 5.6 | 3.4 | | | | | 0 | 0 | 0 | 0 | 0 | 0 | 0.01 | 0.01 | 0.08 | | | | | 0.0 | | | 0 | | 0.5 | | | | 9 | | 0 | |
| | | *SYRUPS AND TOPPINGS* | | | | | | | | | | | | | | | | | | | | | | | | | | | | | | | | | | | | | | | | |
| 23069 | 2 Tbs | Butterscotch, avg | 41 | 103 | 32 | 0.6 | 27.0 | 0.4 | 26.5 | 0.1 | 0.0 | 0.0 | 0.0 | 0.0 | 0.00 | 0.00 | 0 | 37 | 11 | | | | 0.00 | 0.04 | 0.02 | 0.01 | 0.04 | 0.8 | 0.06 | 0.1 | 0.0 | 0.0 | 22 | 0.0 | 0.1 | 3 | 0.0 | 19 | 34 | 0.0 | 143 | 0.08 |
| 23280 | 2 Tbs | Butterscotch, Kraft | 41 | 130 | | 1.0 | 28.0 | 0.0 | 18.0 | 10.0 | 1.5 | 1.0 | | | | | 2 | 200 | 40 | | | | | | | | | | | 0.0 | | | 0 | | 0.0 | | | | 40 | | 150 | |
| 23070 | 2 Tbs | Caramel, avg | 41 | 103 | 32 | 0.6 | 27.0 | 0.4 | 26.5 | 0.1 | 0.0 | 0.0 | 0.0 | 0.0 | 0.00 | 0.00 | 0 | 37 | 11 | | | | 0.00 | 0.04 | 0.02 | 0.01 | 0.04 | 0.8 | 0.06 | 0.1 | 0.0 | 0.0 | 22 | 0.0 | 0.1 | 3 | 0.0 | 19 | 34 | 0.0 | 143 | 0.08 |
| 23281 | 2 Tbs | Caramel, Kraft | 41 | 120 | 26 | 2.0 | 28.0 | 0.0 | 19.0 | 9.0 | 0.0 | 0.0 | 0.0 | 0.0 | 0.00 | 0.00 | 0 | 0 | 0 | 0 | 0 | 0 | | | | | | | | 0.0 | | | 60 | | 0.0 | | | | 90 | | 90 | |
| 23056 | 2 Tbs | Chocolate, avg | 38 | 93 | 29 | 0.7 | 25.0 | 0.7 | 19.7 | 4.6 | 0.5 | 0.3 | 0.2 | 0.0 | 0.00 | [illegible] | 0 | 1651 | 494 | | | | 0.00 | 0.31 | 12.77 | 0.01 | 0.00 | 1.5 | 0.00 | 0.3 | 0.0 | | 5 | 0.2 | 5.2 | 25 | 0.1 | 49 | 183 | 0.5 | 58 | 0.28 |
| 23279 | 2 Tbs | Chocolate, Kraft | 39 | 110 | | 2.0 | 26.0 | 1.0 | 20.0 | 5.0 | 0.0 | 0.0 | 0.0 | 0.0 | 0.00 | 0.00 | 0 | 0 | 0 | 0 | 0 | 0 | | | | | | | | 0.0 | | | 20 | | 0.4 | | | | 190 | | 30 | |
| 23014 | 2 Tbs | Chocolate fudge, avg | 42 | 147 | 22 | 1.9 | 26.4 | 1.2 | 17.6 | 7.7 | 3.7 | 1.7 | 1.6 | 0.1 | 0.01 | [illegible] | 1 | 7 | 2 | | | | 0.02 | 0.09 | 0.12 | 0.03 | 0.09 | 1.7 | 0.20 | 0.1 | 0.0 | 0.0 | 34 | 0.1 | 0.5 | 21 | 0.1 | 57 | 152 | 1.6 | 145 | 0.29 |
| 90112 | 2 Tbs | Chocolate Fudge, Kraft | 41 | 140 | 28 | 1.0 | 24.0 | 0.5 | 17.0 | 6.5 | 4.0 | 2.0 | | | | | 0 | 0 | 0 | 0 | 0 | 0 | | | | | | | | 0.0 | | | 40 | | 0.4 | | | | 85 | | 100 | |
| 23384 | 2 Tbs | Choc Fudge, fat free, fruit swtnd, Weight Watchers | 30 | 90 | 18 | 1.0 | 21.0 | 3.0 | 18.0 | 0.0 | 0.5 | 0.0 | | | | | 0 | 0 | 0 | 0 | 0 | 0 | | | | | | | | 0.0 | | | 60 | | 1.8 | | | | | | 40 | |
| 23388 | 2 Tbs | Hazelnut Fudge, fat free, fruit swtnd, Weight Watchers | 30 | 110 | 22 | 1.0 | 17.0 | 2.0 | 15.0 | 0.0 | 4.0 | 0.0 | | | | | 0 | 0 | 0 | 0 | 0 | 0 | | | | | | | | 0.0 | | | 60 | | 1.8 | | | | | | 40 | |
| 23071 | 2 Tbs | Marshmallow Crème, avg | 38 | 122 | 20 | 0.3 | 30.0 | 0.0 | 17.8 | 12.2 | 0.1 | 0.0 | 0.0 | 0.0 | 0.00 | 0.02 | 0 | 0.4 | 0.04 | 0 | 0.04 | | 0.00 | 0.00 | 0.03 | 0.00 | 0.00 | 0.4 | 0.00 | 0.0 | 0.0 | 0.0 | 1 | 0.0 | 0.1 | 1 | 0.0 | 3 | 2 | 0.7 | 19 | 0.02 |
| 23163 | 2 Tbs | Pineapple, avg | 42 | 106 | 33 | 0.0 | 27.9 | 0.4 | 27.5 | 0.0 | 0.0 | 0.0 | 0.0 | 0.0 | 0.00 | 0.02 | 0 | 9 | 0.8 | 0 | 0.8 | | 0.01 | 0.00 | 0.04 | 0.01 | 0.00 | 1.3 | 0.01 | 24.6 | 0.0 | 0.0 | 9 | 0.0 | 0.2 | 1 | 0.3 | 3 | 133 | 1.3 | 26 | 0.20 |
| 23282 | 2 Tbs | Pineapple, Kraft | 40 | 110 | 33 | 0.0 | 28.0 | 0.0 | 19.0 | 9.0 | 0.0 | 0.0 | 0.0 | 0.0 | 0.00 | 0.00 | 0 | 0 | 0 | 0 | 0 | 0 | | | | | | | | 2.9 | | | 0 | | 0.0 | | | | 15 | | 15 | |
| 23164 | 1 Tbs | Strawberry, avg | 21 | 53 | 33 | 0.0 | 13.9 | 0.2 | 13.7 | 0.0 | 0.0 | 0.0 | 0.0 | 0.0 | 0.00 | [illegible] | 0 | 4 | 0.4 | 0 | 0.4 | | 0.00 | 0.00 | 0.05 | 0.00 | 0.00 | 0.4 | 0.02 | 5.2 | 0.0 | | 5 | 0.0 | 0.2 | 1 | 0.0 | 3 | 15 | 0.4 | 4 | 0.10 |
| 23283 | 2 Tbs | Strawberry, Kraft | 41 | 110 | 33 | 0.0 | 29.0 | 0.0 | 22.0 | 7.0 | 0.0 | 0.0 | 0.0 | 0.0 | 0.00 | 0.00 | 0 | 0 | 0 | 0 | 0 | 0 | | | | | | | | 3.6 | | | 0 | | 0.0 | | | | 25 | | 15 | |
| 23162 | 2 Tbs | With Nuts, avg | 41 | 167 | 19 | 1.8 | 21.9 | 0.7 | | | 9.0 | 0.8 | 2.0 | 5.6 | 0.99 | 4.63 | 0 | 17 | 2 | 0 | 2 | | 0.07 | 0.05 | 0.17 | 0.08 | 0.00 | 8.6 | 0.09 | 0.5 | 0.0 | | 16 | 0.2 | 0.4 | 26 | 0.4 | 46 | 86 | 0.6 | 17 | 0.43 |
| | | **EGGS, SUBSTITUTES AND EGG DISHES** | | | | | | | | | | | | | | | | | | | | | | | | | | | | | | | | | | | | | | | | |
| | | Chicken Egg Whites | | | | | | | | | | | | | | | | | | | | | | | | | | | | | | | | | | | | | | | | |
| 19522 | 1 ea | Cooked, avg | 33 | 17 | 87 | 3.5 | 0.3 | 0.0 | 0.3 | 0.0 | 0.0 | 0.0 | 0.0 | 0.0 | 0.00 | 0.00 | 0 | 0 | 0 | 0 | 0 | 0 | 0.00 | 0.14 | 0.03 | 0.00 | 0.06 | 0.7 | 0.04 | 0.0 | 0.0 | 0.0 | 2 | 0.0 | 0.0 | 4 | 0.0 | 4 | 47 | 5.8 | 105 | 0.00 |
| 19609 | 1/4 cup | Dried, avg | 27 | 103 | 6 | 21.9 | 2.1 | 0.0 | 2.1 | 0.0 | 0.0 | 0.0 | 0.0 | 0.0 | 0.00 | 0.00 | 0 | 0 | 0 | 0 | 0 | 0 | 0.00 | 0.68 | 0.23 | 0.01 | 0.05 | 4.9 | 0.21 | 0.0 | 0.0 | 0.0 | 17 | 0.0 | 0.0 | 24 | 0.0 | 30 | 304 | 33.8 | 346 | 0.03 |
| 19506 | 1 ea | Raw, avg | 33 | 17 | 88 | 3.5 | 0.3 | 0.0 | 0.3 | 0.0 | 0.0 | 0.0 | 0.0 | 0.0 | 0.00 | 0.00 | 0 | 0 | 0 | 0 | 0 | 0 | 0.00 | 0.15 | 0.03 | 0.00 | 0.07 | 1.0 | 0.04 | 0.0 | 0.0 | 0.0 | 2 | 0.0 | 0.0 | 4 | 0.0 | 4 | 47 | 5.8 | 54 | 0.00 |
| 19608 | 1 ea | Raw, fzn, avg | 33 | 16 | 89 | 3.2 | 0.3 | 0.0 | 0.3 | 0.0 | 0.0 | 0.0 | 0.0 | 0.0 | 0.00 | 0.00 | 0 | 0 | 0 | 0 | 0 | 0 | 0.00 | 0.13 | 0.03 | 0.00 | 0.02 | 1.0 | 0.05 | 0.0 | 0.0 | 0.0 | 2 | 0.0 | 0.0 | 3 | 0.0 | 4 | 45 | 5.8 | 52 | 0.01 |
| 19584 | 1/4 cup | Raw, Whipped, Fleischmann's | 33 | 15 | | 4.0 | 0.0 | 0.0 | 0.0 | 0.0 | 0.0 | 0.0 | 0.0 | 0.0 | 0.00 | 0.00 | 0 | | | | | | | | | | | | | | | | | | | | | | 50 | | 55 | |
| | | Chicken Egg Yolks | | | | | | | | | | | | | | | | | | | | | | | | | | | | | | | | | | | | | | | | |
| 19523 | 1 ea | Cooked, avg | 17 | 61 | 49 | 2.8 | 0.3 | 0.0 | 0.3 | 0.0 | 5.2 | 1.6 | 2.0 | 0.7 | 0.04 | 0.67 | [illegible] | 329 | 39 | 99 | 0 | | 0.02 | 0.10 | 0.00 | 0.06 | 0.45 | 18.5 | 0.58 | 0.0 | 0.6 | | 23 | 0.0 | 0.6 | 2 | 0.0 | 83 | 16 | 7.7 | 33 | 0.53 |

| Code | Amount | Description | Basic Components | | | | | | | | | Additional Fats | | | | | | Vit A & Components | | | | | Vitamins | | | | | | | | | | Minerals | | | | | | | | | |
|---|---|---|---|---|---|---|---|---|---|---|---|---|---|---|---|---|---|---|---|---|---|---|---|---|---|---|---|---|---|---|---|---|---|---|---|---|---|---|---|---|---|---|
| | | | Weight (g) | Calories | % Water | Protein (g) | Carbs (g) | Fiber (g) | Sugar (g) | Other Carbs (g) | Fat (g) | Sat Fat (g) | Mono Fat (g) | Poly Fat (g) | Omega 3 (g) | Omega 6 (g) | Choles (mg) | Vit A (IU) | Vit A (RE) | Retinol (RE) | Carotenoids (RE) | Beta Carotene (mcg) | Thiamin (mg) | Riboflavin (mg) | Niacin (NE) | Vit B6 (mg) | Vit B12 (mcg) | Folate (mcg) | Panto (mg) | Vit C (mg) | Vit D (mg) | Vit E (α TE) | Calcium (mg) | Copper (mg) | Iron (mg) | Magnes (mg) | Mang (mg) | Phos (mg) | Potassium (mg) | Selenium (mcg) | Sodium (mg) | Zinc (mg) |
| 19571 | 1/4 cup | Dried, avg | 17 | 113 | 3 | 5.8 | 0.6 | 0.0 | 0.1 | 0.5 | 9.5 | 2.9 | 3.6 | 1.3 | 0.10 | 1.23 | 397 | 224 | 67 | 67 | 0 | | 0.05 | 0.32 | 0.02 | 0.11 | 0.91 | 41.5 | 1.32 | 0.0 | 1.2 | | 48 | 0.0 | 0.9 | 2 | 0.0 | 156 | 41 | 14.8 | 23 | 0.84 |
| 19572 | 1 oz | Frozen, avg | 28 | 85 | 56 | 4.3 | 0.3 | 0.0 | 0.3 | 0.0 | 7.2 | 2.2 | 2.7 | 1.0 | 0.06 | 0.94 | 301 | 395 | 118 | 118 | 0 | | 0.04 | 0.15 | 0.01 | 0.10 | 0.51 | 32.5 | 0.99 | 0.0 | 0.6 | | 39 | 0.0 | 0.9 | 3 | 0.0 | 117 | 33 | 11.7 | 19 | 0.81 |
| 19532 | 1/4 cup | Frozen, salted, avg | 61 | 167 | 51 | 8.5 | 1.0 | 0.0 | 0.9 | 0.1 | 14.0 | 4.3 | 5.4 | 1.9 | 0.17 | 1.75 | 583 | 726 | 218 | 218 | 0 | | 0.08 | 0.26 | 0.02 | 0.16 | 1.54 | 65.3 | 1.97 | 0.0 | 0.0 | | 70 | 0.1 | 2.3 | 6 | 0.0 | 263 | 71 | 23.0 | 2306 | 1.73 |
| 19566 | 1 oz | Frozen, sugared, avg | 28 | 86 | 51 | 3.9 | 3.0 | 0.0 | 3.0 | 0.0 | 6.4 | 2.0 | 2.4 | 0.9 | 0.07 | 0.83 | 269 | 368 | 111 | 111 | 0 | | 0.04 | 0.15 | 0.01 | 0.08 | 0.50 | 38.9 | 0.90 | 0.0 | 0.5 | | 34 | 0.0 | 0.9 | 3 | 0.0 | 108 | 29 | 10.6 | 19 | 0.79 |
| 19508 | 1/4 cup | Raw, avg | 61 | 218 | 49 | 10.2 | 1.1 | 0.0 | 1.1 | 0.0 | 18.8 | 5.8 | 7.1 | 2.6 | 0.14 | 2.42 | 781 | 1186 | 356 | 356 | 0 | | 0.10 | 0.39 | 0.01 | 0.24 | 1.90 | 89.1 | 2.32 | 0.0 | 2.3 | | 84 | 0.0 | 2.2 | 5 | 0.0 | 298 | 57 | 27.6 | 26 | 1.90 |
| | | Chicken Whole Eggs | | | | | | | | | | | | | | | | | | | | | | | | | | | | | | | | | | | | | | | | |
| 19538 | 1/4 cup | Creamed, avg | 60 | 95 | 74 | 4.7 | 3.2 | 0.1 | 1.7 | 1.4 | 7.0 | 2.2 | 2.8 | 1.4 | 0.11 | 1.26 | 116 | 301 | 90 | 86 | 4 | | 0.03 | 0.19 | 0.12 | 0.05 | 0.40 | 13.6 | 0.48 | 0.2 | 0.7 | | 52 | 0.0 | 0.4 | 7 | 0.0 | 76 | 80 | 7.5 | 200 | 0.40 |
| 19539 | 1 ea | Deviled, avg | 31 | 63 | 69 | 3.6 | 0.4 | 0.0 | 0.4 | 0.0 | 5.1 | 1.2 | 1.7 | 1.5 | 0.13 | 1.34 | 121 | 164 | 49 | 49 | 0 | | 0.02 | 0.14 | 0.02 | 0.05 | 0.32 | 12.9 | 0.40 | 0.0 | 0.4 | | 15 | 0.0 | 0.3 | 3 | 0.0 | 49 | 37 | 7.0 | 94 | 0.30 |
| 19527 | 1/4 cup | Dried, avg | 21 | 125 | 3 | 10.0 | 1.0 | 0.0 | 1.0 | 0.0 | 8.6 | 2.7 | 3.2 | 1.2 | 0.12 | 1.09 | 360 | 189 | 57 | 57 | 0 | | 0.04 | 0.32 | 0.06 | 0.08 | 0.83 | 35.9 | 1.24 | 0.0 | 1.1 | | 49 | 0.0 | 1.4 | 9 | 0.0 | 175 | 104 | 25.2 | 110 | 1.11 |
| 19509 | 1 ea | Fried, avg | 46 | 92 | 69 | 6.2 | 0.6 | 0.0 | 0.6 | 0.0 | 6.9 | 1.9 | 2.7 | 1.3 | 0.06 | 1.22 | 211 | 394 | 114 | 114 | 0 | | 0.03 | 0.24 | 0.04 | 0.07 | 0.42 | 17.5 | 0.56 | 0.0 | 0.6 | | 25 | 0.0 | 0.7 | 5 | 0.0 | 89 | 61 | 12.4 | 162 | 0.55 |
| 19604 | 1 ea | Frozen, avg | 50 | 74 | 76 | 6.0 | 0.5 | 0.0 | 0.5 | 0.0 | 5.1 | 1.6 | 1.9 | 0.7 | 0.08 | 0.62 | 216 | 263 | 79 | 79 | 0 | | 0.03 | 0.23 | 0.04 | 0.08 | 0.54 | 36.5 | 0.74 | 0.0 | 0.6 | | 30 | 0.0 | 0.9 | 6 | 0.0 | 101 | 65 | 15.4 | 66 | 0.69 |
| 19510 | 1 ea | Hard Cooked/Boiled, avg | 50 | 78 | 75 | 6.3 | 0.6 | 0.0 | 0.6 | 0.0 | 5.3 | 1.6 | 2.0 | 0.7 | 0.04 | 0.67 | 212 | 280 | 84 | 84 | 0 | | 0.03 | 0.26 | 0.03 | 0.06 | 0.56 | 22.0 | 0.70 | 0.0 | 0.6 | | 25 | 0.0 | 0.6 | 5 | 0.0 | 86 | 63 | 15.4 | 62 | 0.52 |
| 19534 | 1 ea | Omelet, plain, w/milk & butter, avg | 61 | 93 | 76 | 6.3 | 0.6 | 0.0 | 0.6 | 0.0 | 7.0 | 1.9 | 2.8 | 1.3 | 0.06 | 1.24 | 214 | 399 | 114 | 112 | 2 | | 0.03 | 0.24 | 0.04 | 0.07 | 0.43 | 17.7 | 0.57 | 0.0 | 0.8 | | 26 | 0.0 | 0.7 | 5 | 0.0 | 90 | 62 | 13.7 | 165 | 0.56 |
| 19619 | 1 ea | Omelet, w/cheese & ham, avg | 78 | 142 | 71 | 9.8 | 0.8 | 0.0 | | | 10.8 | 3.9 | 4.1 | 1.6 | | | 231 | 495 | 138 | 133 | 5 | | 0.08 | 0.29 | 0.41 | 0.10 | 0.54 | 19.0 | | 0.0 | | | 70 | 0.0 | 0.8 | 9 | | 163 | 98 | | 368 | 0.98 |
| 19614 | 1 ea | Omelet, w/chicken, avg | 95 | 148 | 74 | 12.7 | 0.8 | 0.0 | 0.8 | 0.0 | 10.1 | 3.7 | 4.0 | 1.9 | 0.10 | 1.01 | 287 | 518 | 148 | 145 | 3 | | 0.04 | 0.34 | 1.09 | 0.13 | 0.58 | 23.6 | 0.95 | 0.0 | 1.0 | | 35 | 0.0 | 1.1 | 10 | 0.0 | 141 | 109 | 16.0 | 222 | 1.06 |
| 19611 | 1 ea | Omelet, w/dark green vegs, avg | 84 | 95 | 80 | 6.7 | 1.9 | 0.7 | 0.9 | 0.3 | 6.7 | 2.2 | 3.0 | 1.4 | 0.07 | 1.34 | 202 | 1279 | 198 | 105 | 93 | | 0.04 | 0.27 | 0.19 | 0.11 | 0.40 | 38.4 | 0.72 | 16.5 | 0.8 | | 45 | 0.0 | 1.2 | 16 | 0.2 | 101 | 152 | 11.4 | 201 | 0.67 |
| 19610 | 1 ea | Omelet, w/fish, avg | 88 | 132 | 75 | 10.4 | 0.8 | 0.0 | 0.8 | 0.0 | 9.3 | 3.4 | 3.6 | 1.9 | 0.30 | 0.75 | 267 | 492 | 141 | 138 | 3 | | 0.04 | 0.32 | 0.95 | 0.12 | 1.13 | 23.6 | 0.78 | 0.0 | 3.1 | | 61 | 0.0 | 1.0 | 11 | 0.0 | 156 | 120 | 23.3 | 277 | 0.81 |
| 19580 | 1 ea | Omelet, w/Ham & Cheese, Weight Watchers | 113 | 229 | 55 | 13.0 | 29.9 | 3.0 | 4.0 | 22.9 | 6.0 | 3.0 | | | | | 35 | 299 | 60 | | | | | | | | | | | 2.4 | | | 60 | | 1.1 | | | | 199 | | 468 | |
| 19612 | 1 ea | Omelet, w/mushrooms, avg | 69 | 91 | 78 | 6.2 | 1.1 | 0.1 | 0.7 | 0.2 | 6.7 | 2.6 | 2.7 | 1.3 | 0.06 | 0.60 | 204 | 381 | 109 | 106 | 3 | | 0.04 | 0.28 | 0.48 | 0.07 | 0.41 | 19.2 | 0.85 | 0.4 | 0.9 | | 25 | 0.1 | 0.8 | 6 | 0.0 | 97 | 99 | 11.0 | 157 | 0.61 |
| 19536 | 1 ea | Omelet, w/onion, pep, tom & mush, avg | 145 | 125 | 84 | 5.4 | 7.2 | 1.6 | | | 8.8 | 2.0 | 3.6 | 2.3 | | | 126 | 680 | 147 | 119 | 28 | | 0.09 | 0.34 | 1.89 | 0.15 | 0.26 | 27.8 | | 13.6 | | | 28 | 0.3 | 1.2 | 15 | | 117 | 325 | | 251 | 0.74 |
| 19613 | 1 ea | Omelet, w/sausage, avg | 95 | 172 | 71 | 10.7 | 1.3 | 0.2 | 0.9 | 0.2 | 13.4 | 4.9 | 5.6 | 2.1 | 0.17 | 1.28 | 254 | 447 | 128 | 125 | 2 | | 0.17 | 0.32 | 0.99 | 0.14 | 0.79 | 21.2 | 0.92 | 0.4 | 1.3 | | 35 | 0.1 | 1.1 | 10 | 0.0 | 140 | 145 | 15.2 | 454 | 1.14 |
| 19517 | 1 ea | Poached, avg | 50 | 74 | 75 | 6.2 | 0.6 | 0.0 | 0.6 | 0.0 | 5.0 | 1.5 | 1.9 | 0.7 | 0.04 | 0.64 | 212 | 316 | 95 | 95 | 0 | | 0.02 | 0.22 | 0.03 | 0.06 | 0.40 | 17.5 | 0.56 | 0.0 | 0.6 | | 24 | 0.0 | 0.7 | 5 | 0.0 | 88 | 60 | 15.4 | 140 | 0.55 |
| 19501 | 1 ea | Raw, avg | 50 | 74 | 75 | 6.3 | 0.6 | 0.0 | 0.6 | 0.0 | 5.0 | 1.5 | 1.9 | 0.7 | 0.04 | 0.64 | 212 | 318 | 96 | 96 | 0 | | 0.03 | 0.25 | 0.04 | 0.07 | 0.50 | 23.5 | 0.63 | 0.0 | 0.6 | | 24 | 0.0 | 0.7 | 5 | 0.0 | 89 | 60 | 15.4 | 63 | 0.55 |
| 19516 | 1 ea | Scrambled, avg | 61 | 101 | 73 | 6.8 | 1.3 | 0.0 | 1.3 | 0.0 | 7.4 | 2.2 | 2.9 | 1.3 | 0.07 | 1.24 | 215 | 416 | 119 | 101 | 18 | | 0.03 | 0.27 | 0.05 | 0.07 | 0.47 | 18.3 | 0.62 | 0.1 | 1.0 | | 43 | 0.0 | 0.7 | 7 | 0.0 | 104 | 84 | 13.7 | 171 | 0.61 |
| 19620 | 1/2 cup | Scrambled, no choles, avg | 70 | 127 | 69 | 9.0 | 2.5 | 0.0 | 2.5 | 0.0 | 8.8 | 1.5 | 1.9 | 5.0 | 0.05 | 4.91 | 1 | 1074 | 107 | 0 | 107 | | 0.08 | 0.29 | 0.11 | 0.10 | 0.23 | 9.8 | 1.32 | 0.3 | 0.8 | | 58 | 0.0 | 1.6 | 12 | 0.0 | 57 | 169 | | 159 | 0.78 |
| 19621 | 1/2 cup | Scrambled, no choles, w/cheese, avg | 70 | 59 | 81 | 9.0 | 1.9 | 0.0 | 1.9 | 0.0 | 1.4 | 0.9 | 0.4 | 0.0 | | | 3 | 52 | 12 | 11 | 1.5 | | 0.01 | 0.34 | 0.07 | 0.01 | 0.14 | 2.1 | 0.08 | 0.0 | 0.8 | | 60 | 0.0 | 0.1 | 10 | 0.0 | 80 | 124 | | 248 | 0.26 |
| 19540 | 1/2 cup | Scrambled, prep f/dry, avg | 107 | 238 | 68 | 9.9 | 1.2 | 0.0 | 1.2 | 0.0 | 21.3 | 5.1 | 9.3 | 5.1 | 0.31 | 4.75 | 411 | 1061 | 291 | 278 | 13 | | 0.06 | 0.24 | 0.05 | 0.08 | 1.83 | 29.7 | 1.37 | 0.0 | 1.1 | | 51 | 0.1 | 1.7 | 11 | 0.0 | 149 | 111 | 28.6 | 469 | 1.19 |
| 19551 | 1/2 cup | Scrambled, prep f/fzn, avg | 70 | 92 | 73 | 9.2 | 5.3 | 0.0 | 5.3 | 0.0 | 3.9 | 0.7 | 1.6 | 1.2 | | | 45 | 1718 | 172 | 0 | 172 | | 0.01 | 0.21 | 0.06 | 0.01 | 0.12 | 11.9 | 1.12 | 0.0 | 0.7 | | 12 | 0.0 | 0.2 | 7 | 0.0 | 21 | 103 | 16.0 | 113 | 0.10 |
| 19552 | 1/2 cup | Scrambled, prep f/liquid, avg | 105 | 101 | 80 | 14.3 | 0.8 | 0.0 | 0.8 | 0.0 | 3.9 | 0.8 | 1.1 | 1.9 | 0.22 | 1.68 | 1 | 2577 | 258 | 0 | 258 | | 0.11 | 0.34 | 0.12 | 0.00 | 0.30 | 13.3 | 3.22 | 0.0 | 1.1 | | 63 | 0.0 | 2.5 | 10 | 0.0 | 145 | 394 | 17.3 | 211 | 1.55 |
| 19591 | 1 oz | Scrambled, raw, fzn, low choles, MG Waldbaum | 28 | 18 | 85 | 3.0 | 0.4 | 0.1 | 0.3 | 0.0 | 0.5 | 0.2 | 0.2 | 0.1 | | | 25 | 28 | 8 | 8 | 0 | | | | | | | | | 0.1 | | | 12 | | 0.1 | | | | | | 57 | |
| | | Other Eggs | | | | | | | | | | | | | | | | | | | | | | | | | | | | | | | | | | | | | | | | |
| 19575 | 1 oz | Ant, raw, avg | 28 | 36 | 72 | 4.9 | 1.4 | | | | 1.1 | | | | | | | | | | | | 0.12 | 0.21 | | | | | | | | | 20 | | 0.6 | | | 61 | | | | |
| 19528 | 1 ea | Duck, raw, avg | 70 | 129 | 71 | 9.0 | 1.0 | 0.0 | 1.0 | 0.0 | 9.7 | 2.6 | 4.6 | 0.9 | 0.07 | 0.61 | 619 | 930 | 279 | 268 | 11 | | 0.11 | 0.28 | 0.14 | 0.17 | 3.78 | 56.0 | 1.30 | 0.0 | 3.5 | | 45 | 0.0 | 2.7 | 11 | 0.0 | 154 | 155 | 25.5 | 102 | 0.99 |
| 19529 | 1 ea | Goose,raw, avg | 144 | 266 | 70 | 20.0 | 1.9 | 0.0 | 1.9 | 0.0 | 19.2 | 5.2 | 8.3 | 2.4 | 0.80 | 1.38 | 1227 | 1843 | 553 | | | | 0.21 | 0.55 | 0.27 | 0.34 | 7.34 | 108.9 | 2.53 | 0.0 | 1.9 | | 86 | 0.1 | 5.2 | 23 | 0.1 | 300 | 302 | 53.1 | 199 | 1.92 |
| 19574 | 1 oz | Lizard, raw, avg | 28 | 55 | 68 | 4.5 | 0.0 | 0.0 | 0.0 | 0.0 | 3.9 | | | | | | | | | | | | 0.04 | 0.07 | 0.03 | | | | | | | | 101 | | 0.5 | | | 45 | | | | |
| 19530 | 1 ea | Quail, raw, avg | 9 | 14 | 74 | 1.2 | 0.0 | 0.0 | 0.0 | 0.0 | 1.0 | 0.3 | 0.4 | 0.1 | 0.00 | 0.10 | 76 | 27 | 8 | | | | 0.01 | 0.07 | 0.01 | 0.01 | 0.14 | 6.0 | 0.16 | 0.0 | 0.1 | | 6 | 0.0 | 0.3 | 1 | 0.0 | 20 | 12 | 2.9 | 13 | 0.13 |
| 19576 | 1 oz | Tortoise, raw, avg | 28 | 40 | 77 | 3.4 | 0.0 | 0.0 | 0.0 | 0.0 | 2.9 | | | | | | | | | | | | 0.03 | 0.13 | | | | | | | | | 24 | | 0.4 | | | 54 | | | | |
| 19531 | 1 ea | Turkey, raw, avg | 79 | 135 | 72 | 10.8 | 0.9 | 0.0 | 0.9 | 0.0 | 9.4 | 2.9 | 3.6 | 1.3 | 0.06 | 1.02 | 737 | 438 | 131 | 131 | 0 | | 0.09 | 0.37 | 0.02 | 0.10 | 1.34 | 56.2 | 1.49 | 0.0 | 1.0 | | 78 | 0.0 | 3.2 | 10 | 0.0 | 134 | 112 | 27.1 | 119 | 1.25 |
| | | Substitutes | | | | | | | | | | | | | | | | | | | | | | | | | | | | | | | | | | | | | | | | |
| 19524 | 1/4 cup | Frozen, avg | 60 | 96 | 73 | 6.8 | 1.9 | 0.0 | 1.9 | 0.0 | 6.7 | 1.2 | 1.5 | 3.7 | 0.04 | 3.71 | 1 | 810 | 81 | 81 | 0 | | 0.07 | 0.23 | 0.08 | 0.08 | 0.20 | 9.8 | 1.00 | 0.3 | 0.6 | | 44 | 0.0 | 1.2 | 9 | 0.0 | 43 | 128 | 24.8 | 119 | 0.59 |
| 7736 | 1/4 cup | Frozen, Scramblers, Morningstar Farms | 57 | 37 | 83 | 6.2 | 2.2 | 0.3 | 1.3 | 0.6 | 0.4 | | | | | | 2 | 311 | 31 | 0 | 31 | | 0.28 | 0.39 | 0.00 | 0.13 | 1.77 | | 1.85 | 0.0 | | | 31 | | 1.1 | | | 60 | 50 | | 97 | 0.80 |
| 19525 | 1/4 cup | Liquid, avg | 63 | 53 | 83 | 7.6 | 0.4 | 0.0 | 0.4 | 0.0 | 2.1 | 0.4 | 0.6 | 1.0 | 0.12 | 0.89 | 1 | 1361 | 136 | 136 | 0 | | 0.07 | 0.19 | 0.07 | 0.00 | 0.19 | 9.4 | 1.70 | 0.0 | 0.6 | | 33 | 0.0 | 1.3 | 6 | 0.0 | 76 | 208 | 15.7 | 112 | 0.82 |
| 7772 | 1/4 cup | Liquid, Better 'n Eggs | 50 | 25 | 88 | 5.2 | 0.5 | 0.0 | 0.5 | 0.0 | 0.0 | 0.0 | 0.0 | 0.0 | 0.00 | 0.00 | 0 | 0 | 0 | 0 | 0 | 0 | 0.00 | 0.25 | 0.00 | 0.06 | 0.24 | | | 0.0 | 0.0 | | 3 | | 0.0 | | | 6 | 70 | | 81 | |
| 19581 | 1/4 cup | Liquid, Egg Beaters | 61 | 30 | | 6.0 | 1.0 | 0.0 | 1.0 | 0.0 | 0.0 | 0.0 | 0.0 | 0.0 | 0.00 | 0.00 | 0 | 200 | 40 | | | | | | | | | | | | | | 40 | | 1.1 | | | | 85 | | 100 | |
| 19526 | 1 oz | Powder, avg | 28 | 124 | 4 | 15.5 | 6.1 | 0.0 | 6.1 | 0.0 | 3.6 | 1.1 | 1.5 | 0.5 | 0.02 | 0.43 | 160 | 344 | 103 | 103 | 0 | | 0.06 | 0.49 | 0.16 | 0.04 | 0.99 | 35.0 | 0.95 | 0.2 | 1.0 | | 91 | 0.1 | 0.9 | 18 | 0.0 | 134 | 208 | 35.8 | 224 | 0.51 |
| 19625 | 1 oz | Prep f/Dry Mix, Bateman's | 28 | 31 | 71 | 3.9 | 2.0 | 0.6 | 0.0 | 1.5 | 0.6 | 0.0 | | | | | 0 | 325 | 65 | | | | | | | | | | | 67.2 | | | 12 | | 0.4 | | | | | | 73 | |
| | | **FAST FOODS** | | | | | | | | | | | | | | | | | | | | | | | | | | | | | | | | | | | | | | | | |
| | | *GENERIC FAST FOOD* | | | | | | | | | | | | | | | | | | | | | | | | | | | | | | | | | | | | | | | | |
| | | Breakfast Items | | | | | | | | | | | | | | | | | | | | | | | | | | | | | | | | | | | | | | | | |
| 56600 | 1 ea | Biscuit w/Egg | 136 | 316 | 51 | 11.1 | 24.2 | 0.3 | | | 20.3 | 6.2 | 8.2 | 4.2 | | | 233 | 649 | 178 | 159 | 20 | | 0.34 | 0.34 | 0.71 | 0.08 | 0.75 | 61.2 | 1.05 | 0.0 | | | 154 | 0.1 | 3.1 | 20 | 0.3 | 185 | 160 | 27.3 | 654 | 1.10 |
| 56601 | 1 ea | Biscuit w/Egg & Bacon | 150 | 458 | 47 | 17.0 | 28.7 | 0.8 | | | 31.1 | 8.0 | 13.4 | 7.5 | 0.53 | 6.93 | 352 | 191 | 53 | 47 | 6 | | 0.14 | 0.23 | 2.40 | 0.14 | 1.03 | 60.0 | 1.22 | 2.7 | | | 189 | 0.1 | 3.7 | 24 | 0.3 | 238 | 250 | 30.9 | 999 | 1.63 |
| 56602 | 1 ea | Biscuit w/Egg & Ham | 192 | 442 | 55 | 20.4 | 30.3 | 0.8 | | | 27.1 | 5.9 | 11.0 | 7.7 | 0.50 | 7.20 | 300 | 874 | 240 | 113 | 127 | | 0.67 | 0.60 | 2.00 | 0.27 | 1.19 | 65.3 | 1.67 | 0.0 | | | 221 | 0.1 | 4.6 | 31 | 0.3 | 317 | 319 | 36.9 | 1382 | 2.23 |
| 66028 | 1 ea | Biscuit w/Egg & Sausage | 180 | 581 | 43 | 19.1 | 41.2 | 0.9 | | | 38.7 | 15.0 | 16.4 | 4.4 | 0.25 | 4.20 | 302 | 635 | 164 | 146 | 18 | | 0.50 | 0.45 | 3.60 | 0.20 | 1.37 | 64.8 | 1.53 | 0.0 | | | 155 | 0.1 | 4.0 | 25 | 0.3 | 490 | 320 | 34.2 | 1141 | 2.16 |
| 56603 | 1 ea | Biscuit w/Egg & Steak | 148 | 410 | 52 | 17.9 | 21.3 | | | | 28.4 | 8.6 | 11.7 | 5.8 | | | 272 | 704 | 191 | 170 | 21 | | 0.36 | 0.52 | 3.06 | 0.18 | 1.41 | 56.2 | 1.08 | 0.1 | | | 138 | 0.1 | 5.3 | 25 | 0.2 | 225 | 306 | 31.4 | 888 | 2.80 |
| 66029 | 1 ea | Biscuit w/Egg, Cheese & Bacon | 144 | 477 | 41 | 16.3 | 33.4 | 0.3 | | | 31.4 | 11.4 | 14.2 | 3.5 | 0.15 | 3.35 | 261 | 648 | 166 | 147 | 18 | | 0.30 | 0.43 | 2.30 | 0.10 | 1.05 | 53.3 | 1.18 | 1.6 | | | 164 | 0.1 | 2.5 | 20 | 0.3 | 459 | 230 | 35.6 | 1260 | 1.54 |
| 56604 | 1 ea | Biscuit w/Ham | 113 | 386 | 28 | 13.4 | 43.8 | 0.8 | | | 18.4 | 11.4 | 4.8 | 1.0 | 0.09 | 0.95 | 25 | 133 | 34 | 30 | 4 | | 0.51 | 0.32 | 3.48 | 0.14 | 0.03 | 38.4 | 0.41 | 0.1 | | | 160 | 0.0 | 2.7 | 23 | 0.4 | 554 | 197 | 19.3 | 1433 | 1.65 |
| 66030 | 1 ea | Biscuit w/Sausage | 124 | 485 | 29 | 12.1 | 40.1 | 1.4 | | | 31.7 | 14.3 | 12.8 | 3.0 | 0.27 | 2.76 | 35 | 56 | 14 | 12 | 2 | | 0.40 | 0.29 | 3.27 | 0.11 | 0.51 | 45.9 | 0.36 | 0.1 | | | 128 | 0.0 | 2.6 | 20 | 0.4 | 446 | 198 | 23.2 | 1071 | 1.55 |
| 56605 | 1 ea | Biscuit w/Steak | 141 | 455 | 33 | 13.1 | 44.4 | | | | 25.9 | 6.9 | 11.1 | 6.4 | | | 25 | 65 | 16 | 14 | 2 | | 0.35 | 0.39 | 4.16 | 0.16 | 0.94 | 63.4 | 0.41 | 0.1 | | | 116 | 0.1 | 4.3 | 27 | 0.4 | 204 | 234 | 32.9 | 795 | 2.66 |
| 56606 | 1 ea | Croissant w/Egg & Cheese | 127 | 368 | 46 | 12.8 | 24.3 | | | | 24.8 | 14.1 | 7.5 | 1.4 | | | 216 | 1001 | 255 | 184 | 72 | | 0.19 | 0.38 | 1.51 | 0.10 | 0.77 | 47.0 | 1.05 | 0.1 | | | 244 | 0.1 | 2.2 | 22 | 0.2 | 348 | 174 | 24.5 | 551 | 1.75 |
| 56607 | 1 ea | Croissant w/Egg, Cheese & Bacon | 129 | 413 | 44 | 16.3 | 23.6 | | | | 28.4 | 15.5 | 9.2 | 1.8 | | | 215 | 472 | 120 | 86 | 34 | | 0.35 | 0.34 | 2.19 | 0.12 | 0.86 | 45.1 | 1.07 | 2.2 | | | 151 | 0.1 | 2.2 | 23 | 0.2 | 276 | 201 | 24.5 | 889 | 1.90 |
| 56608 | 1 ea | Croissant w/Egg, Cheese & Ham | 152 | 474 | 51 | 19.0 | 24.2 | | | | 33.6 | 17.5 | 11.4 | 2.4 | | | 213 | 451 | 117 | 84 | 33 | | 0.52 | 0.30 | 3.19 | 0.23 | 1.00 | 45.6 | 1.25 | 11.4 | | | 144 | 0.1 | 2.1 | 26 | 0.2 | 336 | 272 | 27.2 | 1081 | 2.17 |
| 56609 | 1 ea | Croissant w/Egg, Cheese & Sausage | 160 | 523 | 46 | 20.3 | 24.8 | | | | 38.2 | 18.2 | 14.3 | 3.0 | | | 216 | 422 | 109 | 78 | 31 | | 0.99 | 0.32 | 4.00 | 0.11 | 0.90 | 43.2 | 1.31 | 0.2 | | | 144 | 0.1 | 3.0 | 24 | 0.3 | 290 | 283 | 20.6 | 1115 | 2.14 |
| 66031 | 1 ea | English Muffins w/Cheese & Sausage | 115 | 393 | 38 | 15.3 | 29.2 | 1.5 | | | 24.3 | 9.9 | 10.1 | 2.7 | 0.15 | 2.54 | 59 | 380 | 86 | 76 | 10 | | 0.70 | 0.25 | 4.14 | 0.15 | 0.68 | 66.7 | 0.53 | 1.3 | | | 168 | 0.1 | 2.3 | 24 | 0.2 | 186 | 215 | 21.3 | 1036 | 1.68 |
| 66033 | 1 ea | English Muffins w/Egg, Cheese & Sausage | 165 | 487 | 47 | 21.6 | 31.0 | 0.4 | | | 30.9 | 12.4 | 12.8 | 3.3 | 0.11 | 3.21 | 274 | 660 | 172 | 160 | 12 | | 0.84 | 0.50 | 4.45 | 0.20 | 1.37 | 54.5 | 1.40 | 1.5 | | | 196 | 0.1 | 3.5 | 30 | 0.3 | 287 | 294 | 31.0 | 1135 | 2.36 |
| 66032 | 1 ea | English Muffins w/Egg, Cheese & Canadian Bacon | 146 | 308 | 57 | 17.8 | 28.5 | 1.6 | 2.9 | 23.9 | 13.4 | 5.0 | 5.0 | 1.7 | 0.12 | 1.54 | 250 | 625 | 166 | 155 | 12 | | 0.53 | 0.48 | 3.55 | 0.16 | 0.72 | 46.7 | 0.95 | 1.9 | | | 161 | 0.1 | 2.6 | 25 | 0.0 | 288 | 212 | 36.2 | 777 | 1.66 |
| 19533 | 1 ea | Scrambled Eggs | 47 | 100 | 67 | 6.5 | 1.0 | 0.0 | 1.0 | 0.0 | 7.6 | 2.9 | 2.8 | 0.9 | 0.06 | 0.87 | 200 | 418 | 126 | 121 | 5 | | 0.04 | 0.24 | 0.10 | 0.09 | 0.47 | 26.3 | 0.44 | 1.6 | | | 27 | 0.0 | 1.2 | 7 | 0.0 | 114 | 69 | 10.6 | 105 | 0.78 |
| | | Chicken Items | | | | | | | | | | | | | | | | | | | | | | | | | | | | | | | | | | | | | | | | |
| 15065 | 1 pce | Pieces, breaded, fried | 17 | 46 | 51 | 2.9 | 2.4 | 0.0 | 0.0 | 2.4 | 2.8 | 0.6 | 1.2 | 0.6 | 0.02 | 0.36 | 10 | 0 | 0 | 0 | 0 | 0 | 0.02 | 0.03 | 1.20 | 0.05 | 0.05 | 4.9 | 0.14 | 0.0 | 0.1 | | 2 | 0.0 | 0.2 | 4 | 0.0 | 46 | 49 | 2.8 | 82 | 0.16 |
| 15066 | 6 pce | Pieces, breaded, fried w/barbeque sauce | 130 | 330 | 52 | 17.2 | 25.1 | 2.2 | 9.4 | 13.5 | 17.9 | 5.6 | 8.8 | 2.4 | 0.15 | 2.25 | 61 | 342 | 47 | 37 | 10 | | 0.10 | 0.16 | 7.02 | 0.34 | 0.30 | 29.9 | 0.96 | 0.8 | 0.4 | | 21 | 0.2 | 1.5 | 25 | 0.2 | 214 | 318 | 17.2 | 829 | 1.12 |
| 15180 | 6 pce | Pieces, breaded, fried w/honey | 115 | 329 | 45 | 16.8 | 26.9 | | | | 17.6 | 5.5 | 8.6 | 2.2 | 0.10 | 2.13 | 61 | 101 | 30 | 29.5 | 0.5 | | 0.09 | 0.15 | 6.81 | 0.31 | 0.30 | 29.9 | 0.91 | 0.5 | | | 17 | 0.2 | 1.3 | 20 | 0.1 | 202 | 255 | 16.6 | 537 | 1.08 |

| Code | Amount | Description | Weight (g) | Calories | % Water | Protein (g) | Carbs (g) | Fiber (g) | Sugar (g) | Other Carbs (g) | Fat (g) | Sat Fat (g) | Mono Fat (g) | Poly Fat (g) | Omega 3 (g) | Omega 6 (g) | Choles (mg) |
|---|---|---|---|---|---|---|---|---|---|---|---|---|---|---|---|---|---|
| | | | Basic Components | | | | | | | | | Additional Fats | | | | | |
| 15067 | 6 pce | Pieces, breaded, fried w/mustard sauce | 130 | 322 | 54 | 17.4 | 20.8 | 1.2 | 11.0 | 8.6 | 13.0 | 5.7 | 9.0 | 2.9 | 0.24 | 2.57 | 61 |
| 15068 | 6 pce | Pieces, breaded, fried w/sweet & sour sauce | 130 | 346 | 49 | 16.9 | 29.0 | 1.0 | 16.3 | 11.7 | 17.9 | 5.5 | 8.6 | 2.2 | 0.10 | 2.14 | 61 |
| 15187 | 1 ea | Wing, hot and spicy | 61 | 220 | 38 | 14.0 | 5.0 | | | | 16.0 | 4.0 | | | | | 65 |
| 15177 | 1 ea | Wing, hot wings | 135 | 471 | 38 | 27.0 | 18.0 | | | | 33.0 | | | | | | 150 |
| | | Dessert Items | | | | | | | | | | | | | | | |
| 47150 | 1 ea | Brownie, w/out nuts | 60 | 243 | 13 | 2.7 | 39.0 | | | | 10.1 | 3.1 | 3.8 | 2.6 | | | 10 |
| 66034 | 1 ea | Caramel Sundae | 155 | 304 | 56 | 7.3 | 49.3 | 0.0 | | | 9.3 | 4.5 | 3.0 | 1.3 | 0.11 | 0.90 | 25 |
| 45588 | 1 ea | Danish Pastry, cheese | 91 | 353 | 34 | 5.8 | 28.7 | | | | 24.7 | 5.1 | 15.6 | 2.4 | 0.00 | 2.42 | 20 |
| 45512 | 1 ea | Danish Pastry, cinnamon | 88 | 349 | 21 | 4.8 | 46.8 | 0.3 | | | 16.7 | 3.5 | 10.6 | 1.5 | 0.00 | 1.65 | 27 |
| 45513 | 1 ea | Danish Pastry, fruit | 94 | 335 | 29 | 4.8 | 45.0 | | | | 16.0 | 3.3 | 10.1 | 1.6 | 0.00 | 1.57 | 19 |
| 2035 | 1/2 cup | Frozen Yogurt, chocolate, soft serve | 72 | 115 | 64 | 2.9 | 17.9 | 1.6 | 14.3 | 2.0 | 4.3 | 2.6 | 1.3 | 0.2 | 0.05 | 0.10 | 4 |
| 2064 | 1/2 cup | Frozen Yogurt, vanilla, soft serve | 72 | 114 | 65 | 2.9 | 17.4 | 0.0 | 17.3 | 0.1 | 4.0 | 2.5 | 1.1 | 0.2 | 0.06 | 0.09 | 1 |
| 2032 | 1 ea | Hot Fudge Sundae | 158 | 284 | 60 | 5.6 | 47.7 | 0.0 | | | 8.6 | 5.0 | 2.3 | 0.8 | 0.08 | 0.73 | 21 |
| 2031 | 1 ea | Ice Milk Cone, soft serve, svg | 103 | 164 | 66 | 3.9 | 24.1 | 0.1 | | | 6.1 | 3.5 | 1.8 | 0.4 | 0.08 | 0.28 | 28 |
| 49117 | 1 ea | Lemon Pie | 128 | 404 | 38 | 3.8 | 54.5 | 3.3 | 15.4 | 35.8 | 20.6 | 3.1 | 9.5 | 6.9 | 0.73 | 6.16 | 0 |
| 2033 | 1 ea | Strawberry sundae | 153 | 268 | 61 | 6.3 | 44.7 | 0.0 | | | 7.8 | 3.7 | 2.7 | 1.0 | 0.08 | 0.94 | 21 |
| 7208 | 1 ea | French Fries, medium svg | 76 | 232 | 40 | 3.3 | 29.3 | 2.7 | 0.0 | 26.7 | 11.2 | 1.9 | 5.0 | 2.8 | 0.11 | 1.77 | 0 |
| 56666 | 5 pce | Hushpuppies | 78 | 257 | 32 | 4.9 | 34.9 | 2.7 | | | 11.6 | 2.7 | 7.8 | 0.4 | 0.03 | 0.35 | 135 |
| | | Milkshakes | | | | | | | | | | | | | | | |
| 2020 | 1 cup | Chocolate | 166 | 211 | 72 | 5.6 | 34.0 | 1.3 | 29.2 | 3.5 | 6.1 | 3.8 | 1.8 | 0.2 | 0.09 | 0.14 | 22 |
| 2022 | 1 cup | Strawberry | 226 | 255 | 74 | 7.7 | 42.7 | 0.9 | 41.8 | 0.0 | 6.3 | 3.9 | 1.8 | 0.3 | 0.00 | 0.14 | 25 |
| 2024 | 1 cup | Vanilla | 166 | 184 | 75 | 5.8 | 29.7 | 0.7 | 29.0 | 0.0 | 5.0 | 3.1 | 1.4 | 0.2 | 0.07 | 0.11 | 18 |
| 6176 | 8 1/2 pce | Onion Rings | 83 | 276 | 37 | 3.7 | 31.3 | | | | 15.5 | 7.0 | 6.6 | 0.7 | 0.11 | 0.56 | 14 |
| | | Potatoes | | | | | | | | | | | | | | | |
| 6177 | 1 ea | Baked w/Cheese Sauce | 296 | 474 | 66 | 14.6 | 46.5 | | | | 28.7 | 10.5 | 10.7 | 6.0 | | | 18 |
| 6178 | 1 ea | Baked w/Cheese Sauce & Bacon | 299 | 451 | 65 | 18.4 | 44.6 | | | | 25.9 | 10.1 | 9.7 | 4.8 | | | 30 |
| 6179 | 1 ea | Baked w/Cheese sauce & Broccoli | 339 | 403 | 70 | 13.7 | 46.4 | | | | 21.4 | 8.5 | 7.7 | 4.2 | | | 20 |
| 6180 | 1 ea | Baked w/Cheese Sauce & Chili | 395 | 482 | 70 | 23.2 | 55.7 | | | | 21.3 | 13.0 | 6.8 | 0.9 | | | 32 |
| 5463 | 1/2 cup | Hash Browns | 72 | 151 | 60 | 1.9 | 16.1 | | | | 9.2 | 4.3 | 3.9 | 0.5 | 0.07 | 0.40 | 9 |
| 6185 | 1/3 cup | Mashed | 80 | 66 | 79 | 1.8 | 12.9 | | | | 1.0 | 0.4 | 0.3 | 0.2 | | | 2 |
| | | Salads | | | | | | | | | | | | | | | |
| 56628 | 1 1/2 cup | Chef Style, w/turkey, ham & cheese | 326 | 267 | 82 | 26.0 | 4.7 | | | | 16.1 | 8.2 | 5.2 | 1.4 | | | 140 |
| 5461 | 3/4 cup | Coleslaw | 99 | 147 | 74 | 1.5 | 12.8 | 1.7 | | | 11.0 | 1.6 | 2.4 | 6.4 | 0.77 | 5.62 | 5 |
| 6173 | 1/3 cup | Potato | 95 | 108 | 79 | 1.5 | 12.8 | | | | 5.7 | 1.0 | 1.6 | 2.9 | 0.28 | 2.58 | 57 |
| 56623 | 1 1/2 cup | Tossed Vegetable, w/o dressing | 207 | 33 | 96 | 2.6 | 6.7 | | | | 0.1 | 0.0 | 0.0 | 0.1 | | | 0 |
| | | Sandwiches, Cheeseburger | | | | | | | | | | | | | | | |
| 66016 | 1 ea | Double, plain | 155 | 457 | 42 | 27.7 | 22.0 | | | | 28.5 | 13.0 | 11.0 | 1.9 | | | 110 |
| 66013 | 1 ea | Double, w/condiments & vegetables | 166 | 417 | 51 | 21.2 | 35.2 | | | | 21.1 | 8.7 | 7.8 | 2.7 | | | 60 |
| 66012 | 1 ea | Double, w/condiments & vegetables, large | 258 | 704 | 51 | 37.9 | 39.7 | | | | 43.6 | 17.7 | 17.4 | 4.7 | | | 142 |
| 56654 | 1 ea | Double, w/double deck bun, condiments & vegs | 228 | 650 | 47 | 29.6 | 53.1 | | | | 35.3 | 12.8 | 12.6 | 6.4 | 0.65 | 5.71 | 93 |
| 56653 | 1 ea | Double, w/double deck bun, plain | 160 | 461 | 43 | 22.1 | 44.3 | | | | 21.6 | 9.5 | 8.3 | 1.8 | | | 80 |
| 66014 | 1 ea | Plain | 102 | 319 | 37 | 14.8 | 31.7 | | | | 15.2 | 6.5 | 5.8 | 1.5 | | | 50 |
| 56648 | 1 ea | Plain, large | 185 | 609 | 39 | 30.2 | 47.4 | | | | 32.9 | 14.8 | 12.7 | 2.4 | | | 96 |
| 56651 | 1 ea | With Bacon & Condiments, large | 195 | 608 | 44 | 32.0 | 37.0 | | | | 36.9 | 16.2 | 14.5 | 2.7 | | | 111 |
| 56647 | 1 ea | With Condiments | 113 | 295 | 48 | 15.9 | 26.6 | | | | 14.1 | 6.3 | 5.3 | 1.1 | 0.18 | 0.91 | 37 |
| 66015 | 1 ea | With Condiments & Vegetables | 154 | 359 | 55 | 17.9 | 28.2 | | | | 19.9 | 9.2 | 7.2 | 1.5 | 0.55 | 0.92 | 52 |
| 56649 | 1 ea | With condiments & Vegetables, large | 219 | 563 | 52 | 28.3 | 38.3 | | | | 32.9 | 15.0 | 12.6 | 2.0 | 0.39 | 1.64 | 88 |
| 56650 | 1 ea | With Ham, Condiments & Vegetables, large | 254 | 744 | 50 | 39.6 | 37.6 | | | | 48.3 | 21.1 | 18.9 | 3.9 | | | 122 |
| 56652 | 1 ea | With Triple Meat, plain | 304 | 796 | 54 | 55.9 | 26.7 | | | | 51.1 | 21.7 | 21.5 | 3.2 | | | 161 |
| 56000 | 1 ea | Sandwiches, Chicken fillet | 182 | 515 | 47 | 24.2 | 38.8 | 1.3 | 6.0 | 31.5 | 29.5 | 8.5 | 10.4 | 8.4 | 0.96 | 7.42 | 60 |
| 56656 | 1 ea | Sandwiches, Chicken fillet w/cheese | 228 | 632 | 46 | 29.4 | 41.5 | | | | 38.8 | 12.4 | 13.7 | 9.9 | | | 73 |
| 56657 | 1 ea | Sandwiches, Egg & cheese | 146 | 340 | 56 | 15.6 | 26.0 | | | | 19.4 | 6.6 | 8.3 | 2.6 | | | 231 |
| 56665 | 1 ea | Sandwiches, Egg, ham, & cheese | 143 | 347 | 51 | 19.3 | 30.9 | | | | 16.3 | 7.4 | 5.7 | 1.7 | | | 246 |
| | | Sandwiches, Hamburger | | | | | | | | | | | | | | | |
| 66007 | 1 ea | Plain | 90 | 274 | 38 | 12.3 | 30.5 | | | | 11.8 | 4.1 | 5.5 | 0.9 | 0.07 | 0.84 | 35 |
| 56660 | 1 ea | Plain, large | 137 | 426 | 42 | 22.6 | 31.8 | | | | 22.9 | 8.4 | 9.9 | 2.1 | | | 71 |
| 56658 | 1 ea | With Condiments | 107 | 275 | 45 | 12.4 | 34.6 | 2.4 | 6.8 | 25.4 | 9.9 | 3.6 | 3.4 | 1.3 | 0.11 | 0.90 | 30 |
| 56659 | 1 ea | With Condiment & Vegetables | 110 | 279 | 49 | 12.9 | 27.3 | | | | 13.5 | 4.1 | 5.3 | 2.5 | | | 26 |
| 56661 | 1 ea | With Condiments & Vegetables, large | 218 | 512 | 56 | 25.9 | 40.1 | | | | 27.5 | 10.4 | 11.4 | 2.2 | 0.24 | 1.96 | 37 |
| 66009 | 1 ea | Double, plain | 176 | 544 | 41 | 29.9 | 42.9 | | | | 28.0 | 10.4 | 12.1 | 2.3 | | | 19 |
| 66006 | 1 ea | Double, w/condiments | 215 | 576 | 50 | 31.8 | 38.7 | | | | 32.5 | 12.0 | 14.1 | 2.8 | | | 143 |
| 56662 | 1 ea | Double, w/condiments & vegetables, large | 226 | 540 | 54 | 34.4 | 40.2 | | | | 26.7 | 10.5 | 10.3 | 2.8 | | | 122 |
| 56663 | 1 ea | With Triple Meat & Condiments | 259 | 692 | 52 | 50.0 | 28.5 | | | | 41.4 | 15.9 | 18.2 | 2.7 | | | 142 |
| 66004 | 1 ea | Sandwiches, Hotdog, plain | 98 | 242 | 54 | 10.4 | 18.0 | | | | 14.5 | 5.1 | 6.9 | 1.7 | 0.42 | 1.28 | 44 |
| 56667 | 1 ea | Sandwiches, Hotdog w/chili | 114 | 296 | 48 | 13.6 | 31.4 | | | | 13.5 | 4.9 | 6.6 | 1.2 | 0.14 | 1.04 | 51 |
| | | *ARBY'S* | | | | | | | | | | | | | | | |
| | | Breakfast Items | | | | | | | | | | | | | | | |
| 57031 | 1 ea | Bacon Platter | 201 | 537 | 52 | 18.1 | 46.2 | | | | 29.9 | 8.3 | 13.3 | 5.8 | | | 415 |
| 42435 | 1 ea | Cinnamon Nut Danish | 100 | 360 | 22 | 6.0 | 60.0 | | | | 11.0 | 1.0 | 7.0 | 2.0 | | | 0 |
| 42432 | 1 ea | Croissant, plain | 63 | 260 | 20 | 6.0 | 28.0 | | | | 15.6 | 10.4 | 4.6 | 0.6 | | | 49 |

| Code | Vit A (IU) | Vit A (RE) | Retinol (RE) | Carotenoids (RE) | Beta Carotene (mcg) | Thiamin (mg) | Riboflavin (mg) | Niacin (NE) | Vit B6 (mg) | Vit B12 (mcg) | Folate (mcg) | Panto (mg) | Vit C (mg) | Vit D (mg) | Vit E (α TE) | Calcium (mg) | Copper (mg) | Iron (mg) | Magnes (mg) | Mang (mg) | Phos (mg) | Potassium (mg) | Selenium (mcg) | Sodium (mg) | Zinc (mg) |
|---|---|---|---|---|---|---|---|---|---|---|---|---|---|---|---|---|---|---|---|---|---|---|---|---|---|
| | Vit A & Components | | | | | Vitamins | | | | | | | | | | Minerals | | | | | | | | | |
| 15067 | 109 | 32.5 | 32.1 | 0.4 | | 0.12 | 0.16 | 6.94 | 0.31 | 0.31 | 29.9 | 0.92 | 0.4 | 0.4 | | 25 | 0.2 | 1.5 | 26 | 0.2 | 218 | 279 | 26.5 | 790 | 1.14 |
| 15068 | 242 | 73 | 72 | 1 | | 0.10 | 0.20 | 6.86 | 0.32 | 0.36 | 29.9 | 0.92 | 0.8 | 0.4 | | 21 | 0.2 | 1.5 | 23 | 0.2 | 211 | 277 | 16.9 | 677 | 1.09 |
| 15187 | 100 | 30 | | | | | | | | | | | | | | 20 | | 0.7 | | | | | | 440 | |
| 15177 | 50 | 15 | | | | | | | | | | | 6.0 | | | 40 | | 3.2 | | | | | | 1230 | |
| | | | | | | | | | | | | | | | | | | | | | | | | | |
| 47150 | 11 | 2.4 | 2.2 | 0.2 | | 0.07 | 0.13 | 0.58 | 0.02 | 0.16 | 17.4 | 0.33 | 3.2 | | | 25 | 0.0 | 1.3 | 16 | 0.1 | 88 | 83 | 3.8 | 153 | 0.55 |
| 66034 | 264 | 68 | 53 | 15 | | 0.06 | 0.29 | 0.95 | 0.05 | 0.60 | 12.4 | 0.37 | 3.4 | | 0.9 | 189 | 0.1 | 0.2 | 28 | 0.1 | 217 | 318 | 5.0 | 195 | 0.82 |
| 45588 | 155 | 43 | 38 | 5 | | 0.26 | 0.21 | 2.55 | 0.05 | 0.23 | 54.6 | 0.57 | 2.6 | | | 70 | 0.1 | 1.8 | 15 | 0.4 | 80 | 116 | 17.2 | 319 | 0.63 |
| 45512 | 18 | 5.3 | 4.7 | 0.6 | | 0.26 | 0.19 | 2.20 | 0.05 | 0.22 | 54.6 | 0.55 | 2.6 | | | 37 | 0.1 | 1.8 | 14 | 0.4 | 74 | 96 | 15.0 | 326 | 0.48 |
| 45513 | 86 | 24 | 21 | 4 | | 0.29 | 0.21 | 1.80 | 0.06 | 0.23 | 31.0 | 0.59 | 1.6 | | | 22 | 0.1 | 1.4 | 14 | 0.2 | 69 | 110 | 13.9 | 333 | 0.48 |
| 2035 | 115 | 31 | 30 | 1 | | 0.03 | 0.15 | 0.22 | 0.05 | 0.21 | 7.9 | 0.49 | 0.2 | 0.0 | | 106 | 0.1 | 0.9 | 19 | 0.1 | 100 | 188 | 1.7 | 71 | 0.35 |
| 2064 | 153 | 41 | 36 | 5 | | 0.03 | 0.16 | 0.21 | 0.06 | 0.21 | 4.3 | 0.46 | 0.6 | 0.0 | | 103 | 0.0 | 0.2 | 10 | 0.0 | 93 | 152 | 1.8 | 63 | 0.30 |
| 2032 | 221 | 57 | 52 | 5 | | 0.06 | 0.30 | 1.07 | 0.13 | 0.65 | 9.5 | 0.33 | 2.4 | | 0.7 | 207 | 0.1 | 0.6 | 33 | 0.1 | 228 | 395 | 5.2 | 182 | 0.95 |
| 2031 | 211 | 52 | 40 | 11 | | 0.05 | 0.26 | 0.31 | 0.06 | 0.21 | 12.4 | 0.27 | 1.1 | | 0.4 | 153 | 0.0 | 0.2 | 15 | 0.0 | 139 | 169 | 3.8 | 92 | 0.57 |
| 49117 | 41 | 3.9 | 3.5 | 0.4 | | 0.18 | 0.14 | 1.83 | 0.04 | 0.10 | 23.0 | 0.14 | 0.0 | 0.0 | 0.6 | 28 | 0.1 | 1.6 | 13 | 0.3 | 55 | 83 | 3.1 | 479 | 0.29 |
| 2033 | 222 | 58 | 53 | 5 | | 0.06 | 0.28 | 0.90 | 0.08 | 0.64 | 18.4 | 0.44 | 2.0 | | 0.8 | 161 | 0.1 | 0.3 | 24 | 0.2 | 155 | 271 | 4.4 | 92 | 0.66 |
| 7208 | 0 | 0 | 0 | 0 | 0 | 0.06 | 0.03 | 2.17 | 0.27 | 0.00 | 28.9 | 0.38 | 8.8 | | | 11 | 0.1 | 0.6 | 30 | 0.2 | 98 | 524 | 0.5 | 150 | 0.36 |
| 56666 | 94 | 27 | 20 | 6 | | 0.00 | 0.02 | 2.03 | 0.10 | 0.17 | 13.3 | 0.22 | 0.0 | | | 69 | 0.2 | 1.4 | 16 | 0.3 | 190 | 188 | 8.0 | 965 | 0.43 |
| | | | | | | | | | | | | | | | | | | | | | | | | | |
| 2020 | 154 | 38 | 27 | 11 | | 0.10 | 0.41 | 0.27 | 0.08 | 0.56 | 5.8 | 0.65 | 0.7 | 0.7 | | 188 | 0.1 | 0.5 | 28 | 0.1 | 169 | 332 | 2.8 | 161 | 0.68 |
| 2022 | 271 | 56 | 47 | 19 | | 0.10 | 0.44 | 0.40 | 0.10 | 0.70 | 6.8 | 1.11 | 1.8 | 0.5 | | 255 | 0.0 | 0.2 | 29 | 0.0 | 226 | 411 | 4.7 | 188 | 0.81 |
| 2024 | 216 | 53 | 38 | 15 | | 0.07 | 0.30 | 0.31 | 0.09 | 0.60 | 5.5 | 0.69 | 1.3 | 0.3 | | 203 | 0.1 | 0.1 | 20 | 0.0 | 169 | 289 | 3.5 | 136 | 0.60 |
| 6176 | 8 | 1 | 0 | 1 | 5 | 0.08 | 0.10 | 0.92 | 0.06 | 0.12 | 54.8 | 0.20 | 0.6 | | 0.3 | 73 | 0.1 | 0.8 | 16 | 0.3 | 86 | 129 | 2.9 | 430 | 0.35 |
| | | | | | | | | | | | | | | | | | | | | | | | | | |
| 6177 | 835 | 228 | 205 | 23 | 137 | 0.24 | 0.21 | 3.34 | 0.71 | 0.18 | 26.6 | 1.30 | 26.0 | | | 311 | 0.6 | 3.0 | 65 | 0.5 | 320 | 1166 | 7.7 | 332 | 1.89 |
| 6178 | 628 | 173 | 156 | 17 | 104 | 0.27 | 0.24 | 3.98 | 0.75 | 0.33 | 29.9 | 1.29 | 28.7 | | | 308 | 0.6 | 3.1 | 69 | 0.5 | 347 | 1178 | 9.6 | 972 | 2.15 |
| 6179 | 1595 | 278 | 200 | 78 | 467 | 0.27 | 0.27 | 3.59 | 0.78 | 0.34 | 61.0 | 1.42 | 48.5 | | | 336 | 0.6 | 3.3 | 78 | 0.8 | 346 | 1441 | 5.8 | 435 | 2.03 |
| 6180 | 756 | 174 | 137 | 36 | 213 | 0.28 | 0.36 | 4.19 | 0.95 | 0.24 | 47.4 | 2.57 | 31.6 | | | 411 | 0.8 | 6.1 | 111 | 0.7 | 498 | 1572 | 5.5 | 699 | 3.79 |
| 5463 | 18 | 3 | 0 | 3 | 17 | 0.03 | 0.01 | 1.07 | 0.17 | 0.01 | 7.9 | 0.34 | 5.5 | | 0.1 | 7 | 0.1 | 0.5 | 16 | 0.1 | 69 | 267 | 0.2 | 290 | 0.22 |
| 6185 | 33 | 8 | 7 | 1 | 5 | 0.07 | 0.04 | 0.96 | 0.18 | 0.04 | 6.4 | 0.38 | 0.3 | | | 17 | 0.1 | 0.4 | 14 | 0.1 | 44 | 235 | 0.4 | 182 | 0.26 |
| | | | | | | | | | | | | | | | | | | | | | | | | | |
| 56628 | 1053 | 137 | 6 | 131 | | 0.39 | 0.39 | 5.97 | 0.42 | 0.85 | 101.1 | 0.91 | 16.3 | | | 235 | 0.2 | 2.0 | 49 | 0.4 | 401 | 401 | 36.8 | 743 | 3.13 |
| 5461 | 338 | 50 | 6 | 43 | 260 | 0.04 | 0.03 | 0.08 | 0.11 | 0.18 | 38.6 | 0.15 | 8.3 | | | 34 | 0.0 | 0.7 | 9 | 0.1 | 36 | 177 | 1.0 | 267 | 0.20 |
| 6173 | 95 | 16 | 14 | 2 | | 0.07 | 0.10 | 0.26 | 0.14 | 0.11 | 23.8 | 0.35 | 1.0 | | | 13 | 0.1 | 0.7 | 8 | 0.1 | 53 | 256 | 0.9 | 312 | 0.19 |
| 56623 | 2352 | 236 | 0 | 236 | | 0.06 | 0.10 | 1.14 | 0.17 | 0.00 | 76.6 | 0.25 | 48.0 | | | 27 | 0.1 | 1.3 | 23 | 0.3 | 81 | 356 | 0.8 | 54 | 0.43 |
| | | | | | | | | | | | | | | | | | | | | | | | | | |
| 66016 | 332 | 79 | 69 | 10 | | 0.25 | 0.37 | 6.01 | 0.25 | 2.31 | 68.2 | 0.62 | 0.0 | | 1.2 | 232 | 0.1 | 3.4 | 33 | 0.2 | 374 | 308 | 32.1 | 635 | 4.96 |
| 66013 | 398 | 65 | 43 | 22 | | 0.35 | 0.28 | 8.05 | 0.18 | 1.93 | 61.4 | 0.43 | 1.7 | | | 171 | 0.1 | 3.4 | 30 | 0.3 | 242 | 335 | 23.6 | 1051 | 3.49 |
| 66012 | 348 | 54 | 36 | 18 | | 0.36 | 0.49 | 7.25 | 0.41 | 3.41 | 74.8 | 0.85 | 1.0 | | | 240 | 0.2 | 5.9 | 52 | 0.3 | 395 | 596 | 28.9 | 1148 | 6.68 |
| 56654 | 372 | 84 | 59 | 25 | | 0.57 | 0.43 | 8.34 | 0.27 | 2.07 | 91.2 | 0.64 | 2.7 | | 2.0 | 169 | 0.2 | 4.7 | 36 | 0.3 | 349 | 390 | 39.4 | 921 | 4.13 |
| 56653 | 277 | 65 | 43 | 22 | | 0.34 | 0.38 | 6.02 | 0.22 | 1.92 | 70.4 | 0.66 | 0.0 | | | 224 | 0.1 | 3.7 | 34 | 0.3 | 338 | 285 | 34.1 | 891 | 4.35 |
| 66014 | 153 | 37 | 32 | 5 | | 0.40 | 0.40 | 3.70 | 0.09 | 0.97 | 54.1 | 0.43 | 0.0 | | | 141 | 0.1 | 2.4 | 21 | 0.2 | 196 | 164 | 22.6 | 500 | 2.37 |
| 56648 | 616 | 143 | 129 | 19 | | 0.48 | 0.57 | 11.17 | 0.28 | 2.53 | 74.0 | 0.74 | 0.0 | | | 91 | 0.2 | 5.5 | 39 | 0.3 | 422 | 644 | 38.9 | 1589 | 5.55 |
| 56651 | 406 | 80 | 53 | 27 | | 0.31 | 0.41 | 6.63 | 0.31 | 2.34 | 85.8 | 0.35 | 2.1 | | | 162 | 0.2 | 4.7 | 45 | 0.3 | 400 | 332 | 33.0 | 1043 | 6.83 |
| 56647 | 452 | 94 | 82 | 12 | | 0.25 | 0.23 | 3.72 | 0.11 | 0.94 | 54.2 | 0.32 | 1.9 | | 0.5 | 111 | 0.1 | 2.4 | 20 | 0.2 | 176 | 223 | 19.8 | 616 | 2.09 |
| 66015 | 431 | 7 | 52 | 18 | | 0.32 | 0.23 | 6.38 | 0.15 | 1.23 | 64.7 | 0.34 | 2.3 | | | 182 | 0.1 | 2.6 | 26 | 0.3 | 216 | 229 | 20.5 | 976 | 2.62 |
| 56649 | 613 | 129 | 95 | 34 | | 0.39 | 0.46 | 7.38 | 0.28 | 2.56 | 81.0 | 0.72 | 7.9 | | 1.2 | 206 | 0.2 | 4.7 | 44 | 0.3 | 311 | 445 | 37.4 | 1108 | 4.60 |
| 56650 | 505 | 104 | 65 | 40 | | 0.53 | 0.56 | 9.17 | 0.38 | 2.87 | 78.7 | 1.04 | 7.4 | | | 302 | 0.2 | 5.0 | 51 | 0.4 | 531 | 538 | 32.5 | 1712 | 6.63 |
| 56652 | 359 | 85 | 74 | 11 | | 0.61 | 0.64 | 11.46 | 0.61 | 5.90 | 69.9 | 1.16 | 2.7 | | | 283 | 0.3 | 8.3 | 61 | 0.4 | 541 | 821 | 25.5 | 1213 | 10.88 |
| 56000 | 100 | 31 | [illegible] | 0 | | 0.33 | 0.24 | 6.81 | 0.20 | 0.38 | 100.1 | 0.60 | 8.9 | 0.3 | | 60 | 0.2 | 4.7 | 35 | 0.5 | 233 | 353 | 40.4 | 957 | 1.87 |
| 56656 | 620 | 128 | 115 | 13 | | 0.41 | 0.46 | 9.07 | 0.41 | 0.46 | 109.4 | 1.35 | 3.0 | | | 258 | 0.2 | 3.6 | 43 | 0.4 | 406 | 333 | 48.1 | 1238 | 2.90 |
| 56657 | 669 | 181 | 172 | 9 | | 0.26 | 0.57 | 2.07 | 0.13 | 1.14 | 97.8 | 0.88 | 1.5 | | | 225 | 0.1 | 3.0 | 22 | 0.2 | 302 | 188 | 33.7 | 804 | 1.65 |
| 56665 | 562 | 149 | 142 | 7 | | 0.43 | 0.56 | 4.20 | 0.16 | 1.23 | 75.8 | 0.94 | 2.7 | | | 212 | 0.1 | 3.1 | 26 | 0.2 | 346 | 210 | 32.5 | 1005 | 1.99 |
| | | | | | | | | | | | | | | | | | | | | | | | | | |
| 66007 | 0 | 0 | [illegible] | 0 | 0 | 0.33 | 0.27 | 3.72 | 0.06 | 0.89 | 53.1 | 0.37 | 0.0 | | 0.5 | 63 | 0.1 | 2.4 | 19 | 0.2 | 103 | 145 | 21.7 | 387 | 2.00 |
| 56660 | 0 | 0 | [illegible] | 0 | 0 | 0.29 | 0.29 | 6.25 | 0.23 | 2.06 | 60.3 | 0.53 | 0.0 | | 0.7 | 74 | 0.1 | 3.6 | 27 | 0.2 | 175 | 267 | 27.1 | 474 | 4.11 |
| 56658 | 75 | 10 | [illegible] | 10 | 58 | 0.29 | 0.24 | 3.95 | 0.12 | 1.10 | 52.4 | 0.28 | 2.2 | | 0.4 | 127 | 0.2 | 2.7 | 24 | 0.4 | 116 | 254 | 20.9 | 539 | 2.27 |
| 56659 | 83 | 9 | [illegible] | 9 | | 0.23 | 0.20 | 3.68 | 0.12 | 0.88 | 51.7 | 0.30 | 1.7 | | | 63 | 0.1 | 2.6 | 22 | 0.3 | 124 | 227 | 20.6 | 504 | 2.06 |
| 56661 | 312 | 33 | [illegible] | 33 | | 0.41 | 0.37 | 7.28 | 0.33 | 2.38 | 82.8 | 0.72 | 2.6 | | 1.2 | 96 | 0.2 | 4.9 | 44 | 0.3 | 233 | 480 | 33.6 | 824 | 4.88 |
| 66009 | 0 | 0 | [illegible] | 0 | 0 | 0.33 | 0.37 | 8.25 | 0.32 | 2.92 | 77.4 | 0.67 | 0.0 | | 1.3 | 86 | 0.2 | 4.6 | 37 | 0.3 | 234 | 363 | 39.6 | 554 | 5.72 |
| 66006 | 54 | 4 | 0 | 4 | | 0.34 | 0.41 | 6.73 | 0.37 | 3.33 | 83.9 | 0.77 | 1.1 | | | 92 | 0.2 | 5.5 | 45 | 0.3 | 284 | 527 | 44.9 | 742 | 5.81 |
| 56662 | 102 | 11 | 0 | 11 | | 0.36 | 0.38 | 7.57 | 0.54 | 4.07 | 76.8 | 0.54 | 1.1 | | | 102 | 0.2 | 5.9 | 50 | 0.2 | 314 | 570 | 25.5 | 791 | 5.67 |
| 56663 | 153 | 16 | 0 | 16 | | 0.31 | 0.54 | 10.96 | 0.52 | 4.92 | 75.1 | 0.67 | 1.3 | | | 65 | 0.2 | 8.3 | 54 | 0.2 | 394 | 785 | 55.7 | 712 | 10.75 |
| 66004 | 0 | 0 | 0 | 0 | 0 | 0.24 | 0.27 | 3.65 | 0.05 | 0.51 | 48.0 | 0.51 | 0.1 | | | 24 | 0.1 | 2.3 | 13 | 0.1 | 97 | 143 | 26.0 | 670 | 1.98 |
| 56667 | 58 | 6 | 0 | 6 | | 0.22 | 0.40 | 3.74 | 0.05 | 0.30 | 73.0 | 0.55 | 2.7 | | | 19 | 0.1 | 3.3 | 10 | 0.1 | 192 | 166 | 13.0 | 480 | 0.78 |
| | | | | | | | | | | | | | | | | | | | | | | | | | |
| | | | | | | | | | | | | | | | | | | | | | | | | | |
| 57031 | 362 | 72 | | | | | | | | | | | 3.3 | | | 54 | | 3.3 | | | | 445 | | 797 | |
| 42435 | | | | | | 0.38 | 0.26 | 1.20 | | | | | | | | 20 | | 1.8 | | | | 130 | | 105 | 1.20 |
| 42432 | | | | | | 0.15 | 0.14 | 2.00 | | | | | | | | 40 | | 2.7 | | | | 95 | | 300 | 0.30 |

| Code | Amount | Description | Basic Components | | | | | | | | Additional Fats | | | | | | | Vit A & Components | | | | | Vitamins | | | | | | | | | | Minerals | | | | | | | | | |
|---|---|---|---|---|---|---|---|---|---|---|---|---|---|---|---|---|---|---|---|---|---|---|---|---|---|---|---|---|---|---|---|---|---|---|---|---|---|---|---|---|---|---|
| | | | Weight (g) | Calories | % Water | Protein (g) | Carbs (g) | Fiber (g) | Sugar (g) | Other Carbs (g) | Fat (g) | Sat Fat (g) | Mono Fat (g) | Poly Fat (g) | Omega 3 (g) | Omega 6 (g) | Choles (mg) | Vit A (IU) | Vit A (RE) | Retinol (RE) | Carotenoids (RE) | Beta Carotene (mcg) | Thiamin (mg) | Riboflavin (mg) | Niacin (NE) | Vit B6 (mg) | Vit B12 (mcg) | Folate (mcg) | Panto (mg) | Vit C (mg) | Vit D (mg) | Vit E (α TE) | Calcium (mg) | Copper (mg) | Iron (mg) | Magnes (mg) | Mang (mg) | Phos (mg) | Potassium (mg) | Selenium (mcg) | Sodium (mg) | Zinc (mg) |
| 57030 | 1 ea | Egg Platter | 201 | 460 | 58 | 15.0 | 44.9 | | | | 24.0 | 7.2 | 11.0 | 5.1 | | | 346 | 400 | 80 | | | | | | | | | | | 3.6 | | | 60 | | 3.6 | | | | 412 | | 591 | |
| 57032 | 1 ea | Ham Platter | 258 | 518 | 62 | 24.4 | 45.3 | | | | 26.2 | 7.9 | 12.2 | 5.4 | | | 374 | 400 | 80 | | | | 0.68 | 0.43 | 4.00 | | | | | 3.6 | | | 60 | | 3.6 | | | | 578 | | 1177 | 2.10 |
| 57033 | 1 ea | Sausage Platter | 238 | 640 | 54 | 21.0 | 45.9 | | | | 41.0 | 13.3 | 20.2 | 6.8 | | | 406 | 400 | 80 | | | | 0.45 | 0.34 | 3.00 | | | | | 3.6 | | | 80 | | 3.6 | | | | 507 | | 861 | 0.90 |
| 42435 | 1 ea | Desserts, Danish, Cinnamon Nut | 100 | 360 | 22 | 6.0 | 60.0 | | | | 11.0 | 1.0 | 7.0 | 2.0 | | | 0 | | | | | | 0.38 | 0.26 | 1.20 | | | | | | | | 20 | | 1.8 | | | | 130 | | 105 | 1.20 |
| | | Desserts, Ice Cream | | | | | | | | | | | | | | | | | | | | | | | | | | | | | | | | | | | | | | | | |
| 2246 | 1 ea | Butterfinger Polar Swirl, svg | 329 | 457 | 72 | 12.1 | 61.6 | | | | 18.1 | 8.4 | 6.1 | 3.6 | | | 28 | 200 | 40 | | | | 0.09 | 0.68 | 1.20 | | | | | | | | 250 | | | | | | 690 | | 318 | |
| 2245 | 1 ea | Heath Polar Swirl, svg | 329 | 543 | 66 | 10.6 | 76.3 | | | | 21.8 | 5.2 | 13.3 | 2.6 | | | 39 | 200 | 40 | | | | 0.09 | 0.68 | 0.80 | | | | | | | | 250 | | | | | | 520 | | 346 | |
| 2242 | 1 ea | Peanut Butter Cup Polar Swirl, svg | 329 | 517 | 68 | 14.0 | 61.4 | | | | 24.0 | 8.1 | 11.0 | 4.8 | | | 34 | 200 | 40 | | | | 0.09 | 0.68 | 1.20 | | | | | | | | 250 | | | | | | 612 | | 385 | |
| | | Desserts, Turnovers | | | | | | | | | | | | | | | | | | | | | | | | | | | | | | | | | | | | | | | | |
| 48161 | 1 ea | Apple | 85 | 303 | 39 | 4.4 | 27.5 | | | | 18.3 | 6.9 | 8.0 | 3.3 | | | 0 | 100 | 20 | | | | 0.03 | 0.03 | 0.40 | | | | | 1.2 | | | | | 0.7 | | | | 51 | | 178 | |
| 45612 | 1 ea | Blueberry | 85 | 320 | 34 | 3.0 | 32.0 | | | | 19.0 | 6.3 | 7.9 | 3.2 | | | 0 | | | | | | 0.03 | 0.03 | 0.40 | | | | | 6.0 | | | | | 0.7 | | | | 150 | | 240 | |
| 48162 | 1 ea | Cherry | 85 | 280 | 42 | 4.6 | 25.4 | | | | 17.8 | 5.3 | 8.9 | 3.6 | | | 0 | | | | | | 0.03 | 0.07 | 0.40 | | | | | 4.8 | | | | | 0.7 | | | | 68 | | 200 | |
| | | French Fries | | | | | | | | | | | | | | | | | | | | | | | | | | | | | | | | | | | | | | | | |
| 57015 | 5 oz | Cheddar | 142 | 399 | 45 | 6.2 | 46.2 | | | | 21.9 | 9.0 | 10.0 | 1.7 | | | 9 | | | | | | 0.06 | 0.14 | 2.00 | | 0.00 | | | | | | 80 | | 1.4 | | | | 742 | | 443 | 0.90 |
| 6432 | 3 1/2 oz | Curly | 99 | 337 | 31 | 4.2 | 43.2 | | | | 17.7 | 7.4 | 7.6 | 1.5 | | | 0 | 0 | 0 | 0 | 0 | 0 | 0.06 | 0.07 | 2.00 | | 0.00 | | | | | | 20 | | 1.4 | | | | 724 | | 167 | 0.60 |
| 6140 | 1 ea | Medium, svg | 71 | 246 | 41 | 2.1 | 29.8 | 1.2 | | | 13.2 | 3.0 | 5.5 | 4.7 | | | 0 | 0 | 0 | 0 | 0 | 0 | 0.06 | | 2.00 | | 0.00 | | | 3.6 | | | 3 | | 1.1 | | | | 240 | | 114 | |
| | | Milkshakes | | | | | | | | | | | | | | | | | | | | | | | | | | | | | | | | | | | | | | | | |
| 2124 | 1 ea | Chocolate, svg | 340 | 451 | 74 | 10.2 | 76.5 | 0.3 | | | 11.6 | 2.8 | 7.0 | 1.7 | | | 36 | 300 | 60 | | | | 0.12 | 0.68 | 0.80 | 0.14 | | 14.0 | | 4.8 | | | 250 | | 0.7 | 48 | | 350 | 410 | | 341 | 1.50 |
| 2126 | 1 ea | Vanilla, svg | 312 | 330 | 77 | 10.5 | 46.2 | 0.0 | | | 11.5 | 3.9 | 5.3 | 2.3 | | | 32 | 300 | 60 | | | | 0.12 | 0.68 | 4.00 | 0.14 | | 37.0 | | 2.4 | | | 300 | | 2.7 | 36 | | 350 | 686 | | 281 | 1.50 |
| | | Potatoes | | | | | | | | | | | | | | | | | | | | | | | | | | | | | | | | | | | | | | | | |
| 6429 | 1 ea | Baked, Broccoli 'N Cheddar | 340 | 417 | 75 | 10.5 | 55.0 | | | | 17.9 | 6.9 | 6.6 | 3.3 | | | 22 | 300 | 60 | | | | 0.09 | 0.17 | 3.00 | | 0.00 | | | 45.0 | | | 100 | | 2.7 | | | | 1455 | | 361 | |
| 6428 | 1 ea | Baked, Deluxe | 348 | 621 | 65 | 17.2 | 58.9 | | | | 36.4 | 18.1 | 11.1 | 3.9 | | | 58 | 500 | 100 | | | | 0.09 | 0.14 | 3.00 | | 0.00 | | | 33.0 | | | 700 | | 2.7 | | | | 1520 | | 605 | |
| 6430 | 1 ea | Baked, Mushroom & Cheese | 347 | 515 | 71 | 15.0 | 57.5 | | | | 26.7 | 5.8 | 10.7 | 8.7 | | | 47 | 750 | 150 | | | | 0.15 | 0.25 | 3.00 | | 0.00 | | | 33.0 | | | 250 | | | | | | 1445 | | 923 | |
| 6426 | 1 ea | Baked, Plain | 241 | 240 | 75 | 5.8 | 50.2 | | | | 1.9 | 0.0 | 0.5 | 1.0 | | | 0 | 0 | 0 | 0 | 0 | 0 | 0.09 | 0.14 | 3.00 | | 0.00 | | | 33.0 | | | | | 2.7 | | | | 1333 | | 58 | |
| 6139 | 2 ea | Cakes | 85 | 204 | 58 | 1.8 | 19.8 | 1.2 | | | 12.0 | 2.2 | 5.5 | 4.3 | | | 0 | 0 | 0 | 0 | 0 | 0 | 0.06 | | 1.60 | | 0.00 | | | 9.0 | | | | | 1.4 | | | | 289 | | 397 | |
| | | Salads | | | | | | | | | | | | | | | | | | | | | | | | | | | | | | | | | | | | | | | | |
| 52075 | 1 ea | Chef | 411 | 205 | 89 | 18.5 | 13.0 | | | | 9.5 | 3.9 | 1.4 | 1.0 | | | 126 | 5000 | 500 | | | | 0.39 | 0.37 | 7.00 | | | | | 52.8 | | | 170 | | 5.0 | | | | 819 | | 796 | 2.25 |
| 52074 | 1 ea | Garden | 330 | 117 | 92 | 7.0 | 11.4 | | | | 5.2 | 2.7 | 0.0 | 0.5 | | | 12 | 4900 | 490 | | | | 0.17 | 0.19 | 1.20 | | | | | 51.6 | | | 160 | | 1.6 | | | | 600 | | 134 | 0.90 |
| 6431 | 1 ea | Roast Chicken | 400 | 204 | 88 | 24.0 | 12.2 | | | | 7.2 | 3.3 | 0.9 | 0.9 | | | 43 | 4850 | 485 | | | | 0.33 | 0.54 | 5.60 | | 0.00 | | | 51.0 | | | 170 | | 2.0 | | | | 877 | | 508 | |
| 52076 | 1 ea | Side | 150 | 25 | 94 | 2.0 | 4.0 | | | | 0.3 | 0.0 | 0.0 | 0.2 | | | 0 | 1250 | 125 | | | | 0.08 | 0.05 | 0.40 | | | | | 11.4 | | | 30 | | 0.7 | | | | 249 | | 30 | 0.60 |
| | | Sandwiches, Beef | | | | | | | | | | | | | | | | | | | | | | | | | | | | | | | | | | | | | | | | |
| 69045 | 1 ea | Arby Q | 190 | 389 | 55 | 17.6 | 48.2 | | | | 15.2 | 5.4 | 6.3 | 3.5 | | | 29 | | | | | | 0.27 | 0.39 | 9.20 | | | | | | | | 70 | | 9.2 | | | | 456 | | 1268 | |
| 56335 | 1 ea | Bacon 'n Cheddar | 231 | 512 | 59 | 21.2 | 38.9 | 0.3 | | | 31.5 | 8.7 | 12.7 | 10.1 | | | 38 | 200 | 40 | | | | 0.34 | 0.46 | 9.60 | | | | | 10.8 | | | 110 | | 4.3 | | | | 491 | | 1094 | 3.00 |
| 69056 | 1 ea | Beef 'n Cheddar | 194 | 508 | 50 | 24.6 | 43.2 | | | | 26.5 | 7.7 | 12.0 | 6.8 | | | 52 | | | | | | 0.42 | 0.63 | 9.80 | | | | | 1.2 | | | 150 | | 6.1 | | | | 321 | | 1166 | 3.00 |
| 69043 | 1 ea | French Dip | 154 | 368 | 52 | 22.0 | 35.0 | | | | 15.4 | 5.5 | 7.5 | 2.4 | | | 43 | | | | | | 0.19 | 0.48 | 8.40 | | | | | | | | 50 | | 4.1 | | | | 367 | | 1018 | |
| 56340 | 1 ea | French Dip' n Swiss | 179 | 429 | 51 | 28.7 | 35.5 | 1.1 | | | 19.0 | 8.8 | 9.1 | 1.2 | | | 67 | 0 | 0 | 0 | 0 | 0 | 0.21 | 0.54 | 8.60 | 0.22 | | 19.0 | | 0.0 | | | 270 | | 4.1 | 24 | | 260 | 390 | | 1438 | 3.75 |
| 69051 | 1 ea | Roast Beef, Deluxe, light | 182 | 294 | 65 | 18.0 | 33.0 | | | | 10.0 | 3.4 | 4.6 | 2.0 | | | 42 | 200 | 40 | | | | 0.27 | 0.49 | 8.40 | | | | | 7.8 | | | 130 | | 4.5 | | | | 392 | | 826 | |
| 69054 | 1 ea | Roast Beef, Giant | 228 | 544 | 53 | 33.2 | 45.6 | | | | 26.3 | 10.9 | 12.6 | 2.8 | | | 72 | | | | | | 0.41 | 0.75 | 16.80 | | | | | 1.2 | | | 90 | | 7.9 | | | | 599 | | 1433 | 6.00 |
| 56337 | 1 ea | Roast Beef, Junior | 89 | 233 | 48 | 11.5 | 22.8 | 0.5 | | | 10.8 | 3.8 | 4.8 | 2.3 | | | 22 | | | | | | 0.18 | 0.25 | 6.60 | 0.10 | | 7.0 | 0.01 | | | | 40 | | 2.7 | 8 | | 60 | 201 | | 519 | 1.50 |
| 56336 | 1 ea | Roast Beef, Regular | 155 | 383 | 47 | 22.0 | 35.4 | 1.1 | | | 18.2 | 6.9 | 7.9 | 3.4 | | | 43 | 0 | 0 | 0 | 0 | 0 | 0.28 | 0.48 | 11.00 | 0.20 | | 14.0 | | 1.2 | | | 60 | | 4.9 | 16 | | 120 | 422 | | 936 | 3.75 |
| 69049 | 1 ea | Roast Beef, Sub | 305 | 623 | 60 | 37.7 | 46.8 | | | | 32.0 | 11.5 | 13.0 | 6.8 | | | 73 | 500 | 100 | | | | 0.56 | 0.71 | 10.14 | | | | | 9.0 | | | 410 | | 7.7 | | | | 708 | | 1847 | |
| 56338 | 1 ea | Roast Beef, Super | 254 | 552 | 58 | 23.7 | 54.1 | 1.1 | | | 28.3 | 7.6 | 12.2 | 8.4 | | | 43 | 150 | 30 | | | | 0.39 | 0.58 | 12.40 | 0.30 | | 21.0 | | 9.0 | | | 90 | | 6.5 | 25 | | 190 | 533 | | 1174 | 3.75 |
| 69055 | 1 ea | Philly Beef 'n Swiss | 197 | 467 | 53 | 24.1 | 38.2 | | | | 25.3 | 9.6 | 10.6 | 5.1 | | | 53 | | | | | | 0.28 | 0.46 | 8.80 | | | | | 19.2 | | | 290 | | 4.1 | | | | 409 | | 1144 | 3.75 |
| | | Sandwiches, Chicken | | | | | | | | | | | | | | | | | | | | | | | | | | | | | | | | | | | | | | | | |
| 56341 | 1 ea | Breast Fillet | 204 | 445 | 52 | 22.2 | 52.1 | 1.1 | | | 22.5 | 3.0 | 9.6 | 10.0 | | | 45 | | | | | | 0.22 | 0.54 | 9.00 | 0.38 | | 18.0 | | 5.4 | | | 60 | | 2.9 | 30 | | 180 | 330 | | 1019 | 0.15 |
| 69046 | 1 ea | Grilled Deluxe | 230 | 430 | 62 | 23.6 | 41.8 | | | | 19.9 | 3.5 | 5.1 | 4.4 | | | 44 | 400 | 80 | | | | 0.31 | 0.29 | 13.60 | | | | | 8.4 | | | 70 | | 2.5 | | | | 659 | | 901 | |
| 69047 | 1 ea | Grilled w/bbq sauce | 201 | 386 | 58 | 23.4 | 46.7 | | | | 13.1 | 3.6 | 5.2 | 4.4 | | | 43 | 250 | 50 | | | | 0.30 | 0.27 | 13.60 | | | | | 3.0 | | | 70 | | 4.0 | | | | 596 | | 1002 | |
| 69042 | 1 ea | Roasted Club | 238 | 503 | 60 | 30.5 | 36.6 | | | | 27.0 | 6.9 | 9.8 | 10.4 | | | 46 | | | | | | 0.51 | 0.71 | 10.60 | | | | | 7.8 | | | 180 | | 2.9 | | | | 534 | | 1143 | 2.25 |
| 69052 | 1 ea | Roasted Deluxe, light | 195 | 276 | 66 | 24.0 | 33.0 | | | | 7.0 | 1.7 | 2.9 | 2.5 | | | 33 | 200 | 40 | | | | 0.44 | 0.75 | 9.40 | | | | | 7.2 | | | 130 | | 2.9 | | | | 392 | | 326 | |
| 69053 | 1 ea | Sandwiches, Fish Fillet | 223 | 526 | 54 | 23.0 | 50.0 | | | | 27.0 | 7.0 | 9.2 | 10.6 | | | 44 | | | | | | 0.34 | 0.31 | 5.60 | | | | | 1.2 | | | 90 | | 3.8 | | | | 450 | | 872 | 2.25 |
| 56342 | 1 ea | Sandwiches, Ham 'n Cheese | 169 | 355 | 54 | 24.6 | 34.5 | 0.3 | | | 14.2 | 4.9 | 5.6 | 3.7 | | | 55 | 200 | 40 | | | | 0.82 | 0.37 | 7.80 | 0.31 | | 26.0 | | 24.0 | | | 170 | | 2.7 | 31 | | 405 | 382 | | 1400 | 0.90 |
| 69048 | 1 ea | Sandwiches, Italian Sub | 297 | 671 | 58 | 34.1 | 47.4 | | | | 38.8 | 12.8 | 15.7 | 8.5 | | | 69 | 500 | 100 | | | | 0.92 | 0.49 | 8.20 | | | | | 11.4 | | | 410 | | 4.3 | | | | 565 | | 2062 | |
| 69050 | 1 ea | Sandwiches, Tuna Sub | 284 | 663 | 42 | 74.0 | 50.2 | | | | 37.0 | 8.2 | 11.8 | 17.0 | | | 43 | 500 | 100 | | | | 0.56 | 0.71 | 14.20 | | | | | 9.0 | | | 410 | | 7.7 | | | | 708 | | 1847 | |
| 56343 | 1 ea | Sandwiches, Turkey, light roasted | 195 | 260 | 69 | 20.0 | 33.0 | 0.3 | | | 6.0 | 1.5 | 2.2 | 2.3 | | | 33 | 200 | 40 | | | | 0.08 | 0.41 | 15.40 | 0.52 | | 20.0 | | 12.0 | | | 130 | | 3.4 | 30 | | 250 | 353 | | 1262 | 1.50 |
| 69044 | 1 ea | Sandwiches, Turkey Sub | 277 | 486 | 62 | 32.8 | 46.5 | | | | 19.0 | 5.3 | 6.0 | 7.0 | | | 51 | 100 | 20 | | | | 13.20 | 0.54 | 18.80 | | | | | | | | 400 | | 4.7 | | | | 500 | | 2033 | |
| | | *BURGER KING* | | | | | | | | | | | | | | | | | | | | | | | | | | | | | | | | | | | | | | | | |
| | | Breakfast Items | | | | | | | | | | | | | | | | | | | | | | | | | | | | | | | | | | | | | | | | |
| 69071 | 1 ea | Biscuit w/Bacon, Egg & Cheese | 171 | 510 | 45 | 19.0 | 39.0 | 1.0 | 3.0 | 35.0 | 31.0 | 10.0 | | | | | 225 | 400 | 80 | | | | | | | | | | | 0.0 | | | 150 | | 2.7 | | | | | | 1530 | |
| 69070 | 1 ea | Biscuit w/Sausage | 151 | 590 | 33 | 16.0 | 41.0 | 1.0 | 2.0 | 38.0 | 40.0 | 13.0 | | | | | 45 | 0 | 0 | 0 | 0 | 0 | | | | | | | | 0.0 | | | 60 | | 3.6 | | | | | | 1390 | |
| 56346 | 1 ea | Croissant w/Egg, Sausage & Cheese | 176 | 600 | 46 | 22.0 | 25.0 | 1.0 | 3.0 | 21.0 | 46.0 | 16.0 | | | | | 260 | 400 | 80 | | | | | | | | | | | 0.0 | | | 150 | | 3.6 | | | | | | 1140 | |
| 15158 | 1 ea | Chicken Tenders, svg | 88 | 230 | 50 | 16.0 | 14.0 | 2.0 | 0.0 | 12.0 | 12.0 | 3.0 | | | | | 35 | 0 | 0 | 0 | 0 | 0 | | | | | | | | 0.0 | | | 0 | | 0.7 | | | | | | 530 | |
| 6141 | 1 ea | French Fries, medium | 116 | 370 | 40 | 5.0 | 43.0 | 3.0 | 0.0 | 40.0 | 20.0 | 5.0 | | | | | 0 | 0 | 0 | 0 | 0 | 0 | | | | | 0.00 | | | 3.6 | | | 0 | | 1.1 | | | | | | 240 | |
| | | Milkshakes | | | | | | | | | | | | | | | | | | | | | | | | | | | | | | | | | | | | | | | | |
| 2127 | 1 ea | Chocolate, medium | 284 | 320 | 75 | 9.0 | 54.0 | 3.0 | 48.0 | 3.0 | 7.0 | 4.0 | | | | | 20 | 300 | 60 | | | | 0.13 | 0.55 | 0.13 | | | | | 0.0 | | | 200 | | 1.8 | | | | | | 230 | |
| 2221 | 1 ea | Strawberry, large | 341 | 420 | 71 | 9.0 | 83.0 | 1.0 | 78.0 | 4.0 | 6.0 | 4.0 | | | | | 20 | 300 | 60 | | | | | | | | | | | 3.6 | | | 300 | | 0.0 | | | | | | 260 | |
| 2129 | 1 ea | Vanilla, medium | 284 | 300 | 75 | 9.0 | 53.0 | 1.0 | 47.0 | 5.0 | 6.0 | 4.0 | | | | | 20 | 300 | 60 | | | | 0.11 | 0.57 | 0.13 | | | | | 3.6 | | | 300 | | 0.0 | | | | | | 230 | |
| | | Salads | | | | | | | | | | | | | | | | | | | | | | | | | | | | | | | | | | | | | | | | |
| 52098 | 1 ea | Broiled Chicken | 302 | 200 | 87 | 21.0 | 7.0 | 3.0 | 4.0 | 0.0 | 10.0 | 4.0 | | | | | 60 | 5000 | 1000 | | | | | | | | | | | 15.0 | | | 150 | | 3.6 | | | | | | 110 | |
| 52099 | 1 ea | Garden | 215 | 100 | 91 | 6.0 | 7.0 | 3.0 | 4.0 | 0.0 | 5.0 | 3.0 | | | | | 15 | 5500 | 1100 | | | | | | | | | | | 30.0 | | | 150 | | 1.1 | | | | | | 110 | |
| 56364 | 1 ea | Side | 133 | 60 | 91 | 3.0 | 5.0 | 2.0 | 3.0 | 0.0 | 3.0 | 2.0 | | | | | 5 | 2500 | 250 | | | | | | | | | | | 12.0 | | | 80 | | 0.7 | | | | | | 55 | |

| Code | Amount | Description | Weight (g) | Calories | % Water | Protein (g) | Carbs (g) | Fiber (g) | Sugar (g) | Other Carbs (g) | Fat (g) | Sat Fat (g) | Mono Fat (g) | Poly Fat (g) | Omega 3 (g) | Omega 6 (g) | Choles (mg) |
|---|---|---|---|---|---|---|---|---|---|---|---|---|---|---|---|---|---|
| | | Sandwiches, Beef | | | | | | | | | | | | | | | |
| 56352 | 1 ea | Cheeseburger | 138 | 380 | 48 | 23.0 | 28.0 | 1.0 | 5.0 | 22.0 | 19.0 | 9.0 | | | | | 65 |
| 56353 | 1 ea | Double Cheeseburger w/Bacon | 218 | 640 | 48 | 44.0 | 28.0 | 1.0 | 5.0 | 22.0 | 39.0 | 18.0 | | | | | 145 |
| 56351 | 1 ea | Hamburger | 126 | 330 | 48 | 20.0 | 28.0 | 1.0 | 4.0 | 23.0 | 15.0 | 6.0 | | | | | 55 |
| 56354 | 1 ea | Whopper | 270 | 640 | 58 | 27.0 | 45.0 | 3.0 | 8.0 | 34.0 | 39.0 | 11.0 | | | | | 90 |
| 56356 | 1 ea | Whopper, Double Beef | 351 | 870 | 57 | 46.0 | 45.0 | 3.0 | 8.0 | 34.0 | 56.0 | 19.0 | | | | | 170 |
| 56355 | 1 ea | Whopper, w/Cheese | 294 | 730 | 57 | 33.0 | 46.0 | 3.0 | 8.0 | 35.0 | 46.0 | 16.0 | | | | | 115 |
| 56357 | 1 ea | Whopper, Double Beef & Cheese | 375 | 960 | 56 | 52.0 | 46.0 | 3.0 | 8.0 | 35.0 | 63.0 | 24.0 | | | | | 195 |
| 56360 | 1 ea | Sandwiches, Chicken | 229 | 710 | 45 | 26.0 | 54.0 | 2.0 | 4.0 | 48.0 | 43.0 | 9.0 | | | | | 60 |
| 56362 | 1 ea | Sandwiches, Fish, Big | 255 | 700 | 51 | 26.0 | 56.0 | 3.0 | 4.0 | 49.0 | 41.0 | 6.0 | | | | | 90 |
| | | *DAIRY QUEEN* | | | | | | | | | | | | | | | |
| | | Desserts | | | | | | | | | | | | | | | |
| 2131 | 1 ea | Banana Split | 369 | 510 | 68 | 8.0 | 96.0 | 3.0 | 82.0 | 11.0 | 12.0 | 8.0 | | | | | 30 |
| 2431 | 1 ea | Blizzard, Butterfinger, med | 376 | 750 | 57 | 16.0 | 115.0 | 1.0 | 92.0 | 22.0 | 26.0 | 16.0 | | | | | 50 |
| 2370 | 1 ea | Blizzard, Chocolate Chip Cookie Dough, med | 439 | 950 | 55 | 17.0 | 143.0 | 2.0 | 106.0 | 35.0 | 36.0 | 19.0 | | | | | 75 |
| 2368 | 1 ea | Blizzard, Chocolate Sandwich Cookie, med | 326 | 640 | 59 | 12.0 | 97.0 | 1.0 | 74.0 | 22.0 | 23.0 | 11.0 | | | | | 45 |
| 2379 | 1 ea | Blizzard, Heath, med | 404 | 820 | 58 | 14.0 | 119.0 | 1.0 | 106.0 | 12.0 | 33.0 | 20.0 | | | | | 60 |
| 2372 | 1 ea | Blizzard, Reese's Peanut Butter Cup, med | 376 | 790 | 58 | 19.0 | 105.0 | 2.0 | 88.0 | 15.0 | 33.0 | 17.0 | | | | | 55 |
| 2227 | 1 ea | Blizzard, Strawberry, med | 383 | 570 | 68 | 12.0 | 95.0 | 1.0 | 82.0 | 12.0 | 16.0 | 11.0 | | | | | 50 |
| 2230 | 1 pce | Cake Slice, fzn | 172 | 350 | 57 | 7.0 | 54.0 | 1.0 | 39.0 | 14.0 | 12.0 | 7.0 | | | | | 20 |
| 2231 | 1 ea | Frozen Yogurt, cone, med | 213 | 280 | 66 | 9.0 | 59.0 | 0.0 | 39.0 | 20.0 | 1.0 | 0.5 | | | | | 5 |
| 2233 | 1 ea | Frozen Yogurt, cup, med | 198 | 230 | 69 | 8.0 | 49.0 | 0.0 | 38.0 | 11.0 | 0.5 | 0.0 | | | | | 5 |
| 2239 | 1 ea | Frozen Yogurt, Heath Breeze, med | 404 | 710 | 60 | 15.0 | 123.0 | 1.0 | 103.0 | 19.0 | 18.0 | 11.0 | | | | | 20 |
| 2349 | 1/2 cup | Frozen Yogurt, nonfat | 85 | 100 | 71 | 3.0 | 21.0 | 0.3 | 16.0 | 5.0 | 0.0 | 0.0 | 0.0 | 0.0 | 0.00 | 0.00 | |
| 2237 | 1 ea | Frozen Yogurt, Strawberry Breeze, med | 383 | 460 | 70 | 13.0 | 99.0 | 1.0 | 79.0 | 19.0 | 1.0 | 1.0 | 0.0 | 0.0 | 0.00 | 0.00 | 10 |
| 2235 | 1 ea | Frozen Yogurt, Strawberry Sundae, med | 255 | 300 | 69 | 9.0 | 66.0 | 1.0 | 53.0 | 12.0 | 0.5 | 0.5 | 0.0 | 0.0 | 0.00 | 0.00 | 5 |
| 2141 | 1 ea | Hot Fudge Brownie Delight | 305 | 710 | 52 | 11.0 | 102.0 | 0.6 | | | 29.0 | 14.0 | 12.0 | 2.0 | | | 35 |
| 2241 | 1 ea | Ice Cream, Chocolate, big scoop | 113 | 250 | 58 | 4.0 | 28.0 | 0.0 | 24.0 | 4.0 | 14.0 | 9.0 | 4.0 | 1.0 | | | 55 |
| 2222 | 1 ea | Ice Cream, Chocolate, cone, med | 213 | 360 | 64 | 9.0 | 56.0 | 0.0 | 37.0 | 19.0 | 11.0 | 8.0 | | | | | 30 |
| 2136 | 1 ea | Ice Cream, Chocolate, dipped cone, med | 234 | 510 | 59 | 9.0 | 63.0 | 1.0 | 46.0 | 16.0 | 25.0 | 13.0 | | | | | 30 |
| 2348 | 1/2 cup | Ice Cream, Chocolate, soft serve | 94 | 150 | 66 | 4.0 | 22.0 | 0.0 | 17.0 | 5.0 | 5.0 | 3.5 | | | | | 15 |
| 2240 | 1 ea | Ice Cream, Vanilla, big scoop | 113 | 250 | 59 | 4.0 | 27.0 | 0.0 | 22.0 | 5.0 | 14.0 | 9.0 | 4.0 | 1.0 | | | 55 |
| 2143 | 1 ea | Ice Cream, Vanilla, cone, med | 213 | 350 | 64 | 8.0 | 57.0 | 0.0 | 41.0 | 16.0 | 10.0 | 7.0 | | | | | 30 |
| 2347 | 1/2 cup | Ice Cream, Vanilla, soft serve | 94 | 140 | 68 | 3.0 | 22.0 | 0.0 | 19.0 | 3.0 | 4.5 | 3.0 | | | | | 15 |
| 2134 | 1 ea | Ice Cream Sandwich | 61 | 150 | 46 | 3.0 | 24.0 | 1.0 | 13.0 | 10.0 | 5.0 | 2.0 | | | | | 5 |
| 2352 | 1 ea | Misty Slush, med | 595 | 290 | 88 | 0.0 | 74.0 | 0.0 | 74.0 | 0.0 | 0.0 | 0.0 | 0.0 | 0.0 | 0.00 | 0.00 | 0 |
| 2147 | 1 ea | Mr Misty, med | 330 | 250 | 81 | 0.0 | 63.0 | 0.0 | | | 0.0 | 0.0 | 0.0 | 0.0 | 0.00 | 0.00 | 0 |
| 2151 | 1 ea | Peanut Buster Parfait, svg | 305 | 730 | 51 | 16.0 | 99.0 | 2.0 | 85.0 | 12.0 | 31.0 | 17.0 | | | | | 35 |
| 2359 | 1 ea | Starkiss, svg | 85 | 80 | 75 | 0.0 | 21.0 | 0.0 | 21.0 | 0.0 | 0.0 | 0.0 | 0.0 | 0.0 | 0.00 | 0.00 | 0 |
| 2353 | 1 ea | Strawberry Misty Cooler, svg | 340 | 190 | 86 | 0.0 | 49.0 | 1.0 | 49.0 | | 0.0 | 0.0 | 0.0 | 0.0 | 0.00 | 0.00 | 0 |
| 2154 | 1 ea | Sundae, Chocolate, med | 241 | 410 | 62 | 8.0 | 73.0 | 0.0 | 63.0 | 10.0 | 10.0 | 6.0 | | | | | 30 |
| 2225 | 1 ea | Sundae, Nutty Double Fudge | 276 | 570 | 57 | 10.0 | 85.0 | | | | 22.0 | 10.0 | 9.0 | 3.0 | | | 35 |
| 2374 | 1 pce | Treatzza Pizza, Heath | 65 | 180 | 41 | 3.0 | 28.0 | 1.0 | 18.0 | 9.0 | 7.0 | 3.5 | | | | | 5 |
| 2375 | 1 pce | Treatzza Pizza, M & M | 68 | 190 | 42 | 3.0 | 29.0 | 1.0 | 20.0 | 8.0 | 7.0 | 4.0 | | | | | 5 |
| 2373 | 1 pce | Treatzza Pizza, Strawberry-Banana | 76 | 180 | 50 | 3.0 | 29.0 | 1.0 | 19.0 | 9.0 | 6.0 | 3.0 | | | | | 5 |
| 2376 | 1 pce | Treatzza Pizza, Peanut Butter Fudge | 79 | 220 | 47 | 4.0 | 28.0 | 1.0 | 18.0 | 9.0 | 10.0 | 4.5 | | | | | 5 |
| 2364 | 1 ea | Vanilla Orange Bar | 66 | 60 | 70 | 2.0 | 17.0 | 0.0 | 2.0 | 15.0 | 0.0 | 0.0 | 0.0 | 0.0 | 0.00 | 0.00 | 0 |
| | | French Fries | | | | | | | | | | | | | | | |
| 57370 | 1 ea | Regular | 99 | 300 | 41 | 4.0 | 40.0 | 4.0 | 36.0 | 0.0 | 14.0 | 3.0 | | | | | 0 |
| 6144 | 1 ea | Large | 128 | 390 | 40 | 5.0 | 52.0 | 6.0 | 0.0 | 46.0 | 18.0 | 4.0 | 8.0 | 6.0 | | | 0 |
| | | Milkshakes | | | | | | | | | | | | | | | |
| 2224 | 1 ea | Chocolate, med | 539 | 770 | 69 | 17.0 | 130.0 | 0.0 | 113.0 | 17.0 | 20.0 | 13.0 | | | | | 70 |
| 2355 | 1 ea | Chocolate Malt, med | 567 | 880 | 66 | 19.0 | 153.0 | 0.0 | 131.0 | 22.0 | 22.0 | 14.0 | | | | | 70 |
| 2153 | 1 ea | Vanilla, med | 397 | 520 | 71 | 12.0 | 88.0 | 0.3 | | | 14.0 | 8.0 | 2.0 | 2.0 | | | 45 |
| 2145 | 1 ea | Vanilla Malt, med | 418 | 610 | 68 | 13.0 | 106.0 | 0.3 | | | 14.0 | 8.0 | 2.0 | 2.0 | | | 45 |
| | | Salads | | | | | | | | | | | | | | | |
| 52072 | 1 ea | Garden | 284 | 200 | 87 | 13.0 | 7.0 | | | | 13.0 | 7.0 | 5.0 | 1.0 | | | 185 |
| 52071 | 1 ea | Side | 135 | 25 | 94 | 1.0 | 4.0 | | | | 0.0 | 0.0 | 0.0 | 0.0 | 0.00 | 0.00 | 0 |
| | | Sandwiches, Beef | | | | | | | | | | | | | | | |
| 69068 | 1 ea | Bacon Double Cheeseburger, Homestyle | 255 | 610 | 56 | 41.0 | 31.0 | 2.0 | 6.0 | 23.0 | 36.0 | 18.0 | | | | | 130 |
| 56371 | 1 ea | Cheeseburger, Homestyle | 152 | 340 | 55 | 20.0 | 29.0 | 2.0 | 5.0 | 22.0 | 17.0 | 8.0 | | | | | 55 |
| 69067 | 1 ea | Double Cheeseburger, Deluxe, Homestyle | 241 | 540 | 58 | 36.0 | 31.0 | 2.0 | 6.0 | 23.0 | 31.0 | 16.0 | | | | | 115 |
| 56372 | 1 ea | Double Cheeseburger, Homestyle | 219 | 540 | 55 | 35.0 | 30.0 | 2.0 | 5.0 | 23.0 | 31.0 | 16.0 | | | | | 115 |
| 56369 | 1 ea | Double Hamburger, Deluxe, Homestyle | 212 | 440 | 62 | 30.0 | 29.0 | 2.0 | 6.0 | 21.0 | 22.0 | 10.0 | | | | | 30 |
| 56368 | 1 ea | Hamburger, Homestyle | 138 | 290 | 56 | 17.0 | 29.0 | 2.0 | 5.0 | 22.0 | 12.0 | 5.0 | 6.0 | 1.0 | | | 35 |
| 69027 | 1 ea | Ultimate Burger, Double Bacon Cheeseburger | 269 | 670 | 58 | 40.0 | 29.0 | 2.0 | 6.0 | 21.0 | 43.0 | 19.0 | | | | | 135 |
| | | Sandwiches, Chicken | | | | | | | | | | | | | | | |
| 56379 | 1 ea | Breaded Fillet | 191 | 430 | 56 | 24.0 | 37.0 | 2.0 | 5.0 | 30.0 | 20.0 | 4.0 | | | | | 55 |
| 56380 | 1 ea | Breaded Fillet w/Cheese | 205 | 480 | 55 | 27.0 | 38.0 | 2.0 | 5.0 | 31.0 | 25.0 | 7.0 | | | | | 70 |
| 69029 | 1 ea | Grilled Fillet | 184 | 310 | 64 | 24.0 | 30.0 | 3.0 | 5.0 | 22.0 | 10.0 | 2.5 | | | | | 50 |

| Code | Vit A (IU) | Vit A (RE) | Retinol (RE) | Carotenoids (RE) | Beta Carotene (mcg) | Thiamin (mg) | Riboflavin (mg) | Niacin (NE) | Vit B6 (mg) | Vit B12 (mcg) | Folate (mcg) | Panto (mg) | Vit C (mg) | Vit D (mg) | Vit E (α TE) | Calcium (mg) | Copper (mg) | Iron (mg) | Magnes (mg) | Mang (mg) | Phos (mg) | Potassium (mg) | Selenium (mcg) | Sodium (mg) | Zinc (mg) |
|---|---|---|---|---|---|---|---|---|---|---|---|---|---|---|---|---|---|---|---|---|---|---|---|---|---|
| 56352 | 300 | 60 | | | | | | | | | | | 0.0 | | | 100 | | 2.7 | | | | | | 770 | |
| 56353 | 400 | 80 | | | | 0.31 | 0.42 | 6.00 | | | | | 0.0 | | | 200 | | 4.5 | | | | | | 1240 | |
| 56351 | 100 | 20 | | | | 0.28 | 0.31 | 4.89 | | | | | 0.0 | | | 40 | | 1.8 | | | | | | 530 | |
| 56354 | 500 | 00 | | | | 0.33 | 0.41 | 7.00 | 0.35 | | | | 9.0 | | | 80 | | 4.5 | | | | | | 370 | |
| 56356 | 500 | 00 | | | | 0.34 | 0.56 | 10.00 | | | | | 9.0 | | | 80 | | 7.2 | | | | | | 940 | |
| 56355 | 750 | 50 | | | | 0.34 | 0.48 | 7.00 | 0.33 | | | | 9.0 | | | 250 | | 4.5 | | | | | | 1350 | |
| 56357 | 750 | 50 | | | | 0.35 | 0.63 | 10.00 | | | | | 9.0 | | | 250 | | 7.2 | | | | | | 1420 | |
| 56360 | 0 | 0 | 0 | 0 | 0 | | | | | | | | 0.0 | | | 100 | | 3.6 | | | | | | 1400 | |
| 56362 | 100 | 20 | | | | | | | | | | | 1.2 | | | 60 | | 2.7 | | | | | | 980 | |
| 2131 | 1000 | 200 | | | | 0.15 | 0.25 | 0.40 | 0.20 | | | | 15.0 | | | 250 | | 1.8 | | | 40 | 860 | | 180 | |
| 2431 | 1250 | 250 | | | | 0.14 | 0.71 | | 0.15 | | | | 1.2 | | | 450 | | 2.7 | | | 418 | 679 | | 360 | |
| 2370 | 1750 | 350 | | | | | | | | | | | 1.2 | | | 450 | | 2.7 | | | | | | 660 | |
| 2368 | 250 | 50 | | | | | | | | | | | 1.2 | | | 400 | | 2.7 | | | | | | 500 | |
| 2379 | 1500 | 300 | | | | 0.15 | 0.76 | | | | | | 1.2 | | | 450 | | 1.8 | | | 450 | 730 | | 580 | |
| 2372 | 1250 | 250 | | | | | | | | | | | 1.2 | | | 450 | | 2.7 | | | | | | 430 | |
| 2227 | 1500 | 300 | | | | 0.15 | 0.68 | | | | | | 9.0 | | | 450 | | 1.8 | | | 350 | 700 | | 260 | |
| 2230 | 500 | 100 | | | | 0.06 | 0.35 | 0.42 | | | | | 0.0 | | | 200 | | 1.4 | | | 209 | 367 | | 270 | |
| 2231 | 0 | 0 | 0 | 0 | 0 | 0.09 | 0.38 | | | | | | 2.4 | | | 300 | | 1.8 | | | 225 | 285 | | 170 | |
| 2233 | 0 | 0 | 0 | 0 | 0 | 0.08 | 0.47 | | | | | | 1.2 | | | 300 | | 1.4 | | | 209 | 278 | | 160 | |
| 2239 | 100 | 20 | | | | 0.13 | 0.81 | | | | | | 2.4 | | | 450 | | 2.7 | | | 479 | 575 | | 580 | |
| 2349 | 0 | 0 | 0 | 0 | 0 | | | | | | | | 0.0 | | | 100 | | 0.7 | | | | | | 70 | |
| 2237 | 0 | 0 | 0 | 0 | 0 | 0.13 | 0.73 | | | | | | 9.0 | | | 450 | | 2.7 | | | 378 | 530 | | 270 | |
| 2235 | 0 | 0 | 0 | 0 | 0 | 0.09 | 0.49 | | | | | | 6.0 | | | 300 | | 1.8 | | | 220 | 352 | | 130 | |
| 2141 | 400 | 80 | | | | 0.15 | 0.68 | 0.30 | 0.18 | | | | 0.9 | | | 300 | | 5.4 | | | 600 | 510 | | 340 | |
| 2241 | 500 | 100 | | | | 0.05 | 0.23 | | | | | | 0.0 | | | 150 | | 0.0 | | | 133 | 249 | | 95 | |
| 2222 | 1000 | 200 | | | | 0.09 | 0.38 | | | | | | 1.2 | | | 250 | | 1.8 | | | 300 | 525 | | 180 | |
| 2136 | 750 | 150 | | | | 0.09 | 0.38 | 0.17 | 0.14 | | | | 2.4 | | | 300 | | 1.8 | | | 225 | 435 | | 200 | |
| 2348 | 500 | 100 | | | | | | | | | | | 0.0 | | | 100 | | 0.7 | | | | | | 75 | |
| 2240 | 500 | 100 | | | | 0.05 | 0.23 | | | | | | 0.0 | | | 150 | | 0.0 | | | 89 | 204 | | 100 | |
| 2143 | 750 | 150 | | | | 0.09 | 0.38 | 0.17 | 0.14 | | | | 2.4 | | | 300 | | 1.8 | | | 225 | 390 | | 170 | |
| 2347 | 500 | 100 | | | | | | | | | | | 0.0 | | | 150 | | 0.7 | | | | | | 70 | |
| 2134 | 200 | 40 | | | | 0.03 | 0.25 | 0.40 | 0.05 | | | | 0.0 | | | 60 | | 0.7 | | | 60 | 105 | | 115 | |
| 2352 | 0 | 0 | 0 | 0 | 0 | | | | | | | | 0.0 | | | 0 | | 0.0 | | | | | | 30 | |
| 2147 | 0 | 0 | 0 | 0 | 0 | 0.00 | 0.00 | | 0.00 | | | | 2.0 | | | 0 | | 0.0 | | | | | | 10 | |
| 2151 | 750 | 150 | | | | 0.15 | 0.51 | 3.00 | 0.22 | | | | 1.2 | | | 300 | | 1.8 | | | 450 | 660 | | 400 | |
| 2359 | 0 | 0 | 0 | 0 | 0 | | | | | | | | 0.0 | | | 0 | | 0.0 | | | | | | 10 | |
| 2353 | 0 | 0 | 0 | 0 | 0 | | | | | | | | 4.8 | | | 0 | | 0.0 | | | | | | 25 | |
| 2154 | 750 | 150 | | | | 0.08 | 0.35 | 0.40 | 0.19 | | | | 0.0 | | | 250 | | 1.4 | | | 204 | 394 | | 210 | |
| 2225 | 300 | 60 | | | | 0.12 | 0.60 | | | | | | | | | 300 | | 3.6 | | | 300 | 450 | | 170 | |
| 2374 | 200 | 40 | | | | | | | | | | | 0.0 | | | 60 | | 0.7 | | | | | | 160 | |
| 2375 | 200 | 40 | | | | | | | | | | | 0.0 | | | 60 | | 0.7 | | | | | | 160 | |
| 2373 | 200 | 40 | | | | | | | | | | | 2.4 | | | 60 | | 0.7 | | | | | | 140 | |
| 2376 | 200 | 40 | | | | | | | | | | | 0.0 | | | 60 | | 0.7 | | | | | | 200 | |
| 2364 | 100 | 20 | | | | | | | | | | | 0.0 | | | 60 | | 0.0 | | | | | | 40 | |
| 57370 | 0 | 0 | 0 | 0 | 0 | | | | | 0.00 | | | 6.0 | | | 0 | | 1.1 | | | | | | 160 | |
| 6144 | 0 | 0 | 0 | 0 | 0 | 0.15 | 0.07 | 3.00 | | 0.00 | | | 9.0 | | | 0 | | 1.4 | | | 150 | 780 | | 200 | |
| 2224 | 2000 | 400 | | | | 0.16 | 0.80 | 1.08 | | | | | 2.4 | | | 600 | | 2.7 | | | 543 | 814 | | 420 | |
| 2355 | 2000 | 400 | | | | | | | | | | | 2.4 | | | 600 | | 2.7 | | | | | | 500 | |
| 2153 | 400 | 80 | | | | 0.12 | 0.60 | 0.80 | 0.19 | | | | 0.0 | | | 400 | | 1.4 | | | 350 | 570 | | 230 | |
| 2145 | 400 | 80 | | | | 0.12 | 0.60 | 0.80 | 0.19 | | | | 0.0 | | | 400 | | 1.4 | | | 350 | 570 | | 230 | |
| 52072 | 3000 | 600 | | | | 0.15 | 0.34 | 4.00 | | | | | 21.0 | | | 250 | | 1.8 | | | 250 | 460 | | 240 | |
| 52071 | 500 | 50 | 0 | 50 | | 0.06 | 0.10 | | | | | | 15.0 | | | 20 | | 0.7 | | | 40 | 240 | | 15 | |
| 69068 | 750 | 150 | | | | | | | | | | | 6.0 | | | 250 | | 4.5 | | | | | | 1380 | |
| 56371 | 500 | 60 | | | | 0.29 | 0.33 | 3.89 | | | | | 3.6 | | | 150 | | 3.6 | | | 243 | 263 | | 850 | |
| 69067 | 750 | 150 | | | | | | | | | | | 6.0 | | | 250 | | 4.5 | | | | | | 1130 | |
| 56372 | 750 | 150 | | | | 0.29 | 0.49 | 6.78 | | | | | 3.6 | | | 250 | | 4.5 | | | 387 | 426 | | 1130 | |
| 56369 | 300 | 60 | | | | 0.32 | 0.46 | 7.49 | | | | | 6.0 | | | 60 | | 4.5 | | | 267 | 444 | | 680 | |
| 56368 | 200 | 40 | | | | 0.29 | 0.25 | 3.88 | | | | | 3.6 | | | 60 | | 2.7 | | | 145 | 252 | | 630 | |
| 69027 | 200 | 40 | | | | 0.43 | 0.49 | 7.70 | | | | | 3.6 | | | 600 | | 2.7 | | | 389 | 467 | | 1210 | |
| 56379 | 0 | 0 | 0 | 0 | 0 | 0.38 | 0.34 | 11.00 | | | | | 0.0 | | | 40 | | 1.8 | | | 350 | 350 | | 760 | |
| 56380 | 400 | 80 | | | | 0.38 | 0.34 | 11.00 | | | | | 0.0 | | | 100 | | 1.8 | | | 400 | 360 | | 980 | |
| 69029 | 0 | 0 | 0 | 0 | 0 | 0.30 | 1.02 | 12.00 | | | | | 0.0 | | | 200 | | 2.7 | | | 350 | 330 | | 1040 | |

| Code | Amount | Description | Weight (g) | Calories | % Water | Protein (g) | Carbs (g) | Fiber (g) | Sugar (g) | Other Carbs (g) | Fat (g) | Sat Fat (g) | Mono Fat (g) | Poly Fat (g) | Omega 3 (g) | Omega 6 (g) | Choles (mg) |
|---|---|---|---|---|---|---|---|---|---|---|---|---|---|---|---|---|---|
| | | | **Basic Components** | | | | | | | | | **Additional Fats** | | | | | |
| 56381 | 1 ea | Sandwiches, Fish Fillet | 170 | 370 | 58 | 16.0 | 39.0 | 2.0 | 5.0 | 32.0 | 16.0 | 3.5 | | | | | 45 |
| 56382 | 1 ea | Sandwiches, Fish Sandwich w/Cheese | 184 | 420 | 56 | 19.0 | 40.0 | 2.0 | 5.0 | 33.0 | 21.0 | 6.0 | 7.0 | 8.0 | | | 60 |
| 56374 | 1 ea | Sandwiches, Hotdog | 99 | 240 | 57 | 9.0 | 19.0 | 1.0 | 4.0 | 14.0 | 14.0 | 5.0 | | | | | 25 |
| 56375 | 1 ea | Sandwiches, Hotdog, Cheese Dog | 113 | 290 | 55 | 12.0 | 20.0 | 1.0 | 4.0 | 15.0 | 18.0 | 8.0 | 8.0 | 2.0 | | | 40 |
| 56376 | 1 ea | Sandwiches, Hotdog, Chili Dog | 128 | 280 | 61 | 12.0 | 21.0 | 2.0 | 4.0 | 15.0 | 16.0 | 6.0 | | | | | 35 |
| 69069 | 1 ea | Sandwiches, Hotdog, Chili N' Cheese Dog | 142 | 330 | 58 | 14.0 | 22.0 | 2.0 | 4.0 | 16.0 | 21.0 | 9.0 | | | | | 45 |
| | | *DOMINO'S PIZZA* | | | | | | | | | | | | | | | |
| | | Cheese | | | | | | | | | | | | | | | |
| 57024 | 2 pce | Deep Dish, 12" | 205 | 558 | 44 | 23.6 | 63.1 | 3.1 | 4.3 | 55.8 | 23.8 | 9.0 | | | | | 31 |
| 56386 | 2 pce | Hand Tossed, 12" | 147 | 344 | 47 | 14.8 | 49.8 | 2.4 | 1.0 | 46.5 | 9.4 | 4.4 | | | | | 19 |
| 57018 | 1/3 ea | Thin Crust, 12" | 141 | 365 | 46 | 16.2 | 40.2 | 1.8 | 2.3 | 36.1 | 15.5 | 6.3 | | | | | 25 |
| | | Ham | | | | | | | | | | | | | | | |
| 57027 | 2 pce | Deep Dish, 12" | 219 | 576 | 46 | 25.8 | 63.5 | 3.1 | 4.6 | 55.8 | 24.5 | 9.2 | | | | | 39 |
| 56392 | 2 pce | Hand Tossed, 12" | 161 | 362 | 49 | 17.2 | 50.4 | 2.4 | 1.1 | 46.9 | 10.3 | 4.7 | | | | | 26 |
| 57021 | 1/3 ea | Thin Crust, 12" | 158 | 387 | 49 | 19.3 | 40.4 | 1.9 | 2.5 | 36.0 | 16.4 | 6.6 | | | | | 35 |
| | | Italian Sausage & Mushroom | | | | | | | | | | | | | | | |
| 57028 | 2 pce | Deep Dish,12" | 236 | 618 | 47 | 26.2 | 65.6 | 3.8 | 4.7 | 57.1 | 28.3 | 10.9 | | | | | 42 |
| 56388 | 2 pce | Hand Tossed, 12" | 176 | 403 | 50 | 17.4 | 52.3 | 3.0 | 1.2 | 48.0 | 13.9 | 6.2 | | | | | 30 |
| 57022 | 1/3 ea | Thin Crust,12" | 179 | 442 | 50 | 19.7 | 43.1 | 2.5 | 2.7 | 37.9 | 21.5 | 8.6 | | | | | 41 |
| | | Pepperoni | | | | | | | | | | | | | | | |
| 57025 | 2 pce | Deep Dish, 12" | 218 | 621 | 43 | 26.2 | 63.4 | 3.3 | 4.4 | 55.8 | 29.4 | 11.3 | | | | | 44 |
| 57026 | 2 pce | Deep Dish w/extra cheese, 12" | 235 | 672 | 44 | 29.6 | 63.7 | 3.3 | 4.5 | 55.9 | 33.1 | 13.4 | | | | | 54 |
| 57016 | 2 pce | Hand Tossed, 12" | 159 | 405 | 45 | 17.5 | 50.1 | 2.5 | 1.0 | 46.6 | 15.1 | 6.5 | | | | | 32 |
| 56391 | 2 pce | Hand Tossed w/extra cheese, 12" | 175 | 455 | 46 | 20.8 | 50.4 | 2.5 | 1.1 | 46.9 | 18.7 | 8.6 | | | | | 42 |
| 57019 | 1/3 ea | Thin Crust, 12" | 157 | 447 | 44 | 19.8 | 40.5 | 2.0 | 2.4 | 36.1 | 23.1 | 9.3 | | | | | 42 |
| | | Veggie | | | | | | | | | | | | | | | |
| 57029 | 2 pce | Deep Dish, 12" | 236 | 576 | 50 | 24.1 | 65.1 | 3.8 | 4.5 | 56.9 | 24.8 | 9.2 | | | | | 31 |
| 57017 | 2 pce | Hand Tossed, 12" | 176 | 361 | 54 | 15.3 | 51.7 | 3.0 | 1.2 | 47.5 | 10.4 | 4.6 | | | | | 19 |
| 57023 | 1/3 ea | Thin Crust, 12" | 179 | 387 | 55 | 16.8 | 42.6 | 2.7 | 2.5 | 37.4 | 16.8 | 6.4 | | | | | 25 |
| | | *HARDEES* | | | | | | | | | | | | | | | |
| | | Breakfast Biscuits | | | | | | | | | | | | | | | |
| 56395 | 1 ea | Bacon & Egg | 124 | 490 | 29 | 15.0 | 44.0 | | | | 27.0 | 8.7 | 13.5 | 4.8 | | | 155 |
| 56396 | 1 ea | Bacon, Egg & Cheese | 137 | 530 | 29 | 18.0 | 45.0 | | | | 31.0 | 11.0 | 15.0 | 5.0 | | | 155 |
| 56398 | 1 ea | Country Ham | 108 | 430 | 41 | 15.0 | 25.0 | | | | 22.0 | 7.7 | 10.5 | 3.8 | | | 45 |
| 56400 | 1 ea | Ham | 114 | 400 | 32 | 9.0 | 47.0 | | | | 20.0 | 7.3 | 9.1 | 3.6 | | | 15 |
| 56402 | 1 ea | Ham, Egg & Cheese | 159 | 500 | 40 | 18.0 | 48.0 | | | | 27.0 | 10.0 | 13.0 | 4.0 | | | 170 |
| 56403 | 1 ea | Sausage | 118 | 510 | 24 | 13.0 | 44.0 | | | | 31.0 | 10.0 | 16.0 | 5.0 | | | 25 |
| 56404 | 1 ea | Sausage & Egg | 149 | 580 | 34 | 18.0 | 44.0 | | | | 35.0 | 11.0 | 18.0 | 6.0 | | | 170 |
| | | Chicken | | | | | | | | | | | | | | | |
| 15200 | 1 ea | Breast | 148 | 370 | 51 | 29.0 | 29.0 | | | | 15.0 | 4.0 | | | | | 75 |
| 15203 | 1 ea | Leg | 69 | 170 | 48 | 13.0 | 15.0 | | | | 7.0 | 2.0 | | | | | 45 |
| 15202 | 1 ea | Thigh | 121 | 330 | 46 | 19.0 | 30.0 | | | | 15.0 | | | | | | 60 |
| 15201 | 1 ea | Wing | 66 | 200 | 37 | 10.0 | 23.0 | | | | 8.0 | 2.0 | | | | | 30 |
| | | Cool Twist Desserts | | | | | | | | | | | | | | | |
| 2180 | 1 ea | Chocolate Cone | 118 | 180 | 64 | 5.0 | 34.0 | | | | 2.0 | 0.7 | 1.3 | 0.0 | 0.00 | 0.00 | 15 |
| 2158 | 1 ea | Hot Fudge Sundae | 156 | 290 | 59 | 7.0 | 51.0 | | | | 6.0 | 3.0 | 1.6 | 0.2 | | | 20 |
| 2159 | 1 ea | Strawberry Sundae | 164 | 210 | 69 | 5.0 | 43.0 | | | | 2.0 | 0.7 | 1.1 | 0.1 | | | 10 |
| 2179 | 1 ea | Vanilla Cone | 118 | 170 | 65 | 4.0 | 34.0 | | | | 2.0 | 0.7 | 1.3 | 0.0 | 0.00 | 0.00 | 10 |
| 2247 | 1 ea | Vanilla/Chocolate Cone | 118 | 180 | 65 | 4.0 | 34.0 | | | | 2.0 | 0.7 | 1.3 | 0.0 | 0.00 | 0.00 | 10 |
| 6147 | 1 ea | French Fries, med | 142 | 350 | 50 | 5.0 | 49.0 | | | | 15.0 | 3.3 | 6.7 | 5.0 | | | 0 |
| | | Milkshakes | | | | | | | | | | | | | | | |
| 2160 | 1 ea | Chocolate, svg | 349 | 370 | 75 | 13.0 | 67.0 | | | | 5.0 | 2.7 | 2.1 | 0.2 | | | 30 |
| 2250 | 1 ea | Peach, svg | 345 | 390 | 74 | 10.0 | 77.0 | | | | 4.0 | 3.0 | | | | | 25 |
| 2161 | 1 ea | Strawberry, svg | 363 | 420 | 73 | 11.0 | 83.0 | | | | 4.0 | 2.3 | 1.6 | 0.2 | | | 20 |
| 2162 | 1 ea | Vanilla, svg | 349 | 350 | 76 | 12.0 | 65.0 | | | | 5.0 | 2.9 | 1.9 | 0.2 | | | 20 |
| | | Potatoes | | | | | | | | | | | | | | | |
| 6487 | 1/2 cup | Mashed | 113 | 70 | 85 | 2.0 | 14.0 | | | | 0.7 | | | | | | 0 |
| 6145 | 1 ea | Hash Rounds, svg | 79 | 230 | 46 | 3.0 | 24.0 | | | | 14.0 | 3.0 | 7.0 | 4.0 | | | 0 |
| | | Salads | | | | | | | | | | | | | | | |
| 52086 | 1/2 cup | Cole Slaw | 113 | 240 | 67 | 2.0 | 13.0 | | | | 20.0 | 3.0 | | | | | 10 |
| 56429 | 1 ea | Garden | 292 | 210 | 88 | 12.0 | 10.0 | | | | 13.0 | 7.8 | 4.3 | 0.9 | | | 40 |
| 52087 | 1 ea | Grilled Chicken | 278 | 120 | 91 | 18.0 | 2.0 | | | | 4.0 | 1.0 | | | | | 60 |
| 56426 | 1 ea | Side | 131 | 25 | 96 | 1.0 | 14.0 | | | | 0.0 | 0.0 | 0.0 | 0.0 | 0.00 | 0.00 | 0 |
| | | Sandwiches, Beef | | | | | | | | | | | | | | | |
| 56416 | 1 ea | Bacon Cheeseburger | 228 | 600 | 54 | 32.0 | 35.0 | | | | 36.0 | 14.2 | 16.1 | 5.7 | | | 50 |
| 56414 | 1 ea | Cheeseburger | 120 | 300 | 47 | 15.0 | 34.0 | | | | 13.0 | 6.5 | 4.6 | 1.9 | | | 25 |
| 56415 | 1 ea | Cheeseburger, 1/4 pound | 184 | 490 | 51 | 27.0 | 37.0 | | | | 25.0 | 11.5 | 11.5 | 1.9 | | | 35 |
| 56412 | 1 ea | Hamburger | 107 | 260 | 49 | 11.0 | 33.0 | | | | 9.0 | 3.6 | 3.6 | 1.8 | | | 20 |
| 69061 | 1 ea | Hamburger, Frisco | 242 | 760 | 46 | 36.0 | 43.0 | | | | 50.0 | 18.0 | | | | | 70 |
| 56417 | 1 ea | Hamburger, w/mushrooms & swiss cheese | 203 | 520 | 53 | 30.0 | 37.0 | | | | 27.0 | 13.0 | 12.0 | 2.0 | | | 45 |

| Code | Vit A (IU) | Vit A (RE) | Retinol (RE) | Carotenoids (RE) | Beta Carotene (mcg) | Thiamin (mg) | Riboflavin (mg) | Niacin (NE) | Vit B6 (mg) | Vit B12 (mcg) | Folate (mcg) | Panto (mg) | Vit C (mg) | Vit D (mg) | Vit E (α TE) | Calcium (mg) | Copper (mg) | Iron (mg) | Magnes (mg) | Mang (mg) | Phos (mg) | Potassium (mg) | Selenium (mcg) | Sodium (mg) | Zinc (mg) |
|---|---|---|---|---|---|---|---|---|---|---|---|---|---|---|---|---|---|---|---|---|---|---|---|---|---|
| | **Vit A & Components** | | | | | **Vitamins** | | | | | | | | | | **Minerals** | | | | | | | | | |
| 56381 | 0 | 0 | 0 | 0 | 0 | 0.30 | 0.22 | 3.00 | | | | | 0.0 | | | 40 | | 1.8 | | | 150 | 280 | | 630 | |
| 56382 | 400 | 80 | | | | 0.30 | 0.25 | 5.00 | | | | | 0.0 | | | 100 | | 1.8 | | | 250 | 290 | | 850 | |
| 56374 | 100 | 20 | | | | 0.22 | 0.14 | 2.00 | | | | | 3.6 | | | 60 | | 1.8 | | | 60 | 170 | | 730 | |
| 56375 | 300 | 60 | | | | 0.22 | 0.17 | 2.00 | | | | | 3.6 | | | 150 | | 1.8 | | | 150 | 180 | | 950 | |
| 56376 | 400 | 80 | | | | 0.23 | 0.14 | 3.00 | | | | | 3.6 | | | 60 | | 1.8 | | | 60 | 262 | | 870 | |
| 69069 | 750 | 150 | | | | | | | | | | | 3.6 | | | 150 | | 1.8 | | | | | | 1090 | |
| 57024 | 763 | 153 | | | | | | | | | | | 3.1 | | | 451 | | 4.7 | | | | | | 1183 | |
| 56386 | 455 | 91 | | | | 0.71 | 0.63 | 6.82 | 0.18 | | | | 2.6 | | | 276 | | 4.0 | | | | | | 978 | |
| 57018 | 568 | 114 | | | | | | | | | | | 3.5 | | | 423 | | 1.6 | | | | | | 1012 | |
| 57027 | 763 | 153 | | | | | | | | | | | 3.1 | | | 451 | | 4.8 | | | | | | 1345 | |
| 56392 | 457 | 91 | | | | 0.97 | 0.63 | 9.34 | | | | | 2.7 | | | 280 | | 4.2 | | | | | | 1145 | |
| 57021 | 566 | 113 | | | | | | | | | | | 3.6 | | | 423 | | 1.7 | | | | | | 1225 | |
| 57028 | 792 | 158 | | | | | | | | | | | 3.5 | | | 460 | | 5.2 | | | | | | 1357 | |
| 56388 | 483 | 97 | | | | 1.07 | 1.11 | 10.68 | | | | | 3.2 | | | 287 | | 4.6 | | | | | | 1151 | |
| 57022 | 604 | 121 | | | | | | | | | | | 4.3 | | | 435 | | 2.1 | | | | | | 1242 | |
| 57025 | 775 | 155 | | | | | | | | | | | 3.1 | | | 456 | | 5.0 | | | | | | 1382 | |
| 57026 | 887 | 177 | | | | | | | | | | | 3.1 | | | 585 | | 5.2 | | | | | | 1509 | |
| 57016 | 466 | 93 | | | | | | | | | | | 2.7 | | | 281 | | 4.3 | | | | | | 1177 | |
| 56391 | 578 | 116 | | | | 1.00 | 1.09 | 9.96 | | | | | 2.6 | | | 411 | | 4.4 | | | | | | 1302 | |
| 57019 | 584 | 117 | | | | | | | | | | | 3.6 | | | 429 | | 1.9 | | | | | | 1280 | |
| 57029 | 803 | 161 | | | | | | | | | | | 13.0 | | | 460 | | 5.2 | | | | | | 1234 | |
| 57017 | 494 | 99 | | | | | | | | | | | 12.7 | | | 285 | | 4.4 | | | | | | 1028 | |
| 57023 | 618 | 124 | | | | | | | | | | | 16.8 | | | 433 | | 2.0 | | | | | | 1078 | |
| 56395 | | | | | | | | | | | | | | | | 139 | | 3.0 | | | | 180 | | 1250 | |
| 56396 | | | | | | | | | | | | | | | | 207 | | 3.0 | | | | 200 | | 1470 | |
| 56398 | | | | | | | | | | | | | | | | 121 | | 3.0 | | | | 210 | | 1930 | |
| 56400 | | | | | | | | | | | | | | | | 119 | | 2.0 | | | | 170 | | 1340 | |
| 56402 | | | | | | | | | | | | | | | | 206 | | 3.0 | | | | 230 | | 1620 | |
| 56403 | | | | | | | | | | | | | | | | 125 | | 3.0 | | | | 190 | | 1380 | |
| 56404 | | | | | | | | | | | | | | | | 144 | | 4.0 | | | | 240 | | 1400 | |
| 15200 | | | | | | | | | | | | | | | | | | | | | | | | 1190 | |
| 15203 | | | | | | | | | | | | | | | | | | | | | | | | 570 | |
| 15202 | | | | | | | | | | | | | | | | | | | | | | | | 1000 | |
| 15201 | | | | | | | | | | | | | | | | | | | | | | | | 740 | |
| 2180 | | | | | | | | | | | | | | | | 123 | | 2.0 | | | | 220 | | 110 | |
| 2158 | | | | | | | | | | | | | | | | 152 | | 0.4 | | | | 173 | | 310 | |
| 2159 | | | | | | | | | | | | | | | | 187 | | 0.4 | | | | 220 | | 140 | |
| 2179 | | | | | | | | | | | | | | | | 122 | | | | | | 105 | | 130 | |
| 2247 | | | | | | | | | | | | | | | | 123 | | 2.0 | | | | 180 | | 120 | |
| 6147 | 0 | 0 | 0 | 0 | 0 | | | | | 0.00 | | | | | | 19 | | 1.0 | | | | 560 | | 150 | |
| 2160 | | | | | | | | | | | | | | | | 389 | | 1.4 | | | | 616 | | 270 | |
| 2250 | | | | | | | | | | | | | | | | | | | | | | | | 290 | |
| 2161 | | | | | | | | | | | | | | | | 387 | | 0.1 | | | | 475 | | 270 | |
| 2162 | | | | | | | | | | | | | | | | 339 | | 0.1 | | | | 532 | | 300 | |
| 6487 | | | | | | | | | | 0.00 | | | | | | | | | | | | | | 330 | |
| 6145 | 0 | 0 | 0 | 0 | 0 | | | | | 0.00 | | | | | | 10 | | 1.0 | | | | 400 | | 560 | |
| 52086 | | | | | | | | | | | | | | | | | | | | | | | | 340 | |
| 56429 | | | | | | | | | | | | | | | | 289 | | 1.0 | | | | 430 | | 350 | |
| 52087 | | | | | | | | | | | | | | | | | | | | | | | | 520 | |
| 56426 | | | | | | | | | | | | | | | | 22 | | | | | | 170 | | 45 | |
| 56416 | | | | | | | | | | | | | | | | 181 | | 6.0 | | | | 460 | | 950 | |
| 56414 | | | | | | | | | | | | | | | | 178 | | 3.0 | | | | 210 | | 690 | |
| 56415 | | | | | | | | | | | | | | | | 248 | | 5.0 | | | | 350 | | 980 | |
| 56412 | | | | | | | | | | | | | | | | 111 | | 3.0 | | | | 200 | | 460 | |
| 69061 | | | | | | | | | | | | | | | | | | | | | | | | 1280 | |
| 56417 | | | | | | | | | | | | | | | | 294 | | 5.0 | | | | 370 | | 890 | |

| Code | Amount | Description | Basic Components | | | | | | | | Additional Fats | | | | | | | V t A & Components | | | | | Vitamins | | | | | | | | | | Minerals | | | | | | | | | |
|---|---|---|---|---|---|---|---|---|---|---|---|---|---|---|---|---|---|---|---|---|---|---|---|---|---|---|---|---|---|---|---|---|---|---|---|---|---|---|---|---|---|---|
| | | | Weight (g) | Calories | % Water | Protein (g) | Carbs (g) | Fiber (g) | Sugar (g) | Other Carbs (g) | Fat (g) | Sat Fat (g) | Mono Fat (g) | Poly Fat (g) | Omega 3 (g) | Omega 6 (g) | Choles (mg) | Vit A (IU) | Vit A (RE) | Retinol (RE) | Carotenoids (RE) | Beta Carotene (mcg) | Thiamin (mg) | Riboflavin (mg) | Niacin (NE) | Vit B6 (mg) | Vit B12 (mcg) | Folate (mcg) | Panto (mg) | Vit C (mg) | Vit D (mg) | Vit E (α TE) | Calcium (mg) | Copper (mg) | Iron (mg) | Magnes (mg) | Mang (mg) | Phos (mg) | Potassium (mg) | Selenium (mcg) | Sodium (mg) | Zinc (mg) |
|56419|1 ea|Roast Beef, big|169|370|57|21.0|34.0||||16.0|7.0|5.0|2.0|||40||||||||||||||||106||5.0||||320||1050||
|56418|1 ea|Roast Beef, regular|124|270|55|15.0|28.0||||11.0|5.0|4.0|2.0|||25||||||||||||||||105||4.0||||260||780||
|56422|1 ea|Sandwiches, Chicken Fillet|187|400|56|19.0|48.0||||14.0|3.0|4.0|5.0|||55||||||||||||||||123||3.0||||290||1100||
|56423|1 ea|Sandwiches, Fisherman's Fillet|217|500|52|24.0|51.0||||22.0|7.0|9.7|5.3|||60||||||||||||||||209||3.0||||410||1170||
|56420|1 ea|Sandwiches, Ham 'n Cheese, hot|201|530|50|18.0|49.0||||30.0|9.0|||||65||||||||||||||||288||3.0||||300||1710||
|||*HAAGEN-DAZS*|||||||||||||||||||||||||||||||||||||||||
|||Ice Cream|||||||||||||||||||||||||||||||||||||||||
|70664|1/2 cup|Belgian Chocolate|106|329|51|5.0|28.9||||17.9||||||90|353|106|||||0.14|||||||||106|||||159|219||79||
|70661|1/2 cup|Brandied Cherry|106|249|59|4.0|23.9||||14.9|0.5|7.5|7.0|||100|529|159||||0.16|0.18|||||||||106|||||106|170||79||
|2389|1/2 cup|Butter Pecan|106|322|52|5.1|20.1|0.7|18.9|0.5|24.4|10.3|||||106|562|112|||||||||||0.8|||130||0.5||||||144||
|70672|1/2 cup|Cappuccino|106|269|57|5.0|21.9||||17.9|8.0|9.5|0.5|||120|706|212||||0.03|0.18|||||||||159|||||106|189||85||
|2390|1/2 cup|Chocolate Chocolate Chip|106|299|50|5.0|26.3|1.3|23.5|1.0|19.8|12.0|||||103|293|101|||||||||||0.6|||118||1.3||||||59||
|2391|1/2 cup|Chocolate Chocolate Mint|106|302|49|4.8|26.1|1.5|23.3|1.3|21.0|11.3|||||100|493|99|||||||||||0.6|||114||1.3||||||58||
|2394|1/2 cup|Deep Chocolate Peanut Butter|106|359|42|8.3|26.7|3.7|22.3|0.7|24.8|11.4|||||86|445|39|||||||||||0.5|||113||1.6||||||101||
|70663|1/2 cup|Chocolate Swiss Almond|106|299|52|6.0|23.9||||20.9|1.0|11.0|9.0|||105|529|159||||0.03|0.18|||||||||106|||||106|219||74||
|2392|1/2 cup|Coffee|106|266|57|4.9|21.1|0.1|20.7|0.3|18.0|10.3|||||120|515|123|||||||||||0.8|||143||0.3||||||35||
|70671|1/2 cup|Coffee Chip|106|299|52|5.0|25.9||||19.9|10.0|9.5|0.5|||105|529|159|||||0.18|||||||||106||0.4|||159|199||79||
|2393|1/2 cup|Cookies & Cream|106|280|54|4.9|24.0|0.3|21.2|2.4|18.0|10.3|||||113|500|120|||||||||||0.7|||137||0.7||||||119||
|2395|1/2 cup|Macadamia Brittle|106|299|52|4.3|24.8|0.2|22.6|2.0|20.1|11.2|||||109|588|178|||||||||||1.0|||129||0.3||||||119||
|70669|1/2 cup|Macadamia Nut|106|329|50|5.0|23.9||||23.9|||||||353|106||||0.06|0.18|1.27||||||||106||0.4|||106|||||
|70662|1/2 cup|Maple Walnut|106|329|53|6.0|17.9||||25.9|6.0|10.9|9.0|||124|706|212||||0.06|0.18|||||||||106|||||159|199||74||
|2396|1/2 cup|Midnight Cookies & Cream|106|302|48|4.9|29.8|1.3|25.0|3.5|18.7|11.3|||||94|430|96|||||||||||0.6|||118||1.4||||||139||
|70660|1/2 cup|Pralines & Cream|106|288|53|5.0|26.9||||17.9|2.0|8.0|8.0|||100|529|159||||0.03|0.18||||||1.3|||106|||||106|199||179||
|2397|1/2 cup|Rum Raisin|106|271|56|4.0|21.9|0.3|21.3|0.3|17.3|10.4|||||108|555|163|||||||||||0.8|||120||0.3||||||74||
|2398|1/2 cup|Strawberry|106|257|58|4.2|22.7|0.7|21.3|0.6|16.4|9.3|||||96|572|174|||||||||||9.5|||131||0.3||||||78||
|2399|1/2 cup|Vanilla|106|267|58|4.8|20.9|0.0|20.9|0.0|18.1|10.3|||||120|517|123|||||||||||0.8|||140||0.2||||||85||
|70670|1/2 cup|Vanilla Chip|106|299|52|5.0|25.9||||19.9|10.0|9.5|0.5|||105|529|159||||0.03|0.18|||||||||106||0.4|||159|199||79||
|2400|1/2 cup|Vanilla Fudge|106|284|54|4.6|24.9|0.1|24.8|0.0|18.2|11.4|||||104|550|170|||||||||||0.7|||137||0.4||||||107||
|2401|1/2 cup|Vanilla Swiss Almond|106|305|52|6.0|22.6|1.3|21.2|0.1|21.1|11.3|||||107|565|173|||||||||||1.2|||142||0.8||||||77||
|||Ice Cream Bars|||||||||||||||||||||||||||||||||||||||||
|2420|100 g|Chocolate|100|247|56|4.6|20.9|1.1|19.3|0.5|16.8|10.[illegible]|||||108|533|107|||||||||||0.7|||120||1.0||||||73||
|2421|100 g|Coffee|100|249|57|4.5|19.8|0.1|19.4|0.3|16.9|10.2|||||111|577|115|||||||||||0.8|||134||0.3||||||81||
|2422|100 g|Vanilla|100|251|58|4.4|19.8|0.0|19.8|0.0|16.9|10.2|||||111|578|116|||||||||||0.8|||134||0.3||||||81||
|||Ice Cream Extraas|||||||||||||||||||||||||||||||||||||||||
|2402|100 g|Brownie a la Mode|100|284|50|5.2|25.1|0.5|23.6|1.0|18.0|11.3|||||103|417|83|||||||||||0.5|||117||0.8||||||134||
|2416|100 g|Brownie Nut Blast|100|215|54|7.7|28.6|1.1|21.0|6.5|7.9|3.2|||||41|140|28|||||||||||0.6|||195||0.8||||||66||
|2403|100 g|Caramel Cone Explosion|100|298|48|4.8|25.9|0.8|22.2|2.9|19.5|11.9|||||93|500|100|||||||||||0.9|||120||0.5||||||127||
|2404|100 g|Cookie Dough Dynamo|100|298|48|4.2|27.7|0.4|23.3|4.0|18.8|11.3|||||92|487|97|||||||||||0.6|||109||0.6||||||134||
|2405|100 g|Peanut Butter Burst|100|314|46|6.1|25.0|1.1|21.9|2.0|20.9|11.0|||||91|491|98|||||||||||0.6|||113||0.5||||||144||
|2406|100 g|Strawberry Cheesecake|100|273|52|3.9|26.5|0.5|23.7|2.3|16.8|9.6|||||97|520|104|||||||||||2.4|||103||0.5||||||151||
|2407|100 g|Triple Brownie Overload|100|298|48|4.7|26.1|1.3|23.8|1.0|19.9|10.9|||||91|484|97|||||||||||0.6|||103||1.3||||||101||
|||Sorbet|||||||||||||||||||||||||||||||||||||||||
|70645|1/2 cup|Lemon|113|140|69|0.0|34.9||||0.0|0.0|0.0|0.0|0.00|0.00|0|||||||||||||6.8|||||||||29||20||
|2410|1/2 cup|Lemonade, soft serve|113|128|72|0.1|31.8|0.6|28.0|3.2|0.0|0.0|0.0|0.0|0.00|0.00|0|0|0|0|0|0||||||||3.1|||2||0.0||||||6||
|2408|1/2 cup|Mango|113|121|73|0.2|29.7|0.8|27.1|1.3|0.1|0.0|||0.00|0.00|0|1624|325|||||||||||11.5|||5||0.1||||||1||
|2411|1/2 cup|Mango, soft serve|113|121|73|0.2|29.7|0.8|27.1|1.3|0.1|0.0|||0.00|0.00|0|1080|216|||||||||||11.5|||5||0.1||||||1||
|70647|1/2 cup|Orange|113|140|68|0.0|35.9||||0.0|0.0|0.0|0.0|0.00|0.00|0|||||||||||||20.3|||||||||80||20||
|70646|1/2 cup|Raspberry|113|110|76|0.0|27.0||||0.0|0.0|0.0|0.0|0.00|0.00|0|||||||||||||6.8|||||||||60||15||
|2412|1/2 cup|Raspberry, soft serve|113|122|73|0.3|29.6|2.7|25.1|1.8|0.2|0.0|||0.00|0.00|0|16|3|||||||||||6.3|||10||0.2||||||3||
|2409|1/2 cup|Strawberry|113|133|70|0.2|33.0|1.2|29.6|2.1|0.2|0.0|||0.00|0.00|0|18|4|||||||||||14.8|||7||0.2||||||1||
|||Yogurt, Frozen|||||||||||||||||||||||||||||||||||||||||
|70674|1/2 cup|Chocolate, soft serve|95|120|68|4.0|25.9||||0.0|0.0|0.0|0.0|0.00|0.00||127|38||||0.03|0.16|||||||||142|||||95|330||65||
|2418|100 g|Chocolate Mousse, nonfat, soft serve|100|86|68|4.8|25.7|1.2|7.6|16.9|0.3|0.2|||||2|178|36|||||||||||0.7|||148||0.9||||||70||
|70676|1/2 cup|Coffee, soft serve|95|140|67|5.0|21.9||||4.0|2.0|||||35|253|75||||0.03|0.16|||||||||142|||||95|210||75||
|2413|100 g|Pina Colada|100|139|67|3.5|26.9|0.4|22.1|4.4|1.8|1.0|||||25|103|21|||||||||||7.6|||99||0.3||||||27||
|70677|1/2 cup|Raspberry, soft serve|95|140|69|4.0|21.0||||4.0|2.0|||||35|253|75||||0.03|0.16||||||1.1|||142|||||95|190||70||
|2414|100 g|Strawberry Duet|100|135|68|2.8|27.1|0.8|23.1|3.2|1.8|0.9|||||25|119|24|||||||||||10.5|||78||0.2||||||24||
|70675|1/2 cup|Strawberry, soft serve|95|120|68|4.0|25.9||||0.0|0.0|0.0|0.0|0.00|0.00|5|127|33||||0.03|0.16||||||3.4|||142|||||95|210||70||
|2415|100 g|Vanilla Almond Crunch|100|198|55|8.5|29.5|0.5|22.3|6.7|5.0|1.6|||||41|130|20|||||||||||0.6|||227||0.3||||||88||
|2419|100 g|Vanilla Mousse, nonfat, soft serve|100|78|71|4.1|24.1|0.1|7.7|16.3|0.1|0.1|0.0|0.0|0.00|0.00|2|178|35|||||||||||0.7|||143||0.0||||||66||
|70673|1/2 cup|Vanilla, soft serve|95|110||5.0|22.0||||0.0|0.0|0.0|0.0|0.00|0.00|5|130|57||||0.03|0.16|||||||||142|||||95|219||75||
|||*JACK IN THE BOX*|||||||||||||||||||||||||||||||||||||||||
|1215|1 ea|Beef Teriyaki Bowl|440|640|62|28.0|124.0|7.0|21.0|96.0|3.0|1.0|||||25|5000|1000|||||||||||6.0|||150||4.5||||430||930||
|||Breakfast Items|||||||||||||||||||||||||||||||||||||||||
|6149|1 ea|Hash browns, svg|57|160|53|1.0|14.0|1.0|0.0|13.0|11.0|2.5|6.8|0.3|||0|0|0|0|0|0|0.05||1.00||0.00|||6.0|||0||0.4||||190||310||
|56430|1 ea|Jack Sandwich|121|300|49|18.0|30.0|0.0|5.0|25.0|12.0|4.8|4.8|2.4|||185|400|80||||0.47|0.41|3.00|||||9.0|||200||2.7||||220||890||
|56431|1 ea|Sausage Crescent|156|580|39|22.0|28.0|0.0|4.0|24.0|43.0|16.0|||||185|500|100||||0.60|0.51|4.60|||||0.0|||150||2.7||||260||1010||
|19578|1 ea|Scrambled Egg Platter|213|560|52|18.0|50.0|0.0|2.0|48.0|32.0|9.0|15.6|4.4|||380|750|150|||||0.66|5.00|||||9.0|||150||4.5||||450||1060||
|56365|1 ea|Scrambled Egg Pocket|183|430|55|29.0|31.0|0.0|||21.0|8.0|7.4|2.3|||355|1000|200||||0.68|0.68|4.60|||||0.0|||200||3.6||||340||1060||
|69040|1 ea|Sourdough Sandwich|147|380|49|21.0|31.0|0.0|2.0|29.0|20.0|7.0|||||235|750|150|||||||||||9.0|||250||3.6||||260||1120||

| Code | Amount | Description | Basic Components | | | | | | | | | Additional Fats | | | | | | Vit A & Components | | | | | Vitamins | | | | | | | | | | Minerals | | | | | | | | | |
|---|---|---|---|---|---|---|---|---|---|---|---|---|---|---|---|---|---|---|---|---|---|---|---|---|---|---|---|---|---|---|---|---|---|---|---|---|---|---|---|---|---|---|
| | | | Weight (g) | Calories | % Water | Protein (g) | Carbs (g) | Fiber (g) | Sugar (g) | Other Carbs (g) | Fat (g) | Sat Fat (g) | Mono Fat (g) | Poly Fat (g) | Omega 3 (g) | Omega 6 (g) | Choles (mg) | Vit A (IU) | Vit A (RE) | Retinol (RE) | Carotenoids (RE) | Beta Carotene (mcg) | Thiamin (mg) | Riboflavin (mg) | Niacin (NE) | Vit B6 (mg) | Vit B12 (mcg) | Folate (mcg) | Panto (mg) | Vit C (mg) | Vit D (mg) | Vit E (α TE) | Calcium (mg) | Copper (mg) | Iron (mg) | Magnes (mg) | Mang (mg) | Phos (mg) | Potassium (mg) | Selenium (mcg) | Sodium (mg) | Zinc (mg) |
| 56432 | 1 ea | Supreme Crescent | 153 | 530 | 40 | 23.0 | 34.0 | 0.0 | 5.0 | 29.0 | 33.0 | 9.0 | 17.0 | 7.0 | | | 210 | 750 | 150 | | | | 0.65 | 0.54 | 4.20 | | | | | 12.0 | | | 150 | | 3.6 | | | | 270 | | 930 | |
| 69065 | 1 ea | Ultimate Sandwich | 242 | 620 | 53 | 36.0 | 39.0 | | 4.0 | | 35.0 | 11.0 | | | | | 455 | 750 | 150 | | | | | | | | | | | 9.0 | | | 250 | | 4.5 | | | | 450 | | 1800 | |
| 15159 | 1 ea | Chicken Strips, 6 pcs/svg | 177 | 450 | 50 | 39.0 | 28.0 | 0.0 | | | 20.0 | 5.0 | 12.5 | 1.1 | | | 80 | 0 | 0 | 0 | 0 | 0 | 0.18 | 0.17 | 17.60 | | | | | 0.0 | | | 0 | | 1.1 | | | | 600 | | 1100 | |
| 56370 | 1 ea | Chicken Taquitos, 8 pcs/svg | 218 | 560 | 50 | 30.0 | 54.0 | 6.0 | 1.0 | 47.0 | 25.0 | 5.0 | 11.8 | 2.6 | | | 65 | 400 | 80 | | | | 0.14 | 0.17 | 3.20 | | | | | 2.4 | | | 200 | | 2.7 | | | | 440 | | 900 | |
| | | Desserts | | | | | | | | | | | | | | | | | | | | | | | | | | | | | | | | | | | | | | | | |
| 48135 | 1 ea | Apple Turnover | 110 | 350 | 34 | 3.0 | 48.0 | 0.0 | 13.0 | 35.0 | 19.0 | 4.0 | 10.6 | 1.5 | | | 0 | 0 | 0 | 0 | 0 | 0 | 0.20 | 0.12 | 1.80 | | | | | 9.0 | | | 0 | | 1.8 | | | | 80 | | 460 | |
| 2137 | 1 pce | Cheesecake | 99 | 310 | 42 | 8.0 | 29.0 | 2.0 | 22.0 | 5.0 | 18.0 | 9.0 | 7.0 | 1.0 | | | 65 | 0 | 0 | 0 | 0 | 0 | 0.05 | 0.24 | 2.00 | | | | | 0.0 | | | 100 | | 0.4 | | | | 15 | | 210 | |
| 56373 | 1 ea | Egg Rolls, 5 pcs/svg | 285 | 750 | 51 | 5.0 | 92.0 | 7.0 | 10.0 | 75.0 | 41.0 | 12.0 | 21.5 | 4.5 | | | 50 | 0 | 0 | 0 | 0 | 0 | 1.00 | 0.58 | 10.20 | | | | | 6.0 | | | 150 | | 3.6 | | | | 870 | | 1640 | |
| | | French Fries | | | | | | | | | | | | | | | | | | | | | | | | | | | | | | | | | | | | | | | | |
| 6150 | 1 ea | Medium | 109 | 350 | 38 | 4.0 | 45.0 | 4.0 | 0.0 | 41.0 | 17.0 | 4.0 | | | | | 0 | 0 | 0 | 0 | 0 | 0 | 0.18 | 0.03 | 3.80 | | 0.00 | | | 24.0 | | | 0 | | 1.1 | | | | 690 | | 190 | |
| 6425 | 1 ea | Seasoned Curly, svg | 109 | 360 | 38 | 5.0 | 39.0 | 4.0 | 0.0 | 35.0 | 20.0 | 5.0 | | | | | 0 | 0 | 0 | 0 | 0 | 0 | | | | | 0.00 | | | 4.8 | | | 20 | | 1.4 | | | | 560 | | 1070 | |
| | | Milkshakes | | | | | | | | | | | | | | | | | | | | | | | | | | | | | | | | | | | | | | | | |
| 2163 | 1 ea | Chocolate, svg | 322 | 390 | 72 | 9.0 | 74.0 | 0.0 | 66.0 | 8.0 | 6.0 | 3.5 | 2.1 | 0.4 | | | 25 | 0 | 0 | 0 | 0 | 0 | 0.15 | 0.60 | 0.40 | | | | | 0.0 | | | 300 | | 0.7 | | | | 680 | | 210 | |
| 2164 | 1 ea | Strawberry, svg | 298 | 330 | 74 | 9.0 | 60.0 | 0.0 | 52.0 | 8.0 | 7.0 | 4.0 | 2.0 | 1.0 | | | 30 | 0 | 0 | 0 | 0 | 0 | 0.15 | 0.43 | 0.40 | | | | | 0.0 | | | 300 | | 0.0 | | | | 550 | | 180 | |
| 2165 | 1 ea | Vanilla, svg | 304 | 350 | 73 | 9.0 | 62.0 | 0.0 | 55.0 | 7.0 | 7.0 | 4.0 | 1.8 | 1.2 | | | 30 | 0 | 0 | 0 | 0 | 0 | 0.15 | 0.34 | 0.40 | | | | | 0.0 | | | 300 | | 0.0 | | | | 570 | | 180 | |
| | | Salads | | | | | | | | | | | | | | | | | | | | | | | | | | | | | | | | | | | | | | | | |
| 52088 | 1 ea | Garden Chicken | 253 | 200 | 84 | 23.0 | 8.0 | 3.0 | 4.0 | 1.0 | 9.0 | 4.0 | | | | | 65 | 3500 | 700 | | | | | | | | | | | 0.0 | | | 200 | | 0.7 | | | | 560 | | 420 | |
| 56448 | 1 ea | Side | 110 | 70 | 90 | 4.0 | 3.0 | 2.0 | 1.0 | 0.0 | 4.0 | 2.5 | 1.0 | 0.0 | 0.00 | 0.00 | 10 | 1250 | 250 | | | | 0.06 | 0.10 | | | | | | 0.0 | | | 100 | | 0.4 | | | | 190 | | 80 | |
| | | Sandwiches, Beef | | | | | | | | | | | | | | | | | | | | | | | | | | | | | | | | | | | | | | | | |
| 56434 | 1 ea | Cheeseburger | 110 | 330 | 41 | 16.0 | 32.0 | 0.0 | 5.0 | 27.0 | 15.0 | 6.0 | 5.9 | 2.3 | | | 35 | 300 | 60 | | | | 0.23 | 0.23 | 3.00 | | | | | 1.2 | | | 200 | | 2.7 | | | | 200 | | 510 | |
| 69032 | 1 ea | Cheeseburger w/Bacon | 242 | 710 | 49 | 35.0 | 41.0 | 0.0 | 5.0 | 36.0 | 45.0 | 15.0 | 15.7 | 8.7 | | | 110 | 400 | 80 | | | | 0.24 | 0.48 | 8.80 | 0.39 | | | | 9.0 | | | 250 | | 5.4 | | | | 540 | | 1240 | |
| 56366 | 1 ea | Cheeseburger, Double | 152 | 450 | 44 | 24.0 | 35.0 | 0.0 | 6.0 | 29.0 | 24.0 | 10.8 | 10.4 | 2.8 | | | 75 | 500 | 100 | | | | 0.15 | 0.34 | 6.00 | | | | | 0.0 | | | 250 | | 3.6 | | | | 320 | | 900 | |
| 56437 | 1 ea | Cheeseburger, Jumbo Jack | 242 | 610 | 55 | 29.0 | 41.0 | 0.0 | 6.0 | 35.0 | 36.0 | 12.0 | 15.0 | 9.0 | | | 80 | 300 | 60 | | | | 0.36 | 0.44 | 1.60 | | | | | 6.0 | | | 200 | | 5.4 | | | | 460 | | 780 | |
| 69034 | 1 ea | Cheeseburger, Ultimate | 280 | 830 | 50 | 47.0 | 33.0 | 0.0 | 4.0 | 29.0 | 57.0 | 21.7 | 20.2 | 15.1 | | | 130 | 750 | 150 | | | | 0.30 | 0.51 | 8.00 | 0.50 | | | | 0.0 | | | 300 | | 6.3 | | | | 650 | | 1180 | |
| 69036 | 1 ea | Country Fried Steak | 153 | 450 | 46 | 14.0 | 42.0 | 0.0 | 3.0 | 39.0 | 25.0 | 7.0 | | | | | 35 | 100 | 20 | | | | | | | | | | | 4.8 | | | 60 | | 2.7 | | | | 270 | | 890 | |
| 56433 | 1 ea | Hamburger | 97 | 280 | 42 | 13.0 | 31.0 | 0.0 | 5.0 | 26.0 | 11.0 | 4.0 | 4.9 | 2.0 | | | 25 | 100 | 20 | | | | 0.15 | 0.26 | 2.00 | | | | | 1.2 | | | 100 | | 2.7 | | | | 190 | | 430 | |
| 69038 | 1 ea | Hamburger, 1/4 lb w/Cheese | 172 | 510 | 45 | 26.0 | 39.0 | 0.0 | 8.0 | 31.0 | 27.0 | 10.0 | | | | | 65 | 300 | 60 | | | | | | | | | | | 0.0 | | | 150 | | 3.6 | | | | 170 | | 1030 | |
| 69039 | 1 ea | Hamburger, Colossus | 272 | 940 | 40 | 52.0 | 48.0 | 0.0 | 5.0 | 43.0 | 60.0 | 25.0 | | | | | 165 | 500 | 100 | | | | | | | | | | | 3.6 | | | 300 | | 6.3 | | | | 630 | | 1670 | |
| 69033 | 1 ea | Hamburger, Grilled Sourdough | 223 | 670 | 48 | 32.0 | 39.0 | 0.0 | 4.0 | 35.0 | 43.0 | 16.0 | 17.8 | 7.9 | | | 110 | 750 | 150 | | | | 0.65 | 0.48 | 8.00 | 0.33 | | | | 6.0 | | | 200 | | 4.5 | | | | 510 | | 1140 | |
| 56436 | 1 ea | Hamburger, Jumbo Jack | 229 | 560 | 55 | 26.0 | 41.0 | 0.0 | 6.0 | 35.0 | 32.0 | 10.0 | 13.0 | 8.0 | | | 65 | 200 | 40 | | | | 0.36 | 0.29 | 1.80 | | | | | 6.0 | | | 100 | | 4.5 | | | | 450 | | 700 | |
| 69064 | 1 ea | Monterey Roast Beef | 238 | 540 | 57 | 30.0 | 40.0 | 3.0 | 4.0 | 33.0 | 30.0 | 9.0 | | | | | 75 | 400 | 80 | | | | | | | | | | | 4.8 | | | 300 | | 3.6 | | | | 500 | | 1270 | |
| | | Sandwiches, Chicken | | | | | | | | | | | | | | | | | | | | | | | | | | | | | | | | | | | | | | | | |
| 69063 | 1 ea | Caesar Pita | 237 | 520 | 59 | 27.0 | 44.0 | 4.0 | 5.0 | 35.0 | 26.0 | 6.0 | | | | | 55 | 400 | 80 | | | | | | | | | | | 2.4 | | | 250 | | 2.7 | | | | 490 | | 1050 | |
| 56442 | 1 ea | Grilled Fillet | 211 | 430 | 59 | 29.0 | 36.0 | 0.0 | 7.0 | 29.0 | 19.0 | 5.0 | 4.6 | 6.0 | | | 65 | 300 | 60 | | | | 0.27 | 0.37 | 14.40 | | | | | 6.0 | | | 150 | | 6.3 | | | | 540 | | 1070 | |
| 69035 | 1 ea | Regular | 160 | 400 | 52 | 20.0 | 38.0 | 0.0 | | | 18.0 | 4.0 | | | | | 45 | 200 | 40 | | | | | | | | | | | 0.0 | | | 150 | | 1.8 | | | | 180 | | 1290 | |
| 90092 | 1 ea | Smoked w/Cheddar & Bacon | 223 | 540 | 55 | 30.0 | 37.0 | 0.0 | 2.0 | 35.0 | 30.0 | 11.0 | | | | | 80 | 500 | 100 | | | | | | | | | | | 9.0 | | | 300 | | 2.7 | | | | 450 | | 1520 | |
| 90093 | 1 ea | Sourdough Ranch | 225 | 490 | 57 | 29.0 | 45.0 | 1.0 | 6.0 | 38.0 | 21.0 | 6.0 | | | | | 65 | | | | | | | | | | | | | 0.0 | | | 150 | | 1.8 | | | | 340 | | 1060 | |
| 69037 | 1 ea | Spicy Crispy | 224 | 560 | 52 | 24.0 | 55.0 | 0.0 | 5.0 | 50.0 | 27.0 | 5.0 | | | | | 50 | 200 | 40 | | | | | | | | | | | 4.8 | | | 100 | | 2.7 | | | | 470 | | 1020 | |
| 56443 | 1 ea | Supreme | 245 | 620 | 55 | 25.0 | 48.0 | 0.0 | 5.0 | 43.0 | 36.0 | 10.6 | 14.3 | 11.0 | | | 75 | 500 | 100 | | | | 0.39 | 0.32 | 11.00 | | | | | 2.4 | | | 200 | | 2.7 | | | | 190 | | 1520 | |
| 56439 | 1 ea | Sandwiches, Fish Supreme | 245 | 590 | 56 | 22.0 | 51.0 | 0.0 | 5.0 | 46.0 | 32.0 | 8.0 | 11.4 | 7.7 | | | 60 | 500 | 100 | | | | 0.39 | 0.24 | 4.20 | | | | | 4.8 | | | 200 | | 3.6 | | | | 200 | | 1170 | |
| | | *KENTUCKY FRIED CHICKEN* | | | | | | | | | | | | | | | | | | | | | | | | | | | | | | | | | | | | | | | | |
| 7139 | 1/3 cup | Beans, Baked | 110 | 132 | 70 | 5.1 | 24.0 | 4.0 | 9.0 | 11.0 | 2.0 | 1.0 | 0.5 | 0.3 | | | 3 | 250 | 25 | 0 | 25 | 144 | 0.06 | 0.04 | 0.50 | 0.07 | 0.02 | 32.2 | 0.09 | 2.1 | | | 40 | 0.1 | 1.4 | 29 | 0.3 | 90 | 229 | | 535 | 1.29 |
| 56682 | 1 ea | Beans, Mean, svg | 111 | 52 | 86 | 3.0 | 8.0 | 3.0 | 1.0 | 4.0 | 2.0 | 1.0 | | | | | 6 | 2150 | 215 | 0 | 215 | 1240 | | | | | 0.00 | | | 4.8 | | | 140 | | 1.6 | | | | | | 477 | |
| | | Chicken | | | | | | | | | | | | | | | | | | | | | | | | | | | | | | | | | | | | | | | | |
| 15185 | 1 ea | Breast, Center, Hot & Spicy | 125 | 360 | 48 | 28.0 | 13.0 | | | | 22.0 | 5.0 | | | | | 80 | 50 | 15 | | | | | | | | | | | 6.0 | | | 20 | | 0.7 | | | | | | 750 | |
| 15164 | 1 ea | Breast, Center, Original | 103 | 260 | 52 | 25.0 | 8.8 | 0.1 | 1.8 | 6.9 | 14.0 | 3.8 | 7.8 | 2.0 | | | 92 | 50 | 15 | 15 | 0 | 0 | 0.09 | 0.17 | 11.50 | | | | | | 0.3 | | 30 | | 0.7 | | | | | | 609 | |
| 15169 | 1 ea | Breast, Crispy | 118 | 330 | 48 | 26.0 | 14.0 | 0.1 | 3.3 | 10.6 | 19.7 | 4.8 | 10.8 | 2.1 | | | 75 | 50 | 15 | 15 | 0 | 0 | 0.11 | 0.13 | 13.10 | | | | | | 0.3 | | 33 | | 0.8 | | | | | | 740 | |
| 15168 | 1 ea | Breast, Side, Crispy | 116 | 400 | 40 | 21.0 | 19.0 | 0.2 | 3.4 | 15.4 | 27.0 | 5.5 | 12.9 | 2.3 | | | 75 | 50 | 15 | 15 | 0 | 0 | 0.09 | 0.10 | 8.50 | | | | | | 0.2 | | 20 | | 0.7 | | | | | | 710 | |
| 15186 | 1 ea | Breast, Side, Hot & Spicy | 120 | 400 | 43 | 22.0 | 16.0 | | | | 28.0 | 6.0 | | | | | 80 | 50 | 15 | | | | | | | | | | | 6.0 | | | 40 | | 1.1 | | | | | | 850 | |
| 15163 | 1 ea | Breast, Side, Original | 83 | 245 | 47 | 18.0 | 9.0 | 0.2 | 1.7 | 7.2 | 15.0 | 4.1 | 8.7 | 2.2 | | | 78 | 50 | 15 | 15 | 0 | 0 | 0.06 | 0.13 | 6.90 | | | | | | 0.2 | | 68 | | 1.2 | | | | | | 604 | |
| 15184 | 1 ea | Drumstick, Hot & Spicy | 63 | 180 | 46 | 14.0 | 6.0 | | | | 12.0 | 3.0 | | | | | 55 | 50 | 15 | | | | | | | | | | | 6.0 | | | | | | | | | | | 320 | |
| 15173 | 1 ea | Kentucky Nuggets, 6 pcs/svg | 95 | 284 | 48 | 16.0 | 15.0 | 0.1 | | | 18.0 | 4.0 | | | | | 66 | 50 | 15 | 15 | 0 | 0 | 0.02 | 0.02 | 1.00 | 0.05 | | | | 0.1 | | | 2 | | 0.1 | | | | | | 865 | |
| 15170 | 1 ea | Leg, Crispy | 65 | 190 | 50 | 13.6 | 6.1 | 0.1 | 1.2 | 4.8 | 12.0 | 3.2 | 7.2 | 1.6 | | | 65 | 100 | 30 | 30 | 0 | 0 | 0.06 | 0.12 | 3.70 | | | | | | 0.2 | | 20 | | 0.4 | | | | | | 310 | |
| 15165 | 1 ea | Leg, Original | 57 | 152 | 54 | 14.0 | 3.0 | 0.2 | 0.6 | 2.2 | 8.5 | 2.2 | 4.1 | 1.3 | | | 75 | 50 | 15 | 15 | 0 | 0 | 0.05 | 0.12 | 3.20 | | | | | | 0.2 | | 21 | | 1.1 | | | | | | 269 | |
| 56450 | 1 ea | Sandwich, Chicken Little | 47 | 169 | 35 | 5.7 | 13.8 | 0.4 | | | 10.1 | 2.0 | 4.7 | 3.4 | | | 18 | 17 | 5 | 5 | 0 | 0 | 0.16 | 0.12 | 2.20 | | | | | | | | 23 | | 1.7 | | | | | | 331 | |
| 15171 | 1 ea | Thigh, Crispy | 109 | 380 | 43 | 23.0 | 7.0 | 0.2 | 3.0 | 3.8 | 29.8 | 7.7 | 16.0 | 4.2 | | | 90 | 100 | 30 | 30 | 0 | 0 | 0.10 | 0.21 | 6.50 | | | | | | 0.3 | | 49 | | 1.2 | | | | | | 520 | |
| 15183 | 1 ea | Thigh, Hot & Spicy | 119 | 370 | 47 | 24.0 | 10.0 | | | | 27.0 | 6.0 | | | | | 100 | 50 | 15 | | | | | | | | | | | 6.0 | | | 20 | | 1.1 | | | | | | 670 | |
| 15166 | 1 ea | Thigh, Original | 95 | 287 | 49 | 17.9 | 8.0 | 0.2 | 1.6 | 6.2 | 21.0 | 5.3 | 9.4 | 3.1 | | | 112 | 104 | 31 | 31 | 0 | 0 | 0.08 | 0.30 | 5.50 | | | | | | 0.3 | | 40 | | 1.1 | | | | | | 591 | |
| 15172 | 1 ea | Wing, Crispy | 59 | 240 | 34 | 13.0 | 8.0 | 0.1 | 2.1 | 5.8 | 17.0 | 4.2 | 10.3 | 2.4 | | | 65 | 100 | 30 | 30 | 0 | 0 | | 0.04 | 0.06 | 3.30 | | | | | 0.1 | | 20 | | 0.4 | | | | | | 320 | |
| 15167 | 1 ea | Wing, Original | 53 | 172 | 45 | 12.2 | 5.0 | 0.3 | 1.0 | 3.7 | 11.7 | 3.0 | 6.0 | 1.8 | | | 59 | 50 | 15 | 15 | 0 | 0 | 0.03 | 0.08 | 3.70 | | | | | | 0.1 | | 30 | | 0.5 | | | | | | 383 | |
| 56451 | 1 ea | Coleslaw, svg | 90 | 114 | 75 | 1.5 | 13.2 | 0.5 | 6.2 | 6.5 | 6.0 | 1.0 | 1.7 | 3.3 | | | 5 | 310 | 32 | 2 | 30 | 180 | 0.03 | 0.03 | 0.20 | | 0.00 | | | 27.0 | 0.1 | | 30 | | 0.4 | | | | | | 177 | |
| 6152 | 1 ea | Corn on the Cob | 151 | 222 | 70 | 4.0 | 27.0 | 8.0 | 4.0 | 15.0 | 12.0 | 2.0 | 1.0 | 1.5 | | | 0 | 200 | 20 | 0 | 20 | 80 | 0.14 | 0.11 | 1.80 | | 0.00 | | | 1.8 | 0.0 | | 0 | | 0.4 | | | | | | 76 | |
| 56453 | 1 ea | Mashed Potatoes & Gravy, svg | 120 | 103 | 80 | 1.0 | 16.0 | 0.4 | | | 5.0 | 0.4 | 0.5 | 0.2 | | | 0 | 50 | 15 | 15 | 0 | 0 | | 0.04 | 1.20 | | 0.00 | | | | | | 20 | | 0.4 | | | | | | 388 | |
| 56454 | 1/3 cup | Potato Salad | 125 | 180 | 74 | 3.0 | 18.0 | 2.0 | 7.0 | 9.0 | 11.0 | 2.0 | 2.8 | 4.8 | | | 11 | 400 | 80 | | | | 0.07 | 0.02 | 0.60 | 0.19 | | 7.2 | 0.37 | | | | 10 | 0.1 | 2.2 | 15 | | 32 | 256 | | 423 | 0.29 |
| | | *LONG JOHN SILVERS* | | | | | | | | | | | | | | | | | | | | | | | | | | | | | | | | | | | | | | | | |
| 47363 | 1 ea | Dessert, Walnut Brownie | 97 | 440 | 15 | 5.0 | 54.0 | | | | 22.0 | 5.4 | 11.7 | 4.9 | | | 20 | | | | | | 0.12 | 0.34 | 4.00 | | | | | | | | 20 | | 1.8 | | | | 190 | | 150 | 1.20 |
| | | Dinners | | | | | | | | | | | | | | | | | | | | | | | | | | | | | | | | | | | | | | | | |
| 57005 | 1 ea | Chicken | 452 | 590 | 72 | 32.0 | 82.0 | | | | 15.0 | 3.3 | 5.5 | 6.3 | | | 75 | 1250 | 250 | | | | 0.75 | 0.85 | 6.00 | | | | | 6.0 | | | 200 | | 5.4 | | | | 760 | | 1620 | 2.25 |
| 15198 | 1 ea | Chicken, Light Herb | 100 | 120 | 74 | 22.0 | | | | | 4.0 | 1.2 | 1.7 | 1.1 | | | 60 | | | | | | 0.09 | 0.25 | | | | | | | | | | | 0.7 | | | | 270 | | 570 | 0.60 |
| 57006 | 1 ea | Chicken Plank, 2 pc | 197 | 490 | 52 | 19.0 | 50.0 | | | | 26.0 | 5.6 | 15.3 | 5.0 | | | 30 | | | | | | 0.22 | 0.25 | 8.00 | | | | | 9.0 | | | 20 | | 1.8 | | | | 690 | | 1290 | 0.90 |

| Code | Amount | Description | Basic Components | | | | | | | | | Additional Fats | | | | | | Vit A & Components | | | | | Vitamins | | | | | | | | | | Minerals | | | | | | | | | |
|---|---|---|---|---|---|---|---|---|---|---|---|---|---|---|---|---|---|---|---|---|---|---|---|---|---|---|---|---|---|---|---|---|---|---|---|---|---|---|---|---|---|---|
| | | | Weight (g) | Calories | % Water | Protein (g) | Carbs (g) | Fiber (g) | Sugar (g) | Other Carbs (g) | Fat (g) | Sat Fat (g) | Mono Fat (g) | Poly Fat (g) | Omega 3 (g) | Omega 6 (g) | Choles (mg) | Vit A (IU) | Vit A (RE) | Retinol (RE) | Carotenoids (RE) | Beta Carotene (mcg) | Thiamin (mg) | Riboflavin (mg) | Niacin (NE) | Vit B6 (mg) | Vit B12 (mcg) | Folate (mcg) | Panto (mg) | Vit C (mg) | Vit D (mg) | Vit E (α TE) | Calcium (mg) | Copper (mg) | Iron (mg) | Magnes (mg) | Mang (mg) | Phos (mg) | Potassium (mg) | Selenium (mcg) | Sodium (mg) | Zinc (mg) |
| 56455 | 1 ea | Chicken Plank, 3pc | 399 | 890 | 56 | 32.0 | 101.0 | | | | 44.0 | 9.5 | 24.8 | 9.4 | | | 55 | 200 | 40 | | | | 0.52 | 0.51 | 16.00 | | | | | 9.0 | | | 200 | | 4.5 | | | | 1170 | | 2000 | 3.00 |
| 56459 | 1 ea | Clam | 361 | 990 | 46 | 24.0 | 114.0 | | | | 52.0 | 10.9 | 31.3 | 9.9 | | | 75 | 200 | 40 | | | | 0.75 | 0.43 | 12.00 | | | | | 12.0 | | | 200 | | 4.5 | | | | 910 | | 1830 | 3.00 |
| 56461 | 1 ea | Fish, batter dipped | 88 | 180 | 59 | 12.0 | 12.0 | | | | 11.0 | 2.7 | 8.1 | 0.2 | | | 30 | | | | | | 0.15 | 0.17 | 3.00 | | | | | | | | | | 0.4 | | | | 260 | | 490 | 0.30 |
| 56463 | 1 ea | Fish & Chicken, w/fries & coleslaw | 431 | 950 | 55 | 36.0 | 102.0 | | | | 49.0 | 10.5 | 28.8 | 9.5 | | | 75 | 200 | 40 | | | | 0.60 | 0.60 | 14.00 | | | | | 9.0 | | | 200 | | 4.5 | | | | 1280 | | 2090 | 3.00 |
| 57007 | 1 ea | Fish & Chicken, w/fries, small | 229 | 550 | 49 | 23.0 | 51.0 | | | | 32.0 | 6.8 | 19.5 | 5.2 | | | 45 | | | | | | 0.30 | 0.25 | 8.00 | | | | | 9.0 | | | 20 | | 1.8 | | | | 800 | | 1380 | 1.20 |
| 56462 | 1 ea | Fish & More, 2 pc w/fries & coleslaw | 407 | 890 | 57 | 31.0 | 92.0 | | | | 48.0 | 10.1 | 28.5 | 9.5 | | | 75 | 200 | 40 | | | | 0.52 | 0.51 | 12.00 | | | | | 9.0 | | | 200 | | 3.6 | | | | 1230 | | 1790 | 2.25 |
| 56467 | 1 ea | Fish & Fryes, 2pc, batter fried | 261 | 610 | 54 | 27.0 | 52.0 | | | | 37.0 | 7.9 | 23.5 | 5.3 | | | 60 | | | | | | 0.38 | 0.34 | 8.00 | | | | | 9.0 | | | 40 | | 1.8 | | | | 900 | | 1480 | 1.20 |
| 56468 | 1 ea | Fish & Fryes, 3pc, batter fried | 384 | 980 | 54 | 31.0 | 92.0 | | | | 50.0 | 11.3 | 28.4 | 9.7 | | | 70 | 200 | 40 | | | | 0.45 | 0.43 | 8.00 | | | | | 15.0 | | | 200 | | 4.5 | | | | 1120 | | 1530 | 3.00 |
| 57008 | 1 ea | Fish & Shrimp | 487 | 1140 | 55 | 40.0 | 108.0 | | | | 65.0 | 14.1 | 40.6 | 9.5 | | | 145 | 200 | 40 | | | | 0.75 | 0.68 | 14.00 | | | | | 9.0 | | | 20 | | 4.5 | | | | 1340 | | 2440 | 3.75 |
| 57009 | 1 ea | Fish, Shrimp, & Chicken | 513 | 1160 | 56 | 45.0 | 113.0 | | | | 65.0 | 14.2 | 40.3 | 9.6 | | | 135 | 200 | 40 | | | | 0.75 | 0.68 | 16.00 | | | | | 9.0 | | | 200 | | 4.5 | | | | 1450 | | 2590 | 3.75 |
| 57010 | 1 ea | Fish, Shrimp, & Clams | 512 | 1240 | 74 | 44.0 | 123.0 | | | | 70.0 | 15.2 | 44.2 | 9.9 | | | 140 | 200 | 40 | | | | 0.90 | 0.68 | 16.00 | | | | | 9.0 | | | 200 | | 5.4 | | | | 1390 | | 2630 | 3.75 |
| 57003 | 1 ea | Fish w/Lemon Crumb, 3 pc | 493 | 610 | 71 | 39.0 | 86.0 | | | | 13.0 | 2.2 | 3.9 | 5.3 | | | 125 | 3500 | 700 | | | | 0.75 | 0.60 | 24.00 | | | | | 6.0 | | | 200 | | 5.4 | | | | 990 | | 1420 | 2.25 |
| 57004 | 1 ea | Fish w/Lemon Crumb, 2 pc, light portion | 334 | 330 | 77 | 24.0 | 46.0 | | | | 5.0 | 0.9 | 1.6 | 1.2 | | | 75 | 5000 | 1000 | | | | 0.30 | 0.25 | 14.00 | | | | | 18.0 | | | 80 | | 1.8 | | | | 440 | | 640 | 0.90 |
| | | Kid's Meal | | | | | | | | | | | | | | | | | | | | | | | | | | | | | | | | | | | | | | | | |
| 57012 | 1 ea | Chicken Plank | 221 | 560 | 50 | 21.0 | 60.0 | | | | 29.0 | 6.3 | 17.2 | 5.3 | | | 30 | | | | | | 0.30 | 0.25 | 9.00 | | | | | 9.0 | | | 60 | | 2.7 | | | | 750 | | 1310 | 1.20 |
| 57429 | 1 ea | Fish & Chicken | 253 | 620 | 49 | 24.0 | 61.0 | | | | 34.0 | 7.4 | 21.1 | 5.4 | | | 45 | | | | | | 0.38 | 0.34 | 9.00 | | | | | 9.0 | | | 80 | | 2.7 | | | | 860 | | 1400 | 1.50 |
| 57011 | 1 ea | Fish & Fries | 197 | 500 | 52 | 16.0 | 50.0 | | | | 28.0 | 5.3 | 16.9 | 5.3 | | | 30 | | | | | | 0.30 | 0.25 | 6.00 | | | | | 9.0 | | | 60 | | 1.8 | | | | 700 | | 1010 | 1.20 |
| | | Salads | | | | | | | | | | | | | | | | | | | | | | | | | | | | | | | | | | | | | | | | |
| 56476 | 1 ea | Cole slaw | 98 | 140 | 70 | 1.0 | 20.0 | 1.0 | | | 6.0 | 1.0 | 1.5 | 3.5 | | | 15 | 200 | 40 | 5 | 35 | 208 | 0.06 | 0.07 | 2.00 | | 0.00 | | | | | | 60 | | 0.7 | | | | 190 | | 260 | 0.60 |
| 56474 | 1 ea | Ocean Chef | 234 | 110 | 89 | 12.0 | 13.0 | 2.0 | | | 1.0 | 0.1 | 0.4 | 0.2 | | | 40 | 5000 | 500 | | | | 0.12 | 0.14 | 3.00 | | | | | 21.0 | | | 100 | | 3.6 | | | | 95 | | 730 | 0.30 |
| 56475 | 1 ea | Seafood | 278 | 380 | 79 | 15.0 | 12.0 | 2.0 | | | 31.0 | 5.1 | 8.2 | 17.5 | | | 55 | 2000 | 200 | | | | 0.15 | 0.25 | 3.00 | | | | | 21.0 | | | 150 | | 4.5 | | | | 130 | | 930 | 0.90 |
| 52073 | 1 ea | Side | 126 | 25 | 92 | 1.0 | 6.0 | | | | | | | | | | 0 | 3000 | 600 | | | | 0.09 | 0.68 | 0.40 | | | | | 15.0 | | | 40 | | 0.7 | | | | | | 20 | |
| | | Sandwiches | | | | | | | | | | | | | | | | | | | | | | | | | | | | | | | | | | | | | | | | |
| 69031 | 1 ea | Chicken, batter dipped | 127 | 280 | 51 | 14.0 | 39.0 | | | | 8.0 | 2.0 | 5.1 | 0.9 | | | 15 | | | | | | 0.38 | 0.34 | 7.00 | | | | | 1.2 | | | 80 | | 3.6 | | | | 260 | | 790 | 1.20 |
| 69030 | 1 ea | Fish, batter dipped | 159 | 340 | 54 | 18.0 | 40.0 | | | | 13.0 | 3.1 | 8.9 | 1.0 | | | 30 | | | | | | 0.33 | 0.34 | 6.00 | | | | | 1.2 | | | 80 | | 3.6 | | | | 370 | | 890 | 1.50 |
| | | Vegetables | | | | | | | | | | | | | | | | | | | | | | | | | | | | | | | | | | | | | | | | |
| 6423 | 1 pce | Corn Cobette | 94 | 140 | 68 | 3.0 | 18.0 | | | | 8.0 | | | | | | 0 | 300 | 60 | 0 | 60 | 241 | 0.09 | 0.10 | 1.20 | | 0.00 | | | 9.0 | | | | | 0.4 | | | | | | 0 | |
| 6424 | 3 1/2 oz | Green Beans | 99 | 20 | 96 | 1.0 | 3.0 | | | | | | | | | | 0 | 400 | 40 | 0 | 40 | 231 | 0.30 | 0.17 | 0.14 | | 0.00 | | | 2.4 | | | 40 | | 0.7 | | | | 115 | | 320 | |
| | | *McDONALDS* | | | | | | | | | | | | | | | | | | | | | | | | | | | | | | | | | | | | | | | | |
| | | Breakfast Items | | | | | | | | | | | | | | | | | | | | | | | | | | | | | | | | | | | | | | | | |
| 69002 | 1 ea | Biscuit w/Bacon, Egg & Cheese | 152 | 450 | 46 | 17.3 | 33.2 | 1.1 | 3.5 | 28.5 | 27.3 | 8.7 | 8.9 | 2.3 | | | 238 | 497 | 99 | | | | 0.39 | 0.58 | 3.32 | 0.13 | 0.99 | 29.9 | 1.17 | 0.0 | 0.0 | | 103 | 0.1 | 2.6 | 20 | 0.0 | 555 | 245 | 10.6 | 1315 | 1.64 |
| 69003 | 1 ea | Biscuit w/Sausage | 119 | 433 | 37 | 10.1 | 32.3 | 1.1 | 2.6 | 28.5 | 29.3 | 8.6 | 10.1 | 2.8 | | | 33 | 11 | 2 | | | | 0.43 | 0.29 | 3.93 | 0.12 | 0.43 | 4.9 | 0.55 | 0.0 | | | 75 | 0.1 | 2.4 | 15 | | 413 | 207 | | 1128 | 1.08 |
| 69004 | 1 ea | Biscuit w/Sausage & Egg | 170 | 518 | 48 | 16.4 | 32.8 | 1.1 | 3.2 | 28.5 | 35.4 | 10.4 | 12.7 | 3.7 | | | 245 | 293 | 59 | | | | 0.51 | 0.55 | 3.96 | 0.18 | | 27.0 | 1.25 | 0.0 | 0.6 | | 100 | 0.1 | 2.9 | 20 | 0.0 | 499 | 270 | 10.6 | 1199 | 1.61 |
| 69005 | 1 ea | Egg McMuffin | 137 | 289 | 57 | 16.7 | 26.7 | 1.5 | 2.8 | 22.5 | 12.6 | 0.7 | 4.5 | 1.6 | | | 234 | 586 | 100 | 95 | 0 | | 0.49 | 0.45 | 3.33 | 0.15 | 0.67 | 33.2 | 0.89 | 1.8 | 0.6 | | 151 | 0.1 | 2.4 | 24 | 0.0 | 270 | 199 | 10.6 | 730 | 1.56 |
| 6155 | 1 ea | Hashbrown Potatoes, svg | 53 | 130 | 55 | 1.3 | 13.5 | 1.4 | 0.0 | 12.1 | 7.9 | 1.3 | 2.3 | 1.9 | | | 0 | 0 | 0 | 0 | 0 | 0 | 0.08 | 0.02 | 0.90 | 0.08 | 0.00 | 8.3 | | 2.7 | 0.0 | | 7 | 0.0 | 0.3 | 11 | | 51 | 212 | | 332 | 0.15 |
| 69006 | 1 ea | Sausage McMuffin | 112 | 361 | 42 | 12.6 | 26.3 | 1.5 | 1.9 | 22.3 | 22.8 | 8.3 | 8.2 | 2.8 | | | 46 | 238 | 48 | 48 | 0 | 0 | 0.56 | 0.27 | 3.76 | 0.14 | 0.51 | 15.7 | 0.48 | 0.0 | | | 132 | 0.1 | 2.1 | 22 | | 156 | 191 | | 751 | 1.51 |
| 69007 | 1 ea | Sausage McMuffin w/Egg | 163 | 443 | 52 | 18.8 | 26.9 | 1.5 | 2.6 | 22.3 | 23.6 | 10.0 | 10.7 | 3.6 | | | 257 | 586 | 117 | 117 | 0 | | 0.59 | 0.49 | 3.79 | 0.19 | | 33.2 | 1.04 | 0.0 | 0.0 | | 156 | 0.1 | 2.8 | 26 | 0.0 | 275 | 251 | 10.6 | 821 | 2.07 |
| 19579 | 1 ea | Scrambled eggs, svg | 102 | 170 | 73 | 12.6 | 1.1 | 0.0 | 1.1 | 0.0 | 12.2 | 3.6 | 5.3 | 1.7 | | | 424 | 624 | 168 | 168 | 0 | | 0.07 | 0.51 | 0.06 | 0.12 | 1.11 | 44.0 | 1.40 | 0.0 | 1.3 | | 50 | 0.0 | 1.2 | 10 | 0.0 | 172 | 126 | 21.3 | 143 | 1.06 |
| 15174 | 4 pce | Chicken McNuggets, svg | 73 | 198 | 51 | 12.4 | 10.4 | 0.0 | 0.0 | 10.4 | 11.8 | 2.5 | 3.7 | 2.4 | | | 42 | 0 | 0 | 0 | 0 | 0 | 0.08 | 0.11 | 5.15 | 0.21 | 0.21 | | 0.58 | 0.0 | 0.2 | | 9 | 0.0 | 0.7 | 17 | | 199 | 210 | | 353 | 0.69 |
| | | Desserts | | | | | | | | | | | | | | | | | | | | | | | | | | | | | | | | | | | | | | | | |
| 42335 | 1 ea | Danish, Apple | 105 | 360 | 31 | 4.5 | 50.6 | 1.5 | 29.0 | 20.2 | 16.6 | 5.3 | | | | | 42 | 493 | 100 | | | | 0.30 | 0.17 | 2.00 | | | | | 0.5 | | | 78 | | 1.0 | | | 0 | 113 | | 291 | |
| 42337 | 1 ea | Danish, Cheese | 105 | 412 | 26 | 6.7 | 46.8 | 0.1 | 26.3 | 20.5 | 22.2 | 8.4 | | | | | 71 | 696 | 139 | | | | 0.30 | 0.26 | 2.00 | | | | | 0.3 | | | 88 | | 0.9 | | | 0 | 111 | | 343 | |
| 42336 | 1 ea | Danish, Cinnamon Raisin | 105 | 435 | 19 | 5.4 | 55.7 | 1.4 | 30.1 | 24.1 | 22.0 | 7.3 | | | | | 51 | 499 | 100 | | | | 0.30 | 0.26 | 3.00 | | | | | 0.5 | | | 92 | | 1.6 | | | 0 | 112 | | 280 | |
| 42338 | 1 ea | Danish, Raspberry | 105 | 396 | 22 | 4.7 | 58.5 | 1.4 | 36.9 | 20.3 | 16.5 | 5.3 | | | | | 44 | 504 | 101 | | | | 0.30 | 0.17 | 2.00 | | | | | 0.5 | | | 86 | | 1.0 | | | 0 | 93 | | 296 | |
| 2170 | 1 ea | Frozen Yogurt Sundae, Hot Caramel, lowfat | 182 | 307 | 56 | 7.0 | 62.5 | 0.9 | 46.1 | 15.5 | 3.2 | 2.0 | 0.3 | 0.9 | | | 7 | 88 | 18 | | | | 0.09 | 0.34 | 0.27 | | | | | 1.6 | 0.3 | | 246 | | 0.2 | | | 215 | 344 | | 197 | |
| 2171 | 1 ea | Frozen Yogurt Sundae, Hot Fudge, lowfat | 179 | 292 | 60 | 8.0 | 53.5 | 1.8 | 45.9 | 5.3 | 5.2 | 4.7 | 0.1 | 0.4 | | | 5 | 36 | 7 | | | 0 | 0.09 | 0.34 | 0.29 | | | | | 1.6 | 0.5 | | 258 | | 0.6 | | | 238 | 441 | | 190 | |
| 2172 | 1 ea | Frozen Yogurt Sundae, Strawberry, lowfat | 178 | 239 | 65 | 6.1 | 51.4 | 1.1 | 44.5 | 5.3 | 1.0 | 0.7 | 0.1 | 0.2 | | | 5 | 30 | 6 | | | | 0.06 | 0.34 | 0.25 | | | | | 1.7 | 0.9 | | 221 | | 0.3 | | | 171 | 325 | | 115 | |
| 2166 | 1 ea | Frozen Yogurt Sundae, Vanilla, lowfat | 90 | 118 | 68 | 4.1 | 23.7 | 0.4 | 16.0 | 7.3 | 0.7 | 0.5 | 0.2 | 0.0 | | | 3 | 22 | 4 | | | 0 | 0.00 | 0.01 | 0.23 | | | | | 1.0 | 0.2 | | 132 | | 0.2 | | | 101 | 175 | | 85 | |
| | | French Fries | | | | | | | | | | | | | | | | | | | | | | | | | | | | | | | | | | | | | | | | |
| 6157 | 1 ea | Medium | 97 | 320 | 38 | 4.0 | 36.0 | 1.7 | | | 17.0 | 3.5 | 12.0 | 1.5 | | | 0 | 0 | 0 | 0 | 0 | 0 | 0.23 | 0.00 | 3.00 | | 0.00 | | | 12.0 | | | 14 | | 0.7 | | | | | | 150 | |
| 5462 | 1 ea | Large | 147 | 448 | 40 | 6.3 | 56.7 | 5.1 | 0.0 | 51.6 | 21.8 | 3.8 | 6.7 | 5.4 | | | 0 | 0 | 0 | 0 | 0 | 0 | 0.12 | 0.00 | 4.19 | 0.53 | 0.00 | 55.3 | 0.74 | 17.0 | | | 20 | 0.2 | 1.1 | 57 | | 190 | 1013 | | 291 | 0.69 |
| | | Milkshakes | | | | | | | | | | | | | | | | | | | | | | | | | | | | | | | | | | | | | | | | |
| 2167 | 1 ea | Chocolate, small | 295 | 348 | 76 | 12.6 | 62.4 | 0.9 | 58.1 | 3.4 | 5.5 | 3.5 | 0.1 | 0.7 | | | 24 | 190 | 45 | | | | 0.12 | 0.51 | 0.40 | 0.10 | | | | 2.9 | 1.2 | | 372 | | 1.0 | | | 354 | 543 | | 241 | |
| 2168 | 1 ea | Strawberry, small | 294 | 343 | 72 | 11.8 | 62.9 | 0.3 | 59.3 | 3.3 | 5.0 | 3.4 | 0.1 | 0.6 | | | 24 | 190 | 45 | | | | 0.12 | 0.51 | 0.40 | 0.11 | | | | 2.9 | 0.6 | | 366 | | 0.3 | | | 329 | 542 | | 170 | |
| 2169 | 1 ea | Vanilla, small | 293 | 308 | 75 | 11.6 | 54.4 | 0.3 | 50.8 | 3.3 | 5.0 | 3.3 | 0.1 | 0.6 | | | 24 | 185 | 45 | | | | 0.12 | 0.51 | 0.31 | | | | | 2.9 | 0.6 | | 360 | | 0.3 | | | 327 | 533 | | 194 | |
| | | Salads | | | | | | | | | | | | | | | | | | | | | | | | | | | | | | | | | | | | | | | | |
| 52000 | 1 ea | Chef | 313 | 206 | 86 | 19.5 | 8.8 | 2.8 | 5.7 | 0.3 | 10.7 | 4.2 | 3.0 | 1.2 | | | 179 | 5898 | 1180 | | | | 0.33 | 0.37 | 4.32 | 0.36 | 0.96 | 100.0 | 1.05 | 22.2 | 0.4 | | 157 | 0.1 | 1.8 | 40 | 2.9 | 334 | 606 | 9.3 | 727 | 2.16 |
| 52070 | 1 ea | Chunky Chicken | 296 | 164 | 88 | 22.6 | 8.4 | 3.2 | 5.2 | 0.0 | 5.0 | 1.3 | 1.6 | 1.0 | | | 76 | 9865 | 1973 | | | | 0.51 | 0.21 | 8.46 | 0.52 | 0.28 | 82.9 | 1.03 | 30.2 | 0.0 | | 54 | 0.2 | 1.6 | 44 | 0.3 | 276 | 673 | 0.9 | 318 | 1.52 |
| 56479 | 1 ea | Garden | 234 | 84 | 92 | 6.1 | 6.9 | 2.7 | 4.2 | 0.0 | 3.9 | 1.1 | 1.4 | 0.7 | | | 139 | 11140 | 1114 | | | | 0.12 | 0.24 | 0.65 | 0.16 | 0.36 | 96.1 | 0.70 | 21.7 | 0.4 | | 53 | 0.1 | 1.3 | 24 | 0.3 | 103 | 407 | 9.2 | 61 | 0.73 |
| 56480 | 1 ea | Side | 139 | 46 | 92 | 3.3 | 4.2 | 1.7 | 2.3 | 0.2 | 2.0 | 0.6 | 0.7 | 0.4 | | | 70 | 2415 | 483 | | | | 0.07 | 0.13 | 0.39 | 0.09 | 0.18 | 58.9 | 0.36 | 11.9 | 0.2 | | 31 | 0.1 | 0.8 | 14 | 0.2 | 56 | 244 | 4.7 | 33 | 0.41 |
| | | Sandwiches, Beef | | | | | | | | | | | | | | | | | | | | | | | | | | | | | | | | | | | | | | | | |
| 69010 | 1 ea | Big Mac | 216 | 511 | 53 | 25.0 | 46.1 | 3.3 | 7.9 | 35.0 | 25.7 | 9.3 | 7.5 | 4.1 | | | 76 | 328 | 65 | | | | 0.49 | 0.44 | 6.08 | 0.25 | 2.26 | 49.4 | 0.61 | 2.8 | 0.0 | | 202 | 0.3 | 4.3 | 46 | 0.2 | 267 | 456 | 0.1 | 932 | 4.81 |
| 69009 | 1 ea | Cheeseburger | 122 | 318 | 46 | 15.0 | 36.0 | 1.9 | 5.9 | 28.2 | 13.0 | 5.6 | 3.8 | 1.1 | | | 42 | 318 | 64 | | | | 0.33 | 0.31 | 3.81 | 0.15 | 1.20 | 23.7 | 0.39 | 2.5 | 0.0 | | 134 | 0.2 | 2.7 | 27 | 0.1 | 178 | 281 | 1.0 | 766 | 2.62 |
| 69008 | 1 ea | Hamburger | 108 | 265 | 49 | 12.4 | 35.4 | 1.9 | 5.6 | 27.9 | 8.7 | 3.2 | 2.8 | 0.9 | | | 29 | 112 | 22 | | | | 0.33 | 0.26 | 3.81 | 0.14 | 1.04 | 20.8 | 0.34 | 2.5 | 0.0 | | 126 | 0.2 | 2.7 | 24 | 0.1 | 113 | 260 | 1.0 | 532 | 2.25 |
| 69011 | 1 ea | Quarter-Pounder | 171 | 415 | 52 | 22.6 | 36.0 | 1.7 | 7.1 | 27.2 | 20.4 | 7.8 | 6.7 | 1.3 | | | 70 | 165 | 33 | | | | 0.39 | 0.32 | 6.78 | 0.24 | 2.58 | 27.4 | 0.60 | 2.9 | 0.0 | | 127 | 0.3 | 4.3 | 34 | 0.0 | 207 | 405 | 1.4 | 692 | 4.66 |

| Code | Amount | Description | Weight (g) | Calories | % Water | Protein (g) | Carbs (g) | Fiber (g) | Sugar (g) | Other Carbs (g) | Fat (g) | Sat Fat (g) | Mono Fat (g) | Poly Fat (g) | Omega 3 (g) | Omega 6 (g) | Choles (mg) |
|---|---|---|---|---|---|---|---|---|---|---|---|---|---|---|---|---|---|
| 69012 | 1 ea | Quarter-Pounder w/Cheese | 199 | 520 | 50 | 27.9 | 37.2 | 1.7 | 7.7 | 27.8 | 29.1 | 12.6 | 8.7 | 1.7 | | | 97 |
| 69013 | 1 ea | Sandwiches, Filet-O-Fish | 145 | 364 | 49 | 13.7 | 40.8 | 1.5 | 5.5 | 33.8 | 16.2 | 3.7 | 3.8 | 5.6 | | | 37 |
| 69041 | 1 ea | Sandwiches, McChicken | 189 | 491 | 52 | 17.1 | 41.6 | 1.7 | 5.5 | 34.4 | 28.8 | 5.4 | 8.5 | 10.2 | | | 52 |
| 69014 | 1 ea | Sandwiches, McGrilled Chicken | 188 | 254 | 67 | 23.9 | 32.7 | 2.0 | 5.7 | 25.0 | 3.2 | 0.7 | 0.5 | 1.1 | | | 47 |
| | | *PIZZA HUT* | | | | | | | | | | | | | | | |
| | | Beef | | | | | | | | | | | | | | | |
| 57373 | 1 pce | Hand Tossed | 120 | 259 | 54 | 15.0 | 28.9 | 2.0 | | | 9.0 | 4.0 | | | | | 26 |
| 57384 | 1 pce | Pan | 120 | 285 | 52 | 14.0 | 27.9 | 2.0 | | | 13.0 | 5.0 | | | | | 26 |
| 57394 | 1 pce | Thin 'N Crispy | 99 | 229 | 54 | 13.0 | 21.0 | 2.0 | | | 11.0 | 5.0 | | | | | 26 |
| | | Cheese | | | | | | | | | | | | | | | |
| 56489 | 1 pce | Hand Tossed | 108 | 235 | 53 | 13.0 | 29.0 | 2.0 | | | 7.0 | 4.0 | | | | | 25 |
| 56481 | 1 pce | Pan | 108 | 261 | 52 | 12.0 | 28.0 | 2.0 | | | 11.0 | 5.0 | 3.4 | 1.7 | | | 25 |
| 56485 | 1 pce | Thin 'N Crispy | 87 | 205 | 52 | 11.0 | 21.0 | 2.0 | | | 8.0 | 4.0 | 2.2 | 1.2 | | | 25 |
| | | Ham | | | | | | | | | | | | | | | |
| 57372 | 1 pce | Hand Tossed | 105 | 213 | 54 | 12.0 | 29.1 | 2.0 | | | 5.0 | 3.0 | | | | | 21 |
| 57375 | 1 pce | Pan | 105 | 239 | 52 | 11.0 | 28.1 | 2.0 | | | 9.0 | 3.0 | | | | | 21 |
| 57393 | 1 pce | Thin 'N Crispy | 85 | 183 | 54 | 10.0 | 20.9 | 1.0 | | | 7.0 | 3.0 | | | | | 22 |
| | | Italian Sausage | | | | | | | | | | | | | | | |
| 57377 | 1 pce | Hand Tossed | 116 | 268 | 52 | 13.0 | 29.1 | 2.0 | | | 11.0 | 5.0 | | | | | 31 |
| 57385 | 1 pce | Pan | 116 | 294 | 51 | 12.0 | 27.1 | 2.0 | | | 15.1 | 5.0 | | | | | 31 |
| 57374 | 1 pce | Thin 'N Crispy | 94 | 235 | 52 | 11.0 | 20.9 | 2.0 | | | 12.0 | 5.0 | | | | | 31 |
| | | Meat Lover's | | | | | | | | | | | | | | | |
| 57378 | 1 pce | Hand Tossed | 130 | 313 | 54 | 16.9 | 28.9 | 2.0 | | | 11.0 | 6.0 | | | | | 38 |
| 57383 | 1 pce | Pan | 130 | 339 | 50 | 16.0 | 27.9 | 2.0 | | | 17.9 | 7.0 | | | | | 38 |
| 57395 | 1 pce | Thin 'N Crispy | 110 | 288 | 54 | 15.0 | 21.0 | 2.0 | | | 13.0 | 6.0 | | | | | 39 |
| | | Pepperoni | | | | | | | | | | | | | | | |
| 57387 | 1 pce | Bigfoot | 79 | 205 | 46 | 10.0 | 25.0 | 2.0 | | | 7.0 | 3.0 | | | | | 20 |
| 57386 | 1 pce | Bigfoot, w/Mushrooms & Italian Sausage | 90 | 214 | 49 | 11.0 | 25.0 | 2.0 | | | 8.0 | 4.0 | | | | | 21 |
| 56482 | 1 pce | Pan | 104 | 266 | 49 | 11.0 | 28.1 | 2.0 | | | 12.0 | 4.0 | 5.0 | 1.9 | | | 24 |
| 56493 | 1 ea | Personal Pan | 255 | 637 | 50 | 27.0 | 68.9 | 5.0 | | | 28.0 | 10.0 | 11.8 | 4.5 | | | 55 |
| 56486 | 1 pce | Thin 'N Crispy | 84 | 215 | 48 | 11.0 | 21.0 | 1.0 | | | 10.0 | 4.0 | | | | | 25 |
| | | Pepperoni Lover's | | | | | | | | | | | | | | | |
| 57380 | 1 pce | Hand Tossed | 123 | 305 | 50 | 16.0 | 29.9 | 2.0 | | | 14.0 | 6.0 | | | | | 40 |
| 57381 | 1 pce | Pan | 123 | 331 | 50 | 15.0 | 27.9 | 2.0 | | | 17.0 | 7.0 | | | | | 40 |
| 57391 | 1 pce | Thin 'N Crispy | 105 | 290 | 48 | 15.0 | 22.0 | 2.0 | | | 16.0 | 7.0 | | | | | 42 |
| | | Pork | | | | | | | | | | | | | | | |
| 57376 | 1 pce | Hand Tossed | 120 | 267 | 54 | 13.9 | 28.9 | 2.0 | | | 10.0 | 5.0 | | | | | 26 |
| 57389 | 1 pce | Pan | 120 | 293 | 53 | 12.9 | 27.9 | 2.0 | | | 13.9 | 5.0 | | | | | 26 |
| 57392 | 1 pce | Thin 'N Crispy | 99 | 237 | 53 | 12.0 | 21.0 | 2.0 | | | 12.0 | 5.0 | | | | | 26 |
| | | Super Supreme | | | | | | | | | | | | | | | |
| 56492 | 1 pce | Hand Tossed | 143 | 296 | 57 | 16.0 | 30.0 | 3.0 | | | 13.0 | 5.0 | | | | | 34 |
| 56484 | 1 pce | Pan | 143 | 323 | 56 | 15.0 | 28.0 | 3.0 | | | 17.0 | 6.0 | | | | | 34 |
| 56488 | 1 pce | Thin 'N Crispy | 123 | 269 | 57 | 14.0 | 21.9 | 2.0 | | | 14.0 | 6.0 | | | | | 35 |
| | | Supreme | | | | | | | | | | | | | | | |
| 56491 | 1 pce | Hand Tossed | 136 | 283 | 56 | 16.0 | 29.9 | 3.0 | | | 12.0 | 5.0 | | | | | 30 |
| 56494 | 1 ea | Personal Pan | 327 | 721 | 58 | 33.0 | 69.9 | 6.0 | | | 34.0 | 12.0 | 14.7 | 5.6 | | | 66 |
| 56487 | 1 pce | Thin 'N Crispy | 116 | 257 | 57 | 14.0 | 21.0 | 2.0 | | | 13.0 | 5.0 | | | | | 31 |
| | | Veggie Lover's | | | | | | | | | | | | | | | |
| 57379 | 1 pce | Hand Tossed | 132 | 215 | 62 | 10.9 | 29.8 | 3.0 | | | 6.0 | 3.0 | | | | | 17 |
| 57382 | 1 pce | Pan | 133 | 243 | 61 | 10.0 | 29.0 | 3.0 | | | 10.0 | 3.0 | | | | | 17 |
| 57390 | 1 pce | Thin 'N Crispy | 112 | 187 | 64 | 9.0 | 22.1 | 2.0 | | | 7.0 | 3.0 | | | | | 17 |
| | | *SUBWAY* | | | | | | | | | | | | | | | |
| | | Salads | | | | | | | | | | | | | | | |
| 52128 | 1 ea | B L T | 276 | 140 | 91 | 7.0 | 10.0 | 2.0 | 1.0 | 7.0 | 8.0 | 3.0 | | | | | 16 |
| 52119 | 1 ea | Chicken Breast, rstd | 331 | 162 | 89 | 20.0 | 13.0 | 1.0 | 2.0 | 10.0 | 4.0 | 1.0 | | | | | 48 |
| 52127 | 1 ea | Chicken Taco | 370 | 250 | 87 | 18.0 | 15.0 | 2.0 | 3.0 | 10.0 | 14.0 | 5.0 | | | | | 52 |
| 52115 | 1 ea | Club | 331 | 126 | 91 | 14.0 | 12.0 | 1.0 | 2.0 | 9.0 | 3.0 | 1.0 | | | | | 26 |
| 52120 | 1 ea | Cold Cut Trio | 330 | 191 | 89 | 13.0 | 11.0 | 1.0 | 1.0 | 9.0 | 11.0 | 3.0 | | | | | 64 |
| 52123 | 1 ea | Ham | 316 | 116 | 91 | 12.0 | 11.0 | 1.0 | 2.0 | 8.0 | 3.0 | 1.0 | | | | | 28 |
| 52129 | 1 ea | Meatball | 345 | 233 | 88 | 12.0 | 16.0 | 2.0 | 3.0 | 11.0 | 14.0 | 5.0 | | | | | 33 |
| 52121 | 1 ea | Pizza | 335 | 277 | 86 | 12.0 | 13.0 | 2.0 | 3.0 | 8.0 | 20.0 | 8.0 | | | | | 50 |
| 52126 | 1 ea | Roast Beef | 316 | 117 | 92 | 12.0 | 11.0 | 1.0 | 2.0 | 8.0 | 3.0 | 1.0 | | | | | 20 |
| 52117 | 1 ea | Seafood & Crab | 331 | 244 | 88 | 13.0 | 10.0 | 2.0 | 1.0 | 7.0 | 17.0 | 3.0 | | | | | 34 |
| 52116 | 1 ea | Seafood & Crab, w/light mayo | 331 | 161 | 90 | 13.0 | 11.0 | 2.0 | 1.0 | 8.0 | 8.0 | 1.0 | | | | | 32 |
| 52130 | 1 ea | Steak & Cheese | 342 | 212 | 87 | 22.0 | 13.0 | 1.0 | 3.0 | 9.0 | 8.0 | 5.0 | | | | | 70 |
| 52122 | 1 ea | Tuna | 331 | 356 | 84 | 12.0 | 10.0 | 1.0 | 1.0 | 8.0 | 30.0 | 5.0 | | | | | 36 |
| 52118 | 1 ea | Tuna, w/light mayo | 331 | 205 | 89 | 12.0 | 11.0 | 1.0 | 1.0 | 9.0 | 13.0 | 2.0 | | | | | 32 |
| 52114 | 1 ea | Turkey Breast | 316 | 102 | 92 | 11.0 | 12.0 | 1.0 | 1.0 | 10.0 | 2.0 | 1.0 | | | | | 19 |
| 52125 | 1 ea | Turkey Breast & Ham | 316 | 109 | 92 | 11.0 | 11.0 | 1.0 | 2.0 | 8.0 | 3.0 | 1.0 | | | | | 24 |
| 52113 | 1 ea | Veggie Delite | 260 | 51 | 94 | 2.0 | 10.0 | 1.0 | 1.0 | 8.0 | 1.0 | 0.0 | | | 0.00 | 0.00 | 0 |

| Code | Description | Vit A (IU) | Vit A (RE) | Retinol (RE) | Carotenoids (RE) | Beta Carotene (mcg) | Thiamin (mg) | Riboflavin (mg) | Niacin (NE) | Vit B6 (mg) | Vit B12 (mcg) | Folate (mcg) | Panto (mg) | Vit C (mg) | Vit D (mg) | Vit E (α TE) |
|---|---|---|---|---|---|---|---|---|---|---|---|---|---|---|---|---|
| 69012 | Quarter-Pounder w/Cheese | 576 | 115 | | | | 0.39 | 0.43 | 6.78 | 0.26 | 2.89 | 33.2 | 0.70 | 2.9 | 0.0 | |
| 69013 | Sandwiches, Filet-O-Fish | 103 | 21 | | | | 0.32 | 0.23 | 2.58 | 0.07 | 0.58 | 29.6 | 0.38 | 0.0 | 0.0 | |
| 69041 | Sandwiches, McChicken | 146 | 29 | | | | 0.91 | 0.24 | 7.74 | 0.38 | 0.05 | 36.8 | 0.85 | 1.1 | 0.1 | |
| 69014 | Sandwiches, McGrilled Chicken | 230 | 46 | | | | 0.43 | 0.28 | 12.12 | 0.55 | 0.16 | 37.7 | 0.30 | 5.3 | | |
| | *PIZZA HUT* | | | | | | | | | | | | | | | |
| | Beef | | | | | | | | | | | | | | | |
| 57373 | Hand Tossed | 44 | 87 | | | | | | | | | | | | | |
| 57384 | Pan | 444 | 89 | | | | | | | | | | | | | |
| 57394 | Thin 'N Crispy | 457 | 91 | | | | | | | | | | | | | |
| | Cheese | | | | | | | | | | | | | | | |
| 56489 | Hand Tossed | 496 | 99 | | | | 0.24 | 0.24 | 2.65 | | | | | 4.9 | | |
| 56481 | Pan | 527 | 105 | | | | 0.30 | 0.32 | 2.74 | 0.09 | | | | 3.7 | | |
| 56485 | Thin 'N Crispy | 542 | 108 | | | | 0.23 | 0.23 | 2.83 | 0.09 | | | | 2.9 | | |
| | Ham | | | | | | | | | | | | | | | |
| 57372 | Hand Tossed | 426 | 85 | | | | | | | | | | | | | |
| 57375 | Pan | 433 | 87 | | | | | | | | | | | | | |
| 57393 | Thin 'N Crispy | 444 | 89 | | | | | | | | | | | | | |
| | Italian Sausage | | | | | | | | | | | | | | | |
| 57377 | Hand Tossed | 433 | 87 | | | | | | | | | | | | | |
| 57385 | Pan | 441 | 88 | | | | | | | | | | | | | |
| 57374 | Thin 'N Crispy | 451 | 90 | | | | | | | | | | | | | |
| | Meat Lover's | | | | | | | | | | | | | | | |
| 57378 | Hand Tossed | 462 | 92 | | | | | | | | | | | | | |
| 57383 | Pan | 470 | 94 | | | | | | | | | | | | | |
| 57395 | Thin 'N Crispy | 488 | 98 | | | | | | | | | | | | | |
| | Pepperoni | | | | | | | | | | | | | | | |
| 57387 | Bigfoot | 369 | 74 | | | | | | | | | | | | | |
| 57386 | Bigfoot, w/Mushrooms & Italian Sausage | 366 | 73 | | | | | | | | | | | | | |
| 56482 | Pan | 476 | 95 | | | | 0.31 | 0.24 | 2.66 | 0.08 | | 0.0 | | 3.9 | | |
| 56493 | Personal Pan | 1164 | 233 | | | | 0.56 | 0.66 | 8.16 | 0.20 | | | | 10.0 | | |
| 56486 | Thin 'N Crispy | 497 | 99 | | | | 0.24 | 0.25 | 2.98 | | | | | 3.5 | | |
| | Pepperoni Lover's | | | | | | | | | | | | | | | |
| 57380 | Hand Tossed | 614 | 123 | | | | | | | | | | | | | |
| 57381 | Pan | 620 | 124 | | | | | | | | | | | | | |
| 57391 | Thin 'N Crispy | 653 | 131 | | | | | | | | | | | | | |
| | Pork | | | | | | | | | | | | | | | |
| 57376 | Hand Tossed | 446 | 89 | | | | | | | | | | | | | |
| 57389 | Pan | 454 | 91 | | | | | | | | | | | | | |
| 57392 | Thin 'N Crispy | 467 | 93 | | | | | | | | | | | | | |
| | Super Supreme | | | | | | | | | | | | | | | |
| 56492 | Hand Tossed | 495 | 99 | | | | 0.42 | 0.34 | 4.35 | | | | | 7.1 | | |
| 56484 | Pan | 502 | 100 | | | | 0.42 | 0.37 | 3.57 | | | | | 6.1 | | |
| 56488 | Thin 'N Crispy | 519 | 104 | | | | 0.36 | 0.27 | 3.27 | | | | | 4.5 | | |
| | Supreme | | | | | | | | | | | | | | | |
| 56491 | Hand Tossed | 479 | 96 | | | | 0.41 | 0.33 | 4.21 | | | | | 6.8 | | |
| 56494 | Personal Pan | 1199 | 240 | | | | 0.73 | 0.82 | 9.91 | 0.40 | | | | 13.6 | | |
| 56487 | Thin 'N Crispy | 493 | 99 | | | | 0.35 | 0.28 | 3.13 | | | | | 5.8 | | |
| | Veggie Lover's | | | | | | | | | | | | | | | |
| 57379 | Hand Tossed | 471 | 94 | | | | | | | | | | | | | |
| 57382 | Pan | 482 | 96 | | | | | | | | | | | | | |
| 57390 | Thin 'N Crispy | 496 | 99 | | | | | | | | | | | | | |
| | *SUBWAY* | | | | | | | | | | | | | | | |
| | Salads | | | | | | | | | | | | | | | |
| 52128 | B L T | 1363 | 273 | | | | | | | | | | | 32.0 | | |
| 52119 | Chicken Breast, rstd | 1379 | 276 | | | | | | | | | | | 32.0 | | |
| 52127 | Chicken Taco | 1806 | 361 | | | | | | | | | | | 35.0 | | |
| 52115 | Club | 1363 | 273 | | | | | | | | | | | 32.0 | | |
| 52120 | Cold Cut Trio | 1412 | 282 | | | | | | | | | | | 33.0 | | |
| 52123 | Ham | 1363 | 273 | | | | | | | | | | | 32.0 | | |
| 52129 | Meatball | 1474 | 295 | | | | | | | | | | | 33.0 | | |
| 52121 | Pizza | 1952 | 390 | | | | | | | | | | | 33.0 | | |
| 52126 | Roast Beef | 1363 | 273 | | | | | | | | | | | 32.0 | | |
| 52117 | Seafood & Crab | 1366 | 273 | | | | | | | | | | | 32.0 | | |
| 52116 | Seafood & Crab, w/light mayo | 1418 | 284 | | | | | | | | | | | 32.0 | | |
| 52130 | Steak & Cheese | 1639 | 328 | | | | | | | | | | | 35.0 | | |
| 52122 | Tuna | 1389 | 278 | | | | | | | | | | | 32.0 | | |
| 52118 | Tuna, w/light mayo | 1490 | 298 | | | | | | | | | | | 32.0 | | |
| 52114 | Turkey Breast | 1363 | 273 | | | | | | | | | | | 32.0 | | |
| 52125 | Turkey Breast & Ham | 1363 | 273 | | | | | | | | | | | 32.0 | | |
| 52113 | Veggie Delite | 1363 | 136 | | | | | | | | | | | 32.0 | | |

| Code | Description | Calcium (mg) | Copper (mg) | Iron (mg) | Magnes (mg) | Mang (mg) | Phos (mg) | Potassium (mg) | Selenium (mcg) | Sodium (mg) | Zinc (mg) |
|---|---|---|---|---|---|---|---|---|---|---|---|
| 69012 | Quarter-Pounder w/Cheese | 143 | 0.3 | 4.5 | | | | | | 1161 | |
| 69013 | Sandwiches, Filet-O-Fish | 124 | 0.1 | 1.8 | 32 | 0.0 | 183 | 266 | 0.0 | 708 | 0.71 |
| 69041 | Sandwiches, McChicken | 128 | 0.2 | 2.5 | 33 | 0.0 | 223 | 319 | 0.4 | 797 | 1.06 |
| 69014 | Sandwiches, McGrilled Chicken | 117 | 0.1 | 2.4 | 42 | 0.1 | 327 | 433 | 0.1 | 506 | 0.89 |
| | *PIZZA HUT* | | | | | | | | | | |
| | Beef | | | | | | | | | | |
| 57373 | Hand Tossed | 113 | | 2.1 | | | | | | 794 | |
| 57384 | Pan | 114 | | 2.1 | | | | | | 675 | |
| 57394 | Thin 'N Crispy | 116 | | 1.6 | | | | | | 708 | |
| | Cheese | | | | | | | | | | |
| 56489 | Hand Tossed | 142 | | 1.5 | 35 | | | 194 | | 621 | 2.30 |
| 56481 | Pan | 144 | | 1.5 | 32 | | | 168 | | 501 | 2.16 |
| 56485 | Thin 'N Crispy | 145 | | 1.0 | 28 | | | 153 | | 535 | 2.11 |
| | Ham | | | | | | | | | | |
| 57372 | Hand Tossed | 100 | | 1.6 | | | | | | 658 | |
| 57375 | Pan | 101 | | 1.6 | | | | | | 538 | |
| 57393 | Thin 'N Crispy | 103 | | 1.1 | | | | | | 588 | |
| | Italian Sausage | | | | | | | | | | |
| 57377 | Hand Tossed | 104 | | 1.7 | | | | | | 740 | |
| 57385 | Pan | 105 | | 1.7 | | | | | | 619 | |
| 57374 | Thin 'N Crispy | 107 | | 1.2 | | | | | | 648 | |
| | Meat Lover's | | | | | | | | | | |
| 57378 | Hand Tossed | 110 | | 2.1 | | | | | | 955 | |
| 57383 | Pan | 111 | | 2.1 | | | | | | 835 | |
| 57395 | Thin 'N Crispy | 113 | | 1.6 | | | | | | 893 | |
| | Pepperoni | | | | | | | | | | |
| 57387 | Bigfoot | 105 | | 1.6 | | | | | | 589 | |
| 57386 | Bigfoot, w/Mushrooms & Italian Sausage | 106 | | 1.7 | | | | | | 665 | |
| 56482 | Pan | 103 | | 1.6 | 28 | | | 199 | | 570 | 2.07 |
| 56493 | Personal Pan | 250 | | 4.0 | 60 | | | 407 | | 1339 | 3.80 |
| 56486 | Thin 'N Crispy | 104 | | 1.1 | 25 | | | 165 | | 628 | 2.01 |
| | Pepperoni Lover's | | | | | | | | | | |
| 57380 | Hand Tossed | 145 | | 1.8 | | | | | | 895 | |
| 57381 | Pan | 147 | | 1.8 | | | | | | 775 | |
| 57391 | Thin 'N Crispy | 149 | | 1.3 | | | | | | 864 | |
| | Pork | | | | | | | | | | |
| 57376 | Hand Tossed | 115 | | 2.1 | | | | | | 794 | |
| 57389 | Pan | 116 | | 2.1 | | | | | | 674 | |
| 57392 | Thin 'N Crispy | 118 | | 1.6 | | | | | | 708 | |
| | Super Supreme | | | | | | | | | | |
| 56492 | Hand Tossed | 116 | | 2.2 | 45 | | | 304 | | 945 | 2.83 |
| 56484 | Pan | 118 | | 2.2 | 40 | | | 296 | | 825 | 3.00 |
| 56488 | Thin 'N Crispy | 119 | | 1.7 | 36 | | | 280 | | 878 | 2.72 |
| | Supreme | | | | | | | | | | |
| 56491 | Hand Tossed | 116 | | 2.3 | 43 | | | 293 | | 881 | 2.73 |
| 56494 | Personal Pan | 276 | | 5.2 | 74 | | | 603 | | 1758 | 4.69 |
| 56487 | Thin 'N Crispy | 119 | | 1.8 | 39 | | | 315 | | 796 | 2.70 |
| | Veggie Lover's | | | | | | | | | | |
| 57379 | Hand Tossed | 107 | | 1.8 | | | | | | 628 | |
| 57382 | Pan | 109 | | 1.8 | | | | | | 512 | |
| 57390 | Thin 'N Crispy | 111 | | 1.3 | | | | | | 547 | |
| | *SUBWAY* | | | | | | | | | | |
| | Salads | | | | | | | | | | |
| 52128 | B L T | 24 | | 1.0 | | | | | | 672 | |
| 52119 | Chicken Breast, rstd | 32 | | 2.0 | | | | | | 693 | |
| 52127 | Chicken Taco | 115 | | 3.0 | | | | | | 990 | |
| 52115 | Club | 26 | | 2.0 | | | | | | 1067 | |
| 52120 | Cold Cut Trio | 46 | | 2.0 | | | | | | 1127 | |
| 52123 | Ham | 25 | | 2.0 | | | | | | 1034 | |
| 52129 | Meatball | 30 | | 2.0 | | | | | | 761 | |
| 52121 | Pizza | 100 | | 2.0 | | | | | | 1336 | |
| 52126 | Roast Beef | 23 | | 2.0 | | | | | | 654 | |
| 52117 | Seafood & Crab | 25 | | 2.0 | | | | | | 575 | |
| 52116 | Seafood & Crab, w/light mayo | 25 | | 2.0 | | | | | | 599 | |
| 52130 | Steak & Cheese | 86 | | 3.0 | | | | | | 832 | |
| 52122 | Tuna | 29 | | 2.0 | | | | | | 601 | |
| 52118 | Tuna, w/light mayo | 29 | | 2.0 | | | | | | 654 | |
| 52114 | Turkey Breast | 28 | | 2.0 | | | | | | 1117 | |
| 52125 | Turkey Breast & Ham | 27 | | 2.0 | | | | | | 1076 | |
| 52113 | Veggie Delite | 23 | | 1.0 | | | | | | 308 | |

| Code | Amount | Description | Weight (g) | Calories | % Water | Protein (g) | Carbs (g) | Fiber (g) | Sugar (g) | Other Carbs (g) | Fat (g) | Sat Fat (g) | Mono Fat (g) | Poly Fat (g) | Omega 3 (g) | Omega 6 (g) | Choles (mg) | Vit A (IU) | Vit A (RE) | Retinol (RE) | Carotenoids (RE) | Beta Carotene (mcg) | Thiamin (mg) | Riboflavin (mg) | Niacin (NE) | Vit B6 (mg) | Vit B12 (mcg) | Folate (mcg) | Panto (mg) | Vit C (mg) | Vit D (mg) | Vit E (α TE) | Calcium (mg) | Copper (mg) | Iron (mg) | Magnes (mg) | Mang (mg) | Phos (mg) | Potassium (mg) | Selenium (mcg) | Sodium (mg) | Zinc (mg) |
|---|---|---|---|---|---|---|---|---|---|---|---|---|---|---|---|---|---|---|---|---|---|---|---|---|---|---|---|---|---|---|---|---|---|---|---|---|---|---|---|---|---|---|
| | | Sandwiches | | | | | | | | | | | | | | | | | | | | | | | | | | | | | | | | | | | | | | | | |
| 69135 | 1 ea | B.L.T. on white 6" | 191 | 311 | 67 | 14.0 | 38.0 | 3.0 | 2.0 | 33.0 | 10.0 | 3.0 | | | | | 16 | 601 | 120 | | | | | | | | | | | 15.0 | | | 27 | | 3.0 | | | | | | 945 | |
| 69136 | 1 ea | B.L.T. on wheat 6" | 198 | 327 | 65 | 14.0 | 44.0 | 3.0 | 2.0 | 39.0 | 10.0 | 3.0 | | | | | 16 | 601 | 120 | | | | | | | | | | | 15.0 | | | 33 | | 3.0 | | | | | | 557 | |
| 69104 | 1 ea | Bologna, deli style | 171 | 292 | 64 | 10.0 | 38.0 | 2.0 | 3.0 | 33.0 | 12.0 | 4.0 | | | | | 20 | 565 | 113 | | | | | | | | | | | 14.0 | | | 39 | | 3.0 | | | | | | 744 | |
| 69125 | 1 ea | Chicken Breast Roasted on white 6" | 246 | 332 | 70 | 26.0 | 41.0 | 3.0 | 2.0 | 36.0 | 6.0 | 1.0 | | | | | 48 | 617 | 123 | | | | | | | | | | | 15.0 | | | 35 | | 3.0 | | | | | | 967 | |
| 69126 | 1 ea | Chicken Breast Roasted on wheat 6" | 253 | 348 | 68 | 27.0 | 47.0 | 3.0 | 3.0 | 41.0 | 6.0 | 1.0 | | | | | 48 | 617 | 123 | | | | | | | | | | | 15.0 | | | 42 | | 3.0 | | | | | | 978 | |
| 69131 | 1 ea | Chicken Taco Sub on white 6" | 286 | 421 | 70 | 24.0 | 43.0 | 3.0 | 4.0 | 36.0 | 16.0 | 5.0 | | | | | 52 | 1044 | 209 | | | | | | | | | | | 18.0 | | | 118 | | 4.0 | | | | | | 1264 | |
| 69132 | 1 ea | Chicken Taco Sub on wheat 6" | 293 | 436 | 69 | 25.0 | 49.0 | 4.0 | 4.0 | 41.0 | 16.0 | 5.0 | | | | | 52 | 1044 | 209 | | | | | | | | | | | 18.0 | | | 124 | | 4.0 | | | | | | 1275 | |
| 69117 | 1 ea | Club on white 6" | 246 | 297 | 73 | 21.0 | 40.0 | 3.0 | 3.0 | 34.0 | 5.0 | 1.0 | | | | | 26 | 601 | 120 | | | | | | | | | | | 15.0 | | | 29 | | 4.0 | | | | | | 1341 | |
| 69118 | 1 ea | Club on wheat 6" | 253 | 312 | 71 | 21.0 | 46.0 | 3.0 | 3.0 | 40.0 | 5.0 | 1.0 | | | | | 26 | 601 | 120 | | | | | | | | | | | 15.0 | | | 35 | | 4.0 | | | | | | 1352 | |
| 69113 | 1 ea | Coldcut Trio on white 6" | 246 | 362 | 71 | 19.0 | 39.0 | 3.0 | 2.0 | 34.0 | 13.0 | 4.0 | | | | | 64 | 649 | 130 | | | | | | | | | | | 16.0 | | | 49 | | 4.0 | | | | | | 1401 | |
| 69114 | 1 ea | Coldcut Trio on wheat 6" | 253 | 378 | 68 | 20.0 | 46.0 | 3.0 | 2.0 | 41.0 | 13.0 | 4.0 | | | | | 64 | 650 | 130 | | | | | | | | | | | 16.0 | | | 55 | | 4.0 | | | | | | 1412 | |
| 69102 | 1 ea | Ham, Deli Style | 171 | 234 | 69 | 11.0 | 37.0 | 2.0 | 3.0 | 32.0 | 4.0 | 1.0 | | | | | 14 | 565 | 113 | | | | | | | | | | | 14.0 | | | 24 | | 3.0 | | | | | | 773 | |
| 69115 | 1 ea | Ham on white 6" | 232 | 287 | 73 | 18.0 | 39.0 | 3.0 | 3.0 | 33.0 | 5.0 | 1.0 | | | | | 28 | 601 | 120 | | | | | | | | | | | 15.0 | | | 28 | | 3.0 | | | | | | 1308 | |
| 69116 | 1 ea | Ham on wheat 6" | 239 | 302 | 71 | 19.0 | 45.0 | 3.0 | 3.0 | 39.0 | 5.0 | 1.0 | | | | | 28 | 601 | 120 | | | | | | | | | | | 15.0 | | | 35 | | 3.0 | | | | | | 1319 | |
| 69139 | 1 ea | Italian B.M.T. on white 6" | 246 | 445 | 66 | 21.0 | 39.0 | 3.0 | 3.0 | 33.0 | 21.0 | 8.0 | | | | | 56 | 753 | 151 | | | | | | | | | | | 15.0 | | | 44 | | 4.0 | | | | | | 1652 | |
| 69140 | 1 ea | Italian B.M.T. on wheat 6" | 253 | 460 | 64 | 21.0 | 45.0 | 3.0 | 3.0 | 39.0 | 22.0 | 7.0 | | | | | 56 | 754 | 151 | | | | | | | | | | | 15.0 | | | 50 | | 4.0 | | | | | | 1664 | |
| 69129 | 1 ea | Meatball on white 6" | 260 | 404 | 70 | 18.0 | 44.0 | 3.0 | 4.0 | 37.0 | 16.0 | 6.0 | | | | | 33 | 712 | 142 | | | | | | | | | | | 16.0 | | | 32 | | 4.0 | | | | | | 1035 | |
| 69130 | 1 ea | Meatball on wheat 6" | 267 | 419 | 67 | 19.0 | 51.0 | 3.0 | 4.0 | 44.0 | 16.0 | 6.0 | | | | | 33 | 712 | 142 | | | | | | | | | | | 16.0 | | | 39 | | 4.0 | | | | | | 1046 | |
| 69127 | 1 ea | Melt Turkey, Ham, Bacon & Cheese on white 6" | 251 | 366 | 70 | 22.0 | 40.0 | 3.0 | 3.0 | 34.0 | 12.0 | 5.0 | | | | | 42 | 777 | 155 | | | | | | | | | | | 15.0 | | | 93 | | 4.0 | | | | | | 1735 | |
| 69128 | 1 ea | Melt Turkey, Ham, Bacon&Cheese on wheat 6" | 258 | 382 | 68 | 23.0 | 46.0 | 3.0 | 3.0 | 40.0 | 12.0 | 5.0 | | | | | 42 | 778 | 156 | | | | | | | | | | | 15.0 | | | 100 | | 3.0 | | | | | | 1746 | |
| 69133 | 1 ea | Pizza Sub on white 6" | 250 | 448 | 66 | 19.0 | 41.0 | 3.0 | 4.0 | 34.0 | 22.0 | 9.0 | | | | | 50 | 1130 | 238 | | | | | | | | | | | 16.0 | | | 103 | | 4.0 | | | | | | 1639 | |
| 69134 | 1 ea | Pizza Sub on wheat 6" | 257 | 464 | 65 | 19.0 | 48.0 | 3.0 | 4.0 | 41.0 | 22.0 | 9.0 | | | | | 50 | 1131 | 238 | | | | | | | | | | | 16.0 | | | 110 | | 3.0 | | | | | | 1621 | |
| 69103 | 1 ea | Roast Beef, deli style | 180 | 245 | 69 | 13.0 | 38.0 | 2.0 | 4.0 | 32.0 | 4.0 | 1.0 | | | | | 13 | 565 | 113 | | | | | | | | | | | 14.0 | | | 23 | | 3.0 | | | | | | 638 | |
| 69121 | 1 ea | Roast Beef on white 6" | 232 | 288 | 72 | 19.0 | 39.0 | 3.0 | 3.0 | 33.0 | 5.0 | 1.0 | | | | | 20 | 601 | 120 | | | | | | | | | | | 15.0 | | | 25 | | 4.0 | | | | | | 928 | |
| 69122 | 1 ea | Roast Beef on wheat 6" | 239 | 303 | 70 | 20.0 | 45.0 | 3.0 | 3.0 | 39.0 | 5.0 | 1.0 | | | | | 20 | 601 | 120 | | | | | | | | | | | 15.0 | | | 32 | | 3.0 | | | | | | 939 | |
| 69105 | 1 ea | Seafood & Crab, deli style | 178 | 298 | 66 | 12.0 | 37.0 | 2.0 | 3.0 | 32.0 | 11.0 | 2.0 | | | | | 17 | 566 | 113 | | | | | | | | | | | 14.0 | | | 24 | | 3.0 | | | | | | 544 | |
| 69106 | 1 ea | Seafood & Crab, w/light mayo, deli style | 178 | 256 | 68 | 12.0 | 37.0 | 2.0 | 3.0 | 32.0 | 7.0 | 2.0 | | | | | 16 | 592 | 118 | | | | | | | | | | | 14.0 | | | 24 | | 3.0 | | | | | | 556 | |
| 69145 | 1 ea | Seafood & Crab on white 6" | 246 | 415 | 69 | 19.0 | 38.0 | 3.0 | 2.0 | 33.0 | 19.0 | 3.0 | | | | | 34 | 604 | 121 | | | | | | | | | | | 15.0 | | | 28 | | 3.0 | | | | | | 849 | |
| 69146 | 1 ea | Seafood & Crab on wheat 6" | 253 | 430 | 67 | 20.0 | 44.0 | 3.0 | 2.0 | 39.0 | 19.0 | 3.0 | | | | | 34 | 605 | 121 | | | | | | | | | | | 15.0 | | | 34 | | 3.0 | | | | | | 860 | |
| 69147 | 1 ea | Seafood & Crab, w/light mayo on white 6" | 246 | 332 | 72 | 19.0 | 39.0 | 3.0 | 2.0 | 34.0 | 10.0 | 2.0 | | | | | 32 | 656 | 131 | | | | | | | | | | | 15.0 | | | 28 | | 3.0 | | | | | | 873 | |
| 69148 | 1 ea | Seafood & Crab, w/light mayo on wheat 6" | 253 | 347 | 70 | 20.0 | 45.0 | 3.0 | 2.0 | 40.0 | 10.0 | 2.0 | | | | | 32 | 657 | 131 | | | | | | | | | | | 15.0 | | | 34 | | 3.0 | | | | | | 884 | |
| 69123 | 1 ea | Spicy Italian on white 6" | 232 | 467 | 64 | 20.0 | 38.0 | 3.0 | 2.0 | 33.0 | 24.0 | 9.0 | | | | | 57 | 845 | 169 | | | | | | | | | | | 15.0 | | | 40 | | 4.0 | | | | | | 1592 | |
| 69124 | 1 ea | Spicy Italian on wheat 6" | 239 | 482 | 62 | 21.0 | 44.0 | 3.0 | 2.0 | 39.0 | 25.0 | 9.0 | | | | | 57 | 846 | 169 | | | | | | | | | | | 15.0 | | | 47 | | 4.0 | | | | | | 1604 | |
| 69119 | 1 ea | Steak & Cheese on white 6" | 257 | 383 | 68 | 29.0 | 41.0 | 3.0 | 3.0 | 35.0 | 10.0 | 6.0 | | | | | 70 | 877 | 175 | | | | | | | | | | | 18.0 | | | 88 | | 5.0 | | | | | | 1106 | |
| 69120 | 1 ea | Steak & Cheese on wheat 6" | 264 | 398 | 67 | 30.0 | 47.0 | 3.0 | 4.0 | 40.0 | 10.0 | 6.0 | | | | | 70 | 878 | 176 | | | | | | | | | | | 18.0 | | | 95 | | 5.0 | | | | | | 1117 | |
| 69108 | 1 ea | Tuna, Deli Style | 178 | 354 | 63 | 11.0 | 37.0 | 2.0 | 3.0 | 32.0 | 18.0 | 3.0 | | | | | 18 | 578 | 116 | | | | | | | | | | | 14.0 | | | 26 | | 3.0 | | | | | | 557 | |
| 69107 | 1 ea | Tuna, w/light mayo, deli style | 178 | 279 | 67 | 11.0 | 38.0 | 2.0 | 3.0 | 33.0 | 9.0 | 2.0 | | | | | 16 | 628 | 126 | | | | | | | | | | | 14.0 | | | 26 | | 3.0 | | | | | | 583 | |
| 69141 | 1 ea | Tuna on white 6" | 246 | 527 | 62 | 18.0 | 38.0 | 3.0 | 2.0 | 33.0 | 32.0 | 5.0 | | | | | 36 | 627 | 125 | | | | | | | | | | | 15.0 | | | 32 | | 3.0 | | | | | | 875 | |
| 69142 | 1 ea | Tuna on wheat 6" | 253 | 542 | 62 | 19.0 | 44.0 | 3.0 | 2.0 | 39.0 | 32.0 | 5.0 | | | | | 36 | 628 | 126 | | | | | | | | | | | 15.0 | | | 38 | | 3.0 | | | | | | 886 | |
| 69143 | 1 ea | Tuna, w/light mayo on white 6" | 246 | 376 | 70 | 18.0 | 39.0 | 3.0 | 2.0 | 34.0 | 15.0 | 2.0 | | | | | 32 | 728 | 146 | | | | | | | | | | | 15.0 | | | 32 | | 3.0 | | | | | | 928 | |
| 69144 | 1 ea | Tuna, w/light mayo on wheat 6" | 253 | 391 | 68 | 19.0 | 46.0 | 3.0 | 2.0 | 41.0 | 15.0 | 2.0 | | | | | 32 | 729 | 146 | | | | | | | | | | | 15.0 | | | 38 | | 3.0 | | | | | | 940 | |
| 69137 | 1 ea | Turkey Breast & Ham on white 6" | 232 | 280 | 73 | 18.0 | 39.0 | 3.0 | 3.0 | 33.0 | 5.0 | 1.0 | | | | | 24 | 601 | 120 | | | | | | | | | | | 15.0 | | | 29 | | 3.0 | | | | | | 1350 | |
| 69138 | 1 ea | Turkey Breast & Ham on wheat 6" | 239 | 295 | 71 | 18.0 | 46.0 | 3.0 | 3.0 | 40.0 | 5.0 | 1.0 | | | | | 24 | 601 | 120 | | | | | | | | | | | 15.0 | | | 36 | | 3.0 | | | | | | 1361 | |
| 69101 | 1 ea | Turkey, deli style | 180 | 235 | 69 | 12.0 | 38.0 | 2.0 | 3.0 | 33.0 | 4.0 | 1.0 | | | | | 12 | 565 | 113 | | | | | | | | | | | 14.0 | | | 26 | | 3.0 | | | | | | 944 | |
| 69111 | 1 ea | Turkey on white 6" | 232 | 273 | 73 | 17.0 | 40.0 | 3.0 | 2.0 | 35.0 | 4.0 | 1.0 | | | | | 19 | 601 | 120 | | | | | | | | | | | 15.0 | | | 30 | | 4.0 | | | | | | 1391 | |
| 69112 | 1 ea | Turkey on wheat 6" | 239 | 289 | 71 | 18.0 | 46.0 | 3.0 | 2.0 | 41.0 | 4.0 | 1.0 | | | | | 19 | 601 | 120 | | | | | | | | | | | 15.0 | | | 37 | | 3.0 | | | | | | 1403 | |
| 69109 | 1 ea | Veggie Delite on white 6" | 175 | 222 | 71 | 9.0 | 38.0 | 3.0 | 2.0 | 33.0 | 3.0 | 0.0 | | | | | 0 | 601 | 120 | | | | | | | | | | | 15.0 | | | 25 | | 3.0 | | | | | | 582 | |
| 69110 | 1 ea | Veggie Delite on wheat 6" | 182 | 237 | 69 | 9.0 | 44.0 | 3.0 | 2.0 | 39.0 | 3.0 | 0.0 | | | | | 0 | 601 | 120 | | | | | | | | | | | 15.0 | | | 32 | | 3.0 | | | | | | 593 | |
| | | *TACO BELL* | | | | | | | | | | | | | | | | | | | | | | | | | | | | | | | | | | | | | | | | |
| | | Breakfast Items | | | | | | | | | | | | | | | | | | | | | | | | | | | | | | | | | | | | | | | | |
| 56698 | 1 ea | Burrito, Country Breakfast | 113 | 220 | 55 | 8.0 | 26.0 | 2.0 | 1.0 | 23.0 | 14.0 | 5.0 | | | | | 95 | 1250 | 250 | | | | | | | | | | | 0.0 | | | 80 | | 1.1 | | | | | | 690 | |
| 57684 | 1 ea | Burrito, Double Bacon & Egg | 177 | 480 | 51 | 18.0 | 39.0 | 2.0 | 8.0 | 29.0 | 27.0 | 9.0 | | | | | 100 | 2250 | 450 | | | | | | | | | | | 0.0 | | | 150 | | 1.8 | | | | | | 1240 | |
| 56697 | 1 ea | Burrito, Fiesta Breakfast | 92 | 280 | 44 | 9.0 | 25.0 | 2.0 | 1.0 | 22.0 | 16.0 | 6.0 | | | | | 25 | 750 | 150 | | | | | | | | | | | 0.0 | | | 80 | | 0.7 | | | | | | 580 | |
| 56696 | 1 ea | Burrito, Grande Breakfast | 177 | 420 | 56 | 13.0 | 43.0 | 3.0 | 2.0 | 38.0 | 22.0 | 7.0 | | | | | 205 | 2500 | 500 | | | | | | | | | | | 0.0 | | | 100 | | 1.8 | | | | | | 1050 | |
| 57688 | 1 ea | Quesadilla w/Bacon | 170 | 450 | 51 | 19.0 | 33.0 | 2.0 | 1.0 | 30.0 | 27.0 | 11.0 | | | | | 250 | 2250 | 450 | | | | | | | | | | | 0.0 | | | 300 | | 2.7 | | | | | | 1200 | |
| 57687 | 1 ea | Quesadilla w/Sausage | 170 | 430 | 58 | 17.0 | 33.0 | 1.0 | 1.0 | 31.0 | 18.0 | 5.0 | | | | | 285 | 2250 | 450 | | | | | | | | | | | 0.0 | | | 300 | | 2.7 | | | | | | 1090 | |
| | | Burritos | | | | | | | | | | | | | | | | | | | | | | | | | | | | | | | | | | | | | | | | |
| 57675 | 1 ea | Bacon Cheeseburger | 241 | 570 | 55 | 27.0 | 46.0 | 6.0 | 5.0 | 35.0 | 31.0 | 12.0 | | | | | 70 | 1500 | 300 | | | | | | | | | | | 4.8 | | | 200 | | 2.7 | | | | | | 1460 | |
| 56519 | 1 ea | Bean w/red sauce | 198 | 380 | 58 | 13.0 | 55.0 | 13.0 | 3.0 | 39.0 | 12.0 | 4.0 | | | | | 10 | 2250 | 450 | | | | 0.04 | 2.02 | 1.98 | 0.31 | | | | 0.0 | | | 150 | | 2.7 | | | | 495 | | 1100 | |
| 56690 | 1 ea | Big Beef Supreme | 298 | 520 | 64 | 24.0 | 54.0 | 11.0 | 4.0 | 39.0 | 23.0 | 10.0 | | | | | 55 | 3000 | 600 | | | | | | | | | | | 4.8 | | | 150 | | 2.7 | | | | | | 1520 | |
| 56688 | 1 ea | Chicken | 171 | 345 | 58 | 17.0 | 41.0 | | | | 13.0 | 5.0 | | | | | 57 | 2200 | 440 | | | | | | | | | | | 1.2 | | | 140 | | 2.5 | | | | | | 854 | |
| 57678 | 1 ea | Chicken Grilled | 202 | 400 | 57 | 19.0 | 50.0 | 3.0 | 2.0 | 45.0 | 14.0 | 4.0 | | | | | 40 | 3500 | 700 | | | | | | | | | | | 2.4 | | | 150 | | 1.4 | | | | | | 1250 | |
| 57679 | 1 ea | Chicken Big Supreme | 248 | 500 | 58 | 27.0 | 51.0 | 3.0 | 3.0 | 45.0 | 20.0 | 7.0 | | | | | 70 | 1750 | 350 | | | | | | | | | | | 2.4 | | | 150 | | 1.4 | | | | | | 1660 | |
| 57676 | 1 ea | Chicken Club | 227 | 540 | 56 | 20.0 | 43.0 | 4.0 | 5.0 | 34.0 | 32.0 | 10.0 | | | | | 80 | 750 | 150 | | | | | | | | | | | 4.8 | | | 100 | | 1.4 | | | | | | 1250 | |

The column headings are grouped under Basic Components (Weight to Sat Fat), Additional Fats (Mono Fat to Choles), Vit A & Components (Vit A (IU) to Beta Carotene), Vitamins (Thiamin to Vit E) and Minerals (Calcium to Zinc).

| Code | Amount | Description | Basic Components: Weight (g) | Calories | % Water | Protein (g) | Carbs (g) | Fiber (g) | Sugar (g) | Other Carbs (g) | Fat (g) | Sat Fat (g) | Additional Fats: Mono Fat (g) | Poly Fat (g) | Omega 3 (g) | Omega 6 (g) | Choles (mg) |
|---|---|---|---|---|---|---|---|---|---|---|---|---|---|---|---|---|---|
| 57677 | 1 ea | Chili Cheese Burrito | 142 | 330 | 53 | 14.0 | 37.0 | 5.0 | 2.0 | 30.0 | 13.0 | 6.0 | | | | | 35 |
| 56691 | 1 ea | 7 Layer Burrito | 283 | 530 | 61 | 16.0 | 66.0 | 13.0 | 4.0 | 49.0 | 23.0 | 7.0 | | | | | 25 |
| 56522 | 1 ea | Supreme w/red sauce | 255 | 440 | 64 | 17.0 | 51.0 | 10.0 | 4.0 | 37.0 | 19.0 | 8.0 | | | | | 35 |
| 45585 | 1 ea | Cinnamon Twists, svg | 28 | 140 | 6 | 1.0 | 19.0 | 0.0 | 0.0 | 19.0 | 6.0 | 0.0 | | | | | 0 |
| | | Fajita Wraps | | | | | | | | | | | | | | | |
| 57682 | 1 ea | Chicken | 220 | 460 | 57 | 19.0 | 51.0 | 3.0 | 3.0 | 45.0 | 20.0 | 5.0 | | | | | 45 |
| 57683 | 1 ea | Chicken Supreme | 255 | 510 | 60 | 20.0 | 53.0 | 3.0 | 4.0 | 46.0 | 24.0 | 8.0 | | | | | 55 |
| 57680 | 1 ea | Steak | 227 | 470 | 58 | 20.0 | 50.0 | 3.0 | 3.0 | 44.0 | 21.0 | 6.0 | | | | | 40 |
| 57681 | 1 ea | Steak Supreme | 255 | 510 | 60 | 21.0 | 52.0 | 3.0 | 4.0 | 45.0 | 25.0 | 8.0 | | | | | 50 |
| 57690 | 1 ea | Veggie | 227 | 420 | 63 | 10.0 | 53.0 | 3.0 | 3.0 | 47.0 | 19.0 | 5.0 | | | | | 20 |
| 57691 | 1 ea | Veggie Supreme | 255 | 470 | 65 | 11.0 | 55.0 | 3.0 | 4.0 | 48.0 | 22.0 | 7.0 | | | | | 30 |
| | | Gorditas | | | | | | | | | | | | | | | |
| 57667 | 1 ea | Chicken Supreme | 153 | 300 | 60 | 17.0 | 28.0 | 3.0 | 4.0 | 21.0 | 14.0 | 5.0 | | | | | 45 |
| 57663 | 1 ea | Fiesta Beef | 139 | 290 | 62 | 13.0 | 29.0 | 4.0 | 3.0 | 22.0 | 13.0 | 4.5 | | | | | 25 |
| 57668 | 1 ea | Fiesta Chicken | 139 | 260 | 59 | 16.0 | 28.0 | 3.0 | 3.0 | 22.0 | 10.0 | 2.5 | | | | | 30 |
| 57664 | 1 ea | Fiesta Steak | 139 | 270 | 59 | 17.0 | 27.0 | 3.0 | 3.0 | 21.0 | 10.0 | 3.0 | | | | | 25 |
| 57666 | 1 ea | Santa Fe Beef | 153 | 390 | 53 | 14.0 | 32.0 | 5.0 | 3.0 | 24.0 | 23.0 | 6.0 | | | | | 30 |
| 57669 | 1 ea | Santa Fe Chicken | 153 | 370 | 54 | 17.0 | 30.0 | 3.0 | 3.0 | 24.0 | 20.0 | 4.0 | | | | | 40 |
| 57662 | 1 ea | Santa Fe Steak | 153 | 370 | 54 | 18.0 | 29.0 | 3.0 | 3.0 | 23.0 | 21.0 | 4.5 | | | | | 35 |
| 57665 | 1 ea | Supreme Beef | 139 | 291 | 58 | 12.7 | 27.3 | 3.6 | 3.6 | 20.0 | 15.4 | 6.4 | | | | | 32 |
| 57661 | 1 ea | Supreme Steak | 153 | 310 | 60 | 17.0 | 27.0 | 3.0 | 4.0 | 20.0 | 14.0 | 5.0 | | | | | 35 |
| 56530 | 1 ea | Guacamole, svg | 21 | 35 | 80 | 0.0 | 1.0 | 1.0 | 1.0 | 0.0 | 3.0 | 0.0 | | | | | 0 |
| | | Nachos | | | | | | | | | | | | | | | |
| 56534 | 1 ea | Bellgrande, svg | 312 | 770 | 52 | 21.0 | 84.0 | 17.0 | 4.0 | 63.0 | 39.0 | 11.0 | | | | | 35 |
| 56533 | 1 ea | Regular, svg | 99 | 320 | 40 | 5.0 | 34.0 | 3.0 | 2.0 | 29.0 | 18.0 | 4.0 | | | | | 5 |
| 56684 | 1 ea | Supreme, svg | 198 | 450 | 56 | 14.0 | 45.0 | 9.0 | 3.0 | 33.0 | 24.0 | 8.0 | | | | | 30 |
| 56639 | 7 pce | With Cheese | 113 | 346 | 40 | 9.1 | 36.4 | | | | 19.0 | 7.8 | 8.0 | 2.2 | 0.20 | 2.03 | 18 |
| 56640 | 7 pce | With Cheese & Jalapeno Peppers | 204 | 608 | 43 | 16.8 | 60.2 | | | | 34.1 | 14.0 | 14.4 | 4.0 | 0.35 | 3.67 | 84 |
| 56641 | 7 pce | With Cheese, Beans, Beef & Peppers | 225 | 502 | 56 | 17.5 | 49.3 | | | | 27.0 | 11.0 | 9.7 | 5.0 | 0.21 | 4.81 | 18 |
| 56531 | 1 ea | Mexican Pizza | 220 | 570 | 53 | 21.0 | 42.0 | 8.0 | 1.0 | 33.0 | 35.0 | 10.0 | | | | | 45 |
| 56532 | 1 ea | Meximelt | 135 | 290 | 58 | 16.0 | 23.0 | 4.0 | 2.0 | 17.0 | 15.0 | 7.0 | | | | | 45 |
| 56536 | 1 ea | Pintos & Cheese, w/red sauce, svg | 120 | 190 | 68 | 9.0 | 18.0 | 10.0 | 1.0 | 7.0 | 9.0 | 4.0 | | | | | 15 |
| | | Quesadillas | | | | | | | | | | | | | | | |
| 57686 | 1 ea | Bacon & Cheese | 149 | 380 | 52 | 15.0 | 33.0 | 1.0 | 1.0 | 31.0 | 21.0 | 9.0 | | | | | 280 |
| 57685 | 1 ea | Cheese | 120 | 350 | 42 | 16.0 | 32.0 | 2.0 | 1.0 | 29.0 | 18.0 | 9.0 | | | | | 50 |
| 57689 | 1 ea | Chicken | 163 | 163 | 51 | 9.9 | 13.1 | 0.8 | 0.4 | 11.9 | 7.6 | 4.0 | | | | | 30 |
| | | Tacos | | | | | | | | | | | | | | | |
| 57670 | 1 ea | Double Decker | 163 | 340 | 57 | 14.0 | 38.0 | 9.0 | 2.0 | 27.0 | 15.0 | 5.0 | | | | | 25 |
| 57671 | 1 ea | Double Decker Supreme | 198 | 390 | 60 | 15.0 | 40.0 | 9.0 | 3.0 | 28.0 | 19.0 | 8.0 | | | | | 35 |
| 56377 | 1 ea | Regular | 78 | 190 | 58 | 7.0 | 15.0 | 2.0 | 0.0 | 13.0 | 11.0 | 4.0 | | | | | 20 |
| 56525 | 1 ea | Soft | 90 | 220 | 64 | 9.0 | 12.0 | 3.0 | 1.0 | 8.0 | 10.0 | 4.0 | | | | | 25 |
| 57673 | 1 ea | Soft BLT | 128 | 340 | 54 | 11.0 | 22.0 | 2.0 | 3.0 | 17.0 | 23.0 | 8.0 | | | | | 40 |
| 56689 | 1 ea | Soft Chicken | 121 | 200 | 63 | 14.0 | 21.0 | 2.0 | 2.0 | 17.0 | 7.0 | 2.5 | | | | | 35 |
| 56693 | 1 ea | Soft Steak | 128 | 230 | 63 | 15.0 | 20.0 | 2.0 | 1.0 | 17.0 | 10.0 | 2.5 | | | | | 25 |
| 57672 | 1 ea | Soft Steak Supreme | 163 | 290 | 65 | 16.0 | 24.0 | 3.0 | 4.0 | 17.0 | 14.0 | 5.0 | | | | | 35 |
| 56526 | 1 ea | Soft Supreme | 142 | 260 | 64 | 12.0 | 23.0 | 3.0 | 3.0 | 17.0 | 14.0 | 7.0 | | | | | 35 |
| 56378 | 1 ea | Super | 126 | 280 | 59 | 12.0 | 22.0 | 3.0 | 1.0 | 18.0 | 17.0 | 6.0 | | | | | 30 |
| 56692 | 1 ea | Supreme | 113 | 220 | 65 | 10.0 | 14.0 | 3.0 | 2.0 | 9.0 | 14.0 | 7.0 | | | | | 35 |
| 56537 | 1 ea | Taco Salad, w/salsa & shell | 539 | 850 | 71 | 30.0 | 65.0 | 16.0 | 9.0 | 40.0 | 52.0 | 15.0 | | | | | 60 |
| 57674 | 1 ea | Taco Salad, w/salsa, w/o shell | 468 | 420 | 82 | 24.0 | 32.0 | 15.0 | 9.0 | 8.0 | 22.0 | 11.0 | | | | | 60 |
| 56528 | 1 ea | Tostada, w/red sauce | 177 | 300 | 67 | 10.0 | 31.0 | 12.0 | 2.0 | 17.0 | 15.0 | 5.0 | | | | | 15 |
| | | *TACO JOHNS* | | | | | | | | | | | | | | | |
| | | Burritos | | | | | | | | | | | | | | | |
| 57576 | 1 ea | Bean | 170 | 340 | 56 | 14.8 | 45.2 | | 0.4 | | 11.1 | 3.0 | | | | | 15 |
| 57577 | 1 ea | Beef | 170 | 415 | 51 | 22.4 | 39.4 | | 0.4 | | 18.9 | 6.4 | | | | | 43 |
| 57580 | 1 ea | Chicken Fajita | 227 | 360 | 67 | 20.4 | 41.4 | | 3.3 | | 11.9 | 5.0 | | | | | 49 |
| 57578 | 1 ea | Combination | 170 | 378 | 52 | 18.1 | 46.1 | | 0.4 | | 13.4 | 5.6 | | | | | 30 |
| 57579 | 1 ea | Super | 241 | 424 | 64 | 19.6 | 45.0 | | 2.3 | | 18.8 | 6.7 | | | | | 35 |
| 57595 | 1 ea | Chili, Texas Style with 2 crackers | 262 | 297 | 75 | 22.6 | 26.6 | | 1.9 | | 14.3 | 6.5 | | | | | 46 |
| 57581 | 1 ea | Fajita, Chicken, Soft-shell | 120 | 215 | 64 | 13.2 | 20.2 | | 0.5 | | 8.3 | 3.1 | | | | | 33 |
| | | Kid's Meals | | | | | | | | | | | | | | | |
| 57582 | 1 ea | Crispy Taco | 227 | 576 | 55 | 12.5 | 54.7 | | 3.5 | | 33.3 | 9.5 | | | | | 30 |
| 57583 | 1 ea | Soft-shell Taco | 241 | 623 | 52 | 15.0 | 65.7 | | 3.5 | | 32.7 | 9.7 | | | | | 32 |
| 57584 | 1 ea | Taco Burger | 248 | 668 | 50 | 17.7 | 70.3 | | 6.3 | | 34.1 | 10.1 | | | | | 35 |
| | | Mexi Rolls | | | | | | | | | | | | | | | |
| 57589 | 1 ea | With Guacamole | 276 | 838 | 44 | 29.7 | 78.2 | | 1.0 | | 45.5 | 11.8 | | | | | 46 |
| 57590 | 1 ea | With Nacho Cheese | 276 | 812 | 45 | 29.7 | 77.2 | | 1.0 | | 42.9 | 10.5 | | | | | 46 |
| 57591 | 1 ea | With Salsa | 276 | 753 | 48 | 28.5 | 76.4 | | 1.0 | | 37.0 | 10.5 | | | | | 46 |
| 57592 | 1 ea | With Sour Cream | 276 | 853 | 45 | 29.7 | 74.2 | | 1.0 | | 46.9 | 10.5 | | | | | 46 |
| 57597 | 1 ea | Mexican Pizza | 276 | 635 | 58 | 25.8 | 53.0 | | 4.1 | | 35.8 | 13.5 | | | | | 55 |

| Code | Description | Vit A & Components: Vit A (IU) | Vit A (RE) | Retinol (RE) | Carotenoids (RE) | Beta Carotene (mcg) | Vitamins: Thiamin (mg) | Riboflavin (mg) | Niacin (NE) | Vit B6 (mg) | Vit B12 (mcg) | Folate (mcg) | Panto (mg) | Vit C (mg) | Vit D (mg) | Vit E (α TE) | Minerals: Calcium (mg) | Copper (mg) | Iron (mg) | Magnes (mg) | Mang (mg) | Phos (mg) | Potassium (mg) | Selenium (mcg) | Sodium (mg) | Zinc (mg) |
|---|---|---|---|---|---|---|---|---|---|---|---|---|---|---|---|---|---|---|---|---|---|---|---|---|---|---|
| 57677 | Chili Cheese Burrito | 300 | 60 | | | | | | | | | | | 0.0 | | | 200 | | 1.4 | | | | | | 870 | |
| 56691 | 7 Layer Burrito | 1500 | 300 | | | | | | | | | | | 6.0 | | | 200 | | 3.6 | | | | | | 1280 | |
| 56522 | Supreme w/red sauce | 2500 | 500 | | | | 0.40 | 2.10 | 2.89 | 0.35 | | | | 4.8 | | | 150 | | 9.0 | 50 | | | 422 | | 1230 | |
| 45585 | Cinnamon Twists, svg | 200 | 40 | | | | 0.08 | 0.03 | 0.57 | 0.03 | | | | 0.0 | | | 0 | | 0.4 | | | | 22 | | 190 | |
| | Fajita Wraps | | | | | | | | | | | | | | | | | | | | | | | | | |
| 57682 | Chicken | 1500 | 300 | | | | | | | | | | | 3.6 | | | 150 | | 1.4 | | | | | | 1170 | |
| 57683 | Chicken Supreme | 1500 | 300 | | | | | | | | | | | 6.0 | | | 150 | | 1.4 | | | | | | 1180 | |
| 57680 | Steak | 1500 | 300 | | | | | | | | | | | 3.6 | | | 150 | | 1.8 | | | | | | 1190 | |
| 57681 | Steak Supreme | 1500 | 300 | | | | | | | | | | | 6.0 | | | 150 | | 1.8 | | | | | | 1200 | |
| 57690 | Veggie | 1750 | 350 | | | | | | | | | | | 3.6 | | | 150 | | 1.4 | | | | | | 980 | |
| 57691 | Veggie Supreme | 1750 | 350 | | | | | | | | | | | 6.0 | | | 150 | | 1.4 | | | | | | 990 | |
| | Gorditas | | | | | | | | | | | | | | | | | | | | | | | | | |
| 57667 | Chicken Supreme | 200 | 40 | | | | | | | | | | | 3.6 | | | 150 | | 1.4 | | | | | | 540 | |
| 57663 | Fiesta Beef | 500 | 100 | | | | | | | | | | | 0.0 | | | 150 | | 1.8 | | | | | | 680 | |
| 57668 | Fiesta Chicken | 200 | 40 | | | | | | | | | | | 1.2 | | | 150 | | 1.4 | | | | | | 580 | |
| 57664 | Fiesta Steak | 100 | 20 | | | | | | | | | | | 0.0 | | | 150 | | 1.8 | | | | | | 600 | |
| 57666 | Santa Fe Beef | 500 | 100 | | | | | | | | | | | 3.6 | | | 150 | | 1.8 | | | | | | 710 | |
| 57669 | Santa Fe Chicken | 200 | 50 | | | | | | | | | | | 3.6 | | | 150 | | 1.8 | | | | | | 610 | |
| 57662 | Santa Fe Steak | 200 | 40 | | | | | | | | | | | 3.6 | | | 150 | | 2.7 | | | | | | 630 | |
| 57665 | Supreme Beef | 454 | 91 | | | | | | | | | | | 3.3 | | | 136 | | 1.6 | | | | | | 572 | |
| 57661 | Supreme Steak | 100 | 20 | | | | | | | | | | | 3.6 | | | 150 | | 1.8 | | | | | | 550 | |
| 56530 | Guacamole, svg | 0 | 0 | 0 | 0 | 0 | | | | | 0.00 | | | 1.2 | | | 0 | | 0.0 | | | | | | 79 | |
| | Nachos | | | | | | | | | | | | | | | | | | | | | | | | | |
| 56534 | Bellgrande, svg | 750 | 150 | | | | 0.11 | 0.37 | 2.36 | | | | | 3.6 | | | 200 | | 3.6 | | | | 733 | | 1310 | |
| 56533 | Regular, svg | 300 | 60 | | | | 0.16 | 0.15 | 0.64 | 0.18 | | 9.2 | | 0.0 | | | 100 | | 0.7 | | | | 149 | | 570 | 1.57 |
| 56684 | Supreme, svg | 500 | 100 | | | | | | | | | | | 3.6 | | | 150 | | 2.7 | | | | | | 810 | |
| 56639 | With Cheese | 559 | 92 | 61 | 30 | | 0.19 | 0.37 | 1.54 | 0.20 | 0.82 | 10.2 | 1.31 | 1.2 | | | 272 | 0.1 | 1.3 | 55 | 0.2 | 276 | 172 | 15.7 | 816 | 1.79 |
| 56640 | With Cheese & Jalapeno Peppers | 4062 | 471 | 386 | 85 | | 0.12 | 0.49 | 2.84 | 0.37 | 1.02 | 18.4 | 2.45 | 1.0 | | | 620 | 0.2 | 2.4 | 108 | 0.4 | 394 | 294 | 14.1 | 1736 | 2.90 |
| 56641 | With Cheese, Beans, Beef & Peppers | 3002 | 414 | 340 | 74 | | 0.20 | 0.61 | 2.95 | 0.36 | 0.90 | 33.8 | 2.23 | 4.3 | | | 340 | 0.7 | 2.5 | 86 | 0.4 | 342 | 398 | 12.2 | 1588 | 3.22 |
| 56531 | Mexican Pizza | 2000 | 400 | | | | 0.32 | 0.33 | 2.92 | 1.10 | | 59.0 | | 4.8 | | | 250 | | 3.6 | 79 | | | 403 | | 1040 | 5.30 |
| 56532 | Meximelt | 1250 | 250 | | | | | | | | | | | 3.6 | | | 200 | | 1.1 | | | | | | 850 | |
| 56536 | Pintos & Cheese, w/red sauce, svg | 2500 | 250 | | | | 0.05 | 0.14 | 0.40 | 0.20 | 0.00 | 64.0 | | 0.0 | | | 150 | | 1.8 | 103 | | | 360 | | 650 | 2.03 |
| | Quesadillas | | | | | | | | | | | | | | | | | | | | | | | | | |
| 57686 | Bacon & Cheese | 2250 | 450 | | | | | | | | | | | 0.0 | | | 300 | | 2.7 | | | | | | 1010 | |
| 57685 | Cheese | 400 | 80 | | | | | | | | | | | 0.0 | | | 450 | | 1.8 | | | | | | 860 | |
| 57689 | Chicken | 199 | 40 | | | | | | | | | | | 1.0 | | | 179 | | 0.7 | | | | | | 413 | |
| | Tacos | | | | | | | | | | | | | | | | | | | | | | | | | |
| 57670 | Double Decker | 500 | 100 | | | | | | | | | | | 0.0 | | | 100 | | 1.8 | | | | | | 750 | |
| 57671 | Double Decker Supreme | 750 | 150 | | | | | | | | | | | 3.6 | | | 150 | | 1.8 | | | | | | 760 | |
| 56377 | Regular | 0 | 0 | 0 | 0 | 0 | 0.07 | 0.17 | 1.00 | 0.13 | 0.48 | | | 0.0 | | | 100 | 0.1 | 1.1 | 35 | | 146 | 240 | | 410 | 1.20 |
| 56525 | Soft | 500 | 100 | | | | 0.38 | 0.22 | 2.68 | 0.98 | | | | 0.0 | | | 80 | | 1.1 | | | | 192 | | 330 | |
| 57673 | Soft BLT | 200 | 40 | | | | | | | | | | | 3.6 | | | 100 | | 0.7 | | | | | | 610 | |
| 56689 | Soft Chicken | 300 | 60 | | | | | | | | | | | 1.2 | | | 80 | | 0.7 | | | | | | 540 | |
| 56693 | Soft Steak | 200 | 40 | | | | | | | | | | | 0.0 | | | 80 | | 1.4 | | | | | | 1020 | |
| 57672 | Soft Steak Supreme | 400 | 80 | | | | | | | | | | | 12.0 | | | 100 | | 1.4 | | | | | | 1040 | |
| 56526 | Soft Supreme | 750 | 150 | | | | | | | | | | | 3.6 | | | 100 | | 1.8 | | | | | | 590 | |
| 56378 | Super | 0 | 0 | 0 | 0 | 0 | 0.12 | 0.08 | 1.40 | 0.18 | 0.74 | | | 2.4 | | | 150 | 0.2 | 1.8 | 45 | | 198 | 370 | | 720 | 1.80 |
| 56692 | Supreme | 750 | 150 | | | | | | | | | | | 0.0 | | | 100 | | 1.1 | | | | | | 350 | |
| 56537 | Taco Salad, w/salsa & shell | 8000 | 1600 | | | | 0.47 | 0.70 | 4.42 | 0.51 | | 9.1 | | 24.0 | | | 300 | | 6.3 | | | | 966 | | 1780 | 1.54 |
| 57674 | Taco Salad, w/salsa, w/o shell | 8000 | 1600 | | | | | | | | | | | 21.0 | | | 250 | | 4.5 | | | | | | 1520 | |
| 56528 | Tostada, w/red sauce | 2500 | 500 | | | | 0.06 | 0.19 | 0.71 | 0.29 | | | | 1.2 | | | 150 | | 1.8 | | | | 455 | | 650 | |
| | *TACO JOHNS* | | | | | | | | | | | | | | | | | | | | | | | | | |
| | Burritos | | | | | | | | | | | | | | | | | | | | | | | | | |
| 57576 | Bean | 133 | 27 | | | | | | | | | | | 0.7 | | | 260 | | 6.3 | | | | | | 654 | |
| 57577 | Beef | 133 | 27 | | | | | | | | | | | 0.9 | | | 250 | | 6.0 | | | | | | 703 | |
| 57580 | Chicken Fajita | 52 | 10 | | | | | | | | | | | 34.0 | | | 148 | | 2.2 | | | | | | 1202 | |
| 57578 | Combination | 0 | 0 | 0 | 0 | 0 | | | | | | | | 1.5 | | | 155 | | 2.9 | | | | | | 659 | |
| 57579 | Super | 226 | 45 | | | | | | | | | | | 8.8 | | | 298 | | 6.8 | | | | | | 736 | |
| 57595 | Chili, Texas Style with 2 crackers | 1248 | 250 | | | | | | | | | | | 12.1 | | | 130 | | 3.5 | | | | | | 1424 | |
| 57581 | Fajita, Chicken, Soft-shell | 65 | 13 | | | | | | | | | | | 5.1 | | | 110 | | 1.5 | | | | | | 1079 | |
| | Kid's Meals | | | | | | | | | | | | | | | | | | | | | | | | | |
| 57582 | Crispy Taco | 53 | 10 | | | | | | | | | | | 5.0 | | | 88 | | 2.3 | | | | | | 774 | |
| 57583 | Soft-shell Taco | 53 | 11 | | | | | | | | | | | 6.0 | | | 125 | | 3.3 | | | | | | 1021 | |
| 57584 | Taco Burger | 13 | 3 | | | | | | | | | | | 1.2 | | | 140 | | 3.6 | | | | | | 1081 | |
| | Mexi Rolls | | | | | | | | | | | | | | | | | | | | | | | | | |
| 57589 | With Guacamole | 139 | 28 | | | | | | | | | | | 3.3 | | | 238 | | 4.1 | | | | | | 1052 | |
| 57590 | With Nacho Cheese | 120 | 24 | | | | | | | | | | | 1.1 | | | 288 | | 3.6 | | | | | | 1199 | |
| 57591 | With Salsa | 100 | 20 | | | | | | | | | | | 12.9 | | | 247 | | 3.8 | | | | | | 1386 | |
| 57592 | With Sour Cream | 180 | 36 | | | | | | | | | | | 1.1 | | | 308 | | 3.6 | | | | | | 851 | |
| 57597 | Mexican Pizza | 105 | 21 | | | | | | | | | | | 12.5 | | | 235 | | 2.5 | | | | | | 1332 | |

| Code | Amount | Description | Weight (g) | Calories | % Water | Protein (g) | Carbs (g) | Fiber (g) | Sugar (g) | Other Carbs (g) | Fat (g) | Sat Fat (g) | Mono Fat (g) | Poly Fat (g) | Omega 3 (g) | Omega 6 (g) | Choles (mg) | Vit A (IU) | Vit A (RE) | Retinol (RE) | Carotenoids (RE) | Beta Carotene (mcg) | Thiamin (mg) | Riboflavin (mg) | Niacin (NE) | Vit B6 (mg) | Vit B12 (mcg) | Folate (mcg) | Panto (mg) | Vit C (mg) | Vit D (mg) | Vit E (α TE) | Calcium (mg) | Copper (mg) | Iron (mg) | Magnes (mg) | Mang (mg) | Phos (mg) | Potassium (mg) | Selenium (mcg) | Sodium (mg) | Zinc (mg) |
|---|---|---|---|---|---|---|---|---|---|---|---|---|---|---|---|---|---|---|---|---|---|---|---|---|---|---|---|---|---|---|---|---|---|---|---|---|---|---|---|---|---|---|
| | | **Basic Components** | | | | | | | | | | | **Additional Fats** | | | | | **Vit A & Components** | | | | | **Vitamins** | | | | | | | | | | **Minerals** | | | | | | | | | |
| 57594 | 1 ea | Mexican Rice | 227 | 567 | 47 | 7.9 | 94.0 | | 2.0 | | 17.7 | 4.7 | | | | | 0 | 1634 | 327 | | | | | | | | | | | 0.0 | | | 118 | | 3.2 | | | | | | 1294 | |
| 57593 | 1 ea | Nachos Regular | 99 | 293 | 50 | 1.8 | 30.8 | | 0.9 | | 16.8 | 3.8 | | | | | 6 | 88 | 18 | | | | | | | | | | | | | | | | | | | | | | 446 | |
| 57598 | 1 ea | Nachos Super | 368 | 847 | 60 | 18.8 | 76.8 | | 3.6 | | 49.8 | 15.4 | | | | | 50 | 218 | 44 | | | | | | | | | | | 8.1 | | | 173 | | 2.0 | | | | | | 1230 | |
| | | Platters | | | | | | | | | | | | | | | | | | | | | | | | | | | | | | | | | | | | | | | | |
| 57585 | 1 ea | Chimichanga Platter | 524 | 921 | 64 | 32.4 | 118.9 | | 3.3 | | 35.2 | 13.5 | | | | | 50 | 932 | 136 | | | | | | | | | | | 19.6 | | | 375 | | 6.9 | | | | | | 2345 | |
| 57586 | 1 ea | Double Enchilada Platter | 524 | 900 | 65 | 41.8 | 102.9 | | 2.9 | | 36.5 | 13.0 | | | | | 73 | 1302 | 250 | | | | | | | | | | | 13.3 | | | 324 | | 7.6 | | | | | | 2098 | |
| 57587 | 1 ea | Sampler Platter (Taco, Burrito, Enchilada) | 709 | 1277 | 63 | 57.7 | 149.1 | | 3.8 | | 51.0 | 18.5 | | | | | 97 | 1344 | 259 | | | | | | | | | | | 17.6 | | | 479 | | 9.4 | | | | | | 2738 | |
| 57588 | 1 ea | Smothered Burrito Platter | 539 | 973 | 63 | 38.1 | 123.1 | | 3.7 | | 37.5 | 14.6 | | | | | 61 | 1359 | 272 | | | | | | | | | | | 11.9 | | | 360 | | 7.7 | | | | | | 2183 | |
| 57603 | 1 ea | Potato Oles with Nacho Cheese | 523 | 523 | 83 | 5.1 | 49.8 | | 0.9 | | 33.7 | 8.6 | | | | | 6 | 99 | 20 | | | | | | | | | | | 1.3 | | | 17 | | 1.9 | | | | | | 832 | |
| 57596 | 1 pce | Taco Burger | 142 | 276 | 61 | 14.5 | 29.0 | | 3.8 | | 11.2 | 4.3 | | | | | 26 | 40 | 8 | | | | | | | | | | | 4.0 | | | 141 | | 2.5 | | | | | | 567 | |
| 57599 | 1 ea | Taco Salad, No Dressing | 298 | 470 | 72 | 11.2 | 39.8 | | 5.3 | | 30.5 | 8.5 | | | | | 22 | 316 | 53 | | | | | | | | | | | 38.2 | | | 257 | | 4.0 | | | | | | 648 | |
| | | Tacos | | | | | | | | | | | | | | | | | | | | | | | | | | | | | | | | | | | | | | | | |
| 57602 | 1 ea | Bravo | 170 | 332 | 61 | 14.7 | 37.7 | | 0.5 | | 13.6 | 4.4 | | | | | 22 | 40 | 8 | | | | | | | | | | | 4.9 | | | 127 | | 2.5 | | | | | | 654 | |
| 57600 | 1 ea | Crispy | 85 | 178 | 58 | 9.0 | 12.5 | | 0.5 | | 10.3 | 3.7 | | | | | 22 | 40 | 8 | | | | | | | | | | | 3.9 | | | 75 | | 0.9 | | | | | | 256 | |
| 57601 | 1 ea | Soft-shell | 128 | 279 | 55 | 13.6 | 32.1 | | 1.3 | | 11.3 | 4.2 | | | | | 22 | 40 | 8 | | | | | | | | | | | 4.3 | | | 170 | | 1.4 | | | | | | 558 | |
| | | *TACO TIME* | | | | | | | | | | | | | | | | | | | | | | | | | | | | | | | | | | | | | | | | |
| | | Burritos | | | | | | | | | | | | | | | | | | | | | | | | | | | | | | | | | | | | | | | | |
| 56538 | 1 ea | Casita | 340 | 638 | 64 | 30.0 | 54.0 | 4.0 | | | 34.0 | 15.0 | 17.0 | 2.0 | | | 73 | 1275 | 213 | | | | 0.48 | 0.50 | 5.00 | 0.70 | | 93.0 | | 11.0 | | | 379 | | 7.0 | | | 486 | 888 | | 993 | 5.00 |
| 56539 | 1 ea | Chicken Fajita | 170 | 394 | 53 | 26.0 | 38.0 | 2.0 | | | 15.0 | 5.0 | 5.0 | 3.0 | | | 63 | 281 | 47 | | | | 0.24 | 0.35 | 9.00 | 0.41 | | 42.0 | | 7.0 | | | 163 | | 2.0 | | | 252 | 299 | | 143 | 2.00 |
| 56540 | 1 ea | Crispy Bean | 149 | 354 | 55 | 11.0 | 34.0 | 4.0 | | | 21.0 | 4.0 | 11.0 | 6.0 | | | 11 | 119 | 12 | | | | 0.33 | 0.20 | 2.00 | 0.35 | | 13.0 | | | | | 143 | | 4.0 | | | 216 | 347 | | 302 | 2.00 |
| 56541 | 1 ea | Crispy Beef | 149 | 466 | 44 | 22.0 | 32.0 | 1.0 | | | 28.0 | 10.0 | 12.0 | 6.0 | | | 52 | 275 | 28 | | | | 0.24 | 0.37 | 5.00 | 0.33 | | 68.0 | | 2.0 | | | 180 | | 4.0 | | | 253 | 463 | | 571 | 4.00 |
| 56542 | 1 ea | Soft Bean | 255 | 420 | 66 | 18.0 | 50.0 | 6.0 | | | 18.0 | 4.0 | 13.0 | 1.0 | | | 21 | 429 | 51 | | | | 0.51 | 0.30 | 2.00 | 0.60 | | 22.0 | | 3.0 | | | 251 | | 6.0 | | | 361 | 593 | | 586 | 3.00 |
| 56544 | 1 ea | Soft Combination | 255 | 520 | 60 | 27.0 | 48.0 | 4.0 | | | 25.0 | 10.0 | 14.0 | 1.0 | | | 54 | 543 | 30 | | | | 0.45 | 0.44 | 5.00 | 0.60 | | 70.0 | | 5.0 | | | 271 | | 7.0 | | | 392 | 713 | | 826 | 5.00 |
| 56543 | 1 ea | Soft Meat | 255 | 557 | 60 | 34.0 | 36.0 | 1.0 | | | 30.0 | 15.0 | 14.0 | 1.0 | | | 87 | 655 | 33 | | | | 0.33 | 0.51 | 7.00 | 0.58 | | 110.0 | | 6.0 | | | 276 | | 7.0 | | | 407 | 803 | | 1066 | 6.00 |
| 56551 | 1 ea | Chimichanga | 290 | 599 | 63 | 23.0 | 43.0 | 3.0 | | | 39.0 | 16.0 | 19.0 | 4.0 | | | 63 | 1548 | 221 | | | | 0.35 | 0.47 | 4.00 | 0.38 | | 69.0 | | 18.0 | | | 387 | | 5.0 | | | 388 | 622 | | 977 | 3.00 |
| 49038 | 1 ea | Crustos, svg | 99 | 398 | 26 | 4.0 | 45.0 | 1.0 | | | 24.0 | 3.0 | 8.0 | 13.0 | | | 2 | 13 | 1 | | | | 0.14 | 0.18 | 2.00 | 0.03 | | 20.0 | | 2.0 | | | 83 | | 3.0 | | | 43 | 95 | | 2 | 0.00 |
| 45586 | 1 ea | Empanada, Berry | 113 | 387 | 26 | 5.0 | 66.0 | 3.0 | | | 12.0 | 1.0 | 5.0 | 6.0 | | | 2 | 79 | 1 | | | | 0.16 | 0.20 | 2.00 | 0.05 | | 20.0 | | 10.0 | | | 84 | | 3.0 | | | 56 | 170 | | 1 | 0.00 |
| 45587 | 1 ea | Empanada, Cherry | 113 | 323 | 40 | 5.0 | 51.0 | 2.0 | | | 12.0 | 1.0 | 5.0 | 6.0 | | | 2 | 87 | 1 | | | | 0.16 | 0.20 | 2.00 | 49.00 | | 24.0 | | 3.0 | | | 63 | | 2.0 | | | 52 | 159 | | 2 | 0.00 |
| 56552 | 1 ea | Enchilada | 226 | 442 | 63 | 22.0 | 39.0 | 1.0 | | | 21.0 | 10.0 | 9.0 | 2.0 | | | 55 | 1142 | 142 | | | | 0.28 | 0.39 | 5.00 | 0.46 | | 89.0 | | 13.0 | | | 265 | | 5.0 | | | 321 | 636 | | 825 | 4.00 |
| 56554 | 1 ea | Nachos, svg | 297 | 808 | 48 | 26.0 | 78.0 | 3.0 | | | 46.0 | 16.0 | 22.0 | 8.0 | | | 70 | 1607 | 230 | | | | 0.46 | 0.46 | 3.00 | 0.74 | | 46.0 | | 16.0 | | | 670 | | 6.0 | | | 668 | 697 | | 1237 | 3.00 |
| 56553 | 1 ea | Mexi-Fries, svg | 130 | 330 | 58 | 3.0 | 31.0 | 1.0 | | | 20.0 | 7.0 | 9.0 | 4.0 | | | | 0 | 0 | 0 | 0 | 0 | 0.06 | 0.01 | 1.00 | | 0.00 | | | 4.0 | | | 13 | | 1.0 | | | 46 | 315 | | 360 | |
| 7141 | 1 ea | Refritos, svg | 198 | 253 | 75 | 11.0 | 24.0 | 3.0 | | | 13.0 | 4.0 | 8.0 | 1.0 | | | 21 | 430 | 43 | 0 | 43 | 248 | 0.24 | 0.15 | 1.00 | 0.36 | 0.00 | 13.0 | | 3.0 | | | 215 | | 3.0 | | | 253 | 336 | | 425 | 2.00 |
| 56555 | 1 ea | Salad, Chicken Fajita | 297 | 541 | 66 | 28.0 | 39.0 | 2.0 | | | 31.0 | 7.0 | 10.0 | 11.0 | | | 73 | 889 | 127 | | | | 0.26 | 0.36 | 9.00 | 0.44 | | 66.0 | | 20.0 | | | 177 | | 3.0 | | | 267 | 442 | | 490 | 2.00 |
| 56556 | 1 ea | Salad, Taco w/ranch dressing | 262 | 603 | 63 | 23.0 | 29.0 | 1.0 | | | 44.0 | 13.0 | 17.0 | 14.0 | | | 65 | 594 | 74 | | | | 0.23 | 0.37 | 4.00 | 0.32 | | 94.0 | | 5.0 | | | 235 | | 4.0 | | | 280 | 516 | | 837 | 4.00 |
| 56550 | 1 ea | Taco Burger | 233 | 651 | 50 | 26.0 | 48.0 | 3.0 | | | 40.0 | 13.0 | 15.0 | 12.0 | | | 53 | 623 | 103 | | | | 0.47 | 0.46 | 5.00 | 0.30 | | 84.0 | | 4.0 | | | 307 | | 5.0 | | | 365 | 565 | | 1227 | 4.00 |
| | | Tacos | | | | | | | | | | | | | | | | | | | | | | | | | | | | | | | | | | | | | | | | |
| 56545 | 1 ea | Regular | 113 | 260 | 59 | 14.0 | 16.0 | 0.0 | | | 15.0 | 7.0 | 6.0 | 2.0 | | | 37 | 377 | 53 | | | | 0.12 | 0.18 | 2.00 | 0.29 | | 47.0 | | 3.0 | | | 176 | | 3.0 | | | 220 | 339 | | 443 | 2.00 |
| 56546 | 1 ea | Natural Super | 283 | 575 | 61 | 28.0 | 49.0 | 4.0 | | | 31.0 | 13.0 | 17.0 | 1.0 | | | 66 | 754 | 107 | | | | 0.46 | 0.48 | 5.00 | 0.58 | | 74.0 | | 5.0 | 0.1 | | 300 | | 7.0 | | | 414 | 749 | | 763 | 5.00 |
| 56547 | 1 ea | Soft Flour | 184 | 397 | 59 | 22.0 | 32.0 | 1.0 | | | 20.0 | 10.0 | 9.0 | 1.0 | | | 54 | 533 | 76 | | | | 0.25 | 0.39 | 4.00 | 0.31 | | 72.0 | | 4.0 | | | 233 | | 4.0 | | | 281 | 472 | | 562 | 4.00 |
| 56548 | 1 ea | Tostada | 212 | 492 | 56 | 26.0 | 38.0 | 3.0 | | | 28.0 | 10.0 | 14.0 | 4.0 | | | 53 | 419 | 52 | | | | 0.39 | 0.30 | 4.00 | 0.54 | | 57.0 | | 2.0 | | | 276 | | 6.0 | | | 418 | 625 | | 749 | 5.00 |
| 56549 | 1 ea | Tostada Delight | 276 | 627 | 60 | 27.0 | 43.0 | 4.0 | | | 39.0 | 15.0 | 21.0 | 3.0 | | | 66 | 793 | 99 | | | | 0.43 | 0.45 | 4.00 | 0.57 | | 77.0 | | 5.0 | | | 295 | | 6.0 | | | 408 | 753 | | 754 | 5.00 |
| | | *WENDY'S* | | | | | | | | | | | | | | | | | | | | | | | | | | | | | | | | | | | | | | | | |
| 15176 | 5 pce | Chicken Nuggets | 75 | 210 | 52 | 14.0 | 7.0 | 0.0 | 0.0 | 7.0 | 14.0 | 3.0 | | | | | 45 | 0 | 0 | 0 | 0 | 0 | 0.12 | 0.11 | 7.18 | | | | | 1.2 | | | 20 | | 0.4 | | | | 185 | | 460 | |
| 2177 | 1 ea | Dessert, Frosty Dairy, med | 298 | 440 | 68 | 11.0 | 73.0 | 0.0 | 56.0 | 17.0 | 11.0 | 7.0 | | | | | 50 | 1000 | 200 | | | | 0.14 | 0.62 | 0.42 | 0.16 | 1.10 | 22.9 | 1.00 | 0.0 | | | 410 | 0.2 | 1.4 | 60 | | 328 | 714 | | 239 | 1.27 |
| | | French Fries | | | | | | | | | | | | | | | | | | | | | | | | | | | | | | | | | | | | | | | | |
| 6169 | 1 ea | Biggies | 159 | 470 | 41 | 7.0 | 61.0 | 6.0 | 0.0 | 55.0 | 23.0 | 3.5 | | | | | 0 | 0 | 0 | 0 | 0 | 0 | 0.22 | 0.05 | 4.44 | 0.39 | 0.00 | 49.2 | 0.41 | 9.0 | | | 30 | 0.2 | 1.3 | 68 | | 296 | 1034 | | 150 | 0.76 |
| 6168 | 1 ea | Medium | 130 | 390 | 41 | 5.0 | 50.0 | 5.0 | 0.0 | 45.0 | 19.0 | 3.0 | 11.9 | 2.5 | | | 0 | 0 | 0 | 0 | 0 | 0 | 0.18 | 0.04 | 3.60 | 0.33 | 0.00 | 40.2 | 0.34 | 6.0 | | | 20 | 0.2 | 1.1 | 55 | | 242 | 845 | | 120 | 0.62 |
| 56590 | 1 ea | Kid's Meal Cheeseburger | 123 | 320 | 46 | 17.0 | 33.0 | 2.0 | 7.0 | 24.0 | 13.0 | 6.0 | | | | | 45 | 300 | 60 | | | | 0.40 | 1.43 | 4.21 | | | | | 0.0 | | | 170 | | 3.2 | | | | 205 | | 830 | |
| 56589 | 1 ea | Kid's Meal Hamburger | 111 | 270 | 47 | 15.0 | 33.0 | 2.0 | 7.0 | 24.0 | 10.0 | 3.5 | | | | | 30 | 100 | 20 | | | | 0.43 | 0.29 | 4.49 | | | | | 0.0 | | | 110 | | 3.1 | | | | 219 | | 610 | |
| | | Potatoes | | | | | | | | | | | | | | | | | | | | | | | | | | | | | | | | | | | | | | | | |
| 6167 | 1 ea | Baked, plain | 284 | 310 | 71 | 7.0 | 71.0 | 7.0 | 5.0 | 59.0 | 0.0 | 0.0 | 0.0 | 0.0 | 0.00 | 0.00 | 0 | 0 | 0 | 0 | 0 | 0 | 0.31 | 0.12 | 4.30 | 0.80 | 0.17 | 31.2 | 1.27 | 36.0 | | | 30 | 0.4 | 3.8 | 76 | | 162 | 1187 | 2.4 | 25 | 0.74 |
| 56580 | 1 ea | Baked, w/broccoli & cheese | 411 | 470 | 74 | 9.0 | 80.0 | 9.0 | 6.0 | 65.0 | 14.0 | 2.5 | 8.0 | 2.5 | | | 5 | 1750 | 350 | | | | 0.34 | 0.29 | 4.50 | 0.97 | 0.40 | 74.0 | 1.72 | 72.0 | | | 210 | 0.8 | 4.5 | 94 | | 420 | 1745 | 2.5 | 470 | 0.97 |
| 56582 | 1 ea | Baked, w/sour cream & chives | 314 | 380 | 71 | 8.0 | 74.0 | 8.0 | 6.0 | 60.0 | 6.0 | 4.0 | | | | | 15 | 1500 | 300 | | | | 0.23 | 0.14 | 3.04 | 0.80 | 0.20 | 32.4 | 1.50 | 48.0 | | | 80 | 0.6 | 4.3 | 71 | 0.6 | 187 | 1438 | | 40 | 0.91 |
| | | Salads | | | | | | | | | | | | | | | | | | | | | | | | | | | | | | | | | | | | | | | | |
| 52080 | 1 ea | Caesar, Side | 89 | 100 | 77 | 8.0 | 8.0 | 1.0 | 1.0 | 6.0 | 4.0 | 1.5 | | | | | 10 | 1750 | 350 | | | | | | | | | | | 15.0 | | | 30 | | 1.3 | | | | | | 620 | |
| 52082 | 1 ea | Chicken, Grilled | 338 | 200 | 87 | 25.0 | 9.0 | 3.0 | 6.0 | 0.0 | 8.0 | 1.5 | | | | | 50 | 6000 | 1200 | | | | | | | | | | | 36.0 | | | 190 | | 2.0 | | | | | | 720 | |
| 52112 | 1 ea | Chicken Caesar, Grilled | 262 | 260 | 80 | 26.0 | 17.0 | 2.0 | 2.0 | 13.0 | 9.0 | 3.0 | | | | | 60 | 4000 | 800 | | | | | | | | | | | 36.0 | | | 70 | | 3.1 | | | | | | 1170 | |
| 56583 | 1/2 cup | Coleslaw | 72 | 90 | 76 | 0.0 | 10.0 | 2.0 | 8.0 | 0.0 | 6.0 | 0.0 | | | | | 10 | 0 | 0 | 0 | 0 | 0 | | | | | | | | 54.0 | | | 40 | | 0.7 | | | | 120 | | 130 | |
| 52081 | 1 ea | Deluxe Garden | 270 | 110 | 92 | 7.0 | 9.0 | 3.0 | 6.0 | 0.0 | 6.0 | 1.0 | | | | | 0 | 6000 | 1200 | | | | | | | | | | | 36.0 | | | 180 | | 1.4 | | | | | | 350 | |
| 56586 | 1/2 cup | Pasta | 70 | 70 | 81 | 2.0 | 8.0 | 2.0 | 2.0 | 4.0 | 3.0 | 0.0 | | | 0.00 | 0.00 | 0 | 200 | 40 | | | | | 0.04 | 5.00 | | | | | 4.8 | | | 20 | | 0.7 | | | | | | 350 | |
| 52078 | 1/2 cup | Potato | 72 | 160 | 65 | 0.0 | 10.0 | 0.0 | 0.0 | 10.0 | 14.0 | 5.0 | | | | | 10 | 0 | 0 | 0 | 0 | 0 | | | | | | | | 7.2 | | | 0 | | 0.0 | | | | | | 350 | |
| 52079 | 1/2 cup | Seafood | 74 | 140 | 66 | 6.0 | 10.0 | 0.0 | | | 8.0 | 1.0 | | | | | 0 | 0 | 0 | 0 | 0 | 0 | | | | | | | | 2.4 | | | 300 | | 0.7 | | | | | | 600 | |
| 52083 | 1 ea | Side | 155 | 60 | 90 | 4.0 | 5.0 | 2.0 | 3.0 | 0.0 | 3.0 | 0.0 | | | 0.00 | 0.00 | 0 | 3000 | 600 | | | | | | | | | | | 18.0 | | | 100 | | 0.9 | | | | | | 130 | |
| 56588 | 1 ea | Taco | 468 | 380 | 84 | 26.0 | 28.0 | 7.0 | 9.0 | 12.0 | 19.0 | 10.0 | | | | | 65 | 2250 | 450 | | | | 0.27 | 0.46 | 2.94 | 0.43 | 1.20 | 81.0 | 0.44 | 27.0 | | | 370 | 0.4 | 4.1 | 85 | | 341 | 787 | | 1040 | 4.60 |
| | | Sandwiches, Beef | | | | | | | | | | | | | | | | | | | | | | | | | | | | | | | | | | | | | | | | |
| 56571 | 1 ea | Bacon Cheeseburger, Junior | 166 | 380 | 55 | 20.0 | 34.0 | 2.0 | 7.0 | 25.0 | 19.0 | 7.0 | 10.3 | 1.4 | | | 60 | 400 | 80 | | | | 0.30 | 0.31 | 6.43 | 0.26 | 1.99 | 28.2 | 0.29 | 6.0 | | | 170 | 0.1 | 3.4 | 38 | | 334 | 375 | | 850 | 5.90 |
| 56574 | 1 ea | Big Bacon Classic Hamburger | 282 | 580 | 59 | 34.0 | 46.0 | 3.0 | 11.0 | 32.0 | 30.0 | 12.0 | | | | | 100 | 750 | 150 | | | | 0.45 | 1.52 | 5.98 | | | | | 15.0 | | | 250 | | 5.4 | | | | 578 | | 1450 | |
| 56570 | 1 ea | Cheeseburger, Junior | 130 | 320 | 48 | 17.0 | 34.0 | 2.0 | 7.0 | 25.0 | 13.0 | 6.0 | | | | | 45 | 300 | 60 | | | | 0.40 | 1.40 | 4.20 | | | | | 1.2 | | | 170 | | 3.2 | | | | 220 | | 830 | |
| 69058 | 1 ea | Cheeseburger Deluxe, Junior | 180 | 360 | 58 | 18.0 | 36.0 | 3.0 | 8.0 | 25.0 | 17.0 | 6.0 | | | | | 50 | 500 | 100 | | | | | | | | | | | 6.0 | | | 180 | | 3.4 | | | | | | 890 | |
| 69057 | 1 ea | Hamburger, Junior | 118 | 270 | 48 | 15.0 | 34.0 | 2.0 | 7.0 | 25.0 | 10.0 | 3.5 | | | | | 30 | 100 | 20 | | | | | | | | | | | 1.2 | | | 110 | | 3.1 | | | | | | 610 | |

| Code | Amount | | Description | Basic Components | | | | | | | | | Additional Fats | | | | | | Vit A & Components | | | | | Vitamins | | | | | | | | | | Minerals | | | | | | | | | |
|---|---|---|---|---|---|---|---|---|---|---|---|---|---|---|---|---|---|---|---|---|---|---|---|---|---|---|---|---|---|---|---|---|---|---|---|---|---|---|---|---|---|---|---|
| | | | | Weight (g) | Calories | % Water | Protein (g) | Carbs (g) | Fiber (g) | Sugar (g) | Other Carbs (g) | Fat (g) | Sat Fat (g) | Mono Fat (g) | Poly Fat (g) | Omega 3 (g) | Omega 6 (g) | Choles (mg) | Vit A (IU) | Vit A (RE) | Retinol (RE) | Carotenoids (RE) | Beta Carotene (mcg) | Thiamin (mg) | Riboflavin (mg) | Niacin (NE) | Vit B6 (mg) | Vit B12 (mcg) | Folate (mcg) | Panto (mg) | Vit C (mg) | Vit D (mg) | Vit E (α TE) | Calcium (mg) | Copper (mg) | Iron (mg) | Magnes (mg) | Mang (mg) | Phos (mg) | Potassium (mg) | Selenium (mcg) | Sodium (mg) | Zinc (mg) |
| 56564 | 1 | ea | Hamburger, Single, Plain | 133 | 360 | 44 | 24.0 | 31.0 | 2.0 | 5.0 | 24.0 | 16.0 | 6.0 | | | | | 65 | 0 | 0 | 0 | 0 | 0 | 0.43 | 0.38 | 6.71 | | | | | 0.0 | | | 110 | | 4.1 | | | | 296 | | 580 | |
| 56566 | 1 | ea | Hamburger, Single, w/everything | 219 | 420 | 62 | 25.0 | 37.0 | 3.0 | 9.0 | 25.0 | 20.0 | 7.0 | | | | | 70 | 300 | 60 | | | | 0.43 | 0.33 | 5.79 | | | | | 6.0 | | | 130 | | 4.7 | | | | 468 | | 920 | |
| | | | Sandwiches, Chicken | | | | | | | | | | | | | | | | | | | | | | | | | | | | | | | | | | | | | | | | |
| 56577 | 1 | ea | Breaded | 208 | 440 | 56 | 28.0 | 44.0 | 2.0 | 6.0 | 36.0 | 18.0 | 3.5 | | | | | 60 | 200 | 40 | | | | 0.43 | 0.32 | 13.30 | | | | | 6.0 | | | 100 | | 2.9 | | | | 437 | | 840 | |
| 69060 | 1 | ea | Club | 216 | 470 | 56 | 31.0 | 44.0 | 2.0 | 6.0 | 36.0 | 20.0 | 4.0 | | | | | 70 | 200 | 40 | | | | | | | | | | | 6.0 | | | 110 | | 3.1 | | | | | | 970 | |
| 69059 | 1 | ea | Grilled | 189 | 310 | 62 | 27.0 | 35.0 | 2.0 | 8.0 | 25.0 | 8.0 | 1.5 | | | | | 65 | 200 | 40 | | | | | | | | | | | 6.0 | | | 100 | | 2.7 | | | | | | 790 | |
| | | | **FATS, OILS, MARGARINES, AND SHORTENING** | | | | | | | | | | | | | | | | | | | | | | | | | | | | | | | | | | | | | | | | |
| | | | *FATS AND OILS, ANIMAL* | | | | | | | | | | | | | | | | | | | | | | | | | | | | | | | | | | | | | | | | |
| | | | Beef Fat | | | | | | | | | | | | | | | | | | | | | | | | | | | | | | | | | | | | | | | | |
| 8340 | 1 | oz | All cuts, raw, avg | 28 | 189 | 20 | 2.3 | 0.0 | 0.0 | 0.0 | 0.0 | 19.9 | 8.3 | 8.7 | 0.7 | 0.30 | 0.42 | 28 | 0 | 0 | 0 | 0 | 0 | 0.01 | 0.02 | 0.40 | 0.05 | 0.41 | 0.8 | 0.04 | 0.0 | | 0.7 | 3 | 0.0 | 0.2 | 1 | 0.0 | 19 | 18 | | 8 | 0.28 |
| 8688 | 1 | Tbs | Drippings, avg | 13 | 23 | 63 | 0.2 | 3.7 | 0.2 | 2.5 | 0.9 | 0.9 | 0.2 | 0.4 | 0.3 | 0.02 | 0.28 | 0 | 41 | 11 | 10 | 1 | | 0.01 | 0.01 | 0.08 | 0.01 | 0.00 | 0.3 | 0.01 | 0.5 | 0.0 | | 3 | 0.0 | 0.1 | 1 | 0.0 | 3 | 17 | 0.5 | 11 | 0.02 |
| 8004 | 1 | Tbs | Tallow, avg | 13 | 117 | 0 | 0.0 | 0.0 | 0.0 | 0.0 | 0.0 | 13.0 | 6.5 | 5.4 | 0.5 | 0.08 | 0.40 | 14 | 0 | 0 | 0 | 0 | 0 | 0.00 | 0.00 | 0.00 | 0.00 | 0.00 | 0.0 | 0.00 | 0.0 | 0.1 | | 0 | 0.0 | 0.0 | 0 | 0.0 | 0 | 0 | 0.0 | 0 | 0.00 |
| | | | Butter | | | | | | | | | | | | | | | | | | | | | | | | | | | | | | | | | | | | | | | | |
| 8000 | 1 | tsp | Salted, avg | 5 | 36 | 16 | 0.0 | 0.0 | 0.0 | 0.0 | 0.0 | 4.1 | 2.5 | 1.2 | 0.2 | 0.06 | 0.09 | 11 | 153 | 38 | 35 | 3 | | 0.00 | 0.00 | 0.00 | 0.00 | 0.01 | 0.2 | 0.01 | 0.0 | 0.1 | 0.1 | 1 | 0.0 | 0.0 | 0 | 0.0 | 1 | 1 | 0.1 | 41 | 0.00 |
| 8160 | 1 | tsp | Salted, lightly, avg | 5 | 36 | 16 | 0.0 | 0.0 | 0.0 | 0.0 | 0.0 | 4.1 | 2.5 | 1.2 | 0.2 | 0.06 | 0.09 | 11 | 153 | 38 | 34 | 4 | | 0.00 | 0.00 | 0.00 | 0.00 | 0.01 | 0.2 | 0.01 | 0.0 | 0.1 | 0.1 | 1 | 0.0 | 0.0 | 0 | 0.0 | 1 | 1 | | 37 | 0.00 |
| 8025 | 1 | tsp | Unsalted, avg | 5 | 36 | 18 | 0.0 | 0.0 | 0.0 | 0.0 | 0.0 | 4.1 | 2.5 | 1.2 | 0.2 | 0.06 | 0.09 | 11 | 153 | 38 | 35 | 3 | | 0.00 | 0.00 | 0.00 | 0.00 | 0.01 | 0.1 | 0.01 | 0.0 | 0.1 | 0.1 | 1 | 0.0 | 0.0 | 0 | 0.0 | 1 | 1 | 0.1 | 1 | 0.00 |
| 8142 | 1 | tsp | Whipped, salted, avg | 5 | 36 | 16 | 0.0 | 0.0 | 0.0 | 0.0 | 0.0 | 4.1 | 2.5 | 1.2 | 0.2 | 0.06 | 0.09 | 11 | 153 | 38 | 35 | 3 | | 0.00 | 0.00 | 0.00 | 0.00 | 0.01 | 0.1 | 0.01 | 0.0 | 0.1 | 0.1 | 1 | 0.0 | 0.0 | 0 | 0.0 | 1 | 1 | 0.1 | 41 | 0.00 |
| | | | Butter Blends | | | | | | | | | | | | | | | | | | | | | | | | | | | | | | | | | | | | | | | | |
| 8002 | 1 | ea | Butter Spray, 1/3 sec Spray, Pam | 0 | 0 | | 0.0 | 0.0 | | | | 0.0 | 0.0 | | | | | 0 | | | | | | | | | | | | | | | | | | | | | | | | 0 | |
| 8698 | 1 | tsp | I Can't Believe It's Not Butter | 5 | 32 | 27 | 0.0 | 0.0 | 0.0 | 0.0 | 0.0 | 3.6 | 0.7 | 0.5 | 1.6 | | | 0 | 179 | 36 | | | | | | | | | | | 0.0 | 0.0 | | 0 | | 0.0 | | | | | | 34 | |
| 8610 | 1 | tsp | Touch of Butter, 64% Veg Oil, Dairy Spread, Squeeze | 5 | 29 | | 0.0 | 0.0 | 0.0 | 0.0 | 0.0 | 3.2 | 0.5 | | | | | 0 | 179 | 36 | | | | | | | | | | | 0.0 | | | 0 | | 0.0 | | | | 0 | | 41 | |
| 8602 | 1 | tsp | Touch of Butter, 47% Veg Oil, Dairy Spread Tub | 5 | 21 | | 0.0 | 0.0 | 0.0 | 0.0 | 0.0 | 2.5 | 0.5 | 1.1 | 0.5 | | | 0 | 179 | 36 | | | | | | | | | | | 0.0 | | | 0 | | 0.0 | | | | 0 | | 39 | |
| 8175 | 1 | tsp | Touch of Butter, Spread Stick | 5 | 32 | 27 | 0.0 | 0.0 | 0.0 | 0.0 | 0.0 | 3.6 | 0.7 | | | | | 0 | 179 | 44 | | | | | | | | | | | 0.0 | | | 0 | | 0.0 | | | | 0 | | 39 | |
| 8076 | 1 | Tbs | Duck Fat, avg | 13 | 117 | 0 | 0.0 | 0.0 | 0.0 | 0.0 | 0.0 | 13.0 | 4.3 | 6.4 | 1.7 | 0.13 | 1.55 | 13 | 0 | 0 | 0 | 0 | 0 | 0.00 | 0.00 | 0.00 | 0.00 | 0.00 | 0.0 | 0.00 | 0.0 | 0.1 | 0.4 | 0 | 0.0 | 0.0 | 0 | 0.0 | 0 | 0 | 0.0 | 0 | 0.00 |
| | | | Fish Oils | | | | | | | | | | | | | | | | | | | | | | | | | | | | | | | | | | | | | | | | |
| 8067 | 1 | Tbs | Cod liver, avg | 14 | 127 | 0 | 0.0 | 0.0 | 0.0 | 0.0 | 0.0 | 14.0 | 3.2 | 6.5 | 3.2 | 2.63 | 0.26 | 80 | 13986 | 4200 | 4200 | 0 | 0 | 0.00 | 0.00 | 0.00 | 0.00 | 0.00 | 0.0 | 0.00 | 0.0 | 35.0 | | 0 | 0.0 | 0.0 | 0 | 0.0 | 0 | 0 | 0.0 | 0 | 0.00 |
| 8071 | 1 | Tbs | Herring, avg | 14 | 126 | 0 | 0.0 | 0.0 | 0.0 | 0.0 | 0.0 | 14.0 | 3.0 | 7.9 | 2.2 | 1.57 | 0.20 | 107 | 0 | 0 | 0 | 0 | 0 | 0.00 | 0.00 | 0.00 | 0.00 | 0.00 | 0.0 | 0.00 | 0.0 | 21.0 | 1.3 | 0 | 0.0 | 0.0 | 0 | 0.0 | 0 | 0 | 0.0 | 0 | 0.00 |
| 8072 | 1 | Tbs | Menhaden, avg | 14 | 126 | 0 | 0.0 | 0.0 | 0.0 | 0.0 | 0.0 | 14.0 | 4.3 | 3.7 | 4.8 | 3.25 | 0.46 | 73 | 0 | 0 | 0 | 0 | 0 | 0.00 | 0.00 | 0.00 | 0.00 | 0.00 | 0.0 | 0.00 | 0.0 | | 1.0 | 0 | 0.0 | 0.0 | 0 | 0.0 | 0 | 0 | 0.0 | 0 | 0.00 |
| 8073 | 1 | Tbs | Salmon, avg | 14 | 126 | 0 | 0.0 | 0.0 | 0.0 | 0.0 | 0.0 | 14.0 | 2.8 | 4.1 | 5.6 | 4.52 | 0.31 | 68 | 0 | 0 | 0 | 0 | 0 | 0.00 | 0.00 | 0.00 | 0.00 | 0.00 | 0.0 | 0.00 | 0.0 | 14.0 | 2.7 | 0 | 0.0 | 0.0 | 0 | 0.0 | 0 | 0 | 0.0 | 0 | 0.00 |
| 8074 | 1 | Tbs | Sardine, avg | 14 | 126 | 0 | 0.0 | 0.0 | 0.0 | 0.0 | 0.0 | 14.0 | 4.2 | 4.7 | 4.5 | 3.10 | 0.53 | 99 | 0 | 0 | 0 | 0 | 0 | 0.00 | 0.00 | 0.00 | 0.00 | 0.00 | 0.0 | 0.00 | 0.0 | 14.0 | | 0 | 0.0 | 0.0 | 0 | 0.0 | 0 | 0 | 0.0 | 0 | 0.00 |
| 8100 | 1 | Tbs | Shark, avg | 14 | 126 | 0 | 0.0 | 0.0 | 0.0 | 0.0 | 0.0 | 13.9 | 5.3 | 3.6 | 3.5 | 2.78 | 0.04 | | | | | | | | | | | | | | | | 7.0 | | | | | | | | | | |
| 8077 | 1 | Tbs | Goose Fat, avg | 13 | 117 | 0 | 0.0 | 0.0 | 0.0 | 0.0 | 0.0 | 13.0 | 3.6 | 7.4 | 1.4 | 0.06 | 1.27 | 13 | 0 | 0 | 0 | 0 | 0 | 0.00 | 0.00 | 0.00 | 0.00 | 0.00 | 0.0 | 0.00 | 0.0 | 0.1 | 0.4 | 0 | 0.0 | 0.0 | 0 | 0.0 | 0 | 0 | 0.0 | 0 | 0.00 |
| 8040 | 1 | Tbs | Mutton Tallow | 13 | 117 | 0 | 0.0 | 0.0 | 0.0 | 0.0 | 0.0 | 13.0 | 6.1 | 5.3 | 1.0 | 0.30 | 0.71 | 13 | 0 | 0 | 0 | 0 | 0 | 0.00 | 0.00 | 0.00 | 0.00 | 0.00 | 0.0 | 0.00 | 0.0 | | 0.4 | 0 | 0.0 | 0.0 | 0 | 0.0 | 0 | 0 | 0.0 | 0 | 0.00 |
| | | | Pork Fat | | | | | | | | | | | | | | | | | | | | | | | | | | | | | | | | | | | | | | | | |
| 8003 | 1 | Tbs | Bacon grease/meat fat drippings, avg | 14 | 124 | 0 | 0.0 | 0.0 | 0.0 | 0.0 | 0.0 | 13.8 | 6.3 | 5.9 | 1.1 | 0.10 | 0.98 | 14 | 0 | 0 | 0 | 0 | 0 | 0.00 | 0.00 | 0.00 | 0.00 | 0.00 | 0.0 | 0.00 | 0.0 | 0.1 | | 0 | 0.0 | 0.0 | 0 | 0.0 | 0 | 0 | 0.0 | 76 | 0.01 |
| 8341 | 1 | oz | Fresh, raw, avg | 28 | 179 | 25 | 1.8 | 0.0 | 0.0 | 0.0 | 0.0 | 19.0 | 6.6 | 8.4 | 2.0 | 0.17 | 1.76 | 26 | 3 | 1 | 1 | 0 | | 0.06 | 0.03 | 0.50 | 0.01 | 0.09 | 0.6 | 0.07 | 0.0 | | | 13 | 0.0 | 0.1 | 1 | 0.0 | 25 | 34 | 2.2 | 5 | 0.20 |
| 8006 | 1 | Tbs | Lard, avg | 13 | 117 | 0 | 0.0 | 0.0 | 0.0 | 0.0 | 0.0 | 13.0 | 5.1 | 5.5 | 1.8 | 0.08 | 1.71 | 12 | 0 | 0 | 0 | 0 | 0 | 0.00 | 0.00 | 0.00 | 0.00 | 0.00 | 0.0 | 0.00 | 0.0 | 0.0 | 0.2 | 0 | 0.0 | 0.0 | 0 | 0.0 | 0 | 0 | 0.0 | 0 | 0.01 |
| 8036 | 1 | Tbs | Turkey Fat, avg | 13 | 117 | 0 | 0.0 | 0.0 | 0.0 | 0.0 | 0.0 | 13.0 | 3.8 | 5.6 | 3.0 | 0.18 | 2.79 | 13 | 0 | 0 | 0 | 0 | 0 | 0.00 | 0.00 | 0.00 | 0.00 | 0.00 | 0.0 | 0.00 | 0.0 | 0.1 | 0.4 | 0 | 0.0 | 0.0 | 0 | 0.0 | 0 | 0 | 0.0 | 0 | 0.00 |
| | | | *OILS, VEGETABLE* | | | | | | | | | | | | | | | | | | | | | | | | | | | | | | | | | | | | | | | | |
| 8078 | 1 | Tbs | Almond, avg | 14 | 124 | 0 | 0.0 | 0.0 | 0.0 | 0.0 | 0.0 | 14.0 | 1.1 | 9.8 | 2.4 | 0.00 | 2.44 | 0 | 0 | 0 | 0 | 0 | 0 | 0.00 | 0.00 | 0.00 | 0.00 | 0.00 | 0.0 | 0.00 | 0.0 | 0.0 | 5.5 | 0 | 0.0 | 0.0 | 0 | 0.0 | 0 | 0 | 0.0 | 0 | 0.00 |
| 8079 | 1 | Tbs | Apricot kernel, avg | 14 | 124 | 0 | 0.0 | 0.0 | 0.0 | 0.0 | 0.0 | 14.0 | 0.9 | 8.4 | 4.1 | 0.00 | 4.10 | 0 | 0 | 0 | 0 | 0 | 0 | 0.00 | 0.00 | 0.00 | 0.00 | 0.00 | 0.0 | 0.00 | 0.0 | 0.0 | | 0 | 0.0 | 0.0 | 0 | 0.0 | 0 | 0 | 0.0 | 0 | 0.00 |
| 8342 | 1 | Tbs | Avocado, avg | 14 | 124 | 0 | 0.0 | 0.0 | 0.0 | 0.0 | 0.0 | 14.0 | 1.6 | 9.9 | 1.9 | 0.13 | 1.75 | | 0 | 0 | 0 | 0 | 0 | 0.00 | 0.00 | 0.00 | 0.00 | 0.00 | 0.0 | 0.00 | 0.0 | | | 0 | 0.0 | 0.0 | 0 | 0.0 | 0 | 0 | 0.0 | 0 | 0.00 |
| 8084 | 1 | Tbs | Canola, avg | 14 | 124 | 0 | 0.0 | 0.0 | 0.0 | 0.0 | 0.0 | 14.0 | 1.0 | 8.2 | 4.1 | 1.30 | 2.84 | 0 | 0 | 0 | 0 | 0 | 0 | 0.00 | 0.00 | 0.00 | 0.00 | 0.00 | 0.0 | 0.00 | 0.0 | 0.0 | 2.7 | 0 | 0.0 | 0.0 | 0 | 0.0 | 0 | 0 | 0.0 | 0 | 0.00 |
| 8326 | 1 | Tbs | Carob seed, avg | 14 | 124 | 0 | 0.0 | 0.0 | 0.0 | 0.0 | 0.0 | 14.0 | 3.1 | 4.5 | 5.8 | 0.23 | 5.56 | 0 | | | | | | | | | | | | | | | | | | | | | | | | | |
| 8080 | 1 | Tbs | Cocoa butter, avg | 14 | 124 | 0 | 0.0 | 0.0 | 0.0 | 0.0 | 0.0 | 14.0 | 8.4 | 4.6 | 0.4 | 0.01 | 0.39 | 0 | 0 | 0 | 0 | 0 | 0 | 0.00 | 0.00 | 0.00 | 0.00 | 0.00 | 0.0 | 0.00 | 0.0 | 0.0 | 0.3 | 0 | 0.0 | 0.0 | 0 | 0.0 | 0 | 0 | 0.0 | 0 | 0.00 |
| 8037 | 1 | Tbs | Coconut, avg | 14 | 121 | 0 | 0.0 | 0.0 | 0.0 | 0.0 | 0.0 | 14.0 | 12.1 | 0.8 | 0.3 | 0.00 | 0.25 | 0 | 0 | 0 | 0 | 0 | 0 | 0.00 | 0.00 | 0.00 | 0.00 | 0.00 | 0.0 | 0.00 | 0.0 | 0.0 | | 0 | 0.0 | 0.0 | 0 | 0.0 | 0 | 0 | 0.0 | 0 | 0.00 |
| 8009 | 1 | Tbs | Corn, avg | 14 | 124 | 0 | 0.0 | 0.0 | 0.0 | 0.0 | 0.0 | 14.0 | 1.8 | 3.4 | 8.2 | 0.10 | 8.12 | 0 | 0 | 0 | 0 | 0 | 0 | 0.00 | 0.00 | 0.00 | 0.00 | 0.00 | 0.0 | 0.00 | 0.0 | 0.0 | 2.0 | 0 | 0.0 | 0.0 | 0 | 0.0 | 0 | 0 | 0.0 | 0 | 0.00 |
| 8081 | 1 | Tbs | Cottonseed, avg | 14 | 124 | 0 | 0.0 | 0.0 | 0.0 | 0.0 | 0.0 | 14.0 | 3.6 | 2.5 | 7.3 | 0.03 | 7.22 | 0 | 0 | 0 | 0 | 0 | 0 | 0.00 | 0.00 | 0.00 | 0.00 | 0.00 | 0.0 | 0.00 | 0.0 | 0.0 | 4.9 | 0 | 0.0 | 0.0 | 0 | 0.0 | 0 | 0 | 0.0 | 0 | 0.00 |
| 8047 | 1 | Tbs | Grapeseed, avg | 14 | 124 | 0 | 0.0 | 0.0 | 0.0 | 0.0 | 0.0 | 14.0 | 1.3 | 2.3 | 9.8 | 0.01 | 9.74 | 0 | 0 | 0 | 0 | 0 | 0 | 0.00 | 0.00 | 0.00 | 0.00 | 0.00 | 0.0 | 0.00 | 0.0 | 0.0 | 4.0 | 0 | 0.0 | 0.0 | 0 | 0.0 | 0 | 0 | 0.0 | 0 | 0.00 |
| 8048 | 1 | Tbs | Hazelnut, avg | 14 | 124 | 0 | 0.0 | 0.0 | 0.0 | 0.0 | 0.0 | 14.0 | 1.0 | 10.9 | 1.4 | 0.00 | 1.41 | 0 | 0 | 0 | 0 | 0 | 0 | 0.00 | 0.00 | 0.00 | 0.00 | 0.00 | 0.0 | 0.00 | 0.0 | 0.0 | 6.6 | 0 | 0.0 | 0.0 | 0 | 0.0 | 0 | 0 | 0.0 | 0 | 0.00 |
| 8070 | 1 | Tbs | Oat, avg | 14 | 124 | 0 | 0.0 | 0.0 | 0.0 | 0.0 | 0.0 | 14.0 | 2.7 | 4.9 | 5.7 | 0.25 | 5.47 | 0 | 0 | 0 | 0 | 0 | 0 | 0.00 | 0.00 | 0.00 | 0.00 | 0.00 | 0.0 | 0.00 | 0.0 | 0.0 | 1.3 | 0 | 0.0 | 0.0 | 0 | 0.0 | 0 | 0 | 0.0 | 0 | 0.00 |
| 8008 | 1 | Tbs | Olive, avg | 14 | 124 | 0 | 0.0 | 0.0 | 0.0 | 0.0 | 0.0 | 14.0 | 1.9 | 10.3 | 1.2 | 0.08 | 1.09 | 0 | 0 | 0 | 0 | 0 | 0 | 0.00 | 0.00 | 0.00 | 0.00 | 0.00 | 0.0 | 0.00 | 0.0 | 0.0 | | 0 | 0.0 | 0.1 | 0 | 0.0 | 0 | 0 | 0.0 | 0 | 0.01 |
| 8361 | 1 | Tbs | Olive, Extra Virgin, Natural Oils International | 14 | 126 | 0 | 0.0 | 0.0 | 0.0 | 0.0 | 0.0 | 14.0 | 2.0 | 10.8 | 1.3 | 0.10 | 1.12 | | | | | | | | | | | | | | | | | | | | | | | | | | |
| 8082 | 1 | Tbs | Palm, avg | 14 | 124 | 0 | 0.0 | 0.0 | 0.0 | 0.0 | 0.0 | 14.0 | 6.9 | 5.2 | 1.3 | 0.03 | 1.27 | 0 | 0 | 0 | 0 | 0 | 0 | 0.00 | 0.00 | 0.00 | 0.00 | 0.00 | 0.0 | 0.00 | 0.0 | 0.0 | 2.7 | 0 | 0.0 | 0.0 | 0 | 0.0 | 0 | 0 | 0.0 | 0 | 0.00 |
| 8083 | 1 | Tbs | Palm kernel, avg | 14 | 121 | 0 | 0.0 | 0.0 | 0.0 | 0.0 | 0.0 | 14.0 | 11.4 | 1.6 | 0.2 | 0.00 | 0.22 | 0 | 0 | 0 | 0 | 0 | 0 | 0.00 | 0.00 | 0.00 | 0.00 | 0.00 | 0.0 | 0.00 | 0.0 | 0.0 | 0.1 | 0 | 0.0 | 0.0 | 0 | 0.0 | 0 | 0 | 0.0 | 0 | 0.00 |
| 8332 | 1 | Tbs | Peach kernel, avg | 14 | 124 | 0 | 0.0 | 0.0 | 0.0 | 0.0 | 0.0 | 14.0 | 5.1 | 4.2 | 4.1 | 0.00 | 4.09 | 0 | | | | | | | | | | | | | | | 1.9 | | | | | | | | | | |
| 8026 | 1 | Tbs | Peanut, avg | 14 | 124 | 0 | 0.0 | 0.0 | 0.0 | 0.0 | 0.0 | 14.0 | 2.4 | 6.5 | 4.5 | 0.00 | 4.48 | 0 | 0 | 0 | 0 | 0 | 0 | 0.00 | 0.00 | 0.00 | 0.00 | 0.00 | 0.0 | 0.00 | 0.0 | 0.0 | 1.6 | 0 | 0.0 | 0.0 | 0 | 0.0 | 0 | 0 | 0.0 | 0 | 0.00 |
| 8334 | 1 | Tbs | Pistachio nut kernel, avg | 14 | 124 | 0 | 0.0 | 0.0 | 0.0 | 0.0 | 0.0 | 14.0 | 1.9 | 6.9 | 4.6 | 0.00 | 4.55 | 0 | | | | | | | | | | | | | | | | | | | | | | | | | |
| 8049 | 1 | Tbs | Poppyseed, avg | 14 | 124 | 0 | 0.0 | 0.0 | 0.0 | 0.0 | 0.0 | 14.0 | 1.9 | 2.8 | 8.7 | 0.00 | 8.74 | 0 | 0 | 0 | 0 | 0 | 0 | 0.00 | 0.00 | 0.00 | 0.00 | 0.00 | 0.0 | 0.00 | 0.0 | 0.0 | 1.6 | 0 | | 0.0 | 0 | 0.0 | 0 | 0 | 0.0 | 0 | 0.00 |
| 8097 | 1 | Tbs | Pumpkin seed, avg | 14 | 123 | 0 | 0.0 | 0.0 | 0.0 | 0.0 | 0.0 | 13.9 | 2.8 | 3.3 | 7.2 | 0.07 | 7.14 | | | | | | | | | | | | | | | | | | | | | | | | | | |
| 8050 | 1 | Tbs | Rice bran, avg | 14 | 124 | 0 | 0.0 | 0.0 | 0.0 | 0.0 | 0.0 | 14.0 | 2.8 | 5.5 | 4.9 | 0.22 | 4.68 | 0 | 0 | 0 | 0 | 0 | 0 | 0.00 | 0.00 | 0.00 | 0.00 | 0.00 | 0.0 | 0.00 | 0.0 | 0.0 | 5.1 | 0 | | 0.0 | 0 | 0.0 | 0 | 0 | 0.0 | 0 | 0.00 |
| 8010 | 1 | Tbs | Safflower, avg | 14 | 124 | 0 | 0.0 | 0.0 | 0.0 | 0.0 | 0.0 | 14.0 | 1.3 | 1.7 | 10.4 | 0.06 | 10.37 | 0 | 0 | 0 | 0 | 0 | 0 | 0.00 | 0.00 | 0.00 | 0.00 | 0.00 | 0.0 | 0.00 | 0.0 | 0.0 | | 0 | 0.0 | 0.0 | 0 | 0.0 | 0 | 0 | 0.0 | 0 | 0.00 |
| 8027 | 1 | Tbs | Sesame, avg | 14 | 124 | 0 | 0.0 | 0.0 | 0.0 | 0.0 | 0.0 | 14.0 | 2.0 | 5.6 | 5.8 | 0.04 | 5.78 | 0 | 0 | 0 | 0 | 0 | 0 | 0.00 | 0.00 | 0.00 | 0.00 | 0.00 | 0.0 | 0.00 | 0.0 | 0.0 | 0.2 | 0 | 0.0 | 0.0 | 0 | 0.0 | 0 | 0 | 0.0 | 0 | 0.00 |
| | | | Soybean Oil | | | | | | | | | | | | | | | | | | | | | | | | | | | | | | | | | | | | | | | | |
| 8108 | 1 | Tbs | Average | 14 | 124 | 0 | 0.0 | 0.0 | 0.0 | 0.0 | 0.0 | 14.0 | 2.0 | 3.3 | 8.1 | 0.95 | 7.14 | 0 | 0 | 0 | 0 | 0 | 0 | 0.00 | 0.00 | 0.00 | 0.00 | 0.00 | 0.0 | 0.00 | 0.0 | 0.0 | 1.5 | 0 | 0.0 | 0.0 | 0 | 0.0 | 0 | 0 | 0.0 | 0 | 0.00 |

| Code | Amount | Description | Weight (g) | Calories | % Water | Protein (g) | Carbs (g) | Fiber (g) | Sugar (g) | Other Carbs (g) | Fat (g) | Sat Fat (g) | Mono Fat (g) | Poly Fat (g) | Omega 3 (g) | Omega 6 (g) | Choles (mg) | Vit A (IU) | Vit A (RE) | Retinol (RE) | Carotenoids (RE) | Beta Carotene (mcg) | Thiamin (mg) | Riboflavin (mg) | Niacin (NE) | Vit B6 (mg) | Vit B12 (mcg) | Folate (mcg) | Panto (mg) | Vit C (mg) | Vit D (mg) | Vit E (α TE) | Calcium (mg) | Copper (mg) | Iron (mg) | Magnes (mg) | Mang (mg) | Phos (mg) | Potassium (mg) | Selenium (mcg) | Sodium (mg) | Zinc (mg) |
|---|---|---|---|---|---|---|---|---|---|---|---|---|---|---|---|---|---|---|---|---|---|---|---|---|---|---|---|---|---|---|---|---|---|---|---|---|---|---|---|---|---|---|
| | | | Basic Components | | | | | | | | | Additional Fats | | | | | | Vit A & Components | | | | | Vitamins | | | | | | | | | | Minerals | | | | | | | | | |
| 8028 | 1 Tbs | Hydrogenated & cottonseed oil, avg | 14 | 124 | 0 | 0.0 | 0.0 | 0.0 | 0.0 | 0.0 | 14.0 | 2.5 | 4.1 | 6.7 | 0.39 | 6.34 | 0 | 0 | 0 | 0 | 0 | 0 | 0.00 | 0.00 | 0.00 | 0.00 | 0.00 | 0.0 | 0.00 | 0.0 | 0.0 | | 0 | 0.0 | 0.0 | 0 | 0.0 | 0 | 0 | 0.0 | 0 | 0.00 |
| 8661 | 1 Tbs | Hydrogenated Oil, Archer Daniels Midland | 14 | 124 | 0 | 0.0 | 0.0 | 0.0 | 0.0 | 0.0 | 14.0 | 2.9 | 10.8 | 0.3 | | | | 0 | 0 | 0 | 0 | 0 | 0.00 | 0.00 | 0.00 | | | | | 0.0 | | | 0 | | 0.0 | | | | 0 | | 0 | |
| 8011 | 1 Tbs | Sunflower oil, avg | 14 | 124 | 0 | 0.0 | 0.0 | 0.0 | 0.0 | 0.0 | 14.0 | 1.4 | 2.7 | 9.2 | 0.00 | 9.20 | 0 | 0 | 0 | 0 | 0 | 0 | 0.00 | 0.00 | 0.00 | 0.00 | 0.00 | 0.0 | 0.00 | 0.0 | 0.0 | | 0 | 0.0 | 0.0 | 0 | 0.0 | 0 | 0 | 0.0 | 0 | 0.00 |
| 8351 | 1 Tbs | Tomato seed oil, avg | 14 | 124 | 0 | 0.0 | 0.0 | 0.0 | 0.0 | 0.0 | 14.0 | 2.8 | 3.2 | 7.4 | 0.32 | 7.11 | 0 | 0 | 0 | 0 | 0 | 0 | 0.00 | 0.00 | 0.00 | 0.00 | 0.00 | 0.0 | 0.00 | 0.0 | | 0.6 | 0 | | 0.0 | 0 | | 0 | 0 | 0.0 | 0 | 0.00 |
| | | Unspecifed Oil | | | | | | | | | | | | | | | | | | | | | | | | | | | | | | | | | | | | | | | | |
| 8086 | 1 Tbs | Hot Oil, China Bowl Trading Co | 14 | 120 | 0 | 0.0 | 0.0 | 0.0 | 0.0 | 0.0 | 14.0 | 2.0 | | | | | 0 | 0 | 0 | 0 | 0 | 0 | 0.00 | 0.00 | 0.00 | 0.00 | 0.00 | 0.0 | 0.00 | 0.0 | | | 0 | | 0.0 | 0 | 0.0 | 0 | 0 | | 0 | 0.00 |
| 8092 | 1 Tbs | Nutra-Clear, Bunge Foods | 14 | 130 | 0 | 0.0 | 0.0 | 0.0 | 0.0 | 0.0 | 14.0 | 1.0 | 8.0 | 4.0 | | | 0 | | | | | | | | | | 0.00 | | | | | | | | | | | | | | 0 | |
| 8093 | 1 Tbs | Nutra-Fry, Bunge Foods | 14 | 130 | 0 | 0.0 | 0.0 | 0.0 | 0.0 | 0.0 | 14.0 | 1.0 | 8.0 | 2.0 | | | 0 | | | | | | | | | | 0.00 | | | | | | | | | | | | | | 0 | |
| 8672 | 1 Tbs | Popcorn Oil, China Bowl Trading Co | 14 | 130 | 0 | 0.0 | 0.0 | 0.0 | 0.0 | 0.0 | 14.0 | 2.0 | 3.0 | 9.0 | | | | | | | | | | | | | | | | | | | | | | | | | | | 0 | |
| 8671 | 1 Tbs | Wok, China Bowl Trading Co | 14 | 130 | 0 | 0.0 | 0.0 | 0.0 | 0.0 | 0.0 | 14.0 | 2.0 | | | | | | | | | | | | | | | | | | | | | | | | | | | | | 5 | |
| 8085 | 1 Tbs | Walnut oil, avg | 14 | 124 | 0 | 0.0 | 0.0 | 0.0 | 0.0 | 0.0 | 14.0 | 1.3 | 3.2 | 8.9 | 1.46 | 7.41 | 0 | 0 | 0 | 0 | 0 | 0 | 0.00 | 0.00 | 0.00 | 0.00 | 0.00 | 0.0 | 0.00 | 0.0 | 0.0 | 0.1 | 0 | 0.0 | 0.0 | 0 | 0.0 | 0 | 0 | 0.0 | 0 | 0.00 |
| 8335 | 1 Tbs | Watermelon seed oil, avg | 14 | 124 | 0 | 0.0 | 0.0 | 0.0 | 0.0 | 0.0 | 14.0 | 3.4 | 1.6 | 8.3 | 0.00 | 8.35 | 0 | | | | | | | | | | | | | | | | | | | | | | | | | |
| 8038 | 1 Tbs | Wheat germ oil, avg | 14 | 124 | 0 | 0.0 | 0.0 | 0.0 | 0.0 | 0.0 | 14.0 | 2.6 | 2.1 | 8.5 | 0.97 | 7.67 | 0 | 0 | 0 | 0 | 0 | 0 | 0.00 | 0.00 | 0.00 | 0.00 | 0.00 | 0.0 | 0.00 | 0.0 | 0.0 | | 0 | 0.0 | 0.0 | 0 | 0.0 | 0 | 0 | 0.0 | 0 | 0.00 |
| | | *MARGARINES* | | | | | | | | | | | | | | | | | | | | | | | | | | | | | | | | | | | | | | | | |
| | | Corn oil | | | | | | | | | | | | | | | | | | | | | | | | | | | | | | | | | | | | | | | | |
| 8052 | 1 tsp | Hard, avg | 5 | 36 | 16 | 0.0 | 0.0 | 0.0 | 0.0 | 0.0 | 4.0 | 0.7 | 1.9 | 1.2 | 0.02 | 1.19 | 0 | 179 | 40 | 34 | 6 | | 0.00 | 0.00 | 0.00 | 0.00 | 0.00 | 0.1 | 0.00 | 0.0 | | | 2 | 0.0 | 0.0 | 0 | | 1 | 2 | 0.0 | 47 | 0.00 |
| 8061 | 1 tsp | Soft, avg | 5 | 36 | 16 | 0.0 | 0.0 | 0.0 | 0.0 | 0.0 | 4.0 | 0.7 | 1.6 | 1.5 | 0.04 | 1.51 | 0 | 179 | 40 | 35 | 5 | | 0.00 | 0.00 | 0.00 | 0.00 | 0.00 | 0.1 | 0.00 | 0.0 | 0.5 | 0.5 | 1 | | 0.0 | 0 | 0.0 | 1 | 2 | 0.0 | 54 | 0.00 |
| 8053 | 1 tsp | With Soybean/cottonseed oils, hard, avg | 5 | 36 | 16 | 0.0 | 0.0 | 0.0 | 0.0 | 0.0 | 4.0 | 0.8 | 1.8 | 1.3 | 0.02 | 1.24 | 0 | 179 | 40 | 34 | 6 | | 0.00 | 0.00 | 0.00 | 0.00 | 0.00 | 0.1 | 0.00 | 0.0 | 0.1 | 0.6 | 2 | 0.0 | 0.0 | 0 | 0.0 | 1 | 2 | 0.0 | 47 | 0.00 |
| 8344 | 1 tsp | With Soybean/cottonseed oils, w/o salt, hard, avg | 5 | 36 | 18 | 0.0 | 0.0 | 0.0 | 0.0 | 0.0 | 4.0 | 0.8 | 1.8 | 1.3 | 0.02 | 1.24 | 0 | 179 | 40 | 34 | 6 | | 0.00 | 0.00 | 0.00 | 0.00 | 0.00 | 0.0 | 0.00 | 0.0 | | | 1 | 0.0 | 0.0 | 0 | 0.0 | 1 | 1 | 0.0 | 0 | 0.00 |
| 8263 | 1 tsp | Coconut/safflower/palm oils, hard, avg | 5 | 36 | 16 | 0.0 | 0.0 | 0.0 | 0.0 | 0.0 | 4.0 | 2.8 | 0.4 | 0.6 | 0.01 | 0.57 | 0 | 179 | 40 | 34 | 6 | | 0.00 | 0.00 | 0.00 | 0.00 | 0.00 | 0.1 | 0.00 | 0.0 | | 0.4 | 2 | | 0.0 | 0 | | 1 | 2 | 0.0 | 47 | |
| 8241 | 1 tsp | Lard, hard, avg | 5 | 37 | 16 | 0.0 | 0.0 | 0.0 | 0.0 | 0.0 | 4.0 | 1.6 | 1.9 | 0.4 | 0.02 | 0.35 | 3 | 0 | 0 | 0 | 0 | 0 | 0.00 | 0.00 | 0.00 | 0.00 | 0.00 | 0.0 | 0.00 | 0.0 | | | 0 | | 0.0 | 0 | | 0 | 2 | 0.0 | 47 | 0.00 |
| 8249 | 1 tsp | Palm oil, hard, imitation, avg | 5 | 17 | 58 | 0.0 | 0.0 | 0.0 | 0.0 | 0.0 | 1.9 | 0.5 | 0.7 | 0.6 | 0.04 | 0.61 | 0 | 179 | 40 | 35 | 5 | | 0.00 | 0.00 | 0.00 | 0.00 | 0.00 | 0.0 | 0.00 | 0.0 | | | 1 | | 0.0 | 0 | | 1 | 1 | 0.0 | 48 | 0.00 |
| | | Safflower oil | | | | | | | | | | | | | | | | | | | | | | | | | | | | | | | | | | | | | | | | |
| 8058 | 1 tsp | Soft, avg | 5 | 36 | 16 | 0.0 | 0.0 | 0.0 | 0.0 | 0.0 | 4.0 | 0.5 | 1.2 | 2.2 | 0.00 | 2.23 | 0 | 179 | 40 | 35 | 5 | | 0.00 | 0.00 | 0.00 | 0.00 | 0.00 | 0.1 | 0.00 | 0.0 | | 0.6 | 1 | | 0.0 | 0 | | 1 | 2 | 0.0 | 54 | 0.00 |
| 8057 | 1 tsp | With Cottonseed/peanut oils, soft, avg | 5 | 36 | 16 | 0.0 | 0.0 | 0.0 | 0.0 | 0.0 | 4.0 | 0.7 | 0.7 | 2.5 | 0.00 | 2.48 | 0 | 179 | 40 | 35 | 5 | | 0.00 | 0.00 | 0.00 | 0.00 | 0.00 | 0.1 | 0.00 | 0.0 | | 0.3 | 1 | | 0.0 | 0 | | 1 | 2 | 0.0 | 54 | 0.00 |
| 8055 | 1 tsp | With Cottonseed/soybean oils, hard, avg | 5 | 36 | 16 | 0.0 | 0.0 | 0.0 | 0.0 | 0.0 | 4.0 | 0.7 | 1.5 | 1.6 | 0.01 | 1.60 | 0 | 179 | 40 | 34 | 6 | | 0.00 | 0.00 | 0.00 | 0.00 | 0.00 | 0.1 | 0.00 | 0.0 | | 0.8 | 2 | | 0.0 | 0 | | 1 | 2 | 0.0 | 47 | 0.00 |
| 8054 | 1 tsp | With Soybean oil, hard, avg | 5 | 36 | 16 | 0.0 | 0.0 | 0.0 | 0.0 | 0.0 | 4.0 | 0.7 | 1.6 | 1.6 | 0.01 | 1.56 | 0 | 179 | 40 | 34 | 6 | | 0.00 | 0.00 | 0.00 | 0.00 | 0.00 | 0.1 | 0.00 | 0.0 | | 0.9 | 2 | | 0.0 | 0 | | 1 | 2 | 0.0 | 47 | 0.00 |
| | | Soybean oil | | | | | | | | | | | | | | | | | | | | | | | | | | | | | | | | | | | | | | | | |
| 8179 | 1 tsp | Hard, avg | 5 | 36 | 16 | 0.0 | 0.0 | 0.0 | 0.0 | 0.0 | 4.0 | 0.7 | 1.9 | 1.3 | 0.09 | 1.22 | 0 | 179 | 40 | 34 | 6 | | 0.00 | 0.00 | 0.00 | 0.00 | 0.00 | 0.1 | 0.00 | 0.0 | | 0.2 | 2 | 0.0 | 0.0 | 0 | 0.0 | 1 | 2 | 0.0 | 47 | |
| 8247 | 1 tsp | Soft, avg | 5 | 36 | 16 | 0.0 | 0.0 | 0.0 | 0.0 | 0.0 | 4.0 | 0.8 | 1.5 | 1.5 | 0.14 | 1.37 | 0 | 179 | 40 | 35 | 5 | | 0.00 | 0.00 | 0.00 | 0.00 | 0.00 | 0.1 | 0.00 | 0.0 | | 0.4 | 1 | | 0.0 | 0 | | 1 | 2 | 0.0 | 54 | 0.00 |
| 8234 | 1 tsp | With Cottonseed oil, hard, avg | 5 | 36 | 16 | 0.0 | 0.0 | 0.0 | 0.0 | 0.0 | 4.0 | 1.0 | 1.6 | 1.3 | 0.08 | 1.18 | 0 | 179 | 40 | 34 | 6 | | 0.00 | 0.00 | 0.00 | 0.00 | 0.00 | 0.1 | 0.00 | 0.0 | | 0.6 | 2 | | 0.0 | 0 | | 1 | 2 | 0.0 | 47 | 0.00 |
| 8250 | 1 tsp | With Cottonseed oil, hard, imitation, avg | 5 | 17 | 58 | 0.0 | 0.0 | 0.0 | 0.0 | 0.0 | 1.9 | 0.4 | 0.9 | 0.6 | 0.04 | 0.54 | 0 | 179 | 40 | 35 | 5 | | 0.00 | 0.00 | 0.00 | 0.00 | 0.00 | 0.0 | 0.00 | 0.0 | | | 1 | | 0.0 | 0 | | 1 | 1 | 0.0 | 48 | 0.00 |
| 8243 | 1 tsp | With Cottonseed oil, soft, avg | 5 | 36 | 16 | 0.0 | 0.0 | 0.0 | 0.0 | 0.0 | 4.0 | 0.8 | 1.6 | 1.5 | 0.08 | 1.38 | 0 | 179 | 40 | 35 | 5 | | 0.00 | 0.00 | 0.00 | 0.00 | 0.00 | 0.1 | 0.00 | 0.0 | | 0.4 | 1 | | 0.0 | 0 | | 1 | 2 | 0.0 | 54 | 0.00 |
| 8239 | 1 tsp | With Palm oil, hard, avg | 5 | 36 | 16 | 0.0 | 0.0 | 0.0 | 0.0 | 0.0 | 4.0 | 0.9 | 1.6 | 1.4 | 0.12 | 1.29 | 0 | 179 | 40 | 34 | 6 | | 0.00 | 0.00 | 0.00 | 0.00 | 0.00 | 0.1 | 0.00 | 0.0 | | 0.6 | 2 | | 0.0 | 0 | | 1 | 2 | 0.0 | 47 | 0.00 |
| 8345 | 1 tsp | With Palm oil, soft, avg | 5 | 27 | 37 | 0.0 | 0.0 | 0.0 | 0.0 | 0.0 | 3.0 | 0.7 | 1.2 | 1.0 | 0.08 | 0.94 | 0 | 179 | 40 | 35 | 5 | | 0.00 | 0.00 | 0.00 | 0.00 | 0.00 | 0.0 | 0.00 | 0.0 | | 0.3 | 1 | 0.0 | 0.0 | 0 | | 1 | 2 | 0.0 | 50 | 0.00 |
| 8265 | 1 tsp | With Safflower oil, soft, avg | 5 | 36 | 16 | 0.0 | 0.0 | 0.0 | 0.0 | 0.0 | 4.0 | 0.5 | 1.6 | 1.8 | 0.06 | 1.72 | 0 | 179 | 40 | 35 | 5 | | 0.00 | 0.00 | 0.00 | 0.00 | 0.00 | 0.1 | 0.00 | 0.0 | 0.0 | 0.6 | 1 | 0.0 | 0.0 | 0 | 0.0 | 1 | 2 | 0.0 | 54 | 0.00 |
| 8242 | 1 tsp | Without salt, soft, avg | 5 | 36 | 18 | 0.0 | 0.0 | 0.0 | 0.0 | 0.0 | 4.0 | 0.7 | 1.8 | 1.3 | 0.04 | 1.29 | 0 | 179 | 40 | 35 | 5 | | 0.00 | 0.00 | 0.00 | 0.00 | 0.00 | 0.1 | 0.00 | 0.0 | | 0.1 | 1 | | 0.0 | 0 | | 1 | 2 | 0.0 | 1 | 0.00 |
| 8262 | 1 tsp | Sunflower oil, hard, avg | 5 | 36 | 16 | 0.0 | 0.0 | 0.0 | 0.0 | 0.0 | 4.0 | 0.6 | 1.4 | 1.8 | 0.01 | 1.83 | 0 | 179 | 40 | 34 | 6 | | 0.00 | 0.00 | 0.00 | 0.00 | 0.00 | 0.1 | 0.00 | 0.0 | | | 2 | 0.0 | 0.0 | 0 | | 1 | 2 | 0.0 | 47 | 0.00 |
| 8059 | 1 tsp | Sunflower/cottonseed/peanut oils, soft, avg | 5 | 36 | 16 | 0.0 | 0.0 | 0.0 | | | 4.0 | 0.6 | 0.8 | 2.4 | 0.02 | 2.38 | 0 | 179 | 40 | 35 | 5 | | 0.00 | 0.00 | 0.00 | 0.00 | 0.00 | 0.1 | 0.00 | 0.0 | | | 1 | | 0.0 | 0 | | 1 | 2 | 0.0 | 54 | 0.00 |
| | | Unspecified Oils | | | | | | | | | | | | | | | | | | | | | | | | | | | | | | | | | | | | | | | | |
| 8042 | 1 tsp | Hard, avg | 5 | 36 | 16 | 0.0 | 0.0 | 0.0 | 0.0 | 0.0 | 4.0 | 0.8 | 1.8 | 1.3 | 0.06 | 1.22 | 0 | 179 | 40 | 34 | 6 | | 0.00 | 0.00 | 0.00 | 0.00 | 0.00 | 0.1 | 0.00 | 0.0 | | 0.5 | 2 | 0.0 | 0.0 | 0 | | 1 | 2 | 0.0 | 47 | 0.00 |
| 8041 | 1 tsp | Hard, imitation, avg | 5 | 17 | 58 | 0.0 | 0.0 | 0.0 | 0.0 | 0.0 | 1.9 | 0.4 | 0.8 | 0.7 | 0.03 | 0.66 | 0 | 179 | 40 | 35 | 5 | | 0.00 | 0.00 | 0.00 | 0.00 | 0.00 | 0.0 | 0.00 | 0.0 | | | 1 | 0.0 | 0.0 | 0 | | 1 | 1 | 0.0 | 48 | 0.00 |
| 8244 | 1 tsp | Soft, avg | 5 | 36 | 18 | 0.0 | 0.0 | 0.0 | 0.0 | 0.0 | 4.0 | 0.7 | 1.9 | 1.2 | 0.06 | 1.16 | 0 | 179 | 40 | 35 | 5 | | 0.00 | 0.00 | 0.00 | 0.00 | 0.00 | 0.1 | 0.00 | 0.0 | | 0.4 | 1 | | 0.0 | 0 | | 1 | 2 | 0.0 | 1 | 0.00 |
| | | Light | | | | | | | | | | | | | | | | | | | | | | | | | | | | | | | | | | | | | | | | |
| 8484 | 1 tsp | Sodium free, Weight Watchers | 5 | 16 | | 0.0 | 0.7 | 0.0 | 0.0 | 0.7 | 1.4 | 0.4 | | | | | 0 | 176 | 18 | | | | | | | | | | | 0.0 | | | 0 | | 0.0 | | | | 0 | | 0 | |
| 8155 | 1 tsp | Tub, Fleishmann's | 5 | 17 | 58 | 0.0 | 0.0 | 0.0 | 0.0 | 0.0 | 1.9 | 0.3 | 0.7 | 0.8 | 0.01 | 0.81 | 0 | 179 | 40 | | | | 0.00 | 0.00 | 0.00 | 0.00 | 0.00 | 0.0 | 0.00 | 0.0 | 0.5 | 0.3 | 1 | | 0.0 | 0 | 0.0 | 1 | 1 | 0.0 | 48 | 0.00 |
| 8392 | 1 tsp | Weight Watchers | 5 | 16 | 56 | 0.0 | 0.7 | 0.0 | 0.0 | 0.7 | 1.4 | 0.4 | 0.4 | 0.7 | | | 0 | 176 | 18 | | | | | | | | | | | 0.0 | | | 0 | | 0.0 | | | | 2 | | 25 | |
| 8407 | 1 tsp | Liquid, Blue Bonnet | 5 | 36 | | 0.0 | 0.0 | 0.0 | 0.0 | 0.0 | 3.9 | 0.7 | 0.9 | 2.1 | | | 0 | 179 | 36 | | | | | | | | | | | | 0.5 | | | | | | | | 0 | | 45 | |
| 8165 | 1 tsp | Liquid, Parkay | 5 | 36 | 16 | 0.1 | 0.0 | 0.0 | 0.0 | 0.0 | 4.0 | 0.7 | 1.4 | 1.8 | 0.12 | 1.67 | 0 | 179 | 40 | 35 | 5 | | 0.00 | 0.00 | 0.00 | 0.00 | 0.01 | 0.1 | 0.01 | 0.0 | 0.0 | 0.2 | 3 | 0.0 | 0.0 | 0 | 0.0 | 3 | 5 | 0.0 | 39 | 0.00 |
| 8391 | 1 tsp | Reduced fat, stick, Weight Watchers | 5 | 21 | 49 | 0.0 | 0.0 | 0.0 | 0.0 | 0.0 | 2.5 | 0.5 | | | | | 0 | 176 | 18 | | | | | | | | | | | 0.0 | | | 0 | | 0.0 | | | | 2 | | 46 | |
| 8486 | 1 tsp | Reduced fat, Saffola | 5 | 21 | 37 | 0.0 | 0.0 | 0.0 | 0.0 | 0.0 | 3.0 | 0.5 | 1.0 | 1.6 | | | | 183 | 18 | | | | | | | | | | | 0.0 | | | 0 | | 0.0 | | | | | | 41 | |
| | | Soft | | | | | | | | | | | | | | | | | | | | | | | | | | | | | | | | | | | | | | | | |
| 8406 | 1 tsp | Blue Bonnet | 5 | 36 | | 0.0 | 0.0 | 0.0 | 0.0 | 0.0 | 3.9 | 0.7 | 1.8 | 0.0 | 0.00 | 0.00 | 0 | 179 | 36 | | | | | | | | | | | 0.0 | | | | | | | | | 0 | | 39 | |
| 8606 | 1 tsp | Diet, Parkay | 5 | 18 | | 0.0 | 0.0 | 0.0 | 0.0 | 0.0 | 2.1 | 0.4 | | | | | 0 | 179 | 36 | | | | | | | | | | | 0.0 | | | 0 | | 0.0 | | | | 0 | | 39 | |
| 8408 | 1 tsp | Fleischmann's | 5 | 39 | | 0.0 | 0.0 | 0.0 | 0.0 | 0.0 | 4.6 | 0.9 | 1.1 | 1.4 | | | 0 | 179 | 36 | | | | | | | | | | | 0.0 | | | | | | | | | 0 | | 39 | |
| 8600 | 1 tsp | Kraft | 5 | 36 | | 0.0 | 0.0 | 0.0 | 0.0 | 0.0 | 3.9 | 0.7 | | | | | 0 | 179 | 36 | | | | | | | | | | | 0.0 | | | 0 | | 0.0 | | | | 4 | | 38 | |
| 8168 | 1 tsp | Parkay | 5 | 36 | 16 | 0.0 | 0.0 | 0.0 | 0.0 | 0.0 | 4.0 | 0.7 | 1.8 | 1.3 | 0.04 | 1.30 | 0 | 179 | 40 | 35 | 5 | | 0.00 | 0.00 | 0.00 | 0.00 | 0.00 | 0.1 | 0.00 | 0.0 | 0.0 | 0.1 | 1 | 0.0 | 0.0 | 0 | 0.0 | 1 | 2 | 0.0 | 54 | 0.00 |
| 8487 | 1 tsp | Saffola | 5 | 36 | 17 | 0.0 | 0.0 | 0.0 | 0.0 | 0.0 | 4.0 | 0.7 | 1.1 | 1.6 | | | | 183 | 18 | | | | | | | | | | | 0.0 | | | 0 | | 0.0 | | | | | | 34 | |
| 8176 | 1 tsp | Spread, Shedd's | 5 | 21 | 58 | 0.0 | 0.0 | 0.0 | 0.0 | 0.0 | 1.9 | 0.3 | 0.8 | 0.8 | | | 0 | 165 | 50 | 46 | 4 | | 0.00 | 0.00 | 0.00 | 0.00 | 0.00 | 0.0 | 0.00 | 0.0 | 0.0 | 0.0 | 1 | | 0.0 | 0 | 0.0 | 1 | 1 | | 38 | 0.00 |
| 8609 | 1 tsp | Stick, Parkay | 5 | 32 | | 0.0 | 0.0 | 0.0 | 0.0 | 0.0 | 3.6 | 0.7 | | | | | 0 | 179 | 36 | | | | | | | | | | | 0.0 | | | 0 | | 0.0 | | | | 2 | | 39 | |
| 8485 | 1 tsp | Unsalted, soft, Saffola | 5 | 36 | 20 | 0.0 | 0.0 | 0.0 | 0.0 | 0.0 | 4.0 | 0.7 | 1.1 | 1.6 | | | | 183 | 18 | | | | | | | | | | | 0.0 | | | 0 | | 0.0 | | | | | | 0 | |
| 8601 | 1 tsp | Whipped, soft, Kraft | 3 | 23 | | 0.0 | 0.0 | 0.0 | 0.0 | 0.0 | 2.3 | 0.5 | | | | | 0 | 100 | 20 | | | | | | | | | | | 0.0 | | | 0 | | 0.0 | | | | 0 | | 23 | |
| 8607 | 1 tsp | Whipped, soft, Parkay | 3 | 23 | | 0.0 | 0.0 | 0.0 | 0.0 | 0.0 | 2.3 | 0.5 | | | | | 0 | 100 | 20 | | | | | | | | | | | 0.0 | | | 0 | | 0.0 | | | | 2 | | 23 | |
| | | *SHORTENINGS* | | | | | | | | | | | | | | | | | | | | | | | | | | | | | | | | | | | | | | | | |
| 8271 | 1 Tbs | Cake, soybean oil, avg | 13 | 115 | 0 | 0.0 | 0.0 | 0.0 | 0.0 | 0.0 | 13.0 | 3.5 | 7.0 | 1.8 | 0.14 | 1.69 | 0 | 0 | 0 | 0 | 0 | 0 | 0.00 | 0.00 | 0.00 | 0.00 | 0.00 | 0.0 | 0.00 | 0.0 | | | 0 | 0.0 | 0.0 | 0 | | 0 | 0 | 0.0 | 0 | 0.00 |

| Code | Amount | | Description | Basic Components | | | | | | | | | Additional Fats | | | | | | Vit A & Components | | | | | Vitamins | | | | | | | | | | Minerals | | | | | | | | | |
|---|---|---|---|---|---|---|---|---|---|---|---|---|---|---|---|---|---|---|---|---|---|---|---|---|---|---|---|---|---|---|---|---|---|---|---|---|---|---|---|---|---|---|---|
| | | | | Weight (g) | Calories | % Water | Protein (g) | Carbs (g) | Fiber (g) | Sugar (g) | Other Carbs (g) | Fat (g) | Sat Fat (g) | Mono Fat (g) | Poly Fat (g) | Omega 3 (g) | Omega 6 (g) | Choles (mg) | Vit A (IU) | Vit A (RE) | Retinol (RE) | Carotenoids (RE) | Beta Carotene (mcg) | Thiamin (mg) | Riboflavin (mg) | Niacin (NE) | Vit B6 (mg) | Vit B12 (mcg) | Folate (mcg) | Panto (mg) | Vit C (mg) | Vit D (mg) | Vit E (α TE) | Calcium (mg) | Copper (mg) | Iron (mg) | Magnes (mg) | Mang (mg) | Phos (mg) | Potassium (mg) | Selenium (mcg) | Sodium (mg) | Zinc (mg) |
| 8274 | 1 | Tbs | Confectioner shortening, coconut/palm oils, avg | 13 | 115 | 0 | 0.0 | 0.0 | 0.0 | 0.0 | 0.0 | 13.0 | 11.9 | 0.3 | 0.1 | 0.00 | 0.13 | 0 | 0 | 0 | 0 | 0 | 0 | 0.00 | 0.00 | 0.00 | 0.00 | 0.00 | 0.0 | 0.00 | 0.0 | | | 0 | 0.0 | 0.0 | 0 | | 0 | 0 | 0.0 | 0 | 0.00 |
| 8275 | 1 | Tbs | Frying, heavy duty, soybean oil, avg | 13 | 115 | 0 | 0.0 | 0.0 | 0.0 | 0.0 | 0.0 | 13.0 | 2.4 | 5.7 | 4.4 | 0.31 | 4.04 | 0 | 0 | 0 | 0 | 0 | 0 | 0.00 | 0.00 | 0.00 | 0.00 | 0.00 | 0.0 | 0.00 | 0.0 | | 1.1 | 0 | | 0.0 | 0 | | 0 | 0 | 0.0 | 0 | 0.00 |
| 8270 | 1 | Tbs | Frying, regular, soybean/cottonseed oils, avg | 13 | 115 | 0 | 0.0 | 0.0 | 0.0 | 0.0 | 0.0 | 13.0 | 2.0 | 7.6 | 2.9 | 0.10 | 2.76 | 0 | 0 | 0 | 0 | 0 | 0 | 0.00 | 0.00 | 0.00 | 0.00 | 0.00 | 0.0 | 0.00 | 0.0 | | 1.0 | 0 | | 0.0 | 0 | | 0 | 0 | 0.0 | 0 | 0.00 |
| 8317 | 1 | Tbs | Liquid, soybean oil, avg | 13 | 117 | 0 | 0.0 | 0.0 | 0.0 | 0.0 | 0.0 | 13.0 | 2.5 | 9.5 | 1.1 | | | 0 | 0 | 0 | 0 | 0 | 0 | | | | | | | | 0.0 | | | 0 | | 0.0 | | | | | | | |
| | | | Multipurpose Shortening | | | | | | | | | | | | | | | | | | | | | | | | | | | | | | | | | | | | | | | | |
| 8278 | 1 | Tbs | Cottonseed oil, avg | 13 | 115 | 0 | 0.0 | 0.0 | 0.0 | 0.0 | 0.0 | 13.0 | 3.3 | 5.5 | 3.5 | 0.19 | 3.27 | 0 | 0 | 0 | 0 | 0 | 0 | 0.00 | 0.00 | 0.00 | 0.00 | 0.00 | 0.0 | 0.00 | 0.0 | | | 0 | 0.0 | 0.0 | 0 | 0.0 | 0 | 0 | 0.0 | 0 | 0.00 |
| 8007 | 1 | Tbs | Soybean/Cottonseed, oils, avg | 13 | 115 | 0 | 0.0 | 0.0 | 0.0 | 0.0 | 0.0 | 13.0 | 3.3 | 5.8 | 3.4 | 0.21 | 3.18 | 0 | 0 | 0 | 0 | 0 | 0 | 0.00 | 0.00 | 0.00 | 0.00 | 0.00 | 0.0 | 0.00 | 0.0 | 0.0 | | 0 | 0.0 | 0.0 | 0 | 0.0 | 0 | 0 | 0.0 | 0 | 0.00 |
| 8283 | 1 | Tbs | Unspecified oils, avg | 13 | 115 | 0 | 0.0 | 0.0 | 0.0 | 0.0 | 0.0 | 13.0 | 4.0 | 6.6 | 1.8 | 0.08 | 1.77 | 0 | 0 | 0 | 0 | 0 | 0 | 0.00 | 0.00 | 0.00 | 0.00 | 0.00 | 0.0 | 0.00 | 0.0 | | 1.8 | 0 | 0.0 | 0.0 | 0 | 0.0 | 0 | 0 | 0.0 | 0 | 0.00 |
| 8120 | 1 | Tbs | Soybean/Palm oils, Proctor & Gamble | 12 | 106 | 0 | 0.0 | 0.0 | 0.0 | 0.0 | 0.0 | 12.0 | 3.1 | 4.0 | 1.2 | | | 0 | 0 | 0 | 0 | 0 | 0 | | | | | | | | 0.0 | | | 0 | | 0.0 | | | | | | 0 | |
| | | | **FISH, SEAFOOD AND SHELLFISH** | | | | | | | | | | | | | | | | | | | | | | | | | | | | | | | | | | | | | | | | |
| | | | *FINFISH* | | | | | | | | | | | | | | | | | | | | | | | | | | | | | | | | | | | | | | | | |
| 17309 | 3 | oz | Ackee, canned, avg | 85 | 128 | 77 | 2.5 | 3.0 | 2.3 | | | 12.9 | | | | | | | | | | | | 0.03 | 0.06 | 0.94 | | 0.00 | 34.9 | | 25.5 | | | 30 | 0.2 | 0.6 | 34 | | | 230 | | 204 | 0.51 |
| 17288 | 1 | ea | Anchovy, canned in oil, drained, avg | 45 | 94 | 50 | 13.0 | 0.0 | 0.0 | 0.0 | 0.0 | 4.4 | 1.0 | 1.7 | 1.2 | 0.93 | 0.17 | 38 | 32 | 9 | 9 | 0 | 0 | 0.04 | 0.16 | 8.95 | 0.09 | 0.40 | 5.6 | 0.41 | 0.0 | 0.4 | | 104 | 0.2 | 2.1 | 31 | 0.0 | 113 | 245 | 30.6 | 1651 | 1.10 |
| 17188 | 3 | oz | Anchovy, European, raw, avg | 85 | 111 | 73 | 17.3 | 0.0 | 0.0 | 0.0 | 0.0 | 4.1 | 1.1 | 1.0 | 1.4 | 1.24 | 0.09 | 51 | 43 | 13 | 13 | 0 | 0 | 0.05 | 0.22 | 11.90 | 0.12 | 0.53 | 7.5 | 0.55 | 0.0 | | | 125 | 0.2 | 2.8 | 35 | 0.1 | 148 | 326 | 31.0 | 88 | 1.46 |
| | | | Bass | | | | | | | | | | | | | | | | | | | | | | | | | | | | | | | | | | | | | | | | |
| 17029 | 1 | ea | Freshwater, mixed species, bkd/brld, fillet, avg | 62 | 91 | 69 | 15.0 | 0.0 | 0.0 | 0.0 | 0.0 | 2.9 | 0.6 | 1.1 | 0.8 | 0.56 | 0.18 | 54 | 71 | 22 | 22 | 0 | 0 | 0.05 | 0.06 | 0.94 | 0.09 | 1.43 | 10.5 | 0.54 | 1.3 | 0.6 | | 64 | 0.1 | 1.2 | 24 | 0.7 | 159 | 283 | 10.0 | 56 | 0.51 |
| 17028 | 1 | ea | Freshwater, raw, fillet, avg | 79 | 90 | 76 | 14.9 | 0.0 | 0.0 | 0.0 | 0.0 | 2.9 | 0.6 | 1.1 | 0.8 | 0.56 | 0.18 | 54 | 79 | 24 | 24 | 0 | 0 | 0.06 | 0.06 | 0.99 | 0.09 | 1.58 | 11.9 | 0.59 | 1.6 | 0.8 | | 63 | 0.1 | 1.2 | 24 | 0.7 | 158 | 281 | 10.0 | 55 | 0.51 |
| 17086 | 1 | ea | Sea bass, mixed species, bkd/brld, fillet, avg | 101 | 125 | 72 | 23.8 | 0.0 | 0.0 | 0.0 | 0.0 | 2.6 | 0.7 | 0.5 | 1.0 | 0.77 | 0.03 | 54 | 215 | 65 | 65 | 0 | 0 | 0.13 | 0.15 | 1.92 | 0.46 | 0.30 | 5.9 | 0.88 | 0.0 | | | 13 | 0.0 | 0.4 | 54 | 0.0 | 250 | 331 | 47.3 | 88 | 0.53 |
| 17225 | 1 | ea | Sea bass, mixed species, raw, fillet, avg | 129 | 125 | 78 | 23.7 | 0.0 | 0.0 | 0.0 | 0.0 | 2.6 | 0.7 | 0.5 | 1.0 | 0.77 | 0.03 | 53 | 237 | 71 | 71 | 0 | 0 | 0.14 | 0.15 | 2.06 | 0.52 | 0.39 | 6.4 | 0.97 | 0.0 | | | 13 | 0.0 | 0.4 | 53 | 0.0 | 250 | 330 | 47.1 | 88 | 0.52 |
| 17104 | 1 | ea | Striped, baked/broiled, fillet, avg | 124 | 154 | 73 | 28.1 | 0.0 | 0.0 | 0.0 | 0.0 | 3.7 | 0.8 | 1.0 | 1.3 | 1.10 | 0.09 | 128 | 129 | 38 | 38 | 0 | 0 | 0.14 | 0.05 | 3.17 | 0.43 | 5.47 | 12.4 | 1.07 | 0.0 | 1.2 | | 24 | 0.0 | 1.3 | 63 | 0.0 | 315 | 407 | 58.0 | 109 | 0.63 |
| 17226 | 1 | ea | Striped, raw, fillet, avg | 159 | 154 | 79 | 28.1 | 0.0 | 0.0 | 0.0 | 0.0 | 3.7 | 0.8 | 1.0 | 1.2 | 1.22 | 0.02 | 127 | 143 | 43 | 43 | 0 | 0 | 0.16 | 0.05 | 3.34 | 0.48 | 6.07 | 14.3 | 1.19 | 0.0 | | | 24 | 0.0 | 1.3 | 64 | 0.0 | 315 | 407 | 58.0 | 110 | 0.64 |
| 17031 | 1 | ea | Bluefish, baked/broiled, fillet, avg | 117 | 186 | 63 | 30.1 | 0.0 | 0.0 | 0.0 | 0.0 | 6.4 | 1.4 | 2.7 | 1.6 | 0.97 | 0.08 | 89 | 537 | 161 | 161 | 0 | 0 | 0.08 | 0.11 | 8.48 | 0.54 | 7.28 | 2.3 | 1.12 | 0.0 | 1.2 | | 11 | 0.1 | 0.7 | 49 | 0.0 | 340 | 558 | 54.8 | 90 | 1.22 |
| 17030 | 1 | ea | Bluefish, raw, fillet, avg | 150 | 186 | 71 | 30.0 | 0.0 | 0.0 | 0.0 | 0.0 | 6.4 | 1.4 | 2.7 | 1.6 | 1.16 | 0.09 | 88 | 597 | 179 | 179 | 0 | 0 | 0.09 | 0.12 | 8.92 | 0.60 | 8.09 | 2.4 | 1.24 | 0.0 | 1.5 | | 10 | 0.1 | 0.7 | 50 | 0.0 | 340 | 558 | 54.8 | 90 | 1.22 |
| 17105 | 1 | ea | Burbot, baked/broiled, fillet, avg | 90 | 103 | 73 | 22.3 | 0.0 | 0.0 | 0.0 | 0.0 | 0.9 | 0.2 | 0.2 | 0.3 | 0.20 | 0.12 | 69 | 15 | 5 | 5 | 0 | 0 | 0.39 | 0.15 | 1.77 | 0.31 | 0.83 | 0.9 | 0.16 | 0.0 | 1.0 | | 58 | 0.2 | 1.0 | 37 | 0.8 | 230 | 466 | 14.6 | 112 | 0.87 |
| 17191 | 1 | ea | Burbot, raw, fillet, avg | 116 | 104 | 79 | 22.4 | 0.0 | 0.0 | 0.0 | 0.0 | 0.9 | 0.2 | 0.2 | 0.3 | 0.20 | 0.12 | 70 | 17 | 5 | 5 | 0 | 0 | 0.43 | 0.16 | 1.88 | 0.35 | 0.93 | 1.2 | 0.17 | 0.0 | | | 58 | 0.2 | 1.0 | 37 | 0.8 | 232 | 469 | 14.6 | 113 | 0.88 |
| 17106 | 1 | ea | Butterfish, baked/broiled, fillet, avg | 25 | 47 | 67 | 5.6 | 0.0 | 0.0 | 0.0 | 0.0 | 2.6 | 0.8 | 0.9 | 0.8 | 0.47 | 0.20 | 21 | 27 | 8 | 8 | 0 | 0 | 0.04 | 0.05 | 1.44 | 0.09 | 0.46 | 4.3 | 0.22 | 0.0 | | | 7 | 0.0 | 0.2 | 8 | 0.0 | 77 | 120 | 11.7 | 28 | 0.25 |
| 17192 | 1 | ea | Butterfish, raw, fillet, avg | 32 | 47 | 74 | 5.5 | 0.0 | 0.0 | 0.0 | 0.0 | 2.6 | 1.1 | 1.1 | 0.2 | 0.12 | 0.05 | 21 | 32 | 10 | 10 | 0 | | 0.04 | 0.05 | 1.44 | 0.10 | 0.61 | 4.8 | 0.24 | 0.0 | | | 7 | 0.0 | 0.2 | 8 | 0.0 | 77 | 120 | 11.7 | 28 | 0.25 |
| | | | Carp | | | | | | | | | | | | | | | | | | | | | | | | | | | | | | | | | | | | | | | | |
| 17087 | 1 | ea | Baked/broiled, avg | 170 | 275 | 70 | 38.9 | 0.0 | 0.0 | 0.0 | 0.0 | 12.2 | 2.4 | 5.1 | 3.1 | 1.35 | 1.46 | 143 | 54 | 15 | 15 | 0 | 0 | 0.24 | 0.12 | 3.57 | 0.37 | 2.50 | 29.4 | 1.48 | 2.7 | 1.7 | | 88 | 0.1 | 2.7 | 65 | 0.1 | 903 | 726 | 27.5 | 107 | 3.23 |
| 17129 | 3 | oz | Breaded, fried, avg | 85 | 235 | 50 | 17.6 | 10.2 | 0.6 | 0.5 | 9.1 | 13.4 | 3.1 | 5.7 | 3.4 | | | 85 | 66 | 20 | 20 | 0 | | 0.12 | 0.12 | 1.97 | 0.16 | 1.22 | 18.1 | 0.68 | 1.1 | 0.9 | | 57 | 0.1 | 1.7 | 31 | 0.1 | 381 | 311 | | 440 | 1.41 |
| 17032 | 1 | ea | Raw, fillet, avg | 218 | 277 | 76 | 38.8 | 0.0 | 0.0 | 0.0 | 0.0 | 12.2 | 2.4 | 5.1 | 3.1 | 1.35 | 1.46 | 144 | 63 | 20 | 20 | 0 | | 0.25 | 0.12 | 3.58 | 0.41 | 3.34 | 32.7 | 1.63 | 3.5 | 2.2 | | 89 | 0.1 | 2.7 | 63 | 0.1 | 905 | 726 | 27.5 | 107 | 3.23 |
| | | | Catfish | | | | | | | | | | | | | | | | | | | | | | | | | | | | | | | | | | | | | | | | |
| 17127 | 3 | oz | Breaded/battered, baked, avg | 85 | 257 | 47 | 15.4 | 10.2 | 0.6 | 0.5 | 9.1 | 16.8 | 3.7 | 7.5 | 4.5 | | | 67 | 564 | 148 | 138 | 10 | | 0.31 | 0.14 | 2.38 | 0.15 | 1.89 | 14.6 | 0.76 | 0.4 | 10.6 | | 33 | 0.1 | 1.1 | 26 | 0.1 | 201 | 281 | | 547 | 0.77 |
| 17126 | 1 | ea | Breaded/floured, fried, fillet, avg | 332 | 953 | 49 | 61.3 | 40.2 | 2.3 | 2.0 | 36.0 | 59.2 | 14.6 | 26.6 | 13.9 | | | 269 | 320 | 96 | 96 | 0.13 | | 1.16 | 0.54 | 9.89 | 0.61 | 7.53 | 56.5 | 2.99 | 1.6 | 41.5 | | 120 | 0.4 | 4.2 | 100 | 0.1 | 793 | 1106 | | 1756 | 3.09 |
| 17179 | 1 | ea | Channel, farmed, baked/broiled, fillet, avg | 143 | 217 | 72 | 26.7 | 0.0 | 0.0 | 0.0 | 0.0 | 11.5 | 2.6 | 5.9 | 2.0 | 0.35 | 1.45 | 92 | 72 | 21 | 21 | 0 | 0 | 0.60 | 0.10 | 3.59 | 0.23 | 4.00 | 10.0 | 0.88 | 1.1 | | | 13 | 0.2 | 1.2 | 37 | 0.0 | 350 | 459 | 20.7 | 114 | 1.50 |
| 17178 | 1 | ea | Channel, farmed, raw, fillet, avg | 159 | 215 | 75 | 24.8 | 0.0 | 0.0 | 0.0 | 0.0 | 12.1 | 2.8 | 5.7 | 2.5 | 0.59 | 1.53 | 75 | 80 | 24 | 24 | 0 | 0 | 0.57 | 0.12 | 3.66 | 0.30 | 3.93 | 15.9 | 0.95 | 1.0 | | | 14 | 0.2 | 0.8 | 37 | 0.0 | 321 | 475 | 20.0 | 84 | 1.18 |
| 17305 | 1 | ea | Channel, wild, baked/broiled, fillet, avg | 143 | 150 | 78 | 26.5 | 0.0 | 0.0 | 0.0 | 0.0 | 4.1 | 1.1 | 1.6 | 0.9 | 0.48 | 0.33 | 103 | 72 | 21 | 21 | 0 | 0 | 0.32 | 0.10 | 3.42 | 0.15 | 4.15 | 14.3 | 1.30 | 1.1 | | | 16 | 0.1 | 0.5 | 40 | 0.0 | 435 | 599 | 20.4 | 71 | 0.87 |
| 17088 | 1 | ea | Channel, wild, breaded, fried, fillet, avg | 87 | 199 | 59 | 15.7 | 7.0 | 0.7 | 0.3 | 6.0 | 11.6 | 2.9 | 4.9 | 2.9 | 0.45 | 2.36 | 70 | 24 | 7 | 7 | 0 | 0 | 0.06 | 0.12 | 1.98 | 0.17 | 1.65 | 26.1 | 0.64 | 0.0 | 10.9 | | 38 | 0.1 | 1.2 | 23 | 0.0 | 188 | 296 | 12.1 | 244 | 0.75 |
| 17033 | 1 | ea | Channel, wild, raw, steamed/poached, fillet, avg | 159 | 151 | 80 | 26.1 | 0.0 | 0.0 | 0.0 | 0.0 | 4.5 | 1.1 | 1.3 | 1.4 | 0.69 | 0.40 | 92 | 80 | 24 | 24 | 0 | 0 | 0.33 | 0.11 | 3.04 | 0.18 | 3.55 | 15.9 | 1.22 | 1.1 | 19.9 | | 22 | 0.1 | 0.5 | 37 | 0.0 | 332 | 569 | 20.0 | 68 | 0.81 |
| 17128 | 3 | oz | Steamed/poached, avg | 85 | 144 | 69 | 16.5 | 0.0 | 0.0 | 0.0 | 0.0 | 8.1 | 1.9 | 3.8 | 1.7 | | | 50 | 43 | 13 | 13 | 0 | 0 | 0.31 | 0.07 | 2.08 | 0.16 | 2.23 | 8.5 | 0.85 | 0.5 | 10.6 | | 9 | 0.1 | 0.5 | 22 | 0.0 | 193 | 270 | | 51 | 0.79 |
| 17034 | 1 | Tbs | Caviar, black/red, sturgeon roe, granular, avg | 16 | 40 | 48 | 3.9 | 0.6 | 0.0 | 0.0 | 0.6 | 2.9 | 0.6 | 0.7 | 1.2 | 1.05 | 0.09 | 94 | 299 | 90 | 90 | 0 | 0 | 0.03 | 0.10 | 0.02 | 0.05 | 3.20 | 8.0 | 0.56 | 0.0 | 1.1 | | 44 | 0.0 | 1.9 | 48 | 0.0 | 57 | 29 | 10.5 | 240 | 0.15 |
| | | | Cod | | | | | | | | | | | | | | | | | | | | | | | | | | | | | | | | | | | | | | | | |
| 17037 | 1 | ea | Atlantic, baked/broiled, fillet, avg | 180 | 189 | 76 | 41.0 | 0.0 | 0.0 | 0.0 | 0.0 | 1.5 | 0.3 | 0.2 | 0.5 | 0.29 | 0.06 | 99 | 83 | 25 | 25 | 0 | 0 | 0.16 | 0.14 | 4.52 | 0.51 | 1.89 | 14.6 | 0.32 | 1.8 | 2.5 | | 25 | 0.1 | 0.9 | 76 | 0.0 | 248 | 439 | 67.7 | 140 | 1.04 |
| 17089 | 1 | ea | Atlantic, canned w/liquid, avg | 312 | 328 | 76 | 71.1 | 0.0 | 0.0 | 0.0 | 0.0 | 2.7 | 0.5 | 0.4 | 0.9 | 0.49 | 0.11 | 172 | 144 | 44 | 44 | 0 | 0 | 0.27 | 0.25 | 7.83 | 0.88 | 3.28 | 25.3 | 0.53 | 3.1 | 3.4 | | 66 | 0.1 | 1.5 | 128 | 0.1 | 811 | 1647 | 118.9 | 680 | 1.81 |
| 17038 | 1 | pce | Atlantic, dried & salted, avg | 80 | 232 | 16 | 50.2 | 0.0 | 0.0 | 0.0 | 0.0 | 1.9 | 0.4 | 0.3 | 0.6 | 0.35 | 0.08 | 122 | 113 | 34 | 34 | 0 | 0 | 0.21 | 0.19 | 6.00 | 0.69 | 8.00 | 19.8 | 1.34 | 2.8 | 4.1 | | 128 | 0.1 | 2.0 | 106 | 0.0 | 760 | 1166 | 118.4 | 5622 | 1.27 |
| 17036 | 1 | ea | Atlantic, raw, fillet, avg | 231 | 189 | 81 | 41.1 | 0.0 | 0.0 | 0.0 | 0.0 | 1.5 | 0.3 | 0.2 | 0.5 | 0.43 | 0.06 | 99 | 92 | 28 | 28 | 0 | 0 | 0.18 | 0.15 | 4.76 | 0.57 | 2.10 | 16.2 | 0.35 | 2.3 | 2.5 | | 37 | 0.1 | 0.9 | 74 | 0.0 | 469 | 954 | 76.5 | 125 | 1.04 |
| 17107 | 1 | ea | Pacific, baked/broiled, fillet, avg | 90 | 94 | 76 | 20.7 | 0.0 | 0.0 | 0.0 | 0.0 | 0.7 | 0.1 | 0.1 | 0.3 | 0.25 | 0.03 | 42 | 29 | 9 | 9 | 0 | 0 | 0.02 | 0.05 | 2.24 | 0.42 | 0.94 | 7.2 | 0.15 | 2.7 | 1.3 | | 8 | 0.0 | 0.3 | 28 | 0.0 | 201 | 465 | 42.1 | 82 | 0.46 |
| 17166 | 1 | ea | Pacific, raw, fillet, avg | 116 | 95 | 81 | 20.8 | 0.0 | 0.0 | 0.0 | 0.0 | 0.7 | 0.1 | 0.1 | 0.3 | 0.25 | 0.03 | 43 | 32 | 9 | 9 | 0 | 0 | 0.03 | 0.05 | 2.37 | 0.46 | 1.04 | 7.7 | 0.16 | 3.4 | 1.2 | | 8 | 0.0 | 0.3 | 28 | 0.0 | 202 | 467 | 42.3 | 82 | 0.46 |
| 17001 | 3 | oz | Steamed/poached, avg | 85 | 87 | 77 | 18.9 | 0.0 | 0.0 | 0.0 | 0.0 | 0.7 | 0.1 | 0.1 | 0.2 | | | 46 | 34 | 10 | 10 | 0 | 0 | 0.06 | 0.06 | 1.86 | 0.21 | 0.82 | 6.0 | | 0.8 | | | 17 | 0.0 | 0.4 | 31 | | 194 | 373 | 32.0 | 52 | 0.48 |
| | | | Croaker | | | | | | | | | | | | | | | | | | | | | | | | | | | | | | | | | | | | | | | | |
| 17070 | 1 | ea | Atlantic, breaded, fried, fillet, avg | 87 | 192 | 60 | 15.8 | 6.6 | 0.4 | 0.3 | 5.9 | 11.0 | 3.0 | 4.6 | 2.5 | 0.31 | 2.15 | 73 | 65 | 19 | 19 | 0 | 0 | 0.08 | 0.11 | 3.74 | 0.23 | 1.83 | 29.6 | 0.64 | 0.0 | | | 28 | 0.1 | 0.7 | 37 | 0.1 | 189 | 296 | 33.8 | 303 | 0.45 |
| 17194 | 1 | ea | Atlantic, raw, fillet, avg | 79 | 82 | 78 | 14.1 | 0.0 | 0.0 | 0.0 | 0.0 | 2.5 | 0.9 | 0.9 | 0.4 | 0.18 | 0.11 | 48 | 47 | 14 | 14 | 0 | 0 | 0.06 | 0.08 | 3.32 | 0.24 | 1.98 | 11.9 | 0.59 | 0.0 | | | 12 | 0.0 | 0.3 | 32 | 0.0 | 166 | 273 | 28.8 | 44 | 0.33 |
| 17241 | 3 | oz | Baked, avg | 85 | 239 | 47 | 17.9 | 11.9 | 0.7 | 0.6 | 10.6 | 12.9 | 3.5 | 5.4 | 3.0 | | | 85 | 96 | 29 | 29 | 0 | 0 | 0.10 | 0.17 | 4.20 | 0.24 | 1.96 | 19.2 | | 0.0 | | | 39 | 0.1 | 1.1 | 41 | | 214 | 326 | | 513 | 0.55 |
| 17108 | 1 | ea | Cusk, baked/broiled, fillet, avg | 95 | 106 | 70 | 23.2 | 0.0 | 0.0 | 0.0 | 0.0 | 0.8 | 0.2 | 0.2 | 0.4 | | | 50 | 66 | 20 | 20 | 0 | 0 | 0.05 | 0.15 | 3.11 | 0.42 | 1.14 | 1.9 | 0.31 | 0.0 | 1.0 | | 12 | 0.0 | 1.0 | 38 | 0.0 | 249 | 478 | 44.5 | 38 | 0.47 |
| 17195 | 1 | ea | Cusk, raw, fillet, avg | 122 | 106 | 76 | 23.2 | 0.0 | 0.0 | 0.0 | 0.0 | 0.8 | 0.2 | 0.1 | 0.3 | | | 50 | 73 | 22 | 22 | 0 | 0 | 0.05 | 0.16 | 3.28 | 0.47 | 1.27 | 2.4 | 0.34 | 0.0 | | | 12 | 0.0 | 1.0 | 38 | 0.0 | 249 | 478 | 44.5 | 38 | 0.46 |
| 19099 | 3 | oz | Cuttlefish, mixed species, raw, avg | 85 | 67 | 81 | 13.8 | 0.7 | 0.0 | | | 0.6 | 0.1 | 0.1 | 0.1 | 0.09 | 0.01 | 95 | 319 | 95 | 95 | 0 | 0 | 0.01 | 0.77 | 1.04 | 0.13 | 2.55 | 13.6 | 0.43 | 4.5 | | | 77 | 0.5 | 5.1 | 26 | 0.1 | 329 | 301 | 38.1 | 316 | 1.47 |
| 19085 | 3 | oz | Cuttlefish, steamed/boiled, avg | 85 | 134 | 61 | 27.6 | 1.4 | 0.0 | | | 1.2 | 0.2 | 0.1 | 0.2 | 0.18 | 0.03 | 190 | 574 | 173 | 173 | 0 | 0 | 0.01 | 1.47 | 1.86 | 0.23 | 4.59 | 20.4 | 0.76 | 7.2 | | | 153 | 0.8 | 9.2 | 51 | 0.2 | 493 | 541 | 76.2 | 632 | 2.94 |
| 17110 | 1 | ea | Drumfish, baked/broiled, fillet, avg | 154 | 236 | 71 | 34.6 | 0.0 | 0.0 | 0.0 | 0.0 | 9.7 | 2.2 | 4.3 | 2.3 | 1.25 | 0.75 | 126 | 302 | 91 | 91 | 0 | 0 | 0.12 | 0.32 | 4.40 | 0.53 | 3.56 | 26.2 | 1.33 | 1.5 | | | 119 | 0.5 | 1.8 | 59 | 1.4 | 356 | 544 | 24.9 | 148 | 1.31 |
| 17231 | 1 | ea | Drumfish, freshwater, raw, fillet, avg | 198 | 236 | 77 | 34.7 | 0.0 | 0.0 | 0.0 | 0.0 | 9.8 | 2.2 | 4.3 | 2.3 | 1.25 | 0.75 | 127 | 337 | 101 | 101 | 0 | 0 | 0.14 | 0.34 | 4.65 | 0.59 | 3.96 | 29.7 | 1.49 | 2.0 | | | 119 | 0.5 | 1.8 | 59 | 1.4 | 356 | 545 | 24.9 | 149 | 1.31 |
| 17040 | 1 | ea | Fish Cakes, fried, breaded, fzn, baked, avg | 85 | 230 | 53 | 7.8 | 14.6 | 0.9 | 0.4 | 13.3 | 15.2 | 6.0 | 3.4 | 3.4 | 0.00 | 3.40 | 22 | 57 | 17 | 17 | 0 | 0 | 0.03 | 0.06 | 1.36 | 0.04 | 0.85 | 10.5 | 0.21 | 0.0 | 0.9 | | 9 | 0.1 | 0.3 | 15 | 0.0 | 142 | 296 | 14.1 | 150 | 0.34 |
| 17267 | 1 | pce | Fish Fillets, breaded, Healthy Treasures | 85 | 130 | | 11.0 | 16.0 | 1.0 | 3.0 | 12.0 | 3.0 | 1.0 | | | | | 25 | 0 | 0 | 0 | 0 | 0 | | | | | | | | 2.4 | | | 20 | | 1.1 | | | | | | 220 | |
| 18817 | 1 | ea | Fish Fillets, fried, entrée, Weight Watchers | 218 | 230 | 78 | 15.0 | 25.0 | 2.0 | 3.0 | 20.0 | 8.0 | 2.1 | 4.2 | 1.7 | | | 25 | 200 | 40 | | | | 0.09 | 0.14 | 1.60 | | | | | 0.0 | | | 20 | | 1.4 | | | | 370 | | 450 | |
| | | | Fish Sticks/Portions | | | | | | | | | | | | | | | | | | | | | | | | | | | | | | | | | | | | | | | | |
| 17002 | 1 | ea | Breaded, fzn, baked, avg | 28 | 76 | 46 | 4.4 | 6.7 | 0.0 | 0.4 | 6.3 | 3.4 | 0.9 | 1.4 | 0.9 | 0.11 | 0.77 | 31 | 30 | 9 | 9 | 0 | 0 | 0.04 | 0.05 | 0.60 | 0.02 | 0.50 | 5.1 | 0.09 | 0.0 | 0.0 | | 6 | 0.0 | 0.2 | 7 | 0.1 | 51 | 73 | 4.6 | 163 | 0.18 |
| 17261 | 1 | pce | Battered, fzn, Van de Kamps | 71 | 175 | 54 | 6.5 | 13.0 | 0.0 | 2.5 | 10.5 | 11.0 | 1.8 | 4.0 | 0.8 | | | 18 | 0 | 0 | 0 | 0 | 0 | | | | | | | | 0.0 | | | 20 | | 0.4 | | | | | | 355 | |
| 17263 | 1 | pce | Battered, Mrs Paul's | 52 | 125 | | 4.5 | 10.0 | 1.0 | 2.0 | 7.0 | 8.0 | 2.5 | | | | | 15 | 0 | 0 | 0 | 0 | 0 | | | | | | | | 0.0 | | | 10 | | 0.4 | | | | | | 215 | |
| 17271 | 1 | pce | Breaded fish shapes, Sea Pals | 16 | 37 | | 1.8 | 3.5 | 0.2 | 0.4 | 2.9 | 1.8 | 0.5 | | | | | 4 | 0 | 0 | 0 | 0 | 0 | | | | | | | | 0.0 | | | 4 | | 0.1 | | | | | | 62 | |
| 17265 | 1 | pce | Breaded, Minis, Mrs Paul's | 8 | 19 | | 0.9 | 1.7 | 0.2 | 0.2 | 1.4 | 0.9 | 0.2 | | | | | 3 | 0 | 0 | 0 | 0 | 0 | | | | | | | | 0.0 | | | 2 | | 0.0 | | | | | | 28 | |
| 17264 | 1 | ea | Breaded, Mrs Paul's | 42 | 94 | | 4.4 | 7.9 | 0.5 | 1.0 | 6.4 | 4.9 | 1.5 | | | | | 7 | 0 | 0 | 0 | 0 | 0 | | | | | | | | 0.0 | | | 10 | | 0.4 | | | | | | 138 | |
| 17330 | 3 | oz | Gefilte, avg | 85 | 95 | 76 | 14.8 | 0.9 | 0.1 | | | 3.2 | 0.6 | 1.1 | 1.0 | | | 56 | 73 | 22 | 22 | 0 | 0 | 0.07 | 0.08 | 1.62 | 0.13 | 1.00 | 11.7 | | 1.2 | | | 35 | 0.1 | 0.5 | 22 | | 194 | 200 | | 222 | 0.76 |

| Code | Amount | | Description | Weight (g) | Calories | % Water | Protein (g) | Carbs (g) | Fiber (g) | Sugar (g) | Other Carbs (g) | Fat (g) | Sat Fat (g) | Mono Fat (g) | Poly Fat (g) | Omega 3 (g) | Omega 6 (g) | Choles (mg) | Vit A (IU) | Vit A (RE) | Retinol (RE) | Carotenoids (RE) | Beta Carotene (mcg) | Thiamin (mg) | Riboflavin (mg) | Niacin (NE) | Vit B6 (mg) | Vit B12 (mcg) | Folate (mcg) | Panto (mg) | Vit C (mg) | Vit D (mg) | Vit E (α TE) | Calcium (mg) | Copper (mg) | Iron (mg) | Magnes (mg) | Mang (mg) | Phos (mg) | Potassium (mg) | Selenium (mcg) | Sodium (mg) | Zinc (mg) |
|---|---|---|---|---|---|---|---|---|---|---|---|---|---|---|---|---|---|---|---|---|---|---|---|---|---|---|---|---|---|---|---|---|---|---|---|---|---|---|---|---|---|---|---|
| | | | **Basic Components** | | | | | | | | | | **Additional Fats** | | | | | | **Vit A & Components** | | | | | **Vitamins** | | | | | | | | | | **Minerals** | | | | | | | | | |
| 17103 | 3 | oz | Gefilte, sweet, avg | 85 | 71 | 80 | 7.7 | 6.3 | 0.0 | | | 1.5 | 0.4 | 0.7 | 0.2 | 0.10 | 0.10 | 26 | 76 | 23 | 23 | 0 | 0 | 0.06 | 0.05 | 0.85 | 0.07 | 0.72 | 2.4 | 0.17 | 0.7 | | | 20 | 0.2 | 2.1 | 8 | 0.1 | 62 | 77 | 8.9 | 445 | 0.70 |
| 17071 | 1 | ea | Grouper, baked/broiled, fillet, avg | 202 | 238 | 73 | 50.1 | 0.0 | 0.0 | 0.0 | 0.0 | 2.6 | 0.6 | 0.5 | 0.3 | 0.54 | 0.15 | 95 | 333 | 101 | 101 | 0 | 0 | 0.16 | 0.01 | 0.77 | 0.71 | 1.40 | 20.6 | 1.76 | 0.0 | | | 42 | 0.1 | 2.3 | 75 | 0.0 | 289 | 959 | 94.5 | 107 | 1.03 |
| 17196 | 1 | ea | Grouper, raw, fillet, avg | 202 | 186 | 79 | 39.2 | 0.0 | 0.0 | 0.0 | 0.0 | 2.1 | 0.5 | 0.4 | 0.5 | 0.52 | 0.09 | 75 | 289 | 87 | 87 | 0 | 0 | 0.14 | 0.01 | 0.63 | 0.61 | 1.21 | 17.8 | 1.51 | 0.0 | | | 55 | 0.0 | 1.8 | 63 | 0.0 | 327 | 976 | 73.7 | 107 | 0.97 |
| | | | Haddock | | | | | | | | | | | | | | | | | | | | | | | | | | | | | | | | | | | | | | | | |
| 17090 | 1 | ea | Baked/broiled, fillet, avg | 150 | 168 | 74 | 36.3 | 0.0 | 0.0 | 0.0 | 0.0 | 1.4 | 0.3 | 0.2 | 0.5 | 0.36 | 0.06 | 111 | 95 | 29 | 29 | 0 | 0 | 0.06 | 0.07 | 6.95 | 0.52 | 2.09 | 20.0 | 0.23 | 0.0 | 1.5 | | 63 | 0.0 | 2.0 | 75 | 0.0 | 362 | 598 | 60.8 | 130 | 0.72 |
| 17007 | 1 | ea | Floured/breaded, fried, fillet, avg | 81 | 190 | 55 | 15.7 | 10.1 | 0.6 | 0.5 | 9.0 | 9.2 | 2.3 | 3.8 | 2.4 | | | 69 | 78 | 24 | 23 | 0 | | 0.06 | 0.10 | 3.22 | 0.20 | 0.81 | 13.9 | 0.14 | 0.0 | 0.8 | | 45 | 0.0 | 1.4 | 33 | 0.0 | 163 | 247 | 32.8 | 374 | 0.42 |
| 17043 | 1 | ea | Raw, fillet, avg | 193 | 168 | 80 | 36.5 | 0.0 | 0.0 | 0.0 | 0.0 | 1.4 | 0.3 | 0.2 | 0.5 | 0.36 | 0.06 | 110 | 106 | 33 | 33 | 0 | 0 | 0.07 | 0.07 | 7.33 | 0.58 | 2.32 | 22.2 | 0.25 | 0.0 | 1.9 | | 64 | 0.1 | 2.0 | 75 | 0.0 | 363 | 600 | 58.3 | 131 | 0.71 |
| 17010 | 3 | oz | Smoked, avg | 85 | 99 | 72 | 21.4 | 0.0 | 0.0 | 0.0 | 0.0 | 0.8 | 0.1 | 0.1 | 0.3 | 0.21 | 0.04 | 65 | 62 | 19 | 19 | 0 | 0 | 0.04 | 0.04 | 4.31 | 0.34 | 1.36 | 13.0 | 0.14 | 0.0 | 0.9 | | 42 | 0.0 | 1.2 | 46 | 0.0 | 213 | 353 | 36.5 | 649 | 0.43 |
| 17008 | 3 | oz | Steamed/poached, avg | 85 | 93 | 75 | 20.1 | 0.0 | 0.0 | 0.0 | 0.0 | 0.8 | 0.1 | 0.1 | 0.3 | | | 60 | 47 | 14 | 14 | 0 | | 0.03 | 0.04 | 3.43 | 0.26 | 1.09 | 9.8 | 0.10 | 0.0 | 0.9 | | 35 | 0.0 | 1.1 | 37 | 0.0 | 180 | 281 | 34.4 | 65 | 0.39 |
| | | | Halibut | | | | | | | | | | | | | | | | | | | | | | | | | | | | | | | | | | | | | | | | |
| 17291 | 1 | ea | Atlantic/Pacific, baked/broiled, fillet, avg | 318 | 445 | 72 | 84.9 | 0.0 | 0.0 | 0.0 | 0.0 | 9.3 | 1.3 | 3.1 | 3.0 | 1.74 | 0.69 | 130 | 569 | 172 | 172 | 0 | 0 | 0.22 | 0.29 | 22.64 | 1.26 | 4.36 | 43.9 | 1.21 | 0.0 | 3.2 | | 191 | 0.1 | 3.4 | 340 | 0.1 | 906 | 1832 | 148.8 | 219 | 1.69 |
| 17044 | 1 | ea | Atlantic/Pacific, raw, fillet, avg | 408 | 449 | 78 | 84.9 | 0.0 | 0.0 | 0.0 | 0.0 | 9.3 | 1.3 | 3.1 | 3.0 | 1.75 | 0.69 | 131 | 632 | 192 | 192 | 0 | 0 | 0.24 | 0.31 | 23.87 | 1.40 | 4.81 | 49.0 | 1.34 | 0.0 | 20.4 | | 192 | 0.1 | 3.4 | 339 | 0.1 | 906 | 1836 | 148.9 | 220 | 1.71 |
| 17111 | 1 | ea | Greenland, baked/broiled, fillet, avg | 318 | 760 | 62 | 58.5 | 0.0 | 0.0 | 0.0 | 0.0 | 56.3 | 9.9 | 34.0 | 5.5 | 3.92 | 0.75 | 188 | 191 | 57 | 57 | 0 | 0 | 0.23 | 0.33 | 6.11 | 1.54 | 3.05 | 3.2 | 0.92 | 0.0 | 47.7 | | 13 | 0.1 | 2.7 | 105 | 0.0 | 668 | 1094 | 148.8 | 328 | 1.62 |
| 17227 | 1 | ea | Greenland, raw, fillet, avg | 408 | 759 | 70 | 58.8 | 0.0 | 0.0 | 0.0 | 0.0 | 56.3 | 9.9 | 34.2 | 5.5 | 3.92 | 0.75 | 188 | 224 | 69 | 69 | 0 | 0 | 0.24 | 0.33 | 6.12 | 1.71 | 4.08 | 4.1 | 1.02 | 0.0 | | | 12 | 0.1 | 2.7 | 106 | 0.0 | 669 | 1093 | 148.9 | 326 | 1.63 |
| | | | Herring | | | | | | | | | | | | | | | | | | | | | | | | | | | | | | | | | | | | | | | | |
| 17047 | 1 | ea | Atlantic, baked/broiled, fillet, avg | 143 | 290 | 64 | 32.9 | 0.0 | 0.0 | 0.0 | 0.0 | 16.6 | 3.7 | 6.8 | 3.9 | 3.08 | 0.35 | 110 | 146 | 44 | 44 | 0 | 0 | 0.16 | 0.43 | 5.89 | 0.50 | 18.73 | 16.4 | 1.06 | 1.0 | 74.6 | | 106 | 0.2 | 2.0 | 59 | 0.1 | 433 | 599 | 66.9 | 164 | 1.82 |
| 17012 | 3 | oz | Atlantic, pickled, avg | 85 | 223 | 55 | 12.1 | 8.2 | 0.0 | 8.2 | 0.0 | 15.3 | 2.0 | 10.1 | 1.4 | 1.18 | 0.18 | 11 | 732 | 219 | 219 | 0 | 0 | 0.03 | 0.12 | 2.81 | 0.14 | 3.63 | 2.0 | 0.07 | 0.0 | 14.5 | | 65 | 0.1 | 1.0 | 7 | 0.0 | 76 | 59 | 49.7 | 740 | 0.45 |
| 17045 | 1 | ea | Atlantic, raw, fillet, avg | 184 | 291 | 72 | 33.1 | 0.0 | 0.0 | 0.0 | 0.0 | 15.6 | 3.8 | 6.9 | 3.9 | 3.08 | 0.35 | 110 | 173 | 52 | 52 | 0 | 0 | 0.17 | 0.43 | 5.92 | 0.56 | 25.21 | 18.4 | 1.19 | 1.3 | 74.9 | | 105 | 0.2 | 2.0 | 59 | 0.1 | 434 | 602 | 67.2 | 166 | 1.82 |
| 17014 | 1 | ea | Atlantic, smoked, kippered, fillet, avg | 65 | 141 | 60 | 16.0 | 0.0 | 0.0 | 0.0 | 0.0 | 8.1 | 1.8 | 3.3 | 1.9 | 1.49 | 0.17 | 53 | 83 | 25 | 25 | 0 | 0 | 0.08 | 0.21 | 2.86 | 0.27 | 12.15 | 8.9 | 0.57 | 0.6 | 1.9 | | 55 | 0.1 | 1.0 | 30 | 0.0 | 211 | 291 | 34.2 | 597 | 0.88 |
| 17112 | 1 | ea | Pacific, baked/broiled, fillet, avg | 144 | 360 | 64 | 30.2 | 0.0 | 0.0 | 0.0 | 0.0 | 25.6 | 6.0 | 12.7 | 4.5 | 3.16 | 0.53 | 143 | 167 | 50 | 50 | 0 | 0 | 0.11 | 0.37 | 4.06 | 0.75 | 13.85 | 8.6 | 1.66 | 0.0 | 44.6 | | 153 | 0.1 | 2.1 | 59 | 0.1 | 420 | 780 | 67.4 | 137 | 0.98 |
| 17046 | 1 | ea | Pacific, raw, fillet, avg | 184 | 359 | 72 | 30.2 | 0.0 | 0.0 | 0.0 | 0.0 | 25.6 | 6.0 | 12.6 | 4.5 | 3.15 | 0.53 | 142 | 195 | 59 | 59 | 0 | 0 | 0.11 | 0.37 | 4.05 | 0.83 | 18.40 | 9.2 | 1.84 | 0.0 | 57.0 | | 153 | 0.1 | 2.1 | 59 | 0.1 | 420 | 778 | 67.2 | 136 | 0.98 |
| 17312 | 3 | oz | Hilsa, raw, avg | 85 | 232 | 54 | 18.5 | 2.5 | 0.0 | | | 16.5 | | | | | | | | | | | | | | 2.38 | | | | | 20.4 | | | 153 | | 1.8 | | | | | | | |
| | | | Hoki | | | | | | | | | | | | | | | | | | | | | | | | | | | | | | | | | | | | | | | | |
| 17246 | 1 | ea | Baked, avg | 244 | 244 | 76 | 53.7 | 0.0 | 0.0 | 0.0 | 0.0 | 3.2 | 0.7 | 1.0 | 0.7 | | | 132 | 122 | 37 | 37 | 0 | 0 | 0.07 | 0.02 | | 0.12 | 2.20 | 43.9 | | 0.5 | | | 22 | | 0.5 | | | | 800 | 168.4 | 137 | 0.73 |
| 17245 | 1 | ea | Deep dried, avg | 238 | 407 | 66 | 56.6 | 0.0 | 0.0 | 0.0 | 0.0 | 20.0 | 3.8 | 7.9 | 6.4 | | | 138 | 71 | 21 | 21 | 0 | 0 | 0.05 | | | 0.19 | 2.62 | 66.6 | | 0.5 | | | 31 | | 1.2 | | | | 1240 | 138.0 | 181 | 0.95 |
| 17243 | 1 | ea | Grilled, avg | 244 | 276 | 72 | 61.2 | 0.0 | 0.0 | 0.0 | 0.0 | 3.4 | 0.7 | 1.2 | 0.7 | | | 168 | 106 | 32 | 32 | 0 | 0 | 0.05 | 0.02 | | 0.10 | 2.39 | 53.7 | | 0.5 | | | 32 | | 0.7 | | | | 961 | 183.0 | 220 | 0.98 |
| 17244 | 1 | ea | Microwaved, avg | 276 | 257 | 77 | 56.9 | 0.0 | 0.0 | 0.0 | 0.0 | 3.3 | 0.6 | 1.1 | 0.8 | | | 135 | 101 | 30 | 30 | 0 | 0 | 0.03 | | | 0.14 | 2.21 | 71.8 | | 0.6 | | | 28 | | 0.6 | | | | 977 | 162.8 | 130 | 0.83 |
| 17113 | 1 | ea | Ling, baked/broiled, fillet, avg | 151 | 168 | 74 | 36.8 | 0.0 | 0.0 | 0.0 | 0.0 | 1.2 | 0.3 | 0.3 | 0.5 | | | 77 | 174 | 53 | 53 | 0 | 0 | 0.19 | 0.35 | 4.23 | 0.53 | 0.98 | 12.1 | 0.56 | 0.0 | 1.7 | | 66 | 0.2 | 1.3 | 122 | 0.1 | 384 | 734 | 70.7 | 261 | 1.51 |
| 17197 | 1 | ea | Ling, raw, fillet, avg | 193 | 168 | 80 | 36.7 | 0.0 | 0.0 | 0.0 | 0.0 | 1.2 | 0.2 | 0.2 | 0.4 | | | 77 | 193 | 58 | 58 | 0 | 0 | 0.21 | 0.37 | 4.44 | 0.59 | 1.08 | 13.5 | 0.62 | 0.0 | | 0.6 | 66 | 0.2 | 1.3 | 122 | 0.1 | 382 | 731 | 70.4 | 261 | 1.51 |
| 17114 | 1 | ea | Lingcod, baked/broiled, fillet, avg | 302 | 329 | 76 | 68.3 | 0.0 | 0.0 | 0.0 | 0.0 | 4.1 | 0.8 | 1.3 | 1.2 | 0.79 | 0.31 | 202 | 175 | 51 | 51 | 0 | 0 | 0.11 | 0.42 | 6.98 | 1.04 | 12.53 | 30.2 | 2.61 | 0.0 | 3.3 | | 54 | 0.1 | 1.2 | 100 | 0.1 | 779 | 1691 | 141.3 | 230 | 1.75 |
| 17198 | 1 | ea | Lingcod, raw, fillet, avg | 386 | 328 | 81 | 68.3 | 0.0 | 0.0 | 0.0 | 0.0 | 4.1 | 0.8 | 1.4 | 1.2 | 0.00 | 0.00 | 201 | 193 | 58 | 58 | 0 | 0 | 0.12 | 0.44 | 7.33 | 1.16 | 13.90 | 34.7 | 2.89 | 0.0 | | | 54 | 0.1 | 1.2 | 100 | 0.1 | 776 | 1687 | 140.9 | 228 | 1.74 |
| | | | Mackerel | | | | | | | | | | | | | | | | | | | | | | | | | | | | | | | | | | | | | | | | |
| 17049 | 1 | ea | Atlantic, baked/broiled, fillet, avg | 88 | 231 | 53 | 21.0 | 0.0 | 0.0 | 0.0 | 0.0 | 15.7 | 3.7 | 6.2 | 3.3 | 1.16 | 0.17 | 66 | 158 | 48 | 48 | 0 | 0 | 0.14 | 0.36 | 6.03 | 0.40 | 16.72 | 1.3 | 0.87 | 0.4 | 10.2 | | 13 | 0.1 | 1.4 | 85 | 0.0 | 245 | 353 | 45.4 | 73 | 0.83 |
| 17048 | 1 | ea | Atlantic, raw, fillet, avg | 112 | 230 | 64 | 20.8 | 0.0 | 0.0 | 0.0 | 0.0 | 15.6 | 3.7 | 6.1 | 3.3 | 2.75 | 0.45 | 78 | 185 | 56 | 56 | 0 | 0 | 0.20 | 0.35 | 10.17 | 0.45 | 9.76 | 1.5 | 0.96 | 0.4 | 10.1 | | 13 | 0.1 | 1.8 | 85 | 0.0 | 243 | 352 | 49.4 | 101 | 0.71 |
| 17321 | 3 | oz | Atlantic/Pacific, cooked, avg | 85 | 212 | 58 | 21.3 | 0.0 | 0.0 | 0.0 | 0.0 | 13.2 | 1.5 | | | | | 61 | 0 | 0 | 0 | 0 | 0 | | | | | | | | 0.0 | | | 0 | | 0.9 | | | | 405 | | 101 | |
| 17293 | 1 | ea | Jack, canned, drained, avg | 361 | 563 | 69 | 83.8 | 0.0 | 0.0 | 0.0 | 0.0 | 22.7 | 6.7 | 8.1 | 6.0 | 4.59 | 0.61 | 285 | 1567 | 469 | 469 | 0 | 0 | 0.14 | 0.77 | 22.31 | 0.76 | 25.05 | 18.0 | 1.10 | 3.2 | 40.4 | | 870 | 0.5 | 7.4 | 134 | 0.1 | 1087 | 700 | 136.1 | 1368 | 3.68 |
| 17115 | 1 | ea | King, baked/broiled, fillet, avg | 308 | 413 | 69 | 80.1 | 0.0 | 0.0 | 0.0 | 0.0 | 7.9 | 1.4 | 3.0 | 1.3 | 1.20 | 0.23 | 209 | 2584 | 776 | 776 | 0 | 0 | 0.35 | 1.79 | 32.34 | 1.57 | 55.44 | 27.7 | 2.98 | 4.9 | | | 123 | 0.1 | 7.0 | 126 | 0.0 | 979 | 1719 | 144.1 | 625 | 2.22 |
| 17228 | 1 | ea | King, raw, fillet, avg | 396 | 416 | 76 | 80.4 | 0.0 | 0.0 | 0.0 | 0.0 | 7.9 | 1.4 | 3.0 | 1.3 | 1.20 | 0.24 | 210 | 2879 | 863 | 863 | 0 | 0 | 0.40 | 1.88 | 34.02 | 1.75 | 61.78 | 30.1 | 3.32 | 6.3 | | | 123 | 0.1 | 7.0 | 127 | 0.0 | 982 | 1723 | 144.5 | 626 | 2.22 |
| 17092 | 1 | ea | Spanish, baked/broiled, fillet, avg | 146 | 231 | 68 | 34.5 | 0.0 | 0.0 | 0.0 | 0.0 | 9.2 | 2.6 | 3.1 | 2.5 | 1.96 | 0.38 | 107 | 159 | 48 | 48 | 0 | 0 | 0.19 | 0.31 | 7.30 | 0.67 | 10.22 | 1.8 | 1.27 | 2.3 | 13.1 | | 19 | 0.1 | 1.1 | 55 | 0.0 | 396 | 809 | 59.3 | 96 | 0.91 |
| 17229 | 1 | ea | Spanish, raw, fillet, avg | 187 | 260 | 72 | 36.1 | 0.0 | 0.0 | 0.0 | 0.0 | 11.8 | 3.4 | 2.9 | 3.3 | 2.57 | 0.49 | 142 | 187 | 56 | 56 | 0 | 0 | 0.24 | 0.32 | 4.30 | 0.75 | 4.49 | 1.9 | 1.40 | 3.0 | 16.8 | | 21 | 0.1 | 0.8 | 62 | 0.0 | 383 | 834 | 68.3 | 110 | 0.92 |
| 17131 | 1 | ea | Pacific/Jack, mixed species, bkd/brld, fillet, avg | 176 | 354 | 62 | 45.2 | 0.0 | 0.0 | 0.0 | 0.0 | 17.8 | 5.1 | 5.9 | 4.4 | 3.37 | 0.45 | 106 | 83 | 25 | 25 | 0 | 0 | 0.24 | 0.95 | 18.83 | 0.67 | 7.44 | 3.5 | 0.64 | 3.7 | 15.8 | | 51 | 0.2 | 2.6 | 63 | 0.0 | 282 | 917 | 82.4 | 194 | 1.51 |
| 17051 | 1 | ea | Pacific/Jack, raw, fillet, avg | 225 | 356 | 70 | 45.2 | 0.0 | 0.0 | 0.0 | 0.0 | 17.8 | 5.1 | 5.9 | 4.4 | 3.35 | 0.44 | 106 | 97 | 29 | 29 | 0 | 0 | 0.25 | 0.95 | 18.72 | 0.74 | 9.90 | 4.5 | 0.71 | 4.5 | 2.3 | | 52 | 0.2 | 2.6 | 63 | 0.0 | 281 | 914 | 82.1 | 194 | 1.51 |
| 17109 | 1 | ea | Mahi Mahi, dolphin fish, baked/broiled, fillet, avg | 159 | 173 | 71 | 37.7 | 0.0 | 0.0 | 0.0 | 0.0 | 1.4 | 0.4 | 0.2 | 0.3 | 0.23 | 0.08 | 149 | 331 | 99 | 99 | 0 | 0 | 0.04 | 0.14 | 11.81 | 0.73 | 1.10 | 9.5 | 1.38 | 0.0 | 1.7 | | 30 | 0.1 | 2.3 | 60 | 0.0 | 291 | 847 | 74.4 | 180 | 0.94 |
| 17240 | 1 | ea | Mahi Mahi, dolphin fish, raw, fillet, avg | 204 | 173 | 78 | 37.7 | 0.0 | 0.0 | 0.0 | 0.0 | 1.4 | 0.4 | 0.2 | 0.3 | 0.23 | 0.08 | 149 | 367 | 110 | 110 | 0 | 0 | 0.04 | 0.14 | 12.44 | 0.82 | 1.22 | 10.2 | 1.53 | 0.0 | | | 31 | 0.1 | 2.3 | 61 | 0.0 | 292 | 849 | 74.5 | 180 | 0.94 |
| 17116 | 3 | oz | Milkfish, baked/broiled, avg | 85 | 162 | 63 | 22.4 | 0.0 | 0.0 | 0.0 | 0.0 | 7.3 | 1.8 | 2.8 | 2.0 | | | 57 | 93 | 28 | 28 | 0 | 0 | 0.01 | 0.06 | 7.02 | 0.41 | 2.78 | 15.3 | 0.74 | 0.0 | | | 55 | 0.0 | 0.3 | 32 | 0.0 | 177 | 318 | 13.8 | 78 | 0.89 |
| 17199 | 3 | oz | Milkfish, raw, avg | 85 | 126 | 71 | 17.4 | 0.0 | 0.0 | 0.0 | 0.0 | 5.7 | 1.4 | 2.2 | 1.5 | | | 44 | 85 | 26 | 26 | 0 | 0 | 0.01 | 0.05 | 5.47 | 0.36 | 2.89 | 13.6 | 0.64 | 0.0 | | | 43 | 0.0 | 0.3 | 26 | 0.0 | 138 | 248 | 10.7 | 61 | 0.70 |
| 17117 | 3 | oz | Monkfish, baked/broiled, avg | 85 | 82 | 78 | 15.8 | 0.0 | 0.0 | 0.0 | 0.0 | 1.7 | 0.5 | 0.3 | 0.3 | | | 27 | 39 | 12 | 12 | 0 | 0 | 0.02 | 0.06 | 2.18 | 0.24 | 0.88 | 6.8 | 0.15 | 0.9 | | | 9 | 0.0 | 0.3 | 23 | 0.0 | 218 | 436 | 39.8 | 20 | 0.45 |
| 17200 | 3 | oz | Monkfish, raw, avg | 85 | 65 | 83 | 12.3 | 0.0 | 0.0 | 0.0 | 0.0 | 1.3 | 0.3 | 0.2 | 0.5 | | | 21 | 34 | 10 | 10 | 0 | 0 | 0.02 | 0.05 | 1.78 | 0.20 | 0.76 | 6.0 | 0.13 | 0.9 | | | 7 | 0.0 | 0.3 | 18 | 0.0 | 170 | 340 | 31.0 | 15 | 0.35 |
| 17150 | 1 | Tbs | Moochim, Korean style, dried, avg | 5 | 17 | 23 | 1.8 | 0.5 | 0.0 | 0.5 | 0.0 | 0.8 | 0.1 | 0.3 | 0.3 | | | 4 | 4 | 1 | 1 | 0 | 0 | 0.01 | 0.01 | 0.25 | 0.03 | 0.28 | 1.0 | | 0.1 | | | 7 | 0.0 | 0.1 | 5 | | 29 | 44 | | 252 | 0.06 |
| 17072 | 1 | ea | Mullet, striped, baked/broiled, fillet, avg | 93 | 140 | 70 | 23.1 | 0.0 | 0.0 | 0.0 | 0.0 | 4.5 | 1.3 | 1.3 | 0.9 | 0.33 | 0.18 | 59 | 131 | 39 | 39 | 0 | | 0.09 | 0.09 | 5.86 | 0.46 | 0.23 | 9.1 | 0.82 | 1.1 | | | 29 | 0.1 | 1.3 | 31 | 0.0 | 227 | 426 | 43.5 | 66 | 0.82 |
| 17201 | 1 | ea | Mullet, striped, raw, fillet, avg | 119 | 139 | 77 | 23.1 | 0.0 | 0.0 | 0.0 | 0.0 | 4.5 | 1.3 | 1.3 | 0.9 | 0.42 | 0.22 | 58 | 145 | 44 | 44 | 0 | 0 | 0.11 | 0.10 | 6.19 | 0.51 | 0.26 | 10.1 | 0.90 | 1.4 | | | 49 | 0.1 | 1.2 | 35 | 0.0 | 263 | 425 | 43.4 | 77 | 0.62 |
| 17121 | 3 | oz | Orange Roughy, baked/broiled, avg | 85 | 76 | 69 | 16.1 | 0.0 | 0.0 | 0.0 | 0.0 | 0.8 | 0.0 | 0.5 | 0.0 | 0.00 | 0.01 | 22 | 69 | 20 | 20 | 0 | 0 | 0.10 | 0.16 | 3.10 | 0.29 | 1.96 | 6.8 | 0.54 | 0.0 | | | 32 | 0.2 | 0.2 | 32 | 0.0 | 218 | 327 | 39.8 | 69 | 0.82 |
| 17207 | 3 | oz | Orange Roughy, raw, avg | 85 | 59 | 76 | 12.5 | 0.0 | 0.0 | 0.0 | 0.0 | 0.6 | 0.0 | 0.4 | 0.0 | 0.00 | 0.01 | 7 | 60 | 18 | 18 | 0 | 0 | 0.09 | 0.13 | 2.55 | 0.26 | 1.70 | 6.0 | 0.47 | 0.0 | | | 26 | 0.1 | 0.2 | 26 | 0.0 | 170 | 255 | 31.0 | 54 | 0.64 |
| | | | Perch | | | | | | | | | | | | | | | | | | | | | | | | | | | | | | | | | | | | | | | | |
| 17093 | 1 | ea | Atlantic Ocean, baked/broiled, fillet, avg | 50 | 60 | 73 | 11.9 | 0.0 | 0.0 | 0.0 | 0.0 | 1.0 | 0.2 | 0.4 | 0.3 | 0.22 | 0.02 | 27 | 23 | 7 | 7 | 0 | 0 | 0.06 | 0.07 | 1.22 | 0.14 | 0.57 | 5.2 | 0.21 | 0.4 | 0.5 | | 68 | 0.0 | 0.6 | 20 | 0.0 | 138 | 175 | 27.8 | 48 | 0.31 |
| 17052 | 1 | ea | Atlantic Ocean, redfish, raw, fillet, avg | 64 | 60 | 79 | 11.9 | 0.0 | 0.0 | 0.0 | 0.0 | 1.0 | 0.2 | 0.4 | 0.3 | 0.22 | 0.02 | 27 | 26 | 8 | 8 | 0 | 0 | 0.07 | 0.07 | 1.28 | 0.15 | 0.64 | 5.8 | 0.23 | 0.5 | 1.5 | | 68 | 0.0 | 0.6 | 19 | 0.0 | 138 | 175 | 27.7 | 48 | 0.31 |
| 17094 | 1 | ea | Mixed species, baked/broiled, fillet, avg | 46 | 54 | 73 | 11.5 | 0.0 | 0.0 | 0.0 | 0.0 | 0.5 | 0.1 | 0.1 | 0.2 | 0.16 | 0.04 | 53 | 15 | 5 | 5 | 0 | 0 | 0.04 | 0.06 | 0.87 | 0.06 | 1.01 | 2.7 | 0.40 | 0.8 | 0.5 | | 47 | 0.1 | 0.5 | 17 | 0.4 | 118 | 158 | 7.4 | 36 | 0.66 |
| 17239 | 1 | ea | Mixed species, raw, fillet, avg | 60 | 55 | 79 | 11.6 | 0.0 | 0.0 | 0.0 | 0.0 | 0.6 | 0.1 | 0.1 | 0.2 | 0.16 | 0.04 | 54 | 17 | 5 | 5 | 0 | 0 | 0.04 | 0.06 | 0.91 | 0.07 | 1.14 | 3.0 | 0.45 | 1.0 | | | 48 | 0.1 | 0.5 | 18 | 0.4 | 120 | 161 | 7.6 | 37 | 0.67 |
| 17015 | 3 | oz | Ocean, floured/breaded, fried, avg | 85 | 187 | 59 | 16.9 | 6.7 | 0.4 | 0.3 | 6.0 | 10.0 | 2.4 | 4.3 | 2.5 | | | 54 | 58 | 17 | 17 | 0 | | 0.10 | 0.14 | 2.02 | 0.18 | 0.77 | 11.1 | 0.33 | 0.5 | 0.9 | | 102 | 0.0 | 1.2 | 28 | 0.1 | 197 | 243 | 28.9 | 325 | 0.50 |
| | | | Pike | | | | | | | | | | | | | | | | | | | | | | | | | | | | | | | | | | | | | | | | |
| 17095 | 1 | ea | Northern, baked/broiled, fillet, avg | 310 | 350 | 73 | 76.6 | 0.0 | 0.0 | 0.0 | 0.0 | 2.7 | 0.5 | 0.6 | 0.8 | 0.51 | 0.24 | 155 | 251 | 74 | 74 | 0 | 0 | 0.21 | 0.24 | 8.68 | 0.42 | 7.13 | 53.6 | 2.70 | 11.8 | | | 226 | 0.2 | 2.2 | 124 | 1.0 | 874 | 1026 | 50.2 | 152 | 2.67 |
| 17160 | 1 | ea | Northern, raw, fillet, avg | 396 | 348 | 79 | 76.4 | 0.0 | 0.0 | 0.0 | 0.0 | 2.7 | 0.5 | 0.6 | 0.8 | 0.51 | 0.24 | 154 | 277 | 83 | 83 | 0 | 0 | 0.23 | 0.25 | 9.11 | 0.46 | 7.92 | 59.4 | 2.97 | 15.0 | | | 226 | 0.2 | 2.2 | 123 | 1.0 | 871 | 1026 | 49.9 | 154 | 2.65 |
| 17118 | 1 | ea | Walleye, baked/broiled, fillet, avg | 124 | 148 | 74 | 30.4 | 0.0 | 0.0 | 0.0 | 0.0 | 1.9 | 0.4 | 0.5 | 0.7 | 0.52 | 0.13 | 136 | 100 | 30 | 30 | 0 | 0 | 0.39 | 0.24 | 3.47 | 0.17 | 2.86 | 21.1 | 1.07 | 0.0 | | | 175 | 0.3 | 2.1 | 47 | 1.3 | 334 | 619 | 20.1 | 81 | 0.98 |
| 17202 | 1 | ea | Walleye, raw, fillet, avg | 159 | 148 | 79 | 30.4 | 0.0 | 0.0 | 0.0 | 0.0 | 1.9 | 0.4 | 0.5 | 0.7 | 0.52 | 0.13 | 137 | 111 | 33 | 33 | 0 | 0 | 0.43 | 0.25 | 3.66 | 0.19 | 3.18 | 23.9 | 1.19 | 0.0 | | | 175 | 0.3 | 2.1 | 48 | 1.3 | 334 | 619 | 20.0 | 81 | 0.99 |
| | | | Pollock | | | | | | | | | | | | | | | | | | | | | | | | | | | | | | | | | | | | | | | | |
| 17168 | 1 | ea | Atlantic, baked/broiled, fillet, avg | 302 | 356 | 72 | 75.2 | 0.0 | 0.0 | 0.0 | 0.0 | 3.8 | 0.5 | 0.4 | 1.9 | 1.64 | 0.14 | 275 | 121 | 36 | 36 | 0 | 0 | 0.16 | 0.68 | 12.02 | 1.00 | 11.11 | 9.1 | 1.25 | 0.0 | | | 233 | 0.2 | 1.8 | 260 | 0.1 | 855 | 1377 | 141.3 | 332 | 1.81 |
| 17053 | 1 | ea | Atlantic, raw, fillet, avg | 386 | 355 | 78 | 74.9 | 0.0 | 0.0 | 0.0 | 0.0 | 3.8 | 0.5 | 0.4 | 1.9 | 1.63 | 0.14 | 274 | 135 | 42 | 42 | 0 | 0 | 0.18 | 0.71 | 12.62 | 1.11 | 12.31 | 11.6 | 1.38 | 0.0 | 3.9 | | 232 | 0.2 | 1.8 | 259 | 0.1 | 853 | 1374 | 140.9 | 332 | 1.81 |
| 17096 | 1 | ea | Walleye, baked/broiled, fillet, avg | 60 | 68 | 74 | 14.1 | 0.0 | 0.0 | 0.0 | 0.0 | 0.7 | 0.1 | 0.1 | 0.3 | 0.29 | 0.02 | 58 | 46 | 14 | 14 | 0 | 0 | 0.04 | 0.05 | 0.99 | 0.04 | 2.52 | 2.2 | 0.10 | 0.0 | 0.6 | | 4 | 0.0 | 0.2 | 44 | 0.0 | 289 | 232 | 26.0 | 70 | 0.36 |
| 17167 | 1 | ea | Walleye, raw, fillet, avg | 77 | 62 | 82 | 13.2 | 0.0 | 0.0 | 0.0 | 0.0 | 0.6 | 0.1 | 0.1 | 0.3 | 0.29 | 0.02 | 55 | 51 | 15 | 15 | 0 | 0 | 0.05 | 0.04 | 0.99 | 0.05 | 2.39 | 2.4 | 0.11 | 0.0 | 0.8 | | 4 | 0.0 | 0.2 | 44 | 0.0 | 290 | 251 | 16.9 | 76 | 0.34 |
| 17073 | 1 | ea | Pompano, baked/broiled, fillet, avg | 88 | 186 | 63 | 20.9 | 0.0 | 0.0 | 0.0 | 0.0 | 10.6 | 4.0 | 2.9 | 1.3 | 0.31 | 0.17 | 56 | 106 | 32 | 32 | 0 | 0 | 0.60 | 0.13 | 3.34 | 0.20 | 1.06 | 15.2 | 0.77 | 0.0 | | | 38 | 0.1 | 0.6 | 27 | 0.0 | 300 | 560 | 41.2 | 67 | 0.61 |

| Code | Amount | | Description | Weight (g) | Calories | % Water | Protein (g) | Carbs (g) | Fiber (g) | Sugar (g) | Other Carbs (g) | Fat (g) | Sat Fat (g) | Mono Fat (g) | Poly Fat (g) | Omega 3 (g) | Omega 6 (g) | Choles (mg) | Vit A (IU) | Vit A (RE) | Retinol (RE) | Carotenoids (RE) | Beta Carotene (mcg) | Thiamin (mg) | Riboflavin (mg) | Niacin (NE) | Vit B6 (mg) | Vit B12 (mcg) | Folate (mcg) | Panto (mg) | Vit C (mg) | Vit D (mg) | Vit E (α TE) | Calcium (mg) | Copper (mg) | Iron (mg) | Magnes (mg) | Mang (mg) | Phos (mg) | Potassium (mg) | Selenium (mcg) | Sodium (mg) | Zinc (mg) |
|---|---|---|---|---|---|---|---|---|---|---|---|---|---|---|---|---|---|---|---|---|---|---|---|---|---|---|---|---|---|---|---|---|---|---|---|---|---|---|---|---|---|---|---|
| | | | | Basic Components | | | | | | | | | Additional Fats | | | | | | Vit A & Components | | | | | Vitamins | | | | | | | | | | Minerals | | | | | | | | | |
| 17203 | 1 | ea | Pompano, raw, fillet, avg | 112 | 184 | 71 | 20.7 | 0.0 | 0.0 | 0.0 | 0.0 | 10.6 | 3.9 | 2.9 | 1.3 | 0.64 | 0.41 | 56 | 123 | 37 | 37 | 0 | 0 | 0.63 | 0.13 | 3.36 | 0.22 | 1.46 | 16.8 | 0.84 | 0.0 | | | 25 | 0.0 | 0.7 | 30 | 0.0 | 218 | 427 | 40.9 | 73 | 0.81 |
| 17119 | 1 | ea | Pout, ocean, baked/broiled, fillet, avg | 274 | 279 | 76 | 58.4 | 0.0 | 0.0 | 0.0 | 0.0 | 3.2 | 1.1 | 1.2 | 0.1 | 0.00 | 0.11 | 184 | 126 | 38 | 38 | 0 | 0 | 0.25 | 0.20 | 7.01 | 0.76 | 2.85 | 21.9 | 0.47 | 0.0 | | | 36 | 0.1 | 1.0 | 47 | 0.1 | 701 | 1406 | 128.2 | 214 | 3.62 |
| 17204 | 1 | ea | Pout, ocean, raw, fillet, avg | 352 | 278 | 81 | 58.4 | 0.0 | 0.0 | 0.0 | 0.0 | 3.2 | 1.1 | 1.2 | 0.1 | 0.00 | 0.11 | 183 | 141 | 42 | 42 | 0 | 0 | 0.28 | 0.21 | 7.39 | 0.84 | 3.17 | 24.6 | 0.53 | 0.0 | | | 35 | 0.1 | 1.0 | 46 | 0.1 | 704 | 1408 | 128.5 | 215 | 3.63 |
| 17174 | 1 | ea | Pumpkinseed Sunfish, baked/broiled, fillet, avg | 37 | 42 | 74 | 9.2 | 0.0 | 0.0 | 0.0 | 0.0 | 0.3 | 0.1 | 0.1 | 0.1 | 0.06 | 0.04 | 32 | 21 | 6 | 6 | 0 | 0 | 0.03 | 0.03 | 0.54 | 0.05 | 0.85 | 6.3 | 0.32 | 0.4 | | | 38 | 0.1 | 0.6 | 14 | 0.3 | 85 | 166 | 6.0 | 38 | 0.74 |
| 17216 | 1 | ea | Pumpkinseed Sunfish, raw, fillet, avg | 48 | 43 | 80 | 9.3 | 0.0 | 0.0 | 0.0 | 0.0 | 0.3 | 0.1 | 0.1 | 0.1 | 0.06 | 0.05 | 32 | 24 | 7 | 7 | 0 | 0 | 0.04 | 0.03 | 0.58 | 0.06 | 0.96 | 7.2 | 0.36 | 0.5 | | | 38 | 0.1 | 0.6 | 14 | 0.3 | 86 | 168 | 6.0 | 38 | 0.74 |
| 17074 | 1 | ea | Rockfish, Pacific, mixed species, bkd/brld, avg | 149 | 180 | 73 | 35.8 | 0.0 | 0.0 | 0.0 | 0.0 | 3.0 | 0.7 | 0.7 | 0.9 | 0.69 | 0.09 | 66 | 326 | 98 | 98 | 0 | 0 | 0.07 | 0.13 | 5.84 | 0.40 | 1.79 | 15.5 | 1.30 | 0.0 | | | 18 | 0.1 | 0.8 | 51 | 0.0 | 340 | 775 | 69.7 | 115 | 0.79 |
| 17205 | 1 | ea | Rockfish, Pacific, mixed species, raw, fillet, avg | 191 | 180 | 79 | 35.9 | 0.0 | 0.0 | 0.0 | 0.0 | 3.0 | 0.7 | 0.6 | 0.9 | 0.69 | 0.09 | 67 | 363 | 109 | 109 | 0 | 0 | 0.07 | 0.13 | 6.15 | 0.44 | 1.91 | 17.2 | 1.43 | 0.0 | | | 17 | 0.1 | 0.8 | 50 | 0.0 | 340 | 774 | 69.7 | 115 | 0.78 |
| | | | Roe | | | | | | | | | | | | | | | | | | | | | | | | | | | | | | | | | | | | | | | | |
| 17146 | 1 | Tbs | Cod & Shad, cooked, avg | 12 | 23 | 58 | 3.1 | 0.3 | 0.0 | 0.0 | 0.3 | 1.3 | 0.3 | 0.4 | 0.5 | | | 51 | 57 | 16 | 15 | 1 | | 0.03 | 0.10 | 0.24 | 0.02 | 1.30 | 9.4 | 0.36 | 2.0 | 0.3 | | 3 | 0.0 | 0.1 | 3 | 0.0 | 53 | 31 | | 61 | 0.14 |
| 17148 | 1 | Tbs | Herring, avg | 14 | 20 | 68 | 3.1 | 0.2 | 0.0 | 0.0 | 0.2 | 0.9 | 0.2 | 0.2 | 0.4 | | | 52 | 33 | 10 | 10 | 0 | 0 | 0.03 | 0.10 | 0.25 | 0.02 | 1.12 | 10.6 | 0.08 | 1.9 | 0.3 | | 3 | 0.0 | 0.1 | 3 | 0.0 | 56 | 31 | | 13 | 0.14 |
| 17120 | 1/2 | oz | Mixed species, baked/broiled, avg | 14 | 29 | 59 | 4.0 | 0.3 | 0.0 | 0.0 | 0.3 | 1.2 | 0.3 | 0.3 | 0.5 | 0.42 | 0.04 | 67 | 42 | 13 | 13 | 0 | 0 | 0.04 | 0.13 | 0.31 | 0.03 | 1.61 | 12.9 | 0.16 | 2.3 | 0.4 | | 4 | 0.0 | 0.1 | 4 | 0.0 | 72 | 40 | 7.2 | 16 | 0.18 |
| 17206 | 1 | Tbs | Mixed species, raw, avg | 14 | 20 | 68 | 3.1 | 0.2 | 0.0 | | | 0.9 | 0.2 | 0.2 | 0.4 | 0.33 | 0.03 | 52 | 37 | 11 | 11 | 0 | 0 | 0.03 | 0.10 | 0.25 | 0.02 | 1.40 | 11.2 | 0.14 | 2.2 | 0.3 | | 3 | 0.0 | 0.1 | 3 | 0.0 | 56 | 31 | 5.6 | 13 | 0.14 |
| | | | Sablefish | | | | | | | | | | | | | | | | | | | | | | | | | | | | | | | | | | | | | | | | |
| 17122 | 1 | ea | Baked/broiled, fillet, avg | 302 | 755 | 63 | 51.9 | 0.0 | 0.0 | 0.0 | 0.0 | 59.2 | 12.4 | 31.1 | 7.9 | 5.77 | 1.04 | 190 | 1021 | 305 | 305 | 0 | 0 | 0.37 | 0.35 | 15.49 | 1.04 | 4.35 | 51.3 | 2.61 | 0.0 | | | 136 | 0.1 | 5.0 | 214 | 0.1 | 649 | 1386 | 141.3 | 217 | 1.24 |
| 17208 | 1 | ea | Raw, fillet, avg | 386 | 753 | 71 | 51.7 | 0.0 | 0.0 | 0.0 | 0.0 | 59.1 | 12.4 | 31.1 | 7.9 | 5.75 | 1.04 | 189 | 1197 | 359 | 359 | 0 | 0 | 0.39 | 0.35 | 15.44 | 1.16 | 5.79 | 57.9 | 2.89 | 0.0 | | | 135 | 0.1 | 4.9 | 212 | 0.1 | 648 | 1382 | 140.9 | 216 | 1.24 |
| 17075 | 3 | oz | Smoked, avg | 85 | 218 | 60 | 15.0 | 0.0 | 0.0 | 0.0 | 0.0 | 17.1 | 3.6 | 9.0 | 2.3 | 1.67 | 0.30 | 54 | 347 | 104 | 104 | 0 | 0 | 0.11 | 0.10 | 4.51 | 0.33 | 1.70 | 16.7 | 0.84 | 0.0 | | | 43 | 0.0 | 1.4 | 63 | 0.0 | 189 | 400 | 42.7 | 626 | 0.37 |
| | | | Salmon | | | | | | | | | | | | | | | | | | | | | | | | | | | | | | | | | | | | | | | | |
| 17152 | 3 | oz | Chinook, smoked, avg | 85 | 99 | 72 | 15.6 | 0.0 | 0.0 | 0.0 | 0.0 | 3.7 | 0.8 | 1.7 | 0.8 | 0.35 | 0.39 | 20 | 75 | 22 | 22 | 0 | 0 | 0.02 | 0.09 | 4.01 | 0.24 | 2.77 | 1.6 | 0.74 | 0.0 | 6.8 | | 9 | 0.2 | 0.7 | 15 | 0.0 | 139 | 149 | 32.4 | 1700 | 0.26 |
| 17016 | 1 | ea | Coho, wild, steamed/poached, fillet, avg | 310 | 570 | 65 | 84.9 | 0.0 | 0.0 | 0.0 | 0.0 | 23.3 | 5.0 | 8.4 | 7.8 | 4.88 | 1.33 | 177 | 335 | 99 | 99 | 0 | 0 | 0.36 | 0.49 | 24.12 | 1.72 | 13.89 | 27.9 | 2.59 | 3.1 | 15.5 | | 143 | 0.2 | 2.2 | 108 | 0.1 | 924 | 1410 | 143.2 | 164 | 1.61 |
| 17306 | 3 | oz | Nuggets, breaded, fzn, heated, avg | 85 | 180 | 60 | 10.8 | 11.9 | 0.0 | | | 9.9 | 1.3 | 3.9 | 2.6 | 0.53 | 2.03 | 22 | 37 | 5 | 5 | 0 | 0 | 0.18 | 0.13 | 3.85 | 0.19 | 1.76 | 7.7 | 0.44 | 0.0 | | | 7 | 0.1 | 1.1 | 17 | 0.1 | 150 | 140 | | 147 | 0.44 |
| 17171 | 1 | ea | Pink, baked/broiled, fillet, avg | 248 | 370 | 70 | 63.5 | 0.0 | 0.0 | 0.0 | 0.0 | 11.0 | 1.8 | 3.0 | 4.3 | 3.30 | 0.41 | 166 | 337 | 102 | 102 | 0 | 0 | 0.49 | 0.18 | 21.15 | 0.57 | 8.58 | 12.4 | 2.15 | 0.0 | | | 42 | 0.2 | 2.5 | 82 | 0.0 | 732 | 1027 | 141.9 | 213 | 1.76 |
| 17056 | 1 | ea | Pink, raw, fillet, avg | 318 | 369 | 76 | 63.3 | 0.0 | 0.0 | 0.0 | 0.0 | 11.0 | 1.8 | 3.0 | 4.3 | 3.30 | 0.41 | 165 | 375 | 111 | 111 | 0 | 0 | 0.54 | 0.19 | 22.26 | 0.64 | 9.54 | 12.7 | 2.38 | 0.0 | 37.6 | | 41 | 0.2 | 2.4 | 83 | 0.0 | 731 | 1027 | 141.8 | 213 | 1.75 |
| 17154 | 3 | oz | Pink, unsalted, canned w/liquid, avg | 85 | 118 | 70 | 16.8 | 0.0 | 0.0 | 0.0 | 0.0 | 5.1 | 1.3 | 1.6 | 1.7 | 1.45 | 0.11 | 47 | 47 | 14 | 14 | 0 | 0 | 0.02 | 0.16 | 5.56 | 0.26 | 3.74 | 13.1 | 0.47 | 0.0 | 13.3 | | 181 | 0.1 | 0.7 | 29 | 0.0 | 280 | 277 | 28.2 | 64 | 0.78 |
| 17017 | 3 | oz | Pink, w/bone, canned w/liquid, avg | 85 | 118 | 69 | 16.8 | 0.0 | 0.0 | 0.0 | 0.0 | 5.1 | 1.3 | 1.5 | 1.7 | 1.45 | 0.11 | 47 | 47 | 14 | 14 | 0 | 0 | 0.02 | 0.16 | 5.56 | 0.26 | 3.74 | 13.1 | 0.47 | 0.0 | 13.3 | | 181 | 0.1 | 0.7 | 29 | 0.0 | 280 | 277 | 28.2 | 471 | 0.78 |
| 17058 | 3 | oz | Sockeye, w/bone, canned, drained, avg | 85 | 130 | 69 | 17.4 | 0.0 | 0.0 | 0.0 | 0.0 | 6.2 | 1.4 | 2.7 | 1.6 | 1.06 | 0.39 | 37 | 150 | 45 | 45 | 0 | 0 | 0.01 | 0.16 | 4.66 | 0.26 | 0.26 | 8.3 | 0.47 | 0.0 | 4.8 | | 203 | 0.1 | 0.9 | 25 | 0.0 | 277 | 320 | 30.1 | 457 | 0.87 |
| 17155 | 3 | oz | Sockeye, w/bone, unsalted, cnd, drained, avg | 85 | 130 | 69 | 17.4 | 0.0 | 0.0 | 0.0 | 0.0 | 6.2 | 1.4 | 2.4 | 1.9 | 1.06 | 0.39 | 37 | 150 | 45 | 45 | 0 | 0 | 0.01 | 0.16 | 4.66 | 0.26 | 0.26 | 8.3 | 0.47 | 0.0 | 4.8 | | 203 | 0.1 | 0.9 | 25 | 0.0 | 277 | 320 | 30.1 | 64 | 0.87 |
| | | | Sardines | | | | | | | | | | | | | | | | | | | | | | | | | | | | | | | | | | | | | | | | |
| 17297 | 1 | ea | Atlantic, w/bones in oil, canned, drained, avg | 12 | 25 | 60 | 3.0 | 0.0 | 0.0 | 0.0 | 0.0 | 1.4 | 0.2 | 0.5 | 0.6 | 0.18 | 0.42 | 17 | 27 | 8 | 8 | 0 | 0 | 0.01 | 0.03 | 0.63 | 0.02 | 1.07 | 1.4 | 0.08 | 0.0 | 0.8 | | 46 | 0.0 | 0.4 | 5 | 0.0 | 59 | 48 | 6.3 | 61 | 0.16 |
| 17298 | 1 | ea | Pacific, w/bone in tomato sce, cnd, drained, avg | 38 | 68 | 68 | 6.2 | 0.0 | 0.0 | 0.0 | 0.0 | 4.6 | 1.2 | 2.1 | 0.9 | 0.71 | 0.18 | 23 | 139 | 27 | | | | 0.02 | 0.09 | 1.60 | 0.05 | 3.42 | 9.2 | 0.28 | 0.4 | 4.6 | | 91 | 0.1 | 0.9 | 13 | 0.1 | 139 | 130 | 15.4 | 157 | 0.53 |
| 17133 | 1 | ea | Skinless, w/o bones in water, avg | 21 | 46 | 60 | 5.2 | 0.0 | 0.0 | 0.0 | 0.0 | 2.6 | 0.6 | 1.1 | 0.6 | | | 17 | 27 | 8 | 8 | 0 | 0 | 0.03 | 0.07 | 0.92 | 0.09 | 3.93 | 2.9 | 0.19 | 0.2 | 2.5 | | 18 | 0.0 | 0.3 | 10 | 0.0 | 68 | 94 | | 193 | 0.29 |
| 17021 | 3 | oz | With mustard, canned, avg | 85 | 167 | 64 | 16.1 | 1.4 | 0.0 | 1.1 | 0.3 | 10.2 | 3.3 | 3.6 | 2.4 | | | 94 | 26 | 8 | 8 | 0 | 0 | 0.03 | 0.17 | 4.59 | 0.10 | 5.95 | 13.6 | 0.62 | 0.0 | 10.2 | | 258 | 0.1 | 4.4 | 9 | 0.9 | 301 | 221 | 48.5 | 646 | 0.45 |
| 17172 | 1 | ea | Scup fish, baked/broiled, fillet, avg | 50 | 68 | 68 | 12.1 | 0.0 | 0.0 | 0.0 | 0.0 | 1.8 | 0.4 | 0.4 | 0.7 | | | 34 | 52 | 16 | 16 | 0 | 0 | 0.06 | 0.06 | 2.49 | 0.17 | 0.81 | 8.5 | 0.43 | 0.0 | | | 26 | 0.0 | 0.3 | 14 | 0.0 | 118 | 184 | 23.4 | 27 | 0.31 |
| 17210 | 1 | ea | Scup fish, raw, fillet, avg | 64 | 67 | 75 | 12.1 | 0.0 | 0.0 | 0.0 | 0.0 | 1.7 | 0.4 | 0.4 | 0.7 | 0.00 | 0.00 | 33 | 58 | 17 | 17 | 0 | 0 | 0.07 | 0.06 | 2.62 | 0.19 | 0.90 | 9.6 | 0.48 | 0.0 | | | 26 | 0.0 | 0.3 | 15 | 0.0 | 118 | 184 | 23.4 | 27 | 0.31 |
| 17211 | 1 | ea | Shad, American, raw, fillet, avg | 184 | 362 | 68 | 31.1 | 0.0 | 0.0 | 0.0 | 0.0 | 25.4 | 5.8 | 10.5 | 6.0 | 4.73 | 0.54 | 138 | 202 | 61 | 61 | 0 | 0 | 0.28 | 0.44 | 15.46 | 0.74 | 0.28 | 27.6 | 1.38 | 0.0 | | | 86 | 0.1 | 1.8 | 55 | 0.1 | 500 | 707 | 67.2 | 94 | 0.68 |
| 17062 | 1 | ea | Shad, baked/broiled, fillet, avg | 144 | 363 | 59 | 31.2 | 0.0 | 0.0 | 0.0 | 0.0 | 25.5 | 6.5 | 11.8 | 6.8 | 5.29 | 0.60 | 138 | 173 | 52 | 52 | 0 | 0 | 0.26 | 0.44 | 15.55 | 0.67 | 0.20 | 24.5 | 1.25 | 0.0 | 1.4 | | 86 | 0.1 | 1.8 | 55 | 0.1 | 503 | 708 | 67.4 | 94 | 0.68 |
| | | | Shark | | | | | | | | | | | | | | | | | | | | | | | | | | | | | | | | | | | | | | | | |
| 17134 | 3 | oz | Baked/broiled, avg | 85 | 152 | 65 | 20.9 | 0.3 | 0.0 | 0.3 | 0.0 | 7.0 | 1.4 | 2.6 | 2.3 | | | 51 | 328 | 93 | 90 | 3 | | 0.04 | 0.06 | 2.92 | 0.36 | 1.11 | 3.3 | 0.51 | 1.5 | | | 35 | 0.0 | 0.8 | 49 | 0.0 | 209 | 164 | | 341 | 0.43 |
| 17076 | 3 | oz | Batter fried, mixed species, avg | 85 | 194 | 60 | 15.8 | 5.4 | 0.0 | 0.3 | 5.2 | 11.7 | 2.7 | 5.0 | 3.1 | 0.75 | 2.29 | 50 | 153 | 46 | 46 | 0 | 0 | 0.06 | 0.08 | 2.36 | 0.26 | 1.03 | 12.8 | 0.53 | 0.0 | | | 43 | 0.0 | 0.9 | 37 | 0.0 | 165 | 132 | 28.9 | 104 | 0.41 |
| 17212 | 3 | oz | Raw, mixed species, avg | 85 | 111 | 74 | 17.9 | 0.0 | 0.0 | 0.0 | 0.0 | 3.8 | 0.8 | 1.5 | 1.0 | 0.74 | 0.16 | 43 | 198 | 60 | 60 | 0 | 0 | 0.04 | 0.05 | 2.50 | 0.34 | 1.27 | 2.7 | 0.59 | 0.0 | | | 29 | 0.0 | 0.7 | 42 | 0.0 | 179 | 136 | 31.0 | 67 | 0.37 |
| 17077 | 1 | ea | Sheepshead fish, baked/broiled, fillet, avg | 186 | 234 | 69 | 48.4 | 0.0 | 0.0 | 0.0 | 0.0 | 3.0 | 0.7 | 0.7 | 0.7 | 0.35 | 0.28 | 119 | 214 | 65 | 65 | 0 | | 0.02 | 0.09 | 3.35 | 0.65 | 4.28 | 32.2 | 1.62 | 0.0 | | | 69 | 0.2 | 1.2 | 65 | 0.0 | 651 | 952 | 95.4 | 136 | 1.17 |
| 17213 | 1 | ea | Sheepshead fish, raw, fillet, avg | 238 | 257 | 78 | 48.1 | 0.0 | 0.0 | 0.0 | 0.0 | 5.7 | 1.4 | 1.7 | 1.2 | 0.64 | 0.36 | 119 | 238 | 71 | 71 | 0 | 0 | 0.02 | 0.10 | 3.57 | 0.71 | 4.76 | 35.7 | 1.79 | 0.0 | | | 50 | 0.1 | 1.1 | 76 | 0.0 | 745 | 962 | 86.9 | 169 | 0.93 |
| | | | Smelt | | | | | | | | | | | | | | | | | | | | | | | | | | | | | | | | | | | | | | | | |
| 17137 | 1 | ea | Floured/breaded, fried, avg | 29 | 72 | 52 | 6.0 | 3.5 | 0.2 | 0.2 | 3.1 | 3.7 | 0.9 | 1.5 | 1.0 | | | 30 | 28 | 8 | 8 | 0 | | 0.02 | 0.06 | 0.62 | 0.04 | 0.91 | 3.4 | 0.17 | 0.0 | 0.3 | | 25 | 0.0 | 0.5 | 11 | 0.2 | 77 | 94 | | 155 | 0.53 |
| 17100 | 3 | oz | Rainbow, baked/broiled, avg | 85 | 105 | 73 | 19.2 | 0.0 | 0.0 | 0.0 | 0.0 | 2.6 | 0.5 | 0.7 | 1.0 | 0.81 | 0.11 | 77 | 49 | 14 | 14 | 0 | 0 | 0.01 | 0.12 | 1.50 | 0.14 | 3.37 | 3.9 | 0.63 | 0.0 | 0.9 | | 65 | 0.2 | 1.0 | 32 | 0.8 | 251 | 316 | 39.8 | 65 | 1.80 |
| 17063 | 3 | oz | Rainbow, raw, avg | 85 | 82 | 79 | 15.0 | 0.0 | 0.0 | 0.0 | 0.0 | 2.1 | 0.4 | 0.5 | 0.8 | 0.63 | 0.09 | 60 | 43 | 13 | 13 | 0 | 0 | 0.01 | 0.10 | 1.23 | 0.13 | 2.92 | 3.4 | 0.54 | 0.0 | 0.9 | | 51 | 0.1 | 0.8 | 26 | 0.6 | 196 | 247 | 31.0 | 51 | 1.40 |
| 17022 | 1 | ea | Snapper, mixed species, baked/broiled, fillet, avg | 170 | 218 | 70 | 44.7 | 0.0 | 0.0 | 0.0 | 0.0 | 2.9 | 0.6 | 0.5 | 1.0 | 0.55 | 0.12 | 80 | 196 | 60 | 60 | 0 | 0 | 0.09 | 0.01 | 0.59 | 0.78 | 5.95 | 9.9 | 1.48 | 2.7 | 1.7 | | 68 | 0.1 | 0.4 | 63 | 0.0 | 342 | 887 | 83.3 | 97 | 0.75 |
| 17064 | 1 | ea | Snapper, mixed species, raw, fillet, avg | 218 | 218 | 77 | 44.7 | 0.0 | 0.0 | 0.0 | 0.0 | 2.9 | 0.6 | 0.5 | 1.0 | 0.69 | 0.15 | 81 | 218 | 65 | 65 | 0 | 0 | 0.10 | 0.01 | 0.62 | 0.87 | 6.54 | 10.9 | 1.63 | 3.5 | 2.2 | | 70 | 0.1 | 0.4 | 70 | 0.0 | 432 | 909 | 83.3 | 140 | 0.78 |
| | | | Sole/Flounder | | | | | | | | | | | | | | | | | | | | | | | | | | | | | | | | | | | | | | | | |
| 17068 | 1 | ea | Baked/broiled, fillet, avg | 127 | 149 | 73 | 30.7 | 0.0 | 0.0 | 0.0 | 0.0 | 1.9 | 0.5 | 0.3 | 0.8 | 0.66 | 0.08 | 86 | 48 | 14 | 14 | 0 | 0 | 0.10 | 0.14 | 2.77 | 0.30 | 3.19 | 11.7 | 0.74 | 0.0 | 1.9 | | 23 | 0.0 | 0.4 | 74 | 0.0 | 367 | 437 | 73.9 | 133 | 0.80 |
| 17005 | 4 | pce | Batter fried, avg | 64 | 121 | 65 | 13.0 | 4.5 | 0.1 | 0.5 | 3.9 | 5.2 | 1.0 | 2.0 | 1.8 | | | 31 | 240 | 66 | 63 | 3 | | 0.07 | 0.08 | 3.66 | 0.18 | 0.70 | 8.6 | 0.37 | 0.0 | 1.0 | | 44 | 0.0 | 0.8 | 50 | 0.0 | 145 | 277 | 24.8 | 105 | 0.34 |
| 17004 | 1 | ea | Floured/breaded, fried, fillet, avg | 81 | 177 | 59 | 16.2 | 6.4 | 0.4 | 0.3 | 5.8 | 9.2 | 2.3 | 3.8 | 2.4 | | | 56 | 50 | 15 | 15 | 0 | | 0.08 | 0.11 | 2.62 | 0.15 | 1.10 | 9.9 | 0.48 | 1.1 | 1.4 | | 28 | 0.0 | 0.7 | 28 | 0.0 | 164 | 300 | 34.6 | 313 | 0.46 |
| 17042 | 1 | ea | Raw, fillet, avg | 163 | 148 | 79 | 30.6 | 0.0 | 0.0 | 0.0 | 0.0 | 1.9 | 0.5 | 0.4 | 0.5 | 0.34 | 0.07 | 78 | 54 | 16 | 16 | 0 | 0 | 0.15 | 0.12 | 4.73 | 0.34 | 2.48 | 13.0 | 0.82 | 2.8 | 2.4 | | 29 | 0.1 | 0.6 | 51 | 0.0 | 300 | 588 | 53.3 | 132 | 0.73 |
| 17006 | 3 | oz | Steamed/poached, fillet, avg | 85 | 97 | 74 | 20.0 | 0.0 | 0.0 | 0.0 | 0.0 | 1.3 | 0.3 | 0.2 | 0.3 | | | 51 | 28 | 9 | 9 | 0 | 0 | 0.08 | 0.07 | 2.62 | 0.18 | 1.37 | 6.8 | 0.58 | 1.4 | 1.5 | | 19 | 0.0 | 0.4 | 30 | 0.0 | 176 | 326 | 49.5 | 77 | 0.48 |
| 17190 | 1 | ea | Spot fish, baked/broiled, fillet, avg | 50 | 79 | 69 | 11.9 | 0.0 | 0.0 | 0.0 | 0.0 | 3.1 | 0.9 | 0.9 | 0.7 | 0.42 | 0.10 | 38 | 58 | 18 | | | | 0.09 | 0.13 | 4.26 | 0.23 | 1.73 | 3.0 | 0.43 | 0.0 | | | 9 | 0.0 | 0.2 | 27 | 0.0 | 119 | 318 | 23.4 | 18 | 0.32 |
| 17189 | 1 | ea | Spot fish, raw, fillet, avg | 64 | 79 | 76 | 11.8 | 0.0 | 0.0 | 0.0 | 0.0 | 3.1 | 0.9 | 0.9 | 0.7 | 0.42 | 0.10 | 38 | 64 | 19 | 19 | 0 | 0 | 0.10 | 0.14 | 4.48 | 0.26 | 1.92 | 3.2 | 0.48 | 0.0 | | | 9 | 0.0 | 0.2 | 27 | 0.0 | 119 | 317 | 23.4 | 19 | 0.33 |
| 19140 | 3 | oz | Sprats, dried, avg | 85 | 143 | 50 | 21.5 | 0.0 | 0.0 | 0.0 | 0.0 | 6.3 | | | | | | | | | | | | | 0.09 | 2.55 | | 5.87 | 12.8 | | | | | 171 | 3.5 | 1.6 | 62 | | | 128 | | 4429 | 1.62 |
| 17308 | 3 | oz | Sprats, fresh, raw, avg | 85 | 85 | 77 | 16.7 | 0.0 | 0.0 | 0.0 | 0.0 | 1.5 | | | | | | | 57 | 17 | | | | 0.03 | 0.26 | 6.38 | | | | | | | | 33 | | 2.7 | | | | 435 | | 162 | |
| | | | Steelhead | | | | | | | | | | | | | | | | | | | | | | | | | | | | | | | | | | | | | | | | |
| 17023 | 1 | ea | Sea trout, mixed species, baked/broiled, avg | 186 | 247 | 72 | 40.0 | 0.0 | 0.0 | 0.0 | 0.0 | 8.6 | 2.4 | 2.1 | 1.7 | 0.89 | 0.62 | 197 | 214 | 65 | 65 | 0 | 0 | 0.13 | 0.39 | 5.43 | 0.86 | 6.44 | 11.2 | 1.61 | 0.0 | 1.9 | | 41 | 0.1 | 0.7 | 74 | 0.0 | 597 | 813 | 87.0 | 138 | 1.08 |
| 17067 | 1 | ea | Sea trout, mixed species, raw, fillet, avg | 238 | 248 | 78 | 39.7 | 0.0 | 0.0 | 0.0 | 0.0 | 8.6 | 2.4 | 2.1 | 1.7 | 0.89 | 0.62 | 198 | 238 | 71 | 71 | 0 | 0 | 0.14 | 0.40 | 5.71 | 0.95 | 7.14 | 11.9 | 1.79 | 0.0 | 2.4 | | 40 | 0.1 | 0.6 | 74 | 0.0 | 595 | 812 | 86.9 | 138 | 1.07 |
| 17333 | 3 | oz | Sea trout, smoked, avg | 85 | 150 | 63 | 24.2 | 0.0 | 0.0 | 0.0 | 0.0 | 5.3 | 1.5 | 1.3 | 1.1 | | | 121 | 145 | 44 | 44 | 0 | 0 | 0.09 | 0.25 | 3.49 | 0.58 | 4.35 | 7.3 | 1.09 | 0.0 | 1.5 | | 25 | 0.0 | 0.4 | 45 | 0.0 | 363 | 495 | 145.4 | 1700 | 0.65 |
| | | | Sturgeon | | | | | | | | | | | | | | | | | | | | | | | | | | | | | | | | | | | | | | | | |
| 17078 | 1 | cup | Baked/broiled, avg | 136 | 184 | 70 | 28.2 | 0.0 | 0.0 | 0.0 | 0.0 | 7.0 | 1.6 | 3.4 | 1.2 | 0.67 | 0.23 | 105 | 1099 | 329 | 329 | 0 | 0 | 0.11 | 0.12 | 13.74 | 0.31 | 3.40 | 23.5 | 1.18 | 0.0 | | | 23 | 0.1 | 1.2 | 61 | 0.0 | 369 | 495 | 22.0 | 94 | 0.73 |
| 17135 | 3 | oz | Floured/breaded, fried, avg | 85 | 196 | 57 | 14.9 | 6.7 | 0.4 | 0.3 | 6.0 | 11.9 | 2.9 | 5.3 | 2.8 | | | 68 | 514 | 154 | 154 | 0 | | 0.07 | 0.11 | 7.14 | 0.16 | 1.65 | 15.5 | 0.85 | 0.0 | | | 26 | 0.1 | 1.0 | 32 | 0.1 | 194 | 252 | | 307 | 0.45 |
| 17214 | 3 | oz | Raw, mixed species, avg | 85 | 89 | 77 | 13.7 | 0.0 | 0.0 | 0.0 | 0.0 | 3.4 | 0.8 | 1.6 | 0.6 | 0.33 | 0.11 | 51 | 595 | 179 | 179 | 0 | 0 | 0.06 | 0.06 | 7.06 | 0.17 | 1.87 | 12.8 | 0.64 | 0.0 | | | 11 | 0.0 | 0.6 | 30 | 0.0 | 179 | 241 | 10.7 | 46 | 0.36 |
| 17079 | 3 | oz | Smoked, mixed species, avg | 85 | 147 | 62 | 26.5 | 0.0 | 0.0 | 0.0 | 0.0 | 3.7 | 0.9 | 2.0 | 0.4 | 0.25 | 0.10 | 68 | 793 | 238 | 238 | 0 | 0 | 0.08 | 0.08 | 9.44 | 0.23 | 2.47 | 17.0 | 0.85 | 0.0 | | | 14 | 0.0 | 0.8 | 40 | 0.0 | 239 | 322 | 17.1 | 628 | 0.48 |
| 17173 | 1 | ea | Sucker fish, white, baked/broiled, fillet, avg | 124 | 148 | 74 | 26.7 | 0.0 | 0.0 | 0.0 | 0.0 | 3.7 | 0.7 | 1.1 | 1.3 | 0.85 | 0.27 | 66 | 243 | 73 | 73 | 0 | 0 | 0.01 | 0.11 | 1.81 | 0.29 | 2.86 | 21.1 | 1.07 | 0.0 | | | 112 | 0.3 | 2.1 | 47 | 1.0 | 334 | 604 | 20.1 | 63 | 1.19 |
| 17215 | 1 | ea | Sucker fish, white, raw, fillet, avg | 159 | 146 | 80 | 26.7 | 0.0 | 0.0 | 0.0 | 0.0 | 3.7 | 0.7 | 1.1 | 1.3 | 0.84 | 0.27 | 65 | 270 | 81 | 81 | 0 | 0 | 0.02 | 0.11 | 1.91 | 0.32 | 3.18 | 23.9 | 1.19 | 0.0 | | | 111 | 0.3 | 2.1 | 48 | 1.0 | 334 | 604 | 20.0 | 64 | 1.19 |
| | | | Swordfish | | | | | | | | | | | | | | | | | | | | | | | | | | | | | | | | | | | | | | | | |
| 17066 | 1 | pce | Baked/broiled, avg | 106 | 164 | 69 | 26.9 | 0.0 | 0.0 | 0.0 | 0.0 | 5.4 | 1.5 | 2.1 | 1.3 | 1.12 | 0.13 | 53 | 145 | 43 | 43 | 0 | 0 | 0.05 | 0.12 | 12.51 | 0.40 | 2.14 | 2.4 | 0.40 | 1.2 | 1.1 | | 6 | 0.2 | 1.1 | 36 | 0.0 | 357 | 391 | 65.4 | 122 | 1.56 |

| Code | Amount | | Description | Basic Components | | | | | | | | | Additional Fats | | | | | | Vit A & Components | | | | | Vitamins | | | | | | | | | | Minerals | | | | | | | | | |
|---|---|---|---|---|---|---|---|---|---|---|---|---|---|---|---|---|---|---|---|---|---|---|---|---|---|---|---|---|---|---|---|---|---|---|---|---|---|---|---|---|---|---|---|
| | | | | Weight (g) | Calories | % Water | Protein (g) | Carbs (g) | Fiber (g) | Sugar (g) | Other Carbs (g) | Fat (g) | Sat Fat (g) | Mono Fat (g) | Poly Fat (g) | Omega 3 (g) | Omega 6 (g) | Choles (mg) | Vit A (IU) | Vit A (RE) | Retinol (RE) | Carotenoids (RE) | Beta Carotene (mcg) | Thiamin (mg) | Riboflavin (mg) | Niacin (NE) | Vit B6 (mg) | Vit B12 (mcg) | Folate (mcg) | Panto (mg) | Vit C (mg) | Vit D (mg) | Vit E (α TE) | Calcium (mg) | Copper (mg) | Iron (mg) | Magnes (mg) | Mang (mg) | Phos (mg) | Potassium (mg) | Selenium (mcg) | Sodium (mg) | Zinc (mg) |
| 17065 | 1 | pce | Raw, avg | 136 | 165 | 76 | 26.9 | 0.0 | 0.0 | 0.0 | 0.0 | 5.5 | .5 | 2.1 | 1.3 | 1.12 | 0.13 | 53 | 162 | 49 | 49 | 0 | 0 | 0.05 | 0.13 | 13.16 | 0.45 | 2.38 | 2.7 | 0.56 | 1.5 | 1.4 | | 5 | 0.2 | 1.1 | 37 | 0.0 | 358 | 392 | 65.4 | 122 | 1.56 |
| 17136 | 3 | oz | Steamed/poached, avg | 85 | 130 | 69 | 21.3 | 0.0 | 0.0 | 0.0 | 0.0 | 4.3 | .2 | 1.7 | 1.0 | | | 42 | 109 | 33 | 33 | 0 | 0 | 0.03 | 0.09 | 8.86 | 0.28 | 1.60 | 1.7 | 0.34 | 0.9 | 0.9 | | 4 | 0.1 | 0.9 | 26 | 0.0 | 255 | 264 | 42.5 | 87 | 1.24 |
| 17248 | 3 | oz | Tarpon, raw, avg | 85 | 79 | 78 | 17.7 | 0.0 | 0.0 | 0.0 | 0.0 | 0.4 | | | | | | | 495 | 49 | 149 | 0 | 0 | 0.02 | 0.11 | 3.57 | | | | | | | | 67 | | 0.5 | | | 173 | | | | |
| 90068 | 3 | oz | Terripin, raw, avg | 85 | 94 | 77 | 15.8 | 0.0 | 0.0 | 0.0 | 0.0 | 3.0 | 0.0 | | | | 0.00 | 43 | 145 | 43 | 43 | 0 | 0 | 0.01 | 0.03 | 1.28 | | | | | 0.9 | | | 43 | | 2.7 | | | 215 | 243 | | 43 | |
| 17081 | 1 | ea | Tilefish, baked/broiled, fillet, avg | 300 | 441 | 70 | 73.5 | 0.0 | 0.0 | 0.0 | 0.0 | 14.1 | .6 | 4.0 | 3.8 | 2.71 | 0.59 | 192 | 207 | 63 | 63 | 0 | 0 | 0.42 | 0.57 | 10.50 | 0.90 | 7.50 | 51.9 | 2.61 | 0.0 | | | 78 | 0.2 | 0.9 | 99 | 0.0 | 708 | 1536 | 154.5 | 177 | 1.59 |
| 17217 | 1 | ea | Tilefish, raw, fillet, avg | 386 | 371 | 79 | 67.5 | 0.0 | 0.0 | 0.0 | 0.0 | 8.9 | .7 | 2.2 | 2.3 | 1.66 | 0.40 | 193 | 232 | 69 | 69 | 0 | 0 | 0.46 | 0.62 | 11.19 | 1.00 | 8.49 | 57.9 | 2.89 | 0.0 | | | 100 | 0.2 | 1.0 | 108 | 0.0 | 722 | 1671 | 140.9 | 205 | 1.43 |
| | | | Trout | | | | | | | | | | | | | | | | | | | | | | | | | | | | | | | | | | | | | | | | |
| 17138 | 1 | ea | Floured/breaded, fried, avg | 125 | 334 | 51 | 28.7 | 11.8 | 0.7 | 0.6 | 10.6 | 18.4 | .0 | 7.4 | 5.5 | | | 106 | 114 | 34 | 34 | 0 | | 0.41 | 0.48 | 6.25 | 0.24 | 8.74 | 22.8 | 1.00 | 0.5 | 1.3 | | 80 | 0.3 | 2.6 | 34 | 1.0 | 341 | 484 | | 530 | 1.01 |
| 17218 | 1 | ea | Mixed Species, raw, fillet, avg | 79 | 117 | 71 | 16.4 | 0.0 | 0.0 | 0.0 | 0.0 | 5.2 | .9 | 2.6 | 1.2 | 0.70 | 0.29 | 46 | 46 | 13 | 13 | 0 | 0 | 0.28 | 0.26 | 3.56 | 0.16 | 6.15 | 10.5 | 1.53 | 0.4 | | | 34 | 0.1 | 1.2 | 17 | 0.7 | 194 | 285 | 10.0 | 41 | 0.52 |
| 17175 | 1 | ea | Mixed species, baked/broiled, fillet, avg | 62 | 118 | 63 | 16.5 | 0.0 | 0.0 | 0.0 | 0.0 | 5.3 | .9 | 2.6 | 1.2 | 0.70 | 0.29 | 46 | 39 | 12 | 12 | 0 | 0 | 0.26 | 0.26 | 3.58 | 0.14 | 4.64 | 9.3 | 1.39 | 0.3 | 0.6 | | 34 | 0.1 | 1.2 | 17 | 0.7 | 195 | 287 | 10.0 | 42 | 0.53 |
| 17332 | 3 | oz | Rainbow, farmed, smoked, avg | 85 | 157 | 63 | 23.8 | 0.0 | 0.0 | 0.0 | 0.0 | 6.2 | .8 | 1.8 | 2.7 | | | 67 | 317 | 95 | 95 | 0 | 0 | 0.23 | 0.08 | 9.35 | 0.71 | 4.30 | 12.6 | 1.64 | 3.3 | | | | 0.1 | 0.3 | 37 | 0.0 | 321 | 514 | | 1700 | 0.47 |
| | | | Tuna | | | | | | | | | | | | | | | | | | | | | | | | | | | | | | | | | | | | | | | | |
| 17140 | 3 | oz | Floured/breaded, fresh, fried, avg | 85 | 199 | 51 | 20.7 | 6.7 | 0.4 | 0.3 | 5.0 | 9.4 | .4 | 3.9 | 2.4 | | | 56 | 71 | 21 | 21 | 0 | | 0.33 | 0.09 | 8.36 | 0.67 | 0.42 | 5.9 | 0.76 | 0.7 | 3.4 | | 28 | 0.1 | 1.0 | 45 | 0.1 | 177 | 383 | | 293 | 0.53 |
| 17024 | 1 | ea | Light, canned in oil, drained, avg | 171 | 339 | 60 | 49.8 | 0.0 | 0.0 | 0.0 | 0.0 | 14.0 | .6 | 5.0 | 4.9 | 0.35 | 4.58 | 31 | 133 | 39 | 39 | 0 | 0 | 0.06 | 0.21 | 21.20 | 0.19 | 3.76 | 9.1 | 0.63 | 0.0 | 10.1 | | 22 | 0.1 | 2.4 | 53 | 0.0 | 532 | 354 | 130.0 | 605 | 1.54 |
| 17156 | 1 | ea | Light, canned in oil, drained, unsalted, avg | 171 | 339 | 60 | 49.8 | 0.0 | 0.0 | 0.0 | 0.0 | 14.0 | .6 | 5.0 | 4.9 | 0.35 | 4.58 | 31 | 133 | 39 | 39 | 0 | 0 | 0.06 | 0.21 | 21.20 | 0.19 | 3.76 | 9.1 | 0.63 | 0.0 | 10.1 | | 22 | 0.1 | 2.4 | 53 | 0.0 | 532 | 354 | 130.0 | 86 | 1.54 |
| 17027 | 1 | cup | Light, canned in water, drained, avg | 154 | 179 | 74 | 39.3 | 0.0 | 0.0 | 0.0 | 0.0 | 1.3 | .4 | 0.2 | 0.5 | 0.42 | 0.07 | 46 | 86 | 26 | 26 | 0 | 0 | 0.05 | 0.11 | 20.48 | 0.54 | 4.60 | 6.2 | 0.33 | 0.0 | 6.2 | | 17 | 0.1 | 2.4 | 42 | 0.0 | 251 | 365 | 123.8 | 521 | 1.19 |
| 17157 | 1 | ea | Light, canned in water, drained, unsalted, avg | 165 | 191 | 75 | 42.1 | 0.0 | 0.0 | 0.0 | 0.0 | 1.4 | .4 | 0.3 | 0.6 | 0.45 | 0.07 | 49 | 92 | 28 | 28 | 0 | 0 | 0.05 | 0.12 | 21.94 | 0.58 | 4.93 | 6.6 | 0.35 | 0.0 | 6.6 | | 18 | 0.1 | 2.5 | 45 | 0.0 | 269 | 391 | 132.7 | 82 | 1.27 |
| 17141 | 3 | oz | Smoked, fresh, avg | 85 | 186 | 59 | 20.2 | 0.0 | 0.0 | 0.0 | 0.0 | 11.1 | .9 | 4.3 | 3.0 | | | 81 | 133 | 40 | 40 | 0 | 0 | 0.02 | 0.24 | 2.81 | 0.43 | 5.95 | 8.5 | 0.26 | 0.0 | 3.4 | | 56 | 0.1 | 1.2 | 26 | 0.0 | 216 | 255 | | 238 | 0.60 |
| 17083 | 1 | ea | White, canned in oil, drained, avg | 178 | 331 | 64 | 47.2 | 0.0 | 0.0 | 0.0 | 0.0 | 14.4 | .9 | 4.4 | 6.0 | 1.76 | 4.03 | 55 | 142 | 43 | 43 | 0 | 0 | 0.03 | 0.14 | 20.83 | 0.77 | 3.92 | 8.2 | 0.66 | 0.0 | 8.9 | | 7 | 0.2 | 1.2 | 61 | 0.0 | 475 | 593 | 107.0 | 705 | 0.84 |
| 17158 | 1 | ea | White, canned in oil, drained, unsalted, avg | 178 | 331 | 64 | 47.2 | 0.0 | 0.0 | 0.0 | 0.0 | 14.4 | .9 | 4.4 | 6.0 | 1.76 | 4.03 | 55 | 142 | 43 | 43 | 0 | 0 | 0.03 | 0.14 | 20.83 | 0.77 | 3.92 | 8.2 | 0.66 | 0.0 | 8.9 | | 7 | 0.2 | 1.2 | 61 | 0.0 | 475 | 593 | 107.0 | 89 | 0.84 |
| 17151 | 1 | ea | White, canned in water, drained, avg | 172 | 220 | 73 | 40.6 | 0.0 | 0.0 | 0.0 | 0.0 | 5.1 | .4 | 1.3 | 1.9 | 1.60 | 0.18 | 72 | 33 | 10 | 10 | 0 | 0 | 0.01 | 0.08 | 9.98 | 0.37 | 2.01 | 3.4 | 0.21 | 0.0 | 6.9 | | 24 | 0.1 | 1.7 | 57 | 0.0 | 373 | 408 | 113.0 | 648 | 0.83 |
| 17159 | 1 | ea | White, canned in water, drained, unsalted, avg | 172 | 220 | 74 | 40.6 | 0.0 | 0.0 | 0.0 | 0.0 | 5.1 | .4 | 1.3 | 1.9 | 1.60 | 0.18 | 72 | 33 | 10 | 10 | 0 | 0 | 0.01 | 0.08 | 9.98 | 0.37 | 2.01 | 3.4 | 0.21 | 0.0 | 6.9 | | 24 | 0.1 | 1.7 | 57 | 0.0 | 373 | 408 | 113.0 | 86 | 0.83 |
| 17177 | 3 | oz | Yellowfin, fresh, baked/broiled, avg | 85 | 118 | 63 | 25.5 | 0.0 | 0.0 | 0.0 | 0.0 | 1.0 | .3 | 0.2 | 0.3 | 0.25 | 0.04 | 49 | 58 | 17 | 17 | 0 | 0 | 0.43 | 0.05 | 10.11 | 0.88 | 0.51 | 1.7 | 0.74 | 0.9 | | | 18 | 0.1 | 0.8 | 54 | 0.0 | 208 | 484 | 39.8 | 40 | 0.57 |
| 17233 | 3 | oz | Yellowfin, fresh, boneless, raw, avg | 85 | 92 | 71 | 19.9 | 0.0 | 0.0 | 0.0 | 0.0 | 0.8 | .2 | 0.1 | 0.2 | 0.20 | 0.03 | 38 | 50 | 15 | 15 | 0 | 0 | 0.37 | 0.04 | 8.33 | 0.76 | 0.44 | 1.6 | 0.64 | 0.9 | | | 14 | 0.1 | 0.6 | 43 | 0.0 | 162 | 377 | 31.0 | 31 | 0.44 |
| 17161 | 1 | ea | Turbot, baked/broiled, fillet, avg | 318 | 388 | 70 | 65.5 | 0.0 | 0.0 | 0.0 | 0.0 | 12.0 | | | | | | 197 | 127 | 38 | 38 | 0 | 0 | 0.24 | 0.31 | 8.52 | 0.77 | 8.08 | 28.6 | 2.09 | 5.4 | | | 73 | 0.1 | 1.5 | 207 | 0.1 | 525 | 970 | 148.8 | 611 | 0.89 |
| 17220 | 1 | ea | Turbot, raw, fillet, avg | 408 | 388 | 77 | 65.7 | 0.0 | 0.0 | 0.0 | 0.0 | 12.0 | 3.1 | 2.5 | 3.6 | | | 196 | 143 | 45 | 45 | 0 | 0 | 0.27 | 0.33 | 8.98 | 0.86 | 8.98 | 32.6 | 2.33 | 6.9 | | | 73 | 0.2 | 1.5 | 208 | 0.1 | 526 | 971 | 148.9 | 612 | 0.90 |
| 90071 | 3 | oz | Whale, meat, raw, avg | 85 | 133 | 71 | 17.5 | 0.0 | 0.0 | 0.0 | 0.0 | 6.4 | .1 | 3.5 | 1.4 | | 0.17 | 43 | 1581 | 475 | 475 | 0 | 0 | 0.08 | 0.07 | 6.97 | | | | | 5.1 | | | 10 | | 0.9 | | | 122 | 19 | | 66 | |
| | | | Whitefish | | | | | | | | | | | | | | | | | | | | | | | | | | | | | | | | | | | | | | | | |
| 17162 | 1 | ea | Baked/broiled, fillet, avg | 154 | 265 | 65 | 37.7 | 0.0 | 0.0 | 0.0 | 0.0 | 11.6 | .8 | 3.9 | 4.3 | 2.85 | 0.98 | 119 | 202 | 60 | 60 | 0 | 0 | 0.26 | 0.24 | 5.93 | 0.53 | 1.48 | 26.2 | 1.33 | 0.0 | | | 51 | 0.1 | 0.7 | 65 | 0.1 | 533 | 625 | 24.9 | 100 | 1.96 |
| 17221 | 1 | ea | Mixed species, raw, fillet, avg | 158 | 265 | 73 | 37.8 | 0.0 | 0.0 | 0.0 | 0.0 | 11.6 | .8 | 4.0 | 4.3 | 2.85 | 0.98 | 119 | 238 | 71 | 71 | 0 | 0 | 0.28 | 0.24 | 5.94 | 0.59 | 1.98 | 29.7 | 1.49 | 0.0 | | | 51 | 0.1 | 0.7 | 65 | 0.1 | 535 | 628 | 24.9 | 101 | 1.96 |
| 17084 | 1 | cup | Smoked, avg | 136 | 147 | 71 | 31.8 | 0.0 | 0.0 | 0.0 | 0.0 | 1.3 | 0.3 | 0.4 | 0.4 | 0.28 | 0.11 | 45 | 258 | 78 | 78 | 0 | 0 | 0.04 | 0.14 | 3.26 | 0.53 | 4.43 | 9.9 | 0.14 | 0.0 | 1.4 | | 24 | 0.4 | 0.7 | 31 | 0.0 | 180 | 575 | 18.4 | 1386 | 0.67 |
| | | | Whiting | | | | | | | | | | | | | | | | | | | | | | | | | | | | | | | | | | | | | | | | |
| 17144 | 1 | ea | Baked/broiled, mixed species, fillet, avg | 72 | 84 | 75 | 16.9 | 0.0 | 0.0 | 0.0 | 0.0 | 1.2 | 0.3 | 0.3 | 0.4 | 0.38 | 0.03 | 60 | 82 | 24 | 24 | 0 | 0 | 0.05 | 0.04 | 1.20 | 0.13 | 1.87 | 10.8 | 0.18 | 0.0 | | | 45 | 0.0 | 0.3 | 19 | 0.1 | 205 | 312 | 29.6 | 95 | 0.38 |
| 17142 | 1 | ea | Breaded/battered, baked, fillet, avg | 81 | 166 | 61 | 16.2 | 6.6 | 0.4 | 0.3 | 5.9 | 7.9 | .6 | 3.2 | 2.4 | | | 71 | 419 | 113 | 106 | 6 | | 0.08 | 0.09 | 1.45 | 0.13 | 1.87 | 16.7 | 0.24 | 0.0 | | | 55 | 0.0 | 0.7 | 21 | 0.1 | 198 | 220 | | 382 | 0.80 |
| 17222 | 1 | ea | Raw, mixed species, fillet, avg | 92 | 83 | 80 | 16.8 | 0.0 | 0.0 | 0.0 | 0.0 | 1.2 | 0.2 | 0.3 | 0.4 | 0.24 | 0.09 | 62 | 91 | 28 | 28 | 0 | 0 | 0.05 | 0.04 | 1.20 | 0.14 | 2.12 | 12.0 | 0.20 | 0.0 | | | 44 | 0.0 | 0.3 | 19 | 0.1 | 204 | 229 | 29.5 | 66 | 0.81 |
| 17163 | 1 | ea | Wolfish, Atlantic, baked/broiled, fillet, avg | 238 | 293 | 74 | 53.3 | 0.0 | 0.0 | 0.0 | 0.0 | 7.3 | .1 | 2.5 | 2.6 | 1.92 | 0.33 | 140 | 1031 | 309 | 309 | 0 | 0 | 0.50 | 0.23 | 6.19 | 1.10 | 5.59 | 14.3 | 1.57 | 0.0 | | | 19 | 0.1 | 0.3 | 90 | 0.0 | 609 | 916 | 111.4 | 259 | 2.38 |
| 17223 | 1 | ea | Wolfish, Atlantic, raw, fillet, avg | 306 | 294 | 80 | 53.5 | 0.0 | 0.0 | 0.0 | 0.0 | 7.3 | .1 | 2.6 | 2.6 | 1.93 | 0.33 | 141 | 1148 | 346 | 346 | 0 | 0 | 0.55 | 0.24 | 6.52 | 1.22 | 6.21 | 15.3 | 1.74 | 0.0 | | | 18 | 0.1 | 0.3 | 92 | 0.0 | 612 | 918 | 111.7 | 260 | 2.39 |
| 17164 | 1 | ea | Yellowtail fish, baked/broiled, fillet, avg | 292 | 546 | 67 | 86.7 | 0.0 | 0.0 | 0.0 | 0.0 | 19.6 | | | | | | 207 | 304 | 91 | 91 | 0 | 0 | 0.51 | 0.15 | 25.46 | 0.54 | 3.65 | 11.7 | 1.99 | 8.5 | | | 85 | 0.2 | 1.8 | 111 | 0.1 | 587 | 1571 | 136.7 | 146 | 1.96 |
| 17224 | 1 | ea | Yellowtail fish, raw, fillet, avg | 374 | 546 | 74 | 86.4 | 0.0 | 0.0 | 0.0 | 0.0 | 19.6 | .8 | 7.4 | 5.3 | | | 206 | 355 | 108 | 108 | 0 | 0 | 0.54 | 0.15 | 25.43 | 0.60 | 4.86 | 13.8 | 2.21 | 10.5 | | 0.7 | 86 | 0.2 | 1.8 | 112 | 0.1 | 587 | 1571 | 136.5 | 146 | 1.94 |
| | | | *SHELLFISH AND OTHER FISH* | | | | | | | | | | | | | | | | | | | | | | | | | | | | | | | | | | | | | | | | |
| | | | Abalone | | | | | | | | | | | | | | | | | | | | | | | | | | | | | | | | | | | | | | | | |
| 17311 | 3 | oz | Canned, drained, avg | 85 | 123 | 65 | 21.1 | 4.4 | 0.0 | | | 1.7 | | | | | | | 283 | 85 | | | | 0.01 | 0.03 | 2.21 | | | | | | | | 9 | | 7.5 | | | | 94 | | 842 | |
| 19041 | 3 | oz | Fried, avg | 85 | 161 | 60 | 16.7 | 9.4 | 0.0 | 0.2 | 9.2 | 5.8 | .4 | 2.3 | 1.4 | 0.13 | 1.25 | 80 | 4 | 2 | | | | 0.19 | 0.11 | 1.62 | 0.13 | 0.59 | 11.9 | 2.44 | 1.5 | 0.1 | | 31 | 0.2 | 3.2 | 48 | 0.1 | 184 | 241 | 44.0 | 502 | 0.81 |
| 19018 | 3 | oz | Raw, avg | 85 | 89 | 75 | 14.5 | 5.1 | 0.0 | 2.6 | 2.6 | 0.6 | 0.1 | 0.1 | 0.1 | 0.04 | 0.01 | 72 | 4 | 2 | | | | 0.16 | 0.09 | 1.28 | 0.13 | 0.62 | 4.3 | 2.55 | 1.7 | 0.1 | | 26 | 0.2 | 2.7 | 41 | 0.0 | 162 | 213 | 38.1 | 256 | 0.70 |
| 19086 | 3 | oz | Steamed/poached, avg | 85 | 179 | 49 | 29.1 | 10.2 | 0.0 | | | 1.3 | 0.3 | 0.2 | 0.2 | | | 145 | 8 | 3 | 3 | 0 | 0 | 0.29 | 0.13 | 1.91 | 0.22 | 0.74 | 6.4 | 3.83 | 2.6 | 0.2 | | 50 | 0.3 | 4.9 | 70 | 0.1 | 226 | 298 | 57.8 | 435 | 1.39 |
| | | | Clams | | | | | | | | | | | | | | | | | | | | | | | | | | | | | | | | | | | | | | | | |
| 19049 | 15 | ea | Baked/broiled, avg | 150 | 208 | 72 | 22.5 | 4.6 | 0.0 | | | 10.5 | 1.9 | 4.1 | 3.3 | | | 60 | 908 | 253 | 243 | 10 | | 0.13 | 0.30 | 2.94 | 0.10 | 82.41 | 26.8 | 0.45 | 21.7 | 0.2 | | 84 | 0.6 | 24.5 | 16 | 0.8 | 298 | 555 | 72.9 | 621 | 2.40 |
| 19081 | 1 | cup | Breaded, fried, avg | 150 | 303 | 62 | 21.3 | 15.5 | 0.2 | | | 15.8 | .0 | 6.8 | 4.3 | 0.44 | 3.76 | 92 | 453 | 135 | 135 | 0 | 0 | 0.15 | 0.37 | 3.09 | 0.09 | 60.45 | 54.0 | 0.64 | 15.0 | 0.3 | | 94 | 0.5 | 20.8 | 21 | 0.8 | 282 | 489 | 43.3 | 546 | 2.19 |
| 19002 | 1 | cup | Canned, drained, avg | 160 | 237 | 64 | 41.0 | 8.2 | 0.0 | 4.1 | 4.1 | 3.1 | 0.3 | 0.3 | 0.9 | 0.47 | 0.18 | 107 | 912 | 274 | 274 | 0 | 0 | 0.24 | 0.68 | 5.36 | 0.18 | 158.24 | 46.1 | 1.09 | 35.4 | 0.3 | | 147 | 1.1 | 44.8 | 29 | 1.6 | 541 | 1005 | 77.8 | 179 | 4.37 |
| 17325 | 10 | ea | Cooked, small, avg | 70 | 83 | 68 | 18.3 | 0.0 | 0.0 | 0.0 | 0.0 | 1.3 | 0.0 | | | | | 46 | 417 | 125 | 125 | 0 | 0 | | | | | | | | 0.0 | | | 50 | | 9.0 | | | | 442 | | 79 | |
| 19110 | 1 | cup | Fried in crumbs, avg | 153 | 600 | 29 | 17.1 | 51.7 | | | | 35.2 | 3.8 | 15.2 | 9.0 | | | 116 | 162 | 49 | 49 | 0 | 0 | 0.28 | 0.35 | 3.81 | 0.05 | 1.47 | 56.6 | 0.40 | 0.0 | | | 28 | 0.1 | 4.1 | 41 | 0.4 | 317 | 353 | 12.7 | 1109 | 2.17 |
| 19105 | 3 | oz | Raw, razor, avg | 85 | 37 | 88 | 6.8 | 1.2 | | | | 0.3 | | | | | | | | | | | | | 0.05 | 1.53 | | | | | | | | 131 | | 6.9 | | | 86 | | | | |
| 19051 | 10 | ea | Smoked, in oil, avg | 100 | 175 | 69 | 14.2 | 2.9 | 0.0 | 1.4 | 1.4 | 11.6 | 2.7 | 4.8 | 3.1 | | | 38 | 334 | 100 | 100 | 0 | 0 | 0.09 | 0.24 | 1.96 | 0.07 | 54.98 | 17.8 | 0.40 | 13.7 | 0.1 | | 51 | 0.4 | 15.6 | 10 | 0.5 | 188 | 349 | | 321 | 1.52 |
| 19000 | 10 | ea | Steamed, avg | 95 | 141 | 64 | 24.3 | 4.9 | 0.0 | 2.4 | 2.4 | 1.9 | 0.2 | 0.2 | 0.5 | 0.28 | 0.11 | 64 | 542 | 162 | 162 | 0 | 0 | 0.14 | 0.40 | 3.18 | 0.10 | 93.96 | 27.4 | 0.65 | 21.0 | 0.2 | | 87 | 0.7 | 26.6 | 17 | 0.9 | 321 | 597 | 60.8 | 106 | 2.59 |
| 19119 | 1 | cup | Minced, Progresso | 240 | 100 | 88 | 16.0 | 8.0 | 0.0 | 0.0 | 8.0 | 0.0 | 0.0 | 0.0 | 0.0 | 0.00 | 0.00 | 40 | 0 | 0 | 0 | 0 | 0 | | | | | | | | 0.0 | | | 0 | | 2.9 | | | | | | 1000 | |
| | | | Crab | | | | | | | | | | | | | | | | | | | | | | | | | | | | | | | | | | | | | | | | |
| 19094 | 1 | ea | Alaskan king, leg, raw, avg | 172 | 144 | 80 | 31.5 | 0.0 | 0.0 | 0.0 | 0.0 | 1.0 | 0.2 | 0.1 | 0.2 | 0.18 | 0.03 | 72 | 41 | 12 | 12 | 0 | 0 | 0.07 | 0.07 | 1.89 | 0.26 | 15.48 | 75.7 | 0.60 | 12.0 | | | 79 | 1.6 | 1.0 | 84 | 0.1 | 377 | 351 | 62.6 | 1438 | 10.23 |
| 19036 | 1 | ea | Alaskan king, leg, steamed/boiled, avg | 134 | 130 | 78 | 26.0 | 0.0 | 0.0 | 0.0 | 0.0 | 2.1 | 0.2 | 0.2 | 0.7 | 0.57 | 0.08 | 71 | 39 | 12 | 12 | 0 | 0 | 0.07 | 0.07 | 1.80 | 0.24 | 15.41 | 63.3 | 0.54 | 10.2 | 0.1 | | 79 | 1.6 | 1.0 | 84 | 0.1 | 375 | 351 | 53.6 | 1436 | 10.21 |
| 19052 | 1 | cup | Baked/broiled, sauteed, avg | 118 | 163 | 73 | 22.5 | 0.1 | 0.0 | | | 7.5 | 1.3 | 2.8 | 2.5 | | | 111 | 297 | 77 | 71 | 6 | | 0.11 | 0.06 | 3.65 | 0.20 | 8.07 | 56.2 | 0.48 | 3.7 | 0.1 | | 117 | 0.7 | 1.0 | 37 | 0.2 | 229 | 361 | 47.4 | 637 | 4.66 |
| 19124 | 1 | cup | Blue, canned, drained, avg | 135 | 134 | 76 | 27.7 | 0.0 | 0.0 | 0.0 | 0.0 | 1.7 | 0.3 | 0.3 | 0.5 | 0.49 | 0.10 | 120 | 7 | 3 | | | | 0.11 | 0.11 | 1.85 | 0.20 | 0.62 | 57.4 | 0.49 | 3.6 | 0.1 | | 136 | 1.0 | 1.1 | 53 | 0.3 | 351 | 505 | 42.9 | 450 | 5.43 |
| 19095 | 1 | ea | Blue, raw, avg | 21 | 18 | 79 | 3.8 | 0.0 | 0.0 | | | 0.2 | 0.0 | 0.0 | 0.1 | 0.07 | 0.01 | 16 | 1 | 0.4 | | | | 0.02 | 0.01 | 0.57 | 0.03 | 1.89 | 9.2 | 0.07 | 0.6 | | | 19 | 0.1 | 0.2 | 7 | 0.0 | 48 | 69 | 7.9 | 62 | 0.74 |
| 19033 | 1 | cup | Blue, steamed/boiled, avg | 118 | 120 | 77 | 23.8 | 0.0 | 0.0 | 0.0 | 0.0 | 2.1 | 0.3 | 0.3 | 0.3 | 0.58 | 0.13 | 118 | 7 | 2 | 2 | 0 | 0 | 0.12 | 0.06 | 3.89 | 0.21 | 8.61 | 59.9 | 0.51 | 3.9 | 0.1 | | 123 | 0.8 | 1.1 | 39 | 0.2 | 243 | 382 | 47.4 | 329 | 4.98 |
| 19079 | 1 | cup | Deviled, avg | 175 | 343 | 61 | 22.4 | 24.7 | 1.4 | | | 17.2 | 3.5 | 7.0 | 5.2 | | | 163 | 1168 | 242 | 189 | 53 | | 0.22 | 0.25 | 4.11 | 0.24 | 6.34 | 61.6 | | 11.7 | | | 140 | 0.7 | 2.2 | 46 | | 252 | 511 | | 1153 | 3.98 |
| 19096 | 1 | ea | Dungeness, raw, avg | 163 | 140 | 79 | 28.4 | 1.2 | 0.0 | | | 1.6 | 0.2 | 0.3 | 0.5 | 0.50 | 0.00 | 96 | 147 | 44 | 44 | 0 | 0 | 0.08 | 0.27 | 5.12 | 0.24 | 14.67 | 71.7 | 0.57 | 5.7 | | | 75 | 1.1 | 0.6 | 73 | 0.1 | 297 | 577 | 60.5 | 481 | 6.96 |
| 19004 | 1 | ea | Dungeness, steamed/boiled, avg | 127 | 140 | 73 | 28.3 | 1.2 | 0.0 | 0.6 | 0.6 | 1.6 | 0.2 | 0.3 | 0.5 | 0.50 | 0.00 | 97 | 132 | 39 | 39 | 0 | 0 | 0.07 | 0.26 | 4.60 | 0.22 | 13.21 | 53.3 | 0.51 | 4.6 | 0.1 | | 75 | 0.9 | 0.5 | 74 | 0.1 | 222 | 518 | 60.5 | 480 | 6.95 |
| 19097 | 3 | oz | Queen, raw, avg | 85 | 77 | 81 | 15.7 | 0.0 | 0.0 | 0.0 | 0.0 | 1.0 | 0.1 | 0.2 | 0.4 | 0.32 | 0.03 | 47 | 128 | 38 | 38 | 0 | 0 | 0.07 | 0.17 | 2.13 | 0.13 | 7.65 | 37.4 | 0.30 | 6.0 | | | 22 | 0.5 | 2.1 | 42 | 0.0 | 113 | 147 | 29.4 | 458 | 2.38 |
| 19083 | 3 | oz | Queen, steamed/boiled, avg | 85 | 98 | 75 | 20.1 | 0.0 | 0.0 | 0.0 | 0.0 | 1.3 | 0.2 | 0.3 | 0.5 | 0.41 | 0.04 | 60 | 147 | 44 | 44 | 0 | 0 | 0.08 | 0.21 | 2.46 | 0.15 | 8.84 | 35.7 | 0.34 | 6.1 | 0.0 | | 28 | 0.5 | 2.4 | 54 | 0.0 | 109 | 170 | 37.7 | 587 | 3.05 |
| 19055 | 1 | ea | Soft shell, floured/breaded, fried, avg | 65 | 217 | 41 | 13.2 | 11.3 | 0.5 | 0.6 | 10.3 | 13.0 | 3.2 | 5.4 | 3.4 | | | 80 | 47 | 14 | 14 | 0 | | 0.13 | 0.12 | 2.43 | 0.10 | 3.34 | 28.0 | 0.32 | 1.4 | 0.1 | | 71 | 0.4 | 1.2 | 23 | 0.2 | 141 | 203 | | 335 | 2.41 |
| 19087 | 10 | ea | Crayfish, mixed species, raw, avg | 34 | 24 | 84 | 5.1 | 0.0 | 0.0 | 0.0 | 0.0 | 0.3 | 0.1 | 0.1 | 0.1 | 0.06 | 0.04 | 36 | 17 | 5 | 5 | 0 | 0 | 0.02 | 0.01 | 0.64 | 0.03 | 0.71 | 10.2 | 0.19 | 0.2 | | | 9 | 0.1 | 0.2 | 10 | 0.0 | 74 | 89 | 9.7 | 21 | 0.34 |
| 19088 | 3 | oz | Crayfish, mixed species, steamed/boiled, avg | 85 | 74 | 81 | 14.9 | 0.0 | 0.0 | 0.0 | 0.0 | 1.1 | 0.2 | 0.2 | 0.4 | 0.16 | 0.19 | 116 | 43 | 13 | 13 | 0 | 0 | 0.04 | 0.07 | 1.42 | 0.11 | 2.63 | 9.4 | 0.44 | 0.4 | | | 43 | 0.5 | 0.9 | 28 | 0.2 | 205 | 202 | 29.1 | 82 | 1.26 |

| Code | Amount | Description | Basic Components | | | | | | | | | Additional Fats | | | | | | Vit A & Components | | | | | Vitamins | | | | | | | | | | Minerals | | | | | | | | | |
|---|---|---|---|---|---|---|---|---|---|---|---|---|---|---|---|---|---|---|---|---|---|---|---|---|---|---|---|---|---|---|---|---|---|---|---|---|---|---|---|---|---|---|
| | | | Weight (g) | Calories | % Water | Protein (g) | Carbs (g) | Fiber (g) | Sugar (g) | Other Carbs (g) | Fat (g) | Sat Fat (g) | Mono Fat (g) | Poly Fat (g) | Omega 3 (g) | Omega 6 (g) | Choles (mg) | Vit A (IU) | Vit A (RE) | Retinol (RE) | Carotenoids (RE) | Beta Carotene (mcg) | Thiamin (mg) | Riboflavin (mg) | Niacin (NE) | Vit B6 (mg) | Vit B12 (mcg) | Folate (mcg) | Panto (mg) | Vit C (mg) | Vit D (mg) | Vit E (α TE) | Calcium (mg) | Copper (mg) | Iron (mg) | Magnes (mg) | Mang (mg) | Phos (mg) | Potassium (mg) | Selenium (mcg) | Sodium (mg) | Zinc (mg) |
| | | Eel | | | | | | | | | | | | | | | | | | | | | | | | | | | | | | | | | | | | | | | | |
| 17102 | 1 ea | Baked/broiled, fillet, avg | 159 | 375 | 59 | 37.7 | 0.0 | 0.0 | 0.0 | 0.0 | 23.9 | 4.8 | 14.7 | 1.9 | 1.18 | 0.59 | 256 | 6021 | 1806 | 1806 | 0 | 0 | 0.29 | 0.08 | 7.14 | 0.12 | 4.60 | 27.5 | 0.45 | 2.9 | 8.0 | | 41 | 0.0 | 1.0 | 41 | 0.1 | 440 | 555 | 13.2 | 103 | 3.31 |
| 17232 | 1 ea | Raw, fillet, avg | 204 | 375 | 68 | 37.5 | 0.0 | 0.0 | 0.0 | 0.0 | 23.9 | 4.8 | 14.7 | 1.9 | 1.18 | 0.59 | 257 | 7089 | 2128 | 2128 | 0 | 0 | 0.31 | 0.08 | 7.14 | 0.14 | 6.12 | 30.6 | 0.49 | 3.7 | | | 41 | 0.0 | 1.0 | 41 | 0.1 | 441 | 555 | 13.3 | 104 | 3.30 |
| 17041 | 3 oz | Smoked, avg | 85 | 281 | 50 | 15.8 | 0.0 | 0.0 | 0.0 | 0.0 | 23.6 | 5.5 | 12.6 | 3.8 | | | 54 | 1368 | 411 | 411 | 0 | 0 | 0.19 | 0.31 | 1.19 | 0.34 | 6.80 | 7.7 | 0.13 | 0.0 | 76.5 | | 15 | 0.1 | 0.6 | 21 | 0.0 | 172 | 359 | 17.0 | 88 | 3.40 |
| 17130 | 1 cup | Steamed/poached, avg | 123 | 283 | 60 | 28.4 | 0.0 | 0.0 | 0.0 | 0.0 | 17.9 | 3.6 | 11.1 | 1.5 | | | 194 | 4541 | 1363 | 1363 | 0 | 0 | 0.00 | 0.06 | 4.57 | 0.08 | 3.92 | 18.5 | 0.25 | 2.1 | 6.2 | | 31 | 0.0 | 0.8 | 27 | 0.0 | 299 | 355 | | 70 | 2.49 |
| 19107 | 1 oz | Jelly fish, dry, avg | 28 | 20 | 68 | 2.0 | 2.5 | | | | 0.1 | | | | | | | | | | | | 0.00 | 0.01 | | | | | | | | | 52 | | 0.4 | | | 17 | | | | |
| 19071 | 1 cup | Jelly fish, pickled, avg | 58 | 21 | 68 | 3.2 | 0.0 | 0.0 | 0.0 | 0.0 | 0.8 | 0.2 | 0.1 | 0.3 | | | 3 | 3 | 1 | 1 | 0 | 0 | 0.01 | 0.01 | 0.12 | 0.01 | 0.01 | 0.6 | | 0.0 | | | 1 | 0.1 | 1.3 | 1 | | 12 | 2 | | 5620 | 0.24 |
| | | Lobster | | | | | | | | | | | | | | | | | | | | | | | | | | | | | | | | | | | | | | | | |
| 19057 | 1 cup | Baked/broiled, avg | 145 | 168 | 74 | 28.8 | 1.8 | 0.0 | | | 4.4 | 2.4 | 1.2 | 0.3 | | | 110 | 255 | 69 | 66 | 4 | | 0.01 | 0.09 | 1.50 | 0.11 | 4.35 | 15.6 | 0.40 | 0.0 | 0.2 | | 87 | 2.7 | 0.6 | 49 | 0.1 | 260 | 493 | 111.7 | 902 | 4.08 |
| 19076 | 1 cup | Battered, fried, avg | 145 | 306 | 60 | 27.6 | 11.3 | 0.3 | 0.7 | 10.3 | 16.1 | 3.9 | 6.7 | 4.4 | | | 116 | 129 | 39 | 39 | 0 | | 0.09 | 0.16 | 1.90 | 0.10 | 3.45 | 16.0 | 0.39 | 0.1 | | | 109 | 2.4 | 1.1 | 48 | 0.1 | 265 | 474 | | 557 | 3.82 |
| 19023 | 1 ea | Northern, raw, avg | 150 | 135 | 77 | 28.2 | 0.8 | 0.0 | | | 1.3 | 0.3 | 0.4 | 0.2 | 0.00 | 0.00 | 142 | 107 | 32 | 32 | 0 | 0 | 0.01 | 0.07 | 2.19 | 0.09 | 1.39 | 13.7 | 2.44 | 0.0 | 0.2 | | 72 | 2.5 | 0.5 | 40 | 0.1 | 216 | 412 | 62.1 | 444 | 4.53 |
| 19006 | 1 cup | Northern, steamed/boiled, avg | 145 | 142 | 76 | 29.7 | 1.9 | 0.0 | | | 0.9 | 0.2 | 0.2 | 0.1 | 0.12 | 0.01 | 104 | 126 | 38 | 38 | 0 | 0 | 0.01 | 0.10 | 1.55 | 0.11 | 4.51 | 16.1 | 0.41 | 0.0 | 0.1 | | 88 | 2.8 | 0.6 | 51 | 0.1 | 268 | 510 | 61.9 | 551 | 4.23 |
| 19098 | 1 ea | Spiny, raw, avg | 209 | 234 | 74 | 43.1 | 5.1 | 0.0 | | | 3.2 | 0.5 | 0.6 | 1.2 | 0.80 | 0.35 | 146 | 36 | 10 | 10 | 0 | 0 | 0.01 | 0.10 | 8.88 | 0.31 | 7.31 | 1.3 | 0.73 | 4.2 | | | 102 | 0.8 | 2.5 | 84 | 0.0 | 497 | 376 | 96.6 | 370 | 11.85 |
| 19084 | 1 ea | Spiny, steamed/boiled, avg | 163 | 233 | 67 | 43.0 | 5.1 | 0.0 | | | 3.2 | 0.5 | 0.6 | 1.2 | 0.80 | 0.35 | 147 | 33 | 10 | 10 | 0 | 0 | 0.01 | 0.09 | 7.99 | 0.28 | 6.59 | 1.6 | 0.66 | 3.4 | | | 103 | 0.7 | 2.3 | 83 | 0.0 | 373 | 339 | 96.5 | 370 | 11.85 |
| | | Mussels | | | | | | | | | | | | | | | | | | | | | | | | | | | | | | | | | | | | | | | | |
| 19024 | 1 cup | Blue, raw, avg | 150 | 129 | 81 | 17.8 | 5.5 | 0.0 | 2.8 | 2.8 | 3.4 | 0.6 | 0.8 | 0.9 | 0.69 | 0.13 | 42 | 240 | 72 | 72 | 0 | 0 | 0.24 | 0.31 | 2.40 | 0.08 | 18.00 | 63.0 | 0.75 | 12.0 | 0.0 | | 39 | 0.1 | 5.9 | 51 | 5.1 | 296 | 480 | 67.2 | 429 | 2.40 |
| 19044 | 3 oz | Blue, steamed/boiled, avg | 85 | 146 | 61 | 20.2 | 6.3 | 0.0 | 3.1 | 3.1 | 3.8 | 0.7 | 0.9 | 1.0 | 0.70 | 0.15 | 48 | 258 | 77 | 77 | 0 | 0 | 0.26 | 0.36 | 2.55 | 0.09 | 20.40 | 64.3 | 0.81 | 11.6 | | | 28 | 0.1 | 5.7 | 31 | 5.8 | 242 | 228 | 76.2 | 314 | 2.27 |
| 19102 | 1 cup | Smoked, canned in oil, drained, avg | 150 | 292 | 62 | 31.2 | 6.6 | 0.0 | 0.0 | 6.6 | 15.6 | | | | | | 138 | 1089 | 180 | 107 | 74 | | | 0.72 | 3.45 | | | | | 0.0 | | | 102 | | 14.1 | 147 | | | 207 | | 682 | 5.55 |
| | | Octopus | | | | | | | | | | | | | | | | | | | | | | | | | | | | | | | | | | | | | | | | |
| 19072 | 1 cup | Dried, avg | 53 | 179 | 20 | 30.4 | 6.0 | 0.0 | | | 2.7 | 0.7 | 0.2 | 1.0 | | | 454 | 58 | 18 | 18 | 0 | 0 | 0.04 | 0.80 | 4.24 | 0.10 | 2.41 | 9.1 | | 7.8 | | | 63 | 3.7 | 1.3 | 64 | 0.1 | 431 | 480 | | 313 | 2.98 |
| 19058 | 1 cup | Dried, boiled, avg | 107 | 196 | 57 | 33.1 | 6.6 | 0.0 | | | 2.9 | 0.8 | 0.2 | 1.1 | 0.73 | 0.22 | 495 | 63 | 19 | 19 | 0 | 0 | 0.04 | 0.88 | 4.63 | 0.11 | 2.63 | 9.9 | | 8.5 | | | 68 | 4.0 | 1.4 | 71 | 0.1 | 471 | 523 | | 341 | 3.26 |
| 19025 | 3 oz | Raw, avg | 85 | 70 | 80 | 12.7 | 1.9 | 0.0 | | | 0.9 | 0.2 | 0.1 | 0.2 | 0.13 | 0.04 | 41 | 128 | 38 | 38 | 0 | 0 | 0.03 | 0.03 | 1.78 | 0.31 | 17.00 | 13.6 | 0.43 | 4.3 | 0.0 | | 45 | 0.4 | 4.5 | 26 | 0.0 | 158 | 298 | 38.1 | 196 | 1.43 |
| 19059 | 3 oz | Smoked, avg | 85 | 119 | 66 | 21.6 | 3.2 | 0.0 | | | 1.5 | 0.3 | 0.2 | 0.3 | 0.23 | 0.07 | 70 | 196 | 59 | 59 | 0 | 0 | 0.04 | 0.06 | 3.04 | 0.50 | 27.51 | 22.0 | 0.60 | 6.2 | 0.0 | | 77 | 0.6 | 7.7 | 43 | 0.0 | 269 | 507 | | 333 | 2.43 |
| 19048 | 3 oz | Steamed/boiled, avg | 85 | 139 | 60 | 25.3 | 3.7 | 0.0 | | | 1.8 | 0.4 | 0.3 | 0.4 | 0.27 | 0.08 | 82 | 230 | 69 | 69 | 0 | 0 | 0.05 | 0.06 | 3.21 | 0.55 | 30.60 | 20.4 | 0.76 | 6.8 | | | 90 | 0.6 | 8.1 | 51 | 0.0 | 237 | 536 | 76.2 | 391 | 2.86 |
| | | Oysters | | | | | | | | | | | | | | | | | | | | | | | | | | | | | | | | | | | | | | | | |
| 19027 | 10 ea | Eastern, boiled/steamed, avg | 70 | 96 | 70 | 9.9 | 5.5 | 0.0 | 0.0 | 5.5 | 3.4 | 1.1 | 0.4 | 1.4 | 0.85 | 0.19 | 73 | 126 | 38 | 38 | 0 | 0 | 0.13 | 0.13 | 1.74 | 0.08 | 24.50 | 9.8 | 0.25 | 4.2 | 11.2 | | 63 | 5.3 | 8.4 | 66 | 0.5 | 142 | 197 | 50.1 | 295 | 127.40 |
| 19135 | 1 ea | Eastern, canned w/liquid, avg | 272 | 3152 | 85 | 19.2 | 10.6 | 0.0 | 0.0 | 10.6 | 6.7 | 1.7 | 0.7 | 2.0 | 1.29 | 0.32 | 150 | 816 | 245 | 245 | 0 | 0 | 0.41 | 0.45 | 3.37 | 0.26 | 51.95 | 24.2 | 0.49 | 13.6 | 21.8 | | 122 | 12.1 | 18.2 | 147 | 1.2 | 378 | 623 | 97.4 | 305 | 247.52 |
| 19090 | 10 ea | Eastern, medium, baked/broiled, avg | 98 | 77 | 82 | 6.9 | 7.1 | 0.0 | | | 2.1 | 0.7 | 0.2 | 0.7 | 0.49 | 0.09 | 37 | 62 | 19 | 19 | 0 | 0 | 0.13 | 0.05 | 1.75 | 0.07 | 23.81 | 23.5 | 0.19 | 5.9 | | | 55 | 1.4 | 7.6 | 32 | 0.4 | 113 | 149 | 76.0 | 160 | 44.30 |
| 19009 | 10 ea | Eastern, medium, breaded, fried, avg | 147 | 290 | 65 | 12.9 | 17.1 | 0.2 | 0.7 | 16.2 | 18.5 | 4.7 | 6.9 | 4.9 | 0.85 | 3.69 | 119 | 444 | 132 | 132 | 0 | 0 | 0.22 | 0.30 | 2.43 | 0.09 | 22.93 | 45.6 | 0.40 | 5.6 | 19.4 | | 91 | 6.3 | 10.2 | 85 | 0.7 | 234 | 359 | 97.8 | 613 | 128.04 |
| 19089 | 10 ea | Eastern, medium, raw, avg | 142 | 84 | 86 | 7.4 | 7.9 | 0.0 | | | 2.2 | 0.6 | 0.2 | 0.8 | 0.62 | 0.09 | 35 | 36 | 11 | 11 | 0 | 0 | 0.15 | 0.09 | 1.80 | 0.09 | 23.00 | 25.6 | 0.22 | 6.7 | | | 62 | 1.0 | 8.2 | 47 | 0.6 | 132 | 176 | 90.5 | 253 | 53.82 |
| 19045 | 1 ea | Pacific, raw, avg | 50 | 40 | 82 | 4.7 | 2.5 | 0.0 | 0.0 | 2.5 | 1.1 | 0.3 | 0.2 | 0.4 | 0.36 | 0.04 | 25 | 135 | 41 | 41 | 0 | | 0.03 | 0.12 | 1.00 | 0.03 | 8.00 | 5.0 | 0.25 | 4.0 | 4.0 | | 4 | 0.8 | 2.6 | 11 | 0.3 | 81 | 84 | 38.5 | 53 | 8.30 |
| 19008 | 1 ea | Pacific, steamed/boiled, avg | 25 | 41 | 64 | 4.7 | 2.5 | 0.0 | | | 1.1 | 0.3 | 0.2 | 0.4 | 0.36 | 0.04 | 25 | 122 | 37 | 37 | 0 | | 0.03 | 0.11 | 0.90 | 0.02 | 7.20 | 3.8 | 0.22 | 3.2 | 3.9 | | 4 | 0.7 | 2.3 | 11 | 0.3 | 61 | 76 | 38.5 | 53 | 8.30 |
| 17149 | 1 Tbs | Roe, sea urchin, avg | 12 | 17 | 74 | 2.0 | 0.0 | 0.0 | 0.0 | 0.0 | 1.0 | 0.2 | 0.3 | 0.4 | | | 37 | 12 | 4 | 4 | 0 | 0 | 0.01 | 0.09 | 0.17 | 0.02 | 1.20 | 9.6 | 0.12 | 1.7 | | | 4 | 0.0 | 0.1 | 2 | 0.0 | 48 | 16 | | 9 | 0.12 |
| | | Scallops | | | | | | | | | | | | | | | | | | | | | | | | | | | | | | | | | | | | | | | | |
| 19061 | 4 ea | Baked/broiled, avg | 100 | 133 | 70 | 21.2 | 2.9 | 0.0 | | | 4.0 | 0.7 | 1.4 | 1.3 | 0.97 | 0.13 | 40 | 210 | 56 | 53 | 3 | | 0.01 | 0.06 | 1.32 | 0.17 | 1.75 | 18.4 | 0.14 | 3.4 | 0.1 | | 30 | 0.1 | 0.4 | 68 | 0.1 | 265 | 390 | | 511 | 1.14 |
| 19070 | 10 ea | Battered, fried, avg | 80 | 184 | 55 | 14.1 | 10.6 | 0.4 | 0.6 | 9.6 | 9.1 | 2.2 | 3.7 | 2.3 | | | 66 | 96 | 29 | 29 | 0 | 0 | 0.07 | 0.14 | 1.34 | 0.11 | 0.98 | 15.1 | 0.16 | 1.6 | 0.2 | | 29 | 0.1 | 0.9 | 42 | 0.1 | 182 | 247 | | 374 | 0.84 |
| 19030 | 4 ea | Breaded, fried, avg | 62 | 133 | 58 | 11.2 | 6.3 | 0.1 | 0.2 | 6.0 | 6.8 | 1.7 | 2.8 | 1.8 | 0.21 | 1.53 | 38 | 47 | 14 | 14 | 0 | 0 | 0.03 | 0.07 | 0.94 | 0.09 | 0.82 | 22.9 | 0.12 | 1.4 | 0.1 | | 26 | 0.0 | 0.5 | 37 | 0.1 | 146 | 206 | 16.7 | 288 | 0.66 |
| 19137 | 4 ea | Raw, avg | 60 | 53 | 79 | 10.1 | 1.4 | 0.0 | | | 0.5 | 0.0 | 0.0 | 0.2 | 0.12 | 0.02 | 20 | 30 | 9 | 9 | 0 | 0 | 0.01 | 0.04 | 0.69 | 0.09 | 0.92 | 9.6 | 0.09 | 1.8 | 0.1 | | 14 | 0.0 | 0.2 | 34 | 0.1 | 131 | 193 | 13.3 | 97 | 0.57 |
| 19011 | 1 cup | Steamed/boiled, avg | 120 | 127 | 76 | 19.4 | 2.8 | 0.0 | | | 3.8 | 0.7 | 1.3 | 1.2 | 0.93 | 0.13 | 38 | 204 | 55 | 51 | 3 | | 0.01 | 0.07 | 1.20 | 0.17 | 1.59 | 13.9 | 0.21 | 2.8 | 0.1 | | 29 | 0.1 | 0.3 | 65 | 0.1 | 191 | 337 | 97.9 | 492 | 1.10 |
| | | Shrimp | | | | | | | | | | | | | | | | | | | | | | | | | | | | | | | | | | | | | | | | |
| 19065 | 4 ea | Baked/broiled, sauteed, avg | 20 | 31 | 67 | 4.9 | 0.2 | 0.0 | | | 1.0 | 0.2 | 0.3 | 0.4 | 0.26 | 0.06 | 37 | 69 | 19 | 19 | 1 | | 0.01 | 0.01 | 0.58 | 0.02 | 0.27 | 0.7 | 0.06 | 0.5 | 0.7 | | 13 | 0.1 | 0.6 | 9 | 0.0 | 50 | 45 | 7.9 | 99 | 0.27 |
| 19012 | 4 ea | Boiled, avg | 22 | 22 | 77 | 4.6 | 0.0 | 0.0 | 0.0 | 0.0 | 0.2 | 0.1 | 0.0 | 0.1 | 0.07 | 0.02 | 43 | 48 | 15 | 15 | 0 | 0 | 0.01 | 0.01 | 0.57 | 0.03 | 0.33 | 0.8 | 0.07 | 0.5 | 0.8 | | 9 | 0.0 | 0.7 | 7 | 0.0 | 30 | 40 | 8.7 | 49 | 0.34 |
| 19014 | 4 ea | Breaded, fried, avg | 30 | 73 | 53 | 6.4 | 3.5 | 0.1 | 0.1 | 3.2 | 3.7 | 0.6 | 1.1 | 1.5 | 0.15 | 1.37 | 53 | 57 | 17 | 17 | 0 | 0 | 0.04 | 0.04 | 0.92 | 0.03 | 0.56 | 2.4 | 0.11 | 0.5 | 1.2 | | 20 | 0.1 | 0.4 | 12 | 0.0 | 65 | 68 | 12.5 | 103 | 0.41 |
| 19120 | 1 ea | Breaded, Garlic & Herb, Mrs Paul's | 156 | 340 | | 19.0 | 33.0 | 3.0 | 4.0 | 26.0 | 15.0 | 3.0 | | | | | 110 | 0 | 0 | 0 | 0 | 0 | | | | | | | | 0.0 | | | 250 | | 0.7 | | | | | | 910 | |
| 19127 | 1 ea | Canned, drained, avg | 128 | 154 | 73 | 29.6 | 1.3 | 0.0 | | | 2.5 | 0.5 | 0.4 | 1.0 | 0.72 | 0.17 | 221 | 77 | 23 | 23 | 0 | 0 | 0.03 | 0.05 | 3.53 | 0.14 | 1.43 | 2.3 | 0.28 | 2.9 | 5.5 | | 76 | 0.4 | 3.5 | 52 | 0.1 | 298 | 269 | 50.7 | 216 | 1.61 |
| 19077 | 20 ea | Dried, avg | 10 | 30 | 31 | 5.8 | 0.3 | 0.0 | | | 0.5 | 0.1 | 0.1 | 0.2 | | | 44 | 15 | 5 | 5 | 0 | 0 | 0.01 | 0.01 | 0.70 | 0.03 | 0.28 | 0.5 | 0.07 | 0.6 | 1.0 | | 15 | 0.1 | 0.7 | 10 | 0.0 | 59 | 53 | | 43 | 0.32 |
| 19125 | 4 ea | Raw, avg | 24 | 25 | 76 | 4.9 | 0.2 | 0.0 | | | 0.4 | 0.1 | 0.1 | 0.2 | 0.12 | 0.03 | 36 | 43 | 13 | 13 | 0 | 0 | 0.01 | 0.01 | 0.61 | 0.02 | 0.28 | 0.7 | 0.07 | 0.5 | 0.9 | | 12 | 0.1 | 0.6 | 9 | 0.0 | 49 | 44 | 9.1 | 36 | 0.27 |
| 19067 | 4 ea | Snails, steamed, avg | 20 | 36 | 58 | 6.4 | 0.8 | 0.0 | 0.4 | 0.4 | 0.6 | 0.2 | 0.2 | 0.1 | | | 20 | 36 | 11 | 11 | 0 | 0 | 0.00 | 0.04 | 0.42 | 0.04 | 0.12 | 1.8 | 0.04 | 0.0 | | | 4 | 0.1 | 1.3 | 85 | 0.1 | 76 | 107 | | 24 | 0.40 |
| | | Squid | | | | | | | | | | | | | | | | | | | | | | | | | | | | | | | | | | | | | | | | |
| 19068 | 1 cup | Baked/broiled, avg | 140 | 193 | 70 | 26.3 | 5.2 | 0.0 | | | 6.6 | 1.4 | 2.1 | 2.2 | | | 393 | 269 | 71 | 67 | 5 | | 0.03 | 0.56 | 3.49 | 0.09 | 2.09 | 7.9 | 0.70 | 7.5 | | | 56 | 3.2 | 1.2 | 56 | 0.1 | 374 | 417 | | 518 | 2.58 |
| 19103 | 3 oz | Boiled, avg | 85 | 72 | 80 | 14.8 | 0.0 | 0.0 | 0.0 | 0.0 | 1.0 | | | | | | | 354 | 106 | | | 0 | 0.01 | 0.03 | 1.45 | | | | | | | | 41 | | 1.4 | | | 134 | | | | |
| 19074 | 1 cup | Canned, avg | 187 | 198 | 75 | 33.5 | 6.6 | 0.0 | | | 3.0 | 0.8 | 0.2 | 1.1 | | | 501 | 60 | 18 | 18 | 0 | 0 | 0.03 | 0.71 | 3.74 | 0.09 | 2.09 | 7.9 | 0.75 | 7.1 | | | 69 | 3.9 | 1.4 | 64 | 0.1 | 380 | 423 | | 585 | 3.29 |
| 19073 | 3 oz | Dried, avg | 85 | 287 | 20 | 48.7 | 9.6 | 0.0 | | | 4.3 | 1.1 | 0.3 | 1.6 | | | 728 | 93 | 28 | 28 | 0 | 0 | 0.06 | 1.29 | 6.80 | 0.17 | 3.86 | 14.6 | | 12.5 | | | 100 | 5.9 | 2.1 | 103 | | 691 | 769 | | 502 | 4.78 |
| 19047 | 1 cup | Fried in flour, avg | 105 | 184 | 64 | 18.8 | 8.2 | 0.0 | 0.2 | 8.0 | 7.9 | 2.0 | 2.9 | 2.2 | 0.67 | 1.55 | 273 | 37 | 12 | 12 | 0 | 0 | 0.06 | 0.48 | 2.73 | 0.06 | 1.29 | 14.7 | 0.54 | 4.4 | 0.1 | | 41 | 2.2 | 1.1 | 40 | 0.1 | 264 | 293 | 54.4 | 321 | 1.83 |
| 19069 | 3 oz | Pickled, avg | 85 | 78 | 75 | 12.7 | 3.6 | 0.0 | | | 1.1 | 0.3 | 0.1 | 0.4 | | | 190 | 24 | 7 | 7 | 0 | 0 | 0.01 | 0.34 | 1.69 | 0.04 | 1.01 | 3.4 | 0.34 | 3.1 | | | 27 | 1.6 | 0.6 | 27 | 0.0 | 172 | 205 | | 1188 | 1.25 |
| 19093 | 3 oz | Raw, avg | 85 | 78 | 79 | 13.3 | 2.6 | 0.0 | | | 1.2 | 0.3 | 0.1 | 0.4 | 0.42 | 0.01 | 198 | 28 | 9 | 9 | 0 | 0 | 0.02 | 0.35 | 1.85 | 0.05 | 1.11 | 4.2 | 0.43 | 4.0 | | | 27 | 1.6 | 0.6 | 28 | 0.0 | 188 | 209 | 38.1 | 37 | 1.30 |
| | | Surimi | | | | | | | | | | | | | | | | | | | | | | | | | | | | | | | | | | | | | | | | |
| 19037 | 3 oz | Imitation crab, Alaskan king, avg | 85 | 87 | 74 | 10.2 | 8.7 | 0.0 | 4.3 | 4.3 | 1.1 | 0.2 | 0.2 | 0.6 | 0.52 | 0.03 | 17 | 56 | 17 | 17 | 0 | 0 | 0.03 | 0.02 | 0.15 | 0.03 | 1.36 | 1.4 | 0.06 | 0.0 | | | 11 | 0.0 | 0.3 | 37 | 0.0 | 240 | 77 | 19.0 | 715 | 0.28 |
| 17080 | 3 oz | Imitation pollock, avg | 85 | 84 | 76 | 12.9 | 5.8 | 0.0 | | | 0.8 | 0.2 | 0.1 | 0.4 | 0.36 | 0.02 | 26 | 56 | 17 | 17 | 0 | 0 | 0.02 | 0.02 | 0.19 | 0.03 | 1.36 | 1.4 | 0.06 | 0.0 | | | 8 | 0.0 | 0.2 | 37 | 0.0 | 240 | 95 | 23.9 | 122 | 0.28 |
| 19046 | 3 oz | Imitation scallop, avg | 85 | 84 | 74 | 10.9 | 9.0 | 0.0 | 4.5 | 4.5 | 0.3 | 0.1 | 0.1 | 0.2 | 0.15 | 0.01 | 19 | 56 | 17 | 17 | 0 | 0 | 0.01 | 0.01 | 0.26 | 0.03 | 1.36 | 1.4 | 0.06 | 0.0 | | | 7 | 0.0 | 0.3 | 37 | 0.0 | 240 | 88 | 20.1 | 676 | 0.28 |
| 19039 | 3 oz | Imitation shrimp, avg | 85 | 86 | 75 | 10.5 | 7.8 | 0.0 | 3.9 | 3.9 | 1.2 | 0.2 | 0.2 | 0.6 | 0.55 | 0.05 | 31 | 56 | 17 | 17 | 0 | 0 | 0.02 | 0.03 | 0.14 | 0.03 | 1.36 | 1.4 | 0.06 | 0.0 | | | 16 | 0.0 | 0.5 | 37 | 0.0 | 240 | 76 | 19.5 | 599 | 0.28 |
| 19100 | 3 oz | Whelk, mollusks, raw, avg | 85 | 116 | 66 | 20.2 | 6.6 | 0.0 | | | 0.3 | 0.0 | 0.0 | 0.0 | 0.01 | 0.01 | 55 | 72 | 22 | 22 | 0 | 0 | 0.02 | 0.09 | 0.89 | 0.29 | 7.71 | 5.4 | 0.18 | 3.4 | | | 48 | 0.9 | 4.3 | 73 | 0.4 | 120 | 295 | 38.1 | 175 | 1.39 |
| 19040 | 3 oz | Whelk, mollusks, steamed/boiled, avg | 85 | 234 | 32 | 40.5 | 13.2 | 0.0 | 6.6 | 6.6 | 0.7 | 0.1 | 0.0 | 0.0 | 0.02 | 0.02 | 111 | 138 | 42 | 42 | 0 | 0 | 0.04 | 0.18 | 1.70 | 0.55 | 15.39 | 9.7 | 0.34 | 5.8 | | | 96 | 1.8 | 8.6 | 146 | 0.8 | 240 | 590 | 76.2 | 350 | 2.77 |
| | | **FRUIT, VEGETABLE AND BLENDED JUICES** | | | | | | | | | | | | | | | | | | | | | | | | | | | | | | | | | | | | | | | | |
| | | *BLENDED JUICES* | | | | | | | | | | | | | | | | | | | | | | | | | | | | | | | | | | | | | | | | |
| 3319 | 1/2 cup | Apple-cherry, avg | 125 | 59 | 88 | 0.4 | 14.6 | 0.4 | 14.3 | 0.0 | 0.2 | 0.0 | 0.0 | 0.1 | 0.03 | 0.05 | 0 | 67 | 7 | 0 | 7 | 40 | 0.03 | 0.03 | 0.25 | 0.04 | 0.00 | 1.8 | 0.10 | 1.7 | 0.0 | | 10 | 0.0 | 0.5 | 6 | 0.1 | 12 | 154 | 0.4 | 2 | 0.06 |
| 3321 | 1/2 cup | Apple-grape, avg | 122 | 65 | 86 | 0.3 | 15.8 | 0.1 | 15.7 | 0.0 | 0.1 | 0.0 | 0.0 | 0.0 | 0.01 | 0.03 | 0 | 5 | 0.5 | 0 | 0.5 | 3 | 0.03 | 0.03 | 0.20 | 0.05 | 0.00 | 1.3 | 0.07 | 0.7 | 0.0 | | 10 | 0.0 | 0.4 | 7 | 0.3 | 11 | 151 | 0.6 | 4 | 0.05 |
| 3322 | 1/2 cup | Apple-grape-raspberry, avg | 125 | 65 | 86 | 0.6 | 15.9 | 0.1 | 15.7 | 0.0 | 0.3 | 0.0 | 0.0 | 0.1 | | | 0 | 58 | 6 | 0 | 6 | 38 | 0.04 | 0.06 | 0.52 | 0.06 | 0.00 | 11.3 | | 5.4 | 0.0 | | 16 | 0.0 | 0.5 | 12 | 0.3 | 12 | 168 | | 2 | 0.23 |
| 3320 | 1/2 cup | Apple-raspberry, avg | 120 | 54 | 89 | 0.1 | 13.1 | 0.1 | 12.9 | 0.0 | 0.2 | 0.0 | 0.0 | 0.1 | | | 0 | 37 | 4 | 0 | 4 | 22 | 0.03 | 0.02 | 0.17 | 0.04 | 0.00 | 2.7 | | 3.3 | 0.0 | | 10 | 0.0 | 0.6 | 8 | 0.2 | 10 | 155 | | 4 | 0.07 |
| 20071 | 1/2 cup | Cranberry apple drink, low cal, avg | 120 | 23 | 95 | 0.1 | 5.6 | 0.1 | 5.5 | 0.0 | 0.0 | 0.0 | 0.0 | 0.0 | 0.00 | 0.00 | 0 | 4 | 0.4 | 0 | 0.4 | 2 | 0.00 | 0.02 | 0.07 | 0.02 | 0.00 | 0.0 | | 38.4 | 0.0 | 0.0 | 8 | 0.0 | 0.1 | 2 | 0.2 | 4 | 32 | | 2 | 0.05 |

| Code | Amount | Description | Basic Components | | | | | | | | | Additional Fats | | | | | | Vit A & Components | | | | | Vitamins | | | | | | | | | | Minerals | | | | | | | | | |
|---|---|---|---|---|---|---|---|---|---|---|---|---|---|---|---|---|---|---|---|---|---|---|---|---|---|---|---|---|---|---|---|---|---|---|---|---|---|---|---|---|---|---|
| | | | Weight (g) | Calories | % Water | Protein (g) | Carbs (g) | Fiber (g) | Sugar (g) | Other Carbs (g) | Fat (g) | Sat Fat (g) | Mono Fat (g) | Poly Fat (g) | Omega 3 (g) | Omega 6 (g) | Choles (mg) | Vit A (IU) | Vit A (RE) | Retinol (RE) | Carotenoids (RE) | Beta Carotene (mcg) | Thiamin (mg) | Riboflavin (mg) | Niacin (NE) | Vit B6 (mg) | Vit B12 (mcg) | Folate (mcg) | Panto (mg) | Vit C (mg) | Vit D (mg) | Vit E (α TE) | Calcium (mg) | Copper (mg) | Iron (mg) | Magnes (mg) | Mang (mg) | Phos (mg) | Potassium (mg) | Selenium (mcg) | Sodium (mg) | Zinc (mg) |
| 3223 | 1/2 cup | Cranberry-apple drink, w/vit C, bottled, avg | 122 | 82 | 83 | 0.1 | 20.9 | 0.1 | 20.7 | 0.0 | 0.0 | 0.0 | 0.0 | 0.0 | 0.00 | 0.00 | 0 | 4 | 0.4 | 0 | 0.4 | 2 | 0.01 | 0.02 | 0.07 | 0.03 | 0.00 | 0.2 | 0.07 | 39.0 | 0.0 | 0.0 | 9 | 0.0 | 0.1 | 2 | 0.2 | 4 | 33 | 0.0 | 2 | 0.05 |
| 3274 | 1/2 cup | Cranberry-apricot, avg | 122 | 78 | 84 | 0.2 | 19.8 | 0.1 | 19.6 | 0.0 | 0.0 | 0.0 | 0.0 | 0.0 | 0.00 | 0.00 | 0 | 565 | 56 | 0 | 56 | 337 | 0.01 | 0.01 | 0.15 | 0.02 | 0.00 | 0.7 | 0.04 | 0.0 | 0.0 | | 11 | 0.0 | 0.2 | 4 | 0.2 | 6 | 74 | 0.0 | 2 | 0.05 |
| 3275 | 1/2 cup | Cranberry-grape, avg | 122 | 68 | 86 | 0.2 | 17.1 | 0.1 | 17.0 | 0.0 | 0.1 | 0.0 | 0.0 | 0.0 | 0.00 | 0.02 | 0 | 6 | 0.6 | 0 | 0.6 | 4 | 0.01 | 0.02 | 0.15 | 0.03 | 0.00 | 0.9 | 0.06 | 39.0 | 0.0 | | 10 | 0.0 | 0.0 | 4 | 0.2 | 5 | 29 | 0.0 | 4 | 0.05 |
| 3317 | 1/2 cup | Orange-banana, avg | 125 | 71 | 85 | 1.0 | 17.4 | 0.7 | 16.7 | 0.0 | 0.2 | 0.1 | 0.0 | 0.0 | 0.01 | 0.03 | 0 | 98 | 10 | 0 | 10 | 19 | 0.09 | 0.05 | 0.36 | 0.22 | 0.00 | 47.0 | 0.23 | 39.3 | 0.0 | | 10 | 0.1 | 0.2 | 19 | 0.1 | 21 | 302 | 0.5 | 1 | 0.10 |
| 3170 | 1/2 cup | Orange-grapefruit, canned, avg | 124 | 53 | 89 | 0.7 | 12.8 | 0.1 | 12.6 | 0.0 | 0.1 | 0.0 | 0.0 | 0.0 | 0.01 | 0.02 | 0 | 148 | 15 | 0 | 15 | 28 | 0.07 | 0.04 | 0.42 | 0.03 | 0.00 | 17.7 | 0.17 | 36.1 | 0.0 | | 10 | 0.1 | 0.6 | 12 | 0.0 | 17 | 196 | 0.1 | 4 | 0.09 |
| 3302 | 1/2 cup | Pineapple-orange-banana, avg | 125 | 64 | 87 | 0.7 | 15.5 | 0.3 | 14.9 | 0.4 | 0.1 | 0.0 | 0.0 | 0.0 | 0.01 | 0.01 | 0 | 55 | 6 | 0 | 6 | 33 | 0.09 | 0.03 | 0.27 | 0.11 | 0.00 | 32.5 | 0.18 | 29.9 | 0.0 | | 12 | 0.1 | 0.3 | 12 | 0.6 | 15 | 216 | 0.4 | 1 | 0.11 |
| | | *FRUIT JUICES* | | | | | | | | | | | | | | | | | | | | | | | | | | | | | | | | | | | | | | | | |
| 3238 | 1/2 cup | Acerola, fresh, avg | 121 | 28 | 94 | 0.5 | 5.8 | 0.4 | 5.4 | 0.0 | 0.4 | 0.1 | 0.1 | 0.1 | 0.05 | 0.06 | 0 | 616 | 62 | 0 | 62 | 370 | 0.02 | 0.07 | 0.48 | 0.00 | 0.00 | 16.9 | 0.25 | 1936.0 | 0.0 | | 12 | 0.1 | 0.6 | 15 | | 11 | 117 | 0.1 | 4 | 0.12 |
| | | Apple | | | | | | | | | | | | | | | | | | | | | | | | | | | | | | | | | | | | | | | | |
| 3008 | 1/2 cup | Canned/bottled, avg | 124 | 58 | 88 | 0.1 | 14.5 | 0.1 | 13.8 | 0.6 | 0.1 | 0.0 | 0.0 | 0.0 | 0.01 | 0.03 | 0 | 1 | 0.1 | 0 | 0.1 | 1 | 0.03 | 0.02 | 0.12 | 0.04 | 0.00 | 0.1 | 0.08 | 1.1 | 0.0 | 0.0 | 9 | 0.0 | 0.5 | 4 | 0.1 | 9 | 148 | 0.1 | 4 | 0.04 |
| 3328 | 1/2 cup | Canned/bottled, w/vit C, avg | 124 | 58 | 88 | 0.1 | 14.5 | 0.1 | 13.8 | 0.6 | 0.1 | 0.0 | 0.0 | 0.0 | 0.01 | 0.03 | 0 | 1 | 0.1 | 0 | 0.1 | 1 | 0.03 | 0.02 | 0.12 | 0.04 | 0.00 | 0.1 | 0.08 | 51.6 | 0.0 | 0.0 | 9 | 0.0 | 0.5 | 4 | 0.1 | 9 | 148 | 0.1 | 4 | 0.04 |
| 3150 | 1/4 cup | Concentrate, avg | 70 | 116 | 57 | 0.4 | 28.7 | 0.3 | 27.3 | 1.1 | 0.3 | 0.0 | 0.0 | 0.1 | 0.01 | 0.06 | 0 | 0 | 0 | 0 | 0 | 0 | 0.01 | 0.04 | 0.09 | 0.08 | 0.00 | 0.7 | 0.16 | 1.5 | 0.0 | | 14 | 0.0 | 0.6 | 12 | 0.2 | 17 | 314 | 0.3 | 17 | 0.09 |
| 3010 | 1/2 cup | Concentrate, prep w/water, avg | 120 | 56 | 88 | 0.2 | 13.8 | 0.1 | 13.2 | 0.5 | 0.1 | 0.0 | 0.0 | 0.0 | 0.00 | 0.03 | 0 | 0 | 0 | 0 | 0 | 0 | 0.00 | 0.02 | 0.05 | 0.04 | 0.00 | 0.4 | 0.08 | 0.7 | 0.0 | 0.0 | 7 | 0.0 | 0.3 | 6 | 0.1 | 8 | 151 | 0.1 | 8 | 0.05 |
| 3329 | 1/4 cup | Concentrate, w/vit C, avg | 70 | 116 | 57 | 0.4 | 28.7 | 0.3 | 27.4 | 1.1 | 0.3 | 0.0 | 0.0 | 0.1 | 0.01 | 0.06 | 0 | 0 | 0 | 0 | 0 | 0 | 0.01 | 0.04 | 0.09 | 0.08 | 0.00 | 0.7 | 0.16 | 62.2 | 0.0 | | 14 | 0.0 | 0.6 | 12 | 0.2 | 17 | 314 | 0.3 | 17 | 0.09 |
| 3015 | 1/2 cup | Apricot nectar, canned, avg | 126 | 71 | 85 | 0.5 | 18.1 | 0.8 | 17.4 | 0.0 | 0.1 | 0.0 | 0.0 | 0.0 | 0.00 | 0.02 | 0 | 1658 | 166 | 0 | 166 | 992 | 0.01 | 0.02 | 0.33 | 0.03 | 0.00 | 1.6 | 0.12 | 0.8 | 0.0 | | 9 | 0.1 | 0.5 | 6 | 0.0 | 11 | 144 | 0.3 | 4 | 0.11 |
| 3218 | 1/2 cup | Apricot nectar, w/vit C, canned, avg | 126 | 71 | 85 | 0.5 | 18.1 | 0.8 | 17.4 | 0.0 | 0.1 | 0.0 | 0.0 | 0.0 | 0.00 | 0.02 | 0 | 1658 | 166 | 0 | 166 | 992 | 0.01 | 0.02 | 0.33 | 0.03 | 0.00 | 1.6 | 0.12 | 68.5 | 0.0 | | 9 | 0.1 | 0.5 | 6 | 0.0 | 11 | 144 | 0.3 | 4 | 0.11 |
| 3325 | 1/2 cup | Banana nectar, avg | 125 | 89 | 81 | 0.5 | 22.7 | 0.7 | 20.8 | 1.3 | 0.2 | 0.1 | 0.0 | 0.0 | 0.02 | 0.02 | 0 | 35 | 4 | 0 | 4 | 21 | 0.02 | 0.05 | 0.24 | 0.25 | 0.00 | 8.4 | 0.11 | 4.0 | 0.0 | | 4 | 0.1 | 0.1 | 14 | 0.1 | 9 | 174 | 0.5 | 2 | 0.09 |
| 3300 | 1/2 cup | Black currant nectar, avg | 125 | 69 | 85 | 0.5 | 16.8 | 0.0 | 16.8 | 0.0 | 0.0 | | | | | | 0 | 33 | 3 | 0 | 3 | 20 | 0.01 | 0.00 | 0.04 | | 0.00 | | | 37.5 | 0.0 | | 19 | 0.0 | 0.4 | | | 12 | 122 | | 6 | |
| 3326 | 1/2 cup | Cantaloupe nectar, avg | 125 | 75 | 84 | 0.4 | 19.2 | 0.4 | 18.7 | 0.1 | 0.1 | 0.1 | 0.0 | 0.0 | 0.00 | 0.01 | 0 | 1209 | 121 | 0 | 121 | 720 | 0.02 | 0.01 | 0.26 | 0.05 | 0.00 | 4.3 | 0.06 | 14.8 | 0.0 | | 6 | 0.0 | 0.1 | 6 | 0.0 | 9 | 140 | 0.3 | 6 | 0.10 |
| | | Cranberry | | | | | | | | | | | | | | | | | | | | | | | | | | | | | | | | | | | | | | | | |
| 3042 | 1/2 cup | Cocktail, avg | 126 | 72 | 86 | 0.0 | 18.1 | 0.1 | 18.0 | 0.0 | 0.1 | 0.0 | 0.0 | 0.1 | 0.02 | 0.03 | 0 | 5 | 1 | 0 | 1 | 3 | 0.01 | 0.01 | 0.04 | 0.02 | 0.00 | 0.3 | 0.07 | 44.6 | 0.0 | 0.0 | 4 | 0.0 | 0.2 | 3 | 0.2 | 3 | 23 | 0.0 | 3 | 0.09 |
| 20114 | 1/4 cup | Cocktail, concentrate, avg | 72 | 145 | 48 | 0.0 | 37.1 | 0.1 | 30.6 | 6.3 | 0.0 | 0.0 | 0.0 | 0.0 | 0.00 | 0.00 | 0 | 24 | 2 | 0 | 2 | 13 | 0.02 | 0.02 | 0.03 | 0.04 | 0.00 | 0.0 | 0.35 | 33.0 | 0.0 | | 8 | 0.0 | 0.2 | 4 | 0.1 | 4 | 35 | 0.0 | 3 | 0.05 |
| 3276 | 1/2 cup | Cocktail, low cal, bottled, avg | 118 | 22 | 95 | 0.0 | 5.5 | 0.0 | 5.4 | 0.1 | 0.0 | 0.0 | 0.0 | 0.0 | 0.00 | 0.00 | 0 | 5 | 0.5 | 0 | 0.5 | 3 | 0.01 | 0.01 | 0.04 | 0.02 | 0.00 | 0.2 | 0.07 | 38.0 | 0.0 | 0.0 | 11 | 0.0 | 0.0 | 2 | 0.2 | 1 | 26 | 0.0 | 4 | 0.02 |
| 20115 | 1/2 cup | Cocktail, reconstituted, avg | 125 | 69 | 86 | 0.0 | 17.5 | 0.1 | 17.1 | 0.3 | 0.0 | 0.0 | 0.0 | 0.0 | 0.00 | 0.00 | 0 | 13 | 1 | 0 | 1 | 7 | 0.01 | 0.01 | 0.02 | 0.02 | 0.00 | 0.0 | 0.18 | 12.4 | 0.0 | | 6 | 0.0 | 0.1 | 2 | 0.1 | 1 | 18 | 0.0 | 4 | 0.05 |
| | | Grape | | | | | | | | | | | | | | | | | | | | | | | | | | | | | | | | | | | | | | | | |
| 3062 | 1/2 cup | Canned/bottled, avg | 126 | 77 | 84 | 0.7 | 18.9 | 0.1 | 18.8 | 0.0 | 0.1 | 0.0 | 0.0 | 0.0 | 0.01 | 0.02 | 0 | 10 | 1 | 0 | 1 | 7 | 0.03 | 0.05 | 0.33 | 0.08 | 0.00 | 3.3 | 0.05 | 0.1 | 0.0 | 0.0 | 11 | 0.0 | 0.3 | 13 | 0.5 | 14 | 166 | 0.1 | 4 | 0.06 |
| 3233 | 1/4 cup | Concentrate, sweetened, w/vit C, avg | 71 | 127 | 54 | 0.5 | 31.5 | 0.2 | | | 0.2 | 0.1 | 0.0 | 0.1 | 0.01 | 0.05 | 0 | 19 | 2 | 0 | 2 | 13 | 0.04 | 0.06 | 0.31 | 0.10 | 0.00 | 3.1 | 0.06 | 59.0 | 0.0 | | 9 | 0.0 | 0.3 | 11 | 0.4 | 11 | 53 | 0.3 | 5 | 0.09 |
| 3064 | 1/2 cup | Concentrate, sweetened, w/vit C, prep w/water, avg | 125 | 64 | 87 | 0.2 | 16.0 | 0.1 | | | 0.1 | 0.0 | 0.0 | 0.0 | 0.01 | 0.02 | 0 | 10 | 1 | 0 | 1 | 7 | 0.02 | 0.03 | 0.16 | 0.05 | 0.00 | 1.6 | 0.03 | 29.9 | 0.0 | | 5 | 0.0 | 0.1 | 5 | 0.2 | 5 | 26 | 0.1 | 2 | 0.05 |
| | | Grapefruit | | | | | | | | | | | | | | | | | | | | | | | | | | | | | | | | | | | | | | | | |
| 3052 | 1/2 cup | Canned, avg | 124 | 47 | 90 | 0.6 | 11.1 | 0.1 | 11.0 | 0.0 | 0.1 | 0.0 | 0.0 | 0.0 | 0.01 | 0.02 | 0 | 9 | 1 | 0 | 1 | 7 | 0.05 | 0.02 | 0.29 | 0.02 | 0.00 | 12.9 | 0.16 | 36.2 | 0.0 | 0.0 | 9 | 0.0 | 0.2 | 12 | 0.0 | 14 | 190 | 0.1 | 1 | 0.11 |
| 3219 | 1/4 cup | Concentrate, avg | 68 | 99 | 62 | 1.3 | 23.5 | 0.3 | 23.3 | 0.0 | 0.3 | 0.0 | 0.0 | 0.1 | 0.02 | 0.06 | 0 | 21 | 2 | 0 | 2 | 12 | 0.10 | 0.05 | 0.52 | 0.10 | 0.00 | 8.7 | 0.46 | 81.6 | 0.0 | | 18 | 0.1 | 0.3 | 26 | 0.0 | 33 | 329 | 0.2 | 2 | 0.12 |
| 3053 | 1/2 cup | Concentrate, prep w/water, avg | 124 | 51 | 89 | 0.7 | 12.1 | 0.1 | 11.9 | 0.0 | 0.2 | 0.0 | 0.0 | 0.0 | 0.01 | 0.03 | 0 | 11 | 1 | 0 | 1 | 7 | 0.05 | 0.03 | 0.27 | 0.05 | 0.00 | 4.5 | 0.23 | 41.8 | 0.0 | 0.0 | 10 | 0.0 | 0.2 | 14 | 0.0 | 17 | 169 | 0.1 | 1 | 0.06 |
| 3051 | 1/2 cup | Fresh, avg | 124 | 48 | 90 | 0.6 | 11.4 | 0.1 | 11.3 | 0.0 | 0.1 | 0.0 | 0.0 | 0.0 | 0.01 | 0.02 | 0 | 12 | 1 | 0 | 1 | 7 | 0.05 | 0.02 | 0.25 | 0.05 | 0.00 | 12.6 | 0.23 | 47.1 | 0.0 | 0.0 | 11 | 0.0 | 0.2 | 15 | 0.0 | 19 | 201 | 0.1 | 1 | 0.06 |
| 3887 | 1/2 cup | Pink, canned, avg | 124 | 47 | 90 | 0.6 | 11.1 | 0.1 | 11.0 | 0.0 | 0.1 | 0.0 | 0.0 | 0.0 | | | 0 | 546 | 55 | 0 | 55 | 327 | 0.05 | 0.02 | 0.29 | 0.02 | 0.00 | 12.9 | 0.16 | 36.2 | 0.0 | | 9 | 0.0 | 0.2 | 12 | 0.0 | 14 | 190 | 0.3 | 1 | 0.11 |
| 3889 | 1/2 cup | Pink, canned, sweetened, avg | 124 | 57 | 87 | 0.7 | 13.8 | 0.1 | 13.6 | 0.0 | 0.1 | 0.0 | 0.0 | 0.0 | | | 0 | 546 | 55 | 0 | 55 | 327 | 0.05 | 0.03 | 0.40 | 0.02 | 0.00 | 12.9 | 0.16 | 33.4 | 0.0 | | 10 | 0.1 | 0.4 | 12 | 0.0 | 14 | 201 | 0.2 | 2 | 0.07 |
| 3165 | 1/2 cup | Sweetened, canned, avg | 125 | 58 | 87 | 0.7 | 13.9 | 0.1 | 13.8 | 0.0 | 0.1 | 0.0 | 0.0 | 0.0 | 0.01 | 0.02 | 0 | 0 | 0 | 0 | 0 | 0 | 0.05 | 0.03 | 0.40 | 0.02 | 0.00 | 13.0 | 0.16 | 33.6 | 0.0 | 0.0 | 10 | 0.1 | 0.5 | 12 | 0.0 | 14 | 202 | 0.1 | 2 | 0.07 |
| 3305 | 1/2 cup | Guava drink, w/vit C, avg | 126 | 66 | 86 | 0.1 | 16.8 | 1.0 | 15.7 | 0.1 | 0.1 | 0.0 | 0.0 | 0.0 | 0.01 | 0.03 | 0 | 145 | 14 | 0 | 14 | 83 | 0.01 | 0.01 | 0.22 | 0.03 | 0.00 | 2.6 | 0.03 | 42.3 | 0.0 | | 5 | 0.0 | 0.1 | 3 | 0.0 | 5 | 52 | | 4 | 0.07 |
| 3304 | 1/2 cup | Guava nectar, avg | 125 | 75 | 84 | 0.1 | 19.0 | 1.0 | 17.9 | 0.1 | 0.1 | 0.0 | 0.0 | 0.0 | 0.01 | 0.03 | 0 | 108 | 11 | 0 | 11 | 62 | 0.01 | 0.01 | 0.20 | 0.02 | 0.00 | 1.3 | 0.03 | 23.3 | 0.0 | | 5 | 0.0 | 0.1 | 2 | 0.0 | 5 | 46 | | 4 | 0.07 |
| 3301 | 1/2 cup | Granadilla, fresh, avg | 125 | 75 | 82 | 1.0 | 17.1 | 0.3 | 16.8 | 0.0 | 0.5 | | | | | | 0 | 2084 | 209 | 0 | 209 | 1253 | 0.02 | 0.14 | 2.50 | | 0.00 | | | 37.5 | 0.0 | | 11 | | 0.4 | | | 25 | 269 | | 1 | |
| | | Lemon | | | | | | | | | | | | | | | | | | | | | | | | | | | | | | | | | | | | | | | | |
| 3069 | 1/2 cup | Bottled, avg | 122 | 26 | 92 | 0.5 | 7.9 | 0.5 | 3.1 | 4.3 | 0.4 | 0.0 | 0.0 | 0.1 | 0.03 | 0.07 | 0 | 18 | 2 | 0 | 2 | 15 | 0.05 | 0.01 | 0.24 | 0.05 | 0.00 | 12.3 | 0.11 | 30.3 | 0.0 | | 13 | 0.0 | 0.2 | 10 | 0.0 | 11 | 124 | 0.1 | 26 | 0.07 |
| 3068 | 1/2 cup | Fresh, avg | 122 | 31 | 91 | 0.5 | 10.5 | 0.5 | 4.1 | 5.9 | 0.0 | 0.0 | 0.0 | 0.0 | 0.00 | 0.00 | 0 | 24 | 2 | 0 | 2 | 15 | 0.04 | 0.01 | 0.12 | 0.06 | 0.00 | 15.7 | 0.13 | 56.1 | 0.0 | | 9 | 0.0 | 0.0 | 7 | 0.0 | 7 | 151 | 0.1 | 1 | 0.06 |
| 3070 | 1/2 cup | Frozen, avg | 122 | 27 | 92 | 0.6 | 7.9 | 0.5 | 3.1 | 4.4 | 0.4 | 0.1 | 0.0 | 0.1 | 0.04 | 0.08 | 0 | 16 | 1 | 0 | 1 | 7 | 0.07 | 0.02 | 0.17 | 0.07 | 0.00 | 11.6 | 0.15 | 38.4 | 0.0 | | 10 | 0.0 | 0.1 | 10 | 0.0 | 10 | 109 | 0.1 | 1 | 0.06 |
| 3073 | 1/2 cup | Lime, bottled, avg | 123 | 26 | 92 | 0.3 | 8.2 | 0.5 | 3.2 | 4.5 | 0.3 | 0.0 | 0.0 | 0.1 | 0.03 | 0.05 | 0 | 20 | 2 | 0 | 2 | 14 | 0.04 | 0.00 | 0.20 | 0.03 | 0.00 | 3.7 | 0.08 | 7.9 | 0.0 | | 15 | 0.0 | 0.3 | 9 | 0.0 | 12 | 92 | 0.1 | 20 | 0.07 |
| 3072 | 1/2 cup | Lime, fresh, avg | 123 | 33 | 90 | 0.5 | 11.1 | 0.5 | 4.4 | 6.2 | 0.1 | 0.0 | 0.0 | 0.0 | 0.01 | 0.02 | 0 | 12 | 1 | 0 | 1 | 7 | 0.02 | 0.01 | 0.12 | 0.05 | 0.00 | 10.1 | 0.17 | 36.0 | 0.0 | | 11 | 0.0 | 0.0 | 7 | 0.0 | 9 | 134 | 0.1 | 1 | 0.07 |
| 3303 | 1/2 cup | Mango nectar, avg | 125 | 74 | 84 | 0.3 | 19.1 | 1.0 | 18.0 | 0.1 | 0.1 | 0.0 | 0.1 | 0.0 | 0.02 | 0.01 | 0 | 1460 | 146 | 0 | 146 | 875 | 0.02 | 0.03 | 0.26 | 0.06 | 0.00 | 3.5 | 0.08 | 9.7 | 0.0 | | 6 | 0.1 | 0.1 | 5 | 0.0 | 6 | 70 | | 2 | 0.04 |
| | | Orange | | | | | | | | | | | | | | | | | | | | | | | | | | | | | | | | | | | | | | | | |
| 3093 | 1/2 cup | Canned, avg | 124 | 52 | 89 | 0.7 | 12.2 | 0.2 | 12.0 | 0.0 | 0.2 | 0.0 | 0.0 | 0.0 | 0.01 | 0.03 | 0 | 217 | 22 | 0 | 22 | 42 | 0.07 | 0.03 | 0.39 | 0.11 | 0.00 | 22.4 | 0.19 | 42.7 | 0.0 | | 10 | 0.1 | 0.5 | 14 | 0.0 | 17 | 217 | 0.1 | 2 | 0.09 |
| 3092 | 1/2 cup | Chilled, avg | 124 | 55 | 88 | 1.0 | 12.5 | 0.2 | 12.3 | 0.0 | 0.3 | 0.0 | 0.1 | 0.1 | 0.02 | 0.06 | 0 | 97 | 10 | 0 | 10 | 18 | 0.14 | 0.03 | 0.35 | 0.07 | 0.00 | 22.4 | 0.24 | 40.8 | 0.0 | | 12 | 0.0 | 0.2 | 14 | 0.0 | 14 | 236 | 0.2 | 1 | 0.05 |
| 3094 | 1/4 cup | Concentrate, avg | 70 | 111 | 58 | 1.7 | 26.7 | 0.6 | 26.2 | 0.0 | 0.1 | 0.0 | 0.0 | 0.0 | 0.01 | 0.02 | 0 | 193 | 20 | 0 | 20 | 36 | 0.20 | 0.04 | 0.50 | 0.11 | 0.00 | 103.5 | 0.39 | 96.6 | 0.0 | | 22 | 0.1 | 0.2 | 24 | 0.0 | 40 | 472 | 0.3 | 2 | 0.13 |
| 3091 | 1/2 cup | Concentrate, prep w/water, avg | 124 | 56 | 88 | 0.8 | 13.4 | 0.2 | 13.1 | 0.0 | 0.1 | 0.0 | 0.0 | 0.0 | 0.00 | 0.01 | 0 | 97 | 10 | 0 | 10 | 18 | 0.10 | 0.02 | 0.25 | 0.05 | 0.00 | 54.3 | 0.20 | 48.2 | 0.0 | | 11 | 0.1 | 0.1 | 12 | 0.0 | 20 | 236 | 0.1 | 1 | 0.06 |
| 3090 | 1/2 cup | Fresh, avg | 124 | 56 | 88 | 0.9 | 12.9 | 0.2 | 12.6 | 0.0 | 0.2 | 0.0 | 0.0 | 0.0 | 0.01 | 0.04 | 0 | 248 | 25 | 0 | 25 | 46 | 0.11 | 0.04 | 0.50 | 0.05 | 0.00 | 37.6 | 0.24 | 62.0 | 0.0 | 0.0 | 14 | 0.1 | 0.2 | 14 | 0.0 | 21 | 248 | 0.1 | 1 | 0.06 |
| 3095 | 1/2 cup | Papaya nectar, canned, avg | 125 | 71 | 85 | 0.2 | 18.1 | 0.8 | 15.4 | 2.0 | 0.2 | 0.1 | 0.1 | 0.0 | 0.04 | 0.01 | 0 | 139 | 14 | 0 | 14 | 24 | 0.01 | 0.01 | 0.19 | 0.01 | 0.00 | 2.6 | 0.07 | 3.8 | 0.0 | | 12 | 0.0 | 0.4 | 4 | 0.0 | 0 | 39 | 0.4 | 6 | 0.19 |
| 3200 | 1/2 cup | Passion Fruit, purple, fresh, avg | 124 | 63 | 86 | 0.5 | 16.9 | 0.2 | 16.6 | 0.0 | 0.1 | 0.0 | 0.0 | 0.0 | 0.00 | 0.04 | 0 | 889 | 89 | 0 | 89 | 134 | 0.00 | 0.16 | 1.81 | 0.06 | 0.00 | 3.7 | | 37.0 | 0.0 | | 5 | 0.1 | 0.3 | 21 | | 16 | 345 | 0.1 | 7 | 0.06 |
| 3201 | 1/2 cup | Passion Fruit, yellow, avg | 124 | 74 | 84 | 0.8 | 18.0 | 0.2 | 17.7 | 0.0 | 0.2 | 0.0 | 0.0 | 0.1 | 0.00 | 0.13 | 0 | 2988 | 299 | 0 | 299 | 448 | 0.00 | 0.13 | 2.78 | 0.07 | 0.00 | 3.9 | | 22.6 | 0.0 | | 5 | 0.1 | 0.4 | 21 | | 31 | 345 | 0.1 | 7 | 0.07 |
| 3101 | 1/2 cup | Peach nectar, canned, avg | 124 | 67 | 86 | 0.3 | 17.2 | 0.7 | 16.5 | 0.0 | 0.0 | 0.0 | 0.0 | 0.0 | 0.00 | 0.01 | 0 | 320 | 32 | 0 | 32 | 156 | 0.00 | 0.02 | 0.36 | 0.01 | 0.00 | 1.7 | 0.08 | 6.6 | 0.0 | | 6 | 0.1 | 0.2 | 5 | 0.0 | 7 | 50 | 0.2 | 9 | 0.10 |
| 3110 | 1/2 cup | Pear nectar, canned, avg | 125 | 75 | 84 | 0.1 | 19.8 | 0.8 | 19.0 | 0.0 | 0.0 | 0.0 | 0.0 | 0.0 | 0.00 | 0.00 | 0 | 1 | 0.1 | 0 | 0.1 | 1 | 0.00 | 0.02 | 0.16 | 0.02 | 0.00 | 1.5 | 0.03 | 1.4 | 0.0 | | 6 | 0.1 | 0.3 | 4 | 0.0 | 4 | 16 | 0.6 | 5 | 0.09 |
| | | Pineapple | | | | | | | | | | | | | | | | | | | | | | | | | | | | | | | | | | | | | | | | |
| 3120 | 1/2 cup | Canned, avg | 125 | 70 | 86 | 0.4 | 17.3 | 0.3 | 17.0 | 0.0 | 0.1 | 0.0 | 0.0 | 0.0 | 0.02 | 0.02 | 0 | 6 | 1 | 0 | 1 | 4 | 0.07 | 0.03 | 0.32 | 0.12 | 0.00 | 23.9 | 0.13 | 13.4 | 0.0 | | 21 | 0.1 | 0.3 | 16 | 1.2 | 10 | 168 | 0.1 | 1 | 0.14 |
| 3189 | 1/4 cup | Concentrate, avg | 71 | 127 | 53 | 0.9 | 31.5 | 0.5 | 31.0 | 0.0 | 0.1 | 0.0 | 0.0 | 0.0 | 0.01 | 0.01 | 0 | 36 | 4 | 0 | 4 | 21 | 0.16 | 0.04 | 0.64 | 0.18 | 0.00 | 25.1 | 0.31 | 29.8 | 0.0 | | 28 | 0.2 | 0.6 | 25 | 2.4 | 20 | 335 | 0.3 | 2 | 0.28 |
| 3119 | 1/2 cup | Concentrate, prep w/water, avg | 125 | 65 | 86 | 0.5 | 16.0 | 0.3 | 15.8 | 0.0 | 0.0 | 0.0 | 0.0 | 0.0 | 0.01 | 0.01 | 0 | 13 | 1 | 0 | 1 | 7 | 0.09 | 0.02 | 0.25 | 0.09 | 0.00 | 13.3 | 0.16 | 15.0 | 0.0 | | 14 | 0.1 | 0.4 | 11 | 1.2 | 10 | 170 | 0.1 | 1 | 0.14 |
| 3976 | 1/2 cup | Pomegranate, fresh, avg | 125 | 55 | 85 | 0.3 | 14.5 | 0.0 | 7.9 | 6.6 | 0.0 | | | | | | 0 | 0 | 0 | 0 | 0 | 0 | 0.02 | 0.04 | 0.25 | | 0.00 | | | 10.0 | 0.0 | | 4 | 0.1 | 0.3 | 4 | | 10 | 250 | | 1 | |
| 3128 | 1/2 cup | Prune, Bottled, avg | 128 | 91 | 81 | 0.8 | 22.4 | 1.3 | 16.6 | 4.5 | 0.0 | 0.0 | 0.0 | 0.0 | 0.00 | 0.01 | 0 | 4 | 0.4 | 0 | 0.4 | 2 | 0.02 | 0.09 | 1.00 | 0.28 | 0.00 | 0.5 | 0.14 | 5.2 | 0.0 | | 15 | 0.1 | 1.5 | 18 | 0.2 | 32 | 353 | 0.8 | 5 | 0.27 |
| 3559 | 1/2 cup | Prune, 100% juice, reconstituted, Chef America | 127 | 90 | | 0.0 | 22.0 | 0.0 | 18.0 | 4.0 | 0.0 | 0.0 | 0.0 | 0.0 | 0.00 | 0.00 | 0 | 0 | 0 | 0 | 0 | 0 | | | | | 0.00 | | | 60.0 | | | 0 | | 0.0 | | | 22 | 300 | | 0 | |
| 3299 | 1/2 cup | Red currant nectar, avg | 125 | 68 | 86 | 0.5 | 16.5 | 0.0 | 16.5 | 0.0 | 0.0 | | | | | | 0 | 33 | 3 | 0 | 3 | 20 | 0.00 | 0.00 | | | 0.00 | | | 7.5 | 0.0 | | 9 | 0.0 | 0.4 | | | 9 | 138 | | | |
| 3324 | 1/2 cup | Strawberry, avg | 118 | 35 | 92 | 0.7 | 8.3 | 0.1 | 8.1 | 0.0 | 0.5 | 0.0 | 0.1 | 0.2 | 0.09 | 0.13 | 0 | 24 | 2 | 0 | 2 | 13 | 0.02 | 0.07 | 0.25 | 0.06 | 0.00 | 10.6 | | 33.5 | 0.0 | | 17 | 0.1 | 0.4 | 12 | | 22 | 196 | | 1 | 0.15 |
| 3273 | 1/2 cup | Tangelo, fresh, avg | 125 | 51 | 89 | 0.6 | 12.1 | 0.0 | 12.1 | 0.0 | 0.1 | 0.0 | | | | 0.00 | 0 | 525 | 53 | 0 | 53 | 98 | 0.07 | 0.02 | 0.13 | | 0.00 | | | 33.8 | 0.0 | | 22 | | 0.3 | | | 18 | 222 | | 1 | |
| | | Tangerine | | | | | | | | | | | | | | | | | | | | | | | | | | | | | | | | | | | | | | | | |
| 3347 | 1/2 cup | Fresh, avg | 124 | 53 | 89 | 0.6 | 12.5 | 0.2 | 12.3 | 0.0 | 0.2 | 0.0 | 0.0 | 0.0 | 0.01 | 0.04 | 0 | 521 | 52 | 0 | 52 | 118 | 0.07 | 0.02 | 0.12 | 0.05 | 0.00 | 5.7 | 0.16 | 38.4 | 0.0 | | 22 | 0.0 | 0.2 | 10 | 0.0 | 17 | 221 | 0.1 | 1 | 0.04 |
| 3141 | 1/2 cup | Concentrate, prep w/water, sweetened, avg | 124 | 57 | 88 | 0.5 | 13.8 | 0.2 | 13.5 | 0.0 | 0.1 | 0.0 | 0.0 | 0.0 | 0.00 | 0.01 | 0 | 711 | 71 | 0 | 71 | 159 | 0.06 | 0.02 | 0.12 | 0.05 | 0.00 | 5.7 | 0.16 | 30.0 | 0.0 | 0.0 | 10 | 0.0 | 0.1 | 10 | 0.0 | 10 | 140 | 0.3 | 1 | 0.04 |

| Code | Amount | Description | Basic Components | | | | | | | | | Additional Fats | | | | | | Vit A & Components | | | | | Vitamins | | | | | | | | | | Minerals | | | | | | | | | |
|---|---|---|---|---|---|---|---|---|---|---|---|---|---|---|---|---|---|---|---|---|---|---|---|---|---|---|---|---|---|---|---|---|---|---|---|---|---|---|---|---|---|---|
| | | | Weight (g) | Calories | % Water | Protein (g) | Carbs (g) | Fiber (g) | Sugar (g) | Other Carbs (g) | Fat (g) | Sat Fat (g) | Mono Fat (g) | Poly Fat (g) | Omega 3 (g) | Omega 6 (g) | Choles (mg) | Vit A (IU) | Vit A (RE) | Retinol (RE) | Carotenoids (RE) | Beta Carotene (mcg) | Thiamin (mg) | Riboflavin (mg) | Niacin (NE) | Vit B6 (mg) | Vit B12 (mcg) | Folate (mcg) | Panto (mg) | Vit C (mg) | Vit D (mg) | Vit E (α TE) | Calcium (mg) | Copper (mg) | Iron (mg) | Magnes (mg) | Mang (mg) | Phos (mg) | Potassium (mg) | Selenium (mcg) | Sodium (mg) | Zinc (mg) |
| 3421 | 1/4 cup | Concentrate, sweetened, avg | 71 | 114 | 58 | 1.1 | 27.6 | 0.4 | 27.2 | 0.0 | 0.3 | 0.0 | 0.0 | 0.0 | 0.01 | 0.03 | 0 | 1430 | 143 | 0 | 143 | 322 | 0.13 | 0.05 | 0.23 | 0.10 | 0.00 | 11.5 | 0.31 | 60.4 | 0.0 | 0.1 | 19 | 0.1 | 0.2 | 20 | 0.1 | 21 | 282 | | 2 | 0.06 |
| 3140 | 1/2 cup | Canned, sweetened, avg | 124 | 62 | 87 | 0.6 | 14.9 | 0.2 | 14.6 | 0.0 | 0.2 | 0.0 | 0.0 | 0.0 | 0.01 | 0.02 | 0 | 521 | 52 | 0 | 52 | 117 | 0.07 | 0.02 | 0.12 | 0.04 | 0.00 | 5.7 | 0.16 | 27.3 | 0.0 | 0.0 | 22 | 0.0 | 0.2 | 10 | 0.0 | 17 | 221 | 0.1 | 1 | 0.04 |
| | | *VEGETABLE JUICES* | | | | | | | | | | | | | | | | | | | | | | | | | | | | | | | | | | | | | | | | |
| | | Tomato | | | | | | | | | | | | | | | | | | | | | | | | | | | | | | | | | | | | | | | | |
| 20057 | 1/2 cup | & beef broth, canned, avg | 122 | 45 | 90 | 0.7 | 10.4 | 0.1 | 1.2 | 9.0 | 0.1 | 0.0 | 0.0 | 0.0 | 0.00 | 0.03 | 0 | 156 | 16 | 0 | 16 | | 0.00 | 0.04 | 0.20 | 0.03 | 0.06 | 5.2 | 0.04 | 1.1 | 0.0 | | 13 | 0.0 | 0.7 | 4 | 0.0 | 16 | 117 | 0.9 | 160 | 0.02 |
| 20042 | 1/2 cup | & clam juice, canned, avg | 122 | 59 | 87 | 0.7 | 13.4 | 0.2 | 1.6 | 11.6 | 0.2 | 0.1 | 0.0 | 0.0 | 0.00 | 0.02 | 0 | 262 | 27 | 4 | 23 | 135 | 0.05 | 0.04 | 0.23 | 0.10 | 37.33 | 19.4 | 0.31 | 5.0 | 0.0 | | 15 | 0.4 | 0.7 | 27 | 0.1 | 95 | 110 | 0.2 | 442 | 1.32 |
| 5397 | 1/2 cup | Canned, unsalted, avg | 122 | 21 | 94 | 0.9 | 5.2 | 1.0 | 4.0 | 0.2 | 0.1 | 0.0 | 0.0 | 0.0 | 0.00 | 0.03 | 0 | 678 | 68 | 0 | 68 | 401 | 0.06 | 0.04 | 0.82 | 0.14 | 0.00 | 24.3 | 0.31 | 22.3 | 0.0 | | 11 | 0.1 | 0.7 | 13 | 0.5 | 23 | 268 | 0.6 | 12 | 0.17 |
| 5188 | 1/2 cup | Canned, w/salt, avg | 122 | 21 | 94 | 0.9 | 5.2 | 0.5 | 4.0 | 0.6 | 0.1 | 0.0 | 0.0 | 0.0 | 0.00 | 0.03 | 0 | 678 | 68 | 0 | 68 | 401 | 0.06 | 0.04 | 0.82 | 0.14 | 0.00 | 24.3 | 0.31 | 22.3 | 0.0 | | 11 | 0.1 | 0.7 | 13 | 0.1 | 23 | 268 | 0.6 | 440 | 0.17 |
| | | Vegetable | | | | | | | | | | | | | | | | | | | | | | | | | | | | | | | | | | | | | | | | |
| 20080 | 1/2 cup | Cocktail, canned, avg | 121 | 23 | 94 | 0.8 | 5.5 | 1.0 | 4.0 | 0.5 | 0.1 | 0.0 | 0.0 | 0.0 | 0.00 | 0.04 | 0 | 1416 | 142 | 0 | 142 | 830 | 0.05 | 0.03 | 0.88 | 0.17 | 0.00 | 25.5 | 0.32 | 33.5 | 0.0 | | 13 | 0.2 | 0.5 | 13 | 0.1 | 21 | 234 | 0.6 | 327 | 0.24 |
| 6500 | 1/2 cup | V 8, Lightly Tangy, Cambell's | 122 | 30 | 93 | 1.0 | 5.5 | 0.5 | 4.5 | 0.5 | 0.0 | 0.0 | 0.0 | 0.0 | 0.00 | 0.00 | 0 | 1506 | 151 | 0 | 151 | 904 | | | | | 0.00 | | | 30.1 | | | 20 | | 0.5 | | | | | | 171 | |
| 6502 | 1/2 cup | V 8, Low Sodium, Cambell's | 122 | 30 | 93 | 1.0 | 5.5 | 1.0 | 4.5 | 0.0 | 0.0 | 0.0 | 0.0 | 0.0 | 0.00 | 0.00 | 0 | 1255 | 126 | 0 | 126 | 753 | | | | | 0.00 | | | 30.1 | | | 20 | | 0.5 | | | | | | 70 | |
| 6507 | 1/2 cup | V 8, 100%, Cambell's | 122 | 25 | 94 | 0.5 | 5.0 | 0.5 | 4.0 | 0.5 | 0.0 | 0.0 | 0.0 | 0.0 | 0.00 | 0.00 | 0 | 1004 | 100 | 0 | 100 | 602 | | | | | 0.00 | | | 30.1 | | | 20 | | 0.5 | | | | | | 311 | |
| 6505 | 1/2 cup | V 8, Picante, Cambell's | 122 | 25 | 94 | 1.0 | 5.0 | 0.5 | 3.5 | 1.0 | 0.0 | 0.0 | 0.0 | 0.0 | 0.00 | 0.00 | 0 | 1004 | 100 | 0 | 100 | 602 | | | | | 0.00 | | | 30.1 | | | 20 | | 0.5 | | | | | | 341 | |
| 6506 | 1/2 cup | V 8, Spicy Hot, Cambell's | 122 | 25 | 94 | 1.0 | 5.0 | 0.5 | 3.5 | 1.0 | 0.0 | 0.0 | 0.0 | 0.0 | 0.00 | 0.00 | 0 | 1004 | 100 | 0 | 100 | 602 | | | | | 0.00 | | | 18.1 | | | 10 | | 0.4 | | | | | | 392 | |
| | | **FRUITS** | | | | | | | | | | | | | | | | | | | | | | | | | | | | | | | | | | | | | | | | |
| 3387 | 1/2 cup | Acerola, raw, avg | 49 | 16 | 91 | 0.2 | 3.8 | 0.5 | 2.2 | 1.0 | 0.1 | 0.0 | 0.0 | 0.0 | 0.02 | 0.02 | 0 | 376 | 38 | 0 | 38 | 226 | 0.01 | 0.03 | 0.20 | 0.00 | 0.00 | 6.9 | 0.15 | 821.7 | 0.0 | | 6 | 0.0 | 0.1 | 9 | | 5 | 72 | 0.3 | 3 | 0.05 |
| | | Apples | | | | | | | | | | | | | | | | | | | | | | | | | | | | | | | | | | | | | | | | |
| 3308 | 1 ea | Baked, unsweetened, avg | 161 | 101 | 83 | 0.3 | 26.4 | 3.8 | 21.6 | 1.0 | 0.6 | 0.1 | 0.0 | 0.2 | 0.03 | 0.15 | 0 | 78 | 7 | 0 | 7 | 30 | 0.02 | 0.02 | 0.12 | 0.08 | 0.00 | 2.9 | 0.10 | 7.9 | 0.0 | 1.0 | 11 | 0.1 | 0.3 | 8 | 0.1 | 13 | 179 | 0.7 | 0 | 0.07 |
| 3388 | 1/2 cup | Boiled, avg | 86 | 46 | 86 | 0.2 | 11.7 | 2.1 | 9.2 | 0.4 | 0.3 | 0.0 | 0.0 | 0.1 | 0.02 | 0.07 | 0 | 38 | 3 | 0 | 3 | 14 | 0.01 | 0.01 | 0.08 | 0.04 | 0.00 | 0.5 | 0.04 | 0.2 | 0.0 | | 4 | 0.0 | 0.2 | 3 | 0.1 | 7 | 76 | 0.3 | 1 | 0.03 |
| 3318 | 1 ea | Candied, avg | 184 | 254 | 65 | 2.3 | 56.0 | 3.6 | 52.2 | 0.2 | 4.2 | 3.1 | 0.4 | 0.2 | 0.03 | 0.19 | 4 | 88 | 11 | 3 | 8 | 32 | 0.03 | 0.10 | 0.22 | 0.08 | 0.00 | 6.1 | 0.35 | 8.1 | | | 72 | 0.1 | 0.3 | 15 | 0.1 | 61 | 256 | 2.2 | 110 | 0.25 |
| 3389 | 1/2 cup | Canned, avg | 102 | 68 | 82 | 0.2 | 17.1 | 2.0 | 15.3 | 0.0 | 0.4 | 0.1 | 0.0 | 0.1 | 0.02 | 0.11 | 0 | 57 | 6 | 0 | 6 | 25 | 0.01 | 0.01 | 0.08 | 0.04 | 0.00 | 0.1 | 0.03 | 0.2 | 0.0 | | 4 | 0.1 | 0.2 | 3 | 0.2 | 6 | 71 | 0.3 | 3 | 0.05 |
| 3148 | 1/2 cup | Canned, slices, sweetened, avg | 102 | 68 | 82 | 0.2 | 17.0 | 1.7 | 15.3 | 0.0 | 0.5 | 0.1 | 0.0 | 0.1 | 0.03 | 0.12 | 0 | 52 | 5 | 0 | 5 | 21 | 0.01 | 0.01 | 0.07 | 0.04 | 0.00 | 0.3 | 0.03 | 0.4 | 0.0 | | 4 | 0.1 | 0.2 | 2 | 0.2 | 5 | 69 | 0.3 | 3 | 0.03 |
| 3009 | 1/2 cup | Cooked, slices, peeled, avg | 85 | 48 | 85 | 0.2 | 12.2 | 2.4 | 9.4 | 0.5 | 0.4 | 0.1 | 0.0 | 0.1 | 0.02 | 0.09 | 0 | 34 | 3 | 0 | 3 | 14 | 0.01 | 0.01 | 0.05 | 0.04 | 0.00 | 0.5 | 0.04 | 0.3 | 0.0 | | 4 | 0.0 | 0.1 | 3 | 0.1 | 7 | 79 | 0.3 | 1 | 0.03 |
| 3656 | 1/2 cup | Dried, rings, avg | 43 | 104 | 32 | 0.4 | 28.3 | 3.7 | 23.5 | 1.1 | 0.1 | 0.0 | 0.0 | 0.0 | 0.01 | 0.03 | 0 | 0 | 0 | 0 | 0 | 0 | 0.00 | 0.07 | 0.40 | 0.05 | 0.00 | 0.0 | 0.11 | 1.7 | 0.0 | | 6 | 0.1 | 0.6 | 7 | 0.0 | 16 | 194 | 0.6 | 37 | 0.09 |
| 3145 | 1/2 cup | Dried, w/o sugar, avg | 128 | 73 | 84 | 0.3 | 19.6 | 2.6 | 16.3 | 0.7 | 0.1 | 0.0 | 0.0 | 0.0 | 0.01 | 0.02 | 0 | 22 | 3 | 0 | 3 | 10 | 0.01 | 0.02 | 0.17 | 0.06 | 0.00 | 0.0 | 0.07 | 1.3 | 0.0 | | 4 | 0.1 | 0.4 | 5 | 0.0 | 12 | 134 | 0.4 | 26 | 0.06 |
| 3146 | 1/2 cup | Dried, w/sugar, avg | 140 | 116 | 79 | 0.3 | 29.0 | 2.7 | 25.6 | 0.7 | 0.1 | 0.0 | 0.0 | 0.0 | 0.01 | 0.02 | 0 | 22 | 3 | 0 | 3 | 11 | 0.01 | 0.03 | 0.17 | 0.07 | 0.00 | 0.0 | 0.08 | 1.3 | 0.0 | 0.3 | 4 | 0.1 | 0.4 | 4 | 0.0 | 11 | 137 | 0.7 | 27 | 0.06 |
| 3392 | 1/2 cup | Frozen, unsweetened, avg | 86 | 41 | 87 | 0.2 | 10.6 | 1.6 | 8.7 | 0.2 | 0.3 | 0.0 | 0.0 | 0.1 | 0.01 | 0.07 | 0 | 29 | 3 | 0 | 3 | 11 | 0.01 | 0.01 | 0.04 | 0.03 | 0.00 | 0.6 | 0.05 | 0.1 | 0.0 | 0.9 | 3 | 0.0 | 0.2 | 3 | 0.1 | 7 | 66 | 0.2 | 3 | 0.04 |
| 3315 | 1 ea | Pickled, avg | 19 | 25 | 65 | 0.0 | 6.5 | 0.3 | 6.1 | 0.0 | 0.0 | 0.0 | 0.0 | 0.0 | 0.00 | 0.01 | 0 | 7 | 0.6 | 0 | 0.6 | 3 | 0.00 | 0.00 | 0.01 | 0.01 | 0.00 | 0.3 | 0.01 | 0.7 | 0.0 | | 1 | 0.0 | 0.0 | 1 | 0.0 | 1 | 18 | 0.1 | 0 | 0.01 |
| 3512 | 1 ea | Raw, golden delicious, w/peel, avg | 138 | 59 | 85 | 0.4 | 17.0 | 2.5 | 14.5 | 0.0 | 0.0 | 0.0 | 0.0 | 0.0 | 0.00 | 0.00 | 0 | 41 | 4 | 0 | 4 | 14 | 0.03 | 0.01 | 0.14 | | 0.00 | | | 6.9 | | | 4 | | 0.3 | 6 | | | 103 | | 3 | 0.14 |
| 3509 | 1 ea | Raw, granny smith, w/peel, avg | 138 | 61 | 85 | 0.4 | 17.1 | 2.6 | 14.2 | 0.3 | 0.0 | 0.0 | 0.0 | 0.0 | 0.00 | 0.00 | 0 | 14 | 1 | 0 | 1 | 1 | 0.04 | 0.01 | 0.14 | | 0.00 | | | 6.9 | | | 7 | | 0.3 | 6 | | | 152 | | 1 | 0.14 |
| 3264 | 1/2 cup | Raw, rose, avg | 68 | 17 | 93 | 0.4 | 3.9 | 0.9 | 3.0 | 0.0 | 0.2 | | | | | | 0 | 231 | 23 | 0 | 23 | 95 | 0.01 | 0.02 | 0.54 | | 0.00 | | | 15.2 | 0.0 | | 20 | 0.0 | 0.0 | 3 | 0.0 | 5 | 84 | | 0 | 0.04 |
| 3003 | 1 ea | Raw, w/o peel, avg | 128 | 73 | 84 | 0.2 | 18.9 | 2.4 | 15.8 | 0.7 | 0.4 | 0.1 | 0.0 | 0.1 | 0.02 | 0.10 | 0 | 56 | 5 | 0 | 5 | 21 | 0.02 | 0.01 | 0.12 | 0.06 | 0.00 | 0.5 | 0.07 | 5.1 | 0.0 | | 5 | 0.0 | 0.1 | 4 | 0.0 | 9 | 145 | 0.4 | 0 | 0.05 |
| 3000 | 1 ea | Raw, w/peel, avg | 138 | 81 | 84 | 0.3 | 21.1 | 3.7 | 16.6 | 0.8 | 0.5 | 0.1 | 0.0 | 0.1 | 0.02 | 0.12 | 0 | 73 | 7 | 0 | 7 | 28 | 0.02 | 0.02 | 0.11 | 0.07 | 0.00 | 3.9 | 0.08 | 7.9 | 0.0 | | 10 | 0.1 | 0.2 | 7 | 0.1 | 10 | 159 | 0.4 | 0 | 0.06 |
| | | Applesauce | | | | | | | | | | | | | | | | | | | | | | | | | | | | | | | | | | | | | | | | |
| 3006 | 1/2 cup | Canned, avg | 122 | 52 | 88 | 0.2 | 13.8 | 1.5 | 11.8 | 0.5 | 0.1 | 0.0 | 0.0 | 0.0 | 0.00 | 0.01 | 0 | 35 | 4 | 0 | 4 | 15 | 0.02 | 0.03 | 0.23 | 0.03 | 0.00 | 0.7 | 0.12 | 1.5 | 0.0 | 0.1 | 4 | 0.0 | 0.1 | 4 | 0.1 | 9 | 92 | 0.4 | 2 | 0.04 |
| 3330 | 1/2 cup | Canned, w/vit C, avg | 122 | 52 | 88 | 0.2 | 13.8 | 1.5 | 11.4 | 0.9 | 0.1 | 0.0 | 0.0 | 0.0 | 0.00 | 0.01 | 0 | 35 | 4 | 0 | 4 | 15 | 0.02 | 0.03 | 0.23 | 0.03 | 0.00 | 0.7 | 0.12 | 25.9 | 0.0 | | 4 | 0.0 | 0.1 | 4 | 0.1 | 9 | 92 | 0.4 | 2 | 0.04 |
| 3331 | 1/2 cup | Sweetened, avg | 128 | 97 | 80 | 0.2 | 25.5 | 1.5 | 23.9 | 0.0 | 0.2 | 0.0 | 0.0 | 0.1 | 0.01 | 0.06 | 0 | 14 | 1 | 0 | 1 | 5 | 0.02 | 0.04 | 0.24 | 0.03 | 0.00 | 0.8 | 0.07 | 2.2 | 0.0 | | 5 | 0.1 | 0.4 | 4 | 0.1 | 9 | 78 | 0.4 | 36 | 0.05 |
| 3147 | 1/2 cup | Sweetened, w/o salt, avg | 128 | 97 | 80 | 0.2 | 25.5 | 1.5 | 23.9 | 0.0 | 0.2 | 0.0 | 0.0 | 0.1 | 0.01 | 0.06 | 0 | 14 | 1 | 0 | 1 | 5 | 0.02 | 0.04 | 0.24 | 0.03 | 0.00 | 0.8 | 0.07 | 2.2 | 0.0 | | 5 | 0.1 | 0.4 | 4 | 0.1 | 9 | 78 | 0.4 | 4 | 0.05 |
| | | Apricots | | | | | | | | | | | | | | | | | | | | | | | | | | | | | | | | | | | | | | | | |
| 3457 | 1 oz | Candied, avg | 28 | 95 | 12 | 0.2 | 24.2 | | | | 0.1 | 0.0 | | | 0.00 | 0.00 | 0 | 756 | 76 | 0 | 76 | 451 | 0.01 | 0.01 | 0.17 | | 0.00 | | | 2.8 | 0.0 | | 5 | | 0.1 | | | 6 | 79 | | 0 | |
| 3398 | 1/2 cup | Canned in extra heavy syrup, w/o skin & pit, avg | 123 | 118 | 74 | 0.7 | 30.6 | 2.0 | 28.3 | 0.4 | 0.0 | 0.0 | 0.0 | 0.0 | 0.00 | 0.01 | 0 | 1809 | 181 | 0 | 181 | 1078 | 0.02 | 0.03 | 0.42 | 0.07 | 0.00 | 2.0 | 0.11 | 3.0 | 0.0 | 0.4 | 10 | 0.1 | 0.8 | 10 | 0.1 | 18 | 155 | | 16 | 0.12 |
| 3396 | 1/2 cup | Canned in heavy syrup, w/o skin & pit, avg | 129 | 107 | 78 | 0.7 | 27.7 | 2.1 | 25.7 | 0.0 | 0.1 | 0.0 | 0.0 | 0.0 | 0.00 | 0.02 | 0 | 1600 | 160 | 0 | 160 | 954 | 0.02 | 0.03 | 0.54 | 0.07 | 0.00 | 2.2 | 0.12 | 3.6 | 0.0 | 1.1 | 12 | 0.1 | 0.6 | 10 | 0.1 | 17 | 173 | | 14 | 0.13 |
| 3011 | 1/2 cup | Canned in heavy syrup, w/skin, avg | 120 | 100 | 78 | 0.6 | 25.8 | 1.9 | 23.9 | 0.0 | 0.1 | 0.0 | 0.0 | 0.0 | 0.00 | 0.02 | 0 | 1476 | 148 | 0 | 148 | 880 | 0.02 | 0.03 | 0.45 | 0.06 | 0.00 | 2.0 | 0.11 | 3.7 | 0.0 | 1.1 | 11 | 0.1 | 0.4 | 8 | 0.1 | 14 | 168 | 0.4 | 5 | 0.13 |
| 3151 | 1/2 cup | Canned in juice, w/skin, halves, avg | 122 | 59 | 87 | 0.8 | 15.0 | 2.0 | 13.1 | 0.0 | 0.0 | 0.0 | 0.0 | 0.0 | 0.00 | 0.01 | 0 | 2063 | 206 | 0 | 206 | 1230 | 0.02 | 0.02 | 0.42 | 0.07 | 0.00 | 2.1 | 0.11 | 6.0 | 0.0 | | 15 | 0.1 | 0.4 | 12 | 0.1 | 24 | 201 | 0.4 | 5 | 0.13 |
| 3153 | 1/2 cup | Canned in light syrup, w/skin, avg | 126 | 79 | 83 | 0.7 | 20.8 | 2.0 | 18.8 | 0.0 | 0.1 | 0.0 | 0.0 | 0.0 | 0.00 | 0.01 | 0 | 1666 | 166 | 0 | 166 | 992 | 0.02 | 0.03 | 0.38 | 0.07 | 0.00 | 2.1 | 0.12 | 3.4 | 0.0 | | 14 | 0.1 | 0.5 | 10 | 0.1 | 16 | 174 | 0.4 | 5 | 0.14 |
| 3333 | 1/2 cup | Canned in water, w/o skin, avg | 114 | 25 | 93 | 0.8 | 6.2 | 1.3 | 4.9 | 0.1 | 0.0 | 0.0 | 0.0 | 0.0 | 0.00 | 0.01 | 0 | 2063 | 206 | 0 | 206 | 1231 | 0.02 | 0.03 | 0.50 | 0.06 | 0.00 | 1.9 | 0.10 | 2.1 | 0.0 | | 9 | 0.1 | 0.6 | 10 | 0.1 | 18 | 176 | | 13 | 0.13 |
| 3632 | 1/2 cup | Canned in water, w/skin, avg | 122 | 33 | 92 | 0.9 | 7.8 | 2.0 | 5.8 | 0.0 | 0.2 | 0.0 | 0.1 | 0.0 | 0.00 | 0.04 | 0 | 1577 | 157 | 0 | 157 | 938 | 0.03 | 0.03 | 0.48 | 0.07 | 0.00 | 2.1 | 0.11 | 4.1 | 0.0 | | 10 | 0.1 | 0.4 | 9 | 0.1 | 16 | 234 | 0.4 | 4 | 0.13 |
| 3014 | 1/2 cup | Dried, sulfured, uncooked, avg | 65 | 155 | 31 | 2.4 | 40.2 | 5.8 | 34.3 | 0.0 | 0.3 | 0.0 | 0.1 | 0.1 | 0.00 | 0.06 | 0 | 4706 | 471 | 0 | 471 | 2807 | 0.01 | 0.10 | 1.95 | 0.10 | 0.00 | 6.7 | 0.49 | 1.6 | 0.0 | | 29 | 0.3 | 3.1 | 31 | 0.2 | 76 | 896 | 1.4 | 6 | 0.48 |
| 3155 | 1/2 cup | Frozen, sweetened, avg | 121 | 119 | 73 | 0.8 | 30.4 | 2.7 | 27.7 | 0.0 | 0.1 | 0.0 | 0.1 | 0.0 | 0.00 | 0.02 | 0 | 2033 | 203 | 0 | 203 | 1212 | 0.02 | 0.05 | 0.97 | 0.07 | 0.00 | 2.1 | 0.24 | 10.9 | 0.0 | | 12 | 0.1 | 1.1 | 11 | 0.1 | 23 | 277 | 1.1 | 5 | 0.12 |
| 3657 | 1/2 cup | Raw, pitted, fresh, sliced, avg | 82 | 39 | 86 | 1.1 | 9.1 | 2.0 | 7.1 | 0.0 | 0.3 | 0.0 | 0.1 | 0.1 | 0.00 | 0.06 | 0 | 2142 | 214 | 0 | 214 | 1277 | 0.02 | 0.03 | 0.49 | 0.04 | 0.00 | 7.1 | 0.20 | 8.2 | 0.0 | | 11 | 0.1 | 0.4 | 7 | 0.1 | 16 | 243 | 0.3 | 1 | 0.21 |
| 3401 | 1/2 cup | Stewed, dried, halves, sulfured, w/sugar, avg | 135 | 153 | 68 | 1.6 | 39.6 | 5.5 | 33.6 | 0.4 | 0.2 | 0.0 | 0.1 | 0.0 | 0.00 | 0.04 | 0 | 2888 | 289 | 0 | 289 | 1723 | 0.01 | 0.04 | 1.15 | 0.14 | 0.00 | 0.0 | 0.26 | 1.9 | 0.0 | 0.8 | 20 | 0.2 | 2.1 | 20 | 0.1 | 51 | 598 | | 4 | 0.32 |
| 3217 | 1/2 cup | Stewed, dried, sulfured, stewed, avg | 125 | 106 | 76 | 1.6 | 27.4 | 4.0 | 23.1 | 0.3 | 0.2 | 0.0 | 0.1 | 0.0 | 0.00 | 0.04 | 0 | 2954 | 295 | 0 | 295 | 1760 | 0.01 | 0.04 | 1.18 | 0.14 | 0.00 | 0.0 | 0.26 | 2.0 | 0.0 | | 20 | 0.2 | 2.1 | 21 | 0.1 | 51 | 611 | 0.5 | 4 | 0.32 |
| | | Avocado | | | | | | | | | | | | | | | | | | | | | | | | | | | | | | | | | | | | | | | | |
| 3213 | 1/2 cup | Average | 115 | 129 | 80 | 1.8 | 10.2 | 6.1 | 1.0 | 3.1 | 10.2 | 2.0 | 5.6 | 1.7 | 0.10 | 1.60 | 0 | 704 | 70 | 0 | 70 | 376 | 0.12 | 0.14 | 2.21 | 0.32 | 0.00 | 61.3 | 1.12 | 9.1 | 0.0 | | 13 | 0.3 | 0.6 | 39 | 0.2 | 45 | 561 | 0.0 | 6 | 0.48 |
| 3211 | 1/2 cup | California, pureed, avg | 115 | 204 | 73 | 2.4 | 7.9 | 5.6 | 1.0 | 1.3 | 19.9 | 3.0 | 12.9 | 2.3 | 0.13 | 2.21 | 0 | 704 | 70 | 0 | 70 | 376 | 0.12 | 0.14 | 2.21 | 0.32 | 0.00 | 75.3 | 1.12 | 9.1 | 0.0 | 1.5 | 13 | 0.3 | 1.4 | 47 | 0.3 | 48 | 729 | 0.0 | 14 | 0.48 |
| 3658 | 1/2 cup | Sliced, avg | 73 | 118 | 74 | 1.4 | 5.4 | 3.7 | 0.7 | 1.1 | 11.2 | 1.8 | 7.0 | 1.4 | 0.08 | 1.35 | 0 | 447 | 45 | 0 | 45 | 239 | 0.08 | 0.09 | 1.40 | 0.20 | 0.00 | 45.2 | 0.71 | 5.8 | 0.0 | 1.0 | 8 | 0.2 | 0.7 | 28 | 0.2 | 30 | 437 | 0.3 | 7 | 0.31 |
| | | Bananas | | | | | | | | | | | | | | | | | | | | | | | | | | | | | | | | | | | | | | | | |
| 3307 | 1/2 cup | Dried, chips, avg | 46 | 239 | 4 | 1.1 | 26.9 | 3.5 | 17.9 | 5.4 | 15.5 | 13.3 | 0.9 | 0.3 | 0.00 | 0.29 | 0 | 38 | 4 | 0 | 4 | 22 | 0.04 | 0.01 | 0.33 | 0.12 | 0.00 | 6.4 | 0.29 | 2.9 | 0.0 | | 8 | 0.1 | 0.6 | 35 | 0.7 | 26 | 247 | 0.7 | 3 | 0.34 |
| 3361 | 1 ea | Fried, green, avg | 90 | 158 | 64 | 0.9 | 21.5 | 1.5 | 13.5 | 6.5 | 8.8 | 1.2 | 2.1 | 5.0 | | | 0 | 74 | 7 | 0 | 7 | 44 | 0.03 | 0.09 | 0.47 | 0.50 | 0.00 | 13.1 | 0.22 | 6.7 | 0.0 | | 5 | 0.1 | 0.3 | 27 | 0.1 | 18 | 363 | 0.9 | 1 | 0.15 |
| 3306 | 1 ea | Fried, ripe, avg | 91 | 184 | 60 | 1.2 | 23.8 | 1.6 | 19.4 | 2.8 | 10.6 | 2.2 | 4.8 | 3.4 | 0.27 | 3.13 | 0 | 590 | 142 | 125 | 17 | 104 | 0.04 | 0.10 | 0.49 | 0.53 | 0.01 | 9.8 | 0.27 | 6.5 | 0.0 | | 9 | 0.1 | 0.3 | 30 | 0.2 | 23 | 366 | 1.0 | 120 | 0.16 |
| 3458 | 1/2 cup | Raw, red, avg | 75 | 68 | 74 | 0.9 | 17.5 | | | | 0.2 | 0.1 | 0.0 | 0.0 | 0.01 | 0.02 | 0 | 300 | 30 | 0 | 30 | 180 | 0.04 | 0.03 | 0.45 | | 0.00 | | | 7.5 | 0.0 | 0.1 | 8 | | 0.6 | | | 14 | 278 | | 1 | |
| 3021 | 1/2 cup | Raw, slices, avg | 75 | 69 | 74 | 0.8 | 17.5 | 1.8 | 13.9 | 1.9 | 0.4 | 0.1 | 0.0 | 0.1 | 0.02 | 0.04 | 0 | 61 | 6 | 0 | 6 | 36 | 0.03 | 0.08 | 0.41 | 0.43 | 0.00 | 14.3 | 0.19 | 6.8 | 0.0 | 0.2 | 4 | 0.1 | 0.2 | 22 | 0.1 | 15 | 297 | 0.8 | 1 | 0.12 |
| | | Blackberries | | | | | | | | | | | | | | | | | | | | | | | | | | | | | | | | | | | | | | | | |
| 3027 | 1/2 cup | Canned, w/heavy syrup, avg | 128 | 118 | 75 | 1.7 | 29.6 | 4.4 | 25.2 | 0.0 | 0.2 | 0.0 | 0.0 | 0.1 | 0.03 | 0.07 | 0 | 280 | 28 | 0 | 28 | 84 | 0.03 | 0.05 | 0.37 | 0.05 | 0.00 | 33.9 | 0.19 | 3.6 | 0.0 | | 27 | 0.2 | 0.8 | 22 | 0.9 | 18 | 127 | 0.5 | 4 | 0.23 |
| 3024 | 1/2 cup | Fresh, avg | 72 | 37 | 86 | 0.5 | 9.2 | 3.8 | 5.4 | 0.0 | 0.3 | 0.0 | 0.0 | 0.2 | 0.05 | 0.11 | 0 | 119 | 12 | 0 | 12 | 35 | 0.02 | 0.03 | 0.29 | 0.04 | 0.00 | 24.5 | 0.17 | 15.1 | 0.0 | | 23 | 0.1 | 0.4 | 14 | 0.9 | 15 | 141 | 0.4 | 0 | 0.19 |
| 3028 | 1/2 cup | Frozen, unsweetened, avg | 76 | 49 | 82 | 0.9 | 11.9 | 3.8 | 8.1 | 0.0 | 0.3 | 0.0 | 0.0 | 0.2 | 0.06 | 0.12 | 0 | 87 | 8 | 0 | 8 | 25 | 0.02 | 0.03 | 0.92 | 0.05 | 0.00 | 25.8 | 0.11 | 2.4 | 0.0 | | 22 | 0.1 | 0.6 | 17 | 0.9 | 23 | 106 | 0.5 | 1 | 0.19 |
| | | Blueberries | | | | | | | | | | | | | | | | | | | | | | | | | | | | | | | | | | | | | | | | |
| 3030 | 1/2 cup | Canned in heavy syrup, avg | 128 | 113 | 77 | 0.8 | 28.3 | 1.9 | 26.4 | 0.0 | 0.4 | 0.0 | 0.1 | 0.2 | 0.07 | 0.11 | 0 | 82 | 8 | 0 | 8 | 46 | 0.04 | 0.07 | 0.14 | 0.05 | 0.00 | 2.0 | 0.11 | 1.4 | 0.0 | | 6 | 0.1 | 0.4 | 5 | 0.3 | 13 | 51 | 0.5 | 4 | 0.09 |
| 3282 | 1 oz | Dehydrated, Basic Vegetable Products | 28 | 99 | 3 | 1.2 | 24.9 | 2.3 | 22.6 | 0.0 | 0.7 | | | | | | 0 | 176 | 18 | 0 | 18 | 106 | 0.07 | 0.09 | 0.64 | 0.05 | 0.00 | 11.3 | 0.16 | 22.9 | | | 11 | | 0.3 | 9 | | 18 | 157 | | 11 | 0.19 |

| Code | Amount | Description | Basic Components | | | | | | | | | Additional Fats | | | | | | Vit A & Components | | | | | Vitamins | | | | | | | | | | Minerals | | | | | | | | | |
|---|---|---|---|---|---|---|---|---|---|---|---|---|---|---|---|---|---|---|---|---|---|---|---|---|---|---|---|---|---|---|---|---|---|---|---|---|---|---|---|---|---|---|
| | | | Weight (g) | Calories | % Water | Protein (g) | Carbs (g) | Fiber (g) | Sugar (g) | Other Carbs (g) | Fat (g) | Sat Fat (g) | Mono Fat (g) | Poly Fat (g) | Omega 3 (g) | Omega 6 (g) | Choles (mg) | Vit A (IU) | Vit A (RE) | Retinol (RE) | Carotenoids (RE) | Beta Carotene (mcg) | Thiamin (mg) | Riboflavin (mg) | Niacin (NE) | Vit B6 (mg) | Vit B12 (mcg) | Folate (mcg) | Panto (mg) | Vit C (mg) | Vit D (mg) | Vit E (α TE) | Calcium (mg) | Copper (mg) | Iron (mg) | Magnes (mg) | Mang (mg) | Phos (mg) | Potassium (mg) | Selenium (mcg) | Sodium (mg) | Zinc (mg) |
| 3592 | 1 oz | Freeze Dried Blueberries, Mercer Processing | 28 | 99 | 3 | 1.2 | 24.9 | 2.3 | | | 0.7 | | | | | | | 161 | 16 | 0 | 16 | 97 | | | | | 0.00 | 11.3 | | 22.5 | | | 24 | | 1.6 | | | 21 | 130 | | 2 | |
| 3029 | 1/2 cup | Fresh, avg | 72 | 40 | 85 | 0.5 | 10.2 | 1.9 | 8.2 | 0.0 | 0.3 | 0.0 | 0.0 | 0.1 | 0.05 | 0.07 | 0 | 72 | 7 | 0 | 7 | 43 | 0.03 | 0.04 | 0.26 | 0.03 | 0.00 | 4.6 | 0.07 | 9.4 | 0.0 | | 4 | 0.0 | 0.1 | 4 | 0.2 | 7 | 64 | 0.4 | 4 | 0.08 |
| 3031 | 1/2 cup | Frozen, avg | 78 | 40 | 87 | 0.3 | 9.5 | 2.1 | 7.4 | 0.0 | 0.5 | 0.0 | 0.1 | 0.2 | 0.09 | 0.13 | 0 | 63 | 6 | 0 | 6 | 37 | 0.02 | 0.03 | 0.41 | 0.05 | 0.00 | 5.2 | 0.10 | 1.9 | 0.0 | | 6 | 0.0 | 0.1 | 4 | 0.1 | 9 | 42 | 0.5 | 1 | 0.05 |
| 3231 | 1/2 cup | Frozen, sweetened, thawed, avg | 115 | 93 | 77 | 0.5 | 25.3 | 2.4 | 22.9 | 0.0 | 0.1 | 0.0 | 0.0 | 0.1 | 0.03 | 0.04 | 0 | 51 | 5 | 0 | 5 | 28 | 0.02 | 0.06 | 0.29 | 0.07 | 0.00 | 7.7 | 0.14 | 1.1 | 0.0 | | 7 | 0.0 | 0.4 | 2 | 0.3 | 8 | 69 | 0.7 | 1 | 0.07 |
| 3034 | 1/2 cup | Boysenberries, frozen, avg | 66 | 33 | 86 | 0.7 | 8.1 | 2.5 | 5.5 | 0.0 | 0.2 | 0.0 | 0.0 | 0.1 | 0.03 | 0.06 | 0 | 44 | 5 | 0 | 5 | 14 | 0.03 | 0.02 | 0.51 | 0.04 | 0.00 | 41.8 | 0.17 | 2.0 | 0.0 | | 18 | 0.1 | 0.6 | 11 | 0.4 | 18 | 92 | 0.4 | 1 | 0.15 |
| 3032 | 1/2 cup | Boysenberries/Loganberries, cnd in hvy syrup, avg | 128 | 113 | 76 | 1.3 | 28.5 | 3.3 | 25.2 | 0.0 | 0.2 | 0.0 | 0.0 | 0.1 | 0.03 | 0.06 | 0 | 51 | 5 | 0 | 5 | 15 | 0.03 | 0.04 | 0.29 | 0.05 | 0.00 | 44.0 | 0.17 | 7.9 | 0.0 | | 23 | 0.1 | 0.6 | 14 | 0.3 | 13 | 115 | 0.5 | 4 | 0.24 |
| 3239 | 1/2 cup | Breadfruit, raw, avg | 110 | 113 | 71 | 1.2 | 29.8 | 5.4 | 3.5 | 20.9 | 0.3 | 0.1 | 0.0 | 0.1 | 0.02 | 0.05 | 0 | 44 | 4 | 0 | 4 | 26 | 0.12 | 0.03 | 0.99 | 0.11 | 0.00 | 15.4 | 0.50 | 31.9 | 0.0 | | 19 | 0.1 | 0.6 | 28 | 0.1 | 33 | 539 | 0.7 | 2 | 0.13 |
| 3665 | 1/2 cup | Carambola/Starfruit, raw, slices, avg | 54 | 18 | 91 | 0.3 | 4.2 | 1.5 | 2.8 | 0.0 | 0.2 | 0.0 | 0.0 | 0.1 | 0.02 | 0.09 | 0 | 266 | 26 | 0 | 26 | 107 | 0.02 | 0.01 | 0.22 | 0.05 | 0.00 | 7.6 | | 11.4 | 0.0 | | 2 | 0.1 | 0.1 | 5 | 0.0 | 9 | 88 | 0.3 | 1 | 0.06 |
| 3867 | 1/2 cup | Carambola/Starfruit, dried, Freida's Specialty Produce | 61 | 183 | 21 | 3.0 | 44.2 | | | | 0.0 | 0.0 | 0.0 | 0.0 | 0.00 | 0.00 | 0 | 1525 | 153 | 0 | 153 | 619 | | | | | 0.00 | | | | | | 30 | | 1.1 | | | | | | 8 | |
| 3668 | 1/2 cup | Carissa/Natal Plum, raw slices, avg | 75 | 46 | 84 | 0.4 | 10.2 | | | | 1.0 | | | | | | 0 | 30 | 3 | 0 | 3 | 18 | 0.03 | 0.04 | 0.15 | | 0.00 | | | 28.5 | 0.0 | | 8 | 0.2 | 1.0 | 12 | | 5 | 195 | | 2 | |
| 5414 | 1/2 cup | Chayote, chopped, boiled, avg | 80 | 19 | 93 | 0.5 | 4.1 | 2.2 | | | 0.4 | 0.1 | 0.0 | 0.2 | 0.10 | 0.06 | 0 | 38 | 4 | 0 | 4 | 24 | 0.02 | 0.03 | 0.34 | 0.09 | 0.00 | 14.5 | 0.33 | 6.4 | 0.0 | | 10 | 0.1 | 0.2 | 10 | 0.1 | 23 | 138 | 0.2 | 1 | 0.25 |
| 5413 | 1 ea | Chayote, raw, avg | 203 | 39 | 94 | 1.7 | 9.1 | 3.5 | | | 0.3 | 0.1 | 0.0 | 0.1 | 0.07 | 0.04 | 0 | 114 | 12 | 0 | 12 | 73 | 0.05 | 0.06 | 0.95 | 0.15 | 0.00 | 188.8 | 0.51 | 15.6 | 0.0 | | 35 | 0.2 | 0.7 | 24 | 0.4 | 37 | 254 | 0.4 | 4 | 1.50 |
| | | Cherries, Sour | | | | | | | | | | | | | | | | | | | | | | | | | | | | | | | | | | | | | | | | |
| 3335 | 1/2 cup | Canned, in extra heavy syrup, avg | 131 | 149 | 70 | 0.9 | 38.3 | 1.0 | 36.5 | 0.7 | 0.1 | 0.0 | 0.0 | 0.0 | 0.02 | 0.02 | 0 | 912 | 92 | 0 | 92 | 506 | 0.02 | 0.05 | 0.21 | 0.06 | 0.00 | 9.7 | 0.14 | 2.5 | 0.0 | | 13 | 0.1 | 1.7 | 7 | 0.1 | 12 | 119 | | 9 | 0.08 |
| 3403 | 1/2 cup | Canned in heavy syrup, avg | 128 | 116 | 76 | 0.9 | 29.8 | 1.4 | 28.8 | 0.0 | 0.1 | 0.0 | 0.0 | 0.0 | 0.02 | 0.02 | 0 | 914 | 91 | 0 | 91 | 502 | 0.02 | 0.05 | 0.22 | 0.06 | 0.00 | 9.7 | 0.13 | 2.6 | 0.0 | | 13 | 0.1 | 1.7 | 8 | 0.1 | 13 | 119 | 0.4 | 9 | 0.08 |
| 3402 | 1/2 cup | Canned in light syrup, avg | 126 | 94 | 80 | 0.9 | 24.3 | 1.0 | 23.3 | 0.0 | 0.1 | 0.0 | 0.0 | 0.0 | 0.02 | 0.02 | 0 | 915 | 92 | 0 | 92 | 508 | 0.02 | 0.05 | 0.21 | 0.06 | 0.00 | 9.7 | 0.13 | 2.5 | 0.0 | 0.1 | 13 | 0.1 | 1.7 | 8 | 0.1 | 13 | 120 | | 9 | 0.09 |
| 3035 | 1/2 cup | Canned in water, avg | 122 | 44 | 90 | 0.9 | 10.9 | 1.3 | 9.3 | 0.3 | 0.1 | 0.0 | 0.0 | 0.0 | 0.02 | 0.02 | 0 | 920 | 92 | 0 | 92 | 505 | 0.02 | 0.05 | 0.22 | 0.05 | 0.00 | 9.8 | 0.13 | 2.6 | 0.0 | | 13 | 0.1 | 1.7 | 7 | 0.1 | 12 | 120 | 0.4 | 9 | 0.09 |
| 3159 | 1/2 cup | Frozen, unsweetened, avg | 78 | 36 | 87 | 0.7 | 8.6 | 1.2 | 7.3 | 0.0 | 0.3 | 0.1 | 0.1 | 0.1 | 0.05 | 0.05 | 0 | 579 | 68 | 0 | 68 | 374 | 0.03 | 0.03 | 0.11 | 0.05 | 0.00 | 3.5 | 0.14 | 1.3 | 0.0 | | 10 | 0.1 | 0.4 | 7 | 0.0 | 12 | 97 | 0.3 | 1 | 0.08 |
| 3283 | 1 oz | Dried, Dehydrated, Basic Vegetable Products | 28 | 98 | 3 | 2.0 | 23.8 | 0.4 | 23.4 | 0.0 | 0.6 | | | | | | 0 | 2511 | 251 | 0 | 251 | 1386 | 0.06 | 0.08 | 0.78 | 0.09 | 0.00 | 14.7 | 0.28 | 19.6 | | | 31 | | 0.6 | 18 | | 29 | 339 | | 6 | 0.20 |
| 3593 | 1 oz | Dried, Freeze Dried, Mercer Processing | 28 | 99 | 3 | 1.8 | 24.1 | 0.5 | | | 0.7 | | | | | | | 1799 | 180 | 0 | 180 | 993 | 0.07 | 0.12 | 0.54 | | 0.00 | | | 9.0 | | | 24 | | 1.3 | | | 39 | 338 | | 4 | |
| 3609 | 1/2 cup | Raw, Basic Vegetable Products | 78 | 39 | 86 | 0.8 | 9.5 | 0.2 | | | 0.2 | | | | | | | 1001 | 100 | 0 | 100 | 552 | 0.02 | 0.03 | 0.31 | 0.03 | 0.00 | 5.8 | 0.11 | 7.8 | | | 12 | | 0.2 | 7 | | 12 | 135 | | 2 | 0.08 |
| | | Cherries, Sweet | | | | | | | | | | | | | | | | | | | | | | | | | | | | | | | | | | | | | | | | |
| 3406 | 1/2 cup | Canned in extra heavy syrup, avg | 131 | 134 | 73 | 0.8 | 34.3 | 2.0 | 32.1 | 0.2 | 0.2 | 0.0 | 0.1 | 0.1 | 0.03 | 0.03 | 0 | 198 | 20 | 0 | 20 | 108 | 0.03 | 0.05 | 0.51 | 0.04 | 0.00 | 5.5 | 0.17 | 4.7 | 0.0 | 0.1 | 12 | 0.2 | 0.5 | 10 | 0.1 | 22 | 186 | | 4 | 0.13 |
| 3336 | 1/2 cup | Canned in juice, avg | 125 | 68 | 85 | 1.1 | 17.3 | 1.9 | 14.9 | 0.5 | 0.0 | 0.0 | 0.0 | 0.0 | 0.00 | 0.00 | 0 | 156 | 16 | 0 | 16 | 90 | 0.02 | 0.03 | 0.51 | 0.04 | 0.00 | 5.3 | 0.16 | 3.1 | 0.0 | | 18 | 0.1 | 0.7 | 15 | 0.1 | 28 | 164 | 0.4 | 4 | 0.13 |
| 3405 | 1/2 cup | Canned in light syrup, avg | 126 | 84 | 82 | 0.8 | 21.8 | 1.9 | 19.7 | 0.2 | 0.2 | 0.0 | 0.1 | 0.1 | 0.03 | 0.03 | 0 | 198 | 20 | 0 | 20 | 111 | 0.03 | 0.05 | 0.51 | 0.04 | 0.00 | 5.3 | 0.16 | 4.7 | 0.0 | | 11 | 0.2 | 0.5 | 11 | 0.1 | 23 | 186 | 0.4 | 4 | 0.13 |
| 3038 | 1/2 cup | Canned in heavy syrup, avg | 127 | 105 | 78 | 0.8 | 27.1 | 1.9 | 24.9 | 0.2 | 0.2 | 0.0 | 0.1 | 0.1 | 0.03 | 0.03 | 0 | 196 | 19 | 0 | 19 | 105 | 0.03 | 0.05 | 0.50 | 0.04 | 0.00 | 5.3 | 0.16 | 4.6 | 0.0 | | 11 | 0.2 | 0.4 | 11 | 0.1 | 23 | 184 | 0.4 | 4 | 0.13 |
| 3404 | 1/2 cup | Canned in water, avg | 124 | 57 | 87 | 1.0 | 14.6 | 1.9 | 12.5 | 0.2 | 0.2 | 0.0 | 0.0 | 0.0 | 0.02 | 0.02 | 0 | 198 | 20 | 0 | 20 | 110 | 0.03 | 0.05 | 0.51 | 0.04 | 0.00 | 5.2 | 0.16 | 2.7 | 0.0 | | 14 | 0.1 | 0.4 | 11 | 0.1 | 19 | 162 | 0.4 | 1 | 0.10 |
| 3459 | 1/2 cup | Canned, maraschino, avg | 80 | 93 | 70 | 0.2 | 23.5 | | | | 0.1 | 0.0 | 0.0 | 0.0 | 0.02 | 0.02 | 0 | 0 | 0 | 0 | 0 | 0 | 0.00 | 0.00 | 0.00 | | 0.00 | | | 0.0 | 0.0 | 0.1 | 12 | | 0.2 | | | 10 | 101 | | 1 | |
| 3158 | 1/2 cup | Frozen, sweetened, avg | 130 | 116 | 76 | 1.5 | 29.1 | 2.7 | 26.4 | 0.0 | 0.2 | 0.0 | 0.0 | 0.1 | 0.03 | 0.03 | 0 | 246 | 25 | 0 | 25 | 135 | 0.04 | 0.06 | 0.23 | 0.05 | 0.00 | 5.5 | 0.17 | 1.3 | 0.0 | | 16 | 0.0 | 0.5 | 13 | 0.1 | 21 | 259 | 0.5 | 1 | 0.05 |
| 3037 | 1/2 cup | Raw, w/o pits, avg | 72 | 52 | 81 | 0.9 | 12.0 | 1.7 | 10.3 | 0.0 | 0.7 | 0.2 | 0.2 | 0.2 | 0.10 | 0.11 | 0 | 154 | 15 | 0 | 15 | 83 | 0.04 | 0.04 | 0.29 | 0.03 | 0.00 | 3.0 | 0.09 | 5.0 | 0.0 | 0.1 | 11 | 0.1 | 0.3 | 8 | 0.1 | 14 | 161 | 0.4 | 0 | 0.04 |
| | | Cranberries | | | | | | | | | | | | | | | | | | | | | | | | | | | | | | | | | | | | | | | | |
| 3460 | 1 oz | Dried, dehydrated, avg | 28 | 103 | 5 | 0.8 | 23.6 | 7.0 | 16.6 | 0.0 | 1.8 | 0.2 | 0.5 | 1.1 | | | 0 | 34 | 8 | 0 | 8 | 43 | 0.05 | 0.03 | 0.22 | | 0.00 | | | 9.0 | 0.0 | 0.8 | 23 | | 1.0 | | | 6 | 180 | | 4 | |
| 3487 | 1/2 cup | Dried, craisins, sweetened, Ocean Spray | 67 | 216 | 12 | 0.2 | 52.1 | 5.9 | 46.2 | 0.0 | 0.8 | 0.2 | | | | | 0 | 0 | 0 | 0 | 0 | 0 | 0.01 | 0.06 | 0.02 | | 0.00 | | | 0.3 | | | 12 | 0.1 | 0.3 | 5 | | 9 | 58 | | 2 | 0.08 |
| 3865 | 1/2 cup | Dried, Frieda's Specialty Produce | 67 | 201 | 28 | 0.0 | 46.9 | 5.0 | 41.9 | 0.0 | 0.0 | 0.0 | 0.0 | 0.0 | 0.00 | 0.00 | 0 | 0 | 0 | 0 | 0 | 0 | | | | | 0.00 | | | 0.0 | | | 0 | | 0.0 | | | | | | 0 | |
| 3039 | 1/2 cup | Raw, whole, avg | 48 | 24 | 86 | 0.2 | 6.1 | 2.0 | 4.1 | 0.0 | 0.1 | 0.0 | 0.0 | 0.0 | 0.02 | 0.03 | 0 | 22 | 2 | 0 | 2 | 14 | 0.01 | 0.01 | 0.05 | 0.03 | 0.00 | 0.8 | 0.11 | 6.5 | 0.0 | | 3 | 0.0 | 0.1 | 2 | 0.1 | 4 | 34 | 0.3 | 0 | 0.06 |
| 3040 | 1/2 cup | Sauce, sweetened, canned, avg | 138 | 208 | 61 | 0.3 | 53.7 | 1.4 | 52.3 | 0.0 | 0.2 | 0.0 | 0.0 | 0.1 | 0.04 | 0.06 | 0 | 28 | 3 | 0 | 3 | 15 | 0.02 | 0.03 | 0.14 | 0.02 | 0.00 | 1.4 | 0.12 | 2.8 | 0.0 | | 6 | 0.0 | 0.3 | 4 | 0.1 | 8 | 36 | 0.7 | 40 | 0.07 |
| | | Currants | | | | | | | | | | | | | | | | | | | | | | | | | | | | | | | | | | | | | | | | |
| 3190 | 1/2 cup | Black, fresh, avg | 56 | 35 | 82 | 0.8 | 8.6 | 4.1 | 4.5 | 0.0 | 0.2 | 0.0 | 0.0 | 0.1 | 0.04 | 0.06 | 0 | 129 | 13 | 0 | 13 | 77 | 0.03 | 0.03 | 0.17 | 0.04 | 0.00 | 1.9 | 0.22 | 101.4 | 0.0 | | 31 | 0.0 | 0.9 | 13 | 0.1 | 33 | 180 | 0.2 | 1 | 0.15 |
| 3504 | 1/2 cup | Black, stewed w/o sugar, avg | 129 | 36 | 81 | 1.0 | 7.2 | 9.5 | 7.2 | | 0.5 | | 0.1 | 0.3 | | | 0 | 361 | 36 | 0 | 36 | 213 | 0.04 | 0.06 | | 0.08 | 0.00 | 2.6 | | 193.5 | | | 66 | | 1.4 | | | | 413 | 0.5 | 4 | 0.39 |
| 3503 | 1/2 cup | Black, stewed w/sugar, avg | 135 | 85 | 73 | 1.1 | 20.3 | 9.2 | 20.3 | | 0.5 | | 0.1 | 0.3 | | | 0 | 365 | 36 | 0 | 36 | 215 | 0.03 | 0.07 | | 0.07 | 0.00 | 2.7 | | 189.0 | | | 63 | | 1.4 | | | | 392 | 0.5 | 3 | 0.41 |
| 3192 | 1/2 cup | Dried, avg | 72 | 204 | 19 | 2.9 | 53.4 | 4.9 | 48.5 | 0.0 | 0.2 | 0.0 | 0.0 | 0.1 | 0.00 | 0.13 | 0 | 53 | 5 | 0 | 5 | 30 | 0.12 | 0.10 | 1.17 | 0.21 | 0.00 | 7.3 | 0.03 | 3.4 | 0.0 | 0.1 | 62 | 0.3 | 2.3 | 30 | 0.3 | 90 | 642 | 0.5 | 6 | 0.48 |
| 3191 | 1/2 cup | Red/White, fresh, avg | 56 | 31 | 84 | 0.8 | 7.7 | 2.4 | 5.3 | 0.0 | 0.1 | 0.0 | 0.0 | 0.0 | 0.02 | 0.03 | 0 | 67 | 7 | 0 | 7 | 40 | 0.02 | 0.03 | 0.06 | 0.04 | 0.00 | 4.5 | 0.04 | 23.0 | 0.0 | 0.1 | 18 | 0.1 | 0.6 | 7 | 0.1 | 25 | 154 | 0.3 | 1 | 0.13 |
| 3674 | 1/2 cup | Cherimoya, raw, avg | 113 | 106 | 74 | 1.5 | 27.1 | 2.7 | 14.8 | 9.6 | 0.5 | | | | | | 0 | 11 | 1 | 0 | 1 | 7 | 0.11 | 0.12 | 1.47 | | 0.00 | | | 10.2 | 0.0 | | 26 | | 0.6 | | | 45 | | | 3 | |
| 3043 | 1/2 cup | Dates, chopped, pitted, avg | 89 | 245 | 22 | 1.8 | 65.4 | 6.7 | 57.1 | 1.6 | 0.4 | 0.2 | 0.1 | 0.0 | 0.00 | 0.02 | 0 | 45 | 4.5 | 0 | 4.5 | 27 | 0.03 | 0.09 | 1.96 | 0.17 | 0.00 | 11.2 | 0.69 | 0.0 | 0.0 | | 28 | 0.3 | 1.0 | 31 | 0.3 | 36 | 580 | 1.7 | 3 | 0.26 |
| 3310 | 1/2 cup | Elderberries, cooked/canned, avg | 128 | 152 | 68 | 0.6 | 38.8 | 6.5 | 32.2 | 0.1 | 0.5 | 0.0 | 0.1 | 0.2 | 0.10 | 0.13 | 0 | 421 | 42 | 0 | 42 | 253 | 0.05 | 0.06 | 0.42 | 0.19 | 0.00 | 2.8 | 0.12 | 23.6 | 0.0 | | 35 | 0.1 | 1.5 | 5 | 0.0 | 37 | 236 | | 6 | 0.11 |
| 3245 | 1/2 cup | Elderberries, raw, avg | 72 | 53 | 80 | 0.5 | 13.2 | 5.0 | 8.2 | 0.0 | 0.4 | 0.0 | 0.1 | 0.2 | 0.06 | 0.12 | 0 | 432 | 43 | 0 | 43 | 259 | 0.05 | 0.04 | 0.36 | 0.17 | 0.00 | 4.3 | 0.10 | 25.9 | 0.0 | | 27 | 0.0 | 1.2 | 4 | 0.0 | 28 | 202 | 0.4 | 4 | 0.08 |
| | | Figs | | | | | | | | | | | | | | | | | | | | | | | | | | | | | | | | | | | | | | | | |
| 3461 | 1 oz | Candied, avg | 28 | 84 | 21 | 1.0 | 20.6 | | | | 0.1 | 0.0 | 0.0 | 0.0 | 0.00 | 0.03 | 0 | 22 | 2 | 0 | 2 | 13 | 0.03 | 0.03 | 0.20 | | 0.00 | | | 0.0 | 0.0 | | 35 | | 0.8 | | | 22 | 179 | | 10 | |
| 3410 | 1/2 cup | Canned in extra heavy syrup, avg | 130 | 139 | 71 | 0.5 | 36.3 | 2.9 | 33.4 | 0.0 | 0.1 | 0.0 | 0.0 | 0.1 | 0.00 | 0.06 | 0 | 47 | 5 | 0 | 5 | 31 | 0.03 | 0.05 | 0.54 | 0.09 | 0.00 | 2.6 | 0.09 | 1.3 | 0.0 | 0.0 | 34 | 0.1 | 0.4 | 13 | 0.1 | 13 | 126 | | 1 | 0.14 |
| 57486 | 1/2 cup | Canned in heavy syrup, avg | 130 | 114 | 76 | 0.5 | 29.8 | 2.9 | 26.9 | 0.0 | 0.1 | 0.0 | 0.0 | 0.1 | 0.00 | 0.06 | 0 | 48 | 5 | 0 | 5 | 31 | 0.03 | 0.05 | 0.56 | 0.09 | 0.00 | 2.6 | 0.09 | 1.3 | 0.0 | | 35 | 0.1 | 0.4 | 13 | 0.1 | 13 | 129 | 0.5 | 1 | 0.14 |
| 3408 | 1/2 cup | Canned in light syrup, avg | 126 | 87 | 81 | 0.5 | 22.7 | 2.3 | 20.4 | 0.0 | 0.1 | 0.0 | 0.0 | 0.1 | 0.00 | 0.06 | 0 | 47 | 5 | 0 | 5 | 30 | 0.03 | 0.05 | 0.55 | 0.09 | 0.00 | 2.5 | 0.09 | 1.3 | 0.0 | | 34 | 0.1 | 0.4 | 13 | 0.1 | 13 | 129 | 0.5 | 1 | 0.14 |
| 3678 | 1/2 cup | Canned in water, avg | 124 | 66 | 85 | 0.5 | 17.4 | 2.7 | 14.6 | 0.0 | 0.1 | 0.0 | 0.0 | 0.1 | 0.00 | 0.06 | 0 | 47 | 5 | 0 | 5 | 30 | 0.03 | 0.05 | 0.55 | 0.09 | 0.00 | 2.5 | 0.09 | 1.2 | 0.0 | | 35 | 0.1 | 0.4 | 12 | 0.1 | 12 | 128 | 0.5 | 1 | 0.15 |
| 3314 | 1/2 cup | Dried, cooked, unsweetened, avg | 130 | 140 | 70 | 1.7 | 35.9 | 6.6 | 29.6 | 0.0 | 0.6 | 0.1 | 0.1 | 0.3 | 0.00 | 0.31 | 0 | 207 | 21 | 0 | 21 | 125 | 0.01 | 0.14 | 0.83 | 0.17 | 0.00 | 1.3 | 0.17 | 5.7 | 0.0 | | 79 | 0.2 | 1.2 | 32 | 0.2 | 38 | 391 | 1.2 | 6 | 0.27 |
| 3679 | 1/2 cup | Dried, uncooked, avg | 100 | 255 | 28 | 3.0 | 65.4 | 12.2 | 56.1 | 0.0 | 1.2 | 0.2 | 0.3 | 0.6 | 0.00 | 0.56 | 0 | 133 | 13 | 0 | 13 | 78 | 0.07 | 0.09 | 0.69 | 0.22 | 0.00 | 7.5 | 0.44 | 0.8 | 0.0 | | 144 | 0.3 | 2.2 | 59 | 0.4 | 68 | 712 | 1.3 | 11 | 0.51 |
| 3160 | 1 ea | Raw, medium, avg | 50 | 37 | 79 | 0.4 | 9.6 | 1.6 | 7.9 | 0.0 | 0.2 | 0.0 | 0.0 | 0.1 | 0.00 | 0.07 | 0 | 71 | 7 | 0 | 7 | 42 | 0.03 | 0.03 | 0.20 | 0.06 | 0.00 | 3.0 | 0.15 | 1.0 | 0.0 | | 18 | 0.0 | 0.2 | 8 | 0.1 | 7 | 116 | 0.3 | 0 | 0.08 |
| | | Fruit Cocktail | | | | | | | | | | | | | | | | | | | | | | | | | | | | | | | | | | | | | | | | |
| 3412 | 1/2 cup | Canned in extra heavy syrup, avg | 130 | 114 | 76 | 0.5 | 29.8 | 1.4 | 28.3 | 0.0 | 0.1 | 0.0 | 0.0 | 0.0 | 0.01 | 0.03 | 0 | 261 | 26 | 0 | 26 | 156 | 0.02 | 0.02 | 0.48 | 0.06 | 0.00 | 3.4 | 0.08 | 2.5 | 0.0 | | 8 | 0.1 | 0.4 | 6 | 0.2 | 14 | 112 | | 8 | 0.10 |
| 3411 | 1/2 cup | Canned in extra light syrup, avg | 123 | 55 | 88 | 0.5 | 14.3 | 1.4 | 12.9 | 0.0 | 0.1 | 0.0 | 0.0 | 0.0 | 0.00 | 0.03 | 0 | 287 | 28 | 0 | 28 | 170 | 0.04 | 0.01 | 0.62 | 0.06 | 0.00 | 3.3 | 0.08 | 3.7 | 0.0 | | 10 | 0.1 | 0.4 | 7 | 0.2 | 15 | 128 | | 5 | 0.10 |
| 3045 | 1/2 cup | Canned in heavy syrup, avg | 124 | 91 | 80 | 0.5 | 23.4 | 1.2 | 22.1 | 0.1 | 0.1 | 0.0 | 0.0 | 0.0 | 0.00 | 0.03 | 0 | 254 | 25 | 0 | 25 | 149 | 0.02 | 0.02 | 0.46 | 0.06 | 0.00 | 3.2 | 0.07 | 2.4 | 0.0 | | 7 | 0.1 | 0.4 | 6 | 0.2 | 14 | 109 | 0.6 | 7 | 0.10 |
| 3164 | 1/2 cup | Canned in juice, avg | 118 | 54 | 87 | 0.5 | 14.0 | 1.2 | 12.7 | 0.1 | 0.0 | 0.0 | 0.0 | 0.0 | 0.00 | 0.00 | 0 | 360 | 37 | 0 | 37 | 219 | 0.01 | 0.02 | 0.48 | 0.06 | 0.00 | 2.9 | 0.07 | 3.2 | 0.0 | | 9 | 0.1 | 0.2 | 8 | 0.2 | 17 | 112 | 0.6 | 5 | 0.11 |
| 3163 | 1/2 cup | Canned in light syrup, avg | 121 | 69 | 84 | 0.5 | 18.0 | 1.2 | 16.7 | 0.1 | 0.1 | 0.0 | 0.0 | 0.0 | 0.00 | 0.03 | 0 | 252 | 25 | 0 | 25 | 152 | 0.02 | 0.02 | 0.46 | 0.06 | 0.00 | 3.3 | 0.07 | 2.3 | 0.0 | | 7 | 0.1 | 0.4 | 6 | 0.2 | 13 | 108 | 0.6 | 7 | 0.11 |
| 3313 | 1/2 cup | Canned in water, w/o sugar, avg | 118 | 38 | 91 | 0.5 | 10.0 | 1.2 | 8.8 | 0.1 | 0.1 | 0.0 | 0.0 | 0.0 | 0.00 | 0.02 | 0 | 295 | 29 | 0 | 29 | 177 | 0.02 | 0.01 | 0.43 | 0.06 | 0.00 | 3.2 | 0.07 | 2.5 | 0.0 | | 6 | 0.1 | 0.3 | 8 | 0.2 | 13 | 111 | 0.6 | 5 | 0.11 |
| | | Fruit Salad | | | | | | | | | | | | | | | | | | | | | | | | | | | | | | | | | | | | | | | | |
| 3415 | 1/2 cup | Canned in extra heavy syrup, avg | 130 | 114 | 77 | 0.4 | 29.6 | 1.3 | 28.2 | 0.1 | 0.1 | 0.0 | 0.0 | 0.0 | 0.00 | 0.03 | 0 | 828 | 83 | 0 | 83 | 499 | 0.02 | 0.03 | 0.46 | 0.04 | 0.00 | 3.3 | 0.07 | 2.7 | 0.0 | | 8 | 0.1 | 0.4 | 6 | 0.2 | 12 | 104 | | 6 | 0.09 |
| 3414 | 1/2 cup | Canned in heavy syrup, avg | 128 | 93 | 80 | 0.4 | 24.4 | 1.3 | 23.0 | 0.1 | 0.1 | 0.0 | 0.0 | 0.0 | 0.00 | 0.03 | 0 | 645 | 64 | 0 | 64 | 384 | 0.02 | 0.03 | 0.44 | 0.04 | 0.00 | 3.2 | 0.07 | 3.1 | 0.0 | | 8 | 0.1 | 0.4 | 6 | 0.2 | 12 | 102 | 0.6 | 8 | 0.09 |
| 3355 | 1/2 cup | Canned in heavy syrup, tropical, avg | 129 | 111 | 77 | 0.5 | 28.9 | 1.7 | 26.6 | 0.5 | 0.1 | 0.0 | 0.0 | 0.0 | 0.02 | 0.02 | 0 | 164 | 17 | 0 | 17 | 101 | 0.07 | 0.06 | 0.72 | 0.15 | 0.00 | 11.6 | 0.19 | 22.6 | 0.0 | | 17 | 0.1 | 0.7 | 17 | 0.2 | 9 | 169 | 0.6 | 3 | 0.14 |
| 3413 | 1/2 cup | Canned in water, avg | 123 | 37 | 92 | 0.4 | 9.7 | 1.2 | 8.3 | 0.1 | 0.1 | 0.0 | 0.0 | 0.0 | 0.00 | 0.03 | 0 | 541 | 54 | 0 | 54 | 325 | 0.02 | 0.03 | 0.46 | 0.04 | 0.00 | 3.2 | 0.07 | 2.3 | 0.0 | | 9 | 0.1 | 0.4 | 6 | 0.2 | 11 | 96 | | 4 | 0.10 |
| 3654 | 1/2 cup | Feijoa, raw, pureed, avg | 122 | 60 | 87 | 1.5 | 12.9 | 5.1 | 7.8 | 0.0 | 1.0 | 0.3 | 0.1 | 0.4 | | | 0 | 0 | 0 | 0 | 0 | 0 | 0.01 | 0.04 | 0.35 | 0.06 | 0.00 | 46.4 | 0.28 | 24.8 | 0.0 | | 21 | 0.1 | 0.1 | 11 | 0.1 | 24 | 189 | | 4 | 0.05 |
| 3204 | 1/2 cup | Gooseberries, canned in light syrup, avg | 126 | 92 | 80 | 0.8 | 23.7 | 3.0 | 20.7 | 0.0 | 0.3 | 0.0 | 0.0 | 0.1 | 0.02 | 0.12 | 0 | 174 | 18 | 0 | 18 | 106 | 0.03 | 0.07 | 0.19 | 0.02 | 0.00 | 4.0 | 0.17 | 12.6 | 0.0 | | 20 | 0.3 | 0.4 | 8 | 0.2 | 9 | 97 | 0.5 | 3 | 0.14 |
| 3203 | 1/2 cup | Gooseberries, fresh, avg | 75 | 33 | 88 | 0.7 | 7.6 | 3.2 | 4.4 | 0.0 | 0.4 | 0.0 | 0.0 | 0.2 | 0.03 | 0.20 | 0 | 218 | 22 | 0 | 22 | 131 | 0.03 | 0.02 | 0.23 | 0.06 | 0.00 | 4.5 | 0.21 | 20.8 | 0.0 | 0.3 | 19 | 0.1 | 0.2 | 8 | 0.1 | 20 | 148 | 0.5 | 1 | 0.09 |

| Code | Amount | Description | Basic Components | | | | | | | | | Additional Fats | | | | | | Vit A & Components | | | | | Vitamins | | | | | | | | | | Minerals | | | | | | | | | |
|---|---|---|---|---|---|---|---|---|---|---|---|---|---|---|---|---|---|---|---|---|---|---|---|---|---|---|---|---|---|---|---|---|---|---|---|---|---|---|---|---|---|---|
| | | | Weight (g) | Calories | % Water | Protein (g) | Carbs (g) | Fiber (g) | Sugar (g) | Other Carbs (g) | Fat (g) | Sat Fat (g) | Mono Fat (g) | Poly Fat (g) | Omega 3 (g) | Omega 6 (g) | Choles (mg) | Vit A (IU) | Vit A (RE) | Retinol (RE) | Carotenoids (RE) | Beta Carotene (mcg) | Thiamin (mg) | Riboflavin (mg) | Niacin (NE) | Vit B6 (mg) | Vit B12 (mcg) | Folate (mcg) | Panto (mg) | Vit C (mg) | Vit D (mg) | Vit E (α TE) | Calcium (mg) | Copper (mg) | Iron (mg) | Magnes (mg) | Mang (mg) | Phos (mg) | Potassium (mg) | Selenium (mcg) | Sodium (mg) | Zinc (mg) |
| | | Grapes | | | | | | | | | | | | | | | | | | | | | | | | | | | | | | | | | | | | | | | | |
| 3059 | 1/2 cup | American type/slip skin, w/o seeds, avg | 46 | 31 | 81 | 0.3 | 7.9 | 0.5 | 7.4 | 0.1 | 0.2 | 0.1 | 0.0 | 0.0 | 0.01 | 0.04 | 0 | 46 | 5 | 0 | 5 | 27 | 0.04 | 0.03 | 0.14 | 0.05 | 0.00 | 1.8 | 0.01 | 1.8 | 0.0 | | 6 | 0.0 | 0.1 | 2 | 0.3 | 5 | 88 | 0.1 | 1 | 0.02 |
| 3058 | 1/2 cup | European type/adherent skin, avg | 80 | 57 | 81 | 0.5 | 14.2 | 0.8 | 13.4 | 0.0 | 0.5 | 0.2 | 0.0 | 0.1 | 0.03 | 0.10 | 0 | 58 | 6 | 0 | 6 | 33 | 0.07 | 0.05 | 0.24 | 0.09 | 0.00 | 3.1 | 0.02 | 8.6 | 0.0 | | 9 | 0.1 | 0.2 | 5 | 0.0 | 10 | 148 | 0.2 | 2 | 0.04 |
| 3206 | 1/2 cup | Thompson, seedless, canned in heavy syrup, avg | 128 | 93 | 80 | 0.6 | 25.2 | 0.5 | 24.7 | 0.0 | 0.1 | 0.0 | 0.0 | 0.0 | 0.01 | 0.03 | 0 | 82 | 8 | 0 | 8 | 45 | 0.04 | 0.03 | 0.16 | 0.08 | 0.00 | 3.3 | 0.05 | 1.3 | 0.0 | | 13 | 0.1 | 1.2 | 8 | 0.0 | 22 | 132 | 0.1 | 6 | 0.06 |
| 3417 | 1/2 cup | Thompson, seedless, canned in water, avg | 123 | 49 | 89 | 0.6 | 12.7 | 1.2 | 11.4 | 0.0 | 0.1 | 0.0 | 0.0 | 0.0 | 0.01 | 0.03 | 0 | 81 | 9 | 0 | 9 | 51 | 0.04 | 0.03 | 0.16 | 0.08 | 0.00 | 3.2 | 0.05 | 1.2 | 0.0 | | 12 | 0.1 | 1.2 | 7 | 0.0 | 22 | 132 | 0.1 | 7 | 0.06 |
| | | Grapefruit | | | | | | | | | | | | | | | | | | | | | | | | | | | | | | | | | | | | | | | | |
| 3342 | 1/2 cup | Canned in juice, avg | 124 | 46 | 90 | 0.9 | 11.4 | 0.5 | 10.9 | 0.0 | 0.1 | 0.0 | 0.0 | 0.0 | 0.00 | 0.02 | 0 | 0 | 0 | 0 | 0 | 0 | 0.04 | 0.02 | 0.31 | 0.02 | 0.00 | 10.9 | 0.15 | 42.0 | 0.0 | 0.3 | 19 | 0.0 | 0.3 | 14 | 0.0 | 15 | 210 | 1.1 | 9 | 0.10 |
| 3050 | 1/2 cup | Canned in light syrup, avg | 127 | 76 | 84 | 0.7 | 19.6 | 0.5 | 19.0 | 0.0 | 0.1 | 0.0 | 0.0 | 0.0 | 0.01 | 0.02 | 0 | 0 | 0 | 0 | 0 | 0 | 0.05 | 0.03 | 0.31 | 0.03 | 0.00 | 10.8 | 0.15 | 27.1 | 0.0 | 0.3 | 18 | 0.1 | 0.5 | 13 | 0.0 | 13 | 164 | 1.1 | 3 | 0.10 |
| 3416 | 1/2 cup | Canned in water, avg | 122 | 44 | 90 | 0.7 | 11.2 | 0.5 | 10.7 | 0.0 | 0.1 | 0.0 | 0.0 | 0.0 | 0.01 | 0.02 | 0 | 0 | 0 | 0 | 0 | 0 | 0.05 | 0.03 | 0.30 | 0.02 | 0.00 | 10.7 | 0.15 | 26.6 | 0.0 | 0.3 | 18 | 0.1 | 0.5 | 12 | 0.0 | 12 | 161 | 1.1 | 2 | 0.11 |
| 3048 | 1/2 cup | Fresh, sections, avg | 115 | 37 | 91 | 0.7 | 9.3 | 1.3 | 8.0 | 0.0 | 0.1 | 0.0 | 0.0 | 0.0 | 0.01 | 0.02 | 0 | 143 | 14 | 0 | 14 | 80 | 0.04 | 0.02 | 0.29 | 0.05 | 0.00 | 11.7 | 0.33 | 39.6 | 0.0 | 0.3 | 14 | 0.1 | 0.1 | 9 | 0.0 | 9 | 160 | 1.6 | 0 | 0.08 |
| 3817 | 1/2 cup | Pink/red, sections, avg | 115 | 34 | 91 | 0.6 | 8.8 | 1.6 | 7.3 | 0.0 | 0.1 | 0.0 | 0.0 | 0.0 | 0.01 | 0.02 | 0 | 298 | 30 | 0 | 30 | 179 | 0.04 | 0.02 | 0.22 | 0.05 | 0.00 | 14.0 | 0.33 | 43.8 | 0.0 | 0.3 | 13 | 0.1 | 0.1 | 9 | 0.0 | 10 | 148 | 1.0 | 0 | 0.08 |
| 3686 | 1/2 cup | White, avg | 115 | 38 | 90 | 0.8 | 9.7 | 1.3 | 8.4 | 0.0 | 0.1 | 0.0 | 0.0 | 0.0 | 0.01 | 0.02 | 0 | 12 | 1 | 0 | 1 | 7 | 0.04 | 0.02 | 0.31 | 0.05 | 0.00 | 11.5 | 0.33 | 38.3 | 0.0 | 0.3 | 14 | 0.1 | 0.1 | 10 | 0.0 | 9 | 170 | 1.6 | 0 | 0.08 |
| | | Guava | | | | | | | | | | | | | | | | | | | | | | | | | | | | | | | | | | | | | | | | |
| 3870 | 1 oz | Paste, avg | 28 | 79 | 27 | 0.0 | 20.4 | 0.3 | | | 0.0 | 0.0 | 0.0 | 0.0 | | | 0 | 12 | 1 | 0 | 1 | 7 | 0.00 | 0.00 | 0.03 | 0.01 | 0.00 | 0.2 | | 2.5 | | 0.0 | 1 | 0.0 | 0.0 | 1 | | 1 | 19 | | 1 | 0.02 |
| 3634 | 1/2 cup | Raw, avg | 82 | 42 | 86 | 0.7 | 9.8 | 4.4 | 4.9 | 0.4 | 0.5 | 0.1 | 0.0 | 0.2 | 0.06 | 0.15 | 0 | 649 | 65 | 0 | 65 | 373 | 0.04 | 0.04 | 0.98 | 0.12 | 0.00 | 11.5 | 0.12 | 150.9 | 0.0 | | 16 | 0.1 | 0.3 | 8 | 0.1 | 20 | 233 | 0.5 | 2 | 0.19 |
| 3635 | 1/2 cup | Raw, strawberry, avg | 122 | 84 | 81 | 0.7 | 21.2 | 7.7 | 7.3 | 6.2 | 0.7 | 0.2 | 0.1 | 0.3 | 0.09 | 0.22 | 0 | 110 | 11 | 0 | 11 | 63 | 0.04 | 0.04 | 0.73 | 0.09 | 0.00 | 8.5 | 0.09 | 45.1 | 0.0 | | 26 | 0.1 | 0.3 | 21 | 0.2 | 33 | 356 | | 45 | 0.26 |
| 3208 | 1/2 cup | Sauce, cooked, avg | 119 | 43 | 90 | 0.4 | 11.3 | 4.3 | 7.0 | 0.0 | 0.2 | 0.0 | 0.0 | 0.1 | 0.02 | 0.05 | 0 | 337 | 33 | 0 | 33 | 192 | 0.03 | 0.02 | 0.50 | 0.11 | 0.00 | 6.0 | 0.06 | 173.7 | 0.0 | | 8 | 0.1 | 0.2 | 8 | 0.1 | 13 | 268 | 0.6 | 5 | 0.20 |
| 3861 | 1/2 cup | Jackfruit, dried, avg | 61 | 183 | 18 | 3.0 | 45.8 | 1.5 | 35.1 | 9.1 | 0.0 | 0.0 | 0.0 | 0.0 | 0.00 | 0.00 | 0 | 1525 | 153 | 0 | 153 | 915 | | | | | 0.00 | | | 0.0 | | | 30 | | 0.5 | | | | | | 0 | |
| 3636 | 1/2 cup | Jackfruit, raw, avg | 82 | 77 | 73 | 1.2 | 19.7 | 1.3 | 15.1 | 3.3 | 0.2 | 0.1 | 0.0 | 0.1 | 0.02 | 0.05 | 0 | 244 | 25 | 0 | 25 | 148 | 0.02 | 0.09 | 0.33 | 0.09 | 0.00 | 11.5 | | 5.5 | 0.0 | | 28 | 0.2 | 0.5 | 30 | 0.2 | 30 | 248 | 0.5 | 2 | 0.34 |
| 3695 | 1 oz | Jujube fruit, dried, avg | 28 | 80 | 20 | 1.0 | 20.6 | 0.8 | 11.4 | 8.4 | 0.3 | | | | | | 0 | 0 | 0 | 0 | 0 | 0 | 0.06 | 0.10 | 0.14 | 0.06 | 0.00 | | | 3.6 | 0.0 | | 22 | 0.1 | 0.5 | 10 | 0.1 | 28 | 149 | | 3 | 0.05 |
| 3250 | 1 oz | Jujube fruit, raw, avg | 28 | 22 | 78 | 0.3 | 5.7 | 0.3 | 5.3 | 0.0 | 0.1 | | | | | | 0 | 11 | 1 | 0 | 1 | 7 | 0.01 | 0.01 | 0.25 | 0.02 | 0.00 | | | 19.3 | 0.0 | | 6 | 0.0 | 0.1 | 3 | 0.0 | 6 | 70 | | 1 | 0.01 |
| 3858 | 1 ea | Kiwi, raw, medium, avg | 74 | 50 | 81 | 1.0 | 12.0 | 2.0 | 8.0 | 2.0 | 0.5 | 0.0 | 0.0 | 0.0 | 0.00 | 0.00 | 0 | 50 | 5 | 0 | 5 | 30 | | | | | 0.00 | | | 72.0 | | | 30 | | 0.4 | | | | 240 | | 0 | |
| 3367 | 1 ea | Kiwi, dried, EH Worley & Company | 10 | 28 | 10 | 0.4 | 8.0 | 1.8 | 4.3 | 1.9 | 0.3 | 0.1 | 0.0 | 0.1 | | | 0 | | | | | | | | | | 0.00 | | | 26.4 | 0.0 | | 14 | | | | | | 203 | | 2 | |
| 3831 | 1 oz | Kumquats, canned, avg | 28 | 39 | 62 | 0.1 | 9.9 | | | | 0.1 | | | | | | | 0 | 0 | 0 | 0 | 0 | 0.03 | 0.02 | 0.14 | | 0.00 | | | 11.2 | | | 4 | | 0.2 | | | | 44 | | 31 | |
| 3252 | 1 ea | Kumquats, raw, avg | 19 | 12 | 82 | 0.2 | 3.1 | 1.3 | | | 0.0 | 0.0 | 0.0 | 0.0 | 0.00 | 0.00 | 0 | 57 | 6 | 0 | 6 | 34 | 0.02 | 0.02 | 0.09 | 0.01 | 0.00 | 3.0 | | 7.1 | 0.0 | | 8 | 0.0 | 0.1 | 2 | 0.0 | 4 | 37 | 0.1 | 1 | 0.02 |
| | | Lemon | | | | | | | | | | | | | | | | | | | | | | | | | | | | | | | | | | | | | | | | |
| 3066 | 1 ea | Fresh, w/o peel, avg | 58 | 17 | 89 | 0.6 | 5.4 | 1.6 | 1.6 | 2.2 | 0.2 | 0.0 | 0.0 | 0.1 | 0.02 | 0.04 | 0 | 17 | 2 | 0 | 2 | 10 | 0.02 | 0.01 | 0.06 | 0.05 | 0.00 | 6.1 | 0.11 | 30.7 | 0.0 | | 15 | 0.0 | 0.3 | 5 | 0.0 | 9 | 80 | 0.2 | 1 | 0.03 |
| 3418 | 1 ea | Fresh, w/peel, avg | 108 | 22 | 87 | 1.3 | 11.6 | 5.1 | 1.9 | 4.6 | 0.3 | 0.0 | 0.0 | 0.1 | 0.03 | 0.07 | 0 | 32 | 3 | 0 | 3 | 19 | 0.05 | 0.04 | 0.22 | 0.12 | 0.00 | 7.6 | 0.25 | 83.2 | 0.0 | | 66 | 0.3 | 0.8 | 13 | 0.0 | 16 | 157 | | 3 | 0.11 |
| 3463 | 1 oz | Peel, candied, avg | 28 | 88 | 17 | 0.1 | 22.6 | | | | 0.1 | 0.0 | | | | 0.00 | 0 | 0 | 0 | 0 | 0 | 0 | 0.00 | 0.00 | 0.00 | | 0.00 | | | 0.0 | 0.0 | | 0 | | 0.0 | | | 0 | 0 | | 0 | |
| 3071 | 1 ea | Lime, fresh, w/o peel, avg | 67 | 20 | 88 | 0.5 | 7.0 | 1.9 | 1.3 | 3.9 | 0.1 | 0.0 | 0.0 | 0.0 | 0.01 | 0.02 | 0 | 7 | 0.7 | 0 | 0.7 | 4 | 0.02 | 0.01 | 0.13 | 0.03 | 0.00 | 5.5 | 0.15 | 19.5 | 0.0 | | 22 | 0.0 | 0.4 | 4 | 0.0 | 12 | 68 | 0.3 | 1 | 0.07 |
| 3074 | 1/2 cup | Loganberries, frozen, avg | 74 | 41 | 85 | 1.1 | 9.6 | 3.6 | 6.0 | 0.0 | 0.2 | 0.0 | 0.0 | 0.1 | 0.04 | 0.09 | 0 | 26 | 3 | 0 | 3 | 9 | 0.04 | 0.03 | 0.62 | 0.05 | 0.00 | 19.0 | 0.18 | 11.3 | 0.0 | | 19 | 0.1 | 0.5 | 16 | 0.9 | 19 | 107 | 0.4 | 1 | 0.25 |
| | | Longans | | | | | | | | | | | | | | | | | | | | | | | | | | | | | | | | | | | | | | | | |
| 3832 | 1 oz | Canned, whole, avg | 28 | 18 | 82 | 0.1 | 4.6 | | | | 0.1 | | | | | | | 0 | 0 | 0 | 0 | 0 | | 0.01 | 0.03 | | 0.00 | | | 17.6 | | | 1 | | 0.1 | | | | 31 | | 11 | |
| 3255 | 10 ea | Dried, avg | 30 | 86 | 18 | 1.5 | 22.2 | 1.6 | 20.4 | 0.2 | 0.1 | | | | | | 0 | 0 | 0 | 0 | 0 | 0 | 0.01 | 0.15 | 0.30 | | 0.00 | | | 8.4 | 0.0 | | 14 | 0.2 | 1.6 | 14 | 0.1 | 59 | 197 | | 14 | 0.07 |
| 3254 | 10 ea | Raw, avg | 30 | 18 | 83 | 0.4 | 4.5 | 0.3 | 4.2 | 0.0 | 0.0 | | | | | | 0 | 0 | 0 | 0 | 0 | 0 | 0.01 | 0.04 | 0.09 | | 0.00 | | | 25.2 | 0.0 | | 0 | 0.1 | 0.0 | 3 | 0.0 | 6 | 80 | | 0 | 0.02 |
| 3833 | 1 oz | Loquats, canned, avg | 28 | 24 | 77 | 0.1 | 6.2 | | | | 0.0 | | | | | | | 0 | 0 | 0 | 0 | 0 | 0.00 | 0.00 | 0.14 | | 0.00 | | | 0.0 | | | 6 | | 0.0 | | | | | | | |
| 3639 | 1 ea | Loquats, raw, medium, avg | 16 | 8 | 87 | 0.1 | 1.9 | 0.3 | 1.0 | 0.6 | 0.0 | 0.0 | 0.0 | 0.0 | 0.00 | 0.01 | 0 | 244 | 24 | 0 | 24 | 107 | 0.00 | 0.00 | 0.03 | 0.02 | 0.00 | 2.2 | | 0.2 | 0.0 | | 3 | 0.0 | 0.0 | 2 | 0.0 | 4 | 43 | 0.1 | 0 | 0.01 |
| | | Lychees | | | | | | | | | | | | | | | | | | | | | | | | | | | | | | | | | | | | | | | | |
| 3834 | 1 oz | Canned in syrup, avg | 28 | 19 | 79 | 0.1 | 5.1 | 0.1 | | | | | | | | | | 0 | 0 | 0 | 0 | 0 | 0.01 | 0.01 | 0.08 | | 0.00 | | | 2.2 | | | 1 | 0.0 | 0.2 | 2 | | | 21 | | 1 | 0.06 |
| 3166 | 1 oz | Cooked/canned, sweetened, avg | 28 | 25 | 76 | 0.1 | 6.5 | 0.1 | 6.4 | 0.0 | 0.1 | 0.0 | 0.0 | 0.0 | | | 0 | 0 | 0 | 0 | 0 | 0 | 0.00 | 0.01 | 0.10 | 0.02 | 0.00 | 1.3 | | 9.0 | 0.0 | | 1 | 0.0 | 0.1 | 2 | 0.0 | 6 | 28 | 0.0 | 0 | 0.02 |
| 3258 | 15 ea | Dried, avg | 30 | 83 | 22 | 1.1 | 21.2 | 1.4 | 19.8 | 0.0 | 0.4 | 0.1 | 0.1 | 0.1 | 0.05 | 0.06 | 0 | 0 | 0 | 0 | 0 | 0 | 0.00 | 0.17 | 0.93 | 0.03 | 0.00 | 3.6 | | 54.9 | 0.0 | | 10 | 0.2 | 0.5 | 13 | 0.1 | 54 | 333 | 0.4 | 1 | 0.08 |
| 3257 | 3 ea | Raw, avg | 30 | 20 | 82 | 0.2 | 5.0 | 0.4 | 4.6 | 0.0 | 0.1 | 0.0 | 0.0 | 0.0 | 0.02 | 0.02 | 0 | 0 | 0 | 0 | 0 | 0 | 0.00 | 0.02 | 0.18 | 0.03 | 0.00 | 4.2 | | 21.5 | 0.0 | | 2 | 0.0 | 0.1 | 3 | 0.0 | 9 | 51 | 0.2 | 0 | 0.02 |
| 3259 | 1 ea | Mammy Apple, raw, avg | 846 | 431 | 86 | 4.2 | 105.8 | 25.4 | 80.3 | 0.1 | 4.2 | 1.2 | 1.7 | 0.7 | 0.00 | 0.67 | 0 | 1946 | 195 | 0 | 195 | 1167 | 0.17 | 0.34 | 3.38 | 0.85 | 0.00 | 118.4 | 0.87 | 118.4 | 0.0 | | 93 | 0.7 | 5.9 | 135 | | 93 | 398 | 5.1 | 127 | 0.85 |
| 3089 | 1/2 cup | Mandarin Orange sections, canned, avg | 125 | 46 | 90 | 0.8 | 12.0 | 0.9 | 11.1 | 0.0 | 0.0 | 0.0 | 0.0 | 0.0 | 0.00 | 0.01 | 0 | 1065 | 106 | 0 | 106 | 198 | 0.10 | 0.04 | 0.56 | 0.05 | 0.00 | 5.8 | 0.16 | 42.8 | 0.0 | 0.6 | 14 | 0.0 | 0.3 | 14 | 0.0 | 12 | 166 | 0.5 | 6 | 0.64 |
| | | Mangos | | | | | | | | | | | | | | | | | | | | | | | | | | | | | | | | | | | | | | | | |
| 3866 | 3 pce | Dried, Frieda's Specialty Produce | 30 | 98 | | 0.0 | 24.0 | 0.0 | 24.0 | 0.0 | 0.8 | 0.0 | | | 0.00 | 0.00 | 0 | 750 | 75 | 0 | 75 | 450 | | | | | 0.00 | | | 0.0 | | | 4 | | 0.8 | | | | | | 26 | |
| 3221 | 1 ea | Fresh, whole, avg | 207 | 135 | 82 | 1.1 | 35.2 | 3.7 | 30.6 | 0.8 | 0.6 | 0.1 | 0.2 | 0.1 | 0.08 | 0.03 | 0 | 8061 | 805 | 0 | 805 | 4831 | 0.12 | 0.12 | 1.21 | 0.28 | 0.00 | 29.0 | 0.33 | 57.3 | 0.0 | 2.3 | 21 | 0.2 | 0.3 | 19 | 0.1 | 23 | 323 | 1.2 | 4 | 0.08 |
| 3836 | 1 oz | Canned in juice, avg | 28 | 12 | 88 | 0.0 | 3.3 | | | | 0.1 | | | | | | | 0 | 0 | 0 | 0 | 0 | | | 0.25 | | 0.00 | | | 7.0 | | | 1 | | 0.4 | | | | 5 | | 3 | |
| 3835 | 1 oz | Canned in syrup, avg | 28 | 22 | 75 | 0.1 | 6.0 | 0.3 | | | | | | | | | | 0 | 0 | 0 | 0 | 0 | 0.01 | 0.01 | 0.06 | | 0.00 | | | 2.8 | | | 3 | 0.0 | 0.1 | 2 | | | 28 | | 1 | 0.08 |
| 44099 | 1 oz | Chips, dry, avg | 28 | 90 | 9 | 0.4 | 24.5 | | | | 0.3 | | | | | | | | | | | | 0.03 | 0.04 | 0.22 | | 0.00 | | | 16.5 | | | 8 | | 0.1 | | | 8 | | | | |
| | | Melons | | | | | | | | | | | | | | | | | | | | | | | | | | | | | | | | | | | | | | | | |
| 3075 | 1/2 cup | Cantaloupe, cubes, avg | 80 | 28 | 90 | 0.7 | 6.7 | 0.6 | 6.0 | 0.0 | 0.2 | 0.1 | 0.0 | 0.1 | 0.05 | 0.04 | 0 | 2579 | 258 | 0 | 258 | 1536 | 0.03 | 0.02 | 0.46 | 0.09 | 0.00 | 13.6 | 0.10 | 33.8 | 0.0 | 0.1 | 9 | 0.0 | 0.2 | 9 | 0.0 | 14 | 247 | 0.3 | 7 | 0.13 |
| 3843 | 1/4 ea | Cantaloupe, fresh, medium, avg | 134 | 50 | 90 | 1.0 | 12.0 | 1.0 | 11.0 | 0.0 | 0.0 | 0.0 | 0.0 | 0.0 | 0.00 | 0.00 | 0 | 5000 | 500 | 0 | 500 | 2982 | | | | | 0.00 | | | 48.0 | | | 20 | | 0.4 | | | | 280 | | 25 | |
| 3078 | 1/2 cup | Casaba, cubes, avg | 85 | 22 | 92 | 0.8 | 5.3 | 0.7 | 4.6 | 0.0 | 0.1 | 0.0 | 0.0 | 0.0 | 0.02 | 0.01 | 0 | 26 | 3 | 0 | 3 | 15 | 0.05 | 0.02 | 0.34 | 0.10 | 0.00 | 14.5 | 0.12 | 13.6 | 0.0 | | 4 | 0.0 | 0.3 | 7 | 0.0 | 6 | 179 | 0.3 | 10 | 0.14 |
| 3080 | 1/2 cup | Honeydew, fresh, cubes, avg | 42 | 15 | 90 | 0.2 | 3.9 | 0.3 | 3.6 | 0.0 | 0.0 | 0.0 | 0.0 | 0.0 | 0.01 | 0.01 | 0 | 17 | 2 | 0 | 2 | 10 | 0.03 | 0.01 | 0.25 | 0.02 | 0.00 | 2.5 | 0.09 | 10.4 | 0.0 | | 3 | 0.0 | 0.0 | 3 | 0.0 | 4 | 114 | 0.2 | 4 | 0.03 |
| 3850 | 1/4 ea | Honeydew, fresh, medium, avg | 34 | 13 | 89 | 0.3 | 3.3 | 0.3 | 3.0 | 0.0 | 0.0 | 0.0 | 0.0 | 0.0 | 0.00 | 0.00 | 0 | 25 | 3 | 0 | 3 | 15 | | | | | 0.00 | | | 6.9 | | | 0 | | 0.1 | | | | 79 | | 9 | |
| 3168 | 1/2 cup | Mixed Fruit, dried, avg | 68 | 165 | 31 | 1.7 | 43.6 | 5.3 | 38.3 | 0.0 | 0.3 | 0.0 | 0.2 | 0.1 | 0.00 | 0.07 | 0 | 1661 | 166 | 0 | 166 | 996 | 0.03 | 0.11 | 1.31 | 0.11 | 0.00 | 2.7 | 0.30 | 2.6 | 0.0 | | 26 | 0.3 | 1.8 | 27 | 0.2 | 52 | 541 | 0.3 | 12 | 0.34 |
| 3169 | 1/2 cup | Mixed Fruit, frozen, sweetened, thawed, avg | 125 | 122 | 74 | 1.8 | 30.3 | 2.4 | 27.9 | 0.0 | 0.2 | 0.0 | 0.0 | 0.1 | 0.01 | 0.09 | 0 | 403 | 40 | 0 | 40 | 240 | 0.02 | 0.04 | 0.50 | 0.03 | 0.00 | 9.5 | 0.12 | 93.8 | 0.0 | | 9 | 0.0 | 0.3 | 8 | 0.1 | 15 | 164 | 0.3 | 4 | 0.06 |
| 3309 | 1/2 cup | Mulberries, raw, avg | 35 | 15 | 88 | 0.5 | 3.4 | 0.6 | 2.3 | 0.5 | 0.1 | 0.0 | 0.0 | 0.1 | 0.00 | 0.07 | 0 | 9 | 1 | 0 | 1 | 6 | 0.01 | 0.04 | 0.22 | 0.02 | 0.00 | 2.1 | 0.08 | 12.7 | 0.0 | | 14 | 0.0 | 0.6 | 6 | 0.3 | 13 | 68 | 0.2 | 3 | 0.04 |
| 3216 | 1/2 cup | Nectarines, fresh, avg | 69 | 34 | 86 | 0.6 | 8.1 | 1.1 | 6.8 | 0.2 | 0.3 | 0.0 | 0.1 | 0.2 | 0.00 | 0.16 | 0 | 508 | 51 | 0 | 51 | 253 | 0.01 | 0.03 | 0.68 | 0.02 | 0.00 | 2.6 | 0.11 | 3.7 | 0.0 | | 3 | 0.1 | 0.1 | 6 | 0.0 | 11 | 146 | 0.3 | 0 | 0.06 |
| 3260 | 1/2 cup | Oheloberries, raw, avg | 70 | 20 | 92 | 0.3 | 4.8 | 0.9 | 3.9 | 0.0 | 0.2 | 0.1 | 0.0 | 0.0 | | | 0 | 581 | 58 | 0 | 58 | 349 | 0.01 | 0.03 | 0.19 | 0.04 | 0.00 | 18.0 | 0.17 | 4.2 | 0.0 | | 5 | 0.1 | 0.1 | 4 | | 7 | 27 | | 1 | 0.24 |
| | | Oranges | | | | | | | | | | | | | | | | | | | | | | | | | | | | | | | | | | | | | | | | |
| 3715 | 1/2 cup | California navel, avg | 82 | 38 | 87 | 0.8 | 9.5 | 2.0 | 7.5 | 0.0 | 0.1 | 0.0 | 0.0 | 0.0 | 0.00 | 0.01 | 0 | 150 | 15 | 0 | 15 | 27 | 0.07 | 0.03 | 0.24 | 0.06 | 0.00 | 27.6 | 0.20 | 47.0 | 0.0 | 0.1 | 33 | 0.0 | 0.1 | 8 | 0.0 | 16 | 146 | 0.7 | 1 | 0.05 |
| 3714 | 1/2 cup | California valencia, avg | 90 | 44 | 86 | 0.9 | 10.7 | 2.3 | 8.5 | 0.0 | 0.3 | 0.0 | 0.0 | 0.1 | 0.01 | 0.04 | 0 | 207 | 21 | 0 | 21 | 39 | 0.08 | 0.04 | 0.25 | 0.06 | 0.00 | 34.7 | 0.22 | 43.6 | 0.0 | 0.3 | 36 | 0.0 | 0.1 | 9 | 0.0 | 15 | 161 | 0.8 | 0 | 0.05 |
| 3088 | 1 Tbs | Peel, fresh, grated, avg | 6 | 6 | 72 | 0.1 | 1.5 | 0.6 | 0.0 | 0.9 | 0.0 | 0.0 | 0.0 | 0.0 | 0.00 | 0.00 | 0 | 25 | 3 | 0 | 3 | 15 | 0.01 | 0.01 | 0.05 | 0.01 | 0.00 | 1.8 | 0.03 | 8.2 | 0.0 | | 10 | 0.0 | 0.0 | 1 | | 1 | 13 | 0.1 | 0 | 0.01 |
| 3528 | 1/2 cup | Segments, Orville Kent | 105 | 60 | | 1.0 | 14.0 | 0.0 | 11.0 | 3.0 | 0.0 | 0.0 | 0.0 | 0.0 | 0.00 | 0.00 | 0 | 0 | 0 | 0 | 0 | 0 | | | | | 0.00 | | | 48.0 | | | 20 | | 0.0 | | | | | | 15 | |
| 3420 | 1/2 cup | With peel, avg | 85 | 34 | 82 | 1.1 | 13.2 | 3.8 | 4.9 | 4.4 | 0.3 | 0.0 | 0.0 | 0.1 | 0.01 | 0.04 | 0 | 213 | 21 | 0 | 21 | 128 | 0.09 | 0.04 | 0.43 | 0.08 | 0.00 | 25.5 | 0.28 | 60.4 | 0.0 | | 60 | 0.0 | 0.7 | 12 | 0.0 | 19 | 167 | 0.6 | 2 | 0.09 |
| | | Papayas | | | | | | | | | | | | | | | | | | | | | | | | | | | | | | | | | | | | | | | | |
| 3502 | 1/2 cup | Canned, avg | 66 | 43 | 80 | 0.1 | 11.2 | 0.3 | 11.2 | | 0.1 | | | | | | 0 | 548 | 55 | 0 | 55 | 97 | 0.01 | 0.01 | | 0.01 | 0.00 | 2.0 | | 9.9 | | | 15 | | 0.3 | | | | 73 | | 5 | 0.20 |
| 3362 | 1 pce | Dried, avg | 23 | 59 | 26 | 0.9 | 14.9 | 2.6 | 9.1 | 3.2 | 0.2 | 0.1 | 0.1 | 0.0 | 0.04 | 0.01 | 0 | 216 | 21 | 0 | 21 | 38 | 0.03 | 0.04 | 0.46 | 0.03 | 0.00 | 28.9 | | 18.8 | 0.0 | | 37 | 0.0 | 0.2 | 15 | | 8 | 391 | | 5 | 0.11 |

| Code | Amount | Description | Weight (g) | Calories | % Water | Protein (g) | Carbs (g) | Fiber (g) | Sugar (g) | Other Carbs (g) | Fat (g) | Sat Fat (g) | Mono Fat (g) | Poly Fat (g) | Omega 3 (g) | Omega 6 (g) | Choles (mg) | Vit A (IU) | Vit A (RE) | Retinol (RE) | Carotenoids (RE) | Beta Carotene (mcg) | Thiamin (mg) | Riboflavin (mg) | Niacin (NE) | Vit B6 (mg) | Vit B12 (mcg) | Folate (mcg) | Panto (mg) | Vit C (mg) | Vit D (mg) | Vit E (α TE) | Calcium (mg) | Copper (mg) | Iron (mg) | Magnes (mg) | Mang (mg) | Phos (mg) | Potassium (mg) | Selenium (mcg) | Sodium (mg) | Zinc (mg) |
|---|---|---|---|---|---|---|---|---|---|---|---|---|---|---|---|---|---|---|---|---|---|---|---|---|---|---|---|---|---|---|---|---|---|---|---|---|---|---|---|---|---|---|
| | | | **Basic Components** | | | | | | | | | **Additional Fats** | | | | | | **Vit A & Components** | | | | | **Vitamins** | | | | | | | | | | **Minerals** | | | | | | | | | |
| 3171 | 1 ea | Fresh, whole, medium, avg | 304 | 119 | 89 | 1.9 | 29.8 | 5.5 | 17.9 | 6.4 | 0.4 | 0.1 | 0.1 | 0.1 | 0.08 | 0.02 | 0 | 353 | 35 | 0 | 85 | 151 | 0.08 | 0.10 | 1.03 | 0.06 | 0.00 | 115.5 | 0.66 | 187.9 | 0.0 | | 73 | 0.0 | 0.3 | 30 | 0.0 | 15 | 781 | 1.8 | 9 | 0.21 |
| 3722 | 1/2 cup | Passion Fruit, purple, fresh, avg | 118 | 114 | 73 | 2.6 | 27.6 | 12.3 | 15.3 | 0.0 | 0.8 | 0.1 | 0.1 | 0.5 | 0.00 | 0.48 | 0 | 326 | 33 | 0 | 83 | 124 | 0.00 | 0.15 | 1.77 | 0.12 | 0.00 | 16.5 | | 35.4 | 0.0 | | 14 | 0.1 | 1.9 | 34 | | 80 | 411 | 0.7 | 33 | 0.12 |
| | | Peaches | | | | | | | | | | | | | | | | | | | | | | | | | | | | | | | | | | | | | | | | |
| 3427 | 1/2 cup | Canned in extra heavy syrup, halves, avg | 131 | 126 | 73 | 0.6 | 34.2 | 1.3 | 32.5 | 0.4 | 0.0 | 0.0 | 0.0 | 0.0 | 0.00 | 0.02 | 0 | 172 | 7 | 0 | 17 | 83 | 0.01 | 0.03 | 0.68 | 0.02 | 0.00 | 4.1 | 0.07 | 1.6 | 0.0 | | 4 | 0.1 | 0.4 | 7 | 0.1 | 14 | 109 | | 10 | 0.12 |
| 3728 | 1/2 cup | Canned in extra light syrup, halves, avg | 124 | 52 | 88 | 0.5 | 13.8 | 1.2 | 12.2 | 0.4 | 0.1 | 0.0 | 0.0 | 0.1 | 0.00 | 0.06 | 0 | 335 | 33 | 0 | 33 | 162 | 0.02 | 0.02 | 0.99 | 0.02 | 0.00 | 4.1 | 0.06 | 3.7 | 0.0 | | 6 | 0.1 | 0.4 | 6 | 0.1 | 14 | 92 | | 6 | 0.11 |
| 3098 | 1/2 cup | Canned in heavy syrup, avg | 131 | 97 | 79 | 0.6 | 26.1 | 1.7 | 24.4 | 0.0 | 0.1 | 0.0 | 0.0 | 0.1 | 0.00 | 0.06 | 0 | 435 | 43 | 0 | 43 | 210 | 0.01 | 0.03 | 0.80 | 0.02 | 0.00 | 4.2 | 0.07 | 3.7 | 0.0 | | 4 | 0.1 | 0.4 | 7 | 0.1 | 14 | 121 | 0.4 | 8 | 0.12 |
| 3348 | 1/2 cup | Canned in heavy syrup, spiced, avg | 121 | 91 | 79 | 0.5 | 24.3 | 1.6 | 22.7 | 0.0 | 0.1 | 0.0 | 0.0 | 0.1 | 0.00 | 0.06 | 0 | 334 | 39 | 0 | 39 | 183 | 0.01 | 0.04 | 0.65 | 0.02 | 0.00 | 3.9 | 0.06 | 6.4 | 0.0 | | 7 | 0.1 | 0.3 | 8 | 0.1 | 11 | 103 | 0.4 | 5 | 0.10 |
| 3727 | 1/2 cup | Canned in juices, halves, avg | 124 | 55 | 88 | 0.8 | 14.4 | 1.6 | 12.8 | 0.0 | 0.0 | 0.0 | 0.0 | 0.0 | 0.00 | 0.02 | 0 | 472 | 47 | 0 | 47 | 223 | 0.01 | 0.02 | 0.72 | 0.02 | 0.00 | 4.2 | 0.06 | 4.5 | 0.0 | | 7 | 0.1 | 0.3 | 9 | 0.1 | 21 | 159 | 0.4 | 5 | 0.14 |
| 3173 | 1/2 cup | Canned in light syrup, halves, avg | 126 | 68 | 85 | 0.6 | 18.4 | 1.6 | 16.8 | 0.0 | 0.0 | 0.0 | 0.0 | 0.0 | 0.00 | 0.02 | 0 | 446 | 44 | 0 | 44 | 214 | 0.01 | 0.03 | 0.75 | 0.02 | 0.00 | 4.2 | 0.06 | 3.0 | 0.0 | | 4 | 0.1 | 0.5 | 6 | 0.1 | 14 | 122 | 0.4 | 6 | 0.11 |
| 3423 | 1/2 cup | Canned in water, halves, avg | 122 | 29 | 93 | 0.5 | 7.5 | 1.6 | 5.9 | 0.0 | 0.1 | 0.0 | 0.0 | 0.0 | 0.00 | 0.03 | 0 | 649 | 65 | 0 | 65 | 314 | 0.01 | 0.02 | 0.64 | 0.02 | 0.00 | 4.1 | 0.06 | 3.5 | 0.0 | | 2 | 0.1 | 0.4 | 6 | 0.1 | 12 | 121 | 0.4 | 4 | 0.11 |
| 3729 | 1/2 cup | Dried, cooked, dehydrated, sulfured, stewed, avg | 121 | 289 | 32 | 4.4 | 74.2 | 9.9 | 62.4 | 1.9 | 0.9 | 0.1 | 0.3 | 0.4 | 0.01 | 0.43 | 0 | 2617 | 261 | 0 | 261 | 1543 | 0.00 | 0.26 | 5.30 | 0.08 | 0.00 | 0.4 | 0.68 | 5.8 | 0.0 | 0.0 | 34 | 0.4 | 4.9 | 51 | 0.4 | 144 | 1205 | 2.7 | 8 | 0.69 |
| 3430 | 1/2 cup | Dried, cooked, stewed w/sugar, avg | 135 | 139 | 71 | 1.4 | 35.9 | 3.2 | 30.1 | 2.6 | 0.3 | 0.0 | 0.1 | 0.1 | 0.00 | 0.14 | 0 | 243 | 24 | 0 | 24 | 144 | 0.01 | 0.03 | 1.88 | 0.05 | 0.00 | 0.1 | 0.22 | 4.6 | 0.0 | | 11 | 0.1 | 1.6 | 16 | 0.1 | 47 | 394 | 0.9 | 3 | 0.23 |
| 3428 | 1/2 cup | Dried, dehydrated, sulfured, uncooked, avg | 58 | 188 | 8 | 2.8 | 48.3 | 6.4 | 40.7 | 1.2 | 0.6 | 0.1 | 0.2 | 0.3 | 0.01 | 0.28 | 0 | 822 | 82 | 0 | 82 | 483 | 0.02 | 0.06 | 2.80 | 0.09 | 0.00 | 3.8 | 0.30 | 6.1 | 0.0 | | 22 | 0.3 | 3.2 | 33 | 0.2 | 94 | 784 | | 6 | 0.45 |
| 3729 | 1/2 cup | Dried, halves, avg | 80 | 191 | 32 | 2.9 | 49.0 | 6.6 | 41.2 | 1.2 | 0.6 | 0.1 | 0.2 | 0.3 | 0.01 | 0.25 | 0 | 1730 | 173 | 0 | 173 | 1023 | 0.00 | 0.17 | 3.50 | 0.05 | 0.00 | 0.2 | 0.45 | 3.8 | 0.0 | 0.0 | 22 | 0.3 | 3.2 | 34 | 0.2 | 95 | 797 | 1.8 | 6 | 0.46 |
| 3096 | 1 ea | Fresh, whole, medium, avg | 98 | 42 | 88 | 0.7 | 10.9 | 2.0 | 8.6 | 0.3 | 0.1 | 0.0 | 0.0 | 0.0 | 0.00 | 0.04 | 0 | 524 | 53 | 0 | 53 | 263 | 0.02 | 0.04 | 0.97 | 0.02 | 0.00 | 3.3 | 0.17 | 6.5 | 0.0 | | 5 | 0.1 | 0.1 | 7 | 0.0 | 12 | 193 | 0.4 | 0 | 0.14 |
| 57481 | 1/2 cup | Frozen, slices, sweetened, thawed, avg | 125 | 118 | 75 | 0.8 | 30.0 | 2.3 | 27.8 | 0.0 | 0.2 | 0.0 | 0.1 | 0.1 | 0.00 | 0.05 | 0 | 355 | 35 | 0 | 35 | 23 | 0.02 | 0.04 | 0.82 | 0.02 | 0.00 | 4.0 | 0.16 | 117.8 | 0.0 | | 4 | 0.0 | 0.5 | 6 | 0.0 | 14 | 162 | 0.5 | 8 | 0.06 |
| | | Pears | | | | | | | | | | | | | | | | | | | | | | | | | | | | | | | | | | | | | | | | |
| 3434 | 1/2 cup | Canned in extra heavy syrup, avg | 133 | 129 | 74 | 0.3 | 33.6 | 2.1 | 28.6 | 2.9 | 0.2 | 0.0 | 0.0 | 0.0 | 0.00 | 0.04 | 0 | 0 | 0 | 0 | 0 | 0 | 0.01 | 0.03 | 0.32 | 0.02 | 0.00 | 1.6 | 0.03 | 1.5 | 0.0 | | 7 | 0.1 | 0.3 | 5 | 0.0 | 9 | 85 | | 7 | 0.11 |
| 3432 | 1/2 cup | Canned in extra light syrup, halves, avg | 124 | 58 | 87 | 0.4 | 15.1 | 2.0 | 10.4 | 2.7 | 0.1 | 0.0 | 0.0 | 0.0 | 0.00 | 0.03 | 0 | 0 | 0 | 0 | 0 | 0 | 0.01 | 0.02 | 0.50 | 0.02 | 0.00 | 1.5 | 0.03 | 2.5 | 0.0 | | 9 | 0.1 | 0.2 | 6 | 0.0 | 9 | 56 | | 2 | 0.09 |
| 3107 | 1/2 cup | Canned in heavy syrup, avg | 133 | 98 | 80 | 0.3 | 25.5 | 2.1 | 20.5 | 2.9 | 0.2 | 0.0 | 0.0 | 0.0 | 0.00 | 0.04 | 0 | 0 | 0 | 0 | 0 | 0 | 0.01 | 0.03 | 0.32 | 0.02 | 0.00 | 1.6 | 0.03 | 1.5 | 0.0 | | 7 | 0.1 | 0.3 | 5 | 0.0 | 9 | 86 | 0.5 | 7 | 0.11 |
| 3179 | 1/2 cup | Canned in juice, avg | 124 | 62 | 86 | 0.4 | 16.0 | 2.0 | 11.3 | 2.7 | 0.1 | 0.0 | 0.0 | 0.0 | 0.00 | 0.02 | 0 | 7 | 1 | 0 | 1 | 7 | 0.01 | 0.01 | 0.25 | 0.02 | 0.00 | 1.5 | 0.03 | 2.0 | 0.0 | 0.6 | 11 | 0.1 | 0.4 | 9 | 0.0 | 15 | 119 | 0.5 | 5 | 0.11 |
| 3177 | 1/2 cup | Canned in light syrup, avg | 126 | 72 | 84 | 0.2 | 19.2 | 2.0 | 14.4 | 2.8 | 0.0 | 0.0 | 0.0 | 0.0 | 0.00 | 0.01 | 0 | 0 | 0 | 0 | 0 | 0 | 0.01 | 0.02 | 0.19 | 0.02 | 0.00 | 1.5 | 0.03 | 0.9 | 0.0 | 0.6 | 6 | 0.1 | 0.4 | 5 | 0.0 | 9 | 83 | 0.5 | 6 | 0.10 |
| 3645 | 1/2 cup | Canned in water, halves, avg | 122 | 35 | 92 | 0.2 | 9.5 | 2.0 | 5.7 | 1.8 | 0.0 | 0.0 | 0.0 | 0.0 | 0.00 | 0.01 | 0 | 0 | 0 | 0 | 0 | 0 | 0.01 | 0.01 | 0.07 | 0.02 | 0.00 | 1.5 | 0.03 | 1.2 | 0.0 | | 5 | 0.1 | 0.3 | 5 | 0.0 | 9 | 65 | 0.5 | 2 | 0.11 |
| 3435 | 1/2 cup | Dried, cooked w/sugar, avg | 140 | 196 | 61 | 1.2 | 51.9 | 8.1 | 42.0 | 1.8 | 0.4 | 0.0 | 0.1 | 0.1 | 0.00 | 0.09 | 0 | 56 | 6 | 0 | 6 | 34 | 0.01 | 0.03 | 0.47 | 0.05 | 0.00 | 0.0 | 0.10 | 5.3 | 0.0 | | 21 | 0.2 | 1.4 | 21 | 0.2 | 38 | 343 | 3.4 | 4 | 0.25 |
| 3350 | 1/2 cup | Dried, cooked w/o sugar, avg | 128 | 163 | 64 | 1.2 | 43.3 | 8.2 | 35.1 | 0.0 | 0.4 | 0.0 | 0.1 | 0.1 | 0.00 | 0.09 | 0 | 54 | 5 | 0 | 5 | 31 | 0.01 | 0.03 | 0.45 | 0.04 | 0.00 | 0.0 | 0.09 | 5.1 | 0.0 | 0.0 | 20 | 0.2 | 1.3 | 20 | 0.2 | 36 | 330 | 2.8 | 4 | 0.24 |
| 3730 | 1/2 cup | Dried, halves, avg | 90 | 236 | 27 | 1.7 | 62.7 | 6.8 | 47.1 | 8.9 | 0.6 | 0.0 | 0.1 | 0.1 | 0.00 | 0.13 | 0 | 3 | 0.3 | 0 | 0.3 | 2 | 0.01 | 0.13 | 1.23 | 0.06 | 0.00 | 0.0 | 0.14 | 6.3 | 0.0 | 0.0 | 31 | 0.3 | 1.9 | 30 | 0.3 | 53 | 480 | 4.0 | 5 | 0.35 |
| 3104 | 1/2 cup | Fresh, avg | 82 | 48 | 84 | 0.3 | 12.4 | 2.0 | 8.6 | 1.8 | 0.3 | 0.0 | 0.1 | 0.1 | 0.00 | 0.08 | 0 | 16 | 2 | 0 | 2 | 10 | 0.02 | 0.03 | 0.08 | 0.01 | 0.00 | 6.0 | 0.06 | 3.3 | 0.0 | 0.4 | 9 | 0.1 | 0.2 | 5 | 0.1 | 9 | 102 | 0.8 | 0 | 0.10 |
| 3272 | 1 ea | Fresh, Asian, avg | 122 | 51 | 88 | 0.6 | 13.1 | 4.4 | 8.7 | 0.0 | 0.3 | 0.0 | 0.1 | 0.1 | 0.00 | 0.07 | 0 | 0 | 0 | 0 | 0 | 0 | 0.01 | 0.01 | 0.27 | 0.03 | 0.00 | 9.8 | 0.09 | 4.6 | 0.0 | | 5 | 0.1 | 0.0 | 10 | 0.1 | 13 | 148 | 0.7 | 0 | 0.02 |
| | | Persimmons | | | | | | | | | | | | | | | | | | | | | | | | | | | | | | | | | | | | | | | | |
| 3351 | 1 ea | Dried, Japanese, avg | 34 | 93 | 23 | 0.5 | 25.0 | 4.9 | 19.6 | 0.4 | 0.2 | 0. | 0.0 | 0.1 | 0.00 | 0.05 | 0 | 190 | 19 | 0 | 19 | 114 | | 0.01 | 0.06 | 0.04 | 0.00 | 3.0 | | 0.0 | 0.0 | | 9 | 0.2 | 0.3 | 11 | 0.5 | 28 | 273 | | 1 | 0.14 |
| 3193 | 1 ea | Fresh, Japanese, large, avg | 168 | 118 | 80 | 1.0 | 31.2 | 6.0 | 24.7 | 0.5 | 0.3 | 0.0 | 0.1 | 0.1 | 0.01 | 0.07 | 0 | 3641 | 365 | 0 | 365 | 2187 | 0.05 | 0.03 | 0.17 | 0.17 | 0.00 | 12.6 | | 12.6 | 0.0 | | 13 | 0.2 | 0.3 | 15 | 0.6 | 29 | 270 | 1.0 | 2 | 0.18 |
| 3194 | 1 ea | Fresh, native, small, avg | 25 | 32 | 64 | 0.2 | 8.4 | 0.4 | 8.0 | 0.0 | 0.1 | | | | | | 0 | 0 | 0 | 0 | 0 | 0 | | | | | 0.00 | 2.0 | | 16.5 | 0.0 | | 7 | | 0.6 | | | 6 | 78 | | 0 | |
| 7371 | 1/2 cup | Fuyu, Dried, Frieda's Specialty Produce | 61 | 213 | | 1.5 | 53.4 | 4.6 | 41.2 | 7.6 | 0.0 | 0.0 | 0.0 | 0.0 | 0.00 | 0.00 | 0 | 610 | 61 | 0 | 61 | 37 | | | | | 0.00 | | | 109.8 | | | 30 | | 0.5 | | | | | | 15 | |
| | | Pineapple | | | | | | | | | | | | | | | | | | | | | | | | | | | | | | | | | | | | | | | | |
| 3440 | 1/2 cup | Canned in extra heavy syrup, chunks, avg | 130 | 108 | 78 | 0.4 | 27.9 | 1.0 | 27.0 | 0.0 | 0.1 | 0.0 | 0.0 | 0.0 | 0.02 | 0.03 | 0 | 18 | 1 | 0 | 1 | 8 | 0.12 | 0.03 | 0.37 | 0.10 | 0.00 | 6.0 | 0.13 | 9.5 | 0.0 | | 18 | 0.1 | 0.5 | 19 | 1.4 | 9 | 133 | | 1 | 0.14 |
| 3114 | 1/2 cup | Canned in heavy syrup, pieces, avg | 127 | 99 | 79 | 0.4 | 25.7 | 1.0 | 24.6 | 0.0 | 0.1 | 0.0 | 0.0 | 0.1 | 0.02 | 0.03 | 0 | 18 | 1 | 0 | 1 | 7 | 0.11 | 0.03 | 0.36 | 0.09 | 0.00 | 5.8 | 0.13 | 9.4 | 0.0 | 0.1 | 18 | 0.1 | 0.5 | 20 | 1.4 | 9 | 132 | 0.5 | 1 | 0.15 |
| 3183 | 1/2 cup | Canned in juice, avg | 125 | 75 | 84 | 0.5 | 19.6 | 1.0 | 15.6 | 3.0 | 0.1 | 0.0 | 0.0 | 0.0 | 0.02 | 0.02 | 0 | 48 | 5 | 0 | 5 | 29 | 0.12 | 0.02 | 0.36 | 0.09 | 0.00 | 6.0 | 0.13 | 11.9 | 0.0 | | 18 | 0.1 | 0.3 | 18 | 1.4 | 8 | 152 | 0.5 | 1 | 0.13 |
| 3181 | 1/2 cup | Canned in light syrup, avg | 126 | 66 | 86 | 0.5 | 17.0 | 1.0 | 16.0 | 0.0 | 0.2 | 0.0 | 0.0 | 0.1 | 0.02 | 0.03 | 0 | 19 | 1 | 0 | 1 | 7 | 0.11 | 0.03 | 0.37 | 0.09 | 0.00 | 5.9 | 0.13 | 9.4 | 0.0 | | 18 | 0.1 | 0.5 | 20 | 1.4 | 9 | 132 | 0.5 | 1 | 0.15 |
| 3738 | 1/2 cup | Canned in water, slices, avg | 123 | 39 | 91 | 0.5 | 10.2 | 1.0 | 9.4 | 0.0 | 0.1 | 0.0 | 0.0 | 0.0 | 0.02 | 0.02 | 0 | 18 | 2 | 0 | 2 | 14 | 0.11 | 0.03 | 0.37 | 0.09 | 0.00 | 5.9 | 0.12 | 9.5 | 0.0 | | 18 | 0.1 | 0.5 | 22 | 1.4 | 5 | 156 | 0.5 | 1 | 0.15 |
| 3284 | 1 pce | Dried, dehydrated, Basic Vegetable Products | 28 | 99 | 3 | 0.8 | 24.9 | 1.1 | 23.8 | 0.0 | 0.9 | | | | | | 0 | 46 | 5 | 0 | 5 | 27 | 0.13 | 0.06 | 0.85 | 0.16 | 0.00 | 21.3 | 0.32 | 31.0 | | | 14 | | 0.7 | 28 | | 14 | 227 | | 2 | 0.16 |
| 3535 | 1 oz | Dried, rings, World Variety Produce | 28 | 89 | 20 | 1.0 | 20.7 | | | | 0.5 | | | | | | | 307 | 31 | 0 | 31 | 179 | 0.25 | 0.24 | 0.91 | | 0.00 | | | 8.1 | | | 94 | | 1.6 | | | | | | | |
| 3111 | 1/2 cup | Fresh, chunks, avg | 78 | 38 | 86 | 0.3 | 9.7 | 0.9 | 8.7 | 0.0 | 0.3 | 0.0 | 0.0 | 0.1 | 0.05 | 0.07 | 0 | 18 | 2 | 0 | 2 | 9 | 0.07 | 0.03 | 0.33 | 0.07 | 0.00 | 8.3 | 0.12 | 12.0 | 0.0 | 0.1 | 5 | 0.1 | 0.3 | 11 | 1.3 | 5 | 88 | 0.5 | 1 | 0.06 |
| 3118 | 1/2 cup | Frozen, sweetened, avg | 123 | 105 | 77 | 0.5 | 27.3 | 1.4 | 26.0 | 0.0 | 0.1 | 0.0 | 0.0 | 0.0 | 0.02 | 0.02 | 0 | 37 | 4 | 0 | 4 | 22 | 0.12 | 0.04 | 0.37 | 0.09 | 0.00 | 13.0 | 0.13 | 9.8 | 0.0 | | 11 | 0.1 | 0.5 | 12 | 1.3 | 5 | 123 | 0.7 | 2 | 0.14 |
| | | Plantain | | | | | | | | | | | | | | | | | | | | | | | | | | | | | | | | | | | | | | | | |
| 44062 | 32 pce | Chips, avg | 35 | 182 | 4 | 0.8 | 20.4 | 2.7 | | | 11.8 | 10. | 0.7 | 0.2 | | | 0 | 29 | 3 | 0 | 3 | 17 | 0.03 | 0.01 | 0.25 | 0.09 | 0.00 | 4.9 | | 2.2 | | | 6 | 0.1 | 0.4 | 27 | | 20 | 188 | | 2 | 0.26 |
| 3196 | 1/2 cup | Cooked, slices, avg | 77 | 89 | 67 | 0.6 | 24.0 | 1.8 | 4.3 | 17.3 | 0.1 | 0. | 0.0 | 0.0 | 0.01 | 0.02 | 0 | 700 | 70 | 0 | 70 | 420 | 0.04 | 0.04 | 0.58 | 0.18 | 0.00 | 20.0 | 0.18 | 8.4 | 0.0 | | 2 | 0.1 | 0.4 | 25 | 0.0 | 22 | 358 | 1.1 | 4 | 0.10 |
| 5631 | 1/2 cup | Fried, green, avg | 56 | 133 | 48 | 0.8 | 20.1 | 1.4 | | | 6.6 | 0.9 | 1.6 | 3.8 | | | 0 | 532 | 53 | 0 | 53 | 320 | 0.03 | 0.03 | 0.39 | 0.17 | 0.00 | 6.9 | 0.11 | 8.1 | 0.0 | | 3 | 0.0 | 0.4 | 24 | 0.0 | 21 | 283 | | 414 | 0.10 |
| 5632 | 1/2 cup | Fried, ripe, avg | 84 | 215 | 48 | 1.2 | 30.2 | 2.2 | | | 11.6 | 1.3 | 2.6 | 6.6 | | | 0 | 799 | 80 | 0 | 80 | 481 | 0.04 | 0.05 | 0.58 | 0.25 | 0.00 | 10.4 | 0.17 | 12.2 | 0.0 | | 3 | 0.1 | 0.6 | 35 | 0.1 | 32 | 425 | | 4 | 0.13 |
| 3195 | 1/2 cup | Raw, slices, avg | 74 | 90 | 65 | 1.0 | 23.6 | 1.7 | 4.2 | 17.7 | 0.3 | 0. | 0.0 | 0.1 | 0.02 | 0.03 | 0 | 834 | 84 | 0 | 84 | 502 | 0.04 | 0.04 | 0.51 | 0.22 | 0.00 | 16.3 | 0.19 | 13.6 | 0.0 | | 2 | 0.1 | 0.4 | 27 | 0.0 | 25 | 369 | 1.1 | 3 | 0.10 |
| | | Plums | | | | | | | | | | | | | | | | | | | | | | | | | | | | | | | | | | | | | | | | |
| 3124 | 1/2 cup | Canned in heavy syrup, avg | 129 | 115 | 76 | 0.5 | 29.9 | 1.3 | 26.6 | 2.1 | 0.1 | 0. | 0.1 | 0.0 | 0.00 | 0.03 | 0 | 334 | 34 | 0 | 34 | 201 | 0.02 | 0.05 | 0.38 | 0.03 | 0.00 | 3.2 | 0.09 | 0.5 | 0.0 | | 12 | 0.0 | 1.1 | 6 | 0.0 | 17 | 117 | 0.4 | 25 | 0.09 |
| 3185 | 1/2 cup | Canned in juice, avg | 126 | 73 | 84 | 0.6 | 19.2 | 1.3 | 15.9 | 2.0 | 0.0 | 0. | 0.0 | 0.0 | 0.00 | 0.01 | 0 | 1271 | 127 | 0 | 127 | 764 | 0.03 | 0.07 | 0.60 | 0.03 | 0.00 | 3.3 | 0.09 | 3.5 | 0.0 | | 13 | 0.1 | 0.4 | 10 | 0.0 | 19 | 194 | 0.4 | 1 | 0.14 |
| 3187 | 1/2 cup | Canned in light syrup, avg | 126 | 79 | 83 | 0.5 | 20.5 | 1.3 | 19.3 | 0.0 | 0.1 | 0. | 0.1 | 0.0 | 0.00 | 0.03 | 0 | 333 | 33 | 0 | 33 | 197 | 0.02 | 0.05 | 0.37 | 0.03 | 0.00 | 3.3 | 0.09 | 0.5 | 0.0 | | 11 | 0.0 | 1.1 | 6 | 0.0 | 16 | 117 | 0.4 | 25 | 0.10 |
| 3444 | 1/2 cup | Canned in water, avg | 124 | 51 | 88 | 0.5 | 13.6 | 1.2 | 12.4 | 0.0 | 0.0 | 0. | 0.0 | 0.0 | 0.00 | 0.00 | 0 | 1133 | 113 | 0 | 113 | 677 | 0.03 | 0.05 | 0.46 | 0.03 | 0.00 | 3.2 | 0.09 | 3.3 | 0.0 | | 9 | 0.0 | 0.2 | 6 | 0.0 | 16 | 156 | 0.4 | 1 | 0.10 |
| 3123 | 1/2 cup | Fresh, slices, avg | 82 | 45 | 85 | 0.6 | 10.7 | 1.2 | 8.3 | 1.2 | 0.5 | 0. | 0.3 | 0.1 | 0.00 | 0.11 | 0 | 265 | 26 | 0 | 26 | 157 | 0.04 | 0.08 | 0.41 | 0.07 | 0.00 | 1.8 | 0.15 | 7.8 | 0.0 | | 3 | 0.0 | 0.1 | 6 | 0.0 | 8 | 141 | 0.4 | 0 | 0.08 |
| 3197 | 1 ea | Pomegranate, fresh, avg | 154 | 105 | 81 | 1.5 | 26.5 | 0.9 | 21.1 | 4.5 | 0.5 | 0. | 0.1 | 0.1 | 0.00 | 0.10 | 0 | 0 | 0 | 0 | 0 | 0 | 0.05 | 0.05 | 0.46 | 0.16 | 0.00 | 9.2 | 0.92 | 9.4 | 0.0 | | 5 | 0.1 | 0.5 | 5 | 0.9 | 12 | 399 | 0.9 | 5 | 0.18 |
| 3646 | 1/2 cup | Prickly Pear, raw, avg | 74 | 30 | 88 | 0.5 | 7.1 | 2.7 | | | 0.4 | 0. | 0.1 | 0.2 | 0.02 | 0.14 | 0 | 38 | 4 | 0 | 4 | 22 | 0.01 | 0.04 | 0.34 | 0.04 | 0.00 | 4.4 | | 10.4 | 0.0 | | 41 | 0.1 | 0.2 | 63 | | 18 | 163 | 0.4 | 4 | 0.09 |
| | | Prunes | | | | | | | | | | | | | | | | | | | | | | | | | | | | | | | | | | | | | | | | |
| 3352 | 1/2 cup | Canned in heavy syrup, avg | 117 | 123 | 71 | 1.0 | 32.5 | 4.4 | 28.1 | 0.0 | 0.2 | 0. | 0.2 | 0.1 | 0.00 | 0.05 | 0 | 932 | 94 | 0 | 94 | 505 | 0.04 | 0.14 | 1.01 | 0.24 | 0.00 | 0.1 | 0.12 | 3.3 | 0.0 | | 20 | 0.1 | 0.5 | 18 | 0.1 | 30 | 264 | | 4 | 0.22 |
| 3449 | 1/2 cup | Cooked, f/dry, w/sugar, avg | 124 | 154 | 65 | 1.4 | 40.8 | 4.7 | 28.6 | 7.4 | 0.3 | 0. | 0.2 | 0.1 | 0.00 | 0.06 | 0 | 353 | 36 | 0 | 36 | 194 | 0.03 | 0.12 | 0.84 | 0.25 | 0.00 | 0.1 | 0.12 | 3.3 | 0.0 | | 26 | 0.2 | 1.3 | 24 | 0.1 | 41 | 387 | 1.2 | 2 | 0.27 |
| 3448 | 1/2 cup | Cooked, f/dehydrated, avg | 140 | 158 | 68 | 1.7 | 41.6 | 9.2 | 23.9 | 8.4 | 0.3 | 0. | 0.2 | 0.1 | 0.00 | 0.07 | 0 | 732 | 73 | 0 | 73 | 393 | 0.06 | 0.04 | 1.38 | 0.27 | 0.00 | 0.3 | 0.15 | 0.0 | 0.0 | | 34 | 0.3 | 1.6 | 29 | 0.1 | 52 | 494 | | 3 | 0.35 |
| 3127 | 1/2 cup | Cooked, stewed f/dry, w/o sugar, avg | 124 | 133 | 70 | 1.5 | 34.8 | 8.2 | 19.6 | 7.0 | 0.3 | 0. | 0.2 | 0.1 | 0.00 | 0.06 | 0 | 379 | 38 | 0 | 38 | 208 | 0.03 | 0.12 | 0.90 | 0.27 | 0.00 | 0.1 | 0.13 | 3.6 | 0.0 | | 29 | 0.2 | 1.4 | 25 | 0.1 | 43 | 414 | 1.2 | 2 | 0.30 |
| 3647 | 1/2 cup | Dried, avg | 85 | 203 | 32 | 2.2 | 53.3 | 6.0 | 36.5 | 10.3 | 0.4 | 0. | 0.3 | 0.1 | 0.00 | 0.10 | 0 | 1689 | 169 | 0 | 169 | 914 | 0.07 | 0.14 | 1.67 | 0.22 | 0.00 | 3.1 | 0.39 | 2.8 | 0.0 | | 43 | 0.4 | 2.1 | 38 | 0.2 | 67 | 633 | 2.0 | 3 | 0.45 |
| 3447 | 1/2 cup | Dried, dehydrated, uncooked, avg | 66 | 224 | 4 | 2.4 | 58.8 | 6.7 | 40.3 | 11.3 | 0.5 | 0. | 0.3 | 0.1 | 0.00 | 0.10 | 0 | 1163 | 116 | 0 | 116 | 627 | 0.08 | 0.11 | 1.98 | 0.49 | 0.00 | 1.3 | 0.28 | 0.0 | 0.0 | | 48 | 0.4 | 2.3 | 42 | 0.2 | 74 | 698 | | 3 | 0.50 |
| 3879 | 1 oz | Raw, California Prune Board | 28 | 76 | 30 | 0.8 | 18.1 | 1.7 | 9.2 | 7.2 | 0.1 | 0. | | | | | 0 | 328 | 33 | 0 | 33 | 177 | | | | | 0.00 | | | 1.6 | | | 5 | | 0.4 | | | | 203 | | 3 | |
| 3262 | 1/2 cup | Pummelo, fresh, sections, avg | 95 | 36 | 89 | 0.7 | 9.1 | 0.9 | 8.2 | 0.0 | 0.0 | | | | | | 0 | 0 | 0 | 0 | 0 | 0 | 0.03 | 0.03 | 0.21 | 0.03 | 0.00 | 24.7 | 0.27 | 58.0 | 0.0 | | 4 | 0.0 | 0.1 | 6 | 0.0 | 16 | 205 | | 1 | 0.08 |
| 3263 | 1 ea | Quince, raw, avg | 92 | 52 | 84 | 0.4 | 14.1 | 1.7 | 12.3 | 0.0 | 0.1 | 0. | 0.0 | 0.0 | 0.00 | 0.05 | 0 | 37 | 4 | 0 | 4 | 22 | 0.02 | 0.03 | 0.18 | 0.04 | 0.00 | 2.8 | 0.07 | 13.8 | 0.0 | | 10 | 0.1 | 0.6 | 7 | | 16 | 181 | 0.6 | 4 | 0.04 |
| | | Raisins | | | | | | | | | | | | | | | | | | | | | | | | | | | | | | | | | | | | | | | | |
| 3828 | 1 oz | Cooked, avg | 28 | 61 | 40 | 0.4 | 16.1 | 0.7 | | | 0.1 | 0. | 0.0 | 0.0 | | | 0 | 1 | 0.1 | 0 | 0.1 | 0.6 | 0.02 | 0.01 | 0.10 | 0.03 | 0.00 | 0.2 | | 0.3 | | | 6 | 0.0 | 0.3 | 4 | | 13 | 88 | | 2 | 0.04 |
| 3597 | 1 oz | Freeze Dried, Vacu-Dry Sales | 28 | 95 | 4 | 1.1 | 25.5 | 1.4 | 19.0 | 5.0 | 0.3 | 0. | | | | | 0 | 7 | 1 | 0 | 1 | 4 | | | | | 0.00 | | | 0.6 | | | 15 | | 1.1 | | | | 249 | | 3 | |

| Code | Amount | Description | Basic Components | | | | | | | | | Additional Fats | | | | | | Vit A & Components | | | | | Vitamins | | | | | | | | | | Minerals | | | | | | | | | |
|---|---|---|---|---|---|---|---|---|---|---|---|---|---|---|---|---|---|---|---|---|---|---|---|---|---|---|---|---|---|---|---|---|---|---|---|---|---|---|---|---|---|---|
| | | | Weight (g) | Calories | % Water | Protein (g) | Carbs (g) | Fiber (g) | Sugar (g) | Other Carbs (g) | Fat (g) | Sat Fat (g) | Mono Fat (g) | Poly Fat (g) | Omega 3 (g) | Omega 6 (g) | Choles (mg) | Vit A (IU) | Vit A (RE) | Retinol (RE) | Carotenoids (RE) | Beta Carotene (mcg) | Thiamin (mg) | Riboflavin (mg) | Niacin (NE) | Vit B6 (mg) | Vit B12 (mcg) | Folate (mcg) | Panto (mg) | Vit C (mg) | Vit D (mg) | Vit E (α TE) | Calcium (mg) | Copper (mg) | Iron (mg) | Magnes (mg) | Mang (mg) | Phos (mg) | Potassium (mg) | Selenium (mcg) | Sodium (mg) | Zinc (mg) |
| 3450 | 1/2 cup | Seeded raisins, avg | 72 | 213 | 17 | 1.8 | 56.5 | 4.9 | 51.6 | 0.0 | 0.4 | 0.1 | 0.0 | 0.1 | 0.03 | 0.09 | 0 | 0 | 0 | 0 | 0 | 0 | 0.08 | 0.13 | 0.80 | 0.14 | 0.00 | 2.4 | 0.03 | 3.9 | 0.0 | | 20 | 0.2 | 1.9 | 22 | 0.2 | 54 | 594 | 0.4 | 20 | 0.13 |
| 3202 | 1/2 cup | Seedless, golden, packed, avg | 82 | 248 | 15 | 2.8 | 65.2 | 3.3 | 53.3 | 8.6 | 0.4 | 0.1 | 0.0 | 0.1 | 0.03 | 0.09 | 0 | 36 | 3 | 0 | 3 | 20 | 0.01 | 0.16 | 0.93 | 0.26 | 0.00 | 2.7 | 0.11 | 2.6 | 0.0 | | 43 | 0.3 | 1.5 | 29 | 0.3 | 94 | 612 | 0.6 | 10 | 0.26 |
| 3546 | 1/2 cup | Seedless, plumped, avg | 80 | 207 | 27 | 2.2 | 54.6 | 2.8 | | | 0.3 | 0.1 | 0.0 | 0.1 | 0.02 | 0.07 | 0 | 6 | 1 | 0 | 1 | 3 | 0.11 | 0.06 | 0.56 | 0.17 | 0.00 | 2.3 | 0.03 | 2.3 | 0.0 | | 34 | 0.2 | 1.4 | 22 | 0.2 | 67 | 518 | 4.6 | 8 | 0.19 |
| 3130 | 1/2 cup | Seedless, unpacked, avg | 72 | 216 | 15 | 2.3 | 57.0 | 2.9 | 46.8 | 7.3 | 0.3 | 0.1 | 0.0 | 0.1 | 0.02 | 0.07 | 0 | 6 | 1 | 0 | 1 | 4 | 0.11 | 0.06 | 0.59 | 0.18 | 0.00 | 2.4 | 0.03 | 2.4 | 0.0 | | 35 | 0.2 | 1.5 | 24 | 0.2 | 70 | 541 | 0.5 | 9 | 0.19 |
| | | Raspberries | | | | | | | | | | | | | | | | | | | | | | | | | | | | | | | | | | | | | | | | |
| 3132 | 1/2 cup | Canned in heavy syrup, avg | 128 | 116 | 75 | 1.1 | 30.0 | 4.2 | 25.7 | 0.0 | 0.2 | 0.0 | 0.0 | 0.1 | 0.03 | 0.06 | 0 | 42 | 4 | 0 | 4 | 12 | 0.03 | 0.04 | 0.57 | 0.05 | 0.00 | 13.4 | 0.31 | 11.1 | 0.0 | 0.1 | 14 | 0.1 | 0.5 | 15 | 0.3 | 12 | 120 | 0.5 | 4 | 0.20 |
| 3285 | 1 oz | Dehydrated, Basic Vegetable Products | 28 | 99 | 3 | 1.8 | 23.4 | 6.1 | 17.3 | 0.0 | 1.1 | | | | | | 0 | 263 | 26 | 0 | 26 | 79 | 0.06 | 0.18 | 1.82 | 0.10 | 0.00 | | 0.48 | 50.5 | | | 45 | | 1.2 | 36 | | 24 | 307 | | 0 | 0.93 |
| 3131 | 1/2 cup | Fresh, avg | 62 | 30 | 87 | 0.6 | 7.2 | 4.2 | 3.0 | 0.0 | 0.3 | 0.0 | 0.0 | 0.2 | 0.07 | 0.13 | 0 | 81 | 8 | 0 | 8 | 24 | 0.02 | 0.06 | 0.56 | 0.04 | 0.00 | 16.1 | 0.15 | 15.5 | 0.0 | 0.2 | 14 | 0.0 | 0.4 | 11 | 0.6 | 7 | 94 | 0.4 | 0 | 0.29 |
| 3235 | 1/2 cup | Frozen, sweetened, avg | 125 | 129 | 73 | 0.9 | 32.8 | 5.5 | 27.3 | 0.0 | 0.2 | 0.0 | 0.0 | 0.1 | 0.04 | 0.07 | 0 | 75 | 8 | 0 | 8 | 23 | 0.02 | 0.06 | 0.29 | 0.04 | 0.00 | 32.5 | 0.19 | 20.6 | 0.0 | 0.4 | 19 | 0.1 | 0.8 | 16 | 0.8 | 21 | 142 | 0.8 | 1 | 0.23 |
| 3133 | 1/2 cup | Rhubarb, Cooked from frozen, w/sugar, avg | 120 | 139 | 68 | 0.5 | 37.4 | 2.4 | 35.0 | 0.0 | 0.1 | 0.0 | 0.0 | 0.0 | 0.00 | 0.03 | 0 | 83 | 8 | 0 | 8 | 50 | 0.02 | 0.03 | 0.24 | 0.02 | 0.00 | 6.4 | 0.06 | 4.0 | 0.0 | | 174 | 0.0 | 0.3 | 14 | 0.1 | 10 | 115 | 1.1 | 1 | 0.10 |
| 3209 | 1/2 cup | Rhubarb, Raw, diced, avg | 61 | 13 | 94 | 0.5 | 2.8 | 1.1 | 1.7 | 0.0 | 0.1 | 0.0 | 0.0 | 0.1 | 0.00 | 0.06 | 0 | 61 | 6 | 0 | 6 | 37 | 0.01 | 0.02 | 0.18 | 0.01 | 0.00 | 4.3 | 0.05 | 4.9 | 0.0 | | 52 | 0.0 | 0.1 | 7 | 0.1 | 9 | 176 | 0.7 | 2 | 0.06 |
| 3649 | 1/2 ea | Sapodillas, raw, avg | 120 | 100 | 78 | 0.5 | 24.0 | 6.4 | 16.4 | 1.2 | 1.3 | 0.2 | 0.6 | 0.0 | 0.00 | 0.01 | 0 | 72 | 7 | 0 | 7 | 29 | 0.00 | 0.02 | 0.24 | 0.04 | 0.00 | 16.8 | 0.30 | 17.6 | 0.0 | | 25 | 0.1 | 1.0 | 14 | | 14 | 232 | 0.7 | 14 | 0.12 |
| 3267 | 1 ea | Sapotes, raw, avg | 225 | 302 | 62 | 4.8 | 76.0 | 5.8 | 47.3 | 22.9 | 1.4 | 0.2 | 0.6 | 0.0 | 0.00 | 0.01 | 0 | 923 | 92 | 0 | 92 | 554 | 0.02 | 0.04 | 4.05 | 0.13 | 0.00 | 54.0 | 0.97 | 45.0 | 0.0 | | 88 | 0.3 | 2.3 | 68 | | 63 | 774 | | 22 | 0.27 |
| | | Strawberries | | | | | | | | | | | | | | | | | | | | | | | | | | | | | | | | | | | | | | | | |
| 3534 | 1 oz | Dried, World Variety Produce | 28 | 95 | 16 | 0.5 | 22.7 | | | | 0.2 | | | | | | | | | | | | | | | | 0.00 | | | | | | | | | | | | | | | |
| 3135 | 1/2 cup | Fresh, slices, avg | 83 | 25 | 92 | 0.5 | 5.8 | 1.9 | 3.9 | 0.0 | 0.3 | 0.0 | 0.0 | 0.2 | 0.06 | 0.09 | 0 | 22 | 2 | 0 | 2 | 13 | 0.02 | 0.05 | 0.19 | 0.05 | 0.00 | 14.7 | 0.28 | 47.1 | 0.0 | 0.1 | 12 | 0.0 | 0.3 | 8 | 0.2 | 16 | 138 | 0.6 | 1 | 0.11 |
| 3236 | 1/2 cup | Frozen, sliced, sweetened, avg | 128 | 123 | 73 | 0.7 | 33.2 | 2.4 | 30.7 | 0.0 | 0.2 | 0.0 | 0.0 | 0.1 | 0.03 | 0.05 | 0 | 31 | 3 | 0 | 3 | 14 | 0.02 | 0.07 | 0.51 | 0.04 | 0.00 | 19.1 | 0.14 | 53.0 | 0.0 | | 14 | 0.0 | 0.8 | 9 | 0.3 | 17 | 125 | 0.9 | 4 | 0.08 |
| 3783 | 1/2 cup | Frozen, thawed, unsweetened, avg | 110 | 39 | 90 | 0.5 | 10.0 | 2.3 | 7.7 | 0.1 | 0.1 | 0.0 | 0.0 | 0.1 | 0.03 | 0.03 | 0 | 50 | 4 | 0 | 4 | 24 | 0.02 | 0.04 | 0.51 | 0.03 | 0.00 | 18.5 | 0.12 | 45.3 | 0.0 | 0.2 | 18 | 0.1 | 0.8 | 12 | 0.3 | 14 | 163 | 0.8 | 2 | 0.14 |
| 3525 | 1/2 cup | Halves, in light syrup, Birds Eye | 130 | 68 | 86 | 0.6 | 17.3 | 0.0 | 15.0 | 2.3 | 0.1 | 0.0 | | | | | 0 | 46 | 9 | | | | 0.03 | 0.06 | 0.26 | 0.06 | 0.00 | 18.5 | 0.35 | 42.9 | | | 16 | 0.1 | 0.8 | 10 | | 19 | 173 | | 3 | |
| 3453 | 1/2 cup | In heavy syrup, avg | 127 | 117 | 75 | 0.7 | 29.8 | 2.2 | 27.7 | 0.0 | 0.3 | 0.0 | 0.0 | 0.2 | 0.07 | 0.10 | 0 | 33 | 4 | 0 | 4 | 21 | 0.03 | 0.04 | 0.07 | 0.06 | 0.00 | 35.6 | 0.23 | 40.3 | 0.0 | | 17 | 0.1 | 0.6 | 10 | 0.3 | 15 | 109 | 0.5 | 5 | 0.11 |
| | | Tamarinds | | | | | | | | | | | | | | | | | | | | | | | | | | | | | | | | | | | | | | | | |
| 3545 | 1/2 cup | Pods, World Variety Produce | 60 | 185 | 20 | 2.2 | 42.2 | 6.8 | | | 0.9 | | | | | | 0 | 6 | 1 | 0 | 1 | 4 | | | | | 0.00 | | | 3.3 | | | 51 | | 1.0 | | | | | | 7 | |
| 3364 | 1/2 cup | Pulp, dried, sweetened , avg | 110 | 279 | 28 | 2.8 | 72.9 | 5.0 | | | 0.6 | 0.3 | 0.2 | 0.1 | | | 0 | 15 | 1 | 0 | 1 | 9 | 0.30 | 0.14 | 1.73 | 0.06 | 0.00 | 6.9 | | 0.7 | 0.0 | | 74 | 0.1 | 2.8 | 91 | | 112 | 622 | | 28 | 0.10 |
| 3653 | 1/2 cup | Pulp, raw, avg | 60 | 143 | 31 | 1.7 | 37.5 | 3.1 | | | 0.4 | 0.2 | 0.1 | 0.0 | 0.00 | 0.04 | 0 | 18 | 2 | 0 | 2 | 11 | 0.26 | 0.09 | 1.16 | 0.04 | 0.00 | 8.4 | 0.09 | 2.1 | 0.0 | | 44 | 0.1 | 1.7 | 55 | 0.3 | 68 | 377 | 0.8 | 17 | 0.06 |
| 3237 | 1/2 cup | Tangerines, canned in light syrup, avg | 126 | 77 | 83 | 0.6 | 20.4 | 0.9 | 19.5 | 0.0 | 0.1 | 0.0 | 0.0 | 0.0 | 0.01 | 0.02 | 0 | 1058 | 106 | 0 | 106 | 239 | 0.07 | 0.06 | 0.56 | 0.05 | 0.00 | 5.8 | 0.16 | 24.9 | 0.0 | | 9 | 0.1 | 0.5 | 10 | 0.0 | 13 | 98 | 0.5 | 8 | 0.30 |
| 3139 | 1/2 cup | Tangerines, fresh, sections, avg | 98 | 43 | 88 | 0.6 | 11.0 | 2.3 | 8.7 | 0.0 | 0.2 | 0.0 | 0.0 | 0.0 | 0.01 | 0.03 | 0 | 902 | 90 | 0 | 90 | 541 | 0.10 | 0.02 | 0.16 | 0.07 | 0.00 | 20.0 | 0.20 | 30.2 | 0.0 | 0.2 | 14 | 0.0 | 0.1 | 12 | 0.0 | 10 | 154 | 0.5 | 1 | 0.24 |
| 3142 | 1/2 cup | Watermelon, fresh, diced, avg | 76 | 24 | 92 | 0.5 | 5.5 | 0.4 | 5.1 | 0.0 | 0.3 | 0.0 | 0.1 | 0.1 | 0.00 | 0.11 | 0 | 278 | 28 | 0 | 28 | 168 | 0.06 | 0.02 | 0.15 | 0.11 | 0.00 | 1.7 | 0.16 | 7.3 | 0.0 | | 6 | 0.0 | 0.1 | 8 | 0.0 | 7 | 88 | 0.1 | 2 | 0.05 |
| | | **GRAINS, FLOURS AND FRACTIONS** | | | | | | | | | | | | | | | | | | | | | | | | | | | | | | | | | | | | | | | | |
| | | Amaranth | | | | | | | | | | | | | | | | | | | | | | | | | | | | | | | | | | | | | | | | |
| 38453 | 1/4 cup | Flour, Arrowhead Mills | 30 | 110 | 12 | 4.0 | 19.0 | 2.0 | 1.0 | 16.0 | 1.5 | 0.0 | | | | | 0 | 0 | 0 | 0 | 0 | 0 | | 0.07 | 0.40 | | | | | 0.0 | | | 40 | | 7.2 | | | | 110 | | 0 | |
| 38243 | 1/4 cup | Flour, whole grain, American Amaranth | 31 | 115 | 12 | 4.7 | 19.8 | 3.1 | 0.6 | 16.1 | 1.9 | | | | | | | | | | | | | | | | | | | | | | 51 | | 3.1 | | | | 112 | | 7 | |
| 38070 | 1/4 cup | Grain, avg | 49 | 183 | 10 | 7.1 | 32.4 | 7.4 | 0.9 | 24.1 | 3.2 | 0.8 | 0.7 | 1.4 | 0.03 | 1.39 | 0 | 0 | 0 | 0 | 0 | 0 | 0.04 | 0.10 | 0.63 | 0.11 | 0.00 | 24.0 | 0.51 | 2.1 | 0.0 | | 75 | 0.4 | 3.7 | 130 | 1.1 | 223 | 179 | | 10 | 1.56 |
| 38242 | 1/4 cup | Grain, whole, American Amaranth | 31 | 115 | 10 | 5.0 | 18.8 | 2.8 | 0.6 | 15.3 | 2.4 | 0.5 | 0.4 | 0.9 | 0.02 | 0.88 | 0 | | | | | | 0.02 | 0.06 | 0.40 | 0.07 | 0.00 | 15.2 | 0.33 | 1.3 | | | 47 | 0.2 | 2.4 | 82 | 0.7 | 141 | 113 | | 7 | 0.99 |
| 38244 | 1 oz | Puffed, whole grain, American Amaranth | 28 | 104 | 4 | 4.6 | 19.6 | 2.8 | 0.6 | 16.2 | 1.8 | | | | | | | | | | | | | | | | | | | | | | 46 | | 2.8 | | | | 101 | | 6 | |
| 4771 | 1/4 cup | Seeds, Arrowhead Mills | 47 | 170 | 10 | 7.0 | 29.0 | 3.0 | 0.0 | 26.0 | 2.0 | 0.5 | | | | | 0 | 0 | 0 | 0 | 0 | 0 | | 0.10 | 0.80 | | 0.00 | | | 0.0 | | | 80 | | 10.8 | | | | 170 | | 0 | |
| 38071 | 1/4 cup | Arrowroot Flour, avg | 32 | 114 | 11 | 0.1 | 28.2 | 1.1 | 0.0 | 27.1 | 0.0 | 0.0 | 0.0 | 0.0 | 0.00 | 0.01 | 0 | 0 | 0 | 0 | 0 | 0 | 0.00 | 0.00 | 0.00 | 0.00 | 0.00 | 2.2 | 0.04 | 0.0 | 0.0 | | 13 | 0.0 | 0.1 | 1 | 0.2 | 2 | 4 | | 1 | 0.02 |
| | | Barley | | | | | | | | | | | | | | | | | | | | | | | | | | | | | | | | | | | | | | | | |
| 38130 | 1/4 cup | Bran Flour, Barley's Best | 21 | 24 | 4 | 3.7 | 14.2 | 14.2 | | | 1.4 | | | | | | 0 | | | | | | 0.01 | 0.02 | 0.97 | 0.03 | 0.00 | 3.4 | 0.07 | | | | 119 | 0.4 | 3.4 | 57 | 1.0 | 163 | 23 | 840.0 | 3 | 1.89 |
| 38418 | 1/4 cup | Flakes, rolled, Arrowhead Mills | 28 | 83 | 9 | 3.0 | 21.2 | 3.8 | 0.0 | 17.4 | 0.8 | 0.0 | | | | | 0 | 0 | 0 | 0 | 0 | 0 | 0.07 | 0.03 | 0.91 | | | | | 0.0 | | | 0 | | 0.8 | | | | 144 | | 0 | |
| 38452 | 1/4 cup | Flour, Arrowhead Mills | 25 | 75 | 9 | 3.0 | 19.0 | 3.0 | 0.0 | 16.0 | 0.5 | 0.0 | | | | | 0 | 0 | 0 | 0 | 0 | 0 | 0.06 | 0.03 | 0.80 | | | | | 0.0 | | | 0 | | 0.7 | | | | 125 | | 0 | |
| 38138 | 1/4 cup | Groats, avg | 41 | 125 | 13 | 3.2 | 31.3 | | | | 0.6 | | | | | | 0 | | | | | | 0.08 | 0.03 | 1.27 | 0.12 | | 7.8 | 0.20 | 0.0 | 0.0 | | 7 | 0.0 | 0.8 | 27 | 0.5 | 77 | 66 | 0.4 | 1 | 0.52 |
| 38215 | 1 oz | Malted, avg | 28 | 92 | 12 | 3.2 | 20.5 | 0.7 | | | 0.4 | | | | | | | 7 | 1 | 0 | 1 | | 0.09 | | | | | | | 0.0 | 0.0 | 0.0 | 7 | | 1.0 | | | 79 | | | | |
| 38216 | 1 oz | Meal, roasted, avg | 28 | 101 | 12 | 3.0 | 20.5 | 0.7 | | | 0.6 | | | | | | | 10 | 1 | 0 | 1 | | 0.07 | 0.02 | 1.40 | | | | | 0.0 | 0.0 | 0.0 | 9 | | 0.6 | | | 98 | | | 1 | |
| 38003 | 1/4 cup | Pearled, cooked, avg | 39 | 48 | 69 | 0.9 | 11.0 | 1.5 | 0.3 | 9.2 | 0.2 | 0.0 | 0.0 | 0.1 | 0.01 | 0.08 | 0 | 3 | 0.4 | 0 | 0.4 | | 0.03 | 0.02 | 0.80 | 0.04 | 0.00 | 6.2 | 0.05 | 0.0 | 0.0 | 0.0 | 4 | 0.0 | 0.5 | 9 | 0.1 | 21 | 36 | 3.4 | 1 | 0.32 |
| 38002 | 1/4 cup | Pearled, dry, avg | 50 | 176 | 10 | 5.0 | 38.8 | 7.8 | 0.9 | 30.1 | 0.6 | 0.1 | 0.1 | 0.3 | 0.03 | 0.25 | 0 | 11 | 1 | 0 | 1 | | 0.10 | 0.06 | 2.30 | 0.13 | 0.00 | 11.5 | 0.14 | 0.0 | 0.0 | 0.0 | 14 | 0.2 | 1.3 | 40 | 0.7 | 110 | 140 | 18.9 | 4 | 1.07 |
| 38001 | 1/4 cup | Whole, cooked, avg | 50 | 68 | 65 | 1.9 | 14.9 | 3.4 | 0.3 | 11.1 | 0.5 | 0.1 | 0.1 | 0.3 | | | 0 | 0 | 0 | 0 | 0 | 0 | 0.04 | 0.01 | 0.71 | 0.05 | 0.00 | 4.0 | 0.13 | 0.0 | 0.0 | 0.1 | 6 | 0.2 | 0.5 | 11 | 0.2 | 58 | 58 | 9.1 | 0 | 0.39 |
| 38000 | 1/4 cup | Whole, dry, avg | 46 | 163 | 9 | 5.8 | 33.8 | 8.0 | 0.8 | 25.1 | 1.1 | 0.2 | 0.1 | 0.5 | 0.05 | 0.46 | 0 | 10 | 1 | 0 | 1 | | 0.30 | 0.13 | 2.12 | 0.15 | 0.00 | 8.7 | 0.13 | 0.0 | 0.0 | | 15 | 0.2 | 1.7 | 61 | 0.9 | 121 | 208 | 23.7 | 6 | 1.27 |
| | | Buckwheat | | | | | | | | | | | | | | | | | | | | | | | | | | | | | | | | | | | | | | | | |
| 38217 | 1/4 cup | Flour, dark, avg | 24 | 87 | 12 | 2.6 | 17.7 | 0.1 | | | 0.5 | | | | | | | 0 | 0 | 0 | 0 | 0 | 0.07 | 0.02 | 0.36 | | | | | 0.0 | 0.0 | | 5 | | 0.7 | | | 72 | | | 5 | |
| 38053 | 1/4 cup | Flour, whole, avg | 30 | 101 | 11 | 3.8 | 21.2 | 3.0 | 0.8 | 17.4 | 0.9 | 0.2 | 0.3 | 0.3 | 0.02 | 0.26 | 0 | 0 | 0 | 0 | 0 | 0 | 0.13 | 0.06 | 1.85 | 0.17 | 0.00 | 16.2 | 0.13 | 0.0 | 0.0 | 0.1 | 12 | 0.2 | 1.2 | 75 | 0.6 | 101 | 173 | 1.7 | 3 | 0.94 |
| 38278 | 1/4 cup | Groats, dry roasted, avg | 41 | 142 | 8 | 4.8 | 30.8 | 4.2 | 1.2 | 25.3 | 1.1 | 0.2 | 0.3 | 0.3 | 0.03 | 0.31 | 0 | 0 | 0 | 0 | 0 | 0 | 0.09 | 0.11 | 2.11 | 0.14 | 0.00 | 17.2 | 0.50 | 0.0 | 0.0 | | 7 | 0.3 | 1.0 | 91 | 0.7 | 131 | 131 | 3.4 | 5 | 0.99 |
| 38073 | 1/4 cup | Groats, dry roasted, cooked, avg | 42 | 39 | 76 | 1.4 | 8.4 | 1.1 | 0.4 | 6.8 | 0.3 | 0.1 | 0.1 | 0.1 | 0.01 | 0.07 | 0 | 0 | 0 | 0 | 0 | 0 | 0.02 | 0.02 | 0.39 | 0.03 | 0.00 | 5.9 | 0.15 | 0.0 | 0.0 | | 3 | 0.1 | 0.3 | 21 | 0.2 | 29 | 37 | 0.9 | 2 | 0.26 |
| 38100 | 1/4 cup | Kasha, cooked, avg | 50 | 173 | 8 | 5.8 | 37.5 | 4.8 | 0.4 | 32.3 | 1.4 | 0.3 | 0.4 | 0.4 | 0.03 | 0.38 | 0 | 0 | 0 | 0 | 0 | 0 | 0.11 | 0.14 | 2.57 | 0.18 | 0.00 | 21.0 | 0.62 | 0.0 | | | 8 | 0.3 | 1.2 | 110 | 0.8 | 160 | 160 | | 6 | 1.22 |
| 38101 | 1/4 cup | Kasha, raw, avg | 82 | 75 | 76 | 2.8 | 16.3 | 1.9 | 0.7 | 13.7 | 0.5 | 0.1 | 0.2 | 0.2 | 0.01 | 0.14 | 0 | 0 | 0 | 0 | 0 | 0 | 0.03 | 0.03 | 0.77 | 0.06 | 0.00 | 11.5 | 0.29 | 0.0 | 0.0 | | 6 | 0.1 | 0.7 | 42 | 0.3 | 57 | 72 | | 3 | 0.50 |
| 38222 | 1/4 cup | Korean Mook, prep, avg | 42 | 26 | 85 | 1.1 | 5.1 | 0.1 | | | 0.1 | | | | | | | | | | | | 0.00 | 0.08 | 3.11 | | | | | 0.0 | 0.0 | | 5 | | 0.2 | | | 66 | | | | |
| | | Corn | | | | | | | | | | | | | | | | | | | | | | | | | | | | | | | | | | | | | | | | |
| 38074 | 1/4 cup | Bran, crude, avg | 19 | 43 | 5 | 1.6 | 16.3 | 16.2 | 0.0 | 0.0 | 0.2 | 0.0 | 0.0 | 0.1 | 0.00 | 0.08 | 0 | 13 | 1 | 0 | 1 | | 0.00 | 0.02 | 0.52 | 0.03 | 0.00 | 0.8 | 0.12 | 0.0 | 0.0 | | 8 | 0.0 | 0.5 | 12 | 0.0 | 14 | 8 | 3.1 | 1 | 0.30 |
| 38005 | 1/4 cup | Flour, masa, enriched, avg | 28 | 102 | 9 | 2.6 | 21.4 | 2.7 | 0.0 | 18.6 | 1.1 | 0.1 | 0.3 | 0.5 | 0.01 | 0.47 | 0 | 0 | 0 | 0 | 0 | 0 | 0.40 | 0.21 | 2.76 | 0.10 | 0.00 | 52.4 | 0.18 | 0.0 | 0.0 | | 39 | 0.0 | 2.0 | 31 | 0.1 | 62 | 83 | 4.2 | 1 | 0.50 |
| 38161 | 1/4 cup | Flour, masa, enriched, yellow, avg | 28 | 102 | 9 | 2.6 | 21.4 | 3.8 | 0.0 | 17.6 | 1.1 | 0.1 | 0.3 | 0.5 | 0.01 | 0.47 | 0 | 131 | 13 | 0 | 13 | | 0.40 | 0.21 | 2.76 | 0.10 | 0.00 | 52.4 | 0.18 | 0.0 | 0.0 | 0.1 | 39 | 0.0 | 2.0 | 31 | 0.1 | 62 | 83 | 4.2 | 1 | 0.50 |
| 38096 | 1/4 cup | Flour, white, whole grain, avg | 29 | 105 | 11 | 2.0 | 22.3 | 2.8 | 0.0 | 19.5 | 1.1 | 0.2 | 0.3 | 0.5 | 0.02 | 0.50 | 0 | 0 | 0 | 0 | 0 | 0 | 0.07 | 0.02 | 0.55 | 0.11 | 0.00 | 7.3 | 0.19 | 0.0 | 0.0 | | 2 | 0.1 | 0.7 | 27 | 0.1 | 79 | 91 | 4.5 | 1 | 0.50 |
| 38049 | 1/4 cup | Flour, yellow, whole grain, avg | 29 | 105 | 11 | 2.0 | 22.3 | 3.9 | 0.0 | 18.4 | 1.1 | 0.2 | 0.3 | 0.5 | 0.02 | 0.50 | 0 | 136 | 14 | 0 | 14 | | 0.07 | 0.02 | 0.55 | 0.11 | 0.00 | 7.3 | 0.19 | 0.0 | 0.0 | | 2 | 0.1 | 0.7 | 27 | 0.1 | 79 | 91 | 4.5 | 1 | 0.50 |
| 38253 | 1/4 cup | Meal, white, self rising, enriched, avg | 30 | 100 | 13 | 2.5 | 21.1 | 2.0 | 0.0 | 19.1 | 1.0 | 0.1 | 0.3 | 0.5 | 0.01 | 0.45 | 0 | 0 | 0 | 0 | 0 | 0 | 0.20 | 0.12 | 1.59 | 0.16 | 0.00 | 56.1 | 0.13 | 0.0 | 0.0 | 0.1 | 108 | 0.0 | 1.7 | 26 | 0.2 | 241 | 77 | | 374 | 0.60 |
| 38059 | 1/4 cup | Meal, yellow, whole grain, avg | 30 | 109 | 10 | 2.4 | 23.1 | 2.2 | 0.0 | 20.9 | 1.1 | 0.2 | 0.3 | 0.5 | 0.01 | 0.48 | 0 | 141 | 14 | 0 | 14 | | 0.12 | 0.06 | 1.09 | 0.09 | 0.00 | 7.6 | 0.13 | 0.0 | 0.0 | 0.1 | 2 | 0.1 | 1.0 | 38 | 0.1 | 72 | 86 | 4.7 | 11 | 0.55 |
| 38280 | 1/4 cup | Meal, yellow, self rising, enriched, avg | 30 | 100 | 13 | 2.5 | 21.1 | 2.0 | 0.0 | 19.1 | 1.0 | 0.1 | 0.3 | 0.5 | 0.01 | 0.45 | 0 | 141 | 14 | 0 | 14 | | 0.20 | 0.12 | 1.59 | 0.16 | 0.00 | 56.1 | 0.13 | 0.0 | 0.0 | 0.1 | 108 | 0.0 | 1.7 | 26 | 0.1 | 241 | 77 | | 374 | 0.60 |
| 38128 | 1/4 cup | Meal, Blue, Arrowhead Mills | 35 | 130 | 12 | 3.0 | 25.0 | 3.0 | 0.0 | 22.0 | 1.5 | 0.0 | | | | | 0 | 0 | 0 | 0 | 0 | 0 | 0.09 | 0.03 | 0.40 | | 0.00 | | | 0.0 | | | 0 | | 0.7 | | | 65 | 40 | | 0 | |
| 38449 | 1/4 cup | Meal, White, Arrowhead Mills | 32 | 120 | 12 | 3.0 | 23.0 | 3.0 | 0.0 | 20.0 | 1.0 | 0.0 | | | | | 0 | 0 | 0 | 0 | 0 | 0 | 0.22 | 0.10 | 0.80 | | | | | 0.0 | | | 0 | | 0.7 | | | | 95 | | 0 | |
| 38252 | 1/4 cup | White, dry, avg | 42 | 153 | 10 | 4.0 | 31.2 | 3.9 | 0.0 | 27.2 | 2.0 | 0.3 | 0.5 | 0.9 | 0.03 | 0.88 | 0 | 0 | 0 | 0 | 0 | 0 | 0.16 | 0.08 | 1.52 | 0.26 | 0.00 | 11.8 | 0.18 | 0.0 | 0.0 | 0.2 | 3 | 0.1 | 1.1 | 53 | 0.2 | 88 | 121 | 6.5 | 15 | 0.93 |
| 38279 | 1/4 cup | Yellow, dry, avg | 42 | 153 | 10 | 4.0 | 31.2 | 5.6 | 0.1 | 25.5 | 2.0 | 0.3 | 0.5 | 0.9 | 0.03 | 0.88 | 0 | 197 | 20 | 0 | 20 | | 0.16 | 0.08 | 1.52 | 0.26 | 0.00 | 8.0 | 0.18 | 0.0 | 0.0 | | 3 | 0.1 | 1.1 | 53 | 0.2 | 88 | 121 | 6.5 | 15 | 0.93 |
| | | Millet | | | | | | | | | | | | | | | | | | | | | | | | | | | | | | | | | | | | | | | | |
| 38052 | 1/4 cup | Cooked, avg | 60 | 71 | 71 | 2.1 | 14.2 | 0.8 | 0.1 | 13.4 | 0.6 | 0.1 | 0.1 | 0.3 | 0.02 | 0.29 | 0 | 0 | 0 | 0 | 0 | 0 | 0.06 | 0.05 | 0.80 | 0.06 | 0.00 | 11.4 | 0.10 | 0.0 | 0.0 | 0.0 | 2 | 0.1 | 0.4 | 26 | 0.2 | 60 | 37 | 0.5 | 1 | 0.55 |

| Code | Amount | Description | Weight (g) | Calories | % Water | Protein (g) | Carbs (g) | Fiber (g) | Sugar (g) | Other Carbs (g) | Fat (g) | Sat Fat (g) | Mono Fat (g) | Poly Fat (g) | Omega 3 (g) | Omega 6 (g) | Choles (mg) |
|---|---|---|---|---|---|---|---|---|---|---|---|---|---|---|---|---|---|
| | | | Basic Components | | | | | | | | | Additional Fats | | | | | |
| 38282 | 1/4 cup | Dry millet, avg | 50 | 189 | 9 | 5.5 | 36.5 | 4.3 | 0.2 | 32.0 | 2.1 | 0.4 | 0.4 | 1.1 | 0.06 | 1.01 | 0 |
| 38446 | 1/4 cup | Flour, Arrowhead Mills | 35 | 110 | 9 | 4.0 | 26.0 | 2.0 | 0.0 | 24.0 | 1.0 | 0.0 | | | | | 0 |
| | | Oat | | | | | | | | | | | | | | | |
| 38078 | 1/4 cup | Bran, cooked, avg | 55 | 22 | 84 | 1.8 | 6.3 | 1.4 | 0.2 | 4.6 | 0.5 | 0.1 | 0.2 | 0.2 | 0.01 | 0.18 | 0 |
| 38064 | 1/4 cup | Bran, dry, avg | 24 | 59 | 7 | 4.2 | 15.9 | 3.7 | 0.6 | 11.6 | 1.7 | 0.3 | 0.6 | 0.7 | 0.03 | 0.64 | 0 |
| 38417 | 1/4 cup | Flakes, rolled, Arrowhead Mills | 26 | 99 | 9 | 3.8 | 17.6 | 3.1 | 0.8 | 13.8 | 1.9 | 0.4 | | | | | 0 |
| 38445 | 1/4 cup | Flour, Arrowhead Mills | 22 | 88 | 8 | 3.7 | 14.7 | 2.9 | 0.0 | 11.7 | 1.5 | 0.0 | | | | | 0 |
| 38080 | 1/4 cup | Grain, dry, avg | 39 | 152 | 8 | 6.6 | 25.9 | 4.1 | 0.7 | 21.0 | 2.7 | 0.5 | 0.9 | 1.0 | 0.04 | 0.94 | 0 |
| 38422 | 1/4 cup | Groats, whole, Arrowhead Mills | 42 | 160 | 10 | 6.0 | 29.0 | 4.0 | 1.0 | 24.0 | 3.0 | 0.5 | | | | | 0 |
| 38008 | 1/4 cup | Rolled, dry, avg | 20 | 77 | 9 | 3.2 | 13.4 | 2.1 | 0.4 | 10.9 | 1.3 | 0.2 | 0.4 | 0.5 | 0.02 | 0.44 | 0 |
| 38079 | 1/4 cup | Quinoa, grain, dry, avg | 42 | 157 | 9 | 5.5 | 28.9 | 2.5 | | | 2.4 | 0.2 | 0.6 | 1.0 | 0.06 | 0.93 | 0 |
| | | Rice | | | | | | | | | | | | | | | |
| 38050 | 1/4 cup | Bran, crude, avg | 30 | 95 | 6 | 4.0 | 14.9 | 6.3 | 0.3 | 8.3 | 6.3 | 1.3 | 2.3 | 2.2 | 0.09 | 2.14 | 0 |
| 38158 | 1/4 cup | Flour, white, avg | 40 | 146 | 12 | 2.4 | 32.0 | 1.0 | 0.0 | 31.1 | 0.6 | 0.2 | 0.2 | 0.2 | 0.03 | 0.12 | 0 |
| 38443 | 1/4 cup | Flour, Brown, Arrowhead Mills | 35 | 120 | 10 | 3.0 | 27.0 | 2.0 | 0.0 | 25.0 | 1.0 | 0.0 | | | | | 0 |
| 30118 | 1/4 cup | Flour, Sweet, California Natural Products | 41 | 146 | 11 | 3.4 | 32.4 | 0.4 | 0.0 | 32.0 | 0.5 | 0.2 | | | | | 0 |
| 38226 | 1 oz | Germ, Taiwan, avg | 28 | 100 | 13 | 1.7 | 21.6 | 0.3 | | | 0.6 | | | | | | |
| 38051 | 1/4 cup | Polishings, avg | 26 | 69 | 10 | 3.1 | 15.0 | 1.8 | 0.1 | 13.1 | 3.3 | 0.5 | 1.3 | 1.2 | | | 0 |
| | | Rye | | | | | | | | | | | | | | | |
| 38416 | 1/4 cup | Flakes, Rolled, Arrowhead Mills | 25 | 83 | 9 | 3.0 | 18.2 | 3.0 | 0.0 | 15.2 | 0.4 | 0.0 | | | | | 0 |
| 38022 | 1/4 cup | Flour, dark, avg | 32 | 104 | 11 | 4.5 | 22.0 | 7.2 | 1.5 | 13.3 | 0.9 | 0.1 | 0.1 | 0.4 | 0.05 | 0.33 | 0 |
| 38023 | 1/4 cup | Flour, light, avg | 26 | 95 | 9 | 2.2 | 20.9 | 3.8 | 1.4 | 15.7 | 0.4 | 0.0 | 0.0 | 0.1 | 0.02 | 0.13 | 0 |
| 38056 | 1/4 cup | Flour, medium, avg | 26 | 92 | 10 | 2.4 | 20.1 | 3.8 | 1.2 | 15.2 | 0.5 | 0.1 | 0.1 | 0.2 | 0.03 | 0.17 | 0 |
| 38442 | 1/4 cup | Flour, Whole, Arrowhead Mills | 30 | 100 | 11 | 5.0 | 20.0 | 4.0 | 0.0 | 16.0 | 1.0 | 0.0 | | | | | 0 |
| 38142 | 1/4 cup | Germ, avg | 28 | 95 | 12 | 10.9 | 9.2 | | | | 3.1 | | | | | | |
| 38084 | 1/4 cup | Grain, avg | 42 | 141 | 11 | 6.2 | 29.3 | 6.1 | 1.7 | 21.5 | 1.0 | 0.1 | 0.1 | 0.5 | 0.07 | 0.40 | 0 |
| 38420 | 1/4 cup | Whole, Arrowhead Mills | 47 | 160 | 11 | 6.0 | 34.0 | 6.0 | 0.0 | 28.0 | 1.0 | 0.0 | | | | | 0 |
| 38233 | 1 oz | Sorghum, grain, milled, avg | 28 | 100 | 14 | 2.2 | 20.9 | 0.2 | 0.4 | 20.4 | 0.7 | | | | | | |
| 38085 | 1/4 cup | Sorghum, grain, whole, avg | 48 | 163 | 9 | 5.4 | 35.8 | 4.8 | 0.6 | 30.4 | 1.6 | 0.2 | 0.5 | 0.7 | 0.03 | 0.63 | 0 |
| 38139 | 1 oz | Spelt, grain, avg | 28 | 89 | 12 | 3.0 | 20.2 | | | | 0.8 | | | | | | 0 |
| 38439 | 1/4 cup | Spelt Flour, Arrowhead Mills | 35 | 100 | 13 | 4.0 | 24.0 | 5.0 | 0.0 | 19.0 | 0.5 | 0.0 | | | | | 0 |
| | | Tapioca | | | | | | | | | | | | | | | |
| 38375 | 1 Tbs | Granulated, dry, Bascom's | 10 | 35 | 10 | 1.0 | 8.0 | 0.0 | 0.0 | 8.0 | 0.0 | 0.0 | 0.0 | 0.0 | 0.00 | 0.00 | |
| 38374 | 1 Tbs | Large pearl, dry, Bascom's | 10 | 35 | 10 | 0.0 | 9.0 | | | | 0.0 | 0.0 | 0.0 | 0.0 | 0.00 | 0.00 | |
| 38373 | 1 Tbs | Small pearl, dry, Bascom's | 10 | 35 | 10 | 1.0 | 8.0 | | | | 0.0 | 0.0 | 0.0 | 0.0 | 0.00 | 0.00 | |
| 38087 | 1/4 cup | Triticale, flour, avg | 32 | 108 | 10 | 4.2 | 23.4 | 4.7 | 1.0 | 17.7 | 0.5 | 0.1 | 0.1 | 0.3 | 0.02 | 0.24 | 0 |
| 38086 | 1/4 cup | Triticale, grain, dry, avg | 48 | 161 | 10 | 6.3 | 34.6 | 8.7 | 1.4 | 24.5 | 1.0 | 0.2 | 0.1 | 0.4 | 0.03 | 0.41 | 0 |
| | | Wheat | | | | | | | | | | | | | | | |
| 38491 | 1/4 cup | Bisquick, dry, General Mills | 30 | 121 | 16 | 2.1 | 18.3 | 0.5 | 0.5 | 17.2 | 4.5 | 1.2 | 1.9 | 0.4 | | | 0 |
| 38024 | 1/4 cup | Bran, crude, avg | 14 | 30 | 10 | 2.2 | 9.0 | 6.0 | 0.6 | 2.4 | 0.5 | 0.1 | 0.1 | 0.3 | 0.02 | 0.29 | 0 |
| 38493 | 1 oz | Bran, Kretschmer, toasted, Quaker | 28 | 101 | 5 | 5.6 | 14.6 | 11.3 | | | 2.2 | 0.3 | 0.3 | 0.9 | | | 0 |
| 38028 | 1/4 cup | Bulgur, cooked, avg | 46 | 38 | 78 | 1.4 | 8.6 | 2.1 | 0.1 | 6.4 | 0.1 | 0.0 | 0.0 | 0.0 | 0.00 | 0.04 | 0 |
| 38027 | 1/4 cup | Bulgur, dry, avg | 35 | 120 | 9 | 4.3 | 26.6 | 6.4 | 0.3 | 19.8 | 0.5 | 0.1 | 0.1 | 0.2 | 0.01 | 0.18 | 0 |
| 38329 | 1/4 cup | Cracked, dry, avg | 30 | 102 | 10 | 4.1 | 21.8 | 3.5 | 0.6 | 17.7 | 0.5 | 0.1 | 0.1 | 0.2 | 0.01 | 0.22 | 0 |
| 38123 | 1/4 cup | Durum, enriched, Arrowhead Mills | 42 | 143 | 10 | 5.6 | 29.1 | 5.1 | 0.3 | 23.7 | 1.2 | | | | | | 0 |
| 38415 | 1/4 cup | Flakes, Rolled, Arrowhead Mills | 26 | 84 | 9 | 3.1 | 18.4 | 3.8 | 0.0 | 14.5 | 0.4 | 0.0 | | | | | 0 |
| 38030 | 1/4 cup | Flour, all purpose, white, enr, bleached, avg | 31 | 113 | 12 | 3.2 | 23.7 | 0.8 | 0.5 | 22.3 | 0.3 | 0.0 | 0.0 | 0.1 | 0.01 | 0.12 | 0 |
| 38271 | 1/4 cup | Flour, all purpose, white, unenriched, avg | 31 | 113 | 12 | 3.2 | 23.7 | 0.8 | 0.5 | 22.3 | 0.3 | 0.0 | 0.0 | 0.1 | 0.01 | 0.12 | 0 |
| 46086 | 1/4 cup | Flour, cake, white, enriched, avg | 34 | 123 | 12 | 2.8 | 26.5 | 0.6 | 0.6 | 25.4 | 0.3 | 0.0 | 0.0 | 0.1 | 0.01 | 0.12 | 0 |
| 38065 | 1/4 cup | Flour, gluten, avg | 35 | 132 | 8 | 14.5 | 16.5 | 0.3 | 0.4 | 15.9 | 0.7 | 0.0 | 0.0 | 0.0 | 0.00 | 0.00 | 0 |
| 38434 | 1/4 cup | Flour, Pastry, white, unbleached, Arrowhead Mills | 30 | 100 | 11 | 3.0 | 23.0 | 4.0 | 0.0 | 19.0 | 0.5 | 0.0 | | | | | 0 |
| 38353 | 1/4 cup | Flour, Self Rising, bleached, Pillsbury | 30 | 100 | 12 | 2.6 | 21.6 | 0.6 | 0.3 | 20.7 | 0.4 | 0.1 | | | | | 0 |
| 38354 | 1/4 cup | Flour, Self Rising, unbleached, Pillsbury | 30 | 99 | 13 | 2.3 | 21.6 | 0.6 | 0.3 | 20.7 | 0.4 | 0.1 | | | | | 0 |
| 38054 | 1/4 cup | Flour, semolina, enriched, avg | 42 | 151 | 13 | 5.3 | 30.6 | 1.6 | 0.8 | 28.2 | 0.4 | 0.1 | 0.1 | 0.2 | 0.02 | 0.17 | 0 |
| 38270 | 1/4 cup | Flour, semolina, unenriched, avg | 42 | 151 | 13 | 5.3 | 30.6 | 1.6 | 0.8 | 28.2 | 0.4 | 0.1 | 0.1 | 0.2 | 0.02 | 0.17 | 0 |
| 38173 | 1/4 cup | Flour, Shake & Blend, Pillsbury | 31 | 109 | 14 | 3.3 | 22.7 | 0.8 | 0.5 | 21.4 | 0.5 | 0.2 | | | | | 0 |
| 38098 | 1/4 cup | Flour tortilla mix, white, enriched, avg | 28 | 113 | 10 | 2.7 | 18.8 | 0.5 | 0.4 | 17.3 | 3.0 | 1.1 | 1.3 | 0.4 | 0.03 | 0.39 | 0 |
| 38025 | 1/4 cup | Germ, crude, avg | 29 | 104 | 11 | 6.7 | 15.0 | 3.8 | 3.5 | 7.7 | 2.3 | 0.5 | 0.4 | 1.7 | 0.21 | 1.53 | 0 |
| 38026 | 1/4 cup | Germ, toasted, avg | 28 | 107 | 6 | 8.1 | 13.9 | 3.6 | 3.4 | 6.9 | 3.0 | 0.5 | 0.4 | 1.9 | 0.22 | 1.63 | 0 |
| 38143 | 1/4 cup | Grits, avg | 39 | 125 | 13 | 3.7 | 29.6 | 2.8 | | | 0.3 | | | | | | |
| 38459 | 1/4 cup | Kamut, Bread Mix, dry, Arrowhead Mills | 34 | 106 | 8 | 5.3 | 23.4 | 3.8 | 0.0 | 19.5 | 0.3 | 0.0 | | | | | 0 |
| 38447 | 1/4 cup | Kamut, Flour, Arrowhead Mills | 35 | 110 | 10 | 4.0 | 25.0 | 4.0 | 0.0 | 21.0 | 0.5 | 0.0 | | | | | 0 |
| 38068 | 1/4 cup | Sprouted, avg | 27 | 53 | 48 | 2.0 | 11.5 | 0.3 | | | 0.3 | 0.1 | 0.0 | 0.2 | 0.01 | 0.14 | 0 |
| | | Wheat, Whole | | | | | | | | | | | | | | | |
| 38032 | 1/4 cup | Flour, whole, avg | 30 | 102 | 10 | 4.1 | 21.8 | 3.7 | 0.6 | 17.5 | 0.6 | 0.1 | 0.1 | 0.2 | 0.01 | 0.22 | 0 |
| 38436 | 1/4 cup | Flour, Whole, Stone Ground, Arrowhead Mills | 35 | 130 | 10 | 5.0 | 25.0 | 4.0 | 0.0 | 21.0 | 0.5 | 0.0 | | | | | 0 |
| 38090 | 1/4 cup | Grain, durum, avg | 48 | 163 | 11 | 6.6 | 34.1 | 6.0 | 0.4 | 27.7 | 1.2 | 0.2 | 0.2 | 0.5 | 0.02 | 0.45 | 0 |
| 38287 | 1/4 cup | Grain, hard, red, spring, dry, avg | 48 | 158 | 13 | 7.4 | 32.6 | 5.9 | 0.4 | 26.4 | 0.9 | 0.2 | 0.1 | 0.4 | 0.02 | 0.35 | 0 |
| 38029 | 1/4 cup | Grain, hard, red, winter, dry, avg | 48 | 157 | 13 | 6.0 | 34.2 | 5.9 | 0.4 | 27.3 | 0.7 | 0.1 | 0.1 | 0.3 | 0.01 | 0.29 | 0 |
| 38088 | 1/4 cup | Grain, hard, white, dry, avg | 48 | 164 | 10 | 5.4 | 36.4 | 6.0 | 0.4 | 30.0 | 0.8 | 0.1 | 0.1 | 0.4 | 0.02 | 0.34 | 0 |

| Code | Vit A (IU) | Vit A (RE) | Retinol (RE) | Carotenoids (RE) | Beta Carotene (mcg) | Thiamin (mg) | Riboflavin (mg) | Niacin (NE) | Vit B6 (mg) | Vit B12 (mcg) | Folate (mcg) | Panto (mg) | Vit C (mg) | Vit D (mg) | Vit E (α TE) | Calcium (mg) | Copper (mg) | Iron (mg) | Magnes (mg) | Mang (mg) | Phos (mg) | Potassium (mg) | Selenium (mcg) | Sodium (mg) | Zinc (mg) |
|---|---|---|---|---|---|---|---|---|---|---|---|---|---|---|---|---|---|---|---|---|---|---|---|---|---|
| | Vit A & Components | | | | | Vitamins | | | | | | | | | | Minerals | | | | | | | | | |
| 38282 | 0 | 0 | 0 | 0 | 0 | 0.21 | 0.14 | 2.36 | 0.19 | 0.00 | 42.5 | 0.42 | 0.0 | 0.0 | | 4 | 0.4 | 1.5 | 57 | 0.8 | 142 | 98 | 1.4 | 2 | 0.84 |
| 38446 | 0 | 0 | 0 | 0 | 0 | 0.22 | 0.14 | 0.80 | | | | | 0.0 | | | 0 | | 2.7 | | | | 150 | | 0 | |
| 38078 | 0 | 0 | 0 | 0 | 0 | 0.09 | 0.02 | 0.08 | 0.01 | 0.00 | 3.3 | 0.12 | 0.0 | 0.0 | 0.0 | 6 | 0.0 | 0.5 | 22 | 0.5 | 65 | 51 | 4.2 | 1 | 0.29 |
| 38064 | 0 | 0 | 0 | 0 | 0 | 0.28 | 0.05 | 0.22 | 0.04 | 0.00 | 12.5 | 0.36 | 0.0 | 0.0 | 0.2 | 14 | 0.1 | 1.3 | 56 | 1.4 | 176 | 136 | 10.8 | 1 | 0.75 |
| 38417 | 0 | 0 | 0 | 0 | 0 | 0.17 | 0.03 | 0.31 | | | | | 0.0 | | | 0 | | 1.1 | | | | 92 | | 0 | |
| 38445 | 0 | 0 | 0 | 0 | 0 | 0.17 | | | | | | | 0.0 | | | 15 | | 1.1 | | | | 73 | | 0 | |
| 38080 | 0 | 0 | 0 | 0 | 0 | 0.30 | 0.05 | 0.37 | 0.05 | 0.00 | 21.8 | 0.53 | 0.0 | 0.0 | | 21 | 0.2 | 1.8 | 69 | 1.9 | 204 | 167 | | 1 | 1.55 |
| 38422 | 0 | 0 | 0 | 0 | 0 | 0.22 | 0.07 | 0.40 | | | | | 0.0 | | | 20 | | 1.8 | | | | 150 | | 0 | |
| 38008 | 20 | 2 | 0 | 2 | | 0.15 | 0.03 | 0.16 | 0.02 | 0.00 | 6.4 | 0.25 | 0.0 | 0.0 | | 10 | 0.1 | 0.8 | 30 | 0.7 | 95 | 70 | 6.8 | 1 | 0.61 |
| 38079 | 0 | 0 | 0 | 0 | 0 | 0.08 | 0.17 | 1.23 | 0.09 | 0.00 | 20.6 | 0.44 | 0.0 | 0.0 | 2.0 | 25 | 0.3 | 3.9 | 88 | 0.9 | 172 | 311 | | 9 | 1.39 |
| 38050 | 0 | 0 | 0 | 0 | 0 | 0.83 | 0.09 | 10.20 | 1.22 | 0.00 | 18.9 | 2.22 | 0.0 | 0.0 | | 17 | 0.2 | 5.6 | 234 | 4.3 | 503 | 446 | 4.7 | 2 | 1.81 |
| 38158 | 0 | 0 | 0 | 0 | 0 | 0.06 | 0.01 | 1.04 | 0.17 | 0.00 | 1.6 | 0.33 | 0.0 | 0.0 | | 4 | 0.1 | 0.1 | 14 | 0.5 | 39 | 30 | 6.0 | 0 | 0.32 |
| 38443 | 0 | 0 | 0 | 0 | 0 | 0.12 | | 1.60 | | | | | 0.0 | | | 0 | | 0.7 | | | | 75 | | 0 | |
| 30118 | 0 | 0 | 0 | 0 | 0 | | | | | 0.00 | | | 0.0 | | | 7 | | 0.0 | | | | | | 1 | |
| 38226 | | | | | | | | | 0.45 | 0.00 | 120.4 | 0.84 | 0.0 | 0.0 | | 2 | | 0.3 | | | 29 | 56 | | 25 | |
| 38051 | 0 | 0 | 0 | 0 | 0 | 0.48 | 0.05 | 7.33 | 0.11 | 0.00 | 28.6 | 0.91 | 0.0 | 0.0 | | 18 | 0.3 | 2.8 | 156 | 1.2 | 288 | 186 | 7.9 | 0 | 2.13 |
| 38416 | 0 | 0 | 0 | 0 | 0 | 0.11 | 0.05 | 0.30 | | | | | 0.0 | | | 0 | | 0.8 | | | | 114 | | 0 | |
| 38022 | 0 | 0 | 0 | 0 | 0 | 0.10 | 0.08 | 1.37 | 0.14 | 0.00 | 19.2 | 0.47 | 0.0 | 0.0 | | 18 | 0.2 | 2.1 | 79 | 2.2 | 202 | 234 | 11.4 | 0 | 1.80 |
| 38023 | 0 | 0 | 0 | 0 | 0 | 0.09 | 0.02 | 0.21 | 0.06 | 0.00 | 5.7 | 0.17 | 0.0 | 0.0 | | 5 | 0.1 | 0.5 | 18 | 0.5 | 50 | 61 | 9.3 | 1 | 0.45 |
| 38056 | 0 | 0 | 0 | 0 | 0 | 0.07 | 0.03 | 0.45 | 0.07 | 0.00 | 4.9 | 0.13 | 0.0 | 0.0 | 0.2 | 6 | 0.1 | 0.6 | 19 | 1.4 | 54 | 88 | 9.3 | 1 | 0.52 |
| 38442 | 0 | 0 | 0 | 0 | 0 | 0.15 | 0.07 | 0.80 | | | | | 0.0 | | | 20 | | 1.4 | | | | 260 | | 0 | |
| 38142 | | | | | | 0.28 | 0.24 | 0.64 | | 0.00 | | 0.22 | 0.0 | 0.0 | | | 0.2 | | | | | | | | 5.82 |
| 38084 | 0 | 0 | 0 | 0 | 0 | 0.13 | 0.11 | 1.79 | 0.12 | 0.00 | 25.2 | 0.61 | 0.0 | 0.0 | | 14 | 0.2 | 1.1 | 51 | 1.1 | 157 | 111 | 14.8 | 3 | 1.57 |
| 38420 | 0 | 0 | 0 | 0 | 0 | 0.22 | 0.10 | 0.80 | | | | | 0.0 | | | 20 | | 1.8 | | | | 220 | | 0 | |
| 38233 | | | | | | 0.03 | 0.01 | 0.84 | | | | | 0.0 | 0.0 | 0.0 | 5 | | 1.0 | | | 55 | | | 1 | |
| 38085 | 0 | 0 | 0 | 0 | 0 | 0.11 | 0.07 | 1.41 | | 0.00 | | | 0.0 | 0.0 | | 13 | | 2.1 | | | 138 | 168 | | 3 | |
| 38139 | | | | | | | | | | | | | | 0.0 | | 6 | 0.1 | 1.2 | 36 | | 115 | 125 | | 1 | |
| 38439 | 0 | 0 | 0 | 0 | 0 | 0.15 | 0.03 | 1.20 | | | | | 0.0 | | | 0 | | 1.1 | | | | 150 | | 0 | |
| 38375 | | | | | | | | | | | | | 6.0 | | | | | 1.1 | | | | | | 0 | |
| 38374 | | | | | | | | | | | | | | | | | | | | | | | | 0 | |
| 38373 | | | | | | | | | | | | | 6.0 | | | 20 | | 1.1 | | | | | | 0 | |
| 38087 | 0 | 0 | 0 | 0 | 0 | 0.12 | 0.04 | 0.92 | 0.13 | 0.00 | 23.7 | 0.69 | 0.0 | 0.0 | | 11 | 0.2 | 0.8 | 49 | 1.3 | 103 | 149 | | 1 | 0.85 |
| 38086 | 0 | 0 | 0 | 0 | 0 | 0.20 | 0.06 | 0.69 | 0.07 | 0.00 | 35.0 | 0.63 | 0.0 | 0.0 | 0.4 | 18 | 0.2 | 1.2 | 62 | 1.5 | 172 | 159 | | 2 | 1.66 |
| 38491 | 0 | 0 | 0 | 0 | 0 | 0.15 | 0.11 | 1.26 | | | | | 0.0 | | | 45 | | 1.1 | | | | 38 | | 374 | |
| 38024 | 0 | 0 | 0 | 0 | 0 | 0.07 | 0.08 | 1.90 | 0.18 | 0.00 | 11.1 | 0.31 | 0.0 | 0.0 | 0.2 | 10 | 0.1 | 1.5 | 86 | 1.6 | 142 | 165 | 10.9 | 0 | 1.02 |
| 38493 | 0 | 0 | 0 | 0 | 0 | 0.31 | 0.09 | 5.80 | 0.19 | 0.06 | 54.0 | 0.82 | 0.0 | | | 25 | 0.3 | 3.6 | 178 | 4.8 | 372 | 394 | | 2 | 3.14 |
| 38028 | 0 | 0 | 0 | 0 | 0 | 0.03 | 0.01 | 0.46 | 0.04 | 0.00 | 8.3 | 0.16 | 0.0 | 0.0 | 0.0 | 5 | 0.0 | 0.4 | 15 | 0.3 | 18 | 31 | 0.3 | 2 | 0.26 |
| 38027 | 0 | 0 | 0 | 0 | 0 | 0.03 | 0.04 | 1.79 | 0.12 | 0.00 | 9.4 | 0.37 | 0.0 | 0.0 | 0.0 | 12 | 0.1 | 0.9 | 57 | 1.1 | 105 | 143 | 0.8 | 6 | 0.68 |
| 38329 | 0 | 0 | 0 | 0 | 0 | 0.13 | 0.06 | 1.91 | 0.10 | 0.00 | 13.2 | 0.30 | 0.0 | 0.0 | 0.1 | 10 | 0.1 | 1.2 | 41 | 1.1 | 104 | 122 | 21.2 | 2 | 0.88 |
| 38123 | | | | | | 0.23 | 0.05 | 1.65 | | 0.00 | | | 0.0 | 0.0 | | 15 | | 2.0 | | | 156 | | | 1 | |
| 38415 | 0 | 0 | 0 | 0 | 0 | 0.11 | 0.03 | 1.22 | | | | | 0.0 | | | 15 | | 0.8 | | | | 96 | | 0 | |
| 38030 | 0 | 0 | 0 | 0 | 0 | 0.24 | 0.15 | 1.83 | 0.01 | 0.00 | 47.7 | 0.14 | 0.0 | 0.0 | 0.0 | 5 | 0.0 | 1.4 | 7 | 0.2 | 33 | 33 | 10.5 | 1 | 0.22 |
| 38271 | 0 | 0 | 0 | 0 | 0 | 0.04 | 0.01 | 0.39 | 0.01 | 0.00 | 8.1 | 0.14 | 0.0 | 0.0 | | 5 | 0.0 | 0.4 | 7 | 0.2 | 33 | 33 | 10.5 | 1 | 0.22 |
| 46086 | 0 | 0 | 0 | 0 | 0 | 0.30 | 0.15 | 2.31 | 0.01 | 0.00 | 52.4 | 0.16 | 0.0 | 0.0 | 0.0 | 5 | 0.0 | 2.5 | 5 | 0.2 | 29 | 36 | 1.7 | 1 | 0.21 |
| 38065 | 0 | 0 | 0 | 0 | 0 | 0.01 | 0.01 | 0.17 | | 0.00 | 7.5 | | 0.0 | 0.0 | | 14 | | 0.1 | | | 49 | 21 | | 1 | |
| 38434 | 0 | 0 | 0 | 0 | 0 | 0.12 | 0.03 | 1.60 | | | | | 0.0 | | | 0 | | 1.4 | | | | 130 | | 0 | |
| 38353 | 0 | 0 | 0 | 0 | 0 | 0.13 | 0.12 | 1.50 | | | | | 0.0 | | | 91 | | 1.3 | | | | | | 356 | |
| 38354 | 0 | 0 | 0 | 0 | 0 | 0.13 | 0.12 | 1.50 | | | | | 0.0 | | | 91 | | 1.3 | | | | | | 356 | |
| 38054 | 0 | 0 | 0 | 0 | 0 | 0.34 | 0.24 | 2.52 | 0.04 | 0.00 | 64.7 | 0.24 | 0.0 | 0.0 | | 7 | 0.1 | 1.8 | 20 | 0.3 | 57 | 78 | 5.0 | 0 | 0.44 |
| 38270 | 0 | 0 | 0 | 0 | 0 | 0.12 | 0.03 | 1.39 | 0.04 | 0.00 | 30.2 | 0.24 | 0.0 | 0.0 | 0.1 | 7 | 0.1 | 0.5 | 20 | 0.3 | 57 | 78 | | 0 | 0.44 |
| 38173 | 0 | 0 | 0 | 0 | 0 | 0.19 | 0.12 | 1.64 | | | | | 0.0 | | | 6 | | 1.4 | | | | | | 0 | |
| 38098 | 0 | 0 | 0 | 0 | 0 | 0.21 | 0.14 | 1.63 | 0.01 | 0.00 | 38.1 | 0.11 | 0.0 | 0.0 | | 57 | 0.0 | 2.0 | 6 | 0.2 | 59 | 28 | | 190 | 0.18 |
| 38025 | 0 | 0 | 0 | 0 | 0 | 0.55 | 0.14 | 1.97 | 0.38 | 0.00 | 81.5 | 0.66 | 0.0 | 0.0 | 4.1 | 11 | 0.2 | 1.8 | 69 | 3.9 | 244 | 259 | 23.0 | 3 | 3.57 |
| 38026 | 0 | 0 | 0 | 0 | 0 | 0.47 | 0.23 | 1.57 | 0.27 | 0.00 | 98.6 | 0.39 | 1.7 | 0.0 | 4.3 | 13 | 0.2 | 2.5 | 90 | 5.6 | 321 | 265 | 18.2 | 1 | 4.68 |
| 38143 | | | | | | 0.05 | 0.01 | 0.51 | 0.03 | 0.00 | | | | 0.0 | | 7 | | 0.4 | | | | 44 | | 0 | |
| 38459 | 0 | 0 | 0 | 0 | 0 | 0.09 | 0.03 | | | | | | 0.0 | | | 0 | | 0.8 | | | | 144 | | 144 | |
| 38447 | 0 | 0 | 0 | 0 | 0 | 0.09 | 0.03 | 0.80 | | | | | 0.0 | | | 0 | | 0.7 | | | | 150 | | 0 | |
| 38068 | 0 | 0 | 0 | 0 | 0 | 0.06 | 0.04 | 0.83 | 0.07 | 0.00 | 10.3 | 0.26 | 0.7 | 0.0 | | 8 | 0.1 | 0.6 | 22 | 0.5 | 54 | 46 | 11.5 | 4 | 0.45 |
| 38032 | 0 | 0 | 0 | 0 | 0 | 0.13 | 0.06 | 1.91 | 0.10 | 0.00 | 13.2 | 0.30 | 0.0 | 0.0 | 0.1 | 10 | 0.1 | 1.2 | 41 | 1.1 | 104 | 122 | 21.2 | 2 | 0.88 |
| 38436 | 0 | 0 | 0 | 0 | 0 | 0.15 | 0.07 | 1.60 | | | | | 0.0 | | | 20 | | 1.1 | | | | 130 | | 0 | |
| 38090 | 0 | 0 | 0 | 0 | 0 | 0.20 | 0.06 | 3.24 | 0.20 | 0.00 | 20.8 | 0.45 | 0.0 | 0.0 | 0.4 | 16 | 0.3 | 1.7 | 69 | 1.4 | 244 | 207 | 42.9 | 1 | 2.00 |
| 38287 | 0 | 0 | 0 | 0 | 0 | 0.24 | 0.05 | 2.74 | 0.16 | 0.00 | 20.6 | 0.45 | 0.0 | 0.0 | | 12 | 0.2 | 1.7 | 60 | 1.9 | 159 | 163 | 33.9 | 1 | 1.33 |
| 38029 | 0 | 0 | 0 | 0 | 0 | 0.18 | 0.06 | 2.62 | 0.14 | 0.00 | 18.2 | 0.46 | 0.0 | 0.0 | | 14 | 0.2 | 1.5 | 60 | 1.9 | 138 | 174 | 33.9 | 1 | 1.27 |
| 38088 | 0 | 0 | 0 | 0 | 0 | 0.19 | 0.05 | 2.10 | 0.18 | 0.00 | 18.0 | 0.46 | 0.0 | 0.0 | 0.6 | 15 | 0.2 | 2.2 | 45 | 1.8 | 170 | 207 | 37.9 | 1 | 1.60 |

| Code | Amount | Description | Basic Components | | | | | | | | | Additional Fats | | | | | | Vit A & Components | | | | | Vitamins | | | | | | | | | | Minerals | | | | | | | | | |
|---|---|---|---|---|---|---|---|---|---|---|---|---|---|---|---|---|---|---|---|---|---|---|---|---|---|---|---|---|---|---|---|---|---|---|---|---|---|---|---|---|---|---|
| | | | Weight (g) | Calories | % Water | Protein (g) | Carbs (g) | Fiber (g) | Sugar (g) | Other Carbs (g) | Fat (g) | Sat Fat (g) | Mono Fat (g) | Poly Fat (g) | Omega 3 (g) | Omega 6 (g) | Choles (mg) | Vit A (IU) | Vit A (RE) | Retinol (RE) | Carotenoids (RE) | Beta Carotene (mcg) | Thiamin (mg) | Riboflavin (mg) | Niacin (NE) | Vit B6 (mg) | Vit B12 (mcg) | Folate (mcg) | Panto (mg) | Vit C (mg) | Vit D (mg) | Vit E (α TE) | Calcium (mg) | Copper (mg) | Iron (mg) | Magnes (mg) | Mang (mg) | Phos (mg) | Potassium (mg) | Selenium (mcg) | Sodium (mg) | Zinc (mg) |
| 38288 | 1/4 cup | Grain, soft, red winter wheat, dry, avg | 42 | 139 | 12 | 4.4 | 31.2 | 5.3 | 0.3 | 25.6 | 0.7 | 0.1 | 0.1 | 0.3 | 0.01 | 0.26 | 0 | 0 | 0 | 0 | 0 | 0 | 0.17 | 0.04 | 2.02 | 0.11 | 0.00 | 17.2 | 0.36 | 0.0 | 0.0 | | 11 | 0.2 | 1.3 | 53 | 1.8 | 207 | 167 | 33.2 | 1 | 1.10 |
| 38089 | 1/4 cup | Grain, soft white wheat, dry, avg | 42 | 143 | 10 | 4.5 | 31.7 | 5.3 | 0.4 | 26.0 | 0.8 | 0.2 | 0.1 | 0.4 | 0.02 | 0.34 | 0 | 0 | 0 | 0 | 0 | 0 | 0.17 | 0.04 | 2.00 | 0.16 | 0.00 | 17.1 | 0.36 | 0.0 | 0.0 | | 14 | 0.2 | 2.3 | 38 | 1.4 | 169 | 183 | 33.2 | 1 | 1.45 |
| | | **GRAIN PRODUCTS, BREADS, MIXES, CRACKERS, BAKED GOODS, PANCAKES, PASTA, RICE, TORTILLAS** ||||||||||||||||||||||||||||||||||||||||
| | | *BAGELS* ||||||||||||||||||||||||||||||||||||||||
| 42594 | 1 ea | Cinnamon Raisin, large, avg | 118 | 323 | 32 | 11.6 | 65.1 | 2.7 | 2.4 | 60.1 | 2.0 | 0.3 | 0.2 | 0.8 | 0.05 | 0.75 | 0 | 86 | 9 | | | | 0.45 | 0.33 | 3.63 | 0.07 | 0.00 | 106.2 | 0.60 | 0.8 | 0.0 | | 22 | 0.2 | 4.5 | 33 | 1.0 | 118 | 175 | 36.6 | 380 | 1.33 |
| 42592 | 1 ea | Egg, large, avg | 110 | 306 | 33 | 11.7 | 58.3 | 2.5 | 1.7 | 54.1 | 2.3 | 0.5 | 0.5 | 0.7 | 0.03 | 0.67 | 26 | 120 | 36 | | | | 0.59 | 0.26 | 3.78 | 0.10 | 0.18 | 96.8 | 0.74 | 0.7 | 0.1 | | 14 | 0.1 | 4.4 | 28 | 0.5 | 92 | 75 | 33.7 | 556 | 0.85 |
| 42319 | 1 ea | Onion, small, Arnie's Bagelicious | 55 | 143 | 35 | 5.1 | 29.1 | 1.3 | 3.6 | 24.1 | 0.7 | 0.0 | | | | | 0 | 0 | 0 | 0 | 0 | 0 | | | | | | | | 0.0 | | | 12 | | 1.2 | | | | | | 245 | |
| 42321 | 1 ea | Plain, small, Arnie's Bagelicious | 55 | 144 | 35 | 5.0 | 29.3 | 1.3 | 3.7 | 24.3 | 0.8 | 0.0 | | | | | 0 | 0 | 0 | 0 | 0 | 0 | | | | | | | | 0.0 | | | 9 | | 2.0 | | | | | | 252 | |
| 42320 | 1 ea | Sesame Seed, small, Arnie's Bagelicious | 55 | 147 | 35 | 5.2 | 28.0 | 1.6 | 3.6 | 22.9 | 1.6 | 0.0 | | | | | 0 | 0 | 0 | 0 | 0 | 0 | | | | | | | | 0.0 | | | 32 | | 2.1 | | | | | | 232 | |
| 42092 | 1 ea | Whole Wheat, small, avg | 55 | 145 | 28 | 6.0 | 31.0 | 5.4 | 1.1 | 24.5 | 0.8 | 0.1 | 0.1 | 0.3 | | | 0 | 0 | 0 | 0 | 0 | 0 | 0.17 | 0.14 | 2.85 | 0.18 | 0.00 | 39.7 | 0.50 | 0.0 | 0.0 | | 16 | 0.2 | 1.8 | 59 | 1.5 | 159 | 190 | | 271 | 1.28 |
| | | *BISCUITS* ||||||||||||||||||||||||||||||||||||||||
| | | Dough ||||||||||||||||||||||||||||||||||||||||
| 42236 | 1 ea | Buttermilk, Pillsbury | 21 | 51 | 40 | 1.4 | 9.5 | 0.3 | 0.9 | 8.2 | 0.8 | 0.0 | | | | | 0 | 0 | 0 | 0 | 0 | 0 | | | | | | | | 0.0 | | | 6 | | 0.5 | | | | | | 163 | |
| 42107 | 1 ea | Chilled, avg | 30 | 95 | 34 | 1.9 | 13.1 | 0.5 | 1.2 | 11.5 | 4.1 | 1.0 | 2.3 | 0.5 | 0.03 | 0.51 | 0 | 0 | 0 | 0 | 0 | 0 | 0.12 | 0.07 | 0.94 | 0.01 | 0.00 | 16.8 | 0.15 | 0.0 | 0.1 | | 6 | 0.0 | 0.7 | 4 | 0.1 | 106 | 44 | 6.2 | 332 | 0.11 |
| 42109 | 1 ea | Chilled, low fat, avg | 23 | 59 | 38 | 1.5 | 10.9 | 0.4 | 1.0 | 9.6 | 1.0 | 0.3 | 0.6 | 0.2 | 0.01 | 0.15 | 0 | 0 | 0 | 0 | 0 | 0 | 0.10 | 0.05 | 0.76 | 0.01 | 0.00 | 19.6 | 0.08 | 0.0 | 0.1 | | 4 | 0.0 | 0.6 | 3 | 0.1 | 92 | 37 | 4.3 | 287 | 0.09 |
| 42111 | 1 ea | Chilled, mixed grain, avg | 44 | 116 | 38 | 2.7 | 20.9 | 3.5 | 1.7 | 15.7 | 2.5 | 0.6 | 1.3 | 0.4 | 0.02 | 0.37 | 0 | 0 | 0 | 0 | 0 | 0 | 0.17 | 0.09 | 1.50 | 0.03 | 0.00 | 36.5 | 0.14 | 0.0 | 0.1 | | 7 | 0.1 | 1.2 | 13 | 0.3 | 104 | 201 | | 295 | 0.26 |
| 42248 | 1 ea | Cinnamon Raisin, Grands | 57 | 186 | 31 | 3.5 | 26.3 | 0.9 | 9.7 | 15.7 | 7.4 | 1.8 | | | | | 0 | 1 | 0.1 | | | | | | | | | | | 0.0 | | | 32 | | 1.1 | | | | | | 541 | |
| 42241 | 1 ea | Extra Lights Oven Ready, Ballard | 21 | 50 | 41 | 1.4 | 9.4 | 0.3 | 0.9 | 8.2 | 0.7 | 0.1 | | | | | 0 | 0 | 0 | 0 | 0 | 0 | | | | | | | | 0.0 | | | 6 | | 0.5 | | | | | | 163 | |
| 42249 | 1 ea | Flaky, Grands | 57 | 181 | 36 | 3.8 | 22.4 | 0.7 | 2.5 | 19.3 | 8.5 | 1.8 | | | | | 0 | 0 | 0 | 0 | 0 | 0 | | | | | | | | 0.0 | | | 11 | | 1.3 | | | | | | 516 | |
| 42231 | 1 ea | Fluffy, Hungry Jack | 28 | 87 | 36 | 1.7 | 11.2 | 0.4 | 1.5 | 9.4 | 4.1 | 1.0 | | | | | 0 | 0 | 0 | 0 | 0 | 0 | | | | | | | | 0.0 | | | 6 | | 0.6 | | | | | | 282 | |
| | | Dry Mixes ||||||||||||||||||||||||||||||||||||||||
| 42274 | 1 oz | Cinnamon Raisin, Gold Medal | 28 | 118 | | 1.7 | 18.2 | 0.4 | 2.0 | 15.8 | 4.2 | 1.3 | 1.2 | 0.3 | | | 0 | | | | | | 0.14 | 0.11 | 1.26 | | | | | | | | 38 | | 1.0 | | | | 34 | | 252 | |
| 42273 | 1 oz | Old Fashioned, Baking Powder, General Mills | 28 | 108 | 16 | 2.8 | 17.4 | 0.5 | 0.6 | 16.3 | 3.1 | 0.8 | 1.3 | 0.2 | | | 0 | | | | | | 0.15 | 0.09 | 0.08 | | | | | | | | 36 | | 1.0 | | | | 21 | | 315 | |
| 42106 | 2 Tbs | Plain/Buttermilk, avg | 30 | 128 | 9 | 2.4 | 19.0 | 0.6 | 1.7 | 16.7 | 4.6 | 1.2 | 2.6 | 0.6 | 0.03 | 0.57 | 1 | 1 | 1 | | | | 0.17 | 0.13 | 1.36 | 0.02 | 0.12 | 31.2 | 0.27 | 0.1 | 0.0 | | 54 | 0.0 | 0.8 | 8 | 0.1 | 176 | 49 | 2.3 | 383 | 0.18 |
| 42272 | 1 oz | Plain, General Mills | 28 | 120 | 13 | 2.5 | 16.2 | 0.5 | 1.7 | 14.1 | 5.0 | 1.4 | 2.2 | 0.4 | | | 0 | | | | | | 0.13 | 0.10 | 1.05 | | | | | | | | 20 | | 0.9 | | | | 45 | | 310 | |
| | | Prepared ||||||||||||||||||||||||||||||||||||||||
| 42598 | 1 ea | Buttermilk, f/mix, avg | 77 | 280 | 27 | 4.8 | 37.3 | 1.0 | 3.4 | 33.0 | 12.7 | 1.9 | 5.3 | 4.8 | 0.33 | 4.44 | 1 | 2 | 1 | | | | 0.33 | 0.22 | 2.58 | 0.04 | 0.11 | 45.4 | 0.23 | 0.0 | 0.2 | | 38 | 0.1 | 2.5 | 13 | 0.3 | 331 | 172 | 14.5 | 810 | 0.37 |
| 42543 | 1 ea | Buttermilk, f/chilled dough, Grands | 61 | 201 | 35 | 3.9 | 23.3 | 0.7 | 3.2 | 19.3 | 10.3 | 2.7 | | | | | 0 | 5 | 1 | | | | | | | | | | | 0.0 | | | 35 | | 1.4 | | | | | | 573 | |
| 42206 | 1 ea | Cheese, avg | 30 | 115 | 27 | 2.9 | 11.8 | 0.4 | 0.9 | 10.5 | 6.2 | 2.2 | 2.4 | 1.2 | | | 6 | 72 | 17 | 15 | 2 | | 0.10 | 0.10 | 0.78 | 0.01 | 0.04 | 3.4 | 0.09 | 0.1 | 0.1 | | 80 | 0.0 | 0.7 | 6 | 0.1 | 70 | 41 | | 197 | 0.29 |
| 42577 | 1 ea | Cinnamon Raisin, f/mix, Gold Medal | 63 | 262 | | 4.0 | 41.3 | 1.0 | 4.0 | 36.2 | 9.1 | 3.0 | 2.5 | 0.5 | | | 0 | 0 | 0 | 0 | 0 | 0 | 0.30 | 0.17 | 2.01 | | | | | 0.0 | | | 81 | | 1.8 | | | | 75 | | 564 | |
| 42522 | 1 ea | Garlic & Cheese, Pepperidge Farm | 50 | 170 | | 4.0 | 24.0 | 2.0 | 4.0 | 18.0 | 6.0 | 2.5 | 3.0 | 0.5 | | | 10 | 0 | 0 | 0 | 0 | 0 | 0.15 | 0.10 | 1.60 | | | | | 0.0 | | | 60 | | 1.1 | | | | | | 510 | |
| 42001 | 1 ea | Homemade, avg | 60 | 212 | 29 | 4.2 | 26.8 | 0.9 | 1.7 | 24.1 | 9.8 | 2.6 | 4.2 | 2.5 | 0.16 | 2.34 | 2 | 49 | 14 | 13 | 1 | | 0.21 | 0.19 | 1.77 | 0.02 | 0.05 | 36.6 | 0.17 | 0.1 | 0.3 | | 141 | 0.0 | 1.7 | 11 | 0.2 | 98 | 73 | 11.7 | 348 | 0.32 |
| 42579 | 1 ea | Old Fashioned, Baking Powder, f/mix, Gen Mills | 40 | 158 | 14 | 4.0 | 24.7 | 0.5 | 1.0 | 23.2 | 4.9 | 1.0 | 2.0 | 0.0 | 0.00 | 0.00 | 0 | 0 | 0 | 0 | 0 | 0 | 0.15 | 0.10 | 1.58 | | | | | 0.0 | | | 40 | | 1.4 | | | | 30 | | 454 | |
| 42108 | 1 ea | Plain, f/chilled dough, avg | 27 | 93 | 28 | 1.8 | 12.8 | 0.4 | 1.2 | 11.2 | 4.0 | 1.0 | 2.2 | 0.5 | 0.03 | 0.50 | 0 | 0 | 0 | 0 | 0 | 0 | 0.09 | 0.06 | 0.83 | 0.01 | 0.00 | 11.6 | 0.10 | 0.0 | 0.1 | | 5 | 0.0 | 0.7 | 4 | 0.1 | 104 | 42 | 4.8 | 325 | 0.10 |
| 42545 | 1 ea | Plain, f/chilled dough, Grands | 61 | 198 | 36 | 3.9 | 22.9 | 0.7 | 3.2 | 18.9 | 10.2 | 2.7 | | | | | 0 | 0.6 | 0.1 | | | | | | | | | | | 0.0 | | | 37 | | 1.3 | | | | | | 573 | |
| 42110 | 1 ea | Plain, f/chilled dough, low fat, avg | 21 | 63 | 28 | 1.6 | 11.6 | 0.4 | 1.1 | 10.2 | 1.1 | 0.3 | 0.6 | 0.2 | 0.01 | 0.16 | 0 | 0 | 0 | 0 | 0 | 0 | 0.09 | 0.05 | 0.72 | 0.01 | 0.00 | 14.5 | 0.06 | 0.0 | 0.1 | | 4 | 0.0 | 0.6 | 4 | 0.1 | 98 | 39 | 3.7 | 305 | 0.10 |
| 42112 | 1 ea | Plain, f/chilled dough, mixed grains, avg | 41 | 125 | 28 | 2.9 | 22.6 | 1.1 | 1.8 | 19.7 | 2.7 | 0.7 | 1.4 | 0.4 | 0.02 | 0.38 | 0 | 0 | 0 | 0 | 0 | 0 | 0.15 | 0.09 | 1.46 | 0.02 | 0.00 | 4.1 | 0.10 | 0.0 | 0.1 | | 8 | 0.1 | 1.3 | 14 | 0.3 | 158 | 217 | 7.4 | 319 | 0.30 |
| 42546 | 1 ea | Plain, Fluffy, f/chilled dough, Hungry Jack | 28 | 87 | 36 | 1.7 | 11.2 | 0.4 | 1.5 | 9.4 | 4.1 | 1.0 | | | | | 0 | 0 | 0 | 0 | 0 | 0 | | | | | | | | 0.0 | | | 6 | | 0.6 | | | | | | 282 | |
| 42205 | 1 ea | Whole Wheat, avg | 63 | 200 | 28 | 6.2 | 29.2 | 4.8 | 2.1 | 22.3 | 7.6 | 2.2 | 3.0 | 1.9 | | | 4 | 37 | 9 | 8 | 1 | | 0.14 | 0.12 | 2.20 | 0.13 | 0.06 | 12.9 | 0.38 | 0.2 | 0.3 | | 120 | 0.1 | 1.5 | 57 | 1.3 | 176 | 200 | 26.5 | 468 | 1.22 |
| | | *BREADS & ROLLS* ||||||||||||||||||||||||||||||||||||||||
| | | *BREADS* ||||||||||||||||||||||||||||||||||||||||
| 42218 | 1 oz | Apple Cinnamon Quick Bread, dry mix, Pillsbury | 28 | 107 | 8 | 1.4 | 23.1 | 0.8 | 13.0 | 9.3 | 1.0 | 0.2 | | | | | 0 | 1 | 0.1 | | | | | | | | | | | 0.1 | | | 18 | | 0.8 | | | | | | 125 | |
| 42392 | 1 pce | Apple Walnut Swirl Bread, Pepperidge Farm | 28 | 80 | | 2.0 | 14.0 | 1.0 | 4.0 | 9.0 | 2.0 | 0.5 | 1.0 | 0.0 | 0.00 | 0.00 | 0 | 0 | 0 | 0 | 0 | 0 | 0.06 | 0.07 | 0.40 | | | | | 0.0 | | | 0 | | 0.0 | | | | | | 120 | |
| 42171 | 1 pce | Armenian Bread, avg | 20 | 55 | 34 | 1.8 | 10.3 | 0.6 | 0.2 | 9.5 | 0.7 | 0.1 | 0.1 | 0.3 | | | 0 | 0 | 0 | 0 | 0 | 0 | 0.08 | 0.05 | 0.66 | 0.01 | 0.00 | 5.2 | 0.08 | 0.0 | | | 16 | 0.0 | 0.6 | 5 | 0.1 | 15 | 15 | 5.4 | 117 | 0.16 |
| 42039 | 1 pce | Banana Bread, prep f/recipe, w/marg, avg | 60 | 196 | 29 | 2.6 | 32.8 | 0.7 | 20.4 | 11.7 | 6.3 | 1.3 | 2.7 | 1.9 | 0.09 | 1.79 | 26 | 278 | 72 | 60 | 12 | | 0.10 | 0.12 | 0.87 | 0.09 | 0.06 | 19.8 | 0.16 | 1.0 | 0.1 | | 13 | 0.0 | 0.8 | 8 | 0.1 | 35 | 80 | 7.3 | 181 | 0.21 |
| 42219 | 1 oz | Banana Quick Bread, dry mix, Pillsbury | 28 | 106 | 8 | 1.6 | 22.4 | 0.6 | 11.4 | 10.3 | 1.1 | 0.3 | | | | | 0 | 2 | 0 | | | | | | | | | | | 0.0 | | | 11 | | 0.8 | | | | | | 160 | |
| 42221 | 1 oz | Blueberry Quick Bread, dry mix, Pillsbury | 28 | 105 | 9 | 1.5 | 22.6 | 0.4 | 12.3 | 9.8 | 1.1 | 0.3 | | | | | 0 | 2 | 0 | | | | | | | | | | | 0.6 | | | 17 | | 0.7 | | | | | | 123 | |
| 42191 | 1 pce | Barley Bread, avg | 26 | 69 | 37 | 2.1 | 13.0 | 1.2 | 1.1 | 10.7 | 1.0 | 0.3 | 0.3 | 0.3 | | | 1 | 8 | 2 | 1 | 0.3 | | 0.09 | 0.08 | 1.06 | 0.03 | 0.01 | 9.3 | 0.16 | 0.0 | 0.1 | | 10 | 0.1 | 0.7 | 8 | 0.2 | 31 | 39 | | 96 | 0.25 |
| 42175 | 1 oz | Batter Bread, avg | 28 | 79 | 37 | 2.3 | 12.9 | 0.5 | 2.0 | 10.5 | 1.9 | 0.6 | 0.7 | 0.4 | | | 11 | 29 | 8 | 8 | 0.3 | | 0.10 | 0.11 | 0.89 | 0.03 | 0.04 | 11.1 | 0.14 | 0.1 | 0.1 | | 17 | 0.0 | 0.8 | 6 | 0.1 | 35 | 42 | | 108 | 0.20 |
| | | Bread Sticks ||||||||||||||||||||||||||||||||||||||||
| 42509 | 1 ea | Brown & Serve, Pepperidge Farm | 57 | 150 | 34 | 7.0 | 28.0 | 1.0 | 2.0 | 25.0 | 1.5 | 0.5 | 0.5 | 0.5 | | | 0 | 0 | 0 | 0 | 0 | 0 | 0.22 | 0.10 | 1.60 | | | | | 0.0 | | | 60 | | 2.7 | | | | | | 290 | |
| 42400 | 1 oz | Cheddar Cheese, Thin, Pepperidge Farm | 28 | 122 | 5 | 3.5 | 17.5 | 0.9 | 0.0 | 16.6 | 4.4 | 1.8 | 2.6 | 0.0 | 0.00 | 0.00 | 9 | 0 | 0 | 0 | 0 | 0 | 0.21 | 0.12 | 2.10 | | | | | 0.0 | | | 35 | | 1.9 | | | | | | 210 | |
| 42402 | 1 oz | Onion, Thin, Pepperidge Farm | 28 | 122 | 4 | 3.5 | 19.3 | 0.9 | 1.8 | 16.6 | 3.5 | 0.0 | 2.6 | 0.9 | | | 0 | 0 | 0 | 0 | 0 | 0 | 0.16 | 0.12 | 1.40 | | | | | 0.0 | | | 0 | | 1.9 | | | | | | 201 | |
| 42035 | 1 ea | Plain, w/salt coating, avg | 35 | 134 | 5 | 4.2 | 26.4 | 0.8 | 2.7 | 22.8 | 1.0 | 0.2 | 0.4 | 0.3 | 0.00 | 0.30 | 1 | 0 | 0 | 0 | 0 | 0 | 0.23 | 0.18 | 2.25 | 0.01 | 0.00 | 4.0 | 0.05 | 0.0 | 0.0 | | 10 | 0.0 | 1.5 | 7 | 0.2 | 35 | 32 | 9.0 | 586 | 0.20 |
| 42036 | 1 ea | Plain, w/o salt coating, avg | 10 | 41 | 6 | 1.2 | 6.8 | 0.3 | 0.5 | 6.0 | 0.9 | 0.1 | 0.4 | 0.4 | 0.02 | 0.34 | 0 | 0 | 0 | 0 | 0 | 0 | 0.06 | 0.06 | 0.53 | 0.01 | 0.00 | 12.2 | 0.05 | 0.0 | 0.0 | | 2 | 0.0 | 0.4 | 3 | 0.1 | 12 | 12 | 3.8 | 66 | 0.09 |
| 42398 | 1 oz | Sesame, Thin, Pepperidge Farm | 28 | 105 | | 12.3 | 19.3 | 1.8 | 3.5 | 14.0 | 2.6 | 0.0 | 0.9 | 0.9 | | | 0 | 0 | 0 | 0 | 0 | 0 | 0.10 | 0.06 | 0.70 | | | | | 0.0 | | | 35 | | 1.9 | | | | | | 508 | |
| | | Brown Bread ||||||||||||||||||||||||||||||||||||||||
| 42052 | 1 pce | Boston, canned, avg | 45 | 88 | 47 | 2.3 | 19.5 | 2.1 | 9.0 | 8.4 | 0.7 | 0.1 | 0.1 | 0.3 | 0.02 | 0.23 | 0 | 39 | 5 | 2 | 3 | | 0.01 | 0.05 | 0.50 | 0.04 | 0.00 | 4.9 | 0.25 | 0.0 | 0.2 | 0.0 | 31 | 0.0 | 0.9 | 28 | 0.5 | 50 | 143 | 9.9 | 284 | 0.22 |
| 42452 | 1 pce | Plain, B & M | 56 | 130 | 39 | 3.0 | 29.0 | 2.0 | 9.0 | 18.0 | 0.5 | 0.0 | 0.0 | 0.0 | 0.00 | 0.00 | 0 | 0 | 0 | 0 | 0 | 0 | | | | | | | | 0.0 | | | 40 | | 1.4 | | | | | | 390 | |
| 42451 | 1 pce | Raisin, B & M | 56 | 130 | 39 | 3.0 | 29.0 | 2.0 | 11.0 | 16.0 | 0.5 | 0.0 | 0.0 | 0.0 | 0.00 | 0.00 | 0 | 0 | 0 | 0 | 0 | 0 | | | | | | | | 0.0 | | | 40 | | 1.4 | | | | | | 360 | |
| 42194 | 1 pce | Buckwheat Bread, avg | 27 | 71 | 37 | 2.3 | 13.1 | 1.0 | 1.2 | 11.0 | 1.1 | 0.3 | 0.4 | 0.3 | | | 1 | 7 | 2 | 2 | 0.2 | | 0.10 | 0.08 | 1.17 | 0.04 | 0.01 | 10.5 | 0.11 | 0.0 | 0.1 | | 11 | 0.1 | 0.8 | 18 | 0.1 | 38 | 57 | | 100 | 0.32 |
| 42526 | 1 oz | Carrot Quick Bread, dry mix, Pillsbury | 28 | 107 | 7 | 1.7 | 22.4 | 0.9 | 12.2 | 9.4 | 1.2 | 0.3 | | | | | 0 | 805 | 161 | | | | | | | | | | | 1.2 | | | 22 | | 0.9 | | | | | | 148 | |
| | | Cheese Bread ||||||||||||||||||||||||||||||||||||||||
| 42086 | 1 pce | Average | 26 | 71 | 37 | 2.3 | 12.2 | 0.6 | 1.1 | 10.6 | 1.3 | 0.5 | 0.4 | 0.3 | | | 2 | 14 | 4 | 4 | 0.3 | | 0.12 | 0.09 | 0.97 | 0.01 | 0.01 | 8.6 | 0.05 | 0.0 | 0.1 | | 38 | 0.0 | 0.7 | 6 | 0.1 | 32 | 30 | | 144 | 0.19 |
| 42521 | 1 pce | Monterey Jack w/Jalapeno, Pepperidge Farm | 56 | 200 | 31 | 5.0 | 22.0 | 1.0 | 2.0 | 19.0 | 10.0 | 4.0 | | | | | 40 | 0 | 0 | 0 | 0 | 0 | 0.15 | 0.10 | 1.20 | | | | | 0.0 | | | 60 | | 1.1 | | | | | | 280 | |
| 42520 | 1 pce | Two Cheddar, Pepperidge Farm | 56 | 210 | 31 | 5.0 | 21.0 | 1.0 | 2.0 | 18.0 | 11.0 | 5.0 | | | | | 50 | 0 | 0 | 0 | 0 | 0 | 0.15 | 0.10 | 1.60 | | | | | 0.0 | | | 60 | | 1.1 | | | | | | 280 | |
| 42391 | 1 pce | Cinnamon Swirl Bread, Pepperidge Farm | 28 | 80 | | 3.0 | 14.0 | 2.0 | 4.0 | 8.0 | 2.5 | 0.5 | 1.5 | 0.0 | 0.00 | 0.00 | 0 | 0 | 0 | 0 | 0 | 0 | 0.09 | 0.07 | 0.80 | | | | | 0.0 | | | 0 | | 0.7 | | | | | | 115 | |
| | | Cornbread ||||||||||||||||||||||||||||||||||||||||
| 42672 | 1 pce | Average | 65 | 161 | 48 | 4.2 | 23.1 | 1.9 | 3.4 | 17.7 | 5.6 | 2.1 | 2.1 | 1.0 | | | 40 | 167 | 39 | 23 | 15 | | 0.09 | 0.15 | 0.73 | 0.06 | 0.17 | 7.2 | 0.20 | 0.3 | 0.4 | | 61 | 0.0 | 0.8 | 16 | 0.1 | 188 | 94 | | 369 | 0.40 |
| 49012 | 1 ea | Hush Puppies, avg | 22 | 74 | 29 | 1.7 | 10.1 | 0.6 | | | 3.0 | 0.5 | 0.7 | 1.6 | 0.18 | 1.41 | 10 | 31 | 9 | | | | 0.08 | 0.07 | 0.61 | 0.02 | 0.04 | 16.3 | 0.08 | 0.0 | | | 61 | 0.0 | 0.7 | 5 | 0.0 | 42 | 32 | 3.5 | 147 | 0.15 |

| Code | Amount | Description | Basic Components | | | | | | | | | Additional Fats | | | | | | Vit A & Components | | | | | Vitamins | | | | | | | | | | Minerals | | | | | | | | | |
|---|---|---|---|---|---|---|---|---|---|---|---|---|---|---|---|---|---|---|---|---|---|---|---|---|---|---|---|---|---|---|---|---|---|---|---|---|---|---|---|---|---|---|
| | | | Weight (g) | Calories | % Water | Protein (g) | Carbs (g) | Fiber (g) | Sugar (g) | Other Carbs (g) | Fat (g) | Sat Fat (g) | Mono Fat (g) | Poly Fat (g) | Omega 3 (g) | Omega 6 (g) | Choles (mg) | Vit A (IU) | Vit A (RE) | Retinol (RE) | Carotenoids (RE) | Beta Carotene (mcg) | Thiamin (mg) | Riboflavin (mg) | Niacin (NE) | Vit B6 (mg) | Vit B12 (mcg) | Folate (mcg) | Panto (mg) | Vit C (mg) | Vit D (mg) | Vit E (α TE) | Calcium (mg) | Copper (mg) | Iron (mg) | Magnes (mg) | Mang (mg) | Phos (mg) | Potassium (mg) | Selenium (mcg) | Sodium (mg) | Zinc (mg) |
| 42580 | 1 pce | Cornbread, prepared f/mix, Honey, General Mills | 35 | 138 | 11 | 2.0 | 25.7 | 0.0 | 7.9 | 17.8 | 3.0 | 1.0 | 1.5 | 0.0 | 0.00 | 0.00 | [illegible] | 0 | 0 | 0 | 0 | 0 | 0.09 | 0.15 | 0.79 | | | | | 0.0 | | | 20 | | 0.7 | | | | 35 | | 287 | |
| 42116 | 1 pce | Prepared f/recipe w/2% milk, avg | 65 | 173 | 39 | 4.4 | 28.3 | 1.9 | 4.2 | 22.2 | 4.6 | 1.0 | 1.2 | 2.1 | 0.23 | 1.85 | 26 | 180 | 35 | 28 | 7 | | 0.19 | 0.19 | 1.46 | 0.07 | 0.10 | 41.6 | 0.22 | 0.2 | 0.3 | | 162 | 0.0 | 1.6 | 16 | 0.1 | 110 | 96 | 6.6 | 428 | 0.39 |
| 42117 | 1 pce | Prepared f/recipe w/whole milk, avg | 65 | 176 | 39 | 4.4 | 28.3 | 2.3 | 4.2 | 21.8 | 5.0 | 1.3 | 1.3 | 2.1 | 0.23 | 1.87 | 28 | 158 | 28 | 18 | 10 | | 0.19 | 0.19 | 1.46 | 0.07 | 0.10 | 12.3 | 0.22 | 0.2 | 0.3 | | 161 | 0.0 | 1.6 | 16 | 0.1 | 109 | 95 | 5.9 | 428 | 0.38 |
| 42176 | 1 pce | Corn & Molasses Bread, avg | 32 | 86 | 37 | 2.1 | 15.1 | 0.6 | 2.8 | 11.7 | 1.9 | 0.6 | 0.7 | 0.4 | | | 2 | 30 | 6 | 4 | 2 | | 0.11 | 0.11 | 0.95 | 0.05 | 0.03 | 11.2 | 0.13 | 0.1 | 0.1 | | 27 | 0.1 | 0.9 | 15 | 0.1 | 35 | 100 | | 261 | 0.20 |
| 42042 | 1 pce | Cracked Wheat Bread, avg | 25 | 65 | 36 | 2.2 | 12.4 | 1.4 | 1.0 | 10.0 | 1.0 | 0.2 | 0.5 | 0.2 | 0.01 | 0.16 | 0 | 0 | 0 | 0 | 0 | 0 | 0.09 | 0.06 | 0.92 | 0.08 | 0.00 | 15.3 | 0.13 | 0.0 | 0.0 | | 11 | 0.1 | 0.7 | 13 | 0.3 | 38 | 44 | 6.3 | 134 | 0.31 |
| 42483 | 1 pce | Cracked Wheat Bread, Thin, Pepperidge Farm | 25 | 70 | 38 | 2.0 | 12.0 | 0.5 | 1.0 | 10.5 | 1.0 | 0.0 | 0.5 | 0.5 | | | 0 | 0 | 0 | 0 | 0 | 0 | 0.09 | 0.07 | 0.80 | | | | | 0.0 | | | 0 | | 0.7 | | | | | | 140 | |
| 42220 | 1 oz | Cranberry Quick Bread, dry mix, Pillsbury | 28 | 106 | 8 | 1.5 | 22.7 | 0.7 | 12.3 | 9.7 | 1.1 | 0.3 | | | | | 0 | 1 | 0.1 | | | | | | | | | | | 0.0 | | | 11 | | 0.7 | | | | | | 114 | |
| 42173 | 1 pce | Cuban Bread, avg | 20 | 58 | 31 | 1.8 | 11.1 | 0.5 | 0.3 | 10.3 | 0.6 | 0.1 | 0.2 | 0.2 | | | 0 | 0 | 0 | 0 | 0 | 0 | 0.08 | 0.05 | 0.66 | 0.01 | 0.00 | 6.0 | 0.06 | 0.0 | | | 9 | 0.0 | 0.6 | 4 | 0.1 | 17 | 18 | 6.3 | 116 | 0.13 |
| 42222 | 1 oz | Date Quick Bread, dry mix, Pillsbury | 28 | 108 | 7 | 1.4 | 23.0 | 0.9 | 13.0 | 9.1 | 1.1 | 0.3 | | | | | 0 | 3 | 0.3 | | | | | | | | | | | 0.0 | | | 11 | | 0.7 | | | | | | 108 | |
| 42090 | 1 pce | Egg/Challah Bread, avg | 40 | 115 | 35 | 3.8 | 19.1 | 0.9 | 0.5 | 17.7 | 2.4 | 0.6 | 0.9 | 0.4 | 0.02 | 0.42 | 20 | 30 | 9 | 9 | 0 | | 0.18 | 0.17 | 1.94 | 0.03 | 0.04 | 42.0 | 0.11 | 0.0 | 0.0 | | 37 | 0.1 | 1.2 | 8 | 0.2 | 42 | 46 | 12.0 | 197 | 0.32 |
| | | English Muffins | | | | | | | | | | | | | | | | | | | | | | | | | | | | | | | | | | | | | | | | |
| 42214 | 1 ea | Cheese, avg | 63 | 147 | 45 | 5.6 | 25.4 | 1.5 | 2.1 | 21.8 | 2.4 | 1.0 | 0.7 | 0.5 | | | 3 | 33 | 10 | 9 | 1 | | 0.26 | 0.27 | 2.98 | 0.10 | 0.02 | 55.3 | | 0.0 | | | 118 | 0.1 | 1.8 | 14 | | 77 | 80 | | 184 | 0.56 |
| 42149 | 1 ea | Mixed grain, avg | 66 | 155 | 40 | 6.0 | 30.6 | 1.8 | 2.3 | 26.4 | 1.2 | 0.2 | 0.5 | 0.4 | 0.02 | 0.35 | 0 | 0 | 0 | 0 | 0 | 0 | 0.28 | 0.21 | 2.36 | 0.03 | 0.00 | 52.8 | 0.27 | 0.0 | 0.0 | | 129 | 0.2 | 2.0 | 27 | 0.4 | 53 | 103 | 16.8 | 275 | 0.92 |
| 42289 | 1 ea | Plain, enriched, avg | 57 | 134 | 42 | 4.4 | 26.2 | 1.5 | 2.0 | 22.7 | 1.0 | 0.1 | 0.2 | 0.5 | 0.04 | 0.46 | 0 | 0 | 0 | 0 | 0 | 0 | 0.25 | 0.16 | 2.21 | 0.02 | 0.02 | 42.2 | 0.25 | 0.0 | 0.0 | | 30 | 0.1 | 1.4 | 12 | 0.2 | 76 | 75 | 11.5 | 264 | 0.40 |
| 42290 | 1 ea | Plain, unenriched, avg | 57 | 134 | 42 | 4.4 | 26.2 | 1.5 | 2.0 | 22.7 | 1.0 | 0.1 | 0.2 | 0.5 | 0.04 | 0.46 | 0 | 0 | 0 | 0 | 0 | 0 | 0.10 | 0.09 | 0.89 | 0.02 | 0.02 | 21.1 | 0.25 | 0.0 | 0.0 | | 99 | 0.1 | 0.5 | 12 | 0.2 | 76 | 75 | 11.5 | 264 | 0.40 |
| 42151 | 1 ea | Raisin cinnamon, avg | 57 | 139 | 39 | 4.3 | 27.8 | 1.7 | 2.1 | 24.0 | 1.5 | 0.2 | 0.3 | 0.8 | 0.08 | 0.70 | 0 | 1 | 0.1 | | | | 0.22 | 0.17 | 2.02 | 0.04 | 0.00 | 46.2 | 0.30 | 0.2 | 0.0 | | 84 | 0.1 | 1.4 | 9 | 0.2 | 39 | 119 | 9.1 | 255 | 0.57 |
| 42393 | 1 ea | Seven Grain, Pepperidge Farm | 57 | 130 | 42 | 5.0 | 26.0 | 2.0 | 1.0 | 23.0 | 1.0 | 0.0 | 1.0 | 0.0 | 0.00 | 0.00 | 0 | 0 | 0 | 0 | 0 | 0 | 0.22 | 0.14 | 1.60 | | | | | 0.0 | | | 60 | | 1.4 | | | | | | 230 | |
| 42060 | 1 ea | Sourdough, avg | 57 | 134 | 42 | 4.4 | 26.2 | 1.5 | 2.0 | 22.7 | 1.0 | 0.1 | 0.2 | 0.5 | 0.04 | 0.46 | 0 | 0 | 0 | 0 | 0 | 0 | 0.25 | 0.16 | 2.21 | 0.02 | 0.02 | 46.2 | 0.25 | 0.0 | 0.0 | | 99 | 0.1 | 1.4 | 12 | 0.2 | 76 | 75 | 11.5 | 264 | 0.40 |
| 42082 | 1 ea | Whole wheat, avg | 66 | 134 | 46 | 5.8 | 26.7 | 4.4 | 2.0 | 20.2 | 1.4 | 0.8 | 0.5 | 0.1 | 0.00 | 0.05 | 0 | 0 | 0 | 0 | 0 | 0 | 0.20 | 0.09 | 2.25 | 0.11 | 0.00 | 27.7 | 0.46 | 0.0 | 0.0 | | 175 | 0.1 | 1.6 | 47 | 1.2 | 186 | 139 | 26.6 | 420 | 1.06 |
| 42043 | 1 pce | French Bread, avg | 25 | 68 | 34 | 2.2 | 13.0 | 0.8 | 0.3 | 11.9 | 0.8 | 0.2 | 0.3 | 0.2 | 0.01 | 0.17 | 0 | 0 | 0 | 0 | 0 | 0 | 0.13 | 0.08 | 1.19 | 0.01 | 0.00 | 23.8 | 0.10 | 0.0 | 0.0 | | 19 | 0.0 | 0.6 | 7 | 0.1 | 26 | 28 | 7.9 | 152 | 0.22 |
| 42210 | 1 pce | Fruit Bread, w/o nuts, avg | 41 | 150 | 24 | 2.0 | 22.6 | 0.5 | 12.9 | 9.2 | 5.9 | 1.5 | 2.5 | 1.5 | | | 22 | 41 | 11 | 10 | 1 | | 0.08 | 0.09 | 0.70 | 0.08 | 0.04 | 5.4 | 0.12 | 1.0 | 0.1 | | 34 | 0.0 | 0.7 | 7 | 0.1 | 32 | 62 | | 109 | 0.16 |
| 42211 | 1 pce | Fruit & Nut Bread, avg | 56 | 217 | 22 | 3.2 | 29.6 | 0.8 | 16.6 | 12.2 | 10.1 | 2.2 | 3.8 | 3.5 | | | 29 | 58 | 14 | 13 | 1.5 | | 0.12 | 0.12 | 0.93 | 0.12 | 0.05 | 9.0 | 0.17 | 1.3 | 0.1 | | 47 | 0.1 | 1.0 | 15 | 0.1 | 54 | 100 | | 140 | 0.32 |
| | | Garlic Bread | | | | | | | | | | | | | | | | | | | | | | | | | | | | | | | | | | | | | | | | |
| 42519 | 1 pce | Mozzarella, Pepperidge Farm | 56 | 200 | 31 | 6.0 | 21.0 | 1.0 | 2.0 | 18.0 | 10.0 | 5.0 | 3.5 | 1.5 | | | 40 | 0 | 0 | 0 | 0 | 0 | 0.15 | 0.10 | 1.20 | | | | | 0.0 | | | 80 | | 1.1 | | | | | | 280 | |
| 42367 | 1 pce | Parmesan, Pepperidge Farm | 47 | 160 | 30 | 6.0 | 19.0 | 2.0 | 3.0 | 14.0 | 7.0 | 2.0 | 3.0 | 1.0 | | | 10 | 0 | 0 | 0 | 0 | 0 | 0.15 | 0.10 | 1.20 | | | | | 0.0 | | | 20 | | 2.7 | | | | | | 260 | |
| 42368 | 1 pce | Plain, Pepperidge Farm | 47 | 160 | 37 | 5.0 | 14.0 | 1.0 | 2.0 | 11.0 | 10.0 | 3.0 | 4.0 | 1.5 | | | 30 | 0 | 0 | 0 | 0 | 0 | 0.22 | 0.14 | 1.60 | | | | | 0.0 | | | 0 | | 3.6 | | | | | | 250 | |
| 42671 | 1 pce | Greek Bread, avg | 20 | 55 | 34 | 1.8 | 10.3 | 0.6 | 0.2 | 9.5 | 0.7 | 0.1 | 0.1 | 0.3 | | | 0 | 0 | 0 | 0 | 0 | 0 | 0.08 | 0.05 | 0.66 | 0.01 | 0.00 | 5.2 | 0.08 | 0.0 | | | 16 | 0.0 | 0.6 | 5 | 0.1 | 15 | 15 | 5.4 | 117 | 0.16 |
| 42132 | 1 pce | High Calcium Bread, dark Hollywood, avg | 18 | 39 | 41 | 1.6 | 7.9 | 1.4 | | | 0.4 | 0.1 | 0.1 | 0.2 | 0.01 | 0.16 | 0 | 0.5 | 0.05 | 0 | 0.05 | | 0.08 | 0.07 | 0.72 | 0.03 | 0.00 | 5.0 | 0.05 | 0.0 | | | 139 | 0.1 | 0.6 | 12 | 0.3 | 29 | 36 | | 92 | 0.27 |
| 42134 | 1 pce | High Calcium Bread, light Hollywood, avg | 18 | 41 | 41 | 1.5 | 8.0 | 0.3 | | | 0.4 | 0.1 | 0.1 | 0.2 | 0.00 | 0.15 | 0 | 0.7 | 0.07 | 0 | 0.07 | | 0.08 | 0.06 | 0.74 | 0.01 | 0.01 | 3.8 | 0.09 | 0.0 | | | 130 | 0.0 | 0.6 | 7 | 0.1 | 15 | 34 | | 124 | 0.20 |
| 42118 | 1 pce | Indian/Navajo Fry Bread | 90 | 296 | 26 | 6.4 | 48.0 | 1.5 | | | 8.6 | 2.1 | 3.6 | 2.3 | 0.14 | 2.19 | 0 | 0 | 0 | 0 | 0 | 0 | 0.39 | 0.27 | 3.28 | 0.02 | 0.00 | 66.6 | 0.18 | 0.0 | | | 210 | 0.1 | 3.2 | 14 | 0.4 | 141 | 67 | 21.0 | 625 | 0.45 |
| 42202 | 1 pce | Injera Bread, Ethiopian, avg | 127 | 173 | 63 | 5.6 | 37.8 | 1.3 | | | 1.1 | 0.3 | 0.2 | 0.6 | | | 0 | 0 | 0 | 0 | 0 | 0 | 0.13 | 0.10 | 1.52 | 0.08 | 0.00 | 35.6 | | 0.0 | 0.0 | | 74 | 0.1 | 37.0 | 14 | | 145 | 72 | | 254 | 0.42 |
| 42119 | 1 pce | Irish Soda Bread, prep f/recipe, avg | 60 | 174 | 30 | 4.0 | 33.6 | 1.5 | 14.4 | 17.6 | 3.0 | 0.7 | 1.2 | 0.9 | 0.05 | 0.84 | 11 | 116 | 30 | 26 | 4 | | 0.18 | 0.16 | 1.45 | 0.05 | 0.03 | 6.0 | 0.15 | 0.5 | 0.0 | | 49 | 0.1 | 1.6 | 14 | 0.2 | 68 | 160 | | 239 | 0.34 |
| 42046 | 1 pce | Italian Bread, avg | 30 | 81 | 36 | 2.6 | 15.0 | 0.3 | 1.4 | 12.8 | 1.1 | 0.3 | 0.2 | 0.4 | 0.03 | 0.39 | 0 | 0 | 0 | 0 | 0 | 0 | 0.14 | 0.09 | 1.31 | 0.01 | 0.00 | 28.5 | 0.11 | 0.0 | 0.0 | | 23 | 0.1 | 0.9 | 8 | 0.1 | 31 | 33 | 8.2 | 175 | 0.26 |
| 42178 | 1 pce | Milk & Honey Bread, avg | 28 | 74 | 37 | 2.1 | 14.7 | 0.5 | 1.4 | 12.7 | 0.6 | 0.2 | 0.1 | 0.2 | | | 1 | 7 | 2 | 2 | 0.2 | | 0.12 | 0.10 | 1.03 | 0.02 | 0.01 | 13.2 | 0.11 | 0.0 | 0.1 | | 10 | 0.0 | 0.9 | 6 | 0.1 | 29 | 35 | | 53 | 0.17 |
| | | Multi-Grain Breads | | | | | | | | | | | | | | | | | | | | | | | | | | | | | | | | | | | | | | | | |
| 42513 | 1 pce | Crunchy Grain, Pepperidge Farm | 34 | 90 | 36 | 4.0 | 16.0 | 2.0 | 2.0 | 12.0 | 1.0 | 0.0 | 0.5 | 0.5 | | | 0 | 0 | 0 | 0 | 0 | 0 | 0.09 | 0.07 | 0.80 | | | | | 0.0 | | | 20 | | 0.7 | | | | | | 170 | |
| 42097 | 1 pce | Low Calorie, high fiber, avg | 23 | 46 | 42 | 2.0 | 10.2 | 2.3 | | | 0.5 | 0.0 | 0.0 | 0.1 | | | 2 | 0 | 0 | 0 | 0 | 0 | 0.10 | 0.07 | 0.89 | 0.03 | 0.00 | 13.6 | 0.12 | 0.0 | 0.0 | | 18 | 0.1 | 0.6 | 20 | 0.3 | 57 | 40 | | 117 | 0.46 |
| 42047 | 1 pce | Mixed, avg | 26 | 65 | 38 | 2.6 | 12.1 | 1.7 | 1.7 | 8.7 | 1.0 | 0.2 | 0.4 | 0.2 | 0.02 | 0.22 | 0 | 0 | 0 | 0 | 0 | 0 | 0.11 | 0.09 | 1.14 | 0.09 | 0.02 | 20.8 | 0.13 | 0.1 | 0.0 | | 24 | 0.1 | 0.9 | 14 | 0.4 | 46 | 53 | 7.7 | 127 | 0.33 |
| 42512 | 1 pce | Nine Grain, Pepperidge Farm | 34 | 90 | 36 | 4.0 | 16.0 | 2.0 | 2.0 | 12.0 | 1.0 | 0.0 | 0.5 | 0.5 | | | 0 | 0 | 0 | 0 | 0 | 0 | 0.09 | 0.07 | 0.80 | | | | | 0.0 | | | 20 | | 0.7 | | | | | | 170 | |
| 42467 | 1 pce | Seven Grain, Hearty Slice, Pepperidge Farm | 38 | 100 | 39 | 3.0 | 18.0 | 2.0 | 2.0 | 14.0 | 1.5 | 0.0 | 0.5 | 0.0 | 0.00 | 0.00 | 0 | 0 | 0 | 0 | 0 | 0 | 0.12 | 0.07 | 1.20 | | | | | 0.0 | | | 0 | | 0.7 | | | | | | 180 | |
| 42403 | 1 pce | Seven Grain, Light Style, Pepperidge Farm | 17 | 48 | | 2.0 | 9.5 | 1.7 | 1.0 | 6.8 | 0.3 | 0.0 | 0.2 | 0.2 | 0.00 | 0.00 | 0 | 0 | 0 | 0 | 0 | 0 | 0.08 | 0.05 | 0.54 | | | | | 0.0 | | | 14 | | 0.5 | | | | | | 109 | |
| 42223 | 1 oz | Nut Quick Bread, dry mix, Pillsbury | 28 | 115 | 7 | 1.9 | 20.7 | 0.8 | 11.3 | 8.6 | 2.7 | 0.4 | | | | | 0 | 3 | 0.25 | | | | | | | | | | | 0.0 | | | 18 | | 0.8 | | | | | | 140 | |
| 42069 | 1 pce | Oat Bran Bread, avg | 30 | 71 | 44 | 3.1 | 11.9 | 1.4 | 1.2 | 9.4 | 1.3 | 0.2 | 0.5 | 0.5 | 0.03 | 0.48 | 0 | 2 | 0.15 | 0 | 0.15 | | 0.15 | 0.10 | 1.45 | 0.02 | 0.00 | 24.3 | 0.17 | 0.0 | 0.0 | | 20 | 0.0 | 0.9 | 11 | 0.2 | 42 | 44 | 9.0 | 122 | 0.27 |
| 42076 | 1 pce | Oat Bran Bread, low cal, avg | 23 | 46 | 46 | 1.8 | 9.5 | 2.8 | 0.9 | 5.8 | 0.7 | 0.1 | 0.2 | 0.4 | 0.02 | 0.36 | 0 | 0.5 | 0.05 | 0 | 0.05 | | 0.08 | 0.05 | 0.86 | 0.02 | 0.00 | 15.2 | 0.11 | 0.0 | 0.0 | | 13 | 0.1 | 0.7 | 13 | 0.3 | 32 | 23 | 4.7 | 31 | 0.24 |
| | | Oatmeal Breads | | | | | | | | | | | | | | | | | | | | | | | | | | | | | | | | | | | | | | | | |
| 42049 | 1 pce | Average | 27 | 73 | 37 | 2.3 | 13.1 | 1.1 | 1.1 | 11.0 | 1.2 | 0.2 | 0.4 | 0.5 | 0.03 | 0.43 | 0 | 4 | 1 | 0 | 0 | | 0.11 | 0.06 | 0.85 | 0.02 | 0.01 | 16.7 | 0.09 | 0.0 | 0.0 | | 18 | 0.1 | 0.7 | 10 | 0.3 | 34 | 38 | 6.6 | 152 | 0.28 |
| 42468 | 1 pce | Hearty Crunchy, Pepperidge Farm | 38 | 100 | 37 | 4.0 | 17.0 | 2.0 | 2.0 | 13.0 | 2.0 | 0.0 | 1.0 | 0.0 | 0.00 | 0.00 | 0 | 0 | 0 | 0 | 0 | 0 | 0.15 | 0.10 | 1.20 | | | | | 0.0 | | | 20 | | 0.7 | | | | | | 130 | |
| 42373 | 1 pce | Light Style, Pepperidge Farm | 19 | 47 | | 2.3 | 9.0 | 1.7 | 1.0 | 6.3 | 0.3 | 0.0 | 0.3 | 0.0 | 0.00 | 0.00 | 0 | 0 | 0 | 0 | 0 | 0 | 0.08 | 0.05 | 0.67 | | | | | 0.0 | | | 13 | | 0.5 | | | | | | 103 | |
| 42125 | 1 pce | Low Calorie, avg | 23 | 48 | 44 | 1.7 | 10.0 | | 0.9 | | 0.8 | 0.1 | 0.2 | 0.3 | 0.01 | 0.30 | 0 | 1 | 0.2 | | | | 0.08 | 0.06 | 0.70 | 0.01 | 0.02 | 12.7 | 0.10 | 0.0 | 0.0 | | 26 | 0.0 | 0.5 | 6 | 0.1 | 23 | 29 | 5.3 | 39 | 0.19 |
| 42495 | 1 pce | Soft, Pepperidge Farm | 25 | 60 | 40 | 2.0 | 12.0 | 0.0 | 2.0 | 10.0 | 0.5 | 0.0 | | | | | 0 | 0 | 0 | 0 | 0 | 0 | 0.15 | 0.10 | 1.60 | | | | | 0.0 | | | 40 | | 1.1 | | | | | | 2 | |
| 42479 | 1 pce | Thin Sliced, Pepperidge Farm | 25 | 60 | 42 | 2.0 | 11.0 | 1.0 | 1.0 | 9.0 | 1.0 | 0.0 | 0.5 | 0.5 | | | 0 | 0 | 0 | 0 | 0 | 0 | 0.09 | 0.07 | 0.80 | | | | | 0.0 | | | 20 | | 0.7 | | | | | | 150 | |
| 42190 | 1 pce | Pannetone Bread, sweet Italian style, avg | 27 | 86 | 28 | 2.1 | 14.6 | 0.7 | 5.2 | 8.6 | 2.2 | 1.2 | 0.6 | 0.2 | | | 19 | 87 | 22 | 21 | 2 | | 0.10 | 0.12 | 0.95 | 0.05 | 0.05 | 24.0 | 0.22 | 0.3 | 0.1 | | 16 | 0.1 | 0.8 | 6 | 0.1 | 39 | 53 | | 96 | 0.23 |
| | | Pita Breads | | | | | | | | | | | | | | | | | | | | | | | | | | | | | | | | | | | | | | | | |
| 42007 | 1 ea | White, avg | 60 | 165 | 32 | 5.5 | 33.4 | 1.3 | 0.8 | 31.3 | 0.7 | 0.1 | 0.1 | 0.3 | 0.01 | 0.31 | 0 | 0 | 0 | 0 | 0 | 0 | 0.36 | 0.20 | 2.78 | 0.02 | 0.00 | 57.0 | 0.24 | 0.0 | 0.0 | | 52 | 0.1 | 1.6 | 16 | 0.3 | 58 | 72 | 16.3 | 322 | 0.50 |
| 42080 | 1 ea | Whole wheat, avg | 64 | 170 | 31 | 6.3 | 35.2 | 4.7 | 1.0 | 29.5 | 1.7 | 0.3 | 0.2 | 0.7 | 0.03 | 0.64 | 0 | 0 | 0 | 0 | 0 | 0 | 0.22 | 0.05 | 1.82 | 0.17 | 0.00 | 32.0 | 0.53 | 0.0 | 0.0 | | 10 | 0.2 | 2.0 | 44 | 1.1 | 115 | 109 | 28.2 | 340 | 0.97 |
| 42406 | 1 ea | Wholesome Choice, Mini, Pepperidge Farm | 28 | 70 | 31 | 3.0 | 15.0 | 0.5 | 0.5 | 14.0 | 0.0 | 0.0 | 0.0 | 0.0 | 0.00 | 0.00 | 0 | 0 | 0 | 0 | 0 | 0 | 0.12 | 0.07 | 0.80 | | | | | 0.0 | | | 20 | | 0.7 | | | | | | 140 | |
| 42180 | 1 pce | Potato Bread, avg | 26 | 69 | 37 | 2.1 | 12.8 | 0.6 | 1.0 | 11.3 | 0.9 | 0.2 | 0.3 | 0.3 | | | 0 | 0 | 0 | 0 | 0 | 0 | 0.12 | 0.09 | 1.02 | 0.01 | 0.00 | 8.8 | 0.05 | 0.0 | | | 30 | 0.0 | 0.8 | 6 | 0.1 | 27 | 30 | 7.8 | 143 | 0.16 |
| 42473 | 1 pce | Potato Bread, Russet, Pepperidge Farm | 38 | 90 | 36 | 4.0 | 18.0 | 3.0 | 3.0 | 12.0 | 1.5 | 0.5 | | | | | 2 | 0 | 0 | 0 | 0 | 0 | 0.12 | 0.10 | 1.20 | | | | | 0.0 | | | 20 | | 1.4 | | | | | | 250 | |
| 42122 | 1 pce | Protein Bread, avg | 19 | 47 | 40 | 2.3 | 8.3 | 0.6 | 0.7 | 7.0 | 0.4 | 0.1 | 0.0 | 0.2 | 0.01 | 0.18 | 0 | 0.4 | 0.1 | | | | 0.07 | 0.07 | 0.82 | 0.01 | 0.00 | 19.6 | 0.08 | 0.0 | 0.1 | | 24 | 0.1 | 0.8 | 12 | 0.3 | 35 | 61 | 6.3 | 104 | 0.35 |
| | | Pumpernickel Breads | | | | | | | | | | | | | | | | | | | | | | | | | | | | | | | | | | | | | | | | |
| 42006 | 1 pce | Average | 26 | 65 | 38 | 2.3 | 12.3 | 1.7 | 1.2 | 9.5 | 0.8 | 0.1 | 0.2 | 0.3 | 0.02 | 0.30 | 0 | 0 | 0 | 0 | 0 | 0 | 0.09 | 0.08 | 0.80 | 0.03 | 0.00 | 20.8 | 0.11 | 0.0 | 0.0 | | 18 | 0.1 | 0.7 | 14 | 0.3 | 46 | 54 | 6.4 | 174 | 0.38 |
| 42484 | 1 pce | Classic Dark, Pepperidge Farm | 32 | 80 | 38 | 3.0 | 15.0 | 1.0 | 0.5 | 13.5 | 1.0 | 0.5 | 0.0 | 0.5 | | | 0 | 0 | 0 | 0 | 0 | 0 | 0.12 | 0.07 | 1.20 | | | | | 0.0 | | | 20 | | 1.1 | | | | | | 230 | |
| 42489 | 1 pce | Party, Pepperidge Farm | 16 | 37 | 36 | 2.0 | 7.3 | 1.3 | 0.7 | 5.3 | 0.5 | 0.0 | 0.2 | 0.3 | | | 0 | 0 | 0 | 0 | 0 | 0 | 0.08 | 0.05 | 0.53 | | | | | 0.0 | | | 13 | | 0.6 | | | | | | 107 | |
| 42124 | 1 pce | Prepared f/recipe, avg | 60 | 199 | 31 | 2.4 | 30.7 | 0.8 | 19.6 | 10.3 | 7.7 | 1.2 | 1.9 | 4.1 | 0.48 | 3.64 | 26 | 3259 | 334 | 23 | 311 | | 0.09 | 0.10 | 0.79 | 0.02 | 0.05 | 6.6 | 0.17 | 0.6 | 0.2 | | 11 | 0.0 | 1.0 | 8 | 0.1 | 32 | 55 | | 188 | 0.20 |
| 42527 | 1 oz | Pumpkin Quick Bread, dry mix, Pillsbury | 28 | 106 | 8 | 1.6 | 22.5 | 0.7 | 12.1 | 9.7 | 1.1 | 0.3 | | | | | 0 | 136 | 27 | | | | | | | | | | | 0.9 | | | 19 | | 0.7 | | | | | | 162 | |
| | | Raisin Breads | | | | | | | | | | | | | | | | | | | | | | | | | | | | | | | | | | | | | | | | |
| 42051 | 1 pce | Average | 26 | 71 | 34 | 2.1 | 13.6 | 1.1 | 3.5 | 8.9 | 1.1 | 0.3 | 0.6 | 0.2 | 0.01 | 0.17 | 0 | 0 | 0 | 0 | 0 | 0 | 0.09 | 0.10 | 0.90 | 0.02 | 0.00 | 22.6 | 0.10 | 0.0 | 0.1 | | 17 | 0.1 | 0.8 | 7 | 0.1 | 28 | 59 | 5.2 | 101 | 0.19 |
| 42582 | 1 pce | Cinnamon, Pepperidge Farm | 28 | 80 | 32 | 3.0 | 14.0 | 1.0 | 6.0 | 7.0 | 1.5 | 0.0 | 0.5 | 0.0 | 0.00 | 0.00 | 0 | 0 | 0 | 0 | 0 | 0 | 0.09 | 0.07 | 0.80 | | | | | 0.0 | | | 0 | | 1.8 | | | | | | 105 | |
| 42390 | 1 pce | Cinnamon Swirl, Pepperidge Farm | 28 | 80 | | 3.0 | 14.0 | 1.0 | 6.0 | 7.0 | 1.5 | 0.0 | 0.5 | 0.0 | 0.00 | 0.00 | 0 | 0 | 0 | 0 | 0 | 0 | 0.09 | 0.07 | 0.80 | | | | | 0.0 | | | 20 | | 1.8 | | | | | | 105 | |
| 42200 | 1 pce | Rice Bread | 25 | 79 | 36 | 1.7 | 9.8 | 0.6 | 0.3 | 8.9 | 3.9 | 0.4 | 0.5 | 2.7 | | | 0 | 0 | 0 | | | | 0.05 | 0.04 | 0.87 | 0.08 | 0.00 | 19.2 | | 0.0 | 0.0 | | 3 | 0.1 | 0.3 | 14 | | 52 | 93 | | 70 | 0.27 |

| Code | Amount | Description | Basic Components | | | | | | | | | Additional Fats | | | | | | Vit A & Components | | | | | Vitamins | | | | | | | | | | Minerals | | | | | | | | | |
|---|---|---|---|---|---|---|---|---|---|---|---|---|---|---|---|---|---|---|---|---|---|---|---|---|---|---|---|---|---|---|---|---|---|---|---|---|---|---|---|---|---|---|
| | | | Weight (g) | Calories | % Water | Protein (g) | Carbs (g) | Fiber (g) | Sugar (g) | Other Carbs (g) | Fat (g) | Sat Fat (g) | Mono Fat (g) | Poly Fat (g) | Omega 3 (g) | Omega 6 (g) | Choles (mg) | Vit A (IU) | Vit A (RE) | Retinol (RE) | Carotenoids (RE) | Beta Carotene (mcg) | Thiamin (mg) | Riboflavin (mg) | Niacin (NE) | Vit B6 (mg) | Vit B12 (mcg) | Folate (mcg) | Panto (mg) | Vit C (mg) | Vit D (mg) | Vit E (α TE) | Calcium (mg) | Copper (mg) | Iron (mg) | Magnes (mg) | Mang (mg) | Phos (mg) | Potassium (mg) | Selenium (mcg) | Sodium (mg) | Zinc (mg) |
| 42129 | 1 pce | Rice Bran Bread | 27 | 66 | 41 | 2.4 | 11.7 | 1.3 | 0.9 | 9.5 | 1.2 | 0.2 | 0.4 | 0.5 | 0.03 | 0.45 | 0 | 0.8 | 0.08 | 0 | 0.08 | | 0.18 | 0.08 | 1.84 | 0.07 | 0.00 | 17.6 | 0.21 | 0.0 | 0.1 | | 19 | 0.0 | 1.0 | 22 | 0.4 | 48 | 58 | 7.7 | 119 | 0.35 |
| | | Rye Breads | | | | | | | | | | | | | | | | | | | | | | | | | | | | | | | | | | | | | | | | |
| 42005 | 1 pce | Average | 32 | 83 | 37 | 2.7 | 15.5 | 1.9 | 2.6 | 11.0 | 1.1 | 0.2 | 0.4 | 0.3 | 0.02 | 0.24 | 0 | 2 | 0.3 | | | | 0.14 | 0.11 | 1.22 | 0.02 | 0.00 | 27.5 | 0.14 | 0.1 | 0.0 | | 23 | 0.1 | 0.9 | 13 | 0.3 | 40 | 53 | 9.9 | 211 | 0.36 |
| 42581 | 1 pce | Dijon Rye, Thin, Pepperidge Farm | 20 | 49 | 38 | 2.0 | 8.8 | 1.0 | 0.2 | 7.6 | 0.7 | 0.2 | 0.0 | 0.2 | | | 0 | 0 | 0 | 0 | 0 | 0 | 0.06 | 0.07 | 0.78 | | | | | 0.0 | | | 20 | | 0.5 | | | | | | 166 | |
| 42485 | 1 pce | Jewish Seeded, Pepperidge Farm | 32 | 80 | 38 | 3.0 | 15.0 | 1.0 | 0.5 | 13.5 | 1.0 | 0.5 | | | | | 0 | 0 | 0 | 0 | 0 | 0 | 0.15 | 0.10 | 1.20 | | | | | 0.0 | | | 20 | | 1.1 | | | | | | 210 | |
| 42486 | 1 pce | Jewish Seedless, Pepperidge Farm | 32 | 80 | 38 | 3.0 | 15.0 | 1.0 | 0.5 | 13.5 | 1.0 | 0.5 | | | | | 0 | 0 | 0 | 0 | 0 | 0 | 0.15 | 0.10 | 1.20 | | | | | 0.0 | | | 20 | | 1.1 | | | | | | 210 | |
| 42127 | 1 pce | Low Calorie, avg | 23 | 47 | 46 | 2.1 | 9.3 | 2.8 | 1.8 | 4.7 | 0.7 | 0.1 | 0.2 | 0.2 | 0.01 | 0.16 | 0 | 1 | 0.1 | 0 | 0.1 | | 0.08 | 0.06 | 0.58 | 0.02 | 0.01 | 11.0 | 0.07 | 0.1 | 0.0 | | 17 | 0.0 | 0.7 | 5 | 0.1 | 18 | 23 | 6.4 | 93 | 0.15 |
| 42470 | 1 pce | Onion, Pepperidge Farsm | 32 | 80 | 38 | 3.0 | 15.0 | 1.0 | 0.5 | 13.5 | 1.0 | 0.5 | 0.0 | 0.0 | 0.00 | 0.00 | 0 | 0 | 0 | 0 | 0 | 0 | 0.15 | 0.10 | 1.20 | | | | | 0.0 | | | 20 | | 1.1 | | | | | | 210 | |
| 42487 | 1 pce | Party Slices, Pepperidge Farm | 16 | 37 | 36 | 2.0 | 7.3 | 1.0 | 0.7 | 5.7 | 0.5 | 0.0 | 0.2 | 0.3 | | | 0 | 0 | 0 | 0 | 0 | 0 | 0.08 | 0.05 | 0.67 | | | | | 0.0 | | | 13 | | 0.6 | | | | | | 137 | |
| | | Sourdough Breads | | | | | | | | | | | | | | | | | | | | | | | | | | | | | | | | | | | | | | | | |
| 42045 | 1 pce | Average | 25 | 68 | 34 | 2.2 | 13.0 | 0.8 | 0.3 | 11.9 | 0.8 | 0.2 | 0.3 | 0.2 | 0.01 | 0.17 | 0 | 0 | 0 | 0 | 0 | 0 | 0.13 | 0.08 | 1.19 | 0.01 | 0.00 | 23.8 | 0.10 | 0.0 | 0.0 | | 19 | 0.0 | 0.6 | 7 | 0.1 | 26 | 28 | 7.9 | 152 | 0.22 |
| 42517 | 1 pce | Garlic, Pepperidge Farm | 47 | 180 | 26 | 5.0 | 20.0 | 2.0 | 2.0 | 16.0 | 9.0 | 2.5 | | | | | 10 | 0 | 0 | 0 | 0 | 0 | 0.15 | 0.10 | 1.20 | | | | | 0.0 | | | 0 | | 1.8 | | | | | | 220 | |
| 42493 | 1 pce | Light Style, Pepperidge Farm | 20 | 44 | 40 | 2.0 | 9.2 | 1.4 | 1.0 | 6.8 | 0.3 | 0.0 | | | | | 0 | 0 | 0 | 0 | 0 | 0 | 0.10 | 0.06 | 1.02 | | | | | 0.0 | | | 27 | | 0.6 | | | | | | 108 | |
| 42196 | 1 pce | Soy Bread, avg | 26 | 69 | 37 | 3.3 | 11.5 | 0.7 | 1.8 | 9.0 | 1.1 | 0.4 | 0.4 | 0.3 | | | 1 | 14 | 3.3 | 3 | 0.4 | | 0.10 | 0.08 | 0.93 | 0.03 | 0.02 | 12.3 | 0.16 | 0.1 | 0.1 | | 23 | 0.2 | 0.9 | 14 | 0.2 | 44 | 109 | | 74 | 0.23 |
| 42198 | 1 pce | Sunflower Meal Bread, avg | 27 | 75 | 36 | 3.1 | 12.2 | 0.5 | 1.4 | 10.4 | 1.4 | 0.5 | 0.5 | 0.4 | | | 1 | 14 | 3.3 | 3 | 0.4 | | 0.15 | 0.09 | 1.16 | 0.03 | 0.02 | 9.7 | 0.14 | 0.1 | 0.1 | | 17 | 0.1 | 0.8 | 13 | 0.1 | 40 | 34 | | 61 | 0.28 |
| 42182 | 1 pce | Sweet Potato Bread, avg | 25 | 72 | 33 | 2.0 | 12.5 | 0.6 | 2.5 | 9.4 | 1.5 | 0.3 | 0.6 | 0.4 | | | 14 | 367 | 50 | 19 | 30 | | 0.09 | 0.10 | 0.86 | 0.03 | 0.03 | 13.8 | 0.13 | 0.9 | 0.0 | | 5 | 0.0 | 0.8 | 5 | 0.1 | 28 | 40 | | 228 | 0.17 |
| 42192 | 1 pce | Triticale Bread, avg | 25 | 63 | 38 | 2.3 | 11.8 | 1.6 | 1.2 | 8.9 | 0.9 | 0.2 | 0.2 | 0.4 | | | 0 | 0 | 0 | 0 | 0 | 0 | 0.07 | 0.04 | 0.70 | 0.03 | 0.00 | 12.1 | 0.10 | 0.0 | 0.0 | | 22 | 0.1 | 0.7 | 17 | 0.3 | 47 | 52 | | 136 | 0.36 |
| | | Vienna Bread | | | | | | | | | | | | | | | | | | | | | | | | | | | | | | | | | | | | | | | | |
| 42044 | 1 pce | Average | 25 | 68 | 34 | 2.2 | 13.0 | 0.8 | 0.3 | 11.9 | 0.8 | 0.2 | 0.3 | 0.2 | 0.01 | 0.17 | 0 | 0 | 0 | 0 | 0 | 0 | 0.13 | 0.08 | 1.19 | 0.01 | 0.00 | 23.8 | 0.10 | 0.0 | 0.0 | | 19 | 0.0 | 0.6 | 7 | 0.1 | 26 | 28 | 7.9 | 152 | 0.22 |
| 42404 | 1 pce | Light, Pepperidge Farm | 20 | 44 | | 2.0 | 9.5 | 1.7 | 1.0 | 6.8 | 0.3 | 0.2 | 0.2 | 0.0 | 0.00 | 0.00 | 0 | 0 | 0 | 0 | 0 | 0 | 0.08 | 0.05 | 0.68 | | | | | 0.0 | | | 20 | | 0.6 | | | | | | 102 | |
| 42491 | 1 ea | Thick Sliced, enriched, Pepperidge Farm | 25 | 70 | 34 | 3.0 | 12.0 | 0.5 | 0.5 | 11.0 | 1.0 | 0.0 | | | | | 0 | 0 | 0 | 0 | 0 | 0 | 0.15 | 0.10 | 1.20 | | | | | 0.0 | | | 40 | | 1.1 | | | | | | 150 | |
| | | Wheat Breads | | | | | | | | | | | | | | | | | | | | | | | | | | | | | | | | | | | | | | | | |
| 42136 | 1 pce | Bran, avg | 36 | 89 | 38 | 3.2 | 17.2 | 1.4 | 1.5 | 14.3 | 1.2 | 0.3 | 0.6 | 0.2 | 0.01 | 0.22 | 0 | 0 | 0 | 0 | 0 | 0 | 0.14 | 0.10 | 1.58 | 0.06 | 0.00 | 24.8 | 0.19 | 0.0 | 0.0 | | 27 | 0.1 | 1.1 | 29 | 0.6 | 67 | 82 | 11.2 | 175 | 0.49 |
| 42388 | 1 pce | Bran, Old Fashioned, Pepperidge Farm | 34 | 90 | 36 | 3.0 | 17.0 | 2.0 | 2.0 | 13.0 | 1.0 | 0.0 | 0.5 | 0.0 | 0.00 | 0.00 | 0 | 0 | 0 | 0 | 0 | 0 | 0.15 | 0.10 | 1.20 | | | | | 0.0 | | | 0 | | 1.1 | | | | | | 160 | |
| 42528 | 1 oz | Bread Machine Mix, Dry, Pillsbury | 28 | 103 | 12 | 3.2 | 19.2 | 1.1 | 2.1 | 16.0 | 1.5 | 0.3 | | | | | 0 | 0 | 0 | 0 | 0 | 0 | | | | | | | | 0.6 | | | 6 | | 1.2 | | | | | | 197 | |
| 42599 | 1 pce | Germ, avg | 28 | 73 | 37 | 2.7 | 13.5 | 0.6 | 1.2 | 11.7 | 0.8 | 0.2 | 0.4 | 0.2 | 0.01 | 0.17 | 0 | 0.3 | 0.03 | 0 | 0.03 | | 0.10 | 0.11 | 1.26 | 0.02 | 0.02 | 26.3 | 0.15 | 0.1 | 0.1 | | 25 | 0.1 | 1.0 | 8 | 0.2 | 34 | 71 | 7.6 | 155 | 0.27 |
| 42095 | 1 pce | Low calorie, avg | 23 | 46 | 43 | 2.1 | 10.0 | 2.8 | 0.5 | 6.8 | 0.5 | 0.1 | 0.1 | 0.2 | 0.01 | 0.21 | 0 | 0 | 0 | 0 | 0 | 0 | 0.10 | 0.07 | 0.89 | 0.03 | 0.00 | 16.3 | 0.14 | 0.0 | 0.0 | | 18 | 0.0 | 0.7 | 9 | 0.2 | 23 | 28 | 7.0 | 118 | 0.26 |
| 356 | 1 ea | Part whole wheat, loaf, avg | 454 | 899 | 43 | 41.3 | 197.9 | 54.5 | 10.0 | 133.5 | 10.4 | 1.6 | 1.1 | 4.4 | 0.23 | 4.17 | 0 | 0 | 0 | 0 | 0 | 0 | 1.92 | 1.34 | 17.66 | 0.57 | 0.00 | 322.3 | 2.86 | 0.5 | 0.9 | | 363 | 0.6 | 13.4 | 177 | 3.9 | 463 | 554 | 138.0 | 2320 | 5.08 |
| 42078 | 1 pce | Sprouted, avg | 26 | 68 | 37 | 2.2 | 12.5 | 1.4 | 1.0 | 10.1 | 1.1 | 0.2 | 0.3 | 0.4 | | | 0 | 0 | 0 | 0 | 0 | 0 | 0.09 | 0.06 | 0.83 | 0.02 | 0.00 | 7.0 | 0.13 | 0.0 | 0.0 | | 23 | 0.1 | 0.7 | 13 | 0.3 | 33 | 35 | | 138 | 0.36 |
| 42490 | 1 pce | Very Thin, Pepperidge Farm | 16 | 37 | 38 | 1.4 | 7.5 | 1.4 | 0.7 | 5.4 | 0.7 | 0.2 | 0.3 | 0.2 | | | 0 | 0 | 0 | 0 | 0 | 0 | 0.08 | 0.05 | 0.54 | | | | | 0.0 | | | 14 | | 0.4 | | | | | | 78 | |
| | | White Breads | | | | | | | | | | | | | | | | | | | | | | | | | | | | | | | | | | | | | | | | |
| 42216 | 1 pce | Average | 30 | 80 | 37 | 2.5 | 14.9 | 0.7 | 1.2 | 13.0 | 1.1 | 0.2 | 0.5 | 0.2 | 0.01 | 0.21 | 0 | 0 | 0 | 0 | 0 | 0 | 0.14 | 0.10 | 1.19 | 0.02 | 0.01 | 28.5 | 0.12 | 0.0 | 0.1 | | 32 | 0.0 | 0.9 | 7 | 0.1 | 28 | 36 | 8.5 | 161 | 0.19 |
| 42529 | 1 oz | Bread Machine Mix, Dry, Pillsbury | 28 | 103 | 12 | 3.1 | 19.4 | 0.6 | 3.1 | 15.7 | 1.5 | 0.3 | | | | | 0 | 0 | 0 | 0 | 0 | 0 | | | | | | | | 0.6 | | | 5 | | 1.2 | | | | | | 196 | |
| 42472 | 1 pce | Hearty Country, Pepperidge Farm | 38 | 90 | 37 | 3.0 | 19.0 | 2.0 | 2.0 | 15.0 | 1.0 | 0.0 | | | 0.00 | 0.00 | 0 | 0 | 0 | 0 | 0 | 0 | 0.15 | 0.10 | 1.20 | | | | | 0.0 | | | 20 | | 0.7 | | | | | | 190 | |
| 42084 | 1 pce | Low calorie, avg | 23 | 48 | 43 | 2.0 | 10.2 | 2.2 | 0.5 | 7.5 | 0.6 | 0.1 | 0.2 | 0.1 | 0.01 | 0.12 | 0 | 0.7 | 0.2 | | | | 0.09 | 0.07 | 0.84 | 0.01 | 0.06 | 21.9 | 0.11 | 0.1 | 0.0 | | 22 | 0.1 | 0.7 | 5 | 0.1 | 28 | 17 | 5.0 | 104 | 0.31 |
| 42606 | 1 pce | Prepared f/recipe, w/whole milk, avg | 38 | 110 | 35 | 3.0 | 18.8 | 0.8 | 1.8 | 16.3 | 2.4 | 0.6 | 0.6 | 1.1 | 0.12 | 0.94 | 2 | 19 | 5 | 4 | 0.3 | | 0.15 | 0.15 | 1.36 | 0.02 | 0.03 | 16.0 | 0.14 | 0.1 | 0.2 | | 21 | 0.0 | 1.1 | 7 | 0.2 | 44 | 55 | | 136 | 0.24 |
| 42073 | 1 pce | Very low sodium, avg | 25 | 67 | 37 | 2.0 | 12.4 | 0.6 | 1.0 | 10.8 | 0.9 | 0.2 | 0.4 | 0.2 | 0.01 | 0.18 | 0 | 0 | 0 | 0 | 0 | 0 | 0.12 | 0.09 | 0.99 | 0.02 | 0.01 | 23.8 | 0.10 | 0.0 | 0.0 | | 27 | 0.0 | 0.8 | 6 | 0.1 | 24 | 30 | 5.7 | 7 | 0.16 |
| | | Whole Wheat Breads | | | | | | | | | | | | | | | | | | | | | | | | | | | | | | | | | | | | | | | | |
| 42014 | 1 pce | Average | 28 | 69 | 38 | 2.7 | 12.9 | 1.9 | 1.1 | 9.8 | 1.2 | 0.3 | 0.5 | 0.3 | 0.01 | 0.27 | 0 | 0 | 0 | 0 | 0 | 0 | 0.10 | 0.06 | 1.08 | 0.05 | 0.00 | 14.0 | 0.15 | 0.0 | 0.1 | | 20 | 0.1 | 0.9 | 24 | 0.6 | 64 | 71 | 10.2 | 148 | 0.54 |
| 42476 | 1 pce | Hearty Honey Wheatberry, Pepperidge Farm | 38 | 100 | 38 | 3.0 | 18.0 | 2.0 | 3.0 | 13.0 | 1.5 | 0.0 | 0.5 | 1.0 | | | 0 | 0 | 0 | 0 | 0 | 0 | 0.12 | 0.07 | 0.80 | | | | | 0.0 | | | 20 | | 0.7 | | | | | | 200 | |
| 42469 | 1 pce | Hearty Sesame, Pepperidge Farm | 38 | 100 | 38 | 4.0 | 17.0 | 2.0 | 2.0 | 13.0 | 1.5 | 0.0 | 0.5 | 0.0 | 0.00 | 0.00 | 0 | | | | | | 0.15 | 0.10 | 1.20 | | | | | | | | 20 | | 0.7 | | | | | | 180 | |
| 42142 | 1 pce | Prep f/recipe, avg | 46 | 128 | 33 | 3.9 | 23.6 | 2.8 | 2.2 | 18.7 | 2.5 | 0.4 | 0.5 | 1.4 | 0.15 | 1.21 | 0 | 0 | 0 | 0 | 0 | 0 | 0.14 | 0.10 | 1.84 | 0.09 | 0.00 | 28.1 | 0.22 | 0.0 | 0.1 | | 15 | 0.1 | 1.4 | 37 | 0.9 | 86 | 144 | 17.8 | 159 | 0.69 |
| 42477 | 1 pce | Thin Sliced, Pepperidge Farm | 25 | 60 | 38 | 3.0 | 11.0 | 0.5 | 1.0 | 9.5 | 1.0 | 0.0 | 0.5 | 0.5 | | | 0 | 0 | 0 | 0 | 0 | 0 | 0.09 | 0.07 | 0.80 | | | | | 0.0 | | | 20 | | 0.7 | | | | | | 120 | |
| | | ***ROLLS*** | | | | | | | | | | | | | | | | | | | | | | | | | | | | | | | | | | | | | | | | |
| 42185 | 1 ea | Bolillo Roll, Mexican, avg | 117 | 295 | 39 | 9.9 | 58.4 | 2.2 | 1.7 | 54.5 | 1.8 | 0.5 | 0.2 | 0.6 | | | 1 | 15 | 3.8 | 3.4 | 0.4 | | 0.67 | 0.45 | 6.33 | 0.06 | 0.00 | 47.3 | 0.35 | 0.0 | 0.0 | | 14 | 0.2 | 3.7 | 22 | 0.5 | 88 | 96 | | 347 | 0.76 |
| 42183 | 1 ea | Cheese Roll, avg | 41 | 124 | 32 | 3.7 | 20.7 | 0.7 | 3.9 | 16.0 | 2.9 | 1.0 | 1.3 | 0.4 | | | 2 | 22 | 6.2 | 5.8 | 0.4 | | 0.15 | 0.10 | 1.29 | 0.02 | 0.01 | 15.1 | 0.08 | 0.0 | 0.0 | | 54 | 0.0 | 1.1 | 9 | 0.2 | 43 | 39 | 11.1 | 210 | 0.34 |
| 42366 | 1 ea | Cheese & Garlic Roll, Pepperidge Farm | 40 | 130 | | 6.0 | 16.0 | 2.0 | 2.0 | 12.0 | 5.0 | 1.5 | 2.5 | 0.0 | 0.00 | 0.00 | 15 | 200 | 40 | | | | 0.22 | 0.10 | 1.60 | | | | | 0.0 | | | 40 | | 0.7 | | | | | | 280 | |
| | | Dinner Rolls | | | | | | | | | | | | | | | | | | | | | | | | | | | | | | | | | | | | | | | | |
| 42503 | 1 ea | Butter Crescent, Heat & Serve, Pepperidge Farm | 30 | 110 | 28 | 3.0 | 13.0 | 1.0 | 0.5 | 11.5 | 5.0 | 3.0 | | | | | 15 | 0 | 0 | 0 | 0 | 0 | 0.12 | 0.07 | 0.80 | | | | | 0.0 | | | 20 | | 0.7 | | | | | | 160 | |
| 42254 | 1 ea | Butterflake, dough, prep, Pillsbury | 47 | 134 | 37 | 3.1 | 19.4 | 0.7 | 2.7 | 16.1 | 4.9 | 1.1 | | | | | 0 | 2 | 0.2 | | | | | | | | | | | 0.0 | | | 13 | | 1.1 | | | | | | 525 | |
| 42262 | 1 ea | Caramel, dough, prep, Pillsbury | 49 | 171 | 28 | 2.3 | 24.5 | 0.5 | 6.9 | 17.2 | 7.1 | 1.6 | | | | | 0 | 57 | 6 | | | | | | | | | | | 0.0 | | | 11 | | 0.9 | | | | | | 325 | |
| 42255 | 1 ea | Crescent, dough, prep, Pillsbury | 28 | 101 | 31 | 1.8 | 10.9 | 0.3 | 1.7 | 8.9 | 5.6 | 1.3 | | | | | 0 | 0 | 0 | 0 | 0 | 0 | | | | | | | | 0.0 | | | 6 | | 0.6 | | | | | | 214 | |
| 42159 | 1 ea | Egg, avg | 35 | 107 | 30 | 3.3 | 18.2 | 1.3 | | | 2.2 | 0.6 | 1.0 | 0.4 | 0.02 | 0.37 | 17 | 9 | 3 | 2.6 | 0.2 | | 0.18 | 0.18 | 1.15 | 0.02 | 0.08 | 36.8 | 0.23 | 0.0 | | | 21 | 0.0 | 1.2 | 9 | 0.2 | 35 | 36 | 10.4 | 191 | 0.39 |
| 42377 | 1 ea | Finger Roll, w/Poppy Seeds, enr, Pepperidge Farm | 18 | 51 | | 2.4 | 6.8 | 0.3 | 1.4 | 5.1 | 1.5 | 0.5 | 0.7 | 0.2 | | | 2 | 0 | 0 | 0 | 0 | 0 | 0.08 | 0.05 | 0.68 | | | | | 0.0 | | | 14 | | 0.5 | | | | | | 78 | |
| 42378 | 1 ea | Finger Roll, w/Sesame Seeds, enr, Pepperidge Farm | 18 | 51 | | 2.4 | 6.8 | 0.3 | 1.4 | 5.1 | 1.5 | 0.5 | 0.7 | 0.2 | | | 2 | 0 | 0 | 0 | 0 | 0 | 0.08 | 0.05 | 0.68 | | | | | 0.0 | | | 14 | | 0.5 | | | | | | 8 | |
| 42502 | 1 ea | Golden Twists, Heat & Serve, Pepperidge Farm | 30 | 110 | 35 | 2.0 | 13.0 | 1.0 | 1.0 | 11.0 | 4.0 | 1.5 | 1.5 | 0.5 | | | 2 | 0 | 0 | 0 | 0 | 0 | 0.12 | 0.07 | 0.80 | | | | | 0.0 | | | 0 | | 0.7 | | | | | | 160 | |
| 42022 | 1 ea | Hard, white, enriched, avg | 57 | 167 | 31 | 5.6 | 30.0 | 1.3 | 2.9 | 25.9 | 2.5 | 0.3 | 0.6 | 1.0 | 0.06 | 0.92 | 0 | 0 | 0 | 0 | 0 | 0 | 0.27 | 0.19 | 2.42 | 0.02 | 0.00 | 54.1 | 0.23 | 0.0 | 0.0 | | 54 | 0.1 | 1.9 | 15 | 0.3 | 57 | 62 | 22.3 | 310 | 0.54 |
| 42380 | 1 ea | Hearty Potato Classic, Pepperidge Farm | 28 | 80 | | 3.0 | 12.0 | 1.0 | 2.0 | 9.0 | 2.5 | 0.5 | 1.0 | 0.5 | | | 0 | 0 | 0 | 0 | 0 | 0 | 0.09 | 0.07 | 2.00 | | | | | 0.0 | | | 20 | | 1.1 | | | | | | 110 | |
| 42583 | 1 ea | Lite, Bake-n-Serve, dough, prep, Rhodes | 38 | 89 | 39 | 3.6 | 18.7 | 1.0 | 0.8 | 17.0 | 0.5 | 0.0 | | | | | 0 | 0 | 0 | 0 | 0 | 0 | 0.17 | 0.11 | 1.54 | | | | | 0.0 | | | 14 | | 1.1 | | | | | | 144 | |
| 42379 | 1 ea | Parker House, enr, Pepperidge Farm | 18 | 51 | | 2.4 | 6.8 | 0.3 | 1.4 | 5.1 | 1.5 | 0.5 | 0.7 | 0.2 | | | 2 | 0 | 0 | 0 | 0 | 0 | 0.08 | 0.05 | 0.68 | | | 17.1 | | 0.0 | | | 14 | | 0.5 | | | | | | 78 | |
| 42158 | 1 ea | Prepared f/recipe, w/2% milk, avg | 35 | 111 | 29 | 3.0 | 18.7 | 0.7 | 3.5 | 14.5 | 2.6 | 0.6 | 1.0 | 0.7 | 0.04 | 0.67 | 12 | 118 | 32 | 29 | 2 | | 0.14 | 0.14 | 1.21 | 0.02 | 0.05 | 31.5 | 0.16 | 0.1 | 0.1 | | 21 | 0.0 | 1.0 | 7 | 0.1 | 44 | 53 | 8.0 | 145 | 0.24 |
| 42019 | 1 ea | Prepared f/recipe w/whole milk, avg | 35 | 112 | 29 | 3.0 | 18.7 | 1.0 | 3.5 | 14.1 | 2.7 | 0.7 | 1.1 | 0.7 | 0.04 | 0.67 | 13 | 108 | 28 | 26 | 2 | | 0.14 | 0.14 | 1.21 | 0.02 | 0.05 | 15.1 | 0.16 | 0.1 | 0.2 | | 21 | 0.0 | 1.0 | 7 | 0.1 | 44 | 53 | 9.7 | 145 | 0.24 |
| 42160 | 1 ea | Wheat, avg | 36 | 98 | 37 | 3.1 | 16.6 | 1.4 | 2.6 | 12.6 | 2.3 | 0.5 | 1.1 | 0.4 | 0.02 | 0.38 | 0 | 0 | 0 | 0 | 0 | 0 | 0.16 | 0.10 | 1.47 | 0.03 | 0.00 | 18.4 | 0.13 | 0.0 | 0.1 | | 63 | 0.1 | 1.3 | 13 | 0.4 | 37 | 41 | 11.9 | 122 | 0.32 |
| 42555 | 1 oz | Wheat, dough, prep, Rich's | 28 | 79 | 31 | 3.5 | 14.4 | 0.9 | 1.2 | 12.3 | 0.9 | 0.3 | 0.4 | 0.0 | | | 0 | 1.5 | 0.15 | | | | 0.14 | 0.08 | 1.02 | 0.00 | 0.00 | 0.0 | 0.00 | 0.0 | 0.0 | 0.0 | 5 | 0.0 | 0.8 | 7 | | 29 | 38 | | 132 | 0.00 |
| 42589 | 1 ea | White, Bake-n-Serve, dough, prep, Rhodes | 38 | 104 | 35 | 3.5 | 18.4 | 0.9 | 1.5 | 16.0 | 2.2 | 0.0 | | | | | 0 | 0 | 0 | 0 | 0 | 0 | 0.21 | 0.13 | 1.37 | | | | | 0.0 | | | 8 | | 1.2 | | | | | | 150 | |
| 42057 | 1 ea | Whole wheat, avg | 28 | 74 | 33 | 2.4 | 14.3 | 2.1 | 1.2 | 11.0 | 1.3 | 0.2 | 0.3 | 0.6 | 0.03 | 0.57 | 0 | 0 | 0 | 0 | 0 | 0 | 0.07 | 0.04 | 1.03 | 0.05 | 0.00 | 8.7 | 0.14 | 0.0 | 0.0 | | 30 | 0.1 | 0.7 | 24 | 0.6 | 63 | 76 | 13.8 | 134 | 0.56 |
| | | Hamburger/Hotdog Rolls | | | | | | | | | | | | | | | | | | | | | | | | | | | | | | | | | | | | | | | | |
| 42020 | 1 ea | Average | 43 | 123 | 34 | 3.7 | 21.6 | 1.2 | 3.2 | 17.3 | 2.2 | 0.5 | 0.4 | 1.1 | 0.02 | 1.07 | 0 | 0 | 0 | 0 | 0 | 0 | 0.21 | 0.13 | 1.69 | 0.02 | 0.03 | 40.9 | 0.23 | 0.0 | 0.0 | | 60 | 0.0 | 1.4 | 9 | 0.1 | 38 | 61 | 11.4 | 241 | 0.27 |
| 42501 | 1 ea | Frankfurter, Dijon, Pepperidge Farm | 50 | 140 | 34 | 6.0 | 23.0 | 2.0 | 3.0 | 18.0 | 3.0 | 1.5 | 0.5 | 1.0 | | | 0 | 0 | 0 | 0 | 0 | 0 | 0.15 | 0.17 | 2.00 | | | | | 0.0 | | | 80 | | 0.7 | | | | | | 240 | |
| 42163 | 1 ea | Low calorie, w/extra fiber, avg | 43 | 84 | 46 | 3.6 | 18.1 | 2.7 | 1.6 | 13.8 | 0.9 | 0.1 | 0.2 | 0.3 | 0.02 | 0.31 | 0 | 0.4 | 0.04 | 0 | 0.04 | | 0.17 | 0.08 | 2.12 | 0.02 | 0.04 | 40.9 | 0.16 | 0.1 | 0.0 | | 25 | 0.1 | 1.3 | 9 | 0.2 | 36 | 34 | 10.1 | 190 | 0.29 |

| Code | Amount | Description | Basic Components | | | | | | | | | Additional Fats | | | | | | Vit A & Components | | | | | Vitamins | | | | | | | | | | Minerals | | | | | | | | | |
|---|---|---|---|---|---|---|---|---|---|---|---|---|---|---|---|---|---|---|---|---|---|---|---|---|---|---|---|---|---|---|---|---|---|---|---|---|---|---|---|---|---|---|
| | | | Weight (g) | Calories | % Water | Protein (g) | Carbs (g) | Fiber (g) | Sugar (g) | Other Carbs (g) | Fat (g) | Sat Fat (g) | Mono Fat (g) | Poly Fat (g) | Omega 3 (g) | Omega 6 (g) | Choles (mg) | Vit A (IU) | Vit A (RE) | Retinol (RE) | Carotenoids (RE) | Beta Carotene (mcg) | Thiamin (mg) | Riboflavin (mg) | Niacin (NE) | Vit B6 (mg) | Vit B12 (mcg) | Folate (mcg) | Panto (mg) | Vit C (mg) | Vit D (mg) | Vit E (α TE) | Calcium (mg) | Copper (mg) | Iron (mg) | Magnes (mg) | Mang (mg) | Phos (mg) | Potassium (mg) | Selenium (mcg) | Sodium (mg) | Zinc (mg) |
| 42162 | 1 ea | Multigrain, avg | 43 | 113 | 38 | 4.1 | 19.2 | 1.6 | 1.6 | 15.9 | 2.6 | 0.4 | 0.8 | 0.4 | 0.02 | 0.38 | 0 | 0.4 | 0.04 | 0 | 0.04 | | 0.20 | 0.13 | 1.92 | 0.04 | 0.00 | 40.9 | 0.21 | 0.0 | 0.0 | | 41 | 0.1 | 1.7 | 19 | 0.4 | 52 | 69 | 13.7 | 197 | 0.45 |
| 42070 | 1 ea | Oat Bran Roll, avg | 33 | 78 | 44 | 3.1 | 13.3 | 1.4 | | | 1.5 | 0.2 | 0.5 | 0.5 | 0.03 | 0.49 | 0 | 1.7 | 0.2 | 0 | 0.2 | | 0.15 | 0.10 | 1.63 | 0.01 | 0.00 | 31.4 | 0.14 | 0.0 | 0.0 | | 28 | 0.0 | 1.4 | 11 | 0.2 | 38 | 40 | 9.7 | 136 | 0.34 |
| 42058 | 1 ea | Rye Roll, avg | 28 | 80 | 30 | 2.9 | 14.9 | 1.4 | 1.6 | 11.9 | 1.0 | 0.2 | 0.3 | 0.2 | 0.01 | 0.18 | 0 | 2 | 0 | | | | 0.11 | 0.08 | 1.09 | 0.02 | 0.00 | 24.1 | 0.11 | 0.0 | 0.0 | | 8 | 0.1 | 0.8 | 15 | 0.2 | 45 | 50 | 7.8 | 250 | 0.27 |
| | | Sandwich Rolls | | | | | | | | | | | | | | | | | | | | | | | | | | | | | | | | | | | | | | | | |
| 42524 | 1 ea | French Style, enriched, Pepperidge Farm | 50 | 130 | 37 | 4.0 | 25.0 | 1.0 | 0.5 | 23.5 | 1.5 | 1.0 | | | | | 0 | 0 | 0 | 0 | 0 | 0 | 0.22 | 0.17 | 2.00 | | | | | 0.0 | | | 60 | | 1.8 | | | | | | 230 | |
| 42497 | 1 ea | Multigrain, Pepperidge Farm | 54 | 150 | 37 | 6.0 | 24.0 | 3.0 | 4.0 | 17.0 | 3.0 | 0.5 | 1.5 | 0.5 | | | 0 | 0 | 0 | 0 | 0 | 0 | 0.38 | 0.25 | 0.00 | | | | | 0.0 | | | 20 | | 1.8 | | | | | | 230 | |
| 42510 | 1 ea | Multigrain Hoagie, Pepperidge Farm | 69 | 200 | 35 | 7.0 | 32.0 | 2.0 | 2.0 | 28.0 | 4.5 | 2.5 | 1.0 | 1.0 | | | 0 | 0 | 0 | 0 | 0 | 0 | 0.15 | 0.17 | 3.00 | | | | | 0.0 | | | 80 | | 1.1 | | | | | | 340 | |
| 42500 | 1 ea | Onion, Pepperidge Farm | 53 | 150 | 34 | 5.0 | 26.0 | 1.0 | 2.0 | 23.0 | 3.0 | 1.5 | 0.5 | 1.0 | | | 0 | 0 | 0 | 0 | 0 | 0 | 0.22 | 0.17 | 2.00 | | | | | 0.0 | | | 60 | | 1.4 | | | | | | 270 | |
| 42507 | 1 ea | Potato, Pepperidge Farm | 60 | 160 | 38 | 4.0 | 28.0 | 0.5 | 0.5 | 27.0 | 4.0 | 0.5 | 2.0 | 1.5 | | | 0 | 0 | 0 | 0 | 0 | 0 | 0.45 | 0.14 | 5.00 | | | | | 0.0 | | | 0 | | 1.1 | | | | | | 260 | |
| 42504 | 1 ea | Sesame Seed, Pepperidge Farm | 46 | 140 | 31 | 5.0 | 23.0 | 1.0 | 3.0 | 19.0 | 3.0 | 1.5 | 0.5 | 1.0 | | | 0 | 0 | 0 | 0 | 0 | 0 | 0.30 | 0.17 | 1.60 | | | | | 0.0 | | | 40 | | 1.4 | | | | | | 240 | |
| 42539 | 1 ea | Seven Grain, Pepperidge Farm | 38 | 80 | 32 | 4.0 | 19.0 | 2.0 | 3.0 | 14.0 | 2.0 | 0.0 | | | | | 0 | 0 | 0 | 0 | 0 | 0 | 0.15 | 0.10 | 1.20 | | | | | 0.0 | | | 40 | | 1.1 | | | | | | 270 | |
| 42498 | 1 ea | Sourdough, Pepperidge Farm | 57 | 170 | 32 | 6.0 | 28.0 | 1.0 | 3.0 | 24.0 | 3.5 | 1.5 | 0.5 | 1.0 | | | 0 | 0 | 0 | 0 | 0 | 0 | 0.38 | 0.17 | 2.00 | | | | | 0.0 | | | 0 | | 1.8 | | | | | | 290 | |
| 42355 | 1 ea | Sourdough Roll, avg | 47 | 128 | 34 | 4.0 | 24.0 | 1.0 | 0.0 | 23.0 | 2.0 | 0.0 | | | | | 0 | 0 | 0 | 0 | 0 | 0 | | | | | | | | 0.0 | | | 40 | | 1.1 | | | | | | 236 | |
| | | *BREAD CRUMBS, CROUTONS AND SEASONING MIXES* | | | | | | | | | | | | | | | | | | | | | | | | | | | | | | | | | | | | | | | | |
| | | Bread Crumbs | | | | | | | | | | | | | | | | | | | | | | | | | | | | | | | | | | | | | | | | |
| 42440 | 1/4 cup | Italian Style, Progresso | 28 | 110 | 6 | 4.0 | 20.0 | 1.0 | 1.0 | 18.0 | 1.5 | 0.0 | | | | | 0 | 0 | 0 | 0 | 0 | 0 | | | | | | | | 0.0 | | | 40 | | 1.4 | | | | | | 430 | |
| 42004 | 1/4 cup | Plain, dry, grated, avg | 27 | 107 | 6 | 3.4 | 19.6 | 0.6 | 0.7 | 18.3 | 1.5 | 0.3 | 0.6 | 0.3 | 0.02 | 0.28 | 0 | 0.3 | 0.03 | 0 | 0.03 | | 0.21 | 0.12 | 1.85 | 0.03 | 0.01 | 29.4 | 0.08 | 0.0 | 0.1 | | 61 | 0.0 | 1.7 | 12 | 0.2 | 40 | 60 | 10.2 | 233 | 0.33 |
| 42144 | 1/4 cup | Seasoned, dry, grated, avg | 27 | 99 | 6 | 3.8 | 19.0 | 1.1 | 0.8 | 17.1 | 0.7 | 0.2 | 0.3 | 0.2 | 0.01 | 0.17 | 0 | 4 | 1 | | | | 0.04 | 0.05 | 0.74 | 0.04 | 0.01 | 29.4 | 0.08 | 0.1 | 0.0 | | 27 | 0.0 | 0.9 | 10 | 0.2 | 36 | 73 | 9.5 | 716 | 0.25 |
| | | Croutons | | | | | | | | | | | | | | | | | | | | | | | | | | | | | | | | | | | | | | | | |
| 42426 | 10 pce | Caesar Homestyle, Pepperidge Farm | 12 | 60 | | 1.7 | 6.9 | 0.0 | 0.0 | 6.9 | 2.5 | 0.0 | 1.7 | 0.0 | 0.00 | 0.00 | 0 | 0 | 0 | 0 | 0 | 0 | 0.00 | 0.00 | 0.00 | | | | | 0.0 | | | 0 | | 0.0 | | | | | | 154 | |
| 42422 | 10 pce | Cheddar & Romano Cheese, Pepperidge Farm | 8 | 34 | | 1.1 | 4.6 | 0.0 | 0.0 | 4.6 | 1.1 | 0.0 | 0.6 | 0.0 | 0.00 | 0.00 | 0 | 0 | 0 | 0 | 0 | 0 | 0.03 | 0.00 | 0.00 | | | | | 0.0 | | | 0 | | 0.4 | | | | | | 109 | |
| 42423 | 10 pce | Cheese & Garlic, Pepperidge Farm | 8 | 40 | | 2.3 | 4.6 | 0.0 | 0.0 | 4.6 | 1.7 | 0.0 | 1.1 | 0.0 | 0.00 | 0.00 | 0 | 0 | 0 | 0 | 0 | 0 | 0.00 | 0.00 | 0.00 | | | | | 0.0 | | | 0 | | 0.0 | | | | | | 91 | |
| 42541 | 10 pce | Cracked Pepper & Parmesan, Pepperidge Farm | 12 | 60 | 5 | 1.7 | 6.9 | 0.0 | 0.0 | 6.9 | 2.5 | 0.0 | 1.7 | 0.9 | | | 0 | 0 | 0 | 0 | 0 | 0 | 0.00 | 0.00 | 0.00 | | | | | 0.0 | | | 0 | | 0.0 | | | | | | 154 | |
| 42420 | 10 pce | Onion & Garlic, Pepperidge Farm | 8 | 34 | | 1.1 | 5.7 | 0.0 | 0.0 | 5.7 | 1.1 | 0.0 | 1.1 | 0.0 | 0.00 | 0.00 | 0 | 0 | 0 | 0 | 0 | 0 | 0.03 | 0.00 | 0.00 | | | | | 0.0 | | | 0 | | 0.0 | | | | | | 91 | |
| 42016 | 1/4 cup | Plain, avg | 8 | 33 | 6 | 1.0 | 5.9 | 0.4 | 0.2 | 5.3 | 0.5 | 0.1 | 0.2 | 0.1 | 0.01 | 0.10 | 0 | 0 | 0 | 0 | 0 | 0 | 0.05 | 0.02 | 0.44 | 0.00 | 0.00 | 10.6 | 0.03 | 0.0 | 0.0 | | 6 | 0.0 | 0.3 | 2 | 0.0 | 9 | 10 | 3.0 | 56 | 0.07 |
| 42542 | 10 pce | Ranch, Pepperidge Farm | 8 | 40 | 5 | 1.1 | 4.6 | 0.0 | 1.1 | 3.4 | 1.7 | 0.6 | 0.6 | 0.6 | | | 6 | 0 | 0 | 0 | 0 | 0 | 0.03 | 0.00 | 0.00 | | | | | 0.0 | | | 46 | | 0.0 | | | | | | 74 | |
| 42148 | 1/4 cup | Seasoned, avg | 10 | 47 | 4 | 1.1 | 6.3 | 0.5 | 0.0 | 5.8 | 1.3 | 0.5 | 0.5 | 0.2 | 0.01 | 0.22 | 1 | 4 | 1 | | | | 0.05 | 0.04 | 0.47 | 0.01 | 0.01 | 8.8 | 0.08 | 0.0 | 0.0 | | 10 | 0.0 | 0.3 | 4 | 0.1 | 14 | 18 | 2.9 | 124 | 0.09 |
| 42425 | 10 pce | Sourdough Cheese Homestyle, Pepperidge Farm | 12 | 51 | | 1.7 | 6.9 | 0.0 | 0.0 | 6.9 | 1.7 | 0.0 | 1.7 | 0.0 | 0.00 | 0.00 | 3 | 0 | 0 | 0 | 0 | 0 | 0.05 | 0.00 | 0.69 | | | | | 0.0 | | | 0 | | 0.0 | | | | | | 137 | |
| 42424 | 10 pce | Zesty Italian Homestyle, Pepperidge Farm | 8 | 40 | | 1.1 | 4.6 | 0.0 | 0.6 | 4.0 | 1.7 | 0.6 | 0.6 | 0.0 | 0.00 | 0.00 | 2 | 0 | 0 | 0 | 0 | 0 | 0.03 | 0.00 | 0.00 | | | | | 0.0 | | | 46 | | 0.0 | | | | | | 74 | |
| | | Seasoning Mixes | | | | | | | | | | | | | | | | | | | | | | | | | | | | | | | | | | | | | | | | |
| 43514 | 1 oz | Batter mix, chicken, avg | 28 | 90 | 18 | 2.2 | 18.8 | | | | 0.6 | | | | | | | 50 | 15 | 15 | 0 | | 0.04 | 0.02 | 0.34 | | | | | 0.0 | | | 5 | | 0.4 | | | | 29 | | 1229 | |
| 43517 | 1 oz | Batter mix, fish, avg | 28 | 95 | 14 | 2.5 | 20.7 | | | | 0.6 | | | | | | | 44 | 13 | 13 | 0 | | 0.04 | 0.03 | 0.36 | | | | | 0.0 | | | 12 | | 0.4 | | | | 42 | | 330 | |
| 43523 | 1 oz | Crumbs, coating, avg | 28 | 101 | 12 | 2.8 | 20.2 | | | | 0.8 | | | | | | | 0 | 0 | 0 | 0 | 0 | 0.03 | 0.01 | 0.34 | | | | | 0.0 | | | 4 | | 0.3 | | | | 28 | | 431 | |
| 43577 | 1/4 cup | Crumbs, Corn Flake, Kellogg's | 22 | 80 | 3 | 2.0 | 18.0 | 0.0 | 2.0 | 16.0 | 0.0 | 0.0 | 0.0 | 0.0 | 0.00 | 0.00 | 0 | 0 | 0 | 0 | 0 | 0 | 0.24 | 0.27 | 3.20 | 0.32 | | 64.0 | | 10.0 | | | 0 | 0.0 | 5.4 | 2 | | 8 | 28 | | 240 | 0.14 |
| 43550 | 1/4 cup | Cracker meal, avg | 29 | 111 | 8 | 2.7 | 23.5 | 0.7 | 0.5 | 22.2 | 0.5 | 0.1 | 0.0 | 0.2 | 0.01 | 0.20 | 0 | 0 | 0 | 0 | 0 | 0 | 0.20 | 0.14 | 1.66 | 0.01 | 0.00 | 33.3 | 0.14 | 0.0 | 0.0 | | 7 | 0.1 | 1.3 | 7 | 0.3 | 30 | 33 | 12.3 | 8 | 0.20 |
| 43521 | 1 oz | Cracker meal, fine, avg | 28 | 101 | 12 | 2.8 | 21.3 | | | | 0.3 | | | | | | 0 | 0 | 0 | 0 | 0 | 0 | 0.03 | 0.01 | 0.36 | | | | | 0.0 | | | 4 | | 0.3 | | | | 29 | | 0 | |
| 43522 | 1 oz | Cracker meal, medium, avg | 28 | 101 | 12 | 2.8 | 21.3 | | | | 0.3 | | | | | | 0 | 0 | 0 | 0 | 0 | 0 | 0.03 | 0.01 | 0.36 | | | | | 0.0 | | | 4 | | 0.3 | | | | 29 | | 0 | |
| | | *CRACKERS* | | | | | | | | | | | | | | | | | | | | | | | | | | | | | | | | | | | | | | | | |
| 43647 | 7 ea | Amaranth Graham, Health Valley | 28 | 97 | 4 | 3.9 | 22.2 | 2.9 | 4.8 | 14.5 | 0.0 | 0.0 | 0.0 | 0.0 | 0.00 | 0.00 | 0 | 97 | 19 | | | | | | | | | | | 0.0 | | | 1 | | 0.7 | | | | | | 29 | |
| 1034 | 4 ea | Armenian cracker bread, avg | 28 | 105 | 37 | 8.0 | 0.9 | 0.0 | 0.9 | 0.0 | 7.7 | 5.0 | 2.0 | 0.3 | 0.10 | 0.17 | 26 | 237 | 71 | 69 | 2 | | 0.01 | 0.10 | 0.03 | 0.02 | 0.47 | 1.8 | 0.12 | 0.0 | 0.3 | | 269 | 0.0 | 0.0 | 10 | 0.0 | 169 | 31 | 3.6 | 73 | 1.09 |
| 43543 | 9 ea | Butter flavored, snack type, avg | 27 | 136 | 4 | 2.0 | 16.5 | 0.4 | 1.4 | 14.7 | 6.8 | 1.0 | 2.9 | 2.5 | 0.18 | 1.39 | 0 | 0 | 0 | 0 | 0 | 0 | 0.11 | 0.09 | 1.09 | 0.01 | 0.00 | 20.8 | 0.07 | 0.0 | 0.0 | | 32 | 0.1 | 1.0 | 7 | 0.2 | 62 | 36 | 1.8 | 229 | 0.18 |
| 43603 | 7 ea | Butter flavored, Thin Crackers, Pepperidge Farm | 28 | 131 | 4 | 1.9 | 18.7 | 0.0 | 1.9 | 16.3 | 5.6 | 1.9 | 2.8 | 0.0 | 0.00 | 0.00 | 19 | 0 | 0 | 0 | 0 | 0 | 0.11 | 0.06 | 1.49 | | | | | 0.0 | | | 0 | | 1.3 | | | | | | 177 | |
| | | Cheese crackers | | | | | | | | | | | | | | | | | | | | | | | | | | | | | | | | | | | | | | | | |
| 43500 | 30 ea | Average | 30 | 151 | 3 | 3.0 | 17.5 | 0.7 | 0.6 | 16.1 | 7.6 | 2.8 | 3.6 | 0.7 | 0.04 | 0.70 | 4 | 49 | 9 | 8 | 1 | | 0.17 | 0.13 | 1.40 | 0.17 | 0.14 | 24.0 | 0.16 | 0.0 | 0.0 | | 45 | 0.1 | 1.4 | 11 | 0.2 | 65 | 44 | 2.6 | 299 | 0.34 |
| 43597 | 55 ea | Goldfish, Cheddar, Tiny, Pepperidge Farm | 30 | 140 | 2 | 4.0 | 19.0 | 0.5 | 0.0 | 18.5 | 6.0 | 1.5 | 3.0 | 0.5 | | | 10 | 0 | 0 | 0 | 0 | 0 | 0.22 | 0.14 | 1.60 | | | | | 0.0 | | | 20 | | 1.4 | | | | | | 200 | |
| 43602 | 55 ea | Goldfish, Low Sodium, Pepperidge Farm | 30 | 150 | | 3.0 | 18.0 | 0.5 | 0.0 | 17.5 | 6.0 | 1.5 | 3.0 | 0.5 | | | 10 | 0 | 0 | 0 | 0 | 0 | 0.15 | 0.10 | 1.20 | | | | | 0.0 | | | 40 | | 0.7 | | | | | | 140 | |
| 43598 | 55 ea | Goldfish, Parmesan, Pepperidge Farm | 30 | 140 | | 4.0 | 19.0 | 1.0 | 0.0 | 18.0 | 5.0 | 1.5 | 2.5 | 0.0 | 0.00 | 0.00 | 0 | 0 | 0 | 0 | 0 | 0 | 0.14 | 0.07 | 1.20 | | | | | 0.0 | | | 40 | | 0.7 | | | | | | 300 | |
| 43663 | 30 ea | Low sodium, avg | 30 | 151 | 3 | 3.0 | 17.5 | 0.7 | 0.6 | 16.1 | 7.6 | 2.9 | 3.6 | 0.7 | 0.06 | 0.68 | 4 | 49 | 9 | 8 | 1 | | 0.17 | 0.13 | 1.40 | 0.17 | 0.14 | 24.0 | 0.16 | 0.0 | 0.0 | | 45 | 0.1 | 1.4 | 11 | 0.2 | 65 | 32 | 2.6 | 137 | 0.34 |
| 43501 | 4 ea | Peanut butter filling, avg | 28 | 135 | 4 | 3.5 | 16.0 | 0.8 | 1.9 | 13.2 | 6.5 | 1.5 | 3.3 | 1.3 | 0.03 | 1.28 | 1 | 89 | 10 | 9 | 1 | | 0.11 | 0.10 | 1.83 | 0.42 | 0.00 | 24.6 | 0.14 | 0.1 | 0.0 | | 22 | 0.1 | 0.8 | 16 | 0.2 | 91 | 69 | 5.1 | 278 | 0.31 |
| 43594 | 1 ea | Reduced Fat, Snackwells | 30 | 125 | 2 | 3.6 | 23.3 | 0.9 | 0.4 | 21.9 | 2.0 | 0.6 | 0.7 | 0.2 | | | 2 | 63 | 13 | | | | 0.12 | 0.17 | 1.93 | 0.03 | 0.01 | | | 0.1 | | | 20 | 0.0 | 1.5 | 8 | | 47 | 45 | | 339 | 0.31 |
| 43582 | 30 ea | Ritz Bits, Nabisco | 30 | 160 | | 2.0 | 18.0 | 0.0 | 2.0 | 16.0 | 8.0 | 1.0 | 3.0 | 1.0 | | | 0 | | | | | | | | | | | | | | | | 80 | | 1.4 | | | | 30 | | 280 | |
| | | Chili Flavored | | | | | | | | | | | | | | | | | | | | | | | | | | | | | | | | | | | | | | | | |
| 43646 | 15 ea | Fire Hot, w/Cheese, fat free, Health Valley | 30 | 100 | 4 | 4.0 | 22.0 | 4.0 | 2.0 | 16.0 | 0.0 | 0.0 | 0.0 | 0.0 | 0.00 | 0.00 | 0 | 200 | 40 | | | | | | | | | | | 2.4 | | | 0 | | 0.0 | | | | | | 160 | |
| 43645 | 15 ea | Fire Med Jalepeno&Cheese, fat free, Hlth Valley | 30 | 100 | 4 | 4.0 | 22.0 | 4.0 | 2.0 | 16.0 | 0.0 | 0.0 | 0.0 | 0.0 | 0.00 | 0.00 | 0 | 200 | 40 | | | | | | | | | | | 2.4 | | | 0 | | 0.0 | | | | | | 160 | |
| 43644 | 15 ea | Fire Mild, w/Cheese, fat free, Health Valley | 30 | 100 | 4 | 4.0 | 22.0 | 4.0 | 2.0 | 16.0 | 0.0 | 0.0 | 0.0 | 0.0 | 0.00 | 0.00 | 0 | 200 | 40 | | | | | | | | | | | 2.4 | | | 0 | | 0.0 | | | | | | 160 | |
| 43551 | 6 ea | Cuban, avg | 30 | 120 | 7 | 2.3 | 23.0 | 0.6 | 5.9 | 16.4 | 2.0 | 0.5 | 1.1 | 0.3 | | | 0 | 0 | 0 | 0 | 0 | 0 | 0.02 | 0.01 | 0.28 | 0.03 | 0.00 | 4.0 | 0.06 | 0.0 | 0.0 | | 23 | 0.1 | 0.4 | 14 | 0.1 | 28 | 77 | | 77 | 0.17 |
| | | Graham crackers | | | | | | | | | | | | | | | | | | | | | | | | | | | | | | | | | | | | | | | | |
| 43527 | 2 ea | Chocolate coated, avg | 28 | 136 | 3 | 1.6 | 18.6 | 0.9 | 9.8 | 8.0 | 6.5 | 3.8 | 2.2 | 0.3 | 0.02 | 0.27 | 0 | 4 | 0.4 | | | | 0.04 | 0.06 | 0.61 | 0.02 | 0.00 | 4.8 | 0.07 | 0.0 | 0.0 | | 16 | 0.1 | 1.0 | 16 | 0.2 | 38 | 59 | 4.0 | 81 | 0.27 |
| 43640 | 1 ea | Honey, Enriched w/Fiber, Keebler | 21 | 83 | | 1.4 | 16.2 | 1.9 | 5.7 | 8.6 | 2.0 | 0.4 | | | | | 0 | 0 | 0 | 0 | 0 | 0 | | | | | | | | 0.0 | | | 19 | | 0.7 | | | | | | 123 | |
| 43648 | 7 ea | Oat Bran, Fat Free, Healthy Valley | 28 | 97 | 4 | 3.9 | 22.2 | 2.9 | 4.8 | 14.5 | 0.0 | 0.0 | 0.0 | 0.0 | 0.00 | 0.00 | 0 | 97 | 19 | | | | | | | | | | | 0.0 | | | 19 | | 0.7 | | | | | | 29 | |
| 43502 | 4 ea | Plain/Honey, avg | 28 | 118 | 4 | 1.9 | 21.5 | 0.8 | 5.2 | 15.5 | 2.8 | 0.4 | 1.1 | 1.1 | 0.07 | 1.00 | 0 | 0 | 0 | 0 | 0 | 0 | 0.06 | 0.09 | 1.15 | 0.02 | 0.00 | 16.8 | 0.15 | 0.0 | 0.0 | | 7 | 0.1 | 1.0 | 8 | 0.2 | 29 | 38 | 2.9 | 169 | 0.23 |
| 47167 | 4 ea | Plain/Honey, Honey Maid | 28 | 118 | | 2.0 | 21.7 | | | | 2.0 | 0.5 | | | | | | | | | | | | | | | | | | | | | | | | | | | | | 177 | |
| | | Matzoh | | | | | | | | | | | | | | | | | | | | | | | | | | | | | | | | | | | | | | | | |
| 43535 | 1 ea | Egg, avg | 28 | 109 | 6 | 3.4 | 22.0 | 0.8 | 0.3 | 20.9 | 0.6 | 0.2 | 0.2 | 0.1 | 0.01 | 0.13 | 23 | 12 | 4 | 4 | 0 | | 0.22 | 0.17 | 1.42 | 0.02 | 0.05 | 32.8 | 0.12 | 0.0 | 0.0 | | 11 | 0.0 | 0.8 | 7 | 0.2 | 41 | 42 | 7.8 | 6 | 0.20 |
| 43536 | 1 ea | Egg & onion, avg | 28 | 109 | 7 | 2.8 | 21.6 | 1.4 | 1.0 | 19.2 | 1.1 | 0.3 | 0.3 | 0.3 | 0.02 | 0.26 | 13 | 7 | 2 | 2 | 0 | 0 | 0.16 | 0.12 | 1.37 | 0.03 | 0.06 | 44.2 | 0.16 | 0.1 | 0.0 | | 10 | 0.0 | 1.2 | 8 | 0.2 | 25 | 23 | 10.2 | 80 | 0.20 |
| 43534 | 1 ea | Plain, avg | 28 | 111 | 4 | 2.8 | 23.4 | 0.8 | 0.8 | 21.8 | 0.4 | 0.1 | 0.0 | 0.2 | 0.01 | 0.16 | 0 | 0 | 0 | 0 | 0 | 0 | 0.11 | 0.08 | 1.09 | 0.03 | 0.00 | 32.8 | 0.12 | 0.0 | 0.0 | | 4 | 0.0 | 0.9 | 7 | 0.2 | 25 | 31 | 10.3 | 1 | 0.19 |
| 43510 | 1 ea | Whole wheat, avg | 28 | 98 | 5 | 3.7 | 22.1 | 3.3 | 0.5 | 18.3 | 0.4 | 0.1 | 0.1 | 0.2 | 0.01 | 0.17 | 0 | 0 | 0 | 0 | 0 | 0 | 0.10 | 0.08 | 1.51 | 0.04 | 0.00 | 13.4 | 0.35 | 0.0 | 0.0 | | 6 | 0.1 | 1.3 | 38 | 1.0 | 85 | 88 | 21.0 | 1 | 0.73 |
| | | Melba Toast | | | | | | | | | | | | | | | | | | | | | | | | | | | | | | | | | | | | | | | | |
| 43509 | 6 ea | Plain, avg | 30 | 117 | 5 | 3.6 | 23.0 | 1.9 | 0.8 | 20.3 | 1.0 | 0.1 | 0.2 | 0.4 | 0.02 | 0.36 | 0 | 0 | 0 | 0 | 0 | 0 | 0.12 | 0.08 | 1.23 | 0.03 | 0.00 | 37.2 | 0.21 | 0.0 | 0.0 | | 28 | 0.1 | 1.1 | 18 | 0.3 | 59 | 61 | 10.4 | 249 | 0.60 |
| 43566 | 6 ea | Plain, w/o salt, avg | 30 | 117 | 5 | 3.6 | 23.0 | 1.9 | 0.8 | 20.3 | 1.0 | 0.1 | 0.2 | 0.4 | 0.02 | 0.36 | 0 | 0 | 0 | 0 | 0 | 0 | 0.12 | 0.08 | 1.23 | 0.03 | 0.00 | 37.2 | 0.21 | 0.0 | 0.0 | | 28 | 0.1 | 1.1 | 18 | 0.3 | 59 | 61 | 10.4 | 6 | 0.60 |

| Code | Amount | | Description | Basic Components | | | | | | | | | Additional Fats | | | | | | Vit A & Components | | | | | Vitamins | | | | | | | | | | Minerals | | | | | | | | | |
|---|---|---|---|---|---|---|---|---|---|---|---|---|---|---|---|---|---|---|---|---|---|---|---|---|---|---|---|---|---|---|---|---|---|---|---|---|---|---|---|---|---|---|---|
| | | | | Weight (g) | Calories | % Water | Protein (g) | Carbs (g) | Fiber (g) | Sugar (g) | Other Carbs (g) | Fat (g) | Sat Fat (g) | Mono Fat (g) | Poly Fat (g) | Omega 3 (g) | Omega 6 (g) | Choles (mg) | Vit A (IU) | Vit A (RE) | Retinol (RE) | Carotenoids (RE) | Beta Carotene (mcg) | Thiamin (mg) | Riboflavin (mg) | Niacin (NE) | Vit B6 (mg) | Vit B12 (mcg) | Folate (mcg) | Panto (mg) | Vit C (mg) | Vit D (mg) | Vit E (α TE) | Calcium (mg) | Copper (mg) | Iron (mg) | Magnes (mg) | Mang (mg) | Phos (mg) | Potassium (mg) | Selenium (mcg) | Sodium (mg) | Zinc (mg) |
| 43537 | 6 | ea | Rye, avg | 30 | 117 | 5 | 3.5 | 23.2 | 2.4 | 1.0 | 19.8 | 1.0 | 0.1 | 0.3 | 0.4 | 0.03 | 0.37 | 0 | 0 | 0 | 0 | 0 | 0 | 0.14 | 0.09 | 1.42 | 0.03 | 0.00 | 25.5 | 0.15 | 0.0 | 0.0 | | 23 | 0.1 | 1.1 | 12 | 0.2 | 55 | 58 | 11.6 | 270 | 0.41 |
| 43538 | 6 | ea | Wheat, avg | 30 | 112 | 6 | 3.9 | 22.9 | 2.2 | 0.8 | 20.0 | 0.7 | 0.1 | 0.2 | 0.3 | 0.02 | 0.26 | 0 | 0 | 0 | 0 | 0 | 0 | 0.13 | 0.09 | 1.52 | 0.03 | 0.00 | 39.6 | 0.16 | 0.0 | 0.0 | | 13 | 0.1 | 1.4 | 17 | 0.3 | 50 | 44 | 16.5 | 251 | 0.45 |
| 43539 | 3 | ea | Milk cracker, avg | 33 | 150 | 5 | 2.5 | 23.0 | 0.6 | | | 5.2 | 1.0 | 2.9 | 0.7 | 0.05 | 0.70 | 4 | 8 | 2.3 | 2.1 | 0.2 | | 0.18 | 0.14 | 1.46 | 0.01 | 0.03 | 27.1 | 0.13 | 0.1 | | | 57 | 0.1 | 1.2 | 7 | 0.2 | 100 | 38 | 5.2 | 195 | 0.22 |
| 43528 | 15 | ea | Oat Bran cracker, avg | 30 | 131 | 3 | 2.9 | 21.2 | 1.4 | 3.7 | 16.1 | 4.0 | 0.6 | 1.6 | 1.5 | | | 0 | 9 | 1 | 0.6 | 0.3 | | 0.15 | 0.08 | 0.98 | 0.02 | 0.00 | 5.2 | 0.09 | 0.0 | 0.0 | | 26 | 0.1 | 1.2 | 18 | 0.4 | 83 | 62 | | 181 | 0.38 |
| 43507 | 30 | ea | Oyster cracker, avg | 30 | 130 | 4 | 2.8 | 21.5 | 0.9 | 0.5 | 20.1 | 3.5 | 0.9 | 1.9 | 0.5 | 0.03 | 0.48 | 0 | 0 | 0 | 0 | 0 | 0 | 0.17 | 0.14 | 1.58 | 0.01 | 0.00 | 37.2 | 0.14 | 0.0 | 0.0 | | 36 | 0.1 | 1.6 | 8 | 0.2 | 32 | 38 | 3.5 | 391 | 0.23 |
| 43596 | 2 | ea | Pepper Crackers, Snackwells | 30 | 119 | 2 | 3.0 | 25.1 | 1.0 | 2.4 | 21.7 | 0.7 | 0.2 | 0.1 | 0.3 | | | 0 | 0 | 0.1 | | | | 0.11 | 0.13 | 1.57 | 0.02 | | | | 0.2 | | | 52 | 0.1 | 1.5 | 8 | | 102 | 38 | | 296 | 0.27 |
| 49126 | 10 | ea | Pepper Crackers, Water Biscuit, Pepperidge Farm | 30 | 120 | | 4.0 | 24.0 | 1.0 | 0.0 | 23.0 | 2.0 | 1.0 | | | | | 6 | 0 | 0 | 0 | 0 | 0 | | | | | | | | 0.0 | | | 0 | | 0.0 | | | | | | 180 | |
| | | | Pizza Flavored Crackers | | | | | | | | | | | | | | | | | | | | | | | | | | | | | | | | | | | | | | | | |
| 43642 | 15 | ea | Garlic & Herb, Fat Free, Healthy Valley | 30 | 100 | 4 | 4.0 | 22.0 | 4.0 | 2.0 | 16.0 | 0.0 | 0.0 | 0.0 | 0.0 | 0.00 | 0.00 | 0 | 200 | 40 | | | | | | | | | | | 2.4 | | | 0 | | 0.0 | | | | | | 280 | |
| 43624 | 55 | ea | Goldfish, Pepperidge Farm | 30 | 140 | 1 | 3.0 | 19.0 | 1.0 | 1.0 | 17.0 | 6.0 | 1.5 | | | | | 0 | 0 | 0 | 0 | 0 | 0 | 0.22 | 0.14 | 1.60 | | | | | 0.0 | | | 0 | | 1.4 | | | | | | 160 | |
| 43641 | 15 | ea | Italiano, Fat Free, Healthy Valley | 30 | 100 | 4 | 4.0 | 22.0 | 4.0 | 2.0 | 16.0 | 0.0 | 0.0 | 0.0 | 0.0 | 0.00 | 0.00 | 0 | 200 | 40 | | | | | | | | | | | 2.4 | | | 0 | | 0.0 | | | | | | 280 | |
| 43643 | 15 | ea | Zesty Cheese, Fat Free, Healthy Valley | 30 | 100 | 4 | 4.0 | 22.0 | 4.0 | 2.0 | 16.0 | 0.0 | 0.0 | 0.0 | 0.0 | 0.00 | 0.00 | 0 | 200 | 40 | | | | | | | | | | | 2.4 | | | 0 | | 0.0 | | | | | | 280 | |
| 43540 | 3 | ea | Rusk Toast, avg | 30 | 122 | 6 | 4.1 | 21.7 | 0.6 | 0.8 | 20.3 | 2.2 | 0.4 | 0.8 | 0.7 | 0.05 | 0.64 | 23 | 12 | 4 | 4 | 0 | | 0.12 | 0.12 | 1.39 | 0.01 | 0.05 | 26.1 | 0.18 | 0.0 | 0.0 | | 8 | 0.1 | 0.8 | 11 | 0.1 | 46 | 74 | 6.0 | 76 | 0.33 |
| | | | Rye Crackers | | | | | | | | | | | | | | | | | | | | | | | | | | | | | | | | | | | | | | | | |
| 43504 | 3 | ea | Average | 33 | 110 | 5 | 3.2 | 26.5 | 7.6 | 0.7 | 18.3 | 0.3 | 0.0 | 0.1 | 0.1 | 0.02 | 0.12 | 0 | 2 | 0.2 | 0 | 0.2 | | 0.14 | 0.10 | 0.52 | 0.09 | 0.00 | 4.3 | 0.19 | 0.0 | 0.0 | | 13 | 0.2 | 2.0 | 40 | 1.8 | 110 | 163 | 7.9 | 262 | 0.92 |
| 43541 | 4 | ea | Cheese filled, avg | 28 | 135 | 4 | 2.6 | 17.0 | 1.0 | 1.9 | 14.1 | 6.2 | 1.7 | 3.4 | 0.8 | 0.05 | 0.76 | 3 | 94 | 11 | 10 | 1 | | 0.17 | 0.14 | 1.00 | 0.02 | 0.03 | 22.7 | 0.16 | 0.1 | 0.0 | | 62 | 0.0 | 0.7 | 10 | 0.2 | 95 | 96 | 5.8 | 292 | 0.20 |
| 43532 | 3 | ea | Crispbread, avg | 30 | 110 | 6 | 2.4 | 24.7 | 5.0 | 1.0 | 18.8 | 0.4 | 0.0 | 0.0 | 0.2 | 0.02 | 0.14 | 0 | 0 | 0 | 0 | 0 | 0 | 0.07 | 0.04 | 0.31 | 0.06 | 0.00 | 14.1 | 0.20 | 0.0 | 0.0 | | 9 | 0.1 | 0.7 | 23 | 0.7 | 81 | 96 | 11.0 | 79 | 0.72 |
| 43531 | 4 | ea | Crispbread, low sodium, avg | 28 | 96 | 6 | 3.6 | 21.4 | 4.5 | 1.5 | 15.3 | 0.3 | 0.0 | 0.0 | 0.2 | | | 0 | 0 | 0 | 0 | 0 | 0 | 0.09 | 0.07 | 0.34 | 0.08 | 0.00 | 12.6 | 0.17 | 0.0 | 0.0 | | 15 | 0.1 | 1.1 | 34 | 0.6 | 109 | 168 | 6.7 | 66 | 0.78 |
| 43542 | 1 | ea | Seasoned, avg | 22 | 84 | 4 | 2.0 | 16.2 | 4.6 | 0.4 | 11.2 | 2.0 | 0.3 | 0.7 | 0.8 | 0.07 | 0.72 | 0 | 2 | 0.2 | | | | 0.07 | 0.05 | 0.54 | 0.04 | 0.00 | 2.9 | 0.12 | 0.0 | 0.0 | | 10 | 0.1 | 0.7 | 23 | 0.5 | 68 | 100 | 7.2 | 195 | 0.56 |
| | | | Saltine Crackers | | | | | | | | | | | | | | | | | | | | | | | | | | | | | | | | | | | | | | | | |
| 43506 | 10 | ea | Average | 30 | 130 | 4 | 2.8 | 21.5 | 0.9 | 0.5 | 20.1 | 3.5 | 0.9 | 1.9 | 0.5 | 0.03 | 0.48 | 0 | 0 | 0 | 0 | 0 | 0 | 0.17 | 0.14 | 1.58 | 0.01 | 0.00 | 37.2 | 0.14 | 0.0 | 0.0 | | 36 | 0.1 | 1.6 | 8 | 0.2 | 32 | 38 | 3.5 | 391 | 0.23 |
| 43553 | 10 | ea | Low sodium, avg | 30 | 130 | 4 | 2.8 | 21.5 | 0.9 | 0.5 | 20.1 | 3.5 | 0.9 | 1.9 | 0.5 | 0.03 | 0.48 | 0 | 0 | 0 | 0 | 0 | 0 | 0.17 | 0.14 | 1.58 | 0.01 | 0.00 | 37.2 | 0.14 | 0.0 | 0.0 | | 36 | 0.1 | 1.6 | 8 | 0.2 | 32 | 217 | 5.9 | 191 | 0.23 |
| 43664 | 6 | ea | Low sodium, fat-free, avg | 30 | 118 | 3 | 3.2 | 24.7 | 0.8 | 0.5 | 23.4 | 0.5 | 0.1 | 0.0 | 0.2 | 0.01 | 0.19 | 0 | 0 | 0 | 0 | 0 | 0 | 0.16 | 0.18 | 1.71 | 0.03 | 0.00 | 37.2 | 0.12 | 0.0 | 0.0 | | 7 | 0.0 | 2.3 | 8 | 0.2 | 34 | 35 | 6.4 | 191 | 0.28 |
| 43567 | 10 | ea | Unsalted top, avg | 30 | 130 | 4 | 2.8 | 21.5 | 0.9 | 0.5 | 20.1 | 3.5 | 0.9 | 1.9 | 0.5 | 0.03 | 0.48 | 0 | 0 | 0 | 0 | 0 | 0 | 0.17 | 0.14 | 1.58 | 0.01 | 0.00 | 37.2 | 0.14 | 0.0 | 0.0 | | 36 | 0.1 | 1.6 | 8 | 0.2 | 32 | 38 | 3.5 | 230 | 0.23 |
| 43561 | 10 | ea | Whole wheat, avg | 30 | 131 | 2 | 3.3 | 20.9 | 1.9 | 0.5 | 18.5 | 4.1 | 1.0 | 2.2 | 0.6 | | | 0 | 0 | 0 | 0 | 0 | 0 | 0.14 | 0.10 | 1.54 | 0.04 | 0.00 | 6.6 | 0.12 | 0.0 | 0.0 | | 7 | 0.1 | 1.2 | 20 | 0.5 | 58 | 64 | 4.4 | 311 | 0.45 |
| 43585 | 6 | ea | Sesame Bread Wafers, Meal Mates | 30 | 135 | | 3.0 | 21.0 | 3.0 | 0.0 | 18.0 | 4.5 | 0.0 | 1.5 | 0.0 | 0.00 | 0.00 | 0 | | | | | | | | | | | | | | | | 60 | | 2.2 | | | | 60 | | 405 | |
| 49068 | 10 | ea | Water Biscuit, Original, Pepperidge Farm | 30 | 120 | 5 | 4.0 | 22.0 | 1.0 | 0.0 | 21.0 | 2.0 | 1.0 | | | | | 6 | 0 | 0 | 0 | 0 | 0 | | | | | | | | 0.0 | | | 0 | | 0.0 | | | | | | 200 | |
| | | | Wheat Crackers | | | | | | | | | | | | | | | | | | | | | | | | | | | | | | | | | | | | | | | | |
| 43564 | 15 | ea | Average | 30 | 143 | 3 | 2.2 | 19.3 | 1.7 | 0.4 | 17.2 | 6.7 | 2.6 | 3.0 | 0.8 | | | 7 | 15 | 2 | 2 | 0 | | 0.15 | 0.11 | 1.27 | 0.04 | 0.13 | 5.4 | 0.16 | 0.0 | 0.0 | | 10 | 0.1 | 1.0 | 19 | 0.5 | 54 | 59 | 1.9 | 261 | 0.49 |
| 43548 | 4 | ea | Cheese filled, avg | 28 | 139 | 3 | 2.7 | 16.3 | 0.9 | 2.0 | 13.5 | 7.0 | 1.2 | 2.9 | 2.6 | 0.18 | 2.38 | 2 | 20 | 2.5 | 2.3 | 0.2 | | 0.10 | 0.12 | 0.89 | 0.07 | 0.03 | 17.9 | 0.17 | 0.4 | 0.0 | | 57 | 0.0 | 0.7 | 15 | 0.3 | 107 | 86 | 6.8 | 256 | 0.24 |
| 43606 | 4 | ea | Cracked, Pepperidge Farm | 28 | 140 | | 2.0 | 18.0 | 1.0 | 0.0 | 17.0 | 5.0 | 2.0 | 2.0 | 0.0 | 0.00 | 0.00 | 0 | 0 | 0 | 0 | 0 | 0 | 0.06 | 0.00 | 0.00 | | | | | 0.0 | | | 0 | | 0.0 | | | | | | 300 | |
| 43557 | 5 | ea | Crispbread, avg | 30 | 118 | 4 | 3.3 | 24.7 | 0.9 | 0.8 | 23.0 | 0.3 | 0.0 | 0.0 | 0.1 | | | 0 | 0 | 0 | 0 | 0 | 0 | 0.20 | 0.14 | 1.70 | 0.01 | 0.00 | 5.8 | | 0.0 | 0.0 | | 5 | 0.0 | 1.5 | 7 | | 35 | 34 | 1.9 | 149 | 0.23 |
| 43593 | 15 | ea | Fat Free, Snackwells | 30 | 119 | 1 | 3.0 | 24.6 | 1.3 | 4.1 | 19.2 | 0.9 | 0.3 | 0.2 | 0.3 | | | 0 | 2 | 0.5 | | | | 0.08 | 0.14 | 1.46 | 0.03 | 0.05 | | | 0.0 | | | 56 | 0.1 | 1.2 | 14 | | 123 | 86 | | 339 | 0.42 |
| 43569 | 10 | ea | Low salt, avg | 30 | 142 | 3 | 2.6 | 19.5 | 1.4 | 0.4 | 17.7 | 6.2 | 1.6 | 3.4 | 0.8 | 0.04 | 0.80 | 0 | 0 | 0 | 0 | 0 | 0 | 0.15 | 0.10 | 1.49 | 0.04 | 0.00 | 13.2 | 0.16 | 0.0 | 0.0 | | 15 | 0.1 | 1.3 | 19 | 0.5 | 66 | 61 | 1.9 | 85 | 0.48 |
| 43581 | 15 | ea | Original, Nabisco | 30 | 145 | | 2.1 | 19.7 | 2.1 | 2.1 | 15.5 | 6.2 | 1.0 | 2.1 | 0.5 | | | 0 | | | | | | | | | | | | | | | | 21 | | 1.1 | | | | 62 | | 176 | |
| 43549 | 4 | ea | Peanut Butter filled, avg | 28 | 139 | 3 | 3.8 | 15.1 | 1.2 | 1.7 | 12.2 | 7.5 | 1.3 | 3.3 | 2.5 | 0.12 | 2.36 | 0 | 0 | 0 | 0 | 0 | 0 | 0.11 | 0.08 | 1.65 | 0.04 | 0.00 | 19.6 | 0.16 | 0.0 | 0.0 | | 48 | 0.0 | 0.7 | 11 | 0.2 | 97 | 83 | 6.1 | 226 | 0.23 |
| | | | Whole Wheat Crackers | | | | | | | | | | | | | | | | | | | | | | | | | | | | | | | | | | | | | | | | |
| 43563 | 7 | ea | Bran, avg | 28 | 112 | 7 | 2.4 | 19.1 | 3.0 | 0.4 | 15.6 | 3.8 | 0.7 | 2.1 | 0.6 | | | 0 | 0 | 0 | 0 | 0 | 0 | 0.14 | 0.09 | 1.27 | 0.04 | 0.27 | 7.5 | 0.28 | 0.0 | 0.0 | | 7 | 0.1 | 1.0 | 20 | 0.6 | 57 | 38 | 4.1 | 151 | 0.43 |
| 43571 | 10 | ea | Fat Free, Healthy Valley | 30 | 107 | 5 | 4.3 | 23.6 | 4.3 | 2.1 | 17.1 | 0.0 | 0.0 | 0.0 | 0.0 | 0.00 | 0.00 | 0 | 1071 | 214 | | | | | | | | | | | 3.9 | | | 0 | | 0.0 | | | | | | 171 | |
| 43570 | 7 | ea | Low salt | 28 | 124 | 3 | 2.5 | 19.2 | 2.9 | 0.4 | 15.9 | 4.8 | 0.9 | 1.6 | 1.8 | 0.11 | 0.74 | 0 | 0 | 0 | 0 | 0 | 0 | 0.06 | 0.03 | 1.27 | 0.05 | 0.00 | 11.2 | 0.23 | 0.0 | 0.0 | | 14 | 0.1 | 0.9 | 28 | 0.6 | 83 | 83 | 4.1 | 69 | 0.60 |
| 43562 | 7 | ea | 100% | 28 | 113 | 7 | 2.4 | 19.1 | 2.9 | 0.4 | 15.8 | 3.9 | 0.7 | 2.1 | 0.6 | | | 0 | 0 | 0 | 0 | 0 | 0 | 0.14 | 0.08 | 1.23 | 0.04 | 0.27 | 7.3 | | 0.0 | 0.0 | | 6 | 0.1 | 0.9 | 17 | | 53 | 34 | 4.1 | 153 | 0.40 |
| 43508 | 7 | ea | Triscuits | 28 | 124 | 3 | 2.5 | 19.2 | 2.9 | 0.4 | 15.8 | 4.8 | 0.9 | 1.6 | 1.8 | 0.11 | 1.74 | 0 | 0 | 0 | 0 | 0 | 0 | 0.06 | 0.03 | 1.27 | 0.05 | 0.00 | 11.2 | 0.23 | 0.0 | 0.0 | | 14 | 0.1 | 0.9 | 28 | 0.6 | 83 | 83 | 4.1 | 185 | 0.60 |
| | | | *MUFFINS* | | | | | | | | | | | | | | | | | | | | | | | | | | | | | | | | | | | | | | | | |
| 44650 | 1 | ea | Almond Poppyseed Muffin, Krusteaz | 114 | 425 | 28 | 7.5 | 53.6 | 3.6 | 38.8 | 11.2 | 20.3 | 3.5 | 6.0 | 10.7 | | | 75 | 57 | 11 | | | | | | | | | | | 0.0 | | | 71 | | 2.5 | | | 210 | 125 | | 449 | |
| | | | Apple Cinnamon Muffins | | | | | | | | | | | | | | | | | | | | | | | | | | | | | | | | | | | | | | | | |
| 44591 | 1 | oz | Dry Mix, General Mills | 28 | 99 | 25 | 1.1 | 16.2 | 0.2 | 8.4 | 7.6 | 3.4 | 0.8 | 1.3 | 0.2 | | | 6 | | | | | | 0.06 | 0.05 | 0.45 | | | | | | | | 12 | | 0.5 | | | | 22 | | 134 | |
| 44575 | 1 | ea | Pepperidge Farm | 58 | 160 | 36 | 4.0 | 28.0 | 3.0 | 11.0 | 14.0 | 3.5 | 0.5 | 1.0 | 2.0 | | | 0 | 0 | 0 | 0 | 0 | 0 | 0.09 | 0.10 | 1.20 | | | | | 0.0 | | | 20 | | 1.8 | | | | | | 190 | |
| 44668 | 1 | ea | Prepared f/mix, Krusteaz | 57 | 181 | 29 | 2.0 | 33.2 | 1.0 | 18.1 | 14.1 | 4.5 | 1.5 | 2.0 | 1.0 | | | 0 | 0 | 0 | 0 | 0 | 0 | | | | | | | | 0.0 | | | 22 | | 0.5 | | | 90 | 40 | | 332 | |
| 44658 | 1 | ea | Prepared f/mix, low fat, Krusteaz | 57 | 141 | 39 | 2.0 | 31.2 | 1.0 | 18.1 | 12.1 | 1.0 | 0.0 | 0.9 | 0.1 | 0.00 | 0.00 | 0 | 0 | 0 | 0 | 0 | 0 | | | | | | | | 0.0 | | | 59 | | 0.5 | | | 141 | 40 | | 322 | |
| | | | Banana Muffins | | | | | | | | | | | | | | | | | | | | | | | | | | | | | | | | | | | | | | | | |
| 44625 | 1 | ea | Low Fat, Dunkin Donuts | 95 | 240 | 38 | 3.0 | 54.0 | 1.0 | 34.0 | 19.0 | 1.5 | 0.0 | | | | | 0 | 0 | 0 | 0 | 0 | 0 | | | | | | | | 1.2 | | | 0 | | 0.7 | | | | | | 380 | |
| 44550 | 1 | oz | Nut, dry mix, General Mills | 28 | 120 | 7 | 2.0 | 20.4 | 0.6 | 10.1 | 9.7 | 3.4 | 0.4 | 0.8 | 0.8 | | | 0 | | | | | | 0.08 | 0.06 | 0.88 | | | | | | | | 35 | | 0.8 | | | | 54 | | 157 | |
| 44665 | 1 | ea | Nut, Krusteaz | 57 | 191 | 30 | 3.0 | 29.2 | 1.0 | 14.1 | 14.1 | 7.0 | 1.5 | 3.0 | 2.0 | | | 5 | 0 | 0 | 0 | 0 | 0 | | | | | | | | 0.0 | | | 30 | | 0.6 | | | 111 | 70 | | 372 | |
| 44570 | 1 | ea | Nut, Weight Watchers | 71 | 190 | 40 | 3.0 | 32.0 | 3.0 | 13.0 | 16.0 | 5.0 | 1.5 | | | | | 5 | 0 | 0 | 0 | 0 | 0 | | | | | | | | 0.0 | | | 40 | | 1.1 | | | | 105 | | 280 | |
| | | | Basic Muffins | | | | | | | | | | | | | | | | | | | | | | | | | | | | | | | | | | | | | | | | |
| 44636 | 1 | oz | Dry Mix, Krusteaz | 28 | 121 | 6 | 1.6 | 20.7 | 0.4 | 11.5 | 8.9 | 3.5 | 1.0 | 1.8 | 0.7 | | | 0 | 0 | 0 | 0 | 0 | 0 | | | | | | | | 0.0 | | | 2 | | 0.4 | | | 94 | 22 | | 255 | |
| 44655 | 1 | ea | Low Fat, prep f/dry mix, Krusteaz | 57 | 151 | 37 | 2.0 | 32.2 | 1.0 | 21.1 | 10.1 | 1.0 | 0.5 | 0.5 | 0.0 | 0.00 | 0.00 | 0 | 0 | 0 | 0 | 0 | 0 | | | | | | | | 0.0 | | | 73 | | 0.4 | | | 181 | 40 | | 372 | |
| 44660 | 1 | ea | Prepared f/dry mix, Krusteaz | 57 | 181 | 31 | 2.0 | 31.2 | 1.0 | 17.1 | 13.1 | 5.0 | 1.5 | 2.5 | 1.0 | | | 0 | 0 | 0 | 0 | 0 | 0 | | | | | | | | 0.0 | | | 3 | | 0.7 | | | 141 | 30 | | 382 | |
| 44651 | 1 | ea | Blackberry Muffin, Krusteaz | 114 | 420 | 30 | 6.8 | 51.3 | 1.8 | 35.3 | 14.1 | 20.7 | 3.8 | 6.4 | 10.5 | | | 71 | 57 | 11 | | | | | | | | | | | 0.0 | | | 33 | | 1.6 | | | 160 | 123 | | 427 | |
| | | | Blueberry Muffins | | | | | | | | | | | | | | | | | | | | | | | | | | | | | | | | | | | | | | | | |
| 44516 | 1 | ea | Average | 57 | 158 | 38 | 3.1 | 27.4 | 1.5 | 5.7 | 20.2 | 3.7 | 0.8 | 1.1 | 1.4 | 0.10 | 1.32 | 17 | 19 | 5 | 5 | 0.1 | | 0.08 | 0.07 | 0.63 | 0.01 | 0.33 | 25.6 | 0.19 | 0.6 | 0.2 | | 32 | 0.0 | 0.9 | 9 | 0.3 | 112 | 70 | 6.4 | 255 | 0.28 |
| 44517 | 1 | oz | Dry mix, avg | 28 | 102 | 20 | 1.4 | 17.7 | 0.8 | 4.3 | 12.6 | 2.8 | 0.7 | 1.5 | 0.4 | 0.02 | 0.37 | 0 | 3 | 0.3 | 0.3 | 0.01 | | 0.07 | 0.11 | 0.90 | 0.02 | 0.00 | 25.8 | 0.15 | 0.1 | 0.0 | | 7 | 0.0 | 0.4 | 4 | 0.1 | 62 | 24 | 0.9 | 153 | 0.09 |
| 44578 | 1 | ea | Fat Free, Entenmann's | 57 | 120 | | 2.0 | 26.0 | 0.5 | 14.0 | 11.5 | 0.0 | 0.0 | 0.0 | 0.0 | 0.00 | 0.00 | 0 | 100 | 20 | | | | | | | | | | | 0.0 | | | 20 | | 0.0 | | | | 65 | | 220 | |
| 44505 | 1 | ea | Prepared f/dry mix, avg | 50 | 150 | 36 | 2.5 | 24.4 | 0.6 | 5.9 | 18.0 | 4.4 | 0.7 | 1.8 | 1.5 | 0.11 | 1.43 | 23 | 39 | 11 | 9 | 2 | | 0.07 | 0.16 | 1.12 | 0.04 | 0.05 | 5.5 | 0.20 | 0.5 | 0.2 | | 12 | 0.0 | 0.6 | 6 | 0.1 | 94 | 39 | 5.8 | 218 | 0.19 |
| 44667 | 1 | ea | Prepared f/dry mix, Krusteaz | 57 | 171 | 34 | 2.0 | 30.2 | 1.0 | 18.1 | 11.1 | 4.5 | 1.5 | 2.0 | 1.0 | | | 0 | 0 | 0 | 0 | 0 | 0 | | | | | | | | 0.0 | | | 24 | | 0.5 | | | 90 | 40 | | 322 | |
| 44657 | 1 | ea | Prepared f/dry mix, low fat, Krusteaz | 57 | 131 | 43 | 2.0 | 29.2 | 1.0 | 19.1 | 9.0 | 1.0 | 0.0 | 0.5 | 0.5 | 0.00 | 0.00 | 0 | 0 | 0 | 0 | 0 | 0 | | | | | | | | 0.0 | | | 62 | | 0.4 | | | 131 | 40 | | 302 | |
| 44520 | 1 | ea | Prepared f/recipe w/2% milk, avg | 57 | 162 | 40 | 3.7 | 23.2 | 1.1 | 5.6 | 16.5 | 6.2 | 1.2 | 1.5 | 3.1 | 0.36 | 2.71 | 21 | 80 | 22 | 22 | 0.4 | | 0.16 | 0.16 | 1.26 | 0.02 | 0.08 | 27.4 | 0.19 | 0.9 | 0.2 | | 108 | 0.0 | 1.3 | 9 | 0.2 | 83 | 70 | 9.7 | 251 | 0.31 |
| 44501 | 1 | ea | Prepared f/recipe w/whole milk, avg | 57 | 165 | 39 | 3.7 | 23.1 | 1.0 | 5.6 | 16.5 | 6.4 | 1.4 | 1.6 | 3.1 | 0.36 | 2.73 | 22 | 63 | 16 | 15 | 1 | | 0.16 | 0.16 | 1.26 | 0.02 | 0.08 | 6.8 | 0.19 | 0.9 | 0.2 | | 107 | 0.0 | 1.3 | 9 | 0.2 | 82 | 70 | 6.3 | 251 | 0.31 |
| 44518 | 1 | ea | Toaster, avg | 33 | 103 | 31 | 1.5 | 17.6 | 0.6 | 4.2 | 12.8 | 3.1 | 0.5 | 0.7 | 1.8 | 0.20 | 1.56 | 2 | 105 | 22 | 22 | 0.4 | | 0.08 | 0.10 | 0.67 | 0.01 | 0.01 | 18.2 | 0.08 | 0.0 | 0.1 | | 4 | 0.0 | 0.2 | 4 | 0.1 | 19 | 27 | 5.8 | 158 | 0.13 |
| 44569 | 1 | ea | Weight Watchers | 71 | 250 | 20 | 3.5 | 46.0 | 4.0 | 22.0 | 20.0 | 5.0 | 1.0 | 3.0 | 1.0 | | | 45 | 2700 | 540 | | | | | | | | | | | 0.3 | | | 480 | | 0.1 | | | | 92 | | 384 | |

| Code | Amount | Description | Basic Components | | | | | | | | | Additional Fats | | | | | | Vit A & Components | | | | | Vitamins | | | | | | | | | | Minerals | | | | | | | | | |
|---|---|---|---|---|---|---|---|---|---|---|---|---|---|---|---|---|---|---|---|---|---|---|---|---|---|---|---|---|---|---|---|---|---|---|---|---|---|---|---|---|---|---|
| | | | Weight (g) | Calories | % Water | Protein (g) | Carbs (g) | Fiber (g) | Sugar (g) | Other Carbs (g) | Fat (g) | Sat Fat (g) | Mono Fat (g) | Poly Fat (g) | Omega 3 (g) | Omega 6 (g) | Choles (mg) | Vit A (IU) | Vit A (RE) | Retinol (RE) | Carotenoids (RE) | Beta Carotene (mcg) | Thiamin (mg) | Riboflavin (mg) | Niacin (NE) | Vit B6 (mg) | Vit B12 (mcg) | Folate (mcg) | Panto (mg) | Vit C (mg) | Vit D (mg) | Vit E (α TE) | Calcium (mg) | Copper (mg) | Iron (mg) | Magnes (mg) | Mang (mg) | Phos (mg) | Potassium (mg) | Selenium (mcg) | Sodium (mg) | Zinc (mg) |
| 44629 | 1 ea | Bran Muffin, low fat, Dunkin Donuts | 95 | 260 | 30 | 4.0 | 59.0 | 4.0 | 33.0 | 22.0 | 1.5 | 0.0 | | | | | 0 | 0 | 0 | 0 | 0 | 0 | | | | | | | | 0.0 | | | 60 | | 2.7 | | | | | | 440 | |
| 44532 | 1 ea | Buckwheat Muffin, avg | 47 | 144 | 34 | 3.5 | 20.2 | 1.4 | 5.6 | 13.2 | 5.8 | 1.7 | 2.4 | 1.3 | | | 21 | 52 | 14.4 | 13.8 | 0.6 | | 0.10 | 0.12 | 1.11 | 0.07 | 0.07 | 7.9 | 0.14 | 0.1 | 0.2 | | 88 | 0.1 | 0.9 | 31 | 0.2 | 85 | 106 | | 284 | 0.51 |
| 44537 | 1 ea | Carrot Muffin, avg | 58 | 176 | 35 | 3.5 | 25.8 | 1.0 | 9.6 | 15.2 | 6.7 | 1.1 | 1.6 | 3.6 | | | 18 | 2494 | 253 | 20 | 243 | | 0.15 | 0.15 | 1.22 | 0.04 | 0.07 | 7.2 | 0.12 | 1.0 | 0.2 | | 82 | 0.0 | 1.2 | 10 | 0.2 | 68 | 112 | | 251 | 0.30 |
| 44534 | 1 ea | Cheese Muffin, avg | 58 | 184 | 36 | 5.4 | 22.7 | 0.7 | 4.1 | 18.0 | 7.9 | 3.0 | 2.9 | 1.4 | | | 30 | 139 | 35 | 32 | 3 | | 0.17 | 0.20 | 1.34 | 0.03 | 0.11 | 7.6 | 0.17 | 0.1 | 0.3 | | 111 | 0.0 | 1.3 | 10 | 0.2 | 115 | 80 | | 274 | 0.51 |
| 44621 | 1 ea | Cherry, Dunkin Donuts | 95 | 330 | 26 | 5.0 | 53.0 | 1.0 | 28.0 | 24.0 | 11.0 | 2.5 | | | | | 35 | 0 | 0 | 0 | 0 | 0 | | | | | | | | 1.2 | | | 40 | | 1.8 | | | | | | 210 | |
| 44627 | 1 ea | Cherry, low fat, Dunkin Donuts | 95 | 230 | 39 | 3.0 | 53.0 | 0.0 | 35.0 | 18.0 | 1.5 | 0.0 | | | | | 0 | 0 | 0 | 0 | 0 | 0 | | | | | | | | 1.2 | | | 0 | | 0.7 | | | | | | 330 | |
| | | Chocolate Chip Muffins | | | | | | | | | | | | | | | | | | | | | | | | | | | | | | | | | | | | | | | | |
| 44530 | 1 ea | Average | 58 | 190 | 32 | 4.2 | 26.6 | 1.0 | 7.5 | 18.0 | 7.7 | 2.3 | 3.0 | 1.4 | | | 24 | 64 | 17 | 16 | 1 | | 0.17 | 0.18 | 1.37 | 0.03 | 0.09 | 7.5 | 0.17 | 0.1 | 0.5 | | 74 | 0.1 | 1.4 | 16 | 0.2 | 75 | 92 | | 136 | 0.42 |
| 44577 | 1 ea | Chocolate, Weight Watchers | 71 | 200 | | 4.0 | 39.1 | 1.0 | 23.0 | 15.0 | 4.0 | 1.5 | | | | | 5 | 0 | 0 | 0 | 0 | 0 | | | | | | | | 2.4 | | | 40 | | 1.8 | | | | 240 | | 250 | |
| 44597 | 1 oz | Dry Mix, General Mills | 28 | 129 | 5 | 1.7 | 19.6 | 0.5 | 11.2 | 7.9 | 5.0 | 1.3 | 1.9 | 0.3 | | | 7 | | | | | | 0.06 | 0.05 | 0.45 | | | | | | | | 11 | | 0.6 | | | | 82 | | 144 | |
| 44555 | 1 oz | Cinnamon, dry mix, Redi Mix | 28 | 111 | 7 | 1.6 | 20.7 | 0.6 | | | 2.5 | 0.7 | 1.3 | 0.4 | | | 0 | 23 | 5 | 5 | 0 | | 0.10 | 0.08 | 0.87 | | | 3.7 | 0.10 | 0.1 | | | 28 | 0.0 | 0.8 | 4 | | 114 | 37 | 1.6 | 275 | 0.14 |
| | | Corn Meal Muffins | | | | | | | | | | | | | | | | | | | | | | | | | | | | | | | | | | | | | | | | |
| 44521 | 1 ea | Average | 57 | 174 | 33 | 3.4 | 29.0 | 1.9 | 4.6 | 22.5 | 4.8 | 0.3 | 1.2 | 1.8 | 0.10 | 1.73 | 15 | 119 | 21 | 13 | 7 | | 0.16 | 0.19 | 1.16 | 0.05 | 0.05 | 35.3 | 0.25 | 0.0 | 0.3 | | 42 | 0.2 | 1.6 | 18 | 0.2 | 162 | 39 | 8.7 | 297 | 0.31 |
| 44551 | 1 oz | Cornbread, dry mix, General Mills | 28 | 113 | 10 | 2.0 | 20.2 | 0.4 | 6.2 | 13.6 | 2.8 | 0.3 | 1.2 | 0.2 | | | 6 | 32 | 3 | 0 | 3 | | 0.11 | 0.09 | 0.95 | | | | | | | | 36 | | 0.8 | | | | 34 | | 232 | |
| 44628 | 1 ea | Low Fat, Dunkin Donuts | 95 | 250 | 35 | 4.0 | 55.0 | 1.0 | 24.0 | 30.0 | 2.0 | 0.0 | | | | | 0 | 0 | 0 | 0 | 0 | 0 | | | | | | | | 0.0 | | | 0 | | 1.1 | | | | | | 450 | |
| 44504 | 1 ea | Prepared f/dry mix, avg | 50 | 160 | 30 | 3.7 | 24.5 | 1.2 | 3.9 | 19.5 | 5.1 | 1.4 | 2.6 | 0.6 | 0.04 | 0.59 | 31 | 105 | 23 | 15 | 8 | | 0.12 | 0.14 | 1.05 | 0.05 | 0.08 | 5.5 | 0.23 | 0.1 | 0.3 | | 38 | 0.0 | 1.0 | 10 | 0.1 | 192 | 66 | 7.6 | 398 | 0.32 |
| 44524 | 1 ea | Prepared f/recipe w/2% milk, avg | 57 | 180 | 33 | 4.0 | 25.2 | 1.9 | 4.0 | 19.3 | 7.0 | 1.3 | 1.7 | 3.5 | 0.40 | 3.11 | 24 | 137 | 29 | 19 | 10 | | 0.17 | 0.18 | 1.36 | 0.05 | 0.09 | 35.3 | 0.20 | 0.2 | 0.3 | | 148 | 0.0 | 1.5 | 13 | 0.1 | 101 | 83 | 7.6 | 333 | 0.35 |
| 44503 | 1 ea | Prepared f/recipe w/whole milk, avg | 57 | 183 | 32 | 4.0 | 25.2 | 1.9 | 4.0 | 19.3 | 7.4 | 1.5 | 1.8 | 3.5 | 0.41 | 3.12 | 26 | 117 | 23 | 17 | 6 | | 0.17 | 0.18 | 1.36 | 0.05 | 0.09 | 9.7 | 0.20 | 0.2 | 0.3 | | 147 | 0.0 | 1.5 | 13 | 0.1 | 100 | 82 | 8.4 | 333 | 0.35 |
| 44522 | 1 ea | Toaster, avg | 33 | 114 | 24 | 1.7 | 19.1 | 0.5 | 3.0 | 15.6 | 3.7 | 0.5 | 0.9 | 2.1 | 0.24 | 1.85 | 4 | 32 | 7 | 4 | 2 | | 0.10 | 0.12 | 0.76 | 0.02 | 0.01 | 18.3 | 0.08 | 0.0 | 0.2 | | 6 | 0.0 | 0.5 | 5 | 0.1 | 50 | 30 | 5.0 | 142 | 0.13 |
| 44624 | 1 ea | Cranberry Orange, low fat, Dunkin Donuts | 95 | 230 | 39 | 3.0 | 53.0 | 1.0 | 33.0 | 19.0 | 1.5 | 0.0 | | | | | 0 | 0 | 0 | 0 | 0 | 0 | | | | | | | | 2.4 | | | 0 | | 1.1 | | | | | | 330 | |
| 44617 | 1 ea | Cranberry Orange Nut, Dunkin Donuts | 100 | 310 | 32 | 5.0 | 51.0 | 2.0 | 27.0 | 22.0 | 11.0 | 2.5 | | | | | 30 | 0 | 0 | 0 | 0 | 0 | | | | | | | | 3.6 | | | 40 | | 1.8 | | | | | | 130 | |
| 44549 | 1 oz | Date, dry mix, General Mills | 28 | 111 | 9 | 1.4 | 21.6 | 0.5 | 10.9 | 10.2 | 2.2 | 0.3 | 0.8 | 0.2 | | | 0 | | | | | | 0.08 | 0.05 | 0.72 | | | | | | | | 46 | | 0.7 | | | | 43 | | 160 | |
| 44529 | 1 ea | Fruit Nut Muffin, avg | 58 | 165 | 38 | 4.2 | 25.3 | 0.8 | 7.3 | 17.2 | 5.0 | 1.5 | 2.0 | 1.1 | | | 39 | 34 | 23 | 22 | 1 | | 0.16 | 0.18 | 1.31 | 0.03 | 0.11 | 8.4 | 0.17 | 0.3 | 0.3 | | 81 | 0.0 | 1.2 | 9 | 0.2 | 72 | 71 | | 327 | 0.34 |
| 44571 | 1 ea | Harvest Honey Bran, Weight Watchers | 71 | 220 | 27 | 3.0 | 43.0 | 10.0 | 15.0 | 18.0 | 4.0 | 1.0 | | | | | 0 | 100 | 20 | | | | | | | | | | | 0.0 | | | 20 | | 1.1 | | | | 115 | | 150 | |
| 44664 | 1 ea | Honeybran, prep f/dry mix, Krusteaz | 57 | 171 | 33 | 3.0 | 29.2 | 3.0 | 13.1 | 13.1 | 5.0 | 1.0 | 3.0 | 1.0 | | | 5 | 0 | 0 | 0 | 0 | 0 | | | | | | | | 0.0 | | | 62 | | 1.5 | | | 221 | 251 | | 422 | |
| 44602 | 1 oz | Lemon Poppy Seed, dry mix, General Mills | 28 | 125 | 7 | 1.7 | 19.9 | 0.2 | 10.1 | 9.6 | 4.4 | 1.1 | 1.6 | 0.6 | | | 8 | | | | | | 0.08 | 0.06 | 0.57 | | | | | | | | 27 | | 0.6 | | | | 30 | | 164 | |
| 44620 | 1 ea | Lemon Poppy Seed, Dunkin Donuts | 95 | 360 | 19 | 6.0 | 57.0 | 1.0 | 30.0 | 26.0 | 13.0 | 3.0 | | | | | 40 | 0 | 0 | 0 | 0 | 0 | | | | | | | | 0.0 | | | 150 | | 1.1 | | | | | | 440 | |
| | | Oat Bran Muffins | | | | | | | | | | | | | | | | | | | | | | | | | | | | | | | | | | | | | | | | |
| 44514 | 1 ea | Average | 57 | 154 | 35 | 4.0 | 27.5 | 2.6 | 5.4 | 19.5 | 4.2 | 0.5 | 1.0 | 2.4 | 0.26 | 2.09 | 0 | 0 | 0 | 0 | 0 | 0 | 0.15 | 0.05 | 0.24 | 0.09 | 0.01 | 29.6 | 0.58 | 0.0 | 0.0 | | 36 | 0.2 | 2.4 | 89 | 1.5 | 214 | 289 | 6.3 | 224 | 1.05 |
| 44541 | 1 oz | Dry Mix, General Mills | 28 | 121 | 7 | 2.0 | 19.9 | 1.1 | 8.7 | 10.1 | 3.9 | 1.0 | 1.5 | 0.4 | | | 3 | | | | | | 0.07 | 0.05 | 0.56 | | | | | | | | 10 | | 0.8 | | | | 40 | | 188 | |
| 44659 | 1 ea | Prepared f/dry mix, Krusteaz | 57 | 161 | 34 | 3.0 | 32.2 | 1.0 | 14.1 | 17.1 | 2.0 | 1.0 | 0.5 | 0.5 | | | 0 | 0 | 0 | 0 | 0 | 0 | | | | | | | | 0.0 | | | 30 | | 1.1 | | | 101 | 90 | | 322 | |
| 44533 | 1 ea | Oatmeal, avg | 47 | 112 | 47 | 3.2 | 17.4 | 0.7 | 3.1 | 13.6 | 3.2 | 1.0 | 1.2 | 0.7 | | | 18 | 49 | 13 | 12.5 | 0.6 | | 0.13 | 0.13 | 0.95 | 0.02 | 0.07 | 5.5 | 0.09 | 0.1 | 0.2 | | 69 | 0.0 | 0.9 | 9 | 0.2 | 62 | 58 | | 161 | 0.29 |
| 44547 | 1 oz | Orange Cranberry, dry mix, General Mills | 28 | 121 | 7 | 1.4 | 21.0 | 0.7 | 12.6 | 7.7 | 3.4 | 0.9 | 1.2 | 0.3 | | | 6 | | | | | | 0.03 | 0.09 | 0.86 | | | | | | | | 15 | | 0.6 | | | | 40 | | 132 | |
| 44666 | 1 ea | Orange Raisin, prep f/dry mix, Krusteaz | 57 | 171 | 32 | 3.0 | 31.2 | 1.0 | 14.1 | 16.1 | 3.5 | 1.3 | 1.8 | 0.4 | | | 15 | 0 | 0 | 0 | 0 | 0 | | | | | | | | 0.0 | | | 35 | | 0.5 | | | 151 | 70 | | 362 | |
| | | Plain Muffins | | | | | | | | | | | | | | | | | | | | | | | | | | | | | | | | | | | | | | | | |
| 44539 | 1 oz | Dry Mix, General Mills | 28 | 117 | 9 | 1.4 | 20.4 | 0.3 | 11.2 | 9.0 | 3.3 | 0.9 | 1.3 | 0.3 | | | 9 | | | | | | 0.09 | 0.06 | 0.67 | | | | | | | | 38 | | 0.6 | | | | 25 | | 157 | |
| 44515 | 1 ea | Prepared f/recipe w/2% milk, avg | 57 | 169 | 38 | 3.9 | 23.6 | 1.5 | 4.3 | 17.8 | 6.5 | 1.2 | 1.6 | 3.3 | 0.38 | 2.88 | 22 | 80 | 23 | 22 | 0 | | 0.15 | 0.17 | 1.32 | 0.02 | 0.09 | 29.1 | 0.20 | 0.2 | 0.3 | | 114 | 0.0 | 1.4 | 10 | 0.2 | 87 | 69 | 10.3 | 266 | 0.32 |
| 44500 | 1 ea | Prepared f/recipe w/whole milk, avg | 57 | 172 | 37 | 3.9 | 23.6 | 1.5 | 4.3 | 17.8 | 6.8 | 1.5 | 1.7 | 3.3 | 0.38 | 2.89 | 24 | 61 | 17 | 15 | 1 | | 0.15 | 0.17 | 1.32 | 0.02 | 0.09 | 6.8 | 0.20 | 0.2 | 0.3 | | 113 | 0.0 | 1.4 | 9 | 0.2 | 87 | 68 | 6.5 | 266 | 0.32 |
| 44535 | 1 ea | Pumpkin w/Raisins, avg | 58 | 181 | 28 | 2.5 | 34.2 | 1.1 | 22.6 | 10.5 | 4.3 | 0.8 | 1.0 | 2.1 | | | 27 | 3234 | 331 | 12 | 320 | | 0.10 | 0.11 | 0.82 | 0.03 | 0.05 | 6.4 | 0.12 | 0.7 | 0.1 | | 31 | 0.1 | 1.1 | 9 | 0.2 | 41 | 86 | | 154 | 0.21 |
| 44583 | 1 oz | Raisin Bran, dry mix, Gold Medal | 28 | 115 | | 1.4 | 19.9 | 1.0 | 10.1 | 8.8 | 3.6 | 0.9 | 1.4 | 1.3 | | | 5 | | | | | | 0.07 | 0.05 | 0.93 | | | | | | | | 14 | | 0.8 | | | | 69 | | 193 | |
| 44584 | 1 ea | Raisin Bran, prepared f/dry mix, Gold Medal | 65 | 271 | | 3.0 | 46.1 | 2.0 | 23.1 | 21.1 | 8.0 | 2.0 | 3.5 | 1.5 | | | 10 | 0 | 0 | 0 | 0 | 0 | 0.15 | 0.10 | 0.20 | | | | | 0.0 | | | 20 | | 0.2 | | | | 160 | | 451 | |
| 44554 | 1 oz | Strawberry, dry mix, Redi Mix | 28 | 113 | 8 | 1.7 | 19.8 | 0.6 | | | 3.1 | 0.8 | 1.7 | 1.4 | | | 0 | 23 | 5 | 5 | 0 | | 0.11 | 0.08 | 0.87 | 0.01 | 0.03 | 3.7 | 0.10 | 0.0 | | | 27 | 0.0 | 0.7 | 4 | | 114 | 32 | 1.6 | 275 | 0.13 |
| | | Wheat Bran Muffins | | | | | | | | | | | | | | | | | | | | | | | | | | | | | | | | | | | | | | | | |
| 44525 | 1 oz | Dry mix, avg | 28 | 111 | 5 | 2.0 | 20.4 | 1.8 | 7.2 | 11.4 | 3.4 | 0.8 | 1.8 | 1.5 | 0.03 | 0.50 | 0 | 0 | 0 | 0 | 0 | 0 | 0.10 | 0.08 | 1.40 | 0.08 | 0.00 | 23.8 | 0.19 | 0.0 | 0.0 | | 10 | 0.1 | 1.0 | 24 | 0.7 | 134 | 56 | 5.0 | 196 | 0.42 |
| 44506 | 1 ea | Prepared f/dry mix, avg | 50 | 138 | 35 | 3.3 | 23.3 | 2.1 | 8.3 | 12.9 | 4.6 | 1.2 | 2.3 | 1.7 | 0.04 | 0.58 | 34 | 51 | 16 | 7 | 9 | | 0.10 | 0.12 | 1.43 | 0.09 | 0.06 | 8.0 | 0.22 | 0.0 | 0.3 | | 16 | 0.1 | 1.3 | 28 | 0.8 | 167 | 74 | 14.4 | 234 | 0.57 |
| 44528 | 1 ea | Prepared f/recipe w/2% milk, avg | 57 | 161 | 35 | 4.0 | 23.9 | 2.2 | 8.4 | 13.3 | 7.0 | 1.3 | 1.7 | 3.6 | 0.42 | 3.17 | 19 | 478 | 143 | 142 | 0.6 | | 0.19 | 0.25 | 2.30 | 0.18 | 0.08 | 29.6 | 0.27 | 4.4 | 0.6 | | 107 | 0.0 | 2.4 | 44 | 0.1 | 162 | 181 | | 335 | 1.57 |
| 44502 | 1 ea | Prepared f/recipe w/whole milk, avg | 57 | 164 | 35 | 4.0 | 23.8 | 4.0 | 8.4 | 11.4 | 7.3 | 1.5 | 1.8 | 3.6 | 0.42 | 3.17 | 21 | 459 | 136 | 135 | 1 | | 0.19 | 0.25 | 2.29 | 0.18 | 0.08 | 29.6 | 0.27 | 4.4 | 0.6 | | 106 | 0.0 | 2.4 | 44 | 0.1 | 162 | 181 | 10.9 | 335 | 1.57 |
| 44526 | 1 ea | Toaster, w/raisins, avg | 36 | 106 | 31 | 1.9 | 18.8 | 2.8 | 6.6 | 9.4 | 3.2 | 0.5 | 0.7 | 1.7 | 0.20 | 1.53 | 6 | 64 | 18 | 8 | 10 | | 0.09 | 0.11 | 0.87 | 0.04 | 0.01 | 11.5 | 0.11 | 0.0 | 0.2 | | 13 | 0.0 | 1.0 | 11 | 0.3 | 71 | 60 | 6.9 | 178 | 0.23 |
| 44531 | 1 ea | Whole Wheat Muffin, avg | 47 | 142 | 33 | 4.0 | 20.0 | 2.5 | 5.5 | 12.0 | 5.8 | 1.7 | 2.3 | 1.4 | | | 21 | 52 | 14 | 14 | 0.6 | | 0.08 | 0.09 | 1.17 | 0.07 | 0.07 | 8.5 | 0.23 | 0.1 | 0.2 | | 89 | 0.1 | 0.9 | 31 | 0.8 | 110 | 119 | | 283 | 0.72 |
| 44656 | 1 ea | Whole Wheat, low fat, prep f/dry mix, Krusteaz | 57 | 151 | 35 | 3.0 | 32.2 | 1.0 | 19.1 | 12.1 | 1.0 | [illegible] | 0.5 | 0.5 | 0.00 | 0.00 | 0 | 0 | 0 | 0 | 0 | 0 | | | | | | | | 0.0 | | | 70 | | 0.6 | | | 151 | 70 | | 382 | |
| 44536 | 1 ea | Zucchini, avg | 58 | 209 | 30 | 3.0 | 26.4 | 0.8 | 13.6 | 12.1 | 10.5 | 1.7 | 2.5 | 5.7 | | | 37 | 105 | 22 | 17 | 5 | | 0.12 | 0.12 | 0.93 | 0.03 | 0.07 | 9.0 | 0.15 | 1.3 | 0.1 | | 41 | 0.0 | 1.2 | 8 | 0.2 | 45 | 68 | | 169 | 0.25 |
| | | *PANCAKES, FRENCH TOAST, AND WAFFLES* | | | | | | | | | | | | | | | | | | | | | | | | | | | | | | | | | | | | | | | | |
| | | *FRENCH TOAST* | | | | | | | | | | | | | | | | | | | | | | | | | | | | | | | | | | | | | | | | |
| 42155 | 1 pce | Frozen, ready to heat, avg | 59 | 126 | 53 | 4.4 | 18.9 | 0.7 | 2.6 | 15.7 | 3.6 | [illegible] | 1.2 | 0.7 | 0.05 | 0.67 | 48 | 110 | 32 | | | | 0.16 | 0.22 | 1.60 | 0.29 | 0.99 | 30.7 | 0.55 | 0.2 | 0.1 | | 63 | 0.0 | 1.3 | 10 | 0.1 | 82 | 79 | 9.9 | 292 | 0.45 |
| | | Prepared f/frozen | | | | | | | | | | | | | | | | | | | | | | | | | | | | | | | | | | | | | | | | |
| 45144 | 1 ea | Cinnamon swirl, Krusteaz | 43 | 88 | 52 | 3.4 | 14.2 | 0.7 | 2.2 | 11.3 | 2.0 | 0.5 | 1.0 | 0.5 | | | 36 | 0 | 0 | 0 | 0 | 0 | | | | | | | | 0.0 | | | 47 | | 0.8 | | | 52 | 68 | | 245 | |
| 45143 | 1 ea | Regular cut, Krusteaz | 43 | 88 | 53 | 3.6 | 13.8 | 0.7 | 1.7 | 11.3 | 2.0 | 0.6 | 0.9 | 0.5 | | | 36 | 0 | 0 | 0 | 0 | 0 | | | | | | | | 0.0 | | | 45 | | 0.8 | | | 44 | 56 | | 239 | |
| 45145 | 1 ea | Thick cut, Krusteaz | 57 | 115 | 53 | 4.7 | 18.2 | 1.0 | 2.8 | 14.4 | 2.7 | 0.6 | 1.5 | 0.5 | | | 48 | 0 | 0 | 0 | 0 | 0 | | | | | | | | 0.0 | | | 60 | | 1.3 | | | 69 | 73 | | 271 | |
| 42156 | 1 pce | Prepared f/recipe w/2% milk, avg | 65 | 149 | 55 | 5.0 | 16.3 | 0.6 | 4.4 | 11.3 | 7.0 | [illegible] | 2.9 | 1.7 | 0.08 | 1.60 | 75 | 315 | 86 | | | | 0.13 | 0.21 | 1.06 | 0.05 | 0.20 | 27.9 | 0.36 | 0.2 | 0.2 | | 65 | 0.0 | 1.1 | 11 | 0.1 | 76 | 87 | 13.1 | 311 | 0.44 |
| 42040 | 1 pce | Prepared f/recipe w/whole milk, avg | 65 | 151 | 54 | 5.0 | 16.2 | 0.5 | 2.7 | 13.0 | 7.3 | [illegible] | 3.0 | 1.7 | 0.09 | 1.61 | 76 | 298 | 81 | 80 | 1 | | 0.13 | 0.21 | 1.06 | 0.05 | 0.20 | 14.9 | 0.36 | 0.2 | 0.5 | 0.0 | 64 | 0.0 | 1.1 | 11 | 0.1 | 76 | 86 | 10.1 | 311 | 0.44 |
| | | *PANCAKES* | | | | | | | | | | | | | | | | | | | | | | | | | | | | | | | | | | | | | | | | |
| | | Blueberry Pancakes | | | | | | | | | | | | | | | | | | | | | | | | | | | | | | | | | | | | | | | | |
| 45081 | 1 ea | Frozen, 4", Aunt Jemima | 35 | 82 | 43 | 2.2 | 15.3 | 0.3 | | | 1.3 | 0.5 | 0.5 | 0.3 | | | 5 | 43 | 13 | | | | 0.08 | 0.11 | 0.71 | 0.02 | 0.21 | 18.2 | 0.33 | 0.1 | | | 22 | 0.0 | 0.6 | 7 | | 125 | 45 | | 261 | 0.33 |
| 45085 | 1 ea | Microwave, 4", Aunt Jemima | 38 | 69 | | 1.7 | 13.0 | 0.6 | | | 1.3 | 0.2 | 0.3 | 0.2 | | | 13 | 0 | 0 | 0 | 0 | 0 | 0.09 | 0.07 | 0.67 | 0.03 | 0.25 | 2.7 | 0.11 | 0.0 | | | 15 | 0.0 | 0.6 | 5 | 0.1 | 96 | 32 | | 278 | 0.15 |
| 45078 | 1 ea | Prepared f/batter mix, 4", Aunt Jemima | 38 | 69 | | 1.7 | 13.0 | 0.6 | | | 1.3 | 0.2 | 0.3 | 0.2 | | | 9 | 0 | 0 | 0 | 0 | 0 | 0.09 | 0.07 | 0.67 | 0.03 | 0.25 | 2.7 | 0.11 | 0.0 | | | 15 | 0.0 | 0.6 | 5 | 0.1 | 96 | 32 | | 231 | 0.15 |
| 45023 | 1 ea | Prepared f/recipe, 4", avg | 38 | 84 | 53 | 2.3 | 11.0 | 0.5 | 3.0 | 7.5 | 3.5 | 0.8 | 0.9 | 1.5 | 0.18 | 1.40 | 21 | 76 | 19 | 19 | 1 | | 0.07 | 0.10 | 0.58 | 0.02 | 0.08 | 13.7 | 0.15 | 0.8 | 0.2 | | 78 | 0.0 | 0.7 | 6 | 0.1 | 57 | 52 | 5.3 | 157 | 0.21 |
| 45024 | 1/4 cup | Buckwheat, incomplete dry mix, avg | 30 | 102 | 9 | 3.3 | 21.4 | 2.5 | 4.1 | 14.3 | 0.8 | [illegible] | 0.2 | 0.3 | 0.02 | 0.28 | 0 | 0 | 0 | 0 | 0 | 0 | 0.16 | 0.07 | 1.23 | 0.13 | 0.00 | 15.0 | 0.12 | 0.0 | 0.0 | | 143 | 0.1 | 1.4 | 57 | 0.5 | 274 | 95 | 3.9 | 416 | 0.77 |
| 45000 | 1 ea | Buckwheat, prep f/incomplete mix, avg | 30 | 62 | 54 | 2.4 | 8.5 | 0.7 | 1.6 | 6.2 | 2.3 | 0.6 | 0.6 | 0.9 | 0.09 | 0.76 | 20 | 70 | 20 | 20 | 0.4 | | 0.05 | 0.08 | 0.41 | 0.04 | 0.10 | 5.1 | 0.15 | 0.2 | 0.3 | | 77 | 0.0 | 0.6 | 17 | 0.2 | 122 | 70 | 2.7 | 160 | 0.35 |
| | | Buttermilk Pancakes | | | | | | | | | | | | | | | | | | | | | | | | | | | | | | | | | | | | | | | | |
| 45063 | 1 oz | Dry Mix, Pioneer Foods | 28 | 99 | 11 | 1.9 | 20.7 | 0.0 | 3.7 | 17.0 | 0.9 | 0.2 | | | | | 0 | 0 | 0 | | | | 0.02 | 0.01 | 0.13 | | | 24.1 | | 0.1 | | | 4 | | 0.8 | | | | 78 | | 480 | |

| Code | Amount | Description | Basic Components | | | | | | | | | Additional Fats | | | | | | Vit A & Components | | | | | Vitamins | | | | | | | | | | Minerals | | | | | | | | | |
|---|---|---|---|---|---|---|---|---|---|---|---|---|---|---|---|---|---|---|---|---|---|---|---|---|---|---|---|---|---|---|---|---|---|---|---|---|---|---|---|---|---|---|
| | | | Weight (g) | Calories | % Water | Protein (g) | Carbs (g) | Fiber (g) | Sugar (g) | Other Carbs (g) | Fat (g) | Sat Fat (g) | Mono Fat (g) | Poly Fat (g) | Omega 3 (g) | Omega 6 (g) | Choles (mg) | Vit A (IU) | Vit A (RE) | Retinol (RE) | Carotenoids (RE) | Beta Carotene (mcg) | Thiamin (mg) | Riboflavin (mg) | Niacin (NE) | Vit B6 (mg) | Vit B12 (mcg) | Folate (mcg) | Panto (mg) | Vit C (mg) | Vit D (mg) | Vit E (α TE) | Calcium (mg) | Copper (mg) | Iron (mg) | Magnes (mg) | Mang (mg) | Phos (mg) | Potassium (mg) | Selenium (mcg) | Sodium (mg) | Zinc (mg) |
| 45080 | 1 ea | Frozen Buttermilk Pancake, 4", Aunt Jemima | 35 | 79 | 45 | 2.3 | 14.8 | 0.5 | | | 1.2 | 0.3 | 0.5 | 0.3 | | | 8 | 0 | 0 | 0 | 0 | 0 | 0.09 | 0.11 | 0.71 | 0.01 | 0.19 | 9.6 | 0.33 | 0.0 | | | 25 | 0.0 | 0.7 | 7 | | 102 | 34 | | 257 | 0.33 |
| 45052 | 1 ea | Microwave, 4", Hungry Jack | 39 | 81 | 50 | 1.7 | 15.5 | 0.4 | 4.1 | 11.0 | 1.4 | 0.3 | | | | | 3 | 5 | 0.5 | | | | | | | | | | | 0.0 | | | 30 | | 0.7 | | | | | | 197 | |
| 45107 | 1 ea | Microwave, Mini, Hungry Jack | 10 | 21 | 50 | 0.4 | 4.0 | 0.1 | 1.1 | 2.8 | 0.3 | 0.1 | | | | | 1 | 1 | 0.3 | | | | | | | | | | | 0.0 | | | 8 | | 0.2 | | | | | | 50 | |
| 45025 | 1 ea | Prepared f/recipe, 4", avg | 38 | 86 | 52 | 2.6 | 10.9 | 0.3 | 2.6 | 8.0 | 3.5 | 0.7 | 0.9 | 1.7 | 0.20 | 1.51 | 22 | 40 | 11 | 11 | 0.2 | | 0.08 | 0.11 | 0.60 | 0.02 | 0.07 | 14.4 | 0.16 | 0.2 | 0.1 | | 60. | 0.0 | 0.6 | 6 | 0.1 | 53 | 55 | 5.7 | 198 | 0.24 |
| 45034 | 1 ea | Cornmeal, 4", avg | 21 | 43 | 56 | 1.1 | 6.6 | 0.3 | 0.8 | 5.5 | 1.3 | 0.3 | 0.5 | 0.4 | | | 9 | 83 | 19 | 16 | 3 | | 0.05 | 0.05 | 0.36 | 0.02 | 0.03 | 3.1 | 0.04 | 0.0 | 0.1 | | 25 | 0.0 | 0.4 | 4 | 0.0 | 19 | 21 | | 42 | 0.10 |
| | | Crepes | | | | | | | | | | | | | | | | | | | | | | | | | | | | | | | | | | | | | | | | |
| 45031 | 1 ea | Chocolate filled, avg | 78 | 119 | 68 | 4.3 | 15.2 | 0.6 | 11.3 | 3.2 | 4.7 | 2.0 | 1.7 | 0.7 | | | 58 | 217 | 58 | 54 | 4 | | 0.07 | 0.20 | 0.43 | 0.04 | 0.27 | 7.9 | 0.31 | 0.5 | 0.7 | | 81 | 0.0 | 0.7 | 12 | 0.1 | 89 | 126 | | 148 | 0.45 |
| 45032 | 1 ea | Fruit filled, avg | 78 | 131 | 63 | 3.6 | 20.8 | 0.9 | 13.9 | 5.9 | 4.0 | 1.3 | 1.5 | 0.8 | | | 63 | 234 | 59 | 53 | 6 | | 0.08 | 0.16 | 0.57 | 0.04 | 0.19 | 9.4 | 0.31 | 4.3 | 0.4 | | 38 | 0.0 | 0.7 | 8 | 0.1 | 59 | 90 | | 124 | 0.34 |
| 45006 | 1 ea | No filling, avg | 102 | 239 | 56 | 8.9 | 22.2 | 0.6 | 5.1 | 16.5 | 12.5 | 4.1 | 4.9 | 2.4 | | | 163 | 307 | 88 | 86 | 2 | | 0.17 | 0.37 | 1.30 | 0.08 | 0.48 | 19.3 | 0.63 | 0.5 | 0.8 | | 93 | 0.0 | 1.6 | 16 | 0.2 | 145 | 159 | 14.9 | 273 | 0.79 |
| 45033 | 1 ea | Suzette, avg | 66 | 161 | 55 | 4.1 | 15.5 | 0.3 | | | 9.3 | 4.2 | 3.2 | 1.2 | | | 84 | 288 | 76 | 71 | 5 | | 0.08 | 0.17 | 0.60 | 0.04 | 0.22 | 11.2 | 0.33 | 3.0 | 0.5 | | 45 | 0.0 | 0.8 | 9 | 0.1 | 68 | 84 | | 162 | 0.37 |
| 45045 | 1 ea | Indian, prep f/rice flour & dried peas, avg | 29 | 52 | 56 | 2.2 | 9.8 | 0.7 | | | 0.4 | 0.2 | 0.1 | 0.1 | | | 1 | 10 | 2.4 | 2 | 0.4 | | 0.04 | 0.04 | 0.30 | 0.04 | 0.08 | 9.3 | | 0.2 | 0.0 | | 29 | 0.0 | 0.2 | 10 | | 40 | 84 | | 59 | 0.31 |
| 45065 | 1 oz | Multigrain, dry mix, Millers Price | 28 | 102 | 13 | 1.9 | 19.9 | 0.3 | 4.1 | 15.6 | 1.6 | 0.4 | | | | | 0 | 0 | 0 | | | | 0.49 | 0.65 | 0.85 | | | 22.1 | | 0.1 | | | 0 | | 0.8 | | | | 25 | | 503 | |
| 45124 | 1/4 cup | Oat Bran, dry mix, Arrowhead Mills | 30 | 105 | 14 | 5.3 | 18.8 | 4.5 | 3.0 | 11.3 | 1.1 | 0.0 | | | | | 0 | 0 | 0 | 0 | 0 | 0 | 0.17 | 0.10 | 0.60 | | | | | 0.0 | | | 112 | | 1.3 | | | | 232 | | 120 | |
| | | Plain Pancakes | | | | | | | | | | | | | | | | | | | | | | | | | | | | | | | | | | | | | | | | |
| 45019 | 1/4 cup | Dry mix, complete, avg | 32 | 120 | 9 | 3.2 | 22.8 | 0.9 | 5.2 | 16.8 | 1.6 | 0.3 | 0.5 | 0.5 | 0.03 | 0.48 | 7 | 22 | 6 | 6 | 0.1 | | 0.16 | 0.15 | 1.18 | 0.06 | 0.12 | 32.3 | 0.23 | 0.1 | 0.8 | | 77 | 0.1 | 1.0 | 12 | 0.2 | 208 | 109 | 8.3 | 389 | 0.23 |
| 45026 | 1 oz | Dry mix, low sodium, w/fructose, avg | 28 | 98 | 11 | 2.5 | 20.7 | 0.8 | 4.7 | 15.1 | 0.4 | 0.1 | 0.1 | 0.2 | 0.01 | 0.16 | 0 | 35 | 5 | 5 | 0 | | 0.10 | 0.06 | 0.92 | 0.01 | 0.00 | 30.0 | 0.10 | 0.0 | 0.0 | | 28 | 0.0 | 0.9 | 13 | 0.2 | 167 | 189 | 7.0 | 128 | 0.33 |
| 45049 | 1 oz | Dry Mix, extra light, complete, Pillsbury | 28 | 99 | 11 | 2.4 | 19.3 | 0.6 | 3.3 | 15.5 | 1.4 | 0.3 | | | | | 0 | 27 | 3 | | | | | | | | | | | 0.0 | | | 74 | | 1.2 | | | | | | 382 | |
| 45066 | 1 ea | Frozen, RTE, 4", avg | 36 | 82 | 45 | 1.9 | 15.7 | 0.6 | 3.6 | 11.5 | 1.2 | 0.3 | 0.4 | 0.3 | 0.02 | 0.32 | 3 | 36 | 10 | 10 | 0.2 | | 0.14 | 0.17 | 1.44 | 0.03 | 0.06 | 18.0 | 0.16 | 0.1 | 0.4 | | 22 | 0.0 | 1.3 | 5 | 0.1 | 134 | 26 | 5.7 | 183 | 0.24 |
| 45079 | 1 ea | Frozen, 4", Aunt Jemima | 35 | 81 | 43 | 2.2 | 15.4 | 0.4 | | | 1.2 | 0.4 | 0.5 | 0.3 | | | 5 | 27 | 8 | 8 | 0 | | 0.08 | 0.14 | 0.71 | 0.02 | 8.58 | 0.1 | 0.33 | 0.0 | | | 22 | 0.0 | 0.4 | 6 | | 121 | 440 | | 257 | 0.33 |
| 45084 | 1 ea | Microwave, 4", Aunt Jemima | 38 | 62 | | 1.9 | 12.3 | 0.6 | | | 0.8 | 0.2 | 0.3 | 0.2 | | | 6 | 0 | 0 | 0 | 0 | 0 | 0.09 | 0.07 | 0.69 | 0.01 | 0.10 | 5.0 | 0.13 | 0.0 | | | 18 | 0.0 | 0.6 | 5 | 0.1 | 105 | 34 | | 269 | 0.14 |
| 45002 | 1 ea | Prepared f/complete dry mix, 4", avg | 38 | 74 | 53 | 2.0 | 13.9 | 0.5 | 3.2 | 10.3 | 0.9 | 0.2 | 0.3 | 0.3 | 0.02 | 0.29 | 5 | 12 | 3 | 3 | 0 | | 0.08 | 0.08 | 0.65 | 0.03 | 0.08 | 3.4 | 0.09 | 0.1 | 0.5 | | 48 | 0.0 | 0.6 | 8 | 0.1 | 127 | 66 | 3.4 | 239 | 0.15 |
| 45001 | 1 ea | Prepared f/recipe, 4", avg | 38 | 86 | 53 | 2.4 | 10.8 | 0.6 | 2.4 | 7.8 | 3.7 | 0.8 | 0.9 | 1.7 | 0.20 | 1.49 | 22 | 74 | 21 | 20 | 0.4 | | 0.08 | 0.11 | 0.60 | 0.02 | 0.08 | 14.4 | 0.15 | 0.1 | 0.3 | | 83 | 0.0 | 0.7 | 6 | 0.1 | 60 | 50 | 5.7 | 167 | 0.21 |
| 45009 | 1 oz | Potato, dry griddle mix, DCA Foods | 28 | 95 | 12 | 2.5 | 20.2 | | | | 0.6 | | | | | | | 29 | 9 | 9 | 0 | | 0.15 | 0.08 | 1.18 | | | | | 2.8 | | | 20 | | 2.9 | | | | 255 | | 529 | |
| 45036 | 1 ea | Rye, 4", avg | 21 | 63 | 36 | 1.3 | 9.5 | 0.6 | | | 2.2 | 0.6 | 0.9 | 0.6 | | | 8 | 15 | 4 | 4 | 0.1 | | 0.04 | 0.05 | 0.34 | 0.04 | 0.03 | 2.3 | 0.08 | 0.1 | 0.0 | | 22 | 0.0 | 0.5 | 15 | 0.1 | 24 | 96 | | 54 | 0.17 |
| 45035 | 1 ea | Sourdough, 4", avg | 21 | 46 | 52 | 1.2 | 7.2 | 0.3 | 1.6 | 5.3 | 1.4 | 0.3 | 0.4 | 0.6 | | | 8 | 12 | 4 | 4 | 0 | | 0.06 | 0.06 | 0.55 | 0.02 | 0.02 | 8.3 | 0.08 | 0.0 | 0.0 | | 3 | 0.0 | 0.5 | 3 | 0.0 | 16 | 17 | | 46 | 0.11 |
| 45136 | 1 oz | Swedish, dry mix, Krusteaz | 28 | 101 | 11 | 3.4 | 20.7 | 0.4 | 4.2 | 16.2 | 0.5 | 0.1 | 0.1 | 0.3 | | | 0 | 0 | 0 | 0 | 0 | 0 | | | | | | | | 0.0 | | | 15 | | 0.7 | | | 41 | 79 | | 156 | |
| 45151 | 1 ea | Swedish, prep f/dry mix, 7", Krusteaz | 40 | 75 | 59 | 3.0 | 10.0 | 0.0 | 2.0 | 8.0 | 3.0 | 1.5 | 1.0 | 0.5 | | | 62 | 97 | 29 | | | | | | | | | | | 0.0 | | | 14 | | 0.5 | | | 40 | 50 | | 105 | |
| 45130 | 1/4 cup | Whole Grain, dry mix, Arrowhead Mills | 35 | 120 | 9 | 5.0 | 24.0 | 4.0 | 2.0 | 18.0 | 0.5 | 0.0 | | | | | 0 | 0 | 0 | 0 | 0 | 0 | 0.15 | 0.10 | 1.20 | | | | | 0.0 | | | 100 | | 1.1 | | | | 170 | | 260 | |
| | | Whole Wheat Pancakes | | | | | | | | | | | | | | | | | | | | | | | | | | | | | | | | | | | | | | | | |
| 45028 | 1/4 cup | Dry mix, incomplete, avg | 35 | 120 | 9 | 4.5 | 24.9 | 2.4 | 4.6 | 17.8 | 0.5 | 0.1 | 0.1 | 0.2 | 0.01 | 0.20 | 0 | 11 | 1 | 1 | 0.02 | | 0.20 | 0.38 | 2.37 | 0.08 | 0.00 | 28.7 | 0.26 | 0.0 | 0.0 | | 157 | 0.2 | 2.7 | 36 | 0.8 | 274 | 156 | 13.3 | 497 | 0.69 |
| 45008 | 1 ea | Prep f/dry mix, 4", avg | 44 | 92 | 53 | 3.7 | 12.9 | 1.2 | 2.4 | 9.3 | 2.9 | 0.8 | 0.8 | 1.1 | 0.12 | 0.94 | 27 | 99 | 28 | 28 | 1 | | 0.09 | 0.23 | 1.02 | 0.05 | 0.13 | 9.2 | 0.23 | 0.2 | 0.3 | 0.0 | 110 | 0.0 | 1.4 | 20 | 0.7 | 164 | 123 | 10.4 | 252 | 0.46 |
| 45134 | 1 oz | With honey, dry mix, Krusteaz | 28 | 98 | 11 | 3.9 | 19.3 | 1.4 | 2.5 | 15.4 | 0.9 | 0.2 | 0.3 | 0.4 | | | 3 | 0 | 0 | 0 | 0 | 0 | | | | | | | | 0.0 | | | 84 | | 1.1 | | | 211 | 98 | | 212 | |
| 45149 | 1 ea | With honey, prep f/dry mix, 5", Krusteaz | 53 | 99 | 52 | 4.0 | 19.2 | 1.3 | 2.7 | 15.2 | 0.8 | 0.2 | 0.2 | 0.3 | | | 3 | 0 | 0 | 0 | 0 | 0 | | | | | | | | 0.0 | | | 84 | | 1.1 | | | 212 | 99 | | 212 | |
| | | ***WAFFLES*** | | | | | | | | | | | | | | | | | | | | | | | | | | | | | | | | | | | | | | | | |
| 45098 | 1 ea | Apple Cinnamon, 4", Eggo | 39 | 110 | 38 | 2.5 | 16.5 | 0.0 | 3.5 | 13.0 | 4.0 | 0.8 | | | | | 10 | 500 | 150 | | | | 0.15 | 0.17 | 2.00 | 0.20 | 0.60 | 40.0 | | 0.0 | | | 20 | | 1.8 | | | | 20 | | 225 | |
| | | Belgian Waffles | | | | | | | | | | | | | | | | | | | | | | | | | | | | | | | | | | | | | | | | |
| 45057 | 1 oz | Dry mix, General Mills | 28 | 97 | 14 | 2.2 | 20.7 | 0.6 | 1.1 | 19.0 | 0.5 | 0.1 | 0.1 | 0.3 | | | 0 | | | | | | 0.15 | 0.11 | 0.94 | | | | | | | | 90 | | 0.8 | | | | 44 | | 380 | |
| 45111 | 1 ea | Prepared f/dry mix w/eggs & butter, Gen Mills | 102 | 368 | 29 | 8.0 | 46.8 | 1.0 | 3.0 | 42.8 | 16.9 | 9.0 | 5.0 | 1.0 | | | 129 | 498 | 100 | | | | 0.30 | 0.34 | 1.99 | | | | | 0.0 | | | 199 | | 1.8 | | | | 129 | | 1015 | |
| 45142 | 1 ea | Prepared f/frozen, Krusteaz | 68 | 192 | 40 | 4.5 | 29.2 | 1.6 | 6.8 | 20.9 | 6.5 | 1.4 | 3.5 | 1.6 | | | 40 | 0 | 0 | 0 | 0 | 0 | | | | | | | | 0.0 | | | 27 | | 1.5 | | | 177 | 63 | | 484 | |
| 45094 | 1 ea | Blueberry, 4", Eggo | 39 | 110 | 38 | 2.5 | 16.5 | 0.0 | 3.5 | 13.0 | 4.0 | 0.8 | | | | | 10 | 500 | 150 | | | | 0.15 | 0.17 | 2.00 | 0.20 | 0.60 | 40.0 | | 0.0 | | | 20 | | 1.8 | | | | 20 | | 225 | |
| | | Buttermilk Waffles | | | | | | | | | | | | | | | | | | | | | | | | | | | | | | | | | | | | | | | | |
| 45137 | 1 oz | Dry Mix w/egg, Krusteaz | 28 | 115 | 9 | 3.1 | 18.2 | 1.0 | 4.2 | 13.0 | 3.4 | 0.4 | 1.7 | 1.3 | | | 5 | 0 | 0 | 0 | 0 | 0 | | | | | | | | 0.0 | | | 21 | | 0.7 | | | 221 | 62 | | 442 | |
| 45152 | 1 ea | Prepared f/dry mix w/egg, 7", Krusteaz | 81 | 230 | 36 | 6.0 | 37.0 | 2.0 | 9.0 | 26.0 | 7.0 | 1.0 | 3.5 | 2.5 | | | 10 | 0 | 0 | 0 | 0 | 0 | | | | | | | | 0.0 | | | 43 | | 1.5 | | | 450 | 130 | | 900 | |
| 45030 | 1 ea | Prepared f/recipe, 7", avg | 75 | 217 | 42 | 6.2 | 24.8 | 1.1 | 3.2 | 20.4 | 10.2 | 1.9 | 2.5 | 5.1 | 0.59 | 4.50 | 50 | 91 | 26 | 26 | 1 | | 0.20 | 0.27 | 1.55 | 0.04 | 0.16 | 11.3 | 0.36 | 0.4 | 0.2 | | 136 | 0.0 | 1.6 | 14 | 0.2 | 124 | 128 | | 451 | 0.56 |
| 45041 | 1 ea | Cornmeal, 7", avg | 75 | 209 | 42 | 6.2 | 28.1 | 1.3 | 4.3 | 22.5 | 7.8 | 2.0 | 2.2 | 3.0 | | | 75 | 216 | 50 | 42 | 7 | | 0.21 | 0.27 | 1.56 | 0.08 | 0.27 | 16.0 | 0.30 | 0.4 | 0.6 | | 110 | 0.0 | 1.6 | 16 | 0.2 | 108 | 124 | | 312 | 0.55 |
| 45038 | 1 ea | Fruit, 7", avg | 75 | 186 | 43 | 5.5 | 30.4 | 1.3 | 8.3 | 20.9 | 4.7 | 1.8 | 1.6 | 0.9 | | | 34 | 119 | 29 | 26 | 3 | | 0.15 | 0.23 | 0.99 | 0.06 | 0.20 | 7.5 | 0.23 | 2.3 | 0.5 | | 219 | 0.1 | 1.2 | 16 | 0.2 | 262 | 154 | | 523 | 0.53 |
| 45102 | 1 ea | Multi-Bran, 4", Nutri Grain | 39 | 90 | 42 | 2.5 | 16.0 | 3.0 | 2.0 | 11.0 | 3.0 | 0.5 | 1.8 | 0.8 | | | 0 | 500 | 150 | | | | 0.15 | 0.17 | 2.00 | 0.20 | 0.60 | 40.0 | | 0.0 | | | 20 | | 1.8 | | | | 22 | | 200 | |
| 6308 | 1 ea | Nut & Honey, 4", Eggo | 39 | 120 | 35 | 3.0 | 16.0 | 0.0 | 3.5 | 12.5 | 5.0 | 1.0 | | | | | 12 | 500 | 150 | | | | 0.15 | 0.17 | 2.00 | 0.20 | 0.60 | 40.0 | | 0.0 | | | 20 | | 1.8 | | | | 20 | | 240 | |
| 45095 | 1 ea | Oat Bran, 4", Eggo | 39 | 100 | 46 | 3.0 | 13.5 | 1.5 | 1.5 | 10.5 | 3.5 | 0.8 | 2.3 | 0.5 | | | 0 | 500 | 150 | | | | 0.15 | 0.17 | 2.00 | 0.20 | 0.60 | 40.0 | | 0.0 | | | 20 | | 1.8 | | | | 18 | | 175 | |
| | | Plain Waffles | | | | | | | | | | | | | | | | | | | | | | | | | | | | | | | | | | | | | | | | |
| 45061 | 1 oz | Dry Mix, complete, General Mills | 28 | 111 | 15 | 2.2 | 17.9 | 0.4 | 3.1 | 14.4 | 3.4 | 0.5 | 1.3 | 0.5 | | | 0 | | | | | | 0.13 | 0.10 | 1.02 | | | | | | | | 12 | | 0.9 | | | | 36 | | 349 | |
| 45029 | 1 ea | Frozen, ready to heat, 4", avg | 35 | 88 | 45 | 2.1 | 13.5 | 0.8 | 0.9 | 11.8 | 2.7 | 0.5 | 1.1 | 1.0 | 0.07 | 0.90 | 11 | 448 | 134 | 94 | 40 | | 0.16 | 0.18 | 1.64 | 0.33 | 0.83 | 18.5 | 0.21 | 0.0 | 0.3 | | 77 | 0.0 | 1.5 | 7 | 0.1 | 140 | 43 | 6.5 | 262 | 0.19 |
| 45096 | 1 ea | Nutri Grain, 4", Eggo | 39 | 95 | 44 | 2.5 | 15.0 | 2.0 | 2.0 | 11.0 | 3.0 | 0.5 | 1.8 | 0.8 | | | 0 | 500 | 150 | | | | 0.15 | 0.17 | 2.00 | 0.20 | 0.60 | 40.0 | | 0.0 | | | 20 | | 1.8 | | | | 25 | | 215 | |
| 45004 | 1 ea | Prepared f/complete dry mix, 7", avg | 75 | 218 | 42 | 4.6 | 26.4 | 1.0 | 10.0 | 15.3 | 10.3 | 1.7 | 2.7 | 5.2 | 0.57 | 4.60 | 38 | 68 | 20 | 14 | 6 | | 0.15 | 0.19 | 1.23 | 0.08 | 0.19 | 9.0 | 0.25 | 0.2 | 0.4 | | 93 | 0.1 | 1.2 | 15 | 0.2 | 252 | 134 | 13.7 | 458 | 0.35 |
| 45003 | 1 ea | Prepared f/recipe, 7", avg | 75 | 218 | 42 | 5.9 | 24.7 | 1.1 | 3.2 | 20.4 | 10.6 | 2.2 | 2.6 | 5.1 | 0.59 | 4.50 | 52 | 171 | 49 | 47 | 2 | | 0.20 | 0.26 | 1.55 | 0.04 | 0.19 | 34.5 | 0.36 | 0.3 | 0.6 | | 191 | 0.0 | 1.7 | 14 | 0.2 | 142 | 119 | 34.7 | 383 | 0.51 |
| 45103 | 1 ea | Raisin Bran, 4", Nutri Grain | 41 | 105 | 40 | 2.5 | 18.0 | 2.5 | 5.0 | 10.5 | 3.0 | 0.5 | 1.8 | 0.8 | | | 0 | 500 | 150 | | | | 0.15 | 0.17 | 2.00 | 0.20 | 0.60 | 40.0 | | 0.0 | | | 20 | | 1.8 | | | | 55 | | 195 | |
| 45101 | 1 ea | Special K, 4", Eggo | 29 | 70 | 37 | 3.0 | 14.5 | 0.0 | 2.5 | 12.0 | 0.0 | 0.0 | 0.0 | 0.0 | 0.00 | 0.00 | 0 | 500 | 150 | | | | 0.15 | 0.17 | 2.00 | 0.20 | 0.60 | 40.0 | | 0.0 | | | 20 | | 1.8 | | | | 15 | | 125 | |
| 45100 | 1 ea | Strawberry, 4", Eggo | 39 | 110 | 39 | 2.5 | 16.0 | 0.0 | 3.0 | 13.0 | 4.0 | 0.8 | | | | | 10 | 500 | 150 | | | | 0.15 | 0.17 | 2.00 | 0.20 | 0.60 | 40.0 | | 0.0 | | | 20 | | 1.8 | | | | 20 | | 230 | |
| 45037 | 1 ea | Wheat Bran, 4", avg | 38 | 116 | 32 | 3.3 | 16.7 | 2.1 | 6.2 | 8.4 | 4.7 | 1.2 | 1.2 | 2.0 | | | 27 | 205 | 60 | 59 | 1 | | 0.14 | 0.19 | 1.44 | 0.11 | 0.12 | 22.9 | 0.27 | 2.9 | 0.5 | | 83 | 0.1 | 1.4 | 25 | 0.4 | 104 | 123 | | 146 | 0.91 |
| 45083 | 1 ea | Whole Grain, 4", Aunt Jemima | 36 | 78 | 42 | 3.0 | 14.9 | 1.5 | | | 1.4 | 0.4 | 0.6 | 0.3 | | | 3 | 0 | 0 | 0 | 0 | 0 | 0.18 | 0.24 | 2.28 | 0.38 | 1.58 | | | 0.0 | | | 112 | | 2.9 | 17 | | 206 | 89 | | 343 | 0.28 |
| 45016 | 1 ea | Whole Wheat, 4", avg | 39 | 107 | 43 | 3.6 | 12.7 | 1.0 | 2.4 | 9.3 | 4.8 | 1.6 | 1.9 | 1.0 | | | 39 | 91 | 25 | 24 | 1 | | 0.08 | 0.13 | 0.75 | 0.05 | 0.15 | 7.4 | 0.19 | 0.2 | 0.4 | | 84 | 0.0 | 0.7 | 16 | 0.3 | 83 | 90 | | 150 | 0.45 |
| | | ***PASTA*** | | | | | | | | | | | | | | | | | | | | | | | | | | | | | | | | | | | | | | | | |
| 38355 | 2 oz | Angel Hair, dry, DiGiorno | 56 | 160 | | 7.0 | 31.0 | 1.0 | 1.0 | 29.0 | 1.0 | 0.0 | | | | | 0 | 0 | 0 | 0 | 0 | 0 | 0.38 | 0.17 | 3.00 | | | | | 0.0 | | | 0 | | 1.4 | 400 | | 60 | 105 | | 190 | |
| 38151 | 1 cup | Corn, cooked, avg | 140 | 176 | 68 | 3.7 | 39.1 | 6.7 | | | 1.0 | 0.1 | 0.3 | 0.5 | 0.01 | 0.44 | 0 | 80 | 8 | 0 | 8 | | 0.07 | 0.03 | 0.78 | 0.08 | 0.00 | 8.4 | 0.18 | 0.0 | 0.0 | | 1 | 0.1 | 0.3 | 50 | 0.2 | 106 | 43 | 3.9 | 0 | 0.88 |
| 38290 | 1/2 cup | Corn, dry, avg | 52 | 186 | 10 | 3.9 | 41.2 | 5.7 | | | 1.1 | 0.2 | 0.3 | 0.5 | 0.01 | 0.47 | 0 | 88 | 9 | 0 | 9 | | 0.12 | 0.05 | 1.26 | 0.11 | 0.00 | 13.0 | 0.25 | 0.0 | 0.0 | | 2 | 0.1 | 0.5 | 62 | 0.3 | 132 | 153 | 4.1 | 2 | 0.93 |
| 38076 | 1 cup | Couscous, cooked, avg | 157 | 176 | 73 | 6.0 | 36.4 | 2.2 | 0.9 | 33.3 | 0.3 | 0.0 | 0.0 | 0.1 | 0.00 | 0.09 | 0 | 0 | 0 | 0 | 0 | 0 | 0.10 | 0.04 | 1.54 | 0.08 | 0.00 | 23.6 | 0.58 | 0.0 | 0.0 | | 13 | 0.1 | 0.6 | 13 | 0.1 | 35 | 91 | 43.2 | 8 | 0.41 |
| 38281 | 1/2 cup | Couscous, dry, avg | 86 | 323 | 9 | 11.0 | 66.6 | 4.3 | 1.6 | 60.6 | 0.6 | 0.1 | 0.1 | 0.2 | 0.01 | 0.21 | 0 | 0 | 0 | 0 | 0 | 0 | 0.14 | 0.07 | 3.00 | 0.09 | 0.00 | 17.2 | 1.07 | 0.0 | 0.0 | 0.9 | 21 | 0.2 | 0.9 | 38 | 0.7 | 146 | 143 | | 9 | 0.71 |
| | | Fresh Pasta | | | | | | | | | | | | | | | | | | | | | | | | | | | | | | | | | | | | | | | | |
| 38293 | 2 oz | Plain, avg | 57 | 164 | 31 | 6.4 | 31.2 | 2.2 | 1.0 | 28.0 | 1.3 | 0.2 | 0.2 | 0.5 | 0.05 | 0.49 | 42 | 27 | 5 | | | | 0.40 | 0.25 | 1.91 | 0.05 | 0.18 | 100.3 | 0.30 | 0.0 | 0.0 | | 9 | 0.1 | 1.9 | 26 | 0.3 | 93 | 102 | | 15 | 0.70 |
| 38159 | 2 oz | Prepared f/recipe w/egg, avg | 57 | 74 | 69 | 3.0 | 13.4 | 2.2 | 0.7 | 10.4 | 1.0 | 0.2 | 0.3 | 0.3 | 0.03 | 0.27 | 23 | 33 | 10 | 10 | 0 | | 0.10 | 0.10 | 0.72 | 0.02 | 0.06 | 24.5 | 0.13 | 0.0 | 0.0 | | 6 | 0.0 | 0.7 | 8 | 0.1 | 30 | 12 | 12.1 | 47 | 0.25 |

| Code | Amount | Description | Weight (g) | Calories | % Water | Protein (g) | Carbs (g) | Fiber (g) | Sugar (g) | Other Carbs (g) | Fat (g) | Sat Fat (g) | Mono Fat (g) | Poly Fat (g) | Omega 3 (g) | Omega 6 (g) | Choles (mg) | Vit A (IU) | Vit A (RE) | Retinol (RE) | Carotenoids (RE) | Beta Carotene (mcg) | Thiamin (mg) | Riboflavin (mg) | Niacin (NE) | Vit B6 (mg) | Vit B12 (mcg) | Folate (mcg) | Panto (mg) | Vit C (mg) | Vit D (mg) | Vit E (α TE) | Calcium (mg) | Copper (mg) | Iron (mg) | Magnes (mg) | Mang (mg) | Phos (mg) | Potassium (mg) | Selenium (mcg) | Sodium (mg) | Zinc (mg) |
|---|---|---|---|---|---|---|---|---|---|---|---|---|---|---|---|---|---|---|---|---|---|---|---|---|---|---|---|---|---|---|---|---|---|---|---|---|---|---|---|---|---|---|
| | | | **Basic Components** | | | | | | | | | **Additional Fats** | | | | | | **Vit A & Components** | | | | | **Vitamins** | | | | | | | | | | **Minerals** | | | | | | | | | |
| 38093 | 1 cup | Prepared f/recipe w/o egg, avg | 76 | 94 | 69 | 3.3 | 19.1 | 1.2 | 0.8 | 17.0 | 0.7 | 0.1 | 0.1 | 0.4 | 0.04 | 0.34 | 0 | 0 | 0 | 0 | 0 | 0 | 0.14 | 0.11 | 1.02 | 0.02 | 0.00 | 32.7 | 0.11 | 0.0 | 0.0 | | 5 | 0.0 | 0.9 | 11 | 0.1 | 30 | 14 | 3.6 | 56 | 0.28 |
| 38069 | 2 oz | Spinach, cooked, avg | 57 | 74 | 69 | 2.9 | 14.3 | 1.3 | 0.4 | 12.5 | 0.5 | 0.1 | 0.2 | 0.1 | 0.02 | 0.10 | 19 | 59 | 8 | 1 | 7 | | 0.10 | 0.08 | 0.58 | 0.06 | 0.08 | 36.5 | 0.13 | 0.0 | 0.0 | | 10 | 0.0 | 0.6 | 14 | 0.2 | 32 | 21 | | 3 | 0.36 |
| 38303 | 2 oz | Spinach, dry, avg | 57 | 165 | 30 | 6.4 | 31.7 | 1.3 | 1.0 | 28.9 | 1.2 | 0.3 | 0.4 | 0.3 | 0.04 | 0.23 | 42 | 137 | 19 | 3 | 16 | | 0.35 | 0.23 | 1.97 | 0.18 | 0.18 | 100.9 | 0.39 | 0.0 | 0.0 | | 25 | 0.1 | 1.9 | 36 | 0.4 | 84 | 155 | | 15 | 0.80 |
| 38356 | 2 oz | Fettuccini, dry, DiGiorno | 57 | 155 | | 5.7 | 31.8 | 1.5 | 0.8 | 29.3 | 1.2 | 0.0 | | | | | 0 | 0 | 0 | 0 | 0 | 0 | 0.37 | 0.14 | 3.26 | | | | | 0.0 | | | 0 | | 1.5 | 13 | | 49 | 102 | | 132 | |
| 38366 | 1 ea | Lasagna Pasta Sheets, cooked, Bernardi's | 113 | 250 | | 9.0 | 47.0 | 2.0 | 1.0 | 44.0 | 3.0 | 1.0 | | | | | 5 | 0 | 0 | 0 | 0 | 0 | | | | | | | | 0.0 | | | 0 | | 1.8 | | | | | | 15 | |
| | | **Noodles** | | | | | | | | | | | | | | | | | | | | | | | | | | | | | | | | | | | | | | | | |
| 38218 | 2 oz | Buckwheat, dry, avg | 57 | 207 | 12 | 5.9 | 42.8 | 0.2 | | | 0.9 | | | | | | | | | | | | 0.13 | 0.05 | 0.68 | | | | | 0.0 | | | 17 | | 0.6 | | | 128 | | | | |
| 38219 | 1 cup | Buckwheat, prep f/dry, avg | 140 | 162 | 72 | 4.6 | 33.2 | 0.3 | | | 1.0 | | | | | | | | | | | | 0.08 | 0.04 | 0.56 | | | | | 0.0 | | | 14 | | 1.4 | | | 112 | | | | |
| 38390 | 1/2 cup | Cellophane, dry, China Bowl Trading Co | 20 | 70 | 13 | 0.0 | 17.0 | | | | 0.0 | 0.0 | 0.0 | 0.0 | 0.00 | 0.00 | | | | | | | | | | | | | | | | | | | | | | | | | 0 | |
| 38391 | 1/2 cup | Chinese, dry, China Bowl Trading Co | 45 | 150 | 9 | 5.0 | 34.0 | 6.0 | 0.0 | 28.0 | 1.0 | 0.0 | | | 0.00 | 0.00 | | | | | | | | | | | | | | | | | 20 | | 1.8 | | | | | | 0 | |
| 38048 | 1/2 cup | Chow Mein, dry, avg | 22 | 116 | 1 | 1.8 | 12.6 | 0.9 | 0.3 | 11.5 | 6.8 | 1.0 | 1.7 | 3.8 | 0.43 | 3.37 | 0 | 19 | 2 | 0 | 2 | | 0.13 | 0.09 | 1.31 | 0.02 | 0.00 | 19.8 | 0.12 | 0.0 | 0.0 | | 4 | 0.0 | 1.0 | 11 | 0.3 | 35 | 26 | 9.5 | 97 | 0.31 |
| 38347 | 2 oz | Chow Mein, dry, crispy, wide, La Choy | 57 | 300 | 0 | 4.6 | 34.9 | 2.2 | 0.0 | 32.7 | 15.9 | 3.1 | | | | | 0 | 0 | 0 | 0 | 0 | 0 | | | | | | | | 0.0 | | | 1 | | 6.1 | | | | | | 525 | |
| 38251 | 1 cup | Egg, enriched, cooked w/salt, avg | 160 | 213 | 69 | 7.6 | 39.7 | 1.8 | 1.1 | 36.8 | 2.4 | 0.3 | 0.7 | 0.7 | 0.08 | 0.62 | 53 | 32 | 0 | 10 | 0 | | 0.30 | 0.13 | 2.38 | 0.06 | 0.14 | 102.4 | 0.23 | 0.0 | 0.2 | | 19 | 0.1 | 2.5 | 30 | 0.4 | 110 | 45 | 34.7 | 264 | 0.99 |
| 38273 | 1 cup | Egg, unenenriched, cooked w/salt, avg | 160 | 213 | 69 | 7.6 | 39.7 | 2.3 | 1.1 | 36.2 | 2.4 | 0.3 | 0.7 | 0.7 | 0.08 | 0.62 | 53 | 32 | 0 | 10 | 0 | | 0.05 | 0.03 | 0.64 | 0.06 | 0.14 | 11.2 | 0.23 | 0.0 | 0.2 | | 19 | 0.1 | 1.0 | 30 | 0.4 | 110 | 45 | 34.7 | 264 | 0.99 |
| 38259 | 1/2 cup | Egg, unenriched, dry, avg | 19 | 72 | 10 | 2.7 | 13.5 | 0.5 | 0.4 | 12.6 | 0.8 | 0.1 | 0.2 | 0.2 | 0.01 | 0.21 | 18 | 12 | 3 | 3 | 0 | | 0.03 | 0.02 | 0.40 | 0.02 | 0.08 | 5.5 | 0.13 | 0.0 | 0.0 | | 6 | 0.1 | 0.4 | 11 | 0.1 | 41 | 44 | 11.2 | 4 | 0.30 |
| 38160 | 1 cup | Egg/Spinach, cooked, avg | 160 | 211 | 68 | 8.1 | 38.9 | 3.7 | 1.1 | 34.1 | 2.5 | 0.5 | 0.8 | 0.6 | 0.08 | 0.48 | 53 | 165 | 22 | 22 | 0 | | 0.33 | 0.20 | 2.35 | 0.18 | 0.22 | 102.4 | 0.37 | 0.0 | 0.0 | | 30 | 0.1 | 1.7 | 38 | 0.5 | 91 | 59 | 34.9 | 19 | 1.01 |
| 38302 | 1/2 cup | Egg/Spinach, dry, avg | 19 | 73 | 9 | 2.8 | 13.4 | 1.3 | 0.4 | 11.7 | 0.9 | 0.2 | 0.3 | 0.2 | 0.03 | 0.17 | 18 | 60 | 8 | 1.0 | 7 | | 0.21 | 0.09 | 1.25 | 0.08 | 0.08 | 43.9 | 0.17 | 0.0 | 0.0 | | 11 | 0.0 | 0.8 | 16 | 0.2 | 37 | 67 | | 14 | 0.35 |
| 38407 | 2 oz | Japanese, Udon, cooked, avg | 57 | 58 | 76 | 1.4 | 11.6 | 0.1 | | | 0.3 | | | | | | | 0 | 0 | 0 | 0 | 0 | 0.01 | 0.01 | 0.06 | | | | | 0.0 | | | 4 | | 0.1 | | | 10 | 3 | | 26 | |
| 38406 | 2 oz | Japanese, Udon, fresh, avg | 57 | 160 | 33 | 3.9 | 32.5 | 0.1 | | | 0.7 | | | | | | | 0 | 0 | 1 | 0 | 0 | 0.05 | 0.02 | 0.28 | | | | | 0.0 | | | 9 | | 0.3 | | | 31 | 46 | | 342 | |
| | | **Macaroni** | | | | | | | | | | | | | | | | | | | | | | | | | | | | | | | | | | | | | | | | |
| 38102 | 1 cup | Enriched, cooked, avg | 140 | 197 | 66 | 6.7 | 39.6 | 1.8 | 1.8 | 36.0 | 0.9 | 0.1 | 0.1 | 0.4 | 0.03 | 0.35 | 0 | 0 | 0 | 0 | 0 | 0 | 0.29 | 0.14 | 2.34 | 0.05 | 0.00 | 98.0 | 0.16 | 0.0 | 0.0 | | 10 | 0.1 | 2.0 | 25 | 0.4 | 76 | 43 | 29.8 | 1 | 0.74 |
| 38182 | 1 cup | Enriched, protein fortified, cooked, avg | 115 | 189 | 60 | 10.2 | 35.5 | 1.7 | 1.6 | 32.2 | 0.2 | 0.0 | 0.0 | 0.1 | 0.01 | 0.10 | 0 | 0 | 0 | 0 | 0 | 0 | 0.34 | 0.19 | 2.12 | 0.07 | 0.00 | 94.3 | 0.33 | 0.0 | 0.0 | | 11 | 0.1 | 0.8 | 34 | 0.5 | 57 | 48 | 24.5 | 6 | 0.57 |
| 38258 | 1 cup | Unenriched, cooked, avg | 140 | 197 | 66 | 6.7 | 39.6 | 1.8 | 1.8 | 36.0 | 0.9 | 0.1 | 0.1 | 0.4 | 0.03 | 0.35 | 0 | 0 | 0 | 0 | 0 | 0 | 0.03 | 0.03 | 0.56 | 0.05 | 0.00 | 9.8 | 0.16 | 0.0 | 0.0 | | 10 | 0.1 | 0.7 | 25 | 0.4 | 76 | 43 | 29.8 | 1 | 0.74 |
| 38272 | 1/2 cup | Unenriched, dry, avg | 52 | 193 | 10 | 6.7 | 38.8 | 1.2 | 1.8 | 35.3 | 0.8 | 0.1 | 0.1 | 0.3 | 0.03 | 0.31 | 0 | 0 | 0 | 0 | 0 | 0 | 0.05 | 0.03 | 0.88 | 0.06 | 0.00 | 9.4 | 0.22 | 0.0 | 0.0 | | 9 | 0.1 | 0.7 | 25 | 0.4 | 78 | 84 | 32.3 | 4 | 0.63 |
| 38117 | 1 cup | Vegetable, enriched, cooked, avg | 134 | 172 | 68 | 6.1 | 35.6 | 5.8 | 1.5 | 28.4 | 0.1 | 0.0 | 0.0 | 0.1 | 0.01 | 0.05 | 0 | 71 | 7 | 0 | 7 | | 0.15 | 0.08 | 1.43 | 0.03 | 0.00 | 87.1 | 0.47 | 0.0 | 0.0 | | 15 | 0.1 | 0.7 | 25 | 1.3 | 67 | 42 | 26.5 | 8 | 0.59 |
| 38110 | 1 cup | Whole wheat, cooked, avg | 140 | 174 | 67 | 7.5 | 37.1 | 3.9 | 1.1 | 32.1 | 0.8 | 0.1 | 0.1 | 0.3 | 0.01 | 0.28 | 0 | 0 | 0 | 0 | 0 | 0 | 0.15 | 0.06 | 0.99 | 0.11 | 0.00 | 7.0 | 0.59 | 0.0 | 0.0 | | 21 | 0.2 | 1.5 | 42 | 1.9 | 125 | 62 | 36.3 | 4 | 1.13 |
| 38295 | 1/2 cup | Whole wheat, dry, avg | 28 | 97 | 7 | 4.1 | 21.0 | 2.3 | 1.0 | 17.6 | 0.4 | 0.1 | 0.1 | 0.2 | 0.01 | 0.15 | 0 | 0 | 0 | 0 | 0 | 0 | 0.14 | 0.04 | 1.44 | 0.06 | 0.00 | 16.0 | 0.28 | 0.0 | 0.0 | | 11 | 0.1 | 1.0 | 40 | 0.9 | 72 | 60 | | 2 | 0.66 |
| 38067 | 1 cup | Ramen noodles, cooked, avg | 227 | 157 | 82 | 5.5 | 29.3 | 2.8 | 1.6 | 25.0 | 1.7 | 0.4 | 0.5 | 0.5 | | | 39 | 1994 | 204 | 7 | 197 | | 0.22 | 0.10 | 1.75 | 0.06 | 0.10 | 9.1 | 0.17 | 0.2 | 0.0 | | 20 | 0.1 | 1.9 | 25 | | 82 | 50 | 13.0 | 1348 | 0.76 |
| | | **Rice noodles** | | | | | | | | | | | | | | | | | | | | | | | | | | | | | | | | | | | | | | | | |
| 38146 | 1 cup | Cooked, long, avg | 190 | 160 | 79 | 0.1 | 39.3 | 0.2 | | | 0.0 | 0.0 | 0.0 | 0.0 | | | 0 | 0 | 0 | 0 | 0 | 0 | 0.07 | 0.00 | 0.09 | 0.02 | 0.00 | 0.9 | | 0.0 | 0.0 | | 15 | 0.0 | 1.0 | 2 | | 15 | 4 | | 9 | 0.23 |
| 38209 | 1/2 cup | Dried, avg | 70 | 252 | 13 | 3.4 | 57.3 | 0.2 | | | 0.1 | | | | | | | 0 | 0 | 0 | 0 | 0 | 0.03 | 0.01 | 0.21 | | | | | 0.0 | 0.0 | | 8 | | 1.0 | | | 22 | 3 | | 8 | |
| 38210 | 1 cup | Fresh, avg | 140 | 284 | 51 | 3.6 | 64.4 | 0.7 | | | 0.3 | | | | | | | | | | | | 0.06 | 0.01 | 1.82 | | | | | 0.0 | | | 14 | | 3.4 | | | 52 | | | | |
| 38094 | 1 cup | Soba, Japanese, cooked, avg | 114 | 113 | 73 | 5.8 | 24.4 | 1.3 | 0.0 | 23.1 | 0.1 | 0.0 | 0.0 | 0.0 | 0.00 | 0.03 | 0 | 0 | 0 | 0 | 0 | 0 | 0.11 | 0.03 | 0.58 | 0.05 | 0.00 | 8.0 | 0.27 | 0.0 | 0.0 | | 5 | 0.0 | 0.5 | 10 | 0.4 | 28 | 40 | | 68 | 0.14 |
| 38246 | 2 oz | Soba, Japanese, dry, avg | 57 | 192 | 7 | 8.2 | 42.5 | | 0.0 | | 0.4 | 0.1 | 0.1 | 0.1 | 0.01 | 0.12 | 0 | 0 | 0 | 0 | 0 | 0 | 0.27 | 0.07 | 1.83 | 0.14 | 0.00 | 34.2 | 0.54 | 0.0 | 0.0 | | 20 | 0.1 | 1.5 | 54 | 0.7 | 145 | 144 | | 451 | 0.97 |
| 38095 | 1 cup | Somen, Japanese, cooked, avg | 176 | 231 | 68 | 7.0 | 48.4 | 2.8 | 0.0 | 45.6 | 0.3 | 0.0 | 0.0 | 0.1 | 0.01 | 0.12 | 0 | 0 | 0 | 0 | 0 | 0 | 0.04 | 0.06 | 0.17 | 0.02 | 0.00 | 3.5 | 0.30 | 0.0 | 0.0 | | 14 | 0.0 | 0.9 | 4 | 0.4 | 48 | 51 | | 283 | 0.39 |
| 38247 | 2 oz | Somen, Japanese, dry, avg | 57 | 203 | 9 | 6.5 | 42.2 | 2.5 | 0.0 | 39.8 | 0.5 | 0.1 | 0.1 | 0.2 | 0.02 | 0.17 | 0 | 0 | 0 | 0 | 0 | 0 | 0.06 | 0.01 | 0.50 | 0.03 | 0.00 | 8.0 | 0.28 | 0.0 | 0.0 | | 13 | 0.1 | 0.8 | 16 | 0.3 | 46 | 93 | 4.7 | 1049 | 0.26 |
| | | **Spaghetti noodles** | | | | | | | | | | | | | | | | | | | | | | | | | | | | | | | | | | | | | | | | |
| 38121 | 1 cup | Enriched, cooked, avg | 140 | 197 | 66 | 6.7 | 39.6 | 2.4 | 1.8 | 35.4 | 0.9 | 0.1 | 0.1 | 0.4 | 0.03 | 0.35 | 0 | 0 | 0 | 0 | 0 | 0 | 0.29 | 0.14 | 2.34 | 0.05 | 0.00 | 98.0 | 0.16 | 0.0 | 0.0 | | 10 | 0.1 | 2.0 | 25 | 0.4 | 76 | 43 | 29.8 | 140 | 0.74 |
| 38403 | 1 cup | Enriched, protein fortified, cooked, avg | 140 | 230 | 60 | 11.3 | 44.4 | 2.4 | 1.8 | 40.2 | 0.3 | 0.0 | 0.0 | 0.1 | 0.01 | 0.12 | 0 | 0 | 0 | 0 | 0 | 0 | 0.42 | 0.23 | 2.58 | 0.09 | 0.00 | 114.8 | 0.40 | 0.0 | 0.0 | | 14 | 0.1 | 1.0 | 42 | 0.6 | 70 | 59 | 35.3 | 7 | 0.70 |
| 38066 | 1 cup | Spinach, cooked, avg | 140 | 182 | 68 | 6.4 | 36.7 | 4.9 | 1.7 | 30.1 | 0.9 | 0.1 | 0.1 | 0.4 | 0.04 | 0.32 | 0 | 213 | 21 | 0 | 21 | | 0.14 | 0.14 | 2.14 | 0.13 | 0.00 | 16.8 | 0.26 | 0.0 | 0.0 | | 42 | 0.3 | 1.5 | 87 | 2.1 | 151 | 81 | 30.9 | 20 | 1.51 |
| 38062 | 2 oz | Spinach, dry, avg | 57 | 212 | 8 | 7.6 | 42.6 | 6.0 | 1.9 | 34.7 | 0.9 | 0.1 | 0.1 | 0.4 | 0.04 | 0.32 | 0 | 263 | 26 | 0 | 26 | | 0.21 | 0.11 | 2.59 | 0.18 | 0.00 | 27.4 | 0.69 | 0.0 | 0.0 | | 33 | 0.3 | 1.2 | 99 | 1.5 | 189 | 214 | 36.2 | 21 | 1.57 |
| 38274 | 1 cup | Unenriched, cooked w/salt, avg | 140 | 197 | 66 | 6.7 | 39.6 | 2.1 | 1.8 | 35.7 | 0.9 | 0.1 | 0.1 | 0.4 | 0.03 | 0.35 | 0 | 0 | 0 | 0 | 0 | 0 | 0.03 | 0.03 | 0.56 | 0.05 | 0.00 | 9.8 | 0.16 | 0.0 | 0.0 | | 10 | 0.1 | 0.7 | 25 | 0.4 | 76 | 43 | 29.8 | 140 | 0.74 |
| 38261 | 2 oz | Unenriched, dry, avg | 57 | 211 | 10 | 7.3 | 42.6 | 1.4 | 1.9 | 39.3 | 0.9 | 0.1 | 0.1 | 0.4 | 0.03 | 0.34 | 0 | 0 | 0 | 0 | 0 | 0 | 0.05 | 0.03 | 0.97 | 0.06 | 0.00 | 10.3 | 0.25 | 0.0 | 0.0 | | 10 | 0.1 | 0.7 | 27 | 0.4 | 85 | 92 | 35.5 | 4 | 0.69 |
| 38060 | 1 cup | Whole wheat, cooked, avg | 140 | 174 | 67 | 7.5 | 37.1 | 6.3 | 1.1 | 29.7 | 0.8 | 0.1 | 0.1 | 0.3 | 0.01 | 0.28 | 0 | 0 | 0 | 0 | 0 | 0 | 0.15 | 0.06 | 0.99 | 0.11 | 0.00 | 7.0 | 0.59 | 0.0 | 0.0 | | 21 | 0.2 | 1.5 | 42 | 1.9 | 125 | 62 | 36.3 | 4 | 1.13 |
| 38248 | 2 oz | Whole wheat, dry, avg | 57 | 198 | 7 | 8.3 | 42.8 | 7.2 | 2.1 | 33.4 | 0.8 | 0.1 | 0.1 | 0.3 | 0.02 | 0.30 | 0 | 0 | 0 | 0 | 0 | 0 | 0.28 | 0.08 | 2.92 | 0.13 | 0.00 | 32.5 | 0.56 | 0.0 | 0.0 | | 23 | 0.3 | 2.1 | 82 | 1.7 | 147 | 123 | 41.6 | 5 | 1.35 |
| | | **RICE** | | | | | | | | | | | | | | | | | | | | | | | | | | | | | | | | | | | | | | | | |
| 38341 | 1/4 cup | Basmati, brown organic, dry, Lundberg Family Fds | 49 | 168 | 13 | 3.9 | 36.5 | 2.2 | 0.7 | 33.6 | 1.6 | 0.4 | 0.6 | 0.6 | | | 0 | 0 | 0 | 0 | 0 | 0 | | | | | | | | 0.4 | | | 4 | | 0.7 | | | | | | 3 | |
| 38342 | 1/4 cup | Basmati, white organic, dry, Lundberg Family Fds | 51 | 178 | 14 | 4.0 | 39.0 | 1.1 | 0.2 | 37.6 | 0.7 | | | | | | 0 | 0 | 0 | 0 | 0 | 0 | | | | | | | | 0.8 | | | 4 | | 0.2 | | | | | | 4 | |
| 38231 | 1 oz | Black, glutinous, whole grain, dry, avg | 28 | 101 | 12 | 2.1 | 21.6 | 0.2 | | | 0.6 | | | | | | | 0 | 0 | 0 | 0 | 0 | 0.08 | 0.03 | 1.40 | | | | | 0.0 | 0.0 | | 6 | | 1.0 | | | 68 | 81 | | 3 | |
| 38232 | 1 oz | Black, non glutinous, dry, avg | 28 | 101 | 12 | 2.3 | 21.3 | 0.2 | | | 0.6 | | | | | | | | | | | | 0.10 | 0.04 | 1.43 | | | | | 0.0 | 0.0 | | 4 | | 0.5 | | | 74 | 33 | | 1 | |
| | | **Brown Rice** | | | | | | | | | | | | | | | | | | | | | | | | | | | | | | | | | | | | | | | | |
| 38082 | 1/2 cup | Medium grain, cooked, avg | 98 | 110 | 73 | 2.3 | 23.0 | 1.8 | 0.4 | 20.9 | 0.8 | 0.2 | 0.3 | 0.3 | 0.01 | 0.28 | 0 | 0 | 0 | 0 | 0 | 0 | 0.10 | 0.01 | 1.30 | 0.15 | 0.00 | 3.9 | 0.38 | 0.0 | 0.0 | 0.2 | 10 | 0.1 | 0.5 | 43 | 1.1 | 75 | 77 | 6.9 | 1 | 0.61 |
| 38081 | 1/4 cup | Medium grain, dry, avg | 48 | 174 | 12 | 3.6 | 36.6 | 1.6 | 0.3 | 34.6 | 1.3 | 0.3 | 0.5 | 0.5 | 0.02 | 0.44 | 0 | 0 | 0 | 0 | 0 | 0 | 0.20 | 0.02 | 2.07 | 0.24 | 0.00 | 9.6 | 0.72 | 0.0 | 0.0 | 0.3 | 16 | 0.1 | 0.9 | 69 | 1.8 | 127 | 129 | 11.0 | 2 | 0.97 |
| 38427 | 1/4 cup | Long grain, dry, Arrowhead Mills | 43 | 150 | 10 | 3.0 | 33.0 | 2.0 | 0.0 | 31.0 | 1.0 | 0.0 | | | | | 0 | 0 | 0 | 0 | 0 | 0 | 0.15 | 0.03 | 2.00 | | | | | 0.0 | | | 20 | | 0.7 | | | | 90 | | 0 | |
| 38432 | 1/4 cup | Quick, Original, dry, Arrowhead Mills | 32 | 114 | 10 | 2.3 | 24.4 | 1.5 | 0.0 | 22.9 | 0.8 | 0.0 | | | | | 0 | 0 | 0 | 0 | 0 | 0 | 0.09 | 0.03 | 1.52 | | | | | 0.0 | | | 15 | | 0.5 | | | | 65 | | 0 | |
| 38431 | 1/4 cup | Quick, Spanish, dry, Arrowhead Mills | 30 | 112 | 10 | 3.0 | 22.5 | 1.5 | 0.0 | 21.0 | 0.8 | 0.0 | | | | | 0 | 0 | 0 | 0 | 0 | 0 | 0.04 | 0.05 | 1.20 | | | | | 0.0 | | | 15 | | 0.5 | | | | 64 | | 188 | |
| 38430 | 1/4 cup | Quick, Vegetable Herb, dry, Arrowhead Mills | 30 | 112 | 10 | 3.0 | 22.5 | 2.3 | 0.0 | 20.3 | 0.8 | 0.0 | | | | | 0 | 0 | 0 | 0 | 0 | 0 | 0.04 | 0.05 | 1.20 | | | | | 0.0 | | | 15 | | 0.5 | | | | 60 | | 120 | |
| 38429 | 1/4 cup | Quick, Wild Rice & Herb, dry, Arrowhead Mills | 28 | 103 | 10 | 2.9 | 20.6 | 2.2 | 0.0 | 18.4 | 0.7 | 0.0 | | | | | 0 | 0 | 0 | 0 | 0 | 0 | 0.04 | 0.03 | 1.47 | | | | | 0.0 | | | 15 | | 0.3 | | | | 59 | | 162 | |
| 38425 | 1/4 cup | Short grain, dry, Arrowhead Mills | 43 | 170 | 3 | 4.0 | 36.0 | 2.0 | 0.0 | 34.0 | 1.0 | 0.0 | | | | | 0 | 0 | 0 | 0 | 0 | 0 | 0.15 | 0.03 | 2.00 | | | | | 0.0 | | | 20 | | 0.7 | | | | 100 | | 0 | |
| | | **White Rice** | | | | | | | | | | | | | | | | | | | | | | | | | | | | | | | | | | | | | | | | |
| 38157 | 1/2 cup | Enriched, cooked, avg | 93 | 121 | 68 | 2.2 | 26.7 | 0.9 | 0.2 | 25.6 | 0.2 | 0.0 | 0.1 | 0.0 | 0.01 | 0.04 | 0 | 0 | 0 | 0 | 0 | 0 | 0.15 | 0.01 | 1.39 | 0.05 | 0.00 | 54.9 | 0.37 | 0.0 | 0.0 | 0.0 | 1 | 0.1 | 1.4 | 7 | 0.3 | 31 | 24 | 7.0 | 0 | 0.37 |
| 38083 | 1/2 cup | Glutinous, cooked, avg | 87 | 84 | 77 | 1.8 | 18.4 | 0.9 | 0.1 | 17.4 | 0.2 | 0.0 | 0.1 | 0.1 | 0.00 | 0.06 | 0 | 0 | 0 | 0 | 0 | 0 | 0.02 | 0.01 | 0.25 | 0.02 | 0.00 | 0.9 | 0.19 | 0.0 | 0.0 | 0.0 | 2 | 0.0 | 0.1 | 4 | 0.2 | 7 | 9 | 4.9 | 4 | 0.36 |
| 38285 | 1/4 cup | Glutinous, dry, avg | 46 | 170 | 10 | 3.1 | 37.6 | 1.3 | 0.0 | 36.2 | 0.3 | 0.1 | 0.1 | 0.1 | 0.00 | 0.09 | 0 | 0 | 0 | 0 | 0 | 0 | 0.08 | 0.03 | 0.99 | 0.05 | 0.00 | 3.2 | 0.38 | 0.0 | 0.0 | 0.0 | 5 | 0.1 | 0.7 | 11 | 0.4 | 33 | 35 | 6.9 | 3 | 0.55 |
| 38016 | 1/2 cup | Long grain, enriched, cooked, avg | 88 | 100 | 72 | 2.0 | 21.7 | 0.4 | 0.3 | 21.1 | 0.2 | 0.1 | 0.1 | 0.1 | 0.01 | 0.05 | 0 | 0 | 0 | 0 | 0 | 0 | 0.22 | 0.02 | 1.23 | 0.02 | 0.00 | 44.0 | 0.29 | 0.0 | 0.0 | 0.0 | 17 | 0.1 | 1.0 | 11 | 0.2 | 37 | 33 | 7.2 | 3 | 0.27 |
| 38019 | 1/2 cup | Long grain, instant, cooked, avg | 82 | 80 | 76 | 1.7 | 17.5 | 0.5 | 0.2 | 16.8 | 0.1 | 0.0 | 0.0 | 0.0 | 0.01 | 0.03 | 0 | 0 | 0 | 0 | 0 | 0 | 0.06 | 0.04 | 0.72 | 0.01 | 0.00 | 33.6 | 0.15 | 0.0 | 0.0 | 0.0 | 7 | 0.1 | 0.5 | 4 | 0.2 | 11 | 3 | 3.4 | 2 | 0.20 |

| Code | Amount | Description | Basic Components | | | | | | | | | Additional Fats | | | | | | Vit A & Components | | | | | Vitamins | | | | | | | | | | Minerals | | | | | | | | | |
|---|---|---|---|---|---|---|---|---|---|---|---|---|---|---|---|---|---|---|---|---|---|---|---|---|---|---|---|---|---|---|---|---|---|---|---|---|---|---|---|---|---|---|
| | | | Weight (g) | Calories | % Water | Protein (g) | Carbs (g) | Fiber (g) | Sugar (g) | Other Carbs (g) | Fat (g) | Sat Fat (g) | Mono Fat (g) | Poly Fat (g) | Omega 3 (g) | Omega 6 (g) | Choles (mg) | Vit A (IU) | Vit A (RE) | Retinol (RE) | Carotenoids (RE) | Beta Carotene (mcg) | Thiamin (mg) | Riboflavin (mg) | Niacin (NE) | Vit B6 (mg) | Vit B12 (mcg) | Folate (mcg) | Panto (mg) | Vit C (mg) | Vit D (mg) | Vit E (α TE) | Calcium (mg) | Copper (mg) | Iron (mg) | Magnes (mg) | Mang (mg) | Phos (mg) | Potassium (mg) | Selenium (mcg) | Sodium (mg) | Zinc (mg) |
| | | Wild Rice | | | | | | | | | | | | | | | | | | | | | | | | | | | | | | | | | | | | | | | | |
| 38289 | 1/4 cup | Dry, avg | 40 | 143 | 8 | 5.9 | 30.0 | 2.5 | 1.0 | 26.5 | 0.4 | 0.1 | 0.1 | 0.3 | 0.12 | 0.15 | 0 | 8 | 1 | 0 | 1 | | 0.05 | 0.10 | 2.69 | 0.16 | 0.00 | 38.0 | 0.43 | 0.0 | 0.0 | | 8 | 0.2 | 0.8 | 71 | 0.5 | 173 | 171 | 1.1 | 3 | 2.38 |
| 38021 | 1/2 cup | Cooked, avg | 82 | 83 | 74 | 3.3 | 17.5 | 1.5 | 0.6 | 15.4 | 0.3 | 0.0 | 0.0 | 0.2 | 0.08 | 0.10 | 0 | 0 | 0 | 0 | 0 | 0 | 0.04 | 0.07 | 1.06 | 0.11 | 0.00 | 21.3 | 0.13 | 0.0 | 0.0 | 0.0 | 2 | 0.1 | 0.5 | 26 | 0.2 | 67 | 83 | 0.7 | 2 | 1.10 |
| | | *STUFFING AND MIXES* | | | | | | | | | | | | | | | | | | | | | | | | | | | | | | | | | | | | | | | | |
| | | Bread Stuffing | | | | | | | | | | | | | | | | | | | | | | | | | | | | | | | | | | | | | | | | |
| 42560 | 1/2 cup | Beef, dry mix, Stove Top | 30 | 110 | 8 | 4.0 | 22.0 | 1.0 | 4.0 | 17.0 | 1.0 | 0.0 | | | 0.00 | 0.00 | 0 | 500 | 100 | | | | 0.09 | 0.07 | 0.80 | | | | | 0.0 | | | 20 | | 1.1 | | | | 95 | | 520 | |
| 42561 | 1/2 cup | Chicken, dry mix, low sodium, Stove Top | 28 | 110 | | 4.0 | 21.0 | 0.5 | 3.0 | 17.5 | 1.0 | 0.0 | | | 0.00 | 0.00 | 0 | 0 | 0 | 0 | 0 | 0 | 0.09 | 0.07 | 0.80 | | | | | 0.0 | | | 20 | | 1.1 | | | | 85 | | 270 | |
| 42412 | 1/2 cup | Classic Chicken, dry mix, Pepperidge Farm | 34 | 130 | 8 | 5.0 | 24.0 | 3.0 | 3.0 | 18.0 | 1.5 | 0.0 | 1.0 | 0.0 | 0.00 | 0.00 | 0 | 0 | 0 | 0 | 0 | 0 | 0.22 | 0.10 | 2.00 | | | | | 0.0 | | | 30 | | 1.4 | | | | | | 490 | |
| 42409 | 1/2 cup | Country Garden Herb, dry mix, Pepperidge Farm | 34 | 150 | 5 | 4.0 | 22.0 | 2.0 | 4.0 | 16.0 | 5.0 | 1.0 | 1.5 | 1.0 | | | 0 | 0 | 0 | 0 | 0 | 0 | 0.15 | 0.14 | 0.40 | | | | | 0.0 | | | 40 | | 1.8 | | | | | | 360 | |
| 42418 | 1/2 cup | Country Style, dry mix, Pepperidge Farm | 25 | 95 | 5 | 3.4 | 18.2 | 1.4 | 1.4 | 15.5 | 1.0 | 0.0 | 0.7 | 0.0 | 0.00 | 0.00 | 0 | 0 | 0 | 0 | 0 | 0 | 0.10 | 0.07 | 1.08 | | | | | 0.0 | | | 27 | | 1.0 | | | | | | 257 | |
| 42417 | 1/2 cup | Cube, dry mix, Pepperidge Farm | 25 | 95 | 5 | 2.7 | 18.9 | 1.4 | 1.4 | 16.2 | 1.0 | 0.0 | 0.7 | 0.0 | 0.00 | 0.00 | 0 | 0 | 0 | 0 | 0 | 0 | 0.15 | 0.09 | 1.35 | | | | | 0.0 | | | 27 | | 1.2 | | | | | | 358 | |
| 42410 | 1/2 cup | Harvest Veg & Almond, dry mix, Pepperidge Farm | 34 | 140 | 5 | 5.0 | 23.0 | 2.0 | 3.0 | 18.0 | 3.0 | 0.4 | 1.9 | 0.8 | | | 0 | 0 | 0 | 0 | 0 | 0 | 0.15 | 0.14 | 1.60 | | | | | 6.0 | | | 60 | | 3.6 | | | | | | 300 | |
| 42145 | 1 ea | Plain, dry mix, avg, 6 oz pkg | 170 | 656 | 4 | 18.7 | 129.5 | 5.4 | 11.9 | 112.2 | 5.8 | 1.4 | 2.5 | 1.2 | 0.06 | 1.15 | 2 | 2 | 0.2 | 0 | 0.2 | | 1.01 | 0.69 | 9.81 | 0.26 | 0.03 | 244.8 | 0.68 | 0.0 | 0.0 | | 165 | 0.4 | 6.5 | 68 | 1.0 | 240 | 418 | 81.6 | 2703 | 1.58 |
| 42037 | 1/2 cup | Plain, prep f/dry mix, avg | 100 | 178 | 65 | 3.2 | 21.7 | 2.9 | 2.0 | 16.8 | 8.6 | 1.7 | 3.8 | 2.6 | 0.11 | 2.49 | 0 | 313 | 81 | 81 | 0 | | 0.14 | 0.11 | 1.48 | 0.04 | 0.01 | 101.0 | 0.08 | 0.0 | 0.0 | | 32 | 0.1 | 1.1 | 12 | 0.2 | 42 | 74 | 49.8 | 543 | 0.28 |
| 42638 | 1/2 cup | Plain, prep f/dry mix, Stove Top | 108 | 176 | 67 | 4.5 | 20.7 | 3.1 | 2.4 | 15.2 | 8.9 | 5.0 | 3.0 | 0.7 | | | 21 | 358 | 107 | 107 | 0 | | 0.15 | 0.13 | 1.50 | 0.06 | 0.02 | 22.0 | 0.34 | 1.0 | 0.0 | | 41 | 0.1 | 1.2 | 13 | | 62 | 103 | 12.0 | 632 | 0.27 |
| 42038 | 1/2 cup | Plain, prep f/recipe, avg | 116 | 195 | 65 | 4.4 | 25.8 | 2.3 | 3.7 | 19.7 | 8.4 | 1.7 | 3.7 | 2.5 | 0.11 | 2.34 | 0 | 349 | 80 | 80 | 0 | | 0.20 | 0.17 | 1.84 | 0.06 | 0.00 | 19.7 | 0.19 | 2.0 | 0.2 | | 74 | 0.1 | 1.9 | 17 | 0.2 | 57 | 152 | 8.6 | 535 | 0.37 |
| 42564 | 1/2 cup | Pork, dry mix, Stove Top | 28 | 110 | 8 | 4.0 | 20.0 | 1.0 | 3.0 | 16.0 | 1.0 | 0.0 | | | 0.00 | 0.00 | 0 | 0 | 0 | 0 | 0 | 0 | 0.22 | 0.07 | 1.20 | | | | | 0.0 | | | 20 | | 1.1 | | | | 90 | | 500 | |
| 42416 | 1/2 cup | Sage & Onion, dry mix, Pepperidge Farm | 37 | 150 | 5 | 5.0 | 28.0 | 2.0 | 4.0 | 22.0 | 1.5 | 0.0 | 0.5 | 0.0 | 0.00 | 0.00 | 0 | 0 | 0 | 0 | 0 | 0 | 0.22 | 0.14 | 2.00 | | | | | 0.0 | | | 20 | | 2.7 | | | | | | 520 | |
| 42565 | 1/2 cup | San Francisco Style, dry mix, Stove Top | 28 | 110 | 8 | 4.0 | 20.0 | 1.0 | 2.0 | 17.0 | 1.0 | 0.0 | | | 0.00 | 0.00 | 0 | 100 | 20 | | | | 0.09 | 0.07 | 1.20 | | | | | 0.0 | | | 20 | | 1.1 | | | | 95 | | 510 | |
| 42563 | 1/2 cup | Turkey, dry mix, Stove Top | 28 | 110 | 11 | 3.0 | 20.0 | 0.5 | 3.0 | 16.5 | 1.0 | 0.0 | | | 0.00 | 0.00 | 0 | 0 | 0 | 0 | 0 | 0 | 0.09 | 0.07 | 1.20 | | | | | 0.0 | | | 20 | | 1.1 | | | | 85 | | 490 | |
| | | Cornbread Stuffing | | | | | | | | | | | | | | | | | | | | | | | | | | | | | | | | | | | | | | | | |
| 42146 | 1 ea | Dry mix, avg, 6 oz pkg | 170 | 661 | 5 | 17.0 | 130.4 | 24.3 | 5.7 | 100.4 | 7.1 | 1.6 | 2.8 | 1.8 | 0.08 | 1.74 | 0 | 267 | 27 | 22 | 5 | | 0.87 | 0.59 | 8.28 | 0.25 | 0.02 | 236.3 | 0.48 | 6.0 | 0.0 | | 133 | 0.4 | 5.5 | 75 | 0.9 | 192 | 347 | 50.3 | 2181 | 1.28 |
| 42572 | 1/2 cup | Dry mix, microwave, Stove Top | 28 | 120 | | 3.0 | 20.0 | 1.0 | 3.0 | 16.0 | 3.5 | 0.5 | | | | | 0 | 0 | 0 | 0 | 0 | 0 | 0.06 | 0.07 | 0.80 | | | | | 0.0 | | | 0 | | 1.1 | | | | 65 | | 450 | |
| 42407 | 1/2 cup | Honey Pecan, dry mix, Pepperidge Farm | 34 | 140 | 8 | 3.0 | 23.0 | 0.5 | 5.0 | 17.5 | 5.0 | 0.5 | 0.0 | 1.5 | | | 0 | 750 | 150 | | | | 0.22 | 0.10 | 2.00 | | | | | 3.6 | | | 20 | | 1.1 | | | | | | 400 | |
| 42147 | 1/2 cup | Prepared f/dry mix, avg | 100 | 179 | 65 | 2.9 | 21.9 | 2.9 | 1.0 | 18.0 | 8.8 | 1.8 | 3.9 | 2.7 | 0.12 | 2.59 | 0 | 353 | 85 | 68 | 17 | | 0.12 | 0.09 | 1.25 | 0.04 | 0.01 | 97.0 | 0.06 | 0.8 | 0.2 | | 26 | 0.1 | 0.9 | 13 | 0.1 | 34 | 62 | 30.7 | 455 | 0.23 |
| 42411 | 1/2 cup | Wild Rice & Mushroom, dry mix, Pepperidge Farm | 26 | 130 | 5 | 3.8 | 16.8 | 1.5 | 1.5 | 13.8 | 4.6 | 1.1 | 2.3 | 1.1 | | | 0 | 0 | 0 | 0 | 0 | 0 | 0.11 | 0.10 | 1.22 | | | | | 4.6 | | | 31 | | 1.4 | | | | | | 314 | |
| | | *TORTILLAS* | | | | | | | | | | | | | | | | | | | | | | | | | | | | | | | | | | | | | | | | |
| | | Corn Tortillas | | | | | | | | | | | | | | | | | | | | | | | | | | | | | | | | | | | | | | | | |
| 42023 | 1 ea | 6", avg | 26 | 58 | 44 | 1.5 | 12.1 | 1.4 | 0.2 | 10.6 | 0.6 | 0.1 | 0.2 | 0.3 | 0.01 | 0.28 | 0 | 0 | 0 | 0 | 0 | 0 | 0.03 | 0.02 | 0.39 | 0.06 | 0.00 | 29.6 | 0.05 | 0.0 | 0.0 | | 45 | 0.0 | 0.4 | 17 | 0.1 | 82 | 40 | 1.4 | 42 | 0.24 |
| 42297 | 1 ea | 6", unsalted, avg | 26 | 58 | 44 | 1.5 | 12.1 | 1.4 | 0.2 | 10.6 | 0.6 | 0.1 | 0.2 | 0.3 | 0.01 | 0.28 | 0 | 0 | 0 | 0 | 0 | 0 | 0.03 | 0.02 | 0.39 | 0.06 | 0.00 | 29.6 | 0.05 | 0.0 | 0.0 | | 45 | 0.0 | 0.4 | 17 | 0.1 | 82 | 40 | 1.4 | 3 | 0.24 |
| 42168 | 1 ea | Taco shell, baked, 5", avg | 13 | 61 | 6 | 0.9 | 8.1 | 1.0 | 0.1 | 7.0 | 2.9 | 0.4 | 1.2 | 1.1 | 0.07 | 1.03 | 0 | 0 | 0 | 0 | 0 | 0 | 0.03 | 0.01 | 0.18 | 0.04 | 0.00 | 13.6 | 0.06 | 0.0 | 0.0 | | 21 | 0.0 | 0.3 | 14 | 0.1 | 32 | 23 | 1.6 | 48 | 0.18 |
| 42296 | 1 ea | Taco shell, baked, unsalted, 5", avg | 13 | 61 | 6 | 0.9 | 8.1 | 1.0 | 0.1 | 7.0 | 2.9 | 0.4 | 1.2 | 1.1 | 0.07 | 1.03 | 0 | 0 | 0 | 0 | 0 | 0 | 0.03 | 0.01 | 0.18 | 0.04 | 0.00 | 13.6 | 0.06 | 0.0 | 0.0 | | 21 | 0.0 | 0.3 | 14 | 0.1 | 32 | 23 | | 2 | 0.18 |
| 42442 | 1 ea | Taco Shell, Mini, Old El Paso | 4 | 21 | 2 | 0.3 | 2.3 | 0.3 | 0.0 | 2.1 | 1.3 | 0.2 | 0.3 | 0.1 | | | 0 | 0 | 0 | 0 | 0 | 0 | | | | | | | | 0.0 | | | 5 | | 0.1 | | | | | | 17 | |
| 42443 | 1 ea | Taco Shell, Regular, Old El Paso | 11 | 58 | 5 | 0.7 | 6.2 | 0.7 | 0.0 | 5.5 | 3.4 | 0.5 | 1.0 | 0.2 | | | 0 | 0 | 0 | 0 | 0 | 0 | | | | | | | | 0.0 | | | 14 | | 0.2 | | | | | | 45 | |
| 42444 | 1 ea | Taco Shell, Super, Old El Paso | 18 | 92 | 1 | 1.5 | 10.2 | 1.0 | 0.0 | 9.2 | 5.8 | 1.0 | 1.7 | 0.2 | | | 0 | 0 | 0 | 0 | 0 | 0 | | | | | | | | 0.0 | | | 19 | | 0.5 | | | | | | 73 | |
| 42445 | 1 ea | Taco Shell, White, Old El Paso | 11 | 58 | 5 | 0.7 | 6.2 | 0.7 | 0.0 | 5.5 | 3.4 | 0.5 | 1.0 | 0.2 | | | 0 | 0 | 0 | 0 | 0 | 0 | | | | | | | | 0.0 | | | 14 | | 0.2 | | | | | | 10 | |
| 42446 | 1 ea | Tostaco Shell, Old El Paso | 23 | 130 | | 2.0 | 14.0 | 1.0 | 0.0 | 13.0 | 7.0 | 1.0 | 2.0 | 2.0 | | | 0 | 0 | 0 | 0 | 0 | 0 | | | | | | | | 0.0 | | | 40 | | 1.1 | | | | | | 10 | |
| 42447 | 1 ea | Tostada Shell, Old El Paso | 11 | 55 | 2 | 0.7 | 6.5 | 0.7 | 0.0 | 5.8 | 3.4 | 0.7 | 1.0 | 0.2 | | | 0 | 0 | 0 | 0 | 0 | 0 | | | | | | | | 0.0 | | | 14 | | 0.2 | | | | | | 76 | |
| | | Flour Tortillas | | | | | | | | | | | | | | | | | | | | | | | | | | | | | | | | | | | | | | | | |
| 42025 | 1 ea | 10" Flour Tortilla | 72 | 239 | 27 | 6.3 | 40.0 | 2.4 | 0.9 | 36.8 | 5.1 | 1.3 | 2.7 | 0.8 | 0.04 | 0.72 | 0 | 0 | 0 | 0 | 0 | 0 | 0.38 | 0.21 | 2.57 | 0.04 | 0.00 | 88.6 | 0.42 | 0.0 | 0.0 | 0.7 | 90 | 0.2 | 2.4 | 19 | 0.3 | 89 | 94 | 16.9 | 344 | 0.51 |
| 42449 | 1 ea | Soft Taco, Old El Paso | 25 | 90 | 17 | 2.5 | 16.5 | 0.0 | 0.3 | 16.3 | 1.8 | 0.3 | 0.5 | 0.5 | | | 0 | 0 | 0 | 0 | 0 | 0 | | | | | | | | 0.0 | | | 0 | | 0.9 | | | | | | 205 | |
| 42079 | 1 ea | Whole wheat, avg | 35 | 73 | 31 | 2.9 | 20.0 | 1.9 | | | 0.5 | 0.1 | 0.1 | 0.2 | | | 0 | 0 | 0 | 0 | 0 | 0 | 0.10 | 0.02 | 0.85 | 0.07 | 0.00 | 8.4 | 0.21 | 0.0 | 0.0 | | 10 | 0.1 | 0.7 | 26 | 0.1 | 82 | 82 | | 171 | 0.53 |
| | | **GRANOLA BARS, CEREAL BARS, SCONES, AND TARTS** | | | | | | | | | | | | | | | | | | | | | | | | | | | | | | | | | | | | | | | | |
| | | Cereal Bars | | | | | | | | | | | | | | | | | | | | | | | | | | | | | | | | | | | | | | | | |
| 49089 | 1 ea | Apple Bakes, fat free, Health Valley | 27 | 70 | 26 | 2.0 | 18.0 | 2.0 | 11.0 | 5.0 | 0.0 | 0.0 | 0.0 | 0.0 | 0.00 | 0.00 | 0 | 100 | 20 | | | | | | | | | | | 2.4 | | | 0 | | 0.7 | | | | | | 30 | |
| 40255 | 1 ea | Apple Cinnamon Filling, Snackwell's | 37 | 119 | 16 | 1.1 | 29.2 | 1.4 | 17.4 | 10.4 | 0.3 | 0.1 | 0.0 | 0.1 | | | 0 | 1300 | 260 | | | | 0.39 | 0.44 | 5.20 | 0.52 | 0.01 | | | 0.4 | | | 17 | 0.0 | 5.0 | 6 | | 37 | 68 | | 103 | 3.88 |
| 40254 | 1 ea | Blueberry Filling, Snackwell's | 37 | 121 | 16 | 1.0 | 29.3 | 1.2 | 15.8 | 12.4 | 0.3 | 0.0 | 0.0 | 0.1 | | | 0 | 1300 | 260 | | | | 0.39 | 0.44 | 5.20 | 0.52 | 0.01 | | | 0.2 | | | 14 | 0.0 | 4.8 | 5 | | 35 | 44 | | 107 | 3.85 |
| 49081 | 1 ea | Chocolate Sandwich, all flavors, fat free, Health Valley | 52 | 150 | 42 | 3.0 | 26.0 | 3.0 | 18.0 | 5.0 | 0.0 | 0.0 | 0.0 | 0.0 | 0.00 | 0.00 | 0 | 100 | 20 | | | | | | | | | | | 1.2 | | | 0 | | 0.7 | | | | | | 35 | |
| 49090 | 1 ea | Date Bakes, fat free, Health Valley | 27 | 70 | 26 | 2.0 | 18.0 | 2.0 | 11.0 | 5.0 | 0.0 | 0.0 | 0.0 | 0.0 | 0.00 | 0.00 | 0 | 100 | 20 | | | | | | | | | | | 2.4 | | | 0 | | 0.7 | | | | | | 30 | |
| 23265 | 1 ea | Diet Bar, Apple Cinnamon Spice, Nestle Sweet Success | 33 | 120 | 13 | 2.0 | 22.0 | 3.0 | 7.0 | 12.0 | 4.0 | 1.0 | | | | | 0 | 750 | 150 | | | | 0.23 | 0.26 | 3.00 | 0.30 | 0.90 | 60.0 | 1.50 | 9.0 | 1.5 | | 150 | | 2.7 | 60 | | 150 | | | 65 | 0.60 |
| 62180 | 1 ea | Diet Bar, Chocolate Brownie, Nestle Sweet Success | 33 | 120 | 9 | 2.0 | 23.0 | 3.0 | 13.0 | 7.0 | 4.0 | 2.0 | 0.5 | 0.6 | | | 3 | 750 | 150 | | | | 0.22 | 0.25 | 3.00 | 0.30 | 0.90 | 60.1 | 1.50 | 9.0 | 1.5 | | 150 | | 2.7 | 60 | | 150 | 140 | | 45 | 0.59 |
| 62179 | 1 ea | Diet Bar, Chocolate Chip, Nestle Sweet Success | 33 | 120 | 9 | 2.0 | 23.0 | 3.0 | 10.0 | 10.0 | 4.0 | 2.0 | 0.4 | 0.5 | | | 3 | 750 | 150 | | | | 0.22 | 0.25 | 3.00 | 0.30 | 0.90 | 60.1 | 1.50 | 9.0 | 1.5 | | 150 | | 2.7 | 60 | | 150 | 110 | | 40 | 0.59 |
| 62178 | 1 ea | Diet Bar, Chocolate Peanut Butter, Nestle Sweet Success | 33 | 120 | 9 | 2.0 | 23.0 | 3.0 | 12.0 | 8.0 | 4.0 | 2.0 | 0.6 | 0.6 | | | 3 | 750 | 150 | | | | 0.22 | 0.25 | 3.00 | 0.30 | 0.90 | 60.1 | 1.50 | 9.0 | 1.5 | | 150 | | 2.7 | 60 | | 150 | 125 | | 35 | 0.59 |
| 23266 | 1 ea | Oatmeal Raisin, Nestle Sweet Success | 33 | 120 | 13 | 2.0 | 22.0 | 3.0 | 7.0 | 12.0 | 4.0 | 1.0 | | | | | 0 | 750 | 150 | | | | 0.23 | 0.26 | 3.00 | 0.30 | 0.90 | 60.0 | 1.50 | 9.0 | 1.5 | | 150 | | 2.7 | 60 | | 150 | | | 65 | 0.60 |
| 49078 | 1 ea | Fiber 7 Flakes w/Strawberries, fat free, Health Valley | 37 | 110 | 21 | 2.0 | 26.0 | 3.0 | 13.0 | 10.0 | 0.0 | 0.0 | 0.0 | 0.0 | 0.00 | 0.00 | 0 | 100 | 20 | | | | | | | | | | | 1.2 | | | 0 | | 0.7 | | | | | | 25 | |
| 49087 | 1 ea | Marshmallow Tropical Sandwich, fat free, Health Valley | 30 | 90 | 23 | 1.0 | 22.0 | 1.0 | 11.0 | 10.0 | 0.0 | 0.0 | 0.0 | 0.0 | 0.00 | 0.00 | 0 | 20 | 4 | | | | | | | | | | | 2.4 | | | 20 | | 0.7 | | | | | | 0 | |
| 49079 | 1 ea | Oat Bran Flakes w/Blueberries, fat free, Health Valley | 37 | 110 | 21 | 2.0 | 26.0 | 3.0 | 13.0 | 10.0 | 0.0 | 0.0 | 0.0 | 0.0 | 0.00 | 0.00 | 0 | 100 | 20 | | | | | | | | | | | 1.2 | | | 0 | | 0.7 | | | | | | 25 | |
| 49091 | 1 ea | Raisin Bakes, fat free, Health Valley | 27 | 70 | 26 | 2.0 | 18.0 | 2.0 | 11.0 | 5.0 | 0.0 | 0.0 | 0.0 | 0.0 | 0.00 | 0.00 | 0 | 100 | 20 | | | | | | | | | | | 2.4 | | | 0 | | 0.7 | | | | | | 30 | |
| 49080 | 1 ea | Raisin Bran w/ Raisin Apple, fat free, Health Valley | 37 | 110 | 21 | 2.0 | 26.0 | 3.0 | 13.0 | 10.0 | 0.0 | 0.0 | 0.0 | 0.0 | 0.00 | 0.00 | 0 | 100 | 20 | | | | | | | | | | | 1.2 | | | 0 | | 0.7 | | | | | | 25 | |
| 44289 | 1 ea | Strawberry, Nutri Grain | 37 | 140 | 13 | 2.0 | 27.0 | 1.0 | 13.0 | 13.0 | 3.0 | 0.5 | | | | | 0 | 750 | 225 | | | | 0.38 | 0.43 | 5.00 | 0.50 | | 100.0 | | 0.0 | | | 0 | | 1.8 | 8 | | 40 | | | 60 | 1.50 |
| 40253 | 1 ea | Strawberry Filling, Snackwells | 37 | 120 | 16 | 1.0 | 29.3 | 1.1 | 17.9 | 10.3 | 0.3 | 0.0 | 0.0 | 0.1 | | | 0 | 1300 | 260 | | | | 0.39 | 0.44 | 5.20 | 0.52 | 0.01 | | | 2.1 | | | 14 | 0.0 | 4.8 | 6 | | 34 | 47 | | 101 | 3.83 |
| | | Granola Bars | | | | | | | | | | | | | | | | | | | | | | | | | | | | | | | | | | | | | | | | |
| 23100 | 1 ea | Almond, hard, avg | 24 | 119 | 3 | 1.8 | 14.9 | 1.2 | 7.2 | 6.6 | 6.1 | 3.0 | 1.9 | 0.9 | 0.02 | 0.88 | 0 | 9 | 1 | | | | 0.07 | 0.02 | 0.15 | 0.01 | 0.00 | 2.9 | 0.11 | 0.0 | 0.0 | | 8 | 0.0 | 0.6 | 19 | 0.3 | 55 | 66 | 3.6 | 61 | 0.38 |
| 44290 | 1 ea | Chocolate Chip, chewy, Rice Krispies | 28 | 120 | 9 | 1.0 | 20.0 | 1.0 | 8.0 | 11.0 | 4.0 | 1.5 | | | | | 0 | 500 | 150 | | | | 0.15 | 0.17 | 2.00 | 0.20 | | 40.0 | | 0.0 | | | 0 | 0.1 | 1.8 | 8 | | 40 | | | 60 | |
| 23106 | 1 ea | Chocolate Chip, Graham & Marshmallow, soft, av | 28 | 120 | 6 | 1.7 | 19.8 | 1.1 | 17.0 | 1.7 | 4.3 | 2.6 | 0.8 | 0.7 | 0.04 | 0.67 | 0 | 13 | 1 | | | | 0.04 | 0.04 | 0.28 | 0.01 | 0.00 | 5.9 | 0.11 | 0.0 | 0.0 | | 25 | 0.1 | 0.7 | 20 | 0.4 | 57 | 77 | 4.3 | 88 | 0.36 |
| 23101 | 1 ea | Chocolate Chip, hard, avg | 24 | 105 | 2 | 1.8 | 17.3 | 1.1 | 8.3 | 8.0 | 3.9 | 2.7 | 0.6 | 0.3 | 0.01 | 0.29 | 0 | 10 | 1 | | | | 0.04 | 0.02 | 0.13 | 0.01 | 0.00 | 3.1 | 0.12 | 0.0 | 0.0 | | 18 | 0.1 | 0.7 | 17 | 0.4 | 49 | 60 | 3.0 | 83 | 0.46 |
| 23096 | 1 ea | Chocolate Chip, w/choc coating, soft, avg | 35 | 163 | 4 | 2.0 | 22.3 | 1.2 | 16.4 | 4.8 | 8.7 | 5.0 | 2.7 | 0.6 | 0.04 | 0.60 | 2 | 14 | 2 | | | | 0.03 | 0.09 | 0.25 | 0.04 | 0.20 | 9.1 | 0.18 | 0.0 | 0.0 | | 36 | 0.1 | 0.8 | 23 | 0.3 | 70 | 110 | | 70 | 0.45 |
| 23458 | 1 ea | Chocolate Coated, avg | 34 | 158 | 4 | 2.2 | 22.7 | 1.1 | | | 7.2 | 3.4 | 2.5 | 0.9 | | | 3 | 94 | 26 | 24 | 2 | | 0.08 | 0.09 | 0.45 | 0.05 | 0.08 | 9.8 | | 3.0 | | | 40 | 0.1 | 0.6 | 21 | | 67 | 105 | | 62 | 0.45 |
| 23105 | 1 ea | Chocolate, soft, avg | 42 | 176 | 5 | 3.1 | 29.0 | 2.0 | 24.6 | 2.4 | 7.0 | 4.3 | 1.5 | 0.8 | 0.04 | 0.79 | 0 | 18 | 2 | | | | 0.10 | 0.06 | 0.40 | 0.04 | 0.07 | 9.2 | 0.22 | 0.0 | 0.0 | | 39 | 0.2 | 1.1 | 33 | 0.5 | 97 | 143 | 5.3 | 114 | 0.63 |
| 23107 | 1 ea | Nut & Raisin, uncoated, soft, avg | 28 | 127 | 6 | 2.2 | 17.8 | 1.6 | 14.6 | 1.6 | 5.7 | 2.7 | 1.2 | 1.5 | 0.05 | 1.50 | 0 | 11 | 1 | | | | 0.05 | 0.05 | 0.73 | 0.03 | 0.07 | 8.4 | 0.12 | 0.0 | 0.0 | | 24 | 0.1 | 0.6 | 25 | 0.3 | 67 | 110 | 4.3 | 71 | 0.45 |

| Code | Amount | | Description | Basic Components | | | | | | | | | Additional Fats | | | | | | Vit A & Components | | | | | Vitamins | | | | | | | | | | Minerals | | | | | | | | | |
|---|---|---|---|---|---|---|---|---|---|---|---|---|---|---|---|---|---|---|---|---|---|---|---|---|---|---|---|---|---|---|---|---|---|---|---|---|---|---|---|---|---|---|---|
| | | | | Weight (g) | Calories | % Water | Protein (g) | Carbs (g) | Fiber (g) | Sugar (g) | Other Carbs (g) | Fat (g) | Sat Fat (g) | Mono Fat (g) | Poly Fat (g) | Omega 3 (g) | Omega 6 (g) | Choles (mg) | Vit A (IU) | Vit A (RE) | Retinol (RE) | Carotenoids (RE) | Beta Carotene (mcg) | Thiamin (mg) | Riboflavin (mg) | Niacin (NE) | Vit B6 (mg) | Vit B12 (mcg) | Folate (mcg) | Panto (mg) | Vit C (mg) | Vit D (mg) | Vit E (α TE) | Calcium (mg) | Copper (mg) | Iron (mg) | Magnes (mg) | Mang (mg) | Phos (mg) | Potassium (mg) | Selenium (mcg) | Sodium (mg) | Zinc (mg) |
| 23065 | 1 | ea | Nutty Fudge, snack bar, Kudos | 37 | 201 | 2 | 3.0 | 20.1 | | | | 12.0 | | | | | | | | | | | | | 0.10 | | | | | | | | | 40 | | 0.4 | | | | | | 55 | |
| 23168 | 1 | ea | Oat, Raisin & Coconut granola bar, avg | 40 | 182 | 4 | 3.9 | 26.7 | 1.2 | | | 7.0 | 4.5 | 1.0 | 1.0 | | | 0 | 4 | 0.4 | 0 | 0.4 | | 0.11 | 0.04 | 0.70 | 0.14 | 0.00 | 32.4 | | 0.4 | | | 24 | 0.1 | 1.3 | 40 | | 111 | 130 | | 111 | 0.64 |
| 23102 | 1 | ea | Peanut, hard, avg | 24 | 115 | 2 | 2.6 | 15.3 | 1.0 | 7.3 | 7.0 | 5.1 | 0.5 | 1.4 | 2.9 | 0.01 | 2.85 | 0 | 8 | 1 | | | | 0.05 | 0.02 | 0.35 | 0.02 | 0.00 | 5.5 | 0.14 | 0.0 | 0.0 | | 9 | 0.1 | 0.6 | 26 | 0.3 | 72 | 73 | 3.6 | 67 | 0.50 |
| 23109 | 1 | ea | Peanut Butter w/Chocolate, uncoated, soft, avg | 28 | 121 | 6 | 2.7 | 17.4 | 1.2 | 14.6 | 1.7 | 5.6 | 1.6 | 2.3 | 1.3 | 0.01 | 1.28 | 0 | 3 | 1 | | | | 0.03 | 0.03 | 0.88 | 0.03 | 0.13 | 9.2 | 0.15 | 0.0 | 0.0 | | 22 | 0.1 | 0.5 | 25 | 0.4 | 73 | 106 | | 92 | 0.48 |
| 23103 | 1 | ea | Peanut Butter, Hard, avg | 24 | 116 | 2 | 2.4 | 15.0 | 0.7 | 7.2 | 7.1 | 5.7 | 0.8 | 1.7 | 2.9 | 0.03 | 2.88 | 0 | 4 | 0.5 | | | | 0.05 | 0.02 | 0.47 | 0.02 | 0.00 | 4.3 | 0.09 | 0.0 | 0.0 | | 10 | 0.1 | 0.6 | 13 | 0.2 | 33 | 70 | 3.6 | 68 | 0.30 |
| 23433 | 1 | ea | Peanut Butter, Snack bar, Kudos | 37 | 201 | | 4.0 | 19.1 | | | | 12.0 | | | | | | | | | | | | 0.03 | 0.10 | 1.20 | | | | | | | | 20 | | 0.4 | | | | | | 80 | |
| 23108 | 1 | ea | Peanut Butter, soft, uncoated, avg | 24 | 102 | 7 | 2.5 | 15.5 | 1.0 | 13.0 | 1.5 | 3.8 | 0.9 | 1.6 | 1.0 | 0.01 | 1.02 | 0 | 3 | 0.5 | | | | 0.05 | 0.04 | 0.75 | 0.02 | 0.05 | 7.7 | 0.13 | 0.0 | 0.0 | | 22 | 0.2 | 0.5 | 21 | 0.3 | 60 | 70 | 4.5 | 98 | 0.45 |
| 23095 | 1 | ea | Peanut Butter, soft, w/choc coating, avg | 37 | 188 | 3 | 3.8 | 19.8 | 1.0 | 14.4 | 4.3 | 11.5 | 6.3 | 2.4 | 1.7 | 0.03 | 0.68 | 4 | 48 | 13 | | | | 0.04 | 0.08 | 1.22 | 0.04 | 0.00 | 9.3 | 0.20 | 0.2 | 0.0 | | 40 | 0.1 | 0.5 | 25 | 0.5 | 84 | 125 | | 71 | 0.54 |
| 23059 | 1 | ea | Plain, hard, avg | 24 | 113 | 4 | 2.4 | 15.5 | 1.3 | 7.4 | 6.7 | 4.8 | 0.6 | 1.1 | 2.9 | 0.01 | 2.88 | 0 | 36 | 4 | | | | 0.06 | 0.03 | 0.38 | 0.02 | 0.00 | 5.5 | 0.20 | 0.2 | 0.0 | | 15 | 0.1 | 0.7 | 23 | 0.4 | 66 | 81 | 3.9 | 71 | 0.49 |
| 23104 | 1 | ea | Plain, uncoated, soft, avg | 28 | 124 | 6 | 2.1 | 18.8 | 1.3 | 16.0 | 1.5 | 4.8 | 2.0 | 1.1 | 1.5 | 0.08 | 1.41 | 0 | 0 | 0 | 0 | 0 | 0 | 0.08 | 0.05 | 0.14 | 0.03 | 0.11 | 6.7 | 0.15 | 0.0 | 0.0 | | 29 | 0.1 | 0.7 | 21 | 0.4 | 64 | 91 | 4.5 | 78 | 0.42 |
| 23097 | 1 | ea | Raisin, soft, avg | 42 | 188 | 6 | 3.2 | 27.9 | 1.8 | 23.5 | 2.5 | 7.5 | 4.0 | 1.2 | 1.3 | 0.07 | 1.28 | 0 | 0 | 0 | 0 | 0 | 0 | 0.10 | 0.07 | 0.46 | 0.04 | 0.08 | 8.8 | 0.20 | 0.0 | 0.0 | | 42 | 0.1 | 1.0 | 30 | 0.5 | 92 | 152 | 6.6 | 118 | 0.55 |
| 23170 | 1 | ea | Yogurt Coated, w/high fiber, avg | 28 | 96 | 12 | 2.7 | 18.6 | 2.2 | 5.5 | 10.3 | 2.9 | 1.0 | 1.0 | 0.7 | | | 0 | 4 | 0.4 | 0.3 | 0.1 | | 0.12 | 0.05 | 0.84 | 0.04 | 0.01 | 7.9 | | 0.1 | | | 15 | 0.1 | 0.7 | 36 | | 107 | 107 | | 6 | 0.58 |
| 23169 | 1 | ea | With Nougat, avg | 34 | 140 | 3 | 2.0 | 24.1 | 1.3 | 11.6 | 11.2 | 4.8 | 1.9 | 1.1 | 1.5 | | | 0 | 11 | 2 | 1 | 1 | | 0.07 | 0.05 | 0.30 | 0.05 | 0.01 | 10.1 | | 0.1 | | | 15 | 0.1 | 0.6 | 16 | | 54 | 77 | | 48 | 0.45 |
| 49095 | 1 | ea | Scones, all flavors, fat free, Health Valley | 60 | 80 | 58 | 7.0 | 15.0 | 7.0 | 4.0 | 4.0 | 0.0 | 0.0 | 0.0 | 0.0 | 0.00 | 0.00 | 0 | 1000 | 200 | | | | | | | | | | | 12.0 | | | 20 | | 0.1 | | | | | | 160 | |
| 49075 | 1 | ea | Tarts, all flavors, fat free, Health Valley | 52 | 150 | 26 | 3.0 | 35.0 | 3.0 | 18.0 | 14.0 | 0.0 | 0.0 | 0.0 | 0.0 | 0.00 | 0.00 | 0 | 100 | 20 | | | | | | | | | | | 1.2 | | | 0 | | 0.7 | | | | | | 30 | |
| | | | **INFANT FOODS** | | | | | | | | | | | | | | | | | | | | | | | | | | | | | | | | | | | | | | | | |
| | | | *INFANT CEREAL* | | | | | | | | | | | | | | | | | | | | | | | | | | | | | | | | | | | | | | | | |
| | | | Barley Cereal | | | | | | | | | | | | | | | | | | | | | | | | | | | | | | | | | | | | | | | | |
| 60483 | 1 | Tbs | Dry, avg | 2 | 7 | 7 | 0.2 | 1.5 | 0.2 | | | 0.1 | 0.0 | 0.0 | 0.0 | 0.00 | 0.03 | 0 | 0.3 | 0.04 | | | | 0.05 | 0.05 | 0.72 | 0.01 | 0.00 | 0.6 | 0.01 | 0.0 | | | 16 | 0.0 | 0.9 | 2 | | 9 | 8 | 0.6 | 1 | 0.06 |
| 60065 | 1 | Tbs | Dry, Stage 1, Beechnut | 4 | 17 | 5 | 0.3 | 3.4 | 0.3 | 0.6 | 2.5 | 0.0 | 0.0 | 0.0 | 0.0 | 0.00 | 0.00 | | 0 | 0 | 0 | 0 | 0 | 0.05 | 0.06 | 0.76 | | | | | 0.0 | | 0.0 | 25 | | 1.9 | | | | 14 | | 3 | |
| 60868 | 1 | Tbs | Prepared, avg | 15 | 17 | 75 | 0.7 | 2.4 | | | | 0.5 | | | | | | | 16 | 3 | | | | 0.07 | 0.09 | 0.90 | 0.01 | 0.05 | 1.3 | 0.05 | | | | 35 | 0.0 | 1.8 | 5 | | 23 | 29 | | 7 | 0.12 |
| 60532 | 1 | Tbs | Grits Cereal, w/egg yolk, strained, avg | 14 | 8 | 88 | 0.3 | 1.0 | | | | 0.3 | | | | | | | 17 | 4 | | | | 0.00 | 0.01 | 0.04 | 0.00 | 0.01 | 0.4 | 0.13 | 0.1 | | | 4 | 0.0 | 0.1 | 1 | | 5 | 8 | | 5 | 0.03 |
| | | | Mixed Cereal | | | | | | | | | | | | | | | | | | | | | | | | | | | | | | | | | | | | | | | | |
| 60244 | 1 | ea | Apple, Stage 2, 4 oz jar, Beech Nut | 113 | 70 | 86 | 0.0 | 15.9 | 1.0 | 10.0 | 5.0 | 0.0 | 0.0 | 0.0 | 0.0 | 0.00 | 0.00 | | 30 | 5 | | | | 0.18 | 0.22 | 2.69 | | | | | 15.9 | | | 0 | | 5.2 | | | | 80 | | 0 | |
| 60394 | 1 | Tbs | Apple Banana, strained, Heinz | 16 | 11 | 83 | 0.2 | 2.5 | 0.2 | 1.2 | 1.2 | 0.0 | 0.0 | | | | | | 3 | 1 | | | | 0.04 | 0.04 | 0.59 | 0.03 | | | | 9.2 | | | 2 | 0.0 | 0.8 | | | 4 | 10 | | 0 | 0.02 |
| 60549 | 1 | Tbs | Apple Orange, dry, high protein, avg | 2 | 7 | 5 | 0.5 | 1.2 | 0.1 | | | 0.1 | 0.0 | 0.0 | 0.1 | 0.01 | 0.06 | 0 | 1 | 0.1 | | | | 0.08 | 0.09 | 0.48 | 0.01 | 0.01 | 3.8 | | 0.1 | | | 15 | 0.0 | 0.9 | 3 | | 11 | 27 | 0.6 | 2 | 0.05 |
| 60550 | 1 | Tbs | Apple Orange, prep w/whole milk, hi protein, avg | 15 | 17 | 74 | 1.0 | 2.0 | | | | 0.6 | | | | | | | 20 | 4 | | | | 0.10 | 0.13 | 0.60 | 0.01 | 0.05 | 4.1 | | | | | 33 | 0.0 | 2.2 | 6 | | 25 | 52 | | 9 | 0.11 |
| 60571 | 1 | Tbs | Applesauce Banana, junior, RTE, avg | 15 | 12 | 80 | 0.2 | 2.8 | 0.2 | | | 0.1 | 0.0 | 0.0 | 0.0 | 0.00 | 0.02 | 0 | 3 | 0.3 | | | | 0.04 | 0.05 | 0.61 | 0.02 | 0.00 | 0.6 | 0.03 | 1.4 | | | 1 | 0.0 | 0.8 | 1 | | 4 | 5 | 0.4 | 5 | 0.03 |
| 60572 | 1 | Tbs | Applesauce Banana, strained, RTE, avg | 15 | 12 | 80 | 0.2 | 2.7 | 0.2 | | | 0.1 | 0.0 | 0.0 | 0.0 | 0.00 | 0.03 | 0 | 3 | 0.3 | | | | 0.04 | 0.05 | 0.59 | 0.02 | 0.00 | 0.5 | 0.03 | 3.8 | | | 1 | 0.0 | 1.0 | 1 | | 3 | 6 | 0.4 | 0 | 0.03 |
| 60156 | 1 | Tbs | Applesauce Banana, 2nd Foods, Gerber | 14 | 11 | 80 | 0.2 | 2.5 | 0.2 | 1.5 | 0.9 | 0.1 | | | | | | | 1.4 | 0.11 | 0 | 0.14 | 1 | 0.03 | 0.03 | 0.44 | 0.02 | | | | 1.9 | | | 1 | 0.0 | 0.8 | 1 | 0.0 | 4 | 8 | | 0 | 0.03 |
| 60157 | 1 | Tbs | Applesauce Banana, 3rd Food, Gerber | 14 | 11 | 80 | 0.2 | 2.5 | 0.2 | 1.3 | 1.1 | 0.1 | | | | | | | 0.3 | 0.03 | 0 | 0.03 | 0.2 | 0.02 | 0.02 | 0.30 | 0.02 | | | | 1.3 | | | 1 | 0.0 | 0.4 | 1 | 0.0 | 4 | 8 | | 0 | 0.13 |
| 60007 | 1 | Tbs | Banana, dry, avg | 4 | 16 | 4 | 0.3 | 3.3 | 0.1 | 1.2 | 2.0 | 0.2 | | | | | | | | | | | | 0.06 | 0.07 | 0.53 | 0.02 | | | | 0.0 | | | 24 | 0.0 | 1.8 | 3 | 0.0 | 13 | 15 | | 0 | 0.05 |
| 60564 | 1 | Tbs | Banana, dry, 2nd Foods, Gerber | 2 | 8 | 4 | 0.2 | 1.5 | 0.2 | | | 0.1 | 0.0 | 0.0 | 0.0 | 0.00 | 0.03 | 0 | 3 | 0 | | | | 0.08 | 0.07 | 0.41 | 0.01 | 0.00 | 0.3 | | 0.1 | | | 14 | 0.0 | 0.9 | 2 | | 7 | 13 | 0.4 | 2 | 0.03 |
| 60565 | 1 | Tbs | Banana, prep w/whole milk, avg | 15 | 17 | 74 | 0.7 | 2.5 | 0.2 | | | 0.5 | 0.3 | | | | | 2 | 16 | 1 | | | | 0.10 | 0.11 | 0.52 | 0.02 | 0.05 | 1.1 | | 0.2 | | | 32 | 0.0 | 1.7 | 4 | | 21 | 36 | | 9 | 0.08 |
| 60570 | 1 | Tbs | Honey, dry, avg | 2 | 8 | 4 | 0.3 | 1.5 | | | | 0.1 | | | | | | | 0.5 | 0.04 | | | | 0.05 | 0.05 | 0.75 | 0.00 | 0.00 | 0.9 | 0.02 | 0.0 | | | 24 | 0.0 | 1.4 | 2 | | 13 | 5 | | 1 | 0.05 |
| 60562 | 1 | Tbs | Honey, prep w/whole milk, avg | 15 | 17 | 74 | 0.8 | 2.4 | | | | 0.5 | | | | | | | 20 | 4 | | | | 0.07 | 0.09 | 0.94 | 0.01 | 0.05 | 1.7 | 0.07 | | | | 44 | 0.0 | 1.7 | 4 | | 28 | 26 | | 7 | 0.11 |
| 60815 | 1 | ea | Peaches & Yogurt, 3rd Foods, 6 oz jar, Gerber | 170 | 133 | 81 | 3.2 | 27.7 | 1.4 | 17.2 | 9.2 | 0.9 | | | | | | | 43 | 4 | 0 | 4 | 26 | 0.22 | 0.27 | 3.62 | 0.19 | | | | 15.8 | | | 231 | 0.1 | 4.4 | 20 | 0.3 | 177 | 158 | | 34 | 1.53 |
| 60566 | 1 | Tbs | Plain, dry, avg | 2 | 8 | 7 | 0.2 | 1.5 | 0.1 | | | 0.1 | 0.0 | 0.0 | 0.0 | 0.00 | 0.03 | 0 | 0 | 0 | | | | 0.05 | 0.05 | 0.69 | 0.00 | 0.00 | 0.9 | 0.02 | 0.0 | | | 15 | 0.0 | 0.9 | 2 | | 8 | 9 | 0.5 | 1 | 0.05 |
| 60153 | 1 | Tbs | Plain, dry, Heinz | 2 | 7 | 7 | 0.3 | 1.4 | 0.1 | | | 0.1 | 0.0 | 0.0 | 0.0 | | | 0 | 0 | 0 | 0 | 0 | | 0.05 | 0.07 | 0.81 | 0.00 | 0.00 | 0.9 | 0.00 | 0.0 | | | 23 | 0.0 | 1.3 | 2 | | 22 | 7 | 0.0 | 0 | 0.03 |
| 60006 | 1 | Tbs | Plain, dry, 2nd Foods, Gerber | 4 | 15 | 6 | 0.4 | 3.0 | 0.2 | 0.2 | 2.7 | 0.2 | | | | | | | | | | | | 0.06 | 0.07 | 0.53 | 0.01 | | | | | | | 24 | 0.0 | 1.8 | 3 | 0.1 | 20 | 8 | | 0 | 0.06 |
| 60107 | 1 | Tbs | Plain, dry, high protein, avg | 18 | 22 | 76 | 0.6 | 3.2 | | | | 0.6 | | | | | | | 24 | [illegible] | 7 | 0 | | 0.02 | 0.02 | 0.30 | 0.04 | | | | 0.7 | | | 7 | | 0.9 | | | | | | 3 | |
| 60106 | 1 | Tbs | Plain, prep w/formula, Earth's Best | 18 | 12 | 82 | 0.4 | 2.3 | | | | 0.0 | 0.0 | 0.0 | 0.0 | 0.00 | 0.00 | | | | | | | 0.02 | 0.00 | 0.18 | 0.02 | | | | | | | | | 0.9 | | | | | | 0 | |
| 60563 | 1 | Tbs | Plain, prep w/water, Earth's Best | 15 | 17 | 75 | 0.7 | 2.4 | 0.2 | | | 0.5 | 0.3 | | | | | 2 | 15 | 4 | | | | 0.06 | 0.09 | 0.87 | 0.01 | 0.05 | 1.7 | 0.07 | 0.2 | | | 33 | 0.0 | 1.6 | 4 | | 21 | 30 | | 7 | 0.11 |
| 60539 | 1 | Tbs | Plain, prep w/whole milk, avg | 2 | 7 | 6 | 0.7 | 0.9 | 0.1 | | | 0.1 | 0.0 | 0.0 | 0.1 | 0.01 | 0.05 | 0 | 0 | [illegible] | | | | 0.05 | 0.05 | 0.68 | 0.01 | 0.00 | 3.8 | 0.02 | 0.0 | | | 14 | 0.0 | 0.9 | 5 | | 12 | 27 | 0.6 | 1 | 0.09 |
| 60540 | 1 | Tbs | Plain, prep w/whole milk, high protein, avg | 15 | 17 | 74 | 1.3 | 1.7 | | | | 0.6 | | | | | | | 16 | [illegible] | | | | 0.07 | 0.09 | 0.85 | 0.02 | 0.05 | 5.3 | 0.07 | | | | 33 | 0.0 | 1.8 | 7 | | 27 | 52 | | 7 | 0.16 |
| 60506 | 1 | Tbs | With eggs, strained, avg | 16 | 9 | 87 | 0.4 | 1.3 | | | | 0.2 | 0.1 | 0.1 | 0.1 | 0.00 | 0.05 | 8 | 26 | [illegible] | | | | 0.00 | 0.01 | 0.01 | 0.00 | 0.01 | 1.5 | 0.16 | 0.1 | | | 4 | 0.0 | 0.1 | 0 | | 7 | 7 | | 6 | 0.05 |
| 60505 | 1 | Tbs | With egg yolk, junior, avg | 16 | 8 | 89 | 0.3 | 1.1 | 0.1 | | | 0.3 | 0.1 | 0.1 | 0.0 | 0.00 | 0.05 | 10 | 23 | [illegible] | | | | 0.00 | 0.01 | 0.01 | 0.00 | 0.01 | 0.5 | 0.14 | 0.1 | | | 4 | 0.0 | 0.1 | 0 | | 6 | 6 | | 5 | 0.05 |
| 60504 | 1 | Tbs | With egg yolk, strained, avg | 16 | 8 | 89 | 0.3 | 1.1 | 0.1 | | | 0.3 | 0.1 | 0.1 | 0.0 | 0.00 | 0.05 | 10 | 23 | 6 | | | | 0.00 | 0.01 | 0.01 | 0.00 | 0.01 | 0.5 | 0.14 | 0.1 | | | 4 | 0.0 | 0.1 | 0 | | 6 | 6 | | 5 | 0.05 |
| 60507 | 1 | Tbs | With egg yolk & bacon, junior, avg | 16 | 13 | 86 | 0.4 | 1.0 | 0.1 | | | 0.8 | 0.3 | 0.4 | 0.1 | 0.01 | 0.09 | 15 | 15 | [illegible] | | | | 0.01 | 0.01 | 0.04 | 0.00 | 0.01 | 0.7 | 0.18 | 0.1 | | | 4 | 0.0 | 0.1 | 1 | | 8 | 6 | | 8 | 0.04 |
| 60508 | 1 | Tbs | With egg yolk & bacon, strained avg | 14 | 12 | 85 | 0.3 | 1.0 | 0.1 | | | 0.7 | 0.2 | 0.3 | 0.1 | | | 7 | 9 | [illegible] | | | | 0.00 | 0.01 | 0.02 | 0.00 | 0.01 | 0.6 | 0.16 | 0.2 | | | 4 | 0.0 | 0.1 | 1 | | 8 | 5 | | 6 | 0.04 |
| | | | Oatmeal Cereal | | | | | | | | | | | | | | | | | | | | | | | | | | | | | | | | | | | | | | | | |
| 60729 | 1 | ea | Apple, Stage 2, 4 oz jar, Beechnut | 113 | 70 | 85 | 1.0 | 15.9 | 1.0 | 10.0 | 5.0 | 0.0 | 0.0 | 0.0 | 0.0 | 0.00 | 0.00 | | 30 | 6 | | | | | | | | | | | 15.7 | | | 0 | | 5.2 | | | | 80 | | 0 | |
| 60247 | 1 | ea | Apple Banana, Stage 2, 4 oz jar, Beechnut | 113 | 70 | 86 | 0.0 | 15.9 | 1.0 | 10.0 | 5.0 | 0.0 | 0.0 | 0.0 | 0.0 | 0.00 | 0.00 | | | | | | | 0.18 | 0.22 | 2.69 | | | | | 15.9 | | | 12 | | 4.5 | | | | 80 | | 0 | |
| 60395 | 1 | Tbs | Apple Banana, strained, Heinz | 16 | 12 | 82 | 0.2 | 2.5 | 0.2 | 1.1 | 1.2 | 0.1 | 0.0 | | | | | | 6 | 1 | | | | 0.04 | 0.05 | 0.64 | 0.01 | | | | 8.1 | | | 1 | 0.0 | 0.8 | | | 7 | 11 | | 0 | 0.04 |
| 60833 | 1 | Tbs | Apple Cinnamon, instant, dry, grad, Gerber | 4 | 16 | 5 | 0.4 | 3.0 | 0.3 | 1.1 | 1.6 | 0.3 | 0.1 | | | | | | | | | | | 0.03 | 0.03 | 0.38 | 0.02 | | | | 0.1 | | | 11 | 0.0 | 0.6 | 4 | 0.1 | 17 | 12 | | 8 | 0.23 |
| 60813 | 1 | ea | Apple Cinnamon, 3rd Foods, 6 oz jar, Gerber | 170 | 145 | 80 | 2.4 | 31.1 | 2.7 | 17.0 | 11.4 | 1.2 | | | | | | | 17 | 2 | 0 | 2 | 10 | 0.22 | 0.27 | 3.62 | 0.19 | | | | 15.8 | | | 10 | 0.1 | 4.4 | 20 | 0.7 | 65 | 121 | | 3 | 1.53 |
| 60575 | 1 | Tbs | Applesauce Banana, junior, avg | 15 | 11 | 82 | 0.2 | 2.4 | 0.1 | | | 0.1 | 0.0 | 0.0 | 0.0 | 0.00 | 0.04 | 0 | 4 | 0 | | | | 0.04 | 0.07 | 0.50 | 0.04 | 0.00 | 0.5 | 0.03 | 2.9 | | | 1 | 0.0 | 0.8 | 2 | | 6 | 7 | 0.5 | 5 | 0.05 |
| 60576 | 1 | Tbs | Applesauce Banana, strained, avg | 15 | 11 | 82 | 0.2 | 2.3 | 0.1 | | | 0.1 | 0.0 | 0.0 | 0.0 | 0.00 | 0.04 | 0 | 5 | 0 | | | | 0.06 | 0.05 | 0.76 | 0.03 | 0.00 | 0.5 | 0.03 | 3.3 | | | 1 | 0.0 | 0.8 | 2 | | 6 | 7 | 0.5 | 0 | 0.05 |
| 60163 | 1 | Tbs | Applesauce Banana, 2nd Foods, Gerber | 14 | 12 | 80 | 0.2 | 2.5 | 0.2 | 1.5 | 0.8 | 0.1 | | | | | | | 2 | 0.2 | 0 | 0.2 | 1 | 0.03 | 0.03 | 0.44 | 0.02 | | | | 1.9 | | | 1 | 0.0 | 0.8 | 2 | 0.1 | 5 | 10 | | 0 | 0.04 |
| 60579 | 1 | Tbs | Banana, dry, avg | 2 | 8 | 5 | 0.2 | 1.5 | 0.1 | | | 0.1 | 0.0 | 0.0 | 0.0 | 0.00 | 0.04 | 0 | 1 | 0 | | | | 0.07 | 0.07 | 0.40 | 0.01 | 0.00 | 0.4 | | 0.1 | | | 13 | 0.0 | 0.9 | 2 | | 9 | 15 | 0.4 | 2 | 0.04 |
| 60009 | 1 | Tbs | Banana, dry, 2nd Foods, Gerber | 4 | 16 | 4 | 0.5 | 3.0 | 0.2 | 1.2 | 1.6 | 0.3 | | | | | | | | | | | | 0.06 | 0.07 | 0.53 | 0.02 | | | | 0.0 | | | 24 | 0.0 | 1.8 | 5 | 0.1 | 20 | 19 | | 0 | 0.09 |
| 60580 | 1 | Tbs | Banana, prep w/whole milk, avg | 15 | 17 | 74 | 0.7 | 2.4 | | | | 0.6 | | | | | | | 15 | 4 | | | | 0.09 | 0.11 | 0.51 | 0.02 | 0.05 | 1.1 | | 0.2 | | | 31 | 0.0 | 1.7 | 5 | | 23 | 37 | | 9 | 0.09 |
| 60581 | 1 | Tbs | Honey, dry, avg | 2 | 8 | 6 | 0.3 | 1.4 | | | | 0.1 | | | | | | | 0.5 | 0.04 | | | | 0.06 | 0.06 | 0.73 | 0.00 | 0.00 | 0.7 | 0.03 | 0.0 | | | 23 | 0.0 | 1.3 | 3 | | 15 | 5 | 0.7 | 1 | 0.07 |
| 60582 | 1 | Tbs | Honey, prep w/whole milk, avg | 15 | 17 | 74 | 0.8 | 2.3 | 0.3 | | | 0.6 | 0.2 | 0.2 | 0.1 | | | | 20 | 4 | | | | 0.07 | 0.09 | 0.90 | 0.01 | 0.05 | 1.5 | 0.08 | 0.1 | | | 43 | 0.0 | 1.7 | 5 | | 30 | 26 | | 7 | 0.14 |
| 60109 | 1 | ea | Peaches & Bananas, 4.5 oz jar, Earth's Best | 128 | 60 | 89 | 2.0 | 12.0 | | | | 0.0 | 0.0 | 0.0 | 0.0 | 0.00 | 0.00 | | | | | | | 0.04 | 0.05 | | 0.06 | | | | | | | | | 0.6 | | | | | | 10 | |
| 60834 | 1 | Tbs | Peaches & Vanilla, instant, dry, grad, Gerber | 4 | 16 | 6 | 0.4 | 2.9 | 0.3 | 0.9 | 1.7 | 0.3 | 0.1 | | | | | | 7 | 1 | [illegible] | 1 | 4 | 0.03 | 0.03 | 0.38 | 0.02 | | | | 0.1 | | | 11 | 0.0 | 0.6 | 4 | 0.1 | 17 | 16 | | 8 | 0.23 |
| 60577 | 1 | Tbs | Plain, dry, avg | 2 | 8 | 6 | 0.3 | 1.4 | 0.1 | | | 0.2 | 0.0 | 0.0 | 0.1 | 0.00 | 0.05 | 0 | 0 | 0 | | | | 0.06 | 0.05 | 0.72 | 0.00 | 0.00 | 0.7 | 0.03 | 0.1 | | | 15 | 0.0 | 0.9 | 3 | | 10 | 9 | 0.7 | 1 | 0.07 |
| 60008 | 1 | Tbs | Plain, dry, 1st Foods, Gerber | 4 | 16 | 6 | 0.6 | 2.7 | 0.4 | 0.1 | 2.2 | 0.3 | | | | | | | | | | | | 0.06 | 0.07 | 0.53 | 0.01 | | | | | | | 24 | 0.0 | 1.8 | 5 | 0.2 | 20 | 14 | | 0 | 0.13 |
| 60154 | 1 | Tbs | Plain, dry, Heinz | 2 | 7 | 7 | 0.3 | 1.4 | 0.1 | | | 0.1 | 0.0 | 0.0 | 0.1 | | | 0 | 0 | 0 | [illegible] | 0 | | 0.05 | 0.07 | 0.66 | 0.00 | 0.00 | 0.7 | 0.02 | 0.0 | | | 25 | 0.0 | 1.3 | 3 | | 23 | 8 | 1.0 | 0 | 0.05 |
| 60578 | 1 | Tbs | Plain, prep f/dry, w/milk, avg | 15 | 17 | 74 | 0.8 | 2.3 | 0.2 | | | 0.6 | 0.3 | | | | | 2 | 16 | 4 | | | | 0.08 | 0.08 | 0.90 | 0.01 | 0.05 | 1.5 | 0.08 | 0.2 | | | 33 | 0.0 | 1.8 | 5 | | 24 | 31 | | 7 | 0.14 |

| Code | Amount | | Description | Basic Components | | | | | | | | | Additional Fats | | | | | | Vit A & Components | | | | | Vitamins | | | | | | | | | | Minerals | | | | | | | | | |
|---|---|---|---|---|---|---|---|---|---|---|---|---|---|---|---|---|---|---|---|---|---|---|---|---|---|---|---|---|---|---|---|---|---|---|---|---|---|---|---|---|---|---|---|
| | | | | Weight (g) | Calories | % Water | Protein (g) | Carbs (g) | Fiber (g) | Sugar (g) | Other Carbs (g) | Fat (g) | Sat Fat (g) | Mono Fat (g) | Poly Fat (g) | Omega 3 (g) | Omega 6 (g) | Choles (mg) | Vit A (IU) | Vit A (RE) | Retinol (RE) | Carotenoids (RE) | Beta Carotene (mcg) | Thiamin (mg) | Riboflavin (mg) | Niacin (NE) | Vit B6 (mg) | Vit B12 (mcg) | Folate (mcg) | Panto (mg) | Vit C (mg) | Vit D (mg) | Vit E (α TE) | Calcium (mg) | Copper (mg) | Iron (mg) | Magnes (mg) | Mang (mg) | Phos (mg) | Potassium (mg) | Selenium (mcg) | Sodium (mg) | Zinc (mg) |
| 60108 | 1 | ea | Prunes, 4.5 oz jar, Earths Best | 128 | 100 | 80 | 1.0 | 24.0 | | | | 0.0 | 0.0 | 0.0 | 0.0 | 0.00 | 0.00 | | | | | | | 0.04 | 0.15 | 0.48 | 30.00 | | | | | | | | | 0.4 | | | | | | 20 | |
| 60861 | 1 | Tbs | With fruit, dry, instant, avg | 5 | 20 | 5 | 0.5 | 3.7 | 0.4 | | | 0.4 | 0.1 | 0.2 | 0.1 | 0.00 | 0.11 | 0 | 4 | 0.4 | | | | 0.04 | 0.04 | 0.48 | 0.02 | 0.00 | 0.9 | | 0.1 | | | 14 | 0.0 | 0.7 | 5 | 0.1 | 21 | 17 | 1.0 | 10 | 0.28 |
| | | | Rice Cereal | | | | | | | | | | | | | | | | | | | | | | | | | | | | | | | | | | | | | | | | |
| 60798 | 1 | Tbs | Apple, dry, 2nd Foods, Gerber | 4 | 16 | 3 | 0.2 | 3.4 | 0.1 | 1.0 | 2.4 | 0.1 | | | | | | | | | | | | 0.06 | 0.07 | 0.53 | 0.01 | | | | | | | 24 | 0.0 | 1.8 | 2 | 0.1 | 13 | 9 | | 0 | 0.05 |
| 60072 | 1 | ea | Apple, Stage 2, 4 oz jar, Beechnut | 113 | 70 | 86 | 0.0 | 15.9 | 1.0 | 10.0 | 5.0 | 0.0 | 0.0 | 0.0 | 0.0 | 0.00 | 0.00 | | 30 | 6 | | | | 0.16 | 0.25 | 2.09 | | | | | 15.7 | | | 0 | | 5.2 | | | | 70 | | 0 | |
| 60396 | 1 | Tbs | Apples & Bananas, strained, Heinz | 16 | 11 | 83 | 0.1 | 2.6 | 0.1 | 1.2 | 1.3 | 0.0 | 0.0 | | | | | | 4 | 1 | | | | 0.04 | 0.05 | 0.72 | 0.00 | | | | 8.0 | | | 1 | 0.0 | 0.8 | | | 1 | 6 | | 1 | 0.01 |
| 60617 | 1 | Tbs | Applesauce Banana, strained, RTE, avg | 16 | 13 | 81 | 0.2 | 2.7 | 0.2 | | | 0.1 | 0.0 | 0.0 | 0.0 | 0.00 | 0.01 | 0 | 3 | 0.3 | | | | 0.04 | 0.07 | 0.64 | 0.04 | 0.00 | 0.4 | 0.04 | 5.1 | | | 3 | 0.0 | 1.1 | 0 | | 2 | 4 | 0.3 | 4 | 0.01 |
| 60169 | 1 | Tbs | Applesauce Banana, 2nd Foods, Gerber | 14 | 11 | 80 | 0.1 | 2.6 | 0.1 | 1.2 | 1.3 | 0.0 | | | | | | | 1 | 0.1 | 0 | 0.1 | 1 | 0.03 | 0.03 | 0.44 | 0.02 | | | | 1.9 | | | 2 | 0.0 | 0.8 | 1 | 0.0 | 3 | 8 | | 1 | 0.03 |
| 60618 | 1 | Tbs | Banana, dry, avg | 2 | 8 | 5 | 0.2 | 1.6 | 0.0 | | | 0.1 | 0.0 | 0.0 | 0.0 | 0.00 | 0.03 | 0 | 0.6 | 0.1 | | | | 0.08 | 0.08 | 0.47 | 0.01 | 0.00 | 0.2 | | 0.0 | | | 14 | 0.0 | 0.9 | 3 | | 8 | 15 | 0.2 | 2 | 0.03 |
| 60011 | 1 | Tbs | Banana, dry, 2nd Stage, Gerber | 4 | 16 | 4 | 0.2 | 3.4 | 0.1 | 1.2 | 2.0 | 0.1 | | | | | | | | | | | | 0.06 | 0.07 | 0.53 | 0.02 | | | | 0.0 | | | 24 | 0.0 | 1.8 | 3 | 0.1 | 13 | 15 | | 0 | 0.06 |
| 60615 | 1 | Tbs | Banana, prep w/whole milk, avg | 15 | 18 | 74 | 0.6 | 2.6 | 0.0 | | | 0.5 | 0.3 | | | | | 2 | 4 | 4 | | | | 0.10 | 0.11 | 0.59 | 0.02 | 0.05 | 0.9 | | 0.2 | | | 32 | 0.0 | 1.7 | 5 | | 22 | 38 | | 9 | 0.08 |
| 60248 | 1 | ea | Banana & Applesauce, 4.5 oz jar, Beechnut | 128 | 100 | 80 | 2.0 | 24.0 | | | | 0.0 | 0.0 | 0.0 | 0.0 | 0.00 | 0.00 | | | | | | | 0.18 | 0.22 | 2.70 | | | | | 16.0 | | | 48 | | 4.5 | | | | | | 25 | |
| 60105 | 1 | Tbs | Brown Rice, prep w/formula, Earth's Best | 18 | 22 | 76 | 0.4 | 3.4 | | | | 0.6 | | | | | | | 24 | 7 | 7 | 0 | | 0.03 | 0.02 | 0.49 | 0.05 | | | | 0.7 | | | 7 | | 0.9 | | | | | | 3 | |
| 60104 | 1 | Tbs | Brown Rice, prep w/water, Earth's Best | 18 | 12 | 82 | 0.2 | 2.5 | | | | 0.0 | 0.0 | 0.0 | 0.0 | 0.00 | 0.00 | | | | | | | 0.02 | 0.00 | 0.37 | 0.04 | | | | | | | | | 0.9 | | | | | | 0 | |
| 60071 | 1 | Tbs | Golden Delicious Apples, Stage 2, Beechnut | 4 | 17 | 1 | 0.0 | 3.9 | 0.0 | 0.8 | 3.1 | 0.0 | 0.0 | 0.0 | 0.0 | 0.00 | 0.00 | | 0 | 0 | 0 | 0 | 0 | 0.04 | 0.05 | 0.59 | | | | | 0.0 | | | 25 | | 1.7 | | | | 7 | | 0 | |
| 60620 | 1 | Tbs | Honey, dry, avg | 2 | 8 | 5 | 0.1 | 1.6 | | | | 0.1 | | | | | | | 0.5 | 0.06 | | | | 0.05 | 0.06 | 0.73 | 0.01 | 0.00 | 0.5 | | 0.0 | | | 23 | 0.0 | 1.3 | 4 | | 13 | 2 | | 1 | 0.04 |
| 60621 | 1 | Tbs | Honey, prep w/whole milk, avg | 15 | 17 | 74 | 0.6 | 2.6 | | | | 0.5 | | | | | | | 14 | 4 | | | | 0.07 | 0.09 | 0.91 | 0.02 | 0.05 | 1.2 | | 0.0 | | | 44 | 0.0 | 1.6 | 7 | | 27 | 21 | | 7 | 0.10 |
| 60800 | 1 | Tbs | Mixed Fruit, dry, 2nd Foods, Gerber | 14 | 55 | 3 | 0.9 | 11.8 | 0.2 | 3.4 | 8.2 | 0.5 | | | | | | | | | | | | 0.21 | 0.25 | 1.86 | 0.05 | | | | 1.5 | | | 84 | 0.0 | 6.3 | 9 | 0.2 | 47 | 41 | | 1 | 0.17 |
| 60616 | 1 | Tbs | Mixed Fruit, junior, RTE, avg | 15 | 12 | 80 | 0.1 | 2.7 | 0.1 | | | 0.0 | 0.0 | 0.0 | 0.0 | 0.00 | 0.01 | 0 | 2 | 0.3 | | | | 0.02 | 0.02 | 0.32 | 0.02 | 0.00 | 0.2 | 0.04 | 1.4 | | | 2 | 0.0 | 0.4 | 1 | | 3 | 8 | 0.3 | 2 | 0.02 |
| 60171 | 1 | Tbs | Mixed Fruit, 3rd Foods, Gerber | 14 | 11 | 80 | 0.1 | 2.5 | 0.1 | 1.1 | 1.4 | 0.0 | | | | | | | 0.4 | 0.04 | 0 | 0.04 | 0.3 | 0.02 | 0.02 | 0.30 | 0.02 | | | | 1.3 | | | 2 | 0.0 | 0.4 | 1 | 0.0 | 3 | 7 | | 1 | 0.13 |
| 60619 | 1 | Tbs | Plain, dry, avg | 2 | 8 | 7 | 0.1 | 1.6 | 0.0 | | | 0.1 | 0.0 | 0.0 | 0.0 | 0.00 | 0.04 | 0 | 0.3 | 0.02 | | | | 0.05 | 0.04 | 0.62 | 0.01 | 0.00 | 0.5 | | 0.0 | | | 17 | 0.0 | 0.9 | 4 | | 12 | 8 | 0.2 | 1 | 0.04 |
| 60155 | 1 | Tbs | Plain, dry, Heinz | 2 | 8 | 6 | 0.2 | 1.6 | 0.0 | | | 0.1 | 0.0 | 0.0 | 0.0 | | | 0 | 0 | 0 | 0 | 0 | | 0.05 | 0.06 | 0.85 | 0.00 | 0.00 | 0.5 | 0.01 | 0.0 | | | 24 | 0.0 | 1.3 | 4 | | 20 | 3 | 0.2 | 0 | 0.03 |
| 60063 | 1 | Tbs | Plain, dry, Stage 1, Beechnut | 4 | 17 | 1 | 0.3 | 3.7 | 0.0 | 0.0 | 3.7 | 0.0 | 0.0 | 0.0 | 0.0 | 0.00 | 0.00 | | 0 | 0 | 0 | 0 | 0 | 0.05 | 0.06 | 0.76 | | | | | 0.0 | | | 25 | | 1.9 | | | | 4 | | 0 | |
| 60622 | 1 | Tbs | Plain, prep w/whole milk, avg | 15 | 17 | 75 | 0.6 | 2.5 | 0.0 | | | 0.5 | 0.3 | | | | | 2 | 16 | 4 | | | | 0.07 | 0.08 | 0.78 | 0.02 | 0.05 | 1.2 | | 0.2 | | | 36 | 0.0 | 1.8 | 7 | | 26 | 29 | | 7 | 0.10 |
| 60280 | 1 | ea | Plum & Apples, Stage 2, 4 oz jar, Beechnut | 113 | 90 | 84 | 0.0 | 17.9 | 1.0 | 15.9 | 1.0 | 0.0 | 0.0 | 0.0 | 0.0 | 0.00 | 0.00 | | 224 | 45 | | | | 0.01 | 0.02 | 0.24 | | | | | 15.7 | | | 0 | | 0.0 | | | | 105 | | 10 | |
| 60113 | 1 | ea | Plum & Bananas, 4.5 oz jar, Earth's Best | 128 | 90 | 84 | 1.0 | 19.0 | | | | 1.0 | | | | | | | 120 | 12 | 0 | 12 | | 0.04 | 0.08 | 0.48 | 0.21 | | | | 15.8 | | | | | 0.2 | 18 | | | | | 10 | |
| | | | *INFANT COOKIES AND CRACKERS* | | | | | | | | | | | | | | | | | | | | | | | | | | | | | | | | | | | | | | | | |
| 60634 | 1 | ea | Biscuit, teething, avg | 11 | 43 | 6 | 1.2 | 8.4 | 0.2 | | | 0.5 | 0.2 | 0.2 | 0.1 | 0.01 | 0.09 | 0 | 13 | 1.3 | | | | 0.03 | 0.06 | 0.48 | 0.01 | 0.01 | 5.4 | 0.06 | 1.0 | | | 29 | 0.0 | 0.4 | 4 | | 18 | 36 | 2.6 | 40 | 0.10 |
| 60002 | 1 | ea | Biscuit, Toddler Biter, Gerber | 11 | 43 | 7 | 1.0 | 8.5 | 0.2 | 3.3 | 5.0 | 0.6 | | | | | | | | | | | | 0.02 | 0.05 | 0.32 | 0.01 | | | | 0.1 | | | 10 | 0.0 | 0.3 | 4 | 0.0 | 15 | 37 | | 27 | 0.07 |
| | | | Cookies | | | | | | | | | | | | | | | | | | | | | | | | | | | | | | | | | | | | | | | | |
| 60519 | 1 | ea | Arrowroot, avg | 5 | 22 | 6 | 0.4 | 3.6 | 0.0 | | | 0.7 | 0.2 | 0.4 | 0.0 | 0.00 | 0.04 | 0 | 0 | 0 | 0 | 0 | 0 | 0.02 | 0.02 | 0.29 | 0.00 | 0.00 | 1.8 | 0.03 | 0.3 | | | 2 | 0.0 | 0.2 | 1 | | 6 | 8 | 0.9 | 19 | 0.03 |
| 60001 | 1 | ea | Arrowroot, grad, Gerber | 4 | 18 | 3 | 0.3 | 2.9 | 0.1 | 1.0 | 1.8 | 0.6 | 0.1 | | | | | | 0.2 | 0.02 | 0 | 0.02 | 0.1 | 0.02 | 0.01 | 0.13 | 0.03 | | | | 0.2 | | | 2 | 0.0 | 0.1 | 1 | 0.0 | 5 | 5 | | 12 | 0.03 |
| 60844 | 1 | ea | Banana, grad, Gerger | 8 | 35 | 6 | 0.5 | 5.9 | 0.3 | 1.9 | 3.7 | 1.0 | 0.2 | | | | | | 188 | 19 | 0 | 19 | 113 | 0.04 | 0.03 | 0.29 | 0.02 | | | | 0.1 | | | 7 | 0.0 | 0.2 | 2 | 0.0 | 15 | 34 | | 1 | 0.06 |
| 60520 | 1 | ea | Plain, avg | 6 | 26 | 6 | 0.7 | 4.0 | 0.0 | | | 0.8 | 0.2 | 0.4 | 0.1 | 0.00 | 0.06 | 0 | 1 | 0.1 | | | | 0.09 | 0.19 | 0.96 | 0.35 | 0.28 | 0.6 | 0.03 | 0.4 | | | 6 | 0.0 | 0.3 | 3 | | 11 | 30 | 1.0 | 12 | 0.07 |
| 60843 | 1 | ea | Fruit Bar, Apple Cinnamon, grad, Gerber | 9 | 36 | 11 | 0.5 | 6.6 | 0.3 | 3.2 | 3.1 | 0.9 | 0.2 | | | | | | 0.5 | 0.05 | 0 | 0.05 | 0.3 | 0.03 | 0.02 | 0.20 | 0.01 | | | | | | | 4 | 0.0 | 0.2 | 1 | 0.0 | 8 | 13 | | 7 | 0.02 |
| 60845 | 1 | ea | Fruit Bar, Strawberry, grad, Gerber | 9 | 36 | 11 | 0.5 | 6.5 | 0.3 | 3.2 | 3.1 | 0.9 | 0.2 | | | | | | 0.2 | 0.02 | 0 | 0.02 | 0.1 | 0.03 | 0.02 | 0.18 | 0.01 | | | | 0.2 | | | 4 | 0.0 | 0.2 | 2 | 0.0 | 8 | 14 | | 8 | 0.03 |
| 60611 | 1 | ea | Pretzels, avg | 6 | 24 | 4 | 0.6 | 4.9 | 0.1 | | | 0.1 | 0.0 | 0.0 | 0.0 | 0.00 | 0.05 | 0 | 0.5 | 0.06 | | | | 0.03 | 0.02 | 0.21 | 0.00 | 0.00 | 5.1 | 0.03 | 0.2 | | | 1 | 0.0 | 0.2 | 2 | | 7 | 8 | 0.5 | 16 | 0.05 |
| 60148 | 1 | ea | Pretzels, grad, Gerber | 3 | 12 | 4 | 0.4 | 2.4 | 0.1 | 0.2 | 2.1 | 0.1 | 0.0 | | | | | | | | | | | 0.02 | 0.01 | 0.14 | 0.00 | | | | | | | 1 | 0.0 | 0.1 | 1 | 0.0 | 4 | 4 | | 9 | 0.03 |
| 60149 | 1 | ea | Zwieback Toast, Gerber | 7 | 30 | 5 | 0.9 | 4.9 | 0.3 | 0.9 | 3.7 | 0.8 | | | | | | | | | | | | 0.06 | 0.04 | 0.41 | 0.01 | | | | 0.1 | | | 4 | 0.0 | 0.2 | 2 | 0.0 | 9 | 11 | | 13 | 0.08 |
| | | | *INFANT DESSERTS* | | | | | | | | | | | | | | | | | | | | | | | | | | | | | | | | | | | | | | | | |
| | | | Cottage Cheese | | | | | | | | | | | | | | | | | | | | | | | | | | | | | | | | | | | | | | | | |
| 60525 | 1 | Tbs | With pineapple, stained, avg | 14 | 10 | 83 | 0.4 | 1.8 | 0.0 | | | 0.1 | | | | | | | 4 | 0.4 | | | | 0.00 | 0.01 | 0.01 | 0.00 | 0.01 | 0.6 | 0.01 | 3.3 | | | 4 | 0.0 | 0.0 | 1 | | 5 | 6 | | 7 | 0.02 |
| 60524 | 1 | Tbs | With pineapple, junior, avg | 14 | 11 | 80 | 0.4 | 2.2 | 0.0 | | | 0.1 | 0.1 | 0.0 | 0.0 | | | 0 | 2 | 0.3 | | | | 0.00 | 0.01 | 0.01 | 0.00 | 0.01 | 0.7 | 0.02 | 3.3 | | | 4 | 0.0 | 0.0 | 1 | | 5 | 6 | | 7 | 0.02 |
| 60739 | 1 | ea | With Pears, 4 oz jar, Beechnut | 113 | 120 | 76 | 2.0 | 23.9 | 1.0 | 16.9 | 6.0 | 1.0 | | | | | | | 0 | 0 | 0 | 0 | 0 | | | | | | | | 15.7 | | | 12 | | 0.0 | | | | 75 | | 15 | |
| 60743 | 1 | ea | With Pears, Stage 3, 6 oz jar, Beechnut | 170 | 180 | 75 | 3.0 | 37.0 | 1.0 | 26.0 | 10.0 | 2.0 | | | | | | | 0 | 0 | 0 | 0 | 0 | | | | | | | | 15.8 | | | 12 | | 0.0 | | | | 110 | | 20 | |
| | | | Fruit | | | | | | | | | | | | | | | | | | | | | | | | | | | | | | | | | | | | | | | | |
| 60461 | 1 | Tbs | Apple Betty, junior, avg | 14 | 10 | 80 | 0.1 | 2.7 | 0.1 | | | 0.0 | 0.0 | 0.0 | 0.0 | 0.00 | 0.00 | | 2 | 0.3 | | | | 0.00 | 0.01 | 0.01 | 0.00 | 0.01 | 0.1 | | 3.8 | | | 2 | 0.0 | 0.0 | 0 | | 1 | 7 | | 1 | 0.00 |
| 60462 | 1 | Tbs | Apple Betty, strained, avg | 14 | 10 | 80 | 0.1 | 2.7 | 0.1 | | | 0.0 | 0.0 | 0.0 | 0.0 | 0.00 | 0.00 | | 2 | 0.3 | | | | 0.00 | 0.01 | 0.01 | 0.00 | 0.01 | 0.1 | | 4.9 | | | 3 | 0.0 | 0.0 | 0 | | 0 | 7 | | 1 | 0.00 |
| 60431 | 1 | ea | Apple, Peach, Strawbry, Stg 2, 4 oz jar, Beechnut | 113 | 100 | 81 | 0.0 | 21.9 | 1.0 | 18.9 | 2.0 | 0.0 | 0.0 | 0.0 | 0.0 | 0.00 | 0.00 | | 0 | 0 | 0 | 0 | 0 | 0.02 | 0.03 | 0.12 | | | | | 15.9 | | | 0 | | 0.0 | | | | 120 | | 0 | |
| 60089 | 1 | ea | Apple Strawberry, Stage 2, 4 oz jar, Beechnut | 113 | 100 | 83 | 0.0 | 22.9 | 1.0 | 16.9 | 5.0 | 0.0 | 0.0 | 0.0 | 0.0 | 0.00 | 0.00 | | 0 | 0 | 0 | 0 | 0 | 0.02 | 0.03 | | | | | | 15.7 | | | 0 | | 0.0 | | | | 105 | | 0 | |
| 60450 | 1 | Tbs | Banana Apple, 2nd Foods, Gerber | 14 | 10 | 83 | 0.0 | 2.3 | 0.1 | 1.3 | 0.9 | 0.0 | | | | | | | 2 | 0.2 | 0 | 0.2 | 1 | 0.00 | 0.00 | 0.02 | 0.01 | | | | 1.9 | | | 0 | 0.0 | 0.0 | 1 | 0.0 | 1 | 10 | | 1 | 0.01 |
| 60774 | 1 | ea | Banana Apple, strained, 4 oz jar, Heinz | 113 | 77 | 83 | 0.6 | 18.0 | 0.8 | 9.2 | 8.0 | 0.2 | | | | | | | 26 | 5 | | | | 0.02 | 0.03 | 0.33 | 0.17 | | | | 67.0 | | | 6 | | 0.0 | | | 11 | 158 | | 9 | |
| 60276 | 1 | ea | Banana Pineapple, Stage 2, 4 oz jar, Beechnut | 113 | 100 | 80 | 0.0 | 22.9 | 0.0 | 11.0 | 12.0 | 0.0 | 0.0 | 0.0 | 0.0 | 0.00 | 0.00 | | 30 | 6 | | | | 0.02 | 0.02 | 0.12 | | | | | 44.8 | | | 0 | | 0.0 | | | | 140 | | 15 | |
| 60828 | 1 | ea | Blueberry Buckle, 3rd Foods, 6 oz jar, Gerber | 170 | 124 | 82 | 0.3 | 30.8 | 0.3 | 18.0 | 12.4 | 0.0 | 0.0 | 0.0 | 0.0 | 0.00 | 0.00 | | | | | | | 0.02 | 0.02 | 0.07 | 0.02 | | | | 15.8 | | | 7 | 0.0 | 0.2 | 2 | 0.0 | 5 | 22 | | 68 | |
| 60862 | 1 | Tbs | Cherry Cobbler, junior, avg | 16 | 12 | 80 | 0.0 | 3.1 | 0.0 | | | 0.0 | 0.0 | 0.0 | 0.0 | 0.00 | 0.00 | 0 | 5 | 0.5 | | | | 0.00 | 0.00 | 0.01 | 0.00 | 0.00 | 0.3 | 0.01 | 1.5 | | | 1 | 0.0 | 0.0 | 0 | 0.0 | 1 | 7 | 0.1 | 7 | 0.01 |
| 60829 | 1 | ea | Cherry Cobbler, 3rd Foods, 6 oz jar, Gerber | 170 | 134 | 80 | 0.5 | 32.6 | 0.3 | 19.4 | 12.9 | 0.2 | | | | | | | 53 | 5 | 0 | 5 | 32 | 0.02 | 0.02 | 0.10 | 0.03 | | | | 15.8 | | | 9 | 0.0 | 0.2 | 3 | 0.0 | 10 | 77 | | 73 | |
| 60526 | 1 | Tbs | Dutch Apple, junior, avg | 16 | 13 | 80 | 0.0 | 3.1 | 0.2 | 2.6 | 0.3 | 0.0 | 0.0 | 0.0 | 0.0 | 0.00 | 0.01 | 0 | 3 | 0.3 | 0 | 0.3 | | 0.00 | 0.00 | 0.01 | 0.00 | 0.00 | 0.0 | 0.00 | 2.9 | | | 0 | 0.0 | 0.0 | 1 | 0.0 | 1 | 11 | 0.0 | 0 | 0.00 |
| 60527 | 1 | Tbs | Dutch Apple, strained, avg | 16 | 11 | 82 | 0.0 | 2.7 | 0.1 | | | 0.1 | 0.1 | 0.0 | 0.0 | 0.00 | 0.00 | 0 | 8 | 1 | | | | 0.00 | 0.00 | 0.01 | 0.00 | 0.00 | 0.1 | | 3.4 | | | 1 | 0.0 | 0.0 | 0 | | 0 | 5 | 0.0 | 3 | 0.00 |
| 60179 | 1 | Tbs | Dutch Apple, 2nd Foods, Gerber | 14 | 11 | 79 | 0.0 | 2.8 | 0.2 | 2.5 | 0.1 | 0.0 | | | | | | | 4 | 0.5 | 0 | 0.5 | 3 | 0.00 | 0.00 | 0.01 | 0.00 | | | | 1.9 | | | 0 | 0.0 | 0.0 | 1 | 0.0 | 1 | 9 | | 1 | |
| 60180 | 1 | Tbs | Dutch Apple, 3rd Foods, Gerber | 14 | 11 | 82 | 0.0 | 2.4 | 0.1 | 1.8 | 0.4 | 0.1 | | | | | | | 2 | 0.2 | 0 | 0.2 | 1 | 0.00 | 0.00 | 0.01 | 0.00 | | | | 1.3 | | | 0 | 0.0 | 0.0 | 0 | 0.0 | 1 | 6 | | 2 | |
| 60529 | 1 | Tbs | Fruit, junior, avg | 15 | 9 | 82 | 0.0 | 2.6 | 0.1 | | | 0.0 | 0.0 | 0.0 | 0.0 | 0.00 | 0.00 | 0 | 36 | 4 | | | | 0.00 | 0.00 | 0.02 | 0.00 | 0.00 | 0.5 | 0.02 | 0.5 | | | 1 | 0.0 | 0.0 | 1 | | 1 | 14 | 0.1 | 2 | 0.01 |
| 60530 | 1 | Tbs | Fruit, strained, avg | 15 | 9 | 83 | 0.0 | 2.4 | 0.1 | | | 0.0 | 0.0 | 0.0 | 0.0 | 0.00 | 0.00 | 0 | 38 | 4 | | | | 0.00 | 0.00 | 0.02 | 0.01 | 0.00 | 0.5 | 0.02 | 0.4 | | | 1 | 0.0 | 0.0 | 1 | | 1 | 14 | 0.1 | 2 | 0.01 |
| 60740 | 1 | ea | Fruit, Stage 2, 4 oz jar, Beechnut | 113 | 80 | 83 | 0.0 | 18.9 | 1.0 | 15.9 | 2.0 | 0.0 | 0.0 | 0.0 | 0.0 | 0.00 | 0.00 | | 60 | 12 | | | | | | | | | | | 15.7 | | | 0 | | 0.0 | | | | 140 | | 0 | |
| 60438 | 1 | ea | Fruit, Stage 3, 6 oz jar, Beechnut | 170 | 120 | 87 | 0.0 | 28.0 | 2.0 | 23.0 | 3.0 | 0.0 | 0.0 | 0.0 | 0.0 | 0.00 | 0.00 | | 120 | 12 | | | | 0.02 | 0.04 | 0.02 | | | | | 16.0 | | | 0 | | 0.0 | | | | 200 | | 0 | |
| 60818 | 1 | ea | Fruit Salad, 3rd Foods, 6 oz jar, Gerber | 170 | 155 | 77 | 0.7 | 37.6 | 2.9 | 30.9 | 3.7 | 0.2 | | | | | | | 65 | 6 | 0 | 6 | 39 | 0.03 | 0.05 | 0.43 | 0.10 | | | | 15.8 | | | 10 | 0.1 | 0.3 | 14 | 0.2 | 19 | 206 | | 5 | 0.17 |
| 60446 | 1 | ea | Guava Fruit, Stage 2, 4 oz jar, Beechnut | 113 | 90 | 81 | 0.0 | 21.9 | 2.0 | 14.9 | 5.0 | 0.0 | 0.0 | 0.0 | 0.0 | 0.00 | 0.00 | | 30 | 3 | | | | 0.01 | 0.02 | 0.24 | | | | | 15.9 | | | 0 | | 0.0 | | | | 110 | | 10 | |
| 60362 | 1 | Tbs | Hawaiian Delight, strained, Heinz | 16 | 11 | 83 | 0.0 | 2.6 | 0.0 | 1.4 | 1.2 | 0.0 | 0.0 | | | | | | 3 | 1 | | | | 0.00 | 0.00 | 0.02 | 0.00 | | | | 8.0 | | | 1 | 0.0 | 0.0 | | | 1 | 3 | | 2 | 0.00 |
| 60079 | 1 | Tbs | Hawaiian Delight, 2nd Foods, Gerber | 14 | 12 | 78 | 0.2 | 2.8 | 0.0 | 1.6 | 1.2 | 0.0 | | | | | | | 0.4 | 0.04 | 0 | 0.04 | 0.3 | 0.01 | 0.01 | 0.02 | 0.01 | | | | 1.9 | | | 6 | 0.0 | 0.0 | 1 | 0.0 | 5 | 12 | | 2 | 0.03 |
| 60080 | 1 | Tbs | Hawaiian Delight, 3rd Foods, Gerber | 14 | 12 | 78 | 0.2 | 2.9 | 0.0 | 1.7 | 1.2 | 0.0 | | | | | | | 0.1 | 0.01 | 0 | 0.01 | 0.1 | 0.01 | 0.01 | 0.02 | 0.01 | | | | 1.3 | | | 6 | 0.0 | 0.0 | 1 | 0.0 | 5 | 10 | | 2 | 0.03 |
| 60749 | 1 | ea | Island Fruit Tropical, Stage 3, 4 oz jar, Beechnut | 113 | 100 | 79 | 0.0 | 22.9 | 0.0 | 14.0 | 9.0 | 0.0 | 0.0 | 0.0 | 0.0 | 0.00 | 0.00 | 0 | 224 | 22 | | | | 0.04 | 0.06 | 0.42 | | 0.00 | | | 15.7 | | | 0 | | 0.0 | | | | 110 | | 10 | |

| Code | Amount | Description | Weight (g) | Calories | % Water | Protein (g) | Carbs (g) | Fiber (g) | Sugar (g) | Other Carbs (g) | Fat (g) | Sat Fat (g) | Mono Fat (g) | Poly Fat (g) | Omega 3 (g) | Omega 6 (g) | Choles (mg) | Vit A (IU) | Vit A (RE) | Retinol (RE) | Carotenoids (RE) | Beta Carotene (mcg) | Thiamin (mg) | Riboflavin (mg) | Niacin (NE) | Vit B6 (mg) | Vit B12 (mcg) | Folate (mcg) | Panto (mg) | Vit C (mg) | Vit D (mg) | Vit E (α TE) | Calcium (mg) | Copper (mg) | Iron (mg) | Magnes (mg) | Mang (mg) | Phos (mg) | Potassium (mg) | Selenium (mcg) | Sodium (mg) | Zinc (mg) |
|---|---|---|---|---|---|---|---|---|---|---|---|---|---|---|---|---|---|---|---|---|---|---|---|---|---|---|---|---|---|---|---|---|---|---|---|---|---|---|---|---|---|---|
| | | **Basic Components** | | | | | | | | | | **Additional Fats** | | | | | | **Vit A & Components** | | | | | **Vitamins** | | | | | | | | | | **Minerals** | | | | | | | | | |
| 60447 | 1 ea | Mango, Stage 2, 4.5 oz jar, Beechnut | 128 | 110 | 80 | 0.0 | 26.0 | 1.0 | 15.0 | 10.0 | 0.0 | 0.0 | 0.0 | 0.0 | 0.00 | 0.00 | | 375 | 75 | | | | 0.01 | 0.01 | | | | | | 16.0 | | | 0 | | 0.0 | | | | 55 | | 10 | |
| 60448 | 1 ea | Papaya, Stage 2, 4 oz jar, Beechnut | 113 | 100 | 81 | 0.0 | 21.9 | 0.0 | 15.9 | 6.0 | 0.0 | 0.0 | 0.0 | 0.0 | 0.00 | 0.00 | | 149 | 15 | | | | 0.01 | 0.01 | | | | | | 15.9 | | | 0 | | 0.0 | | | | 110 | | 10 | |
| 60591 | 1 Tbs | Peach Cobbler, junior, avg | 15 | 10 | 81 | 0.0 | 2.7 | 0.1 | | | 0.0 | 0.0 | 0.0 | 0.0 | 0.00 | 0.00 | 0 | 21 | 2 | | | | 0.00 | 0.00 | 0.04 | 0.00 | 0.00 | 0.2 | | 3.1 | | | 1 | 0.0 | 0.0 | 0 | | 1 | 8 | 0.2 | 1 | 0.00 |
| 60592 | 1 Tbs | Peach Cobbler, strained, avg | 15 | 10 | 82 | 0.0 | 2.7 | 0.1 | | | 0.0 | 0.0 | 0.0 | 0.0 | 0.00 | 0.00 | 0 | 21 | 2 | | | | 0.00 | 0.00 | 0.04 | 0.00 | 0.00 | 0.2 | | 3.1 | | | 1 | 0.0 | 0.0 | 0 | | 1 | 8 | 0.2 | 1 | 0.05 |
| 60183 | 1 Tbs | Peach Cobbler, 2nd Foods, Gerber | 14 | 11 | 81 | 0.1 | 2.5 | 0.1 | 1.6 | 0.9 | 0.0 | | | | | | | 22 | 2 | 0 | 2 | 13 | 0.00 | 0.00 | 0.06 | 0.00 | | | | 1.9 | | | 1 | 0.0 | 0.0 | 1 | 0.0 | 1 | 12 | | 1 | 0.01 |
| 60184 | 1 Tbs | Peach Cobbler, 3rd Foods, Gerber | 14 | 11 | 81 | 0.1 | 2.6 | 0.1 | 1.6 | 0.9 | 0.0 | | | | | | | 15 | 2 | 0 | 2 | 9 | 0.00 | 0.00 | 0.06 | 0.00 | | | | 1.3 | | | 1 | 0.0 | 0.0 | 1 | 0.0 | 1 | 12 | | 1 | 0.01 |
| 60593 | 1 Tbs | Peach Melba, junior, avg | 14 | 8 | 83 | 0.0 | 2.3 | | | | 0.0 | 0.0 | 0.0 | 0.0 | 0.00 | 0.00 | | 27 | 3 | | | | 0.00 | 0.00 | 0.04 | 0.00 | 0.00 | 0.3 | | 3.6 | | | 2 | 0.0 | 0.0 | 0 | | 1 | 13 | | 1 | 0.04 |
| 60594 | 1 Tbs | Peach Melba, strained, avg | 14 | 8 | 83 | 0.0 | 2.3 | | | | 0.0 | 0.0 | 0.0 | 0.0 | 0.00 | 0.00 | | 26 | 3 | | | | 0.00 | 0.01 | 0.05 | 0.00 | 0.00 | 0.3 | | 4.4 | | | 1 | 0.0 | 0.0 | 0 | | 1 | 12 | | 1 | 0.04 |
| 60605 | 1 Tbs | Pineapple Orange, strained, avg | 14 | 10 | 80 | 0.0 | 2.7 | 0.1 | | | 0.0 | 0.0 | 0.0 | 0.0 | 0.00 | 0.00 | | 8 | 1 | | | | 0.00 | 0.00 | 0.01 | 0.00 | 0.01 | 0.4 | 0.02 | 2.0 | | | 2 | 0.0 | 0.0 | 1 | | 1 | 7 | | 1 | 0.02 |
| 60830 | 1 ea | Raspberry Cobbler, 3rd Foods, 6 oz jar, Gerber | 170 | 129 | 81 | 0.3 | 31.6 | 0.2 | 17.3 | 14.1 | 0.2 | | | | | | | | | | | | 0.02 | | 0.12 | 0.02 | | | | 15.8 | | | 7 | 0.0 | 0.3 | 3 | 0.0 | 5 | 36 | | 77 | |
| 60414 | 1 Tbs | Tutti Frutti, Heinz | 16 | 11 | 83 | 0.0 | 2.5 | 0.1 | 1.4 | 1.1 | 0.1 | 0.0 | | | | | | 30 | 6 | | | | 0.00 | 0.00 | 0.02 | 0.00 | | | | 6.7 | | | 2 | 0.0 | 0.0 | | | 1 | 7 | | 2 | 0.01 |
| 60363 | 1 Tbs | TuttiFrutti, strained, Heinz | 16 | 11 | 83 | 0.0 | 2.6 | 0.0 | 1.5 | 1.0 | 0.0 | 0.0 | | | | | | 19 | 4 | | | | 0.00 | 0.00 | 0.01 | 0.00 | | | | 8.9 | | | 2 | 0.0 | 0.0 | | | 1 | 6 | | 2 | 0.01 |
| | | Puddings | | | | | | | | | | | | | | | | | | | | | | | | | | | | | | | | | | | | | | | | |
| 60353 | 1 Tbs | Banana, strained, Heinz | 16 | 12 | 82 | 0.1 | 2.6 | 0.1 | 1.5 | 1.0 | 0.1 | 0.0 | | | | | | 7 | 1 | | | | 0.00 | 0.01 | 0.03 | 0.02 | | | | 6.7 | | | 2 | 0.0 | 0.1 | | | 4 | 15 | | 1 | 0.01 |
| 60747 | 1 ea | Banana, Stage 2, 4 oz jar, Beechnut | 113 | 110 | 77 | 0.0 | 25.9 | 0.0 | 14.9 | 11.0 | 0.0 | 0.0 | 0.0 | 0.0 | 0.00 | 0.00 | | 30 | 6 | | | | 0.03 | 0.09 | 0.17 | | | | | 15.6 | | | 0 | 0.0 | 0.0 | 8 | 0.0 | 54 | 120 | 0.0 | 0 | 0.31 |
| 60498 | 1 Tbs | Caramel, junior, avg | 14 | 11 | 80 | 0.2 | 2.4 | | | | 0.1 | | | | | | | 5 | 0.4 | | | | 0.00 | 0.01 | 0.01 | 0.00 | 0.00 | 0.1 | 0.03 | 0.3 | | | 8 | 0.0 | 0.0 | 1 | | 6 | 8 | | 4 | 0.04 |
| 60499 | 1 Tbs | Caramel, strained, avg | 14 | 11 | 80 | 0.2 | 2.4 | | | | 0.1 | | | | | | | 5 | 1 | | | | 0.00 | 0.01 | 0.00 | 0.00 | 0.00 | 0.1 | 0.03 | 0.3 | | | 6 | 0.0 | 0.0 | 1 | | 6 | 7 | | 4 | 0.04 |
| 60510 | 1 Tbs | Cherry Vanilla, junior, avg | 16 | 11 | 81 | 0.0 | 2.9 | 0.0 | | | 0.0 | 0.0 | 0.0 | 0.0 | 0.00 | 0.01 | 2 | 32 | 3 | | | | 0.00 | 0.00 | 0.01 | 0.00 | 0.00 | 0.0 | | 0.2 | | | 1 | 0.0 | 0.0 | 0 | | 1 | 5 | 0.1 | 2 | 0.00 |
| 60509 | 1 Tbs | Cherry Vanilla, strained, avg | 16 | 11 | 82 | 0.0 | 2.8 | 0.0 | | | 0.0 | 0.0 | 0.0 | 0.0 | 0.00 | 0.01 | 2 | 32 | 3 | | | | 0.00 | 0.00 | 0.01 | 0.00 | 0.00 | 0.0 | | 0.2 | | | 1 | 0.0 | 0.0 | 0 | | 1 | 5 | 0.1 | 3 | 0.01 |
| 60176 | 1 Tbs | Cherry Vanilla, 2nd Foods, Gerber | 14 | 10 | 83 | 0.0 | 2.3 | 0.0 | 1.6 | 0.7 | 0.0 | | | | | | | 2 | 0.2 | 0 | 0.2 | 1 | 0.00 | 0.00 | 0.01 | 0.00 | | | | 0.0 | | | 1 | 0.0 | 0.0 | 0 | 0.0 | 1 | 6 | | 1 | |
| 60518 | 1 Tbs | Chocolate Custard, junior, avg | 14 | 12 | 78 | 0.3 | 2.4 | 0.1 | | | 0.2 | | | | | | | 6 | 1 | 0 | 1 | | 0.00 | 0.02 | 0.02 | 0.00 | 0.00 | 0.7 | 0.04 | 0.2 | | | 9 | 0.0 | 0.1 | 1 | | 7 | 12 | | 4 | 0.05 |
| 60517 | 1 Tbs | Chocolate Custard, strained, avg | 14 | 12 | 80 | 0.3 | 2.3 | 0.1 | | | 0.2 | 0.2 | 0.0 | 0.0 | | | 0 | 6 | 1 | 0 | 1 | | 0.00 | 0.01 | 0.01 | 0.00 | 0.00 | 0.6 | 0.04 | 0.2 | | | 9 | 0.0 | 0.1 | 1 | | 7 | 12 | | 3 | 0.04 |
| 60355 | 1 Tbs | Custard, strained, Heinz | 16 | 12 | 82 | 0.3 | 2.2 | 0.1 | 1.2 | 1.0 | 0.2 | 0.1 | | | | | | 7 | 1 | | | | 0.00 | 0.01 | 0.02 | 0.00 | | | | 0.1 | | | 10 | 0.0 | 0.0 | | | 10 | 12 | | 4 | 0.03 |
| 60586 | 1 Tbs | Orange, strained, avg | 16 | 13 | 80 | 0.2 | 2.8 | 0.1 | | | 0.1 | 0.1 | 0.0 | 0.0 | 0.00 | 0.01 | 0 | 18 | 2 | | | | 0.01 | 0.01 | 0.02 | 0.00 | 0.00 | 1.2 | 0.04 | 1.5 | | | 5 | 0.0 | 0.0 | 1 | | 4 | 14 | 0.1 | 3 | 0.03 |
| 60607 | 1 Tbs | Pineapple, junior, avg | 15 | 13 | 76 | 0.2 | 3.2 | 0.1 | | | 0.1 | 0.0 | 0.0 | 0.0 | 0.00 | 0.01 | 0 | 6 | 1 | | | | 0.01 | 0.01 | 0.02 | 0.01 | 0.01 | 0.8 | 0.03 | 4.0 | | | 5 | 0.0 | 0.0 | 1 | | 5 | 14 | 0.2 | 3 | 0.03 |
| 60606 | 1 Tbs | Pineapple, strained, avg | 15 | 12 | 78 | 0.2 | 3.0 | 0.1 | | | 0.0 | 0.0 | 0.0 | 0.0 | 0.00 | 0.01 | 0 | 6 | 1 | | | | 0.01 | 0.01 | 0.02 | 0.01 | 0.01 | 0.8 | 0.03 | 4.1 | | | 5 | 0.0 | 0.0 | 1 | | 5 | 12 | 0.2 | 3 | 0.03 |
| 60742 | 1 ea | Vanilla, Stage 2, 4 oz jar, Beechnut | 113 | 120 | 75 | 2.0 | 22.9 | 0.0 | 14.0 | 9.0 | 3.0 | | | | | | | 0 | 0 | 0 | 0 | 0 | | | | | | | | 0.0 | | | 60 | | 0.0 | | | | 130 | | 60 | |
| 60640 | 1 Tbs | Vanilla Custard, junior, avg | 14 | 12 | 79 | 0.2 | 2.5 | 0.0 | 1.6 | 0.8 | 0.1 | 0.0 | 0.1 | 0.0 | 0.00 | 0.02 | 5 | 7 | 2 | 2 | 0 | 0 | 0.00 | 0.01 | 0.01 | 0.00 | 0.03 | 0.8 | 0.03 | 0.1 | | | 8 | 0.0 | 0.0 | 1 | 0.0 | 8 | 10 | 0.3 | 4 | 0.04 |
| 60641 | 1 Tbs | Vanilla Custard, strained, avg | 14 | 12 | 80 | 0.2 | 2.3 | 0.0 | | | 0.3 | 0.1 | 0.1 | 0.0 | 0.00 | 0.02 | 1 | 9 | 1 | | | | 0.00 | 0.01 | 0.01 | 0.00 | 0.00 | 0.8 | 0.04 | 0.1 | | | 8 | 0.0 | 0.0 | 1 | | 6 | 9 | 0.3 | 4 | 0.04 |
| 60275 | 1 ea | Vanilla Custard, Stage 2, 4 oz jar, Beechnut | 113 | 120 | 75 | 2.0 | 22.9 | 0.0 | 14.0 | 9.0 | 3.0 | | | | | | | 0 | 0 | 0 | 0 | 0 | 0.01 | 0.10 | | | | | | 0.0 | | | 60 | | 0.0 | | | | 130 | | 60 | |
| 60069 | 1 ea | Vanilla Custard, Stage 3, 6 oz jar, Beechnut | 170 | 190 | 76 | 2.0 | 32.0 | 0.0 | 21.0 | 11.0 | 6.0 | | | | | | | 60 | 6 | | | | 0.01 | 0.10 | | | | | | 0.0 | | | 90 | | 0.0 | | | | 180 | | 85 | |
| | | Tapioca pudding desserts | | | | | | | | | | | | | | | | | | | | | | | | | | | | | | | | | | | | | | | | |
| 60415 | 1 Tbs | Apple Cranberry, Heinz | 16 | 11 | 84 | 0.0 | 2.6 | 0.1 | 1.5 | 0.9 | 0.0 | 0.0 | | | | | | 1 | 0.3 | | | | 0.00 | 0.00 | 0.01 | 0.00 | | | | 4.2 | | | 1 | 0.0 | 0.0 | | | 0 | 5 | | 1 | 0.01 |
| 60477 | 1 Tbs | Apricot, junior, avg | 15 | 9 | 82 | 0.0 | 2.6 | 0.2 | | | 0.0 | 0.0 | 0.0 | 0.0 | 0.00 | 0.00 | 0 | 108 | 11 | | | | 0.00 | 0.00 | 0.03 | 0.00 | 0.00 | 0.2 | 0.02 | 2.7 | | | 1 | 0.0 | 0.0 | 1 | | 2 | 19 | 0.0 | 1 | 0.01 |
| 60478 | 1 Tbs | Apricot, strained, avg | 15 | 9 | 83 | 0.0 | 2.4 | 0.2 | | | 0.0 | 0.0 | 0.0 | 0.0 | 0.00 | 0.00 | 0 | 109 | 11 | | | | 0.00 | 0.00 | 0.03 | 0.00 | 0.00 | 0.2 | 0.02 | 3.2 | | | 1 | 0.0 | 0.0 | 1 | | 2 | 18 | 0.0 | 1 | 0.01 |
| 60250 | 1 Tbs | Apricot, 2nd Foods, Gerber | 14 | 9 | 83 | 0.0 | 2.3 | 0.1 | 1.5 | 0.7 | 0.0 | | | | | | | 163 | 16 | 0 | 16 | 98 | 0.00 | 0.00 | 0.03 | 0.01 | | | | 1.9 | | | 1 | 0.0 | 0.0 | 1 | 0.0 | 1 | 17 | | 1 | 0.01 |
| 60251 | 1 Tbs | Apricot, 3rd Foods, Gerber | 14 | 10 | 82 | 0.1 | 2.4 | 0.1 | 1.5 | 0.7 | 0.0 | | | | | | | 120 | 12 | 0 | 12 | 72 | 0.00 | 0.00 | 0.03 | 0.01 | | | | 1.3 | | | 1 | 0.0 | 0.0 | 1 | 0.0 | 1 | 18 | | 1 | 0.01 |
| 60481 | 1 Tbs | Banana, junior, avg | 15 | 10 | 82 | 0.1 | 2.7 | 0.2 | | | 0.0 | 0.0 | 0.0 | 0.0 | 0.00 | 0.00 | 0 | 7 | 0.7 | | | | 0.00 | 0.00 | 0.03 | 0.02 | 0.00 | 1.0 | 0.03 | 3.9 | | | 1 | 0.0 | 0.0 | 2 | | 1 | 16 | 0.1 | 1 | 0.01 |
| 60482 | 1 Tbs | Banana, strained, avg | 15 | 9 | 84 | 0.1 | 2.3 | 0.2 | | | 0.0 | 0.0 | 0.0 | 0.0 | 0.00 | 0.00 | 0 | 6 | 0.7 | | | | 0.00 | 0.00 | 0.03 | 0.02 | 0.00 | 0.8 | 0.02 | 2.5 | | | 1 | 0.0 | 0.0 | 2 | | 1 | 13 | 0.1 | 1 | 0.01 |
| 60254 | 1 Tbs | Banana, 2nd Foods, Gerber | 14 | 11 | 80 | 0.1 | 2.6 | 0.1 | 1.6 | 1.0 | 0.0 | | | | | | | 3 | 0.3 | 0 | 0.3 | 2 | 0.00 | 0.01 | 0.05 | 0.02 | | | | 1.9 | | | 1 | 0.0 | 0.0 | 2 | 0.0 | 1 | 21 | | 1 | 0.01 |
| 60255 | 1 Tbs | Banana, 3rd Foods, Gerber | 14 | 11 | 80 | 0.1 | 2.6 | 0.1 | 1.5 | 1.0 | 0.0 | | | | | | | 3 | 0.3 | 0 | 0.3 | 2 | 0.00 | 0.01 | 0.04 | 0.02 | | | | 1.3 | | | 1 | 0.0 | 0.0 | 2 | 0.0 | 1 | 20 | | 1 | 0.01 |
| 60479 | 1 Tbs | Banana Pineapple, junior, avg | 15 | 10 | 82 | 0.0 | 2.7 | 0.2 | | | 0.0 | 0.0 | 0.0 | 0.0 | 0.00 | 0.00 | 0 | 6 | 0.6 | | | | 0.00 | 0.00 | 0.03 | 0.01 | 0.00 | 0.8 | 0.02 | 2.9 | | | 1 | 0.0 | 0.0 | 1 | | 1 | 10 | 0.1 | 1 | 0.01 |
| 60480 | 1 Tbs | Banana Pineapple, strained, avg | 15 | 10 | 81 | 0.0 | 2.8 | 0.2 | | | 0.0 | 0.0 | 0.0 | 0.0 | 0.00 | 0.00 | 0 | 6 | 0.6 | | | | 0.00 | 0.00 | 0.03 | 0.01 | 0.00 | 0.8 | 0.02 | 3.2 | | | 1 | 0.0 | 0.0 | 1 | | 1 | 12 | 0.1 | 1 | 0.00 |
| 60252 | 1 Tbs | Banana Pineapple, 2nd Foods, Gerber | 14 | 7 | 87 | 0.1 | 1.7 | 0.1 | 0.8 | 0.3 | 0.0 | | | | | | | 2 | 0.2 | 0 | 0.2 | 1 | 0.00 | 0.00 | 0.03 | 0.02 | | | | 1.9 | | | 0 | 0.0 | 0.0 | 2 | 0.0 | 2 | 15 | | 1 | 0.01 |
| 60253 | 1 Tbs | Banana Pineapple, 3rd Foods, Gerber | 14 | 8 | 87 | 0.1 | 1.8 | 0.1 | 0.9 | 0.3 | 0.0 | | | | | | | 4 | 0.4 | 0 | 0.4 | 3 | 0.00 | 0.01 | 0.03 | 0.02 | | | | 1.3 | | | 1 | 0.0 | 0.0 | 1 | 0.0 | 1 | 15 | | 1 | 0.01 |
| 60817 | 1 ea | Banana Strawberry, 3rd Foods, 6 oz jar, Gerber | 170 | 131 | 81 | 0.5 | 32.0 | 0.7 | 21.3 | 10.0 | 0.2 | | | | | | | 39 | 4 | 0 | 4 | 23 | | 0.05 | 0.37 | 0.19 | | | | 15.8 | | | 7 | 0.1 | 0.2 | 17 | 0.3 | 15 | 155 | | 14 | 0.17 |
| 60704 | 1 ea | Banana Vanilla, 4 oz jar, Gerber | 113 | 96 | 80 | 0.6 | 20.9 | 0.5 | 14.4 | 6.1 | 0.9 | | | | | | | 8 | 0.8 | 0 | 0.8 | 5 | 0.01 | 0.06 | 0.19 | 0.10 | | | | 15.7 | | | 16 | 0.0 | 0.1 | 12 | 0.3 | 16 | 97 | | 11 | 0.11 |
| 60534 | 1 Tbs | Guava, strained, avg | 15 | 10 | 81 | 0.0 | 2.7 | 0.3 | | | 0.0 | 0.0 | 0.0 | 0.0 | 0.00 | 0.00 | | 45 | 5 | | | | 0.00 | 0.01 | 0.06 | 0.01 | 0.00 | 0.3 | 0.02 | 11.3 | | | 1 | | 0.0 | 0 | | 1 | 11 | 0.1 | 0 | 0.01 |
| 60533 | 1 Tbs | Guava Papaya, strained, avg | 16 | 10 | 82 | 0.0 | 2.7 | 0.3 | | | 0.0 | 0.0 | 0.0 | 0.0 | | | 0 | 29 | 3 | | | | 0.00 | 0.00 | 0.04 | 0.00 | 0.00 | 0.3 | | 12.9 | | | 1 | | 0.0 | 1 | | 1 | 12 | 0.1 | 1 | 0.01 |
| 60560 | 1 Tbs | Mango, strained, avg | 15 | 12 | 78 | 0.0 | 3.2 | 0.2 | | | 0.0 | 0.0 | 0.0 | 0.0 | 0.00 | 0.00 | 0 | 100 | 10 | | | | 0.00 | 0.00 | 0.04 | 0.02 | 0.00 | 0.3 | 0.03 | 18.6 | | | 1 | 0.0 | 0.0 | 1 | | 1 | 9 | 0.1 | 1 | 0.01 |
| 60326 | 1 Tbs | Mango, Gerber | 14 | 11 | 81 | 0.0 | 2.5 | 0.1 | 1.6 | 0.9 | 0.0 | | | | | | | 81 | 8 | 0 | 8 | 49 | 0.00 | 0.00 | 0.03 | 0.01 | | | | 1.9 | | | 1 | 0.0 | 0.0 | 1 | 0.0 | 1 | 11 | | 1 | |
| 60047 | 1 Tbs | Mango Bananas, w/passion fruit juice, avg | 14 | 10 | 82 | 0.0 | 2.5 | 0.0 | 1.5 | 0.9 | 0.0 | | | | | | | 29 | 3 | 0 | 3 | 18 | 0.00 | 0.00 | 0.03 | 0.01 | | | | 1.9 | | | 1 | 0.0 | 0.0 | 1 | 0.0 | 1 | 10 | | 1 | |
| 60327 | 1 Tbs | Papaya, Gerber | 14 | 9 | 84 | 0.0 | 2.2 | 0.0 | 1.4 | 0.8 | 0.0 | | | | | | | 15 | 1 | 0 | 1 | 9 | 0.00 | 0.00 | 0.01 | 0.00 | | | | 1.9 | | | 1 | 0.0 | 0.0 | 1 | 0.0 | 1 | 9 | | 1 | |
| 60590 | 1 Tbs | Papaya Applesauce, strained, avg | 16 | 11 | 81 | 0.0 | 3.0 | 0.2 | | | 0.0 | 0.0 | 0.0 | 0.0 | | | 0 | 12 | 1 | | | | 0.00 | 0.00 | 0.02 | 0.00 | 0.00 | 0.3 | 0.04 | 18.1 | | | 1 | 0.0 | 0.1 | 1 | | 1 | 13 | 0.1 | 1 | 0.00 |
| 60048 | 1 Tbs | Peach Mango, Gerber | 14 | 10 | 82 | 0.0 | 2.4 | 0.0 | 1.5 | 0.9 | 0.0 | | | | | | | 45 | 4 | 0 | 4 | 27 | 0.00 | 0.00 | 0.04 | 0.01 | | | | 1.9 | | | 1 | 0.0 | 0.0 | 1 | 0.0 | 1 | 9 | | 1 | |
| 60609 | 1 Tbs | Plums, junior, avg | 15 | 11 | 79 | 0.0 | 3.1 | 0.2 | | | 0.0 | 0.0 | 0.0 | 0.0 | 0.00 | 0.00 | 0 | 14 | 1 | | | | 0.00 | 0.00 | 0.03 | 0.00 | 0.00 | 0.1 | 0.02 | 0.1 | | | 1 | 0.0 | 0.0 | 1 | | 1 | 12 | 0.1 | 1 | 0.01 |
| 60608 | 1 Tbs | Plums, strained, avg | 15 | 11 | 80 | 0.0 | 3.0 | 0.2 | | | 0.0 | 0.0 | 0.0 | 0.0 | 0.00 | 0.00 | 0 | 14 | 2 | | | | 0.00 | 0.00 | 0.03 | 0.00 | 0.00 | 0.1 | 0.02 | 0.2 | | | 1 | 0.0 | 0.0 | 1 | | 1 | 13 | 0.1 | 1 | 0.01 |
| 60264 | 1 Tbs | Plums, 2nd Foods, Gerber | 14 | 10 | 81 | 0.0 | 2.5 | 0.1 | 1.5 | 0.9 | 0.0 | | | | | | | 8 | 1 | 0 | 1 | 5 | 0.00 | 0.00 | 0.04 | 0.01 | | | | | | | 1 | 0.0 | 0.0 | 1 | 0.0 | 1 | 14 | | 0 | 0.01 |
| 60265 | 1 Tbs | Plums, 3rd Foods, Gerber | 14 | 11 | 81 | 0.0 | 2.5 | 0.2 | 1.6 | 0.8 | 0.0 | | | | | | | 22 | 2 | 0 | 2 | 13 | 0.00 | 0.01 | 0.04 | 0.01 | | | | | | | 1 | 0.0 | 0.0 | 1 | 0.0 | 1 | 14 | | 0 | 0.01 |
| 60613 | 1 Tbs | Prunes, junior, avg | 15 | 11 | 80 | 0.1 | 2.8 | 0.4 | | | 0.0 | 0.0 | 0.0 | 0.0 | 0.00 | 0.00 | 0 | 61 | 5 | | | | 0.00 | 0.01 | 0.08 | 0.01 | 0.00 | 0.0 | 0.02 | 0.1 | | | 2 | 0.0 | 0.0 | 2 | | 2 | 24 | 0.1 | 0 | 0.02 |
| 60612 | 1 Tbs | Prunes, strained, avg | 15 | 11 | 80 | 0.1 | 2.8 | 0.4 | | | 0.0 | 0.0 | 0.0 | 0.0 | 0.00 | 0.00 | 0 | 68 | 7 | | | | 0.00 | 0.01 | 0.08 | 0.01 | 0.00 | 0.0 | 0.02 | 0.1 | | | 2 | 0.0 | 0.1 | 2 | | 2 | 27 | 0.1 | 1 | 0.01 |
| 60266 | 1 Tbs | Prunes, 2nd Foods, Gerber | 14 | 11 | 81 | 0.1 | 2.5 | 0.3 | 1.1 | 1.2 | 0.0 | | | | | | | 51 | 5 | 0 | 5 | 31 | 0.00 | 0.01 | 0.08 | 0.01 | | | | | | | 2 | 0.0 | 0.0 | 2 | 0.0 | 3 | 28 | | 1 | 0.01 |
| 60049 | 1 Tbs | Tropical Fruits, Gerber | 14 | 9 | 84 | 0.0 | 2.1 | 0.0 | 1.3 | 0.8 | 0.0 | | | | | | | 21 | 2 | 0 | 2 | 13 | 0.00 | 0.00 | 0.01 | 0.01 | | | | 1.9 | | | 1 | 0.0 | 0.0 | 1 | 0.0 | 0 | 5 | | 1 | |
| | | Yogurt | | | | | | | | | | | | | | | | | | | | | | | | | | | | | | | | | | | | | | | | |
| 60738 | 1 ea | Apple, Stage 2, 4 oz jar, Beechnut | 113 | 100 | 79 | 1.0 | 21.9 | 0.0 | 15.9 | 6.0 | 1.0 | | | | | | | 0 | 0 | 0 | 0 | 0 | | | | | | | | 15.7 | | | 36 | | 0.0 | | | | 80 | | 25 | |
| 60814 | 1 ea | Apple, w/Oatmeal, 3rd Foods, 6 oz jar, Gerber | 170 | 131 | 81 | 3.2 | 27.0 | 1.7 | 15.8 | 9.5 | 1.0 | | | | | | | 3 | 0.3 | 0 | 0.3 | 2 | 0.22 | 0.27 | 3.62 | 0.19 | | | | 15.8 | | | 226 | 0.1 | 4.4 | 22 | 0.4 | 145 | 145 | | 27 | 1.53 |
| 60671 | 1 ea | Banana, 2nd Foods, 4 oz jar, Gerber | 113 | 84 | 81 | 1.2 | 19.0 | 0.5 | 12.2 | 6.3 | 0.5 | | | | | | | 23 | 2 | 0 | 2 | 14 | 0.01 | 0.06 | 0.21 | 0.10 | | | | 15.7 | | | 33 | 0.0 | 0.1 | 11 | 0.1 | 34 | 114 | | 18 | 0.23 |
| 60354 | 1 Tbs | Banana, strained, Heinz | 16 | 13 | 80 | 0.2 | 2.9 | 0.1 | 1.7 | 1.0 | 0.1 | 0.0 | | | | | | 10 | 2 | | | | 0.00 | 0.01 | 0.03 | 0.01 | | | | 8.7 | | | 6 | 0.0 | 0.0 | | | 5 | 18 | | 3 | 0.02 |
| 60672 | 1 ea | Mixed Fruit, 2nd Foods, 4 oz jar, Gerber | 113 | 88 | 80 | 1.2 | 20.2 | 0.6 | 12.4 | 7.2 | 0.3 | | | | | | | 122 | 12 | 0 | 12 | 73 | 0.02 | 0.05 | 0.33 | 0.05 | | | | 15.7 | | | 34 | 0.0 | 0.1 | 10 | 0.1 | 35 | 127 | | 17 | 0.23 |
| 60449 | 1 ea | Mixed Fruit, Stage 3, 6 oz jar, Beechnut | 170 | 170 | 76 | 1.0 | 39.0 | 1.0 | 25.0 | 13.0 | 0.0 | 0.0 | 0.0 | 0.0 | 0.00 | 0.00 | | 0 | 0 | 0 | 0 | 0 | 0.03 | 0.08 | 0.12 | | | | | 16.0 | | | 36 | | 0.0 | | | | 180 | | 30 | |

| Code | Amount | | Description | Basic Components: Weight (g) | Calories | % Water | Protein (g) | Carbs (g) | Fiber (g) | Sugar (g) | Other Carbs (g) | Fat (g) | Additional Fats: Sat Fat (g) | Mono Fat (g) | Poly Fat (g) | Omega 3 (g) | Omega 6 (g) | Choles (mg) |
|---|---|---|---|---|---|---|---|---|---|---|---|---|---|---|---|---|---|---|
| 60358 | 1 | Tbs | Mixed Fruit, strained, Heinz | 16 | 12 | 82 | 0.1 | 2.6 | 0.1 | 1.6 | 1.0 | 0.1 | 0.0 | | | | | |
| 60360 | 1 | Tbs | Peach, strained, Heinz | 16 | 13 | 80 | 0.2 | 2.8 | 0.1 | 1.5 | 1.2 | 0.1 | 0.0 | | | | | |
| 60051 | 1 | ea | With Apple Juice, 2nd Foods, 4.5 oz jar, Gerber | 127 | 93 | 82 | 2.5 | 18.3 | 0.8 | 15.1 | 2.4 | 1.0 | | | | | | |
| 60052 | 1 | ea | With Banana Juice, 2nd Fds, 4.5 oz jar, Gerber | 127 | 108 | 79 | 2.8 | 21.6 | 1.0 | 18.2 | 2.4 | 1.1 | | | | | | |
| 60054 | 1 | ea | With Mxd Fruit Juice, 2nd Fds, 4.5 oz jar, Gerber | 127 | 97 | 81 | 2.8 | 19.0 | 0.6 | 15.7 | 2.7 | 1.0 | | | | | | |
| | | | *INFANT DINNERS* | | | | | | | | | | | | | | | |
| 60824 | 1 | ea | Beef & Broccoli, 3rd Foods, 6 oz jar, Gerber | 170 | 92 | 88 | 4.4 | 12.4 | 3.2 | 2.2 | 7.0 | 2.2 | | | | | | |
| 60678 | 1 | ea | Beef & Carrots, 2nd Foods, 4 oz jar, Gerber | 113 | 67 | 87 | 3.8 | 6.4 | 2.9 | 3.8 | | 2.8 | | | | | | |
| 60778 | 1 | ea | Beef & Carrots, strained, 4 oz jar, Heinz | 113 | 63 | 90 | 3.5 | 4.0 | 2.3 | 1.4 | 0.3 | 3.7 | | | | | | |
| | | | Beef & Noodles | | | | | | | | | | | | | | | |
| 60489 | 1 | Tbs | Junior, avg | 16 | 9 | 88 | 0.4 | 1.2 | 0.2 | | | 0.3 | 0.1 | 0.1 | 0.0 | 0.00 | 0.01 | 1 |
| 60492 | 1 | Tbs | Strained, avg | 16 | 10 | 87 | 0.4 | 1.3 | 0.2 | 0.2 | 0.9 | 0.4 | 0.1 | 0.2 | 0.0 | 0.00 | 0.02 | 1 |
| 60193 | 1 | Tbs | 2nd Foods, Gerber | 14 | 9 | 86 | 0.4 | 1.2 | 0.2 | 0.2 | 0.9 | 0.3 | | | | | | |
| 60194 | 1 | Tbs | 3rd Foods, Gerber | 14 | 9 | 87 | 0.3 | 1.2 | 0.2 | 0.1 | 0.9 | 0.3 | | | | | | |
| 60493 | 1 | Tbs | Beef & Rice, toddler, avg | 16 | 13 | 82 | 0.8 | 1.4 | | | | 0.5 | | | | | | |
| | | | Beef & Vegetables | | | | | | | | | | | | | | | |
| 60541 | 1 | Tbs | High meat, junior, avg | 14 | 12 | 83 | 0.9 | 0.7 | 0.1 | | | 0.6 | | | | | | |
| 60542 | 1 | Tbs | High meat, strained, avg | 14 | 11 | 85 | 0.8 | 0.6 | 0.1 | | | 0.6 | | | | | | |
| 60660 | 1 | Tbs | Junior, avg | 16 | 10 | 86 | 0.4 | 1.4 | 0.2 | 0.2 | 1.0 | 0.3 | 0.1 | 0.1 | 0.0 | 0.00 | 0.02 | 1 |
| 60651 | 1 | Tbs | Strained, avg | 16 | 10 | 87 | 0.4 | 1.2 | 0.4 | 0.3 | 0.6 | 0.4 | 0.2 | 0.2 | 0.0 | 0.00 | 0.02 | 1 |
| 60012 | 1 | Tbs | 2nd Foods, Gerber | 14 | 10 | 85 | 0.4 | 1.2 | 0.4 | 0.3 | 0.5 | 0.3 | 0.1 | 0.2 | 0.0 | 0.00 | 0.01 | |
| 60013 | 1 | Tbs | 3rd Foods, Gerber | 14 | 9 | 86 | 0.3 | 1.3 | 0.2 | 0.2 | 0.9 | 0.2 | 0.1 | 0.1 | 0.0 | 0.00 | 0.00 | |
| 60644 | 1 | Tbs | With dumplings, junior, avg | 15 | 7 | 89 | 0.3 | 1.2 | | | | 0.1 | | | | | | |
| 60645 | 1 | Tbs | With dumplings, strained, avg | 15 | 7 | 89 | 0.3 | 1.2 | | | | 0.1 | | | | | | |
| 60086 | 1 | ea | With Macaroni, Stage 2, 4 oz jar, Beechnut | 113 | 110 | 85 | 2.0 | 9.0 | 1.0 | 3.0 | 5.0 | 6.0 | | | | | | |
| 60491 | 1 | Tbs | Beef Stew, toddler, avg | 16 | 8 | 87 | 0.8 | 0.9 | 0.2 | | | 0.2 | 0.1 | 0.1 | 0.0 | 0.00 | 0.01 | 2 |
| 60185 | 1 | ea | Beef Supreme, Stage 2, 4 oz jar, Beechnut | 113 | 130 | 83 | 2.0 | 8.0 | 1.0 | 2.0 | 5.0 | 9.0 | | | | | | |
| 60848 | 1 | ea | Beef Supreme, Stage 3, 7.5 oz jar, Beechnut | 213 | 173 | 84 | 5.8 | 19.4 | | | | 8.1 | | | | | | |
| | | | Beef Vegetable Stew | | | | | | | | | | | | | | | |
| 60722 | 1 | ea | Grad, 6 oz jar, Gerber | 170 | 121 | 83 | 9.5 | 15.6 | 2.4 | 2.9 | 10.4 | 2.4 | 0.9 | | | | | 12 |
| 60783 | 1 | ea | Junior, 6 oz jar, Heinz | 170 | 124 | 84 | 6.8 | 16.0 | 2.4 | 0.7 | 12.9 | 3.7 | 1.4 | | | | | 14 |
| 60217 | 1 | ea | 6 oz jar, Beechnut | 170 | 110 | 86 | 4.0 | 16.0 | 1.0 | 2.0 | 13.0 | 3.0 | | | | | | |
| | | | Carrots & Broccoli | | | | | | | | | | | | | | | |
| 60787 | 1 | ea | With Cheese, 6 oz jar, Heinz | 170 | 85 | 89 | 3.6 | 13.1 | 2.4 | 1.4 | 9.4 | 2.0 | 1.2 | | | | | |
| 60042 | 1 | Tbs | With Cheese, 3rd Foods, Gerber | 14 | 6 | 90 | 0.2 | 1.0 | 0.1 | 0.2 | 0.7 | 0.1 | | | | | | |
| 60803 | 1 | ea | With Cheese & Rice, 2nd Foods, 4 oz jar, Gerber | 113 | 71 | 86 | 3.2 | 10.4 | 1.2 | 3.2 | 6.0 | 1.9 | | | | | | |
| 60804 | 1 | ea | Carrots, Zucc & Egg Ndls, 2nd Fds, 4 oz jar, Gerber | 113 | 68 | 87 | 2.6 | 8.7 | 1.5 | 1.8 | 5.4 | 2.4 | | | | | | |
| 60825 | 1 | ea | Chicken Alfredo, 3rd Foods, 6 oz jar, Gerber | 170 | 95 | 88 | 4.1 | 11.1 | 1.7 | 1.4 | 8.0 | 3.7 | | | | | | |
| 60674 | 1 | ea | Chicken & Apples, 2nd Foods, 4 oz jar, Gerber | 113 | 72 | 85 | 2.6 | 12.2 | 2.3 | 7.9 | 2.0 | 1.6 | | | | | | |
| | | | Chicken & Broccoli | | | | | | | | | | | | | | | |
| 60677 | 1 | ea | 2nd Foods, 4 oz jar, Gerber | 113 | 55 | 91 | 4.4 | 4.0 | 2.6 | 1.4 | 0.0 | 1.7 | | | | | | |
| 60771 | 1 | ea | Strained, 4.7 oz jar, Heinz | 133 | 53 | 90 | 6.0 | 4.8 | 2.7 | 1.2 | 0.9 | 1.2 | | | | | | |
| 60842 | 1 | ea | With Cheese Sauce, grad, 6 oz jar, Gerber | 170 | 105 | 86 | 6.8 | 11.2 | 1.4 | 2.2 | 7.7 | 3.6 | 2.0 | | | | | 14 |
| | | | Chicken & Noodles | | | | | | | | | | | | | | | |
| 60511 | 1 | Tbs | Junior, avg | 16 | 9 | 87 | 0.4 | 1.4 | 0.1 | 0.2 | 1.1 | 0.2 | 0.1 | 0.1 | 0.0 | 0.00 | 0.04 | 1 |
| 60515 | 1 | Tbs | Strained, avg | 16 | 11 | 86 | 0.4 | 1.5 | 0.3 | 0.4 | 0.7 | 0.3 | 0.1 | 0.1 | 0.1 | 0.00 | 0.07 | 3 |
| 60197 | 1 | Tbs | 2nd Foods, Gerber | 14 | 10 | 84 | 0.4 | 1.4 | 0.3 | 0.4 | 0.7 | 0.3 | | | | | | |
| 60198 | 1 | Tbs | 3rd Foods, Gerber | 14 | 8 | 87 | 0.3 | 1.3 | 0.1 | 0.1 | 1.0 | 0.1 | | | | | | |
| 60648 | 1 | Tbs | With vegetables, junior, avg | 16 | 10 | 86 | 0.3 | 1.5 | 0.2 | | | 0.4 | | | | | | |
| 60646 | 1 | Tbs | With vegetables, strained, avg | 16 | 10 | 87 | 0.3 | 1.3 | 0.2 | | | 0.4 | 0.1 | 0.1 | 0.2 | | | 1 |
| 60801 | 1 | ea | Chicken & Pears, 2nd Foods, 4 oz jar, Gerber | 113 | 77 | 84 | 2.9 | 12.4 | 3.6 | 7.1 | 1.7 | 1.7 | | | | | | |
| 60744 | 1 | ea | Chicken & Stars, 6 oz jar, Beechnut | 170 | 150 | 82 | 7.0 | 17.0 | 1.0 | 2.0 | 14.0 | 6.0 | | | | | | |
| | | | Chicken & Vegetables | | | | | | | | | | | | | | | |
| 60537 | 1 | Tbs | High meat, junior, avg | 14 | 13 | 83 | 1.0 | 0.6 | 0.1 | | | 0.8 | | | | | | |
| 60543 | 1 | Tbs | High meat, strained, avg | 14 | 11 | 84 | 0.9 | 0.8 | 0.1 | | | 0.5 | 0.1 | 0.2 | 0.1 | | | 3 |
| 60863 | 1 | Tbs | Junior, avg | 16 | 8 | 88 | 0.3 | 1.4 | 0.2 | 0.2 | 1.0 | 0.2 | 0.0 | 0.1 | 0.0 | 0.00 | 0.04 | 1 |
| 60652 | 1 | Tbs | Strained, avg | 16 | 9 | 87 | 0.4 | 1.3 | 0.3 | 0.3 | 0.8 | 0.3 | 0.1 | 0.1 | 0.1 | 0.00 | 0.05 | 2 |
| 60014 | 1 | Tbs | 2nd Foods, Gerber | 14 | 9 | 86 | 0.4 | 1.2 | 0.3 | 0.3 | 0.6 | 0.3 | | | | | | |
| 60015 | 1 | Tbs | 3rd Foods, Gerber | 14 | 7 | 89 | 0.3 | 1.1 | 0.1 | 0.2 | 0.9 | 0.1 | | | | | | |
| 60404 | 1 | Tbs | With Noodles, junior, Heinz | 16 | 9 | 88 | 0.3 | 1.3 | 0.3 | 0.1 | 1.0 | 0.3 | | | | | | |
| 60781 | 1 | ea | With Rice, junior, 6 oz jar, Heinz | 170 | 105 | 86 | 4.6 | 15.6 | 2.6 | 2.4 | 10.7 | 2.7 | 0.9 | | | | | |
| 60083 | 1 | ea | Chicken Rice, Stage 2, 4 oz jar, Beechnut | 113 | 80 | 88 | 1.0 | 9.0 | 1.0 | 3.0 | 5.0 | 3.0 | | | | | | |
| | | | Chicken Soup | | | | | | | | | | | | | | | |
| 60523 | 1 | Tbs | Creamed, strained, avg | 14 | 8 | 87 | 0.3 | 1.2 | 0.0 | | | 0.2 | 0.1 | 0.1 | 0.0 | | | 1 |
| 60512 | 1 | Tbs | Strained, avg | 14 | 7 | 89 | 0.2 | 1.0 | 0.2 | | | 0.2 | 0.0 | 0.1 | 0.1 | 0.01 | 0.11 | 1 |
| 60736 | 1 | ea | Stage 2, 4 oz jar, Beechnut | 113 | 90 | | 1.0 | 8.0 | 1.0 | 3.0 | 4.0 | 4.0 | | | | | | |
| | | | Chicken Stew | | | | | | | | | | | | | | | |
| 60513 | 1 | Tbs | Toddler, avg | 16 | 12 | 83 | 0.8 | 1.0 | 0.1 | | | 0.6 | 0.2 | 0.3 | 0.1 | 0.00 | 0.12 | 5 |
| 60716 | 1 | ea | With Noodles, grad, 6 oz jar, Gerber | 170 | 117 | 84 | 7.3 | 14.6 | 1.9 | 1.5 | 11.2 | 3.2 | 1.0 | | | | | 17 |
| 60794 | 1 | ea | With Vegetables, junior, 4 oz jar, Heinz | 113 | 67 | 88 | 2.7 | 8.1 | 1.9 | 1.9 | 4.3 | 2.5 | 0.6 | | | | | |

| Code | Vit A & Components: Vit A (IU) | Vit A (RE) | Retinol (RE) | Carotenoids (RE) | Beta Carotene (mcg) | Vitamins: Thiamin (mg) | Riboflavin (mg) | Niacin (NE) | Vit B6 (mg) | Vit B12 (mcg) | Folate (mcg) | Panto (mg) | Vit C (mg) | Vit D (mg) | Vit E (α TE) | Minerals: Calcium (mg) | Copper (mg) | Iron (mg) | Magnes (mg) | Mang (mg) | Phos (mg) | Potassium (mg) | Selenium (mcg) | Sodium (mg) | Zinc (mg) |
|---|---|---|---|---|---|---|---|---|---|---|---|---|---|---|---|---|---|---|---|---|---|---|---|---|---|
| 60358 | 1 | 0 | | | | 0.00 | 0.01 | 0.01 | 0.00 | | | | 12.1 | | | 5 | 0.0 | 0.0 | | | 4 | 12 | | 2 | 0.01 |
| 60360 | 59 | 12 | | | | 0.00 | 0.01 | 0.07 | 0.00 | | | | 9.7 | | | 5 | 0.0 | 0.1 | | | 4 | 17 | | 2 | 0.02 |
| 60051 | 9 | 1 | 0 | 1 | 5 | 0.04 | 0.09 | 0.14 | 0.03 | | | | 35.4 | | | 90 | 0.0 | 0.3 | 11 | 0.1 | 75 | 178 | | 44 | 0.38 |
| 60052 | 15 | 2 | 0 | 2 | 9 | 0.04 | 0.11 | 0.28 | 0.10 | | | | 35.4 | | | 93 | 0.0 | 0.1 | 17 | 0.1 | 80 | 224 | | 41 | 0.38 |
| 60054 | 23 | 2 | 0 | 2 | 14 | 0.05 | 0.11 | 0.20 | 0.04 | | | | 35.4 | | | 93 | 0.0 | 0.1 | 14 | 0.1 | 77 | 193 | | 43 | 0.38 |
| 60824 | 3352 | 335 | 0 | 335 | 2011 | 0.05 | 0.07 | 1.56 | 0.09 | | | | 7.1 | | | 20 | 0.1 | 0.9 | 17 | 0.1 | 58 | 214 | | 332 | 0.68 |
| 60678 | 16331 | 1633 | 0 | 1633 | 9798 | 0.02 | 0.07 | 1.05 | 0.11 | | | | 0.9 | | | 25 | 0.1 | 0.6 | 12 | 0.2 | 54 | 255 | | 66 | 0.90 |
| 60778 | 9153 | 1831 | | | | 0.02 | 0.05 | 0.82 | 0.08 | | | | 0.3 | | | 27 | | 0.5 | | | 38 | 164 | | 16 | |
| 60489 | 105 | 14 | | | | 0.00 | 0.01 | 0.09 | 0.00 | 0.02 | 1.9 | 0.04 | 0.2 | | | 1 | 0.0 | 0.1 | 1 | | 5 | 7 | 0.9 | 3 | 0.06 |
| 60492 | 115 | 12 | 0 | 12 | | 0.01 | 0.01 | 0.10 | 0.01 | 0.03 | 1.3 | 0.02 | 0.0 | | | 2 | 0.0 | 0.1 | 2 | 0.0 | 6 | 14 | 0.6 | 2 | 0.10 |
| 60193 | 93 | 9 | 0 | 9 | 56 | 0.00 | 0.00 | 0.09 | 0.01 | | | | | | | 1 | 0.0 | 0.1 | 1 | 0.0 | 5 | 11 | | 2 | 0.08 |
| 60194 | 218 | 22 | 0 | 22 | 131 | 0.01 | 0.01 | 0.10 | 0.01 | | | | 0.0 | | | 1 | 0.0 | 0.1 | 1 | 0.0 | 5 | 13 | | 14 | 0.07 |
| 60493 | 80 | 13 | 0 | 20 | | 0.00 | 0.01 | 0.21 | 0.02 | 0.08 | 1.0 | | 0.6 | | | 2 | 0.0 | 0.1 | 1 | | 6 | 19 | 1.3 | 57 | 0.15 |
| 60541 | 111 | 14 | 4 | 10 | | 0.01 | 0.01 | 0.20 | 0.01 | 0.08 | 0.9 | 0.04 | 0.3 | | | 2 | 0.0 | 0.1 | 1 | | 7 | 21 | | 5 | 0.20 |
| 60542 | 110 | 15 | 7 | 9 | | 0.00 | 0.01 | 0.19 | 0.01 | 0.07 | 0.8 | 0.03 | 0.3 | | | 2 | 0.0 | 0.1 | 1 | | 7 | 20 | | 5 | 0.18 |
| 60660 | 407 | 41 | 0 | 41 | | 0.00 | 0.01 | 0.10 | 0.01 | 0.03 | 0.6 | 0.02 | 0.0 | | | 2 | 0.0 | 0.1 | 2 | 0.0 | 6 | 20 | 0.3 | 12 | 0.08 |
| 60651 | 467 | 47 | 0 | 47 | | 0.01 | 0.01 | 0.13 | 0.01 | 0.03 | 1.3 | 0.02 | 0.0 | | | 3 | 0.0 | 0.1 | 2 | 0.0 | 7 | 25 | 0.3 | 3 | 0.09 |
| 60012 | 451 | 45 | 0 | 45 | 270 | 0.00 | 0.01 | 0.12 | 0.01 | | | | 0.0 | | | 2 | 0.0 | 0.1 | 2 | 0.0 | 7 | 33 | | 2 | 0.08 |
| 60013 | 347 | 35 | 0 | 35 | 208 | 0.00 | 0.01 | 0.09 | 0.01 | | | | 0.0 | | | 1 | 0.0 | 0.1 | 2 | 0.0 | 5 | 19 | | 14 | 0.07 |
| 60644 | 99 | 13 | | | | 0.01 | 0.01 | 0.07 | 0.01 | 0.01 | 1.1 | 0.03 | 0.1 | | | 2 | 0.0 | 0.1 | 1 | | 4 | 7 | 0.3 | 8 | 0.05 |
| 60645 | 62 | 8 | | | | 0.01 | 0.01 | 0.09 | 0.01 | 0.01 | 1.1 | 0.03 | 0.1 | | | 2 | 0.0 | 0.1 | 1 | | 4 | 7 | 0.3 | 7 | 0.06 |
| 60086 | 4350 | 870 | | | | 0.02 | 0.05 | 0.05 | | | | | 0.0 | | | 24 | | 0.3 | | | | 180 | | 50 | |
| 60491 | 264 | 40 | | | | 0.00 | 0.01 | 0.21 | 0.01 | 0.08 | 1.0 | | 0.5 | | | 1 | 0.0 | 0.1 | 2 | | 7 | 23 | 0.7 | 55 | 0.14 |
| 60185 | 3587 | 717 | | | | 0.01 | 0.05 | 0.90 | | | | | 0.0 | | | 24 | | 0.3 | | | | 169 | | 45 | |
| 60848 | 3131 | 438 | | | | 0.02 | 0.11 | 2.04 | | | | | 3.2 | | | 26 | 0.1 | 0.9 | 23 | 0.3 | 126 | 273 | 6.4 | 77 | 2.92 |
| 60722 | 3774 | 377 | 0 | 377 | 2264 | 0.05 | 0.31 | 2.24 | 0.20 | | | | 0.3 | | | 29 | 0.1 | 1.0 | 26 | 0.1 | 92 | 343 | | 333 | 1.36 |
| 60783 | 1168 | 234 | | | | 0.53 | 0.10 | 1.38 | 0.10 | | | | 0.9 | | | 27 | | 1.2 | | | 82 | 238 | | 24 | |
| 60217 | 3000 | 600 | | | | 0.01 | 0.08 | 0.10 | | | | | 0.0 | | | 0 | | 0.8 | | | | 70 | | 170 | |
| 60787 | 1539 | 308 | | | | 0.03 | 0.09 | 0.66 | 0.10 | | | | 16.1 | | | 75 | | 0.5 | | | 73 | 170 | | 71 | |
| 60042 | 361 | 36 | 0 | 36 | 217 | 0.00 | 0.00 | 0.04 | 0.01 | | | | 1.1 | | | 4 | 0.0 | 0.0 | 1 | 0.0 | 6 | 14 | | 6 | 0.04 |
| 60803 | 883 | 88 | 0 | 88 | 530 | 0.03 | 0.11 | 0.27 | 0.06 | | | | | | | 87 | 0.0 | 0.3 | 14 | 0.1 | 82 | 163 | | 72 | 0.45 |
| 60804 | 3713 | 371 | 0 | 371 | 2228 | 0.06 | 0.08 | 0.63 | 0.07 | | | | | | | 41 | 0.1 | 0.8 | 15 | 0.1 | 68 | 147 | | 49 | 0.45 |
| 60825 | 1693 | 169 | 0 | 169 | 1016 | 0.03 | 0.05 | 0.75 | 0.05 | | | | 0.5 | | | 58 | 0.1 | 0.9 | 14 | 0.1 | 73 | 139 | | 376 | 0.68 |
| 60674 | 10 | 1 | 0 | 1 | 6 | 0.02 | 0.08 | 0.64 | 0.07 | | | | 0.1 | | | 21 | 0.0 | 0.5 | 7 | 0.0 | 38 | 106 | | 15 | 0.45 |
| 60677 | 583 | 58 | 0 | 58 | 350 | 0.02 | 0.09 | 0.82 | 0.09 | | | | 22.5 | | | 47 | 0.0 | 0.7 | 11 | 0.1 | 68 | 200 | | 21 | 0.79 |
| 60771 | 900 | 180 | | | | 0.03 | 0.01 | 1.24 | 0.16 | | | | 29.0 | | | 44 | | 0.6 | | | 77 | 273 | | 23 | |
| 60842 | 357 | 36 | 0 | 36 | 214 | 0.02 | 0.15 | 2.23 | 0.15 | | | | 5.1 | | | 88 | 0.1 | 0.5 | 17 | 0.1 | 150 | 214 | | 321 | 0.85 |
| 60511 | 277 | 117 | 0 | 28 | | 0.01 | 0.01 | 0.11 | 0.01 | 0.00 | 1.1 | 0.03 | 0.0 | | | 3 | 0.0 | 0.1 | 1 | 0.0 | 13 | 6 | 0.6 | 12 | 0.06 |
| 60515 | 349 | 35 | 0 | 35 | | 0.01 | 0.01 | 0.12 | 0.01 | 0.00 | 1.8 | 0.03 | 0.0 | | | 4 | 0.0 | 0.1 | 2 | 0.0 | 7 | 22 | 0.6 | 4 | 0.09 |
| 60197 | 843 | 84 | 0 | 84 | 506 | 0.01 | 0.01 | 0.11 | 0.01 | | | | 0.0 | | | 4 | 0.0 | 0.1 | 2 | 0.0 | 8 | 31 | | 2 | 0.08 |
| 60198 | 285 | 28 | 0 | 28 | 171 | 0.00 | 0.01 | 0.10 | 0.01 | | | | 0.0 | | | 4 | 0.0 | 0.1 | 1 | 0.0 | 5 | 12 | | 15 | 0.06 |
| 60648 | 168 | 21 | | | | 0.01 | 0.01 | 0.11 | 0.00 | 0.01 | 0.5 | 0.03 | 0.1 | | | 4 | 0.0 | 0.1 | 2 | | 5 | 9 | 0.5 | 4 | 0.05 |
| 60646 | 227 | 28 | | | | 0.01 | 0.01 | 0.07 | 0.00 | 0.01 | 0.5 | 0.03 | 0.1 | | | 4 | 0.0 | 0.1 | 2 | | 5 | 9 | 0.5 | 3 | 0.04 |
| 60801 | 3 | 0.3 | 0 | 0.3 | 2 | 0.01 | 0.08 | 0.90 | 0.06 | | | | 0.1 | | | 35 | 0.1 | 0.6 | 11 | 0.0 | 47 | 139 | | 18 | 0.56 |
| 60744 | 1500 | 300 | | | | | | | | | | | 0.0 | | | 12 | | 0.9 | | | | 90 | | 170 | |
| 60537 | 117 | 18 | 10 | 8 | | 0.00 | 0.01 | 0.14 | 0.01 | 0.02 | 0.2 | 0.05 | 0.2 | | | 6 | 0.0 | 0.1 | 1 | | 8 | 9 | | 4 | 0.14 |
| 60543 | 81 | 12 | 5 | 6 | | 0.00 | 0.01 | 0.14 | 0.01 | 0.02 | 0.2 | 0.04 | 0.1 | | | 7 | 0.0 | 0.1 | 1 | | 8 | 8 | | 4 | 0.13 |
| 60863 | 418 | 42 | 0 | 42 | | 0.00 | 0.01 | 0.10 | 0.01 | 0.00 | 0.5 | 0.02 | 0.0 | | | 4 | 0.0 | 0.1 | 1 | 0.0 | 5 | 13 | 0.3 | 12 | 0.05 |
| 60652 | 661 | 66 | 0 | 66 | | 0.01 | 0.01 | 0.12 | 0.01 | 0.00 | 0.8 | 0.02 | 0.0 | | | 4 | 0.0 | 0.1 | 2 | 0.0 | 8 | 25 | 0.4 | 4 | 0.08 |
| 60014 | 941 | 94 | 0 | 94 | 565 | 0.01 | 0.01 | 0.09 | 0.01 | | | | 0.0 | | | 3 | 0.0 | 0.1 | 2 | 0.0 | 7 | 30 | | 3 | 0.07 |
| 60015 | 410 | 41 | 0 | 41 | 246 | 0.00 | 0.00 | 0.08 | 0.01 | | | | | | | 4 | 0.0 | 0.0 | 1 | 0.0 | 5 | 12 | | 15 | 0.04 |
| 60404 | 161 | 32 | | | | 0.01 | 0.01 | 0.10 | 0.00 | | | | 0.0 | | | 4 | 0.0 | 0.1 | | | 5 | 10 | | 3 | 0.03 |
| 60781 | 1295 | 259 | | | | 0.07 | 0.07 | 1.92 | 0.19 | | | | 1.4 | | | 71 | | 1.1 | | | 82 | 255 | | 34 | |
| 60083 | 6278 | 1256 | | | | 0.02 | 0.03 | 0.60 | | | | | 0.0 | | | 36 | | 0.6 | | | | 115 | | 70 | |
| 60523 | 102 | 16 | | | | 0.00 | 0.01 | 0.05 | 0.01 | 0.01 | 0.9 | | 0.2 | | | 5 | 0.0 | 0.0 | 1 | | 4 | 11 | | 3 | 0.04 |
| 60512 | 194 | 24 | | | | 0.00 | 0.00 | 0.04 | 0.01 | 0.02 | 0.7 | | 0.1 | | | 5 | 0.0 | 0.0 | 1 | | 3 | 9 | 0.2 | 2 | 0.03 |
| 60736 | 4783 | 957 | | | | | | | | | | | 0.0 | | | 36 | | 0.3 | | | | 135 | | 50 | |
| 60513 | 162 | 19 | | | | 0.00 | 0.01 | 0.18 | 0.01 | 0.02 | 2.6 | | 0.3 | | | 6 | 0.0 | 0.1 | 2 | | 8 | 15 | 0.9 | 32 | 0.07 |
| 60716 | 2412 | 241 | 0 | 241 | 1447 | 0.09 | 0.15 | 3.09 | 0.20 | | | | 0.5 | | | 24 | 0.1 | 1.2 | 24 | 0.1 | 109 | 206 | | 389 | 0.85 |
| 60794 | 1051 | 210 | | | | 0.03 | 0.06 | 1.21 | 0.09 | | | | 0.0 | | | 44 | | 0.6 | | | 50 | 181 | | 21 | |

| Code | Amount | Description | Basic Components | | | | | | | | | Additional Fats | | | | | | Vit A & Components | | | | | Vitamins | | | | | | | | | | Minerals | | | | | | | | | |
|---|---|---|---|---|---|---|---|---|---|---|---|---|---|---|---|---|---|---|---|---|---|---|---|---|---|---|---|---|---|---|---|---|---|---|---|---|---|---|---|---|---|---|
| | | | Weight (g) | Calories | % Water | Protein (g) | Carbs (g) | Fiber (g) | Sugar (g) | Other Carbs (g) | Fat (g) | Sat Fat (g) | Mono Fat (g) | Poly Fat (g) | Omega 3 (g) | Omega 6 (g) | Choles (mg) | Vit A (IU) | Vit A (RE) | Retinol (RE) | Carotenoids (RE) | Beta Carotene (mcg) | Thiamin (mg) | Riboflavin (mg) | Niacin (NE) | Vit B6 (mg) | Vit B12 (mcg) | Folate (mcg) | Panto (mg) | Vit C (mg) | Vit D (mg) | Vit E (α TE) | Calcium (mg) | Copper (mg) | Iron (mg) | Magnes (mg) | Mang (mg) | Phos (mg) | Potassium (mg) | Selenium (mcg) | Sodium (mg) | Zinc (mg) |
| 60675 | 1 ea | Ham & Apples, 2nd Foods, 4 oz jar, Gerber | 113 | 70 | 85 | 2.9 | 12.3 | 2.0 | 7.6 | 2.7 | 1.0 | | | | | | | 7 | 1 | 0 | 1 | 4 | 0.07 | 0.07 | 0.82 | 0.08 | | | | 0.1 | | | 5 | 0.0 | 0.3 | 8 | 0.0 | 38 | 136 | | 10 | 0.45 |
| 60841 | 1 ea | Ham & Au Gratin Potatoes, grad, 6 oz jar, Gerber | 170 | 131 | 81 | 6.5 | 19.4 | 2.0 | 1.4 | 16.0 | 3.4 | 2.0 | | | | | 12 | 2 | 0 | 0 | 0 | 1 | 0.09 | 0.17 | 2.04 | 0.29 | | | | 0.2 | | | 87 | 0.1 | 0.7 | 24 | 0.1 | 187 | 253 | | 413 | 1.02 |
| | | Ham & Vegetables | | | | | | | | | | | | | | | | | | | | | | | | | | | | | | | | | | | | | | | | |
| 60538 | 1 Tbs | High meat, junior, avg | 14 | 11 | 84 | 0.9 | 0.9 | 0.1 | | | 0.5 | 0.2 | 0.2 | 0.1 | 0.00 | 0.06 | 3 | 36 | 9 | 9 | 1 | | 0.02 | 0.01 | 0.16 | 0.01 | 0.04 | 0.9 | 0.06 | 0.3 | | | 1 | | 0.1 | 1 | | 8 | 23 | | 3 | 0.15 |
| 60544 | 1 Tbs | High meat, strained, avg | 14 | 11 | 84 | 0.9 | 0.8 | 0.1 | | | 0.5 | 0.2 | 0.2 | 0.1 | 0.00 | 0.07 | | 23 | 6 | 5 | 1 | | 0.01 | 0.01 | 0.20 | 0.01 | 0.04 | 0.9 | 0.05 | 0.3 | | | 2 | | 0.1 | 1 | | 8 | 22 | | 3 | 0.14 |
| 60661 | 1 Tbs | Junior, avg | 16 | 10 | 87 | 0.3 | 1.4 | 0.2 | 0.2 | 1.1 | 0.3 | 0.1 | 0.1 | 0.1 | 0.01 | 0.07 | 0 | 227 | 23 | 0 | 23 | | 0.01 | 0.01 | 0.08 | 0.01 | 0.00 | 1.3 | | 0.2 | | | 2 | 0.0 | 0.0 | 1 | 0.0 | 5 | 16 | 0.4 | 14 | 0.05 |
| 60653 | 1 Tbs | Strained, avg | 16 | 9 | 88 | 0.4 | 1.2 | 0.3 | 0.2 | 0.8 | 0.3 | 0.1 | 0.2 | 0.0 | 0.00 | 0.03 | 1 | 460 | 46 | 0 | 46 | | 0.01 | 0.01 | 0.11 | 0.01 | 0.01 | 0.5 | 0.02 | 0.3 | | | 3 | 0.0 | 0.1 | 2 | 0.0 | 5 | 23 | 0.4 | 3 | 0.05 |
| 60654 | 1 Tbs | Toddler, avg | 14 | 10 | 84 | 0.6 | 1.1 | 0.2 | | | 0.4 | 0.1 | 0.2 | 0.0 | 0.00 | 0.04 | 1 | 50 | 7 | | | | 0.01 | 0.01 | 0.10 | 0.01 | 0.02 | 0.7 | | 0.5 | | | 3 | 0.0 | 0.1 | 2 | | 6 | 21 | | 42 | 0.07 |
| 60213 | 1 Tbs | 2nd Foods, Gerber | 14 | 8 | 87 | 0.3 | 1.3 | 0.1 | 0.2 | 1.0 | 0.2 | | | | | | | 113 | 1 | 0 | 11 | 68 | 0.01 | 0.00 | 0.08 | 0.01 | | | | 0.0 | | | 1 | 0.0 | 0.0 | 1 | 0.0 | 4 | 11 | | 1 | 0.04 |
| 60214 | 1 Tbs | 3rd Foods, Gerber | 14 | 9 | 86 | 0.3 | 1.3 | 0.1 | 0.2 | 1.0 | 0.3 | | | | | | | 236 | 24 | 0 | 24 | 141 | 0.00 | 0.01 | 0.07 | 0.01 | | | | 0.2 | | | 2 | 0.0 | 0.0 | 1 | 0.0 | 4 | 15 | | 14 | 0.03 |
| 60551 | 1 Tbs | Lamb & Noodles, junior, avg | 14 | 9 | 86 | 0.3 | 1.2 | | | | 0.3 | | | | | | | 110 | 5 | | | | 0.01 | 0.01 | 0.09 | 0.01 | 0.03 | 0.6 | 0.03 | 0.3 | | | 3 | 0.0 | 0.1 | 1 | | 8 | 11 | | 3 | 0.04 |
| | | Lamb & Vegetables | | | | | | | | | | | | | | | | | | | | | | | | | | | | | | | | | | | | | | | | |
| 60662 | 1 Tbs | Junior, avg | 16 | 8 | 89 | 0.3 | 1.1 | 0.2 | | | 0.3 | 0.1 | 0.1 | 0.0 | 0.00 | 0.02 | 1 | 237 | 32 | | | | 0.00 | 0.01 | 0.09 | 0.01 | 0.03 | 0.6 | 0.03 | 0.3 | | | 2 | 0.0 | 0.1 | 1 | | 8 | 15 | 0.4 | 2 | 0.04 |
| 60655 | 1 Tbs | Strained, avg | 15 | 8 | 89 | 0.3 | 1.0 | 0.2 | | | 0.3 | 0.1 | 0.1 | 0.0 | 0.00 | 0.02 | 1 | 299 | 42 | | | | 0.00 | 0.01 | 0.08 | 0.01 | 0.02 | 0.5 | 0.02 | 0.2 | | | 2 | 0.0 | 0.1 | 1 | | 7 | 14 | 0.4 | 3 | 0.03 |
| 60188 | 1 ea | Stage 2, 4 oz jar, Beechnut | 113 | 80 | 88 | 1.0 | 9.0 | 1.0 | 3.0 | 5.0 | 3.0 | | | | | | | 5082 | 1016 | | | | 0.02 | 0.03 | 0.60 | | | | | 0.0 | | | 24 | | 0.3 | | | | 169 | | 55 | |
| 60490 | 1 Tbs | Lasagna, beef, toddler, avg | 15 | 12 | 82 | 0.6 | 1.5 | 0.1 | | | 0.3 | 0.2 | 0.1 | 0.0 | | | 3 | 74 | 23 | | | | 0.01 | 0.01 | 0.20 | 0.01 | 0.08 | 0.9 | | 0.3 | | | 3 | 0.0 | 0.1 | 2 | | 6 | 18 | 1.3 | 68 | 0.11 |
| 60822 | 1 ea | Lasagna w/Meat Sauce, 3rd Foods, 6 oz jar, Gerber | 170 | 100 | 87 | 3.4 | 15.1 | 1.7 | 4.6 | 8.8 | 2.9 | | | | | | | 1047 | 105 | 0 | 105 | 623 | 0.05 | 0.09 | 0.94 | 0.10 | | | | 0.7 | | | 15 | 0.0 | 0.7 | 17 | 0.1 | 48 | 173 | | 165 | 0.68 |
| 60663 | 1 Tbs | Liver & Vegetables, junior, avg | 14 | 6 | 89 | 0.3 | 1.1 | 0.2 | | | 0.1 | | | | | | | 550 | 100 | 58 | 32 | | 0.00 | 0.03 | 0.16 | 0.01 | 0.25 | 4.5 | | 0.3 | | | 1 | 0.0 | 0.3 | 2 | | 5 | 12 | | 2 | 0.05 |
| 60656 | 1 Tbs | Liver & Vegetables, strained, avg | 14 | 5 | 90 | 0.3 | 1.0 | 0.2 | | | 0.1 | 0.0 | 0.0 | 0.0 | | | 5 | 435 | 103 | 39 | 14 | | 0.00 | 0.04 | 0.17 | 0.01 | 0.25 | 4.0 | | 0.3 | | | 1 | 0.0 | 0.3 | 2 | | 6 | 13 | | 3 | 0.05 |
| | | Macaroni & Beef | | | | | | | | | | | | | | | | | | | | | | | | | | | | | | | | | | | | | | | | |
| 60795 | 1 ea | Junior, 6 oz jar, Heinz | 170 | 104 | 86 | 4.9 | 16.0 | 2.2 | 1.7 | 12.1 | 2.2 | 1.[illegible] | | | | | | 906 | 181 | | | | 0.44 | 0.10 | 1.65 | 0.10 | | | | 0.0 | | | 32 | | 1.1 | | | 61 | 221 | | 27 | |
| 60206 | 1 ea | Stage 3, 6 oz jar, Beechnut | 170 | 130 | 88 | 3.0 | 14.0 | 2.0 | 2.0 | 10.0 | 5.0 | | | | | | | 6000 | 1200 | | | | 0.03 | 0.08 | 0.60 | | | | | 0.0 | | | 36 | | 0.3 | | | | 190 | | 60 | |
| 60555 | 1 Tbs | With tomato, junior, avg | 16 | 9 | 87 | 0.4 | 1.5 | 0.2 | | | 0.2 | 0.1 | 0.1 | 0.0 | 0.00 | 0.01 | 1 | 111 | 17 | | | | 0.01 | 0.01 | 0.12 | 0.01 | 0.04 | 1.4 | | 0.2 | | | 2 | 0.0 | 0.1 | 1 | | 7 | 12 | 1.3 | 3 | 0.06 |
| 60556 | 1 Tbs | With tomato, strained, avg | 16 | 10 | 86 | 0.4 | 1.5 | 0.2 | 0.3 | 1.0 | 0.2 | 0.1 | 0.1 | 0.0 | 0.00 | 0.03 | 1 | 140 | 14 | 0 | 14 | | 0.01 | 0.01 | 0.11 | 0.01 | 0.02 | 1.4 | 0.02 | 0.0 | | | 3 | 0.0 | 0.1 | 2 | 0.0 | 6 | 18 | 1.3 | 6 | 0.09 |
| 60717 | 1 ea | With Tomato, grad, 6 oz jar, Gerber | 170 | 136 | 81 | 8.2 | 18.2 | 2.2 | 5.4 | 10.5 | 3.4 | 1.4 | | | | | 14 | 250 | 25 | 0 | 25 | 150 | 0.09 | 0.26 | 3.01 | 0.22 | | | | 0.9 | | | 27 | 0.1 | 1.5 | 31 | 0.2 | 109 | 389 | | 325 | 1.53 |
| 60204 | 1 Tbs | With Tomato, 2nd Foods, Gerber | 14 | 8 | 86 | 0.3 | 1.3 | 0.2 | 0.3 | 0.9 | 0.2 | | | | | | | 155 | 15 | 0 | 15 | 93 | 0.00 | 0.01 | 0.10 | 0.01 | | | | | | | 2 | 0.0 | 0.1 | 1 | 0.0 | 5 | 18 | | 5 | 0.06 |
| | | Macaroni & Cheese | | | | | | | | | | | | | | | | | | | | | | | | | | | | | | | | | | | | | | | | |
| 60557 | 1 Tbs | Junior, avg | 16 | 10 | 86 | 0.4 | 1.3 | 0.0 | | | 0.3 | 0.2 | 0.1 | 0.0 | 0.00 | 0.02 | 1 | 2 | 0 | | | | 0.01 | 0.01 | 0.09 | 0.00 | 0.00 | 1.8 | | 0.2 | | | 8 | 0.0 | 0.0 | 1 | | 9 | 7 | 0.6 | 12 | 0.05 |
| 60559 | 1 Tbs | Strained, avg | 16 | 11 | 85 | 0.5 | 1.4 | 0.1 | 0.2 | 1.1 | 0.3 | 0.2 | 0.1 | 0.0 | 0.00 | 0.01 | 1 | 14 | 4 | 4 | 0 | 0 | 0.01 | 0.01 | 0.08 | 0.01 | 0.02 | 1.8 | 0.03 | 0.0 | | | 11 | 0.0 | 0.0 | 1 | 0.0 | 14 | 11 | 0.6 | 14 | 0.06 |
| 60201 | 1 Tbs | 2nd Foods, Gerber | 14 | 9 | 86 | 0.4 | 1.2 | 0.1 | 0.2 | 0.9 | 0.3 | | | | | | | 1 | 0.1 | 0 | 0.1 | 1 | 0.00 | 0.01 | 0.07 | 0.00 | | | | 0.0 | | | 8 | 0.0 | 0.0 | 1 | 0.0 | 12 | 8 | | 13 | 0.06 |
| 60558 | 1 Tbs | Macaroni & Ham, junior, avg | 14 | 8 | 86 | 0.4 | 1.2 | | | | 0.2 | | | | | | | 74 | 10 | | | | 0.01 | 0.01 | 0.11 | 0.00 | 0.00 | 0.3 | | 0.3 | | | 11 | 0.0 | 0.1 | 1 | | 8 | 15 | | 7 | 0.05 |
| | | Pasta Shells | | | | | | | | | | | | | | | | | | | | | | | | | | | | | | | | | | | | | | | | |
| 60746 | 1 ea | Seashells w/Tomato Sauce, 6 oz jar, Beechnut | 170 | 150 | 81 | 3.0 | 25.0 | 1.0 | 5.0 | 19.0 | 4.0 | | | | | | | 3300 | 660 | | | | | | | | | | | 0.0 | | | 24 | | 1.2 | | | | 90 | | 170 | |
| 60784 | 1 ea | Vegetables w/Cheese Sce, junior, 4 oz jar, Heinz | 113 | 77 | 61 | 29.4 | 12.5 | 1.5 | 0.8 | 10.3 | 1.7 | 0.8 | | | | | | 814 | 163 | | | | 0.06 | 0.28 | 0.62 | 0.07 | | | | 34.6 | | | 62 | | 0.5 | | | 61 | 113 | | 46 | |
| 60847 | 1 ea | With Cheese, grad, 6 oz jar, Gerber | 170 | 136 | 82 | 6.0 | 18.9 | 1.7 | 2.0 | 15.1 | 4.4 | 2.9 | | | | | 10 | | | | | | 0.07 | 0.17 | 1.38 | 0.10 | | | | | | | 177 | 0.1 | 1.0 | 20 | 0.2 | 228 | 100 | | 396 | 1.02 |
| 60720 | 1 ea | Ravioli & Cheese, grad, 6 oz jar, Gerber | 170 | 156 | 78 | 6.5 | 26.5 | 2.9 | 6.5 | 17.2 | 2.7 | 1.4 | | | | | 9 | 257 | 25 | 0 | 26 | 154 | 0.12 | 0.22 | 4.69 | 0.31 | | | | 0.2 | | | 85 | 0.2 | 1.5 | 36 | 0.2 | 162 | 374 | | 252 | 1.19 |
| | | Spaghetti | | | | | | | | | | | | | | | | | | | | | | | | | | | | | | | | | | | | | | | | |
| 60207 | 1 Tbs | Beef w/Tomato Sauce, 3rd Foods, Gerber | 14 | 9 | 85 | 0.3 | 1.4 | 0.1 | 0.8 | 0.4 | 0.2 | | | | | | | 194 | 19 | 0 | 19 | 117 | 0.00 | 0.01 | 0.07 | 0.01 | | | | 0.1 | | | 4 | 0.0 | 0.0 | 1 | 0.0 | 4 | 19 | | 28 | 0.06 |
| 60219 | 1 ea | Rings w/Meat Sauce, 6 oz jar, Beechnut | 170 | 160 | 80 | 7.0 | 20.0 | 0.0 | 5.0 | 15.0 | 6.0 | | | | | | | 3600 | 720 | | | | 0.02 | 0.08 | 1.20 | | | | | 0.0 | | | 24 | | 1.5 | | | | 100 | | 180 | |
| 60624 | 1 Tbs | With meat & tomato sauce, junior, avg | 16 | 11 | 84 | 0.4 | 1.8 | 0.2 | 0.4 | 1.2 | 0.2 | 0.1 | 0.1 | 0.0 | 0.00 | 0.03 | 1 | 201 | 20 | | | | 0.01 | 0.01 | 0.15 | 0.01 | 0.00 | 4.3 | 0.01 | 0.0 | | | 2 | 0.0 | 0.1 | 2 | 0.0 | 6 | 20 | 1.3 | 12 | 0.08 |
| 60623 | 1 Tbs | With meat & tomato sauce, toddler, avg | 16 | 12 | 82 | 0.8 | 1.7 | | | | 0.2 | | | | | | | 71 | 11 | | | | 0.01 | 0.02 | 0.25 | 0.01 | 0.04 | 5.1 | | 0.7 | | | 4 | 0.0 | 0.1 | 2 | | 7 | 26 | 1.3 | 57 | 0.08 |
| 60718 | 1 ea | With Mini Meatballs & Sauce, 6 oz jar, Gerber | 170 | 151 | 79 | 8.3 | 21.4 | 2.9 | 6.5 | 12.1 | 3.7 | 1.9 | | | | | 12 | 99 | 10 | 0 | 10 | 59 | 0.10 | 0.24 | 2.70 | 0.20 | | | | 0.3 | | | 31 | 0.1 | 1.2 | 29 | 0.2 | 114 | 364 | | 272 | 1.53 |
| 60676 | 1 ea | Turkey & Apples, 2nd Foods, 4 oz jar, Gerber | 113 | 73 | 85 | 3.2 | 11.9 | 2.1 | 7.8 | 1.9 | 1.5 | | | | | | | 10 | 1 | 0 | 1 | 6 | 0.02 | 0.09 | 0.86 | 0.08 | | | | 0.2 | | | 9 | 0.0 | 0.5 | 8 | 0.0 | 46 | 132 | | 15 | 0.56 |
| 60679 | 1 ea | Turkey & Green Beans, 2nd Foods, 4 oz jar, Gerber | 113 | 60 | 89 | 4.4 | 6.6 | 2.6 | 1.7 | 2.3 | 1.7 | | | | | | | 426 | 43 | 0 | 43 | 256 | 0.03 | 0.11 | 1.24 | 0.08 | | | | 2.6 | | | 36 | 0.1 | 0.8 | 20 | 0.2 | 63 | 207 | | 14 | 0.56 |
| 60649 | 1 Tbs | Turkey & Noodles w/vegetables, junior, avg | 16 | 8 | 89 | 0.3 | 1.2 | 0.2 | | | 0.2 | 0.1 | 0.0 | 0.1 | | | 0 | 159 | 2 | | | | 0.00 | 0.01 | 0.05 | 0.00 | 0.02 | 0.4 | 0.03 | 0.1 | | | 5 | 0.0 | 0.0 | 1 | | 5 | 12 | 0.4 | 3 | 0.05 |
| 60647 | 1 Tbs | Turkey & Noodles w/vegetables, strained, avg | 16 | 7 | 90 | 0.2 | 1.1 | 0.2 | | | 0.2 | 0.1 | 0.0 | 0.1 | | | 0 | 159 | 2 | | | | 0.00 | 0.01 | 0.04 | 0.00 | 0.02 | 0.4 | 0.03 | 0.1 | | | 5 | 0.0 | 0.0 | 1 | | 4 | 10 | 0.4 | 3 | 0.04 |
| | | Turkey & Rice | | | | | | | | | | | | | | | | | | | | | | | | | | | | | | | | | | | | | | | | |
| 60636 | 1 Tbs | Junior, avg | 16 | 9 | 87 | 0.4 | 1.5 | 0.2 | 0.2 | 1.2 | 0.1 | 0.0 | 0.0 | 0.0 | 0.00 | 0.03 | 1 | 302 | 30 | 0 | 30 | | 0.01 | 0.01 | 0.11 | 0.01 | 0.00 | 1.3 | 0.03 | 0.0 | | | 4 | 0.0 | 0.1 | 1 | 0.0 | 6 | 14 | 0.5 | 13 | 0.08 |
| 60637 | 1 Tbs | Strained, avg | 16 | 8 | 88 | 0.4 | 1.3 | 0.1 | 0.3 | 0.9 | 0.2 | 0.1 | 0.1 | 0.0 | 0.00 | 0.04 | 1 | 260 | 26 | 0 | 26 | | 0.00 | 0.01 | 0.10 | 0.01 | 0.00 | 0.6 | 0.03 | 0.0 | | | 3 | 0.0 | 0.0 | 1 | 0.0 | 5 | 15 | 0.5 | 3 | 0.06 |
| 60209 | 1 Tbs | 2nd Foods, Gerber | 14 | 7 | 88 | 0.3 | 1.1 | 0.1 | 0.2 | 0.8 | 0.1 | | | | | | | 172 | 17 | 0 | 17 | 103 | 0.00 | 0.01 | 0.10 | 0.01 | | | | | | | 2 | 0.0 | 0.0 | 1 | 0.0 | 5 | 12 | | 3 | 0.06 |
| 60210 | 1 Tbs | 3rd Foods, Gerber | 14 | 8 | 88 | 0.4 | 1.2 | 0.1 | 0.2 | 0.9 | 0.1 | | | | | | | 181 | 36 | | | | 0.00 | 0.01 | 0.10 | 0.01 | | | | 0.1 | | | 2 | | 0.0 | | | 5 | 13 | | 2 | |
| 60867 | 1 Tbs | With vegetables, toddler, avg | 15 | 9 | 86 | 0.6 | 1.1 | 0.1 | | | 0.2 | 0.1 | 0.1 | 0.0 | 0.00 | 0.04 | 1 | 340 | 34 | | | | 0.01 | 0.01 | 0.32 | 0.02 | 0.02 | 0.5 | 0.04 | 0.0 | | | 2 | 0.0 | 0.1 | 2 | 0.0 | 9 | 16 | 0.5 | 27 | 0.09 |
| 60846 | 1 ea | With Vegetables, 3rd Foods, 6 oz jar, Gerber | 170 | 105 | 87 | 4.4 | 14.1 | 1.5 | 2.4 | 10.2 | 3.4 | | | | | | | 3835 | 384 | 0 | 384 | 2302 | 0.03 | 0.09 | 1.22 | 0.10 | | | | 0.5 | | | 36 | 0.1 | 0.7 | 15 | 0.2 | 66 | 179 | | 180 | 0.85 |
| 60802 | 1 ea | Turkey & Sweet Potatoes, 2nd Fds, 4 oz jar, Gerber | 113 | 89 | 82 | 4.0 | 14.4 | 1.9 | 9.2 | 3.3 | 1.8 | | | | | | | 9143 | 914 | 0 | 914 | 5486 | 0.02 | 0.07 | 0.88 | 0.09 | | | | 4.0 | | | 28 | 0.1 | 0.6 | 17 | 0.3 | 59 | 276 | | 21 | 0.79 |
| | | Turkey & Vegetables | | | | | | | | | | | | | | | | | | | | | | | | | | | | | | | | | | | | | | | | |
| 60546 | 1 Tbs | High meat, junior, avg | 14 | 13 | 82 | 0.8 | 0.8 | 0.1 | | | 0.7 | | | | | | | 89 | 16 | 10 | 5 | | 0.00 | 0.01 | 0.11 | 0.01 | 0.06 | 1.4 | | 0.2 | | | 10 | 0.0 | 0.1 | 1 | | 9 | 15 | | 6 | 0.13 |
| 60664 | 1 Tbs | Junior, avg | 16 | 8 | 88 | 0.3 | 1.2 | 0.1 | 0.2 | 0.8 | 0.3 | 0.1 | 0.1 | 0.1 | 0.00 | 0.06 | 1 | 263 | 26 | 0 | 26 | | 0.00 | 0.01 | 0.09 | 0.01 | 0.00 | 1.1 | 0.03 | 0.1 | | | 3 | 0.0 | 0.1 | 1 | 0.0 | 5 | 16 | 0.3 | 14 | 0.05 |
| 60658 | 1 Tbs | Strained, avg | 16 | 8 | 89 | 0.4 | 1.2 | 0.2 | 0.2 | 0.7 | 0.1 | 0.0 | 0.0 | 0.0 | 0.00 | 0.03 | 1 | 703 | 70 | 0 | 70 | | 0.00 | 0.00 | 0.07 | 0.01 | 0.00 | 1.6 | 0.04 | 0.1 | | | 4 | 0.0 | 0.1 | 2 | 0.0 | 7 | 16 | 0.3 | 3 | 0.11 |
| 60657 | 1 Tbs | Toddler, avg | 16 | 13 | 82 | 0.8 | 1.3 | | | | 0.5 | | | | | | | 336 | 43 | | | | 0.00 | 0.01 | 0.09 | 0.01 | 0.07 | 0.5 | | 0.5 | | | 7 | 0.0 | 0.1 | 3 | | 9 | 27 | 0.3 | 53 | 0.05 |
| 60016 | 1 Tbs | 2nd Foods, Gerber | 14 | 7 | 89 | 0.3 | 1.1 | 0.1 | 0.2 | 0.9 | 0.1 | | | | | | | 158 | 16 | 0 | 16 | 95 | 0.00 | 0.00 | 0.06 | 0.01 | | | | 0.1 | | | 1 | 0.0 | 0.0 | 1 | 0.0 | 4 | 9 | | 2 | 0.06 |
| 60017 | 1 Tbs | 3rd Foods, Gerber | 14 | 7 | 88 | 0.3 | 1.1 | 0.2 | 0.2 | 0.8 | 0.2 | | | | | | | 201 | 20 | 0 | 20 | 121 | 0.00 | 0.00 | 0.08 | 0.01 | | | | 0.2 | | | 2 | 0.0 | 0.1 | 1 | 0.0 | 5 | 16 | | 15 | 0.04 |
| 60721 | 1 ea | Turkey Stew w/Rice, grad, 6 oz jar, Gerber | 170 | 102 | 86 | 6.5 | 12.8 | 1.4 | 1.2 | 10.2 | 2.7 | 0.9 | | | | | 15 | 3856 | 386 | 0 | 386 | 2314 | 0.12 | 0.12 | 3.59 | 0.24 | | | | 0.5 | | | 22 | 0.2 | 0.7 | 24 | 0.4 | 107 | 182 | | 318 | 1.02 |
| 60068 | 1 ea | Turkey Stew w/Rice, 6 oz jar, Beechnut | 170 | 150 | 82 | 6.0 | 14.0 | 1.0 | 3.0 | 10.0 | 7.0 | | | | | | | 5000 | 500 | | | | 0.01 | 0.04 | 1.20 | | | | | 0.0 | | | 20 | | 1.1 | | | | 150 | | 200 | |
| 60090 | 1 ea | Turkey Supreme, Stage 2, 4 oz jar, Beechnut | 113 | 90 | 86 | 3.0 | 9.0 | 1.0 | 3.0 | 5.0 | 4.0 | | | | | | | 3587 | 717 | | | | 0.01 | 0.04 | 0.60 | | | | | 0.0 | | | 60 | | 0.6 | | | | 40 | | 45 | |
| 60547 | 1 Tbs | Veal & Vegetables, high meat, junior, avg | 14 | 10 | 84 | 0.9 | 0.8 | 0.1 | | | 0.4 | | | | | | | 60 | 11 | 8 | 3 | | 0.00 | 0.01 | 0.22 | 0.01 | 0.06 | 0.8 | 0.04 | 0.2 | | | 2 | 0.0 | 0.1 | 1 | | 8 | 22 | | 4 | 0.15 |
| 60548 | 1 Tbs | Veal & Vegetables, high meat, strained, avg | 14 | 10 | 85 | 0.8 | 0.9 | 0.1 | | | 0.4 | | | | | | | 38 | 11 | 10 | 1 | | 0.00 | 0.01 | 0.23 | 0.01 | 0.06 | 0.8 | 0.04 | 0.3 | | | 1 | 0.0 | 0.1 | 1 | | 8 | 21 | | 3 | 0.14 |
| 60806 | 1 ea | Vegetable Stew, 2nd Foods, 4 oz jar, Gerber | 113 | 75 | 85 | 2.7 | 11.5 | 1.6 | 2.3 | 7.7 | 1.9 | | | | | | | 1237 | 124 | 0 | 124 | 742 | 0.03 | 0.10 | 0.44 | 0.03 | | | | 0.1 | | | 61 | 0.0 | 0.5 | 19 | 0.2 | 72 | 183 | | 37 | 0.34 |
| | | Vegetables & Bacon | | | | | | | | | | | | | | | | | | | | | | | | | | | | | | | | | | | | | | | | |
| 60659 | 1 Tbs | Junior, avg | 16 | 11 | 86 | 0.3 | 1.2 | 0.2 | | | 0.6 | 0.2 | 0.3 | 0.1 | 0.00 | 0.06 | 0 | 252 | 35 | | | | 0.01 | 0.00 | 0.09 | 0.01 | 0.02 | 1.4 | | 0.2 | | | 2 | 0.0 | 0.1 | 1 | | 6 | 14 | 0.3 | 7 | 0.04 |
| 60650 | 1 Tbs | Strained, avg | 16 | 11 | 86 | 0.3 | 1.4 | 0.3 | 0.3 | 0.9 | 0.5 | 0.2 | 0.2 | 0.1 | 0.01 | 0.05 | 1 | 365 | 36 | 0 | 36 | | 0.01 | 0.01 | 0.08 | 0.01 | 0.01 | 0.5 | 0.03 | 0.0 | | | 2 | 0.0 | 0.0 | 2 | 0.0 | 4 | 19 | 0.3 | 8 | 0.05 |

| Code | Amount | Description | Weight (g) | Calories | % Water | Protein (g) | Carbs (g) | Fiber (g) | Sugar (g) | Other Carbs (g) | Fat (g) | Sat Fat (g) | Mono Fat (g) | Poly Fat (g) | Omega 3 (g) | Omega 6 (g) | Choles (mg) |
|---|---|---|---|---|---|---|---|---|---|---|---|---|---|---|---|---|---|
| 60211 | 1 Tbs | 2nd Foods, Gerber | 14 | 11 | 85 | 0.3 | 1.3 | 0.2 | 0.3 | 0.8 | 0.4 | | | | | | |
| 60212 | 1 Tbs | 3rd Foods, Gerber | 14 | 11 | 84 | 0.3 | 1.3 | 0.3 | 0.2 | 0.8 | 0.5 | | | | | | |
| 60805 | 1 ea | Vegetables & Pasta, 2nd Foods, 4 oz jar, Gerber | 113 | 78 | 84 | 3.1 | 11.9 | 3.1 | 2.6 | 6.2 | 2.0 | | | | | | |
| 60823 | 1 ea | Vegetables & Pasta, 3rd Foods, 6 oz jar, Gerber | 170 | 100 | 86 | 3.7 | 17.9 | 1.9 | 4.3 | 11.7 | 1.7 | | | | | | |
| 60567 | 1 Tbs | Vegetables, mixed, junior, avg | 16 | 5 | 91 | 0.2 | 1.3 | | | | 0.0 | 0.0 | 0.0 | 0.0 | 0.00 | 0.00 | |
| 60574 | 1 Tbs | Vegetables, mixed, strained, avg | 16 | 7 | 89 | 0.2 | 1.5 | | | | 0.0 | | | | | | |
| 60827 | 1 ea | Vegetables Trio, 3rd Foods, 6 oz jar, Gerber | 170 | 97 | 87 | 3.9 | 15.0 | 2.6 | 3.7 | 8.7 | 2.6 | | | | | | |
| | | *INFANT FRUIT JUICES* | | | | | | | | | | | | | | | |
| | | Apple Juice | | | | | | | | | | | | | | | |
| 60465 | 1/2 cup | Average | 125 | 59 | 88 | 0.0 | 14.6 | 0.1 | | | 0.1 | 0.0 | 0.0 | 0.0 | 0.01 | 0.03 | 0 |
| 60377 | 1/2 cup | Strained, Heinz | 125 | 61 | 88 | 0.1 | 14.6 | 0.0 | 12.9 | 1.8 | 0.1 | 0.0 | | | | | |
| 60440 | 1 ea | With added vit C, Stage 1, 4 fl oz, Beechnut | 130 | 60 | 89 | 0.0 | 15.0 | 0.0 | 14.0 | 1.0 | 0.0 | 0.0 | 0.0 | 0.0 | 0.00 | 0.00 | |
| 60427 | 1 ea | With calcium, grad, 6 fl oz jar, Gerber | 189 | 85 | 88 | 0.2 | 21.0 | 0.8 | 17.6 | 2.6 | 0.0 | 0.0 | 0.0 | 0.0 | 0.00 | 0.00 | |
| | | Apple Banana Juice | | | | | | | | | | | | | | | |
| 60859 | 1/2 cup | Average | 125 | 64 | 87 | 0.3 | 15.4 | 0.3 | | | 0.1 | 0.0 | 0.0 | 0.0 | 0.01 | 0.04 | 0 |
| 60172 | 1 ea | 2nd Foods, 4 fl oz jar, Gerber | 127 | 65 | 87 | 0.3 | 15.6 | 0.3 | 14.2 | 1.1 | 0.1 | | | | | | |
| 60379 | 1/2 cup | Strained, Heinz | 125 | 65 | 87 | 0.3 | 15.5 | 0.1 | 12.5 | 2.9 | 0.3 | 0.1 | | | | | |
| 60696 | 1 ea | With calcium, grad, 6 fl oz jar, Gerber | 189 | 94 | 87 | 0.2 | 23.6 | 0.9 | 19.3 | 3.4 | 0.2 | | | | | | |
| 60666 | 1 ea | Apple Carrot, 3rd Foods, 4 fl oz jar, Gerber | 123 | 52 | 89 | 0.2 | 12.4 | 0.6 | 9.8 | 2.0 | 0.1 | | | | | | |
| 60457 | 1/2 cup | Apple Cherry, avg | 125 | 51 | 90 | 0.1 | 12.4 | 0.1 | | | 0.3 | 0.0 | 0.0 | 0.1 | 0.01 | 0.06 | 0 |
| 60380 | 1/2 cup | Apple Cherry, strained, Heinz | 125 | 56 | 89 | 0.1 | 13.5 | 0.0 | 11.6 | 1.9 | 0.1 | 0.0 | | | | | |
| 60860 | 1/2 cup | Apple Cranberry, avg | 125 | 59 | 88 | 0.0 | 14.3 | 0.0 | | | 0.0 | 0.0 | 0.0 | 0.0 | 0.00 | 0.01 | 0 |
| 60799 | 1 ea | Apple Cranberry, 2nd Foods, 4 fl oz jar, Gerber | 127 | 60 | 88 | 0.0 | 14.5 | 0.0 | 12.8 | 1.7 | 0.3 | | | | | | |
| | | Apple Grape Juice | | | | | | | | | | | | | | | |
| 60458 | 1/2 cup | Average | 125 | 58 | 88 | 0.1 | 14.3 | 0.1 | | | 0.3 | 0.0 | 0.0 | 0.1 | 0.01 | 0.06 | 0 |
| 60178 | 1 ea | 2nd Foods, 4 fl oz jar, Gerber | 127 | 61 | 88 | 0.1 | 14.7 | 0.1 | 14.0 | 0.6 | 0.1 | | | | | | |
| 60374 | 1/2 cup | Strained, Heinz | 125 | 58 | 88 | 0.3 | 14.0 | 0.0 | 12.5 | 1.5 | 0.1 | 0.0 | | | | | |
| 60429 | 1 ea | With calcium, grad, 8 fl oz jar, Gerber | 189 | 91 | 88 | 0.2 | 22.1 | 0.6 | 18.3 | 3.2 | 0.2 | | | | | | |
| | | Apple Peach Juice | | | | | | | | | | | | | | | |
| 60469 | 1/2 cup | Average | 125 | 52 | 89 | 0.3 | 13.1 | 0.1 | | | 0.1 | 0.0 | 0.0 | 0.0 | 0.01 | 0.03 | 0 |
| 60174 | 1 ea | 2nd Foods, 4 fl oz jar, Gerber | 127 | 60 | 88 | 0.3 | 14.4 | 0.4 | 12.6 | 1.4 | 0.1 | | | | | | |
| 60375 | 1/2 cup | Strained, Heinz | 125 | 55 | 89 | 0.3 | 13.0 | 0.1 | 10.8 | 2.1 | 0.3 | 0.1 | | | | | |
| 60470 | 1/2 cup | Apple Plum, avg | 125 | 61 | 87 | 0.1 | 15.4 | 0.1 | | | 0.0 | 0.0 | 0.0 | 0.0 | 0.00 | 0.00 | 0 |
| 60195 | 1 ea | Apple Plum, 2nd Foods, 4 fl oz jar, Gerber | 127 | 61 | 88 | 0.3 | 14.9 | 0.1 | 14.0 | 0.8 | 0.1 | | | | | | |
| | | Apple Prune Juice | | | | | | | | | | | | | | | |
| 60459 | 1/2 cup | Average | 125 | 91 | 81 | 0.3 | 22.5 | 0.1 | | | 0.1 | 0.0 | 0.0 | 0.0 | 0.01 | 0.03 | 0 |
| 60087 | 1 ea | 2nd Foods, 4 fl oz jar, Gerber | 127 | 67 | 86 | 0.3 | 16.3 | 0.5 | 12.8 | 2.9 | 0.1 | | | | | | |
| 60370 | 1/2 cup | Strained, Heinz | 125 | 61 | 88 | 0.3 | 14.9 | 0.1 | 12.9 | 1.9 | 0.1 | 0.0 | | | | | |
| 60667 | 1 ea | Apple Sweet Potato, 3rd Foods, 4 fl oz jar, Gerber | 123 | 60 | 88 | 0.5 | 14.5 | 0.6 | 11.7 | 2.2 | 0.1 | | | | | | |
| | | Mixed Fruit Juice | | | | | | | | | | | | | | | |
| 60573 | 1/2 cup | Average | 125 | 59 | 88 | 0.1 | 14.5 | 0.1 | | | 0.1 | 0.0 | 0.0 | 0.0 | 0.00 | 0.04 | 0 |
| 60088 | 1 ea | 2nd Foods, 4 fl oz jar, Gerber | 127 | 62 | 88 | 0.3 | 14.6 | 0.1 | 13.3 | 1.1 | 0.1 | | | | | | |
| 60371 | 1/2 cup | Strained, Heinz | 125 | 61 | 88 | 0.4 | 14.6 | 0.0 | 12.3 | 2.4 | 0.1 | 0.0 | | | | | |
| 60831 | 1 ea | Tropical Fruit, 4 fl oz jar, Gerber | 127 | 71 | 86 | 0.6 | 17.0 | 0.4 | 14.0 | 2.7 | 0.1 | | | | | | |
| 60731 | 1 ea | With added vit C & Iron, 4 fl oz jar, Beechnut | 124 | 100 | 81 | 0.0 | 23.0 | 0.0 | 18.0 | 5.0 | 0.0 | 0.0 | 0.0 | 0.0 | 0.00 | 0.00 | |
| 60430 | 1 ea | With calcium, grad, 8 fl oz jar, Gerber | 189 | 100 | 86 | 0.4 | 24.2 | 0.8 | 18.9 | 4.5 | 0.2 | | | | | | |
| 60699 | 1 ea | With Guava, 4 fl oz jar, Gerber | 125 | 69 | 87 | 0.4 | 16.0 | 0.8 | 11.5 | 3.8 | 0.1 | | | | | | |
| | | Orange Juice | | | | | | | | | | | | | | | |
| 60585 | 1/2 cup | Average | 125 | 55 | 88 | 0.8 | 12.8 | 0.1 | | | 0.4 | 0.0 | 0.1 | 0.1 | 0.02 | 0.06 | 0 |
| 60175 | 1 ea | 2nd Foods, 4 fl oz jar, Gerber | 127 | 60 | 88 | 0.8 | 13.3 | 0.3 | 12.1 | 1.0 | 0.3 | | | | | | |
| 60372 | 1/2 cup | Strained, Heinz | 125 | 58 | 88 | 0.9 | 13.5 | 0.1 | 10.9 | 2.5 | 0.3 | 0.0 | | | | | |
| 60588 | 1/2 cup | Orange Apple, avg | 125 | 54 | 89 | 0.5 | 12.6 | | | | 0.3 | | | | | | |
| 60587 | 1/2 cup | Orange Apple Banana, avg | 125 | 59 | 88 | 0.5 | 14.4 | 0.1 | | | 0.1 | 0.0 | 0.0 | 0.0 | 0.01 | 0.03 | 0 |
| 60589 | 1/2 cup | Orange Apricot, avg | 125 | 58 | 88 | 1.0 | 13.6 | 0.1 | | | 0.1 | 0.0 | 0.0 | 0.0 | 0.01 | 0.02 | 0 |
| 60583 | 1/2 cup | Orange Banana, avg | 125 | 62 | 87 | 0.9 | 14.9 | | | | 0.1 | | | | | | |
| 60832 | 1 ea | Orange Banana Pineapple, 4 fl oz jar, Gerber | 127 | 72 | 86 | 0.8 | 17.0 | 0.5 | 13.8 | 2.7 | 0.1 | | | | | | |
| 60668 | 1 ea | Orange Carrot, 3rd Foods, 4 fl oz jar, Gerber | 123 | 53 | 89 | 0.7 | 11.9 | 0.9 | 9.1 | 2.0 | 0.1 | | | | | | |
| 60584 | 1/2 cup | Orange Pineapple, avg | 125 | 60 | 87 | 0.6 | 14.6 | 0.1 | | | 0.1 | 0.0 | 0.0 | 0.0 | 0.01 | 0.02 | 0 |
| | | Pear Juice | | | | | | | | | | | | | | | |
| 60751 | 1/2 cup | Strained, Heinz | 125 | 60 | 88 | 0.3 | 14.5 | 0.1 | 9.3 | 5.1 | 0.1 | 0.0 | | | | | |
| 60039 | 1 ea | 1st Foods, 4 fl oz jar, Gerber | 127 | 60 | 88 | 0.3 | 14.4 | 0.3 | 12.3 | 1.8 | 0.1 | | | | | | |
| 60075 | 1 ea | Prep f/conc, w/added vit C, 4 fl oz jar, Beech | 124 | 60 | 88 | 0.0 | 15.0 | 0.0 | 13.0 | 2.0 | 0.0 | 0.0 | 0.0 | 0.0 | 0.00 | 0.00 | |
| 60669 | 1 ea | Pineapple Carrot, 3rd Foods, 4 fl oz jar, Gerber | 123 | 57 | 88 | 0.5 | 13.3 | 0.5 | 10.9 | 1.8 | 0.1 | | | | | | |
| 60614 | 1/2 cup | Prune Orange, avg | 125 | 88 | 82 | 0.8 | 21.0 | | | | 0.4 | | | | | | |
| 60076 | 1/2 cup | Tropical Blend, Stage 2, Beechnut | 124 | 70 | 86 | 0.0 | 17.0 | | | | | | | | | | |

| Code | Vit A (IU) | Vit A (RE) | Retinol (RE) | Carotenoids (RE) | Beta Carotene (mcg) | Thiamin (mg) | Riboflavin (mg) | Niacin (NE) | Vit B6 (mg) | Vit B12 (mcg) | Folate (mcg) | Panto (mg) | Vit C (mg) | Vit D (mg) | Vit E (α TE) | Calcium (mg) | Copper (mg) | Iron (mg) | Magnes (mg) | Mang (mg) | Phos (mg) | Potassium (mg) | Selenium (mcg) | Sodium (mg) | Zinc (mg) |
|---|---|---|---|---|---|---|---|---|---|---|---|---|---|---|---|---|---|---|---|---|---|---|---|---|---|
| 60211 | 229 | 23 | 0 | 23 | 138 | 0.00 | 0.00 | 0.06 | 0.01 | | | | 0.2 | | | 2 | 0.0 | 0.0 | 1 | 0.0 | 4 | 18 | | 7 | 0.04 |
| 60212 | 278 | 28 | 0 | 28 | 167 | 0.00 | 0.01 | 0.06 | 0.01 | | | | 0.0 | | | 2 | 0.0 | 0.0 | 1 | 0.0 | 5 | 18 | | 12 | 0.04 |
| 60805 | 2336 | 234 | 0 | 234 | 1401 | 0.07 | 0.12 | 0.46 | 0.08 | | | | 0.2 | | | 53 | 0.1 | 0.8 | 19 | 0.2 | 71 | 217 | | 24 | 0.56 |
| 60823 | 1746 | 175 | 0 | 175 | 1048 | 0.07 | 0.17 | 0.90 | 0.09 | | | | | | | 78 | 0.1 | 0.7 | 27 | 0.3 | 102 | 204 | | 206 | 0.68 |
| 60567 | 391 | 39 | | | | 0.00 | 0.00 | 0.07 | 0.01 | 0.00 | 1.1 | 0.04 | 0.5 | | | 3 | 0.0 | 0.0 | 2 | | 4 | 18 | 0.1 | 1 | 0.04 |
| 60574 | 436 | 44 | | | | 0.00 | 0.00 | 0.08 | 0.01 | 0.00 | 1.3 | 0.04 | 0.4 | | | 4 | 0.0 | 0.1 | 2 | | 4 | 19 | 0.1 | 1 | 0.03 |
| 60827 | 2572 | 257 | 0 | 257 | 1543 | 0.07 | 0.10 | 0.44 | 0.09 | | | | | | | 73 | 0.1 | 0.7 | 20 | 0.1 | 83 | 209 | | 309 | 0.51 |
| 60465 | 23 | 3 | 0 | 3 | | 0.01 | 0.02 | 0.10 | 0.04 | 0.00 | 0.1 | 0.14 | 72.4 | | | 5 | 0.0 | 0.7 | 4 | | 6 | 114 | 0.1 | 4 | 0.04 |
| 60377 | 10 | 1 | | | | 0.00 | 0.01 | 0.13 | 0.01 | | | | 152.3 | | | 14 | 0.0 | 0.3 | | | 10 | 114 | | 6 | 0.06 |
| 60440 | 0 | 0 | 0 | 0 | 0 | | | | | | | | 42.0 | | | 0 | | 0.3 | | | | 105 | | 10 | |
| 60427 | | | | | | 0.02 | 0.04 | 0.15 | 0.06 | | | | 40.1 | | | 161 | 0.0 | 0.4 | 9 | 0.1 | 15 | 170 | | 6 | |
| 60859 | 11 | 1 | 0 | 1 | | 0.01 | 0.01 | 0.17 | 0.07 | 0.00 | 1.3 | 0.16 | 34.9 | | | 9 | 0.0 | 0.3 | 8 | 0.1 | 10 | 154 | 0.4 | 5 | 0.05 |
| 60172 | 11 | 1 | 0 | 1 | 7 | 0.01 | 0.01 | 0.17 | 0.08 | | | | 35.4 | | | 9 | 0.0 | 0.3 | 8 | 0.1 | 10 | 159 | | 5 | |
| 60379 | 11 | 1 | | | | 0.01 | 0.01 | 0.11 | 0.05 | | | | 138.6 | | | 15 | 0.0 | 0.4 | | | 9 | 144 | | 8 | 0.13 |
| 60696 | 2 | 0.2 | 0 | 0.2 | 1 | | 0.06 | 0.25 | 0.11 | | | | 40.1 | | | 161 | 0.0 | 0.6 | 13 | 0.2 | 19 | 215 | | 8 | 0.19 |
| 60666 | 2429 | 243 | 0 | 243 | 1458 | 0.01 | 0.01 | 0.12 | 0.06 | | | | 34.3 | | | 12 | 0.0 | 0.2 | 7 | 0.1 | 12 | 125 | | 12 | 0.25 |
| 60457 | 6 | 1 | | | | 0.01 | 0.02 | 0.12 | 0.04 | 0.00 | 0.4 | 0.13 | 72.9 | | | 6 | 0.1 | 0.8 | 4 | | 8 | 122 | 0.1 | 4 | 0.04 |
| 60380 | 14 | 1 | | | | 0.01 | 0.01 | 0.11 | 0.01 | | | | 120.0 | | | 15 | 0.0 | 0.4 | | | 12 | 124 | | 8 | 0.13 |
| 60860 | 0 | 0 | 0 | 0 | 0 | 0.00 | 0.02 | 0.09 | 0.04 | 0.00 | 0.0 | | 34.9 | | | 8 | 0.0 | 0.3 | 4 | 0.2 | 9 | 121 | 0.1 | 6 | 0.06 |
| 60799 | | | | | | | 0.03 | 0.09 | 0.04 | | | | 35.4 | | | 10 | 0.0 | 0.3 | 4 | 0.2 | 8 | 123 | | 6 | |
| 60458 | 8 | 1 | | | | 0.01 | 0.03 | 0.14 | 0.04 | 0.00 | 0.4 | 0.09 | 67.0 | | | 8 | 0.1 | 0.5 | 4 | | 6 | 112 | 0.1 | 4 | 0.04 |
| 60178 | 4 | 0.4 | 0 | 0.4 | 2 | 0.01 | 0.03 | 0.15 | 0.04 | | | | 35.4 | | | 9 | 0.0 | 0.3 | 6 | 0.1 | 8 | 122 | | 6 | |
| 60374 | 16 | 2 | | | | 0.01 | 0.01 | 0.16 | 0.02 | | | | 117.0 | | | 15 | 0.0 | 0.3 | | | 10 | 130 | | 8 | 0.04 |
| 60429 | | | | | | 0.02 | 0.06 | 0.17 | 0.06 | | | | 40.1 | | | 161 | 0.0 | 0.4 | 9 | 0.1 | 15 | 155 | | 8 | 0.19 |
| 60469 | 79 | 8 | 0 | 8 | | 0.01 | 0.01 | 0.27 | 0.03 | 0.00 | 1.6 | 0.10 | 73.1 | | | 4 | 0.0 | 0.7 | 4 | | 5 | 121 | 0.4 | 1 | 0.03 |
| 60174 | 37 | 4 | 0 | 4 | 22 | 0.01 | 0.03 | 0.27 | 0.03 | | | | 35.4 | | | 9 | 0.0 | 0.4 | 6 | 0.1 | 10 | 146 | | 5 | |
| 60375 | 49 | 5 | | | | 0.01 | 0.01 | 0.20 | 0.02 | | | | 127.1 | | | 15 | 0.0 | 0.5 | | | 14 | 115 | | 9 | 0.07 |
| 60470 | 54 | 5 | 0 | 5 | | 0.02 | 0.02 | 0.24 | 0.04 | 0.00 | 0.3 | 0.15 | 72.8 | | | 6 | 0.1 | 0.8 | 4 | | 4 | 126 | 0.4 | 1 | 0.04 |
| 60195 | 13 | 1 | 0 | 1 | 8 | 0.01 | 0.03 | 0.23 | 0.04 | | | | 35.4 | | | 10 | | 0.3 | | | 9 | 156 | | 6 | |
| 60459 | 20 | 3 | 0 | 3 | | 0.01 | 0.00 | 0.38 | 0.04 | 0.00 | 0.1 | 0.23 | 84.4 | | | 11 | 0.1 | 1.2 | 9 | | 19 | 185 | 0.4 | 6 | 0.06 |
| 60087 | 18 | 2 | 0 | 2 | 11 | 0.01 | 0.10 | 0.30 | 0.05 | | | | 35.4 | | | 11 | 0.0 | 0.4 | 9 | 0.1 | 13 | 170 | | 5 | 0.13 |
| 60370 | 11 | 1 | | | | 0.01 | 0.05 | 0.49 | 0.11 | | | | 197.6 | | | 18 | 0.0 | 0.4 | | | 20 | 144 | | 8 | 0.06 |
| 60667 | 2531 | 253 | 0 | 253 | 1519 | 0.01 | 0.02 | 0.15 | 0.07 | | | | 34.3 | | | 15 | 0.0 | 0.1 | 11 | 0.1 | 17 | 178 | | 9 | 0.25 |
| 60573 | 53 | 5 | 0 | 5 | | 0.03 | 0.02 | 0.15 | 0.05 | 0.00 | 8.4 | 0.14 | 79.5 | | | 10 | 0.0 | 0.4 | 6 | | 6 | 126 | 0.6 | 5 | 0.04 |
| 60088 | 27 | 3 | 0 | 3 | 16 | 0.04 | 0.01 | 0.17 | 0.08 | | | | 35.4 | | | 11 | 0.0 | 0.3 | 9 | 0.2 | 10 | 151 | | 5 | |
| 60371 | 160 | 16 | | | | 0.04 | 0.02 | 0.16 | 0.06 | | | | 178.1 | | | 16 | 0.0 | 0.4 | | | 15 | 168 | | 6 | 0.04 |
| 60831 | 25 | 3 | 0 | 3 | 15 | 0.05 | 0.06 | 0.37 | 0.15 | | | | 35.4 | | | 14 | 0.0 | 0.3 | 22 | 0.3 | 14 | 182 | | 8 | 0.13 |
| 60731 | 0 | 0 | 0 | 0 | 0 | | | | | | | | 42.0 | | | 12 | | 2.3 | | | | 60 | | 10 | |
| 60430 | | | | | | | 0.02 | 0.15 | 0.09 | | | | 40.1 | | | 161 | 0.0 | 0.6 | 11 | 0.1 | 21 | 159 | | 8 | 0.19 |
| 60699 | 85 | 9 | 0 | 9 | 51 | 0.02 | 0.05 | 0.39 | 0.05 | | | | 34.9 | | | 15 | 0.0 | 0.3 | 9 | 0.1 | 18 | 145 | | 6 | 0.13 |
| 60585 | 69 | 8 | 0 | 8 | | 0.06 | 0.04 | 0.30 | 0.07 | 0.00 | 33.0 | 0.17 | 78.1 | | | 15 | 0.1 | 0.2 | 11 | | 14 | 230 | 0.1 | 1 | 0.07 |
| 60175 | 15 | 2 | 0 | 2 | 9 | 0.09 | 0.04 | 0.29 | 0.06 | | | | 35.4 | | | 15 | 0.1 | 0.1 | 14 | 0.0 | 20 | 234 | | 4 | |
| 60372 | 91 | 9 | | | | 0.13 | 0.02 | 0.25 | 0.09 | | | | 154.5 | | | 20 | 0.0 | 0.4 | | | 20 | 214 | | 6 | 0.15 |
| 60588 | 91 | 9 | 0 | 9 | | 0.05 | 0.04 | 0.23 | 0.05 | 0.00 | 15.3 | 0.15 | 96.1 | | | 12 | 0.0 | 0.3 | 6 | | 9 | 172 | 0.1 | 4 | 0.03 |
| 60587 | 34 | 4 | 0 | 4 | | 0.05 | 0.03 | 0.33 | 0.08 | 0.00 | 12.1 | 0.17 | 40.1 | | | 6 | 0.1 | 0.4 | 8 | | 10 | 168 | 0.1 | 5 | 0.03 |
| 60589 | 270 | 28 | 0 | 28 | | 0.07 | 0.04 | 0.33 | 0.07 | 0.00 | 24.9 | 0.12 | 107.4 | | | 8 | 0.1 | 0.5 | 9 | | 15 | 249 | 0.1 | 8 | 0.04 |
| 60583 | 58 | 6 | 0 | 6 | | 0.06 | 0.05 | 0.23 | 0.07 | 0.00 | 30.5 | 0.19 | 42.5 | | | 21 | 0.1 | 0.1 | 18 | | 16 | 250 | 0.1 | 4 | 0.11 |
| 60832 | 11 | 1 | 0 | 1 | 7 | 0.05 | 0.08 | 0.44 | 0.14 | | | | 35.4 | | | 13 | 0.1 | 0.1 | 20 | 0.1 | 23 | 291 | | 8 | 0.13 |
| 60668 | 2496 | 250 | 0 | 250 | 1497 | 0.07 | 0.05 | 0.27 | 0.07 | | | | 34.3 | | | 16 | 0.0 | 0.2 | 14 | 0.1 | 23 | 216 | | 10 | 0.12 |
| 60584 | 39 | 4 | 0 | 4 | | 0.06 | 0.03 | 0.24 | 0.08 | 0.00 | 23.3 | 0.07 | 66.8 | | | 10 | 0.1 | 0.5 | 11 | | 11 | 176 | 0.1 | 2 | 0.05 |
| 60751 | 9 | 1 | | | | 0.01 | 0.02 | 0.28 | 0.05 | | | | 145.0 | | | 19 | | 0.5 | | | 11 | 168 | | 10 | |
| 60039 | | | | | | 0.01 | 0.01 | 0.18 | 0.03 | | | | 35.4 | | | 11 | 0.0 | 0.3 | 8 | 0.4 | 11 | 157 | | 5 | 0.13 |
| 60075 | 0 | 0 | 0 | 0 | 0 | | 0.03 | 0.24 | | | | | 42.0 | | | 0 | | 0.0 | | | | 130 | | 5 | |
| 60669 | 1900 | 190 | 0 | 190 | 1140 | 0.07 | 0.04 | 0.23 | 0.09 | | | | 34.3 | | | 15 | 0.0 | 0.2 | 16 | 0.2 | 14 | 140 | | 10 | 0.12 |
| 60614 | 164 | 16 | 0 | 16 | | 0.05 | 0.15 | 0.50 | 0.08 | 0.00 | 16.4 | 0.17 | 79.8 | | | 15 | 0.1 | 1.1 | 10 | | 12 | 226 | 0.1 | 2 | 0.05 |
| 60076 | 15 | 1.5 | | | | 0.01 | 0.01 | 0.12 | | | | | 42.0 | | | | | | | | | | | 5 | |

| Code | Amount | Description | Weight (g) | Calories | % Water | Protein (g) | Carbs (g) | Fiber (g) | Sugar (g) | Other Carbs (g) | Fat (g) |
|---|---|---|---|---|---|---|---|---|---|---|---|
| | | | Basic Components | | | | | | | | |
| 60733 | 1 ea | Tropical Blend, w/added vit C, 4 fl oz jar, Beech | 124 | 90 | 85 | 0.0 | 19.0 | 0.0 | 15.0 | 4.0 | 0.0 |
| 60040 | 1 ea | White Grape, 1st Foods, 4 fl oz jar, Gerber | 127 | 83 | 84 | 0.4 | 19.8 | | 19.6 | | 0.1 |
| 60750 | 1/2 cup | White Grape, strained, Heinz | 125 | 74 | 85 | 0.5 | 17.6 | 0.1 | 16.6 | 0.9 | 0.1 |
| | | *INFANT FRUITS* | | | | | | | | | |
| | | Apples | | | | | | | | | |
| 60854 | 1 Tbs | Dices, toddler, avg | 16 | 8 | 88 | 0.0 | 1.9 | 0.1 | | | 0.0 |
| 60835 | 1 ea | Dices, grad, 4.5 oz jar, Gerber | 128 | 65 | 88 | 0.3 | 15.5 | 1.2 | 11.8 | 2.6 | 0.1 |
| 60094 | 1 ea | 4.5 oz jar, Earths Best | 128 | 70 | 87 | 0.3 | 17.0 | 1.9 | | | 0.1 |
| | | Apples & Apricots | | | | | | | | | |
| 60286 | 1 ea | Stage 2, 4 oz jar, Beechnut | 113 | 70 | 85 | 0.0 | 16.9 | 1.0 | 10.0 | 6.0 | 0.0 |
| 60392 | 1 Tbs | Strained, Heinz | 16 | 9 | 86 | 0.0 | 2.0 | 0.3 | 1.4 | 0.4 | 0.0 |
| 60098 | 1 ea | 4.5 oz jar, Earths Best | 128 | 70 | 87 | 0.0 | 17.0 | | | | 0.0 |
| | | Apples & Bananas | | | | | | | | | |
| 60289 | 1 ea | Stage 2, 4 oz jar, Beechnut | 113 | 60 | 88 | 0.0 | 14.0 | 1.0 | 12.0 | 1.0 | 0.0 |
| 60112 | 1 ea | 4.5oz jar, Earths Best | 128 | 80 | 86 | 0.0 | 18.0 | | | | |
| 60816 | 1 ea | 3rd Foods, 6 fl oz jar, Gerber | 170 | 126 | 82 | 0.7 | 30.1 | 2.9 | 22.6 | 4.6 | 0.2 |
| 60215 | 1 ea | With Pears, Stage 2, 4 oz jar, Beechnut | 113 | 90 | 81 | 0.0 | 19.9 | 1.0 | 15.9 | 3.0 | 0.0 |
| | | Apples & Blueberries | | | | | | | | | |
| 60463 | 1 Tbs | Junior, avg | 16 | 10 | 83 | 0.0 | 2.7 | 0.3 | | | 0.0 |
| 60464 | 1 Tbs | Strained, avg | 16 | 10 | 83 | 0.0 | 2.6 | 0.3 | | | 0.0 |
| 60241 | 1 Tbs | 2nd Foods, Gerber | 14 | 7 | 88 | 0.0 | 1.7 | 0.2 | 1.3 | 0.2 | 0.0 |
| 60670 | 1 ea | 3rd Foods, 6 oz jar, Gerber | 170 | 85 | 88 | 0.3 | 20.1 | 3.1 | 15.3 | 1.7 | 0.3 |
| 60290 | 1 ea | Apples & Cherries, Stage 2, 4 oz jar, Beechnut | 113 | 80 | 86 | 0.0 | 17.9 | 1.0 | 7.0 | 10.0 | 0.0 |
| 60434 | 1 ea | Apples & Cherries, Stage 3, 6 oz jar, Beechnut | 170 | 110 | 89 | 0.0 | 26.0 | 1.0 | 10.0 | 15.0 | 0.0 |
| 60389 | 1 Tbs | Apples & Cranberries, strained, Heinz | 16 | 11 | 83 | 0.0 | 2.6 | 0.1 | 1.6 | 0.9 | 0.0 |
| 60748 | 1 ea | Apples & Pears, Stage 2, 4 oz jar, Beechnut | 113 | 85 | 83 | 0.0 | 18.9 | 1.0 | 16.9 | 1.0 | 0.1 |
| 60390 | 1 Tbs | Apples & Pears, strained, Heinz | 16 | 9 | 87 | 0.0 | 2.0 | 0.3 | 1.3 | 0.4 | 0.0 |
| 60111 | 1 ea | Apples & Plums, 4.5 oz jar, Earths Best | 128 | 70 | 87 | 0.0 | 17.0 | | | | 0.0 |
| 60466 | 1 Tbs | Apples & Raspberries w/sugar, junior, avg | 16 | 9 | 84 | 0.0 | 2.5 | 0.3 | | | 0.0 |
| 60467 | 1 Tbs | Apples & Raspberries w/sugar, strained, avg | 16 | 9 | 84 | 0.0 | 2.5 | 0.3 | | | 0.0 |
| | | Applesauce | | | | | | | | | |
| 60055 | 1 ea | Golden Delicious, Stage 1, 2.5 oz jar, Beechnut | 71 | 50 | 84 | 0.0 | 12.0 | 1.0 | 8.0 | 3.0 | 0.0 |
| 60249 | 1 Tbs | Golden Delicious, Stage 2, Beechnut | 16 | 10 | 87 | 0.0 | 2.1 | 0.1 | 1.6 | 0.4 | 0.0 |
| 60474 | 1 Tbs | Junior, avg | 16 | 6 | 90 | 0.0 | 1.6 | 0.3 | | | 0.0 |
| 60475 | 1 Tbs | Strained, avg | 16 | 7 | 89 | 0.0 | 1.7 | 0.3 | | | 0.0 |
| 62126 | 1 Tbs | 1st Foods, Gerber | 14 | 8 | 86 | 0.0 | 1.9 | 0.3 | 1.6 | 0.0 | 0.0 |
| 60245 | 1 Tbs | 2nd Foods, Gerber | 14 | 7 | 87 | 0.0 | 1.7 | 0.2 | 1.4 | 0.2 | 0.0 |
| 60246 | 1 Tbs | 3rd Foods, Gerber | 14 | 7 | 87 | 0.0 | 1.7 | 0.2 | 1.3 | 0.2 | 0.0 |
| | | Applesauce & Apricots | | | | | | | | | |
| 60471 | 1 Tbs | Junior, avg | 16 | 8 | 87 | 0.0 | 2.0 | 0.3 | | | 0.0 |
| 60473 | 1 Tbs | Strained, avg | 16 | 7 | 88 | 0.0 | 1.9 | 0.3 | | | 0.0 |
| 60018 | 1 Tbs | 2nd Foods, Gerber | 14 | 7 | 87 | 0.0 | 1.8 | 0.3 | 1.3 | 0.2 | 0.0 |
| 60857 | 1 Tbs | Applesauce & Bananas, junior, avg | 16 | 11 | 83 | 0.1 | 2.6 | 0.3 | | | 0.0 |
| 60472 | 1 Tbs | Applesauce & Cherries, junior, avg | 16 | 9 | 86 | 0.0 | 2.3 | 0.2 | | | 0.0 |
| 60476 | 1 Tbs | Applesauce & Cherries, strained, avg | 16 | 8 | 86 | 0.0 | 2.3 | 0.2 | | | 0.0 |
| 60460 | 1 Tbs | Applesauce & Pineapple, junior, avg | 16 | 6 | 89 | 0.0 | 1.7 | 0.2 | | | 0.0 |
| 60468 | 1 Tbs | Applesauce & Pineapple, strained, avg | 16 | 6 | 90 | 0.0 | 1.6 | 0.2 | | | 0.0 |
| 60292 | 1 ea | Apricots, Pears & Apples, Stage 2, 4 oz jar, Beechnut | 113 | 90 | 82 | 0.0 | 19.9 | 2.0 | 9.0 | 9.0 | 0.0 |
| 60435 | 1 ea | Apricots, Pears & Apples, Stage 3, 6 oz jar, Beechnut | 170 | 130 | 81 | 0.0 | 32.0 | 3.0 | 14.0 | 15.0 | 0.0 |
| 60093 | 1 ea | Bananas, 4.5 oz jar, Earth's Best | 128 | 90 | 84 | 1.0 | 20.0 | 1.4 | | | 0.4 |
| 60728 | 1 ea | Bananas, Stage 1, 4 oz jar, Beechnut | 113 | 110 | 79 | 0.0 | 23.9 | 1.0 | 12.0 | 11.0 | 0.0 |
| 60285 | 1 ea | Bananas, Stage 3, 4 oz jar, Beechnut | 113 | 159 | 70 | 1.0 | 32.9 | 3.0 | 15.9 | 14.0 | 0.0 |
| 60293 | 1 ea | Bananas, Pears & Apples, Stg 2, 4 oz jar, Bchnut | 113 | 90 | 81 | 0.0 | 20.9 | 1.0 | 15.9 | 4.0 | 0.0 |
| 60700 | 1 ea | Mango, w/mixed fruit juice, 4.4 oz jar, Gerber | 125 | 71 | 86 | 0.3 | 17.1 | 0.4 | 14.1 | 2.6 | 0.1 |
| 60836 | 1 ea | Mixed Fruit, diced, grad, 4.5 oz jar, Gerber | 128 | 61 | 88 | 0.4 | 14.6 | 1.4 | 11.0 | 2.2 | 0.1 |
| 60701 | 1 ea | Papaya, w/mixed fruit juice, 4.4 oz jar, Gerber | 125 | 69 | 86 | 0.4 | 16.5 | 0.6 | 13.5 | 2.4 | 0.1 |
| | | Peaches | | | | | | | | | |
| 60858 | 1 Tbs | Dices, toddler, avg | 16 | 8 | 87 | 0.1 | 1.9 | 0.1 | | | 0.0 |
| 60422 | 1 Tbs | Junior, Heinz | 16 | 11 | 83 | 0.2 | 2.5 | 0.3 | 1.9 | 0.3 | 0.0 |
| 60388 | 1 Tbs | Strained, Heinz | 16 | 11 | 83 | 0.2 | 2.4 | 0.3 | 1.8 | 0.3 | 0.0 |
| 60596 | 1 Tbs | With sugar, junior, avg | 16 | 11 | 80 | 0.1 | 3.0 | 0.2 | | | 0.0 |
| 60595 | 1 Tbs | With sugar, strained, avg | 16 | 11 | 80 | 0.1 | 3.0 | 0.2 | | | 0.0 |
| 60318 | 1 Tbs | 1st Foods, Gerber | 14 | 6 | 89 | 0.1 | 1.3 | 0.2 | 0.9 | 0.2 | 0.0 |
| 60019 | 1 Tbs | 2nd Foods, Gerber | 14 | 9 | 83 | 0.1 | 2.2 | 0.2 | 1.7 | 0.3 | 0.0 |
| 60260 | 1 Tbs | 3rd Foods, Gerber | 14 | 9 | 83 | 0.1 | 2.2 | 0.2 | 1.7 | 0.3 | 0.0 |
| 60735 | 1 ea | Peaches & Bananas, 4 oz jar, Beechnut | 113 | 70 | 87 | 0.0 | 14.9 | 3.0 | 8.0 | 4.0 | 0.0 |
| | | Pears | | | | | | | | | |
| 60838 | 1 ea | Dices, grad, 4.5 oz jar, Gerber | 128 | 74 | 86 | 0.4 | 17.4 | 1.5 | 14.8 | 1.0 | 0.1 |
| 60599 | 1 Tbs | Junior, avg | 16 | 7 | 88 | 0.0 | 1.9 | 0.6 | | | 0.0 |
| 60600 | 1 Tbs | Strained, avg | 16 | 7 | 88 | 0.0 | 1.7 | 0.6 | | | 0.0 |

| Code | Sat Fat (g) | Mono Fat (g) | Poly Fat (g) | Omega 3 (g) | Omega 6 (g) | Choles (mg) | Vit A (IU) | Vit A (RE) | Retinol (RE) | Carotenoids (RE) | Beta Carotene (mcg) |
|---|---|---|---|---|---|---|---|---|---|---|---|
| | Additional Fats | | | | | | Vit A & Components | | | | |
| 60733 | 0.0 | 0.0 | 0.0 | 0.00 | 0.00 | | 30 | 3 | | | |
| 60040 | | | | | | | | | | | |
| 60750 | 0.1 | 0.0 | 0.0 | 0.00 | 0.00 | | 18 | 2 | | | |
| 60854 | 0.0 | 0.0 | 0.0 | 0.00 | 0.00 | 0 | 1 | 0.2 | | | |
| 60835 | | | | | | | 8 | 1 | 0 | 1 | 5 |
| 60094 | 0.0 | 0.0 | 0.0 | | | 0 | 0 | 0 | 0 | 0 | 0 |
| 60286 | 0.0 | 0.0 | 0.0 | 0.00 | 0.00 | | 598 | 60 | | | |
| 60392 | 0.0 | | | | | | 90 | 9 | | | |
| 60098 | 0.0 | 0.0 | 0.0 | 0.00 | 0.00 | | 750 | 75 | 0 | 75 | |
| 60289 | 0.0 | 0.0 | 0.0 | 0.00 | 0.00 | | 0 | 0 | 0 | 0 | 0 |
| 60112 | | | | | | | 60 | 6 | 0 | 6 | |
| 60816 | | | | | | | 34 | 3 | 0 | 3 | 20 |
| 60215 | 0.0 | 0.0 | 0.0 | 0.00 | 0.00 | | 0 | 0 | 0 | 0 | 0 |
| 60463 | 0.0 | 0.0 | 0.0 | 0.00 | 0.01 | 0 | 7 | 1 | | | |
| 60464 | 0.0 | 0.0 | 0.0 | 0.00 | 0.01 | 0 | 3 | 0.3 | | | |
| 60241 | | | | | | | 3 | 0.3 | 0 | 0.3 | 2 |
| 60670 | | | | | | | 34 | 3 | 0 | 3 | 20 |
| 60290 | 0.0 | 0.0 | 0.0 | 0.00 | 0.00 | | 30 | 3 | | | |
| 60434 | 0.0 | 0.0 | 0.0 | 0.00 | 0.00 | | 60 | 6 | | | |
| 60389 | 0.0 | | | | | | 1 | 0.2 | | | |
| 60748 | | | | | | 0 | 0 | 0 | 0 | 0 | 0 |
| 60390 | 0.0 | | | | | | 8 | 1 | | | |
| 60111 | 0.0 | 0.0 | 0.0 | 0.00 | 0.00 | | 150 | 15 | 0 | 15 | |
| 60466 | 0.0 | 0.0 | 0.0 | 0.00 | 0.01 | 0 | 5 | 0.5 | | | |
| 60467 | 0.0 | 0.0 | 0.0 | 0.00 | 0.01 | 0 | 4 | 0.3 | | | |
| 60055 | 0.0 | 0.0 | 0.0 | 0.00 | 0.00 | | 0 | 0 | 0 | 0 | 0 |
| 60249 | 0.0 | 0.0 | 0.0 | 0.00 | 0.00 | | 0 | 0 | 0 | 0 | 0 |
| 60474 | 0.0 | 0.0 | 0.0 | 0.00 | 0.00 | 0 | 1 | 0.2 | | | |
| 60475 | 0.0 | 0.0 | 0.0 | 0.00 | 0.01 | 0 | 3 | 0.3 | | | |
| 62126 | | | | | | | 2 | 0.2 | 0 | 0.2 | 1 |
| 60245 | | | | | | | 3 | 0.3 | 0 | 0.3 | 2 |
| 60246 | | | | | | | 4 | 0.4 | 0 | 0.4 | 2 |
| 60471 | 0.0 | 0.0 | 0.0 | 0.00 | 0.01 | 0 | 54 | 5 | | | |
| 60473 | 0.0 | 0.0 | 0.0 | 0.00 | 0.01 | 0 | 62 | 6 | | | |
| 60018 | | | | | | | 91 | 9 | 0 | 9 | 55 |
| 60857 | 0.0 | 0.0 | 0.0 | 0.00 | 0.01 | 0 | 3 | 0 | | | |
| 60472 | 0.0 | 0.0 | 0.0 | 0.00 | 0.00 | 0 | 7 | 0.6 | | | |
| 60476 | 0.0 | 0.0 | 0.0 | 0.00 | 0.00 | 0 | 7 | 0.6 | | | |
| 60460 | 0.0 | 0.0 | 0.0 | 0.00 | 0.00 | 0 | 3 | 0.3 | | | |
| 60468 | 0.0 | 0.0 | 0.0 | 0.00 | 0.00 | 0 | 3 | 0.3 | | | |
| 60292 | 0.0 | 0.0 | 0.0 | 0.00 | 0.00 | | 1196 | 12 | | | |
| 60435 | 0.0 | 0.0 | 0.0 | 0.00 | 0.00 | | 1950 | 195 | | | |
| 60093 | 0.0 | 0.0 | 0.1 | | | 0 | 0 | 0 | 0 | 0 | 0 |
| 60728 | 0.0 | 0.0 | 0.0 | 0.00 | 0.00 | | 30 | 3 | | | |
| 60285 | 0.0 | 0.0 | 0.0 | 0.00 | 0.00 | | 90 | 9 | | | |
| 60293 | 0.0 | 0.0 | 0.0 | 0.00 | 0.00 | | 30 | 3 | | | |
| 60700 | | | | | | | 69 | 7 | 0 | 7 | 41 |
| 60836 | | | | | | | 119 | 12 | 0 | 12 | 71 |
| 60701 | | | | | | | 49 | 5 | 0 | 5 | 29 |
| 60858 | 0.0 | 0.0 | 0.0 | 0.00 | 0.01 | 0 | 22 | 2 | | | |
| 60422 | 0.0 | | | | | | 56 | 5 | | | |
| 60388 | 0.0 | | | | | | 56 | 5 | | | |
| 60596 | 0.0 | 0.0 | 0.0 | 0.00 | 0.01 | 0 | 28 | 3 | | | |
| 60595 | 0.0 | 0.0 | 0.0 | 0.00 | 0.01 | 0 | 26 | 3 | | | |
| 60318 | | | | | | | 12 | 1 | 0 | 1 | 7 |
| 60019 | | | | | | | 32 | 3 | 0 | 3 | 19 |
| 60260 | | | | | | | 12 | 1 | 0 | 1 | 7 |
| 60735 | 0.0 | 0.0 | 0.0 | 0.00 | 0.00 | | 374 | 37 | | | |
| 60838 | | | | | | | 1 | 0.1 | 0 | 0.1 | 1 |
| 60599 | 0.0 | 0.0 | 0.0 | 0.00 | 0.00 | 0 | 5 | 0.5 | | | |
| 60600 | 0.0 | 0.0 | 0.0 | 0.00 | 0.01 | 0 | 5 | 0.5 | | | |

| Code | Thiamin (mg) | Riboflavin (mg) | Niacin (NE) | Vit B6 (mg) | Vit B12 (mcg) | Folate (mcg) | Panto (mg) | Vit C (mg) | Vit D (mg) | Vit E (α TE) | Calcium (mg) | Copper (mg) | Iron (mg) | Magnes (mg) | Mang (mg) | Phos (mg) | Potassium (mg) | Selenium (mcg) | Sodium (mg) | Zinc (mg) |
|---|---|---|---|---|---|---|---|---|---|---|---|---|---|---|---|---|---|---|---|---|
| | Vitamins | | | | | | | | | | Minerals | | | | | | | | | |
| 60733 | | | | | | | | 42.0 | | | 12 | | 0.0 | | | | 105 | | 5 | |
| 60040 | 0.01 | 0.01 | 0.14 | 0.08 | | | | 35.4 | | | 17 | 0.0 | 0.1 | 10 | 0.1 | 22 | 52 | | 8 | |
| 60750 | 0.02 | 0.01 | 0.10 | 0.07 | | | | 190.6 | | | 18 | | 0.2 | | | 20 | 46 | | 8 | |
| 60854 | 0.00 | 0.00 | 0.01 | 0.01 | 0.00 | 0.2 | 0.01 | 5.0 | | | 2 | 0.0 | 0.0 | 1 | 0.0 | 2 | 8 | 0.0 | 2 | 0.01 |
| 60835 | 0.01 | 0.03 | 0.10 | 0.06 | | | | 40.1 | | | 13 | 0.0 | 0.3 | 8 | 0.1 | 17 | 64 | | 15 | |
| 60094 | 0.02 | 0.02 | | 0.09 | | | | 15.8 | | | 4 | | 0.2 | | | | | | 10 | |
| 60286 | 0.02 | 0.02 | | | | | | 15.9 | | | 0 | | 0.0 | | | | 140 | | 0 | |
| 60392 | 0.00 | 0.00 | 0.02 | 0.01 | | | | 7.6 | | | 1 | 0.0 | 0.0 | | | 2 | 19 | | 0 | 0.01 |
| 60098 | 0.02 | 0.02 | 0.20 | 0.12 | | | | 15.8 | | | | | 0.2 | | | | | | 5 | |
| 60289 | 0.02 | 0.36 | | | | | | 15.9 | | | 0 | | 0.0 | | | | 110 | | 0 | |
| 60112 | 0.02 | 0.03 | 0.24 | | | | | 15.8 | | | | | 0.2 | | | | | | 5 | |
| 60816 | 0.02 | 0.07 | 0.41 | 0.17 | | | | 15.8 | | | 7 | 0.1 | 0.3 | 19 | 0.2 | 20 | 248 | | 2 | 0.17 |
| 60215 | 0.02 | 0.03 | | | | | | 15.7 | | | 0 | | 0.0 | | | | 140 | | 0 | |
| 60463 | 0.00 | 0.01 | 0.02 | 0.01 | 0.00 | 0.6 | 0.03 | 2.2 | | | 1 | 0.0 | 0.1 | 0 | | 1 | 10 | 0.1 | 2 | 0.01 |
| 60464 | 0.00 | 0.01 | 0.02 | 0.01 | 0.00 | 0.6 | 0.03 | 4.4 | | | 1 | 0.0 | 0.0 | 0 | | 1 | 11 | 0.1 | 0 | 0.01 |
| 60241 | 0.00 | 0.01 | 0.01 | 0.00 | | | | 1.9 | | | 1 | 0.0 | 0.0 | 1 | 0.0 | 1 | 12 | | 0 | |
| 60670 | 0.03 | 0.07 | 0.20 | 0.07 | | | | 15.8 | | | 7 | | 0.2 | | | 15 | 155 | | 2 | |
| 60290 | 0.02 | 0.36 | | | | | | 15.9 | | | 0 | | 0.3 | | | | 130 | | 0 | |
| 60434 | 0.02 | 0.02 | | | | | | 16.0 | | | 0 | | 0.3 | | | | 200 | | 0 | |
| 60389 | 0.00 | 0.00 | 0.01 | 0.00 | | | | 4.2 | | | 1 | 0.0 | 0.0 | | | 0 | 5 | | 1 | 0.01 |
| 60748 | 0.03 | 0.06 | 0.26 | 0.02 | 0.00 | | | 26.9 | | | 0 | | 0.0 | | | | 120 | | | |
| 60390 | 0.00 | 0.00 | 0.02 | 0.01 | | | | 7.1 | | | 1 | 0.0 | 0.0 | | | 1 | 15 | | 0 | 0.01 |
| 60111 | 0.02 | 0.03 | 0.01 | 0.09 | | | | 15.8 | | | | | 0.2 | | | | | | 10 | |
| 60466 | 0.00 | 0.00 | 0.02 | 0.01 | 0.00 | 0.5 | 0.01 | 4.6 | | | 1 | 0.0 | 0.0 | 1 | | 1 | 12 | 0.0 | 0 | 0.01 |
| 60467 | 0.00 | 0.00 | 0.02 | 0.01 | 0.00 | 0.5 | 0.01 | 4.3 | | | 1 | 0.0 | 0.0 | 1 | | 1 | 13 | 0.0 | 0 | 0.01 |
| 60055 | | 0.01 | | | | | | 12.3 | | | 0 | | 0.0 | | | | 75 | | 0 | |
| 60249 | 0.00 | 0.00 | | | | | | 2.3 | | | 0 | | 0.0 | | | | 16 | | 0 | |
| 60474 | 0.00 | 0.00 | 0.01 | 0.00 | 0.00 | 0.3 | 0.02 | 6.0 | | | 1 | 0.0 | 0.0 | 0 | | 1 | 12 | 0.0 | 0 | 0.01 |
| 60475 | 0.00 | 0.00 | 0.01 | 0.00 | 0.00 | 0.3 | 0.02 | 6.1 | | | 1 | 0.0 | 0.0 | 0 | | 1 | 11 | 0.0 | 0 | 0.00 |
| 62126 | 0.00 | 0.00 | 0.01 | 0.01 | | | | 3.1 | | | 1 | 0.0 | 0.0 | 1 | 0.0 | 1 | 14 | | 0 | |
| 60245 | 0.00 | 0.00 | 0.01 | 0.01 | | | | 1.9 | | | 1 | 0.0 | 0.0 | 1 | 0.0 | 1 | 12 | | 0 | |
| 60246 | 0.00 | 0.00 | 0.01 | 0.01 | | | | 1.3 | | | 1 | 0.0 | 0.0 | 1 | 0.0 | 1 | 13 | | 0 | |
| 60471 | 0.00 | 0.00 | 0.02 | 0.00 | 0.00 | 0.2 | 0.02 | 2.9 | | | 1 | 0.0 | 0.0 | 1 | | 2 | 17 | 0.0 | 0 | 0.00 |
| 60473 | 0.00 | 0.00 | 0.02 | 0.00 | 0.00 | 0.2 | 0.02 | 3.0 | | | 1 | 0.0 | 0.0 | 1 | | 1 | 19 | 0.0 | 0 | 0.01 |
| 60018 | 0.00 | 0.01 | 0.03 | 0.01 | | | | 1.9 | | | 1 | 0.0 | 0.0 | 1 | 0.0 | 2 | 18 | | 0 | |
| 60857 | 0.00 | 0.00 | 0.03 | 0.02 | 0.00 | 0.5 | 0.02 | 2.8 | | | 1 | 0.0 | 0.0 | 1 | 0.0 | 2 | 21 | 0.1 | 0 | 0.01 |
| 60472 | 0.00 | 0.00 | 0.02 | 0.01 | 0.00 | 0.1 | 0.02 | 6.8 | | | 0 | 0.0 | 0.0 | 1 | | 1 | 21 | 0.0 | 0 | 0.00 |
| 60476 | 0.00 | 0.00 | 0.02 | 0.01 | 0.00 | 0.1 | 0.02 | 6.8 | | | 0 | 0.0 | 0.0 | 1 | | 1 | 21 | 0.0 | 0 | 0.00 |
| 60460 | 0.00 | 0.00 | 0.01 | 0.01 | 0.00 | 0.3 | 0.02 | 4.3 | | | 1 | 0.0 | 0.0 | 1 | | 1 | 12 | 0.0 | 0 | 0.00 |
| 60468 | 0.00 | 0.00 | 0.01 | 0.01 | 0.00 | 0.3 | 0.02 | 4.5 | | | 1 | 0.0 | 0.0 | 0 | | 1 | 12 | 0.0 | 0 | 0.00 |
| 60292 | 0.02 | 0.36 | 0.36 | | | | | 15.9 | | | 0 | | 0.3 | | | | 239 | | 0 | |
| 60435 | 0.02 | 0.03 | 0.36 | | | | | 16.0 | | | 12 | | 0.6 | | | | 360 | | 0 | |
| 60093 | 0.01 | 0.10 | 0.04 | 2.10 | | | | 15.8 | | | 5 | | 0.6 | | | | | | 0 | |
| 60728 | | | | | | | | 15.7 | | | 0 | | 0.3 | | | | 279 | | 0 | |
| 60285 | 0.01 | 0.03 | 0.24 | | | | | 15.7 | | | 0 | | 0.3 | | | | 409 | | 0 | |
| 60293 | 0.02 | 0.05 | 0.24 | | | | | 15.9 | | | 0 | | 0.0 | | | | 239 | | 0 | |
| 60700 | 0.02 | 0.04 | 0.34 | 0.07 | | | | 34.9 | | | 14 | 0.0 | 0.3 | 9 | 0.1 | 16 | 120 | | 6 | 0.13 |
| 60836 | 0.03 | 0.04 | 0.41 | 0.06 | | | | 40.1 | | | 12 | 0.0 | 0.3 | 9 | 0.0 | 15 | 69 | | 10 | |
| 60701 | 0.02 | 0.06 | 0.63 | 0.06 | | | | 34.9 | | | 15 | 0.0 | 0.3 | 18 | 0.1 | 16 | 134 | | 8 | 0.13 |
| 60858 | 0.00 | 0.00 | 0.08 | 0.01 | 0.00 | 0.8 | 0.03 | 5.0 | | | 1 | 0.0 | 0.0 | 1 | 0.0 | 3 | 13 | 0.1 | 1 | 0.02 |
| 60422 | 0.00 | 0.01 | 0.10 | 0.00 | | | | 7.6 | | | 1 | 0.0 | 0.0 | | | 3 | 31 | | 1 | 0.01 |
| 60388 | 0.00 | 0.01 | 0.10 | 0.00 | | | | 6.7 | | | 1 | 0.0 | 0.0 | | | 3 | 30 | | 1 | 0.01 |
| 60596 | 0.00 | 0.01 | 0.10 | 0.00 | 0.00 | 0.6 | 0.02 | 3.0 | | | 1 | 0.0 | 0.0 | 1 | | 2 | 25 | 0.1 | 1 | 0.01 |
| 60595 | 0.00 | 0.01 | 0.10 | 0.00 | 0.00 | 0.6 | 0.02 | 5.0 | | | 1 | 0.0 | 0.0 | 1 | | 2 | 26 | 0.1 | 1 | 0.01 |
| 60318 | 0.00 | 0.01 | 0.09 | 0.00 | | | | 3.1 | | | 1 | 0.0 | 0.0 | 1 | 0.0 | 2 | 22 | | 0 | 0.01 |
| 60019 | 0.00 | 0.01 | 0.11 | 0.00 | | | | 1.9 | | | 1 | 0.0 | 0.0 | 1 | 0.0 | 2 | 22 | | 0 | 0.01 |
| 60260 | 0.00 | 0.00 | 0.10 | 0.00 | | | | 1.3 | | | 1 | 0.0 | 0.0 | 1 | 0.0 | 2 | 23 | | 0 | 0.01 |
| 60735 | | | | | | | | 15.7 | | | 0 | | 0.0 | | | | 199 | | 0 | |
| 60838 | 0.01 | 0.03 | 0.17 | 0.05 | | | | 40.1 | | | 12 | 0.1 | 0.3 | 9 | 0.0 | 17 | 65 | | 8 | |
| 60599 | 0.00 | 0.00 | 0.03 | 0.00 | 0.00 | 0.6 | 0.02 | 3.5 | | | 1 | 0.0 | 0.0 | 1 | | 2 | 18 | 0.1 | 0 | 0.01 |
| 60600 | 0.00 | 0.00 | 0.03 | 0.00 | 0.00 | 0.6 | 0.01 | 3.9 | | | 1 | 0.0 | 0.0 | 1 | | 2 | 21 | 0.1 | 0 | 0.01 |

| Code | Amount | Description | Basic Components | | | | | | | | | Additional Fats | | | | | | Vit A & Components | | | | | Vitamins | | | | | | | | | | Minerals | | | | | | | | | |
|---|---|---|---|---|---|---|---|---|---|---|---|---|---|---|---|---|---|---|---|---|---|---|---|---|---|---|---|---|---|---|---|---|---|---|---|---|---|---|---|---|---|---|
| | | | Weight (g) | Calories | % Water | Protein (g) | Carbs (g) | Fiber (g) | Sugar (g) | Other Carbs (g) | Fat (g) | Sat Fat (g) | Mono Fat (g) | Poly Fat (g) | Omega 3 (g) | Omega 6 (g) | Choles (mg) | Vit A (IU) | Vit A (RE) | Retinol (RE) | Carotenoids (RE) | Beta Carotene (mcg) | Thiamin (mg) | Riboflavin (mg) | Niacin (NE) | Vit B6 (mg) | Vit B12 (mcg) | Folate (mcg) | Panto (mg) | Vit C (mg) | Vit D (mg) | Vit E (α TE) | Calcium (mg) | Copper (mg) | Iron (mg) | Magnes (mg) | Mang (mg) | Phos (mg) | Potassium (mg) | Selenium (mcg) | Sodium (mg) | Zinc (mg) |
| 60856 | 1 Tbs | Toddler, diced, avg | 16 | 9 | 86 | 0.0 | 2.2 | 0.2 | | | 0.0 | 0.0 | 0.0 | 0.0 | 0.00 | 0.01 | 0 | 0 | 0 | 0 | 0 | 0 | 0.00 | 0.00 | 0.02 | 0.01 | 0.00 | 0.2 | | 5.0 | | | 2 | 0.0 | 0.0 | 1 | 0.0 | 2 | 8 | 0.1 | 1 | 0.01 |
| 60319 | 1 Tbs | 1st Foods, Gerber | 14 | 8 | 86 | 0.1 | 1.9 | 0.4 | 1.0 | 0.4 | 0.0 | | | | | | | 2 | 0.2 | 0 | 0.2 | 1 | 0.00 | 0.00 | 0.03 | 0.00 | | | | 3.1 | | | 1 | 0.0 | 0.0 | 1 | 0.0 | 2 | 17 | | 0 | 0.01 |
| 60020 | 1 Tbs | 2nd Foods, Gerber | 14 | 8 | 86 | 0.1 | 1.8 | 0.4 | 1.1 | 0.4 | 0.0 | | | | | | | 1 | 0.1 | 0 | 0.1 | 0.4 | 0.00 | 0.00 | 0.04 | 0.00 | | | | 1.9 | | | 1 | 0.0 | 0.0 | 1 | 0.0 | 2 | 16 | | 0 | 0.01 |
| 60261 | 1 Tbs | 3rd Foods, Gerber | 14 | 8 | 86 | 0.1 | 1.8 | 0.4 | 1.1 | 0.3 | 0.0 | | | | | | | 2 | 0.2 | 0 | 0.2 | 1 | 0.00 | 0.00 | 0.03 | 0.00 | | | | 1.3 | | | 1 | 0.0 | 0.0 | 1 | 0.0 | 2 | 17 | | 0 | 0.01 |
| | | Pears & Pineapple | | | | | | | | | | | | | | | | | | | | | | | | | | | | | | | | | | | | | | | | |
| 60597 | 1 Tbs | Junior, avg | 16 | 7 | 88 | 0.0 | 1.8 | 0.4 | | | 0.0 | 0.0 | 0.0 | 0.0 | 0.00 | 0.01 | 0 | 5 | 0.5 | | | | 0.00 | 0.00 | 0.03 | 0.00 | 0.00 | 0.5 | 0.02 | 2.7 | | | 2 | 0.0 | 0.0 | 1 | | 2 | 19 | 0.1 | 0 | 0.02 |
| 60598 | 1 Tbs | Strained, avg | 16 | 7 | 88 | 0.0 | 1.7 | 0.4 | | | 0.0 | 0.0 | 0.0 | 0.0 | 0.00 | 0.00 | 0 | 5 | 0.5 | | | | 0.00 | 0.00 | 0.03 | 0.00 | 0.00 | 0.4 | 0.01 | 4.4 | | | 2 | 0.0 | 0.0 | 1 | | 1 | 19 | 0.1 | 1 | 0.01 |
| 60262 | 1 Tbs | 2nd Foods, Gerber | 14 | 8 | 86 | 0.1 | 1.8 | 0.4 | 1.0 | 0.3 | 0.0 | | | | | | | 2 | 0.2 | 0 | 0.2 | 1 | 0.00 | 0.00 | 0.03 | 0.00 | | | | 1.9 | | | 1 | 0.0 | 0.0 | 1 | 0.0 | 2 | 15 | | 0 | 0.01 |
| 60796 | 1 ea | Plums, junior, 6 oz jar, Heinz | 170 | 116 | 83 | 0.5 | 28.6 | 1.5 | 16.8 | 10.2 | 0.0 | 0.0 | 0.0 | 0.0 | 0.00 | 0.00 | | 88 | 9 | | | | 0.00 | 0.05 | 0.00 | 0.03 | | | | 0.0 | | | 53 | | 0.0 | | | 10 | 129 | | 7 | |
| 60041 | 1 Tbs | Prunes, 1st Foods, Gerber | 14 | 14 | 74 | 0.1 | 3.4 | 0.4 | 2.1 | 0.9 | 0.0 | | | | | | | 54 | 5 | 0 | 5 | 33 | 0.00 | 0.03 | 0.12 | 0.02 | | | | 0.1 | | | 3 | 0.0 | 0.0 | 2 | 0.0 | 4 | 43 | | 1 | 0.03 |
| 60281 | 1 ea | Prunes & Pears, Stage 2, 4 oz jar, Beechnut | 113 | 110 | 79 | 0.0 | 23.9 | 3.0 | 10.0 | 11.0 | 0.0 | 0.0 | 0.0 | 0.0 | 0.00 | 0.00 | | 448 | 45 | | | | 0.02 | 0.05 | 0.48 | | | | | 0.0 | | | 12 | | 0.3 | | | | 199 | | 10 | |
| 60635 | 1 Tbs | Tropical Fruit, junior, avg | 15 | 9 | 83 | 0.0 | 2.5 | | | | 0.0 | 0.0 | 0.0 | 0.0 | 0.00 | 0.00 | | 3 | 0.3 | | | | 0.00 | 0.00 | 0.01 | 0.00 | 0.00 | 0.5 | 0.01 | 2.8 | | | 2 | 0.0 | 0.0 | 1 | | 1 | 9 | 0.1 | 1 | 0.01 |
| | | *INFANT MEATS* | | | | | | | | | | | | | | | | | | | | | | | | | | | | | | | | | | | | | | | | |
| | | Beef | | | | | | | | | | | | | | | | | | | | | | | | | | | | | | | | | | | | | | | | |
| 60494 | 1 Tbs | Junior, avg | 15 | 16 | 80 | 2.2 | 0.0 | 0.0 | 0.0 | 0.0 | 0.7 | 0.4 | 0.3 | 0.0 | 0.00 | 0.02 | 4 | 9 | 5 | | | | 0.00 | 0.02 | 0.49 | 0.02 | 0.22 | 0.9 | 0.05 | 0.3 | | | 1 | 0.0 | 0.2 | 1 | | 11 | 29 | 1.1 | 10 | 0.30 |
| 60495 | 1 Tbs | Strained, avg | 15 | 16 | 81 | 2.0 | 0.0 | 0.0 | 0.0 | 0.0 | 0.8 | 0.4 | 0.3 | 0.0 | 0.01 | 0.02 | 4 | 10 | 3 | | | | 0.00 | 0.02 | 0.43 | 0.02 | 0.21 | 0.8 | 0.05 | 0.3 | | | 1 | 0.0 | 0.2 | 3 | | 13 | 33 | 1.4 | 12 | 0.37 |
| 60496 | 1 Tbs | With Beef Heart, strained, avg | 14 | 13 | 82 | 1.8 | 0.0 | 0.0 | 0.0 | 0.0 | 0.6 | 0.3 | 0.3 | 0.0 | 0.00 | 0.03 | | 18 | 5 | 5 | 0 | | 0.00 | 0.05 | 0.54 | 0.02 | 0.96 | 0.7 | | 0.3 | | | 1 | 0.0 | 0.3 | 2 | | 13 | 28 | | 9 | 0.26 |
| 60078 | 1 ea | With Broth, Stage 1, 2.5 oz jar, Beechnut | 71 | 90 | 80 | 8.0 | 0.0 | 0.0 | 0.0 | 0.0 | 6.0 | | | | | | | 0 | 0 | 0 | 0 | 0 | 0.01 | 0.08 | 1.20 | | | | | 0.0 | | | 0 | | 0.9 | | | | 135 | | 40 | |
| 60807 | 1 ea | With Gravy, 2nd Foods, 2.5 oz jar, Gerber | 71 | 79 | 78 | 8.7 | 2.8 | 0.8 | 0.1 | 1.9 | 3.7 | | | | | | | 4 | 0.4 | 0 | 0.4 | 3 | 0.01 | 0.08 | 1.57 | 0.07 | | | | 0.4 | | | 8 | 0.0 | 0.9 | 10 | 0.0 | 79 | 135 | | 30 | 1.99 |
| | | Chicken | | | | | | | | | | | | | | | | | | | | | | | | | | | | | | | | | | | | | | | | |
| 60516 | 1 Tbs | Junior, avg | 15 | 22 | 76 | 2.2 | 0.0 | 0.0 | 0.0 | 0.0 | 1.4 | 0.4 | 0.6 | 0.3 | 0.01 | 0.34 | 9 | 6 | 2 | | | | 0.00 | 0.02 | 0.51 | 0.03 | 0.06 | 1.7 | 0.11 | 0.2 | | | 8 | 0.0 | 0.1 | 2 | | 14 | 18 | 1.5 | 8 | 0.15 |
| 60514 | 1 ea | Sticks, junior, avg | 10 | 19 | 68 | 1.5 | 0.1 | 0.0 | | | 1.4 | 0.4 | 0.6 | 0.3 | 0.01 | 0.28 | 8 | 1 | 0.3 | 0.3 | 0 | | 0.00 | 0.02 | 0.20 | 0.01 | 0.04 | 1.1 | 0.07 | 0.2 | | | 7 | 0.0 | 0.2 | 1 | | 12 | 11 | 1.0 | 48 | 0.10 |
| 60230 | 1 ea | Sticks, Finger, grad, Gerber | 10 | 14 | 74 | 1.5 | 0.1 | 0.0 | 0.1 | 0.0 | 0.8 | 0.2 | | | | | 9 | | | | | | 0.00 | 0.01 | 0.25 | 0.01 | | | | 0.1 | | | 8 | 0.0 | 0.1 | 1 | 0.0 | 14 | 11 | | 42 | 0.13 |
| 60849 | 1 Tbs | Strained, avg | 15 | 20 | 78 | 2.1 | 0.0 | 0.0 | | | 1.2 | 0.3 | 0.5 | 0.3 | 0.01 | 0.28 | 9 | 8 | 2 | | | | 0.00 | 0.02 | 0.49 | 0.03 | 0.06 | 1.6 | 0.10 | 0.3 | | | 10 | 0.0 | 0.2 | 2 | | 15 | 21 | 1.7 | 7 | 0.18 |
| 60073 | 1 ea | With Broth, Stage 1, 2.5 oz jar, Beechnut | 71 | 70 | 83 | 8.0 | 0.0 | 0.0 | 0.0 | 0.0 | 3.0 | | | | | | | 0 | 0 | 0 | 0 | 0 | 0.02 | 0.08 | 1.20 | | | | | 0.0 | | | 12 | | 0.6 | | | | 120 | | 55 | |
| 60808 | 1 ea | With Gravy, 2nd Foods, 2.5 oz jar, Gerber | 71 | 77 | 79 | 8.1 | 2.6 | 0.4 | 0.1 | 2.1 | 3.9 | | | | | | | | | | | | 0.01 | 0.08 | 2.61 | 0.08 | | | | 0.3 | | | 93 | 0.0 | 0.7 | 10 | 0.0 | 95 | 115 | | 33 | 0.85 |
| 60528 | 1 Tbs | Egg Yolks, strained, avg | 14 | 28 | 71 | 1.4 | 0.1 | 0.0 | | | 2.4 | 0.7 | 1.0 | 0.3 | 0.01 | 0.29 | 103 | 175 | 53 | 53 | 0 | | 0.01 | 0.04 | 0.00 | 0.02 | 0.22 | 12.9 | 0.30 | 0.2 | | | 11 | 0.0 | 0.4 | 1 | | 40 | 11 | | 5 | 0.27 |
| | | Ham | | | | | | | | | | | | | | | | | | | | | | | | | | | | | | | | | | | | | | | | |
| 60535 | 1 Tbs | Junior, avg | 15 | 19 | 78 | 2.3 | 0.0 | 0.0 | 0.0 | 0.0 | 1.0 | 0.3 | 0.5 | 0.1 | 0.00 | 0.13 | 4 | 5 | 2 | | | | 0.02 | 0.03 | 0.43 | 0.03 | 0.02 | 0.3 | 0.08 | 0.3 | | | 1 | 0.0 | 0.2 | 2 | | 13 | 32 | 2.3 | 10 | 0.26 |
| 60536 | 1 Tbs | Strained, avg | 15 | 17 | 79 | 2.1 | 0.0 | 0.0 | 0.0 | 0.0 | 0.9 | 0.3 | 0.4 | 0.1 | 0.00 | 0.11 | 4 | 6 | 2 | | | | 0.02 | 0.02 | 0.39 | 0.04 | 0.02 | 0.3 | 0.08 | 0.3 | | | 1 | 0.0 | 0.2 | 2 | | 12 | 31 | 2.1 | 6 | 0.34 |
| 60809 | 1 ea | With Gravy, 2nd Foods, 2.5 oz jar, Gerber | 71 | 69 | 80 | 7.7 | 3.0 | 0.4 | 0.2 | 2.4 | 2.9 | | | | | | | | | | | | 0.12 | 0.11 | 2.18 | 0.13 | | | | 0.2 | | | 6 | 0.0 | 0.5 | 9 | 0.0 | 81 | 146 | | 25 | 1.28 |
| | | Lamb | | | | | | | | | | | | | | | | | | | | | | | | | | | | | | | | | | | | | | | | |
| 60552 | 1 Tbs | Junior, avg | 15 | 17 | 80 | 2.3 | 0.0 | 0.0 | 0.0 | 0.0 | 0.8 | 0.4 | 0.3 | 0.0 | 0.01 | 0.02 | 6 | 4 | 1 | | | | 0.00 | 0.03 | 0.48 | 0.03 | 0.34 | 0.3 | 0.06 | 0.3 | | | 1 | 0.0 | 0.2 | 2 | | 14 | 32 | 1.1 | 11 | 0.39 |
| 60553 | 1 Tbs | Strained, avg | 15 | 15 | 80 | 2.1 | 0.0 | 0.0 | | | 0.7 | 0.3 | 0.3 | 0.0 | 0.01 | 0.02 | 6 | 5 | 2 | | | | 0.00 | 0.03 | 0.44 | 0.02 | 0.33 | 0.3 | 0.06 | 0.2 | | | 1 | 0.0 | 0.2 | 2 | | 15 | 31 | 1.3 | 9 | 0.41 |
| 60074 | 1 ea | With Broth, Stage 1, 2.5 oz jar, Beechnut | 71 | 60 | 85 | 9.0 | 0.0 | 0.0 | 0.0 | 0.0 | 3.0 | | | | | | | 0 | 0 | 0 | 0 | 0 | 0.02 | 0.10 | 1.50 | | | | | 0.0 | | | 0 | | 0.6 | | | | 130 | | 50 | |
| 60810 | 1 ea | With Gravy, 2nd Foods, 2.5 oz jar, Gerber | 71 | 70 | 80 | 8.6 | 2.4 | 0.3 | 0.2 | 1.9 | 2.9 | | | | | | | | | | | | 0.01 | 0.11 | 1.84 | 0.05 | | | | 0.1 | | | 7 | 0.0 | 0.7 | 9 | 0.0 | 75 | 128 | | 29 | 1.77 |
| 60554 | 1 Tbs | Liver, strained, avg | 14 | 14 | 79 | 2.0 | 0.2 | 0.0 | | | 0.5 | 0.2 | 0.1 | 0.1 | 0.01 | 0.05 | 26 | 5339 | 1603 | | | | 0.01 | 0.25 | 1.17 | 0.05 | 0.30 | 47.2 | | 2.7 | | | 1 | 0.3 | 0.7 | 2 | | 28 | 32 | | 10 | 0.42 |
| 60561 | 1 ea | Meat Sticks, junior, avg | 10 | 18 | 70 | 1.3 | 0.1 | 0.0 | | | 1.5 | 0.6 | 0.6 | 0.2 | 0.01 | 0.15 | 7 | 7 | 2 | | | | 0.01 | 0.02 | 0.15 | 0.01 | 0.03 | 0.9 | 0.05 | 0.2 | | | 3 | 0.0 | 0.1 | 1 | | 10 | 11 | 1.3 | 55 | 0.19 |
| 60235 | 1 ea | Meat Sticks, Finger, grad, Gerber | 10 | 15 | 73 | 1.4 | 0.2 | 0.1 | 0.1 | 0.0 | 0.9 | 0.3 | | | | | 5 | 1 | 0.1 | 0 | 0.1 | 1 | 0.00 | 0.01 | 0.17 | 0.01 | | | | 0.1 | | | 3 | 0.0 | 0.1 | 1 | 0.0 | 11 | 13 | | 49 | 0.30 |
| 60610 | 1 Tbs | Pork, strained, avg | 15 | 19 | 78 | 2.1 | 0.0 | 0.0 | 0.0 | 0.0 | 1.1 | 0.4 | 0.5 | 0.1 | 0.00 | 0.10 | 7 | 6 | 2 | | | | 0.02 | 0.03 | 0.34 | 0.03 | 0.15 | 0.3 | 0.04 | 0.3 | | | 1 | 0.0 | 0.2 | 2 | | 14 | 33 | 1.9 | 6 | 0.34 |
| | | Turkey | | | | | | | | | | | | | | | | | | | | | | | | | | | | | | | | | | | | | | | | |
| 60639 | 1 Tbs | Junior, avg | 15 | 19 | 78 | 2.3 | 0.0 | 0.0 | 0.0 | 0.0 | 1.1 | 0.3 | 0.4 | 0.3 | 0.01 | 0.25 | 8 | 5 | 2 | | | | 0.00 | 0.04 | 0.52 | 0.02 | 0.16 | 1.8 | 0.09 | 0.4 | | | 4 | 0.0 | 0.2 | 2 | | 14 | 27 | 2.6 | 11 | 0.27 |
| 60638 | 1 ea | Sticks, junior, avg | 10 | 18 | 70 | 1.4 | 0.1 | 0.1 | | | 1.4 | 0.4 | 0.5 | 0.4 | 0.02 | 0.33 | 7 | 2 | 1 | | | | 0.00 | 0.02 | 0.17 | 0.01 | 0.10 | 1.1 | 0.06 | 0.2 | | | 7 | 0.0 | 0.1 | 2 | | 10 | 9 | 1.0 | 48 | 0.18 |
| 60238 | 1 ea | Sticks, Finger, grad, Gerber | 10 | 13 | 76 | 1.4 | 0.1 | 0.0 | 0.1 | 0.0 | 0.8 | 0.3 | | | | | 9 | 0.2 | 0.02 | 0 | 0.02 | 0:1 | 0.00 | 0.02 | 0.19 | 0.01 | | | | 0.1 | | | 10 | 0.0 | 0.1 | 1 | 0.0 | 13 | 12 | | 43 | 0.23 |
| 60850 | 1 Tbs | Strained, avg | 15 | 17 | 79 | 2.1 | 0.0 | 0.0 | | | 0.9 | 0.3 | 0.3 | 0.2 | 0.01 | 0.21 | 9 | 7 | 2 | | | | 0.00 | 0.03 | 0.55 | 0.03 | 0.15 | 1.7 | 0.09 | 0.3 | | | 3 | 0.0 | 0.2 | 2 | | 19 | 35 | 2.5 | 8 | 0.27 |
| 60082 | 1 ea | With Broth, Stage 1, 2.5 oz jar, Beechnut | 71 | 90 | 81 | 8.0 | 0.0 | 0.0 | 0.0 | 0.0 | 6.0 | | | | | | | 0 | 0 | 0 | 0 | 0 | 0.01 | 0.10 | 1.20 | | | | | 0.0 | | | 12 | | 0.6 | | | | 90 | | 40 | |
| 60811 | 1 ea | With Gravy, 2nd Foods, 2.5 oz jar, Gerber | 71 | 74 | 80 | 7.4 | 2.8 | 0.2 | 0.2 | 2.4 | 3.8 | | | | | | | 4 | 0.4 | 0 | 0.4 | 3 | 0.01 | 0.11 | 1.33 | 0.08 | | | | 0.9 | | | 61 | 0.0 | 0.6 | 9 | 0.0 | 100 | 110 | | 35 | 1.49 |
| | | Veal | | | | | | | | | | | | | | | | | | | | | | | | | | | | | | | | | | | | | | | | |
| 60642 | 1 Tbs | Junior, avg | 15 | 17 | 80 | 2.3 | 0.0 | 0.0 | 0.0 | 0.0 | 0.8 | 0.4 | 0.3 | 0.0 | 0.00 | 0.02 | 4 | 8 | 2 | | | | 0.00 | 0.03 | 0.57 | 0.02 | 0.20 | 1.0 | 0.07 | 0.3 | | | 1 | 0.0 | 0.2 | 2 | | 15 | 35 | 0.8 | 10 | 0.38 |
| 60643 | 1 Tbs | Strained, avg | 15 | 15 | 81 | 2.0 | 0.0 | 0.0 | 0.0 | 0.0 | 0.7 | 0.3 | 0.3 | 0.0 | 0.00 | 0.02 | 4 | 7 | 2 | | | | 0.00 | 0.02 | 0.53 | 0.02 | 0.20 | 0.9 | 0.06 | 0.3 | | | 1 | 0.0 | 0.2 | 2 | | 15 | 32 | 0.9 | 10 | 0.30 |
| 60081 | 1 ea | With Broth, Stage 1, 2.5 oz jar, Beechnut | 71 | 60 | 85 | 9.0 | 0.0 | 0.0 | 0.0 | 0.0 | 2.0 | | | | | | | 0 | 0 | 0 | 0 | 0 | 0.01 | 0.10 | 2.10 | | | | | 0.0 | | | 0 | | 0.3 | | | | 130 | | 50 | |
| 60812 | 1 ea | With Gravy, 2nd Foods, 2.5 oz jar, Gerber | 71 | 64 | 81 | 8.2 | 2.4 | 0.1 | 0.1 | 2.1 | 2.3 | | | | | | | 1 | 0.1 | 0 | 0.1 | 0.43 | 0.01 | 0.11 | 2.48 | 0.08 | | | | 0.6 | | | 5 | 0.0 | 0.5 | 9 | 0.0 | 79 | 132 | | 37 | 1.49 |
| | | *INFANT VEGETABLES* | | | | | | | | | | | | | | | | | | | | | | | | | | | | | | | | | | | | | | | | |
| | | Beets | | | | | | | | | | | | | | | | | | | | | | | | | | | | | | | | | | | | | | | | |
| 60497 | 1 Tbs | Strained, avg | 14 | 5 | 90 | 0.2 | 1.1 | 0.3 | | | 0.0 | 0.0 | 0.0 | 0.0 | 0.00 | 0.00 | 0 | 5 | 0.4 | | | | 0.00 | 0.01 | 0.02 | 0.00 | 0.00 | 4.3 | 0.01 | 0.3 | | | 2 | 0.0 | 0.0 | 2 | | 2 | 25 | 0.0 | 12 | 0.02 |
| 60345 | 1 Tbs | Strained, Heinz | 16 | 6 | 90 | 0.2 | 1.3 | 0.3 | 1.0 | 0.0 | 0.0 | 0.0 | | | | | | 3 | 1 | | | | 0.00 | 0.00 | 0.02 | 0.00 | | | | 0.5 | | | 2 | 0.0 | 0.1 | | | 4 | 41 | | 5 | 0.03 |
| 60022 | 1 Tbs | 2nd Foods, Gerber | 14 | 5 | 89 | 0.2 | 1.2 | 0.2 | 1.0 | 0.0 | 0.0 | | | | | | | 3 | 0.3 | 0 | 0.3 | 2 | 0.00 | 0.01 | 0.02 | 0.00 | | | | 0.0 | | | 2 | | 0.0 | | | 3 | 42 | | 5 | |
| | | Carrots | | | | | | | | | | | | | | | | | | | | | | | | | | | | | | | | | | | | | | | | |
| 60501 | 1 Tbs | Buttered, junior, avg | 14 | 5 | 91 | 0.1 | 0.9 | | | | 0.1 | | | | | | | 1378 | 138 | | | | 0.00 | 0.01 | 0.07 | | | 1.2 | | 1.1 | | | 5 | | 0.0 | | | | 20 | | 2 | |
| 60503 | 1 Tbs | Buttered, strained, avg | 14 | 5 | 91 | 0.1 | 1.0 | | | | 0.1 | | | | | | | 1516 | 152 | | | | 0.00 | 0.01 | 0.08 | | | 1.3 | | 1.3 | | | 5 | | 0.0 | | | | 32 | | 3 | |
| 60500 | 1 Tbs | Junior, avg | 14 | 4 | 91 | 0.1 | 1.0 | 0.2 | | | 0.0 | 0.0 | 0.0 | 0.0 | 0.00 | 0.01 | 0 | 1653 | 165 | | | | 0.00 | 0.01 | 0.07 | 0.01 | 0.00 | 2.4 | 0.04 | 0.8 | | | 3 | 0.0 | 0.1 | 2 | | 3 | 28 | 0.0 | 7 | 0.02 |
| 60502 | 1 Tbs | Strained, avg | 14 | 4 | 92 | 0.1 | 0.8 | 0.2 | | | 0.0 | 0.0 | 0.0 | 0.0 | 0.00 | 0.01 | 0 | 1605 | 160 | | | | 0.00 | 0.01 | 0.06 | 0.01 | 0.00 | 2.1 | 0.03 | 0.8 | | | 3 | 0.0 | 0.1 | 1 | | 3 | 27 | 0.0 | 5 | 0.02 |
| 60320 | 1 Tbs | 1st Foods, Gerber | 14 | 5 | 91 | 0.1 | 0.9 | 0.3 | 0.6 | 0.0 | 0.1 | | | | | | | 2358 | 236 | 0 | 236 | 1415 | 0.00 | 0.01 | 0.05 | 0.01 | | | | 0.1 | | | 4 | 0.0 | 0.0 | 1 | 0.0 | 4 | 32 | | 6 | 0.03 |
| 60023 | 1 Tbs | 2nd Foods, Gerber | 14 | 4 | 92 | 0.1 | 0.9 | 0.3 | 0.4 | 0.2 | 0.0 | | | | | | | 2197 | 220 | 0 | 220 | 1318 | 0.00 | 0.01 | 0.06 | 0.01 | | | | 0.1 | | | 3 | 0.0 | 0.0 | 1 | 0.0 | 4 | 33 | | 4 | 0.03 |
| 60279 | 1 Tbs | 3rd Foods, Gerber | 14 | 6 | 88 | 0.1 | 1.4 | 0.3 | 0.9 | 0.2 | 0.0 | | | | | | | 2089 | 209 | 0 | 209 | 1253 | 0.00 | 0.01 | 0.06 | 0.01 | | | | 0.0 | | | 3 | 0.0 | 0.0 | 2 | 0.0 | 4 | 30 | | 4 | 0.03 |
| 60101 | 1 ea | 4.5 oz jar, Earth's Best | 128 | 40 | 93 | 1.0 | 8.0 | | | | 0.0 | 0.0 | 0.0 | 0.0 | 0.00 | 0.00 | | 13500 | 1350 | 0 | 1350 | | 0.02 | 0.03 | 0.60 | | | | | | | | 24 | | 0.4 | | | | | | 70 | |
| | | Corn | | | | | | | | | | | | | | | | | | | | | | | | | | | | | | | | | | | | | | | | |
| 60521 | 1 Tbs | Creamed, junior, avg | 15 | 10 | 81 | 0.2 | 2.4 | 0.3 | | | 0.1 | 0.0 | 0.0 | 0.0 | 0.00 | 0.03 | 0 | 12 | 1 | | | | 0.00 | 0.01 | 0.08 | 0.01 | 0.00 | 1.9 | 0.05 | 0.3 | | | 3 | 0.0 | 0.0 | 1 | | 5 | 12 | 0.2 | 8 | 0.03 |
| 60522 | 1 Tbs | Creamed, strained, avg | 15 | 9 | 84 | 0.2 | 2.1 | 0.3 | | | 0.1 | 0.0 | 0.0 | 0.0 | 0.00 | 0.03 | 0 | 11 | 1 | | | | 0.00 | 0.01 | 0.08 | 0.01 | 0.00 | 1.7 | 0.04 | 0.3 | | | 3 | 0.0 | 0.0 | 1 | | 5 | 14 | 0.2 | 6 | 0.03 |
| 60328 | 1 Tbs | Creamed, 2nd Foods, Gerber | 14 | 9 | 85 | 0.3 | 1.8 | 0.1 | 0.1 | 1.6 | 0.1 | | | | | | | 1 | 0.1 | 0 | 0.1 | 0.3 | 0.00 | 0.01 | 0.08 | 0.01 | | | | 0.0 | | | 3 | 0.0 | 0.0 | 2 | 0.0 | 7 | 15 | | 1 | 0.04 |

| Code | Amount | Description | Basic Components | | | | | | | | | Additional Fats | | | | | | Vit A & Components | | | | | Vitamins | | | | | | | | | | Minerals | | | | | | | | | |
|---|---|---|---|---|---|---|---|---|---|---|---|---|---|---|---|---|---|---|---|---|---|---|---|---|---|---|---|---|---|---|---|---|---|---|---|---|---|---|---|---|---|---|
| | | | Weight (g) | Calories | % Water | Protein (g) | Carbs (g) | Fiber (g) | Sugar (g) | Other Carbs (g) | Fat (g) | Sat Fat (g) | Mono Fat (g) | Poly Fat (g) | Omega 3 (g) | Omega 6 (g) | Choles (mg) | Vit A (IU) | Vit A (RE) | Retinol (RE) | Carotenoids (RE) | Beta Carotene (mcg) | Thiamin (mg) | Riboflavin (mg) | Niacin (NE) | Vit B6 (mg) | Vit B12 (mcg) | Folate (mcg) | Panto (mg) | Vit C (mg) | Vit D (mg) | Vit E (α TE) | Calcium (mg) | Copper (mg) | Iron (mg) | Magnes (mg) | Mang (mg) | Phos (mg) | Potassium (mg) | Selenium (mcg) | Sodium (mg) | Zinc (mg) |
| 60531 | 1 Tbs | Garden Vegetables, strained, avg | 15 | 6 | 90 | 0.3 | 1.0 | 0.2 | | | 0.0 | 0.0 | 0.0 | 0.0 | 0.01 | 0.01 | 0 | 910 | 91 | | | | 0.01 | 0.01 | 0.12 | 0.02 | 0.00 | 6.0 | 0.04 | 0.9 | | | 4 | 0.0 | 0.1 | 3 | | 4 | 25 | 0.1 | 5 | 0.04 |
| 60269 | 1 ea | Garden Vegetables, Stage 2, 4 oz jar, Beechnut | 113 | 50 | 91 | 1.0 | 9.0 | 3.0 | 2.0 | 4.0 | 0.0 | 0.0 | 0.0 | 0.0 | 0.00 | 0.00 | | 2392 | 239 | | | | 0.00 | 0.05 | 0.48 | | | | | 0.0 | | | 12 | | 0.6 | | | | 110 | | 10 | |
| | | Green Beans | | | | | | | | | | | | | | | | | | | | | | | | | | | | | | | | | | | | | | | | |
| 60485 | 1 Tbs | Buttered, junior, avg | 14 | 4 | 91 | 0.2 | 0.9 | | | | 0.1 | | | | | | | 53 | 5 | | | | 0.00 | 0.02 | 0.04 | | | 3.8 | | 1.2 | | | 10 | | 0.2 | | | | 24 | | 0 | |
| 60486 | 1 Tbs | Buttered, strained, avg | 14 | 5 | 91 | 0.2 | 0.9 | | | | 0.1 | | | | | | | 64 | 6 | | | | 0.00 | 0.01 | 0.05 | | | 4.0 | | 1.2 | | | 9 | | 0.2 | | | | 22 | | 0 | |
| 60484 | 1 Tbs | Creamed, junior, avg | 15 | 5 | 91 | 0.2 | 1.1 | 0.2 | | | 0.1 | 0.0 | 0.0 | 0.0 | 0.01 | 0.02 | 0 | 23 | 2 | | | | 0.00 | 0.01 | 0.03 | 0.00 | 0.01 | 6.0 | 0.03 | 0.4 | | | 5 | 0.0 | 0.0 | 1 | | 3 | 10 | 0.1 | 2 | 0.02 |
| 60851 | 1 Tbs | Diced, toddler, avg | 16 | 5 | 93 | 0.2 | 0.9 | 0.2 | | | 0.0 | 0.0 | 0.0 | 0.0 | 0.01 | 0.01 | 0 | 56 | 6 | | | | 0.00 | 0.01 | 0.04 | 0.00 | 0.00 | 5.1 | 0.01 | 0.3 | | | 4 | 0.0 | 0.1 | 3 | 0.0 | 4 | 19 | 0.1 | 6 | 0.02 |
| 60713 | 1 ea | Diced, grad, 4.5 oz jar, Gerber | 128 | 37 | 93 | 1.7 | 7.0 | 1.7 | 1.4 | 4.0 | 0.3 | | | | | | | 463 | 46 | 0 | 46 | 278 | 0.03 | 0.05 | 0.29 | 0.04 | | | | 2.2 | | | 35 | 0.0 | 0.5 | 24 | 0.1 | 26 | 148 | | 47 | 0.13 |
| 60487 | 1 Tbs | Junior, avg | 15 | 4 | 92 | 0.2 | 0.9 | 0.3 | | | 0.0 | 0.0 | 0.0 | 0.0 | 0.00 | 0.00 | 0 | 65 | 6 | | | | 0.00 | 0.02 | 0.05 | 0.01 | 0.00 | 4.9 | 0.02 | 1.3 | | | 10 | 0.0 | 0.2 | 3 | | 3 | 19 | 0.0 | 0 | 0.03 |
| 60488 | 1 Tbs | Strained, avg | 15 | 4 | 92 | 0.2 | 0.9 | 0.3 | | | 0.0 | 0.0 | 0.0 | 0.0 | 0.00 | 0.00 | 0 | 67 | 7 | | | | 0.00 | 0.01 | 0.05 | 0.01 | 0.00 | 5.2 | 0.02 | 0.8 | | | 6 | 0.0 | 0.1 | 4 | | 3 | 24 | 0.0 | 0 | 0.03 |
| 60321 | 1 Tbs | 1st Foods, Gerber | 14 | 4 | 92 | 0.2 | 0.8 | 0.3 | 0.3 | 0.2 | 0.0 | | | | | | | 54 | 5 | 0 | 5 | 32 | 0.00 | 0.01 | 0.05 | 0.01 | | | | 0.2 | | | 5 | 0.0 | 0.1 | 3 | 0.0 | 4 | 25 | | 0 | 0.03 |
| 60021 | 1 Tbs | 2nd Foods, Gerber | 14 | 4 | 92 | 0.2 | 0.8 | 0.3 | 0.3 | 0.2 | 0.0 | | | | | | | 55 | 6 | 0 | 6 | 33 | 0.00 | 0.01 | 0.05 | 0.01 | | | | 0.3 | | | 5 | 0.0 | 0.1 | 3 | 0.0 | 4 | 26 | | 0 | 0.03 |
| 60273 | 1 ea | Stage 3, 6 oz jar, Beechnut | 170 | 50 | 94 | 1.0 | 10.0 | 4.0 | 3.0 | 3.0 | 0.0 | 0.0 | 0.0 | 0.0 | 0.00 | 0.00 | | 525 | 53 | | | | 0.02 | 0.10 | 0.36 | | | | | 0.0 | | | 60 | | 1.2 | | | | 180 | | 0 | |
| 60819 | 1 ea | Green Beans & Rice, 3rd Foods, 6 oz jar, Gerber | 170 | 70 | 89 | 2.0 | 14.6 | 2.2 | 3.1 | 9.4 | 0.2 | | | | | | | 371 | 37 | 0 | 37 | 222 | 0.03 | 0.07 | 0.54 | 0.07 | | | | 1.5 | | | 36 | 0.1 | 0.7 | 24 | 0.4 | 41 | 167 | | 162 | 0.51 |
| | | Mixed Vegetables | | | | | | | | | | | | | | | | | | | | | | | | | | | | | | | | | | | | | | | | |
| 60839 | 1 ea | Dices, grad, 2.5 oz jar, Gerber | 71 | 33 | 89 | 1.2 | 6.2 | 1.9 | 1.3 | 2.9 | 0.4 | | | | | | | 7752 | 775 | 0 | 775 | 4651 | 0.01 | 0.01 | 0.16 | 0.04 | | | | 0.9 | | | 13 | 0.0 | 0.3 | 9 | 0.1 | 21 | 80 | | 54 | 0.21 |
| 60569 | 1 Tbs | Junior, avg | 15 | 6 | 89 | 0.2 | 1.2 | 0.2 | | | 0.1 | 0.0 | 0.0 | 0.0 | 0.00 | 0.02 | 0 | 629 | 63 | 0 | 63 | | 0.00 | 0.00 | 0.10 | 0.01 | 0.00 | 0.6 | 0.04 | 0.4 | | | 2 | 0.0 | 0.1 | 2 | | 4 | 26 | 0.1 | 5 | 0.04 |
| 60568 | 1 Tbs | Strained, avg | 15 | 6 | 90 | 0.2 | 1.2 | 0.2 | | | 0.1 | 0.0 | 0.0 | 0.0 | 0.00 | 0.03 | 0 | 599 | 50 | | | | 0.00 | 0.00 | 0.05 | 0.01 | 0.00 | 0.6 | 0.04 | 0.3 | | | 2 | 0.0 | 0.0 | 2 | | 3 | 19 | 0.1 | 2 | 0.02 |
| 60024 | 1 Tbs | 2nd Foods, Gerber | 14 | 6 | 90 | 0.2 | 1.2 | 0.2 | 0.3 | 0.7 | 0.1 | | | | | | | 709 | 71 | 0 | 71 | 425 | 0.00 | 0.00 | 0.05 | 0.01 | | | | 0.0 | | | 2 | 0.0 | 0.0 | 1 | 0.0 | 4 | 19 | | 2 | 0.03 |
| 60283 | 1 Tbs | 3rd Foods, Gerber | 14 | 6 | 88 | 0.2 | 1.3 | 0.2 | 0.3 | 0.8 | 0.0 | | | | | | | 667 | 57 | 0 | 67 | 400 | 0.01 | 0.00 | 0.08 | 0.01 | | | | 0.1 | | | 2 | 0.0 | 0.1 | 2 | 0.0 | 4 | 27 | | 14 | 0.03 |
| | | Peas | | | | | | | | | | | | | | | | | | | | | | | | | | | | | | | | | | | | | | | | |
| 60601 | 1 Tbs | Buttered, junior, avg | 14 | 8 | 84 | 0.5 | 1.6 | | | | 0.2 | | | | | | | 57 | 6 | | | | 0.01 | 0.01 | 0.19 | | | 5.1 | | 1.8 | | | 6 | | 0.1 | | | | 16 | | 1 | |
| 60604 | 1 Tbs | Buttered, strained, avg | 14 | 8 | 84 | 0.5 | 1.5 | | | | 0.2 | | | | | | | 46 | 5 | | | | 0.01 | 0.01 | 0.19 | | | 4.9 | | 1.7 | | | 5 | | 0.2 | | | | 14 | | 1 | |
| 60602 | 1 Tbs | Creamed, strained, avg | 15 | 8 | 86 | 0.3 | 1.3 | 0.3 | | | 0.3 | 0.1 | 0.1 | 0.1 | 0.02 | 0.12 | 1 | 13 | 1 | | | | 0.01 | 0.01 | 0.12 | 0.01 | 0.01 | 3.4 | 0.05 | 0.2 | | | 2 | 0.0 | 0.1 | 2 | | 5 | 13 | 0.1 | 2 | 0.06 |
| 60714 | 1 ea | Diced, grad, 4.5 oz jar, Gerber | 128 | 82 | 85 | 5.0 | 13.2 | 5.0 | 2.7 | 5.5 | 1.0 | | | | | | | 389 | 39 | 0 | 39 | 233 | 0.13 | 0.08 | 1.09 | 0.03 | | | | 7.7 | | | 27 | 0.1 | 1.3 | 24 | 0.2 | 86 | 104 | | 61 | 0.64 |
| 60603 | 1 Tbs | Strained, avg | 15 | 6 | 88 | 0.5 | 1.2 | 0.3 | | | 0.0 | 0.0 | 0.0 | 0.0 | 0.00 | 0.02 | 0 | 85 | 8 | | | | 0.01 | 0.01 | 0.15 | 0.01 | 0.00 | 3.9 | 0.04 | 1.0 | | | 3 | 0.0 | 0.1 | 2 | | 6 | 17 | 0.0 | 1 | 0.05 |
| 60322 | 1 Tbs | 1st Foods, Gerber | 14 | 7 | 88 | 0.4 | 1.1 | 0.4 | 0.3 | 0.3 | 0.1 | | | | | | | 54 | 5 | 0 | 5 | 32 | 0.01 | 0.01 | 0.12 | 0.01 | | | | 0.1 | | | 3 | 0.0 | 0.1 | 3 | 0.0 | 8 | 13 | | 1 | 0.07 |
| 60025 | 1 Tbs | 2nd Foods, Gerber | 14 | 7 | 88 | 0.4 | 1.1 | 0.4 | 0.4 | 0.3 | 0.1 | | | | | | | 48 | 5 | 0 | 5 | 29 | 0.01 | 0.01 | 0.14 | 0.01 | | | | 0.5 | | | 3 | 0.0 | 0.1 | 3 | 0.0 | 8 | 13 | | 1 | 0.06 |
| 60115 | 1 ea | Peas & Brown Rice, 4.5 oz jar, Earth's Best | 128 | 80 | 84 | 5.0 | 16.0 | | | | 0.0 | 0.0 | 0.0 | 0.0 | 0.00 | 0.00 | | 1500 | 150 | 0 | 150 | | 0.12 | 0.05 | 1.80 | | | | | | | | 24 | | 1.0 | 27 | | | | | 10 | |
| 60270 | 1 ea | Peas & Carrots, Stage 2, 4 oz jar, Beechnut | 113 | 50 | 89 | 2.0 | 10.0 | 3.0 | 3.0 | 4.0 | 0.0 | 0.0 | 0.0 | 0.0 | 0.00 | 0.00 | | 4783 | 478 | | | | 0.02 | 0.05 | 0.05 | | | | | 0.0 | | | 12 | | 0.3 | | | | 130 | | 25 | |
| 60820 | 1 ea | Peas & Rice, 3rd Foods, 6 oz jar, Gerber | 170 | 92 | 86 | 4.3 | 17.2 | 3.4 | 2.7 | 11.1 | 0.7 | | | | | | | 338 | 34 | 0 | 34 | 203 | 0.07 | 0.10 | 1.43 | 0.07 | | | | 3.2 | | | 27 | 0.1 | 1.5 | 29 | 0.4 | 83 | 156 | | 151 | 0.85 |
| 60715 | 1 ea | Potatoes, diced, grad, 4.5 oz jar, Gerber | 128 | 65 | 87 | 1.3 | 15.1 | 1.2 | 0.6 | 13.3 | 0.0 | 0.0 | 0.0 | 0.0 | 0.00 | 0.00 | | 1 | 0.1 | 0 | 0.1 | 1 | 0.03 | 0.01 | 0.45 | 0.09 | | | | 13.4 | | | 5 | 0.1 | 0.3 | 19 | 0.1 | 29 | 141 | | 73 | 0.26 |
| 60797 | 1 ea | Potatoes, 1st Foods, 2.5 oz jar, Gerber | 71 | 35 | 87 | 0.8 | 7.9 | 0.7 | 0.2 | 7.0 | 0.1 | | | | | | | | | | | | 0.03 | 0.01 | 0.44 | 0.11 | | | | | | | 4 | 0.0 | 0.3 | 9 | 0.0 | 23 | 109 | | 8 | 0.14 |
| 60625 | 1 Tbs | Spinach, creamed, strained, avg | 15 | 6 | 90 | 0.4 | 0.9 | 0.3 | | | 0.2 | 0.1 | 0.0 | 0.0 | 0.01 | 0.01 | 1 | 626 | 63 | | | | 0.00 | 0.02 | 0.03 | 0.01 | 0.01 | 9.1 | | 1.3 | | | 13 | 0.0 | 0.1 | 8 | | 8 | 29 | 0.4 | 7 | 0.05 |
| 60329 | 1 Tbs | Spinach, creamed, 2nd Foods, Gerber | 14 | 7 | 88 | 0.4 | 1.0 | 0.2 | 0.3 | 0.5 | 0.1 | | | | | | | 557 | 56 | 0 | 56 | 334 | 0.01 | 0.02 | 0.05 | 0.01 | | | | 0.6 | | | 13 | 0.0 | 0.1 | 5 | 0.1 | 9 | 32 | | 4 | 0.08 |
| | | Squash | | | | | | | | | | | | | | | | | | | | | | | | | | | | | | | | | | | | | | | | |
| 60628 | 1 Tbs | Buttered, junior, avg | 14 | 4 | 92 | 0.1 | 0.9 | 0.2 | | | 0.1 | 0.0 | 0.0 | 0.0 | | | 0 | 214 | 21 | | | | 0.00 | 0.01 | 0.04 | 0.01 | | 1.6 | | 1.1 | | | 4 | | 0.1 | | | | 19 | | 0 | |
| 60629 | 1 Tbs | Buttered, strained, avg | 14 | 4 | 92 | 0.1 | 1.0 | | | | 0.0 | | | | | | | 232 | 23 | | | | 0.00 | 0.01 | 0.05 | | | 1.7 | | 1.1 | | | 5 | | 0.1 | | | | 18 | | 0 | |
| 60060 | 1 ea | Butternut, Stage 1, 2.5 oz jar, Beechnut | 71 | 30 | 88 | 1.0 | 7.0 | 2.0 | 2.0 | 3.0 | 0.0 | 0.0 | 0.0 | 0.0 | 0.00 | 0.00 | | 2705 | 270 | | | | 0.02 | 0.01 | 0.24 | | | | | 0.0 | | | 0 | | 0.0 | | | | 170 | | 10 | |
| 60627 | 1 Tbs | Strained, avg | 14 | 3 | 93 | 0.1 | 0.8 | 0.3 | | | 0.0 | 0.0 | 0.0 | 0.0 | 0.01 | 0.00 | 0 | 233 | 28 | | | | 0.00 | 0.01 | 0.05 | 0.01 | 0.00 | 2.2 | 0.03 | 1.1 | | | 3 | 0.0 | 0.0 | 2 | | 2 | 25 | 0.0 | 0 | 0.02 |
| 60102 | 1 ea | Winter, 4.5 oz jar, Earth's Best | 128 | 50 | 90 | 1.0 | 12.0 | | | | 0.0 | 0.0 | 0.0 | 0.0 | 0.00 | 0.00 | | 675 | 67 | 0 | 67 | | 0.04 | 0.10 | 0.60 | | | | | | | | 24 | | 0.6 | 18 | | | | | 10 | |
| 60323 | 1 Tbs | 1st Foods, Gerber | 14 | 5 | 92 | 0.1 | 1.0 | 0.2 | 0.5 | 0.2 | 0.0 | | | | | | | 133 | 13 | 0 | 13 | 80 | 0.00 | 0.01 | 0.07 | 0.01 | | | | 0.4 | | | 4 | 0.0 | 0.0 | 2 | 0.0 | 3 | 28 | | 0 | 0.03 |
| 60287 | 1 Tbs | 2nd Foods, Gerber | 14 | 5 | 92 | 0.1 | 1.0 | 0.2 | 0.5 | 0.3 | 0.0 | | | | | | | 220 | 22 | 0 | 22 | 132 | 0.00 | 0.01 | 0.06 | 0.01 | | | | 0.5 | | | 4 | 0.0 | 0.0 | 2 | 0.0 | 3 | 24 | | 0 | 0.01 |
| 60288 | 1 Tbs | 3rd Foods, Gerber | 14 | 10 | 83 | 0.1 | 2.1 | 0.3 | 1.2 | 0.6 | 0.0 | | | | | | | 436 | 44 | 0 | 44 | 262 | 0.00 | 0.01 | 0.05 | 0.01 | | | | 0.8 | | | 3 | 0.0 | 0.0 | 2 | 0.0 | 3 | 32 | | 8 | 0.01 |
| | | Sweet Potatoes | | | | | | | | | | | | | | | | | | | | | | | | | | | | | | | | | | | | | | | | |
| 60631 | 1 Tbs | Buttered, junior, avg | 14 | 8 | 86 | 0.1 | 1.7 | | | | 0.1 | | | | | | | 846 | 85 | | | | 0.00 | 0.01 | 0.04 | | | 1.9 | | 1.3 | | | 4 | | 0.1 | | | | 30 | | 1 | |
| 60630 | 1 Tbs | Buttered, strained, avg | 14 | 8 | 86 | 0.1 | 1.7 | | | | 0.1 | | | | | | | 954 | 95 | | | | 0.00 | 0.01 | 0.04 | | | 1.8 | | 1.3 | | | 3 | | 0.1 | | | | 29 | | 1 | |
| 60632 | 1 Tbs | Junior, avg | 14 | 8 | 84 | 0.2 | 1.9 | 0.2 | | | 0.0 | 0.0 | 0.0 | 0.0 | 0.00 | 0.01 | 0 | 929 | 93 | | | | 0.00 | 0.00 | 0.05 | 0.02 | 0.00 | 1.4 | 0.06 | 1.3 | | | 2 | 0.0 | 0.1 | 2 | | 3 | 34 | 0.1 | 3 | 0.02 |
| 60633 | 1 Tbs | Strained, avg | 14 | 8 | 85 | 0.2 | 1.8 | 0.2 | | | 0.0 | 0.0 | 0.0 | 0.0 | 0.00 | 0.01 | 0 | 901 | 90 | | | | 0.00 | 0.00 | 0.05 | 0.01 | 0.00 | 1.4 | 0.05 | 1.4 | | | 2 | 0.0 | 0.1 | 2 | | 3 | 37 | 0.1 | 3 | 0.03 |
| 60324 | 1 Tbs | 1st Foods, Gerber | 14 | 9 | 83 | 0.2 | 2.1 | 0.2 | 1.1 | 0.7 | 0.0 | | | | | | | 1124 | 112 | 0 | 112 | 674 | 0.00 | 0.00 | 0.05 | 0.01 | | | | 0.1 | | | 2 | 0.0 | 0.0 | 2 | 0.0 | 4 | 35 | | 2 | 0.03 |
| 60026 | 1 Tbs | 2nd Foods, Gerber | 14 | 9 | 84 | 0.1 | 2.0 | 0.2 | 1.3 | 0.5 | 0.0 | | | | | | | 869 | 87 | 0 | 87 | 522 | 0.00 | 0.01 | 0.05 | 0.02 | | | | 0.2 | | | 2 | 0.0 | 0.0 | 2 | 0.0 | 4 | 35 | | 2 | 0.03 |
| 60291 | 1 Tbs | 3rd Foods, Gerber | 14 | 10 | 82 | 0.1 | 2.2 | 0.2 | 1.1 | 0.9 | 0.1 | | | | | | | 1075 | 108 | 0 | 108 | 645 | 0.00 | 0.01 | 0.05 | 0.02 | | | | 0.4 | | | 2 | 0.0 | 0.1 | 2 | 0.0 | 3 | 40 | | 9 | 0.03 |
| 60103 | 1 ea | 4.5 oz jar, Earth's Best | 128 | 60 | 90 | 1.0 | 12.0 | | | | 1.0 | | | | | | | 1650 | 165 | 0 | 165 | | 0.06 | 0.08 | 0.60 | | | | | 2.1 | | | 24 | | 0.4 | 12 | | | | | 15 | |
| | | **INFANT FORMULAS** | | | | | | | | | | | | | | | | | | | | | | | | | | | | | | | | | | | | | | | | |
| 62072 | 1/2 cup | Alimentum, w/iron, Ready To Feed (RTF) Ross | 122 | 79 | 133 | 2.2 | 8.1 | 0.0 | | | 4.4 | 2.2 | 0.4 | 1.4 | 0.07 | 1.28 | 2 | 239 | 72 | | | | 0.05 | 0.07 | 1.08 | 0.05 | 0.37 | 12.2 | 0.60 | 7.2 | 0.9 | | 85 | 0.1 | 1.4 | 6 | 0.0 | 60 | 94 | 2.2 | 35 | 0.60 |
| 62656 | 1/2 cup | Alsoy, RTF, Carnation | 158 | 79 | 90 | 2.2 | 8.8 | | | | 4.0 | | | | | | | 247 | 49 | | | | 0.05 | 0.07 | 1.04 | 0.05 | 0.25 | 12.8 | 3.74 | 12.8 | 1.3 | | 84 | 0.1 | 1.4 | 9 | 27.1 | 49 | 92 | | 27 | 0.71 |
| 62312 | 1/2 cup | CalciloXD, w/iron, prep f/pwd, Ross | 122 | 80 | 88 | 1.8 | 8.2 | | | | 4.5 | | | | | 1.04 | | 240 | 48 | | | | 0.08 | 0.12 | 0.84 | 0.05 | 0.20 | 12.0 | 0.36 | 7.2 | 0.0 | | 8 | 0.1 | 1.4 | 5 | 0.0 | 20 | 66 | | 17 | 0.60 |
| 62595 | 1/2 cup | Compleat Pediatric, RTF, Novartis Nutrition | 125 | 118 | 80 | 4.5 | 15.4 | 0.5 | | | 4.6 | | | | | | | | | | | | | 0.34 | | | | | | 31.3 | | | 118 | | | 22 | | 118 | 178 | | 80 | |
| 62301 | 1/2 cup | DF Soy, for diarrhea, RTF, Ross | 122 | 80 | 88 | 2.1 | 8.1 | | | | 4.4 | | | | | 1.04 | | 241 | 72 | | | | 0.05 | 0.07 | 1.08 | 0.05 | 0.36 | 12.0 | 0.60 | 7.2 | 1.2 | | 84 | 0.1 | 1.4 | 6 | 0.0 | 60 | 87 | | 35 | 0.60 |
| | | Enfamil | | | | | | | | | | | | | | | | | | | | | | | | | | | | | | | | | | | | | | | | |
| 60294 | 1/2 cup | Low iron, RTF, Mead Johnson | 122 | 81 | 88 | 1.7 | 8.7 | 0.0 | | | 4.2 | 1.8 | 1.6 | 0.8 | 0.07 | 0.73 | 1 | 240 | 72 | | | | 0.06 | 0.11 | 0.80 | 0.05 | 0.24 | 13.4 | 0.36 | 9.6 | | | 62 | 0.1 | 0.6 | 6 | 0.0 | 43 | 87 | 2.2 | 22 | 0.81 |
| 62585 | 1/2 cup | Next Step, milk based, prep f/pwd, Md Johnson | 123 | 81 | 87 | 2.1 | 9.0 | | | | 4.1 | | | 0.7 | 0.00 | 0.69 | | 239 | 48 | | | | 0.08 | 0.12 | 0.85 | 0.05 | 0.20 | 12.1 | 0.36 | 7.3 | 1.2 | | 97 | 0.1 | 1.5 | 6 | 5.6 | 68 | 105 | 2.3 | 33 | 0.73 |
| 62586 | 1/2 cup | Next Step Soy, prep f/pwd, Mead Johnson | 122 | 80 | 87 | 2.6 | 9.4 | | | | 3.5 | | | 0.6 | 0.00 | 0.61 | | 239 | 48 | | | | 0.06 | 0.07 | 0.80 | 0.07 | 0.24 | 12.8 | 0.40 | 9.6 | 1.2 | | 92 | 0.1 | 1.4 | 6 | 0.0 | 72 | 120 | 2.2 | 36 | 0.96 |
| 60296 | 1/2 cup | With iron, RTF, Mead Johnson | 122 | 81 | 88 | 1.7 | 8.7 | 0.0 | | | 4.2 | 1.8 | 1.6 | 0.8 | 0.07 | 0.73 | 1 | 240 | 72 | | | | 0.06 | 0.11 | 0.80 | 0.05 | 0.24 | 12.2 | | 9.6 | | | 62 | 0.1 | 1.4 | 6 | | 43 | 87 | 2.2 | 22 | 0.81 |
| 62356 | 1/2 cup | Follow-Up, w/iron, RTF, Carnation | 150 | 98 | 87 | 2.6 | 12.9 | 0.0 | | | 4.1 | 1.8 | 1.3 | 0.9 | 0.08 | 0.83 | 2 | 240 | 72 | | | | 0.08 | 0.09 | 1.26 | 0.06 | 0.31 | 15.0 | 0.34 | 7.8 | 1.2 | | 132 | 0.1 | 1.8 | 9 | 0.0 | 88 | 132 | | 38 | 0.62 |
| 62658 | 1/2 cup | Follow-Up Soy, RTF, Carnation | 150 | 74 | 90 | 2.3 | 8.7 | | | | 3.2 | | | | | | | 226 | 68 | | | | 0.06 | 0.07 | 0.87 | 0.06 | 0.23 | 11.7 | 0.34 | 11.7 | 1.1 | | 99 | 0.1 | 1.3 | 9 | 0.0 | 66 | 86 | | 30 | 0.87 |
| 62351 | 1/2 cup | Good Start, w/iron, RTF, Carnation | 150 | 99 | 88 | 2.4 | 11.0 | 0.0 | | | 5.1 | 2.2 | 1.6 | 1.1 | 0.09 | 1.02 | 9 | 300 | 90 | | | | 0.06 | 0.14 | 0.74 | 0.08 | 0.21 | 9.0 | 0.35 | 8.0 | 1.2 | | 63 | 0.1 | 1.5 | 6 | 0.0 | 36 | 98 | | 24 | 0.74 |
| 62358 | 1/2 cup | I-Soyalac, w/iron, RTF, Carnation | 122 | 82 | 88 | 2.4 | 8.1 | 0.0 | | | 4.4 | 0.6 | 0.9 | 2.6 | 0.37 | 2.28 | 0 | 250 | 66 | | | | 0.07 | 0.07 | 1.00 | 0.07 | 0.24 | 12.2 | | 9.6 | | | 81 | 0.1 | 1.5 | 9 | | 50 | 94 | | 34 | 0.62 |
| 60299 | 1/2 cup | Isomil, w/iron, Ross | 122 | 80 | 133 | 2.0 | 8.3 | 0.0 | | | 4.4 | 1.4 | 1.7 | 1.0 | 0.10 | 0.92 | 0 | 240 | 72 | | | | 0.05 | 0.07 | 1.08 | 0.05 | 0.37 | 12.2 | 0.60 | 7.2 | 1.2 | | 84 | 0.1 | 1.4 | 6 | 0.0 | 59 | 87 | 1.7 | 35 | 0.60 |
| 60300 | 1/2 cup | Isomil SF, w/iron, Ross | 122 | 80 | 133 | 2.2 | 8.1 | 0.0 | | | 4.4 | 1.5 | 0.7 | 1.2 | 0.18 | 1.01 | 0 | 240 | 72 | | | | 0.05 | 0.07 | 1.09 | 0.05 | 0.37 | 12.2 | 0.60 | 7.3 | 1.2 | | 84 | 0.1 | 1.4 | 6 | 0.0 | 59 | 87 | 1.7 | 35 | 0.60 |

| Code | Amount | Description | Basic Components | | | | | | | | | Additional Fats | | | | | | Vit A & Components | | | | | Vitamins | | | | | | | | | | Minerals | | | | | | | | | |
|---|---|---|---|---|---|---|---|---|---|---|---|---|---|---|---|---|---|---|---|---|---|---|---|---|---|---|---|---|---|---|---|---|---|---|---|---|---|---|---|---|---|---|
| | | | Weight (g) | Calories | % Water | Protein (g) | Carbs (g) | Fiber (g) | Sugar (g) | Other Carbs (g) | Fat (g) | Sat Fat (g) | Mono Fat (g) | Poly Fat (g) | Omega 3 (g) | Omega 6 (g) | Choles (mg) | Vit A (IU) | Vit A (RE) | Retinol (RE) | Carotenoids (RE) | Beta Carotene (mcg) | Thiamin (mg) | Riboflavin (mg) | Niacin (NE) | Vit B6 (mg) | Vit B12 (mcg) | Folate (mcg) | Panto (mg) | Vit C (mg) | Vit D (mg) | Vit E (α TE) | Calcium (mg) | Copper (mg) | Iron (mg) | Magnes (mg) | Mang (mg) | Phos (mg) | Potassium (mg) | Selenium (mcg) | Sodium (mg) | Zinc (mg) |
| 62354 | 1/2 cup | Lactofree, w/iron, RTF, Mead Johnson | 122 | 81 | 87 | 1.8 | 8.4 | 0.0 | | | 4.4 | 1.9 | 1.7 | 0.8 | 0.08 | 0.76 | 1 | 240 | 72 | | | | 0.06 | 0.07 | 0.80 | 0.05 | 0.24 | 13.4 | | 9.6 | | | 66 | 0.1 | 1.4 | 6 | | 44 | 88 | 2.2 | 24 | 0.81 |
| 60301 | 1/2 cup | LoFenalac, w/iron, prep f/pwd, Mead Johnson | 123 | 80 | 87 | 2.6 | 10.4 | 0.0 | | | 3.1 | 0.4 | 0.8 | 1.9 | 0.04 | 1.84 | 0 | 248 | 74 | | | | 0.06 | 0.08 | 1.00 | 0.05 | 0.25 | 12.3 | | 6.5 | | | 75 | 0.1 | 1.5 | 9 | | 57 | 81 | 2.2 | 38 | 0.63 |
| 60302 | 1/2 cup | Nursoy, w/iron, RTF, Wyeth-Ayerst | 122 | 81 | 88 | 2.2 | 8.2 | 0.0 | | | 4.3 | 2.0 | 1.7 | 0.6 | 0.06 | 0.55 | 0 | 240 | 56 | | | | 0.09 | 0.12 | 0.60 | 0.05 | 0.24 | 6.1 | 0.36 | 6.6 | | | 72 | 0.1 | 1.4 | 9 | 24.1 | 50 | 84 | 2.2 | 22 | 0.65 |
| 60303 | 1/2 cup | Nutramigen, w/iron, RTF, Mead Johnson | 123 | 81 | 88 | 2.3 | 8.9 | 0.0 | | | 4.0 | 1.7 | 1.5 | 0.8 | 0.07 | 0.69 | 0 | 242 | 73 | | | | 0.07 | 0.07 | 0.81 | 0.05 | 0.25 | 12.3 | | 9.7 | | | 76 | 0.1 | 1.5 | 9 | | 50 | 89 | 2.2 | 38 | 0.81 |
| 62598 | 1/2 cup | Parents Choice, w/iron, prep f/pwd, Wyeth-Ayerst | 123 | 80 | 87 | 1.8 | 8.5 | | | | 4.2 | | | 0.4 | 0.00 | 0.40 | | 239 | 48 | | | | 0.08 | 0.12 | 0.60 | 0.05 | 0.16 | 6.0 | 0.25 | 6.8 | 1.2 | | 50 | 0.1 | 1.4 | 6 | 0.0 | 34 | 66 | | 18 | 0.64 |
| 62125 | 1/2 cup | Portagen, w/iron, prep f/pwd, Mead Johnson | 124 | 79 | 86 | 2.8 | 9.2 | 0.0 | | | 3.9 | 3.4 | 0.2 | 0.3 | 0.01 | 0.30 | 1 | 622 | 184 | | | | 0.12 | 0.15 | 1.67 | 0.17 | 0.51 | 12.4 | | 6.4 | | | 76 | 0.1 | 1.5 | 16 | | 56 | 99 | 0.4 | 43 | 0.74 |
| 60304 | 1/2 cup | Pregestimil, w/iron, prep f/pwd, Mead Johnson | 123 | 80 | 87 | 2.2 | 8.2 | 0.0 | | | 4.5 | 2.7 | 0.8 | 0.9 | 0.05 | 0.90 | 0 | 304 | 87 | | | | 0.06 | 0.08 | 1.00 | 0.05 | 0.25 | 12.3 | | 9.3 | | | 75 | 0.1 | 1.5 | 9 | | 50 | 87 | 2.2 | 31 | 0.75 |
| 60305 | 1/2 cup | Prosobee, w/iron, RTF, Mead Johnson | 122 | 81 | 88 | 2.4 | 8.0 | 0.0 | | | 4.2 | 1.8 | 1.6 | 0.8 | 0.07 | 0.73 | 0 | 240 | 72 | | | | 0.06 | 0.07 | 0.80 | 0.05 | 0.24 | 13.4 | | 9.6 | | | 84 | 0.1 | 1.4 | 9 | | 66 | 96 | 2.2 | 29 | 0.96 |
| 62579 | 1/2 cup | SandoSource Peptide, RTF, Novartis Nutrition | 127 | 118 | 78 | 5.9 | 19.3 | | | | 2.1 | | | | | | | 676 | 135 | | | | 0.20 | 0.23 | 2.70 | 0.27 | 0.81 | 53.9 | 1.35 | 20.3 | 0.7 | | 68 | 0.1 | 1.2 | 27 | 0.2 | 68 | 189 | 6.8 | 142 | 1.55 |
| | | Similac | | | | | | | | | | | | | | | | | | | | | | | | | | | | | | | | | | | | | | | | |
| 60306 | 1/2 cup | 13, low iron, RTF, Ross | 121 | 52 | 92 | 1.4 | 5.5 | | | | 2.7 | | | | | 0.68 | | 156 | 47 | | | | 0.05 | 0.08 | 0.55 | 0.03 | 0.13 | 7.8 | 0.23 | 4.7 | 0.8 | | 47 | 0.0 | 0.1 | 4 | 0.0 | 37 | 69 | | 18 | 0.39 |
| 60308 | 1/2 cup | 24, low iron, RTF, Ross | 122 | 95 | 84 | 2.6 | 9.9 | | | | 5.0 | | | | | 1.23 | | 284 | 85 | | | | 0.09 | 0.14 | 0.99 | 0.06 | 0.24 | 14.2 | 0.43 | 8.5 | 1.4 | | 85 | 0.1 | 0.2 | 7 | 0.0 | 66 | 125 | | 32 | 0.71 |
| 60456 | 1/2 cup | 24, w/iron, RTF, Ross | 122 | 95 | 84 | 2.6 | 9.9 | | | | 5.0 | | | | | 1.23 | | 284 | 57 | | | | 0.09 | 0.14 | 0.99 | 0.06 | 0.24 | 14.2 | 0.43 | 8.5 | 1.4 | | 85 | 0.1 | 1.7 | 7 | 0.0 | 66 | 125 | | 32 | 0.71 |
| 60309 | 1/2 cup | 27, low iron, RTF, Ross | 124 | 109 | 83 | 2.9 | 11.4 | | | | 5.7 | | | | | 1.41 | | 326 | 98 | | | | 0.11 | 0.16 | 1.14 | 0.07 | 0.27 | 16.3 | 0.49 | 9.8 | 1.6 | | 98 | 0.1 | 0.2 | 8 | 0.0 | 76 | 144 | | 37 | 0.82 |
| 60135 | 1/2 cup | Low Iron, Ross | 126 | 83 | 137 | 1.7 | 8.9 | 0.0 | | | 4.5 | 1.6 | 1.7 | 1.0 | 0.10 | 0.91 | 2 | 248 | 74 | | | | 0.08 | 0.12 | 0.87 | 0.05 | 0.20 | 12.6 | 0.37 | 7.4 | 1.2 | | 66 | 0.1 | 0.2 | 5 | 0.0 | 35 | 87 | 1.8 | 20 | 0.62 |
| 60455 | 1/2 cup | Natural Care, low iron, Ross | 122 | 96 | 109 | 2.6 | 10.0 | 0.0 | | | 5.1 | 3.1 | 0.5 | 1.0 | 0.10 | 0.92 | 3 | 1182 | 355 | | | | 0.24 | 0.59 | 4.73 | 0.24 | 0.52 | 35.4 | 1.79 | 35.0 | 3.5 | | 199 | 0.2 | 0.4 | 11 | 0.0 | 110 | 122 | 1.7 | 41 | 1.41 |
| 62313 | 1/2 cup | PM 60/40, low iron, prep f/pwd, Ross | 122 | 80 | 88 | 1.8 | 8.2 | 0.0 | | | 4.5 | 2.0 | 0.7 | 1.6 | 0.18 | 1.04 | 2 | 240 | 72 | | | | 0.08 | 0.12 | 0.84 | 0.05 | 0.20 | 12.0 | 0.36 | 7.2 | 1.2 | | 45 | 0.1 | 0.2 | 5 | 0.0 | 22 | 69 | | 19 | 0.60 |
| 60310 | 1/2 cup | PM 60/40, low iron, RTF, Ross | 122 | 80 | 134 | 1.8 | 8.2 | 0.0 | | | 4.5 | 2.0 | 0.7 | 1.6 | 0.18 | 1.39 | 2 | 240 | 72 | | | | 0.09 | 0.12 | 0.84 | 0.05 | 0.20 | 12.2 | 0.36 | 7.3 | 1.2 | | 45 | 0.1 | 0.2 | 5 | 0.0 | 22 | 78 | 1.6 | 19 | 0.60 |
| 60311 | 1/2 cup | Special Care 20, low iron, RTF, Ross | 122 | 80 | 87 | 2.2 | 8.5 | | | | 4.3 | | | | | 0.56 | | 542 | 163 | | | | 0.20 | 0.49 | 3.99 | 0.20 | 0.44 | 29.5 | 1.52 | 29.5 | 3.0 | | 144 | 0.2 | 0.3 | 10 | 0.0 | 72 | 103 | | 34 | 1.20 |
| 60312 | 1/2 cup | Special Care 24, low Iron, RTF, Ross | 122 | 95 | 84 | 2.6 | 10.0 | | | | 5.1 | | | | | 0.66 | | 643 | 193 | | | | 0.24 | 0.59 | 4.73 | 0.24 | 0.52 | 35.0 | 1.80 | 35.0 | 3.5 | | 170 | 0.2 | 0.3 | 11 | 0.0 | 85 | 122 | | 41 | 1.42 |
| 60136 | 1/2 cup | Special Care 24, w/iron, RTF, Ross | 122 | 96 | 109 | 2.6 | 10.0 | 0.0 | | | 5.1 | 3.1 | 0.5 | 1.0 | 0.10 | 0.93 | 3 | 1182 | 355 | | | | 0.24 | 0.59 | 4.73 | 0.24 | 0.52 | 35.4 | 1.79 | 35.0 | 3.5 | | 171 | 0.2 | 1.7 | 11 | 0.0 | 96 | 122 | 1.7 | 41 | 1.41 |
| 62355 | 1/2 cup | Toddlers Best, RTF, Ross | 123 | 80 | 87 | 2.8 | 8.8 | 0.0 | | | 3.8 | 1.3 | 1.5 | 0.9 | 0.08 | 0.79 | 2 | 241 | 73 | | | | 0.08 | 0.12 | 0.84 | 0.05 | 0.20 | 12.3 | 0.36 | 7.4 | | | 125 | 0.1 | 1.5 | 7 | 0.0 | 76 | 121 | | 32 | 0.68 |
| 60173 | 1/2 cup | With Iron, Ross | 126 | 83 | 137 | 1.7 | 8.9 | 0.0 | | | 4.5 | 1.6 | 1.7 | 1.0 | 0.10 | 0.91 | 2 | 248 | 74 | | | | 0.08 | 0.12 | 0.87 | 0.05 | 0.20 | 12.6 | 0.37 | 7.4 | 1.2 | | 66 | 0.1 | 1.5 | 5 | 0.0 | 35 | 87 | 1.8 | 20 | 0.62 |
| 62360 | 1/2 cup | SMA, low iron, RTF, Wyeth-Ayerst | 122 | 81 | 88 | 1.7 | 8.5 | 0.0 | | | 4.3 | 2.0 | 1.7 | 0.6 | 0.06 | 0.55 | 5 | 240 | 72 | | | | 0.09 | 0.12 | 0.60 | 0.05 | 0.16 | 6.1 | 0.25 | 6.8 | | | 50 | 0.1 | 0.2 | 6 | 12.1 | 34 | 67 | 2.2 | 17 | 0.65 |
| 60314 | 1/2 cup | SMA, w/iron, RTF, Wyeth-Averst | 122 | 81 | 88 | 1.7 | 8.5 | 0.0 | | | 4.3 | 2.0 | 1.7 | 0.6 | 0.06 | 0.55 | 5 | 240 | 72 | | | | 0.09 | 0.12 | 0.60 | 0.05 | 0.16 | 6.1 | 0.25 | 6.8 | | | 50 | 0.1 | 1.4 | 6 | 12.1 | 34 | 67 | 2.2 | 17 | 0.65 |
| 62597 | 1/2 cup | Soy, w/iron, prep f/pwd, Wyeth-Ayerst | 124 | 80 | 86 | 2.2 | 8.2 | | | | 4.3 | | | 0.4 | 0.00 | 0.40 | | 241 | 48 | | | | 0.08 | 0.12 | 0.60 | 0.05 | 0.00 | 6.0 | 0.36 | 6.7 | 1.2 | | 72 | 0.1 | 1.4 | 8 | 0.0 | 51 | 84 | | 24 | 0.64 |
| 62357 | 1/2 cup | Soyalac, w/iron, RTF, Carnation | 122 | 82 | 88 | 2.4 | 8.1 | 0.0 | | | 4.4 | 0.6 | 0.9 | 2.6 | 0.37 | 2.28 | 0 | 250 | 66 | | | | 0.06 | 0.07 | 1.00 | 0.06 | 0.24 | 12.2 | | 9.6 | | | 76 | 0.1 | 1.5 | 10 | | 44 | 95 | | 35 | 0.62 |
| 62581 | 1/2 cup | Vivonex Pediatric, prep f/pwd, Novartis Nutrition | 127 | 95 | 83 | 2.8 | 14.9 | | | | 2.8 | | | | | | | 296 | 59 | | | | 0.18 | 0.21 | 2.36 | 0.24 | | 23.6 | | 11.8 | 1.5 | | 115 | | 1.2 | | | | 142 | | 47 | 1.42 |
| | | **MEALS, ENTRÉES AND DISHES** | | | | | | | | | | | | | | | | | | | | | | | | | | | | | | | | | | | | | | | | |
| | | *CANNED MEALS, ENTREES AND DISHES* | | | | | | | | | | | | | | | | | | | | | | | | | | | | | | | | | | | | | | | | |
| 56092 | 1 cup | Chicken Chow Mein, avg | 250 | 95 | 89 | 6.5 | 17.8 | 2.0 | 3.0 | 12.8 | 0.9 | 0.0 | 0.1 | 0.8 | | 0.00 | 8 | 150 | 28 | 20 | 9 | | 0.05 | 0.10 | 1.00 | 0.09 | 0.05 | 12.0 | 0.16 | 12.5 | | | 45 | 0.2 | 1.3 | 15 | | 85 | 418 | 1.3 | 725 | 1.30 |
| | | Chili | | | | | | | | | | | | | | | | | | | | | | | | | | | | | | | | | | | | | | | | |
| 56001 | 1 cup | With Beans, avg | 256 | 287 | 76 | 14.6 | 30.5 | 11.3 | 3.1 | 16.1 | 14.1 | 6.0 | 6.0 | 0.9 | 0.39 | 0.53 | 44 | 863 | 87 | 0 | 87 | | 0.12 | 0.27 | 0.92 | 0.34 | 0.00 | 58.1 | 3.64 | 4.4 | 0.0 | | 120 | 0.3 | 8.8 | 115 | 0.3 | 394 | 934 | 3.3 | 1336 | 5.12 |
| 57131 | 1 cup | With Beans, Libby's | 255 | 421 | 70 | 16.0 | 29.0 | 4.0 | 1.0 | 24.0 | 28.0 | 12.8 | | | | | 51 | 750 | 150 | | | | | | | | | | | 0.0 | | | 61 | | 3.6 | | | | | | 1211 | |
| 57132 | 1 cup | Without Beans, Libby's | 253 | 481 | 69 | 21.0 | 16.0 | 1.0 | 2.0 | 13.0 | 38.0 | 17.7 | | | | | 76 | 1250 | 250 | | | | | | | | | | | 0.0 | | | 81 | | 3.6 | | | | | | 1581 | |
| | | Hash | | | | | | | | | | | | | | | | | | | | | | | | | | | | | | | | | | | | | | | | |
| 56070 | 1 cup | Corned Beef, avg | 220 | 398 | 67 | 19.4 | 23.5 | 1.1 | 0.1 | 22.4 | 24.9 | 11.9 | 10.9 | 0.9 | | 0.51 | 73 | 0 | 0 | 0 | 0 | 0 | 0.02 | 0.20 | 4.62 | 0.43 | 1.35 | 20.2 | 1.10 | 0.0 | 0.0 | | 29 | 0.3 | 4.4 | 35 | | 147 | 440 | 16.9 | 1188 | 3.30 |
| 57133 | 1 cup | Corned Beef, Libby's | 252 | 471 | 66 | 21.0 | 25.0 | 8.0 | 1.0 | 16.0 | 35.3 | 15.1 | | | | | 91 | 0 | 0 | 0 | 0 | 0 | | | | | | | | 0.0 | | | 20 | | 1.8 | | | | | | 1200 | |
| 56815 | 1 cup | Corned Beef, Chef-Mate | 253 | 486 | 65 | 24.2 | 29.1 | 6.1 | 2.2 | 20.8 | 30.4 | 13.4 | 14.7 | 1.1 | 0.18 | 0.89 | 89 | 0 | 0 | 0 | 0 | 0 | 0.22 | 0.30 | 6.32 | 0.58 | 2.45 | | 1.23 | 1.5 | | | 46 | 0.3 | 3.0 | 38 | 0.1 | 240 | 536 | | 1594 | 7.51 |
| 57135 | 1 cup | Roast Beef, Libby's | 234 | 461 | 66 | 19.0 | 23.0 | 3.0 | 0.9 | 19.1 | 32.8 | 14.0 | 11.6 | 6.4 | | | 80 | 0 | 0 | 0 | 0 | 0 | 0.19 | 0.23 | 4.66 | 0.61 | | 24.6 | | 0.0 | | | 19 | | 1.8 | 44 | | | 725 | | 1390 | 5.99 |
| | | Sardines | | | | | | | | | | | | | | | | | | | | | | | | | | | | | | | | | | | | | | | | |
| 18828 | 1 ea | With Mustard Sauce, 3.7 oz can, PET | 106 | 160 | | 17.0 | 2.0 | 2.0 | 0.0 | 0.0 | 10.0 | 5.0 | | | | | 105 | 0 | 0 | 0 | 0 | 0 | | | | | | | | 0.0 | | | 250 | | 1.8 | | | | | | 820 | |
| 18827 | 1 ea | With Soy Oil, 2.96 oz can, PET | 84 | 150 | | 18.0 | 1.0 | 0.0 | 0.0 | 1.0 | 8.0 | 4.0 | | | | | 100 | 0 | 0 | 0 | 0 | 0 | | | | | | | | 0.0 | | | 250 | | 1.4 | | | | | | 310 | |
| 18826 | 1 ea | With Tomato Sauce, 3.7 oz can, PET | 106 | 150 | | 16.0 | 5.0 | 2.0 | 3.0 | 0.0 | 8.0 | 4.0 | | | | | 115 | 0 | 0 | 0 | 0 | 0 | | | | | | | | 0.0 | | | 250 | | 1.4 | | | | | | 960 | |
| 56096 | 1 cup | Spaghetti, w/sauce & cheese, avg | 250 | 190 | 80 | 5.5 | 38.5 | 2.5 | | | 1.5 | 0.0 | 0.4 | 0.5 | | 0.00 | 8 | 925 | 120 | 40 | 80 | | 0.35 | 0.28 | 4.50 | 0.13 | 0.00 | 6.0 | 0.45 | 10.0 | | | 40 | 0.2 | 2.8 | 20 | | 88 | 302 | 21.0 | 955 | 1.12 |
| 56099 | 1 cup | Spaghetti, w/sauce & meatballs, avg | 250 | 258 | 78 | 12.3 | 28.5 | 5.8 | | | 10.3 | 2.2 | 3.9 | 3.9 | 0.00 | 3.93 | 22 | 1000 | 100 | 0 | 100 | | 0.15 | 0.17 | 2.25 | 0.12 | 0.82 | 5.0 | 0.29 | 5.0 | | | 52 | 0.3 | 3.3 | 20 | | 112 | 245 | 22.0 | 1220 | 2.39 |
| | | Spreads | | | | | | | | | | | | | | | | | | | | | | | | | | | | | | | | | | | | | | | | |
| 16273 | 1/4 cup | Chunky Chicken, Underwood | 55 | 120 | | 9.0 | 2.0 | 0.0 | 0.5 | 1.5 | 8.0 | 2.5 | | | | | 40 | 0 | 0 | 0 | 0 | 0 | | | | | | | | 0.0 | | | 0 | | 0.7 | | | | | | 470 | |
| 12906 | 1 ea | Deviled Ham, 3.1 oz can, Red Devil | 88 | 310 | | 11.0 | 18.0 | 1.0 | 0.0 | 17.0 | 22.0 | 6.0 | | | | | 50 | 0 | 0 | 0 | 0 | 0 | | | | | | | | 0.0 | | | 20 | | 2.7 | | | | | | 680 | |
| 12908 | 1/4 cup | Deviled Ham, Underwood | 56 | 160 | | 8.0 | 0.0 | 0.0 | 0.0 | 0.0 | 14.0 | 4.5 | | | | | 45 | 0 | 0 | 0 | 0 | 0 | | | | | | | | 0.0 | | | 0 | | 1.1 | | | | | | 440 | |
| 12905 | 1 ea | Honey Ham, 3.1 oz can, Red Devil | 88 | 320 | | 11.0 | 19.0 | 1.0 | 1.0 | 17.0 | 22.0 | 6.0 | | | | | 50 | 0 | 0 | 0 | 0 | 0 | | | | | | | | 0.0 | | | 20 | | 1.8 | | | | | | 560 | |
| 12907 | 1/4 cup | Honey Ham, Underwood | 56 | 170 | | 8.0 | 1.0 | 0.0 | 1.0 | 0.0 | 15.0 | 5.0 | | | | | 25 | 0 | 0 | 0 | 0 | 0 | | | | | | | | 0.0 | | | 0 | | 0.7 | | | | | | 330 | |
| 82035 | 1 ea | Tamales, can, Old El Paso | 69 | 111 | 71 | 2.3 | 10.4 | 1.7 | 0.0 | 8.7 | 6.4 | 2.3 | 2.7 | 0.5 | | | 10 | | | | | | | | | | | | | | | | 13 | | 0.6 | | | | | | 198 | |
| | | *DRY AND PREPARED MEALS, ENTREES AND DISHES* | | | | | | | | | | | | | | | | | | | | | | | | | | | | | | | | | | | | | | | | |
| | | *MEAT DISHES* | | | | | | | | | | | | | | | | | | | | | | | | | | | | | | | | | | | | | | | | |
| | | Beef & Potatoes | | | | | | | | | | | | | | | | | | | | | | | | | | | | | | | | | | | | | | | | |
| 56151 | 1 cup | With Cheese Sauce, avg | 249 | 513 | 62 | 33.9 | 23.3 | 2.4 | | | 31.7 | 14.4 | 12.2 | 2.2 | | | 117 | 589 | 121 | 109 | 12 | | 0.15 | 0.45 | 6.60 | 0.57 | 3.25 | 23.2 | | 7.4 | | | 314 | 0.2 | 3.0 | 55 | | 431 | 759 | | 889 | 6.50 |
| 56148 | 1 cup | With Cream Sauce, avg | 252 | 310 | 75 | 24.5 | 23.5 | 1.7 | | | 12.9 | 4.7 | 4.9 | 1.9 | | | 68 | 394 | 100 | 91 | 9 | | 0.20 | 0.39 | 3.81 | 0.52 | 2.24 | 17.6 | | 6.7 | | | 141 | 0.2 | 2.4 | 50 | | 297 | 685 | | 917 | 5.37 |
| 56147 | 1 cup | With Mushroom Soup, avg | 252 | 328 | 73 | 27.4 | 24.0 | 2.0 | | | 12.9 | 4.3 | 4.1 | 2.9 | | | 78 | 22 | 5 | 5 | 1 | | 0.17 | 0.30 | 4.37 | 0.50 | 2.62 | 18.9 | | 7.3 | | | 53 | 0.3 | 3.4 | 40 | | 272 | 580 | | 645 | 6.99 |
| 57118 | 1 cup | Beef Chili w/beans, prep f/mix, Basic American | 240 | 303 | 74 | 20.0 | 33.0 | 7.5 | 3.1 | 22.4 | 10.2 | 3.6 | | | | | 44 | | | | | | 0.19 | 0.23 | 4.20 | | | | | 24.0 | | | 109 | | 4.0 | | | 265 | 737 | | 967 | |
| | | Chicken | | | | | | | | | | | | | | | | | | | | | | | | | | | | | | | | | | | | | | | | |
| 16180 | 1 cup | With BBQ Sauce, Chef Mate | 254 | 200 | 80 | 18.0 | 22.0 | 4.0 | 8.0 | 10.0 | 6.0 | 2.0 | | | | | 60 | 600 | 120 | | | | | | | | | | | 2.4 | | | 80 | | 2.2 | | | | | | 740 | |
| 15925 | 1 cup | With Cheese Sauce, avg | 241 | 362 | 71 | 41.8 | 10.0 | 0.4 | 1.9 | 7.8 | 16.3 | 6.5 | 5.5 | 2.7 | | | 130 | 233 | 70 | 70 | 0 | | 0.15 | 0.46 | 11.19 | 0.63 | 0.88 | 12.7 | | 1.0 | | | 265 | 0.1 | 1.6 | 51 | | 424 | 530 | | 781 | 2.95 |
| 56213 | 1 cup | With Dumplings, avg | 244 | 373 | 71 | 26.9 | 19.6 | 0.6 | | | 20.0 | 5.7 | 8.1 | 4.5 | | | 95 | 171 | 49 | 48 | 1 | | 0.21 | 0.30 | 9.50 | 0.31 | 0.32 | 10.7 | | 1.9 | | | 110 | 0.1 | 2.3 | 34 | | 249 | 303 | | 1005 | 1.94 |
| 56214 | 1 cup | With Stuffing, avg | 200 | 270 | 70 | 35.1 | 18.0 | 0.7 | | | 5.5 | 1.4 | 1.7 | 1.4 | | | 104 | 62 | 19 | 19 | 0 | | 0.15 | 0.28 | 12.67 | 0.42 | 0.36 | 20.0 | | 2.9 | | | 50 | 0.1 | 2.1 | 44 | | 304 | 384 | | 446 | 2.47 |
| | | Chicken Breast | | | | | | | | | | | | | | | | | | | | | | | | | | | | | | | | | | | | | | | | |
| 15918 | 1 ea | With BBQ Sauce, avg | 123 | 235 | 65 | 28.5 | 2.8 | 0.6 | | | 11.4 | 3.1 | 4.4 | 2.6 | | | 90 | 295 | 52 | 34 | 18 | | 0.07 | 0.18 | 9.53 | 0.46 | 0.31 | 6.3 | | 1.4 | | | 17 | 0.1 | 1.4 | 30 | | 199 | 276 | | 256 | 1.94 |
| 15908 | 1 ea | With Gravy, avg | 129 | 172 | 75 | 19.5 | 3.6 | 0.3 | | | 8.4 | 2.2 | 3.4 | 1.7 | | | 57 | 277 | 83 | 83 | 0 | | 0.05 | 0.14 | 6.06 | 0.30 | 0.27 | 5.1 | | 0.0 | | | 23 | 0.1 | 1.1 | 17 | | 142 | 224 | | 436 | 1.85 |
| 15912 | 1 ea | With Mushroom Soup Sauce, avg | 129 | 188 | 72 | 21.1 | 4.2 | 0.1 | | | 9.2 | 2.6 | 2.7 | 3.0 | | | 63 | 49 | 14 | 14 | 0.3 | | 0.06 | 0.17 | 6.65 | 0.33 | 0.31 | 6.1 | | 0.5 | | | 35 | 0.1 | 1.0 | 21 | | 161 | 217 | | 470 | 1.72 |
| 16226 | 1 cup | Chicken Fajita, prep f/mix, Orval Kent | 212 | 348 | | 30.3 | 9.1 | 3.0 | 3.0 | 3.0 | 21.2 | 4.5 | | | | | 114 | 0 | 0 | 0 | 0 | 0 | | | | | | | | 9.1 | | | 61 | | 2.2 | | | | | | 742 | |

| Code | Amount | Description | Basic Components | | | | | | | | | Additional Fats | | | | | | Vit A & Components | | | | | Vitamins | | | | | | | | | | Minerals | | | | | | | | | |
|---|---|---|---|---|---|---|---|---|---|---|---|---|---|---|---|---|---|---|---|---|---|---|---|---|---|---|---|---|---|---|---|---|---|---|---|---|---|---|---|---|---|---|
| | | | Weight (g) | Calories | % Water | Protein (g) | Carbs (g) | Fiber (g) | Sugar (g) | Other Carbs (g) | Fat (g) | Sat Fat (g) | Mono Fat (g) | Poly Fat (g) | Omega 3 (g) | Omega 6 (g) | Cholest (mg) | Vit A (IU) | Vit A (RE) | Retinol (RE) | Carotenoids (RE) | Beta Carotene (mcg) | Thiamin (mg) | Riboflavin (mg) | Niacin (NE) | Vit B6 (mg) | Vit B12 (mcg) | Folate (mcg) | Panto (mg) | Vit C (mg) | Vit D (mg) | Vit E (α TE) | Calcium (mg) | Copper (mg) | Iron (mg) | Magnes (mg) | Mang (mg) | Phos (mg) | Potassium (mg) | Selenium (mcg) | Sodium (mg) | Zinc (mg) |
| 57536 | 7 oz | Chicken Stir Fry, Chicken Helper | 198 | 330 | | 21.0 | 35.0 | | | | 11.0 | | | | | | | 80 | 16 | | | | 0.15 | 0.34 | 5.00 | | | | | | | | | | | | | | 250 | | 980 | |
| 56246 | 1 ea | Frankfurter, w/sauerkraut, avg | 120 | 158 | 78 | 5.8 | 4.4 | 1.9 | | | 13.2 | 4.9 | 6.2 | 1.3 | | | 23 | 14 | 2 | 0 | 2 | | 0.11 | 0.07 | 1.29 | 0.16 | 0.58 | 19.6 | | 22.7 | | | 28 | 0.1 | 1.6 | 14 | | 54 | 203 | | 1000 | 0.97 |
| 56142 | 1 cup | Frankfurters, w/tomato sauce, avg | 244 | 425 | 72 | 15.3 | 11.9 | 1.8 | | | 35.5 | 13.0 | 16.6 | 3.4 | | | 61 | 1145 | 115 | 0 | 115 | | 0.31 | 0.21 | 4.53 | 0.33 | 1.49 | 12.7 | | 45.2 | | | 32 | 0.3 | 2.3 | 37 | | 144 | 659 | | 2098 | 2.53 |
| 57608 | 1 cup | Ham & Potatoes, w/gravy, avg | 252 | 255 | 78 | 20.5 | 20.9 | 1.8 | | | 9.5 | 3.2 | 4.3 | 1.1 | | | 55 | 2 | 1 | 1 | 0 | | 0.56 | 0.26 | 5.87 | 0.50 | 0.53 | 16.4 | | 25.3 | | | 23 | 0.3 | 1.7 | 40 | | 260 | 816 | | 980 | 2.40 |
| 56182 | 1 cup | Lamb & Potatoes, w/gravy, avg | 252 | 255 | 79 | 20.4 | 19.8 | 1.8 | | | 10.1 | 4.0 | 4.1 | 0.9 | | | 66 | 0 | 0 | 0 | 0 | 0 | 0.14 | 0.22 | 6.43 | 0.34 | 1.95 | 27.1 | | 14.6 | | | 28 | 0.3 | 2.4 | 43 | | 219 | 759 | | 408 | 4.79 |
| 56183 | 1 cup | Lamb & Potatoes, w/tomato sauce, avg | 252 | 265 | 78 | 20.8 | 21.9 | 2.5 | | | 10.2 | 4.0 | 4.1 | 1.0 | | | 66 | 290 | 29 | 0 | 29 | | 0.17 | 0.24 | 6.79 | 0.38 | 1.95 | 30.0 | | 21.8 | | | 38 | 0.4 | 2.7 | 50 | | 229 | 867 | | 489 | 4.84 |
| 19412 | 1 cup | Mussels, w/tomato sauce, avg | 240 | 269 | 73 | 30.1 | 23.7 | 3.5 | | | 5.6 | 1.1 | 1.3 | 1.5 | | | 67 | 754 | 144 | 104 | 41 | | 0.42 | 0.52 | 4.42 | 0.21 | 25.92 | 103.2 | | 25.0 | | | 74 | 0.3 | 9.0 | 89 | | 386 | 912 | | 1488 | 3.94 |
| 56181 | 1 cup | Pork & Potatoes, w/cheese sauce, avg | 249 | 388 | 70 | 26.1 | 20.0 | 1.9 | | | 22.8 | 10.0 | 8.7 | 2.4 | | | 82 | 484 | 99 | 89 | 10 | | 0.53 | 0.43 | 5.14 | 0.49 | 0.78 | 14.9 | | 16.2 | | | 259 | 0.2 | 1.4 | 47 | | 421 | 687 | | 1267 | 3.25 |
| 19414 | 1 cup | Scallops, w/cheese sauce, avg | 244 | 271 | 75 | 33.7 | 14.6 | 0.4 | | | 9.6 | 4.6 | 2.6 | 1.3 | | | 85 | 296 | 89 | 89 | 0 | | 0.18 | 0.33 | 1.61 | 0.18 | 1.99 | 19.4 | | 1.1 | | | 398 | 0.4 | 3.5 | 85 | | 586 | 795 | | 1035 | 3.84 |
| 19410 | 1 cup | Shrimp, w/lobster sauce, avg | 185 | 289 | 68 | 34.8 | 7.3 | 0.6 | | | 12.2 | 2.5 | 3.4 | 5.0 | | | 257 | 137 | 41 | 40 | 0 | | 0.20 | 0.20 | 4.95 | 0.27 | 1.56 | 24.0 | | 3.2 | | | 83 | 0.4 | 3.8 | 59 | | 366 | 420 | | 993 | 2.33 |
| 18803 | 1 cup | Tuna, w/white sauce, avg | 257 | 410 | 69 | 31.7 | 11.8 | 0.4 | | | 25.7 | 7.1 | 10.0 | 6.7 | | | 137 | 808 | 238 | 223 | 15 | | 0.11 | 0.45 | 10.35 | 0.17 | 2.47 | 22.4 | | 0.9 | | | 173 | 0.1 | 1.7 | 43 | | 415 | 382 | | 813 | 1.49 |
| 16901 | 1 cup | Turkey, w/gravy, avg | 244 | 266 | 77 | 38.1 | 6.4 | 0.5 | | | 8.5 | 2.7 | 2.3 | 2.3 | | | 93 | 0 | 0 | 0 | 0 | 0 | 0.10 | 0.32 | 8.10 | 0.56 | 0.57 | 10.8 | | 0.0 | | | 34 | 0.2 | 3.0 | 34 | | 290 | 490 | | 805 | 4.69 |
| 57613 | 1 cup | Turkey & Potatoes, w/gravy, avg | 242 | 283 | 77 | 18.4 | 22.2 | 1.7 | | | 13.0 | 3.8 | 5.4 | 2.9 | | | 53 | 106 | 30 | 28 | 3 | | 0.14 | 0.17 | 5.29 | 0.38 | 0.14 | 14.6 | | 14.6 | | | 24 | 0.3 | 1.8 | 36 | | 143 | 624 | | 1089 | 1.55 |
| 56216 | 1 ea | Turkey Cake, Patty or Croquet, avg | 62 | 161 | 54 | 10.4 | 7.7 | 0.3 | | | 9.6 | 2.6 | 3.9 | 2.5 | | | 30 | 236 | 60 | 55 | 5 | | 0.06 | 0.13 | 2.98 | 0.10 | 0.14 | 5.0 | | 0.7 | | | 43 | 0.0 | 0.7 | 14 | | 93 | 126 | | 228 | 0.77 |
| 56217 | 1 ea | Turkey Meatball, w/breading, avg | 28 | 48 | 65 | 5.7 | 2.0 | 0.1 | | | 1.7 | 0.5 | 0.6 | 0.4 | | | 24 | 50 | 10 | 8 | 2 | | 0.03 | 0.06 | 1.72 | 0.09 | 0.08 | 3.4 | | 1.0 | | | 13 | 0.0 | 0.3 | 6 | | 46 | 62 | | 115 | 0.43 |
| 11901 | 1 pce | Veal, w/gravy, avg | 65 | 94 | 72 | 10.9 | 1.4 | 0.1 | | | 4.7 | 2.0 | 1.9 | 0.3 | | | 38 | 0 | 0 | 0 | 0 | 0 | 0.03 | 0.10 | 2.15 | 0.13 | 0.58 | 5.3 | | 0.0 | | | 6 | 0.1 | 0.5 | 10 | | 92 | 133 | | 185 | 1.35 |
| | | *PASTA AND PASTA/RICE* | | | | | | | | | | | | | | | | | | | | | | | | | | | | | | | | | | | | | | | | |
| | | Beef & Noodles | | | | | | | | | | | | | | | | | | | | | | | | | | | | | | | | | | | | | | | | |
| 56157 | 1 cup | With Cream Sauce, avg | 249 | 408 | 69 | 27.8 | 22.6 | 1.2 | | | 22.3 | 7.1 | 9.0 | 4.3 | | | 90 | 769 | 197 | 180 | 17 | | 0.25 | 0.45 | 4.21 | 0.43 | 2.58 | 17.2 | | 1.0 | | | 164 | 0.1 | 3.1 | 47 | | 331 | 518 | | 779 | 4.20 |
| 56156 | 1 cup | With Gravy, avg | 249 | 306 | 74 | 32.8 | 18.4 | 1.6 | | | 10.6 | 4.0 | 4.4 | 0.6 | | | 97 | 11 | 3 | 3 | 0 | | 0.23 | 0.29 | 5.35 | 0.49 | 2.92 | 15.1 | | 0.0 | | | 17 | 0.2 | 4.1 | 37 | | 289 | 483 | | 807 | 5.68 |
| 56159 | 1 cup | With Mushroom Soup, avg | 249 | 381 | 69 | 33.8 | 22.4 | 1.5 | | | 16.4 | 6.5 | 5.2 | 3.6 | | | 107 | 53 | 14 | 13 | 1 | | 0.21 | 0.38 | 5.51 | 0.51 | 3.04 | 15.9 | | 0.8 | | | 75 | 0.2 | 4.0 | 47 | | 339 | 540 | | 767 | 5.57 |
| 56153 | 1 cup | With Tomato Sauce, avg | 249 | 281 | 75 | 30.1 | 20.8 | 2.7 | | | 8.3 | 2.9 | 3.4 | 0.6 | | | 92 | 971 | 99 | 3 | 96 | | 0.26 | 0.31 | 5.76 | 0.63 | 2.79 | 19.8 | | 12.8 | | | 25 | 0.3 | 4.1 | 55 | | 289 | 779 | | 687 | 4.89 |
| 56152 | 1 cup | Without Sauce, avg | 156 | 270 | 64 | 26.3 | 17.8 | 1.6 | | | 9.6 | 3.0 | 4.0 | 1.2 | | | 89 | 125 | 33 | 30 | 2 | | 0.22 | 0.24 | 4.41 | 0.43 | 2.46 | 13.1 | | 0.0 | | | 14 | 0.1 | 3.3 | 36 | | 240 | 354 | | 668 | 4.19 |
| 56158 | 1 cup | Beef Stroganoff w/noodles, avg | 256 | 343 | 75 | 20.0 | 20.8 | 1.6 | | | 19.8 | 7.7 | 5.5 | 4.9 | | | 74 | 294 | 73 | 65 | 8 | | 0.20 | 0.40 | 4.32 | 0.22 | 1.88 | 19.0 | | 2.1 | | | 69 | 0.3 | 3.3 | 36 | | 253 | 456 | | 453 | 3.74 |
| 57534 | 1 cup | Beef Stroganoff, Hamburger Helper | 124 | 390 | | 22.0 | 30.0 | 2.2 | | | 20.0 | 7.3 | 8.1 | 1.9 | | | 90 | 40 | 12 | | | | 0.30 | 0.34 | 5.00 | 0.18 | | | | 0.0 | | | 100 | | 2.7 | | | | | | 870 | |
| 56197 | 1 cup | Chicken & Noodles, w/cheese sauce, avg | 224 | 334 | 68 | 27.1 | 30.3 | 2.3 | | | 11.1 | 4.4 | 3.6 | 1.9 | | | 101 | 173 | 52 | 52 | 0 | | 0.24 | 0.36 | 5.44 | 0.24 | 0.57 | 14.4 | | 0.9 | | | 199 | 0.1 | 2.3 | 47 | | 300 | 323 | | 674 | 2.17 |
| 56200 | 1 cup | Chicken & Noodles, w/tomato sauce, avg | 224 | 287 | 72 | 20.7 | 28.9 | 3.4 | | | 9.9 | 2.2 | 3.8 | 2.8 | | | 72 | 1239 | 172 | 72 | 100 | | 0.25 | 0.23 | 5.83 | 0.32 | 0.19 | 16.4 | | 12.9 | | | 34 | 0.3 | 2.8 | 47 | | 177 | 513 | | 717 | 1.88 |
| 56227 | 1 cup | Fish & Noodles, w/mushroom soup, avg | 224 | 262 | 75 | 17.6 | 25.6 | 1.8 | | | 9.7 | 2.8 | 2.4 | 3.7 | | | 40 | 148 | 39 | 37 | 2 | | 0.15 | 0.19 | 7.71 | 0.19 | 1.52 | 9.4 | | 0.8 | | | 74 | 0.2 | 2.2 | 34 | | 179 | 231 | | 1093 | 1.26 |
| 56170 | 1 cup | Ham & Noodle Casserole, w/cream sauce, avg | 244 | 400 | 68 | 24.8 | 29.0 | 1.8 | | | 20.3 | 6.8 | 8.1 | 4.3 | | | 71 | 639 | 150 | 136 | 14 | | 0.38 | 0.47 | 4.30 | 0.25 | 0.65 | 12.6 | | 0.7 | | | 195 | 0.2 | 1.9 | 46 | | 329 | 434 | | 1430 | 2.53 |
| 56178 | 1 cup | Ham & Noodles, w/o sauce, avg | 157 | 243 | 66 | 21.0 | 21.4 | 1.9 | | | 7.6 | 2.0 | 3.3 | 1.6 | | | 66 | 156 | 41 | 38 | 3 | | 0.62 | 0.24 | 4.66 | 0.35 | 0.55 | 8.7 | | 0.0 | | | 16 | 0.1 | 2.0 | 31 | | 214 | 239 | | 1118 | 2.26 |
| 56184 | 1 cup | Lamb & Noodles, w/gravy, avg | 249 | 356 | 73 | 22.0 | 26.8 | 2.1 | | | 17.4 | 4.2 | 7.5 | 4.3 | | | 80 | 613 | 158 | 146 | 13 | | 0.27 | 0.28 | 5.46 | 0.13 | 1.58 | 21.9 | | 0.3 | | | 22 | 0.2 | 3.0 | 35 | | 197 | 254 | | 700 | 3.51 |
| 38163 | 1 cup | Rice A Roni, w/pasta, cooked | 202 | 246 | 72 | 5.1 | 43.2 | 5.1 | 3.4 | 34.7 | 5.7 | 1.1 | 2.3 | 1.9 | 0.09 | 1.82 | 2 | 0 | 0 | 0 | 0 | 0 | 0.25 | 0.16 | 3.60 | 0.20 | 0.12 | 88.9 | 0.58 | 0.4 | 0.0 | | 16 | 0.0 | 1.9 | 24 | 0.4 | 75 | 85 | | 1147 | 0.57 |
| 38286 | 1/2 cup | Rice A Roni, w/pasta, dry | 82 | 302 | 7 | 7.7 | 61.7 | 1.5 | 4.9 | 55.3 | 2.0 | 0.4 | 0.5 | 0.8 | 0.04 | 0.75 | 2 | 0 | 0 | 0 | 0 | 0 | 0.62 | 0.22 | 5.75 | 0.12 | 0.16 | 170.6 | 0.55 | 0.5 | 0.0 | | 38 | 0.2 | 3.3 | 33 | 0.9 | 130 | 171 | 26.2 | 1530 | 0.99 |
| 56177 | 1 cup | Sausage & Noodles w/cream sauce, avg | 244 | 398 | 68 | 17.5 | 33.6 | 3.3 | | | 21.4 | 11.7 | 6.8 | 1.5 | | | 78 | 989 | 188 | 134 | 54 | | 0.32 | 0.34 | 2.34 | 0.16 | 0.52 | 31.1 | | 12.3 | | | 290 | 0.2 | 2.2 | 41 | | 393 | 276 | | 1091 | 2.24 |
| 56219 | 1 cup | Scallops & Noodles w/cheese sauce, avg | 224 | 363 | 67 | 30.5 | 26.7 | 1.5 | | | 15.5 | 5.6 | 5.3 | 3.2 | | | 87 | 672 | 179 | 167 | 12 | | 0.22 | 0.29 | 2.34 | 0.14 | 1.47 | 20.7 | | 0.5 | | | 293 | 0.4 | 4.1 | 78 | | 491 | 605 | | 728 | 3.79 |
| 56228 | 1 cup | Shellfish & Noodles w/tomato sauce, avg | 224 | 251 | 75 | 15.2 | 33.5 | 3.4 | | | 6.0 | 1.2 | 2.1 | 1.8 | | | 81 | 497 | 97 | 70 | 26 | | 0.27 | 0.17 | 3.04 | 0.14 | 8.99 | 18.3 | | 9.1 | | | 52 | 0.3 | 5.1 | 47 | | 197 | 284 | | 340 | 1.44 |
| 56220 | 1 cup | Shrimp & Noodles w/cheese sauce, avg | 224 | 349 | 69 | 28.4 | 23.6 | 1.5 | | | 15.2 | 5.7 | 5.4 | 3.2 | | | 220 | 789 | 215 | 202 | 12 | | 0.17 | 0.27 | 3.73 | 0.17 | 1.64 | 15.8 | | 2.4 | | | 222 | 0.3 | 4.2 | 58 | | 302 | 329 | | 697 | 2.44 |
| 70577 | 1 ea | Spaghetti, w/beef, pkg, Dining Lite | 255 | 220 | 82 | 12.0 | 25.0 | | | | 8.0 | | | | | | 20 | 1000 | 200 | | | | 0.15 | 0.17 | 2.00 | | | | | 12.0 | | | 80 | | 2.7 | | | | 570 | | 440 | |
| | | Tuna | | | | | | | | | | | | | | | | | | | | | | | | | | | | | | | | | | | | | | | | |
| 56221 | 1 cup | Casserole, w/cream sauce, avg | 224 | 432 | 62 | 28.4 | 33.2 | 2.1 | | | 20.0 | 5.0 | 7.7 | 5.7 | | | 47 | 682 | 177 | 164 | 13 | | 0.22 | 0.33 | 10.01 | 0.13 | 1.70 | 14.8 | | 0.5 | | | 130 | 0.1 | 2.6 | 47 | | 323 | 284 | | 500 | 1.35 |
| 56222 | 1 cup | Casserole, w/mushroom soup, avg | 224 | 403 | 64 | 27.1 | 31.5 | 2.2 | | | 18.0 | 4.3 | 5.9 | 6.4 | | | 40 | 353 | 93 | 87 | 6 | | 0.18 | 0.26 | 10.10 | 0.11 | 1.65 | 13.6 | | 0.8 | | | 81 | 0.2 | 2.6 | 40 | | 287 | 240 | | 883 | 1.42 |
| 57535 | 1 cup | Creamy Noodle, Tuna Helper | 138 | 300 | | 14.0 | 30.0 | 1.7 | | | 14.0 | 4.2 | 4.7 | 4.9 | | | 5 | 60 | 50 | | | | 0.22 | 0.17 | 6.00 | 0.13 | | | | 0.1 | | | 40 | | 1.1 | | | | | | 960 | |
| | | Turkey & Noodles | | | | | | | | | | | | | | | | | | | | | | | | | | | | | | | | | | | | | | | | |
| 56196 | 1 cup | With Cream Sauce, avg | 224 | 327 | 70 | 22.6 | 28.9 | 1.9 | | | 12.8 | 4.2 | 4.7 | 2.8 | | | 85 | 410 | 106 | 98 | 8 | | 0.24 | 0.34 | 4.91 | 0.20 | 0.39 | 14.3 | | 0.8 | | | 141 | 0.1 | 2.2 | 40 | | 237 | 287 | | 732 | 2.00 |
| 56192 | 1 cup | With Gravy, avg | 224 | 307 | 73 | 19.8 | 24.2 | 1.9 | | | 13.8 | 3.9 | 5.6 | 3.1 | | | 76 | 119 | 34 | 31 | 3 | | 0.21 | 0.20 | 5.03 | 0.17 | 0.19 | 10.7 | | 0.2 | | | 25 | 0.1 | 2.2 | 29 | | 150 | 148 | | 1066 | 1.63 |
| 56194 | 1 cup | With Mushroom Soup, avg | 224 | 314 | 72 | 22.9 | 26.8 | 2.0 | | | 12.2 | 3.6 | 3.2 | 4.1 | | | 83 | 86 | 24 | 23 | 1 | | 0.20 | 0.27 | 5.49 | 0.20 | 0.34 | 12.6 | | 0.9 | | | 74 | 0.2 | 2.3 | 36 | | 202 | 233 | | 588 | 2.20 |
| 56190 | 1 cup | Without Sauce, avg | 157 | 261 | 66 | 21.7 | 22.2 | 2.0 | | | 8.7 | 2.4 | 3.3 | 2.0 | | | 85 | 50 | 15 | 15 | 0 | | 0.20 | 0.18 | 5.25 | 0.20 | 0.22 | 10.1 | | 0.0 | | | 20 | 0.1 | 2.2 | 30 | | 157 | 140 | | 218 | 1.83 |
| 57614 | 1 cup | Turkey Tetrazzini | 246 | 371 | 72 | 19.1 | 28.4 | 1.6 | | | 19.8 | 6.9 | 6.0 | 5.3 | | | 49 | 496 | 115 | 98 | 18 | | 0.19 | 0.25 | 5.02 | 0.20 | 0.31 | 13.2 | | 5.3 | | | 145 | 0.2 | 2.0 | 32 | | 219 | 202 | | 814 | 2.01 |
| 56185 | 1 cup | Veal & Noodles, w/cream sauce, avg | 224 | 390 | 67 | 27.5 | 20.4 | 1.0 | | | 21.5 | 7.0 | 8.5 | 4.1 | | | 112 | 695 | 178 | 163 | 15 | | 0.20 | 0.48 | 5.32 | 0.22 | 1.48 | 18.9 | | 0.7 | | | 168 | 0.2 | 1.9 | 43 | | 307 | 399 | | 726 | 5.06 |
| 56186 | 1 cup | Venison & Noodles, w/cream sauce, avg | 249 | 354 | 72 | 27.2 | 20.9 | 1.1 | | | 17.4 | 5.5 | 6.7 | 4.1 | | | 105 | 711 | 182 | 167 | 15 | | 0.27 | 0.67 | 5.38 | 0.23 | 4.35 | 12.6 | | 0.9 | | | 152 | 0.3 | 4.1 | 42 | | 301 | 428 | | 717 | 2.61 |
| | | *RICE/GRAIN DISHES* | | | | | | | | | | | | | | | | | | | | | | | | | | | | | | | | | | | | | | | | |
| | | Beef & Rice | | | | | | | | | | | | | | | | | | | | | | | | | | | | | | | | | | | | | | | | |
| 56165 | 1/2 cup | With Cream Sauce, avg | 124 | 226 | 66 | 11.7 | 16.5 | 0.4 | | | 12.2 | 4.3 | 5.1 | 1.7 | | | 37 | 217 | 64 | 58 | 6 | | 0.11 | 0.15 | 2.85 | 0.16 | 1.19 | 6.9 | | 0.3 | | | 63 | 0.1 | 1.5 | 19 | | 125 | 186 | | 513 | 2.23 |
| 56164 | 1/2 cup | With Gravy, avg | 111 | 160 | 71 | 10.3 | 14.1 | 0.4 | | | 6.5 | 2.6 | 2.8 | 0.3 | | | 30 | 0 | 0 | 0 | 0 | 0 | 0.10 | 0.08 | 2.73 | 0.13 | 0.97 | 4.9 | | 0.0 | | | 10 | 0.1 | 1.5 | 12 | | 87 | 141 | | 412 | 2.23 |
| 56166 | 1/2 cup | With Mushroom Soup, avg | 124 | 206 | 68 | 10.3 | 16.6 | 0.4 | | | 10.6 | 3.7 | 3.6 | 2.2 | | | 31 | 56 | 14 | 13 | 1 | | 0.08 | 0.13 | 2.77 | 0.13 | 1.00 | 6.3 | | 0.5 | | | 47 | 0.1 | 1.5 | 16 | | 108 | 171 | | 529 | 2.12 |
| 56168 | 1/2 cup | With Soy Sauce, avg | 122 | 172 | 73 | 10.8 | 11.3 | 0.6 | | | 9.0 | 3.2 | 3.4 | 1.4 | | | 34 | 15 | 1 | 0 | 1 | | 0.07 | 0.11 | 2.94 | 0.14 | 1.09 | 9.6 | | 1.5 | | | 23 | 0.1 | 1.6 | 15 | | 96 | 200 | | 495 | 2.28 |
| 56161 | 1/2 cup | With Tomato Sauce, avg | 122 | 168 | 71 | 9.5 | 17.5 | 1.7 | | | 6.8 | 2.9 | 3.0 | 0.3 | | | 24 | 765 | 75 | 0 | 76 | | 0.13 | 0.10 | 2.75 | 0.21 | 0.76 | 8.9 | | 20.2 | | | 17 | 0.2 | 1.7 | 28 | | 115 | 394 | | 387 | 1.47 |
| 56160 | 1/2 cup | Without Sauce, avg | 98 | 197 | 61 | 11.8 | 16.3 | 0.3 | | | 8.8 | 3.2 | 3.8 | 0.7 | | | 38 | 67 | 17 | 16 | 1 | | 0.11 | 0.09 | 3.30 | 0.17 | 1.24 | 5.5 | | 0.0 | | | 12 | 0.1 | 1.7 | 16 | | 100 | 147 | | 364 | 2.46 |
| 57340 | 1/4 cup | Beef Flavored Rice, dry, Golden Saute | 30 | 113 | 12 | 3.0 | 21.1 | 0.5 | 0.5 | 20.2 | 2.0 | 0.7 | | | | | 0 | 0 | 0 | 0 | 0 | 0 | | | | | | | | 0.0 | | | 0 | | 0.5 | | | | | | 457 | |
| 66064 | 1/4 cup | Boil-in-a-Bag Rice, dry, Minute | 22 | 84 | 8 | 1.8 | 18.5 | 0.0 | 0.0 | 13.5 | 0.0 | 0.0 | 0.0 | 0.0 | 0.00 | 0.00 | 0 | 0 | 0 | 0 | 0 | 0 | 0.10 | 0.00 | 0.70 | | | | | 0.0 | | | 0 | | 0.6 | | | | 7 | | 4 | |
| 66068 | 1/4 cup | Brown Rice, instant, dry, Minute | 22 | 87 | | 2.0 | 17.4 | 1.0 | 0.0 | 16.4 | 0.8 | 0.0 | | | 0.00 | 0.00 | 0 | 0 | 0 | 0 | 0 | 0 | 0.03 | 0.00 | 0.82 | | | | | 0.0 | | | 0 | | 0.2 | | | | 20 | | 5 | |
| 57343 | 1/4 cup | Chicken Broth Rice, dry, Golden Saute | 32 | 128 | 10 | 3.0 | 23.1 | 1.0 | 1.5 | 20.7 | 2.2 | 0.7 | | | | | 0 | 0 | 0 | 0 | 0 | 0 | | | | | | | | 2.4 | | | 0 | | 0.5 | | | | | | 394 | |
| 57339 | 1/4 cup | Chicken Flavored Rice, dry, Golden Saute | 31 | 120 | 10 | 3.0 | 22.0 | 0.5 | 1.5 | 20.0 | 2.5 | 1.0 | | | | | 0 | 0 | 0 | 0 | 0 | 0 | | | | | | | | 0.0 | | | 0 | | 0.5 | | | | | | 460 | |
| | | Chicken & Rice | | | | | | | | | | | | | | | | | | | | | | | | | | | | | | | | | | | | | | | | |
| 56210 | 1/2 cup | Teriyaki, Hamburger Helper | 122 | 161 | 70 | 20.8 | 11.0 | 0.1 | | | 3.3 | 0.8 | 0.9 | 0.9 | | | 63 | 37 | 12 | 12 | 0 | | 0.12 | 0.16 | 7.85 | 0.28 | 0.22 | 6.1 | | 1.8 | | | 31 | 0.1 | 1.3 | 33 | | 187 | 266 | | 360 | 1.59 |

| Code | Amount | Description | Basic Components | | | | | | | | | Additional Fats | | | | | | Vit A & Components | | | | | Vitamins | | | | | | | | | | Minerals | | | | | | | | | |
|---|---|---|---|---|---|---|---|---|---|---|---|---|---|---|---|---|---|---|---|---|---|---|---|---|---|---|---|---|---|---|---|---|---|---|---|---|---|---|---|---|---|---|
| | | | Weight (g) | Calories | % Water | Protein (g) | Carbs (g) | Fiber (g) | Sugar (g) | Other Carbs (g) | Fat (g) | Sat Fat (g) | Mono Fat (g) | Poly Fat (g) | Omega 3 (g) | Omega 6 (g) | Choles (mg) | Vit A (IU) | Vit A (RE) | Retinol (RE) | Carotenoids (RE) | Beta Carotene (mcg) | Thiamin (mg) | Riboflavin (mg) | Niacin (NE) | Vit B6 (mg) | Vit B12 (mcg) | Folate (mcg) | Panto (mg) | Vit C (mg) | Vit D (mg) | Vit E (α TE) | Calcium (mg) | Copper (mg) | Iron (mg) | Magnes (mg) | Mang (mg) | Phos (mg) | Potassium (mg) | Selenium (mcg) | Sodium (mg) | Zinc (mg) |
| 56204 | 1/2 cup | With Cream Sauce, avg | 124 | 185 | 70 | 11.2 | 16.2 | 0.6 | | | 8.2 | 2.3 | 3.2 | 2.0 | | | 31 | 318 | 80 | 72 | 8 | | 0.13 | 0.13 | 3.75 | 0.16 | 0.21 | 6.7 | | 0.9 | | | 57 | 0.1 | 1.1 | 17 | | 114 | 157 | | 381 | 1.00 |
| 56206 | 1/2 cup | With Mushroom Soup, avg | 124 | 217 | 66 | 13.1 | 17.2 | 0.4 | | | 10.3 | 2.3 | 3.9 | 3.4 | | | 31 | 462 | 97 | 77 | 21 | | 0.10 | 0.08 | 5.95 | 0.20 | 0.15 | 3.2 | | 0.6 | | | 29 | 0.1 | 1.3 | 20 | | 129 | 187 | | 575 | 0.77 |
| 56208 | 1/2 cup | With Tomato Sauce, avg | 122 | 123 | 75 | 10.2 | 17.5 | 1.7 | | | 1.4 | 0.3 | 0.4 | 0.3 | | | 27 | 781 | 81 | 5 | 76 | | 0.13 | 0.09 | 4.51 | 0.24 | 0.09 | 8.7 | | 20.9 | | | 20 | 0.1 | 1.3 | 29 | | 110 | 361 | | 397 | 0.91 |
| 56202 | 1/2 cup | Without Sauce, avg | 98 | 154 | 67 | 10.8 | 17.5 | 0.3 | | | 3.9 | 1.1 | 1.5 | 0.9 | | | 29 | 17 | 5 | 5 | 0 | | 0.12 | 0.06 | 2.97 | 0.15 | 0.07 | 3.9 | | 0.0 | | | 12 | 0.1 | 1.1 | 16 | | 79 | 84 | | 347 | 0.95 |
| | | Couscous | | | | | | | | | | | | | | | | | | | | | | | | | | | | | | | | | | | | | | | | |
| 56894 | 1/2 cup | Asparagus Au Gratin, Casbah Sahara | 124 | 76 | | 5.5 | 12.0 | 0.3 | | | 1.1 | | | | | | | | | | | | | | | | | | | | | | | | | | | | 147 | | 186 | |
| 56895 | 1/2 cup | Cheddar Broccoli, Meal in a Cup, Casbah Sahara | 124 | 55 | | 2.2 | 9.8 | 0.3 | | | 1.1 | | | | | | | | | | | | | | | | | | | | | | | | | | | | 71 | | 175 | |
| 56896 | 1/2 cup | Hearty Harvest, Casbah Sahara | 124 | 76 | | 2.7 | 15.8 | 1.1 | | | 0.3 | | | | | | | | | | | | | | | | | | | | | | | | | | | | 175 | | 202 | |
| 56828 | 1/2 cup | Moroccan, Spice Hunter | 117 | 72 | | 3.1 | 12.4 | | | | 1.0 | | | | | | | | | | | | | | | | | | | | | | | | | | | | 144 | | 98 | |
| | | Fish & Rice | | | | | | | | | | | | | | | | | | | | | | | | | | | | | | | | | | | | | | | | |
| 56225 | 1/2 cup | With Cream Sauce, avg | 124 | 188 | 70 | 11.2 | 17.6 | 0.4 | | | 7.8 | 2.4 | 3.1 | 2.0 | | | 17 | 370 | 95 | 87 | 8 | | 0.10 | 0.15 | 4.82 | 0.15 | 0.96 | 5.7 | | 0.4 | | | 82 | 0.1 | 1.1 | 22 | | 128 | 182 | | 207 | 0.66 |
| 56226 | 1/2 cup | With Mushroom Soup, avg | 124 | 160 | 73 | 10.2 | 16.4 | 0.4 | | | 5.6 | 1.7 | 1.4 | 2.2 | | | 12 | 85 | 22 | 21 | 2 | | 0.09 | 0.10 | 4.87 | 0.14 | 0.92 | 5.1 | | 0.5 | | | 46 | 0.1 | 1.2 | 19 | | 103 | 149 | | 689 | 0.71 |
| 56224 | 1/2 cup | With Tomato Sauce, avg | 124 | 143 | 73 | 10.2 | 19.2 | 0.5 | | | 2.7 | 0.8 | 0.9 | 0.8 | 0.00 | 0.00 | 11 | 339 | 48 | 21 | 27 | | 0.10 | 0.08 | 5.08 | 0.18 | 0.88 | 7.3 | | 24.4 | | | 38 | 0.1 | 1.6 | 19 | | 99 | 217 | | 641 | 0.58 |
| 38145 | 1/2 cup | Fried Rice, w/bean sprouts & scallions, avg | 83 | 132 | 68 | 2.7 | 17.0 | 0.7 | 0.5 | 15.8 | 5.9 | 0.9 | 1.5 | 3.1 | | | 22 | 47 | 10 | 8 | 2 | | 0.10 | 0.05 | 1.12 | 0.07 | 0.06 | 11.0 | | 2.0 | | | 15 | 0.1 | 0.9 | 12 | | 46 | 67 | | 143 | 0.44 |
| 57346 | 1/4 cup | Fried Rice, dry, Golden Saute | 30 | 120 | 10 | 2.5 | 23.5 | 0.5 | 1.0 | 22.0 | 0.5 | 0.0 | | | | | 0 | 100 | 20 | | | | | | | | | | | 0.0 | | | 0 | | 0.9 | | | | | | 450 | |
| 56171 | 1/2 cup | Ham & Rice, w/mushroom soup, avg | 124 | 167 | 71 | 8.9 | 17.2 | 0.4 | | | 6.7 | 2.1 | 1.9 | 2.2 | | | 16 | 58 | 15 | 13 | 1 | | 0.23 | 0.14 | 2.22 | 0.16 | 0.25 | 4.6 | | 0.5 | | | 46 | 0.1 | 0.9 | 16 | | 112 | 160 | | 940 | 1.14 |
| 56179 | 1/2 cup | Ham & Rice, w/o sauce, avg | 98 | 147 | 66 | 10.8 | 16.5 | 0.3 | | | 3.6 | 1.0 | 1.6 | 0.7 | | | 21 | 75 | 19 | 18 | 2 | | 0.35 | 0.10 | 2.72 | 0.23 | 0.26 | 3.3 | | 0.0 | | | 10 | 0.1 | 1.0 | 16 | | 112 | 140 | | 608 | 1.22 |
| 57355 | 1/4 cup | Herb & Butter Rice, dry, Golden Saute | 30 | 120 | 10 | 3.0 | 21.0 | 0.5 | 1.0 | 19.5 | 2.5 | 1.0 | | | | | 1 | 0 | 0 | 0 | 0 | 0 | | | | | | | | 0.0 | | | 0 | | 0.5 | | | | | | 435 | |
| 66066 | 1/4 cup | Long Grain Rice, dry, Minute | 22 | 85 | 10 | 1.5 | 18.0 | 0.0 | 0.0 | 18.0 | 0.0 | 0.0 | 0.0 | 0.0 | 0.00 | 0.00 | 0 | 0 | 0 | 0 | 0 | 0 | 0.08 | 0.00 | 0.10 | | | | | 0.0 | | | 0 | | 0.5 | | | | 10 | | 2 | |
| 66067 | 1/4 cup | Long Grain/Wild Rice Mix, dry, Minute | 22 | 79 | 10 | 2.1 | 17.2 | 0.3 | 0.7 | 16.2 | 0.2 | 0.0 | | | 0.00 | 0.00 | 0 | 0 | 0 | 0 | 0 | 0 | 0.08 | 0.00 | 0.69 | | | | | 0.0 | | | 7 | | 0.6 | | | | 33 | | 327 | |
| 57345 | 1/4 cup | Onion Mushroom Rice, dry, Golden Saute | 30 | 118 | 8 | 3.0 | 22.1 | 1.0 | 1.0 | 20.2 | 2.0 | 0.7 | | | | | 0 | 0 | 0 | 0 | 0 | 0 | | | | | | | | 0.0 | | | 0 | | 0.5 | | | | | | 418 | |
| 57341 | 1/4 cup | Oriental Rice, dry, Golden Saute | 30 | 118 | 11 | 3.0 | 21.1 | 0.5 | 0.5 | 20.2 | 2.2 | 0.7 | | | | | 0 | 0 | 0 | 0 | 0 | 0 | | | | | | | | 0.6 | | | 0 | | 0.5 | | | | | | 448 | |
| 66065 | 1/4 cup | Original Rice, dry, Minute | 22 | 85 | 8 | 2.0 | 18.5 | 0.0 | 0.0 | 18.5 | 0.0 | 0.0 | 0.0 | 0.0 | 0.00 | 0.00 | 0 | 0 | 0 | 0 | 0 | 0 | 0.08 | 0.00 | 0.60 | | | | | 0.0 | | | 0 | | 0.5 | | | | 5 | | 2 | |
| 56173 | 1/2 cup | Pork & Rice, w/tomato sauce, avg | 122 | 173 | 70 | 12.1 | 18.0 | 0.7 | | | 5.5 | 2.0 | 2.4 | 0.5 | | | 31 | 261 | 27 | 1 | 26 | | 0.42 | 0.13 | 3.03 | 0.26 | 0.24 | 6.0 | | 3.7 | | | 17 | 0.1 | 1.2 | 22 | | 120 | 271 | | 572 | 1.22 |
| | | Sausage & Rice | | | | | | | | | | | | | | | | | | | | | | | | | | | | | | | | | | | | | | | | |
| 56176 | 1/2 cup | With Cheese Sauce, avg | 122 | 224 | 65 | 10.3 | 16.5 | 0.4 | | | 12.8 | 5.2 | 5.1 | 1.5 | | | 35 | 94 | 28 | 28 | 0 | | 0.30 | 0.21 | 1.88 | 0.16 | 0.73 | 4.6 | | 1.1 | | | 150 | 0.1 | 0.8 | 21 | | 174 | 248 | | 734 | 1.10 |
| 56175 | 1/2 cup | With Mushroom Soup, avg | 122 | 220 | 67 | 8.0 | 16.0 | 0.4 | | | 13.5 | 4.5 | 4.9 | 3.0 | | | 26 | 13 | 3 | 3 | 0.3 | | 0.30 | 0.13 | 2.26 | 0.14 | 0.59 | 3.8 | | 1.1 | | | 40 | 0.1 | 1.0 | 13 | | 100 | 172 | | 813 | 1.20 |
| 56174 | 1/2 cup | With Tomato Sauce, avg | 122 | 250 | 60 | 10.2 | 22.1 | 1.7 | | | 13.1 | 4.5 | 5.8 | 1.6 | | | 34 | 338 | 16 | 0 | 16 | | 0.42 | 0.13 | 3.08 | 0.23 | 0.71 | 13.6 | | 4.7 | | | 24 | 0.1 | 1.3 | 17 | | 115 | 260 | | 725 | 1.33 |
| 57344 | 1/4 cup | Savory Herb Rice, dry, Golden Saute | 30 | 118 | 11 | 3.0 | 21.1 | 0.5 | 1.0 | 19.7 | 2.2 | 0.7 | | | | | 0 | 0 | 0 | 0 | 0 | 0 | | | | | | | | 0.0 | | | 0 | | 0.5 | | | | | | 443 | |
| | | Spanish Rice | | | | | | | | | | | | | | | | | | | | | | | | | | | | | | | | | | | | | | | | |
| 56131 | 1/2 cup | Average | 122 | 109 | 78 | 2.5 | 20.8 | 1.9 | | | 1.9 | 0.3 | 0.7 | 0.7 | | | 0 | 581 | 58 | 0 | 58 | | 0.12 | 0.04 | 1.50 | 0.16 | 0.00 | 10.2 | | 19.6 | | | 35 | 0.1 | 1.2 | 21 | | 48 | 272 | | 162 | 0.42 |
| 57342 | 1/4 cup | Dry, Golden Saute | 32 | 123 | 12 | 3.0 | 22.6 | 1.0 | 3.0 | 18.7 | 2.2 | 0.7 | | | | | 0 | 98 | 20 | | | | | | | | | | | 0.6 | | | 0 | | 0.7 | | | | | | 448 | |
| 56998 | 1/2 cup | Old El Paso | 123 | 65 | 85 | 1.5 | 14.0 | 1.0 | 1.0 | 12.0 | 0.5 | | | | | | 0 | | | | | | | | | | | | | | | | | | 0.4 | | | | | | 670 | |
| 57240 | 1/2 cup | Stuffing Mix, long grain/wild rice, Stove Top | 30 | 110 | 8 | 4.0 | 22.0 | 0.5 | 3.0 | 18.5 | 1.0 | 0.0 | | | 0.00 | 0.00 | 0 | 0 | 0 | 0 | 0 | 0 | 0.09 | 0.07 | 0.80 | | | | | 0.0 | | | 20 | | 1.1 | | | | 75 | | 490 | |
| 56223 | 1/2 cup | Tuna & Rice, w/mushroom soup, avg | 124 | 180 | 70 | 11.0 | 16.1 | 0.5 | | | 7.6 | 2.0 | 2.1 | 2.8 | | | 9 | 193 | 34 | 22 | 12 | | 0.08 | 0.11 | 4.50 | 0.08 | 0.68 | 5.4 | | 4.4 | | | 45 | 0.1 | 1.1 | 19 | | 143 | 146 | | 515 | 0.74 |
| | | *OTHER BEAN AND VEGETARIAN DISHES* | | | | | | | | | | | | | | | | | | | | | | | | | | | | | | | | | | | | | | | | |
| | | Chili | | | | | | | | | | | | | | | | | | | | | | | | | | | | | | | | | | | | | | | | |
| 56327 | 1 oz | With Kidney Beans, dry mix, Basic American | 28 | 106 | 6 | 4.6 | 19.6 | 4.5 | 1.8 | 13.3 | 1.0 | 0.1 | 0.1 | 0.5 | | | | 0 | 0 | 0 | 0 | 0 | 0.10 | 0.08 | 0.78 | 0.00 | | | | 14.4 | | | 61 | | 1.7 | | | 107 | 351 | | 553 | |
| 57117 | 1/2 cup | With Kidney Beans, prep f/mix, Basic American | 120 | 88 | 78 | 3.9 | 16.5 | 3.8 | 1.5 | 11.2 | 0.8 | 0.1 | | | | | 0 | | | | | | 0.09 | 0.06 | 0.65 | | | | | 12.0 | | | 52 | | 1.4 | | | 90 | 293 | | 462 | |
| 56911 | 1/2 cup | Mild Veg, w/black beans, fat free, Health Valley | 120 | 80 | 80 | 7.0 | 15.0 | 7.0 | 4.0 | 4.0 | 0.0 | 0.0 | 0.0 | 0.0 | 0.00 | 0.00 | 0 | 5000 | 1000 | | | | | | | | | | | 12.0 | | | 20 | | 1.8 | | | | | | 160 | |
| 56910 | 1/2 cup | Mild Veg, w/3 beans, fat free, Health Valley | 120 | 120 | 81 | 7.0 | 15.0 | 7.0 | 4.0 | 4.0 | 0.0 | 0.0 | 0.0 | 0.0 | 0.00 | 0.00 | 0 | 5000 | 1000 | | | | | | | | | | | 12.0 | | | 20 | | 1.8 | | | | | | 160 | |
| 56909 | 1/2 cup | Spicy Veg, w/black beans, fat free, Health Valley | 120 | 120 | 81 | 7.0 | 15.0 | 7.0 | 4.0 | 4.0 | 0.0 | 0.0 | 0.0 | 0.0 | 0.00 | 0.00 | 0 | 5000 | 1000 | | | | | | | | | | | 12.0 | | | 20 | | 1.8 | | | | | | 160 | |
| 56898 | 1/2 cup | Jambalaya, Meal in a Cup, Casbah Sahara | 124 | 55 | | 1.6 | 12.0 | 1.1 | | | 0.0 | 0.0 | 0.0 | 0.0 | 0.00 | 0.00 | | | | | | | | | | | | | | | | | | | | | | | | | 213 | |
| 56897 | 1/2 cup | La Fiesta, Meal in a Cup, Casbah Sahara | 124 | 76 | | 2.7 | 14.7 | 1.6 | | | 0.3 | | | | | | | | | | | | | | | | | | | | | | | | | | | | | | 175 | |
| 56899 | 1/2 cup | Pasta Fasul, Meal in a Cup, Casbah Sahara | 124 | 71 | | 4.9 | 5.5 | 1.1 | | | 0.0 | 0.0 | 0.0 | 0.0 | 0.00 | 0.00 | | | | | | | | | | | | | | | | | | | | | | | | | 208 | |
| 56900 | 1/2 cup | Thai Yum, Meal in a Cup, Casbah Sahara | 124 | 71 | | 1.6 | 13.1 | 1.1 | | | 0.0 | 0.0 | 0.0 | 0.0 | 0.00 | 0.00 | | | | | | | | | | | | | | | | | | | | | | | | | 208 | |
| | | **FROZEN/REFRIGERATED MEALS, ENTREES, DISHES AND PIZZAS** | | | | | | | | | | | | | | | | | | | | | | | | | | | | | | | | | | | | | | | | |
| | | *BREAKFASTS* | | | | | | | | | | | | | | | | | | | | | | | | | | | | | | | | | | | | | | | | |
| | | Biscuits | | | | | | | | | | | | | | | | | | | | | | | | | | | | | | | | | | | | | | | | |
| 56600 | 1 ea | With Egg, avg | 136 | 316 | 51 | 11.1 | 24.2 | 0.3 | | | 20.3 | 6.2 | 8.2 | 4.2 | | | 233 | 649 | 178 | 159 | 20 | | 0.34 | 0.34 | 0.71 | 0.08 | 0.75 | 61.2 | 1.05 | 0.0 | | | 154 | 0.1 | 3.1 | 20 | 0.3 | 185 | 160 | 27.3 | 654 | 1.10 |
| 56601 | 1 ea | With Egg & Bacon, avg | 150 | 458 | 47 | 17.0 | 28.7 | 0.8 | | | 31.1 | 8.0 | 13.4 | 7.5 | 0.53 | 6.93 | 352 | 191 | 53 | 47 | 6 | | 0.14 | 0.23 | 2.40 | 0.14 | 1.03 | 60.0 | 1.22 | 2.7 | | | 189 | 0.1 | 3.7 | 24 | 0.3 | 238 | 250 | 30.9 | 999 | 1.63 |
| 56602 | 1 ea | With Egg & Ham, avg | 192 | 442 | 55 | 20.4 | 30.3 | 0.8 | | | 27.1 | 5.9 | 11.0 | 7.7 | 0.50 | 7.20 | 300 | 874 | 240 | 113 | 127 | | 0.67 | 0.60 | 2.00 | 0.27 | 1.19 | 65.3 | 1.67 | 0.0 | | | 221 | 0.1 | 4.6 | 31 | 0.3 | 317 | 319 | 36.9 | 1382 | 2.23 |
| 66028 | 1 ea | With Egg & Sausage, avg | 180 | 581 | 43 | 19.1 | 41.2 | 0.9 | | | 38.7 | 15.0 | 16.4 | 4.4 | 0.25 | 4.20 | 302 | 635 | 164 | 146 | 18 | | 0.50 | 0.45 | 3.60 | 0.20 | 1.37 | 64.8 | 1.53 | 0.0 | | | 155 | 0.1 | 4.0 | 25 | 0.3 | 490 | 320 | 34.2 | 1141 | 2.16 |
| 56603 | 1 ea | With Egg & Steak, avg | 148 | 410 | 52 | 17.9 | 21.3 | | | | 28.4 | 8.6 | 11.7 | 5.8 | | | 272 | 704 | 191 | 170 | 21 | | 0.36 | 0.52 | 3.06 | 0.18 | 1.41 | 56.2 | 1.08 | 0.1 | | | 138 | 0.1 | 5.3 | 25 | 0.2 | 225 | 306 | 31.4 | 888 | 2.80 |
| 66029 | 1 ea | With Egg, Cheese & Bacon, avg | 144 | 477 | 41 | 16.3 | 33.4 | 0.3 | | | 31.4 | 11.4 | 14.2 | 3.5 | 0.15 | 3.35 | 261 | 648 | 166 | 147 | 18 | | 0.30 | 0.43 | 2.30 | 0.10 | 1.05 | 53.3 | 1.18 | 1.6 | | | 164 | 0.1 | 2.5 | 20 | 0.3 | 459 | 230 | 35.6 | 1260 | 1.54 |
| 56604 | 1 ea | With Ham, avg | 113 | 386 | 28 | 13.4 | 43.8 | 0.8 | | | 18.4 | 11.4 | 4.8 | 1.0 | 0.09 | 0.95 | 25 | 133 | 34 | 30 | 4 | | 0.51 | 0.32 | 3.48 | 0.14 | 0.03 | 38.4 | 0.41 | 0.1 | | | 160 | 0.0 | 2.7 | 23 | 0.4 | 554 | 197 | 19.3 | 1433 | 1.65 |
| 66030 | 1 ea | With Sausage, avg | 124 | 485 | 29 | 12.1 | 40.1 | 1.4 | | | 31.7 | 14.3 | 12.8 | 3.0 | 0.27 | 2.76 | 35 | 56 | 14 | 12 | 2 | | 0.40 | 0.29 | 3.27 | 0.11 | 0.51 | 45.9 | 0.36 | 0.1 | | | 128 | 0.0 | 2.6 | 20 | 0.4 | 446 | 198 | 23.2 | 1071 | 1.55 |
| 56605 | 1 ea | With Steak, avg | 141 | 455 | 33 | 13.1 | 44.4 | | | | 25.9 | 6.9 | 11.1 | 6.4 | | | 25 | 65 | 16 | 14 | 2 | | 0.35 | 0.39 | 4.16 | 0.16 | 0.94 | 63.4 | 0.41 | 0.1 | | | 116 | 0.1 | 4.3 | 27 | 0.4 | 204 | 234 | 32.9 | 795 | 2.66 |
| | | Burritos | | | | | | | | | | | | | | | | | | | | | | | | | | | | | | | | | | | | | | | | |
| 70756 | 1 ea | With Sausage, Great Starts | 99 | 240 | 53 | 9.0 | 24.0 | 1.0 | 2.0 | 21.0 | 12.0 | 4.0 | | | | | 90 | 100 | 20 | | | | | | | | | | | 1.2 | | | 60 | | 1.4 | | | | | | 500 | |
| 70753 | 1 ea | With Scrambled Eggs, Great Starts | 99 | 200 | 57 | 8.0 | 25.0 | 2.0 | 2.0 | 21.0 | 8.0 | 3.0 | | | | | 60 | 100 | 20 | | | | | | | | | | | 2.4 | | | 80 | | 1.4 | | | | | | 510 | |
| 70752 | 1 ea | With Scrambled Eggs & Bacon, Great Starts | 99 | 250 | 50 | 10.0 | 27.0 | 1.0 | 3.0 | 23.0 | 11.0 | 4.0 | | | | | 90 | 100 | 20 | | | | | | | | | | | 1.2 | | | 80 | | 1.8 | | | | | | 540 | |
| | | Croissants | | | | | | | | | | | | | | | | | | | | | | | | | | | | | | | | | | | | | | | | |
| 56606 | 1 ea | With Egg & Cheese, avg | 127 | 368 | 46 | 12.8 | 24.3 | | | | 24.8 | 14.1 | 7.5 | 1.4 | | | 216 | 1001 | 255 | 184 | 72 | | 0.19 | 0.38 | 1.51 | 0.10 | 0.77 | 47.0 | 1.05 | 0.1 | | | 244 | 0.1 | 2.2 | 22 | 0.2 | 348 | 174 | 24.5 | 551 | 1.75 |
| 56607 | 1 ea | With Egg, Cheese & Bacon, avg | 129 | 413 | 44 | 16.3 | 23.6 | | | | 28.4 | 15.5 | 9.2 | 1.8 | | | 215 | 472 | 120 | 86 | 34 | | 0.35 | 0.34 | 2.19 | 0.12 | 0.86 | 45.1 | 1.07 | 2.2 | | | 151 | 0.1 | 2.2 | 23 | 0.2 | 276 | 201 | 24.5 | 889 | 1.90 |
| 56608 | 1 ea | With Egg, Cheese & Ham, avg | 152 | 474 | 51 | 19.0 | 24.2 | | | | 33.6 | 17.5 | 11.4 | 2.4 | | | 213 | 451 | 117 | 84 | 33 | | 0.52 | 0.30 | 3.19 | 0.23 | 1.00 | 45.6 | 1.25 | 11.4 | | | 144 | 0.1 | 2.1 | 26 | 0.2 | 336 | 272 | 27.2 | 1081 | 2.17 |
| 56609 | 1 ea | With Egg, Cheese & Sausage, avg | 160 | 523 | 46 | 20.3 | 24.8 | | | | 38.2 | 18.2 | 14.3 | 3.0 | | | 216 | 422 | 109 | 78 | 31 | | 0.99 | 0.32 | 4.00 | 0.11 | 0.90 | 43.2 | 1.31 | 0.2 | | | 144 | 0.1 | 3.0 | 24 | 0.3 | 290 | 283 | 20.6 | 1115 | 2.14 |
| | | French Toast | | | | | | | | | | | | | | | | | | | | | | | | | | | | | | | | | | | | | | | | |
| 56775 | 1 pce | Aunt Jemima | 42 | 82 | 54 | 3.3 | 13.1 | 0.6 | | | 2.2 | 0.5 | 0.6 | 0.5 | | | 23 | 72 | 21 | 21 | 0 | | 0.13 | 0.12 | 1.40 | 0.18 | 0.67 | 18.3 | 0.49 | 0.0 | | | 47 | 0.0 | 1.0 | 7 | 0.0 | 49 | 59 | | 274 | 0.30 |
| 57489 | 1 ea | Bagel, w/maple syrup, Sunny French | 71 | 190 | 41 | 14.1 | 21.0 | 0.0 | 5.7 | 15.3 | 5.3 | 1.3 | 1.7 | 1.3 | 0.07 | 1.23 | 129 | 183 | 37 | | | | 0.03 | 0.15 | 0.15 | 0.04 | 0.35 | 19.2 | 0.39 | 0.0 | | | 40 | 0.0 | 0.7 | 4 | 0.0 | 89 | 68 | | 283 | 0.35 |

| Code | Amount | | Description | Basic Components | | | | | | | | | Additional Fats | | | | | | Vit A & Components | | | | | Vitamins | | | | | | | | | | | Minerals | | | | | | | | | | |
|---|---|---|---|---|---|---|---|---|---|---|---|---|---|---|---|---|---|---|---|---|---|---|---|---|---|---|---|---|---|---|---|---|---|---|---|---|---|---|---|---|---|---|---|
| | | | | Weight (g) | Calories | % Water | Protein (g) | Carbs (g) | Fiber (g) | Sugar (g) | Other Carbs (g) | Fat (g) | Sat Fat (g) | Mono Fat (g) | Poly Fat (g) | Omega 3 (g) | Omega 6 (g) | Chols (mg) | Vit A (IU) | Vit A (RE) | Retinol (RE) | Carotenoids (RE) | Beta Carotene (mcg) | Thiamin (mg) | Riboflavin (mg) | Niacin (NE) | Vit B6 (mg) | Vit B12 (mcg) | Folate (mcg) | Panto (mg) | Vit C (mg) | Vit D (mg) | Vit E (α TE) | Calcium (mg) | Copper (mg) | Iron (mg) | Magnes (mg) | Mang (mg) | Phos (mg) | Potassium (mg) | Selenium (mcg) | Sodium (mg) | Zinc (mg) |
| 56776 | 1 | pce | Cinnamon Swirl, Aunt Jemima | 42 | 82 | 53 | 3.3 | 13.1 | 0.6 | | | 2.2 | 0.5 | 0.6 | 0.5 | | | 20 | 72 | 21 | 21 | 0 | | 0.14 | 0.12 | 1.34 | 0.17 | 0.67 | 23.7 | 0.49 | 0.0 | | | 47 | 0.0 | 1.0 | 7 | 0.1 | 55 | 60 | | 255 | 0.30 |
| 56800 | 1 | ea | Cinnamon Swirl, Great Starts | 156 | 440 | 48 | 14.0 | 35.0 | 2.0 | 11.0 | 22.0 | 28.0 | 12.0 | | | | | 150 | 300 | 60 | | | | 0.34 | 0.38 | 3.00 | | | | | 0.0 | | | 80 | | 1.8 | | | | 184 | | 580 | |
| 42354 | 1 | pce | Sticks, avg | 28 | 102 | 30 | 1.6 | 11.5 | 0.5 | | | 5.8 | 0.9 | 2.5 | 2.0 | 0.13 | 1.78 | 15 | 9 | 3 | 2 | 0.2 | | 0.04 | 0.05 | 0.59 | 0.05 | 0.01 | 16.2 | 0.11 | 0.0 | | | 15 | 0.1 | 0.6 | 5 | 0.0 | 24 | 25 | 4.7 | 99 | 0.18 |
| 42353 | 1 | pce | With Butter, avg | 68 | 180 | 51 | 5.2 | 18.2 | 0.3 | | | 9.5 | 3.9 | 3.6 | 1.2 | | | 58 | 238 | 73 | 68 | 6 | | 0.29 | 0.25 | 1.97 | 0.03 | 0.18 | 36.7 | 0.27 | 0.1 | | | 37 | 0.0 | 1.0 | 8 | 0.1 | 73 | 89 | 10.5 | 258 | 0.30 |
| 56799 | 1 | ea | With Sausage, Great Starts | 156 | 410 | 52 | 13.0 | 33.0 | 3.0 | 8.0 | 22.0 | 26.0 | 9.0 | | | | | 110 | 400 | 80 | | | | 0.42 | 0.37 | 3.60 | 0.20 | | | | 0.0 | | | 100 | | 1.8 | | | | 218 | | 580 | |
| 70762 | 1 | ea | Muffin, w/egg, bacon & cheese, Great Starts | 116 | 290 | 51 | 14.0 | 25.0 | 2.0 | 2.0 | 21.0 | 15.0 | 5.0 | | | | | 95 | 0 | 0 | 0 | 0 | 0 | | | | | | | | 0.0 | | | 150 | | 1.8 | | | | | | 750 | |
| | | | Pancakes | | | | | | | | | | | | | | | | | | | | | | | | | | | | | | | | | | | | | | | | |
| 70761 | 1 | ea | Silver Dollar, w/eggs, Great Starts | 120 | 250 | 60 | 9.0 | 22.0 | 1.0 | 6.0 | 15.0 | 14.0 | 5.0 | | | | | 290 | 0 | 0 | 0 | 0 | 0 | | | | | | | | 0.0 | | | 60 | | 1.4 | | | | | | 540 | |
| 70754 | 1 | ea | With Bacon, Great Starts | 128 | 400 | 40 | 12.0 | 42.0 | 1.0 | 13.0 | 28.0 | 20.0 | 7.0 | | | | | 100 | 0 | 0 | 0 | 0 | 0 | | | | | | | | 0.0 | | | 60 | | 1.1 | | | | | | 1030 | |
| 56801 | 1 | ea | With Sausage, Great Starts | 170 | 490 | 44 | 14.0 | 52.0 | 3.0 | 15.0 | 34.0 | 25.0 | 11.0 | | | | | 90 | 0 | 0 | 0 | 0 | 0 | 0.46 | 0.37 | 3.80 | 0.29 | | | | 0.0 | | | 80 | | 1.8 | | | | 258 | | 950 | |
| | | | Potatoes & Meat | | | | | | | | | | | | | | | | | | | | | | | | | | | | | | | | | | | | | | | | |
| 57128 | 1 | cup | Original Flavor, Morning Classics | 172 | 241 | 73 | 8.0 | 22.0 | 1.0 | 0.0 | 21.0 | 13.8 | 5.2 | | | | | 21 | 0 | 0 | 0 | 0 | 0 | | | | | | | | 8.9 | | | 21 | | 1.1 | | | | | | 931 | |
| 57130 | 1 | cup | Sausage Flavor, Morning Classics | 172 | 241 | 73 | 8.0 | 22.0 | 1.0 | 0.0 | 21.0 | 13.8 | 5.2 | | | | | 21 | 0 | 0 | 0 | 0 | 0 | | | | | | | | 8.9 | | | 21 | | 1.1 | | | | | | 1120 | |
| 57129 | 1 | cup | Smoke Flavor, Morning Classics | 172 | 241 | 73 | 8.0 | 22.0 | 1.0 | 0.0 | 21.0 | 13.8 | 5.2 | | | | | 21 | 0 | 0 | 0 | 0 | 0 | | | | | | | | 8.9 | | | 21 | | 1.1 | | | | | | 850 | |
| | | | Scrambled Eggs | | | | | | | | | | | | | | | | | | | | | | | | | | | | | | | | | | | | | | | | |
| 70757 | 1 | ea | With Bacon, Great Starts | 149 | 290 | 66 | 11.0 | 17.0 | 1.0 | 2.0 | 14.0 | 19.0 | 9.0 | | | | | 240 | 0 | 0 | 0 | 0 | 0 | | | | | | | | 0.0 | | | 60 | | 1.4 | | | | | | 700 | |
| 70758 | 1 | ea | With Sausage, Great Starts | 177 | 360 | 64 | 12.0 | 21.0 | 3.0 | 2.0 | 16.0 | 26.0 | 10.0 | | | | | 280 | 0 | 0 | 0 | 0 | 0 | | | | | | | | 0.0 | | | 60 | | 1.8 | | | | | | 800 | |
| 70129 | 1 | ea | With Sausage & Hash Browns, avg | 177 | 419 | 61 | 15.6 | 19.0 | 1.1 | | | 31.5 | 9.2 | 11.8 | 7.9 | | | 257 | 340 | 102 | 102 | 0 | | 0.36 | 0.40 | 2.96 | 0.27 | 1.09 | 23.2 | | 4.1 | | | 60 | 0.1 | 2.0 | 25 | | 216 | 464 | | 843 | 1.69 |
| | | | *CHILDREN'S MEALS* | | | | | | | | | | | | | | | | | | | | | | | | | | | | | | | | | | | | | | | | |
| 70779 | 1 | ea | Beef Patties, Meal Belly Bust, Swanson | 227 | 480 | 56 | 20.0 | 57.0 | 6.0 | 19.0 | 32.0 | 19.0 | 7.0 | | | | | 45 | 0 | 0 | 0 | 0 | 0 | | | | | | | | 6.0 | | | 60 | | 3.6 | | | | | | 640 | |
| | | | Breakfast | | | | | | | | | | | | | | | | | | | | | | | | | | | | | | | | | | | | | | | | |
| 70773 | 1 | ea | Blast, Five Waffle Sticks, Swanson | 78 | 330 | 20 | 4.0 | 39.0 | 1.0 | 32.0 | 6.0 | 17.0 | 7.0 | | | | | 25 | 0 | 0 | 0 | 0 | 0 | | | | | | | | 0.0 | | | 20 | | 1.1 | | | | | | 250 | |
| 70772 | 1 | ea | Blast, French Toast Sticks, Swanson | 106 | 310 | 40 | 7.0 | 41.0 | 2.0 | 17.0 | 22.0 | 14.0 | 4.0 | | | | | 45 | 500 | 100 | | | | | | | | | | | 0.0 | | | 80 | | 0.7 | | | | | | 300 | |
| 70771 | 1 | ea | Blast, Six Mini Pancakes, Swanson | 120 | 320 | 40 | 7.0 | 54.0 | 2.0 | 24.0 | 28.0 | 8.0 | 4.0 | | | | | 45 | 0 | 0 | 0 | 0 | 0 | | | | | | | | 0.0 | | | 60 | | 0.7 | | | | | | 640 | |
| | | | Chicken | | | | | | | | | | | | | | | | | | | | | | | | | | | | | | | | | | | | | | | | |
| 70774 | 1 | ea | Chompin' Chic Drumlets, Swanson | 255 | 490 | 63 | 16.0 | 51.0 | 3.0 | 19.0 | 29.0 | 25.0 | 9.0 | | | | | 55 | 0 | 0 | 0 | 0 | 0 | | | | | | | | 6.0 | | | 40 | | 1.8 | | | | | | 980 | |
| 70781 | 1 | ea | Frazzlin' Fried Chicken, Swanson | 281 | 580 | 61 | 23.0 | 53.0 | 4.0 | 17.0 | 32.0 | 31.0 | 11.0 | | | | | 95 | 100 | 20 | | | | | | | | | | | 4.8 | | | 60 | | 2.7 | | | | | | 1090 | |
| 16248 | 1 | ea | Fried Chicken, Kids Cuisine | 286 | 440 | 69 | 19.0 | 48.0 | 6.0 | 11.0 | 31.0 | 20.0 | 6.0 | | | | | 65 | 0 | 0 | 0 | 0 | 0 | | | | | | | | 4.8 | | | 60 | | 1.4 | | | | | | 710 | |
| 16224 | 1 | ea | Nuggets, Kids Cuisine | 241 | 360 | 69 | 14.0 | 46.0 | 6.0 | 12.0 | 28.0 | 13.0 | 3.0 | | | | | 30 | 100 | 20 | | | | | | | | | | | 0.0 | | | 80 | | 1.8 | | | | | | 500 | |
| 18824 | 1 | ea | Fish Sticks, Kids Cuisine | 241 | 340 | 69 | 11.0 | 54.0 | 7.0 | 26.0 | 21.0 | 9.0 | 2.0 | | | | | 10 | 0 | 0 | 0 | 0 | 0 | | | | | | | | 0.0 | | | 20 | | 1.8 | | | | | | 820 | |
| 70782 | 1 | ea | Fish Sticks, Swanson | 198 | 370 | 61 | 12.0 | 48.0 | 4.0 | 10.0 | 34.0 | 14.0 | 5.0 | | | | | 30 | 100 | 20 | | | | | | | | | | | 2.4 | | | 60 | | 1.4 | | | | | | 610 | |
| 70585 | 1 | ea | Macaroni & Cheese, w/franks, Kids Cuisine | 255 | 380 | 69 | 9.0 | 55.0 | | | | 14.0 | | | | | | 40 | 64 | 19 | | | | 0.27 | 0.26 | 1.00 | | | | | 6.1 | | | 105 | | 2.0 | | | 160 | 320 | | 1000 | |
| | | | Pizza | | | | | | | | | | | | | | | | | | | | | | | | | | | | | | | | | | | | | | | | |
| 81072 | 1 | ea | Cheese, Kids Cuisine | 194 | 320 | 63 | 10.0 | 53.0 | 5.0 | 17.0 | 31.0 | 8.0 | 3.0 | | | | | 25 | 100 | 20 | | | | | | | | | | | 6.0 | | | 80 | | 1.4 | | | | | | 470 | |
| 70780 | 1 | ea | Cheese, Swanson | 224 | 350 | 63 | 11.0 | 57.0 | 5.0 | 27.0 | 25.0 | 9.0 | 4.5 | | | | | 15 | 100 | 20 | | | | | | | | | | | 2.4 | | | 200 | | 1.4 | | | | | | 500 | |
| 69026 | 1 | ea | Hamburger, Kids Cuisine | 194 | 330 | 63 | 12.0 | 50.0 | 5.0 | 23.0 | 22.0 | 9.0 | 2.5 | | | | | 20 | 200 | 40 | | | | | | | | | | | 6.0 | | | 100 | | 1.4 | | | | | | 440 | |
| | | | Sandwiches | | | | | | | | | | | | | | | | | | | | | | | | | | | | | | | | | | | | | | | | |
| 69024 | 1 | ea | Beef Patty, w/cheese, Kids Cuisine | 177 | 270 | 67 | 10.0 | 40.0 | 5.0 | 22.0 | 13.0 | 7.0 | 4.0 | | | | | 20 | 0 | 0 | 0 | 0 | 0 | | | | | | | | 3.6 | | | 100 | | 1.1 | | | | | | 330 | |
| 69025 | 1 | ea | Chicken, Kids Cuisine | 234 | 440 | 60 | 15.0 | 63.0 | 4.0 | 25.0 | 34.0 | 14.0 | 3.0 | | | | | 20 | 100 | 20 | | | | | | | | | | | 0.0 | | | 60 | | 2.7 | | | | | | 680 | |
| 70783 | 1 | ea | Grilled Cheese, Swanson | 184 | 490 | 45 | 12.0 | 60.0 | 4.0 | 16.0 | 40.0 | 22.0 | 10.0 | | | | | 35 | 0 | 0 | 0 | 0 | 0 | | | | | | | | 2.4 | | | 250 | | 2.7 | | | | | | 930 | |
| 70778 | 1 | ea | Wobblin Wheels & Cheese, Swanson | 312 | 370 | 72 | 12.0 | 59.0 | 2.0 | 28.0 | 29.0 | 10.0 | 5.0 | | | | | 20 | 1750 | 350 | | | | | | | | | | | 2.4 | | | 200 | | 1.4 | | | | | | 560 | |
| 70776 | 1 | ea | Spaghetti, Razzlin' Rings, Swanson | 340 | 390 | 74 | 12.0 | 60.0 | 4.0 | 33.0 | 23.0 | 11.0 | 5.0 | | | | | 20 | 300 | 60 | | | | | | | | | | | 24.0 | | | 60 | | 1.8 | | | | | | 710 | |
| | | | *DINNERS AND MEALS* | | | | | | | | | | | | | | | | | | | | | | | | | | | | | | | | | | | | | | | | |
| 11111 | 1 | ea | Beef, Banquet | 255 | 240 | 79 | 26.0 | 19.0 | 4.0 | 12.0 | 3.0 | 7.0 | 3.0 | | | | | 70 | 200 | 40 | | | | | | | | | | | 6.0 | | | 40 | | 3.6 | | | | | | 660 | |
| 70156 | 1 | ea | Beef, Cannelloni, w/pork, low calorie, avg | 273 | 246 | 80 | 18.2 | 24.6 | 2.3 | | | 8.1 | 3.6 | 3.1 | 0.5 | | | 41 | 4816 | 508 | 40 | 468 | | 0.30 | 0.38 | 3.54 | 0.27 | 1.10 | 44.8 | | 3.8 | | | 150 | 0.3 | 3.0 | 52 | | 232 | 453 | | 606 | 3.31 |
| 11117 | 1 | ea | Beef, Cantonese, Healthy Choice | 326 | 270 | 81 | 22.0 | 32.0 | 5.0 | 4.0 | 23.0 | 6.0 | 2.5 | | | | | 55 | 500 | 100 | | | | | | | | | | | 21.0 | | | 40 | | 1.8 | | | | | | 480 | |
| 70026 | 1 | ea | Beef, Hash, corned, w/apple slices & vegs, avg | 284 | 406 | 69 | 19.8 | 43.6 | 4.0 | | | 17.5 | 6.8 | 6.8 | 1.0 | | | 60 | 354 | 36 | 3 | 33 | | 0.20 | 0.19 | 2.75 | 0.29 | 1.08 | 46.1 | | 13.4 | | | 57 | 0.2 | 2.4 | 40 | | 159 | 415 | | 2363 | 2.91 |
| 70025 | 1 | ea | Beef, Meatballs, Swedish, in sauce w/noodles, avg | 284 | 503 | 67 | 24.9 | 36.2 | 2.3 | | | 27.9 | 12.3 | 10.8 | 2.0 | | | 114 | 303 | 77 | 69 | 7 | | 0.28 | 0.45 | 6.09 | 0.35 | 2.12 | 21.4 | | 0.9 | | | 105 | 0.2 | 3.7 | 45 | | 273 | 423 | | 821 | 4.71 |
| 11026 | 1 | ea | Beef, Meatballs, Swedish, Armour | 284 | 300 | 80 | 18.0 | 20.0 | 4.0 | 2.0 | 14.0 | 17.0 | 7.0 | | | | | 40 | 2500 | 500 | | | | 0.30 | 0.26 | 2.00 | | | | | 0.0 | | | 80 | | 1.8 | | | 230 | 460 | | 940 | |
| | | | Beef, Meatloaf | | | | | | | | | | | | | | | | | | | | | | | | | | | | | | | | | | | | | | | | |
| 11024 | 1 | ea | Armour | 319 | 300 | 80 | 19.0 | 33.0 | 7.0 | 4.0 | 22.0 | 10.0 | 5.0 | | | | | 65 | 200 | 40 | | | | 0.30 | 0.26 | 3.00 | | | | | 12.0 | | | 40 | | 1.8 | | | 260 | 590 | | 600 | |
| 11033 | 1 | ea | Banquet | 269 | 280 | 80 | 12.0 | 23.0 | 4.0 | 2.0 | 17.0 | 17.0 | 7.0 | | | | | 40 | 3000 | 600 | | | | 0.21 | 0.31 | 6.90 | | | | | 42.0 | | | 40 | | 1.8 | | | | 900 | | 1100 | |
| 11107 | 1 | ea | Extra Helping, Banquet | 539 | 650 | 78 | 29.0 | 49.0 | 10.0 | 13.0 | 25.0 | 38.0 | 16.0 | | | | | 85 | 4500 | 900 | | | | | | | | | | | 1700.0 | | | 100 | | 3.6 | | | | | | 2140 | |
| 70766 | 1 | ea | Hungry Man | 468 | 640 | 73 | 24.0 | 65.0 | 6.0 | 25.0 | 34.0 | 31.0 | 14.0 | | | | | 45 | 300 | 60 | | | | | | | | | | | 18.0 | | | 150 | | 5.4 | | | | | | 1370 | |
| 11062 | 1 | ea | Swanson | 305 | 380 | 75 | 19.0 | 37.0 | 5.0 | 13.0 | 13.0 | 14.0 | 6.0 | | | | | 35 | 200 | 40 | | | | | | | | | | | 9.0 | | | 40 | | 3.6 | | | | | | 730 | |
| 57470 | 1 | ea | With Gravy & Mashed Pot, Marie Calendar | 380 | 555 | 75 | 23.6 | 45.2 | 7.2 | 9.2 | 23.8 | 30.8 | 11.3 | | | | | 82 | 205 | 41 | | | | | | | | | | | 4.1 | | | 41 | | 1.1 | | | | | | 1264 | |
| 70122 | 1 | ea | With Tomato sce, potatoes & vegs, avg | 312 | 402 | 74 | 22.2 | 35.9 | 3.7 | | | 19.2 | 5.9 | 7.3 | 2.7 | | | 59 | 901 | 115 | 45 | 71 | | 0.22 | 0.33 | 6.01 | 0.31 | 2.02 | 31.8 | | 25.1 | | | 131 | 0.2 | 3.1 | 50 | | 246 | 686 | | 1214 | 3.93 |
| 70123 | 1 | ea | With Tomato sce, potatoes, veg & dessert, avg | 312 | 493 | 66 | 18.7 | 58.3 | 5.5 | | | 21.7 | 7.5 | 9.1 | 2.9 | | | 78 | 1467 | 204 | 86 | 118 | | 0.29 | 0.38 | 6.05 | 0.37 | 1.21 | 49.1 | | 32.5 | | | 81 | 0.4 | 4.2 | 62 | | 237 | 939 | | 1725 | 3.35 |
| 70124 | 1 | ea | With Tomato sce, vegs & applesauce, avg | 312 | 374 | 75 | 18.5 | 38.9 | 3.6 | | | 16.5 | 5.5 | 7.1 | 2.0 | | | 50 | 3775 | 415 | 58 | 358 | | 0.21 | 0.24 | 5.93 | 0.38 | 1.70 | 35.1 | | 18.2 | | | 47 | 0.3 | 2.7 | 44 | | 203 | 602 | | 933 | 3.53 |
| 70027 | 1 | ea | Beef, Oriental, w/vegetables & rice, low cal, avg | 245 | 289 | 73 | 21.0 | 34.9 | 1.3 | | | 6.4 | 2.1 | 2.6 | 0.7 | | | 54 | 3621 | 362 | 0 | 362 | | 0.18 | 0.22 | 3.53 | 0.32 | 1.84 | 25.8 | | 6.9 | | | 37 | 0.2 | 3.7 | 39 | | 206 | 306 | | 1220 | 5.18 |
| 57123 | 1 | cup | Beef, Oriental, w/vegetables, Chef Mate | 253 | 190 | | 9.0 | 25.0 | 1.0 | 5.0 | 13.0 | 6.0 | 3.5 | | | | | 15 | 3500 | 700 | | | | | | | | | | | 3.6 | | | 20 | | 1.1 | | | | | | 1150 | |
| 11110 | 1 | ea | Beef, Patty, Banquet | 269 | 300 | 80 | 11.0 | 21.0 | 3.0 | 2.0 | 15.0 | 20.0 | 8.0 | | | | | 35 | 3000 | 600 | | | | | | | | | | | 3.6 | | | 40 | | | | | | | | 1060 | |
| | | | Beef, Pepper Steak | | | | | | | | | | | | | | | | | | | | | | | | | | | | | | | | | | | | | | | | |
| 70333 | 1 | ea | La Choy | 283 | 93 | 91 | 5.1 | 19.3 | 3.7 | 10.3 | 5.3 | 0.4 | 0.0 | | | | | 0 | 301 | 60 | | | | | | | | | | | 12.7 | | | 6 | | 6.3 | | | | | | 2468 | |
| 11027 | 1 | ea | Lite, Armour | 312 | 210 | 84 | 16.0 | 29.0 | 5.0 | 5.0 | 19.0 | 4.0 | 1.5 | | | | | 60 | 750 | 150 | | | | 0.15 | 0.26 | 1.60 | | | | | 12.0 | | | 40 | | 1.8 | | | 150 | 320 | | 370 | |
| 70030 | 1 | ea | With Rice & vegetables, avg | 284 | 281 | 78 | 21.7 | 27.5 | 1.7 | | | 9.1 | 2.8 | 3.7 | 1.5 | | | 54 | 2722 | 275 | 5 | 270 | | 0.23 | 0.24 | 4.46 | 0.54 | 1.92 | 32.8 | | 70.9 | | | 40 | 0.2 | 3.5 | 45 | | 219 | 568 | | 366 | 3.54 |
| 70438 | 1 | ea | With Rice, Budget Gourmet | 284 | 300 | 77 | 15.0 | 39.0 | | | | 9.0 | | | | | | 25 | 300 | 60 | | | | 0.15 | 0.17 | 3.00 | | | | | 2.4 | | | 40 | | 0.7 | | | | | | 300 | |
| | | | Beef, Pot Roast | | | | | | | | | | | | | | | | | | | | | | | | | | | | | | | | | | | | | | | | |
| 70402 | 1 | ea | Stouffers | 252 | 270 | 78 | 19.0 | 25.0 | 4.0 | 2.0 | 19.0 | 10.0 | 3.0 | | | | | 40 | 1500 | 300 | | | | 0.38 | 0.14 | 3.00 | | | | | 0.6 | | | 40 | | 1.8 | | | | 700 | | 540 | |
| 11118 | 1 | ea | Yankee, Healthy Choice | 312 | 290 | 80 | 19.0 | 38.0 | 4.0 | 25.0 | 9.0 | 7.0 | 3.0 | | | | | 55 | 2250 | 450 | | | | | | | | | | | 6.0 | | | 40 | | 1.8 | | | | | | 460 | |

| Code | Amount | Description | Weight (g) | Calories | % Water | Protein (g) | Carbs (g) | Fiber (g) | Sugar (g) | Other Carbs (g) | Fat (g) | Sat Fat (g) | Mono Fat (g) | Poly Fat (g) | Omega 3 (g) | Omega 6 (g) | Choles (mg) | Vit A (IU) | Vit A (RE) | Retinol (RE) | Carotenoids (RE) | Beta Carotene (mcg) | Thiamin (mg) | Riboflavin (mg) | Niacin (NE) | Vit B6 (mg) | Vit B12 (mcg) | Folate (mcg) | Panto (mg) | Vit C (mg) | Vit D (mg) | Vit E (α TE) | Calcium (mg) | Copper (mg) | Iron (mg) | Magnes (mg) | Mang (mg) | Phos (mg) | Potassium (mg) | Selenium (mcg) | Sodium (mg) | Zinc (mg) |
|---|---|---|---|---|---|---|---|---|---|---|---|---|---|---|---|---|---|---|---|---|---|---|---|---|---|---|---|---|---|---|---|---|---|---|---|---|---|---|---|---|---|---|
| Basic Components / Additional Fats / Vit A & Components / Vitamins / Minerals | | | | | | | | | | | | | | | | | | | | | | | | | | | | | | | | | | | | | | | | | | |
| 70770 | 1 ea | Yankee, Hungry Man |454|360|82|27.0|48.0|6.0|16.0|26.0|6.0|2.0|||||45|3000|600|||||||||||12.0|||80||4.5||||||1140||
| 70793 | 1 ea | Yankee, Swanson |326|250|83|12.0|39.0|5.0|15.0|19.0|4.5|1.5|||||20|7000|1400|||||||||||6.0|||60||1.8||||||850||
| | | Beef, Salisbury Steak ||||||||||||||||||||||||||||||||||||||||||
| 11034 | 1 ea | Banquet |269|310|78|14.0|28.0|5.0|2.0|21.0|16.0|7.0|||||35|0|0|0|0|0|0.18|0.27|6.70|||||3.6|||40||1.8||||590||910||
| 11105 | 1 ea | Con Queso, Patio |312|390|77|18.0|33.0|10.0|7.0|16.0|20.0|11.0|||||40|300|60|||||||||||3.6|||100||2.7||||||1570||
| 11035 | 1 ea | Extra Helping, Banquet |539|740|76|31.0|52.0|11.0|3.0|38.0|46.0|19.0|||||75|100|20||||0.23|0.34|7.00|||||6.0|||100||3.6|||430|1010||1860||
| 11058 | 1 ea | Healthy Choice |326|330|77|18.0|48.0|6.0|24.0|18.0|7.0|3.0|||||50|1000|200||||0.23|0.26|3.00|||||12.0|||40||1.8|||230|610||470||
| 11028 | 1 ea | Lite, Armour |326|260|82|22.0|26.0|6.0|6.0|14.0|7.0|4.0|||||55|300|60||||0.38|0.26|3.00|||||18.0|||60||2.7|||230|660||860||
| 70791 | 1 ea | Beef, Sandwich, Roast Beef, Swanson |291|350|73|16.0|46.0|6.0|21.0|19.0|12.0|4.5|||||30|200|40|||||||||||12.0|||60||2.7||||||770||
| 11031 | 1 ea | Beef, Sandwich, Salisbury Steak, Banquet |142|220|77|9.0|8.0|2.0|1.0|5.0|16.0|7.0|||||25|0|0|0|0|0||||||||1.2|||20||1.1||||||790||
| | | Beef, Sirloin ||||||||||||||||||||||||||||||||||||||||||
| 70001 | 1 ea | Chopped, w/gravy, potatoes & vegetables, avg |347|559|68|26.5|47.4|5.4|||30.0|14.3|11.8|1.9|||139|917|164|108|56||0.41|0.39|5.57|0.66|2.34|74.8||22.8|||49|0.4|4.0|73||323|802||1974|4.85|
| 70008 | 1 ea | With Gravy, potatoes & vegetables, avg |312|278|80|27.2|20.7|3.8|||9.8|4.4|3.7|0.5|||75|10748|1089|20|1068||0.20|0.33|4.74|0.63|2.09|39.7||38.7|||47|0.3|3.7|53||259|774||977|5.79|
| 70456 | 1 ea | With Herb Sauce, Budget Gourmet |284|290|79|19.0|27.0||||12.0||||||25|200|40||||0.15|0.51|9.00|||||2.4|||60||2.7||||||770||
| | | Beef, Sliced ||||||||||||||||||||||||||||||||||||||||||
| 70732 | 1 ea | With Broccoli, Swanson |284|350|74|11.0|53.0|4.0|25.0|24.0|10.0|5.0|||||30|1750|350|||||||||||15.0|||60||1.8||||||830||
| 56138 | 1 ea | With Carrots, low calorie, avg |284|372|76|27.9|14.1|2.3|||22.5|8.8|9.7|1.0|||97|9241|924|0.3|924||0.12|0.38|7.22|0.54|3.24|23.5||31.9|||71|0.3|3.6|48||258|716||824|5.96|
| 70731 | 1 ea | With Gravy, Swanson |312|460|71|17.0|47.0|3.0|13.0|31.0|22.0|10.0|||||45|100|20|||||||||||6.0|||60||2.7||||||910||
| 70018 | 1 ea | With Gravy, potatoes & vegetables, avg |312|462|74|24.0|24.8|3.2|||28.4|9.7|12.3|4.0|||72|10131|1091|117|974||0.15|0.23|4.71|0.58|2.34|22.5||5.9|||34|0.2|3.2|41||243|665||814|3.84|
| 70019 | 1 ea | With Gravy, potatoes, vegs & dessert, avg |326|375|75|28.6|36.9|3.3|||12.3|3.6|5.2|2.0|||78|578|102|67|36||0.32|0.34|5.90|0.67|2.50|47.4||10.6|||33|0.3|3.7|55||293|688||1294|4.63|
| 70020 | 1 ea | With Gravy, pot, vegs, soup & dessert, avg |425|595|70|32.7|60.8|5.4|||25.8|9.8|10.9|2.0|||89|566|63|10|53||0.41|0.46|7.23|0.56|2.14|47.3||18.9|||64|0.3|5.1|64||366|824||1250|5.04|
| 56088 | 1 ea | With Macaroni, tom sce, vegs & dessert, avg |340|422|72|15.8|59.9|7.0|||14.0|3.8|6.2|2.5|||27|1165|127|13|114||0.27|0.31|5.27|0.45|0.77|37.3|0.40|11.1|0.0||78|0.3|2.9|61||194|585|20.0|809|2.56|
| 70023 | 1 ea | With Noodles & vegetables, avg |298|405|68|13.6|58.9|3.7|||14.1|4.8|5.6|2.4|||30|2594|332|109|224||0.25|0.25|3.44|0.20|0.88|38.0||16.5|||116|0.2|2.0|45||209|465||2757|2.25|
| 56136 | 1 ea | With Potatoes, avg |227|547|54|24.7|48.2|5.4|||28.6|11.5|12.1|2.2|||73|0|0|0|0|0|0.25|0.25|7.90|0.50|2.34|34.0||13.0|||43|0.3|4.0|48||257|792||817|4.74|
| 70021 | 1 ea | With Potatoes & vegetable in sauce, avg |284|389|73|27.7|23.5|3.3|||20.2|7.7|7.9|2.0|||85|3260|353|39|314||0.18|0.32|5.03|0.60|1.93|31.1||39.4|||97|0.4|3.4|48||310|713||954|4.66|
| | | Beef, Steak ||||||||||||||||||||||||||||||||||||||||||
| 16236 | 1 ea | Chicken Fried, Banquet |524|800|72|29.0|73.0|6.0|14.0|53.0|44.0|14.0|||||55|0|0|0|0|0||||||||0.0|||250||2.7||||||2050||
| 70004 | 1 ea | Swiss, w/gravy, potatoes, vegs & dessert, avg |326|430|72|23.4|44.3|5.1|||18.0|6.2|7.5|2.0|||65|8499|852|3|849||0.36|0.35|4.98|0.53|1.82|51.7||18.2|||46|0.4|4.1|55||258|681||799|5.03|
| 70017 | 1 ea | With Potatoes & vegetables, avg |312|346|77|29.3|24.1|3.9|||14.7|5.8|6.0|1.6|||75|1038|133|43|90||0.22|0.36|5.49|0.59|2.31|49.2||51.9|||75|0.3|4.1|56||306|792||933|5.77|
| 70032 | 1 ea | With Rice & vegetables, low calorie, avg |284|304|76|25.0|29.0|1.6|||9.3|3.1|3.7|1.6|||65|765|83|10|73||0.16|0.29|4.17|0.54|2.05|22.8||36.5|||48|0.2|3.3|51||239|517||1065|5.34|
| | | Beef, Tips ||||||||||||||||||||||||||||||||||||||||||
| 11116 | 1 ea | Healthy Choice |319|280|82|20.0|32.0|4.0|18.0|10.0|8.0|3.0|||||50|3000|600|||||||||||42.0|||20||1.8||||||480||
| 70768 | 1 ea | Hungry Man |447|440|78|23.0|53.0|7.0|15.0|31.0|15.0|5.0|||||50|5000|1000|||||||||||9.0|||80||1.8||||||890||
| 70006 | 1 ea | With Gravy, potatoes & vegetables, avg |284|344|77|22.6|21.5|3.8|||18.7|7.6|8.5|1.2|||68|2324|232|0|232||0.24|0.29|4.54|0.57|2.18|36.4||22.8|||31|0.4|3.5|51||239|772||753|4.13|
| 70022 | 1 ea | With Gravy, potatoes & vegs in chs sce, avg |326|388|75|31.8|30.1|4.9|||15.8|6.5|6.3|1.5|||78|1855|222|55|168||0.23|0.40|5.56|0.65|2.39|49.0||44.1|||117|0.4|4.3|62||342|802||1125|6.26|
| 11060 | 1 ea | With Noodles & Gravy, Swanson |283|290|77|16.0|34.0|5.0|15.0|14.0|11.0|5.0|||||50|5000|1000|||||||||||2.4|||40||2.7||||||530||
| 70007 | 1 ea | With Potatoes & vegetables, low cal, avg |333|290|80|25.0|33.6|3.1|||5.9|2.2|2.4|0.5|||67|6770|681|6|675||0.16|0.28|4.59|0.52|2.19|18.6||5.1|||33|0.2|3.1|40||230|589||476|5.15|
| 56081 | 1 ea | Chicken, A La King, w/rice, avg |269|441|69|18.7|41.0|1.4|||22.1|8.0|8.2|4.3|||124|1151|259|221|39||0.30|0.27|6.18|0.37|0.47|18.7|0.44|11.2|0.5||105|0.2|2.5|38||239|309|7.0|1028|1.93|
| 16260 | 1 ea | Chicken, Alfredo, w/broccoli, Healthy Choice |343|316|79|26.3|35.8|2.1|3.2|30.5|7.4|3.2|||||53|105|21|||||||||||2.5|||105||1.9||||||558||
| 70059 | 1 ea | Chicken, Barbecue, w/beans, vegs & dessert, avg |333|506|67|27.8|61.2|7.5|||17.6|4.6|6.5|4.9|||77|589|72|18|54||0.23|0.29|5.47|0.32|0.19|74.8||15.7|||50|0.3|3.1|67||253|606||1026|2.97|
| 16261 | 1 ea | Chicken, Barbecue, Healthy Choice |361|290|76|25.0|57.0|7.0|37.0|13.0|5.0|3.0|||||50|2250|450|||||||||||6.0|||40||1.8||||||450||
| 15939 | 1 ea | Chicken, Burgundy, lite, Armour |284|210|83|20.0|20.0|4.0|2.0|14.0|5.0|1.5|||||45|2500|500||||0.15|0.17|6.00|||||9.0|||40||0.7|||180|510||760||
| 70423 | 1 ea | Chicken, Cacciatore, Budget Gourmet |312|300|80|20.0|27.0||||13.0||||||60|200|40||||0.23|0.51|5.00|||||21.0|||150||1.8||||||810||
| 16259 | 1 ea | Chicken, Cantonese, Healthy Choice |319|293|79|23.0|35.6|2.1|15.7|17.8|6.3|3.1|||||52|3138|628|||||||||||6.3|||42||1.9||||||502||
| 70075 | 1 ea | Chicken, Chow Mein, w/rice, low calorie, avg |319|290|79|19.0|38.0|1.9|||6.3|1.8|2.4|1.4|||48|486|54|8|46||0.21|0.19|5.66|0.34|0.12|29.3||20.0|||45|0.2|2.5|38||163|338||1069|1.81|
| 83007 | 1 ea | Chicken, Chow Mein, Banquet |255|210|82|9.0|28.0|3.0|3.0|22.0|7.0|2.0|||||30|500|100|||||||||||9.0|||20||0.7||||||850||
| 70069 | 1 ea | Chicken, Cordon Bleu, w/vegetables & rice, avg |312|493|65|32.1|59.0|4.9|||13.7|5.0|5.0|2.4|||69|10702|1103|48|1055||0.29|0.42|8.66|0.48|0.41|43.5||14.1|||259|0.3|3.4|66||359|421||1220|2.89|
| 16267 | 1 ea | Chicken, Dijon, Healthy Choice |312|270|78|23.0|33.0|6.0|6.0|21.0|5.0|2.0|||||40|4500|900|||||||||||18.0|||80||1.4||||||470||
| 70048 | 1 ea | Chicken, Divan, avg |241|352|74|22.0|14.5|1.0|||22.2|9.2|8.2|3.3|||87|1049|220|172|48||0.13|0.42|4.62|0.27|0.74|36.3||23.0|||268|0.1|1.6|41||299|405||677|2.10|
| 15956 | 1 ea | Chicken, Dumplings, Banquet |284|260|80|13.0|35.0|3.0|16.0|16.0|8.0|2.5|||||35|2000|400||||0.24|0.25|6.00|||||6.7|||60||2.0||||460||780||
| 81000 | 1 ea | Chicken, Fettucini, Armour |284|230|82|16.0|25.0|6.0|7.0|12.0|8.0||||||25|2500|500||||0.15|0.17|3.00|||||9.0|||80||1.1|||330|400||520||
| | | Chicken, Fried ||||||||||||||||||||||||||||||||||||||||||
| 15952 | 1 ea | Banquet |255|470|67|21.0|35.0|6.0|1.0|28.0|27.0|9.0|||||105|0|0|0|0|0|0.14|0.14|5.00|||||4.8|||80||1.1||||480||960||
| 15984 | 1 ea | Dark Meat, Swanson |281|580|60|24.0|54.0|5.0|17.0|32.0|30.0|10.0|||||105|100|20|||||||||||4.8|||60||2.7||||||1430||
| 15954 | 1 ea | Extra Helping, Banquet |510|790|71|37.0|72.0|8.0|14.0|50.0|39.0|9.0|||||110|0|0|0|0|0|0.23|0.26|6.00|||||0.0|||150||1.8|||180|750||1820||
| 70053 | 1 ea | With Potatoes, avg |227|470|62|24.8|31.4|2.4|||27.0|6.2|9.1|8.2|||68|547|127|117|10||0.30|0.29|7.87|0.32|0.25|14.5||6.7|||73|0.1|2.3|43||232|388||1246|1.90|
| 70060 | 1 ea | With Potatoes, vegs, cornbread & dessert, avg |425|672|67|26.8|80.8|9.1|||28.3|7.3|9.3|6.5|||102|7255|780|88|692||0.57|0.45|8.31|0.40|0.37|48.2||21.5|||178|0.2|3.4|72||421|731||1177|2.33|
| 70058 | 1 ea | With Potatoes, vegetables & dessert, avg |326|590|64|32.6|49.4|6.2|||29.6|7.4|10.5|6.9|||111|2941|323|55|268||0.34|0.39|10.30|0.45|0.36|30.4||12.4|||111|0.2|2.7|62||297|603||1548|2.63|
| 70061 | 1 ea | With Potatoes, vegetables, soup & dessert, avg |425|706|66|37.6|69.0|5.2|||31.2|7.7|10.9|7.3|||123|5202|550|57|493||0.48|0.46|12.55|0.53|0.42|36.7||12.6|||98|0.2|3.6|68||340|676||1182|2.92|
| 15983 | 1 ea | White Meat, Swanson |294|630|58|26.0|62.0|5.0|18.0|39.0|31.0|8.0|||||55|200|40|||||||||||2.4|||100||3.6||||||1700||
| 15933 | 1 ea | Chicken, Glazed, Armour |305|280|82|19.0|20.0|4.0|7.0|9.0|14.0|4.0|||||55|300|60||||0.15|0.26|4.00|||||9.0|||20||1.1|||190|400||740||
| 16263 | 1 ea | Chicken, Herb, Healthy Choice |326|294|85|17.1|41.7|2.8|21.8|17.1|5.7|2.4|||||43|1185|237|||||||||||0.0|||38||0.7||||||512||
| 15996 | 1 ea | Chicken, Hungry Man |489|630|72|26.0|80.0|9.0|22.0|49.0|22.0|6.0|||||55|750|150|||||||||||12.0|||80||4.5||||||1680||
| 70070 | 1 ea | Chicken, Kiev, w/rice & vegetables, avg |227|504|61|25.9|30.9|1.9|||30.3|12.5|11.5|4.6|||104|3332|399|99|301||0.25|0.25|8.21|0.35|0.29|16.3||7.6|||57|0.1|2.2|43||209|300||697|1.27|
| 15931 | 1 ea | Chicken, Mesquite, Armour |270|280|72|21.0|39.0|5.0|16.0|18.0|13.0||||||65|200|40||||0.23|0.17|4.00|||||18.0|||20||1.4|||270|810||630||
| 16262 | 1 ea | Chicken, Mesquite Barbecue, Healthy Choice |298|310|74|18.0|48.0|6.0|15.0|27.0|5.0|2.0|||||55|1750|350|||||||||||9.0|||40||1.4||||||480||
| 15953 | 1 ea | Chicken, Nuggets, Banquet |191|410|59|18.0|38.0|4.0|11.0|23.0|21.0|5.0|||||45|0|0|0|0|0||||||||6.0|||20||1.8||||||650||
| 16269 | 1 ea | Chicken, Nuggets, Morton |198|320|69|13.0|30.0|3.0|12.0|15.0|17.0|4.0|||||30|2000|400|||||||||||2.4|||40||1.4||||||460||
| 70082 | 1 ea | Chicken, Orange, w/rice, low calorie, avg |227|302|70|25.7|36.7|1.1|||4.9|1.2|2.0|1.1|||61|2260|232|8|223||0.07|0.13|6.74|0.37|0.18|17.1||7.6|||41|0.2|1.3|41||186|293||676|1.52|
| 70066 | 1 ea | Chicken, Oriental, fried, w/rice & vegs, avg |276|397|69|30.1|38.0|2.0|||13.2|2.3|3.4|6.5|||69|3180|322|5|317||0.26|0.17|13.48|0.68|0.26|27.2||30.9|||44|0.2|2.6|52||276|408||646|1.58|

| Code | Amount | | Description | Basic Components | | | | | | | | | Additional Fats | | | | | | Vit A & Components | | | | | Vitamins | | | | | | | | | | | Minerals | | | | | | | | | |
|---|---|---|---|---|---|---|---|---|---|---|---|---|---|---|---|---|---|---|---|---|---|---|---|---|---|---|---|---|---|---|---|---|---|---|---|---|---|---|---|---|---|---|---|
| | | | | Weight (g) | Calories | % Water | Protein (g) | Carbs (g) | Fiber (g) | Sugar (g) | Other Carbs (g) | Fat (g) | Sat Fat (g) | Mono Fat (g) | Poly Fat (g) | Omega 3 (g) | Omega 6 (g) | Cholest (mg) | Vit A (IU) | Vit A (RE) | Retinol (RE) | Carotenoids (RE) | Beta Carotene (mcg) | Thiamin (mg) | Riboflavin (mg) | Niacin (NE) | Vit B6 (mg) | Vit B12 (mcg) | Folate (mcg) | Panto (mg) | Vit C (mg) | Vit D (mg) | Vit E (α TE) | Calcium (mg) | Copper (mg) | Iron (mg) | Magnes (mg) | Mang (mg) | Phos (mg) | Potassium (mg) | Selenium (mcg) | Sodium (mg) | Zinc (mg) |
| 70073 | 1 | ea | Chicken, Oriental, w/vegs & rice, low cal, avg | 255 | 482 | 57 | 32.3 | 58.5 | 4.7 | | | 14.3 | 2.9 | 5.1 | 4.9 | | | 71 | 4809 | 485 | 6 | 479 | | 0.18 | 0.27 | 13.64 | 1.03 | 0.29 | 33.5 | | 11.5 | | | 115 | 0.3 | 4.7 | 79 | | 319 | 696 | | 632 | 1.96 |
| | | | Chicken, Parmigiana | | | | | | | | | | | | | | | | | | | | | | | | | | | | | | | | | | | | | | | | |
| 81071 | 1 | ea | Banquet | 269 | 290 | 79 | 14.0 | 27.0 | 3.0 | 3.0 | 21.0 | 15.0 | 4.0 | | | | | 50 | 300 | 60 | | | | | | | | | | | 60.0 | | | 60 | | 1.8 | | | | | | 900 | |
| 81068 | 1 | ea | Extra Helping, Banquet | 539 | 650 | 77 | 24.0 | 64.0 | 9.0 | 9.0 | 46.0 | 33.0 | 3.0 | | | | | 65 | 2250 | 450 | | | | | | | | | | | 108.0 | | | 150 | | 2.7 | | | | | | 1770 | |
| 81007 | 1 | ea | Healthy Choice | 326 | 330 | 77 | 19.0 | 46.0 | 3.0 | 23.0 | 20.0 | 8.0 | 3.0 | | | | | 40 | 3000 | 500 | | | | 0.38 | 0.17 | 6.00 | | | | | 9.0 | | | 60 | | 1.1 | | | 260 | 620 | | 490 | |
| 70063 | 1 | ea | With Vegetables, low calorie, avg | 226 | 301 | 75 | 22.7 | 15.0 | 2.5 | | | 16.8 | 6.2 | 5.7 | 3.4 | | | 56 | 1793 | 246 | 98 | 148 | | 0.16 | 0.29 | 3.65 | 0.25 | 0.37 | 36.1 | | 54.1 | | | 271 | 0.1 | 1.8 | 36 | | 271 | 353 | | 936 | 2.21 |
| | | | Chicken, Patty | | | | | | | | | | | | | | | | | | | | | | | | | | | | | | | | | | | | | | | | |
| 70765 | 1 | ea | Hungry Man | 482 | 700 | 68 | 36.0 | 87.0 | 13.0 | 42.0 | 32.0 | 23.0 | 3.0 | | | | | 90 | 500 | 100 | | | | | | | | | | | 6.0 | | | 100 | | 4.5 | | | | | | 1420 | |
| 16270 | 1 | ea | Morton | 191 | 280 | 73 | 11.0 | 24.0 | 4.0 | 12.0 | 8.0 | 15.0 | 3.0 | | | | | 20 | 3000 | 500 | | | | | | | | | | | 0.0 | | | 40 | | 1.1 | | | | | | 840 | |
| 70056 | 1 | ea | With Potatoes & vegetables, avg | 213 | 447 | 55 | 26.7 | 46.8 | 5.9 | | | 18.0 | 4.8 | 5.0 | 7.1 | | | 58 | 352 | 66 | 47 | 20 | | 0.24 | 0.17 | 12.68 | 0.63 | 0.24 | 37.2 | | 8.2 | | | 28 | 0.2 | 1.7 | 55 | | 258 | 743 | | 852 | 1.24 |
| 70057 | 1 | ea | With Tomato sauce, fettucine & vegs, avg | 326 | 394 | 76 | 30.7 | 27.7 | 3.3 | | | 18.0 | 5.6 | 6.4 | 3.6 | | | 111 | 1446 | 251 | 159 | 92 | | 0.23 | 0.28 | 11.93 | 0.57 | 0.37 | 25.7 | | 18.6 | | | 134 | 0.2 | 2.8 | 68 | | 303 | 479 | | 893 | 1.96 |
| 70064 | 1 | ea | With Vegetables, low calorie, avg | 184 | 256 | 74 | 21.1 | 9.7 | 1.7 | | | 14.4 | 3.1 | 5.9 | 4.3 | | | 53 | 3702 | 390 | 30 | 360 | | 0.10 | 0.20 | 6.19 | 0.38 | 0.26 | 26.7 | | 15.4 | | | 52 | 0.1 | 2.0 | 20 | | 136 | 230 | | 979 | 1.45 |
| 15979 | 1 | ea | Chicken, Sweet & Sour, Healthy Choice | 326 | 376 | 74 | 20.9 | 55.4 | 5.2 | 26.1 | 24.0 | 7.3 | 3.1 | | | | | 47 | 2090 | 418 | | | | 0.30 | 0.15 | 5.02 | | | | | 15.7 | | | 42 | | 1.1 | | | 220 | 470 | | 376 | |
| 70065 | 1 | ea | Chicken, Teriyaki, w/rice & vegetables, avg | 284 | 364 | 73 | 23.9 | 34.2 | 3.0 | | | 14.1 | 4.4 | 5.6 | 2.8 | | | 68 | 17685 | 1303 | 53 | 175 | | 0.20 | 0.22 | 8.32 | 0.57 | 0.22 | 21.8 | | 3.0 | | | 57 | 0.3 | 2.8 | 54 | | 227 | 420 | | 1977 | 2.17 |
| 16266 | 1 | ea | Chicken, Teriyaki, Healthy Choice | 347 | 300 | 80 | 18.9 | 41.2 | 3.3 | 12.2 | 25.6 | 6.7 | 3.3 | | | | | 50 | 1112 | 222 | | | | | | | | | | | 13.3 | | | 22 | | 1.2 | | | | | | 667 | |
| | | | Chicken, W/Noodles | | | | | | | | | | | | | | | | | | | | | | | | | | | | | | | | | | | | | | | | |
| 15957 | 1 | ea | Banquet | 227 | 210 | 81 | 10.0 | 24.0 | 2.0 | 2.0 | 20.0 | 9.0 | 3.0 | | | | | 40 | 50 | 10 | | | | 0.18 | 0.19 | 3.80 | | | | | 0.0 | | | 60 | | 1.4 | | | | 250 | | 810 | |
| 70432 | 1 | ea | With Broccoli, Budget Gourmet | 248 | 450 | 67 | 23.0 | 31.0 | | | | 26.0 | | | | | | 130 | 400 | 80 | | | | 0.23 | 0.17 | 4.00 | | | | | 2.4 | | | 250 | | 1.8 | | | | | | 1110 | |
| 70155 | 1 | ea | With Gravy, vegetables & dessert, avg | 298 | 316 | 77 | 15.2 | 40.2 | 4.1 | | | 10.4 | .9 | 4.0 | 3.5 | | | 39 | 378 | 43 | 7 | 35 | | 0.34 | 0.23 | 4.91 | 0.17 | 0.17 | 37.0 | | 4.8 | | | 30 | 0.2 | 2.9 | 36 | | 161 | 253 | | 942 | 1.52 |
| 70051 | 1 | ea | With Vegetables & dessert, avg | 291 | 393 | 71 | 16.8 | 50.1 | 3.2 | | | 14.0 | 3.5 | 5.8 | 3.6 | | | 49 | 97 | 24 | 21 | 3 | | 0.34 | 0.27 | 4.92 | 0.16 | 0.26 | 41.5 | | 0.6 | | | 44 | 0.6 | 3.2 | 55 | | 210 | 439 | | 1083 | 1.27 |
| 70049 | 1 | ea | Chicken, W/Potatoes, vegs & dessert, avg | 539 | 744 | 72 | 45.5 | 61.4 | 5.0 | | | 35.1 | 3.3 | 13.0 | 8.9 | | | 113 | 1393 | 276 | 217 | 60 | | 0.53 | 0.54 | 15.74 | 0.64 | 0.47 | 56.0 | | 16.5 | | | 113 | 0.3 | 4.7 | 75 | | 431 | 803 | | 2129 | 3.59 |
| 70067 | 1 | ea | Chicken, W/Rice & vegetables, low calorie, avg | 241 | 272 | 75 | 25.1 | 24.9 | 1.6 | | | 7.9 | .7 | 1.9 | 2.6 | | | 63 | 157 | 20 | 6 | 14 | | 0.10 | 0.19 | 10.46 | 0.54 | 0.25 | 14.6 | | 4.3 | | | 36 | 0.2 | 1.6 | 39 | | 217 | 345 | | 815 | 1.55 |
| 70072 | 1 | ea | Chicken, W/Vegetables & rice, avg | 284 | 312 | 75 | 19.0 | 40.1 | 3.4 | | | 8.3 | 2.7 | 3.3 | 1.6 | | | 43 | 1022 | 115 | 19 | 96 | | 0.34 | 0.25 | 9.37 | 0.48 | 0.15 | 29.0 | | 32.5 | | | 45 | 0.5 | 3.6 | 48 | | 222 | 483 | | 727 | 1.70 |
| 15934 | 1 | ea | Chicken, W/Wine & Mushrooms, Amour | 284 | 260 | 81 | 20.0 | 20.0 | 4.0 | 4.0 | 12.0 | 11.0 | 5.0 | | | | | 50 | 3000 | 500 | | | | 0.15 | 0.17 | 6.00 | | | | | 12.0 | | | 60 | | 0.7 | | | 250 | 550 | | 540 | |
| 16247 | 1 | ea | Chicken, White Meat, Banquet | 248 | 470 | 66 | 22.0 | 33.0 | 6.0 | 2.0 | 25.0 | 28.0 | 1[illegible].0 | | | | | 100 | 0 | 0 | 0 | 0 | 0 | | | | | | | | 4.8 | | | 40 | | 1.4 | | | | | | 1100 | |
| 70111 | 1 | ea | Fish, Cake, w/potatoes & vegetables, avg | 255 | 449 | 64 | 28.0 | 35.4 | 4.0 | | | 21.8 | 6.7 | 8.9 | 4.9 | | | 76 | 413 | 55 | 20 | 35 | | 0.41 | 0.28 | 5.41 | 0.53 | 1.13 | 57.4 | | 13.0 | | | 84 | 0.2 | 2.8 | 74 | | 367 | 892 | | 1976 | 1.57 |
| 70112 | 1 | ea | Fish, Cake, w/potatoes, vegs & dessert, avg | 298 | 593 | 61 | 24.9 | 58.5 | 6.0 | | | 29.3 | 6.8 | 9.2 | 11.7 | | | 42 | 498 | 59 | 14 | 45 | | 0.34 | 0.18 | 4.65 | 0.45 | 0.80 | 55.6 | | 13.3 | | | 45 | 0.3 | 2.6 | 75 | | 343 | 852 | | 960 | 1.49 |
| 70107 | 1 | ea | Fish, Cod, w/cheese sauce & vegs, low cal, avg | 262 | 283 | 76 | 31.3 | 18.8 | 2.9 | | | 9.1 | 3.4 | 2.9 | 2.0 | | | 68 | 1413 | 187 | 66 | 120 | | 0.18 | 0.32 | 3.76 | 0.41 | 1.12 | 57.4 | | 58.2 | | | 199 | 0.1 | 1.9 | 76 | | 304 | 579 | | 650 | 1.50 |
| 70106 | 1 | ea | Fish, Cod, w/vegetables, low calorie, avg | 191 | 229 | 77 | 20.4 | 9.1 | 2.8 | | | 12.6 | 2.4 | 3.6 | 5.9 | | | 44 | 6034 | 511 | 11 | 599 | | 0.12 | 0.13 | 2.52 | 0.33 | 0.83 | 41.1 | | 23.5 | | | 57 | 0.1 | 1.0 | 46 | | 246 | 567 | | 493 | 0.71 |
| 70099 | 1 | ea | Fish, Flounder, w/chopped broccoli, low cal, avg | 351 | 270 | 82 | 32.2 | 22.8 | 2.7 | | | 5.5 | 2.5 | 1.4 | 0.8 | | | 67 | 1521 | 226 | 110 | 176 | | 0.23 | 0.42 | 4.74 | 0.40 | 2.01 | 61.7 | | 63.1 | | | 274 | 0.1 | 1.8 | 77 | | 442 | 906 | | 649 | 1.54 |
| 70108 | 1 | ea | Fish, Flounder, w/crm sce, pot&carrots, lo cal, avg | 298 | 286 | 78 | 24.9 | 30.3 | 3.0 | | | 6.1 | .5 | 1.4 | 2.5 | | | 60 | 8219 | 344 | 33 | 811 | | 0.21 | 0.23 | 4.66 | 0.42 | 1.54 | 23.1 | | 14.1 | | | 83 | 0.2 | 1.4 | 54 | | 274 | 706 | | 718 | 1.08 |
| 70098 | 1 | ea | Fish, Haddock, w/chopped spinach, low cal, avg | 255 | 196 | 82 | 25.8 | 13.6 | 0.8 | | | 3.9 | .8 | 1.1 | 0.6 | | | 69 | 2090 | 278 | 104 | 174 | | 0.11 | 0.28 | 4.58 | 0.40 | 1.46 | 50.6 | | 2.8 | | | 229 | 0.1 | 2.3 | 79 | | 347 | 632 | | 479 | 1.13 |
| 70101 | 1 | ea | Fish, Sole, w/vegetables, low calorie, avg | 241 | 214 | 77 | 33.5 | 13.5 | 3.3 | | | 2.7 | 0.6 | 0.6 | 0.8 | | | 77 | 74 | 17 | 14 | 2 | | 0.22 | 0.23 | 5.56 | 0.42 | 2.30 | 61.4 | | 35.9 | | | 67 | 0.1 | 1.6 | 65 | | 340 | 769 | | 1762 | 0.96 |
| 70100 | 1 | ea | Fish, Turbot, w/vegetables, low calorie, avg | 241 | 330 | 73 | 21.1 | 18.7 | 4.0 | | | 19.3 | 3.6 | 10.9 | 2.6 | | | 53 | 7572 | 769 | 17 | 752 | | 0.32 | 0.20 | 3.42 | 0.52 | 0.98 | 31.6 | | 7.8 | | | 41 | 0.1 | 2.2 | 51 | | 253 | 480 | | 1186 | 0.98 |
| 70110 | 1 | ea | Fish, W/Lemon Sauce, potatoes & vegs, avg | 284 | 298 | 77 | 17.4 | 31.8 | 2.6 | | | 10.8 | 4.1 | 2.3 | 3.7 | | | 40 | 521 | 78 | 38 | 40 | | 0.32 | 0.14 | 3.63 | 0.35 | 0.56 | 45.7 | | 10.0 | | | 40 | 0.2 | 2.0 | 57 | | 247 | 488 | | 1221 | 1.39 |
| | | | Fish & Chips | | | | | | | | | | | | | | | | | | | | | | | | | | | | | | | | | | | | | | | | |
| 70096 | 1 | ea | Average | 156 | 324 | 58 | 13.3 | 34.8 | 3.9 | | | 14.9 | 4.3 | 4.9 | 4.8 | | | 23 | 64 | 13 | 9 | 3 | | 0.18 | 0.10 | 3.05 | 0.30 | 0.45 | 16.8 | | 7.4 | | | 25 | 0.1 | 1.6 | 41 | | 198 | 554 | | 621 | 0.71 |
| 70097 | 1 | ea | Large portion, avg | 447 | 943 | 57 | 38.2 | 101.3 | 11.1 | | | 43.5 | 1[illegible].1 | 17.3 | 12.2 | | | 67 | 214 | 41 | 30 | 12 | | 0.53 | 0.31 | 8.57 | 0.81 | 1.30 | 46.4 | | 18.6 | | | 76 | 0.4 | 4.6 | 116 | | 572 | 1506 | | 2181 | 2.10 |
| 70109 | 1 | ea | With Potatoes & vegetables, avg | 291 | 474 | 67 | 29.8 | 42.5 | 6.0 | | | 21.5 | 6.3 | 8.5 | 5.3 | | | 111 | 466 | 60 | 19 | 40 | | 0.26 | 0.37 | 6.90 | 0.55 | 3.63 | 34.5 | | 15.8 | | | 113 | 0.2 | 2.3 | 113 | | 390 | 905 | | 212 | 1.24 |
| 70379 | 1 | ea | Swanson | 284 | 490 | 64 | 19.0 | 59.0 | 5.0 | 18.0 | 35.0 | 20.0 | 4.0 | | | | | 45 | 100 | 20 | | | | | | | | | | | 2.4 | | | 60 | | 1.4 | | | | | | 1030 | |
| | | | Lasagna | | | | | | | | | | | | | | | | | | | | | | | | | | | | | | | | | | | | | | | | |
| 70134 | 1 | ea | Tuna, low calorie, avg | 276 | 276 | 77 | 19.2 | 32.4 | 3.6 | | | 7.7 | 3.0 | 2.5 | 1.6 | | | 19 | 6969 | 770 | 108 | 662 | | 0.20 | 0.32 | 5.38 | 0.28 | 1.03 | 71.7 | | 18.2 | | | 298 | 0.2 | 2.4 | 72 | | 273 | 433 | | 925 | 1.71 |
| 70132 | 1 | ea | Veal, low calorie, avg | 291 | 271 | 78 | 22.4 | 29.8 | 3.5 | | | 7.1 | 3.5 | 2.1 | 0.7 | | | 30 | 3207 | 342 | 31 | 372 | | 0.11 | 0.32 | 5.05 | 0.29 | 0.77 | 35.9 | | 14.6 | | | 236 | 0.3 | 2.9 | 47 | | 274 | 506 | | 949 | 2.73 |
| 70133 | 1 | ea | Vegetable, avg | 312 | 371 | 76 | 14.1 | 32.6 | 5.1 | | | 21.7 | 9.4 | 6.7 | 4.3 | | | 41 | 6140 | 713 | 145 | 567 | | 0.23 | 0.40 | 3.31 | 0.28 | 0.20 | 65.1 | | 69.6 | | | 290 | 0.3 | 2.8 | 56 | | 278 | 596 | | 1089 | 1.67 |
| 70135 | 1 | ea | Zucchini, low calorie, avg | 312 | 300 | 77 | 17.5 | 39.8 | 5.3 | | | 8.6 | 5.0 | 2.3 | 0.6 | | | 25 | 5086 | 566 | 81 | 485 | | 0.25 | 0.32 | 2.46 | 0.29 | 0.23 | 38.1 | | 24.6 | | | 362 | 0.3 | 2.2 | 69 | | 356 | 612 | | 899 | 2.22 |
| | | | Lunches | | | | | | | | | | | | | | | | | | | | | | | | | | | | | | | | | | | | | | | | |
| 56938 | 1 | ea | Bologna & American Cheese, Lunchable | 128 | 450 | | 18.0 | 19.0 | 0.0 | 3.0 | 15.0 | 34.0 | 15.0 | | | | | 85 | 300 | 60 | | | | | | | | | | | 0.0 | | | 300 | | 2.7 | | | | | | 1620 | |
| 56927 | 1 | ea | Bologna, w/Wild Cherry, Lunchable | 318 | 530 | | 13.0 | 58.0 | 0.5 | 45.0 | 12.5 | 29.0 | 14.0 | | | | | 60 | 400 | 80 | | | | | | | | | | | | | | 200 | | 1.4 | | | | | | 1120 | |
| 56932 | 1 | ea | Chicken & Turkey, Lunchable | 145 | 380 | | 22.0 | 24.0 | 1.0 | 7.0 | 15.0 | 22.0 | 1[illegible].0 | | | | | 70 | 300 | 60 | | | | | | | | | | | | | | 200 | | 1.8 | | | | | | 1840 | |
| 16189 | 1 | ea | Chicken Alfredo, Lunch Express | 273 | 360 | 74 | 18.0 | 34.0 | 3.0 | 4.0 | 27.0 | 17.0 | 6.0 | | | | | 60 | 1000 | 200 | | | | | | | | | | | 6.0 | | | 150 | | 1.1 | | | | 360 | | 620 | |
| 16188 | 1 | ea | Chicken Chow Mein, w/Rice, Lunch Express | 301 | 260 | 78 | 13.0 | 43.0 | 3.0 | 2.0 | 33.0 | 4.0 | .0 | | | | | 30 | 300 | 60 | | | | | | | | | | | 6.0 | | | 20 | | 1.1 | | | | 280 | | 940 | |
| 16185 | 1 | ea | Chicken Fettucini, Lunch Express | 251 | 250 | 79 | 16.0 | 32.0 | 4.0 | 7.0 | 21.0 | 6.0 | 2.5 | 1.5 | 1.0 | | | 35 | 500 | 100 | | | | | | | | | | | 24.0 | | | 150 | | 0.7 | | | | 430 | | 540 | |
| 16184 | 1 | ea | Chicken Mandarin, Lunch Express | 276 | 270 | 78 | 12.0 | 41.0 | 2.0 | 10.0 | 23.0 | 6.0 | .0 | 2.5 | 1.5 | | | 30 | 400 | 80 | | | | | | | | | | | 36.0 | | | 250 | | 1.1 | | | | 340 | | 520 | |
| 16182 | 1 | ea | Chicken Marinara, Lunch Express | 259 | 270 | 75 | 15.0 | 38.0 | 4.0 | 4.0 | 30.0 | 6.0 | .5 | 2.0 | 1.5 | | | 20 | 1000 | 200 | | | | | | | | | | | 12.0 | | | 40 | | 0.7 | | | | 390 | | 540 | |
| 16186 | 1 | ea | Chicken Oriental, Lunch Express | 276 | 320 | 75 | 14.0 | 45.0 | 2.0 | 12.0 | 31.0 | 9.0 | .5 | | | | | 40 | 750 | 150 | | | | | | | | | | | 9.0 | | | 20 | | 1.1 | | | | 380 | | 930 | |
| 16181 | 1 | ea | Chicken Stir Fry, Lunch Express | 255 | 280 | 75 | 11.0 | 39.0 | 3.0 | 7.0 | 23.0 | 9.0 | .0 | 3.5 | 2.5 | | | 15 | 1750 | 350 | | | | | | | | | | | 15.0 | | | 40 | | 0.7 | | | | 330 | | 590 | |
| 56929 | 1 | ea | Chicken, w/Jack Cheese & Pudding, Lunchable | 176 | 370 | | 19.0 | 33.0 | 0.0 | 16.0 | 17.0 | 18.0 | 9.0 | | | | | 55 | 200 | 40 | | | | | | | | | | | | | | 200 | | 2.7 | | | | | | 1490 | |
| 16183 | 1 | ea | Chicken, w/Rice, mexican style, Lunch Express | 255 | 270 | 76 | 10.0 | 39.0 | 3.0 | 3.0 | 33.0 | 8.0 | .5 | 2.5 | 1.5 | | | 20 | 1500 | 300 | | | | | | | | | | | 12.0 | | | 40 | | 0.7 | | | | 300 | | 590 | |
| 16187 | 1 | ea | Chicken, w/Vegs & Rice, Lunch Express | 280 | 340 | 74 | 15.0 | 45.0 | 2.0 | 6.0 | 37.0 | 11.0 | 2.5 | | | | | 30 | 2000 | 400 | | | | | | | | | | | 3.6 | | | 100 | | 0.7 | | | | 290 | | 750 | |
| 56935 | 1 | ea | Ham & Cheddar Cheese, Lunchable | 128 | 340 | | 21.0 | 19.0 | 0.0 | 4.0 | 15.0 | 20.0 | 1[illegible].0 | | | | | 75 | 300 | 60 | | | | | | | | | | | | | | 250 | | 1.8 | | | | | | 1830 | |
| 56926 | 1 | ea | Ham & Fruit Punch, Lunchable | 318 | 450 | | 15.0 | 53.0 | 0.5 | 39.0 | 13.5 | 20.0 | 1[illegible].0 | | | | | 50 | 400 | 80 | | | | | | | | | | | | | | 200 | | 1.4 | | | | | | 1260 | |
| 56939 | 1 | ea | Ham & Swiss Cheese, Lunchable | 128 | 320 | | 22.0 | 19.0 | 0.0 | 4.0 | 15.0 | 17.0 | 8.0 | | | | | 60 | 400 | 80 | | | | | | | | | | | | | | 300 | | 1.8 | | | | | | 1770 | |
| 56930 | 1 | ea | Ham, w/Amer Cheese & Pudding, Lunchable | 176 | 390 | | 18.0 | 34.0 | 0.5 | 17.0 | 15.5 | 20.0 | 9.0 | | | | | 55 | 200 | 40 | | | | | | | | | | | | | | 250 | | 2.7 | | | | | | 1540 | |
| 56924 | 1 | ea | Ham, w/Cheese & Vegetables, Lunchable | 128 | 380 | | 13.0 | 36.0 | 1.0 | 13.0 | 22.0 | 21.0 | 9.0 | | | | | 45 | 400 | 80 | | | | | | | | | | | 2.4 | | | 40 | | 1.8 | | | | | | 1240 | |
| 56923 | 1 | ea | Ham, w/Herb Chive Cheese, Lunchable | 128 | 390 | | 13.0 | 37.0 | 1.0 | 14.0 | 22.0 | 21.0 | 9.0 | | | | | 45 | 300 | 60 | | | | | | | | | | | | | | 60 | | 1.8 | | | | | | 1270 | |
| 56928 | 1 | ea | Ham, w/Swiss Cheese & Cookies, Lunchable | 119 | 360 | | 18.0 | 29.0 | 0.5 | 5.0 | 23.5 | 19.0 | 8.0 | | | | | 50 | 300 | 60 | | | | | | | | | | | | | | 250 | | 1.4 | | | | | | 1420 | |
| 11092 | 1 | ea | Oriental Beef, Lunch Express | 273 | 260 | 80 | 12.0 | 34.0 | 4.0 | 8.0 | 22.0 | 8.0 | .5 | | | | | 20 | 2000 | 400 | | | | | | | | | | | 12.0 | | | 40 | | 1.8 | | | | 380 | | 1220 | |
| 56940 | 1 | ea | Pepperoni & American Cheese, Lunchable | 128 | 480 | | 20.0 | 19.0 | 0.0 | 3.0 | 15.0 | 36.0 | 17.0 | | | | | 95 | 300 | 60 | | | | | | | | | | | | | | 250 | | 2.7 | | | | | | 1840 | |
| 11091 | 1 | ea | Rigatoni, w/Meat Sauce, Lunch Express | 305 | 340 | 75 | 14.0 | 44.0 | 3.0 | 8.0 | 33.0 | 12.0 | 2.5 | | | | | 30 | 750 | 150 | | | | | | | | | | | 12.0 | | | 60 | | 1.8 | | | | 470 | | 710 | |
| 56936 | 1 | ea | Salami & American Cheese, Lunchable | 128 | 430 | | 18.0 | 18.0 | 0.0 | 3.0 | 15.0 | 32.0 | 15.0 | | | | | 80 | 300 | 60 | | | | | | | | | | | | | | 250 | | 2.7 | | | | | | 1740 | |

| Code | Amount | | Description | Basic Components | | | | | | | | | Additional Fats | | | | | | Vit A & Components | | | | | Vitamins | | | | | | | | | | Minerals | | | | | | | | | |
|---|---|---|---|---|---|---|---|---|---|---|---|---|---|---|---|---|---|---|---|---|---|---|---|---|---|---|---|---|---|---|---|---|---|---|---|---|---|---|---|---|---|---|---|
| | | | | Weight (g) | Calories | % Water | Protein (g) | Carbs (g) | Fiber (g) | Sugar (g) | Other Carbs (g) | Fat (g) | Sat Fat (g) | Mono Fat (g) | Poly Fat (g) | Omega 3 (g) | Omega 6 (g) | Choles (mg) | Vit A (IU) | Vit A (RE) | Retinol (RE) | Carotenoids (RE) | Beta Carotene (mcg) | Thiamin (mg) | Riboflavin (mg) | Niacin (NE) | Vit B6 (mg) | Vit B12 (mcg) | Folate (mcg) | Panto (mg) | Vit C (mg) | Vit D (mg) | Vit E (α TE) | Calcium (mg) | Copper (mg) | Iron (mg) | Magnes (mg) | Mang (mg) | Phos (mg) | Potassium (mg) | Selenium (mcg) | Sodium (mg) | Zinc (mg) |
| 11090 | 1 | ea | Spaghetti, w/Meat Sauce, Lunch Express |273|320|75|15.0|43.0|5.0|7.0|31.0|10.0|3.5| | | | |30|500|100| | | | | | | | | | |6.0| | |60| |1.8| | | |480| |580| |
| 11089 | 1 | ea | Swedish Meatballs, w/Pasta, Lunch Express |291|530|67|19.0|41.0|3.0|3.0|35.0|32.0|11.0| | | | |65| | | | | | | | | | | | |1.2| | |60| |2.7| | | |300| |1010| |
| 56848 | 1 | ea | Teriyaki Stir Fry, Lunch Express |255|260|76|15.0|39.0|4.0|9.0|26.0|5.0|1.0|2.0|1.5| | |30|1000|200| | | | | | | | | | |12.0| | |20| |1.4| | | |330| |550| |
| 18821 | 1 | ea | Tuna Casserole, Lunch Express |273|280|74|18.0|39.0|4.0|6.0|29.0|6.0|2.0|1.5|1.0| | |20|1250|250| | | | | | | | | | |1.2| | |200| |1.8| | | |270| |590| |
| 56933 | 1 | ea | Turkey & Ham, Lunchable |145|360| |23.0|23.0|1.0|6.0|16.0|19.0|10.0| | | | |60|300|60| | | | | | | | | | | | | |300| |1.8| | | | | |1930| |
| 56934 | 1 | ea | Turkey & Jack Cheese, Lunchable |128|350| |20.0|20.0|1.0|5.0|14.0|21.0|10.0| | | | |75|200|40| | | | | | | | | | | | | |250| |1.8| | | | | |1690| |
| 16920 | 1 | ea | Turkey Dijon, w/Pasta, Lunch Express |280|270|77|16.0|37.0|6.0|8.0|23.0|6.0|1.5|2.0|1.5| | |30|1250|250| | | | | | | | | | |18.0| | |100| |1.8| | | |320| |570| |
| 56937 | 1 | ea | Turkey, w/Cheddar Cheese, Lunchable |128|360| |20.0|20.0|1.0|5.0|14.0|22.0|11.0| | | | |70|300|60| | | | | | | | | | | | | |300| |1.8| | | | | |1650| |
| 56931 | 1 | ea | Turkey, w/Cheddar Cheese & Jell-o, Lunchable |163|320| |17.0|27.0|0.5|16.0|10.5|16.0|9.0| | | | |50|400|80| | | | | | | | | | | | | |20| |6.0| | | | | |1360| |
| 56922 | 1 | ea | Turkey, w/Green Onion Cheese, Lunchable |128|380| |14.0|36.0|1.0|12.0|23.0|20.0|9.0| | | | |45|400|80| | | | | | | | | | | | | |60| |1.8| | | | | |1280| |
| 56925 | 1 | ea | Turkey, w/Pacific Cooler, Lunchable |318|460| |16.0|53.0|0.5|39.0|13.5|21.0|10.0| | | | |50|300|60| | | | | | | | | | | | | |200| |1.4| | | | | |1310| |
| 56921 | 1 | ea | Turkey, w/Ranch & Herb Cheese, Lunchable |128|380| |14.0|36.0|1.0|12.0|23.0|20.0|9.0| | | | |45|200|40| | | | | | | | | | | | | |60| |1.8| | | | | |1280| |
| 70733 | 1 | ea | Mexican, Beef Enchilada, Swanson |383|500|71|21.0|68.0|11.0|16.0|41.0|16.0|6.0| | | | |25|750|150| | | | | | | | | | |36.0| | |200| |3.6| | | | | |1220| |
| | | | Mexican, Cheese Enchilada | | | | | | | | | | | | | | | | | | | | | | | | | | | | | | | | | | | | | | | | |
| 70152 | 1 | ea | Average |284|585|56|24.4|67.0|11.9| | |26.1|14.2|8.4|2.0| | |60|1345|235|143|92| |0.26|0.38|2.72|0.43|0.47|154.6| |17.8| | |568|0.4|3.4|97| |594|784| |1877|3.05|
| 82023 | 1 | ea | Banquet |312|360|74|15.0|54.0|9.0|7.0|38.0|10.0|3.0| | | | |20|750|150| | | | | | | | | | |0.0| | |150| |2.7| | | | | |1580| |
| 70153 | 1 | ea | Low Calorie, avg |241|357|69|26.7|28.5|2.5| | |15.3|8.6|4.4|1.2| | |75|4974|583|125|458| |0.11|0.29|4.65|0.40|0.35|23.7| |91.9| | |371|0.2|1.7|58| |415|412| |995|2.22|
| 82006 | 1 | ea | Patio |340|330|78|13.0|52.0|10.0|7.0|35.0|8.0|3.0|2.8|1.2| | |15|500|100| | | |0.26|0.21|1.20|0.17| | | |4.8| | |200| |1.8| | | | | |1570| |
| 70151 | 1 | ea | With Beans & rice, avg |340|517|66|19.1|70.2|13.6| | |18.5|7.9|7.1|2.4| | |31|669|122|79|43| |0.32|0.27|2.21|0.33|0.18|112.7| |5.8| | |289|0.4|4.1|102| |418|653| |1955|2.63|
| 82013 | 1 | ea | Mexican, Chicken Picante, Healthy Choice |319|220|83|19.0|31.0|6.0|25.0|0.0|2.0|1.5| | | | |35|300|60| | | | | | | | | | |30.0| | |100| |1.4| | | | | |330| |
| 82022 | 1 | ea | Mexican, Chimichanga, Banquet |269|470|65|13.0|56.0|9.0|9.0|38.0|23.0|7.0| | | | |15|400|80| | | | | | | | | | |6.0| | |60| |2.7| | | | | |1180| |
| 82007 | 1 | ea | Mexican, Fiesta, Patio |340|340|78|13.0|51.0|11.0|5.0|35.0|9.0|4.0| | | | |15|400|80| | | |0.24|0.21|1.40| | | | |3.6| | |150| |1.8| | | | | |1760| |
| 56794 | 1 | ea | Mexican, Swanson |376|470|74|18.0|59.0|5.0|11.0|43.0|18.0|6.0| | | | |25|1000|200| | | | | | | | | | |30.0| | |200| |2.7| | | | | |1610| |
| 70767 | 1 | ea | Mexican, Hungry Man |567|690|74|26.0|87.0|13.0|19.0|55.0|27.0|9.0| | | | |35|1500|300| | | | | | | | | | |36.0| | |300| |3.6| | | | | |2170| |
| 82015 | 1 | ea | Mexican, Ranchera, Patio |369|410|77|13.0|55.0|14.0|1.0|40.0|15.0|6.0| | | | |25|500|100| | | | | | | | | | |6.0| | |100| |2.7| | | | | |2400| |
| 70037 | 1 | ea | Pork, Ham, glazed, w/sweet potatoes & vegs, avg |284|318|74|16.3|43.8|2.6| | |9.1|2.0|3.4|3.0| | |37|11570|1176|28|1148| |0.63|0.25|3.58|0.49|0.45|21.9| |63.3| | |51|0.2|1.9|37| |185|514| |1588|2.49|
| 70790 | 1 | ea | Pork, Patty, Swanson |298|470|68|16.0|58.0|5.0|28.0|25.0|19.0|7.0| | | | |30|300|60| | | | | | | | | | |6.0| | |80| |2.7| | | | | |900| |
| 70024 | 1 | ea | Pork, Shortribs, w/bbq sce, potatoes & veg, avg |298|387|74|27.8|29.6|4.4| | |17.7|7.6|7.3|1.1| | |77|1173|130|18|112| |0.19|0.26|4.55|0.51|2.55|39.7| |17.4| | |63|0.4|4.4|63| |256|840| |578|6.67|
| 70034 | 1 | ea | Pork, Sliced, w/swt potatoes, vegs & dessert, avg |319|408|71|21.9|55.5|4.2| | |10.9|3.6|4.7|1.6| | |64|16429|1664|31|1633| |0.63|0.41|4.87|0.51|0.48|50.3| |18.5| | |51|0.3|2.2|48| |262|568| |1254|2.57|
| 70035 | 1 | ea | Pork, W/Gravy, potatoes, vegs & dessert, avg |319|459|71|26.8|42.0|3.5| | |20.3|5.4|7.6|4.0| | |67|9691|1037|111|926| |0.97|0.39|6.34|0.52|0.64|20.2| |9.6| | |86|0.1|1.9|48| |284|657| |970|2.38|
| 70036 | 1 | ea | Pork, W/Rice & Vegs, in soy sce, low cal, avg |255|258|77|14.9|33.8|2.5| | |6.7|2.1|2.9|1.2| | |33|327|37|6|31| |0.41|0.27|4.51|0.41|0.76|18.3| |30.5| | |31|0.4|2.1|36| |194|433| |1058|4.35|
| 70118 | 1 | ea | Seafood Newburg, w/rice & vegetables, avg |298|286|79|14.3|34.3|1.8| | |9.6|4.8|2.9|1.2| | |80|737|131|85|46| |0.10|0.18|2.77|0.21|1.12|15.6| |6.8| | |80|0.3|1.9|54| |188|322| |1249|1.42|
| | | | Shrimp | | | | | | | | | | | | | | | | | | | | | | | | | | | | | | | | | | | | | | | | |
| 70115 | 1 | ea | Chow Mein, w/egg roll, avg |369|443|74|15.0|67.9|3.1| | |11.9|2.6|4.9|3.4| | |48|3585|361|4|357| |0.38|0.24|4.76|0.37|0.68|34.7| |43.3| | |55|0.3|3.7|44| |185|465| |590|2.14|
| 70116 | 1 | ea | Creole, w/rice & pep, low cal, avg |284|250|78|9.9|46.5|2.5| | |2.6|0.4|0.5|1.2| | |40|744|77|4|73| |0.27|0.11|3.66|0.34|0.26|21.0| |50.1| | |43|0.3|2.9|43| |145|395| |824|1.13|
| 19426 | 1 | ea | Marinara, Healthy Choice |298|250|81|10.0|44.0|5.0|27.0|12.0|4.0|2.0| | | | |55|300|60| | | | | | | | | | |1.2| | |60| |1.8| | | | | |260| |
| 70114 | 1 | ea | With Potatoes & vegetables, avg |198|376|61|23.6|33.7|4.3| | |16.7|5.1|6.6|3.7| | |182|4061|451|67|384| |0.27|0.19|4.48|0.26|0.94|30.8| |10.7| | |75|0.4|4.0|55| |281|495| |507|1.60|
| 70119 | 1 | ea | With Rice & vegetables, avg |312|287|77|13.3|50.1|3.9| | |3.9|0.8|1.4|1.3| | |53|1263|144|27|117| |0.31|0.21|4.73|0.29|0.39|41.5| |73.4| | |59|0.6|3.7|47| |193|490| |1220|1.43|
| 70140 | 1 | ea | Spaghetti & Meatballs, w/apples & bread, avg |326|447|69|24.6|55.0|4.8| | |14.4|5.2|5.8|1.2| | |55|37|4|0|4| |0.31|0.28|5.91|0.31|1.78|46.3| |1.4| | |42|0.6|3.9|55| |228|489| |2194|3.96|
| 70141 | 1 | ea | Spaghetti & Meatballs, w/vegs & dessert, avg |354|365|76|15.0|56.5|5.5| | |9.3|3.1|3.5|1.6| | |21|1635|205|62|143| |0.40|0.32|4.53|0.30|0.67|47.8| |31.6| | |96|0.3|3.2|57| |219|588| |1012|2.38|
| 70444 | 1 | ea | Turkey, A La King, Budget Gourmet |284|390|74|20.0|36.0| | | |18.0| | | | | |75|500|100| | | |0.15|0.34|5.00| | | | |2.4| | |150| |1.1| | | | | |740| |
| 16904 | 1 | ea | Turkey, Banquet |262|270|78|15.0|31.0|3.0|2.0|26.0|10.0|3.0| | | | |45|0|0|0|0|0|0.14|0.19|5.80| | | | |2.4| | |80| |1.8| | | |500| |1100| |
| | | | Turkey, Breast | | | | | | | | | | | | | | | | | | | | | | | | | | | | | | | | | | | | | | | | |
| 16912 | 1 | ea | Healthy Choice |298|290|78|22.0|40.0|5.0|20.0|15.0|4.5|2.0| | | | |45|400|80| | | |0.45|0.26|6.00| | | | |36.0| | |20| |1.4| | |270|540| |460| |
| 70094 | 1 | ea | With Gravy, rice & veg, avg |319|450|73|26.7|31.2|2.9| | |23.3|4.7|9.5|7.6| | |54|7388|739|0|739| |0.26|0.21|7.39|0.64|0.34|41.5| |38.9| | |57|0.2|2.7|51| |258|552| |1215|2.27|
| 70792 | 1 | ea | With Pasta, Swanson |319|270|81|20.0|31.0|6.0|11.0|14.0|7.0|4.0| | | | |35|7000|1400| | | | | | | | | | |36.0| | |150| |1.8| | | | | |720| |
| 16905 | 1 | ea | Turkey, Extra Helping, Banquet |533|560|78|32.0|63.0|7.0|26.0|30.0|20.0|5.0| | | | |75|0|0|0|0|0|0.45|0.34|5.00|0.34| | | |0.0| | |100| |3.6| | |320|670| |1910| |
| 70093 | 1 | ea | Turkey, Tetrazzini, avg |340|527|72|25.3|37.7|2.7| | |29.3|9.4|12.0|6.1| | |85|414|97|82|14| |0.32|0.40|5.71|0.35|0.38|28.7| |3.8| | |160|0.2|3.3|51| |282|490| |1010|2.70|
| | | | Turkey, W/Dressing | | | | | | | | | | | | | | | | | | | | | | | | | | | | | | | | | | | | | | | | |
| 16902 | 1 | ea | Armour |319|270|81|17.0|34.0|5.0|1.0|28.0|7.0|4.0| | | | |60|2250|450| | | |0.30|0.17|5.00| | | | |6.0| | |60| |1.8| | |210|520| |1020| |
| 70085 | 1 | ea | Gravy & potatoes, avg |376|429|76|31.5|33.2|2.9| | |18.6|4.2|5.5|4.7| | |98|965|145|87|58| |0.24|0.34|7.32|0.42|0.50|21.4| |12.4| | |113|0.2|2.7|53| |320|681| |2948|3.04|
| 70084 | 1 | ea | Gravy & potatoes, x-lrg, avg |248|308|75|16.6|27.4|1.9| | |14.6|3.3|4.5|4.1| | |32|466|103|92|11| |0.14|0.19|5.33|0.17|0.92|14.6| |6.7| | |62|0.1|1.7|30| |226|409| |1535|1.74|
| 70089 | 1 | ea | Gravy, potatoes & vegetables, avg |312|509|67|30.8|46.1|3.6| | |22.6|5.0|8.0|6.2| | |75|6936|787|147|640| |0.26|0.27|7.71|0.56|0.41|39.9| |12.0| | |81|0.2|2.6|53| |296|615| |1248|2.59|
| 70090 | 1 | ea | Gravy, potatoes, vegetables & dessert, avg |326|339|77|26.5|28.0|3.5| | |13.2|3.1|4.2|3.4| | |55|612|90|50|40| |0.26|0.24|7.08|0.48|0.32|47.0| |14.2| | |72|0.2|2.3|55| |277|570| |1793|2.36|
| 70091 | 1 | ea | Gravy, potatoes, vegs, soup & dessert, avg |454|808|64|45.9|79.6|3.7| | |33.9|8.1|12.4|9.3| | |227|1317|301|260|41| |0.36|0.69|8.90|0.59|2.05|67.0| |10.3| | |123|0.4|6.1|68| |418|735| |772|5.33|
| 70086 | 1 | ea | Gravy, vegetables & fruit, avg |298|292|77|21.0|40.1|5.0| | |5.4|1.7|1.5|1.5| | |42|647|67|4|63| |0.32|0.27|5.10|0.40|0.22|49.7| |15.8| | |77|0.2|3.1|45| |215|480| |435|2.40|
| 70087 | 1 | ea | Low calorie, avg |454|372|80|42.9|32.4|6.0| | |7.7|2.4|1.7|2.3| | |95|21465|2147|0|2147| |0.32|0.55|9.03|0.95|0.53|78.8| |65.8| | |168|0.3|4.6|82| |409|999| |1557|4.73|
| 70092 | 1 | ea | Potatoes, vegetables & dessert, avg |524|608|74|35.0|73.8|6.7| | |19.6|4.3|6.5|5.3| | |94|1058|175|113|62| |0.39|0.41|8.36|0.59|0.42|70.7| |21.0| | |121|0.4|4.0|79| |383|802| |1996|3.89|
| 16913 | 1 | ea | Turkey, W/Mostly white meat, Swanson |333|320|78|20.0|42.0|4.0|15.0|23.0|8.0|3.0| | | | |35|500|100| | | | | | | | | | |9.0| | |40| |1.8| | | | | |1030| |
| 70088 | 1 | ea | Turkey, W/Vegetables in sauce, low calorie, avg |269|264|79|22.3|18.3|2.6| | |10.4|3.5|3.5|2.4| | |54|6884|723|52|671| |0.17|0.30|4.38|0.39|0.34|27.3| |4.6| | |156|0.2|2.2|51| |245|476| |880|2.60|
| 70038 | 1 | ea | Veal, Breaded, w/spaghetti & tomato sauce, avg |234|302|73|15.3|27.3|3.0| | |14.8|3.6|6.0|4.0| | |73|2969|308|16|292| |0.21|0.26|3.98|0.27|0.63|27.7| |21.3| | |51|0.2|2.0|37| |171|442| |1718|1.60|
| 70136 | 1 | ea | Veal, W/Macaroni & Cheese, low calorie, avg |369|369|77|27.1|42.0|4.0| | |10.4|5.3|3.2|0.9| | |59|1487|193|62|131| |0.37|0.45|6.48|0.39|1.01|27.0| |21.8| | |273|0.5|3.6|66| |369|694| |590|3.97|
| 70040 | 1 | ea | Veal, W/Peppers in sauce & rice, low calorie, avg |369|306|80|27.0|32.4|3.8| | |8.1|3.2|3.0|1.0| | |81|2744|274|0|274| |0.33|0.39|8.67|0.75|1.49|40.0| |72.0| | |55|0.4|3.1|63| |288|849| |886|4.82|
| | | | Veal, Parmigiana | | | | | | | | | | | | | | | | | | | | | | | | | | | | | | | | | | | | | | | | |
| 70769 | 1 | ea | Hungry Man, Swanson |517|640|73|34.0|74.0|6.0|24.0|44.0|23.0|11.0| | | | |70|500|100| | | | | | | | | | |24.0| | |300| |5.4| | | | | |1990| |
| 11066 | 1 | ea | Swanson |319|440|75|19.0|40.0|5.0|14.0|21.0|18.0|8.0| | | | |85|500|100| | | | | | | | | | |9.0| | |150| |2.7| | | | | |1060| |
| 70046 | 1 | ea | With Potatoes & vegetables, avg |312|440|69|35.5|40.3|4.2| | |15.4|5.1|5.2|2.1| | |115|811|105|40|65| |0.32|0.51|7.77|0.50|1.71|63.4| |21.0| | |162|0.4|2.9|75| |396|792| |1314|6.96|
| 70045 | 1 | ea | With Vegetables & spaghetti, in butter, avg |305|387|74|17.3|38.1|5.8| | |19.3|4.9|8.0|5.0| | |43|7561|866|164|702| |0.23|0.26|4.04|0.37|0.64|37.5| |15.1| | |180|0.3|2.6|64| |256|561| |1229|2.21|
| 70043 | 1 | ea | With Vegetables, fettucini & dessert, avg |361|495|72|22.9|48.6|4.2| | |23.9|8.4|7.9|6.0| | |97|1751|298|169|129| |0.26|0.44|5.34|0.33|0.65|29.5| |25.6| | |282|0.3|3.0|61| |354|621| |1404|2.80|
| 70039 | 1 | ea | With Vegetables, low calorie, avg |255|194|84|20.4|8.6|2.2| | |9.0|4.8|3.0|0.5| | |64|955|119|33|86| |0.13|0.31|5.12|0.32|0.93|24.9| |14.4| | |227|0.3|1.7|51| |321|650| |444|3.16|

| Code | Amount | | Description | Weight (g) | Calories | % Water | Protein (g) | Carbs (g) | Fiber (g) | Sugar (g) | Other Carbs (g) | Fat (g) | Sat Fat (g) | Mono Fat (g) | Poly Fat (g) | Omega 3 (g) | Omega 6 (g) | Choles (mg) | Vit A (IU) | Vit A (RE) | Retinol (RE) | Carotenoids (RE) | Beta Carotene (mcg) | Thiamin (mg) | Riboflavin (mg) | Niacin (NE) | Vit B6 (mg) | Vit B12 (mcg) | Folate (mcg) | Panto (mg) | Vit C (mg) | Vit D (mg) | Vit E (α TE) | Calcium (mg) | Copper (mg) | Iron (mg) | Magnes (mg) | Mang (mg) | Phos (mg) | Potassium (mg) | Selenium (mcg) | Sodium (mg) | Zinc (mg) |
|---|---|---|---|---|---|---|---|---|---|---|---|---|---|---|---|---|---|---|---|---|---|---|---|---|---|---|---|---|---|---|---|---|---|---|---|---|---|---|---|---|---|---|---|
| | | | **Basic Components** | | | | | | | | | | **Additional Fats** | | | | | | **Vit A & Components** | | | | | **Vitamins** | | | | | | | | | | **Minerals** | | | | | | | | | |
| 70042 | 1 | ea | With Vegetables, muffin & dessert, avg | 347 | 545 | 69 | 23.8 | 49.6 | 5.2 | | | 28.4 | 11.6 | 12.0 | 2.5 | | | 87 | 1160 | 158 | 61 | 97 | | 0.34 | 0.40 | 5.00 | 0.32 | 0.67 | 57.7 | | 25.2 | | | 177 | 0.3 | 2.8 | 52 | | 278 | 552 | | 958 | 2.83 |
| 70041 | 1 | ea | With Vegetables & potato wedges, low cal, avg | 312 | 290 | 79 | 23.6 | 25.9 | 4.6 | | | 10.6 | 4.4 | 4.1 | 1.1 | | | 75 | 7672 | 774 | 11 | 764 | | 0.16 | 0.32 | 6.06 | 0.63 | 1.09 | 41.6 | | 38.9 | | | 56 | 0.4 | 2.3 | 53 | | 262 | 727 | | 714 | 2.75 |
| | | | *ENTREES AND DISHES* | | | | | | | | | | | | | | | | | | | | | | | | | | | | | | | | | | | | | | | | |
| 11108 | 1 | ea | Beef, Charbroiled w/gravy, Banquet | 132 | 180 | 78 | 8.0 | 7.0 | 2.0 | 0.0 | 5.0 | 13.0 | 6.0 | | | | | 25 | 0 | 0 | 0 | 0 | 0 | | | | | | | | 0.0 | | | 20 | | 1.1 | | | | | | 640 | |
| 57478 | 1 | ea | Beef, Chicken Fried Steak, Marie Calendar | 425 | 650 | 70 | 23.0 | 69.0 | 7.0 | 9.0 | 53.0 | 31.0 | 10.0 | | | | | 50 | 749 | 150 | | | | | | | | | | | 24.0 | | | 150 | | 2.7 | | | | | | 2258 | |
| 57154 | 1 | oz | Beef, Chop Suey, Nestle | 28 | 16 | 86 | 1.5 | 1.6 | 0.2 | 0.7 | 0.7 | 0.5 | 0.1 | 0.1 | 0.0 | 0.00 | 0.00 | 4 | 140 | 28 | | | | 0.01 | 0.02 | 0.20 | | | | | 2.6 | | | 4 | | 0.1 | | | | 40 | | 84 | |
| | | | Beef, Macaroni | | | | | | | | | | | | | | | | | | | | | | | | | | | | | | | | | | | | | | | | |
| 11109 | 1 | ea | Banquet | 227 | 230 | 80 | 6.0 | 31.0 | 3.0 | 3.0 | 25.0 | 7.0 | 3.0 | | | | | 25 | | | | | | | | | | | | | 1.2 | | | 100 | | | | | | | | 810 | |
| 11112 | 1 | ea | Healthy Choice | 241 | 210 | 79 | 14.0 | 34.0 | 5.0 | 9.0 | 20.0 | 2.0 | 0.5 | | | | | 15 | 500 | 100 | | | | | | | | | | | 54.0 | | | 40 | | 2.7 | | | | | | 450 | |
| 11029 | 1 | ea | Lean Cuisine | 284 | 280 | 77 | 13.0 | 40.0 | 3.0 | 9.0 | 23.0 | 8.0 | 2.0 | 2.0 | 1.0 | | | 25 | 500 | 100 | | | | 0.09 | 0.17 | 3.00 | | | | | 12.0 | | | 60 | | 2.7 | | | | 410 | | 550 | |
| 11103 | 1 | ea | Weight Watchers | 269 | 220 | 81 | 13.0 | 32.0 | 4.0 | 15.0 | 13.0 | 4.5 | 1.5 | | | | | 10 | 1000 | 200 | | | | | | | | | | | 12.0 | | | 60 | | 2.7 | | | | 620 | | 560 | |
| | | | Beef, Meatballs | | | | | | | | | | | | | | | | | | | | | | | | | | | | | | | | | | | | | | | | |
| 11122 | 6 | pce | Bernardis | 84 | 270 | 51 | 12.0 | 5.0 | 2.0 | 0.5 | 2.5 | 22.0 | 10.0 | | | | | 65 | 0 | 0 | 0 | 0 | 0 | | | | | | | | 0.0 | | | 40 | | 1.4 | | | | | | 630 | |
| 11099 | 1 | ea | Lean Cuisine | 259 | 290 | 74 | 22.0 | 32.0 | 3.0 | 2.0 | 27.0 | 8.0 | 3.0 | 2.5 | 1.0 | | | 55 | 100 | 20 | | | | 0.60 | 0.51 | 5.00 | 0.30 | 1.00 | 32.0 | 0.70 | 0.0 | 0.2 | | 40 | 0.2 | 1.8 | 44 | | 207 | 370 | 34.0 | 590 | 3.70 |
| 11055 | 1 | ea | Stouffers | 262 | 440 | 67 | 23.0 | 36.0 | 3.0 | 2.0 | 31.0 | 23.0 | 8.0 | | | | | 85 | 100 | 20 | | | | 0.00 | 0.10 | 1.00 | | | | | 0.4 | | | 40 | | 2.7 | | | | 330 | | 840 | |
| 11104 | 1 | ea | Weight Watchers | 255 | 280 | 76 | 18.0 | 35.0 | 3.0 | 8.0 | 24.0 | 8.0 | 3.0 | | | | | 30 | 750 | 150 | | | | | | | | | | | 3.6 | | | 100 | | 3.6 | | | | 490 | | 510 | |
| | | | Beef, Meatloaf | | | | | | | | | | | | | | | | | | | | | | | | | | | | | | | | | | | | | | | | |
| 11119 | 1 | ea | Healthy Choice | 340 | 320 | 79 | 15.0 | 52.0 | 6.0 | 17.0 | 23.0 | 5.0 | 2.5 | | | | | 35 | 750 | 150 | | | | | | | | | | | 54.0 | | | 40 | | 1.8 | | | | | | 460 | |
| 11093 | 1 | ea | Lean Cuisine | 266 | 270 | 79 | 21.0 | 24.0 | 4.0 | 4.0 | 15.0 | 10.0 | 4.0 | 2.5 | 0.5 | | | 55 | 300 | 60 | | | | | | | | | | | 1.2 | | | 80 | | 1.8 | | | | 520 | | 530 | |
| 11098 | 1 | ea | Stouffers | 280 | 380 | 75 | 20.0 | 24.0 | 3.0 | 2.0 | 13.0 | 24.0 | 8.0 | | | | | 80 | 100 | 20 | | | | | | | | | | | 1.2 | | | 40 | | 2.7 | | | | 450 | | 910 | |
| 11114 | 1 | ea | Beef, Mesquite BBQ, Healthy Choice | 312 | 320 | 77 | 21.0 | 38.0 | 5.0 | 16.0 | 17.0 | 9.0 | 3.0 | | | | | 55 | 1250 | 250 | | | | | | | | | | | 0.0 | | | 40 | | 1.1 | | | | | | 490 | |
| 57455 | 1 | ea | Beef, Patty, charbroiled, Banquet | 255 | 290 | | 11.0 | 26.0 | 6.0 | 3.0 | 17.0 | 16.0 | 7.0 | | | | | 25 | 0 | 0 | 0 | 0 | 0 | | | | | | | | 2.4 | | | 40 | | 1.8 | | | | | | 1209 | |
| 57396 | 1 | ea | Beef, Patty, w/green pepper, Travis Meats | 113 | 256 | 63 | 18.7 | 3.2 | 1.9 | 0.7 | 0.6 | 18.7 | 7.5 | 8.1 | 0.8 | | | 57 | 216 | 43 | | | | 0.23 | 0.23 | 5.20 | | | | | 10.6 | | | 42 | | 4.3 | | | 174 | 425 | | 275 | 6.35 |
| 11023 | 1 | cup | Beef, Pepper Steak, avg | 217 | 332 | 73 | 28.7 | 5.4 | 1.0 | 1.8 | 2.6 | 21.3 | 4.4 | 6.2 | 9.0 | | | 72 | 193 | 19 | 0 | 19 | | 0.13 | 0.25 | 4.59 | 0.48 | 2.98 | 27.1 | 0.65 | 18.8 | 0.7 | | 28 | 0.1 | 3.2 | 37 | 0.2 | 267 | 556 | | 649 | 4.55 |
| 11042 | 1 | ea | Beef, Pepper Steak, Chung King | 369 | 300 | 81 | 15.0 | 50.0 | 5.0 | 15.0 | 30.0 | 4.0 | 1.0 | | | | | 10 | 750 | 150 | | | | 0.15 | 0.26 | 2.00 | | | | | 36.0 | | | 20 | | 1.8 | | | 170 | 370 | | 1610 | |
| 11094 | 1 | ea | Beef, Pot Roast, Lean Cuisine | 255 | 210 | 81 | 16.0 | 21.0 | 3.0 | 6.0 | 12.0 | 7.0 | 1.5 | 2.0 | 1.0 | | | 40 | 480 | 150 | | | | | | | | | | | | | | 100 | | 1.4 | | | | 600 | | 570 | |
| 57469 | 1 | cup | Beef, Pot Roast, w/gravy, Marie Calendar | 213 | 180 | 81 | 14.0 | 21.0 | 3.0 | 3.0 | 15.0 | 5.0 | 1.0 | | | | | 35 | 0 | 0 | 0 | 0 | 0 | | | | | | | | 2.4 | | | 0 | | 0.7 | | | | | | 661 | |
| 11038 | 1 | pce | Beef, Sliced, w/gravy, Banquet | 80 | 50 | 84 | 6.5 | 3.5 | 0.3 | 1.0 | 2.3 | 1.5 | 0.8 | | | | | 20 | 0 | 0 | 0 | 0 | 0 | | | | | | | | 0.0 | | | 0 | | | | | | | | 428 | |
| 57134 | 1 | cup | Beef, Sliced, w/gravy, Libby's | 228 | 210 | 78 | 39.0 | 3.0 | 0.0 | 0.0 | 3.0 | 4.6 | 2.3 | | | | | 105 | 0 | 0 | 0 | 0 | 0 | | | | | | | | 1.8 | | | 0 | | 2.2 | | | | | | 1199 | |
| | | | Beef, Stroganoff | | | | | | | | | | | | | | | | | | | | | | | | | | | | | | | | | | | | | | | | |
| 57122 | 1 | ea | Pepperidge Farm | 156 | 420 | 55 | 13.0 | 27.0 | 5.0 | 1.0 | 21.0 | 29.0 | 12.0 | | | | | 40 | 0 | 0 | 0 | 0 | 0 | | | | | | | | 0.0 | | | 80 | | 0.7 | | | | | | 500 | |
| 70445 | 1 | ea | Slim Selects | 248 | 280 | 77 | 18.0 | 29.0 | | | | 10.0 | | | | | | 60 | 300 | 60 | | | | 0.26 | 0.34 | 4.00 | | | | | 9.0 | | | 60 | | 2.7 | | | | | | 560 | |
| 57474 | 1 | cup | With Noodles, Marie Calendar | 184 | 439 | 59 | 24.0 | 23.0 | 3.0 | 4.0 | 15.0 | 27.0 | 11.0 | | | | | 40 | 100 | 20 | | | | | | | | | | | 6.0 | | | 20 | | 1.4 | | | | | | 779 | |
| 70127 | 1 | ea | Beef, Stuffed Cabbage, w/tomato sce, low cal, avg | 305 | 247 | 83 | 16.1 | 22.2 | 3.8 | | | 10.6 | 3.9 | 4.5 | 0.8 | | | 49 | 3264 | 329 | 3 | 325 | | 0.24 | 0.23 | 4.04 | 0.34 | 1.28 | 31.8 | | 31.7 | | | 49 | 0.2 | 2.1 | 43 | | 168 | 592 | | 692 | 3.20 |
| 11022 | 1 | ea | Beef, Swiss Steak, avg | 170 | 179 | 79 | 19.8 | 6.6 | 1.3 | 1.5 | 3.8 | 7.8 | 2.0 | 2.7 | 2.2 | | | 49 | 2059 | 206 | 0 | 206 | | 0.11 | 0.20 | 3.75 | 0.28 | 1.90 | 12.1 | 0.34 | 9.1 | 0.5 | | 26 | 0.1 | 2.4 | 31 | 0.1 | 202 | 495 | | 413 | 3.13 |
| | | | Beef, Tips | | | | | | | | | | | | | | | | | | | | | | | | | | | | | | | | | | | | | | | | |
| 11113 | 1 | ea | Francais, Healthy Choice | 262 | 280 | 75 | 20.0 | 40.0 | 4.0 | 1.0 | 35.0 | 5.0 | 1.5 | | | | | 30 | 0 | 0 | 0 | 0 | 0 | | | | | | | | 0.0 | | | 20 | | 1.8 | | | | | | 520 | |
| 70426 | 1 | ea | With Burgundy Sauce, Budget Gourmet | 312 | 310 | 80 | 24.0 | 28.0 | | | | 11.0 | | | | | | 65 | 200 | 40 | | | | 0.23 | 0.43 | 6.00 | | | | | 6.0 | | | 60 | | 3.6 | | | | | | 720 | |
| 70440 | 1 | ea | With Country Gravy, Budget Gourmet | 284 | 310 | 80 | 16.0 | 21.0 | | | | 18.0 | | | | | | 40 | 750 | 150 | | | | 0.15 | 0.17 | 4.00 | 0.28 | | | | 2.4 | | | 60 | | 0.4 | | | | | | 570 | |
| 11039 | 1 | cup | Beef, W/Noodles, Banquet | 227 | 150 | 85 | 12.0 | 17.0 | 2.0 | 1.0 | 14.0 | 4.0 | 2.0 | | | | | 40 | | | | | | | | | | | | | 2.4 | | | 20 | | 1.4 | | | | | | 1200 | |
| 11040 | 1 | ea | Beef, W/Onion Gravy, Marie Calendar | 132 | 180 | 78 | 8.0 | 7.0 | 2.0 | 5.0 | 0.0 | 14.0 | 6.0 | | | | | 20 | 0 | 0 | 0 | 0 | 0 | | | | | | | | 0.0 | | | 20 | | 1.1 | | | | | | 630 | |
| 11096 | 1 | ea | Beef, W/Potatoes, Stouffers | 230 | 270 | 74 | 19.0 | 25.0 | 2.0 | 2.0 | 21.0 | 10.0 | 3.0 | | | | | 45 | | | | | | | | | | | | | 6.0 | | | 20 | | 1.8 | | | | 730 | | 900 | |
| | | | Cannelloni | | | | | | | | | | | | | | | | | | | | | | | | | | | | | | | | | | | | | | | | |
| 57428 | 1 | ea | Beef, Bernardis | 85 | 200 | | 9.0 | 19.0 | 1.0 | 2.0 | 15.0 | 10.0 | 5.0 | | | | | 25 | 100 | 20 | | | | | | | | | | | 0.0 | | | 40 | | 1.4 | | | | | | 290 | |
| 70145 | 1 | ea | Cheese, low calorie, avg | 259 | 298 | 76 | 21.9 | 24.3 | 1.7 | | | 12.5 | 7.0 | 3.4 | 1.2 | | | 41 | 1210 | 190 | 99 | 91 | | 0.16 | 0.29 | 1.67 | 0.13 | 0.42 | 19.3 | | 9.9 | | | 269 | 0.1 | 1.5 | 31 | | 262 | 225 | | 1220 | 1.67 |
| 56737 | 1 | ea | Cheese, Lean Cuisine | 259 | 270 | 77 | 21.0 | 28.0 | 3.0 | 5.0 | 20.0 | 8.0 | 3.5 | 1.5 | 0.5 | | | 30 | 400 | 60 | | | | 0.12 | 0.25 | 1.60 | 0.14 | 0.00 | 0.0 | | 12.0 | | | 350 | 0.1 | 1.1 | 36 | | | 400 | | 500 | 1.60 |
| 56833 | 1 | cup | Cantonese Noodle, Spice Hunter | 234 | 82 | | 3.1 | 15.5 | | | | 0.0 | 0.0 | 0.0 | 0.0 | 0.00 | 0.00 | | | | | | | | | | | | | | | | | | | | | | | 144 | | 567 | |
| 15969 | 1 | ea | Chicken, A La King, Stouffers | 269 | 320 | 73 | 15.0 | 43.0 | 3.0 | 4.0 | 35.0 | 10.0 | 3.0 | | | | | 55 | 100 | 20 | | | | 0.10 | 0.10 | 1.50 | | | | | 3.6 | | | 100 | | 0.7 | | | | 290 | | 750 | |
| 70785 | 1 | cup | Chicken, A La King, Swanson | 245 | 320 | | 15.0 | 17.0 | 0.0 | 2.0 | 15.0 | 22.0 | 8.0 | | | | | 60 | 0 | 0 | 0 | 0 | 0 | | | | | | | | 0.0 | | | 80 | | 1.1 | | | | | | 1080 | |
| 15965 | 1 | ea | Chicken, A L' Orange, Lean Cuisine | 255 | 260 | 75 | 19.0 | 40.0 | 1.0 | 10.0 | 23.0 | 2.5 | 0.5 | 0.5 | 0.5 | | | 40 | 1500 | 300 | | | | 0.22 | 0.17 | 10.00 | 0.29 | 0.00 | 0.0 | | 21.0 | | | 40 | 0.2 | 0.7 | 47 | | | 410 | | 260 | 1.00 |
| 70071 | 1 | ea | Chicken, Au Gratin, w/vegetables, avg | 258 | 317 | 74 | 29.5 | 19.1 | 2.0 | | | 13.2 | 7.4 | 3.8 | 1.0 | | | 88 | 3372 | 400 | 93 | 307 | | 0.17 | 0.33 | 10.47 | 0.58 | 0.50 | 71.2 | | 12.7 | | | 279 | 0.2 | 2.9 | 70 | | 348 | 511 | | 1112 | 2.12 |
| 70447 | 1 | ea | Chicken, Au Gratin, Slim Select | 258 | 260 | 80 | 20.0 | 21.0 | | | | 11.0 | | | | | | 70 | 3500 | 700 | | | | 0.12 | 0.34 | 7.00 | | | | | 12.0 | | | 20 | | 1.8 | | | | | | 820 | |
| 16196 | 1 | ea | Chicken, Baked, Lean Cuisine | 227 | 240 | 75 | 18.0 | 31.0 | 3.0 | 6.0 | 22.0 | 5.0 | 0.5 | 2.0 | 1.5 | | | 35 | 200 | 40 | | | | | | | | | | | 1.2 | | | 100 | | 1.4 | | | | 460 | | 480 | |
| 16197 | 1 | ea | Chicken, Baked, Stouffers | 252 | 270 | 78 | 22.0 | 19.0 | 2.0 | 1.0 | 15.0 | 12.0 | 3.0 | | | | | 75 | | | | | | | | | | | | | 1.2 | | | 20 | | 0.7 | | | | 550 | | 750 | |
| | | | Chicken, BBQ | | | | | | | | | | | | | | | | | | | | | | | | | | | | | | | | | | | | | | | | |
| 16245 | 1 | ea | Banquet | 255 | 320 | 74 | 18.0 | 36.0 | 3.0 | 15.0 | 13.0 | 12.0 | 2.5 | | | | | 60 | 300 | 60 | | | | | | | | | | | 6.0 | | | 60 | | 1.8 | | | | | | 800 | |
| 16225 | 1 | cup | Orval Kent | 210 | 360 | | 31.5 | 28.5 | 1.5 | 19.5 | 7.5 | 13.5 | 3.8 | | | | | 128 | 0 | 0 | 0 | 0 | 0 | | | | | | | | 1.8 | | | 60 | | 2.7 | | | | | | 1005 | |
| 16220 | 1 | ea | Weight Watchers | 210 | 190 | 79 | 18.0 | 22.0 | 1.0 | 7.0 | 14.0 | 3.5 | 1.0 | | | | | 20 | 400 | 80 | | | | | | | | | | | 6.0 | | | 40 | | 1.8 | | | | 580 | | 340 | |
| 70076 | 1 | ea | Chicken, Cacciatore, w/noodles, avg | 308 | 290 | 79 | 21.6 | 29.4 | 3.3 | | | 9.7 | 2.4 | 3.5 | 2.5 | | | 59 | 748 | 100 | 37 | 62 | | 0.15 | 0.34 | 7.02 | 0.42 | 0.20 | 31.5 | | 26.6 | | | 31 | 0.4 | 2.5 | 43 | | 219 | 616 | | 933 | 2.56 |
| 81084 | 1 | ea | Chicken, Cacciatore, Healthy Choice | 354 | 270 | 82 | 22.0 | 36.0 | 5.0 | 10.0 | 21.0 | 4.0 | 1.0 | | | | | 35 | 200 | 40 | | | | | | | | | | | 6.0 | | | 40 | | 1.8 | | | | | | 550 | |
| 16221 | 1 | ea | Chicken, Cordon Bleu, Weight Watchers | 255 | 220 | 80 | 17.0 | 27.0 | 3.0 | 1.0 | 23.0 | 6.0 | 2.0 | | | | | 20 | 1000 | 200 | | | | | | | | | | | 6.0 | | | 150 | | 1.4 | | | | 350 | | 500 | |
| 15973 | 1 | ea | Chicken, Creamed, Stouffers | 184 | 280 | 73 | 17.0 | 8.0 | 1.0 | 3.0 | 4.0 | 20.0 | 7.0 | | | | | 80 | 0 | 0 | 0 | 0 | 0 | 0.00 | 0.10 | 1.60 | | | | | 0.0 | | | 80 | | 0.4 | | | | 210 | | 720 | |
| 57449 | 3 | oz | Chicken, Croquettes, Tyson | 85 | 247 | 47 | 9.6 | 17.9 | 1.2 | 3.6 | 13.1 | 15.3 | 3.7 | | | | | 35 | | | | | | | | | | | | | 1.2 | | | 0 | | 5.0 | | | | | | 0 | |
| 15971 | 1 | ea | Chicken, Divan, Stouffers | 227 | 210 | 80 | 21.0 | 10.0 | 1.0 | 6.0 | 3.0 | 10.0 | 4.0 | | | | | 65 | 100 | 20 | | | | 0.10 | 0.10 | 2.10 | | | | | 24.0 | | | 150 | | 0.4 | | | | 500 | | 570 | |
| | | | Chicken, W/Dumplings | | | | | | | | | | | | | | | | | | | | | | | | | | | | | | | | | | | | | | | | |
| 15958 | 1 | cup | Banquet | 211 | 310 | 71 | 13.0 | 32.0 | 2.0 | 2.0 | 23.0 | 15.0 | 5.0 | | | | | 40 | 0 | 0 | 0 | 0 | 0 | | | | | | | | 0.0 | | | 40 | | 1.4 | | | | | | 1360 | |
| 70786 | 1 | cup | Swanson | 247 | 260 | 81 | 11.0 | 22.0 | 0.0 | 1.0 | 21.0 | 14.0 | 5.0 | | | | | 65 | 400 | 80 | | | | | | | | | | | 0.0 | | | 40 | | 1.1 | | | | | | 1120 | |
| 82029 | 1 | ea | Chicken, Fajitas, Healthy Choice | 198 | 260 | 69 | 21.0 | 36.0 | 5.0 | 6.0 | 25.0 | 4.0 | 1.0 | | | | | 30 | 750 | 150 | | | | | | | | | | | 36.0 | | | 20 | | 1.8 | | | | | | 410 | |
| 70433 | 1 | ea | Chicken, Fettucini, Budget Gourmet | 284 | 400 | 74 | 23.0 | 29.0 | | | | 21.0 | | | | | | 100 | 1750 | 350 | | | | 0.15 | 0.43 | 6.00 | | | | | 2.4 | | | 200 | | 1.8 | | | | | | 740 | |
| 15940 | 1 | ea | Chicken, Fiesta, Lean Cuisine | 241 | 240 | 76 | 18.0 | 31.0 | 3.0 | 3.0 | 25.0 | 5.0 | 1.0 | 2.0 | 1.0 | | | 45 | 750 | 150 | | | | 0.22 | 0.14 | 6.00 | | | | | 15.0 | | | 40 | | 1.1 | | | | 420 | | 590 | |

| Code | Amount | | Description | Basic Components | | | | | | | | | Additional Fats | | | | | |
|---|---|---|---|---|---|---|---|---|---|---|---|---|---|---|---|---|---|---|
| | | | | Weight (g) | Calories | % Water | Protein (g) | Carbs (g) | Fiber (g) | Sugar (g) | Other Carbs (g) | Fat (g) | Sat Fat (g) | Mono Fat (g) | Poly Fat (g) | Omega 3 (g) | Omega 6 (g) | Choles (mg) |
| 16257 | 1 | ea | Chicken, Francesca, Healthy Choice | 354 | 330 | 76 | 23.0 | 46.0 | 4.0 | 6.0 | 36.0 | 6.0 | 2.5 | | | | | 30 |
| 70449 | 1 | ea | Chicken, French Recipe, Budget Gourmet | 284 | 260 | 81 | 21.0 | 21.0 | | | | 10.0 | | | | | | 60 |
| | | | Chicken, Fried | | | | | | | | | | | | | | | |
| 16241 | 1 | ea | Country, Banquet | 101 | 269 | 54 | 14.0 | 13.0 | 1.0 | 1.0 | 11.0 | 18.0 | 5.0 | | | | | 65 |
| 16199 | 1 | ea | Homestyle, Stouffers | 202 | 330 | 67 | 18.0 | 29.0 | 3.0 | 2.0 | 24.0 | 16.0 | 4.0 | | | | | 55 |
| 57278 | 1 | pce | Honey BBQ, skinless, Banquet | 90 | 211 | 57 | 18.1 | 7.0 | 2.0 | 1.0 | 4.0 | 13.1 | 3.0 | | | | | 55 |
| 16242 | 1 | ea | Original, Banquet | 101 | 269 | 54 | 14.0 | 13.0 | 1.0 | 1.0 | 11.0 | 18.0 | 5.0 | | | | | 65 |
| 16238 | 1 | ea | Skinless, w/bone, Banquet | 90 | 210 | 57 | 18.0 | 7.0 | 2.0 | 1.0 | 4.0 | 13.0 | 3.0 | | | | | 55 |
| 16223 | 1 | ea | Southern, Weight Watchers | 227 | 280 | 75 | 19.0 | 25.0 | 1.0 | 4.0 | 20.0 | 11.0 | 4.5 | | | | | 65 |
| 57480 | 1 | ea | With Gravy, Marie Calendar | 454 | 611 | 73 | 25.0 | 67.1 | 6.0 | 9.0 | 52.0 | 27.0 | 8.0 | | | | | 55 |
| 16177 | 1 | ea | Chicken, Glazed, Healthy Choice | 241 | 230 | 79 | 17.0 | 30.0 | 3.0 | 6.0 | 21.0 | 4.0 | 1.5 | | | | | 45 |
| 15963 | 1 | ea | Chicken, Glazed, Lean Cuisine | 241 | 240 | 77 | 22.0 | 24.0 | 2.0 | 6.0 | 16.0 | 6.0 | 1.0 | 1.0 | 3.0 | | | 60 |
| 16206 | 1 | ea | Chicken, W/Honey BBQ Sauce, Lean Cuisine | 248 | 250 | 75 | 18.0 | 35.0 | 6.0 | 11.0 | 18.0 | 4.5 | 1.0 | 1.5 | 1.5 | | | 50 |
| | | | Chicken, Honey Mustard | | | | | | | | | | | | | | | |
| 16253 | 1 | ea | Healthy Choice | 269 | 270 | 76 | 21.0 | 38.0 | 2.0 | 7.0 | 29.0 | 4.0 | 1.5 | | | | | 40 |
| 16191 | 1 | ea | Lean Cuisine | 213 | 250 | 72 | 20.0 | 32.0 | 4.0 | 12.0 | 16.0 | 4.5 | 1.0 | 1.5 | 1.0 | | | 50 |
| 16216 | 1 | ea | Weight Watchers | 241 | 200 | 80 | 13.0 | 33.0 | 6.0 | 2.0 | 25.0 | 2.0 | 0.5 | | | | | 30 |
| 15961 | 1 | ea | Chicken, Imperial, Chung King | 369 | 460 | 76 | 17.0 | 59.0 | 5.0 | 17.0 | 37.0 | 10.0 | 3.0 | | | | | 25 |
| 15938 | 1 | ea | Chicken, Italiano, Lean Cuisine | 255 | 270 | 75 | 22.0 | 31.0 | 3.0 | 6.0 | 22.0 | 6.0 | 2.0 | 2.0 | 2.0 | | | 40 |
| 16217 | 1 | ea | Chicken, Lemon Herb Piccata, Weight Watchers | 241 | 190 | | 11.0 | 32.0 | 3.0 | 8.0 | 21.0 | 2.0 | 0.5 | | | | | 25 |
| 16251 | 1 | ea | Chicken, Mandarin, Healthy Choice | 284 | 280 | 76 | 20.0 | 44.0 | 4.0 | 9.0 | 31.0 | 2.5 | 0.0 | | | | | 35 |
| 70454 | 1 | ea | Chicken, Mandarin, Slim Select | 284 | 290 | 77 | 19.0 | 40.0 | | | | 6.0 | | | | | | 25 |
| 15966 | 1 | ea | Chicken, Marsala, Lean Cuisine | 230 | 180 | 81 | 22.0 | 13.0 | 5.0 | 7.0 | 1.0 | 4.0 | 1.0 | 1.0 | 1.0 | | | 60 |
| 16210 | 1 | ea | Chicken, Marsala, Weight Watchers | 255 | 150 | 86 | 10.0 | 22.0 | 6.0 | 3.0 | 13.0 | 2.0 | 0.5 | | | | | 25 |
| 16213 | 1 | ea | Chicken Mirabella, Weight Watchers | 261 | 170 | 85 | 11.0 | 26.0 | 6.0 | 6.0 | 14.0 | 2.0 | 0.5 | | | | | 20 |
| 16201 | 1 | ea | Chicken, Monterey, Stouffers | 266 | 410 | 71 | 23.0 | 35.0 | 4.0 | 4.0 | 27.0 | 20.0 | 9.0 | | | | | 75 |
| | | | Chicken, W/Noodles | | | | | | | | | | | | | | | |
| 70690 | 100 | g | La Choy | 100 | 96 | 77 | 2.7 | 18.6 | 3.5 | 15.2 | 0.0 | 1.2 | | | | | | 4 |
| 57459 | 1 | cup | Marie Calendar | 162 | 270 | 69 | 10.0 | 22.0 | 1.0 | 2.0 | 19.0 | 16.0 | 6.0 | | | | | 20 |
| 70078 | 1 | ea | With Vegetables, avg | 361 | 285 | 82 | 25.9 | 30.2 | 5.3 | | | 7.0 | 2.0 | 2.2 | 1.8 | | | 61 |
| 70083 | 1 | ea | With Vegetables & cream sauce, avg | 284 | 349 | 75 | 25.1 | 29.6 | 3.5 | | | 14.4 | 6.3 | 4.5 | 2.3 | | | 99 |
| 81069 | 1 | ea | Chicken, Parmesan, Banquet | 132 | 240 | 67 | 11.0 | 18.0 | 2.0 | 4.0 | 12.0 | 13.0 | 5.0 | | | | | 20 |
| 15967 | 1 | ea | Chicken, Parmesan, Lean Cuisine | 308 | 220 | 82 | 22.0 | 22.0 | 5.0 | 10.0 | 7.0 | 5.0 | 1.5 | 1.5 | 1.0 | | | 50 |
| | | | Chicken, Pieces | | | | | | | | | | | | | | | |
| 70566 | 1 | ea | Chunks, Banquet | 88 | 270 | 45 | 12.0 | 18.0 | 1.0 | 2.0 | 15.0 | 17.0 | 3.0 | | | | | 20 |
| 16274 | 1 | cup | Chunky Snackers, Red Devil | 220 | 675 | | 32.5 | 50.0 | 2.5 | 1.3 | 46.3 | 40.0 | 8.8 | | | | | 112 |
| 16244 | 1 | ea | Hot Popcorn, Banquet | 85 | 290 | 42 | 11.0 | 18.0 | 2.0 | 0.0 | 16.0 | 19.0 | 4.0 | | | | | 35 |
| 70565 | 1 | ea | Nuggets, Banquet | 94 | 280 | 48 | 14.0 | 16.0 | 1.0 | 2.0 | 13.0 | 18.0 | 4.0 | | | | | 25 |
| 16243 | 4 | pce | Southern Fried Nuggets, Banquet | 85 | 226 | 54 | 10.6 | 14.6 | 1.3 | 0.0 | 13.3 | 13.3 | 2.7 | | | | | 30 |
| 57280 | 1 | ea | Chicken, Primavera, Banquet | 298 | 330 | | 13.0 | 40.0 | 6.0 | 10.0 | 24.0 | 13.0 | 5.0 | | | | | 25 |
| 57475 | 1 | cup | Chicken, Primavera, Marie Calendar | 184 | 309 | 70 | 12.0 | 22.0 | 3.0 | 2.0 | 17.0 | 19.0 | 8.0 | | | | | 25 |
| 70787 | 1 | cup | Chicken, Stew, Swanson | 245 | 180 | 84 | 11.0 | 17.0 | 2.0 | 2.0 | 13.0 | 8.0 | 3.0 | | | | | 35 |
| 57350 | 1 | cup | Chicken, Stir Fry, w/pasta, Lipton | 124 | 440 | 12 | 14.0 | 90.0 | 4.0 | 4.0 | 82.0 | 4.0 | 0.0 | | | | | 0 |
| 70328 | 1 | cup | Chicken, Teriaki, La Choy | 244 | 110 | 89 | 7.3 | 14.8 | 2.9 | 8.5 | 3.4 | 3.0 | 0.9 | | | | | 15 |
| 16219 | 1 | ea | Chicken, Tex-Mex, Weight Watchers | 235 | 260 | 74 | 21.0 | 35.0 | 1.0 | 20.0 | 14.0 | 4.0 | 1.5 | | | | | 35 |
| 57479 | 1 | ea | Chicken, W/Mashed Potatoes, Marie Calendar | 397 | 670 | 70 | 43.0 | 32.0 | 7.0 | 7.0 | 18.0 | 42.0 | 15.0 | | | | | 205 |
| 16193 | 1 | ea | Chicken, W/Peanut Sauce, Lean Cuisine | 255 | 280 | 74 | 23.0 | 33.0 | 3.0 | 5.0 | 25.0 | 6.0 | 1.0 | 2.0 | 2.0 | | | 45 |
| 70160 | 1 | ea | Chicken, W/Vegetables & cream sce, low cal, avg | 255 | 245 | 80 | 26.9 | 15.1 | 1.6 | | | 8.1 | 1.9 | 2.5 | 2.8 | | | 66 |
| 15960 | 1 | ea | Chicken, W/Walnuts, Chun King | 369 | 460 | 74 | 19.0 | 56.0 | 5.0 | 15.0 | 36.0 | 19.0 | 5.0 | | | | | 35 |
| | | | Chicken, Wings | | | | | | | | | | | | | | | |
| 16239 | 4 | pce | BBQ, Banquet | 113 | 189 | 71 | 14.9 | 5.0 | 1.0 | 4.0 | 0.0 | 12.0 | 4.0 | | | | | 70 |
| 15903 | 7 | pce | Buffalo, w/hot pepper sauce, avg | 112 | 343 | 53 | 29.1 | 0.2 | 0.1 | 0.1 | 0.1 | 24.3 | 6.4 | 9.7 | 5.7 | | | 91 |
| 16240 | 4 | pce | Hot & Spicy, Banquet | 113 | 229 | 68 | 14.9 | 5.0 | 1.0 | 0.0 | 4.0 | 15.9 | 5.0 | | | | | 85 |
| | | | Chow Mein | | | | | | | | | | | | | | | |
| 70688 | 1 | cup | Beef, La Choy | 247 | 104 | 88 | 9.2 | 14.9 | 3.5 | 3.0 | 8.4 | 1.7 | 0.8 | | | | | 12 |
| 83002 | 1 | ea | Chicken, Chung King | 369 | 370 | 79 | 16.0 | 45.0 | 4.0 | 6.0 | 35.0 | 14.0 | 5.0 | | | | | 45 |
| 83005 | 1 | ea | Chicken, Weight Watchers | 255 | 200 | 81 | 12.0 | 34.0 | 3.0 | 5.0 | 26.0 | 2.0 | 0.5 | | | | | 25 |
| 15964 | 1 | ea | Chicken, W/Rice, Lean Cuisine | 255 | 210 | 81 | 13.0 | 28.0 | 2.0 | 2.0 | 24.0 | 5.0 | 1.0 | 2.0 | 1.0 | | | 35 |
| 15970 | 1 | ea | Chicken, W/Rice, Stouffers | 301 | 260 | 78 | 13.0 | 43.0 | 3.0 | 2.0 | 38.0 | 4.0 | 1.0 | | | | | 30 |
| 70693 | 100 | g | Pork, La Choy | 100 | 35 | 90 | 2.3 | 4.2 | 1.2 | 0.9 | 2.1 | 1.3 | 0.5 | | | | | 4 |
| 70177 | 1 | cup | Clams, Fried, Mrs Paul | 227 | 748 | 39 | 21.4 | 77.4 | 2.7 | 8.0 | 66.8 | 42.7 | 8.0 | 14.3 | 8.5 | | | 27 |
| 70173 | 5 | pce | Crab, Deviled Miniatures, Mrs Paul's | 82 | 199 | 51 | 6.6 | 22.4 | 1.7 | 4.1 | 16.6 | 9.1 | 2.5 | | | | | 12 |
| | | | Eggrolls | | | | | | | | | | | | | | | |
| 83000 | 5 | pce | Chicken, Chun King | 88 | 174 | 58 | 5.0 | 24.9 | 2.5 | 1.7 | 20.8 | 5.8 | 1.2 | | | | | 8 |
| 83015 | 1 | ea | Lobster, La Choy | 106 | 210 | 55 | 7.0 | 34.0 | 5.0 | 3.0 | 26.0 | 6.0 | 1.0 | | | | | 0 |
| 83012 | 1 | ea | MuSho Pork, La Choy | 57 | 191 | 31 | 6.0 | 25.1 | 2.0 | 8.0 | 15.1 | 7.0 | 1.5 | | | | | 15 |
| 83009 | 1 | ea | Pork, La Choy | 57 | 171 | 36 | 6.0 | 23.1 | 3.0 | 6.0 | 14.1 | 6.0 | 1.5 | | | | | 5 |
| 56704 | 5 | pce | Pork & Shrimp, Chung King | 88 | 183 | 61 | 5.0 | 24.1 | 2.5 | 1.7 | 19.9 | 6.6 | 1.7 | | | | | 8 |
| 83001 | 5 | pce | Shrimp, Chung King | 88 | 158 | 61 | 4.2 | 24.1 | 2.5 | 1.7 | 19.9 | 5.0 | 0.8 | | | | | 8 |
| 83017 | 1 | ea | Shrimp, La Choy | 106 | 240 | 54 | 8.0 | 31.0 | 3.0 | 2.0 | 26.0 | 9.0 | 2.0 | | | | | 10 |

| Code | Vit A & Components | | | | | Vitamins | | | | | | | | | |
|---|---|---|---|---|---|---|---|---|---|---|---|---|---|---|---|
| | Vit A (IU) | Vit A (RE) | Retinol (RE) | Carotenoids (RE) | Beta Carotene (mcg) | Thiamin (mg) | Riboflavin (mg) | Niacin (NE) | Vit B6 (mg) | Vit B12 (mcg) | Folate (mcg) | Panto (mg) | Vit C (mg) | Vit D (mg) | Vit E (α TE) |
| 16257 | 100 | 20 | | | | | | | | | | | 15.0 | | |
| 70449 | 3000 | 600 | | | | 0.15 | 0.34 | 9.00 | | | | | 2.4 | | |
| 16241 | 0 | 0 | 0 | 0 | 0 | | | | | | | | 3.6 | | |
| 16199 | 100 | 20 | | | | | | | | | | | 1.2 | | |
| 57278 | 0 | 0 | 0 | 0 | 0 | | | | | | | | 6.0 | | |
| 16242 | 0 | 0 | 0 | 0 | 0 | | | | | | | | 3.6 | | |
| 16238 | 0 | 0 | 0 | 0 | 0 | | | | | | | | 6.0 | | |
| 16223 | 750 | 150 | | | | | | | | | | | 0.0 | | |
| 57480 | 300 | 60 | | | | | | | | | | | 9.0 | | |
| 16177 | 0 | 0 | 0 | 0 | 0 | 0.15 | 0.14 | 7.00 | | | | | 0.0 | | |
| 15963 | 100 | 20 | | | | 0.15 | 0.17 | 8.00 | 0.31 | 0.00 | 0.0 | | 2.4 | | |
| 16206 | 750 | 150 | | | | 0.15 | 0.17 | 6.00 | | | | | 9.0 | | |
| 16253 | 1000 | 200 | | | | | | | | | | | 0.0 | | |
| 16191 | 1000 | 200 | | | | | | | | | | | 2.4 | | |
| 16216 | 500 | 100 | | | | | | | | | | | 9.0 | | |
| 15961 | 1000 | 200 | | | | 0.15 | 0.43 | 2.00 | | | | | 0.0 | | |
| 15938 | 300 | 60 | | | | 0.15 | 0.25 | 6.00 | | | | | 6.0 | | |
| 16217 | 1750 | 350 | | | | | | | | | | | 9.0 | | |
| 16251 | 750 | 150 | | | | | | | | | | | 15.0 | | |
| 70454 | 1750 | 350 | | | | 0.09 | 0.34 | 0.80 | | | | | 2.4 | | |
| 15966 | 2000 | 400 | | | | 0.22 | 0.17 | 8.00 | | | | | 9.0 | | |
| 16210 | 400 | 80 | | | | | | | | | | | 6.0 | | |
| 16213 | 1250 | 250 | | | | | | | | | | | 9.0 | | |
| 16201 | 500 | 100 | | | | | | | | | | | 9.0 | | |
| 70690 | 56 | 11 | | | | | | | | | | | 3.4 | | |
| 57459 | 300 | 60 | | | | | | | | | | | 2.4 | | |
| 70078 | 4415 | 452 | 16 | 436 | | 0.21 | 0.31 | 6.88 | 0.45 | 0.17 | 56.8 | | 37.8 | | |
| 70083 | 1347 | 184 | 73 | 111 | | 0.11 | 0.28 | 4.19 | 0.28 | 0.36 | 30.5 | | 22.6 | | |
| 81069 | 200 | 40 | | | | | | | | | | | 36.0 | | |
| 15967 | 750 | 150 | | | | 0.22 | 0.25 | 7.00 | | | | | 6.0 | | |
| 70566 | 0 | 0 | 0 | 0 | 0 | | | | | | | | 0.0 | | |
| 16274 | 0 | 0 | 0 | 0 | 0 | | | | | | | | 0.0 | | |
| 16244 | 0 | 0 | 0 | 0 | 0 | | | | | | | | 0.0 | | |
| 70565 | 0 | 0 | 0 | 0 | 0 | | | | | | | | 0.0 | | |
| 16243 | 0 | 0 | 0 | 0 | 0 | | | | | | | | 1.6 | | |
| 57280 | 501 | 100 | | | | | | | | | | | 12.0 | | |
| 57475 | 300 | 60 | | | | | | | | | | | 9.0 | | |
| 70787 | 3500 | 700 | | | | | | | | | | | 2.4 | | |
| 57350 | 400 | 80 | | | | | | | | | | | 4.8 | | |
| 70328 | 54 | 11 | | | | 0.10 | 0.15 | 4.73 | | | | | 11.4 | | |
| 16219 | 1500 | 300 | | | | | | | | | | | 12.0 | | |
| 57479 | 750 | 150 | | | | | | | | | | | 60.0 | | |
| 16193 | 400 | 80 | | | | | | | | | | | 4.8 | | |
| 70160 | 923 | 131 | 58 | 73 | | 0.14 | 0.32 | 6.04 | 0.32 | 0.33 | 31.2 | | 31.5 | | |
| 15960 | 0 | 0 | 0 | 0 | 0 | 1.50 | 0.17 | 2.00 | | | | | 0.0 | | |
| 16239 | 0 | 0 | 0 | 0 | 0 | | | | | | | | 4.8 | | |
| 15903 | 260 | 60 | 51 | 9 | | 0.05 | 0.14 | 7.20 | 0.46 | 0.31 | 3.5 | 1.01 | 0.2 | 0.3 | |
| 16240 | 0 | 0 | 0 | 0 | 0 | | | | | | | | 4.8 | | |
| 70688 | 58 | 12 | | | | | | | | | | | 11.1 | | |
| 83002 | 500 | 100 | | | | 1.50 | 0.17 | 3.00 | | | | | 9.0 | | |
| 83005 | 1499 | 300 | | | | | | | | | | | 36.0 | | |
| 15964 | 100 | 20 | | | | 0.15 | 0.17 | 5.00 | | | | | 6.0 | | |
| 15970 | 300 | 60 | | | | 0.00 | 0.10 | 0.90 | | | | | 6.0 | | |
| 70693 | 17 | 3 | | | | | | | | | | | 1.7 | | |
| 70177 | 53 | 11 | | | | 0.37 | 0.19 | 3.74 | 0.06 | | | | 0.0 | | |
| 70173 | 0 | 0 | 0 | 0 | 0 | 0.13 | 0.26 | 1.16 | | | | | 0.0 | | |
| 83000 | 83 | 2 | | | | 0.08 | 0.05 | 0.58 | | | | | 1.0 | | |
| 83015 | 0 | 0 | 0 | 0 | 0 | | | | | | | | 1.2 | | |
| 83012 | 302 | 60 | | | | | | | | | | | 0.0 | | |
| 83009 | 402 | 80 | | | | | | | | | | | 0.0 | | |
| 56704 | 83 | 17 | | | | 0.16 | 0.07 | 0.58 | | | | | 3.0 | | |
| 83001 | 83 | 17 | | | | 0.07 | 0.02 | 0.33 | | | | | 3.0 | | |
| 83017 | 100 | 20 | | | | | | | | | | | 3.6 | | |

| Code | Minerals | | | | | | | | | |
|---|---|---|---|---|---|---|---|---|---|---|
| | Calcium (mg) | Copper (mg) | Iron (mg) | Magnes (mg) | Mang (mg) | Phos (mg) | Potassium (mg) | Selenium (mcg) | Sodium (mg) | Zinc (mg) |
| 16257 | 100 | | 1.8 | | | | | | 600 | |
| 70449 | 60 | | 1.1 | | | | | | 790 | |
| 16241 | 80 | | 0.7 | | | | | | 619 | |
| 16199 | 20 | | 0.7 | | | | 370 | | 780 | |
| 57278 | 20 | | 0.4 | | | | | | 482 | |
| 16242 | 80 | | 0.7 | | | | | | 619 | |
| 16238 | 20 | | 0.4 | | | | | | 480 | |
| 16223 | 80 | | 1.1 | | | | 550 | | 590 | |
| 57480 | 20 | | 0.4 | | | | | | 1681 | |
| 16177 | 20 | | 0.4 | | | 240 | 370 | | 480 | |
| 15963 | 20 | 0.1 | 0.4 | 38 | | | 370 | | 460 | 0.93 |
| 16206 | 40 | | 1.8 | | | | 820 | | 560 | |
| 16253 | 20 | | 0.4 | | | | | | 520 | |
| 16191 | 40 | | 1.4 | | | | 310 | | 460 | |
| 16216 | 40 | | 1.1 | | | | 320 | | 340 | |
| 15961 | 40 | | 1.8 | | | 150 | 260 | | 1670 | |
| 15938 | 80 | | 1.1 | | | | 600 | | 490 | |
| 16217 | 40 | | 0.7 | | | | 220 | | 590 | |
| 16251 | 20 | | 0.7 | | | | | | 520 | |
| 70454 | 40 | | 0.7 | | | | | | 690 | |
| 15966 | 20 | 0.1 | 1.1 | 42 | | | 520 | | 470 | 0.98 |
| 16210 | 20 | | 1.1 | | | | 330 | | 500 | |
| 16213 | 60 | | 1.8 | | | | 330 | | 410 | |
| 16201 | 350 | | 1.1 | | | | 350 | | 700 | |
| 70690 | 1 | | 0.1 | | | | | | 262 | |
| 57459 | 40 | | 0.7 | | | | | | 670 | |
| 70078 | 69 | 0.4 | 2.7 | 58 | | 245 | 690 | | 812 | 2.38 |
| 70083 | 165 | 0.2 | 1.6 | 51 | | 267 | 335 | | 156 | 2.29 |
| 81069 | 100 | | 1.1 | | | | | | 690 | |
| 15967 | 100 | 0.1 | 1.4 | 59 | | | 820 | | 530 | 1.30 |
| 70566 | 20 | | 1.4 | | | | | | 720 | |
| 16274 | 50 | | 4.5 | | | | | | 1800 | |
| 16244 | 60 | | 1.1 | | | | | | 789 | |
| 70565 | 20 | | 1.4 | | | | | | 620 | |
| 16243 | 13 | | 1.2 | | | | | | 558 | |
| 57280 | 80 | | 1.8 | | | | | | 931 | |
| 57475 | 60 | | 0.7 | | | | | | 449 | |
| 70787 | 40 | | 1.1 | | | | | | 1110 | |
| 57350 | 0 | | 2.9 | | | | | | 1700 | |
| 70328 | 2 | | 10.0 | | | | | | 1220 | |
| 16219 | 40 | | 2.7 | | | | 670 | | 430 | |
| 57479 | 100 | | 1.8 | | | | | | 2101 | |
| 16193 | 80 | | 1.4 | | | | 480 | | 6 | |
| 70160 | 122 | 0.2 | 2.0 | 38 | | 250 | 439 | | 648 | 2.30 |
| 15960 | 60 | | 1.8 | | | 150 | 200 | | 1820 | |
| 16239 | 20 | | 0.4 | | | | | | 538 | |
| 15903 | 17 | 0.1 | 1.4 | 21 | 0.0 | 165 | 205 | | 213 | 1.98 |
| 16240 | 20 | | 0.7 | | | | | | 279 | |
| 70688 | 30 | | 0.6 | | | | | | 756 | |
| 83002 | 40 | | 1.4 | | | 200 | 260 | | 2010 | |
| 83005 | 40 | | 0.7 | | | | 360 | | 430 | |
| 15964 | 20 | 0.2 | 0.4 | 30 | | | 300 | | 510 | 1.10 |
| 15970 | 20 | | 1.1 | | | | 290 | | 940 | |
| 70693 | 1 | | 3.2 | | | | | | 497 | |
| 70177 | 53 | | 3.8 | | | | 304 | | 1442 | |
| 70173 | 66 | | 1.2 | | | | 153 | | 447 | |
| 83000 | 17 | | 0.3 | | | 75 | 100 | | 216 | |
| 83015 | 20 | | | | | | | | 360 | |
| 83012 | 20 | | 1.1 | | | | | | 332 | |
| 83009 | 20 | | 1.4 | | | | | | 392 | |
| 56704 | 17 | | 0.3 | | | 58 | 108 | | 216 | |
| 83001 | 17 | | 0.3 | | | 42 | 66 | | 299 | |
| 83017 | 20 | | 1.1 | | | | | | 350 | |

| Code | Amount | | Description | Basic Components | | | | | | | | | Additional Fats | | | | | | Vit A & Components | | | | | Vitamins | | | | | | | | | | Minerals | | | | | | | | | |
|---|---|---|---|---|---|---|---|---|---|---|---|---|---|---|---|---|---|---|---|---|---|---|---|---|---|---|---|---|---|---|---|---|---|---|---|---|---|---|---|---|---|---|---|
| | | | | Weight (g) | Calories | % Water | Protein (g) | Carbs (g) | Fiber (g) | Sugar (g) | Other Carbs (g) | Fat (g) | Sat Fat (g) | Mono Fat (g) | Poly Fat (g) | Omega 3 (g) | Omega 6 (g) | Choles (mg) | Vit A (IU) | Vit A (RE) | Retinol (RE) | Carotenoids (RE) | Beta Carotene (mcg) | Thiamin (mg) | Riboflavin (mg) | Niacin (NE) | Vit B6 (mg) | Vit B12 (mcg) | Folate (mcg) | Panto (mg) | Vit C (mg) | Vit D (mg) | Vit E (α TE) | Calcium (mg) | Copper (mg) | Iron (mg) | Magnes (mg) | Mang (mg) | Phos (mg) | Potassium (mg) | Selenium (mcg) | Sodium (mg) | Zinc (mg) |
| 83010 | 1 | ea | Sweet & Sour, La Choy | 57 | 181 | 29 | 6.0 | 29.2 | 3.0 | 10.1 | 16.1 | 4.0 | 1.0 | | | | | 5 | 101 | 20 | | | | | | | | | | | 2.4 | | | 20 | | 1.4 | | | | | | 302 | |
| 81038 | 1 | ea | Fettucini Alfredo, Healthy Choice | 227 | 250 | 74 | 11.0 | 39.0 | 2.0 | 4.0 | 33.0 | 5.0 | 2.0 | | | | | 30 | 0 | 0 | 0 | 0 | 0 | 0.23 | 0.17 | 1.20 | | | | | 0.0 | | | 100 | | 0.7 | | | 140 | 70 | | 480 | |
| 81063 | 1 | ea | Fettucini Alfredo, w/Broccoli, Weight Watchers | 241 | 220 | 81 | 15.0 | 24.0 | 6.0 | 1.0 | 17.0 | 6.0 | 2.5 | | | | | 15 | 300 | 50 | | | | | | | | | | | 1.2 | | | 250 | | 2.7 | | | | 510 | | 540 | |
| | | | Finfish | | | | | | | | | | | | | | | | | | | | | | | | | | | | | | | | | | | | | | | | |
| 18818 | 1 | ea | Fish Divan, Lean Cuisine | 294 | 210 | 82 | 25.0 | 15.0 | 3.0 | 7.0 | 5.0 | 6.0 | 1.0 | 1.0 | 2.5 | | | 65 | 300 | 30 | | | | 0.15 | 0.34 | 2.00 | 0.23 | 2.00 | 0.0 | | 18.0 | | | 150 | 0.1 | 0.7 | 63 | | | 710 | | 490 | 1.10 |
| 18822 | 1 | ea | Fish Fillet, w/Macaroni & Cheese, Stouffers | 255 | 430 | 67 | 24.0 | 37.0 | 2.0 | 7.0 | 28.0 | 21.0 | 5.0 | | | | | 70 | 100 | 20 | | | | | | | | | | | | | | 150 | | 1.1 | | | | 440 | | 930 | |
| 18825 | 1 | ea | Lemon Pepper, Healthy Choice | 303 | 320 | 78 | 14.0 | 50.0 | 5.0 | 20.0 | 25.0 | 7.0 | 2.0 | | | | | 30 | 500 | 100 | | | | | | | | | | | 30.0 | | | 20 | | 1.1 | | | | | | 480 | |
| 18831 | 1 | ea | Pollock, w/Broccoli & Cheese, svg, Viking | 124 | 243 | | 14.9 | 15.4 | 0.6 | 0.5 | 14.3 | 13.3 | 2.6 | | | | | 52 | 185 | 37 | | | | | | | | | | | 8.3 | | | 45 | | 0.5 | | | | | | 353 | |
| 18830 | 1 | ea | Pollock, Krunchy-Lite, svg, Viking | 102 | 171 | | 15.9 | 14.7 | 0.6 | 0.8 | 13.3 | 4.8 | 0.4 | | | | | 58 | 28 | 6 | | | | | | | | | | | 0.0 | | | 7 | | 0.7 | | | | | | 247 | |
| 18832 | 1 | ea | Pollock, Krunchy-Lite Fiesta, svg, Viking | 102 | 142 | | 14.4 | 11.3 | 0.5 | 1.1 | 9.7 | 3.8 | 0.6 | | | | | 94 | 75 | 15 | | | | | | | | | | | 2.1 | | | 29 | | 0.7 | | | | | | 256 | |
| | | | Finfish, Fried Fillets | | | | | | | | | | | | | | | | | | | | | | | | | | | | | | | | | | | | | | | | |
| 70223 | 1 | pce | Cod, Mrs Paul's | 127 | 250 | 58 | 14.0 | 24.0 | 2.0 | 5.0 | 17.0 | 11.0 | 3.0 | | | | | 40 | 0 | 0 | 0 | 0 | 0 | 0.12 | 0.15 | 1.60 | | | | | 0.0 | | | 20 | | 0.7 | | | | 347 | | 510 | |
| 70226 | 1 | pce | Battered, Mrs Paul's | 77 | 170 | 53 | 7.0 | 16.0 | 1.0 | 3.0 | 12.0 | 10.0 | 2.5 | | | | | 20 | 0 | 0 | 0 | 0 | 0 | 0.12 | 0.12 | 2.40 | | | | | 0.0 | | | 20 | | 0.4 | | | | 151 | | 420 | |
| 70259 | 1 | ea | Battered, Van De Kamp's | 75 | 180 | 56 | 8.0 | 12.0 | 0.0 | 3.0 | 9.0 | 11.0 | 1.5 | 4.5 | 1.0 | | | 20 | 0 | 0 | 0 | 0 | 0 | 0.12 | 0.10 | 1.20 | 0.07 | | | | 0.0 | | | 0 | | 0.4 | | | 200 | 190 | | 340 | |
| 70176 | 1 | pce | Battered, Crunchy, Mrs Paul's | 56 | 124 | 56 | 5.0 | 11.4 | 1.0 | 2.5 | 7.9 | 6.4 | 1.3 | 1.5 | 3.6 | | | 12 | 0 | 0 | 0 | 0 | 0 | 0.06 | 0.06 | 0.69 | 0.04 | | | | 0.0 | | | 10 | | 0.5 | | | | 82 | | 337 | |
| 70267 | 1 | ea | Breaded, Van De Kamp's | 50 | 141 | 51 | 5.6 | 8.6 | 0.0 | 1.0 | 7.6 | 9.6 | 1.5 | 3.5 | 0.8 | | | 18 | 0 | 0 | 0 | 0 | 0 | 0.08 | 0.05 | 0.81 | | | | | 0.0 | | | 0 | | 0.2 | | | 101 | 71 | | 136 | |
| 70194 | 1 | pce | Breaded, Crunchy, Mrs Paul's | 57 | 110 | 61 | 6.5 | 10.5 | 1.0 | 2.0 | 7.5 | 5.0 | 1.0 | 1.2 | 2.9 | | | 18 | 0 | 0 | 0 | 0 | 0 | 0.05 | 0.06 | 0.75 | 0.04 | | | | 0.0 | | | 10 | | 0.4 | | | | 94 | | 245 | |
| 70189 | 1 | pce | Flounder, Crunchy Batter, Mrs Paul's | 53 | 130 | 56 | 5.5 | 12.0 | 1.0 | 2.0 | 9.0 | 7.0 | 1.5 | | | | | 15 | 0 | 0 | 0 | 0 | 0 | 0.04 | 0.05 | 0.60 | | | | | 0.0 | | | 20 | | 0.4 | | | | 101 | | 270 | |
| 70256 | 1 | ea | Flounder, Van De Kamp's | 113 | 110 | 77 | 22.0 | 0.0 | 0.0 | 0.0 | 0.0 | 2.0 | 0.0 | 0.5 | 0.5 | | | 45 | 0 | 0 | 0 | 0 | 0 | 0.06 | 0.03 | 2.00 | | | | | | | | 0 | | 0.4 | | | 200 | 500 | | 105 | |
| 70190 | 1 | pce | Haddock, Crunchy Batter, Mrs Paul's | 53 | 125 | 52 | 5.0 | 12.5 | 1.0 | 3.5 | 8.0 | 6.0 | 1.3 | | | | | 12 | 0 | 0 | 0 | 0 | 0 | 0.05 | 0.05 | 0.90 | | | | | 0.0 | | | 10 | | 0.4 | | | | 141 | | 315 | |
| 70263 | 1 | ea | Haddock, Battered, Van De Kamp's | 56 | 129 | 56 | 6.4 | 8.9 | 0.0 | 2.5 | 6.4 | 7.9 | 1.2 | 3.5 | 0.5 | | | 15 | 0 | 0 | 0 | 0 | 0 | 0.06 | 0.07 | 0.99 | | | | | 0.0 | | | 20 | | 0.4 | | | 149 | 109 | | 263 | |
| 70264 | 1 | ea | Haddock, Breaded, Van De Kamp's | 50 | 141 | 50 | 6.1 | 9.6 | 0.0 | 0.5 | 9.1 | 8.6 | 1.5 | 3.5 | 0.8 | | | 13 | 0 | 0 | 0 | 0 | 0 | 0.08 | 0.05 | 0.81 | | | | | 0.0 | | | 0 | | 0.5 | | | 101 | 71 | | 157 | |
| 70260 | 1 | ea | Halibut, Battered, Van De Kamp's | 38 | 111 | 48 | 4.4 | 7.4 | 0.0 | 1.3 | 6.1 | 7.1 | 1.0 | 2.7 | 0.5 | | | 7 | 0 | 0 | 0 | 0 | 0 | 0.04 | 0.03 | 1.35 | 0.02 | | | | 0.0 | | | 13 | | 0.4 | | | 67 | 67 | | 175 | |
| 70261 | 1 | ea | Perch, Battered, Van De Kamp's | 56 | 149 | 51 | 5.9 | 9.4 | 0.0 | 1.0 | 8.4 | 9.9 | 1.2 | 3.5 | 0.7 | | | 12 | 0 | 0 | 0 | 0 | 0 | 0.07 | 0.07 | 0.99 | | | | | 0.0 | | | 10 | | 0.4 | | | 149 | 134 | | 238 | |
| 70255 | 1 | ea | Sole, Van De Kamp's | 113 | 110 | 77 | 23.0 | 0.0 | 0.0 | 0.0 | 0.0 | 1.5 | 0.0 | 0.0 | 0.5 | | | 50 | 0 | 0 | 0 | 0 | 0 | 0.06 | 0.03 | 2.00 | | | | | | | | 20 | | 0.4 | | | 200 | 500 | | 125 | |
| 70749 | 1 | ea | Fish, N Chips, Swanson | 156 | 350 | 54 | 16.0 | 38.0 | 4.0 | 6.0 | 28.0 | 15.0 | 4.5 | | | | | 30 | 200 | 40 | | | | | | | | | | | 1.2 | | | 150 | | 1.4 | | | | | | 930 | |
| | | | Fish, Sticks | | | | | | | | | | | | | | | | | | | | | | | | | | | | | | | | | | | | | | | | |
| 70200 | 5 | pce | Battered, Mrs Paul's | 92 | 226 | 54 | 6.7 | 22.6 | 0.8 | 5.0 | 16.7 | 12.5 | 2.9 | 2.2 | 5.2 | | | 21 | 0 | 0 | 0 | 0 | 0 | 0.07 | 0.11 | 0.67 | 0.04 | | | | 0.0 | | | 17 | | 0.6 | | | | 156 | | 560 | |
| 70262 | 5 | ea | Battered, Van de Kamp's | 95 | 219 | 58 | 9.2 | 15.1 | 0.0 | 3.4 | 11.8 | 13.5 | 2.5 | 5.9 | 1.3 | | | 25 | 0 | 0 | 0 | 0 | 0 | 0.10 | 0.08 | 1.01 | 0.05 | | | | 0.0 | | | 17 | | 0.6 | | | 168 | 143 | | 454 | |
| 70265 | 5 | ea | Breaded, Van de Kamp's | 95 | 242 | 51 | 10.8 | 19.2 | 0.0 | 2.5 | 16.7 | 14.2 | 2.1 | 5.8 | 0.8 | | | 29 | 0 | 0 | 0 | 0 | 0 | 0.10 | 0.06 | 1.00 | 0.04 | | | | 0.0 | | | 0 | | 0.6 | | | 83 | 92 | | 325 | |
| | | | Lasagnas | | | | | | | | | | | | | | | | | | | | | | | | | | | | | | | | | | | | | | | | |
| 81064 | 1 | ea | Garden, Weight Watchers | 312 | 230 | 83 | 17.0 | 30.0 | 6.0 | 2.0 | 22.0 | 5.0 | 1.0 | | | | | 5 | 1000 | 200 | | | | | | | | | | | 9.0 | | | 350 | | 5.4 | | | | 730 | | 460 | |
| 81079 | 1 | ea | Healthy Choice | 397 | 290 | 83 | 13.5 | 48.7 | 5.2 | 23.8 | 19.7 | 4.1 | 2.6 | | | | | 10 | 1296 | 259 | | | | | | | | | | | 0.0 | | | 207 | | 1.9 | | | | | | 321 | |
| 70434 | 1 | ea | Italian Sausage, Budget Gourmet | 284 | 420 | 72 | 20.0 | 38.0 | | | | 20.0 | | | | | | 80 | 5000 | 1000 | | | | 0.45 | 0.43 | 4.00 | | | | | | | | 40 | | 2.7 | | | | | | 950 | |
| 70443 | 1 | ea | Three Cheese, Budget Gourmet | 284 | 400 | 73 | 22.0 | 38.0 | | | | 17.0 | | | | | | 65 | 5000 | 1000 | | | | 0.38 | 0.51 | 4.00 | | | | | 2.4 | | | 500 | | 2.7 | | | | | | 760 | |
| 18819 | 1 | ea | Tuna, Lean Cuisine | 276 | 230 | 81 | 14.0 | 29.0 | 3.0 | 9.0 | 17.0 | 6.0 | 1.5 | 1.0 | 1.5 | | | 20 | 2250 | 450 | | | | 0.15 | 0.34 | 3.00 | 0.20 | 0.00 | 0.0 | | 1.2 | | | 250 | 0.1 | 1.1 | 45 | | | 440 | | 540 | 1.40 |
| 57279 | 1 | ea | Vegetable, Banquet | 298 | 260 | | 11.0 | 41.0 | 7.0 | 10.0 | 24.0 | 6.0 | 2.0 | | | | | 10 | 150 | 30 | | | | | | | | | | | 60.1 | | | 150 | | 2.7 | | | | | | 851 | |
| 81003 | 1 | cup | With Meat Sauce, Banquet | 227 | 240 | 77 | 12.0 | 32.0 | 5.0 | 4.0 | 23.0 | 7.0 | 3.0 | | | | | 15 | 750 | 150 | | | | | | | | | | | 72.0 | | | 150 | | 1.8 | | | | | | 650 | |
| 70452 | 1 | ea | With Meat Sauce, Slim Select | 284 | 290 | 78 | 18.0 | 32.0 | | | | 10.0 | | | | | | 25 | 5000 | 1000 | | | | 0.15 | 0.26 | 0.80 | | | | | 2.4 | | | 300 | | 2.7 | | | | | | 890 | |
| | | | Macaroni & Cheese | | | | | | | | | | | | | | | | | | | | | | | | | | | | | | | | | | | | | | | | |
| 66038 | 1 | cup | Banquet | 227 | 220 | 78 | 9.0 | 35.0 | 4.0 | 7.0 | 24.0 | 5.0 | 2.5 | | | | | 10 | 100 | 20 | | | | | | | | | | | | | | 100 | | 1.1 | | | | | | 1380 | |
| 66047 | 1 | ea | Healthy Choice | 255 | 320 | 74 | 15.0 | 50.0 | 4.0 | 13.0 | 33.0 | 7.0 | 2.5 | | | | | 25 | 0 | 0 | 0 | 0 | 0 | | | | | | | | 0.0 | | | 250 | | 1.4 | | | | | | 580 | |
| 66042 | 1 | ea | Weight Watchers | 255 | 260 | 75 | 15.0 | 43.0 | 7.0 | 2.0 | 34.0 | 6.0 | 2.0 | | | | | 20 | 500 | 100 | | | | | | | | | | | 0.0 | | | 250 | | 1.8 | | | | 410 | | 550 | |
| | | | Mexican, Burritos | | | | | | | | | | | | | | | | | | | | | | | | | | | | | | | | | | | | | | | | |
| 82019 | 1 | ea | Bean & Cheese, Patio | 142 | 270 | 57 | 9.0 | 46.0 | 7.0 | 2.0 | 37.0 | 5.0 | 2.0 | | | | | 5 | 200 | 40 | | | | | | | | | | | 3.6 | | | 60 | | 1.1 | | | | | | 530 | |
| 70150 | 1 | ea | Beef & Bean, w/salsa, avg | 305 | 540 | 63 | 23.5 | 61.5 | 6.1 | | | 22.0 | 9.2 | 8.9 | 1.9 | | | 49 | 912 | 131 | 15 | 86 | | 0.49 | 0.45 | 5.70 | 0.31 | 1.08 | 134.4 | | 20.5 | | | 143 | 0.4 | 5.6 | 70 | | 351 | 686 | | 888 | 3.63 |
| 82001 | 1 | ea | Beef & Bean, Patio | 170 | 420 | 52 | 11.0 | 51.0 | 7.0 | 2.0 | 42.0 | 19.0 | 7.0 | 6.3 | 1.1 | | | 20 | 500 | 100 | | | | 0.36 | 0.25 | 2.70 | 0.20 | | | | 2.4 | | | 40 | | 1.4 | | | | | | 800 | |
| 82002 | 1 | ea | Beef & Bean, w/green chili, Patio | 142 | 260 | 58 | 11.0 | 44.0 | 7.0 | 3.0 | 34.0 | 5.0 | 1.5 | | | | | 10 | 0 | 0 | 0 | 0 | 0 | 0.46 | 0.20 | 3.10 | | | | | 1.2 | | | 20 | | 0.7 | | | | | | 890 | |
| 82003 | 1 | ea | Beef & Bean, w/red chili, Patio | 142 | 260 | 59 | 11.0 | 42.0 | 7.0 | 3.0 | 32.0 | 5.0 | 2.0 | | | | | 10 | 200 | 40 | | | | 0.47 | 0.27 | 2.50 | | | | | 4.8 | | | 20 | | 1.8 | | | | | | 640 | |
| 82020 | 1 | ea | Chicken, Patio | 142 | 260 | 57 | 12.0 | 44.0 | 3.0 | 5.0 | 36.0 | 4.0 | 1.5 | | | | | 15 | 0 | 0 | 0 | 0 | 0 | | | | | | | | 1.2 | | | 60 | | 0.7 | | | | | | 740 | |
| 16255 | 1 | ea | Chicken con Queso, Healthy Choice | 306 | 358 | 73 | 14.3 | 61.4 | 6.1 | 11.3 | 44.0 | 6.1 | 2.5 | | | | | 36 | 1535 | 307 | | | | | | | | | | | 15.4 | | | 41 | | 1.8 | | | | | | 604 | |
| 82010 | 1 | ea | Nacho Beef, Patio | 170 | 410 | 53 | 13.0 | 48.0 | 5.0 | 3.0 | 40.0 | 18.0 | 18.0 | | | | | 20 | 100 | 20 | | | | 0.10 | 0.08 | 0.90 | | | | | 1.2 | | | 60 | | 1.4 | | | 126 | 190 | | 520 | |
| 82011 | 1 | ea | Nacho Cheese, Patio | 170 | 360 | 56 | 10.0 | 52.0 | 3.0 | 8.0 | 41.0 | 13.0 | 4.0 | | | | | 15 | 0 | 0 | 0 | 0 | 0 | 0.10 | 0.12 | 0.40 | | | | | 2.4 | | | 150 | | 1.1 | | | 197 | 210 | | 500 | |
| 82032 | 1 | ea | Ranchero, Beef, Healthy Choice | 306 | 290 | 79 | 13.0 | 44.0 | 6.0 | 6.0 | 32.0 | 7.0 | 2.5 | | | | | 15 | 200 | 40 | | | | | | | | | | | 3.6 | | | 20 | | 1.1 | | | | | | 500 | |
| 82031 | 1 | ea | Ranchero, Mild, Healthy Choice | 306 | 300 | 78 | 13.0 | 45.0 | 7.0 | 6.0 | 32.0 | 7.0 | 2.5 | | | | | 15 | 200 | 40 | | | | | | | | | | | 4.8 | | | 20 | | 1.1 | | | | | | 430 | |
| 82004 | 1 | ea | Red Chili, Patio | 142 | 270 | 58 | 11.0 | 42.0 | 6.0 | 4.0 | 32.0 | 6.0 | 2.0 | | | | | 10 | 400 | 30 | | | | 0.49 | 0.30 | 0.80 | | | | | 3.6 | | | 20 | | 2.7 | | | | | | 850 | |
| | | | Mexican, Enchiladas | | | | | | | | | | | | | | | | | | | | | | | | | | | | | | | | | | | | | | | | |
| 82017 | 1 | ea | Beef, Patio | 80 | 84 | 76 | 3.0 | 13.4 | 2.5 | 0.2 | 10.7 | 2.0 | 0.7 | | | | | 5 | 199 | 40 | | | | | | | | | | | 0.6 | | | 50 | | 0.7 | | | | | | 457 | |
| 70322 | 1 | ea | Beef, Shredded, Van De Kamp's | 156 | 360 | 51 | 20.0 | 40.0 | | | | 14.0 | | | | | | 60 | | | | | | | | | | | | | | | | | | | | | | 440 | | 1010 | |
| 70458 | 1 | ea | Beef, Sirloin Ranchero, Slim Select | 255 | 290 | 78 | 19.0 | 20.0 | | | | 15.0 | | | | | | 35 | 1500 | 300 | | | | 0.15 | 0.34 | 7.00 | | | | | 1.2 | | | 200 | | 6.3 | | | | | | 770 | |
| 11036 | 1 | ea | Beef & Cheese, Banquet | 132 | 130 | 78 | 4.0 | 19.0 | 3.0 | 4.0 | 12.0 | 4.0 | 1.5 | | | | | 5 | 500 | 100 | | | | | | | | | | | 1.2 | | | 100 | | 1.1 | | | | | | 630 | |
| 70327 | 1 | ea | Cheese Rancho, Van De Kamp's | 318 | 520 | 68 | 22.0 | 52.0 | | | | 24.0 | | | | | | 60 | 300 | 160 | | | | 0.08 | 0.34 | 4.00 | | | | | 0.0 | | | 400 | | 1.4 | | | 500 | 660 | | 1250 | |
| 82012 | 1 | ea | Chicken, Grande, Weight Watchers | 255 | 290 | 74 | 15.0 | 42.0 | 4.0 | 2.0 | 36.0 | 8.0 | 2.5 | | | | | 20 | 1500 | 300 | | | | | | | | | | | 12.0 | | | 300 | | 1.1 | | | | 600 | | 550 | |
| 16198 | 1 | ea | Chicken, Stouffers | 284 | 370 | 72 | 16.0 | 45.0 | 3.0 | 6.0 | 36.0 | 14.0 | 3.5 | | | | | 30 | 500 | 100 | | | | | | | | | | | 6.0 | | | 250 | | 1.1 | | | | 350 | | 970 | |
| 82030 | 1 | ea | Chicken Suiza, Healthy Choice | 284 | 280 | 76 | 14.0 | 43.0 | 5.0 | 4.0 | 34.0 | 6.0 | 3.0 | | | | | 40 | 300 | 60 | | | | | | | | | | | 6.0 | | | 150 | | 1.1 | | | | | | 440 | |
| 15978 | 1 | ea | Chicken Suiza, Weight Watchers | 255 | 250 | 80 | 15.0 | 28.0 | 4.0 | 5.0 | 19.0 | 8.0 | 3.0 | | | | | 25 | 200 | 40 | | | | 0.15 | 0.26 | 4.00 | | | | | 1.2 | | | 300 | | 1.4 | | | | 470 | | 570 | |
| 56701 | 6 | pce | Mozzerella Cheese Nuggets, Banquet | 27 | 84 | 44 | 3.8 | 6.1 | 0.8 | 0.0 | 5.3 | 4.6 | 1.3 | | | | | 8 | 0 | 0 | 0 | 0 | 0 | 0.05 | 0.08 | 0.14 | | | | | 0.0 | | | 76 | | 0.3 | | | 221 | 46 | | 152 | |
| | | | Oriental | | | | | | | | | | | | | | | | | | | | | | | | | | | | | | | | | | | | | | | | |
| 11047 | 1 | ea | Beef, Lean Cuisine | 255 | 250 | 79 | 14.0 | 30.0 | 4.0 | 5.0 | 21.0 | 8.0 | 3.0 | 3.0 | 0.5 | | | 30 | 750 | 150 | | | | 0.09 | 0.17 | 3.00 | 0.20 | 1.98 | 0.0 | | 18.0 | | | 40 | 0.1 | 1.8 | 27 | | | 410 | | 430 | 3.90 |
| 70455 | 1 | ea | Beef, Slim Select | 284 | 290 | 78 | 17.0 | 36.0 | | | | 9.0 | | | | | | 25 | 375 | 75 | | | | 0.15 | 0.34 | 7.00 | | | | | 9.0 | | | 60 | | 1.8 | | | | | | 810 | |

| Code | Amount | | Description | Basic Components | | | | | | | | | Additional Fats | | | | | |
|---|---|---|---|---|---|---|---|---|---|---|---|---|---|---|---|---|---|---|
| | | | | Weight (g) | Calories | % Water | Protein (g) | Carbs (g) | Fiber (g) | Sugar (g) | Other Carbs (g) | Fat (g) | Sat Fat (g) | Mono Fat (g) | Poly Fat (g) | Omega 3 (g) | Omega 6 (g) | Choles (mg) |
| 83019 | 1 | ea | Beef Broccoli Beijing, Healthy Choice | 340 | 300 | 77 | 21.0 | 45.0 | 5.0 | 11.0 | 29.0 | 4.5 | 1.5 | | | | | 25 |
| 83003 | 1 | ea | Beef Pepper Steak, Healthy Choice | 269 | 250 | 78 | 19.0 | 34.0 | 3.0 | 0.0 | 31.0 | 4.0 | 1.5 | | | | | 35 |
| 83008 | 1 | ea | Chicken, Banquet | 255 | 260 | 78 | 12.0 | 34.0 | 4.0 | 16.0 | 14.0 | 9.0 | 2.5 | | | | | 40 |
| 16256 | 1 | ea | Chicken, Ginger, Healthy Choice | 357 | 380 | 76 | 24.0 | 59.0 | 5.0 | 17.0 | 37.0 | 5.0 | 1.0 | | | | | 30 |
| 16258 | 1 | ea | Chicken, Sesame Shanghai, Healthy Choice | 340 | 300 | 79 | 24.0 | 40.0 | 6.0 | 4.0 | 30.0 | 5.0 | 1.0 | | | | | 40 |
| 70074 | 1 | ea | Chicken, W/Vegetables, avg | 255 | 204 | 80 | 17.3 | 26.2 | 2.9 | | | 4.1 | 1.1 | 1.4 | 1.0 | | | 46 |
| 57124 | 1 | cup | Chicken, W/Vegetables, Chef Mate | 252 | 210 | | 11.0 | 24.0 | 1.0 | 8.0 | 15.0 | 8.0 | 1.5 | | | | | 40 |
| | | | Parmigiana | | | | | | | | | | | | | | | |
| 16200 | 1 | ea | Chicken, Stouffers | 308 | 320 | 78 | 27.0 | 30.0 | 4.0 | 9.0 | 17.0 | 10.0 | 2.0 | | | | | 75 |
| 81067 | 1 | ea | Chicken, Weight Watchers | 258 | 230 | 80 | 19.0 | 25.0 | 2.0 | 2.0 | 21.0 | 6.0 | 3.0 | | | | | 50 |
| 70182 | 1 | cup | Eggplant, Mrs Paul's | 236 | 440 | 67 | 10.0 | 38.0 | 6.0 | 18.0 | 14.0 | 28.0 | 8.0 | | | | | 20 |
| 70044 | 1 | ea | Veal, W/Vegetables & tortellini, avg | 340 | 707 | 60 | 38.1 | 54.7 | 3.1 | | | 37.3 | 16.8 | 12.0 | 5.4 | | | 306 |
| 81004 | 1 | pce | Veal, Banquet | 132 | 230 | 67 | 9.0 | 19.0 | 2.0 | 2.0 | 15.0 | 14.0 | 4.0 | | | | | 20 |
| 57430 | 1 | ea | Pastry, w/Broccoli, Cheese & Vegs, Pepp Farm | 103 | 240 | | 6.0 | 24.0 | 3.0 | 3.0 | 18.0 | 14.0 | 4.5 | | | | | 50 |
| | | | Pork | | | | | | | | | | | | | | | |
| 12909 | 3 | oz | BBQ, Richs | 85 | 167 | 65 | 8.5 | 9.5 | 0.3 | 3.7 | 5.5 | 10.6 | 3.5 | 4.5 | 1.4 | | | 34 |
| 12910 | 3 | oz | Chop, Marinated, Tyson | 85 | 130 | 70 | 16.1 | 0.6 | 0.0 | 0.1 | 0.4 | 7.0 | 2.9 | 3.3 | 0.7 | | | 48 |
| 70451 | 1 | ea | Ham, w/Asparagus Au Gratin, Budget Gourmet | 255 | 280 | 77 | 14.0 | 33.0 | | | | 10.0 | | | | | | 40 |
| | | | Potatoes | | | | | | | | | | | | | | | |
| 53229 | 1 | ea | Casserole, Healthy Choice | 262 | 210 | 82 | 11.0 | 30.0 | 6.0 | 5.0 | 19.0 | 5.0 | 1.5 | | | | | 10 |
| 57287 | 1 | ea | Casserole, Life Choice | 380 | 160 | 84 | 8.0 | 37.1 | 9.0 | 11.0 | 17.0 | 0.5 | 0.0 | | | | | 5 |
| 53230 | 1 | ea | Cheddar Broccoli, Healthy Choice | 298 | 330 | 76 | 13.0 | 53.0 | 6.0 | 8.0 | 39.0 | 7.0 | 3.0 | | | | | 25 |
| | | | Pot Pies | | | | | | | | | | | | | | | |
| 56067 | 1 | ea | Beef, avg | 234 | 449 | 63 | 17.1 | 42.1 | 2.8 | 3.0 | 36.3 | 26.7 | 7.0 | 14.0 | 5.6 | | 2.34 | 42 |
| 11041 | 1 | ea | Beef, Banquet | 227 | 450 | 62 | 17.0 | 44.0 | 4.0 | | | 25.0 | 11.0 | | | | | 30 |
| 11076 | 1 | ea | Beef, Hungry Man, Swanson | 397 | 660 | 67 | 24.0 | 70.0 | 6.0 | 8.0 | 56.0 | 31.0 | 13.0 | | | | | 50 |
| 57460 | 1 | ea | Beef Yankee, Marie Calendar | 284 | 691 | 58 | 16.0 | 57.1 | 3.0 | 4.0 | 50.1 | 44.1 | 10.0 | | | | | 25 |
| 56072 | 1 | ea | Chicken, avg | 230 | 504 | 58 | 15.4 | 51.1 | 3.9 | 6.4 | 40.7 | 26.4 | 6.9 | 13.8 | 4.9 | | 2.30 | 30 |
| 57532 | 1 | ea | Chicken & Broccoli, Marie Calendar | 284 | 781 | | 18.0 | 88.2 | 3.0 | 13.0 | 72.1 | 48.1 | 16.0 | | | | | 20 |
| 57461 | 1 | ea | Chicken, Au Gratin, Marie Calendar | 284 | 721 | 57 | 19.0 | 53.1 | 4.0 | 5.0 | 44.1 | 48.1 | 13.0 | | | | | 25 |
| 15959 | 1 | ea | Chicken, Banquet | 227 | 450 | 63 | 14.0 | 39.0 | 6.0 | | | 30.0 | 12.0 | | | | | 35 |
| 16192 | 1 | ea | Chicken, Lean Cuisine | 269 | 320 | 73 | 18.0 | 39.0 | 3.0 | 13.0 | 23.0 | 10.0 | 2.5 | 2.5 | 1.0 | | | 35 |
| 66045 | 1 | ea | Macaroni & Cheese, Banquet | 198 | 200 | 77 | 7.0 | 35.0 | 2.0 | 2.0 | 31.0 | 3.0 | 1.5 | | | | | 10 |
| 56086 | 1 | ea | Turkey, avg | 233 | 459 | 62 | 13.5 | 46.8 | 4.0 | 6.1 | 36.8 | 32.6 | 9.3 | 16.3 | 6.9 | | 2.33 | 21 |
| 16928 | 1 | ea | Turkey, Banquet | 198 | 370 | 65 | 10.0 | 38.0 | 3.0 | 3.0 | 32.0 | 20.0 | 8.0 | | | | | 45 |
| 16935 | 1 | ea | Turkey, Lean Cuisine | 269 | 300 | 73 | 20.0 | 34.0 | 3.0 | 15.0 | 16.0 | 9.0 | 2.0 | 2.5 | 1.0 | | | 50 |
| 57457 | 1 | ea | Turkey, Marie Calendar | 284 | 711 | 57 | 17.0 | 57.1 | 4.0 | 5.0 | 48.1 | 46.1 | 10.0 | | | | | 20 |
| 53228 | 1 | ea | Vegetable & Cheese, Banquet | 198 | 390 | 61 | 8.0 | 49.0 | 3.0 | 2.0 | 44.0 | 18.0 | 8.0 | | | | | 15 |
| | | | Ravioli entrees | | | | | | | | | | | | | | | |
| 57400 | 1 | cup | Beef, Bernardis | 120 | 270 | | 11.0 | 43.0 | 2.0 | 3.0 | 38.0 | 6.0 | 2.0 | | | | | 25 |
| 11095 | 1 | ea | Beef, Stouffers | 269 | 370 | 71 | 17.0 | 43.0 | 5.0 | 8.0 | 30.0 | 14.0 | 4.0 | | | | | 80 |
| 70446 | 1 | ea | Cheese, Slim Selects | 284 | 260 | 80 | 12.0 | 36.0 | 2.1 | | | 7.0 | 4.5 | 2.0 | 0.4 | | | 45 |
| 81081 | 1 | ea | Cheese Parmigiana, Healthy Choice | 255 | 260 | 76 | 11.0 | 44.0 | 6.0 | 14.0 | 24.0 | 5.0 | 2.5 | | | | | 30 |
| 57401 | 1 | cup | Espanol, Bernardis | 120 | 290 | | 13.0 | 43.0 | 2.0 | 3.0 | 38.0 | 6.0 | 3.0 | | | | | 25 |
| 81061 | 1 | ea | Florentine, Weight Watchers | 241 | 200 | 80 | 9.0 | 37.0 | 4.0 | 10.0 | 23.0 | 2.0 | 0.5 | | | | | 5 |
| | | | Rice entrees | | | | | | | | | | | | | | | |
| 56830 | 1 | cup | Brown & Wild Rice Amandine, Spice Hunter | 234 | 165 | | 5.2 | 30.9 | | | | 2.1 | | | | | | |
| 38321 | 1 | ea | Florentine, Rice Originals | 113 | 145 | 73 | 4.2 | 22.1 | | | | 4.2 | 2.6 | 1.2 | 0.1 | | | 11 |
| 66039 | 1 | ea | Fried, w/Chicken, Chung King | 227 | 270 | 74 | 9.0 | 44.0 | 4.0 | 6.0 | 34.0 | 6.0 | 1.5 | | | | | 25 |
| 66040 | 1 | ea | Fried, w/Pork, Chun King | 227 | 290 | 71 | 11.0 | 48.0 | 5.0 | 2.0 | 41.0 | 6.0 | 2.0 | 1.7 | 1.7 | | | 25 |
| 38320 | 1 | ea | Medley, Rice Originals | 283 | 238 | 80 | 6.5 | 45.8 | 3.1 | 1.7 | 41.0 | 2.8 | 1.7 | | | | | 6 |
| 38323 | 1 | ea | Pilaf, Rice Originals | 113 | 92 | 80 | 2.3 | 17.7 | 1.2 | 1.4 | 15.1 | 1.1 | 0.6 | | | | | 0 |
| 56887 | 1 | ea | Spanish, w/Beans, lofat, low sod, dry, Am Clss | 63 | 210 | 5 | 9.0 | 49.0 | 8.0 | 7.0 | 34.0 | 1.5 | 0.0 | | | 0.00 | 0.00 | 0 |
| 38319 | 1 | ea | White N' Wild, Rice Originals | 283 | 246 | 79 | 5.7 | 45.3 | 2.5 | 3.1 | 39.6 | 5.1 | 5.7 | | | | | 0 |
| 38322 | 1 | ea | With Broccoli, Rice Originals | 113 | 124 | 76 | 3.3 | 17.4 | 0.8 | 0.6 | 16.0 | 4.6 | 1.5 | | | | | 6 |
| 70138 | 1 | ea | With Broccoli & cheese sauce, avg | 128 | 189 | 69 | 6.5 | 22.1 | 1.3 | | | 8.4 | 3.5 | 2.9 | 1.6 | | | 14 |
| 70139 | 1 | ea | With Green beans, water chestnuts & sauce, avg | 284 | 284 | 79 | 7.3 | 40.5 | 2.6 | | | 10.5 | 3.2 | 4.1 | 2.6 | | | 9 |
| | | | Salisbury Steak | | | | | | | | | | | | | | | |
| 11025 | 1 | ea | Armour | 319 | 330 | 80 | 23.0 | 20.0 | 4.0 | 6.0 | 10.0 | 18.0 | 8.0 | | | | | 50 |
| 11037 | 1 | ea | Banquet | 132 | 200 | 74 | 12.0 | 7.0 | 2.0 | 0.0 | 5.0 | 14.0 | 6.0 | | | | | 25 |
| 11115 | 1 | ea | Healthy Choice | 312 | 310 | 82 | 16.0 | 40.0 | 4.0 | 8.0 | 28.0 | 9.0 | 3.0 | | | | | 45 |
| 11054 | 1 | ea | Stouffers | 273 | 370 | 73 | 24.0 | 26.0 | | 4.0 | | 19.0 | | | | | | 50 |
| 11056 | 1 | ea | Weight Watchers | 241 | 250 | 78 | 19.0 | 24.0 | 4.0 | 7.0 | 13.0 | 9.0 | 3.0 | 3.0 | 1.0 | | | 30 |
| | | | Sandwiches | | | | | | | | | | | | | | | |
| 11030 | 1 | ea | Creamed Chipped Beef, Banquet | 113 | 100 | 82 | 9.0 | 8.0 | 0.0 | 1.0 | 7.0 | 3.0 | 1.5 | | | | | 25 |
| 11032 | 1 | ea | Sliced beef, w/gravy, Banquet | 113 | 70 | 86 | 8.0 | 5.0 | 0.5 | 0.5 | 4.0 | 2.0 | 1.0 | | | | | 25 |
| 16903 | 1 | ea | Turkey, w/gravy, Banquet | 142 | 90 | 86 | 8.0 | 7.0 | 0.5 | 1.0 | 5.5 | 4.0 | 1.5 | | | | | 30 |
| 70172 | 10 | pce | Scallops, Fried, Mrs Paul's | 82 | 176 | 56 | 8.4 | 18.4 | 0.8 | 3.3 | 14.2 | 6.7 | 1.7 | | | | | 8 |
| 70113 | 1 | ea | Scallops, W/Potatoes & vegetables, avg | 227 | 413 | 62 | 25.4 | 38.8 | 4.8 | | | 17.3 | 5.4 | 7.0 | 3.6 | | | 61 |
| 70439 | 1 | ea | Seafood Newburg, Budget Gourmet | 284 | 350 | 74 | 17.0 | 43.0 | | | | 12.0 | | | | | | 70 |

| Code | Vit A & Components | | | | | Vitamins | | | | | | | | | | | Minerals | | | | | | | | | |
|---|---|---|---|---|---|---|---|---|---|---|---|---|---|---|---|---|---|---|---|---|---|---|---|---|---|
| | Vit A (IU) | Vit A (RE) | Retinol (RE) | Carotenoids (RE) | Beta Carotene (mcg) | Thiamin (mg) | Riboflavin (mg) | Niacin (NE) | Vit B6 (mg) | Vit B12 (mcg) | Folate (mcg) | Panto (mg) | Vit C (mg) | Vit D (mg) | Vit E (α TE) | Calcium (mg) | Copper (mg) | Iron (mg) | Magnes (mg) | Mang (mg) | Phos (mg) | Potassium (mg) | Selenium (mcg) | Sodium (mg) | Zinc (mg) |
| 83019 | 1000 | 200 | | | | | | | | | | | 12.0 | | | 40 | | 2.7 | | | | | | 420 | |
| 83003 | 200 | 40 | | | | 0.15 | 0.17 | 1.60 | | | | | 9.0 | | | 20 | | 1.1 | | | 130 | 250 | | 470 | |
| 83008 | 1250 | 250 | | | | | | | | | | | 18.0 | | | 40 | | 1.1 | | | | | | 610 | |
| 16256 | 500 | 100 | | | | | | | | | | | 0.0 | | | 60 | | 2.7 | | | | | | 430 | |
| 16258 | 750 | 150 | | | | | | | | | | | 4.8 | | | 40 | | 1.8 | | | | | | 550 | |
| 70074 | 5722 | 578 | 8 | 570 | | 0.13 | 0.22 | 6.17 | 0.44 | 0.17 | 27.0 | | 41.3 | | | 56 | 0.3 | 2.0 | 43 | | 158 | 479 | | 892 | 1.63 |
| 57124 | 1750 | 350 | | | | | | | | | | | 2.4 | | | 20 | | 0.7 | | | | | | 1170 | |
| 16200 | 500 | 100 | | | | | | | | | | | 6.0 | | | 150 | | 1.4 | | | | 770 | | 890 | |
| 81067 | 400 | 80 | | | | | | | | | | | 4.8 | | | 150 | | 1.8 | | | | 620 | | 470 | |
| 70182 | 1000 | 304 | | | | 0.22 | 0.46 | 3.60 | | | | | 9.6 | | | 200 | | 2.2 | | | | 688 | | 1060 | |
| 70044 | 1787 | 361 | 268 | 94 | | 0.51 | 0.85 | 8.12 | 0.39 | 1.34 | 58.6 | | 10.4 | | | 415 | 0.3 | 5.2 | 68 | | 537 | 687 | | 1727 | 3.90 |
| 81004 | 200 | 40 | | | | | | | | | | | 54.0 | | | 40 | | 0.7 | | | | | | 740 | |
| 57430 | 400 | 80 | | | | 0.15 | 0.10 | 1.20 | | | | | 12.0 | | | 80 | | 1.1 | | | | | | 430 | |
| 12909 | 339 | 102 | | | | 0.37 | 0.14 | 2.24 | 0.19 | 0.31 | 1.9 | 0.31 | 2.2 | 0.0 | | 19 | 0.0 | 0.8 | 11 | | 94 | 247 | | 480 | 1.15 |
| 12910 | 0 | 0 | 0 | 0 | 0 | | | | | | | | 0.0 | | | 10 | | 0.4 | | | | 0 | | 261 | |
| 70451 | 100 | 20 | | | | 0.38 | 0.34 | 4.00 | | | | | 4.8 | | | 100 | | 1.1 | | | | | | 1130 | |
| 53229 | 1250 | 250 | | | | | | | | | | | 21.0 | | | 100 | | 0.7 | | | | | | 520 | |
| 57287 | 401 | 80 | | | | | | | | | | | 27.1 | | | 201 | | 1.8 | | | | | | 592 | |
| 53230 | 300 | 60 | | | | | | | | | | | 27.0 | | | 200 | | 1.1 | | | | | | 550 | |
| 56067 | 959 | 187 | 51 | 136 | | 0.07 | 0.14 | 2.81 | 0.27 | 1.30 | 17.0 | 0.29 | 0.0 | 0.1 | | 23 | 0.1 | 2.3 | 7 | | 112 | 218 | 11.6 | 856 | 2.64 |
| 11041 | 500 | 100 | | | | 0.32 | 0.28 | 4.60 | | | | | 1.5 | | | 20 | | 1.8 | | | 137 | 190 | | 930 | |
| 11076 | 3000 | 600 | | | | | | | | | | | 4.8 | | | 40 | | 4.5 | | | | | | 1590 | |
| 57460 | 100 | 20 | | | | | | | | | | | 4.0 | | | 40 | | 1.8 | | | | | | 1392 | |
| 56072 | 2093 | 116 | 3 | 113 | | 0.23 | 0.32 | 3.22 | 0.46 | 0.23 | 29.0 | 1.10 | 9.2 | 0.2 | | 25 | 0.1 | 2.3 | 30 | 0.5 | 115 | 352 | 32.0 | 945 | 1.22 |
| 57532 | 200 | 40 | | | | | | | | | | | 2.4 | | | 80 | | 3.6 | | | | | | 1032 | |
| 57461 | 200 | 40 | | | | | | | | | | | 2.4 | | | 150 | | 2.7 | | | | | | 1042 | |
| 15959 | 750 | 107 | | | | 0.31 | 0.27 | 6.00 | | | | | 1.0 | | | 40 | | 1.4 | | | 143 | 190 | | 1010 | |
| 16192 | 2000 | 400 | | | | | | | | | | | 2.4 | | | 100 | | 1.1 | | | | 450 | | 590 | |
| 66045 | 0 | 0 | 0 | 0 | 0 | | | | | | | | 0.0 | | | 100 | | 1.1 | | | | | | 600 | |
| 56086 | 2074 | 145 | 4 | 141 | | 0.21 | 0.19 | 3.73 | 0.46 | 0.20 | 24.0 | 1.10 | 4.7 | 0.0 | | 28 | 0.3 | 2.1 | 26 | | 130 | 266 | 31.9 | 860 | 1.50 |
| 16928 | 750 | 150 | | | | | | | | | | | 0.0 | | | 40 | | 1.1 | | | | | | 850 | |
| 16935 | 2500 | 500 | | | | | | | | | | | 1.2 | | | 150 | | 1.4 | | | | 400 | | 590 | |
| 57457 | 100 | 20 | | | | | | | | | | | 2.4 | | | 40 | | 1.8 | | | | | | 771 | |
| 53228 | 1250 | 250 | | | | | | | | | | | 0.0 | | | 80 | | 1.1 | | | | | | 1000 | |
| 57400 | 0 | 0 | 0 | 0 | 0 | | | | | | | | 1.2 | | | 60 | | 2.7 | | | | | | 660 | |
| 11095 | 500 | 100 | | | | | | | | | | | 6.0 | | | 80 | | 1.8 | | | | 510 | | 680 | |
| 70446 | 750 | 150 | | | | 0.26 | 0.26 | 2.00 | 0.10 | | | | 3.6 | | | 25 | | 1.8 | | | | | | 960 | |
| 81081 | 300 | 60 | | | | | | | | | | | 0.0 | | | 150 | | 1.8 | | | | | | 290 | |
| 57401 | 0 | 0 | 0 | 0 | 0 | | | | | | | | 1.2 | | | 150 | | 1.8 | | | | | | 840 | |
| 81061 | 1250 | 250 | | | | | | | | | | | 12.0 | | | 150 | | 2.7 | | | | 490 | | 480 | |
| 56830 | | | | | | | | | | | | | | | | | | | | | | 186 | | 93 | |
| 38321 | 1535 | 307 | | | | 0.18 | 0.03 | 1.77 | | | | | 5.1 | | | 206 | | 0.9 | | | 94 | 106 | | 395 | |
| 66039 | 400 | 100 | | | | 0.75 | 0.17 | 1.20 | | | | | 0.0 | | | 20 | | 1.4 | | | 120 | 190 | | 1330 | |
| 66040 | 750 | 150 | | | | 0.30 | 0.17 | 1.20 | 0.21 | | | | 0.0 | | | 20 | | 1.8 | | | 120 | 180 | | 1310 | |
| 38320 | 289 | 58 | | | | | | | | | | | 7.1 | | | 42 | | 3.7 | | | | | | 883 | |
| 38323 | 1548 | 310 | | | | | | | | | | | 2.1 | | | 20 | | 1.5 | | | | | | 408 | |
| 56887 | 2000 | 400 | | | | | | | | | | | 12.0 | | | 60 | | 2.7 | | | | | | 140 | |
| 38319 | 263 | 53 | | | | | | | | | | | 5.1 | | | 57 | | 4.0 | | | | | | 1002 | |
| 38322 | 1807 | 361 | | | | | | | | | | | 7.5 | | | 54 | | 1.5 | | | | | | 400 | |
| 70138 | 804 | 108 | 39 | 69 | | 0.14 | 0.10 | 1.26 | 0.15 | 0.06 | 22.2 | | 34.0 | | | 125 | 0.1 | 1.2 | 22 | | 128 | 156 | | 545 | 0.90 |
| 70139 | 745 | 145 | 98 | 48 | | 0.24 | 0.30 | 3.23 | 0.22 | 0.26 | 32.3 | | 7.6 | | | 131 | 0.3 | 2.6 | 40 | | 168 | 454 | | 630 | 1.26 |
| 11025 | 300 | 60 | | | | 0.23 | 0.34 | 2.00 | | | | | 24.0 | | | 100 | | 1.8 | | | 270 | 530 | | 1310 | |
| 11037 | 0 | 0 | 0 | 0 | 0 | | | | | | | | 0.0 | | | 20 | | 1.1 | | | | | | 610 | |
| 11115 | 1000 | 200 | | | | | | | | | | | 0.0 | | | 20 | | 1.8 | | | | | | 550 | |
| 11054 | 100 | 20 | | | | 0.10 | 0.10 | 1.10 | | | | | 2.1 | | | 200 | | 1.1 | | | | 340 | | 1220 | |
| 11056 | 300 | 60 | | | | 0.23 | 0.26 | 7.00 | 0.22 | | | | 0.0 | | | 100 | | 2.7 | | | | 450 | | 590 | |
| 11030 | 0 | 0 | 0 | 0 | 0 | | | | | | | | 0.0 | | | 8 | | 0.7 | | | | | | 700 | |
| 11032 | 0 | 0 | 0 | 0 | 0 | | | | | | | | 0.0 | | | 0 | | 1.1 | | | | | | 440 | |
| 16903 | 0 | 0 | 0 | 0 | 0 | | | | | | | | 0.0 | | | 20 | | 0.4 | | | | | | 670 | |
| 70172 | 0 | 0 | 0 | 0 | 0 | 0.04 | 0.14 | 1.26 | | | | | 0.0 | | | 50 | | 0.9 | | | | 196 | | 351 | |
| 70113 | 470 | 65 | 27 | 38 | | 0.27 | 0.21 | 3.85 | 0.35 | 1.47 | 62.5 | | 14.4 | | | 66 | 0.3 | 2.5 | 95 | | 368 | 733 | | 608 | 1.95 |
| 70439 | 200 | 40 | | | | 0.23 | 0.26 | 2.00 | | | | | | | | 100 | | 0.7 | | | | | | 660 | |

| Code | Amount | | Description | Basic Components | | | | | | | | | Additional Fats | | | | | | Vit A & Components | | | | | Vitamins | | | | | | | | | | Minerals | | | | | | | | | |
|---|---|---|---|---|---|---|---|---|---|---|---|---|---|---|---|---|---|---|---|---|---|---|---|---|---|---|---|---|---|---|---|---|---|---|---|---|---|---|---|---|---|---|---|
| | | | | Weight (g) | Calories | % Water | Protein (g) | Carbs (g) | Fiber (g) | Sugar (g) | Other Carbs (g) | Fat (g) | Sat Fat (g) | Mono Fat (g) | Poly Fat (g) | Omega 3 (g) | Omega 6 (g) | Choles (mg) | Vit A (IU) | Vit A (RE) | Retinol (RE) | Carotenoids (RE) | Beta Carotene (mcg) | Thiamin (mg) | Riboflavin (mg) | Niacin (NE) | Vit B6 (mg) | Vit B12 (mcg) | Folate (mcg) | Panto (mg) | Vit C (mg) | Vit D (mg) | Vit E (α TE) | Calcium (mg) | Copper (mg) | Iron (mg) | Magnes (mg) | Mang (mg) | Phos (mg) | Potassium (mg) | Selenium (mcg) | Sodium (mg) | Zinc (mg) |
| 70117 | 1 | ea | Seafood Platter, W/Fish, scallops & shrimp, avg | 255 | 523 | 59 | 26.4 | 48.7 | 3.8 | | | 25.4 | 7.8 | 10.8 | 5.2 | | | 94 | 139 | 37 | 35 | 2 | | 0.29 | 0.25 | 5.37 | 0.56 | 1.07 | 25.2 | | 8.6 | | | 69 | 0.3 | 2.7 | 76 | | 319 | 806 | | 954 | 1.42 |
| | | | Shrimp | | | | | | | | | | | | | | | | | | | | | | | | | | | | | | | | | | | | | | | | |
| 70702 | 15 | ea | Breaded, Popcorn, Van De Kamp's | 84 | 202 | 52 | 8.3 | 21.0 | 0.8 | 1.5 | 18.8 | 9.8 | 1.5 | 3.8 | 1.5 | | | 26 | 0 | 0 | 0 | 0 | 0 | | | | | | | | 0.0 | | | 30 | | 1.1 | | | | | | 458 | |
| 57538 | 1 | cup | Breaded, w/Angel Hair Pasta, Banquet | 213 | 301 | | 11.0 | 37.1 | 3.0 | 5.0 | 29.1 | 12.0 | 2.0 | | | | | 30 | 100 | 20 | | | | | | | | | | | 9.0 | | | 80 | | 1.8 | | | | | | 471 | |
| 70703 | 5 | ea | Breaded, Whole, Van De Kamp's | 80 | 171 | 54 | 9.3 | 18.6 | 1.4 | 1.4 | 15.7 | 7.1 | 1.1 | 2.9 | 1.1 | | | 36 | 0 | 0 | 0 | 0 | 0 | | | | | | | | 0.0 | | | 14 | | 1.0 | | | | | | 371 | |
| 70701 | 5 | ea | Butterfly, Breaded, Van De Kamp's | 80 | 200 | 50 | 8.6 | 20.0 | 1.4 | 0.7 | 17.9 | 10.0 | 1.8 | 4.3 | 1.4 | | | 39 | 0 | 0 | 0 | 0 | 0 | | | | | | | | 0.0 | | | 14 | | 0.8 | | | | | | 414 | |
| 19422 | 1 | ea | Creole, Armour | 284 | 220 | 78 | 6.0 | 49.0 | 16.0 | 6.0 | 27.0 | 5.0 | 0.0 | | | | | 20 | 400 | 30 | | | | 0.15 | 0.14 | 1.20 | | | | | 120.0 | | | 40 | | 1.1 | | | 110 | 420 | | 720 | |
| | | | Spaghetti | | | | | | | | | | | | | | | | | | | | | | | | | | | | | | | | | | | | | | | | |
| 57465 | 1 | cup | Marinara, w/Garlic Bread, Marie Calendar | 227 | 270 | 73 | 10.0 | 35.0 | 3.0 | 5.0 | 27.0 | 10.0 | 3.0 | | | | | 10 | 300 | 60 | | | | | | | | | | | 15.0 | | | 80 | | 1.1 | | | | | | 540 | |
| 57463 | 1 | cup | With Meat Sauce & Garlic Bread, Marie Calendar | 193 | 260 | 71 | 11.0 | 32.0 | 3.0 | 5.0 | 24.0 | 10.0 | 3.0 | | | | | 5 | 100 | 20 | | | | | | | | | | | 3.6 | | | 60 | | 1.1 | | | | | | 570 | |
| 56769 | 1 | ea | With Meat Sauce, Weight Watchers | 284 | 250 | 82 | 15.0 | 24.0 | 6.0 | 10.0 | 8.0 | 6.0 | 2.0 | 3.0 | 1.0 | | | 10 | 750 | 150 | | | | 0.45 | 0.85 | 7.00 | 0.20 | | | | 9.0 | | | 100 | | 3.6 | | | | 690 | | 470 | |
| | | | Sweet & Sour | | | | | | | | | | | | | | | | | | | | | | | | | | | | | | | | | | | | | | | | |
| 15941 | 1 | ea | Chicken, Armour | 312 | 220 | 82 | 16.0 | 38.0 | 4.0 | 0.0 | 34.0 | 1.0 | 0.0 | | | | | 30 | 750 | 150 | | | | 0.15 | 0.17 | 4.00 | | | | | 27.0 | | | 40 | | 0.7 | | | 160 | 490 | | 520 | |
| 16190 | 1 | ea | Chicken, Lean Cuisine | 294 | 260 | 78 | 17.0 | 43.0 | 3.0 | 12.0 | 28.0 | 2.5 | 1.0 | 1.0 | 0.5 | | | 45 | 750 | 150 | | | | | | | | | | | 12.0 | | | 20 | | 0.4 | | | | 500 | | 440 | |
| 15948 | 8 | pce | Chicken Nuggets, Banquet | 79 | 201 | 53 | 10.0 | 15.7 | 1.3 | 0.0 | 14.4 | 11.3 | 2.5 | | | | | 28 | 0 | 0 | 0 | 0 | 0 | 0.11 | 0.06 | 4.08 | | | | | 0.8 | | | 13 | | 1.1 | | | 145 | 176 | | 420 | |
| 70442 | 1 | ea | Chicken, w/Rice, Budget Gourmet | 284 | 350 | 72 | 18.0 | 53.0 | | | | 7.0 | | | | | | 40 | 400 | 30 | | | | 0.12 | 0.34 | 3.00 | | | | | 2.4 | | | 60 | | 0.7 | | | | | | 640 | |
| 12902 | 1 | ea | Pork, Chung King | 369 | 450 | 71 | 12.0 | 86.0 | 4.0 | 32.0 | 50.0 | 6.0 | 2.5 | | | | | 20 | 1300 | 200 | | | | 0.45 | 0.17 | 2.00 | | | | | 4.8 | | | 20 | | 1.1 | | | 140 | 330 | | 1180 | |
| 70463 | 1 | ea | Tortellini, Cheese, Budget Gourmet | 156 | 180 | 79 | 7.0 | 25.0 | | | | | | | | | | 15 | 200 | 40 | | | | 0.12 | 0.26 | 1.60 | | | | | 2.4 | | | 100 | | 1.4 | | | | | | 400 | |
| 18820 | 1 | ea | Tuna Noodle Casserole, Stouffers | 284 | 330 | 76 | 19.0 | 31.0 | 3.0 | 9.0 | 19.0 | 14.0 | 2.0 | | | | | 40 | 100 | 20 | | | | 0.00 | 0.10 | 1.40 | | | | | 0.0 | | | 150 | | 1.1 | | | | 390 | | 1130 | |
| 18823 | 1 | ea | Tuna Noodle Casserole, Weight Watchers | 269 | 240 | 80 | 15.0 | 30.0 | 5.0 | 9.0 | 16.0 | 7.0 | 2.5 | | | | | 15 | 750 | 150 | | | | | | | | | | | 12.0 | | | 150 | | 1.4 | | | | 620 | | 580 | |
| 70450 | 1 | ea | Turkey, Glazed, Slim Select | 255 | 270 | 76 | 17.0 | 39.0 | | | | 5.0 | | | | | | 50 | | | | | | 0.09 | 0.17 | 5.00 | | | | | 2.4 | | | 20 | | 1.1 | | | | | | 760 | |
| 16922 | 1 | ea | Turkey, Lean Cuisine | 266 | 230 | 80 | 18.0 | 26.0 | 3.0 | 7.0 | 16.0 | 6.0 | 1.5 | 1.5 | 1.5 | | | 50 | 1500 | 300 | | | | | | | | | | | 1.2 | | | 100 | | 0.7 | | | | 300 | | 590 | |
| 16926 | 4 | ea | Turkey, Nuggets, breaded, Louis Rich | 92 | 254 | 51 | 13.2 | 14.2 | 0.4 | 0.0 | 13.7 | 16.1 | 3.2 | 7.7 | 5.2 | 0.61 | 4.57 | 37 | 0 | 0 | 0 | 0 | 0 | | | | | | | | 0.0 | | | 9 | 0.3 | 0.8 | 19 | | 181 | 162 | | 625 | 1.69 |
| 16924 | 1 | ea | Turkey, Patty, Louis Rich | 113 | 153 | 74 | 19.2 | 0.0 | 0.0 | 0.0 | 0.0 | 8.5 | 2.1 | 3.1 | 3.0 | 0.21 | 2.84 | 70 | 0 | 0 | 0 | 0 | 0 | | | | | | | | 0.0 | | | 9 | 0.2 | 1.0 | 26 | | 232 | 240 | | 450 | 1.86 |
| | | | Turkey, Roasted | | | | | | | | | | | | | | | | | | | | | | | | | | | | | | | | | | | | | | | | |
| 16933 | 1 | ea | Healthy Choice | 284 | 250 | 79 | 20.0 | 28.0 | 4.0 | 16.0 | 8.0 | 6.0 | 2.0 | | | | | 40 | 500 | 100 | | | | | | | | | | | 0.0 | | | 40 | | 1.8 | | | | | | 530 | |
| 16923 | 1 | ea | Stouffers | 223 | 280 | 74 | 19.0 | 25.0 | 1.0 | 4.0 | 20.0 | 11.0 | 2.5 | | | | | 40 | 100 | 20 | | | | | | | | | | | | | | 20 | | 0.7 | | | | 380 | | 950 | |
| 16927 | 1 | ea | Medallions, Weight Watchers | 241 | 190 | 80 | 10.0 | 34.0 | 4.0 | 3.0 | 27.0 | 2.0 | 0.5 | | | | | 20 | 500 | 100 | | | | | | | | | | | 4.8 | | | 20 | | 1.8 | | | | 220 | | 530 | |
| 16930 | 1 | ea | With Mushrooms, Healthy Choice | 241 | 230 | 78 | 19.0 | 26.0 | 2.0 | 3.0 | 21.0 | 5.0 | 1.5 | | | | | 45 | 750 | 150 | | | | | | | | | | | 0.0 | | | 0 | | 0.7 | | | | | | 440 | |
| 16925 | 3 | ea | Turkey, Sticks, breaded, Louis Rich | 85 | 230 | | 12.0 | 12.0 | 0.0 | 0.0 | 12.0 | 15.0 | 3.0 | | | | | 35 | 0 | 0 | 0 | 0 | 0 | | | | | | | | 0.0 | | | 0 | | 0.7 | | | | | | 580 | |
| 16910 | 1 | ea | Turkey, Tetrazzini, Stouffers | 284 | 360 | 76 | 18.0 | 28.0 | 2.0 | 5.0 | 21.0 | 19.0 | 3.0 | | | | | 40 | 40 | 8 | | | | 0.10 | 0.10 | 1.10 | | | | | 0.0 | | | 100 | | 1.1 | | | | 390 | | 1140 | |
| 56820 | 1 | ea | Turkey, W/Dressing, Libby's | 198 | 180 | 81 | 11.0 | 17.0 | 2.0 | 2.0 | 13.0 | 7.9 | 2.0 | | | | | 36 | 1249 | 250 | | | | | | | | | | | 0.0 | | | 20 | | 1.1 | | | | | | 830 | |
| 16906 | 1 | pce | Turkey, W/Gravy, Banquet | 68 | 50 | 85 | 4.0 | 2.5 | 0.3 | 0.0 | 2.3 | 2.5 | 0.3 | | | | | 12 | 0 | 0 | 0 | 0 | 0 | | | | | | | | 0.0 | | | 0 | | 0.2 | | | | | | 295 | |
| 57398 | 1 | ea | Veal, Patty, w/Cheese, Travis Meats | 91 | 227 | 58 | 11.9 | 10.0 | 0.2 | 0.1 | 9.7 | 14.9 | 7.4 | 4.4 | 0.6 | | | 51 | 165 | 33 | | | | 0.08 | 0.14 | 3.57 | | | | | 0.0 | | | 93 | | 0.9 | | | 98 | 145 | | 479 | 1.34 |
| | | | Vegetables | | | | | | | | | | | | | | | | | | | | | | | | | | | | | | | | | | | | | | | | |
| 56915 | 1 | cup | Broccoli, w/Cheese Sauce, Green Giant | 168 | 104 | 85 | 4.4 | 13.4 | 2.9 | 7.2 | 3.4 | 3.9 | 1.2 | | | | | 5 | 1555 | 155 | | | | | | | | | | | 60.5 | | | 84 | | 0.8 | | | | | | 786 | |
| 70698 | 1 | ea | Chop Suey, La Choy | 85 | 11 | 95 | 0.7 | 2.4 | 1.0 | 0.0 | 1.4 | 0.4 | 0.0 | | | | | 0 | 0 | 0 | 0 | 0 | 0 | | | | | | | | 3.2 | | | 15 | | 0.1 | | | | | | 439 | |
| 70162 | 1 | pce | Corn Fritters, Mrs Paul | 63 | 130 | 54 | 3.0 | 16.0 | 1.0 | 4.0 | 11.0 | 7.0 | 2.0 | | | | | 5 | 65 | 13 | | | | 0.16 | 0.12 | 1.40 | | | | | 0.0 | | | 20 | | 0.7 | | | | 98 | | 310 | |
| 81082 | 1 | ea | Pasta Italiano, Healthy Choice | 284 | 250 | 81 | 9.0 | 48.0 | 6.0 | 8.0 | 34.0 | 3.0 | 1.5 | | | | | 10 | 500 | 100 | | | | | | | | | | | 2.4 | | | 60 | | 2.7 | | | | | | 480 | |
| 70476 | 1 | ea | Spring Vegetables, w/Cheese, Budget Gourmet | 156 | 150 | 83 | 6.0 | 10.0 | 2.0 | 5.0 | 3.0 | 10.0 | 5.0 | | | | | 25 | 2500 | 500 | | | | 0.03 | 0.19 | 0.88 | | | | | 30.0 | | | 150 | | 0.7 | | | | | | 450 | |
| 56891 | 1 | ea | With Barley, American Classics | 43 | 150 | 16 | 6.0 | 29.0 | 6.0 | 5.0 | 18.0 | 0.5 | 0.0 | | | 0.00 | 0.00 | 0 | 1500 | 300 | | | | | | | | | | | 15.0 | | | 40 | | 3.6 | | | | | | 470 | |
| 70689 | 1 | cup | With Noodles, La Choy | 266 | 130 | 86 | 4.8 | 26.6 | 2.9 | 10.2 | 13.5 | 1.3 | 0.5 | | | | | 0 | 116 | 23 | | | | | | | | | | | 2.3 | | | 32 | | 0.6 | | | | | | 1311 | |
| 56321 | 1 | cup | With Pasta & cream sauce, avg | 162 | 185 | 76 | 7.9 | 20.7 | 1.3 | | | 8.0 | 2.7 | 3.7 | 1.2 | | | 8 | 5148 | 521 | 0 | 521 | | 0.17 | 0.23 | 1.34 | 0.14 | 0.25 | 27.9 | | 17.9 | | | 162 | 0.1 | 1.2 | 29 | | 149 | 259 | | 442 | 0.81 |
| 70479 | 1 | ea | Ziti, w/Marinara Sauce, Budget Gourmet | 177 | 220 | 75 | 9.0 | 25.0 | 2.0 | 2.0 | 21.0 | 10.0 | 4.0 | | | | | 15 | 500 | 100 | | | | 0.12 | 0.34 | 2.00 | | | | | 9.0 | | | 150 | | 1.1 | | | | | | 720 | |
| | | | *PIZZA* | | | | | | | | | | | | | | | | | | | | | | | | | | | | | | | | | | | | | | | | |
| 56846 | 1 | pce | Artichoke Heart, whole wheat, Spago | 76 | 170 | | 8.0 | 19.0 | | | | 7.0 | | | | | | | | | | | | | | | | | | | | | | | | | | | | 250 | | 12 | |
| | | | Canadian Bacon | | | | | | | | | | | | | | | | | | | | | | | | | | | | | | | | | | | | | | | | |
| 56784 | 1 | ea | For One, Celeste | 220 | 541 | 51 | 27.3 | 49.6 | | | | 26.0 | | | | | | 20 | 1553 | 311 | | | | 0.37 | 0.73 | 2.93 | 0.29 | 2.00 | 141.0 | 0.00 | 0.0 | | | 491 | 0.3 | 1.9 | 62 | | 684 | 444 | | 1533 | 4.00 |
| 57164 | 1 | pce | 1/5 of 12", Tombstone | 125 | 288 | 52 | 16.0 | 28.8 | 1.6 | 5.6 | 21.6 | 12.0 | 5.5 | | | | | 32 | 501 | 120 | | | | | | | | | | | 12.0 | | | 200 | | 1.2 | | | | | | 737 | |
| 57255 | 1 | ea | Two Cheese, Totinos | 418 | 940 | 54 | 50.6 | 90.7 | 4.2 | 11.3 | 75.2 | 42.2 | 15.5 | | | | | 79 | 0 | 0 | 0 | 0 | 0 | | | | | | | | 0.0 | | | 794 | | 6.7 | | | | | | 2433 | |
| | | | Cheese | | | | | | | | | | | | | | | | | | | | | | | | | | | | | | | | | | | | | | | | |
| 56743 | 1 | ea | Double Cheese, Lunch Express | 167 | 421 | 49 | 21.1 | 41.1 | 3.0 | 4.0 | 34.1 | 19.1 | 7.0 | | | | | 35 | 301 | 60 | | | | 0.30 | 0.30 | 2.41 | | | | | 6.0 | | | 401 | | 2.7 | | | | 261 | | 712 | |
| 56774 | 1 | ea | Extra Cheese, Weight Watchers | 163 | 390 | 48 | 23.0 | 49.0 | 6.0 | 3.0 | 40.0 | 12.0 | 4.0 | 3.0 | 1.0 | | | 35 | 400 | 80 | | | | 0.30 | 0.51 | 3.00 | 0.06 | | | | 6.0 | | | 700 | | 1.8 | | | | 290 | | 590 | |
| 57222 | 1 | pce | Extra Cheese, 12", Tombstone | 145 | 370 | 49 | 18.0 | 36.0 | 2.0 | 6.0 | 28.0 | 17.0 | 9.0 | | | | | 30 | 750 | 150 | | | | | | | | | | | 9.0 | | | 350 | | 1.1 | | | | | | 630 | |
| 56782 | 1 | ea | For One, Celeste | 184 | 497 | 46 | 21.2 | 48.0 | 3.6 | | | 24.5 | 11.0 | 5.0 | 2.0 | | | 40 | 927 | 185 | | | | 0.15 | 0.44 | 1.23 | 0.15 | 2.00 | 35.0 | 0.00 | 0.0 | | | 375 | 0.2 | 1.4 | 48 | | 386 | 342 | | 1070 | 4.00 |
| 56843 | 1 | pce | Four Cheese, Spago | 76 | 170 | | 8.0 | 19.0 | | | | 7.0 | | | | | | 12 | | | | | | | | | | | | | | | | | | | | | | | | 250 | |
| 57218 | 1 | ea | Low Fat, 1 1/2 svgs, Tombstone | 184 | 360 | | 23.0 | 45.0 | 3.0 | 8.0 | 34.0 | 10.0 | 4.5 | | | | | 15 | 750 | 150 | | | | | | | | | | | 3.6 | | | 350 | | 1.1 | | | | | | 920 | |
| 66001 | 1 | pce | 1/8 of 12", avg | 63 | 140 | 48 | 7.7 | 20.5 | 1.1 | | | 3.2 | 1.5 | 1.0 | 0.5 | 0.05 | 0.44 | 9 | 382 | 74 | | | | 0.18 | 0.16 | 2.48 | 0.04 | 0.33 | 34.7 | 0.22 | 1.3 | | | 117 | 0.1 | 0.6 | 16 | 0.2 | 113 | 110 | 13.5 | 336 | 0.81 |
| 56789 | 1 | pce | 1/4 each, Celeste | 126 | 317 | 49 | 14.2 | 27.8 | 2.2 | | | 16.6 | 7.0 | 3.0 | 1.0 | | | 20 | 779 | 156 | | | | 0.08 | 0.39 | 1.11 | 0.10 | 1.00 | 14.0 | 0.00 | 0.0 | | | 204 | 0.1 | 1.0 | 30 | | 266 | 268 | | 770 | 3.00 |
| 56741 | 1 | ea | Stouffer's | 294 | 706 | 53 | 29.4 | 82.3 | 4.1 | | | 25.9 | 9.7 | 9.7 | 6.5 | | | 103 | 794 | 159 | | | | 0.88 | 0.88 | 5.88 | 0.11 | | | | 12.1 | | | 412 | | 5.9 | | | | 529 | | 1705 | |
| 81041 | 1 | ea | Three Cheese, Deep Dish, Pappalos | 138 | 344 | 46 | 17.9 | 42.4 | 2.2 | 3.2 | 37.0 | 11.3 | 5.4 | | | | | 23 | 0 | 0 | 0 | 0 | 0 | | | | | | | | 0.0 | | | 284 | | 2.9 | | | | | | 615 | |
| 57274 | 1 | ea | Three Cheese, For One, Pappalos | 204 | 492 | 49 | 29.0 | 50.0 | 2.9 | 4.1 | 43.0 | 19.6 | 10.0 | | | | | 45 | 0 | 0 | 0 | 0 | 0 | | | | | | | | 0.0 | | | 530 | | 3.1 | | | | | | 957 | |
| 57168 | 1 | pce | Three Cheese, 1/4 of 12", Tombstone | 138 | 380 | 50 | 20.0 | 25.0 | 2.0 | 5.0 | 18.0 | 22.0 | 12.0 | | | | | 45 | 1000 | 200 | | | | | | | | | | | 4.8 | | | 450 | | 0.7 | | | | | | 730 | |
| 56847 | 1 | pce | Chicken, Spicy, Spago | 76 | 180 | | 9.0 | 18.0 | | | | 8.0 | | | | | | 23 | | | | | | | | | | | | | | | | | | | | | | | | 320 | |
| 56618 | 1 | pce | Combination, 12", avg | 79 | 184 | 48 | 13.0 | 21.3 | | | | 5.4 | 1.5 | 2.5 | 0.9 | 0.05 | 0.86 | 21 | 524 | 101 | 93 | 8 | | 0.21 | 0.17 | 1.96 | 0.09 | 0.36 | 32.4 | 0.83 | 1.6 | | | 101 | 0.1 | 1.5 | 18 | 0.1 | 131 | 179 | 10.9 | 332 | 1.11 |
| 57247 | 1 | pce | Combination, 1/4, Totinos | 125 | 306 | 52 | 12.0 | 27.9 | 1.5 | 3.3 | 23.1 | 16.4 | 3.3 | | | | | 14 | 0 | 0 | 0 | 0 | 0 | | | | | | | | 0.0 | | | 190 | | 1.8 | | | | | | 738 | |
| | | | Croissant | | | | | | | | | | | | | | | | | | | | | | | | | | | | | | | | | | | | | | | | |
| 70407 | 1 | ea | Deluxe, Pepperidge Farm | 142 | 450 | 41 | 14.0 | 40.0 | 7.0 | 12.0 | 21.0 | 27.0 | 10.0 | 12.0 | 2.0 | | | 85 | 200 | 40 | | | | 0.52 | 0.34 | 4.00 | | | | | 1.2 | | | 200 | | 2.7 | | | | 201 | | 910 | |
| 70404 | 1 | ea | Pastry Cheese, Pepperidge Farm | 124 | 390 | 40 | 12.0 | 39.0 | 6.0 | 11.0 | 22.0 | 20.0 | 4.5 | 5.8 | 9.7 | | | 90 | 300 | 66 | | | | 45.00 | 0.25 | 4.00 | | | | | 2.4 | | | 350 | | 1.8 | | | | 214 | | 770 | |
| 70405 | 1 | ea | Pepperoni Pizza, Pepperidge Farm | 128 | 420 | 38 | 15.0 | 39.0 | 5.0 | 8.0 | 26.0 | 23.0 | 9.0 | 1.5 | 9.0 | | | 90 | 300 | 60 | | | | 0.52 | 0.34 | 4.00 | | | | | 3.6 | | | 150 | | 1.8 | | | | 232 | | 810 | |

| Code | Amount | Description | Basic Components | | | | | | | | | Additional Fats | | | | | | Vit A & Components | | | | | Vitamins | | | | | | | | | | Minerals | | | | | | | | | |
|---|---|---|---|---|---|---|---|---|---|---|---|---|---|---|---|---|---|---|---|---|---|---|---|---|---|---|---|---|---|---|---|---|---|---|---|---|---|---|---|---|---|---|
| | | | Weight (g) | Calories | % Water | Protein (g) | Carbs (g) | Fiber (g) | Sugar (g) | Other Carbs (g) | Fat (g) | Sat Fat (g) | Mono Fat (g) | Poly Fat (g) | Omega 3 (g) | Omega 6 (g) | Choles (mg) | Vit A (IU) | Vit A (RE) | Retinol (RE) | Carotenoids (RE) | Beta Carotene (mcg) | Thiamin (mg) | Riboflavin (mg) | Niacin (NE) | Vit B6 (mg) | Vit B12 (mcg) | Folate (mcg) | Panto (mg) | Vit C (mg) | Vit D (mg) | Vit E (α TE) | Calcium (mg) | Copper (mg) | Iron (mg) | Magnes (mg) | Mang (mg) | Phos (mg) | Potassium (mg) | Selenium (mcg) | Sodium (mg) | Zinc (mg) |
| | | Deluxe | | | | | | | | | | | | | | | | | | | | | | | | | | | | | | | | | | | | | | | | |
| 56772 | 1 ea | Combo, Weight Watchers | 186 | 380 | 56 | 23.0 | 47.0 | 6.0 | 4.0 | 37.0 | 11.0 | 3.5 | 5.0 | 2.0 | | | 40 | 750 | 150 | | | | 0.30 | 0.51 | 3.00 | 0.20 | | | | 4.8 | | | 500 | | 3.6 | | | | 370 | | 550 | |
| 56781 | 1 ea | For One, Celeste | 234 | 582 | 53 | 22.7 | 51.2 | 4.4 | | | 31.8 | 10.0 | 9.0 | 3.0 | | | 20 | 1226 | 245 | | | | 0.30 | 0.82 | 3.53 | 0.26 | 2.00 | 80.0 | 2.00 | 0.0 | | | 332 | 0.3 | 2.6 | 61 | | 480 | 498 | | 1367 | 5.00 |
| 56742 | 1 ea | Lunch Express | 188 | 460 | 52 | 21.0 | 40.0 | 4.0 | 4.0 | 32.0 | 25.0 | 8.0 | | | | | 45 | 300 | 58 | | | | 0.30 | 0.20 | 2.30 | 0.07 | | | | 12.0 | | | 250 | | 2.7 | | | | 340 | | 1001 | |
| 56788 | 1 pce | 1/4 each, Celeste | 158 | 378 | 55 | 15.5 | 29.3 | 3.1 | | | 22.1 | 7.0 | 7.0 | 2.0 | | | 20 | 950 | 190 | | | | 0.20 | 0.55 | 2.65 | 0.17 | 2.00 | 57.0 | 2.00 | 0.0 | | | 267 | 0.2 | 1.9 | 38 | | 357 | 352 | | 903 | 3.00 |
| 57166 | 1 pce | 1/5 of 12", Tombstone | 125 | 299 | 52 | 14.0 | 27.1 | 1.9 | 4.7 | 20.5 | 14.9 | 6.5 | | | | | 28 | 466 | 93 | | | | | | | | | | | 8.4 | | | 233 | | 1.3 | | | | | | 597 | |
| 57199 | 1 pce | Four Meat, 1/6 of 12", Tombstone | 133 | 350 | 48 | 17.0 | 31.0 | 2.0 | 5.0 | 24.0 | 18.0 | 8.0 | | | | | 40 | 500 | 100 | | | | | | | | | | | 6.0 | | | 250 | | 1.1 | | | | | | 810 | |
| | | French Bread | | | | | | | | | | | | | | | | | | | | | | | | | | | | | | | | | | | | | | | | |
| 56878 | 1 ea | Bacon Cheddar, Stouffers | 161 | 440 | 45 | 16.0 | 44.0 | 4.0 | 4.0 | 36.0 | 22.0 | 7.0 | | | | | 30 | 300 | 60 | | | | | | | | | | | 6.0 | | | 250 | | 3.6 | | | | 310 | | 940 | |
| 56733 | 1 ea | Cheese, Lean Cuisine | 145 | 298 | 50 | 18.8 | 40.9 | 3.4 | 6.8 | 30.7 | 6.8 | 3.4 | 1.3 | 0.4 | | | 17 | 256 | 51 | | | | | | | | | | | 5.1 | | | 384 | | 3.1 | | | | 315 | | 341 | |
| 56877 | 1 ea | Cheeseburger, Stouffers | 168 | 440 | 50 | 21.0 | 31.0 | 5.0 | 4.0 | 22.0 | 26.0 | 9.0 | | | | | 55 | 750 | 150 | | | | | | | | | | | 12.0 | | | 250 | | 2.7 | | | | 290 | | 1110 | |
| 56736 | 1 ea | Deluxe, Lean Cuisine | 174 | 330 | 53 | 23.0 | 45.0 | 5.0 | 5.0 | 35.0 | 6.0 | 2.5 | 2.0 | 1.0 | | | 30 | 500 | 100 | | | | | | | | | | | 6.0 | | | 250 | | 3.6 | | | | 380 | | 560 | |
| 56876 | 1 ea | Double Cheese, Stouffers | 167 | 420 | 47 | 19.0 | 44.0 | 5.0 | 3.0 | 36.0 | 19.0 | 7.0 | | | | | 30 | 300 | 60 | | | | | | | | | | | 9.0 | | | 350 | | 2.7 | | | | 260 | | 790 | |
| 56875 | 1 ea | Garden Vegetable, Stouffers | 179 | 340 | 57 | 12.0 | 45.0 | 4.0 | 5.0 | 36.0 | 12.0 | 4.0 | | | | | 15 | 300 | 60 | | | | | | | | | | | 30.0 | | | 200 | | 2.7 | | | | 260 | | 540 | |
| 81077 | 1 ea | Pepperoni, Healthy Choice | 170 | 340 | 53 | 24.0 | 49.0 | 6.0 | 6.0 | 37.0 | 5.0 | 1.5 | | | | | 20 | 300 | 60 | | | | | | | | | | | 0.0 | | | 300 | | 5.4 | | | | | | 580 | |
| 56735 | 1 ea | Pepperoni, Stouffers | 149 | 330 | 47 | 20.0 | 46.0 | 4.0 | 4.0 | 38.0 | 7.0 | 3.0 | 2.5 | 1.0 | | | 25 | 500 | 100 | | | | | | | | | | | 6.0 | | | 250 | | 3.6 | | | | 350 | | 590 | |
| 56746 | 1 ea | Pepperoni & Mushroom, Stouffers | 174 | 430 | 53 | 17.0 | 43.0 | 3.0 | 3.0 | 37.0 | 21.0 | 6.0 | | | | | 30 | 400 | 80 | | | | 0.40 | 0.20 | 2.90 | | | | | 9.0 | | | 250 | | 2.7 | | | | 340 | | 1000 | |
| 81076 | 1 ea | Sausage, Healthy Choice | 170 | 320 | 55 | 21.0 | 48.0 | 5.0 | 5.0 | 38.0 | 5.0 | 1.5 | | | | | 25 | 200 | 40 | | | | | | | | | | | 0.0 | | | 150 | | 2.7 | | | | | | 580 | |
| 56734 | 1 ea | Sausage, Stouffers | 170 | 420 | 53 | 19.0 | 41.0 | 4.0 | 3.0 | 34.0 | 20.0 | 5.0 | 13.9 | 1.1 | | | 35 | 400 | 80 | | | | 0.45 | 0.51 | 5.00 | 0.07 | | | | 6.0 | | | 250 | 0.2 | 2.7 | 39 | | | 340 | | 900 | 2.20 |
| 56874 | 1 ea | Sausage & Pepperoni, Stouffers | 177 | 460 | 44 | 22.0 | 45.0 | 4.0 | 4.0 | 37.0 | 25.0 | 7.0 | | | | | 40 | 400 | 80 | | | | | | | | | | | 6.0 | | | 200 | | 3.6 | | | | 360 | | 1130 | |
| 81075 | 1 ea | Supreme, Healthy Choice | 180 | 330 | 57 | 21.0 | 51.0 | 6.0 | 7.0 | 38.0 | 5.0 | 1.5 | | | | | 20 | 200 | 40 | | | | | | | | | | | 0.0 | | | 200 | | 3.6 | | | | | | 580 | |
| 56749 | 1 ea | Vegetable Deluxe, Stouffers | 181 | 380 | 56 | 18.0 | 43.0 | 5.0 | 3.0 | 35.0 | 17.0 | 6.0 | | | | | 25 | 1250 | 250 | | | | 0.30 | 0.20 | 1.70 | 0.12 | | | | 2.4 | | | 300 | | 2.7 | | | | 220 | | 830 | |
| 56873 | 1 ea | White, Stouffers | 144 | 460 | 36 | 17.0 | 43.0 | 5.0 | 2.0 | 36.0 | 28.0 | 8.0 | | | | | 25 | 250 | 50 | | | | | | | | | | | | | | 350 | | 2.7 | | | | 110 | | 760 | |
| 56744 | 1 ea | Hamburger, Stouffers | 345 | 828 | 54 | 38.0 | 79.3 | | | | 38.0 | | | | | | 138 | 587 | 117 | | | | 0.69 | 0.69 | 7.93 | | | | | 12.1 | | | 414 | | 5.9 | | | | 690 | | 2036 | |
| 57156 | 1 pce | Hamburger & Cheese, 1/5 of 12", Tombstone | 125 | 320 | 52 | 15.0 | 29.0 | 2.0 | 5.0 | 22.0 | 16.0 | 8.0 | | | | | 30 | 500 | 100 | | | | | | | | | | | 6.0 | | | 250 | | 1.4 | | | | | | 660 | |
| 57245 | 1 ea | Mexican Style, Totinos | 310 | 744 | 53 | 30.1 | 68.2 | 4.6 | 6.8 | 56.7 | 38.8 | 8.7 | | | | | 31 | 0 | 0 | 0 | 0 | 0 | | | | | | | | 0.0 | | | 477 | | 4.3 | | | | | | 1500 | |
| 56844 | 1 pce | Mushroom & Spinach, Spago | 77 | 122 | | 9.1 | 21.3 | | | | 4.1 | | | | | | 4 | | | | | | | | | | | | | | | | | | | | | | | | 223 | |
| | | Pepperoni | | | | | | | | | | | | | | | | | | | | | | | | | | | | | | | | | | | | | | | | |
| 57158 | 1 pce | Cheese, 1/5 of 12", Tombstone | 125 | 340 | 47 | 15.0 | 29.0 | 2.0 | 5.0 | 22.0 | 18.0 | 8.0 | | | | | 35 | 500 | 100 | | | | | | | | | | | 6.0 | | | 250 | | 1.1 | | | | | | 750 | |
| 81020 | 1 ea | Deep Dish, Pappalos | 146 | 393 | 45 | 19.1 | 42.3 | 2.3 | 3.1 | 36.9 | 16.4 | 7.2 | | | | | 35 | 0 | 0 | 0 | 0 | 0 | | | | | | | | 0.0 | | | 237 | | 3.1 | | | | | | 828 | |
| 57193 | 1 pce | Dbl Pepperoni & Cheese, 1/6 of 12", Tombstone | 129 | 350 | 49 | 19.0 | 25.0 | 2.0 | 5.0 | 18.0 | 20.0 | 10.0 | | | | | 45 | 500 | 100 | | | | | | | | | | | 6.0 | | | 350 | | 1.1 | | | | | | 850 | |
| 56779 | 1 ea | For One, Celeste | 191 | 546 | 45 | 20.2 | 49.7 | 3.9 | | | 29.6 | 9.0 | 7.0 | 2.0 | | | 20 | 1316 | 263 | | | | 0.25 | 0.71 | 2.58 | 0.21 | 2.00 | 97.0 | 0.00 | 0.0 | | | 336 | 0.3 | 2.0 | 53 | | 443 | 416 | | 1353 | 4.00 |
| 57271 | 1 ea | For One, Pappalos | 218 | 569 | 48 | 30.1 | 51.9 | 3.1 | 4.1 | 44.7 | 26.8 | 12.6 | | | | | 61 | 0 | 0 | 0 | 0 | 0 | | | | | | | | 0.0 | | | 403 | | 3.9 | | | | | | 1277 | |
| 57219 | 1 ea | Low Fat, 1 1/2 svgs, Tombstone | 192 | 400 | 56 | 26.0 | 45.0 | 4.0 | 8.0 | 33.0 | 13.0 | 5.0 | | | | | 35 | 1000 | 200 | | | | | | | | | | | 2.4 | | | 300 | | 1.8 | | | | | | 1040 | |
| 56745 | 1 ea | Lunch Express | 163 | 440 | 48 | 19.0 | 39.0 | 4.0 | 3.0 | 32.0 | 23.0 | 8.0 | | | | | 40 | 50 | 100 | | | | 0.30 | 0.30 | 2.50 | | | | | 12.0 | | | 250 | | 3.6 | | | | 310 | | 960 | |
| 56619 | 1 pce | 1/8 of 12", avg | 71 | 181 | 46 | 10.2 | 19.9 | | | | 7.0 | 2.2 | 3.1 | 1.2 | 0.04 | 1.12 | 14 | 282 | 55 | 50 | 4 | | 0.13 | 0.23 | 3.05 | 0.06 | 0.18 | 36.9 | 0.25 | 1.6 | | | 65 | 0.1 | 0.9 | 9 | 0.1 | 75 | 153 | 13.1 | 267 | 0.52 |
| 56786 | 1 pce | 1/4 each, Celeste | 135 | 368 | 48 | 15.0 | 29.2 | 2.4 | | | 21.3 | 7.0 | 7.0 | 2.0 | | | 15 | 1343 | 270 | | | | 0.14 | 0.57 | 1.63 | 0.18 | 1.00 | 101.0 | 0.00 | 0.0 | | | 186 | 0.2 | 1.4 | 39 | | 386 | 284 | | 1000 | 4.00 |
| 57201 | 1 pce | 1/4 of 12", Tombstone | 128 | 360 | 48 | 16.0 | 31.0 | 2.0 | 5.0 | 24.0 | 19.0 | 9.0 | | | | | 40 | 500 | 100 | | | | | | | | | | | 6.0 | | | 250 | | 1.1 | | | | | | 790 | |
| 56987 | 1 ea | Pizza Pocket, Ore-Ida | 170 | 510 | 43 | 19.0 | 50.0 | 4.0 | 10.0 | 36.0 | 26.0 | 7.0 | | | | | 35 | 750 | 150 | | | | | | | | | | | 0.0 | | | 250 | | 4.5 | | | | 320 | | 1039 | |
| 56095 | 1 pce | Two Cheese, 1/3, Totinos | 136 | 363 | 49 | 16.3 | 29.9 | 1.5 | 3.4 | 25.0 | 19.9 | 7.6 | | | | | 34 | 0 | 0 | 0 | 0 | 0 | | | | | | | | 0.0 | | | 265 | | 2.3 | | | | | | 823 | |
| 56773 | 1 ea | Weight Watchers | 158 | 390 | 48 | 23.0 | 46.0 | 4.0 | 3.0 | 39.0 | 12.0 | 4.0 | 5.0 | 2.0 | | | 45 | 400 | 80 | | | | 0.23 | 0.51 | 3.00 | | | | | 4.8 | | | 450 | | 1.8 | | | | 320 | | 650 | |
| 57191 | 1 pce | With Sausage, 1/3 of 9", Tombstone | 125 | 360 | 47 | 16.0 | 28.0 | 2.0 | 5.0 | 21.0 | 21.0 | 9.0 | | | | | 35 | 500 | 100 | | | | | | | | | | | 6.0 | | | 200 | | 1.4 | | | | | | 820 | |
| | | Pizza Rolls | | | | | | | | | | | | | | | | | | | | | | | | | | | | | | | | | | | | | | | | |
| 81037 | 1 ea | Cheese, pkg, Jenos | 85 | 197 | 46 | 9.2 | 30.1 | 1.4 | | | 5.1 | 1.9 | 2.3 | 0.9 | | | 18 | 111 | 22 | | | | 0.09 | 0.09 | 0.94 | | | | | 0.0 | | | 137 | | 0.7 | | | 177 | 145 | | 375 | |
| 57260 | 1 ea | Cheese & Beef, Nacho, Totinos | 14 | 34 | 51 | 1.3 | 3.7 | 0.2 | 0.3 | 3.2 | 1.6 | 0.6 | | | | | 4 | 0 | 0 | 0 | 0 | 0 | | | | | | | | 0.0 | | | 15 | | 0.2 | | | | | | 73 | |
| 57258 | 1 ea | Combination, Totinos | 14 | 36 | 49 | 1.5 | 3.8 | 0.2 | 0.5 | 3.1 | 1.7 | 0.5 | | | | | 4 | 0 | 0 | 0 | 0 | 0 | | | | | | | | 0.0 | | | 11 | | 0.2 | | | | | | 41 | |
| 81054 | 1 ea | Combo, pkg, Jenos | 85 | 213 | 46 | 9.9 | 25.7 | 1.9 | | | 8.6 | 2.8 | 4.2 | 1.5 | | | 14 | 20 | 4 | | | | 0.05 | 0.12 | 1.50 | | | | | 0.4 | | | 74 | | 0.9 | | | 111 | 199 | | 233 | |
| 81036 | 1 ea | Hamburger, pkg, Jenos | 85 | 211 | 45 | 9.6 | 27.6 | 2.0 | | | 7.8 | 2.7 | 3.9 | 1.1 | | | 20 | 43 | 9 | | | | 0.04 | 0.12 | 1.36 | | | | | 0.1 | | | 77 | | 0.8 | | | 113 | 198 | | 314 | |
| 57259 | 1 ea | Hamburger & Cheese, Totinos | 14 | 34 | 49 | 1.5 | 3.9 | 0.2 | 0.7 | 3.1 | 1.4 | 0.4 | | | | | 4 | 0 | 0 | 0 | 0 | 0 | | | | | | | | 0.0 | | | 12 | | 0.2 | | | | | | 57 | |
| 81035 | 1 ea | Pepperoni, pkg, Jenos | 85 | 210 | 47 | 9.4 | 25.7 | 1.8 | | | 8.5 | 2.8 | 4.3 | 1.4 | | | 20 | 28 | 6 | | | | 0.10 | 0.14 | 1.36 | | | | | 0.0 | | | 69 | | 0.9 | | | 109 | 199 | | 349 | |
| 57261 | 1 ea | Pepperoni & Cheese, Totinos | 14 | 36 | 49 | 1.5 | 3.7 | 0.2 | 0.3 | 3.2 | 1.7 | 0.5 | | | | | 4 | 0 | 0 | 0 | 0 | 0 | | | | | | | | 0.0 | | | 11 | | 0.2 | | | | | | 58 | |
| 81055 | 1 ea | Sausage, pkg, Jenos | 85 | 200 | 48 | 9.2 | 26.1 | 1.6 | | | 7.2 | 2.2 | 3.6 | 1.4 | | | 14 | 14 | 3 | | | | 0.09 | 0.15 | 1.30 | | | | | 0.1 | | | 66 | | 0.8 | | | 106 | 197 | | 335 | |
| 57262 | 1 ea | Sausage & Cheese, Totinos | 14 | 34 | 50 | 1.4 | 3.8 | 0.2 | 0.4 | 3.2 | 1.5 | 0.4 | | | | | 3 | 0 | 0 | 0 | 0 | 0 | | | | | | | | 0.0 | | | 10 | | 0.2 | | | | | | 58 | |
| 57263 | 1 ea | Sausage & Mushroom, Totinos | 14 | 33 | 51 | 1.3 | 3.8 | 0.2 | 0.5 | 3.1 | 1.4 | 0.4 | | | | | 3 | 0 | 0 | 0 | 0 | 0 | | | | | | | | 0.0 | | | 11 | | 0.2 | | | | | | 56 | |
| 57266 | 1 ea | Three Meat, Totinos | 14 | 34 | 50 | 1.5 | 3.7 | 0.2 | 0.5 | 3.0 | 1.5 | 0.5 | | | | | 4 | 0 | 0 | 0 | 0 | 0 | | | | | | | | 0.0 | | | 11 | | 0.2 | | | | | | 62 | |
| | | Sausage | | | | | | | | | | | | | | | | | | | | | | | | | | | | | | | | | | | | | | | | |
| 81021 | 1 ea | Deep Dish, Pappalos | 149 | 381 | 47 | 18.5 | 42.0 | 2.1 | 3.3 | 36.7 | 15.5 | 9.4 | | | | | 27 | 0 | 0 | 0 | 0 | 0 | | | | | | | | 0.0 | | | 231 | | 2.8 | | | | | | 688 | |
| 57197 | 1 pce | Double Saus, Pepp & Chs, 1/6 of 12", Tombstone | 135 | 360 | 51 | 20.0 | 25.0 | 2.0 | 5.0 | 18.0 | 20.0 | 10.0 | | | | | 45 | 500 | 100 | | | | | | | | | | | 6.0 | | | 400 | | 1.1 | | | | | | 800 | |
| 56778 | 1 ea | For One, Celeste | 213 | 571 | 48 | 22.6 | 48.8 | 4.2 | | | 31.7 | 10.0 | 7.0 | 3.0 | | | 20 | 1359 | 272 | | | | 0.30 | 0.77 | 2.85 | 0.23 | 2.00 | 109.0 | 0.00 | 0.0 | | | 371 | 0.3 | 2.3 | 60 | | 505 | 456 | | 1363 | 0.00 |
| 56747 | 1 ea | Lunch Express | 184 | 459 | 51 | 21.0 | 39.9 | 3.0 | 4.0 | 32.9 | 25.0 | 8.0 | | | | | 40 | 399 | 80 | | | | 0.40 | 0.20 | 2.40 | 0.09 | | | | 9.0 | | | 200 | | 3.6 | | | | 399 | | 1088 | |
| 56785 | 1 pce | 1/4 each, Celeste | 142 | 376 | 50 | 15.6 | 29.7 | | | | 21.7 | 7.0 | 6.0 | 2.0 | | | 12 | 1048 | 210 | | | | 0.18 | 0.51 | 1.95 | 1.00 | 89.00 | 0.2 | 0.00 | 0.0 | | | 322 | 0.2 | 1.5 | 40 | | 385 | 311 | | 907 | 3.00 |
| 57205 | 1 pce | Three Sausage, 1/6 of 12", Tombstone | 131 | 340 | 50 | 16.0 | 31.0 | 2.0 | 5.0 | 24.0 | 17.0 | 8.0 | | | | | 35 | 500 | 100 | | | | | | | | | | | 6.0 | | | 250 | | 1.1 | | | | | | 740 | |
| 57160 | 1 pce | With Cheese, 1/5 of 12", Tombstone | 125 | 320 | 52 | 15.0 | 29.0 | 2.0 | 5.0 | 22.0 | 16.0 | 8.0 | | | | | 30 | 500 | 100 | | | | | | | | | | | 6.0 | | | 250 | | 1.4 | | | | | | 650 | |
| 57195 | 1 pce | With Double Cheese, 1/6 of 12", Tombstone | 135 | 350 | 52 | 20.0 | 25.0 | 2.0 | 5.0 | 18.0 | 19.0 | 10.0 | | | | | 40 | 500 | 100 | | | | | | | | | | | 6.0 | | | 400 | | 1.4 | | | | | | 740 | |
| 56780 | 1 ea | With Mushrooms, For One, Celeste | 241 | 592 | 53 | 23.9 | 51.3 | 4.5 | | | 32.3 | 11.0 | 10.0 | 3.0 | | | 20 | 1200 | 240 | | | | 0.34 | 0.87 | 3.93 | 0.34 | 2.00 | 82.0 | 2.00 | 0.0 | | | 362 | 0.3 | 2.4 | 60 | | 504 | 549 | | 1367 | 5.00 |
| 56787 | 1 pce | With Mushrooms, 1/4 each, Celeste | 177 | 387 | 60 | 16.9 | 29.4 | 1.5 | | | 22.4 | 6.4 | 10.6 | 1.5 | | | 15 | 1065 | 213 | | | | 0.24 | 0.51 | 2.91 | 0.19 | 2.00 | 102.0 | 0.00 | 0.0 | | | 310 | 0.2 | 1.6 | 45 | | 407 | 361 | | 1033 | 3.00 |
| 57162 | 1 pce | With Mushrooms & Cheese, 1/5 of 12", Tombstone | 125 | 310 | 52 | 14.5 | 28.1 | 1.9 | 4.8 | 21.3 | 15.5 | 6.8 | | | | | 29 | 484 | 97 | | | | | | | | | | | 5.8 | | | 242 | | 1.0 | | | | | | 610 | |
| 81040 | 1 ea | With Pepperoni, Deep Dish, Pappalos | 151 | 394 | 46 | 19.2 | 42.9 | 2.3 | 3.2 | 37.4 | 16.3 | 8.8 | | | | | 30 | 0 | 0 | 0 | 0 | 0 | | | | | | | | 0.0 | | | 237 | | 3.0 | | | | | | 761 | |
| 57272 | 1 ea | With Pepperoni, For One, Pappalos | 232 | 592 | 49 | 30.9 | 52.9 | 3.0 | 4.4 | 45.5 | 28.5 | 16.5 | | | | | 58 | 0 | 0 | 0 | 0 | 0 | | | | | | | | 0.0 | | | 441 | | 3.7 | | | | | | 1213 | |
| 56748 | 1 ea | With Pepperoni, Lunch Express | 181 | 500 | 47 | 24.0 | 41.0 | 4.0 | 2.0 | 35.0 | 27.0 | 9.0 | | | | | 60 | 750 | 150 | | | | 0.30 | 0.20 | 2.30 | | | | | 12.0 | | | 250 | | 3.6 | | | | 360 | | 1140 | |

| Code | Amount | | Description | Basic Components | | | | | | | | | Additional Fats | | | | | | Vit A & Components | | | | | Vitamins | | | | | | | | | | Minerals | | | | | | | | | |
|---|---|---|---|---|---|---|---|---|---|---|---|---|---|---|---|---|---|---|---|---|---|---|---|---|---|---|---|---|---|---|---|---|---|---|---|---|---|---|---|---|---|---|---|
| | | | | Weight (g) | Calories | % Water | Protein (g) | Carbs (g) | Fiber (g) | Sugar (g) | Other Carbs (g) | Fat (g) | Sat Fat (g) | Mono Fat (g) | Poly Fat (g) | Omega 3 (g) | Omega 6 (g) | Choles (mg) | Vit A (IU) | Vit A (RE) | Retinol (RE) | Carotenoids (RE) | Beta Carotene (mcg) | Thiamin (mg) | Riboflavin (mg) | Niacin (NE) | Vit B6 (mg) | Vit B12 (mcg) | Folate (mcg) | Panto (mg) | Vit C (mg) | Vit D (mg) | Vit E (α TE) | Calcium (mg) | Copper (mg) | Iron (mg) | Magnes (mg) | Mang (mg) | Phos (mg) | Potassium (mg) | Selenium (mcg) | Sodium (mg) | Zinc (mg) |
| 56730 | 1 | ea | With Pepperoni, Stouffers | 357 | 928 | 52 | 39.3 | 82.1 | | | | 46.4 | | | | | | | 1000 | 200 | | | | 1.43 | 0.71 | 10.00 | | | | | 12.1 | | | 393 | | 8.2 | | | | 821 | | 2749 | |
| | | | Supreme | | | | | | | | | | | | | | | | | | | | | | | | | | | | | | | | | | | | | | | | |
| 81042 | 1 | ea | Deep Dish, Pappalos | 153 | 379 | 49 | 18.4 | 41.0 | 2.3 | 3.4 | 35.3 | 15.3 | 8.5 | | | | | 29 | 0 | 0 | 0 | 0 | 0 | | | | | | | | 0.0 | | | 223 | | 2.9 | | | | | | 747 | |
| 56783 | 1 | ea | For One, Celeste | 255 | 678 | 51 | 26.5 | 54.0 | 4.5 | | | 39.3 | 12.0 | 11.0 | 4.0 | | | 20 | 1343 | 339 | | | | 0.33 | 0.92 | 3.72 | 0.28 | 3.00 | 120.0 | 3.00 | 0.0 | | | 454 | 0.4 | 2.7 | 64 | | 602 | 528 | | 1610 | 5.00 |
| 57273 | 1 | ea | For One, Pappalos | 204 | 494 | 52 | 25.7 | 44.5 | 2.9 | 4.1 | 37.5 | 23.7 | 13.9 | | | | | 47 | 0 | 0 | 0 | 0 | 0 | | | | | | | | 0.0 | | | 367 | | 3.3 | | | | | | 1028 | |
| 57220 | 1 | ea | Low Fat, 1 1/2 svgs, Tombstone | 219 | 400 | | 27.0 | 45.0 | 4.0 | 9.0 | 32.0 | 13.0 | 5.0 | | | | | 35 | 1250 | 250 | | | | | | | | | | | 2.4 | | | 300 | | 1.8 | | | | | | 1090 | |
| 56790 | 1 | pce | 1/4 each, Celeste | 163 | 381 | 53 | 16.8 | 29.2 | 3.0 | | | 24.1 | 7.0 | 6.0 | 2.0 | | | 15 | 1167 | 233 | | | | 0.20 | 0.68 | 2.20 | 0.20 | 2.00 | 67.0 | 0.00 | 0.0 | | | 295 | 0.2 | 1.8 | 41 | | 408 | 342 | | 1090 | 3.00 |
| 57179 | 1 | pce | 1/6 of 12", Tombstone | 130 | 330 | 51 | 15.0 | 29.0 | 2.0 | 5.0 | 22.0 | 17.0 | 8.0 | | | | | 35 | 500 | 100 | | | | | | | | | | | 9.0 | | | 250 | | 1.1 | | | | | | 720 | |
| 57172 | 1 | pce | Taco, 1/4 of 12", Tombstone | 145 | 380 | | 16.0 | 26.0 | 2.0 | 5.0 | 19.0 | 23.0 | 11.0 | | | | | 50 | 1250 | 250 | | | | | | | | | | | 9.0 | | | 250 | | 1.4 | | | | | | 850 | |
| 57243 | 1 | ea | Three Meat, Totinos | 298 | 724 | 52 | 29.8 | 66.5 | 3.3 | 7.7 | 55.4 | 37.8 | 8.8 | | | | | 33 | 0 | 0 | 0 | 0 | 0 | | | | | | | | 0.0 | | | 456 | | 4.5 | | | | | | 1836 | |
| 57217 | 1 | pce | Vegetable, light, 1/4, Tombstone | 131 | 240 | 51 | 25.0 | 31.0 | 3.0 | 7.0 | 21.0 | 7.0 | 2.5 | | | | | 10 | 1000 | 200 | | | | | | | | | | | 6.0 | | | 400 | | 1.8 | | | | | | 500 | |
| 57221 | 1 | ea | Vegetable, low fat, 1 1/2 svgs, Tombstone | 206 | 360 | | 22.0 | 46.0 | 5.0 | 8.0 | 33.0 | 10.0 | 4.0 | | | | | 15 | 1500 | 500 | | | | | | | | | | | 3.6 | | | 300 | | 1.8 | | | | | | 730 | |
| 15907 | 1 | cup | Almond Chicken | 242 | 276 | 77 | 19.7 | 18.4 | 3.9 | 3.9 | 10.7 | 14.0 | 2.0 | 5.3 | 5.9 | | | 34 | 738 | 75 | 3 | 73 | | 0.03 | 0.19 | 8.59 | 0.42 | 0.24 | 31.5 | 0.73 | 10.5 | 0.7 | | 80 | 0.3 | 2.0 | 58 | 0.5 | 237 | 552 | | 615 | 1.54 |
| | | | **HOMEMADE AND GENERIC MEALS, ENTREES AND DISHES** | | | | | | | | | | | | | | | | | | | | | | | | | | | | | | | | | | | | | | | | |
| 56087 | 1 | cup | Beef Macaroni, w/tomato sauce | 226 | 255 | 76 | 16.3 | 25.8 | 2.5 | 5.5 | 17.3 | 9.7 | 3.3 | 4.1 | 1.5 | 0.04 | 0.42 | 39 | 971 | 97 | 0 | 97 | | 0.22 | 0.22 | 4.31 | 0.29 | 0.88 | 20.4 | 0.52 | 13.7 | 0.1 | | 26 | 0.3 | 2.7 | 40 | 0.4 | 133 | 522 | 13.6 | 862 | 3.14 |
| 57512 | 3 | oz | Cabbage Leaves, stuffed w/rice & beef | 85 | 103 | 75 | 6.8 | 7.6 | 1.4 | | | 5.2 | 2.0 | 2.2 | 1.3 | | | 34 | 289 | 33 | 6 | 27 | | 0.05 | 0.08 | 1.69 | 0.11 | 0.52 | 18.5 | | 14.8 | | | 22 | 0.1 | 1.1 | 15 | | 65 | 243 | | 247 | 1.36 |
| | | | Chicken | | | | | | | | | | | | | | | | | | | | | | | | | | | | | | | | | | | | | | | | |
| 15901 | 1 | cup | A La King | 245 | 468 | 68 | 27.4 | 12.3 | 1.2 | 2.9 | 8.1 | 34.3 | 12.7 | 14.3 | 5.2 | | 3.33 | 136 | 1127 | 222 | 238 | 34 | | 0.10 | 0.42 | 5.39 | 0.23 | 0.31 | 11.0 | 0.88 | 12.3 | 0.6 | | 127 | 0.3 | 2.5 | 20 | | 358 | 404 | 8.9 | 760 | 1.80 |
| 15904 | 1 | cup | Cacciatore | 244 | 459 | 66 | 41.9 | 12.8 | 2.2 | 4.7 | 5.3 | 25.7 | 6.4 | 9.4 | 7.4 | | | 127 | 1093 | 135 | 38 | 96 | | 0.19 | 0.32 | 13.93 | 0.72 | 0.44 | 16.4 | 1.95 | 24.9 | 0.7 | | 59 | 0.3 | 2.9 | 56 | 0.2 | 305 | 686 | | 590 | 3.13 |
| 15926 | 1 | ea | Cordon Bleu, svg | 229 | 483 | 63 | 46.0 | 8.6 | 0.6 | | | 28.1 | 14.8 | 9.0 | 2.2 | | | 130 | 800 | 201 | 130 | 21 | | 0.26 | 0.40 | 16.87 | 0.75 | 0.77 | 15.8 | | 1.7 | | | 208 | 0.2 | 2.2 | 50 | | 456 | 490 | | 616 | 2.62 |
| 16334 | 3 | oz | Divan | 85 | 114 | 73 | 14.4 | 3.0 | 1.0 | | | 4.8 | 2.1 | 1.6 | 0.7 | | | 48 | 829 | 108 | 37 | 71 | | 0.04 | 0.12 | 3.37 | 0.17 | 0.17 | 13.7 | | 14.5 | 0.3 | | 100 | 0.0 | 0.7 | 20 | | 134 | 156 | | 145 | 0.71 |
| 15911 | 1 | cup | Fricassee | 244 | 317 | 77 | 28.1 | 8.4 | 0.3 | | | 18.1 | 5.2 | 7.5 | 3.9 | | | 33 | 44 | 13 | 13 | 0 | | 0.11 | 0.23 | 7.90 | 0.25 | 0.33 | 9.9 | | 0.0 | | | 20 | 0.1 | 1.8 | 22 | | 185 | 293 | | 691 | 1.98 |
| 15928 | 1 | ea | Kiev, svg | 258 | 640 | 53 | 72.9 | 10.0 | 0.5 | | | 32.4 | 15.9 | 10.3 | 3.5 | | | 231 | 859 | 217 | 137 | 21 | | 0.22 | 0.35 | 31.66 | 1.36 | 0.87 | 15.3 | | 0.0 | | | 54 | 0.1 | 3.1 | 72 | | 555 | 614 | | 1037 | 2.45 |
| 15927 | 1 | pce | Parmigiana | 182 | 317 | 66 | 28.5 | 15.1 | 1.4 | | | 15.6 | 5.4 | 4.4 | 4.3 | | | 138 | 832 | 146 | 91 | 55 | | 0.15 | 0.33 | 8.25 | 0.36 | 0.43 | 18.1 | | 8.7 | | | 189 | 0.2 | 2.1 | 44 | | 317 | 462 | | 768 | 2.32 |
| 56249 | 1 | ea | Pate, w/vegetables, low cal, svg | 85 | 128 | 68 | 24.2 | 0.2 | 0.0 | | | 2.6 | 0.7 | 0.9 | 0.6 | | | 64 | 217 | 25 | 5 | 20 | | 0.04 | 0.10 | 7.04 | 0.28 | 0.19 | 3.0 | | 0.0 | | | 11 | 0.0 | 0.8 | 20 | | 139 | 157 | | 71 | 0.82 |
| 15915 | 1 | ea | Teriyaki, breast | 128 | 175 | 67 | 26.4 | 6.9 | 0.2 | | | 3.6 | 0.9 | 1.0 | 0.9 | | | 31 | 64 | 16 | 14 | 2 | | 0.08 | 0.20 | 8.69 | 0.46 | 0.28 | 12.6 | | 3.1 | | | 27 | 0.1 | 1.8 | 36 | | 198 | 310 | | 1866 | 1.94 |
| 15916 | 1 | ea | Teriyaki, drumstick | 68 | 93 | 67 | 14.0 | 3.6 | 0.1 | | | 1.9 | 0.5 | 0.6 | 0.5 | | | 43 | 34 | 8 | 7 | 1 | | 0.04 | 0.10 | 4.62 | 0.25 | 0.15 | 6.7 | | 1.7 | | | 14 | 0.1 | 0.9 | 19 | | 105 | 165 | | 991 | 1.03 |
| 56090 | 1 | cup | With Noodles | 240 | 367 | 71 | 22.3 | 25.7 | 1.8 | | | 18.5 | 5.9 | 7.1 | 3.5 | 0.00 | 3.53 | 96 | 432 | 10 | 10 | 0 | | 0.05 | 0.17 | 4.32 | 0.19 | 0.25 | 9.6 | 0.63 | 0.0 | 0.0 | | 26 | 0.2 | 2.2 | 26 | 0.3 | 247 | 149 | 27.6 | 600 | 1.53 |
| 56112 | 1 | ea | Chiles Relleno | 143 | 425 | 52 | 22.8 | 6.8 | 1.1 | | | 34.6 | 17.0 | 10.2 | 5.4 | | | 166 | 4912 | 641 | 214 | 428 | | 0.07 | 0.46 | 0.77 | 0.22 | 0.54 | 28.7 | | 88.5 | | | 595 | 0.2 | 1.6 | 39 | | 409 | 337 | | 619 | 2.75 |
| | | | Chili | | | | | | | | | | | | | | | | | | | | | | | | | | | | | | | | | | | | | | | | |
| 56139 | 1 | cup | Con Carne, w/beef | 254 | 351 | 72 | 25.1 | 21.1 | 3.7 | | | 18.8 | 6.7 | 8.0 | 1.7 | | | 81 | 1614 | 162 | 0 | 162 | | 0.18 | 0.30 | 6.54 | 0.35 | 1.97 | 25.8 | | 27.9 | | | 58 | 0.3 | 4.0 | 51 | | 226 | 828 | | 1407 | 5.07 |
| 56154 | 1 | cup | Con Carne, w/beef, beans & macaroni | 253 | 334 | 71 | 20.6 | 37.2 | 5.2 | | | 11.7 | 4.1 | 4.8 | 1.3 | | | 48 | 958 | 96 | 0 | 96 | | 0.26 | 0.27 | 4.99 | 0.24 | 1.17 | 38.4 | | 17.0 | | | 53 | 0.3 | 3.8 | 53 | | 218 | 630 | | 1027 | 3.59 |
| 56163 | 1 | cup | Con Carne, w/beef, beans & rice | 250 | 298 | 73 | 11.2 | 46.0 | 5.8 | | | 8.4 | 3.6 | 3.5 | 0.6 | | | 25 | 500 | 50 | 0 | 50 | | 0.24 | 0.17 | 2.03 | 0.29 | 0.00 | 36.7 | | 2.5 | | | 80 | 0.2 | 6.2 | 80 | | 275 | 580 | | 1162 | 3.43 |
| 56116 | 1 | cup | Con Carne, w/chicken & beans | 254 | 216 | 79 | 17.1 | 26.5 | 5.3 | | | 5.3 | 1.2 | 1.8 | 1.5 | | | 33 | 1195 | 124 | 6 | 118 | | 0.22 | 0.23 | 5.15 | 0.36 | 0.12 | 57.8 | | 21.3 | | | 58 | 0.3 | 2.7 | 53 | | 196 | 681 | | 1222 | 1.49 |
| 56114 | 1 | cup | Con Carne, w/pork & beans | 254 | 274 | 75 | 23.6 | 27.1 | 5.4 | | | 8.3 | 2.5 | 3.5 | 1.4 | | | 51 | 1197 | 121 | 1 | 120 | | 0.67 | 0.35 | 4.69 | 0.44 | 0.44 | 42.7 | | 21.4 | | | 66 | 0.3 | 2.8 | 56 | | 259 | 790 | | 1260 | 2.43 |
| 56115 | 1 | cup | Con Carne, w/venison & beans | 254 | 251 | 75 | 25.5 | 27.2 | 5.4 | | | 4.8 | 1.4 | 1.5 | 1.4 | | | 71 | 1194 | 120 | 0 | 120 | | 0.24 | 0.53 | 5.23 | 0.26 | 2.76 | 41.5 | | 21.2 | | | 56 | 0.5 | 5.0 | 58 | | 264 | 782 | | 1321 | 2.42 |
| 56141 | 1 | ea | Chili Dog | 125 | 234 | 68 | 9.6 | 10.7 | 2.9 | | | 17.5 | 6.7 | 8.0 | 1.5 | | | 36 | 269 | 27 | 0 | 27 | | 0.13 | 0.14 | 1.47 | 0.16 | 0.59 | 19.9 | | 13.1 | | | 42 | 0.1 | 3.3 | 40 | | 162 | 368 | | 922 | 2.43 |
| 56637 | 1 | ea | Chimichanga, w/beef, cheese & red chili peppers | 180 | 364 | 59 | 14.7 | 38.3 | | | | 17.5 | 8.4 | 7.1 | 0.5 | 0.00 | 0.55 | 50 | 702 | 99 | 21 | 78 | | 0.23 | 0.95 | 3.46 | 0.16 | 1.28 | 90.0 | 1.48 | 1.8 | | | 218 | 0.6 | 3.1 | 41 | 0.4 | 146 | 329 | 24.7 | 895 | 4.63 |
| | | | Chow Mein | | | | | | | | | | | | | | | | | | | | | | | | | | | | | | | | | | | | | | | | |
| 56094 | 1 | cup | Beef, w/noodles | 220 | 425 | 63 | 21.6 | 31.1 | 3.4 | | | 24.5 | 5.0 | 8.6 | 9.3 | | | 46 | 631 | 134 | 106 | 28 | | 0.37 | 0.37 | 5.63 | 0.44 | 1.59 | 43.9 | 0.77 | 20.3 | | | 40 | 0.3 | 4.2 | 53 | | 251 | 515 | 23.8 | 818 | 3.52 |
| 57619 | 1 | cup | Beef, w/o noodles | 220 | 275 | 76 | 21.8 | 12.2 | 2.3 | | | 15.8 | 4.0 | 6.8 | 3.6 | | | 53 | 704 | 153 | 125 | 29 | | 0.18 | 0.26 | 4.09 | 0.48 | 1.87 | 42.2 | | 23.8 | | | 37 | 0.2 | 2.9 | 42 | | 224 | 554 | | 774 | 3.53 |
| 56091 | 1 | cup | Chicken, w/noodles | 250 | 255 | 78 | 31.0 | 10.0 | 1.0 | 1.8 | 7.3 | 10.0 | 2.4 | 4.3 | 3.1 | 0.00 | 3.13 | 78 | 275 | 50 | 49 | 1 | | 0.07 | 0.23 | 4.25 | 0.41 | 0.23 | 19.0 | 0.69 | 10.0 | 0.0 | | 58 | 0.4 | 2.5 | 28 | | 292 | 472 | 8.0 | 718 | 2.12 |
| 57622 | 1 | cup | Chicken, w/o noodles | 220 | 194 | 81 | 20.0 | 10.5 | 1.6 | | | 8.2 | 1.8 | 2.5 | 3.1 | | | 48 | 81 | 14 | 9 | 5 | | 0.13 | 0.22 | 6.87 | 0.37 | 0.22 | 50.2 | | 9.9 | | | 37 | 0.2 | 1.7 | 35 | | 185 | 414 | | 968 | 1.63 |
| 57618 | 1 | cup | Pork, w/noodles | 220 | 436 | 63 | 22.0 | 31.2 | 3.4 | | | 25.4 | 5.2 | 9.1 | 9.5 | | | 48 | 636 | 135 | 108 | 28 | | 0.78 | 0.43 | 6.19 | 0.42 | 0.43 | 41.9 | | 20.5 | | | 48 | 0.2 | 3.3 | 53 | | 251 | 493 | | 816 | 2.57 |
| 57621 | 1 | cup | Pork, w/o noodles | 220 | 288 | 75 | 22.3 | 12.2 | 2.3 | | | 16.8 | 4.3 | 7.4 | 3.8 | | | 57 | 709 | 155 | 126 | 29 | | 0.65 | 0.33 | 4.75 | 0.43 | 0.48 | 39.7 | | 24.0 | | | 48 | 0.2 | 1.8 | 40 | | 224 | 528 | | 770 | 2.42 |
| 56238 | 1 | cup | Shrimp, w/noodles | 220 | 277 | 73 | 21.3 | 21.8 | 2.1 | | | 12.0 | 1.8 | 2.9 | 6.4 | | | 121 | 97 | 18 | 3 | 5 | | 0.21 | 0.26 | 5.12 | 0.19 | 0.84 | 37.6 | | 8.1 | | | 66 | 0.4 | 3.9 | 57 | | 268 | 418 | | 937 | 1.60 |
| 57623 | 1 | cup | Shrimp, w/o noodles | 220 | 172 | 82 | 21.7 | 9.3 | 1.3 | | | 5.3 | 0.8 | 1.2 | 2.7 | | | 136 | 84 | 18 | 4 | 4 | | 0.09 | 0.18 | 4.18 | 0.19 | 0.95 | 34.5 | | 9.2 | | | 68 | 0.4 | 3.1 | 51 | | 257 | 438 | | 722 | 1.43 |
| 56169 | 1 | pce | Creamed Dried Beef, on toast | 145 | 241 | 67 | 11.0 | 21.2 | 0.7 | | | 12.3 | 4.1 | 4.8 | 2.7 | | | 22 | 504 | 128 | 117 | 11 | | 0.20 | 0.31 | 2.29 | 0.11 | 0.76 | 16.0 | | 3.4 | | | 160 | 0.1 | 1.8 | 28 | | 161 | 273 | | 867 | 1.48 |
| 56293 | 1 | ea | Crepes, meat filled | 119 | 264 | 60 | 21.1 | 10.8 | 0.4 | 1.7 | 8.7 | 14.7 | 5.1 | 4.7 | 3.5 | 0.43 | 3.10 | 118 | 231 | 62 | 57 | 4 | | 0.19 | 0.33 | 3.19 | 0.30 | 1.86 | 16.9 | 0.54 | 1.1 | 0.6 | 0.6 | 53 | 0.1 | 2.7 | 26 | 0.1 | 210 | 304 | 18.5 | 243 | 4.07 |
| | | | Curry | | | | | | | | | | | | | | | | | | | | | | | | | | | | | | | | | | | | | | | | |
| 15924 | 1 | cup | Chicken | 236 | 293 | 76 | 27.3 | 10.3 | 2.1 | 0.8 | 7.4 | 16.1 | 3.3 | 6.5 | 4.8 | | | 85 | 1322 | 242 | 164 | 78 | | 0.13 | 0.23 | 10.23 | 0.50 | 0.30 | 20.2 | | 18.3 | | | 45 | 0.2 | 2.1 | 52 | | 250 | 623 | | 1189 | 2.14 |
| 57497 | 3 | oz | Herring Fish, oily | 85 | 297 | 50 | 9.2 | 2.7 | | | | 27.7 | | | | | | | 634 | 190 | | | | 0.03 | 0.11 | 3.74 | | 3.06 | 11.1 | | 6.8 | | | 37 | 0.1 | 0.9 | 24 | | | 297 | | 537 | 0.43 |
| 13900 | 1 | cup | Lamb | 236 | 283 | 79 | 27.6 | 2.7 | 0.6 | 1.6 | 0.6 | 17.3 | 4.3 | 5.7 | 5.5 | | | 87 | 6 | 1 | 0 | 1 | | 0.08 | 0.27 | 7.87 | 0.19 | 2.83 | 25.4 | 0.71 | 1.3 | 0.2 | | 31 | 0.2 | 2.6 | 35 | 0.1 | 274 | 472 | | 474 | 6.45 |
| 56883 | 1 | ea | Lentils & Rice, in sauce, svg | 69 | 260 | 11 | 12.0 | 46.0 | 8.0 | 4.0 | 34.0 | 3.0 | 1.5 | | | | | 0 | 1500 | 300 | | | | | | | | | | | 15.0 | | | 40 | | 7.2 | | | | | | 470 | |
| 57504 | 3 | oz | Mutton | 85 | 320 | 44 | 14.2 | 2.0 | | | | 28.3 | | | | | | | 638 | 128 | | | | 0.06 | 0.15 | 5.36 | | 1.19 | 9.4 | | 5.1 | | | 20 | 0.2 | 1.6 | 26 | | | 332 | | 654 | 2.21 |
| 19408 | 1 | cup | Shrimp | 236 | 314 | 74 | 27.4 | 13.9 | 0.4 | | | 16.1 | 5.1 | 5.9 | 3.9 | | | 82 | 728 | 188 | 173 | 15 | | 0.13 | 0.30 | 3.17 | 0.17 | 1.34 | 11.3 | | 3.6 | | | 227 | 0.3 | 3.0 | 61 | | 363 | 437 | | 632 | 1.79 |
| 57499 | 3 | oz | White Haddock Fish | 85 | 216 | 60 | 9.2 | 2.7 | | | | 18.7 | | | | | | | 558 | 167 | | | | 0.06 | 0.07 | 3.74 | | 0.51 | 14.5 | | 6.8 | | | 29 | 0.2 | 0.7 | 20 | | | 276 | | 564 | 0.26 |
| 56229 | 1 | cup | Dumplings, Liver | 250 | 770 | 42 | 56.9 | 35.3 | 1.4 | | | 43.3 | 11.2 | 16.2 | 10.9 | | | 1038 | 30220 | 8750 | 8698 | 53 | | 0.54 | 2.89 | 15.28 | 0.96 | 72.88 | 1111.0 | | 46.7 | | | 105 | 11.4 | 9.9 | 48 | | 638 | 510 | | 1810 | 10.28 |
| 56292 | 1 | ea | Dumplings, Pork, svg | 100 | 340 | 40 | 13.2 | 24.1 | 0.9 | | | 20.9 | 5.7 | 9.1 | 4.9 | | | 29 | 87 | 25 | 23 | 2 | | 0.53 | 0.27 | 3.57 | 0.20 | 0.30 | 8.6 | | 0.3 | | | 32 | 0.1 | 1.8 | 18 | | 131 | 198 | | 346 | 1.11 |
| | | | Egg Foo Young | | | | | | | | | | | | | | | | | | | | | | | | | | | | | | | | | | | | | | | | |
| 56290 | 1 | ea | Beef | 86 | 129 | 74 | 9.2 | 3.1 | 0.4 | | | 8.8 | 2.2 | 3.2 | 2.4 | | | 80 | 319 | 92 | 90 | 2 | | 0.05 | 0.24 | 0.74 | 0.15 | 0.72 | 22.1 | | 2.5 | | | 26 | 0.1 | 1.1 | 11 | | 112 | 144 | | 184 | 1.16 |
| 56287 | 1 | ea | Chicken | 86 | 131 | 74 | 8.8 | 3.9 | 0.5 | | | 8.7 | 2.1 | 3.1 | 2.5 | | | 81 | 329 | 95 | 93 | 2 | | 0.05 | 0.25 | 0.96 | 0.13 | 0.37 | 22.5 | | 2.7 | | | 28 | 0.1 | 0.9 | 11 | | 103 | 144 | | 187 | 0.81 |
| 56288 | 1 | ea | Pork | 86 | 134 | 73 | 9.0 | 3.9 | 0.5 | | | 9.0 | 2.2 | 3.3 | 2.5 | | | 82 | 325 | 98 | 92 | 1 | | 0.14 | 0.27 | 0.85 | 0.15 | 0.43 | 22.5 | | 2.8 | | | 28 | 0.1 | 0.9 | 12 | | 113 | 167 | | 187 | 0.92 |
| 56289 | 1 | ea | Shrimp | 86 | 153 | 70 | 8.2 | 3.6 | 0.7 | | | 11.8 | 2.5 | 5.0 | 3.1 | | | 82 | 1885 | 233 | 75 | 164 | | 0.04 | 0.23 | 0.81 | 0.12 | 0.46 | 19.8 | | 1.8 | | | 34 | 0.1 | 1.1 | 14 | | 115 | 161 | | 474 | 0.69 |
| | | | Egg Roll | | | | | | | | | | | | | | | | | | | | | | | | | | | | | | | | | | | | | | | | |
| 56127 | 1 | ea | With Chicken | 64 | 105 | 69 | 4.2 | 9.2 | 0.6 | | | 5.6 | 1.3 | 2.4 | 1.5 | | | 40 | 75 | 13 | 16 | 2 | | 0.08 | 0.11 | 1.11 | 0.05 | 0.08 | 10.6 | | 2.9 | | | 14 | 0.0 | 0.8 | 8 | | 42 | 72 | | 188 | 0.34 |
| 56291 | 1 | ea | With Meat | 64 | 115 | 66 | 5.0 | 9.4 | 0.7 | | | 6.2 | 1.5 | 2.7 | 1.5 | | | 37 | 55 | 11 | 13 | 1 | | 0.16 | 0.13 | 1.31 | 0.10 | 0.13 | 9.0 | | 2.1 | | | 13 | 0.0 | 0.8 | 10 | | 58 | 124 | | 303 | 0.46 |
| 56126 | 1 | ea | With Shrimp | 64 | 105 | 68 | 3.5 | 10.1 | 0.7 | | | 5.6 | 1.2 | 2.4 | 1.6 | | | 39 | 60 | 15 | 15 | 1 | | 0.08 | 0.10 | 0.92 | 0.06 | 0.12 | 9.0 | | 2.3 | | | 15 | 0.1 | 0.9 | 10 | | 47 | 99 | | 326 | 0.29 |
| 56110 | 1 | ea | Without Meat | 64 | 102 | 70 | 2.5 | 10.0 | 0.7 | | | 5.8 | 1.2 | 2.5 | 1.6 | | | 30 | 57 | 15 | 14 | 1 | | 0.08 | 0.10 | 0.81 | 0.06 | 0.06 | 12.5 | | 3.3 | | | 12 | 0.1 | 0.8 | 9 | | 38 | 98 | | 307 | 0.25 |
| 57513 | 3 | oz | Eggplant Parmesan Casserole, low calorie | 85 | 77 | 80 | 6.2 | 5.4 | 1.5 | | | 3.8 | 2.3 | 1.0 | 0.2 | | | 11 | 362 | 53 | 50 | 27 | | 0.06 | 0.09 | 0.58 | 0.09 | 0.18 | 10.8 | | 3.5 | | | 164 | 0.1 | 0.4 | 16 | | 123 | 220 | | 288 | 0.69 |

| Code | Amount | | Description | Basic Components | | | | | | | | | Additional Fats | | | | | | Vit A & Components | | | | | Vitamins | | | | | | | | | | Minerals | | | | | | | | | |
|---|---|---|---|---|---|---|---|---|---|---|---|---|---|---|---|---|---|---|---|---|---|---|---|---|---|---|---|---|---|---|---|---|---|---|---|---|---|---|---|---|---|---|---|
| | | | | Weight (g) | Calories | % Water | Protein (g) | Carbs (g) | Fiber (g) | Sugar (g) | Other Carbs (g) | Fat (g) | Sat Fat (g) | Mono Fat (g) | Poly Fat (g) | Omega 3 (g) | Omega 6 (g) | Choles (mg) | Vit A (IU) | Vit A (RE) | Retinol (RE) | Carotenoids (RE) | Beta Carotene (mcg) | Thiamin (mg) | Riboflavin (mg) | Niacin (NE) | Vit B6 (mg) | Vit B12 (mcg) | Folate (mcg) | Panto (mg) | Vit C (mg) | Vit D (mg) | Vit E (α TE) | Calcium (mg) | Copper (mg) | Iron (mg) | Magnes (mg) | Mang (mg) | Phos (mg) | Potassium (mg) | Selenium (mcg) | Sodium (mg) | Zinc (mg) |
| 56322 | 1 | cup | Eggplant Parmesan Casserole, regular | 198 | 319 | 71 | 14.5 | 17.4 | 3.2 | | | 22.1 | 9.7 | 7.8 | 3.4 | | | 57 | 953 | 169 | 104 | 65 | | 0.17 | 0.23 | 1.60 | 0.20 | 0.51 | 23.0 | | 8.2 | | | 392 | 0.2 | 1.5 | 36 | | 289 | 449 | | 683 | 1.53 |
| 18804 | 1 | cup | Fish, w/tomato based sauce | 222 | 224 | 78 | 35.0 | 3.9 | 1.3 | | | 6.9 | 1.4 | 2.5 | 2.1 | | | 87 | 838 | 132 | 72 | 59 | | 0.20 | 0.17 | 5.92 | 0.44 | 2.21 | 20.9 | | 16.3 | | | 58 | 0.2 | 1.2 | 67 | | 353 | 857 | | 349 | 0.96 |
| | | | Fish Patty | | | | | | | | | | | | | | | | | | | | | | | | | | | | | | | | | | | | | | | | |
| 18806 | 1 | ea | Codfish | 120 | 239 | 62 | 16.4 | 15.2 | 1.4 | | | 12.6 | 3.3 | 5.3 | 3.2 | | | 66 | 84 | 25 | 25 | 0 | | 0.13 | 0.13 | 2.50 | 0.31 | 0.63 | 12.9 | | 4.5 | | | 34 | 0.1 | 0.8 | 38 | | 205 | 522 | | 334 | 0.65 |
| 18813 | 1 | ea | Haddock | 120 | 239 | 62 | 16.4 | 15.2 | 1.4 | | | 12.6 | 3.3 | 5.3 | 3.2 | | | 66 | 84 | 25 | 25 | 0 | | 0.13 | 0.13 | 2.50 | 0.31 | 0.63 | 12.9 | | 4.5 | | | 34 | 0.1 | 0.8 | 38 | | 205 | 522 | | 334 | 0.65 |
| 18812 | 1 | ea | Mackerel | 120 | 299 | 54 | 19.3 | 15.7 | 1.5 | | | 17.7 | 4.8 | 7.3 | 4.5 | | | 91 | 324 | 97 | 97 | 0 | | 0.12 | 0.24 | 5.41 | 0.30 | 3.76 | 12.0 | | 4.7 | | | 193 | 0.2 | 2.0 | 40 | | 265 | 349 | | 478 | 1.04 |
| 18808 | 1 | ea | Salmon | 120 | 262 | 59 | 16.3 | 14.2 | 1.3 | | | 15.6 | 4.1 | 6.5 | 4.0 | | | 56 | 90 | 27 | 27 | 0 | | 0.09 | 0.18 | 5.44 | 0.37 | 2.19 | 19.6 | | 3.8 | | | 180 | 0.2 | 0.9 | 32 | | 275 | 385 | | 658 | 0.93 |
| 19418 | 1 | ea | Shrimp | 120 | 248 | 60 | 17.5 | 15.0 | 1.3 | | | 13.3 | 3.4 | 5.4 | 3.5 | | | 143 | 95 | 29 | 29 | 0 | | 0.10 | 0.10 | 2.71 | 0.22 | 0.78 | 9.2 | | 5.2 | | | 58 | 0.3 | 2.3 | 40 | | 197 | 329 | | 300 | 1.10 |
| 18810 | 1 | ea | Tuna | 120 | 300 | 53 | 21.9 | 13.9 | 1.3 | | | 17.4 | 4.2 | 7.2 | 4.9 | | | 42 | 99 | 30 | 30 | 0 | | 0.10 | 0.15 | 9.15 | 0.21 | 1.38 | 10.9 | | 3.7 | | | 28 | 0.1 | 1.4 | 32 | | 252 | 325 | | 420 | 0.88 |
| 18834 | 1 | cup | Fish Timbale | 175 | 371 | 68 | 18.8 | 4.3 | 0.1 | | | 31.0 | 18.1 | 9.1 | 1.6 | | | 242 | 1268 | 358 | 347 | 12 | | 0.10 | 0.28 | 2.24 | 0.19 | 1.34 | 17.4 | | 1.4 | | | 86 | 0.0 | 0.8 | 32 | | 234 | 364 | | 434 | 0.82 |
| 56119 | 1 | ea | Flauta, w/beef | 113 | 360 | 49 | 16.5 | 12.8 | 1.7 | | | 27.3 | 4.9 | 11.6 | 9.1 | | | 45 | 148 | 15 | 0 | 15 | | 0.07 | 0.15 | 2.13 | 0.25 | 1.45 | 10.1 | | 13.8 | | | 50 | 0.1 | 2.2 | 29 | | 199 | 292 | | 188 | 4.18 |
| 56120 | 1 | ea | Flauta, w/chicken | 113 | 342 | 52 | 13.9 | 12.8 | 1.7 | | | 26.6 | 4.3 | 11.1 | 9.6 | | | 37 | 170 | 21 | 7 | 15 | | 0.05 | 0.10 | 3.21 | 0.22 | 0.09 | 8.0 | | 13.8 | | | 52 | 0.1 | 1.0 | 27 | | 147 | 243 | | 189 | 1.18 |
| 18811 | 1 | pce | Flounder, stuffed | 210 | 332 | 66 | 42.8 | 13.3 | 0.7 | | | 10.9 | 2.4 | 4.0 | 3.2 | | | 160 | 506 | 125 | 111 | 14 | | 0.28 | 0.27 | 6.80 | 0.42 | 5.34 | 45.2 | | 5.7 | | | 118 | 0.4 | 1.9 | 73 | | 439 | 798 | | 857 | 2.77 |
| 56117 | 4 | ea | Grape Leaves, stuffed w/beef & rice | 84 | 212 | 61 | 6.8 | 7.3 | 0.8 | | | 17.4 | 4.1 | 10.6 | 1.5 | | | 24 | 1466 | 147 | 0 | 147 | | 0.06 | 0.09 | 1.73 | 0.10 | 0.54 | 10.1 | | 9.3 | | | 24 | 0.1 | 1.3 | 16 | | 66 | 176 | | 65 | 1.42 |
| 56236 | 4 | ea | Grape Leaves, stuffed w/lamb & rice | 84 | 212 | 61 | 7.3 | 8.1 | 0.9 | | | 16.9 | 3.6 | 10.7 | 1.7 | | | 23 | 1639 | 164 | 0 | 164 | | 0.08 | 0.09 | 2.10 | 0.10 | 0.61 | 13.9 | | 10.4 | | | 29 | 0.1 | 1.3 | 18 | | 74 | 186 | | 67 | 1.35 |
| 56155 | 1 | cup | Goulash, beef | 249 | 341 | 72 | 29.7 | 23.3 | 2.4 | | | 13.8 | 3.5 | 4.9 | 3.9 | | | 90 | 441 | 47 | 4 | 43 | | 0.25 | 0.31 | 5.69 | 0.40 | 2.65 | 22.6 | | 7.3 | | | 25 | 0.2 | 4.0 | 50 | | 314 | 588 | | 456 | 4.63 |
| 13901 | 1 | cup | Goulash, lamb | 249 | 309 | 76 | 32.6 | 8.1 | 1.3 | | | 15.8 | 4.8 | 5.8 | 3.4 | | | 105 | 591 | 59 | 0 | 59 | | 0.25 | 0.40 | 9.33 | 0.37 | 4.46 | 51.1 | | 10.1 | | | 40 | 0.3 | 3.3 | 50 | | 324 | 623 | | 647 | 7.84 |
| 56242 | 1 | cup | Gumbo, w/rice | 244 | 193 | 83 | 14.0 | 17.0 | 2.3 | | | 7.7 | 1.7 | 2.3 | 2.9 | | | 41 | 562 | 70 | 22 | 49 | | 0.20 | 0.17 | 4.51 | 0.21 | 2.38 | 45.8 | | 14.2 | | | 71 | 0.8 | 2.6 | 41 | | 154 | 454 | | 888 | 14.74 |
| 56259 | 1 | cup | Gumbo, w/o rice | 244 | 181 | 85 | 14.9 | 11.0 | 2.5 | | | 8.5 | 1.8 | 2.5 | 3.2 | | | 46 | 632 | 79 | 25 | 55 | | 0.18 | 0.18 | 4.64 | 0.21 | 2.67 | 50.6 | | 16.0 | | | 76 | 0.9 | 2.6 | 41 | | 159 | 500 | | 605 | 16.43 |
| 12901 | 1 | ea | Ham Croquette | 62 | 152 | 55 | 9.3 | 7.7 | 0.3 | | | 9.1 | 2.5 | 3.9 | 2.2 | | | 20 | 226 | 57 | 52 | 5 | | 0.24 | 0.15 | 1.91 | 0.15 | 0.28 | 4.9 | | 0.4 | | | 42 | 0.0 | 0.7 | 13 | | 104 | 148 | | 543 | 0.92 |
| 16335 | 1 | cup | Kung Pou Chicken | 162 | 408 | 56 | 27.1 | 11.3 | 2.0 | | | 28.6 | 4.8 | 13.0 | 9.1 | | | 60 | 906 | 93 | 4 | 89 | | 0.14 | 0.14 | 12.46 | 0.56 | 0.24 | 40.2 | | 9.3 | | | 47 | 0.2 | 1.9 | 60 | | 249 | 415 | | 988 | 1.42 |
| 57500 | 3 | oz | Lamb Kheema | 85 | 264 | 50 | 16.7 | 1.6 | | | | 21.2 | | | | | | | 650 | 130 | | | | 0.06 | 0.17 | 6.04 | | 1.28 | 9.4 | | 4.3 | | | 19 | 0.2 | 1.5 | 27 | | | 359 | | 694 | 3.23 |
| 13902 | 1 | pce | Lamb Loaf | 108 | 198 | 66 | 14.4 | 8.6 | 0.5 | | | 11.4 | 4.7 | 4.5 | 1.0 | | | 93 | 111 | 29 | 27 | 2 | | 0.07 | 0.24 | 4.02 | 0.10 | 1.46 | 16.3 | | 1.2 | | | 57 | 0.1 | 1.5 | 22 | | 164 | 257 | | 517 | 3.07 |
| 56258 | 1 | cup | Liver, chopped | 208 | 460 | 64 | 26.8 | 5.6 | 0.8 | | | 35.9 | 10.9 | 14.8 | 7.0 | | | 734 | 14876 | 4462 | 4462 | 0 | | 0.18 | 1.75 | 4.09 | 0.62 | 17.77 | 715.7 | | 17.5 | | | 42 | 0.4 | 8.1 | 27 | | 356 | 250 | | 2157 | 4.35 |
| 56230 | 1 | cup | Liver Hash | 225 | 286 | 72 | 31.9 | 23.0 | 1.9 | | | 6.7 | 2.3 | 1.6 | 1.1 | | | 767 | 19895 | 5969 | 5969 | 0 | | 0.46 | 2.15 | 7.07 | 0.91 | 23.56 | 946.4 | | 41.8 | | | 25 | 0.5 | 10.6 | 43 | | 421 | 464 | | 92 | 5.48 |
| 57522 | 3 | oz | Lo Mein, w/meat | 85 | 122 | 70 | 7.2 | 13.4 | 1.0 | | | 4.3 | 0.8 | 1.2 | 1.9 | | | 13 | 16 | 2 | 1 | 1 | | 0.16 | 0.10 | 1.81 | 0.12 | 0.08 | 17.6 | | 3.5 | | | 11 | 0.1 | 0.9 | 17 | | 69 | 105 | | 117 | 0.69 |
| 57521 | 3 | oz | Lo Mein, w/o meat | 85 | 57 | 82 | 2.6 | 11.4 | 1.2 | | | 0.3 | 0.1 | 0.0 | 0.1 | | | 0 | 553 | 55 | 0 | 55 | | 0.10 | 0.10 | 1.20 | 0.08 | 0.00 | 20.7 | | 5.2 | | | 20 | 0.1 | 0.9 | 14 | | 47 | 166 | | 264 | 0.39 |
| 18800 | 1 | cup | Lobster Newberg | 244 | 612 | 61 | 29.8 | 11.7 | 0.2 | 6.1 | 5.5 | 49.8 | 29.6 | 14.7 | 2.3 | | | 368 | 2023 | 523 | 500 | 22 | | 0.10 | 0.41 | 1.59 | 0.17 | 4.02 | 32.4 | 0.98 | 0.8 | 1.5 | | 242 | 2.2 | 1.2 | 56 | 0.1 | 398 | 608 | | 647 | 4.09 |
| 56297 | 1 | ea | Manapua, w/meat, svg | 93 | 214 | 55 | 10.8 | 21.4 | 0.8 | | | 9.0 | 2.7 | 3.4 | 2.1 | | | 28 | 15 | 3 | 2 | 1 | | 0.37 | 0.25 | 3.08 | 0.09 | 0.40 | 10.7 | | 0.4 | | | 16 | 0.1 | 1.8 | 13 | | 102 | 163 | | 101 | 2.08 |
| 56298 | 1 | ea | Manapua, w/o meat, svg | 103 | 237 | 46 | 6.0 | 44.3 | 2.5 | | | 3.9 | 0.5 | 0.9 | 2.2 | | | 0 | 0 | 0 | 0 | 0 | 0 | 0.27 | 0.21 | 2.21 | 0.03 | 0.00 | 25.0 | | 0.3 | | | 31 | 0.1 | 2.2 | 19 | | 81 | 124 | | 414 | 0.48 |
| 56250 | 1 | cup | Moo Goo Gai Pan | 216 | 281 | 77 | 15.2 | 11.9 | 2.7 | | | 19.8 | 4.7 | 6.5 | 7.4 | | | 39 | 1318 | 202 | 97 | 105 | | 0.14 | 0.33 | 4.35 | 0.33 | 0.35 | 44.2 | | 34.1 | | | 130 | 0.2 | 1.6 | 32 | | 197 | 475 | | 326 | 1.57 |
| 56080 | 1 | cup | Moussaka, w/lamb | 250 | 237 | 82 | 16.4 | 12.9 | 3.6 | 6.9 | 2.4 | 13.0 | 4.6 | 5.4 | 1.9 | 0.22 | 1.67 | 97 | 536 | 105 | 74 | 31 | | 0.15 | 0.31 | 4.14 | 0.23 | 1.41 | 44.6 | 0.97 | 6.0 | 0.6 | 0.5 | 68 | 0.2 | 1.8 | 39 | 0.3 | 179 | 557 | 13.6 | 432 | 2.56 |
| 57503 | 3 | oz | Mutton Biriani | 85 | 212 | 53 | 6.8 | 21.1 | | | | 11.6 | | | | | | | 417 | 83 | | | | 0.04 | 0.09 | 2.47 | | 0.34 | 11.1 | | 4.3 | | | 27 | 0.1 | 0.8 | 17 | | | 217 | | 252 | 1.28 |
| 19416 | 1 | ea | Oyster Fritter | 40 | 125 | 40 | 3.8 | 12.7 | 0.4 | | | 6.3 | 1.6 | 2.5 | 1.7 | | | 36 | 132 | 38 | 37 | 1 | | 0.12 | 0.13 | 1.09 | 0.02 | 3.67 | 6.3 | | 0.9 | | | 52 | 1.0 | 2.3 | 16 | | 66 | 75 | | 109 | 20.40 |
| 19403 | 1 | cup | Oysters Rockefeller | 224 | 262 | 75 | 16.5 | 21.2 | 3.6 | 3.6 | 14.0 | 12.5 | 4.7 | 4.2 | 2.0 | | | 78 | 7665 | 847 | 120 | 727 | | 0.38 | 0.42 | 3.56 | 0.24 | 21.13 | 127.9 | 0.45 | 32.9 | 8.1 | | 179 | 5.0 | 10.2 | 123 | 1.3 | 260 | 663 | | 889 | 100.40 |
| 56167 | 1 | ea | Porcupine Balls, w/mushroom soup | 35 | 63 | 66 | 4.0 | 3.9 | 0.1 | | | 3.3 | 1.2 | 1.3 | 0.4 | | | 13 | 0 | 0 | 0 | 0 | 0 | 0.03 | 0.04 | 1.07 | 0.05 | 0.44 | 2.3 | | 0.2 | | | 6 | 0.0 | 0.6 | 5 | | 33 | 58 | | 171 | 0.86 |
| 56162 | 1 | ea | Porcupine Balls, w/tomato based sauce | 35 | 58 | 67 | 3.8 | 4.5 | 0.1 | | | 2.6 | 1.0 | 1.1 | 0.2 | | | 13 | 59 | 6 | 0 | 6 | | 0.03 | 0.03 | 1.07 | 0.06 | 0.41 | 2.8 | | 5.7 | | | 5 | 0.0 | 0.6 | 5 | | 31 | 72 | | 167 | 0.79 |
| | | | Pot Pies | | | | | | | | | | | | | | | | | | | | | | | | | | | | | | | | | | | | | | | | |
| 56068 | 1 | pce | Beef | 210 | 517 | 55 | 21.2 | 39.5 | 2.5 | 2.7 | 34.2 | 30.4 | 8.4 | 14.7 | 7.3 | | 5.96 | 44 | 1722 | 519 | 142 | 377 | | 0.29 | 0.29 | 4.83 | 0.24 | 1.20 | 28.8 | 0.26 | 6.3 | 0.2 | | 29 | 0.1 | 3.8 | 6 | | 149 | 334 | 11.5 | 596 | 3.17 |
| 56093 | 1 | pce | Chicken | 232 | 545 | 57 | 23.4 | 42.5 | 3.5 | 5.6 | 33.4 | 31.3 | 10.9 | 14.5 | 5.8 | | 5.13 | 72 | 3086 | 735 | 102 | 633 | | 0.32 | 0.32 | 4.87 | 0.46 | 0.23 | 29.0 | 1.11 | 4.6 | | | 70 | 0.3 | 3.0 | 26 | | 232 | 343 | 29.9 | 594 | 2.00 |
| 56233 | 1 | ea | Ham | 632 | 1492 | 57 | 55.2 | 115.2 | 7.1 | | | 89.6 | 23.1 | 39.4 | 22.4 | | | 76 | 9556 | 956 | 0 | 956 | | 1.50 | 1.02 | 17.23 | 0.77 | 0.92 | 67.9 | | 25.4 | | | 70 | 0.5 | 8.8 | 95 | | 581 | 1239 | | 3741 | 5.40 |
| 56241 | 1 | ea | Oyster | 656 | 1660 | 56 | 37.8 | 133.8 | 5.2 | | | 108.4 | 34.9 | 42.4 | 24.4 | | | 190 | 2364 | 610 | 574 | 36 | | 1.30 | 1.42 | 10.60 | 0.29 | 33.78 | 67.9 | | 13.8 | | | 446 | 8.5 | 20.2 | 177 | | 663 | 1207 | | 1916 | 177.97 |
| 56240 | 1 | ea | Tuna | 769 | 1746 | 59 | 71.4 | 125.4 | 8.9 | | | 106.0 | 31.2 | 42.4 | 26.3 | | | 92 | 21317 | 2500 | 565 | 1935 | | 1.20 | 1.12 | 31.12 | 0.46 | 3.61 | 84.3 | | 17.6 | | | 192 | 0.6 | 10.5 | 123 | | 877 | 1123 | | 1892 | 3.68 |
| 56122 | 1 | ea | Quesadilla | 54 | 199 | 29 | 6.4 | 20.6 | 1.2 | | | 10.0 | 3.6 | 3.6 | 2.3 | | | 14 | 292 | 55 | 37 | 18 | | 0.15 | 0.15 | 1.20 | 0.03 | 0.06 | 5.1 | | 3.2 | | | 123 | 0.1 | 1.3 | 14 | | 112 | 65 | | 255 | 0.67 |
| | | | Quiche | | | | | | | | | | | | | | | | | | | | | | | | | | | | | | | | | | | | | | | | |
| 57515 | 3 | oz | Cheese | 85 | 258 | 53 | 7.3 | 11.0 | 0.3 | | | 20.7 | 10.0 | 7.0 | 2.4 | | | 106 | 551 | 147 | 144 | 4 | | 0.09 | 0.24 | 0.66 | 0.04 | 0.25 | 9.4 | | 0.3 | | | 147 | 0.0 | 0.8 | 12 | | 139 | 101 | | 190 | 0.76 |
| 56098 | 1 | pce | Lorraine, 1/8 pce | 176 | 509 | 54 | 20.0 | 19.9 | 0.6 | | | 38.7 | 17.6 | 13.8 | 4.9 | | | 204 | 914 | 243 | 237 | 5 | | 0.23 | 0.44 | 4.71 | 0.20 | 0.99 | 17.4 | 0.84 | 2.8 | 1.1 | | 201 | 0.1 | 1.9 | 26 | | 271 | 271 | 15.0 | 549 | 1.66 |
| 57514 | 3 | oz | Spinach | 85 | 200 | 62 | 6.5 | 9.7 | 0.7 | | | 15.1 | 7.2 | 5.1 | 1.8 | | | 92 | 1692 | 240 | 109 | 130 | | 0.10 | 0.23 | 0.66 | 0.08 | 0.23 | 30.4 | | 3.0 | | | 145 | 0.1 | 1.3 | 24 | | 123 | 166 | | 194 | 0.77 |
| 18809 | 1 | ea | Salmon Loaf | 105 | 210 | 60 | 16.5 | 8.9 | 0.4 | | | 11.6 | 3.1 | 4.3 | 3.1 | | | 122 | 464 | 120 | 111 | 9 | | 0.09 | 0.30 | 4.52 | 0.22 | 2.35 | 22.1 | | 2.1 | | | 189 | 0.1 | 1.3 | 30 | | 275 | 289 | | 791 | 0.97 |
| 56231 | 1 | cup | Shepherd's Pie, w/beef | 243 | 287 | 74 | 18.2 | 31.0 | 3.3 | | | 10.3 | 3.0 | 4.3 | 2.1 | | | 41 | 523 | 102 | 74 | 28 | | 0.20 | 0.20 | 3.98 | 0.58 | 1.38 | 20.2 | | 17.4 | | | 41 | 0.3 | 2.3 | 46 | | 202 | 753 | | 702 | 4.19 |
| | | | Shrimp | | | | | | | | | | | | | | | | | | | | | | | | | | | | | | | | | | | | | | | | |
| 19401 | 1 | cup | Cocktail | 230 | 195 | 78 | 25.2 | 19.3 | 4.2 | 9.6 | 5.5 | 2.2 | 0.5 | 0.3 | 0.8 | | | 172 | 603 | 72 | 18 | 54 | | 0.11 | 0.10 | 3.85 | 0.24 | 1.12 | 54.5 | 0.46 | 24.5 | 3.7 | | 85 | 0.4 | 3.5 | 55 | 0.1 | 276 | 554 | | 991 | 1.49 |
| 56239 | 1 | cup | Creole, w/rice | 243 | 306 | 73 | 27.7 | 25.7 | 1.7 | | | 9.6 | 1.9 | 3.6 | 3.2 | | | 185 | 912 | 163 | 108 | 55 | | 0.18 | 0.09 | 4.65 | 0.24 | 1.21 | 10.8 | | 18.1 | | | 102 | 0.5 | 5.5 | 63 | | 316 | 454 | | 656 | 1.81 |
| 19428 | 1 | cup | Scampi | 136 | 219 | 69 | 29.3 | 1.3 | 0.0 | | | 10.1 | 5.2 | 2.6 | 1.2 | | | 239 | 363 | 94 | 86 | 8 | | 0.03 | 0.05 | 3.49 | 0.14 | 1.43 | 2.5 | | 2.9 | | | 78 | 0.4 | 3.5 | 52 | | 296 | 268 | | 291 | 1.60 |
| 19419 | 1 | cup | Stuffed | 140 | 276 | 62 | 28.2 | 8.7 | 0.4 | | | 13.5 | 3.1 | 5.2 | 3.8 | | | 221 | 380 | 107 | 103 | 4 | | 0.15 | 0.17 | 4.19 | 0.21 | 5.53 | 43.5 | | 3.4 | | | 113 | 0.6 | 2.7 | 48 | | 297 | 356 | | 694 | 3.62 |
| 19413 | 1 | cup | Teriyaki | 201 | 249 | 67 | 37.9 | 13.5 | 0.3 | | | 3.0 | 0.6 | 0.4 | 1.2 | | | 259 | 310 | 86 | 83 | 3 | | 0.08 | 0.14 | 6.11 | 0.28 | 1.79 | 17.4 | | 4.5 | | | 115 | 0.5 | 5.6 | 88 | | 384 | 488 | | 3383 | 2.19 |
| | | | Souffles | | | | | | | | | | | | | | | | | | | | | | | | | | | | | | | | | | | | | | | | |
| 56075 | 1 | cup | Cheese | 112 | 196 | 71 | 11.6 | 5.6 | 0.1 | 3.2 | 2.3 | 14.2 | 5.6 | 4.8 | 2.8 | 0.15 | 2.61 | 194 | 578 | 167 | 157 | 10 | | 0.08 | 0.35 | 0.29 | 0.09 | 0.78 | 23.0 | 0.82 | 0.5 | 1.1 | 0.4 | 209 | 0.0 | 0.8 | 17 | 0.0 | 201 | 146 | 11.8 | 298 | 1.01 |
| 15929 | 1 | cup | Chicken | 159 | 289 | 69 | 19.7 | 8.8 | 0.2 | | | 19.1 | 5.4 | 7.6 | 4.4 | | | 223 | 876 | 237 | 224 | 13 | | 0.11 | 0.42 | 4.04 | 0.26 | 0.61 | 21.2 | | 0.4 | | | 113 | 0.0 | 1.4 | 25 | | 226 | 262 | | 528 | 1.59 |
| 18816 | 1 | cup | Seafood | 159 | 258 | 72 | 17.5 | 8.9 | 0.2 | | | 16.6 | 4.7 | 6.6 | 3.9 | | | 224 | 863 | 233 | 221 | 12 | | 0.10 | 0.37 | 2.68 | 0.16 | 1.07 | 25.8 | | 1.1 | | | 130 | 0.2 | 1.6 | 29 | | 232 | 272 | | 606 | 1.59 |
| 56097 | 1 | cup | Spaghetti, w/sauce & cheese | 250 | 260 | 77 | 8.8 | 37.0 | 2.5 | | | 8.8 | 2.0 | 5.4 | 1.2 | | 0.70 | 8 | 1075 | 140 | 48 | 92 | | 0.25 | 0.17 | 2.25 | 0.20 | 0.00 | 8.0 | 0.45 | 12.5 | | | 80 | 0.4 | 2.3 | 25 | | 135 | 408 | 21.0 | 955 | 1.30 |
| 56100 | 1 | cup | Spaghetti, w/sauce & meatballs | 248 | 332 | 70 | 18.6 | 38.7 | 7.7 | | | 11.9 | 3.3 | 6.3 | 2.2 | | 0.89 | 74 | 1587 | 159 | 26 | 133 | | 0.25 | 0.30 | 3.97 | 0.20 | 1.20 | 10.0 | 0.40 | 22.3 | | | 124 | 0.4 | 3.7 | 40 | | 236 | 665 | 22.0 | 1009 | 2.45 |
| 56244 | 1 | cup | Sukiyaki | 162 | 175 | 77 | 19.2 | 6.4 | 1.1 | | | 8.0 | 3.0 | 3.2 | 0.8 | | | 154 | 2276 | 263 | 53 | 210 | | 0.13 | 0.42 | 3.21 | 0.36 | 1.56 | 61.8 | | 4.3 | | | 63 | 0.2 | 3.3 | 47 | | 209 | 468 | | 761 | 3.69 |
| | | | Sushi | | | | | | | | | | | | | | | | | | | | | | | | | | | | | | | | | | | | | | | | |
| 56315 | 1 | cup | With Egg, rolled in seaweed, w/o veg & fish | 166 | 204 | 74 | 9.0 | 23.2 | 0.4 | | | 8.0 | 2.0 | 3.2 | 1.8 | | | 196 | 644 | 133 | 103 | 30 | | 0.14 | 0.27 | 1.58 | 0.14 | 0.41 | 27.6 | | 2.2 | | | 45 | 0.1 | 1.8 | 23 | | 144 | 139 | | 548 | 1.12 |

| Code | Amount | | Description | Basic Components | | | | | | | | | Additional Fats | | | | | | Vit A & Components | | | | | Vitamins | | | | | | | | | | Minerals | | | | | | | | | |
|---|---|---|---|---|---|---|---|---|---|---|---|---|---|---|---|---|---|---|---|---|---|---|---|---|---|---|---|---|---|---|---|---|---|---|---|---|---|---|---|---|---|---|---|
| | | | | Weight (g) | Calories | % Water | Protein (g) | Carbs (g) | Fiber (g) | Sugar (g) | Other Carbs (g) | Fat (g) | Sat Fat (g) | Mono Fat (g) | Poly Fat (g) | Omega 3 (g) | Omega 6 (g) | Choles (mg) | Vit A (IU) | Vit A (RE) | Retinol (RE) | Carotenoids (RE) | Beta Carotene (mcg) | Thiamin (mg) | Riboflavin (mg) | Niacin (NE) | Vit B6 (mg) | Vit B12 (mcg) | Folate (mcg) | Panto (mg) | Vit C (mg) | Vit D (mg) | Vit E (α TE) | Calcium (mg) | Copper (mg) | Iron (mg) | Magnes (mg) | Mang (mg) | Phos (mg) | Potassium (mg) | Selenium (mcg) | Sodium (mg) | Zinc (mg) |
| 56314 | 1 | cup | With Vegetables, rolled in seaweed | 166 | 193 | 71 | 3.7 | 43.2 | 1.0 | | | 0.4 | 0.1 | 0.1 | 0.1 | | | 0 | 656 | 66 | 0 | 66 | | 0.21 | 0.04 | 2.00 | 0.15 | 0.00 | 10.8 | | 2.6 | | | 23 | 0.1 | 1.5 | 23 | | 68 | 111 | | 151 | 0.71 |
| 56312 | 1 | cup | With Vegetables, w/o fish | 166 | 246 | 63 | 5.2 | 54.5 | 1.7 | | | 0.5 | 0.1 | 0.1 | 0.1 | | | 0 | 1912 | 191 | 0 | 191 | | 0.31 | 0.06 | 2.69 | 0.14 | 0.00 | 15.9 | | 4.2 | | | 25 | 0.2 | 2.6 | 25 | | 85 | 174 | | 370 | 0.91 |
| 56313 | 1 | cup | With Vegetables & Fish | 166 | 237 | 64 | 8.9 | 48.2 | 1.5 | | | 0.7 | 0.2 | 0.2 | 0.2 | | | 12 | 1708 | 172 | 2 | 170 | | 0.29 | 0.07 | 3.03 | 0.16 | 0.33 | 15.4 | | 4.1 | | | 27 | 0.2 | 2.4 | 27 | | 110 | 216 | | 344 | 0.85 |
| 56311 | 1 | cup | Without Vegetables & Fish | 145 | 265 | 55 | 4.8 | 59.2 | 0.7 | | | 0.4 | 0.1 | 0.1 | 0.1 | | | 0 | 0 | 0 | 0 | 0 | 0 | 0.31 | 0.03 | 2.79 | 0.10 | 0.00 | 3.7 | | 0.0 | | | 20 | 0.1 | 2.8 | 19 | | 74 | 81 | | 122 | 0.75 |
| | | | Sweet & Sour | | | | | | | | | | | | | | | | | | | | | | | | | | | | | | | | | | | | | | | | |
| 12900 | 1 | cup | Pork | 226 | 231 | 77 | 14.9 | 25.0 | 1.3 | 19.1 | 4.7 | 8.2 | 2.2 | 2.9 | 2.5 | | | 38 | 279 | 28 | 1 | 27 | | 0.55 | 0.21 | 3.60 | 0.41 | 0.35 | 10.5 | 0.45 | 20.2 | 0.7 | | 29 | 0.2 | 1.4 | 34 | 0.9 | 147 | 389 | | 1220 | 1.46 |
| 56235 | 1 | cup | Pork, w/rice | 244 | 268 | 74 | 13.1 | 39.7 | 1.4 | | | 6.3 | 1.7 | 2.2 | 1.9 | | | 29 | 207 | 21 | 1 | 20 | | 0.53 | 0.16 | 3.78 | 0.37 | 0.26 | 10.1 | | 15.0 | | | 29 | 0.2 | 1.8 | 34 | | 146 | 317 | | 908 | 1.43 |
| 19400 | 1 | cup | Shrimp | 176 | 479 | 48 | 17.7 | 41.3 | 0.3 | 35.6 | 5.0 | 28.8 | 4.2 | 6.6 | 16.4 | | | 121 | 418 | 50 | 13 | 38 | | 0.05 | 0.09 | 2.89 | 0.20 | 0.78 | 6.6 | 0.35 | 9.2 | 2.8 | | 58 | 0.3 | 3.0 | 46 | 0.2 | 197 | 366 | | 818 | 1.18 |
| 56916 | 1 | cup | Tabbouleh | 160 | 187 | 78 | 3.2 | 17.0 | 4.7 | | | 13.0 | 1.3 | 9.3 | 1.2 | | | 0 | 1667 | 167 | 0 | 167 | | 0.09 | 0.07 | 1.38 | 0.12 | 0.00 | 58.9 | | 52.0 | | | 54 | 0.1 | 2.4 | 45 | | 74 | 336 | | 642 | 0.68 |
| 56113 | 1 | ea | Tamale, w/meat | 70 | 183 | 51 | 7.3 | 16.0 | 2.9 | | | 10.1 | 3.7 | 4.3 | 1.3 | | | 24 | 168 | 18 | 1 | 16 | | 0.24 | 0.18 | 2.93 | 0.11 | 0.18 | 5.4 | | 3.5 | | | 32 | 0.1 | 1.9 | 29 | | 80 | 154 | | 229 | 1.14 |
| 18803 | 1 | cup | Tuna, w/white sauce | 237 | 410 | 69 | 31.7 | 11.8 | 0.4 | | | 25.7 | 7.1 | 10.0 | 6.7 | | | 137 | 808 | 238 | 223 | 15 | | 0.11 | 0.45 | 10.35 | 0.17 | 2.47 | 22.4 | | 0.9 | | | 173 | 0.1 | 1.7 | 43 | | 415 | 382 | | 813 | 1.49 |
| 56089 | 1 | cup | Tuna Noodle Casserole | 202 | 237 | 75 | 16.7 | 25.4 | 1.4 | 0.9 | 23.0 | 7.3 | 1.3 | 1.5 | 3.2 | 0.16 | 2.99 | 41 | 42 | 13 | 13 | 0 | | 0.18 | 0.15 | 7.78 | 0.20 | 1.52 | 9.7 | 0.37 | 0.7 | 1.9 | | 34 | 0.2 | 2.3 | 31 | 0.4 | 155 | 182 | 54.0 | 772 | 1.20 |
| | | | Turnovers | | | | | | | | | | | | | | | | | | | | | | | | | | | | | | | | | | | | | | | | |
| 56301 | 1 | ea | Chicken, w/gravy | 112 | 321 | 51 | 10.8 | 22.1 | 0.8 | | | 21.0 | 5.5 | 8.9 | 5.5 | | | 26 | 315 | 94 | 86 | 7 | | 0.18 | 0.23 | 2.85 | 0.09 | 0.21 | 8.5 | | 0.3 | | | 64 | 0.1 | 1.4 | 16 | | 106 | 137 | | 440 | 0.83 |
| 56299 | 1 | ea | Meat Filled, w/o gravy | 88 | 334 | 36 | 11.1 | 21.9 | 0.8 | | | 22.2 | 6.7 | 9.7 | 4.1 | | | 29 | 0 | 0 | 0 | 0 | 0 | 0.20 | 0.20 | 2.47 | 0.09 | 0.85 | 7.9 | | 0.0 | | | 9 | 0.1 | 2.3 | 12 | | 96 | 110 | | 370 | 2.25 |
| 56300 | 1 | ea | Meat Filled, w/gravy | 152 | 389 | 55 | 14.1 | 26.3 | 1.1 | | | 25.2 | 7.3 | 10.9 | 4.5 | | | 32 | 0 | 0 | 0 | 0 | 0 | 0.23 | 0.23 | 3.03 | 0.10 | 0.97 | 9.6 | | 0.0 | | | 12 | 0.2 | 2.8 | 14 | | 120 | 164 | | 719 | 2.99 |
| | | | Veal | | | | | | | | | | | | | | | | | | | | | | | | | | | | | | | | | | | | | | | | |
| 11907 | 1 | ea | Cordon Bleu, svg | 229 | 492 | 65 | 35.1 | 3.4 | 0.8 | | | 36.4 | 19.2 | 12.7 | 1.9 | | | 169 | 908 | 204 | 169 | 35 | | 0.23 | 0.38 | 6.62 | 0.33 | 1.62 | 21.8 | | 5.6 | | | 169 | 0.2 | 1.7 | 39 | | 382 | 479 | | 570 | 4.51 |
| 11905 | 1 | pce | Marsala | 96 | 264 | 57 | 12.2 | 5.9 | 0.2 | | | 19.0 | 8.3 | 8.4 | 1.1 | | | 66 | 339 | 83 | 74 | 9 | | 0.08 | 0.17 | 3.97 | 0.17 | 0.56 | 6.8 | | 1.9 | | | 12 | 0.1 | 0.8 | 16 | | 129 | 220 | | 205 | 1.48 |
| 11906 | 1 | pce | Parmigiana | 182 | 349 | 64 | 27.0 | 15.1 | 1.4 | | | 19.9 | 7.7 | 6.5 | 4.1 | | | 138 | 795 | 135 | 79 | 56 | | 0.17 | 0.43 | 6.87 | 0.37 | 1.03 | 21.2 | | 6.9 | | | 187 | 0.2 | 2.0 | 42 | | 344 | 541 | | 755 | 3.10 |
| 11900 | 1 | ea | Patty | 79 | 209 | 53 | 16.4 | 6.4 | 0.4 | 0.3 | 5.8 | 12.6 | 4.4 | 5.1 | 1.9 | | | 81 | 27 | 8 | 8 | 0 | | 0.06 | 0.22 | 5.68 | 0.28 | 0.73 | 11.9 | | 0.0 | 0.2 | | 24 | 0.1 | 0.9 | 19 | 0.1 | 152 | 220 | | 310 | 1.92 |
| 11902 | 1 | pce | Scallopini | 96 | 257 | 58 | 17.6 | 1.0 | 0.2 | | | 19.4 | 5.5 | 8.3 | 4.2 | | | 62 | 541 | 165 | 151 | 14 | | 0.05 | 0.19 | 3.64 | 0.22 | 0.95 | 9.8 | | 0.4 | | | 45 | 0.1 | 0.7 | 19 | | 170 | 228 | | 331 | 1.90 |
| 11904 | 1 | cup | With Butter Sauce | 188 | 321 | 70 | 28.1 | 2.9 | 0.2 | | | 21.5 | 11.5 | 7.2 | 1.1 | | | 128 | 348 | 158 | 110 | 48 | | 0.11 | 0.30 | 6.74 | 0.28 | 1.14 | 14.8 | | 0.4 | | | 24 | 0.2 | 1.4 | 23 | | 205 | 331 | | 1040 | 2.98 |
| 11912 | 1 | cup | With Cream Sauce | 246 | 312 | 76 | 33.8 | 5.0 | 0.7 | | | 16.8 | 6.3 | 6.4 | 1.9 | | | 123 | 906 | 137 | 69 | 67 | | 0.19 | 0.46 | 10.76 | 0.53 | 1.48 | 20.5 | | 1.9 | | | 49 | 0.2 | 1.8 | 47 | | 367 | 610 | | 730 | 3.75 |
| 56111 | 1 | ea | WonTon, fried, meat filled | 19 | 61 | 43 | 2.6 | 4.1 | 0.2 | | | 3.8 | 0.7 | 1.6 | 1.2 | | | 13 | 132 | 22 | 4 | 18 | | 0.08 | 0.06 | 0.59 | 0.03 | 0.06 | 3.5 | | 0.4 | | | 6 | 0.0 | 0.4 | 4 | | 24 | 38 | | 83 | 0.24 |
| | | | **MEATS—BEEF, GAME, GOAT, LAMB, LUNCH MEATS, SAUSAGES, PORK & HAM, VEAL, ORGAN MEATS** | | | | | | | | | | | | | | | | | | | | | | | | | | | | | | | | | | | | | | | | |
| | | | *BEEF* | | | | | | | | | | | | | | | | | | | | | | | | | | | | | | | | | | | | | | | | |
| | | | Commodity Beef | | | | | | | | | | | | | | | | | | | | | | | | | | | | | | | | | | | | | | | | |
| 11499 | 3 | oz | Ground, bulk/coarse, ckd f/fzn | 85 | 194 | 66 | 14.8 | 0.0 | 0.0 | 0.0 | 0.0 | 14.5 | 5.3 | 6.3 | 0.6 | 0.06 | 0.11 | 59 | 0 | 0 | 0 | 0 | 0 | 0.05 | 0.20 | 3.58 | 0.20 | 1.62 | 6.0 | 0.31 | 0.0 | | | 6 | 0.1 | 1.4 | 14 | 0.0 | 104 | 209 | | 48 | 3.05 |
| 11495 | 4 | oz | Ground, bulk/coarse, fzn | 113 | 293 | 56 | 29.5 | 0.0 | 0.0 | 0.0 | 0.0 | 18.4 | 6.5 | 8.5 | 0.7 | 0.10 | 0.55 | 101 | 46 | 14 | 14 | 0 | 0 | 0.08 | 0.14 | 3.82 | 0.15 | 3.46 | 10.2 | 0.65 | 0.0 | | | 10 | 0.2 | 3.4 | 27 | 0.0 | 250 | 376 | | 107 | 7.10 |
| 11496 | 3 | oz | Patties, ckd f/fzn | 85 | 212 | 59 | 19.6 | 0.8 | 0.0 | | | 13.9 | 5.3 | 6.9 | 0.5 | 0.06 | 0.42 | 73 | 30 | 9 | 9 | 0 | 0 | 0.04 | 0.16 | 2.50 | 0.14 | 2.98 | 6.8 | 0.52 | 0.0 | | | 7 | 0.1 | 2.2 | 16 | 0.0 | 156 | 198 | | 56 | 4.47 |
| 11498 | 4 | oz | Patties, fzn, raw | 113 | 231 | 65 | 16.5 | 0.0 | 0.0 | 0.0 | 0.0 | 17.7 | 7.2 | 7.8 | 0.7 | 0.09 | 0.12 | 60 | 0 | 0 | 0 | 0 | 0 | 0.05 | 0.18 | 4.35 | 0.24 | 2.32 | 6.8 | 0.35 | 0.0 | | | 8 | 0.1 | 2.2 | 20 | 0.0 | 164 | 304 | | 84 | 4.66 |
| 11494 | 3 | oz | Patties, w/veg protein, ckd f/fzn | 85 | 210 | 58 | 13.3 | 6.7 | 1.2 | | | 14.4 | 5.3 | 6.6 | 0.5 | 0.08 | 0.43 | 32 | 40 | 12 | 12 | 0 | 0 | 0.22 | 0.18 | 3.27 | 0.22 | 2.44 | 14.5 | 0.99 | 0.0 | | | 33 | 0.2 | 3.1 | 42 | 0.3 | 200 | 276 | | 56 | 7.07 |
| 11497 | 4 | oz | Patties, w/veg protein, fzn, raw | 113 | 254 | 63 | 17.2 | 4.3 | 1.5 | | | 18.6 | 6.5 | 8.6 | 0.6 | 0.08 | 0.55 | 37 | 55 | 17 | 17 | 0 | 0 | 0.35 | 0.25 | 4.84 | 0.50 | 4.06 | | 1.65 | 0.0 | | | 33 | 0.2 | 3.0 | 41 | 0.3 | 215 | 332 | | 62 | 6.15 |
| | | | Dried Beef | | | | | | | | | | | | | | | | | | | | | | | | | | | | | | | | | | | | | | | | |
| 10051 | 1 | ea | Beef Jerky, large pce | 20 | 82 | 23 | 6.6 | 2.2 | 0.4 | 1.8 | 0.0 | 5.1 | 2.2 | 2.3 | 0.2 | 0.04 | 0.17 | 10 | 0 | 0 | 0 | 0 | 0 | 0.03 | 0.03 | 0.35 | 0.04 | 0.20 | 26.8 | 0.03 | 0.0 | 0.1 | | 4 | 0.0 | 1.1 | 10 | 0.0 | 81 | 119 | 2.1 | 443 | 1.62 |
| 10742 | 1 | pce | Beef Jerky, Tombstone | 13 | 36 | | 6.1 | 1.0 | 0.0 | 0.0 | 1.0 | 0.0 | 0.0 | 0.0 | 0.0 | 0.00 | 0.00 | 15 | 0 | 0 | 0 | 0 | 0 | | | | | | | | 3.7 | | | 0 | | 0.7 | | | | | | 315 | |
| 10743 | 1 | pce | Beef Sticks, Tombstone | 21 | 108 | | 3.0 | 0.0 | 0.0 | 0.0 | 0.0 | 9.9 | 4.4 | | | | | 20 | 0 | 0 | 0 | 0 | 0 | | | | | | | | 2.4 | | | 0 | | 0.4 | | | | | | 266 | |
| 10009 | 5 | pce | Cured | 21 | 35 | 56 | 6.1 | 0.3 | 0.0 | 0.3 | 0.0 | 0.8 | 0.3 | 0.3 | 0.0 | 0.01 | 0.03 | 9 | 0 | 0 | 0 | 0 | 0 | 0.02 | 0.04 | 1.14 | 0.07 | 0.56 | 2.3 | 0.13 | 0.0 | 0.1 | | 1 | 0.0 | 0.9 | 7 | 0.0 | 37 | 93 | 13.0 | 729 | 1.10 |
| 10052 | 1 | ea | Meat Sticks, smkd | 20 | 110 | 19 | 4.3 | 1.1 | | | | 9.9 | 4.2 | 4.1 | 0.9 | 0.03 | 0.81 | 27 | 302 | 34 | 34 | 0 | | 0.03 | 0.09 | 0.91 | 0.04 | 0.20 | 0.0 | 0.07 | 1.4 | 0.2 | | 14 | 0.0 | 0.7 | 4 | 0.0 | 36 | 51 | | 296 | 0.48 |
| 10744 | 1 | pce | Snappy Sticks, Tombstone | 21 | 108 | 19 | 3.9 | 1.0 | 0.0 | 0.0 | 1.0 | 9.9 | 4.4 | | | | | 20 | 0 | 0 | 0 | 0 | 0 | | | | | | | | 2.4 | | | 0 | | 0.4 | | | | | | 256 | |
| 10106 | 1 | oz | Fat, cooked | 28 | 190 | 19 | 3.0 | 0.0 | 0.0 | 0.0 | 0.0 | 19.7 | 8.0 | 8.5 | 0.7 | 0.23 | 0.45 | 27 | 0 | 0 | 0 | 0 | 0 | 0.01 | 0.03 | 0.43 | 0.04 | 0.45 | 0.8 | 0.04 | 0.0 | 0.1 | | 4 | 0.0 | 0.3 | 2 | 0.0 | 21 | 33 | | 11 | 0.39 |
| | | | Ground Beef | | | | | | | | | | | | | | | | | | | | | | | | | | | | | | | | | | | | | | | | |
| 10732 | 4 | oz | 9% Fat, raw | 113 | 191 | 69 | 23.2 | 0.0 | 0.0 | 0.0 | 0.0 | 10.2 | 4.7 | 4.4 | 0.4 | | | 41 | 0 | 0 | 0 | 0 | 0 | 0.07 | 0.31 | 5.62 | 0.32 | 2.57 | 9.9 | 0.48 | 0.0 | 0.4 | | 9 | 0.1 | 2.4 | 25 | | 175 | 353 | | 81 | 5.15 |
| 10454 | 3 | oz | 16% Fat, bkd | 85 | 213 | 59 | 20.8 | 0.0 | 0.0 | 0.0 | 0.0 | 13.7 | 5.4 | 6.0 | 0.5 | 0.05 | 0.43 | 70 | 0 | 0 | 0 | 0 | 0 | 0.03 | 0.20 | 3.54 | 0.19 | 1.47 | 7.7 | 0.23 | 0.0 | 0.3 | | 6 | 0.1 | 1.9 | 14 | 0.0 | 105 | 190 | | 42 | 4.54 |
| 10456 | 3 | oz | 16% Fat, brld | 85 | 218 | 57 | 21.6 | 0.0 | 0.0 | 0.0 | 0.0 | 13.9 | 5.5 | 6.1 | 0.5 | 0.05 | 0.44 | 71 | 0 | 0 | 0 | 0 | 0 | 0.05 | 0.23 | 4.22 | 0.23 | 1.84 | 7.7 | 0.30 | 0.0 | 0.3 | | 6 | 0.1 | 2.0 | 18 | 0.0 | 137 | 266 | | 60 | 4.63 |
| 10261 | 3 | oz | 16% Fat, pan fried | 85 | 217 | 58 | 21.3 | 0.0 | 0.0 | 0.0 | 0.0 | 13.9 | 5.5 | 6.1 | 0.5 | 0.05 | 0.44 | 69 | 0 | 0 | 0 | 0 | 0 | 0.05 | 0.22 | 4.00 | 0.23 | 1.70 | 7.7 | 0.21 | 0.0 | 0.3 | | 6 | 0.1 | 2.0 | 18 | 0.0 | 136 | 265 | | 60 | 4.61 |
| 10453 | 4 | oz | 17% Fat, raw | 113 | 264 | 63 | 21.1 | 0.0 | 0.0 | 0.0 | 0.0 | 19.3 | 7.7 | 8.4 | 0.8 | 0.11 | 0.69 | 78 | 0 | 0 | 0 | 0 | 0 | 0.07 | 0.28 | 5.12 | 0.29 | 2.33 | 9.0 | 0.44 | 0.0 | 0.3 | | 8 | 0.1 | 2.2 | 23 | 0.0 | 159 | 321 | 15.7 | 75 | 4.68 |
| 10459 | 3 | oz | 18% Fat, bkd | 85 | 228 | 57 | 20.3 | 0.0 | 0.0 | 0.0 | 0.0 | 15.6 | 6.7 | 6.8 | 0.6 | 0.07 | 0.48 | 66 | 0 | 0 | 0 | 0 | 0 | 0.04 | 0.16 | 3.64 | 0.17 | 1.50 | 7.7 | 0.23 | 0.0 | 0.3 | | 8 | 0.1 | 1.8 | 14 | 0.0 | 109 | 190 | | 48 | 4.34 |
| 10673 | 3 | oz | 19% Fat, brld | 85 | 231 | 56 | 21.0 | 0.0 | 0.0 | 0.0 | 0.0 | 15.7 | 6.2 | 6.9 | 0.6 | 0.07 | 0.49 | 74 | 0 | 0 | 0 | 0 | 0 | 0.04 | 0.18 | 4.39 | 0.22 | 2.00 | 7.7 | 0.32 | 0.0 | 0.3 | | 9 | 0.1 | 1.8 | 18 | 0.0 | 134 | 256 | 24.7 | 65 | 4.56 |
| 8208 | 3 | oz | 19% Fat, fried | 85 | 234 | 56 | 20.6 | 0.0 | 0.0 | 0.0 | 0.0 | 16.2 | 6.4 | 7.1 | 0.6 | 0.07 | 0.51 | 71 | 0 | 0 | 0 | 0 | 0 | 0.04 | 0.19 | 4.07 | 0.24 | 1.93 | 7.7 | 0.27 | 0.0 | 0.3 | | 9 | 0.1 | 1.9 | 17 | 0.0 | 135 | 254 | | 65 | 4.42 |
| 10725 | 3 | oz | 21% Fat, bkd | 85 | 244 | 55 | 19.6 | 0.0 | 0.0 | 0.0 | 0.0 | 17.8 | 7.0 | 7.8 | 0.7 | 0.03 | 0.56 | 74 | 0 | 0 | 0 | 0 | 0 | 0.03 | 0.14 | 4.04 | 0.20 | 1.99 | 7.7 | 0.19 | 0.0 | 0.3 | | 9 | 0.1 | 2.0 | 13 | 0.0 | 116 | 188 | 16.5 | 51 | 4.16 |
| 10700 | 3 | oz | 21% Fat, brld | 85 | 246 | 54 | 20.5 | 0.0 | 0.0 | 0.0 | 0.0 | 17.6 | 6.9 | 7.7 | 0.7 | 0.03 | 0.55 | 77 | 0 | 0 | 0 | 0 | 0 | 0.03 | 0.16 | 4.90 | 0.23 | 2.49 | 7.7 | 0.28 | 0.0 | 0.3 | | 9 | 0.1 | 2.1 | 17 | 0.0 | 145 | 248 | 16.5 | 71 | 4.40 |
| 10458 | 4 | oz | 21% Fat, raw | 113 | 298 | 60 | 20.0 | 0.0 | 0.0 | 0.0 | 0.0 | 23.4 | 9.4 | 10.2 | 1.0 | 0.11 | 0.81 | 85 | 0 | 0 | 0 | 0 | 0 | 0.06 | 0.24 | 5.10 | 0.28 | 2.64 | 9.0 | 0.42 | 0.0 | 0.3 | | 9 | 0.1 | 2.0 | 20 | 0.0 | 154 | 295 | 17.7 | 78 | 4.36 |
| 10464 | 3 | oz | 23% Fat, fried | 85 | 260 | 52 | 20.3 | 0.0 | 0.0 | 0.0 | 0.0 | 19.2 | 7.5 | 8.4 | 0.7 | 0.03 | 0.60 | 76 | 0 | 0 | 0 | 0 | 0 | 0.03 | 0.17 | 4.96 | 0.20 | 2.30 | 7.7 | 0.29 | 0.0 | 0.3 | | 9 | 0.1 | 2.1 | 17 | 0.0 | 145 | 255 | | 71 | 4.31 |
| 10462 | 4 | oz | 27% Fat, raw | 113 | 350 | 56 | 18.8 | 0.0 | 0.0 | 0.0 | 0.0 | 30.1 | 12.2 | 13.1 | 1.2 | 0.13 | 0.99 | 96 | 0 | 0 | 0 | 0 | 0 | 0.04 | 0.17 | 5.06 | 0.27 | 2.99 | 7.9 | 0.39 | 0.0 | 0.3 | | 9 | 0.1 | 2.0 | 18 | 0.0 | 147 | 258 | 14.4 | 77 | 4.01 |
| | | | Ground Beef Patties | | | | | | | | | | | | | | | | | | | | | | | | | | | | | | | | | | | | | | | | |
| 10739 | 3 | oz | Breaded, Kings Command Foods | 85 | 219 | | 16.4 | 11.2 | 0.4 | 0.0 | 10.8 | 11.9 | 3.8 | 5.3 | 1.2 | | | 42 | 74 | 15 | | | | 0.18 | 0.20 | 4.43 | 0.19 | 1.34 | 17.9 | | 0.0 | | | 26 | | 2.1 | | | 123 | 303 | | 58 | 3.97 |
| 10741 | 3 | oz | Kings Command Foods | 85 | 210 | | 17.6 | 2.9 | 0.2 | 0.0 | 2.7 | 14.1 | 5.8 | 6.0 | 0.3 | | | 47 | 128 | 38 | | | | 0.14 | 0.20 | 4.85 | 0.26 | 1.66 | 19.6 | | 0.0 | | | 29 | | 2.3 | | | 136 | 375 | | 345 | 5.64 |
| 10773 | 1 | ea | Tenderflake | 85 | 222 | 60 | 14.7 | 0.8 | 0.7 | 0.0 | 0.1 | 17.8 | 7.2 | 7.7 | 0.7 | | | 50 | 32 | 10 | 10 | 0 | 0 | 0.14 | 0.13 | 2.89 | | | | | 0.0 | | | 18 | | 1.8 | | | 144 | 276 | | 130 | 3.84 |
| 10774 | 1 | ea | Travis Meats | 91 | 236 | 60 | 15.1 | 1.6 | 1.4 | 0.1 | 0.2 | 18.9 | 7.2 | 8.2 | 0.7 | | | 46 | 67 | 20 | 20 | 0 | 0 | 0.20 | 0.15 | 3.40 | | | | | 0.0 | | | 31 | | 2.1 | | | 155 | 329 | | 146 | 4.96 |
| | | | Retail Cuts, all grades, lean & fat, 1/8" trim | | | | | | | | | | | | | | | | | | | | | | | | | | | | | | | | | | | | | | | | |
| 10820 | 3 | oz | Average, ckd | 85 | 247 | 53 | 22.4 | 0.0 | 0.0 | 0.0 | 0.0 | 16.7 | 6.6 | 7.2 | 0.6 | 0.16 | 0.44 | 74 | 0 | 0 | 0 | 0 | 0 | 0.08 | 0.19 | 3.16 | 0.29 | 2.10 | 6.0 | 0.31 | 0.0 | | | 8 | 0.1 | 2.3 | 20 | 0.0 | 177 | 271 | | 54 | 5.10 |
| 10819 | 4 | oz | Average, raw | 113 | 264 | 62 | 21.1 | 0.0 | 0.0 | 0.0 | 0.0 | 19.4 | 7.8 | 8.4 | 0.7 | 0.21 | 0.50 | 75 | 0 | 0 | 0 | 0 | 0 | 0.11 | 0.18 | 3.65 | 0.44 | 3.33 | 6.8 | 0.36 | 0.0 | | | 8 | 0.1 | 2.2 | 21 | 0.0 | 200 | 346 | | 66 | 4.24 |
| 10008 | 1 | cup | Brisket, corned, cnd, ckd | 140 | 350 | 58 | 37.9 | 0.0 | 0.0 | 0.0 | 0.0 | 20.9 | 8.2 | 8.3 | 0.9 | 0.29 | 0.59 | 120 | 0 | 0 | 0 | 0 | 0 | 0.03 | 0.21 | 3.40 | 0.18 | 2.27 | 12.6 | 0.88 | 0.0 | 0.4 | | 17 | 0.1 | 2.9 | 20 | 0.0 | 155 | 190 | 60.1 | 1408 | 5.00 |
| 10787 | 3 | oz | Brisket, corned, ckd | 85 | 213 | 60 | 15.5 | 0.4 | 0.0 | | | 16.1 | 5.4 | 7.8 | 0.6 | 0.17 | 0.46 | 83 | 0 | 0 | 0 | 0 | 0 | 0.02 | 0.14 | 2.58 | 0.20 | 1.39 | 5.1 | 0.36 | 0.0 | 0.3 | | 7 | 0.1 | 1.6 | 10 | 0.0 | 106 | 123 | | 964 | 3.89 |
| 10485 | 4 | oz | Brisket, corned, raw | 113 | 224 | 67 | 16.6 | 0.2 | 0.0 | | | 16.8 | 5.3 | 8.1 | 0.6 | 0.17 | 0.43 | 61 | 0 | 0 | 0 | 0 | 0 | 0.05 | 0.18 | 4.14 | 0.33 | 2.01 | 5.7 | 0.64 | 30.5 | 0.3 | | 8 | 0.1 | 1.9 | 16 | 0.0 | 132 | 336 | | 138 | 3.22 |
| 10828 | 3 | oz | Brisket, whole, brsd | 85 | 281 | 50 | 22.0 | 0.0 | 0.0 | 0.0 | 0.0 | 20.8 | 8.0 | 9.3 | 0.7 | 0.20 | 0.53 | 79 | 0 | 0 | 0 | 0 | 0 | 0.05 | 0.17 | 2.78 | 0.22 | 2.04 | 6.0 | 0.26 | 0.0 | | | 6 | 0.1 | 2.1 | 17 | 0.0 | 176 | 213 | | 54 | 4.90 |
| 10827 | 4 | oz | Brisket, whole, raw | 113 | 284 | 61 | 20.8 | 0.0 | 0.0 | 0.0 | 0.0 | 21.6 | 8.5 | 9.6 | 0.7 | 0.24 | 0.51 | 77 | 0 | 0 | 0 | 0 | 0 | 0.10 | 0.17 | 3.93 | 0.43 | 2.54 | 6.8 | 0.35 | 0.0 | | | 7 | 0.1 | 1.9 | 21 | 0.0 | 200 | 319 | | 78 | 4.19 |
| 10834 | 3 | oz | Chuck, arm pot roast, brsd | 85 | 263 | 50 | 24.2 | 0.0 | 0.0 | 0.0 | 0.0 | 17.6 | 6.9 | 7.5 | 0.7 | 0.20 | 0.48 | 85 | 0 | 0 | 0 | 0 | 0 | 0.06 | 0.21 | 2.79 | 0.25 | 2.58 | 7.7 | 0.29 | 0.0 | | | 9 | 0.1 | 2.8 | 17 | 0.0 | 196 | 217 | | 52 | 6.13 |

| Code | Amount | Description | Weight (g) | Calories | % Water | Protein (g) | Carbs (g) | Fiber (g) | Sugar (g) | Other Carbs (g) | Fat (g) | Sat Fat (g) | Mono Fat (g) | Poly Fat (g) | Omega 3 (g) | Omega 6 (g) | Choles (mg) | Vit A (IU) | Vit A (RE) | Retinol (RE) | Carotenoids (RE) | Beta Carotene (mcg) |
|---|---|---|---|---|---|---|---|---|---|---|---|---|---|---|---|---|---|---|---|---|---|---|
| | | | Basic Components | | | | | | | | | Additional Fats | | | | | | Vit A & Components | | | | |
| 10833 | 4 oz | Chuck, arm pot roast, raw | 113 | 264 | 63 | 21.2 | 0.0 | 0.0 | 0.0 | 0.0 | 19.2 | 7.8 | 8.2 | 0.8 | 0.25 | 0.51 | 76 | 0 | 0 | 0 | 0 | 0 |
| 10840 | 3 oz | Chuck, blade pot roast, brsd | 85 | 290 | 48 | 22.8 | 0.0 | 0.0 | 0.0 | 0.0 | 21.3 | 8.5 | 9.3 | 0.8 | 0.21 | 0.55 | 88 | 0 | 0 | 0 | 0 | 0 |
| 10839 | 4 oz | Chuck, blade pot roast, raw | 113 | 280 | 61 | 19.4 | 0.0 | 0.0 | 0.0 | 0.0 | 21.9 | 8.8 | 9.6 | 0.8 | 0.25 | 0.56 | 80 | 0 | 0 | 0 | 0 | 0 |
| 11487 | 3 oz | Porterhouse Steak, ckd | 85 | 252 | 53 | 20.0 | 0.0 | 0.0 | 0.0 | 0.0 | 18.5 | 7.2 | 8.2 | 0.7 | 0.20 | 0.48 | 60 | 0 | 0 | 0 | 0 | 0 |
| 11486 | 4 oz | Porterhouse Steak, raw | 113 | 279 | 61 | 21.2 | 0.0 | 0.0 | 0.0 | 0.0 | 20.9 | 8.4 | 9.3 | 0.8 | 0.24 | 0.55 | 72 | 0 | 0 | 0 | 0 | 0 |
| 10859 | 3 oz | Ribs, large end 6-9, ckd | 85 | 287 | 49 | 18.4 | 0.0 | 0.0 | 0.0 | 0.0 | 23.1 | 9.4 | 9.8 | 0.9 | 0.26 | 0.62 | 68 | 0 | 0 | 0 | 0 | 0 |
| 10950 | 4 oz | Ribs, large end 6-9, raw | 113 | 357 | 54 | 18.4 | 0.0 | 0.0 | 0.0 | 0.0 | 30.8 | 12.8 | 13.2 | 1.1 | 0.38 | 0.75 | 80 | 0 | 0 | 0 | 0 | 0 |
| 10871 | 3 oz | Ribs, small end 10-12, ckd | 85 | 281 | 49 | 20.3 | 0.0 | 0.0 | 0.0 | 0.0 | 21.4 | 8.7 | 9.2 | 0.7 | 0.22 | 0.52 | 71 | 0 | 0 | 0 | 0 | 0 |
| 10870 | 4 oz | Ribs, small end 10-12, raw | 113 | 329 | 56 | 19.2 | 0.0 | 0.0 | 0.0 | 0.0 | 27.3 | 11.2 | 11.9 | 1.0 | 0.33 | 0.63 | 79 | 0 | 0 | 0 | 0 | 0 |
| 10846 | 3 oz | Ribs, whole 6-12, ckd | 85 | 286 | 48 | 19.0 | 0.0 | 0.0 | 0.0 | 0.0 | 22.8 | 9.3 | 9.7 | 0.8 | 0.25 | 0.59 | 70 | 0 | 0 | 0 | 0 | 0 |
| 10845 | 4 oz | Ribs, whole 6-12, raw | 85 | 260 | 55 | 14.0 | 0.0 | 0.0 | 0.0 | 0.0 | 22.2 | 9.2 | 9.5 | 0.8 | 0.27 | 0.53 | 60 | 0 | 0 | 0 | 0 | 0 |
| 11410 | 3 oz | Round, bottom, ckd | 85 | 218 | 54 | 25.1 | 0.0 | 0.0 | 0.0 | 0.0 | 12.2 | 4.5 | 5.3 | 0.5 | 0.11 | 0.36 | 82 | 0 | 0 | 0 | 0 | 0 |
| 10886 | 4 oz | Round, bottom, raw | 113 | 216 | 66 | 23.4 | 0.0 | 0.0 | 0.0 | 0.0 | 12.9 | 4.9 | 5.7 | 0.5 | 0.11 | 0.36 | 71 | 0 | 0 | 0 | 0 | 0 |
| 11425 | 3 oz | Round, tip, ckd | 85 | 186 | 62 | 23.4 | 0.0 | 0.0 | 0.0 | 0.0 | 9.6 | 3.6 | 4.0 | 0.4 | 0.08 | 0.30 | 70 | 0 | 0 | 0 | 0 | 0 |
| 11424 | 4 oz | Round, tip , raw | 113 | 214 | 66 | 22.1 | 0.0 | 0.0 | 0.0 | 0.0 | 13.2 | 5.2 | 5.7 | 0.5 | 0.15 | 0.37 | 73 | 0 | 0 | 0 | 0 | 0 |
| 11463 | 3 oz | Sirloin, top, ckd | 85 | 211 | 57 | 24.0 | 0.0 | 0.0 | 0.0 | 0.0 | 12.0 | 4.8 | 5.2 | 0.5 | 0.11 | 0.35 | 77 | 0 | 0 | 0 | 0 | 0 |
| 10943 | 4 oz | Sirloin, top, raw | 113 | 231 | 65 | 22.0 | 0.0 | 0.0 | 0.0 | 0.0 | 15.1 | 6.0 | 6.5 | 0.6 | 0.17 | 0.43 | 75 | 0 | 0 | 0 | 0 | 0 |
| 11491 | 3 oz | T-bone Steak, ckd | 85 | 238 | 55 | 20.7 | 0.0 | 0.0 | 0.0 | 0.0 | 16.6 | 6.4 | 7.3 | 0.6 | 0.17 | 0.42 | 53 | 0 | 0 | 0 | 0 | 0 |
| 11490 | 4 oz | T-bone Steak, raw | 113 | 249 | 64 | 21.7 | 0.0 | 0.0 | 0.0 | 0.0 | 17.3 | 6.9 | 7.6 | 0.7 | 0.19 | 0.47 | 64 | 0 | 0 | 0 | 0 | 0 |
| 11451 | 3 oz | Tenderloin, ckd | 85 | 239 | 54 | 21.8 | 0.0 | 0.0 | 0.0 | 0.0 | 16.2 | 6.3 | 6.6 | 0.6 | 0.15 | 0.46 | 73 | 0 | 0 | 0 | 0 | 0 |
| 10931 | 4 oz | Tenderloin, raw | 113 | 308 | 58 | 20.3 | 0.0 | 0.0 | 0.0 | 0.0 | 24.5 | 9.9 | 10.4 | 0.9 | 0.28 | 0.67 | 79 | 0 | 0 | 0 | 0 | 0 |
| 11432 | 3 oz | Top Round, ckd | 85 | 176 | 60 | 25.9 | 0.0 | 0.0 | 0.0 | 0.0 | 7.2 | 2.7 | 2.9 | 0.3 | 0.06 | 0.24 | 72 | 0 | 0 | 0 | 0 | 0 |
| 10907 | 4 oz | Top Round, raw | 113 | 184 | 68 | 24.6 | 0.0 | 0.0 | 0.0 | 0.0 | 8.8 | 3.4 | 3.7 | 0.4 | 0.09 | 0.26 | 68 | 0 | 0 | 0 | 0 | 0 |
| | | Steaks, Prepared | | | | | | | | | | | | | | | | | | | | |
| 10083 | 1 ea | Battered, fried | 243 | 768 | 48 | 57.4 | 13.5 | 0.4 | 3.1 | 10.0 | 52.1 | 18.8 | 22.5 | 5.7 | | | 214 | 74 | 20 | 17 | 3 | |
| 10084 | 1 ea | Battered, fried, lean | 165 | 434 | 52 | 43.3 | 9.2 | 0.3 | 2.1 | 6.8 | 23.7 | 8.0 | 10.2 | 3.5 | | | 145 | 50 | 14 | 12 | 2 | |
| 10080 | 1 ea | Breaded, brld | 243 | 799 | 43 | 59.0 | 25.7 | 1.4 | 1.3 | 22.9 | 49.4 | 16.7 | 19.3 | 8.5 | | | 185 | 22 | 7 | 7 | 0 | 0 |
| 10082 | 1 ea | Breaded, brld, lean | 165 | 455 | 48 | 44.3 | 17.4 | 1.0 | 0.9 | 15.5 | 21.8 | 6.5 | 8.0 | 5.4 | | | 125 | 15 | 5 | 5 | 0 | 0 |
| 11678 | 3 oz | Broiled | 85 | 216 | 55 | 23.7 | 0.0 | 0.0 | 0.0 | 0.0 | 12.8 | 5.0 | 5.4 | 0.5 | | | 71 | 0 | 0 | 0 | 0 | 0 |
| 11679 | 3 oz | Broiled, lean | 85 | 169 | 60 | 25.0 | 0.0 | 0.0 | 0.0 | 0.0 | 6.9 | 2.6 | 2.8 | 0.2 | | | 68 | 0 | 0 | 0 | 0 | 0 |
| 10740 | 3 oz | Cube, Kings Command Foods | 85 | 247 | | 17.3 | 1.9 | 0.2 | 0.0 | 1.7 | 18.5 | 7.9 | 8.0 | 0.7 | | | 59 | 67 | 20 | | | |
| 10072 | 1 ea | Fried | 153 | 441 | 51 | 47.0 | 0.0 | 0.0 | 0.0 | 0.0 | 26.6 | 10.1 | 11.4 | 1.7 | | | 148 | 0 | 0 | 0 | 0 | 0 |
| 10079 | 1 ea | Fried, lean | 117 | 269 | 55 | 39.5 | 0.0 | 0.0 | 0.0 | 0.0 | 11.2 | 4.0 | 4.7 | 1.0 | | | 113 | 0 | 0 | 0 | 0 | 0 |
| 10738 | 3 oz | Pepper, Kings Command Foods | 85 | 255 | | 15.6 | 2.7 | 0.3 | 0.0 | 2.4 | 20.0 | 8.7 | 8.5 | 0.8 | | | 55 | 116 | 35 | | | |
| | | *GAME MEATS* | | | | | | | | | | | | | | | | | | | | |
| 14052 | 4 oz | Antelope, raw | 113 | 129 | 74 | 25.3 | 0.0 | 0.0 | 0.0 | 0.0 | 2.3 | 0.8 | 0.5 | 0.5 | 0.08 | 0.42 | 107 | 0 | 0 | 0 | 0 | 0 |
| 14053 | 3 oz | Antelope, rstd | 85 | 128 | 66 | 25.1 | 0.0 | 0.0 | 0.0 | 0.0 | 2.3 | 0.8 | 0.5 | 0.5 | 0.08 | 0.41 | 107 | 0 | 0 | 0 | 0 | 0 |
| 14006 | 3 oz | Bear, ckd | 85 | 220 | 54 | 27.5 | 0.0 | 0.0 | 0.0 | 0.0 | 11.4 | 3.0 | 4.8 | 2.0 | 0.07 | 1.61 | 83 | 0 | 0 | 0 | 0 | 0 |
| 14054 | 4 oz | Bear, raw | 113 | 182 | 71 | 22.7 | 0.0 | 0.0 | 0.0 | 0.0 | 9.4 | 2.5 | 3.4 | 3.1 | 0.06 | 1.32 | | 0 | 0 | 0 | 0 | 0 |
| 14055 | 4 oz | Beaver, raw | 113 | 165 | 71 | 27.2 | 0.0 | 0.0 | 0.0 | 0.0 | 5.4 | 1.6 | 1.5 | 1.1 | 0.22 | 0.83 | | 0 | 0 | 0 | 0 | 0 |
| 14007 | 3 oz | Beaver, rstd | 85 | 180 | 58 | 29.7 | 0.0 | 0.0 | 0.0 | 0.0 | 5.9 | 1.8 | 1.6 | 1.1 | 0.24 | 0.91 | 99 | 0 | 0 | 0 | 0 | 0 |
| 14067 | 4 oz | Beefalo, raw | 113 | 162 | 71 | 26.3 | 0.0 | 0.0 | 0.0 | 0.0 | 5.4 | 2.3 | 2.3 | 0.2 | 0.05 | 0.12 | 50 | 0 | 0 | 0 | 0 | 0 |
| 14008 | 3 oz | Beefalo, rstd | 85 | 160 | 62 | 26.1 | 0.0 | 0.0 | 0.0 | 0.0 | 5.4 | 2.3 | 2.3 | 0.2 | 0.05 | 0.12 | 49 | 0 | 0 | 0 | 0 | 0 |
| 14056 | 4 oz | Bison, raw | 113 | 123 | 75 | 24.4 | 0.0 | 0.0 | 0.0 | 0.0 | 2.1 | 0.8 | 0.8 | 0.2 | 0.03 | 0.19 | 70 | 0 | 0 | 0 | 0 | 0 |
| 14009 | 3 oz | Bison, rstd | 85 | 122 | 66 | 24.1 | 0.0 | 0.0 | 0.0 | 0.0 | 2.1 | 0.8 | 0.8 | 0.2 | 0.03 | 0.17 | 70 | 0 | 0 | 0 | 0 | 0 |
| 14057 | 4 oz | Boar, raw | 113 | 138 | 72 | 24.3 | 0.0 | 0.0 | 0.0 | 0.0 | 3.8 | 1.1 | 1.5 | 0.5 | 0.02 | 0.52 | 67 | 0 | 0 | 0 | 0 | 0 |
| 14010 | 3 oz | Boar, rstd | 85 | 136 | 64 | 24.1 | 0.0 | 0.0 | 0.0 | 0.0 | 3.7 | 1.1 | 1.5 | 0.5 | 0.03 | 0.52 | 65 | 0 | 0 | 0 | 0 | 0 |
| 14059 | 4 oz | Caribou, raw | 113 | 144 | 72 | 25.5 | 0.0 | 0.0 | 0.0 | 0.0 | 3.8 | 1.5 | 1.1 | 0.5 | 0.09 | 0.42 | 94 | 0 | 0 | 0 | 0 | 0 |
| 14012 | 3 oz | Caribou, rstd | 85 | 142 | 62 | 25.3 | 0.0 | 0.0 | 0.0 | 0.0 | 3.8 | 1.4 | 1.1 | 0.5 | 0.08 | 0.42 | 93 | 0 | 0 | 0 | 0 | 0 |
| 14061 | 4 oz | Elk, raw | 113 | 125 | 74 | 26.0 | 0.0 | 0.0 | 0.0 | 0.0 | 1.6 | 0.6 | 0.4 | 0.3 | 0.05 | 0.29 | 62 | 0 | 0 | 0 | 0 | 0 |
| 14014 | 3 oz | Elk, rstd | 85 | 124 | 66 | 25.7 | 0.0 | 0.0 | 0.0 | 0.0 | 1.6 | 0.6 | 0.4 | 0.3 | 0.05 | 0.29 | 62 | 0 | 0 | 0 | 0 | 0 |
| 14005 | 4 ea | Frog legs, raw | 96 | 70 | 82 | 15.7 | 0.0 | 0.0 | 0.0 | 0.0 | 0.3 | 0.0 | 0.1 | 0.1 | | 0.00 | 48 | 0 | 0 | 0 | 0 | 0 |
| 14029 | 2 ea | Frog legs, stmd | 100 | 106 | 74 | 23.8 | 0.0 | 0.0 | 0.0 | 0.0 | 0.4 | 0.1 | 0.1 | 0.2 | | | 72 | 65 | 20 | 20 | 0 | 0 |
| 14026 | 4 oz | Horse, raw | 113 | 150 | 73 | 24.2 | 0.0 | 0.0 | 0.0 | 0.0 | 5.2 | 1.6 | 1.8 | 0.7 | 0.41 | 0.33 | 59 | 0 | 0 | 0 | 0 | 0 |
| 14018 | 3 oz | Horse, rstd | 85 | 149 | 64 | 23.9 | 0.0 | 0.0 | 0.0 | 0.0 | 5.1 | 1.6 | 1.8 | 0.7 | 0.40 | 0.32 | 58 | 0 | 0 | 0 | 0 | 0 |
| 14062 | 4 oz | Moose, raw | 113 | 115 | 76 | 25.1 | 0.0 | 0.0 | 0.0 | 0.0 | 0.8 | 0.2 | 0.2 | 0.3 | 0.03 | 0.24 | 67 | 0 | 0 | 0 | 0 | 0 |
| 14019 | 3 oz | Moose, rstd | 85 | 114 | 68 | 24.9 | 0.0 | 0.0 | 0.0 | 0.0 | 0.8 | 0.2 | 0.2 | 0.3 | 0.03 | 0.24 | 66 | 0 | 0 | 0 | 0 | 0 |
| 14063 | 4 oz | Muskrat, raw | 113 | 183 | 69 | 23.5 | 0.0 | 0.0 | 0.0 | 0.0 | 9.2 | | | | | | | 0 | 0 | 0 | 0 | 0 |
| 14020 | 3 oz | Muskrat, rstd | 85 | 199 | 56 | 25.6 | 0.0 | 0.0 | 0.0 | 0.0 | 9.9 | | | | | | 103 | 0 | 0 | 0 | 0 | 0 |
| 14021 | 3 oz | Opossum, rstd | 85 | 188 | 58 | 25.7 | 0.0 | 0.0 | 0.0 | 0.0 | 8.7 | 1.0 | 3.2 | 2.5 | 0.06 | 2.48 | 110 | 0 | 0 | 0 | 0 | 0 |
| | | Rabbit | | | | | | | | | | | | | | | | | | | | |
| 14048 | 4 oz | Raw | 113 | 154 | 73 | 22.7 | 0.0 | 0.0 | 0.0 | 0.0 | 6.3 | 1.9 | 1.7 | 1.2 | 0.21 | 0.94 | 64 | 0 | 0 | 0 | 0 | 0 |
| 14004 | 3 oz | Roasted | 85 | 167 | 61 | 24.7 | 0.0 | 0.0 | 0.0 | 0.0 | 6.8 | 2.0 | 1.8 | 1.3 | 0.23 | 1.02 | 70 | 0 | 0 | 0 | 0 | 0 |
| 14049 | 3 oz | Stewed | 85 | 175 | 59 | 25.8 | 0.0 | 0.0 | 0.0 | 0.0 | 7.1 | 2.1 | 1.9 | 1.4 | 0.29 | 1.10 | 73 | 0 | 0 | 0 | 0 | 0 |
| 14023 | 3 oz | Raccoon, rstd | 85 | 217 | 54 | 24.8 | 0.0 | 0.0 | 0.0 | 0.0 | 12.3 | 3.5 | 4.4 | 1.8 | 0.12 | 1.40 | 82 | 0 | 0 | 0 | 0 | 0 |
| 14051 | 4 oz | Squirrel, raw | 113 | 136 | 74 | 24.0 | 0.0 | 0.0 | 0.0 | 0.0 | 3.6 | 0.4 | 1.3 | 1.1 | 0.02 | 1.04 | 94 | 0 | 0 | 0 | 0 | 0 |
| 14024 | 3 oz | Squirrel, rstd | 85 | 147 | 62 | 26.2 | 0.0 | 0.0 | 0.0 | 0.0 | 4.0 | 0.7 | 1.1 | 1.2 | 0.10 | 1.13 | 103 | 0 | 0 | 0 | 0 | 0 |
| | | Venison | | | | | | | | | | | | | | | | | | | | |
| 14043 | 1 ea | Chop, ckd | 89 | 184 | 60 | 25.8 | 0.0 | 0.0 | 0.0 | 0.0 | 8.3 | 2.5 | 3.3 | 2.0 | | | 95 | 0 | 0 | 0 | 0 | 0 |
| 14033 | 2 pce | Jerky | 28 | 95 | 27 | 9.5 | 4.1 | 0.0 | | | 4.3 | 1.7 | 1.8 | 0.6 | | | 38 | 0 | 0 | 0 | 0 | 0 |

| Code | Description | Thiamin (mg) | Riboflavin (mg) | Niacin (NE) | Vit B6 (mg) | Vit B12 (mcg) | Folate (mcg) | Panto (mg) | Vit C (mg) | Vit D (mg) | Vit E (α TE) | Calcium (mg) | Copper (mg) | Iron (mg) | Magnes (mg) | Mang (mg) | Phos (mg) | Potassium (mg) | Selenium (mcg) | Sodium (mg) | Zinc (mg) |
|---|---|---|---|---|---|---|---|---|---|---|---|---|---|---|---|---|---|---|---|---|---|
| | | Vitamins | | | | | | | | | | Minerals | | | | | | | | | |
| 10833 | Chuck, arm pot roast, raw | 0.12 | 0.20 | 3.72 | 0.44 | 3.50 | 7.9 | 0.35 | 0.0 | | | 8 | 0.1 | 2.4 | 23 | 0.0 | 200 | 355 | | 68 | 4.66 |
| 10840 | Chuck, blade pot roast, brsd | 0.06 | 0.20 | 2.07 | 0.22 | 1.95 | 4.3 | 0.26 | 0.0 | | | 11 | 0.1 | 2.7 | 16 | 0.0 | 172 | 198 | | 55 | 7.15 |
| 10839 | Chuck, blade pot roast, raw | 0.11 | 0.19 | 2.46 | 0.41 | 3.84 | 5.7 | 0.33 | 0.0 | | | 11 | 0.1 | 2.3 | 19 | 0.0 | 183 | 306 | | 77 | 5.63 |
| 11487 | Porterhouse Steak, ckd | 0.09 | 0.19 | 3.46 | 0.30 | 1.83 | 6.0 | 0.26 | 0.0 | | | 7 | 0.1 | 2.3 | 20 | 0.0 | 159 | 273 | | 54 | 3.89 |
| 11486 | Porterhouse Steak, raw | 0.11 | 0.19 | 4.00 | 0.43 | 3.07 | 6.8 | 0.35 | 0.0 | | | 7 | 0.1 | 2.2 | 21 | 0.0 | 192 | 338 | | 60 | 3.60 |
| 10859 | Ribs, large end 6-9, ckd | 0.06 | 0.14 | 2.36 | 0.20 | 2.46 | 5.1 | 0.30 | 0.0 | | | 9 | 0.1 | 1.9 | 16 | 0.0 | 155 | 263 | | 54 | 4.31 |
| 10950 | Ribs, large end 6-9, raw | 0.09 | 0.15 | 2.95 | 0.33 | 3.06 | 5.7 | 0.37 | 0.0 | | | 9 | 0.1 | 1.9 | 18 | 0.0 | 173 | 294 | | 62 | 4.24 |
| 10871 | Ribs, small end 10-12, ckd | 0.08 | 0.16 | 3.43 | 0.29 | 2.48 | 6.0 | 0.26 | 0.0 | | | 11 | 0.1 | 1.9 | 19 | 0.0 | 150 | 280 | | 53 | 4.82 |
| 10870 | Ribs, small end 10-12, raw | 0.09 | 0.15 | 3.53 | 0.40 | 3.40 | 5.7 | 0.32 | 0.0 | | | 11 | 0.1 | 2.0 | 19 | 0.0 | 183 | 329 | | 61 | 4.17 |
| 10846 | Ribs, whole 6-12, ckd | 0.07 | 0.14 | 2.78 | 0.23 | 2.46 | 5.1 | 0.28 | 0.0 | | | 9 | 0.1 | 1.9 | 17 | 0.0 | 152 | 268 | | 54 | 4.49 |
| 10845 | Ribs, whole 6-12, raw | 0.07 | 0.11 | 2.38 | 0.26 | 2.40 | 4.3 | 0.26 | 0.0 | | | 8 | 0.1 | 1.5 | 14 | 0.0 | 133 | 231 | | 47 | 3.17 |
| 11410 | Round, bottom, ckd | 0.06 | 0.20 | 3.26 | 0.29 | 2.02 | 8.5 | 0.33 | 0.0 | | | 5 | 0.1 | 2.7 | 20 | 0.0 | 214 | 246 | | 43 | 4.31 |
| 10886 | Round, bottom, raw | 0.12 | 0.20 | 4.40 | 0.60 | 3.16 | 10.2 | 0.47 | 0.0 | | | 6 | 0.1 | 2.5 | 26 | 0.0 | 227 | 389 | | 63 | 3.72 |
| 11425 | Round, tip, ckd | 0.08 | 0.22 | 3.05 | 0.32 | 2.38 | 6.8 | 0.38 | 0.0 | | | 5 | 0.1 | 2.4 | 22 | 0.0 | 196 | 312 | | 54 | 5.67 |
| 11424 | Round, tip , raw | 0.12 | 0.20 | 3.57 | 0.46 | 3.40 | 7.9 | 0.37 | 0.0 | | | 6 | 0.1 | 2.3 | 25 | 0.0 | 218 | 372 | | 66 | 4.98 |
| 11463 | Sirloin, top, ckd | 0.10 | 0.23 | 3.38 | 0.36 | 2.30 | 7.7 | 0.31 | 0.0 | | | 9 | 0.1 | 2.6 | 25 | 0.0 | 192 | 316 | | 54 | 5.07 |
| 10943 | Sirloin, top, raw | 0.14 | 0.24 | 3.70 | 0.45 | 3.32 | 7.9 | 0.37 | 0.0 | | | 8 | 0.1 | 2.7 | 24 | 0.0 | 214 | 363 | | 61 | 4.19 |
| 11491 | T-bone Steak, ckd | 0.09 | 0.19 | 3.52 | 0.30 | 1.84 | 6.0 | 0.26 | 0.0 | | | 7 | 0.1 | 2.4 | 20 | 0.0 | 164 | 286 | | 56 | 3.98 |
| 11490 | T-bone Steak, raw | 0.11 | 0.20 | 4.11 | 0.44 | 3.14 | 6.8 | 0.35 | 0.0 | | | 7 | 0.1 | 2.4 | 23 | 0.0 | 198 | 351 | | 61 | 3.70 |
| 11451 | Tenderloin, ckd | 0.10 | 0.23 | 3.03 | 0.33 | 2.07 | 5.1 | 0.29 | 0.0 | | | 7 | 0.1 | 2.7 | 22 | 0.0 | 182 | 318 | | 51 | 4.22 |
| 10931 | Tenderloin, raw | 0.14 | 0.24 | 3.36 | 0.42 | 2.92 | 6.8 | 0.34 | 0.0 | | | 8 | 0.1 | 2.6 | 21 | 0.0 | 203 | 340 | | 55 | 3.41 |
| 11432 | Top Round, ckd | 0.09 | 0.22 | 4.92 | 0.46 | 2.07 | 10.2 | 0.40 | 0.0 | | | 5 | 0.1 | 2.4 | 26 | 0.0 | 201 | 360 | | 51 | 4.54 |
| 10907 | Top Round, raw | 0.11 | 0.20 | 4.71 | 0.55 | 3.11 | 10.2 | 0.40 | 0.0 | | | 3 | 0.1 | 2.3 | 27 | 0.0 | 236 | 409 | | 56 | 3.11 |
| | Steaks, Prepared | | | | | | | | | | | | | | | | | | | | |
| 10083 | Battered, fried | 0.30 | 0.67 | 7.69 | 0.86 | 6.43 | 21.0 | 0.87 | 0.2 | 0.7 | | 131 | 0.3 | 7.1 | 63 | 0.0 | 576 | 846 | | 812 | 10.81 |
| 10084 | Battered, fried, lean | 0.23 | 0.50 | 5.76 | 0.66 | 4.77 | 15.6 | 0.66 | 0.2 | 0.5 | | 89 | 0.2 | 5.4 | 48 | 0.0 | 429 | 642 | | 558 | 8.32 |
| 10080 | Breaded, brld | 0.33 | 0.67 | 8.72 | 0.85 | 6.33 | 28.1 | 0.86 | 0.1 | 0.7 | | 78 | 0.3 | 7.9 | 68 | 0.0 | 503 | 838 | | 816 | 10.76 |
| 10082 | Breaded, brld, lean | 0.25 | 0.50 | 6.46 | 0.65 | 4.70 | 21.0 | 0.58 | 0.1 | 0.5 | | 51 | 0.2 | 5.9 | 51 | 0.0 | 379 | 637 | | 561 | 8.29 |
| 11678 | Broiled | 0.08 | 0.19 | 3.86 | 0.33 | 2.07 | 7.0 | | 0.0 | 0.3 | | 8 | 0.1 | 2.2 | 21 | | 176 | 309 | | 247 | 4.38 |
| 11679 | Broiled, lean | 0.09 | 0.20 | 4.44 | 0.39 | 2.15 | 7.9 | | 0.0 | 0.3 | | 8 | 0.1 | 2.3 | 25 | | 192 | 348 | | 252 | 4.94 |
| 10740 | Cube, Kings Command Foods | 0.09 | 0.16 | 4.13 | 0.21 | 1.85 | 17.8 | | 0.0 | | | 20 | | 2.2 | | | 121 | 316 | | 38 | 5.00 |
| 10072 | Fried | 0.17 | 0.41 | 6.88 | 0.77 | 5.01 | 16.1 | 0.61 | 0.0 | 0.5 | | 14 | 0.2 | 4.8 | 46 | 0.0 | 387 | 675 | | 459 | 7.42 |
| 10079 | Fried, lean | 0.15 | 0.35 | 5.77 | 0.65 | 4.12 | 13.6 | 0.51 | 0.0 | 0.4 | | 9 | 0.2 | 4.0 | 40 | 0.0 | 326 | 572 | | 356 | 6.28 |
| 10738 | Pepper, Kings Command Foods | 0.10 | 0.15 | 3.85 | 0.21 | 1.69 | 18.8 | | 4.7 | | | 22 | | 2.2 | | | 114 | 325 | | 161 | 4.78 |
| | *GAME MEATS* | | | | | | | | | | | | | | | | | | | | |
| 14052 | Antelope, raw | 0.36 | 0.66 | | | | | | 0.0 | 0.3 | | 3 | 0.2 | 3.6 | 31 | 0.0 | 212 | 399 | | 58 | 1.45 |
| 14053 | Antelope, rstd | 0.22 | 0.62 | | | | | | 0.0 | 0.3 | | 3 | 0.2 | 3.6 | 24 | 0.0 | 179 | 316 | | 46 | 1.43 |
| 14006 | Bear, ckd | 0.09 | 0.70 | 2.85 | 0.25 | 2.10 | 5.1 | | 0.0 | 0.3 | | 4 | 0.1 | 9.1 | 20 | | 145 | 224 | | 60 | 8.76 |
| 14054 | Bear, raw | 0.18 | 0.77 | 3.62 | 0.21 | 1.82 | 4.4 | | 0.0 | 0.3 | | 3 | 0.1 | 7.5 | 17 | | 171 | 193 | | 52 | 7.58 |
| 14055 | Beaver, raw | 0.07 | 0.25 | 2.15 | 0.44 | 7.72 | .10.2 | 0.87 | 2.3 | 0.3 | | 17 | 0.2 | 7.8 | 28 | | 268 | 393 | | 58 | 2.11 |
| 14007 | Beaver, rstd | 0.04 | 0.26 | 1.87 | 0.40 | 7.06 | 9.4 | 0.79 | 2.6 | 0.3 | | 19 | 0.2 | 8.5 | 25 | | 248 | 343 | | 50 | 1.93 |
| 14067 | Beefalo, raw | 0.05 | 0.10 | 5.24 | 0.40 | 2.73 | 17.0 | 0.62 | 7.9 | 0.3 | | 20 | 0.1 | 2.6 | 28 | 0.0 | 253 | 493 | | 88 | 5.49 |
| 14008 | Beefalo, rstd | 0.03 | 0.09 | 4.16 | 0.34 | 2.17 | 15.3 | 0.49 | 7.7 | 0.3 | | 20 | 0.1 | 2.6 | 0 | 0.0 | 213 | 390 | | 70 | 5.44 |
| 14056 | Bison, raw | 0.11 | 0.26 | 3.54 | 0.40 | 2.73 | 8.1 | 0.62 | 0.0 | 0.3 | | 7 | 0.1 | 2.9 | 28 | 0.0 | 211 | 388 | | 61 | 3.16 |
| 14009 | Bison, rstd | 0.09 | 0.23 | 3.15 | 0.34 | 2.43 | 6.8 | 0.49 | 0.0 | 0.3 | | 7 | 0.1 | 2.9 | 22 | 0.0 | 178 | 307 | | 48 | 3.13 |
| 14057 | Boar, raw | 0.44 | 0.12 | 4.52 | 0.45 | 0.63 | 6.2 | 0.88 | 0.0 | 0.3 | | 14 | 0.0 | 1.0 | 24 | 0.0 | 136 | 341 | | 52 | 2.59 |
| 14010 | Boar, rstd | 0.26 | 0.12 | 3.58 | 0.36 | 0.60 | 5.1 | 0.70 | 0.0 | 0.3 | | 14 | 0.0 | 1.0 | 23 | 0.0 | 114 | 337 | | 51 | 2.56 |
| 14059 | Caribou, raw | 0.36 | 0.81 | 6.22 | 0.42 | 7.13 | 4.5 | 2.88 | 0.0 | 0.3 | | 19 | 0.3 | 5.3 | 29 | 0.1 | 235 | 333 | | 64 | 4.52 |
| 14012 | Caribou, rstd | 0.21 | 0.76 | 4.92 | 0.27 | 5.64 | 4.3 | 2.28 | 2.6 | 0.3 | | 19 | 0.2 | 5.2 | 23 | 0.1 | 198 | 264 | | 51 | 4.47 |
| 14061 | Elk, raw | 0.32 | 0.73 | 5.54 | 0.37 | 6.33 | 4.1 | 2.59 | 0.0 | 0.3 | | 5 | 0.1 | 3.1 | 26 | 0.0 | 182 | 353 | | 66 | 2.71 |
| 14014 | Elk, rstd | 0.19 | 0.68 | 4.93 | 0.21 | 5.53 | 3.4 | 1.53 | 0.0 | 0.3 | | 4 | 0.1 | 3.1 | 20 | 0.0 | 153 | 279 | | 52 | 2.69 |
| 14005 | Frog legs, raw | 0.13 | 0.24 | 1.15 | 0.12 | 0.38 | 11.5 | 0.36 | 0.0 | 0.3 | | 17 | 0.2 | 1.4 | 19 | | 141 | 274 | | 56 | 1.34 |
| 14029 | Frog legs, stmd | 0.19 | 0.34 | 1.57 | 0.16 | 0.52 | 16.3 | 0.50 | 0.0 | 0.3 | | 26 | 0.3 | 2.0 | 29 | | 160 | 372 | | 84 | 1.45 |
| 14026 | Horse, raw | 0.15 | 0.11 | 5.20 | 0.43 | 3.39 | 2.3 | 0.16 | 1.1 | 0.3 | | 7 | 0.2 | 4.3 | 27 | 0.0 | 250 | 407 | | 60 | 3.28 |
| 14018 | Horse, rstd | 0.09 | 0.10 | 4.11 | 0.28 | 2.69 | 1.5 | 0.11 | 1.7 | 0.3 | | 7 | 0.1 | 4.3 | 21 | 0.0 | 210 | 322 | | 47 | 3.25 |
| 14062 | Moose, raw | 0.07 | 0.31 | 5.65 | 0.34 | 5.76 | 4.0 | | 4.5 | 0.3 | | 6 | 0.1 | 3.6 | 26 | 0.0 | 179 | 358 | | 73 | 3.16 |
| 14019 | Moose, rstd | 0.04 | 0.29 | 4.47 | 0.31 | 5.36 | 3.4 | | 4.3 | 0.3 | | 5 | 0.1 | 3.6 | 20 | 0.0 | 150 | 284 | | 59 | 3.13 |
| 14063 | Muskrat, raw | 0.10 | 0.59 | 7.01 | 0.40 | 6.89 | 10.2 | 0.79 | 5.7 | 0.3 | | 28 | 0.2 | 5.8 | 25 | 0.0 | 249 | 312 | | 93 | 1.86 |
| 14020 | Muskrat, rstd | 0.07 | 0.60 | 6.11 | 0.40 | 7.06 | 9.4 | 0.79 | 6.0 | 0.3 | | 31 | 0.2 | 6.0 | 22 | 0.0 | 230 | 272 | | 81 | 1.93 |
| 14021 | Opossum, rstd | 0.09 | 0.31 | 7.17 | 0.40 | 7.06 | 8.5 | | 0.0 | 0.3 | | 14 | 0.2 | 3.9 | 29 | | 236 | 372 | | 49 | 1.94 |
| | Rabbit | | | | | | | | | | | | | | | | | | | | |
| 14048 | Raw | 0.11 | 0.17 | 8.22 | 0.56 | 8.09 | 9.0 | 0.90 | 0.0 | 0.3 | | 15 | 0.2 | 1.8 | 21 | 0.0 | 241 | 373 | | 46 | 1.77 |
| 14004 | Roasted | 0.08 | 0.18 | 7.17 | 0.40 | 7.06 | 9.4 | 0.79 | 0.0 | 0.3 | | 16 | 0.2 | 1.9 | 18 | 0.0 | 224 | 326 | 0.9 | 40 | 1.93 |
| 14049 | Stewed | 0.05 | 0.14 | 6.09 | 0.29 | 5.53 | 7.7 | 0.57 | 0.0 | 0.3 | | 17 | 0.1 | 2.0 | 17 | 0.0 | 192 | 255 | | 31 | 2.01 |
| 14023 | Raccoon, rstd | 0.50 | 0.44 | 3.98 | 0.40 | 7.06 | 9.4 | | 0.0 | 0.3 | | 12 | 0.2 | 6.0 | 26 | | 222 | 338 | | 67 | 1.93 |
| 14051 | Squirrel, raw | 0.08 | 0.24 | 4.52 | 0.36 | 6.34 | 8.9 | 0.92 | 0.0 | 0.3 | | 2 | 0.1 | 5.3 | 27 | 0.0 | 194 | 344 | | 116 | 1.73 |
| 14024 | Squirrel, rstd | 0.05 | 0.25 | 3.94 | 0.31 | 5.53 | 7.7 | 0.79 | 0.0 | 0.3 | | 3 | 0.1 | 5.8 | 24 | 0.0 | 179 | 299 | | 101 | 1.51 |
| | Venison | | | | | | | | | | | | | | | | | | | | |
| 14043 | Chop, ckd | 0.17 | 0.49 | 5.73 | 0.25 | 5.67 | 3.8 | | 0.0 | 0.3 | | 6 | 0.3 | 3.6 | 22 | 0.0 | 205 | 303 | | 310 | 2.35 |
| 14033 | Jerky | 0.05 | 0.19 | 1.98 | 0.08 | 1.83 | 1.6 | | 0.0 | 0.1 | | 3 | 0.1 | 1.4 | 8 | 0.0 | 71 | 106 | | 820 | 0.87 |

| Code | Amount | | Description | Basic Components | | | | | | | | | Additional Fats | | | | | | Vit A & Components | | | | | Vitamins | | | | | | | | | | Minerals | | | | | | | | | |
|---|---|---|---|---|---|---|---|---|---|---|---|---|---|---|---|---|---|---|---|---|---|---|---|---|---|---|---|---|---|---|---|---|---|---|---|---|---|---|---|---|---|---|---|
| | | | | Weight (g) | Calories | % Water | Protein (g) | Carbs (g) | Fiber (g) | Sugar (g) | Other Carbs (g) | Fat (g) | Sat Fat (g) | Mono Fat (g) | Poly Fat (g) | Omega 3 (g) | Omega 6 (g) | Choles (mg) | Vit A (IU) | Vit A (RE) | Retinol (RE) | Carotenoids (RE) | Beta Carotene (mcg) | Thiamin (mg) | Riboflavin (mg) | Niacin (NE) | Vit B6 (mg) | Vit B12 (mcg) | Folate (mcg) | Panto (mg) | Vit C (mg) | Vit D (mg) | Vit E (α TE) | Calcium (mg) | Copper (mg) | Iron (mg) | Magnes (mg) | Mang (mg) | Phos (mg) | Potassium (mg) | Selenium (mcg) | Sodium (mg) | Zinc (mg) |
| 14038 | 1 | pce | Loaf | 108 | 148 | 69 | 21.4 | 6.3 | 0.4 | | | 3.5 | 1.4 | 1.1 | 0.6 | | | 99 | 58 | 16 | 16 | 0 | | 0.16 | 0.49 | 5.17 | 0.18 | 4.05 | 8.9 | | 0.6 | | | 39 | 0.2 | 3.3 | 26 | | 207 | 325 | | 372 | 1.96 |
| 14060 | 4 | oz | Raw | 113 | 136 | 74 | 26.0 | 0.0 | 0.0 | 0.0 | 0.0 | 2.7 | 1.1 | 0.8 | 0.5 | 0.08 | 0.45 | 96 | 0 | 0 | 0 | 0 | 0 | 0.25 | 0.54 | 7.20 | 0.42 | 7.13 | 4.5 | 0.31 | 0.0 | 0.3 | | 6 | 0.3 | 3.8 | 26 | 0.0 | 228 | 359 | | 58 | 2.36 |
| 14044 | 3 | oz | Ribs, ckd | 85 | 146 | 62 | 27.5 | 0.0 | 0.0 | 0.0 | 0.0 | 3.1 | 1.2 | 0.9 | 0.6 | | | 102 | 0 | 0 | 0 | 0 | 0 | 0.15 | 0.55 | 5.73 | 0.22 | 5.30 | 4.6 | | 0.0 | 0.3 | | 6 | 0.3 | 4.1 | 24 | 0.0 | 206 | 305 | | 331 | 2.51 |
| 14013 | 3 | oz | Roasted | 85 | 134 | 65 | 25.7 | 0.0 | 0.0 | 0.0 | 0.0 | 2.7 | 1.1 | 0.7 | 0.5 | 0.08 | 0.45 | 95 | 0 | 0 | 0 | 0 | 0 | 0.15 | 0.51 | 5.70 | 0.32 | 2.70 | 4.0 | 0.27 | 0.0 | 0.3 | | 6 | 0.3 | 3.8 | 20 | 0.0 | 192 | 285 | | 46 | 2.34 |
| 14046 | 1 | ea | Steak, breaded, ckd | 101 | 206 | 58 | 22.6 | 10.7 | 0.6 | 0.5 | 9.5 | 7.4 | 1.8 | 2.0 | 3.0 | | | 104 | 46 | 14 | 0 | 14 | 0 | 0.17 | 0.45 | 5.04 | 0.21 | 4.43 | 10.1 | | 0.0 | 0.3 | | 25 | 0.2 | 3.5 | 23 | 0.0 | 191 | 265 | | 192 | 1.98 |
| 14045 | 1 | cup | Stewed | 140 | 241 | 62 | 45.4 | 0.0 | 0.0 | 0.0 | 0.0 | 5.2 | 2.0 | 1.5 | 1.0 | | | 168 | 0 | 0 | 0 | 0 | 0 | 0.20 | 0.81 | 6.92 | 0.26 | 7.48 | 5.1 | | 0.0 | 0.4 | | 8 | 0.5 | 6.7 | 29 | 0.1 | 259 | 346 | | 515 | 4.13 |
| 14037 | 1 | pce | With gravy | 65 | 77 | 72 | 12.6 | 1.4 | 0.1 | | | 2.0 | 0.8 | 0.7 | 0.3 | | | 44 | 0 | 0 | 0 | 0 | 0 | 0.07 | 0.24 | 2.59 | 0.10 | 2.25 | 2.5 | | 0.0 | | | 5 | 0.2 | 1.9 | 10 | | 95 | 151 | | 631 | 1.34 |
| 14036 | 1 | cup | With tomato sauce | 249 | 229 | 78 | 40.1 | 5.7 | 1.2 | | | 4.3 | 1.6 | 1.2 | 0.3 | | | 144 | 732 | 73 | 0 | 73 | 430 | 0.22 | 0.74 | 6.83 | 0.34 | 6.45 | 9.6 | | 9.8 | | | 17 | 0.6 | 6.4 | 40 | | 249 | 590 | | 523 | 3.75 |
| 14058 | 4 | oz | Water Buffalo, raw | 113 | 112 | 76 | 23.1 | 0.0 | 0.0 | 0.0 | 0.0 | 1.5 | 0.5 | 0.5 | 0.3 | 0.05 | 0.26 | 52 | 0 | 0 | 0 | 0 | 0 | 0.05 | 0.23 | 6.75 | 0.60 | 1.88 | 9.0 | 0.18 | 0.0 | 0.3 | | 14 | 0.2 | 1.8 | 36 | | 223 | 336 | | 60 | 2.18 |
| 14011 | 3 | oz | Water Buffalo, rstd | 85 | 111 | 69 | 22.8 | 0.0 | 0.0 | 0.0 | 0.0 | 1.5 | 0.5 | 0.5 | 0.3 | 0.04 | 0.26 | 52 | 0 | 0 | 0 | 0 | 0 | 0.03 | 0.21 | 5.35 | 0.39 | 1.49 | 7.7 | 0.14 | 0.0 | 0.3 | | 13 | 0.2 | 1.8 | 28 | | 187 | 266 | | 48 | 2.16 |
| | | | *GOAT* | | | | | | | | | | | | | | | | | | | | | | | | | | | | | | | | | | | | | | | | |
| 13670 | 3 | oz | Baked | 85 | 134 | 66 | 21.5 | 0.0 | 0.0 | 0.0 | 0.0 | 4.7 | 2.0 | 1.8 | 0.3 | | | 114 | 0 | 0 | 0 | 0 | 0 | 0.06 | 0.27 | 6.84 | 0.21 | 1.60 | 11.8 | | 0.0 | | | 17 | 0.1 | 0.8 | 20 | | 181 | 263 | | 287 | 3.95 |
| 13530 | 3 | oz | Broiled | 85 | 178 | 58 | 27.7 | 0.0 | 0.0 | 0.0 | 0.0 | 6.6 | 2.8 | 2.5 | 0.4 | 0.03 | 0.36 | 144 | 0 | 0 | 0 | 0 | 0 | 0.05 | 0.30 | 8.44 | 0.22 | 1.37 | 13.5 | 0.72 | 0.0 | | | 31 | 0.1 | 1.1 | 23 | 0.0 | 203 | 240 | | 276 | 3.68 |
| 13531 | 3 | oz | Fried | 85 | 155 | 60 | 28.0 | 0.0 | 0.0 | 0.0 | 0.0 | 3.9 | 1.5 | 1.4 | 0.3 | 0.02 | 0.21 | 90 | 0 | 0 | 0 | 0 | 0 | 0.06 | 0.31 | 10.68 | 0.43 | 1.28 | 13.5 | 0.85 | 0.0 | | | 6 | 0.1 | 0.7 | 27 | 0.0 | 245 | 373 | | 262 | 2.86 |
| 13528 | 4 | oz | Raw | 113 | 123 | 76 | 23.3 | 0.0 | 0.0 | 0.0 | 0.0 | 2.6 | 0.8 | 1.2 | 0.2 | 0.02 | 0.17 | 64 | 0 | 0 | 0 | 0 | 0 | 0.12 | 0.55 | 4.24 | | 1.28 | 5.7 | | 0.0 | 0.3 | | 15 | 0.3 | 3.2 | | 0.0 | 203 | 435 | | 93 | 4.52 |
| 13623 | 3 | oz | Roasted | 85 | 122 | 68 | 23.0 | 0.0 | 0.0 | 0.0 | 0.0 | 2.6 | 0.8 | 1.2 | 0.2 | 0.02 | 0.18 | 64 | 0 | 0 | 0 | 0 | 0 | 0.08 | 0.52 | 3.36 | 0.00 | 1.01 | 4.3 | 0.51 | 0.0 | 0.3 | | 14 | 0.3 | 3.2 | 0 | 0.0 | 171 | 344 | | 73 | 4.48 |
| 14016 | 2 | ea | Roasted, ribs | 92 | 132 | 68 | 24.9 | 0.0 | 0.0 | 0.0 | 0.0 | 2.8 | 0.9 | 1.3 | 0.2 | 0.02 | 0.19 | 69 | 0 | 0 | 0 | 0 | 0 | 0.08 | 0.56 | 3.63 | 0.00 | 1.09 | 4.6 | 0.55 | 0.0 | 0.3 | | 16 | 0.3 | 3.4 | 0 | 0.0 | 185 | 373 | | 79 | 4.85 |
| | | | *LAMB* | | | | | | | | | | | | | | | | | | | | | | | | | | | | | | | | | | | | | | | | |
| 13584 | 1 | oz | Fat, ckd | 28 | 164 | 26 | 2.7 | 0.0 | 0.0 | 0.0 | 0.0 | 16.9 | 8.8 | 6.5 | 0.7 | 0.32 | 0.39 | 31 | 0 | 0 | 0 | 0 | 0 | 0.02 | 0.05 | 2.25 | 0.01 | 0.68 | 0.8 | 0.17 | 0.0 | | | 8 | 0.0 | 0.4 | 3 | 0.0 | 38 | 24 | | 10 | 0.33 |
| 13583 | 1 | oz | Fat, raw | 28 | 179 | 26 | 1.9 | 0.0 | 0.0 | 0.0 | 0.0 | 18.9 | 9.5 | 7.3 | 0.8 | 0.36 | 0.44 | 24 | 0 | 0 | 0 | 0 | 0 | 0.02 | 0.05 | 1.84 | 0.01 | 0.48 | 0.8 | 0.17 | 0.0 | | | 6 | 0.0 | 0.3 | 2 | 0.0 | 24 | 14 | 1.1 | 6 | 0.24 |
| 13524 | 3 | oz | Ground, 20% fat, brld | 85 | 241 | 55 | 21.1 | 0.0 | 0.0 | 0.0 | 0.0 | 16.7 | 6.9 | 7.1 | 1.2 | 0.22 | 0.97 | 82 | 0 | 0 | 0 | 0 | 0 | 0.09 | 0.21 | 5.70 | 0.12 | 2.22 | 16.1 | 0.56 | 0.0 | 0.3 | | 19 | 0.1 | 1.5 | 20 | 0.0 | 171 | 288 | | 69 | 3.97 |
| 13578 | 4 | oz | Ground, 23% fat, raw | 113 | 319 | 60 | 18.8 | 0.0 | 0.0 | 0.0 | 0.0 | 26.4 | 11.5 | 10.8 | 2.1 | 0.47 | 1.62 | 82 | 0 | 0 | 0 | 0 | 0 | 0.12 | 0.24 | 6.73 | 0.15 | 2.61 | 20.3 | 0.73 | 0.0 | | | 18 | 0.1 | 1.8 | 24 | 0.0 | 177 | 251 | 4.3 | 67 | 3.85 |
| | | | Retail Cuts, choice, lean & fat, 1/8" trim | | | | | | | | | | | | | | | | | | | | | | | | | | | | | | | | | | | | | | | | |
| 13628 | 3 | oz | Average, ckd | 85 | 230 | 56 | 21.7 | 0.0 | 0.0 | 0.0 | 0.0 | 15.3 | 6.3 | 6.5 | 1.1 | 0.20 | 0.89 | 82 | 0 | 0 | 0 | 0 | 0 | 0.09 | 0.22 | 5.57 | 0.12 | 2.18 | 16.1 | 0.57 | 0.0 | | | 14 | 0.1 | 1.6 | 20 | 0.0 | 164 | 270 | | 61 | 4.03 |
| 13627 | 4 | oz | Average, raw | 113 | 275 | 63 | 19.8 | 0.0 | 0.0 | 0.0 | 0.0 | 21.1 | 9.1 | 8.6 | 1.7 | 0.37 | 1.30 | 79 | 0 | 0 | 0 | 0 | 0 | 0.14 | 0.25 | 6.86 | 0.16 | 2.76 | 21.5 | 0.77 | 0.0 | | | 14 | 0.1 | 1.8 | 25 | 0.0 | 188 | 270 | | 67 | 3.98 |
| 13630 | 3 | oz | Foreshank, brsd | 85 | 207 | 57 | 24.1 | 0.0 | 0.0 | 0.0 | 0.0 | 11.5 | 4.8 | 4.8 | 0.8 | 0.16 | 0.66 | 90 | 0 | 0 | 0 | 0 | 0 | 0.04 | 0.16 | 4.64 | 0.09 | 1.94 | 14.5 | 0.54 | 0.0 | | | 17 | 0.1 | 1.8 | 19 | 0.0 | 141 | 218 | | 61 | 6.54 |
| 13629 | 4 | oz | Foreshank, raw | 113 | 227 | 67 | 21.4 | 0.0 | 0.0 | 0.0 | 0.0 | 15.1 | 6.6 | 6.2 | 1.2 | 0.27 | 0.92 | 81 | 0 | 0 | 0 | 0 | 0 | 0.11 | 0.21 | 6.18 | 0.17 | 2.64 | 21.5 | 0.78 | 0.0 | | | 12 | 0.1 | 1.9 | 25 | 0.0 | 192 | 242 | | 81 | 5.90 |
| 13633 | 4 | oz | Leg, shank, raw | 113 | 209 | 69 | 21.5 | 0.0 | 0.0 | 0.0 | 0.0 | 13.0 | 5.5 | 5.3 | 1.1 | 0.23 | 0.82 | 76 | 0 | 0 | 0 | 0 | 0 | 0.15 | 0.27 | 7.02 | 0.18 | 2.87 | 23.7 | 0.78 | 0.0 | | | 8 | 0.1 | 2.0 | 28 | 0.0 | 206 | 302 | | 66 | 4.05 |
| 13634 | 3 | oz | Leg, shank, rstd | 85 | 184 | 61 | 22.7 | 0.0 | 0.0 | 0.0 | 0.0 | 9.7 | 3.9 | 4.1 | 0.7 | 0.12 | 0.56 | 77 | 0 | 0 | 0 | 0 | 0 | 0.09 | 0.23 | 5.54 | 0.14 | 2.28 | 19.6 | 0.60 | 0.0 | | | 8 | 0.1 | 1.7 | 21 | 0.0 | 170 | 280 | | 55 | 4.01 |
| 13635 | 4 | oz | Leg, sirloin, raw | 113 | 295 | 61 | 19.4 | 0.0 | 0.0 | 0.0 | 0.0 | 23.5 | 10.3 | 9.7 | 1.9 | 0.42 | 1.44 | 80 | 0 | 0 | 0 | 0 | 0 | 0.15 | 0.26 | 7.16 | 0.16 | 2.83 | 21.5 | 0.79 | 0.0 | | | 11 | 0.1 | 1.8 | 26 | 0.0 | 182 | 266 | | 63 | 3.54 |
| 13636 | 3 | oz | Leg, sirloin, rstd | 85 | 241 | 55 | 21.3 | 0.0 | 0.0 | 0.0 | 0.0 | 16.7 | 7.0 | 7.1 | 1.2 | 0.24 | 0.97 | 82 | 0 | 0 | 0 | 0 | 0 | 0.09 | 0.24 | 5.60 | 0.12 | 2.16 | 14.5 | 0.57 | 0.0 | | | 9 | 0.1 | 1.7 | 20 | 0.0 | 157 | 258 | | 58 | 3.57 |
| 13631 | 4 | oz | Leg, whole, raw | 113 | 236 | 66 | 20.9 | 0.0 | 0.0 | 0.0 | 0.0 | 16.3 | 7.0 | 6.7 | 1.3 | 0.28 | 1.02 | 77 | 0 | 0 | 0 | 0 | 0 | 0.15 | 0.27 | 7.06 | 0.17 | 2.87 | 22.6 | 0.79 | 0.0 | | | 9 | 0.1 | 1.9 | 27 | 0.0 | 198 | 292 | | 64 | 3.88 |
| 13632 | 3 | oz | Leg, whole, rstd | 85 | 206 | 59 | 22.3 | 0.0 | 0.0 | 0.0 | 0.0 | 12.2 | 5.0 | 5.2 | 0.9 | 0.16 | 0.71 | 78 | 0 | 0 | 0 | 0 | 0 | 0.09 | 0.24 | 5.55 | 0.13 | 2.21 | 17.0 | 0.59 | 0.0 | | | 9 | 0.1 | 1.7 | 20 | 0.0 | 165 | 271 | | 57 | 3.85 |
| 13638 | 1 | ea | Loin, steak, brld | 53 | 157 | 53 | 13.8 | 0.0 | 0.0 | 0.0 | 0.0 | 10.9 | 4.6 | 4.6 | 0.8 | 0.15 | 0.63 | 52 | 0 | 0 | 0 | 0 | 0 | 0.06 | 0.14 | 3.74 | 0.07 | 1.31 | 10.1 | 0.34 | 0.0 | | | 11 | 0.1 | 1.0 | 13 | 0.0 | 107 | 178 | | 41 | 1.91 |
| 13637 | 1 | ea | Loin, steak, raw | 79 | 220 | 60 | 13.6 | 0.0 | 0.0 | 0.0 | 0.0 | 18.0 | 7.9 | 7.4 | 1.4 | 0.32 | 1.09 | 57 | 0 | 0 | 0 | 0 | 0 | 0.09 | 0.17 | 5.12 | 0.11 | 1.64 | 14.2 | 0.51 | 0.0 | | | 11 | 0.1 | 1.3 | 17 | 0.0 | 126 | 179 | | 47 | 2.09 |
| 13641 | 3 | oz | Rib, brld | 85 | 289 | 49 | 19.6 | 0.0 | 0.0 | 0.0 | 0.0 | 22.8 | 9.7 | 9.4 | 1.8 | 0.39 | 1.46 | 83 | 0 | 0 | 0 | 0 | 0 | 0.08 | 0.20 | 5.88 | 0.09 | 2.18 | 12.8 | 0.52 | 0.0 | | | 15 | 0.1 | 1.6 | 20 | 0.0 | 156 | 235 | | 65 | 3.58 |
| 13640 | 4 | oz | Rib, raw | 113 | 386 | 54 | 17.3 | 0.0 | 0.0 | 0.0 | 0.0 | 34.7 | 15.1 | 14.2 | 2.7 | 0.62 | 2.11 | 84 | 0 | 0 | 0 | 0 | 0 | 0.11 | 0.21 | 6.85 | 0.14 | 2.42 | 17.0 | 0.70 | 0.0 | | | 16 | 0.1 | 1.6 | 21 | 0.0 | 162 | 227 | | 66 | 3.24 |
| 13642 | 3 | oz | Rib, rstd | 85 | 290 | 50 | 18.5 | 0.0 | 0.0 | 0.0 | 0.0 | 23.4 | 9.9 | 9.9 | 1.7 | 0.34 | 1.35 | 82 | 0 | 0 | 0 | 0 | 0 | 0.08 | 0.18 | 5.67 | 0.10 | 1.89 | 13.6 | 0.54 | 0.0 | | | 19 | 0.1 | 1.4 | 17 | 0.0 | 145 | 235 | | 63 | 3.08 |
| 13648 | 3 | oz | Shoulder, arm, steak, brsd | 85 | 286 | 45 | 26.4 | 0.0 | 0.0 | 0.0 | 0.0 | 19.3 | 7.8 | 8.2 | 1.4 | 0.24 | 1.12 | 102 | 0 | 0 | 0 | 0 | 0 | 0.06 | 0.21 | 5.62 | 0.09 | 2.20 | 16.1 | 0.52 | 0.0 | | | 21 | 0.1 | 2.1 | 22 | 0.0 | 179 | 264 | | 61 | 5.30 |
| 13649 | 3 | oz | Shoulder, arm, steak, brld | 85 | 229 | 56 | 21.2 | 0.0 | 0.0 | 0.0 | 0.0 | 15.4 | 6.5 | 6.3 | 1.2 | 0.26 | 0.98 | 82 | 0 | 0 | 0 | 0 | 0 | 0.09 | 0.23 | 5.94 | 0.10 | 2.45 | 16.1 | 0.58 | 0.0 | | | 15 | 0.1 | 1.8 | 23 | 0.0 | 170 | 267 | | 66 | 4.26 |
| 13647 | 1 | ea | Shoulder, arm, steak, raw | 84 | 205 | 63 | 14.4 | 0.0 | 0.0 | 0.0 | 0.0 | 15.9 | 6.9 | 6.5 | 1.3 | 0.29 | 0.97 | 59 | 0 | 0 | 0 | 0 | 0 | 0.09 | 0.18 | 5.11 | 0.11 | 2.07 | 16.0 | 0.58 | 0.0 | | | 12 | 0.1 | 1.3 | 18 | 0.0 | 136 | 205 | | 51 | 2.96 |
| 13652 | 3 | oz | Shoulder, blade, brsd | 85 | 288 | 46 | 24.6 | 0.0 | 0.0 | 0.0 | 0.0 | 20.3 | 8.4 | 8.3 | 1.7 | 0.34 | 1.33 | 99 | 0 | 0 | 0 | 0 | 0 | 0.05 | 0.18 | 5.10 | 0.09 | 2.41 | 15.3 | 0.52 | 0.0 | | | 23 | 0.1 | 2.0 | 20 | 0.0 | 159 | 207 | | 64 | 5.93 |
| 13653 | 3 | oz | Shoulder, blade, brld | 85 | 227 | 57 | 20.0 | 0.0 | 0.0 | 0.0 | 0.0 | 15.7 | 6.4 | 6.7 | 1.1 | 0.19 | 0.91 | 81 | 0 | 0 | 0 | 0 | 0 | 0.08 | 0.21 | 5.38 | 0.13 | 2.33 | 15.3 | 0.57 | 0.0 | | | 20 | 0.1 | 1.5 | 20 | 0.0 | 171 | 290 | | 71 | 4.90 |
| 13651 | 4 | oz | Shoulder, blade, raw | 113 | 276 | 63 | 19.2 | 0.0 | 0.0 | 0.0 | 0.0 | 21.5 | 9.1 | 8.8 | 1.7 | 0.36 | 1.37 | 80 | 0 | 0 | 0 | 0 | 0 | 0.12 | 0.24 | 6.10 | 0.16 | 2.96 | 22.6 | 0.77 | 0.0 | | | 19 | 0.1 | 1.7 | 24 | 0.0 | 184 | 264 | | 71 | 4.97 |
| 13654 | 3 | oz | Shoulder, blade, rstd | 85 | 230 | 57 | 19.2 | 0.0 | 0.0 | 0.0 | 0.0 | 16.3 | 6.8 | 6.7 | 1.3 | 0.27 | 1.07 | 78 | 0 | 0 | 0 | 0 | 0 | 0.08 | 0.20 | 4.96 | 0.11 | 2.28 | 17.9 | 0.60 | 0.0 | | | 18 | 0.1 | 1.7 | 20 | 0.0 | 157 | 211 | | 57 | 4.86 |
| 13644 | 3 | oz | Shoulder, whole, brsd | 85 | 287 | 46 | 25.1 | 0.0 | 0.0 | 0.0 | 0.0 | 20.1 | 8.3 | 8.3 | 1.6 | 0.31 | 1.28 | 99 | 0 | 0 | 0 | 0 | 0 | 0.06 | 0.19 | 5.23 | 0.09 | 2.36 | 15.3 | 0.52 | 0.0 | | | 23 | 0.1 | 2.0 | 21 | 0.0 | 164 | 222 | | 63 | 5.78 |
| 13645 | 3 | oz | Shoulder, whole, brld | 85 | 228 | 57 | 20.2 | 0.0 | 0.0 | 0.0 | 0.0 | 15.6 | 6.4 | 6.6 | 1.1 | 0.21 | 0.93 | 81 | 0 | 0 | 0 | 0 | 0 | 0.09 | 0.22 | 5.52 | 0.12 | 2.36 | 15.3 | 0.58 | 0.0 | | | 20 | 0.1 | 1.6 | 21 | 0.0 | 171 | 285 | | 70 | 4.74 |
| 13643 | 4 | oz | Shoulder, whole, raw | 113 | 276 | 63 | 19.3 | 0.0 | 0.0 | 0.0 | 0.0 | 21.5 | 9.2 | 8.8 | 1.7 | 0.37 | 1.35 | 80 | 0 | 0 | 0 | 0 | 0 | 0.12 | 0.24 | 6.35 | 0.16 | 2.90 | 21.5 | 0.77 | 0.0 | | | 18 | 0.1 | 1.7 | 24 | 0.0 | 184 | 268 | | 71 | 4.66 |
| 13646 | 3 | oz | Shoulder, whole, rstd | 85 | 229 | 57 | 19.3 | 0.0 | 0.0 | 0.0 | 0.0 | 16.2 | 6.8 | 6.6 | 1.3 | 0.27 | 1.05 | 77 | 0 | 0 | 0 | 0 | 0 | 0.08 | 0.20 | 5.13 | 0.11 | 2.25 | 17.9 | 0.60 | 0.0 | | | 17 | 0.1 | 1.7 | 20 | 0.0 | 157 | 213 | | 56 | 4.62 |
| | | | *LUNCHMEATS AND SAUSAGES* | | | | | | | | | | | | | | | | | | | | | | | | | | | | | | | | | | | | | | | | |
| | | | Beef Lunchmeat | | | | | | | | | | | | | | | | | | | | | | | | | | | | | | | | | | | | | | | | |
| 13002 | 1 | pce | Bologna, avg | 23 | 72 | 55 | 2.8 | 0.2 | 0.0 | 0.2 | 0.0 | 6.6 | 2.8 | 3.2 | 0.3 | 0.06 | 0.20 | 13 | 0 | 0 | 0 | 0 | 0 | 0.01 | 0.03 | 0.55 | 0.03 | 0.33 | 1.1 | 0.06 | 0.0 | 0.2 | | 3 | 0.0 | 0.4 | 3 | 0.0 | 20 | 36 | 2.6 | 225 | 0.50 |
| 13069 | 1 | pce | Bologna, lebanon, avg | 23 | 49 | 61 | 4.4 | 0.6 | 0.0 | 0.6 | 0.0 | 3.0 | 1.3 | 1.4 | 0.1 | 0.03 | 0.11 | 16 | 0 | 0 | 0 | 0 | 0 | 0.01 | 0.04 | 1.00 | 0.06 | 0.59 | 0.7 | 0.12 | 0.0 | 0.2 | | 3 | 0.0 | 0.6 | 4 | 0.0 | 35 | 69 | 3.7 | 308 | 0.92 |
| 13176 | 1 | pce | Bologna, light, Oscar Mayer | 28 | 56 | 65 | 3.3 | 1.7 | 0.0 | 0.6 | 1.1 | 4.0 | 1.6 | 2.0 | 0.1 | 0.01 | 0.13 | 13 | 0 | 0 | 0 | 0 | 0 | | | | | | | | 0.0 | | | 4 | 0.1 | 0.3 | 4 | | 50 | 44 | | 314 | 0.53 |
| 13275 | 1 | pce | Bologna, low sod, avg | 23 | 72 | 55 | 2.7 | 0.5 | 0.0 | | | 6.5 | 2.7 | 3.1 | 0.2 | | | 13 | 0 | 0 | 0 | 0 | 0 | 0.01 | 0.03 | 0.60 | 0.04 | 0.32 | 1.1 | | 4.4 | | | 3 | 0.0 | 0.3 | 2 | | 19 | 36 | | 157 | 0.46 |
| 13177 | 1 | pce | Bologna, Oscar Mayer | 28 | 89 | 54 | 3.1 | 0.7 | 0.0 | 0.4 | 0.3 | 8.2 | 3.6 | 4.3 | 0.3 | 0.07 | 0.25 | 20 | 0 | 0 | 0 | 0 | 0 | 0.01 | 0.03 | 0.68 | 0.05 | 0.40 | 3.7 | 0.08 | 0.0 | 9.0 | | 3 | 0.0 | 0.4 | 4 | 4.0 | 31 | 47 | | 310 | 0.57 |
| 13100 | 1 | oz | Jellied, cured, avg | 28 | 31 | 75 | 5.3 | 0.0 | 0.0 | 0.0 | 0.0 | 0.9 | 0.4 | 0.4 | 0.0 | 0.01 | 0.04 | 10 | 0 | 0 | 0 | 0 | 0 | 0.04 | 0.08 | 1.36 | 0.07 | 1.44 | 2.0 | 0.19 | 0.0 | | | 3 | 0.0 | 1.0 | 5 | 0.0 | 39 | 113 | 4.6 | 370 | 0.99 |
| 13039 | 1 | pce | Loaf, corned beef, jellied, avg | 28 | 43 | 69 | 6.4 | 0.0 | 0.0 | 0.0 | 0.0 | 1.7 | 0.7 | 0.8 | 0.1 | 0.02 | 0.07 | 13 | 0 | 0 | 0 | 0 | 0 | 0.00 | 0.03 | 0.49 | 0.03 | 0.36 | 2.2 | 0.05 | 0.0 | 0.1 | | 3 | 0.0 | 0.6 | 3 | 0.0 | 20 | 28 | 4.8 | 267 | 1.15 |
| 13038 | 1 | pce | Loaf, pork barbecue, avg | 23 | 40 | 65 | 3.6 | 1.5 | 0.0 | 0.5 | 0.9 | 2.0 | 0.7 | 1.0 | 0.2 | 0.02 | 0.17 | 9 | 16 | 2 | 0 | 2 | | 0.08 | 0.06 | 0.52 | 0.06 | 0.39 | 2.1 | 0.36 | 0.0 | 0.2 | | 13 | 0.0 | 0.3 | 4 | 0.0 | 30 | 76 | 4.9 | 307 | 0.57 |
| 13067 | 1 | pce | Loaf, slice, avg | 28 | 86 | 52 | 4.0 | 0.8 | 0.0 | 0.8 | 0.0 | 7.3 | 3.1 | 3.4 | 0.2 | 0.06 | 0.18 | 18 | 0 | 0 | 0 | 0 | 0 | 0.03 | 0.06 | 1.02 | 0.05 | 1.09 | 1.4 | 0.15 | 0.0 | 0.3 | | 3 | 0.0 | 0.6 | 4 | 0.0 | 33 | 58 | 6.2 | 372 | 0.71 |
| 13101 | 1 | oz | Pastrami, avg | 28 | 98 | 47 | 4.8 | 0.9 | 0.0 | 0.3 | 0.6 | 8.2 | 2.9 | 4.1 | 0.3 | 0.06 | 0.22 | 26 | 0 | 0 | 0 | 0 | 0 | 0.03 | 0.05 | 1.42 | 0.05 | 0.49 | 2.0 | 0.08 | 0.0 | | | 3 | 0.0 | 0.5 | 5 | 0.0 | 42 | 64 | 2.9 | 344 | 1.19 |
| 13166 | 2 | pce | Roast Beef, pouch, Oscar Mayer | 26 | 30 | 72 | 5.3 | 0.3 | 0.0 | 0.1 | 0.3 | 0.8 | 0.3 | 0.4 | 0.1 | 0.01 | 0.05 | 12 | 0 | 0 | 0 | 0 | 0 | | | | | | | | 0.0 | | | 2 | 0.0 | 0.5 | 6 | | 72 | 85 | | 263 | 0.88 |
| 13035 | 1 | pce | Salami, beerwurst, avg | 23 | 76 | 53 | 2.9 | 0.4 | 0.0 | 0.4 | 0.0 | 6.9 | 3.0 | 3.2 | 0.3 | 0.07 | 0.19 | 14 | 0 | 0 | 0 | 0 | 0 | 0.02 | 0.03 | 0.78 | 0.04 | 0.45 | 0.7 | 0.08 | 0.0 | 0.2 | | 2 | 0.0 | 0.3 | 3 | 0.0 | 22 | 40 | 3.7 | 235 | 0.56 |
| 13023 | 1 | pce | Salami, ckd, avg | 23 | 60 | 58 | 3.5 | 0.6 | 0.0 | 0.3 | 0.4 | 4.8 | 2.1 | 2.2 | 0.2 | 0.05 | 0.18 | 15 | 0 | 0 | 0 | 0 | 0 | 0.02 | 0.04 | 0.75 | 0.04 | 0.70 | 0.5 | 0.22 | 0.0 | 0.2 | | 2 | 0.0 | 0.5 | 3 | 0.0 | 26 | 52 | 3.4 | 270 | 0.50 |
| 13215 | 1 | pce | Salami, cotto, avg | 23 | 48 | 65 | 3.3 | 0.4 | 0.0 | 0.3 | 0.2 | 3.6 | 1.5 | 1.6 | 0.2 | 0.05 | 0.14 | 19 | 23 | [illegible] | | | | | | | | | | | 0.0 | | | 2 | 0.1 | 0.6 | 4 | | 52 | 48 | | 301 | 0.48 |
| 13103 | 1 | oz | Smoked, chopped, cured, avg | 28 | 37 | 69 | 5.7 | 0.5 | 0.0 | 0.5 | 0.0 | 1.2 | 0.5 | 0.5 | 0.1 | 0.01 | 0.05 | 13 | 0 | 0 | 0 | 0 | 0 | 0.02 | 0.05 | 1.28 | 0.10 | 0.48 | 2.2 | 0.17 | 0.0 | | | 2 | 0.0 | 0.8 | 6 | 0.0 | 51 | 106 | 5.5 | 352 | 1.10 |
| 13000 | 6 | pce | Thin Sliced, avg | 25 | 44 | 58 | 7.0 | 1.4 | 0.0 | 1.4 | 0.0 | 1.0 | 0.4 | 0.4 | 0.1 | 0.00 | 0.04 | 10 | 0 | 0 | 0 | 0 | 0 | 0.02 | 0.05 | 1.32 | 0.09 | 0.64 | 2.8 | 0.15 | 0.0 | 0.1 | | 3 | 0.0 | 0.7 | 5 | 0.0 | 42 | 107 | 7.1 | 360 | 1.00 |
| | | | Beef & Pork Lunchmeat | | | | | | | | | | | | | | | | | | | | | | | | | | | | | | | | | | | | | | | | |
| 13032 | 1 | pce | Bologna, avg | 23 | 57 | 61 | 3.5 | 0.2 | 0.0 | 0.2 | 0.0 | 4.6 | 1.6 | 2.2 | 0.3 | 0.06 | 0.42 | 14 | 0 | 0 | 0 | 0 | 0 | 0.12 | 0.04 | 0.90 | 0.06 | 0.21 | 1.1 | 0.17 | 0.0 | 0.3 | | 3 | 0.0 | 0.2 | 3 | 0.0 | 32 | 65 | 2.9 | 272 | 0.47 |
| 13251 | 1 | pce | Bologna, fat free, Oscar Mayer | 28 | 22 | 78 | 3.5 | 1.7 | 0.0 | 0.6 | 1.1 | 0.2 | 0.1 | 0.1 | 0.0 | 0.01 | 0.03 | 7 | 0 | 0 | 0 | 0 | 0 | | | | | | | | 0.0 | | | 4 | 0.1 | 0.3 | 6 | | 43 | 44 | | 274 | 0.32 |

| Code | Amount | | Description | Basic Components | | | | | | | | | Additional Fats | | | | | | Vit A & Components | | | | |
|---|---|---|---|---|---|---|---|---|---|---|---|---|---|---|---|---|---|---|---|---|---|---|---|
| | | | | Weight (g) | Calories | % Water | Protein (g) | Carbs (g) | Fiber (g) | Sugar (g) | Other Carbs (g) | Fat (g) | Sat Fat (g) | Mono Fat (g) | Poly Fat (g) | Omega 3 (g) | Omega 6 (g) | Choles (mg) | Vit A (IU) | Vit A (RE) | Retinol (RE) | Carotenoids (RE) | Beta Carotene (mcg) |
| 13175 | 1 | pce | Bologna, garlic, Oscar Mayer | 41 | 130 | 54 | 4.5 | 1.0 | 0.0 | 0.6 | 0.4 | 12.1 | 4.5 | 4.9 | 1.7 | 0.62 | 1.07 | 42 | 0 | 0 | 0 | 0 | 0 |
| 13048 | 1 | pce | Mortadella, avg | 15 | 47 | 52 | 2.5 | 0.5 | 0.0 | 0.5 | 0.0 | 3.8 | 1.4 | 1.7 | 0.5 | 0.03 | 0.44 | 8 | 0 | 0 | 0 | 0 | 0 |
| 13086 | 1 | pce | Mother's Loaf, avg | 21 | 59 | 55 | 2.5 | 1.6 | 0.0 | | | 4.7 | 1.7 | 2.2 | 0.5 | 0.05 | 0.49 | 9 | 0 | 0 | 0 | 0 | 0 |
| 13087 | 1 | pce | Picnic Loaf, avg | 28 | 65 | 60 | 4.2 | 1.3 | 0.0 | | | 4.6 | 1.7 | 2.2 | 0.5 | 0.06 | 0.47 | 11 | 0 | 0 | 0 | 0 | 0 |
| 13024 | 1 | pce | Salami, ckd, avg | 28 | 70 | 60 | 3.9 | 0.6 | 0.0 | 0.6 | 0.0 | 5.6 | 2.3 | 2.6 | 0.6 | 0.11 | 0.45 | 18 | 0 | 0 | 0 | 0 | 0 |
| 13216 | 1 | pce | Salami, cotto, w/chicken, Oscar Mayer | 23 | 56 | 61 | 3.1 | 0.5 | 0.0 | 0.3 | 0.2 | 4.7 | 1.9 | 2.3 | 0.4 | 0.01 | 0.37 | 18 | 0 | 0 | 0 | 0 | 0 |
| 13026 | 3 | pce | Salami, dry, avg | 30 | 125 | 35 | 6.9 | 0.8 | 0.0 | 0.8 | 0.0 | 10.3 | 3.7 | 5.1 | 1.0 | 0.10 | 0.86 | 24 | 0 | 0 | 0 | 0 | 0 |
| 13046 | 1 | pce | Sausage, avg | 23 | 60 | 59 | 3.5 | 0.4 | 0.0 | 0.4 | 0.0 | 4.8 | 1.8 | 2.3 | 0.5 | 0.06 | 0.41 | 15 | 0 | 0 | 0 | 0 | 0 |
| | | | Chicken Lunchmeat | | | | | | | | | | | | | | | | | | | | |
| 13165 | 2 | pce | Breast, honey glazed, thin, avg | 26 | 28 | 70 | 5.2 | 1.1 | 0.0 | 1.1 | 0.1 | 0.3 | 0.1 | 0.2 | 0.1 | 0.01 | 0.06 | 14 | 0 | 0 | 0 | 0 | 0 |
| 13257 | 2 | pce | Breast, roasted, fat free, Oscar Mayer | 26 | 22 | 76 | 4.8 | 0.4 | 0.0 | 0.3 | 0.2 | 0.2 | 0.1 | 0.0 | 0.0 | 0.00 | 0.01 | 12 | 0 | 0 | 0 | 0 | 0 |
| 13222 | 2 | pce | Breast, roasted, Oscar Mayer | 26 | 20 | | 4.5 | 0.5 | 0.0 | 0.0 | 0.5 | 0.0 | 0.0 | 0.0 | 0.0 | 0.00 | 0.00 | 12 | | | | | |
| 13156 | 1 | pce | Breast, smoked, Louis Rich | 28 | 30 | | 5.0 | 1.0 | 0.0 | 0.0 | 1.0 | 1.0 | 0.0 | | | | | 15 | 0 | 0 | 0 | 0 | 0 |
| 13205 | 1 | pce | Olive Loaf, Oscar Mayer | 28 | 74 | 58 | 2.8 | 1.9 | 0.0 | 0.9 | 1.0 | 6.1 | 2.0 | 3.1 | 0.7 | 0.04 | 0.70 | 20 | 0 | 0 | 0 | 0 | 0 |
| 13094 | 1 | pce | Roll, light meat, avg | 28 | 45 | 69 | 5.5 | 0.7 | 0.0 | | | 2.1 | 0.6 | 0.8 | 0.4 | 0.02 | 0.40 | 14 | 23 | 7 | | | |
| 56967 | 1 | ea | Corn Dog, pork & beef, Bryan Foods | 114 | 361 | | 9.0 | 37.1 | | | | 20.1 | | | | | | | | | | | |
| 56968 | 4 | ea | Corn Dog, turkey, bite size, Bryan Foods | 76 | 214 | | 6.7 | 17.4 | | | | 12.0 | | | | | | | | | | | |
| | | | Frankfurters | | | | | | | | | | | | | | | | | | | | |
| 13008 | 1 | ea | Beef, avg | 57 | 180 | 55 | 6.8 | 1.0 | 0.0 | 1.0 | 0.0 | 16.2 | 6.9 | 7.8 | 0.8 | 0.15 | 0.63 | 35 | 0 | 0 | 0 | 0 | 0 |
| 13197 | 1 | ea | Beef, big & juicy, deli, Oscar Mayer | 76 | 237 | 56 | 8.8 | 1.0 | 0.0 | 0.4 | 0.6 | 22.0 | 9.7 | 11.5 | 0.7 | 0.03 | 0.72 | 49 | 0 | 0 | 0 | 0 | 0 |
| 13194 | 1 | ea | Beef, big & juicy, original, Oscar Mayer | 76 | 236 | 56 | 8.7 | 1.0 | 0.0 | 1.0 | 0.0 | 22.0 | 8.6 | 10.0 | 1.4 | 0.08 | 1.30 | 44 | 0 | 0 | 0 | 0 | 0 |
| 13190 | 1 | ea | Beef, bun length, Oscar Mayer | 57 | 184 | 54 | 6.4 | 1.6 | 0.0 | 1.1 | 0.5 | 16.9 | 7.1 | 8.3 | 0.6 | 0.10 | 0.45 | 33 | 0 | 0 | 0 | 0 | 0 |
| 13250 | 1 | ea | Beef, fat free, Oscar Mayer | 50 | 39 | 78 | 6.6 | 2.6 | 0.0 | 1.9 | 0.7 | 0.3 | 0.1 | 0.1 | 0.1 | 0.01 | 0.05 | 15 | 0 | 0 | 0 | 0 | 0 |
| 13272 | 1 | ea | Beef, light, Oscar Mayer | 57 | 110 | 67 | 6.1 | 2.4 | 0.0 | 1.2 | 1.2 | 8.5 | 3.6 | 4.2 | 0.4 | 0.05 | 0.31 | 28 | 0 | 0 | 0 | 0 | 0 |
| 13191 | 1 | ea | Beef, Oscar Mayer | 45 | 143 | 54 | 5.0 | 1.2 | 0.0 | 0.7 | 0.5 | 13.1 | 3.5 | 9.2 | 0.4 | 0.09 | 0.29 | 29 | 41 | 12 | | | |
| 13193 | 1 | ea | Beef, quarter pound, Oscar Mayer | 114 | 350 | | 15.0 | 2.0 | 0.0 | 2.0 | 0.0 | 32.0 | 13.0 | | | | | 65 | | | | | |
| 13009 | 1 | ea | Beef & Pork, avg | 57 | 182 | 54 | 6.4 | 1.5 | 0.0 | 1.1 | 0.3 | 16.6 | 6.2 | 7.8 | 1.6 | 0.22 | 1.33 | 28 | 0 | 0 | 0 | 0 | 0 |
| 13196 | 1 | ea | Beef & Pork, big & juicy, hot 'n spicy, Oscar Mayer | 76 | 218 | 57 | 9.8 | 0.9 | 0.0 | 0.7 | 0.2 | 19.5 | 7.5 | 9.8 | 2.1 | 0.11 | 2.03 | 47 | 0 | 0 | 0 | 0 | 0 |
| 13195 | 1 | ea | Beef & Pork, big & juicy, original, Oscar Mayer | 76 | 236 | 56 | 8.7 | 0.8 | 0.0 | 0.4 | 0.4 | 22.0 | 9.3 | 10.6 | 1.7 | 0.14 | 1.59 | 45 | 0 | 0 | 0 | 0 | 0 |
| 13198 | 1 | ea | Beef & Pork, big & juicy, smokie links, Oscar Mayer | 76 | 218 | 57 | 9.6 | 1.1 | 0.0 | 0.7 | 0.4 | 19.5 | 17.1 | 2.0 | 0.4 | 0.02 | 0.40 | 51 | 0 | 0 | 0 | 0 | 0 |
| 13276 | 1 | ea | Beef & Pork, light, avg | 57 | 127 | 65 | 7.3 | 0.3 | | | | 10.8 | 3.8 | 5.7 | 1.1 | 0.10 | 1.00 | 30 | | | | | |
| 13274 | 1 | ea | Beef & Pork, low salt, avg | 45 | 142 | 57 | 5.4 | 0.8 | 0.0 | | | 12.8 | 5.4 | 6.1 | 0.6 | | | 27 | 0 | 0 | 0 | 0 | 0 |
| 13260 | 1 | ea | Chicken, avg | 45 | 116 | 58 | 5.8 | 3.1 | 0.0 | | | 8.8 | 2.5 | 3.8 | 1.8 | 0.07 | 1.68 | 45 | 59 | 17 | 17 | 0 | 0 |
| 13012 | 1 | ea | Turkey, avg | 45 | 102 | 63 | 6.4 | 0.7 | 0.0 | 0.7 | 0.0 | 8.0 | 2.7 | 2.5 | 2.3 | 0.16 | 2.09 | 48 | 0 | 0 | 0 | 0 | 0 |
| 13132 | 1 | ea | Turkey, bun length, Louis Rich | 57 | 110 | 63 | 7.0 | 2.0 | 0.0 | 1.0 | 1.0 | 8.0 | 2.5 | | | | | 50 | 0 | 0 | 0 | 0 | 0 |
| 13130 | 1 | ea | Turkey, Louis Rich | 45 | 84 | 67 | 5.0 | 2.4 | 0.0 | 0.7 | 1.7 | 6.1 | 1.9 | 2.7 | 1.6 | 0.08 | 1.48 | 41 | 0 | 0 | 0 | 0 | 0 |
| 13217 | 1 | ea | Turkey & Beef, Healthy Favorites | 57 | 60 | | 9.0 | 2.0 | 0.0 | 2.0 | 0.0 | 1.5 | 0.5 | | | | | 25 | | | | | |
| 13192 | 1 | ea | Turkey & Cheese, Oscar Mayer | 45 | 143 | 53 | 5.4 | 1.2 | 0.0 | 0.8 | 0.4 | 12.9 | 11.2 | 1.3 | 0.4 | 0.02 | 0.36 | 33 | 77 | 23 | | | |
| 13188 | 1 | ea | Turkey & Pork, bun length, Oscar Mayer | 57 | 185 | 53 | 6.3 | 1.7 | 0.0 | 1.1 | 0.6 | 17.0 | 5.7 | 8.5 | 2.7 | 0.14 | 2.54 | 35 | 0 | 0 | 0 | 0 | 0 |
| 13187 | 1 | ea | Turkey & Pork, light, Oscar Mayer | 57 | 111 | 67 | 6.9 | 1.6 | 0.0 | 0.9 | 0.7 | 8.5 | 3.2 | 4.1 | 1.2 | 0.06 | 1.17 | 35 | 0 | 0 | 0 | 0 | 0 |
| 13186 | 3 | ea | Turkey & Pork, little wiener, Oscar Mayer | 28 | 87 | 55 | 3.0 | 0.6 | 0.0 | 0.4 | 0.2 | 8.1 | 3.1 | 4.0 | 0.8 | 0.08 | 0.67 | 15 | 0 | 0 | 0 | 0 | 0 |
| 13189 | 1 | ea | Turkey & Pork, Oscar Mayer | 45 | 145 | 53 | 4.9 | 1.3 | 0.0 | 0.8 | 0.5 | 13.3 | 4.5 | 6.7 | 2.1 | 2.00 | 0.10 | 28 | 0 | 0 | 0 | 0 | 0 |
| | | | Ham/Pork Lunchmeat | | | | | | | | | | | | | | | | | | | | |
| 13221 | 2 | pce | Baked, Oscar Mayer | 26 | 23 | 76 | 4.4 | 0.3 | 0.0 | 0.3 | 0.0 | 0.4 | 0.2 | 0.2 | 0.1 | 0.00 | 0.05 | 12 | 0 | 0 | 0 | 0 | 0 |
| 13170 | 1 | pce | Boiled, Oscar Mayer | 21 | 22 | 75 | 3.4 | 0.2 | 0.0 | 0.1 | 0.2 | 0.8 | 0.3 | 0.4 | 0.1 | 0.01 | 0.07 | 10 | | | | | |
| 13164 | 2 | pce | Boiled, thin, Oscar Mayer | 26 | 25 | | 4.5 | 0.0 | 0.0 | 0.0 | 0.0 | 1.0 | 0.3 | | | | | 12 | | | | | |
| 13042 | 1 | pce | Cheese Loaf, avg | 28 | 73 | 58 | 4.6 | 0.4 | 0.0 | 0.3 | 0.1 | 5.7 | 2.1 | 2.6 | 0.6 | 0.08 | 0.53 | 16 | 21 | 6 | | | |
| 13057 | 1 | pce | Chopped, sliced, avg | 21 | 48 | 64 | 3.6 | 0.0 | 0.0 | 0.0 | 0.0 | 3.6 | 1.2 | 1.7 | 0.4 | 0.06 | 0.38 | 11 | 0 | 0 | 0 | 0 | 0 |
| 13033 | 1 | ea | Cured, patty, grilled, avg | 60 | 205 | 51 | 8.0 | 1.0 | 0.0 | 1.0 | 0.0 | 18.5 | 6.7 | 8.8 | 2.0 | 0.19 | 1.80 | 43 | 0 | 0 | 0 | 0 | 0 |
| 13261 | 1 | pce | Extra Lean, 5% fat, sliced, avg | 28 | 37 | 70 | 5.4 | 0.3 | 0.0 | | | 1.4 | 0.5 | 0.7 | 0.1 | 0.01 | 0.12 | 13 | 0 | 0 | 0 | 0 | 0 |
| 13211 | 1 | pce | Head Cheese, Oscar Mayer | 28 | 52 | 68 | 4.4 | 0.0 | 0.0 | 0.0 | 0.0 | 3.8 | 1.3 | 2.1 | 0.4 | 0.05 | 0.35 | 25 | 28 | 8 | | | 0 |
| 13220 | 2 | pce | Honey, Oscar Mayer | 26 | 28 | 73 | 4.4 | 0.9 | 0.0 | 0.9 | 0.0 | 0.7 | 0.2 | 0.4 | 0.1 | 0.00 | 0.06 | 12 | 0 | 0 | 0 | 0 | 0 |
| 13208 | 1 | pce | Honey Loaf, Oscar Mayer | 28 | 33 | 71 | 5.1 | 1.1 | 0.0 | 1.1 | 0.0 | 1.0 | 0.4 | 0.5 | 0.1 | 0.02 | 0.10 | 15 | 0 | 0 | 0 | 0 | 0 |
| 13076 | 2 | pce | Low Salt, sliced, avg | 28 | 46 | 66 | 6.2 | 0.1 | 0.0 | 0.1 | 0.0 | 2.2 | 0.7 | 1.0 | 0.3 | 0.04 | 0.26 | 16 | 0 | 0 | 0 | 0 | 0 |
| 13013 | 1 | pce | Minced, avg | 21 | 55 | 57 | 3.4 | 0.4 | 0.0 | 0.4 | 0.0 | 4.3 | 1.5 | 2.0 | 0.5 | 0.07 | 0.45 | 15 | 0 | 0 | 0 | 0 | 0 |
| 13168 | 1 | pce | 98% Fat Free, lower sod, Oscar Mayer | 21 | 23 | 73 | 3.5 | 0.6 | 0.0 | 0.4 | 0.2 | 0.7 | 0.3 | 0.4 | 0.1 | 0.00 | 0.07 | 9 | 0 | 0 | 0 | 0 | 0 |
| 13049 | 1 | pce | Olive Loaf, avg | 28 | 66 | 58 | 3.3 | 2.6 | 0.0 | 2.6 | 0.0 | 4.6 | 1.6 | 2.2 | 0.5 | 0.03 | 0.51 | 11 | 56 | 6 | | | |
| 13263 | 1 | pce | Regular, 11% fat, avg | 28 | 51 | 65 | 4.9 | 0.9 | 0.0 | | | 3.0 | 0.9 | 1.4 | 0.3 | 0.05 | 0.29 | 16 | 0 | 0 | 0 | 0 | 0 |
| 13031 | 1 | pce | Salami, beerwurst, avg | 23 | 55 | 62 | 3.3 | 0.5 | 0.0 | 0.5 | 0.0 | 4.3 | 1.4 | 2.1 | 0.5 | 0.10 | 0.45 | 14 | 0 | 0 | 0 | 0 | 0 |
| 13090 | 3 | pce | Salami, dry, avg | 30 | 122 | 36 | 6.8 | 0.5 | 0.0 | 0.5 | 0.0 | 10.1 | 3.6 | 4.8 | 1.1 | 0.08 | 1.03 | 24 | 0 | 0 | 0 | 0 | 0 |
| 13219 | 2 | pce | Smoked, Oscar Mayer | 26 | 24 | 76 | 4.4 | 0.2 | 0.0 | 0.1 | 0.1 | 0.7 | 0.2 | 0.3 | 0.1 | 0.00 | 0.05 | 12 | 0 | 0 | 0 | 0 | 0 |
| 13083 | 1 | pce | Liver Cheese Lunchmeat, avg | 38 | 116 | 54 | 5.8 | 0.8 | 0.0 | | | 9.7 | 3.4 | 4.7 | 1.3 | 0.13 | 1.17 | 66 | 6646 | 1996 | | | |
| 13019 | 1 | pce | Liverwurst Lunchmeat, avg | 18 | 59 | 52 | 2.5 | 0.4 | 0.0 | 0.1 | 0.3 | 5.1 | 1.9 | 2.4 | 0.5 | 0.03 | 0.44 | 28 | 4980 | 1494 | 1494 | 0 | 0 |
| 13206 | 1 | pce | Old Fashioned Loaf Lunchmeat, Oscar Mayer | 28 | 65 | 59 | 3.7 | 2.2 | 0.0 | 1.3 | 0.9 | 4.6 | 1.6 | 2.2 | 0.7 | 0.03 | 0.71 | 17 | 0 | 0 | 0 | 0 | 0 |
| | | | Pepperoni | | | | | | | | | | | | | | | | | | | | |
| 13021 | 5 | pce | Average | 28 | 139 | 27 | 5.9 | 0.8 | 0.0 | 0.8 | 0.0 | 12.3 | 4.5 | 5.9 | 1.2 | 0.11 | 1.09 | 22 | 0 | 0 | 0 | 0 | 0 |
| 13073 | 1 | oz | Bits, Oscar Mayer | 28 | 161 | | 15.4 | 1.4 | | | | 8.6 | | | | | | 32 | | | | | |
| 13253 | 14 | pce | Oscar Mayer | 28 | 133 | 31 | 5.1 | 0.2 | 0.0 | 0.1 | 0.1 | 12.5 | 4.8 | 6.2 | 1.1 | 0.17 | 0.95 | 23 | 0 | 0 | 0 | 0 | 0 |
| 13096 | 1 | Tbs | Pate, Chicken Liver, avg | 13 | 26 | 66 | 1.8 | 0.9 | 0.0 | | | 1.7 | 0.5 | 0.7 | 0.3 | 0.01 | 0.29 | 51 | 94 | 28 | | | |
| 13265 | 1 | Tbs | Pate, Goose Liver, smkd, avg | 13 | 60 | 37 | 1.5 | 0.6 | 0.0 | | | 5.7 | 1.9 | 3.3 | 0.1 | 0.00 | 0.11 | 19 | 433 | 130 | | | |

| Code | Vitamins | | | | | | | | | | Minerals | | | | | | | | | |
|---|---|---|---|---|---|---|---|---|---|---|---|---|---|---|---|---|---|---|---|---|
| | Thiamin (mg) | Riboflavin (mg) | Niacin (NE) | Vit B6 (mg) | Vit B12 (mcg) | Folate (mcg) | Panto (mg) | Vit C (mg) | Vit D (mg) | Vit E (α TE) | Calcium (mg) | Copper (mg) | Iron (mg) | Magnes (mg) | Mang (mg) | Phos (mg) | Potassium (mg) | Selenium (mcg) | Sodium (mg) | Zinc (mg) |
| 13175 | | | | | | | | 0.0 | | | 28 | 0.1 | 0.7 | 9 | | 82 | 63 | | 424 | 0.58 |
| 13048 | 0.02 | 0.02 | 0.40 | 0.02 | 0.22 | 0.5 | 0.07 | 0.0 | 0.0 | | 3 | 0.0 | 0.2 | 2 | 0.0 | 15 | 24 | 3.4 | 187 | 0.31 |
| 13086 | 0.12 | 0.04 | 0.66 | 0.04 | 0.22 | 1.7 | 0.10 | 0.2 | 0.2 | | 9 | 0.0 | 0.3 | 3 | 0.0 | 27 | 47 | 7.4 | 237 | 0.30 |
| 13087 | 0.10 | 0.07 | 0.65 | 0.08 | 0.42 | 0.6 | 0.19 | 0.0 | 0.3 | | 13 | 0.0 | 0.3 | 4 | 0.0 | 35 | 75 | 10.0 | 326 | 0.61 |
| 13024 | 0.07 | 0.11 | 0.99 | 0.06 | 1.02 | 0.6 | 0.24 | 0.0 | 0.3 | | 4 | 0.1 | 0.7 | 4 | 0.0 | 32 | 55 | 4.1 | 298 | 0.60 |
| 13216 | | | | | | | | 0.0 | | | 18 | 0.1 | 0.7 | 7 | | 57 | 50 | | 252 | 0.46 |
| 13026 | 0.18 | 0.09 | 1.46 | 0.15 | 0.57 | 0.6 | 0.32 | 0.0 | 0.5 | | 2 | 0.0 | 0.5 | 5 | 0.0 | 43 | 113 | 7.8 | 558 | 0.97 |
| 13046 | 0.05 | 0.04 | 0.81 | 0.05 | 0.45 | 0.7 | 0.09 | 0.0 | 0.1 | | 3 | 0.0 | 0.3 | 3 | 0.0 | 28 | 56 | 3.5 | 272 | 0.56 |
| 13165 | | | | | | | | 0.0 | | | 2 | 0.0 | 0.3 | 9 | | 75 | 86 | | 360 | 0.18 |
| 13257 | | | | | | | | 0.0 | | | 3 | 0.1 | 0.3 | 10 | | 66 | 82 | | 323 | 0.16 |
| 13222 | | | | | | | | | | | | | 0.4 | | | | | | 310 | |
| 13156 | | | | | | | | 0.0 | | | 0 | | 0.0 | | | | | | 360 | |
| 13205 | | | | | | | | 0.0 | | | 31 | 0.1 | 0.5 | 8 | | 37 | 52 | | 369 | 0.29 |
| 13094 | 0.02 | 0.04 | 1.48 | 0.06 | 0.04 | 0.6 | 0.11 | 0.0 | | | 12 | 0.0 | 0.3 | 5 | 0.0 | 44 | 64 | 3.5 | 164 | 0.20 |
| 56967 | | | | | | | | | | | | | | | | | | | 1024 | |
| 56968 | | | | | | | | | | | | | | | | | | | 830 | |
| 13008 | 0.03 | 0.06 | 1.38 | 0.07 | 0.88 | 2.3 | 0.17 | 0.0 | 0.5 | | 11 | 0.0 | 0.8 | 2 | 0.0 | 50 | 95 | 7.9 | 585 | 1.24 |
| 13197 | | | | | | | | 0.0 | | | 14 | 0.2 | 1.4 | 13 | | 119 | 119 | | 677 | 2.03 |
| 13194 | | | | | | | | 0.0 | | | 15 | 0.2 | 1.5 | 14 | | 123 | 108 | | 697 | 1.95 |
| 13190 | | | | | | | | 0.0 | | | 7 | 0.1 | 0.9 | 8 | | 60 | 90 | | 576 | 1.28 |
| 13250 | | | | | | | | 0.0 | | | 10 | 0.1 | 1.0 | 10 | | 64 | 234 | | 484 | 1.21 |
| 13272 | | | | | | | | 0.0 | | | 12 | 0.1 | 0.9 | 10 | | 93 | 239 | | 615 | 1.20 |
| 13191 | 0.02 | 0.05 | 0.99 | 0.05 | 0.51 | 6.9 | 0.03 | 0.0 | 0.3 | | 5 | 0.0 | 0.5 | 6 | 9.0 | 41 | 77 | | 458 | 0.90 |
| 13193 | | | | | | | | | | | 20 | | 2.7 | | | | | | 1050 | |
| 13009 | 0.11 | 0.07 | 1.50 | 0.07 | 0.74 | 2.3 | 0.20 | 0.0 | 0.5 | | 6 | 0.0 | 0.7 | 6 | 0.0 | 49 | 95 | 7.9 | 638 | 1.05 |
| 13196 | | | | | | | | 0.0 | | | 10 | 0.2 | 1.2 | 13 | | 158 | 140 | | 754 | 1.59 |
| 13195 | | | | | | | | 0.0 | | | 12 | 0.2 | 1.1 | 14 | | 93 | 129 | | 681 | 1.54 |
| 13198 | | | | | | | | 0.0 | | | 15 | 0.2 | 1.3 | 20 | | 152 | 136 | | 767 | 1.66 |
| 13276 | | | | | | | | | | | 7 | | 0.5 | 10 | | 114 | 99 | | 623 | 1.05 |
| 13274 | 0.02 | 0.04 | 1.09 | 0.05 | 0.69 | 1.8 | | 10.8 | | | 9 | 0.0 | 0.6 | 1 | | 39 | 75 | | 140 | 0.98 |
| 13260 | 0.03 | 0.05 | 1.39 | 0.14 | 0.11 | 1.8 | 0.37 | 0.0 | | | 43 | 0.0 | 0.9 | 4 | 0.0 | 48 | 38 | 8.3 | 616 | 0.47 |
| 13012 | 0.02 | 0.08 | 1.86 | 0.10 | 0.13 | 3.6 | 0.32 | 0.0 | 0.1 | | 48 | 0.0 | 0.8 | 6 | 0.0 | 60 | 81 | 6.9 | 642 | 1.40 |
| 13132 | | | | | | | | | | | 80 | | 1.4 | | | | | | 630 | |
| 13130 | | | | | | | | 0.0 | | | 59 | 0.1 | 1.0 | 10 | | 66 | 72 | | 511 | 0.89 |
| 13217 | | | | | | | | | | | | | 0.4 | | | | | | 570 | |
| 13192 | | | | | | | | 0.0 | | | 74 | 0.1 | 0.7 | 11 | | 97 | 59 | | 515 | 0.83 |
| 13188 | | | | | | | | 0.0 | | | 34 | 0.2 | 0.6 | 9 | | 83 | 91 | | 566 | 0.99 |
| 13187 | | | | | | | | 0.0 | | | 22 | 0.1 | 0.7 | 10 | | 96 | 226 | | 591 | 1.01 |
| 13186 | 0.07 | 0.04 | 0.75 | 0.03 | 0.35 | 0.6 | 0.11 | 0.0 | 0.4 | | 3 | 0.0 | 0.4 | 3 | | 27 | 45 | | 291 | 0.52 |
| 13189 | | | | | | | | 0.0 | | | 27 | 0.1 | 0.5 | 8 | | 66 | 73 | | 435 | 0.77 |
| 13221 | | | | | | | | 0.0 | | | 2 | 0.1 | 0.4 | 9 | | 64 | 83 | | 322 | 0.61 |
| 13170 | | | | | | | | 0.0 | | | 2 | 0.1 | 0.3 | 6 | | 50 | 59 | | 283 | 0.39 |
| 13164 | | | | | | | | | | | | | 0.4 | | | | | | 340 | |
| 13042 | 0.17 | 0.05 | 0.97 | 0.07 | 0.23 | 0.8 | 0.15 | 0.0 | 0.3 | | 16 | 0.0 | 0.3 | 4 | 0.0 | 71 | 82 | 9.7 | 376 | 0.56 |
| 13057 | 0.13 | 0.04 | 0.81 | 0.07 | 0.19 | 0.2 | 0.06 | 0.0 | 0.2 | | 1 | 0.0 | 0.2 | 3 | 0.0 | 33 | 67 | 3.7 | 288 | 0.41 |
| 13033 | 0.21 | 0.11 | 1.95 | 0.10 | 0.42 | 1.8 | 0.16 | 0.0 | 0.2 | | 5 | 0.1 | 1.0 | 6 | 0.0 | 61 | 146 | 12.7 | 638 | 1.14 |
| 13261 | 0.26 | 0.06 | 1.36 | 0.13 | 0.21 | 1.1 | 0.13 | 0.0 | | | 2 | 0.0 | 0.2 | 5 | 0.0 | 61 | 98 | 4.5 | 400 | 0.54 |
| 13211 | 0.01 | 0.05 | 0.27 | 0.04 | | | | 0.0 | 0.3 | | 5 | 0.1 | 0.4 | 3 | 5.0 | 17 | 9 | | 355 | 0.32 |
| 13220 | | | | | | | | 0.0 | | | 3 | 0.1 | 0.3 | 9 | | 68 | 72 | | 318 | 0.51 |
| 13208 | 0.19 | 0.08 | 1.02 | 0.11 | 0.26 | 2.3 | 0.18 | 0.0 | 0.3 | | 6 | 0.1 | 0.4 | 6 | 6.0 | 50 | 101 | | 378 | 0.74 |
| 13076 | 0.21 | 0.08 | 1.49 | 0.10 | 0.19 | 0.8 | 0.11 | 6.2 | 0.2 | | 2 | 0.0 | 0.4 | 5 | 0.0 | 69 | 101 | 4.6 | 271 | 0.74 |
| 13013 | 0.15 | 0.04 | 0.87 | 0.05 | 0.20 | 0.2 | 0.04 | 0.0 | 0.1 | | 2 | 0.0 | 0.2 | 3 | 0.0 | 33 | 65 | 4.2 | 261 | 0.40 |
| 13168 | | | | | | | | 0.0 | | | 1 | 0.0 | 0.3 | 5 | | 55 | 197 | | 174 | 0.42 |
| 13049 | 0.08 | 0.07 | 0.52 | 0.06 | 0.35 | 0.6 | 0.22 | 0.0 | 0.3 | | 31 | 0.0 | 0.2 | 5 | 0.0 | 36 | 83 | 4.6 | 416 | 0.39 |
| 13263 | 0.24 | 0.07 | 1.47 | 0.10 | 0.23 | 0.8 | 0.13 | 0.0 | | | 2 | 0.0 | 0.3 | 5 | 0.0 | 69 | 93 | 4.6 | 369 | 0.60 |
| 13031 | 0.13 | 0.04 | 0.75 | 0.08 | 0.20 | 0.7 | 0.11 | 0.0 | 0.2 | | 2 | 0.0 | 0.2 | 3 | 0.0 | 24 | 58 | 4.8 | 285 | 0.40 |
| 13090 | 0.28 | 0.10 | 1.68 | 0.17 | 0.84 | 0.6 | 0.32 | 0.0 | 0.3 | | 4 | 0.0 | 0.4 | 7 | 0.0 | 69 | 113 | 7.6 | 678 | 1.26 |
| 13219 | | | | | | | | 0.0 | | | 26 | 0.1 | 0.3 | 8 | | 62 | 66 | | 318 | 0.49 |
| 13083 | 0.08 | 0.85 | 4.48 | 0.18 | 9.35 | 39.5 | 1.35 | 1.1 | 0.4 | | 3 | 0.1 | 4.1 | 5 | 0.1 | 79 | 86 | 13.9 | 465 | 1.41 |
| 13019 | 0.05 | 0.19 | 0.77 | 0.03 | 2.43 | 5.4 | 0.53 | 0.0 | 0.1 | | 5 | 0.0 | 1.2 | 2 | 0.0 | 41 | 31 | 10.4 | 155 | 0.41 |
| 13206 | | | | | | | | 0.0 | | | 32 | 0.0 | 0.4 | 6 | | 58 | 82 | | 332 | 0.52 |
| 13021 | 0.09 | 0.07 | 1.39 | 0.07 | 0.70 | 1.1 | 0.52 | 0.0 | 0.3 | | 3 | 0.0 | 0.4 | 4 | 0.0 | 33 | 97 | 6.7 | 571 | 0.70 |
| 13073 | | | | | | | | | | | | | | | | | 227 | | 1203 | |
| 13253 | | | | | | | | 0.0 | | | 5 | 0.1 | 0.6 | 6 | | 54 | 84 | | 516 | 0.77 |
| 13096 | 0.01 | 0.18 | 0.98 | 0.03 | 1.05 | 41.7 | 0.34 | 1.3 | | | 1 | 0.0 | 1.2 | 2 | 0.0 | 23 | 12 | 6.0 | 50 | 0.28 |
| 13265 | 0.01 | 0.04 | 0.33 | 0.01 | 1.22 | 7.8 | 0.16 | 0.0 | | | 9 | 0.1 | 0.7 | 2 | 0.0 | 26 | 18 | 5.7 | 91 | 0.12 |

| Code | Amount | Description | Basic Components | | | | | | | | | Additional Fats | | | | | | Vit A & Components | | | | | Vitamins | | | | | | | | | | Minerals | | | | | | | | | |
|---|---|---|---|---|---|---|---|---|---|---|---|---|---|---|---|---|---|---|---|---|---|---|---|---|---|---|---|---|---|---|---|---|---|---|---|---|---|---|---|---|---|---|
| | | | Weight (g) | Calories | % Water | Protein (g) | Carbs (g) | Fiber (g) | Sugar (g) | Other Carbs (g) | Fat (g) | Sat Fat (g) | Mono Fat (g) | Poly Fat (g) | Omega 3 (g) | Omega 6 (g) | Choles (mg) | Vit A (IU) | Vit A (RE) | Retinol (RE) | Carotenoids (RE) | Beta Carotene (mcg) | Thiamin (mg) | Riboflavin (mg) | Niacin (NE) | Vit B6 (mg) | Vit B12 (mcg) | Folate (mcg) | Panto (mg) | Vit C (mg) | Vit D (mg) | Vit E (α TE) | Calcium (mg) | Copper (mg) | Iron (mg) | Magnes (mg) | Mang (mg) | Phos (mg) | Potassium (mg) | Selenium (mcg) | Sodium (mg) | Zinc (mg) |
| 13050 | 1 pce | Peppered Loaf Lunchmeat, avg | 28 | 41 | 67 | 4.8 | 1.3 | 0.0 | 1.3 | 0.0 | 1.8 | 0.5 | 0.8 | 0.1 | 0.02 | 0.12 | 13 | 0 | 0 | 0 | 0 | 0 | 0.11 | 0.08 | 0.86 | 0.08 | 0.55 | 0.6 | 0.15 | 0.0 | 0.2 | | 15 | 0.0 | 0.3 | 6 | 0.0 | 48 | 110 | 5.9 | 426 | 0.90 |
| 13051 | 1 pce | Pickle/Pimiento Loaf Lunchmeat, w/pork, avg | 28 | 73 | 57 | 3.2 | 1.7 | 0.0 | 1.5 | 0.2 | 5.9 | 2.2 | 2.7 | 0.7 | 0.08 | 0.65 | 10 | 20 | 2 | 0 | 2 | | 0.08 | 0.07 | 0.57 | 0.05 | 0.33 | 1.4 | 0.22 | 0.0 | 0.3 | | 27 | 0.0 | 0.3 | 5 | 0.0 | 39 | 95 | 4.1 | 389 | 0.39 |
| 13204 | 1 pce | Pickle/Pimiento Loaf Lunchmeat, w/chick, Oscar Mayer | 28 | 75 | 56 | 2.7 | 2.6 | 0.0 | 1.9 | 0.7 | 6.1 | 2.0 | 2.9 | 0.8 | 0.04 | 0.75 | 22 | 0 | 0 | 0 | 0 | 0 | | | | | | | | 0.0 | | | 31 | 0.1 | 0.6 | 8 | | 42 | 49 | | 357 | 0.33 |
| | | Sausages | | | | | | | | | | | | | | | | | | | | | | | | | | | | | | | | | | | | | | | | |
| 13102 | 1 ea | Beef, link, smoked, avg | 43 | 134 | 54 | 6.1 | 1.0 | 0.0 | 1.0 | 0.0 | 11.6 | 4.3 | 5.6 | 0.5 | 0.04 | 0.41 | 29 | 0 | 0 | 0 | 0 | 0 | 0.02 | 0.06 | 1.37 | 0.05 | 0.80 | 1.7 | 0.08 | 0.0 | | | 3 | 0.0 | 0.8 | 6 | 0.0 | 45 | 76 | 6.3 | 486 | 1.20 |
| 13028 | 1 ea | Beef & Pork, link, smkd, avg | 16 | 54 | 52 | 2.1 | 0.2 | 0.0 | 0.2 | 0.0 | 4.8 | 1.7 | 2.3 | 0.5 | 0.06 | 0.46 | 11 | 0 | 0 | 0 | 0 | 0 | 0.04 | 0.03 | 0.52 | 0.03 | 0.24 | 0.3 | 0.07 | 0.0 | 0.1 | | 2 | 0.0 | 0.2 | 2 | 0.0 | 17 | 30 | 2.1 | 151 | 0.34 |
| 13089 | 1 ea | Beef & Pork, patty, ckd, avg | 27 | 107 | 45 | 3.7 | 0.7 | 0.0 | 0.7 | 0.0 | 9.8 | 3.5 | 4.6 | 1.1 | 0.09 | 0.97 | 19 | 0 | 0 | 0 | 0 | 0 | 0.10 | 0.04 | 0.91 | 0.01 | 0.12 | 0.5 | 0.13 | 0.0 | 0.3 | | 3 | 0.0 | 0.3 | 3 | 0.0 | 29 | 51 | 3.9 | 217 | 0.50 |
| 13199 | 1 pce | Beef Summer, Oscar Mayer | 23 | 71 | 52 | 3.3 | 0.4 | 0.0 | 0.3 | 0.2 | 6.2 | 2.7 | 3.0 | 0.3 | 0.05 | 0.22 | 18 | 23 | 7 | | | | 0.04 | 0.08 | 0.99 | 0.06 | 1.26 | 1.1 | | 0.0 | 0.2 | | 2 | 0.0 | 0.6 | 4 | 7.5 | 28 | 54 | | 328 | 0.54 |
| 13001 | 1 pce | Berliner, avg | 23 | 53 | 61 | 3.5 | 0.6 | 0.0 | 0.5 | 0.1 | 4.0 | 1.3 | 1.8 | 0.4 | 0.04 | 0.32 | 11 | 0 | 0 | 0 | 0 | 0 | 0.09 | 0.05 | 0.72 | 0.05 | 0.61 | 1.1 | 0.16 | 0.0 | 0.1 | | 3 | 0.0 | 0.3 | 3 | 0.0 | 30 | 65 | 3.2 | 298 | 0.57 |
| 13077 | 1 pce | Blood, avg | 25 | 94 | 47 | 3.7 | 0.3 | 0.0 | 0.3 | 0.0 | 8.6 | 3.3 | 4.0 | 0.9 | 0.06 | 0.80 | 30 | 0 | 0 | 0 | 0 | 0 | 0.02 | 0.03 | 0.30 | 0.01 | 0.25 | 1.3 | 0.15 | 0.0 | | | 2 | 0.0 | 1.6 | 2 | 0.0 | 6 | 10 | 3.0 | 170 | 0.32 |
| 13078 | 1 ea | Bockworst, link, avg | 65 | 200 | 56 | 8.6 | 0.3 | 0.0 | 0.3 | 0.0 | 17.9 | 6.5 | 8.4 | 1.9 | 0.16 | 1.72 | 38 | 15 | 4 | 4 | 0 | 0 | 0.27 | 0.11 | 2.68 | 0.15 | 0.53 | 3.9 | 0.44 | 0.0 | | | 10 | 0.0 | 0.4 | 12 | 0.0 | 95 | 175 | 6.9 | 718 | 1.01 |
| 13079 | 1 ea | Bratwurst, link, ckd, avg | 85 | 256 | 56 | 12.0 | 1.8 | 0.0 | 1.8 | 0.0 | 22.0 | 7.9 | 10.4 | 2.3 | 0.22 | 2.11 | 51 | 0 | 0 | 0 | 0 | 0 | 0.43 | 0.16 | 2.72 | 0.18 | 0.81 | 1.7 | 0.27 | 0.9 | 0.9 | | 37 | 0.1 | 1.1 | 13 | 0.0 | 127 | 180 | 18.0 | 473 | 1.96 |
| 13066 | 1 pce | Braunschweiger, avg | 28 | 101 | 48 | 3.8 | 0.9 | 0.0 | 0.9 | 0.0 | 9.0 | 3.1 | 4.2 | 1.0 | 0.11 | 0.94 | 44 | 3934 | 1182 | 1182 | 0 | 0 | 0.07 | 0.43 | 2.34 | 0.09 | 5.63 | 12.3 | 0.95 | 0.0 | 0.1 | | 3 | 0.1 | 2.6 | 3 | 0.0 | 47 | 56 | 16.2 | 320 | 0.79 |
| 13036 | 1 ea | Brotwurst, link, avg | 70 | 226 | 51 | 10.0 | 2.1 | 0.0 | 2.1 | 0.0 | 19.5 | 7.0 | 9.3 | 2.0 | 0.20 | 1.75 | 44 | 0 | 0 | 0 | 0 | 0 | 0.17 | 0.16 | 2.31 | 0.09 | 1.43 | 3.5 | 0.04 | 0.0 | 0.2 | | 34 | 0.1 | 0.7 | 11 | 0.0 | 94 | 197 | 9.4 | 778 | 1.47 |
| 90060 | 1 pce | Capiocola, avg | 21 | 105 | 26 | 4.2 | 0.0 | 0.0 | 0.0 | 0.0 | 9.6 | 3.5 | 4.0 | 0.9 | 0.00 | 0.87 | 14 | 0 | 0 | 0 | 0 | 0 | 0.09 | 0.03 | 0.55 | | | | | 0.0 | | | 2 | | 0.6 | | | 35 | 47 | | 259 | |
| 13181 | 1 ea | Cheese Smokies, Oscar Mayer | 43 | 130 | 55 | 5.6 | 0.8 | 0.0 | 0.7 | 0.1 | 11.6 | 4.1 | 5.6 | 1.2 | 0.15 | 1.01 | 30 | 69 | 21 | | | | | | | | | | | 0.0 | | | 19 | 0.1 | 0.5 | 7 | | 124 | 78 | | 450 | 0.84 |
| 13070 | 1 ea | Chorizo, link, avg | 60 | 273 | 32 | 14.5 | 1.1 | 0.0 | 1.1 | 0.0 | 23.0 | 8.5 | 11.0 | 2.1 | 0.23 | 1.81 | 53 | 0 | 0 | 0 | 0 | 0 | 0.33 | 0.18 | 3.08 | 0.32 | 1.20 | 1.2 | 0.67 | 0.0 | | | 5 | 0.0 | 1.0 | 11 | 0.0 | 90 | 239 | 12.7 | 741 | 2.05 |
| 13015 | 1 ea | Italian, link, ckd, avg | 67 | 216 | 50 | 13.4 | 1.0 | 0.0 | 1.0 | 0.0 | 17.2 | 6.[illegible] | 8.0 | 2.2 | 0.29 | 1.90 | 52 | 0 | 0 | 0 | 0 | 0 | 0.42 | 0.16 | 2.79 | 0.22 | 0.87 | 3.4 | 0.30 | 1.3 | 0.9 | | 16 | 0.1 | 1.0 | 12 | 0.1 | 114 | 204 | 14.7 | 618 | 1.60 |
| 13082 | 1 ea | Italian, link, raw, avg | 102 | 353 | 51 | 14.6 | 0.7 | 0.0 | 0.7 | 0.0 | 31.9 | 11.5 | 14.6 | 4.1 | 0.42 | 3.69 | 78 | 0 | 0 | 0 | 0 | 0 | 0.53 | 0.17 | 3.32 | 0.31 | 0.93 | 8.2 | 0.52 | 2.0 | 1.0 | | 18 | 0.1 | 1.2 | 14 | 0.1 | 145 | 258 | 25.3 | 746 | 1.83 |
| 13043 | 1 pce | Kielbasa, avg | 26 | 81 | 54 | 3.5 | 0.6 | 0.0 | 0.6 | 0.0 | 7.1 | 2.5 | 3.4 | 0.8 | 0.10 | 0.70 | 17 | 0 | 0 | 0 | 0 | 0 | 0.05 | 0.06 | 0.75 | 0.05 | 0.42 | 1.3 | 0.21 | 0.0 | 0.1 | | 11 | 0.0 | 0.4 | 4 | 0.0 | 38 | 70 | 4.6 | 280 | 0.53 |
| 13044 | 1 ea | Knockwurst, link, avg | 68 | 209 | 56 | 8.1 | 1.2 | 0.0 | 1.2 | 0.0 | 18.9 | 6.9 | 8.7 | 2.0 | 0.30 | 1.69 | 39 | 0 | 0 | 0 | 0 | 0 | 0.23 | 0.10 | 1.86 | 0.12 | 0.80 | 1.4 | 0.22 | 0.0 | 0.2 | | 7 | 0.0 | 0.6 | 7 | 0.0 | 67 | 135 | 9.2 | 687 | 1.13 |
| 13065 | 1 ea | Pork, brown & serve, link, unheated, avg | 13 | 51 | 45 | 1.8 | 0.4 | 0.0 | 0.4 | 0.0 | 5.0 | 1.7 | 2.2 | 0.5 | 0.04 | 0.46 | 8 | 0 | 0 | 0 | 0 | 0 | 0.10 | 0.04 | 0.48 | 0.03 | 0.20 | 0.7 | 0.09 | 0.0 | 0.2 | | 1 | 0.0 | 0.3 | 2 | 0.0 | 21 | 35 | 2.0 | 124 | 0.15 |
| 13016 | 1 ea | Pork, link, ckd | 13 | 48 | 45 | 2.6 | 0.1 | 0.0 | 0.1 | 0.0 | 4.1 | 1.4 | 2.0 | 0.4 | 0.01 | 0.34 | 11 | 0 | 0 | 0 | 0 | 0 | 0.10 | 0.03 | 0.59 | 0.04 | 0.23 | 0.3 | 0.09 | 0.2 | 0.4 | | 4 | 0.0 | 0.2 | 2 | 0.0 | 24 | 47 | 2.4 | 168 | 0.33 |
| 13266 | 1 ea | Pork, patty, ckd, avg | 27 | 100 | 45 | 5.3 | 0.3 | 0.0 | | | 8.4 | 2.9 | 3.8 | 1.0 | 0.15 | 0.88 | 22 | 0 | 0 | 0 | 0 | 0 | 0.20 | 0.07 | 1.22 | 0.09 | 0.47 | 0.5 | 0.19 | 0.5 | | | 9 | 0.0 | 0.3 | 5 | 0.0 | 50 | 97 | 4.9 | 349 | 0.68 |
| 13068 | 1 ea | Pork, patty, raw, avg | 57 | 238 | 44 | 6.7 | 0.6 | 0.0 | 0.6 | 0.0 | 23.0 | 8.3 | 10.5 | 3.0 | 0.43 | 2.50 | 39 | 0 | 0 | 0 | 0 | 0 | 0.31 | 0.09 | 1.62 | 0.14 | 0.64 | 2.3 | 0.23 | 1.1 | 0.2 | | 10 | 0.0 | 0.5 | 6 | 0.0 | 67 | 116 | 6.6 | 380 | 0.91 |
| 13285 | 1 oz | Pork, pickled, avg | 28 | 81 | 53 | 4.5 | 0.7 | 0.0 | | | 6.5 | 2.6 | 3.0 | 0.7 | | | 21 | 0 | 0 | 0 | 0 | 0 | 0.03 | 0.12 | 1.15 | 0.07 | 1.18 | 0.6 | | 3.9 | | | 4 | 0.1 | 0.9 | 5 | | 37 | 64 | | 444 | 0.69 |
| 13022 | 1 ea | Pork, polish, avg | 227 | 740 | 53 | 32.0 | 3.7 | 0.0 | 3.7 | 0.0 | 65.1 | 23.4 | 30.6 | 7.0 | 0.65 | 6.33 | 159 | 0 | 0 | 0 | 0 | 0 | 1.14 | 0.34 | 7.81 | 0.43 | 2.22 | 4.5 | 1.02 | 2.3 | 2.9 | | 27 | 0.2 | 3.3 | 32 | 0.1 | 309 | 538 | 40.2 | 1989 | 4.38 |
| 13027 | 1 ea | Pork, smoked, link, avg | 68 | 265 | 39 | 15.1 | 1.4 | 0.0 | 1.4 | 0.0 | 21.6 | 7.7 | 9.9 | 2.6 | 0.25 | 2.31 | 46 | 0 | 0 | 0 | 0 | 0 | 0.43 | 0.17 | 3.08 | 0.24 | 1.11 | 3.4 | 0.53 | 1.4 | 0.9 | | 20 | 0.0 | 0.8 | 13 | 0.0 | 110 | 228 | 14.8 | 1020 | 1.92 |
| 13184 | 1 ea | Pork, smokie links, Oscar Mayer | 43 | 130 | 56 | 5.3 | 0.7 | 0.0 | 0.7 | 0.0 | 11.7 | 4.[illegible] | 5.7 | 1.2 | 0.10 | 1.10 | 27 | 0 | 0 | 0 | 0 | 0 | | | | | | | | 0.0 | | | 4 | 0.1 | 0.5 | 7 | | 103 | 77 | | 433 | 0.90 |
| 13252 | 1 pce | Pork, smokie sausage, little cheese, Oscar May | 10 | 31 | 53 | 1.4 | 0.2 | 0.0 | 0.0 | 0.1 | 2.8 | 1.[illegible] | 1.3 | 0.3 | 0.01 | 0.27 | 7 | 17 | 5 | | | | | | | | | | | 0.0 | | | 7 | 0.0 | 0.1 | 2 | | 25 | 15 | | 104 | 0.20 |
| 13030 | 1 pce | Thuringer Summer, beef & pork, avg | 23 | 77 | 51 | 3.6 | 0.1 | 0.0 | 0.1 | 0.0 | 6.8 | 2.[illegible] | 3.0 | 0.3 | 0.05 | 0.23 | 17 | 0 | 0 | 0 | 0 | 0 | 0.03 | 0.08 | 0.99 | 0.06 | 1.26 | 0.5 | 0.23 | 0.0 | 0.1 | | 3 | 0.0 | 0.6 | 3 | 0.0 | 26 | 62 | 4.7 | 286 | 0.59 |
| 90061 | 1 ea | Thuringer Summer, dry, avg | 150 | 676 | 29 | 36.9 | 2.6 | 0.0 | 2.6 | 0.0 | 56.4 | 24.[illegible] | 24.0 | 3.0 | 0.00 | 3.00 | 98 | 0 | 0 | 0 | 0 | 0 | 0.41 | 0.34 | 8.25 | | | | | 0.0 | | | 21 | | 4.1 | | | 441 | 330 | | 1650 | |
| 13052 | 1 pce | Turkey, breakfast, Louis Rich | 28 | 64 | 60 | 6.1 | 0.0 | 0.0 | 0.0 | 0.0 | 4.6 | 1.6 | 1.8 | 1.2 | 0.05 | 1.15 | 23 | 0 | 0 | 0 | 0 | 0 | 0.03 | 0.08 | 1.40 | 0.08 | 0.49 | 1.0 | 0.09 | 0.0 | 0.1 | | 5 | 0.0 | 0.5 | 6 | 0.0 | 51 | 75 | 5.1 | 188 | 0.96 |
| 13119 | 1 oz | Turkey, cheddar, smoked, Louis Rich | 28 | 46 | 68 | 4.6 | 0.8 | 0.0 | 0.7 | 0.1 | 2.7 | 1.[illegible] | 0.9 | 0.5 | 0.07 | 0.47 | 17 | 50 | 15 | | | | | | | | | | | 0.0 | | | 16 | 0.0 | 0.3 | 5 | | 80 | 51 | | 267 | 0.57 |
| 13116 | 1 oz | Turkey, ground, Louis Rich | 28 | 48 | 69 | 4.7 | 0.2 | 0.0 | 0.2 | 0.0 | 3.2 | 1.[illegible] | 1.1 | 1.0 | 0.05 | 0.93 | 23 | 0 | 0 | 0 | 0 | 0 | | | | | | | | 0.0 | | | 10 | 0.1 | 0.5 | 7 | | 43 | 70 | | 170 | 0.78 |
| 13115 | 1 ea | Turkey, links, Louis Rich | 28 | 46 | 69 | 5.2 | 0.0 | 0.0 | 0.0 | 0.0 | 2.8 | 0.[illegible] | 1.1 | 0.6 | 0.02 | 0.61 | 21 | 0 | 0 | 0 | 0 | 0 | | | | | | | | 0.0 | | | 2 | 0.0 | 0.4 | 6 | | 49 | 80 | | 232 | 0.66 |
| 13104 | 1 oz | Turkey, summer, Louis Rich | 28 | 49 | 67 | 4.7 | 0.3 | 0.0 | 0.3 | 0.0 | 3.4 | 1.[illegible] | 1.3 | 0.9 | | 0.87 | 22 | 0 | 0 | 0 | 0 | 0 | 0.03 | 0.12 | 1.38 | 0.08 | 1.13 | 1.0 | 0.09 | 0.0 | 0.1 | | 4 | 0.0 | 0.5 | 6 | | 67 | 64 | 2.6 | 300 | 0.71 |
| 13054 | 1 ea | Vienna, beef & pork, cnd, avg | 16 | 45 | 60 | 1.6 | 0.3 | 0.0 | 0.3 | 0.0 | 4.0 | 1.5 | 2.0 | 0.3 | 0.05 | 0.21 | 8 | 0 | 0 | 0 | 0 | 0 | 0.01 | 0.02 | 0.26 | 0.02 | 0.16 | 0.6 | 0.06 | 0.0 | 0.1 | | 2 | 0.0 | 0.1 | 1 | 0.0 | 8 | 16 | 2.7 | 152 | 0.26 |
| 13240 | 1 ea | Vienna, chicken, Libby's | 16 | 33 | 68 | 2.0 | 0.0 | 0.0 | 0.0 | 0.0 | 2.7 | 0.[illegible] | | | | | 17 | 0 | 0 | 0 | 0 | 0 | | | | | | | | 0.0 | | | 7 | | 0.2 | | | | | | 150 | |
| 13239 | 1 ea | Vienna, Libby's | 16 | 43 | 62 | 1.7 | 0.0 | 0.0 | 0.0 | 0.0 | 4.0 | 0.[illegible] | | | | | 17 | 0 | 0 | 0 | 0 | 0 | | | | | | | | 0.0 | | | 7 | | 0.2 | | | | | | 100 | |
| 13241 | 1 ea | Vienna, w/barbecue sauce, Libby's | 20 | 47 | 66 | 1.7 | 0.7 | 0.0 | 0.3 | 0.3 | 4.0 | 0.[illegible] | | | | | 17 | 0 | 0 | 0 | 0 | 0 | | | | | | | | 0.0 | | | 11 | | 0.4 | | | | | | 103 | |
| | | Spreads | | | | | | | | | | | | | | | | | | | | | | | | | | | | | | | | | | | | | | | | |
| 13095 | 1 Tbs | Chicken, cnd, avg | 13 | 25 | 66 | 2.0 | 0.7 | 0.0 | | | 1.5 | 0.4 | 0.6 | 0.3 | 0.02 | 0.29 | 7 | 1 | 3 | | | | 0.00 | 0.01 | 0.36 | 0.02 | 0.02 | 0.4 | 0.06 | 0.0 | | | 16 | 0.0 | 0.3 | 2 | 0.0 | 12 | 14 | 1.4 | 50 | 0.15 |
| 13034 | 1 Tbs | Ham Salad, avg | 15 | 32 | 63 | 1.3 | 1.6 | 0.0 | 0.5 | 1.1 | 2.3 | 0.[illegible] | 1.1 | 0.4 | 0.05 | 0.36 | 6 | 0 | 0 | 0 | 0 | 0 | 0.07 | 0.02 | 0.31 | 0.02 | 0.11 | 0.2 | 0.05 | 0.0 | 0.0 | | 1 | 0.0 | 0.1 | 2 | 0.0 | 18 | 23 | 2.7 | 137 | 0.17 |
| 13045 | 1 pce | Luncheon Meat, cnd, avg | 21 | 70 | 52 | 2.6 | 0.4 | 0.0 | 0.4 | 0.0 | 6.4 | 2.3 | 3.0 | 0.7 | 0.10 | 0.65 | 13 | 0 | 0 | 0 | 0 | 0 | 0.08 | 0.04 | 0.66 | 0.04 | 0.19 | 1.3 | 0.10 | 0.2 | 0.1 | | 1 | 0.0 | 0.2 | 2 | 0.0 | 17 | 45 | 5.9 | 271 | 0.31 |
| 13056 | 1 Tbs | Pork & Beef, avg | 15 | 35 | 60 | 1.1 | 1.8 | 0.0 | | | 2.6 | 0.9 | 1.1 | 0.4 | 0.06 | 0.33 | 6 | 3 | 1 | | | | 0.03 | 0.02 | 0.26 | 0.02 | 0.17 | 0.3 | 0.06 | 0.0 | 0.0 | | 2 | 0.0 | 0.1 | 1 | 0.0 | 9 | 17 | 1.5 | 152 | 0.15 |
| 8412 | 1 oz | Pork, Chicken & Beef, Oscar Mayer | 30 | 71 | 59 | 1.9 | 4.6 | 0.1 | 2.4 | 2.1 | 5.0 | 1.9 | 2.3 | 0.3 | 0.03 | 0.73 | 13 | 30 | 9 | | | | | | | | | | | 0.0 | | | 8 | 0.1 | 0.2 | 4 | | 21 | 35 | | 246 | 0.26 |
| 13268 | 1 Tbs | Poultry Salad, avg | 13 | 26 | 66 | 1.5 | 1.0 | 0.0 | | | 1.8 | 0.4 | 0.4 | 0.3 | 0.01 | 0.78 | 4 | 8 | 5 | | | | 0.00 | 0.01 | 0.22 | 0.01 | 0.05 | 0.6 | 0.04 | 0.1 | | | 1 | 0.0 | 0.1 | 1 | 0.0 | 4 | 24 | 1.4 | 49 | 0.14 |
| | | Turkey Lunchmeat | | | | | | | | | | | | | | | | | | | | | | | | | | | | | | | | | | | | | | | | |
| 13007 | 1 pce | Bologna, avg | 28 | 56 | 65 | 3.8 | 0.3 | 0.0 | 0.3 | 0.0 | 4.3 | 1.4 | 1.3 | 1.2 | 0.09 | 1.11 | 28 | 0 | 0 | 0 | 0 | 0 | 0.02 | 0.05 | 0.99 | 0.06 | 0.08 | 2.0 | 0.20 | 0.0 | 0.3 | | 24 | 0.0 | 0.4 | 4 | 0.0 | 37 | 56 | 3.6 | 246 | 0.49 |
| 13149 | 1 pce | Bologna, deluxe, Louis Rich | 56 | 115 | 67 | 6.4 | 1.0 | 0.0 | 0.6 | 0.4 | 9.6 | 2.9 | 3.6 | 2.5 | 0.14 | 2.48 | 44 | 0 | 0 | 0 | 0 | 0 | 0.03 | 0.10 | 2.15 | 0.10 | 0.84 | | | 0.0 | | | 68 | 0.1 | 0.9 | 10 | 0.0 | 99 | 103 | | 484 | 1.14 |
| 13259 | 1 oz | Breast, barbecued, Louis Rich | 28 | 29 | 72 | 5.8 | 0.9 | 0.0 | 0.7 | 0.2 | 0.3 | 0.[illegible] | 0.1 | 0.1 | 0.00 | 0.05 | 12 | 0 | 0 | 0 | 0 | 0 | 0.01 | 0.03 | 2.67 | 0.11 | | 1.0 | | 0.0 | | | 7 | 0.1 | 0.3 | 8 | | 90 | 88 | | 300 | 0.29 |
| 13110 | 1 pce | Breast, honey roasted, deluxe, Louis Rich | 80 | 80 | 73 | 16.0 | 3.0 | 0.0 | 3.0 | 0.0 | 1.0 | 0.5 | | | | | 35 | 0 | 0 | 0 | 0 | 0 | | | | | | | | 0.0 | | | 0 | | 0.7 | | | | | | 940 | |
| 13223 | 1 pce | Breast, roasted, fat free, deli thin, Oscar Mayer | 13 | 10 | 76 | 2.0 | 0.5 | 0.0 | | | 0.0 | 0.0 | 0.0 | 0.0 | 0.00 | 0.00 | 4 | | | | | | | | | | | | | | | | | | 0.2 | | | | | | 152 | |
| 13113 | 1 pce | Breast, roasted, fat free, deli thin, Louis Rich | 13 | 11 | 77 | 1.9 | 0.6 | 0.0 | 0.2 | 0.4 | 0.1 | 0.0 | 0.0 | 0.0 | 0.00 | 0.02 | 4 | 0 | 0 | 0 | 0 | 0 | | | | | | | | 0.0 | | | 1 | 0.0 | 0.1 | 4 | | 30 | 26 | | 155 | 0.11 |
| 13114 | 1 pce | Breast, roasted, fat free, Louis Rich | 28 | 22 | 77 | 4.0 | 1.1 | 0.0 | 0.4 | 0.7 | 0.2 | 0.[illegible] | 0.1 | 0.0 | 0.00 | 0.05 | 9 | 0 | 0 | 0 | 0 | 0 | | | | | | | | 0.0 | | | 3 | 0.1 | 0.3 | 8 | | 65 | 59 | | 387 | 0.24 |
| 13135 | 1 pce | Breast, roasted, thin cut, Louis Rich | 10 | 10 | 74 | 2.1 | 0.1 | 0.0 | 0.0 | 0.0 | 0.1 | 0.0 | 0.0 | 0.0 | 0.00 | 0.02 | 4 | 0 | 0 | 0 | 0 | 0 | | | | | | | | 0.0 | | | 1 | 0.0 | 0.1 | 3 | | 32 | 31 | | 119 | 0.09 |
| 13141 | 1 pce | Breast, smoked, deli thin, Louis Rich | 13 | 12 | 74 | 2.3 | 0.3 | 0.0 | 0.0 | 0.3 | 0.3 | 0.0 | | | 0.00 | 0.00 | 5 | 0 | 0 | 0 | 0 | 0 | | | | | | | | 0.0 | | | 0 | | 0.1 | | | | | | 122 | |
| 13112 | 1 pce | Breast, smoked, fat free, Louis Rich | 28 | 23 | 77 | 4.3 | 1.0 | 0.0 | 0.3 | 0.7 | 0.2 | 0.[illegible] | 0.1 | 0.0 | 0.00 | 0.03 | 10 | 0 | 0 | 0 | 0 | 0 | | | | | | | | 0.0 | | | 3 | 0.1 | 0.3 | 8 | | 69 | 61 | | 300 | 0.25 |
| 13108 | 1 pce | Breast, smoked, dinner slice, Louis Rich | 80 | 80 | 73 | 16.0 | 2.0 | 0.0 | 0.5 | 1.5 | 1.0 | 0.0 | | | 0.00 | 0.00 | 35 | 0 | 0 | 0 | 0 | 0 | | | | | | | | 0.0 | | | 0 | | 0.7 | | | | | | 1060 | |
| 13107 | 1 pce | Ham, chunk, Louis Rich | 56 | 64 | 73 | 10.3 | 0.5 | 0.0 | 0.5 | 0.0 | 2.3 | 0.8 | 0.9 | 0.6 | 0.03 | 0.61 | 41 | 0 | 0 | 0 | 0 | 0 | | | | | | | | 0.0 | | | 3 | 0.1 | 0.8 | 10 | | 156 | 155 | | 608 | 1.38 |
| 13155 | 1 pce | Ham, honey cured, Louis Rich | 21 | 23 | 73 | 3.8 | 0.7 | 0.0 | 0.4 | 0.2 | 0.6 | 0.2 | 0.2 | 0.1 | 0.00 | 0.12 | 14 | 0 | 0 | 0 | 0 | 0 | | | | | | | | 0.0 | | | 1 | 0.0 | 0.3 | 5 | | 63 | 60 | | 217 | 0.53 |
| 13020 | 1 pce | Pastrami, avg | 28 | 39 | 71 | 5.2 | 0.5 | 0.0 | 0.5 | 0.0 | 1.7 | 0.5 | 0.6 | 0.4 | 0.03 | 0.40 | 15 | 0 | 0 | 0 | 0 | 0 | 0.02 | 0.07 | 0.99 | 0.08 | 0.07 | 1.4 | 0.16 | 0.0 | 0.1 | | 3 | 0.0 | 0.5 | 4 | 0.0 | 56 | 73 | 4.5 | 293 | 0.60 |
| 13121 | 1 oz | Pastrami, chunk, Louis Rich | 28 | 33 | 72 | 5.1 | 0.3 | 0.0 | 0.0 | 0.3 | 1.3 | 0.4 | 0.4 | 0.3 | 0.01 | 0.31 | 18 | 0 | 0 | 0 | 0 | 0 | 0.02 | 0.08 | 1.46 | 0.08 | 0.56 | | | 0.0 | | | 2 | 0.0 | 0.4 | 6 | 0.0 | 83 | 86 | | 285 | 0.73 |
| 13248 | 1 pce | Pastrami, Oscar Mayer | 23 | 24 | 74 | 4.2 | 0.2 | 0.0 | 0.1 | 0.2 | 0.8 | 0.2 | 0.2 | 0.2 | 0.01 | 0.18 | 14 | 0 | 0 | 0 | 0 | 0 | | | | | | | | 0.0 | | | 2 | 0.0 | 0.3 | 4 | | 66 | 63 | | 261 | 0.56 |

| Code | Amount | | Description | Basic Components | | | | | | | | | Additional Fats | | | | | | Vit A & Components | | | | | Vitamins | | | | | | | | | | Minerals | | | | | | | | | |
|---|---|---|---|---|---|---|---|---|---|---|---|---|---|---|---|---|---|---|---|---|---|---|---|---|---|---|---|---|---|---|---|---|---|---|---|---|---|---|---|---|---|---|---|
| | | | | Weight (g) | Calories | % Water | Protein (g) | Carbs (g) | Fiber (g) | Sugar (g) | Other Carbs (g) | Fat (g) | Sat Fat (g) | Mono Fat (g) | Poly Fat (g) | Omega 3 (g) | Omega 6 (g) | Choles (mg) | Vit A (IU) | Vit A (RE) | Retinol (RE) | Carotenoids (RE) | Beta Carotene (mcg) | Thiamin (mg) | Riboflavin (mg) | Niacin (NE) | Vit B6 (mg) | Vit B12 (mcg) | Folate (mcg) | Panto (mg) | Vit C (mg) | Vit D (mg) | Vit E (α TE) | Calcium (mg) | Copper (mg) | Iron (mg) | Magnes (mg) | Mang (mg) | Phos (mg) | Potassium (mg) | Selenium (mcg) | Sodium (mg) | Zinc (mg) |
| 13120 | 7 | pce | Salami, chunks, Louis Rich | 28 | 52 | 68 | 3.8 | 0.1 | 0.0 | 0.1 | 0.0 | 4.1 | 1.3 | 1.6 | 1.2 | 0.06 | 1.10 | 24 | 0 | 0 | 0 | 0 | 0 | | | | | | | | 0.0 | | | 25 | 0.1 | 0.4 | 5 | | 48 | 56 | | 251 | 0.63 |
| 13025 | 1 | pce | Salami, ckd, avg | 28 | 55 | 66 | 4.6 | 0.2 | 0.0 | 0.2 | 0.0 | 3.9 | 1.1 | 1.3 | 1.0 | 0.06 | 0.90 | 23 | 0 | 0 | 0 | 0 | 0 | 0.02 | 0.05 | 0.99 | 0.07 | 0.06 | 1.1 | 0.14 | 0.0 | 0.3 | | 6 | 0.0 | 0.5 | 4 | 0.0 | 30 | 68 | 3.7 | 281 | 0.51 |
| 13148 | 1 | pce | Salami, cotto, Louis Rich | 28 | 42 | 71 | 4.2 | 0.3 | 0.0 | 0.1 | 0.2 | 2.7 | 0.8 | 1.1 | 0.6 | 0.03 | 0.62 | 22 | 28 | 8 | | | | | | | | | | | 0.0 | | | 9 | 0.1 | 0.5 | 6 | | 76 | 62 | | 285 | 0.66 |
| | | | *PORK AND HAM* | | | | | | | | | | | | | | | | | | | | | | | | | | | | | | | | | | | | | | | | |
| | | | Bacon | | | | | | | | | | | | | | | | | | | | | | | | | | | | | | | | | | | | | | | | |
| 27096 | 1 | Tbs | Bits, Oscar Mayer | 7 | 24 | 30 | 2.7 | 0.2 | 0.0 | 0.2 | 0.0 | 1.3 | 0.5 | 0.7 | 0.2 | 0.01 | 0.15 | 5 | 0 | 0 | 0 | 0 | 0 | | | | | | | | 0.0 | | | 2 | 0.0 | 0.2 | 5 | | 43 | 39 | | 224 | 0.35 |
| 12002 | 1 | pce | Canadian, grilled | 23 | 43 | 62 | 5.6 | 0.3 | 0.0 | 0.3 | 0.0 | 1.9 | 0.7 | 0.9 | 0.2 | 0.03 | 0.16 | 13 | 0 | 0 | 0 | 0 | 0 | 0.19 | 0.05 | 1.59 | 0.10 | 0.18 | 0.9 | 0.12 | 0.0 | 0.1 | | 2 | 0.0 | 0.2 | 5 | 0.0 | 68 | 90 | 5.7 | 356 | 0.39 |
| 12008 | 1 | pce | Canadian, unheated | 28 | 44 | 67 | 5.8 | 0.5 | 0.0 | 0.5 | 0.0 | 2.0 | 0.6 | 0.9 | 0.2 | 0.03 | 0.15 | 14 | 0 | 0 | 0 | 0 | 0 | 0.21 | 0.05 | 1.74 | 0.11 | 0.19 | 1.1 | 0.15 | 0.0 | 0.1 | | 2 | 0.0 | 0.2 | 5 | 0.0 | 68 | 96 | 7.0 | 395 | 0.39 |
| 12000 | 4 | pce | Cooked | 32 | 184 | 13 | 9.8 | 0.2 | 0.0 | 0.2 | 0.0 | 15.7 | 5.6 | 7.6 | 1.9 | 0.25 | 1.61 | 27 | 0 | 0 | 0 | 0 | 0 | 0.22 | 0.09 | 2.34 | 0.09 | 0.56 | 1.6 | 0.34 | 0.0 | 0.1 | | 4 | 0.1 | 0.5 | 8 | 0.0 | 108 | 156 | 7.9 | 511 | 1.04 |
| 12244 | 5 | pce | Cooked, low sod, Oscar Mayer | 30 | 140 | 20 | 10.0 | 1.5 | 0.0 | 1.0 | 0.5 | 10.5 | 4.0 | 5.2 | 1.2 | 0.15 | 1.05 | 30 | 0 | 0 | 0 | 0 | 0 | | | | | | | | 0.0 | | | 5 | 0.1 | 0.5 | 15 | | 145 | 462 | | 438 | 1.02 |
| 12247 | 3 | pce | Cooked, thick cut, Oscar Mayer | 30 | 150 | | 6.0 | 0.0 | 0.0 | 0.0 | 0.0 | 12.0 | 6.0 | | | | | 30 | | | | | | | | | | | | | | | | | | | | | | | | 750 | |
| 12322 | 1 | oz | Smoked, low sod | 28 | 161 | 13 | 8.5 | 0.2 | 0.0 | | | 13.8 | 4.9 | 6.6 | 1.6 | | | 24 | 0 | 0 | 0 | 0 | 0 | 0.19 | 0.08 | 2.05 | 0.08 | 0.49 | 1.4 | | 9.4 | 0.1 | | 3 | 0.0 | 0.5 | 7 | | 94 | 136 | | 288 | 0.91 |
| 12165 | 2 | pce | Raw, average | 57 | 317 | 32 | 4.9 | 0.1 | 0.0 | 0.1 | 0.0 | 32.8 | 12.1 | 15.0 | 3.8 | 0.43 | 3.42 | 38 | 0 | 0 | 0 | 0 | 0 | 0.21 | 0.06 | 1.58 | 0.08 | 0.53 | 1.1 | 0.20 | 0.0 | | | 4 | 0.0 | 0.3 | 5 | 0.0 | 81 | 87 | 14.3 | 416 | 0.66 |
| | | | Fat | | | | | | | | | | | | | | | | | | | | | | | | | | | | | | | | | | | | | | | | |
| 8003 | 1 | Tbs | Bacon Grease/Meat Fat Drippings | 14 | 124 | 0 | 0.0 | 0.0 | 0.0 | 0.0 | 0.0 | 13.8 | 6.3 | 5.9 | 1.1 | 0.10 | 0.98 | 14 | 0 | 0 | 0 | 0 | 0 | 0.00 | 0.00 | 0.00 | 0.00 | 0.00 | 0.0 | 0.00 | 0.0 | 0.1 | | 0 | 0.0 | 0.0 | 0 | 0.0 | 0 | 0 | 0.0 | 76 | 0.01 |
| 12100 | 1 | Tbs | Cooked | 9 | 57 | 23 | 1.1 | 0.0 | 0.0 | 0.0 | 0.0 | 5.8 | 2.2 | 2.5 | 0.6 | 0.02 | 0.53 | 8 | 1 | 0.4 | 0.4 | 0 | 0 | 0.03 | 0.01 | 0.23 | 0.01 | 0.04 | 0.2 | 0.03 | 0.0 | 0.0 | | 5 | 0.0 | 0.0 | 1 | 0.0 | 15 | 21 | 1.5 | 3 | 0.11 |
| 12153 | 1 | oz | Raw | 28 | 240 | 4 | 0.5 | 0.0 | 0.0 | 0.0 | 0.0 | 26.4 | 12.7 | 10.4 | 2.0 | 0.26 | 1.78 | 31 | 0 | 0 | 0 | 0 | 0 | 0.03 | 0.02 | 0.35 | 0.01 | 0.06 | 0.0 | 0.00 | 0.0 | | | 0 | 0.0 | 0.0 | 0 | 0.0 | 5 | 9 | 2.2 | 1 | 0.05 |
| 12323 | 1 | oz | Salt Pork, ckd | 28 | 200 | 13 | 1.8 | 0.0 | 0.0 | 0.0 | 0.0 | 21.4 | 7.6 | 10.2 | 2.5 | | | 24 | 0 | 0 | 0 | 0 | 0 | 0.03 | 0.02 | 0.47 | 0.01 | 0.06 | 0.2 | | 0.0 | 0.1 | | 2 | 0.0 | 0.2 | 2 | | 12 | 18 | | 358 | 0.31 |
| 12171 | 1 | oz | Salt Pork, raw | 28 | 209 | 11 | 1.4 | 0.0 | 0.0 | 0.0 | 0.0 | 22.5 | 8.2 | 10.6 | 2.6 | 0.18 | 2.44 | 24 | 0 | 0 | 0 | 0 | 0 | 0.06 | 0.02 | 0.45 | 0.02 | 0.08 | 0.3 | 0.06 | 0.0 | | | 2 | 0.0 | 0.1 | 2 | 0.0 | 15 | 18 | 1.6 | 399 | 0.25 |
| | | | Ham, Cured | | | | | | | | | | | | | | | | | | | | | | | | | | | | | | | | | | | | | | | | |
| 13170 | 4 | pce | Boiled, 4% fat, Oscar Mayer | 84 | 87 | 75 | 13.7 | 0.9 | 0.0 | 0.3 | 0.7 | 3.1 | 1.1 | 1.6 | 0.3 | 0.04 | 0.30 | 40 | | | | | | | | | | | | | 0.0 | | | 8 | 0.2 | 1.2 | 25 | | 201 | 237 | | 1132 | 1.56 |
| 12212 | 3 | oz | Boneless, 5% fat, rstd | 85 | 123 | 68 | 17.8 | 1.3 | 0.0 | 1.3 | 0.0 | 4.7 | 1.5 | 2.2 | 0.5 | 0.05 | 0.41 | 45 | 0 | 0 | 0 | 0 | 0 | 0.64 | 0.17 | 3.42 | 0.34 | 0.55 | 2.6 | 0.34 | 0.0 | 0.3 | | 7 | 0.1 | 1.3 | 12 | 0.0 | 167 | 244 | 16.6 | 1023 | 2.45 |
| 12307 | 3 | oz | Boneless, 8% fat, rstd | 85 | 140 | 66 | 18.7 | 0.4 | 0.0 | | | 6.5 | 2.2 | 3.2 | 0.9 | 0.14 | 0.76 | 48 | 0 | 0 | 0 | 0 | 0 | 0.63 | 0.24 | 4.52 | 0.30 | 0.58 | 2.6 | 0.51 | 0.0 | | | 7 | 0.1 | 1.2 | 16 | 0.0 | 211 | 308 | 16.6 | 1177 | 2.24 |
| 12211 | 3 | oz | Boneless, 11% fat, rstd | 85 | 151 | 64 | 19.2 | 0.0 | 0.0 | 0.0 | 0.0 | 7.7 | 2.7 | 3.8 | 1.2 | 0.20 | 0.99 | 50 | 0 | 0 | 0 | 0 | 0 | 0.62 | 0.28 | 5.23 | 0.26 | 0.60 | 2.6 | 0.61 | 0.0 | 0.3 | | 7 | 0.1 | 1.1 | 19 | 0.0 | 239 | 348 | 16.8 | 1275 | 2.10 |
| 12209 | 3 | oz | Canned, 4% fat, rstd | 85 | 116 | 70 | 18.0 | 0.4 | 0.0 | 0.4 | 0.0 | 4.1 | 1.4 | 2.1 | 0.4 | 0.04 | 0.33 | 26 | 0 | 0 | 0 | 0 | 0 | 0.88 | 0.21 | 4.16 | 0.38 | 0.60 | 4.3 | 0.48 | 0.0 | 0.3 | | 5 | 0.0 | 0.8 | 18 | 0.0 | 178 | 296 | 14.8 | 965 | 1.90 |
| 12226 | 3 | oz | Canned, 7% fat, rstd | 85 | 142 | 66 | 17.8 | 0.4 | 0.0 | 0.4 | 0.0 | 7.2 | 2.4 | 3.5 | 0.8 | 0.08 | 0.69 | 35 | 0 | 0 | 0 | 0 | 0 | 0.82 | 0.21 | 4.28 | 0.34 | 0.71 | 4.3 | 0.53 | 0.0 | 0.3 | | 6 | 0.1 | 0.9 | 17 | 0.0 | 188 | 298 | 22.6 | 908 | 1.97 |
| 12168 | 3 | oz | Canned, 13% fat, rstd | 85 | 192 | 61 | 17.4 | 0.4 | 0.0 | 0.4 | 0.0 | 12.9 | 4.3 | 6.0 | 1.5 | 0.14 | 1.38 | 53 | 0 | 0 | 0 | 0 | 0 | 0.70 | 0.22 | 4.51 | 0.26 | 0.90 | 4.3 | 0.62 | 11.9 | 0.3 | | 7 | 0.1 | 1.2 | 14 | 0.0 | 207 | 303 | 30.5 | 800 | 2.13 |
| 12243 | 1 | ea | Dinner Slice, 3% fat, Oscar Mayer | 84 | 83 | 75 | 14.0 | 0.5 | 0.0 | 0.4 | 0.1 | 2.8 | 1.0 | 1.5 | 0.3 | 0.03 | 0.26 | 41 | 0 | 0 | 0 | 0 | 0 | 0.60 | 0.19 | 3.93 | 0.32 | 0.41 | | | 0.0 | | | 4 | 0.1 | 1.0 | 17 | | 203 | 221 | | 1018 | 1.66 |
| 12242 | 1 | ea | Dinner Steak, 3% fat, Oscar Mayer | 57 | 56 | 76 | 9.5 | 0.2 | 0.0 | 0.2 | 0.0 | 1.9 | 0.7 | 1.0 | 0.3 | 0.02 | 0.24 | 30 | 0 | 0 | 0 | 0 | 0 | | | | | | | | 0.0 | | | 3 | 0.1 | 0.6 | 11 | | 147 | 151 | | 753 | 1.09 |
| 13169 | 4 | pce | Honey, 4% fat, Oscar Mayer | 84 | 93 | 73 | 14.0 | 2.5 | 0.0 | 2.5 | 0.0 | 2.9 | 1.1 | 1.6 | 0.3 | 0.01 | 0.28 | 39 | 0 | 0 | 0 | 0 | 0 | | | | | | | | 0.0 | | | 8 | 0.2 | 1.1 | 25 | | 217 | 236 | | 1048 | 1.75 |
| 12091 | 2 | pce | Low sod, 5% fat | 84 | 122 | 68 | 17.6 | 1.3 | 0.0 | 1.3 | 0.0 | 4.6 | 1.5 | 2.2 | 0.5 | 0.05 | 0.40 | 45 | 0 | 0 | 0 | 0 | 0 | 0.63 | 0.17 | 3.38 | 0.34 | 0.55 | 2.5 | 0.42 | 17.6 | 0.3 | | 7 | 0.1 | 1.2 | 12 | 0.0 | 165 | 241 | 17.5 | 814 | 2.42 |
| 12090 | 2 | pce | Low sod, 8% fat | 84 | 144 | 65 | 18.7 | 0.3 | 0.0 | 0.3 | 0.0 | 7.0 | 2.4 | 3.4 | 1.0 | | | 49 | 0 | 0 | 0 | 0 | 0 | 0.61 | 0.26 | 4.82 | 0.28 | 0.58 | 2.5 | 0.42 | 18.8 | 0.3 | | 7 | 0.1 | 1.2 | 18 | 0.0 | 223 | 324 | 21.5 | 814 | 2.14 |
| 13168 | 4 | pce | Low sod, 4% fat, Oscar Mayer | 84 | 91 | 73 | 14.0 | 2.4 | 0.0 | 1.6 | 0.8 | 2.8 | 1.0 | 1.5 | 0.3 | 0.01 | 0.27 | 36 | 0 | 0 | 0 | 0 | 0 | | | | | | | | 0.0 | | | 5 | 0.2 | 1.2 | 20 | | 218 | 788 | | 698 | 1.68 |
| 12169 | 1 | ea | Patty, 28% fat, unheated | 65 | 205 | 54 | 8.3 | 1.1 | 0.0 | | | 18.3 | 6.6 | 8.6 | 2.0 | 0.19 | 1.79 | 45 | 0 | 0 | 0 | 0 | 0 | 0.30 | 0.10 | 1.96 | 0.10 | 0.70 | 1.9 | 0.20 | 0.0 | 0.2 | | 5 | 0.0 | 0.7 | 6 | 0.0 | 97 | 155 | 10.3 | 707 | 1.02 |
| 12175 | 3 | oz | Shoulder arm picnic, 7% fat, rstd | 85 | 145 | 64 | 21.2 | 0.0 | 0.0 | 0.0 | 0.0 | 6.0 | 2.0 | 2.7 | 0.7 | 0.07 | 0.62 | 41 | 0 | 0 | 0 | 0 | 0 | 0.62 | 0.19 | 4.08 | 0.31 | 0.94 | 3.4 | 0.56 | 0.0 | 0.3 | | 9 | 0.1 | 0.9 | 14 | 0.0 | 207 | 248 | 35.1 | 1046 | 2.50 |
| 12174 | 3 | oz | Shoulder arm picnic, 21% fat, rstd | 85 | 238 | 55 | 17.3 | 0.0 | 0.0 | 0.0 | 0.0 | 18.2 | 6.5 | 8.6 | 2.0 | 0.19 | 1.77 | 49 | 0 | 0 | 0 | 0 | 0 | 0.52 | 0.16 | 3.51 | 0.24 | 0.79 | 2.6 | 0.48 | 0.0 | 0.3 | | 9 | 0.1 | 0.8 | 12 | 0.0 | 188 | 219 | 28.6 | 911 | 2.13 |
| 12177 | 3 | oz | Shoulder blade roll, 24% fat, rstd | 85 | 244 | 56 | 14.7 | 0.3 | 0.0 | 0.3 | 0.0 | 20.0 | 7.1 | 9.4 | 2.1 | 0.31 | 1.83 | 57 | 0 | 0 | 0 | 0 | 0 | 0.39 | 0.24 | 2.02 | 0.18 | 0.89 | 2.6 | 0.65 | 2.7 | 0.3 | | 6 | 0.1 | 0.8 | 11 | 0.0 | 133 | 165 | 24.3 | 827 | 2.08 |
| 12006 | 3 | oz | Whole, 6% fat, rstd | 85 | 133 | 66 | 21.3 | 0.0 | 0.0 | 0.0 | 0.0 | 4.7 | 1.6 | 2.2 | 0.5 | 0.05 | 0.48 | 47 | 0 | 0 | 0 | 0 | 0 | 0.58 | 0.22 | 4.27 | 0.40 | 0.60 | 3.4 | 0.42 | 0.0 | 0.3 | | 6 | 0.1 | 0.8 | 19 | 0.0 | 193 | 269 | 21.6 | 1128 | 2.18 |
| 12005 | 3 | oz | Whole, 17% fat, rstd | 85 | 207 | 58 | 18.4 | 0.0 | 0.0 | 0.0 | 0.0 | 14.3 | 5.1 | 6.7 | 1.5 | 0.14 | 1.39 | 53 | 0 | 0 | 0 | 0 | 0 | 0.51 | 0.19 | 3.79 | 0.32 | 0.54 | 2.6 | 0.39 | 0.0 | 0.3 | | 6 | 0.1 | 0.7 | 16 | 0.0 | 182 | 243 | 19.3 | 1009 | 1.97 |
| | | | Pork | | | | | | | | | | | | | | | | | | | | | | | | | | | | | | | | | | | | | | | | |
| 12259 | 4 | oz | Back Ribs, raw | 113 | 319 | 59 | 18.2 | 0.0 | 0.0 | 0.0 | 0.0 | 26.7 | 9.9 | 12.1 | 2.2 | 0.09 | 2.03 | 92 | 11 | 3 | 3 | 0 | | 0.66 | 0.29 | 5.16 | 0.45 | 0.93 | 4.5 | 0.84 | 0.2 | 0.3 | | 36 | 0.1 | 1.0 | 18 | 0.0 | 162 | 263 | 27.1 | 85 | 2.61 |
| 12097 | 3 | oz | Back Ribs, rstd | 85 | 315 | 45 | 20.7 | 0.0 | 0.0 | 0.0 | 0.0 | 25.2 | 9.4 | 11.5 | 2.0 | 0.08 | 1.81 | 100 | 8 | 3 | 3 | 0 | | 0.36 | 0.17 | 3.02 | 0.26 | 0.54 | 2.6 | 0.49 | 0.3 | 0.3 | | 38 | 0.1 | 1.2 | 18 | 0.0 | 166 | 268 | 33.4 | 86 | 2.86 |
| 12081 | 1 | ea | Chop, breaded, bkd | 100 | 259 | 52 | 25.5 | 6.3 | 0.2 | 0.5 | 5.7 | 14.0 | 5.1 | 6.2 | 1.5 | | | 72 | 6 | 2 | 2 | 0 | | 0.81 | 0.30 | 4.75 | 0.42 | 0.63 | 5.8 | 0.57 | 0.5 | 0.3 | | 24 | 0.1 | 1.0 | 27 | 0.1 | 240 | 400 | | 415 | 2.20 |
| 12087 | 3 | oz | Chop, breaded, fried | 85 | 244 | 50 | 19.3 | 7.5 | 0.4 | 0.3 | 6.8 | 14.6 | 4.6 | 5.8 | 2.8 | | | 82 | 38 | 11 | 11 | 0 | | 0.58 | 0.30 | 3.30 | 0.28 | 0.64 | 8.0 | 0.48 | 0.4 | 0.3 | | 33 | 0.1 | 1.3 | 21 | 0.1 | 175 | 258 | | 343 | 2.47 |
| 12046 | 1 | ea | Chop, center rib, raw | 98 | 205 | 65 | 19.8 | 0.0 | 0.0 | 0.0 | 0.0 | 13.3 | 4.6 | 5.9 | 1.4 | 0.09 | 1.26 | 59 | 6 | 2 | 2 | 0 | | 0.86 | 0.23 | 5.21 | 0.42 | 0.60 | 2.9 | 0.58 | 0.3 | 0.3 | | 24 | 0.1 | 0.7 | 20 | 0.0 | 196 | 376 | 28.9 | 41 | 1.49 |
| 12050 | 3 | oz | Chop, center rib, rstd | 85 | 217 | 56 | 23.3 | 0.0 | 0.0 | 0.0 | 0.0 | 13.0 | 5.0 | 5.9 | 1.1 | 0.03 | 1.03 | 62 | 5 | 2 | 2 | 0 | | 0.62 | 0.26 | 5.20 | 0.28 | 0.56 | 2.6 | 0.45 | 0.3 | 0.3 | | 24 | 0.1 | 0.8 | 18 | 0.0 | 196 | 358 | 34.9 | 39 | 1.75 |
| 12910 | 3 | oz | Chop, marinated, Tyson | 85 | 130 | 70 | 16.1 | 0.6 | 0.0 | 0.1 | 0.4 | 7.0 | 2.9 | 3.3 | 0.7 | | | 48 | 0 | 0 | 0 | 0 | 0 | | | | | | | | 0.0 | | | 10 | | 0.4 | | | | 0 | | 261 | |
| 12083 | 1 | ea | Chop, smoked, ckd | 84 | 235 | 55 | 17.2 | 0.0 | 0.0 | 0.0 | 0.0 | 17.9 | 6.4 | 8.5 | 1.9 | | | 49 | 0 | 0 | 0 | 0 | 0 | 0.51 | 0.16 | 3.47 | 0.24 | 0.78 | 2.5 | 0.47 | 0.0 | 0.3 | | 8 | 0.1 | 0.8 | 12 | 0.0 | 186 | 217 | 39.7 | 900 | 2.11 |
| 12309 | 3 | oz | Composite Cuts, ckd | 85 | 232 | 55 | 23.5 | 0.0 | 0.0 | 0.0 | 0.0 | 14.6 | 5.3 | 6.5 | 1.2 | 0.04 | 1.15 | 77 | 7 | 2 | 2 | 0 | 0 | 0.65 | 0.28 | 4.19 | 0.33 | 0.65 | 5.1 | 0.57 | 0.3 | 0.3 | | 21 | 0.1 | 0.9 | 20 | 0.0 | 197 | 301 | 34.5 | 53 | 2.47 |
| 12118 | 3 | oz | Composite Cuts, lean, ckd | 85 | 180 | 60 | 24.9 | 0.0 | 0.0 | 0.0 | 0.0 | 8.2 | 2.9 | 3.7 | 0.6 | 0.02 | 0.60 | 73 | 6 | 2 | 2 | 0 | | 0.72 | 0.29 | 4.39 | 0.37 | 0.64 | 5.1 | 0.58 | 0.3 | 0.3 | | 18 | 0.1 | 0.9 | 22 | 0.0 | 201 | 319 | 38.3 | 50 | 2.52 |
| 12137 | 4 | oz | Composite Cuts, lean, raw | 113 | 162 | 72 | 23.8 | 0.0 | 0.0 | 0.0 | 0.0 | 6.6 | 2.3 | 3.0 | 0.7 | 0.02 | 0.66 | 69 | 7 | 2 | 2 | 0 | 0 | 1.09 | 0.31 | 5.46 | 0.57 | 0.76 | 5.7 | 0.89 | 0.8 | 0.3 | | 18 | 0.1 | 1.0 | 26 | 0.0 | 238 | 429 | 36.5 | 64 | 2.35 |
| 12308 | 4 | oz | Composite Cuts, raw | 113 | 244 | 65 | 21.5 | 0.0 | 0.0 | 0.0 | 0.0 | 17.0 | 6.0 | 7.5 | 1.8 | 0.10 | 1.57 | 76 | 8 | 2 | 2 | 0 | 0 | 0.95 | 0.29 | 5.09 | 0.50 | 0.75 | 5.7 | 0.82 | 0.6 | 0.3 | | 21 | 0.1 | 1.0 | 24 | 0.0 | 226 | 379 | 32.1 | 62 | 2.27 |
| 12330 | 6 | ea | Cubes, prep, Travis Meats | 85 | 210 | 60 | 14.1 | 0.0 | 0.0 | 0.0 | 0.0 | 16.8 | 5.8 | 7.4 | 1.8 | | | 60 | 5 | 2 | 2 | 0 | 0 | 0.61 | 0.22 | 3.36 | | | | | 0.6 | | | 12 | | 0.8 | | | 156 | 246 | | 60 | 2.01 |
| 12099 | 3 | oz | Ground, ckd | 85 | 252 | 53 | 21.8 | 0.0 | 0.0 | 0.0 | 0.0 | 17.7 | 6.6 | 7.9 | 1.6 | 0.06 | 1.46 | 80 | 7 | 2 | 2 | 0 | 0 | 0.60 | 0.19 | 3.58 | 0.33 | 0.46 | 5.1 | 0.44 | 0.6 | 0.3 | | 19 | 0.0 | 1.1 | 20 | 0.0 | 192 | 308 | 30.1 | 62 | 2.73 |
| 12342 | 3 | oz | Ground, roast, prep, Travis Meats | 85 | 147 | 65 | 22.9 | 2.3 | 0.0 | | | 4.6 | | | | | | 36 | 8 | 2 | 2 | 0 | 0 | | | | | | | | 0.9 | | | 28 | | 1.2 | | | | | | 154 | |
| 12336 | 3 | oz | Ground, slab, prep, Travis Meats | 85 | 211 | 65 | 12.6 | 0.0 | 0.0 | 0.0 | 0.0 | 16.8 | 5.8 | 7.4 | 1.8 | | | 60 | 5 | 2 | 2 | 0 | 0 | 0.61 | 0.22 | 3.36 | | | | | 0.6 | | | 12 | | 0.8 | | | 159 | 245 | | 57 | 2.01 |
| 12281 | 4 | oz | Ground, raw | 113 | 297 | 61 | 19.1 | 0.0 | 0.0 | 0.0 | 0.0 | 24.0 | 8.9 | 10.7 | 2.2 | 0.08 | 1.98 | 81 | 8 | 2 | 2 | 0 | 0 | 0.83 | 0.27 | 4.90 | 0.43 | 0.79 | 5.7 | 0.75 | 0.8 | 0.3 | | 16 | 0.1 | 1.0 | 21 | 0.0 | 198 | 324 | 27.8 | 63 | 2.49 |
| 12215 | 4 | oz | Leg, ham, raw | 113 | 277 | 62 | 19.7 | 0.0 | 0.0 | 0.0 | 0.0 | 21.4 | 7.4 | 9.5 | 2.3 | 0.16 | 2.01 | 82 | 8 | 2 | 2 | 0 | 0 | 0.83 | 0.23 | 5.16 | 0.45 | 0.71 | 7.9 | 0.77 | 0.8 | 0.3 | | 6 | 0.1 | 1.0 | 23 | 0.0 | 225 | 356 | 33.2 | 53 | 2.18 |
| 12016 | 3 | oz | Leg, ham, rstd | 85 | 232 | 55 | 22.8 | 0.0 | 0.0 | 0.0 | 0.0 | 15.0 | 5.5 | 6.7 | 1.4 | 0.04 | 1.35 | 80 | 9 | 3 | 3 | 0 | 0 | 0.54 | 0.27 | 3.88 | 0.34 | 0.58 | 8.5 | 0.52 | 0.3 | 0.3 | | 12 | 0.1 | 0.9 | 19 | 0.0 | 224 | 299 | 38.5 | 51 | 2.52 |
| 12182 | 1 | ea | Loin Chop, raw | 110 | 314 | 59 | 17.4 | 0.0 | 0.0 | 0.0 | 0.0 | 26.5 | 9.2 | 11.8 | 2.8 | 0.20 | 2.51 | 79 | 9 | 2 | 2 | 0 | 0 | 0.72 | 0.25 | 4.02 | 0.41 | 0.10 | 3.3 | 0.68 | 0.7 | 0.3 | | 32 | 0.1 | 0.9 | 18 | 0.0 | 180 | 309 | 28.8 | 59 | 2.59 |
| 12022 | 3 | oz | Loin Chop, rstd | 85 | 275 | 51 | 20.1 | 0.0 | 0.0 | 0.0 | 0.0 | 20.9 | 7.8 | 9.0 | 1.8 | 0.06 | 1.69 | 79 | 8 | 3 | 3 | 0 | 0 | 0.45 | 0.25 | 3.60 | 0.32 | 0.62 | 3.4 | 0.41 | 0.2 | 0.3 | | 29 | 0.1 | 0.9 | 17 | 0.0 | 179 | 277 | 31.5 | 26 | 2.81 |
| 12331 | 3 | oz | Patty, cubed, prep, Travis Meats | 85 | 225 | 61 | 13.5 | 0.8 | 0.6 | 0.0 | 0.1 | 18.5 | 6.7 | 8.2 | 1.8 | | | 52 | 37 | 11 | 11 | 0 | 0 | 0.55 | 0.19 | 3.68 | | | | | 0.4 | | | 25 | | 1.1 | | | 147 | 274 | | 153 | 2.89 |
| 12269 | 4 | oz | Ribs, country style, raw | 113 | 272 | 64 | 19.2 | 0.0 | 0.0 | 0.0 | 0.0 | 21.1 | 7.3 | 9.4 | 2.3 | 0.15 | 2.01 | 78 | 9 | 2 | 2 | 0 | 0 | 0.80 | 0.28 | 4.38 | 0.46 | 0.85 | 4.5 | 0.75 | 0.8 | 0.3 | | 31 | 0.1 | 1.0 | 20 | 0.0 | 195 | 341 | 31.9 | 66 | 2.89 |
| 12235 | 3 | oz | Ribs, country style, rstd | 85 | 279 | 51 | 19.9 | 0.0 | 0.0 | 0.0 | 0.0 | 21.5 | 7.8 | 9.4 | 1.7 | 0.05 | 1.58 | 78 | 8 | 3 | 3 | 0 | 0 | 0.76 | 0.29 | 3.67 | 0.38 | 0.67 | 4.3 | 0.64 | 0.3 | 0.3 | | 21 | 0.0 | 0.9 | 20 | 0.0 | 192 | 292 | 31.5 | 44 | 2.01 |
| 12042 | 1 | ea | Roast, center loin, raw | 112 | 224 | 67 | 22.5 | 0.0 | 0.0 | 0.0 | 0.0 | 14.2 | 4.9 | 6.3 | 1.5 | 0.10 | 1.34 | 75 | 8 | 2 | 2 | 0 | 0 | 1.23 | 0.23 | 5.30 | 0.54 | 0.62 | 5.6 | 0.87 | 1.0 | 0.3 | | 27 | 0.1 | 0.9 | 24 | 0.0 | 215 | 372 | 33.0 | 67 | 1.75 |
| 12045 | 3 | oz | Roast, center loin, rstd | 85 | 199 | 60 | 22.4 | 0.0 | 0.0 | 0.0 | 0.0 | 11.5 | 4.3 | 5.0 | 1.0 | 0.03 | 0.93 | 68 | 6 | 2 | 2 | 0 | | 0.73 | 0.22 | 4.44 | 0.30 | 0.48 | 3.4 | 0.56 | 0.8 | 0.3 | | 23 | 0.1 | 0.8 | 17 | 0.0 | 183 | 299 | 34.9 | 54 | 1.72 |
| 12141 | 1 | ea | Roast, sirloin, raw | 107 | 219 | 66 | 20.5 | 0.0 | 0.0 | 0.0 | 0.0 | 14.6 | 5.1 | 6.5 | 1.6 | 0.11 | 1.38 | 72 | 7 | 2 | 2 | 0 | 0 | 1.05 | 0.29 | 4.37 | 0.59 | 0.68 | 5.4 | 0.81 | 0.9 | 0.3 | | 18 | 0.0 | 1.0 | 24 | 0.0 | 210 | 342 | 32.1 | 58 | 1.99 |
| 12106 | 3 | oz | Roast, sirloin, rstd | 85 | 222 | 56 | 23.1 | 0.0 | 0.0 | 0.0 | 0.0 | 13.6 | 4.8 | 6.0 | 1.2 | 0.03 | 1.10 | 74 | 7 | 2 | 2 | 0 | 0 | 0.64 | 0.27 | 4.46 | 0.33 | 0.65 | 5.1 | 0.49 | 0.3 | 0.3 | | 20 | 0.1 | 0.9 | 20 | 0.0 | 187 | 298 | 34.3 | 51 | 2.07 |
| 12285 | 4 | oz | Roast, top loin, raw | 113 | 216 | 67 | 22.8 | 0.0 | 0.0 | 0.0 | 0.0 | 13.1 | 4.5 | 5.9 | 1.4 | 0.09 | 1.24 | 67 | 7 | 2 | 2 | 0 | 0 | 0.90 | 0.28 | 5.32 | 0.48 | 0.58 | 6.8 | 0.81 | 0.3 | 0.3 | | 21 | 0.1 | 0.8 | 24 | 0.0 | 228 | 441 | 33.9 | 49 | 1.74 |
| 12060 | 3 | oz | Roast, top loin, rstd | 85 | 192 | 59 | 24.5 | 0.0 | 0.0 | 0.0 | 0.0 | 9.7 | 3.5 | 4.5 | 0.7 | 0.02 | 0.62 | 66 | 7 | 3 | 3 | 0 | 0 | 0.52 | 0.25 | 4.36 | 0.32 | 0.47 | 6.8 | 0.46 | 0.3 | 0.3 | | 4 | 0.0 | 0.7 | 20 | 0.0 | 183 | 291 | 38.9 | 37 | 1.88 |

| Code | Amount | Description | Weight (g) | Calories | % Water | Protein (g) | Carbs (g) | Fiber (g) | Sugar (g) | Other Carbs (g) | Fat (g) | Sat Fat (g) | Mono Fat (g) | Poly Fat (g) | Omega 3 (g) | Omega 6 (g) | Choles (mg) | Vit A (IU) | Vit A (RE) | Retinol (RE) | Carotenoids (RE) | Beta Carotene (mcg) | Thiamin (mg) | Riboflavin (mg) | Niacin (NE) | Vit B6 (mg) | Vit B12 (mcg) | Folate (mcg) | Panto (mg) | Vit C (mg) | Vit D (mg) | Vit E (α TE) | Calcium (mg) | Copper (mg) | Iron (mg) | Magnes (mg) | Mang (mg) | Phos (mg) | Potassium (mg) | Selenium (mcg) | Sodium (mg) | Zinc (mg) |
|---|---|---|---|---|---|---|---|---|---|---|---|---|---|---|---|---|---|---|---|---|---|---|---|---|---|---|---|---|---|---|---|---|---|---|---|---|---|---|---|---|---|---|
| | | **Basic Components** | | | | | | | | | | **Additional Fats** | | | | | | **Vit A & Components** | | | | | **Vitamins** | | | | | | | | | | **Minerals** | | | | | | | | | |
| 12258 | 4 oz | Spareribs, raw | 113 | 323 | 57 | 19.3 | 0.0 | 0.0 | 0.0 | 0.0 | 26.7 | 10.1 | 11.5 | 2.4 | 0.10 | 2.33 | 88 | 12 | 3 | 3 | 0 | 0 | 0.70 | 0.31 | 5.49 | 0.47 | 0.98 | 4.5 | 0.90 | 0.0 | 0.3 | | 35 | 0.1 | 1.1 | 25 | 0.0 | 270 | 293 | 30.8 | 86 | 3.05 |
| 12010 | 3 oz | Spareribs, brsd | 85 | 337 | 40 | 24.7 | 0.0 | 0.0 | 0.0 | 0.0 | 25.8 | 9.4 | 11.5 | 2.3 | 0.09 | 2.23 | 103 | 9 | 3 | 3 | 0 | 0 | 0.35 | 0.32 | 4.66 | 0.30 | 0.92 | 3.4 | 0.64 | 0.0 | 0.3 | | 40 | 0.1 | 1.6 | 20 | 0.0 | 222 | 272 | 31.8 | 79 | 3.91 |
| 12289 | 1 ea | Steak, boston blade, raw | 228 | 497 | 66 | 40.4 | 0.0 | 0.0 | 0.0 | 0.0 | 36.0 | 12.5 | 16.1 | 3.9 | 0.25 | 3.44 | 162 | 16 | 5 | 5 | 0 | 0 | 1.84 | 0.66 | 8.39 | 0.70 | 1.94 | 13.7 | 1.78 | 1.6 | 0.7 | | 57 | 0.2 | 2.6 | 41 | 0.0 | 399 | 714 | 59.1 | 144 | 6.91 |
| 12115 | 3 oz | Steak, boston blade, rstd | 85 | 229 | 58 | 19.6 | 0.0 | 0.0 | 0.0 | 0.0 | 16.1 | 5.9 | 7.0 | 1.5 | 0.05 | 1.37 | 73 | 6 | 2 | 2 | 0 | 0 | 0.54 | 0.30 | 3.45 | 0.20 | 0.75 | 4.3 | 0.57 | 0.6 | 0.3 | | 24 | 0.1 | 1.2 | 15 | 0.0 | 167 | 282 | 29.2 | 57 | 3.37 |
| 12332 | 1 ea | Steak, breaded, prep, Travis Meats | 113 | 300 | 57 | 13.2 | 12.7 | 0.4 | 0.3 | 12.0 | 21.3 | 7.3 | 9.4 | 2.3 | | | 58 | 6 | 2 | | | | 0.58 | 0.23 | 3.46 | | | | | 0.5 | | | 13 | | 1.3 | | | 148 | 221 | | 339 | 1.78 |
| 12344 | 3 oz | Steak, lean, bkd | 85 | 179 | 61 | 23.4 | 0.0 | 0.0 | 0.0 | 0.0 | 8.8 | 3.1 | 3.9 | 0.8 | | | 76 | 7 | 2 | 2 | 0 | 0 | 0.80 | 0.34 | 4.05 | 0.37 | 0.82 | 5.1 | | 0.6 | 0.3 | | 20 | 0.1 | 1.2 | 22 | | 201 | 328 | | 254 | 3.05 |
| 12001 | 3 oz | Stew Meat, prep, Travis Meats | 85 | 179 | 61 | 23.4 | 0.0 | 0.0 | 0.0 | 0.0 | 8.8 | 3.1 | 3.9 | 0.8 | | | 76 | 7 | 2 | 2 | 0 | 0 | 0.80 | 0.34 | 4.05 | 0.37 | 0.82 | 5.1 | | 0.6 | 0.3 | | 20 | 0.1 | 1.2 | 22 | | 201 | 328 | | 254 | 3.05 |
| 12335 | 4 oz | Tenderloin, raw | 113 | 243 | 65 | 21.6 | 0.0 | 0.0 | 0.0 | 0.0 | 16.7 | 5.3 | 7.5 | 1.8 | | | 68 | 7 | 2 | 2 | 0 | 0 | 0.65 | 0.27 | 5.06 | | | | | 0.3 | | | 24 | | 0.8 | | | 218 | 416 | | 46 | 1.67 |
| 12238 | 3 oz | Tenderloin, rstd | 85 | 147 | 65 | 23.6 | 0.0 | 0.0 | 0.0 | 0.0 | 5.1 | 1.3 | 2.1 | 0.5 | 0.01 | 0.43 | 67 | 6 | 2 | 2 | 0 | 0 | 0.79 | 0.33 | 3.96 | 0.35 | 0.47 | 5.1 | 0.58 | 0.3 | 0.3 | | 5 | 0.0 | 1.2 | 23 | 0.0 | 218 | 368 | 40.3 | 47 | 2.21 |
| 12221 | 4 oz | Whole Shoulder, raw | 113 | 267 | 64 | 19.4 | 0.0 | 0.0 | 0.0 | 0.0 | 20.3 | 7.1 | 9.1 | 2.2 | 0.15 | 1.92 | 80 | 8 | 2 | 2 | 0 | 0 | 0.87 | 0.31 | 4.33 | 0.39 | 0.84 | 5.7 | 0.81 | 0.8 | 0.3 | | 17 | 0.1 | 1.2 | 20 | 0.0 | 206 | 341 | 28.8 | 73 | 3.05 |
| 12109 | 3 oz | Whole Shoulder, rstd | 85 | 248 | 55 | 19.8 | 0.0 | 0.0 | 0.0 | 0.0 | 18.2 | 6.[illegible] | 8.0 | 1.7 | 0.06 | 1.61 | 77 | 7 | 2 | 2 | 0 | 0 | 0.49 | 0.28 | 3.39 | 0.24 | 0.68 | 4.3 | 0.51 | 0.4 | 0.3 | | 20 | 0.1 | 1.1 | 15 | 0.0 | 180 | 280 | 28.4 | 58 | 3.15 |
| | | ***VEAL*** | | | | | | | | | | | | | | | | | | | | | | | | | | | | | | | | | | | | | | | | |
| 11591 | 3 oz | Cube Steak, prep, Kings Command Foods | 85 | 203 | | 18.0 | 1.8 | 0.2 | 0.0 | 1.6 | 13.4 | 5.6 | 5.3 | 1.5 | | | 72 | 63 | 19 | | | | 0.11 | 0.23 | 5.54 | 0.23 | 1.32 | 19.7 | | 0.0 | | | 20 | | 1.3 | | | 160 | 357 | | 60 | 4.42 |
| 11633 | 1 ea | Dinner Steak, prep, Travis | 113 | 292 | 62 | 18.1 | 0.0 | 0.0 | 0.0 | 0.0 | 24.0 | 11.7 | 9.7 | 1.3 | | | 90 | 0 | 0 | 0 | 0 | 0 | 0.07 | 0.25 | 7.01 | | | | | 0.0 | | | 14 | | 0.9 | | | 191 | 296 | | 77 | 2.76 |
| 11553 | 1 oz | Fat, cooked | 28 | 180 | 22 | 2.6 | 0.0 | 0.0 | 0.0 | 0.0 | 18.7 | 9.[illegible] | 7.8 | 0.9 | 0.15 | 0.74 | 20 | 0 | 0 | 0 | 0 | 0 | 0.01 | 0.03 | 0.78 | 0.03 | 0.15 | 1.4 | 0.13 | 0.0 | 0.1 | 0.1 | 1 | 0.0 | 0.3 | 3 | 0.0 | 32 | 48 | | 16 | 0.24 |
| 11534 | 1 oz | Fat, raw | 28 | 179 | 25 | 1.7 | 0.0 | 0.0 | 0.0 | 0.0 | 19.0 | 9.2 | 8.0 | 0.9 | 0.16 | 0.76 | 20 | 0 | 0 | 0 | 0 | 0 | 0.01 | 0.02 | 0.66 | 0.04 | 0.12 | 1.1 | 0.12 | 0.0 | 0.1 | 0.1 | 2 | 0.0 | 0.2 | 1 | 0.0 | 20 | 30 | | 7 | 0.15 |
| 11581 | 4 oz | Ground, 7% fat, raw | 113 | 163 | 73 | 21.9 | 0.0 | 0.0 | 0.0 | 0.0 | 7.7 | 3.2 | 2.9 | 0.5 | 0.05 | 0.49 | 93 | 0 | 0 | 0 | 0 | 0 | 0.09 | 0.31 | 8.48 | 0.46 | 1.51 | 14.7 | 1.48 | 0.0 | 0.3 | 0.3 | 17 | 0.1 | 0.9 | 27 | 0.0 | 229 | 356 | | 93 | 3.46 |
| 11530 | 3 oz | Ground, 8% fat, brld | 85 | 146 | 67 | 20.7 | 0.0 | 0.0 | 0.0 | 0.0 | 6.4 | 2.6 | 2.4 | 0.5 | 0.04 | 0.43 | 88 | 0 | 0 | 0 | 0 | 0 | 0.06 | 0.23 | 6.83 | 0.33 | 1.08 | 9.4 | 0.99 | 0.0 | 0.3 | | 14 | 0.1 | 0.8 | 20 | 0.0 | 184 | 286 | | 71 | 3.29 |
| 11592 | 3 oz | Patty, breaded, prep, Kings Command Foods | 85 | 210 | | 17.1 | 10.8 | 0.4 | 0.0 | 10.4 | 10.7 | 2.6 | 5.0 | 1.6 | | | 48 | 64 | 19 | | | | 0.18 | 0.23 | 5.93 | 0.24 | 1.12 | 15.7 | | 0.0 | | | 24 | | 1.6 | | | 137 | 302 | | 66 | 3.42 |
| 11635 | 1 ea | Patty, breaded, prep, Travis | 113 | 264 | 60 | 14.0 | 12.7 | 0.4 | 0.3 | 12.0 | 17.0 | 7.8 | 6.9 | 0.9 | | | 63 | 121 | 24 | | | | 0.12 | 0.22 | 5.50 | | | | | 0.0 | | | 15 | | 1.2 | | | 106 | 220 | | 345 | 2.04 |
| 11593 | 1 ea | Patty, prep, Tenderflake | 85 | 223 | 61 | 13.1 | 0.8 | 0.7 | 0.0 | 0.1 | 18.5 | 8.6 | 7.5 | 1.0 | | | 56 | 32 | 5 | | | | 0.11 | 0.18 | 4.98 | | | | | 0.0 | | | 22 | | 1.1 | | | 144 | 260 | | 139 | 3.06 |
| | | Retail Cuts | | | | | | | | | | | | | | | | | | | | | | | | | | | | | | | | | | | | | | | | |
| 11531 | 3 oz | Average, ckd | 85 | 196 | 57 | 25.6 | 0.0 | 0.0 | 0.0 | 0.0 | 9.7 | 3.6 | 3.7 | 0.7 | 0.06 | 0.62 | 97 | 0 | 0 | 0 | 0 | 0 | 0.05 | 0.27 | 6.77 | 0.26 | 1.33 | 12.8 | 1.07 | 0.0 | | 0.3 | 19 | 0.1 | 1.0 | 22 | 0.0 | 203 | 276 | | 74 | 4.05 |
| 11552 | 3 oz | Average, lean, ckd | 85 | 167 | 60 | 27.1 | 0.0 | 0.0 | 0.0 | 0.0 | 5.6 | 1.6 | 2.0 | 0.5 | 0.03 | 0.48 | 100 | 0 | 0 | 0 | 0 | 0 | 0.05 | 0.29 | 7.16 | 0.28 | 1.40 | 13.6 | 1.13 | 0.0 | 0.3 | 0.4 | 20 | 0.1 | 1.0 | 24 | 0.0 | 213 | 287 | 11.1 | 76 | 4.34 |
| 11533 | 4 oz | Average, lean, raw | 113 | 127 | 76 | 22.8 | 0.0 | 0.0 | 0.0 | 0.0 | 3.2 | 1.0 | 1.0 | 0.3 | 0.01 | 0.33 | 94 | 0 | 0 | 0 | 0 | 0 | 0.09 | 0.32 | 8.85 | 0.49 | 1.58 | 14.7 | 1.55 | 0.0 | 0.3 | 0.3 | 17 | 0.1 | 1.0 | 28 | 0.0 | 238 | 371 | | 97 | 3.65 |
| 11551 | 4 oz | Average, raw | 113 | 163 | 73 | 21.9 | 0.0 | 0.0 | 0.0 | 0.0 | 7.7 | 3.2 | 2.9 | 0.5 | 0.05 | 0.49 | 93 | 0 | 0 | 0 | 0 | 0 | 0.09 | 0.31 | 8.48 | 0.46 | 1.51 | 14.7 | 1.48 | 0.0 | 0.3 | 0.3 | 17 | 0.1 | 0.9 | 27 | 0.0 | 229 | 356 | | 93 | 3.46 |
| 11687 | 3 oz | Breast, brsd | 85 | 226 | 56 | 23.0 | 0.0 | 0.0 | 0.0 | 0.0 | 14.3 | 5.6 | 6.8 | 1.0 | 0.05 | 0.87 | 96 | | | | | | 0.05 | 0.25 | 6.78 | 0.22 | 1.13 | 11.1 | 0.88 | | | | 8 | 0.1 | 0.7 | 17 | 0.0 | 162 | 231 | | 55 | 3.09 |
| 11690 | 3 oz | Breast, lean, brsd | 85 | 185 | 60 | 25.8 | 0.0 | 0.0 | 0.0 | 0.0 | 8.3 | 3.2 | 3.8 | 0.7 | 0.03 | 0.61 | 99 | | | | | | 0.05 | 0.28 | 7.62 | 0.25 | 1.26 | 12.8 | 0.97 | | | | 8 | 0.1 | 0.7 | 19 | 0.0 | 177 | 246 | | 53 | 3.56 |
| 11686 | 4 oz | Breast, raw | 113 | 235 | 68 | 19.8 | 0.0 | 0.0 | 0.0 | 0.0 | 16.7 | 6.7 | 8.1 | 1.1 | 0.06 | 1.00 | 80 | | | | | | | | | | | | | | | | 8 | 0.1 | 0.6 | 20 | 0.0 | 194 | 323 | | 80 | 2.63 |
| 11682 | 3 oz | Chop, fried | 85 | 224 | 56 | 21.3 | 0.0 | 0.0 | 0.0 | 0.0 | 14.8 | 5.6 | 6.3 | 1.7 | | | 82 | 0 | 0 | 0 | 0 | 0 | 0.06 | 0.20 | 4.35 | 0.16 | 1.01 | 9.7 | | 0.0 | 0.3 | | 9 | 0.1 | 0.8 | 17 | | 181 | 238 | | 240 | 2.70 |
| 11683 | 3 oz | Chop, lean, fried | 85 | 178 | 58 | 27.7 | 0.0 | 0.0 | 0.0 | 0.0 | 6.6 | 2.8 | 2.5 | 0.4 | | | 144 | 0 | 0 | 0 | 0 | 0 | 0.05 | 0.30 | 8.44 | 0.22 | 1.37 | 13.5 | | 0.0 | 0.3 | | 31 | 0.1 | 1.1 | 23 | | 203 | 240 | | 276 | 3.68 |
| 11516 | 3 oz | Leg, lean, rstd | 85 | 128 | 67 | 23.9 | 0.0 | 0.0 | 0.0 | 0.0 | 2.9 | 1.0 | 1.0 | 0.2 | 0.02 | 0.23 | 88 | 0 | 0 | 0 | 0 | 0 | 0.05 | 0.28 | 8.59 | 0.26 | 1.00 | 13.6 | 0.85 | 0.0 | 0.3 | 0.5 | 5 | 0.1 | 0.8 | 24 | 0.0 | 201 | 334 | 11.1 | 58 | 2.62 |
| 11555 | 3 oz | Leg, top round, brsd | 85 | 179 | 56 | 30.8 | 0.0 | 0.0 | 0.0 | 0.0 | 5.4 | 2.2 | 2.0 | 0.4 | 0.03 | 0.37 | 114 | 0 | 0 | 0 | 0 | 0 | 0.05 | 0.30 | 9.01 | 0.31 | 0.99 | 15.3 | 0.87 | 0.0 | 0.3 | 0.4 | 7 | 0.1 | 1.1 | 25 | 0.0 | 212 | 326 | | 57 | 3.37 |
| 11557 | 3 oz | Leg, top round, lean, brsd | 85 | 173 | 56 | 31.2 | 0.0 | 0.0 | 0.0 | 0.0 | 4.3 | 1.6 | 1.6 | 0.3 | 0.03 | 0.32 | 115 | 0 | 0 | 0 | 0 | 0 | 0.05 | 0.31 | 9.10 | 0.31 | 1.01 | 15.3 | 0.88 | 0.0 | 0.3 | 0.4 | 8 | 0.1 | 1.1 | 26 | 0.0 | 214 | 329 | 11.1 | 57 | 3.43 |
| 11556 | 4 oz | Leg, top round, lean, raw | 113 | 121 | 76 | 24.1 | 0.0 | 0.0 | 0.0 | 0.0 | 2.0 | 0.6 | 0.6 | 0.2 | 0.01 | 0.19 | 83 | 0 | 0 | 0 | 0 | 0 | 0.09 | 0.32 | 10.80 | 0.53 | 1.19 | 15.8 | 1.23 | 0.0 | 0.3 | 0.3 | 6 | 0.1 | 0.9 | 31 | 0.0 | 252 | 420 | | 72 | 2.64 |
| 11554 | 4 oz | Leg, top round, raw | 113 | 132 | 75 | 23.7 | 0.0 | 0.0 | 0.0 | 0.0 | 3.5 | 1.3 | 1.3 | 0.3 | 0.02 | 0.25 | 83 | 0 | 0 | 0 | 0 | 0 | 0.09 | 0.31 | 10.64 | 0.52 | 1.18 | 15.8 | 1.21 | 0.0 | 0.3 | | 6 | 0.1 | 0.9 | 29 | 0.0 | 249 | 415 | | 71 | 2.60 |
| 11509 | 3 oz | Leg, top round, rstd | 85 | 136 | 66 | 23.5 | 0.0 | 0.0 | 0.0 | 0.0 | 4.0 | 1.6 | 1.5 | 0.3 | 0.03 | 0.27 | 83 | 0 | 0 | 0 | 0 | 0 | 0.05 | 0.27 | 8.44 | 0.26 | 0.99 | 13.6 | 0.84 | 0.0 | 0.3 | 0.4 | 5 | 0.1 | 0.8 | 24 | 0.0 | 199 | 331 | | 58 | 2.58 |
| 11529 | 3 oz | Leg/Shoulder, lean, cubed, brsd | 85 | 160 | 59 | 29.7 | 0.0 | 0.0 | 0.0 | 0.0 | 3.7 | 1.1 | 1.2 | 0.4 | 0.02 | 0.37 | 123 | 0 | 0 | 0 | 0 | 0 | 0.06 | 0.34 | 7.06 | 0.32 | 1.42 | 13.6 | 1.01 | 0.0 | 0.3 | 0.4 | 25 | 0.1 | 1.2 | 24 | 0.0 | 203 | 291 | 11.1 | 79 | 5.11 |
| 11580 | 4 oz | Leg/Shoulder, lean, cubed, raw | 113 | 123 | 76 | 22.9 | 0.0 | 0.0 | 0.0 | 0.0 | 2.8 | 0.8 | 0.9 | 0.3 | 0.01 | 0.28 | 95 | 0 | 0 | 0 | 0 | 0 | 0.10 | 0.33 | 8.36 | 0.51 | 1.68 | 14.7 | 1.41 | 0.0 | 0.3 | 0.3 | 19 | 0.1 | 1.0 | 28 | 0.0 | 241 | 374 | | 94 | 3.93 |
| 11517 | 1 ea | Loin Chop, brsd | 80 | 227 | 52 | 24.2 | 0.0 | 0.0 | 0.0 | 0.0 | 13.8 | 5.4 | 5.4 | 0.9 | 0.09 | 0.33 | 94 | 0 | 0 | 0 | 0 | 0 | 0.03 | 0.24 | 7.22 | 0.21 | 0.97 | 11.2 | 0.63 | 0.0 | 0.2 | 0.3 | 22 | 0.1 | 0.9 | 19 | 0.0 | 176 | 224 | 12.2 | 64 | 2.90 |
| 11504 | 1 ea | Loin Chop, breaded, fried | 127 | 290 | 51 | 34.7 | 12.5 | 0.4 | 1.1 | 11.0 | 11.7 | 3.9 | 4.3 | 1.9 | 0.18 | 1.70 | 142 | 43 | 13 | 0 | 13 | 0 | 0.20 | 0.44 | 13.08 | 0.51 | 1.57 | 34.3 | 1.36 | 0.0 | 0.4 | 0.7 | 50 | 0.1 | 2.1 | 39 | 0.2 | 317 | 471 | | 577 | 3.49 |
| 11507 | 1 ea | Loin Chop, fried | 105 | 222 | 58 | 33.4 | 0.0 | 0.0 | 0.0 | 0.0 | 8.8 | 3.3 | 3.4 | 0.6 | 0.05 | 0.56 | 110 | 0 | 0 | 0 | 0 | 0 | 0.07 | 0.37 | 12.70 | 0.51 | 1.52 | 15.7 | 1.23 | 0.0 | 0.3 | 0.4 | 6 | 0.1 | 0.9 | 33 | 0.0 | 293 | 446 | | 80 | 3.39 |
| 11518 | 1 ea | Loin Chop, lean, brsd | 69 | 156 | 57 | 23.2 | 0.0 | 0.0 | 0.0 | 0.0 | 6.3 | 1.8 | 2.3 | 0.6 | 0.03 | 0.54 | 86 | 0 | 0 | 0 | 0 | 0 | 0.03 | 0.23 | 6.97 | 0.19 | 0.91 | 10.4 | 0.59 | 0.0 | 0.2 | 0.3 | 22 | 0.1 | 0.8 | 19 | 0.0 | 164 | 205 | 9.0 | 58 | 2.82 |
| 11511 | 1 ea | Loin Chop, lean, breaded, fried | 101 | 208 | 53 | 28.7 | 9.9 | 0.2 | 0.9 | 8.7 | 6.3 | 1.6 | 2.2 | 1.4 | 0.11 | 1.25 | 114 | 34 | 10 | 0 | 10 | 0 | 0.16 | 0.36 | 10.91 | 0.42 | 1.29 | 28.3 | 1.12 | 0.0 | 0.3 | 0.5 | 39 | 0.1 | 1.7 | 32 | 0.1 | 261 | 387 | 13.6 | 460 | 2.90 |
| 11514 | 1 ea | Loin Chop, lean, fried | 85 | 156 | 61 | 28.2 | 0.0 | 0.0 | 0.0 | 0.0 | 3.9 | 1.1 | 1.4 | 0.3 | 0.02 | 0.33 | 91 | 0 | 0 | 0 | 0 | 0 | 0.06 | 0.31 | 10.71 | 0.43 | 1.28 | 13.6 | 1.04 | 0.0 | 0.3 | 0.4 | 6 | 0.1 | 0.7 | 27 | 0.0 | 247 | 376 | 11.1 | 65 | 2.87 |
| 11559 | 1 ea | Loin Chop, lean, raw | 113 | 131 | 75 | 22.8 | 0.0 | 0.0 | 0.0 | 0.0 | 3.8 | 1.1 | 1.2 | 0.4 | 0.01 | 0.37 | 90 | 0 | 0 | 0 | 0 | 0 | 0.08 | 0.29 | 10.26 | 0.63 | 1.33 | 15.8 | 1.57 | 0.0 | 0.3 | 0.3 | 19 | 0.1 | 0.8 | 28 | 0.0 | 238 | 366 | | 103 | 2.81 |
| 11560 | 3 oz | Loin Chop, lean, rstd | 85 | 149 | 65 | 22.4 | 0.0 | 0.0 | 0.0 | 0.0 | 5.9 | 2.2 | 2.1 | 0.5 | 0.03 | 0.45 | 90 | 0 | 0 | 0 | 0 | 0 | 0.05 | 0.26 | 8.04 | 0.31 | 1.11 | 13.6 | 1.08 | 0.0 | 0.3 | 0.4 | 18 | 0.1 | 0.7 | 22 | 0.0 | 189 | 289 | 11.1 | 82 | 2.75 |
| 11558 | 4 oz | Loin Chop, raw | 113 | 184 | 70 | 21.4 | 0.0 | 0.0 | 0.0 | 0.0 | 10.3 | 4.4 | 4.0 | 0.7 | 0.07 | 0.62 | 89 | 0 | 0 | 0 | 0 | 0 | 0.08 | 0.27 | 9.58 | 0.60 | 1.25 | 14.7 | 1.47 | 0.0 | 0.3 | 0.3 | 18 | 0.1 | 0.8 | 26 | 0.0 | 225 | 344 | | 96 | 2.62 |
| 11595 | 1 ea | Loin Chop, rstd | 229 | 497 | 61 | 56.8 | 0.0 | 0.0 | 0.0 | 0.0 | 28.2 | 12.0 | 10.9 | 1.9 | 0.21 | 1.65 | 236 | 0 | 0 | 0 | 0 | 0 | 0.11 | 0.64 | 20.29 | 0.78 | 2.84 | 34.3 | 2.75 | 0.0 | 0.7 | 1.0 | 44 | 0.3 | 2.0 | 57 | 0.1 | 485 | 744 | | 213 | 6.94 |
| 11561 | 3 oz | Ribs, brsd | 85 | 213 | 53 | 27.5 | 0.0 | 0.0 | 0.0 | 0.0 | 10.6 | 4.2 | 4.0 | 0.8 | 0.07 | 0.73 | 118 | 0 | 0 | 0 | 0 | 0 | 0.04 | 0.25 | 6.38 | 0.27 | 1.23 | 13.6 | 0.91 | 0.0 | 0.3 | 0.3 | 19 | 0.1 | 1.2 | 21 | 0.0 | 179 | 260 | | 81 | 4.73 |
| 11563 | 3 oz | Ribs, lean, brsd | 85 | 185 | 56 | 29.2 | 0.0 | 0.0 | 0.0 | 0.0 | 6.6 | 2.2 | 2.2 | 0.6 | 0.03 | 0.60 | 112 | 0 | 0 | 0 | 0 | 0 | 0.05 | 0.26 | 6.72 | 0.29 | 1.30 | 13.6 | 0.96 | 0.0 | 0.3 | 0.3 | 20 | 0.1 | 1.2 | 22 | 0.0 | 185 | 270 | 11.1 | 84 | 5.08 |
| 11562 | 4 oz | Ribs, lean, raw | 113 | 136 | 75 | 22.6 | 0.0 | 0.0 | 0.0 | 0.0 | 4.4 | 1.3 | 1.4 | 0.5 | 0.01 | 0.44 | 94 | 0 | 0 | 0 | 0 | 0 | 0.08 | 0.27 | 7.97 | 0.50 | 1.54 | 14.7 | 1.34 | 0.0 | 0.3 | 0.2 | 16 | 0.1 | 1.0 | 26 | 0.0 | 219 | 346 | | 107 | 3.92 |
| 11520 | 3 oz | Ribs, lean, rstd | 85 | 150 | 65 | 21.9 | 0.0 | 0.0 | 0.0 | 0.0 | 6.3 | 1.8 | 2.3 | 0.6 | 0.03 | 0.54 | 98 | 0 | 0 | 0 | 0 | 0 | 0.05 | 0.25 | 6.38 | 0.23 | 1.34 | 11.9 | 1.17 | 0.0 | 0.3 | 0.3 | 10 | 0.1 | 0.8 | 20 | 0.0 | 176 | 264 | 11.1 | 82 | 3.82 |
| 11597 | 4 oz | Ribs, raw | 113 | 183 | 71 | 21.4 | 0.0 | 0.0 | 0.0 | 0.0 | 10.2 | 4.2 | 3.9 | 0.7 | 0.07 | 0.64 | 93 | 0 | 0 | 0 | 0 | 0 | 0.08 | 0.26 | 7.55 | 0.47 | 1.46 | 13.6 | 1.28 | 0.0 | 0.3 | | 15 | 0.1 | 1.0 | 25 | 0.0 | 208 | 328 | | 101 | 3.66 |
| 11519 | 3 oz | Ribs, rstd | 85 | 194 | 60 | 20.4 | 0.0 | 0.0 | 0.0 | 0.0 | 11.9 | 4.6 | 4.6 | 0.8 | 0.08 | 0.73 | 94 | 0 | 0 | 0 | 0 | 0 | 0.04 | 0.23 | 5.93 | 0.21 | 1.24 | 11.1 | 1.09 | 0.0 | 0.3 | 0.3 | 9 | 0.1 | 0.8 | 19 | 0.0 | 167 | 251 | 10.3 | 78 | 3.48 |
| 11521 | 3 oz | Shoulder, arm/blade, brsd | 85 | 194 | 56 | 27.3 | 0.0 | 0.0 | 0.0 | 0.0 | 8.6 | 3.2 | 3.3 | 0.6 | 0.05 | 0.57 | 107 | 0 | 0 | 0 | 0 | 0 | 0.05 | 0.29 | 5.46 | 0.21 | 1.56 | 12.8 | 1.30 | 0.0 | 0.3 | 0.4 | 30 | 0.1 | 1.2 | 23 | 0.0 | 213 | 263 | | 81 | 5.60 |
| 11522 | 3 oz | Shoulder, arm/blade, lean, brsd | 85 | 169 | 59 | 28.6 | 0.0 | 0.0 | 0.0 | 0.0 | 5.2 | 1.4 | 1.9 | 0.5 | 0.03 | 0.44 | 111 | 0 | 0 | 0 | 0 | 0 | 0.05 | 0.30 | 5.68 | 0.22 | 1.65 | 13.6 | 1.37 | 0.0 | 0.3 | 0.4 | 31 | 0.1 | 1.2 | 24 | 0.0 | 221 | 271 | 11.1 | 82 | 5.95 |
| 11566 | 4 oz | Shoulder, arm/blade, lean, raw | 113 | 127 | 77 | 22.4 | 0.0 | 0.0 | 0.0 | 0.0 | 3.4 | 1.0 | 1.1 | 0.4 | 0.01 | 0.34 | 97 | 0 | 0 | 0 | 0 | 0 | 0.10 | 0.33 | 6.95 | 0.45 | 1.90 | 12.4 | 1.64 | 0.0 | 0.3 | 0.3 | 25 | 0.1 | 1.0 | 27 | 0.0 | 235 | 351 | | 104 | 4.59 |
| 11567 | 3 oz | Shoulder, arm/blade, lean, rstd | 85 | 145 | 67 | 21.9 | 0.0 | 0.0 | 0.0 | 0.0 | 5.6 | 2.1 | 2.0 | 0.5 | 0.03 | 0.42 | 97 | 0 | 0 | 0 | 0 | 0 | 0.06 | 0.29 | 5.47 | 0.22 | 1.58 | 11.1 | 1.12 | 0.0 | 0.3 | 0.4 | 23 | 0.1 | 0.9 | 21 | 0.0 | 185 | 278 | 11.1 | 82 | 4.46 |
| 11564 | 4 oz | Shoulder, arm/blade, raw | 113 | 147 | 75 | 21.8 | 0.0 | 0.0 | 0.0 | 0.0 | 6.0 | 2.3 | 2.2 | 0.5 | 0.03 | 0.42 | 98 | 0 | 0 | 0 | 0 | 0 | 0.10 | 0.33 | 6.99 | 0.44 | 1.89 | 13.6 | 1.60 | 0.0 | 0.3 | 0.3 | 25 | 0.1 | 1.0 | 26 | 0.0 | 229 | 341 | | 103 | 4.44 |
| 11565 | 3 oz | Shoulder, arm/blade, rstd | 85 | 156 | 65 | 21.5 | 0.0 | 0.0 | 0.0 | 0.0 | 7.2 | 2.9 | 2.7 | 0.5 | 0.04 | 0.48 | 95 | 0 | 0 | 0 | 0 | 0 | 0.06 | 0.29 | 5.38 | 0.22 | 1.55 | 10.2 | 1.11 | 0.0 | 0.3 | 0.4 | 23 | 0.1 | 0.9 | 21 | 0.0 | 183 | 274 | | 82 | 4.35 |
| 11692 | 3 oz | Shank, brsd | 85 | 162 | 62 | 26.8 | 0.0 | 0.0 | 0.0 | 0.0 | 5.3 | 1.8 | 2.0 | 0.5 | 0.02 | 0.43 | 105 | | | | | | 0.04 | 0.25 | 8.03 | 0.23 | 1.37 | 14.5 | 1.05 | | | | 28 | 0.1 | 1.1 | 21 | 0.0 | 191 | 259 | | 79 | 5.64 |
| 11694 | 3 oz | Shank, lean, brsd | 85 | 150 | 63 | 27.4 | 0.0 | 0.0 | 0.0 | 0.0 | 3.7 | 1.0 | 1.3 | 0.4 | 0.01 | 0.37 | 107 | 0 | 0 | 0 | 0 | 0 | 0.04 | 0.25 | 8.21 | 0.23 | 1.39 | 14.5 | 1.06 | | | | 29 | 0.1 | 1.1 | 21 | 0.0 | 194 | 263 | | 80 | 5.79 |
| 11693 | 4 oz | Shank, lean, raw | 113 | 122 | 78 | 21.8 | 0.0 | 0.0 | 0.0 | 0.0 | 3.2 | 0.8 | 1.1 | 0.4 | 0.01 | 0.35 | 85 | | | | | | 0.09 | 0.31 | 8.59 | 0.50 | 1.55 | 17.0 | 1.47 | | | | 23 | 0.1 | 0.9 | 24 | 0.0 | 217 | 357 | | 96 | 4.54 |
| 11691 | 4 oz | Shank, raw | 113 | 128 | 77 | 21.7 | 0.0 | 0.0 | 0.0 | 0.0 | 3.9 | 1.2 | 1.4 | 0.4 | 0.02 | 0.39 | 85 | | | | | | 0.09 | 0.30 | 8.43 | 0.49 | 1.54 | 17.0 | 1.46 | | | | 23 | 0.1 | 0.9 | 24 | 0.0 | 216 | 355 | | 95 | 4.51 |
| 11577 | 3 oz | Sirloin, brsd | 85 | 214 | 54 | 26.6 | 0.0 | 0.0 | 0.0 | 0.0 | 11.1 | 4.4 | 4.4 | 0.7 | 0.08 | 0.65 | 92 | 0 | 0 | 0 | 0 | 0 | 0.04 | 0.30 | 5.59 | 0.30 | 1.26 | 12.8 | 0.86 | 0.0 | 0.3 | 0.3 | 14 | 0.1 | 1.0 | 23 | 0.0 | 207 | 273 | | 67 | 3.67 |
| 11576 | 4 oz | Sirloin, raw | 113 | 172 | 72 | 21.6 | 0.0 | 0.0 | 0.0 | 0.0 | 8.8 | 3.8 | 3.4 | 0.6 | 0.07 | 0.51 | 88 | 0 | 0 | 0 | 0 | 0 | 0.09 | 0.34 | 9.54 | 0.55 | 1.44 | 14.7 | 1.54 | 0.0 | 0.3 | 0.3 | 12 | 0.1 | 0.9 | 27 | 0.0 | 236 | 372 | | 86 | 2.88 |
| 11527 | 3 oz | Sirloin, rstd | 85 | 172 | 63 | 21.3 | 0.0 | 0.0 | 0.0 | 0.0 | 8.9 | 3.8 | 3.5 | 0.6 | 0.06 | 0.51 | 87 | 0 | 0 | 0 | 0 | 0 | 0.05 | 0.30 | 7.54 | 0.27 | 1.21 | 12.8 | 1.07 | 0.0 | 0.3 | 0.4 | 11 | 0.1 | 0.8 | 22 | 0.0 | 190 | 298 | | 71 | 2.85 |
| 11579 | 3 oz | Sirloin, lean, brsd | 85 | 173 | 59 | 28.9 | 0.0 | 0.0 | 0.0 | 0.0 | 5.5 | 1.5 | 2.0 | 0.5 | 0.03 | 0.47 | 95 | 0 | 0 | 0 | 0 | 0 | 0.05 | 0.32 | 5.99 | 0.32 | 1.35 | 13.6 | 0.92 | 0.0 | 0.3 | 0.4 | 16 | 0.1 | 1.0 | 25 | 0.0 | 220 | 288 | 11.1 | 69 | 4.04 |
| 11528 | 3 oz | Sirloin, lean, rstd | 85 | 143 | 66 | 22.4 | 0.0 | 0.0 | 0.0 | 0.0 | 5.3 | 2.0 | 1.9 | 0.4 | 0.03 | 0.37 | 88 | 0 | 0 | 0 | 0 | 0 | 0.05 | 0.31 | 7.93 | 0.29 | 1.27 | 13.6 | 1.12 | 0.0 | 0.3 | 0.4 | 12 | 0.1 | 0.8 | 23 | 0.0 | 196 | 310 | 11.1 | 72 | 3.01 |

| Code | Amount | Description | Basic Components | | | | | | | | | Additional Fats | | | | | | Vit A & Components | | | | | Vitamins | | | | | | | | | | Minerals | | | | | | | | | |
|---|---|---|---|---|---|---|---|---|---|---|---|---|---|---|---|---|---|---|---|---|---|---|---|---|---|---|---|---|---|---|---|---|---|---|---|---|---|---|---|---|---|---|
| | | | Weight (g) | Calories | % Water | Protein (g) | Carbs (g) | Fiber (g) | Sugar (g) | Other Carbs (g) | Fat (g) | Sat Fat (g) | Mono Fat (g) | Poly Fat (g) | Omega 3 (g) | Omega 6 (g) | Choles (mg) | Vit A (IU) | Vit A (RE) | Retinol (RE) | Carotenoids (RE) | Beta Carotene (mcg) | Thiamin (mg) | Riboflavin (mg) | Niacin (NE) | Vit B6 (mg) | Vit B12 (mcg) | Folate (mcg) | Panto (mg) | Vit C (mg) | Vit D (mg) | Vit E (α TE) | Calcium (mg) | Copper (mg) | Iron (mg) | Magnes (mg) | Mang (mg) | Phos (mg) | Potassium (mg) | Selenium (mcg) | Sodium (mg) | Zinc (mg) |
| 11578 | 4 oz | Sirloin, lean, raw | 113 | 124 | 76 | 22.8 | 0.0 | 0.0 | 0.0 | 0.0 | 2.9 | 0.9 | 0.9 | 0.3 | 0.01 | 0.29 | 89 | 0 | 0 | 0 | 0 | 0 | 0.09 | 0.35 | 10.14 | 0.59 | 1.51 | 15.8 | 1.64 | 0.0 | 0.3 | 0.3 | 12 | 0.1 | 0.9 | 29 | 0.0 | 249 | 393 | | 90 | 3.08 |
| 11636 | 1 ea | Slices, Italian, breaded, prep, 3 oz svg, Travis | 113 | 266 | 60 | 14.1 | 12.4 | 0.2 | 0.0 | 12.2 | 17.4 | 7.8 | 6.9 | 0.9 | | | 63 | 8 | 2 | | | | 0.11 | 0.21 | 5.42 | | | | | 0.1 | | | 18 | | 1.1 | | | 149 | 222 | | 388 | 2.04 |
| 11634 | 1 ea | Slices, prep, 3 oz svg, Travis | 85 | 220 | 50 | 13.6 | 10.0 | 0.0 | 0.0 | 10.0 | 18.1 | 8.4 | 7.3 | 1.0 | | | 67 | 0 | 0 | 0 | 0 | 0 | 0.05 | 0.19 | 5.28 | | | | | 0.0 | | | 11 | | 0.7 | | | 144 | 223 | | 58 | 2.08 |
| | | *ORGAN MEATS* | | | | | | | | | | | | | | | | | | | | | | | | | | | | | | | | | | | | | | | | |
| | | Beef | | | | | | | | | | | | | | | | | | | | | | | | | | | | | | | | | | | | | | | | |
| 10468 | 3 oz | Brains, ckd | 85 | 136 | 73 | 9.4 | 0.0 | 0.0 | 0.0 | 0.0 | 10.6 | 2.5 | 2.1 | 1.2 | 0.57 | 0.28 | 1746 | 0 | 0 | 0 | 0 | 0 | 0.07 | 0.14 | 1.85 | 0.20 | 7.31 | 6.0 | 0.48 | 0.9 | 0.3 | | 8 | 0.2 | 1.9 | 12 | 0.0 | 299 | 204 | | 102 | 1.06 |
| 10467 | 4 oz | Brains, raw | 85 | 107 | 78 | 8.3 | 0.0 | 0.0 | 0.0 | 0.0 | 7.9 | 1.8 | 1.6 | 0.9 | 0.43 | 0.20 | 1421 | 0 | 0 | 0 | 0 | 0 | 0.13 | 0.23 | 3.89 | 0.22 | 9.27 | 3.4 | 1.04 | 14.1 | 0.3 | | 7 | 0.2 | 1.8 | 11 | 0.0 | 218 | 273 | | 88 | 1.04 |
| 10785 | 3 oz | Heart, ckd | 85 | 149 | 64 | 24.5 | 0.4 | 0.0 | | | 4.8 | 1.4 | 1.1 | 1.2 | 0.02 | 1.15 | 164 | 0 | 0 | 0 | 0 | 0 | 0.12 | 1.31 | 3.46 | 0.18 | 12.16 | 1.7 | 0.74 | 1.3 | 0.3 | | 5 | 0.6 | 6.4 | 21 | 0.1 | 213 | 198 | 18.0 | 54 | 2.66 |
| 10469 | 4 oz | Heart, raw | 113 | 132 | 76 | 19.3 | 2.9 | 0.0 | | | 4.3 | 1.3 | 0.9 | 1.0 | 0.01 | 1.03 | 158 | 0 | 0 | 0 | 0 | 0 | 0.21 | 1.15 | 10.69 | 0.49 | 15.48 | 2.3 | 2.62 | 7.1 | 0.3 | | 2 | 0.4 | 5.2 | 26 | 0.0 | 195 | 301 | | 71 | 2.69 |
| 10034 | 3 oz | Kidney, ckd | 85 | 122 | 69 | 21.7 | 0.8 | 0.0 | | | 2.9 | 0.9 | 0.6 | 0.6 | 0.01 | 0.62 | 329 | 1055 | 317 | 317 | 0 | 0 | 0.16 | 3.45 | 5.12 | 0.44 | 43.60 | 83.3 | 1.44 | 0.7 | 0.3 | | 14 | 0.6 | 6.2 | 15 | 0.2 | 260 | 152 | | 114 | 3.59 |
| 10470 | 4 oz | Kidney, raw | 113 | 121 | 77 | 18.8 | 2.5 | 0.0 | | | 3.5 | 1.1 | 0.7 | 0.8 | 0.01 | 0.75 | 322 | 994 | 298 | 298 | 0 | 0 | 0.43 | 2.88 | 8.98 | 0.58 | 30.51 | 90.4 | 4.11 | 10.1 | 0.3 | | 7 | 0.5 | 8.3 | 19 | 0.1 | 237 | 290 | 168.4 | 202 | 2.09 |
| 10472 | 3 oz | Liver, brsd | 85 | 137 | 66 | 20.7 | 2.9 | 0.0 | 0.0 | 2.9 | 4.2 | 1.6 | 0.6 | 0.9 | 0.21 | 0.63 | 331 | 30327 | 9012 | 8989 | 23 | | 0.17 | 3.49 | 9.10 | 0.77 | 60.35 | 184.5 | 3.88 | 19.6 | 0.3 | | 6 | 3.8 | 5.8 | 17 | 0.4 | 343 | 200 | | 60 | 5.16 |
| 10471 | 4 oz | Liver, raw | 113 | 162 | 69 | 22.6 | 6.6 | 0.0 | 0.0 | 6.6 | 4.4 | 1.7 | 0.6 | 0.9 | 0.23 | 0.66 | 400 | 39941 | 11868 | 11829 | 40 | | 0.29 | 3.14 | 14.46 | 1.06 | 78.20 | 280.2 | 8.61 | 24.9 | 0.3 | | 7 | 3.8 | 7.7 | 21 | 0.3 | 359 | 365 | 46.7 | 82 | 4.43 |
| 10474 | 3 oz | Lungs, brsd | 85 | 102 | 76 | 17.3 | 0.0 | 0.0 | 0.0 | 0.0 | 3.1 | 1.1 | 0.8 | 0.4 | 0.03 | 0.39 | 235 | 33 | 10 | 10 | 0 | 0 | 0.03 | 0.12 | 2.12 | 0.02 | 2.20 | 6.8 | 0.53 | 27.8 | 0.3 | | 9 | 0.2 | 4.6 | 9 | 0.0 | 151 | 147 | | 86 | 1.39 |
| 10473 | 4 oz | Lungs, raw | 113 | 104 | 79 | 18.3 | 0.0 | 0.0 | 0.0 | 0.0 | 2.8 | 1.0 | 0.7 | 0.4 | 0.02 | 0.35 | 273 | 52 | 16 | 16 | 0 | 0 | 0.05 | 0.26 | 4.52 | 0.05 | 4.31 | 12.4 | 1.13 | 43.5 | 0.3 | | 11 | 0.3 | 9.0 | 16 | 0.0 | 253 | 384 | | 224 | 1.82 |
| 10477 | 3 oz | Pancreas, brsd | 85 | 230 | 56 | 23.0 | 0.0 | 0.0 | 0.0 | 0.0 | 14.6 | 5.0 | 5.0 | 2.7 | 0.10 | 2.22 | 223 | 0 | 0 | 0 | 0 | 0 | 0.15 | 0.41 | 3.37 | 0.15 | 14.11 | 2.6 | 3.61 | 17.3 | 0.3 | | 14 | 0.1 | 2.2 | 18 | 0.2 | 385 | 209 | | 51 | 3.91 |
| 10476 | 4 oz | Pancreas, raw | 113 | 266 | 65 | 17.7 | 0.0 | 0.0 | 0.0 | 0.0 | 21.0 | 7.2 | 7.3 | 3.9 | 0.15 | 3.20 | 232 | 0 | 0 | 0 | 0 | 0 | 0.16 | 0.50 | 5.03 | 0.23 | 15.82 | 3.4 | 4.41 | 15.5 | 0.3 | | 10 | 0.1 | 2.5 | 20 | 0.2 | 370 | 312 | | 76 | 2.92 |
| 10479 | 3 oz | Spleen, brsd | 85 | 123 | 70 | 21.3 | 0.0 | 0.0 | 0.0 | 0.0 | 3.6 | 1.2 | 1.0 | 0.3 | 0.00 | 0.26 | 295 | 0 | 0 | 0 | 0 | 0 | 0.04 | 0.26 | 4.73 | 0.03 | 4.27 | 3.4 | 0.74 | 42.8 | 0.3 | | 10 | 0.8 | 33.5 | 16 | 0.1 | 259 | 241 | | 48 | 2.37 |
| 10478 | 4 oz | Spleen, raw | 113 | 119 | 77 | 20.7 | 0.0 | 0.0 | 0.0 | 0.0 | 3.4 | 1.1 | 0.9 | 0.2 | 0.00 | 0.25 | 297 | 0 | 0 | 0 | 0 | 0 | 0.06 | 0.42 | 9.49 | 0.08 | 6.42 | 4.5 | 1.22 | 51.4 | 0.3 | | 10 | 0.2 | 50.4 | 25 | 0.1 | 334 | 485 | | 96 | 2.38 |
| 10482 | 3 oz | Thymus, brsd | 85 | 271 | 53 | 18.6 | 0.0 | 0.0 | 0.0 | 0.0 | 21.3 | 7.3 | 7.3 | 4.0 | 0.14 | 2.31 | 250 | 0 | 0 | 0 | 0 | 0 | 0.07 | 0.19 | 1.56 | 0.07 | 1.28 | 0.9 | 1.67 | 25.7 | 0.3 | | 9 | 0.0 | 1.3 | 9 | 0.1 | 309 | 368 | | 99 | 1.87 |
| 10481 | 4 oz | Thymus, raw | 113 | 267 | 68 | 13.8 | 0.0 | 0.0 | 0.0 | 0.0 | 23.1 | 7.9 | 8.0 | 4.3 | 0.16 | 2.51 | 252 | 0 | 0 | 0 | 0 | 0 | 0.12 | 0.39 | 3.90 | 0.18 | 2.41 | 2.3 | 3.42 | 38.4 | 0.3 | | 8 | 0.1 | 2.4 | 16 | 0.1 | 444 | 407 | | 108 | 2.33 |
| 10011 | 3 oz | Tongue, ckd | 85 | 241 | 56 | 18.8 | 0.3 | 0.0 | | | 17.6 | 7.6 | 8.0 | 0.7 | 0.00 | 0.66 | 91 | 0 | 0 | 0 | 0 | 0 | 0.03 | 0.30 | 1.83 | 0.14 | 5.02 | 4.3 | 0.44 | 0.4 | 0.3 | | 6 | 0.2 | 2.9 | 14 | 0.0 | 121 | 153 | 18.0 | 51 | 4.08 |
| 11606 | 4 pce | Tongue, smkd, cured, pickled, ckd | 80 | 214 | 57 | 15.4 | 0.2 | 0.0 | | | 16.2 | 7.0 | 7.4 | 0.6 | | | 72 | 0 | 0 | 0 | 0 | 0 | 0.10 | 0.23 | 4.00 | 0.11 | 4.17 | 3.2 | | 0.0 | | | 6 | 0.2 | 2.6 | 13 | | 146 | 158 | | 817 | 3.63 |
| 10483 | 4 oz | Tongue, raw | 113 | 253 | 64 | 16.8 | 4.2 | 0.0 | | | 18.2 | 7.9 | 8.2 | 1.0 | 0.00 | 1.01 | 98 | 0 | 0 | 0 | 0 | 0 | 0.14 | 0.38 | 4.79 | 0.35 | 4.28 | 7.9 | 0.74 | 3.5 | 0.3 | | 7 | 0.2 | 3.3 | 18 | 0.0 | 150 | 356 | | 78 | 3.24 |
| 10019 | 3 oz | Tripe, pickled | 85 | 53 | 86 | 10.0 | 0.0 | 0.0 | 0.0 | 0.0 | 1.1 | 0.4 | 0.4 | 0.0 | 0.00 | 0.01 | 58 | 0 | 0 | 0 | 0 | 0 | 0.00 | 0.13 | 1.36 | 0.02 | 0.78 | 0.9 | 0.36 | 0.0 | 0.3 | | 108 | 0.1 | 1.4 | 6 | 0.0 | 73 | 16 | | 39 | 1.47 |
| 10018 | 4 oz | Tripe, raw | 113 | 111 | 81 | 16.5 | 0.0 | 0.0 | 0.0 | 0.0 | 4.5 | 2.3 | 1.5 | 0.1 | 0.02 | 0.06 | 107 | 0 | 0 | 0 | 0 | 0 | 0.01 | 0.19 | 0.07 | 0.05 | 1.74 | 2.3 | 0.64 | 3.8 | 0.3 | | 10 | 0.1 | 2.2 | 9 | 0.0 | 89 | 305 | | 52 | 2.79 |
| | | Chicken | | | | | | | | | | | | | | | | | | | | | | | | | | | | | | | | | | | | | | | | |
| 15106 | 3 oz | Giblets, ckd | 85 | 133 | 68 | 22.0 | 0.8 | 0.0 | 0.0 | 0.8 | 4.1 | 1.3 | 1.0 | 0.9 | 0.05 | 0.84 | 334 | 6316 | 1895 | 1895 | 0 | 0 | 0.07 | 0.81 | 3.49 | 0.29 | 8.59 | 319.6 | 2.52 | 6.8 | 0.3 | | 10 | 0.2 | 5.5 | 17 | 0.1 | 195 | 134 | | 49 | 3.88 |
| 15104 | 4 oz | Giblets, raw | 113 | 140 | 75 | 20.2 | 2.0 | 0.0 | 0.0 | 2.0 | 5.1 | 1.5 | 1.3 | 1.2 | 0.07 | 1.15 | 296 | 9997 | 2999 | 2999 | 0 | 0 | 0.10 | 1.12 | 7.53 | 0.47 | 12.88 | 389.9 | 3.63 | 18.3 | 0.3 | | 11 | 0.3 | 6.6 | 20 | 0.2 | 223 | 258 | | 87 | 3.75 |
| 15025 | 3 oz | Gizzards, ckd | 85 | 130 | 67 | 23.1 | 1.0 | 0.0 | 0.0 | 1.0 | 3.1 | 0.9 | 0.8 | 0.9 | 0.03 | 0.88 | 165 | 160 | 48 | 48 | 0 | 0 | 0.02 | 0.21 | 3.38 | 0.10 | 1.65 | 45.1 | 0.61 | 1.4 | 0.3 | | 9 | 0.1 | 3.5 | 17 | 0.1 | 132 | 152 | 9.9 | 57 | 3.72 |
| 15107 | 4 oz | Gizzards, raw | 113 | 133 | 76 | 20.6 | 0.7 | 0.0 | 0.0 | 0.7 | 4.7 | 1.4 | 1.2 | 1.4 | 0.03 | 1.33 | 147 | 245 | 73 | 73 | 0 | 0 | 0.04 | 0.21 | 5.34 | 0.16 | 2.40 | 58.8 | 0.85 | 3.6 | 0.3 | | 9 | 0.1 | 4.0 | 18 | 0.1 | 153 | 267 | | 86 | 3.39 |
| 15024 | 3 oz | Heart, ckd | 85 | 157 | 65 | 22.4 | 0.1 | 0.0 | 0.0 | 0.1 | 6.7 | 1.9 | 1.7 | 2.0 | 0.05 | 1.90 | 206 | 24 | 8 | 8 | 0 | 0 | 0.06 | 0.63 | 2.38 | 0.27 | 6.20 | 68.0 | 2.25 | 1.5 | 0.3 | 1.4 | 16 | 0.4 | 7.7 | 17 | 0.1 | 169 | 112 | | 41 | 6.21 |
| 15108 | 4 oz | Heart, raw | 113 | 173 | 74 | 17.6 | 0.8 | 0.0 | 0.0 | 0.8 | 10.5 | 3.0 | 2.7 | 3.1 | 0.08 | 2.97 | 154 | 34 | 10 | 10 | 0 | 0 | 0.17 | 0.82 | 5.51 | 0.41 | 8.24 | 81.4 | 2.89 | 3.6 | 0.3 | 1.3 | 14 | 0.4 | 6.7 | 17 | 0.1 | 200 | 199 | | 84 | 7.45 |
| 15215 | 3 oz | Liver, ckd | 85 | 133 | 68 | 20.7 | 0.7 | 0.0 | 0.0 | 0.7 | 4.6 | 1.6 | 1.1 | 0.8 | 0.09 | 0.63 | 536 | 13919 | 4176 | 4176 | 0 | 0 | 0.13 | 1.49 | 3.78 | 0.49 | 16.49 | 654.5 | 4.60 | 13.4 | 0.3 | | 12 | 0.3 | 7.2 | 18 | 0.3 | 265 | 119 | 60.3 | 43 | 3.69 |
| 15109 | 4 oz | Liver, raw | 113 | 141 | 74 | 20.3 | 3.9 | 0.0 | 0.0 | 3.9 | 4.4 | 1.5 | 1.1 | 0.7 | 0.09 | 0.59 | 496 | 23220 | 6966 | 6966 | 0 | 0 | 0.16 | 2.21 | 10.45 | 0.86 | 25.99 | 833.9 | 6.98 | 38.2 | 0.3 | | 12 | 0.4 | 9.7 | 23 | 0.3 | 307 | 258 | 72.4 | 89 | 3.47 |
| | | Lamb | | | | | | | | | | | | | | | | | | | | | | | | | | | | | | | | | | | | | | | | |
| 13506 | 3 oz | Brains, brsd | 85 | 123 | 76 | 10.7 | 0.0 | 0.0 | 0.0 | 0.0 | 8.7 | 2.2 | 1.6 | 0.9 | 0.50 | 0.26 | 1737 | 0 | 0 | 0 | 0 | 0 | 0.09 | 0.20 | 2.10 | 0.09 | 7.86 | 4.3 | 0.84 | 10.2 | 0.3 | | 10 | 0.2 | 1.4 | 12 | 0.1 | 286 | 174 | | 114 | 1.16 |
| 13537 | 4 oz | Brains, raw | 113 | 138 | 79 | 11.8 | 0.0 | 0.0 | 0.0 | 0.0 | 9.7 | 2.5 | 1.8 | 1.0 | 0.55 | 0.29 | 1528 | 0 | 0 | 0 | 0 | 0 | 0.15 | 0.34 | 4.41 | 0.33 | 12.77 | 3.4 | 1.04 | 18.1 | | | 10 | 0.3 | 2.0 | 14 | 0.0 | 305 | 334 | | 127 | 1.32 |
| 13504 | 3 oz | Heart, brsd | 85 | 157 | 64 | 21.3 | 1.6 | 0.0 | | | 6.7 | 2.7 | 1.9 | 0.7 | 0.24 | 0.38 | 212 | 0 | 0 | 0 | 0 | 0 | 0.14 | 1.01 | 3.71 | 0.26 | 9.52 | 1.7 | 1.16 | 6.0 | 0.2 | | 12 | 0.5 | 4.7 | 20 | 0.0 | 216 | 160 | 16.4 | 54 | 3.13 |
| 13539 | 4 oz | Heart, raw | 113 | 138 | 77 | 18.6 | 0.2 | 0.0 | | | 6.4 | 2.5 | 1.8 | 0.6 | 0.22 | 0.37 | 153 | 0 | 0 | 0 | 0 | 0 | 0.42 | 1.12 | 6.94 | 0.44 | 11.64 | 2.3 | 2.97 | 5.7 | | | 7 | 0.4 | 5.2 | 19 | 0.1 | 198 | 357 | | 101 | 2.11 |
| 13541 | 3 oz | Kidneys, brsd | 85 | 116 | 70 | 20.1 | 0.8 | 0.0 | | | 3.1 | 1.0 | 0.7 | 0.6 | 0.16 | 0.37 | 480 | 387 | 116 | 116 | 0 | 0 | 0.30 | 1.76 | 5.09 | 0.10 | 67.07 | 68.8 | 1.73 | 10.2 | | | 15 | 0.3 | 10.5 | 17 | 0.1 | 247 | 151 | | 128 | 3.23 |
| 13540 | 4 oz | Kidneys, raw | 113 | 110 | 79 | 17.7 | 0.9 | 0.0 | | | 3.3 | 1.1 | 0.7 | 0.6 | 0.17 | 0.40 | 381 | 357 | 107 | 107 | 0 | 0 | 0.70 | 2.53 | 8.49 | 0.25 | 59.21 | 31.6 | 4.77 | 12.4 | | | 15 | 0.5 | 7.2 | 19 | 0.1 | 278 | 313 | 143.5 | 176 | 2.53 |
| 13505 | 3 oz | Liver, brsd | 85 | 187 | 57 | 26.0 | 2.2 | 0.0 | 0.0 | 2.2 | 7.5 | 2.9 | 1.6 | 1.1 | 0.10 | 1.01 | 426 | 21203 | 6367 | 6354 | 13 | | 0.20 | 3.43 | 10.37 | 0.42 | 65.03 | 62.1 | 3.37 | 3.4 | 0.4 | | 7 | 6.0 | 7.0 | 19 | 0.4 | 357 | 188 | 68.0 | 48 | 6.71 |
| 13542 | 4 oz | Liver, raw | 113 | 157 | 71 | 23.1 | 2.0 | 0.0 | 0.0 | 2.0 | 5.7 | 2.2 | 1.2 | 0.8 | 0.16 | 0.57 | 419 | 27812 | 8351 | 8326 | 25 | | 0.38 | 4.10 | 18.19 | 1.02 | 101.81 | 259.9 | 6.93 | 4.5 | | | 8 | 7.9 | 8.3 | 21 | 0.2 | 411 | 354 | 93.1 | 79 | 5.27 |
| 13545 | 3 oz | Lungs, brsd | 85 | 96 | 76 | 16.9 | 0.0 | 0.0 | 0.0 | 0.0 | 2.6 | 0.9 | 0.7 | 0.4 | | | 241 | 90 | 27 | 27 | 0 | 0 | 0.03 | 0.12 | 2.07 | 0.05 | 2.14 | 6.8 | | 23.8 | | | 10 | 0.2 | 3.9 | 9 | 0.0 | 160 | 108 | | 71 | 1.64 |
| 13544 | 4 oz | Lungs, raw | 113 | 107 | 80 | 18.9 | 0.0 | 0.0 | 0.0 | 0.0 | 2.9 | 1.0 | 0.8 | 0.4 | | | 269 | 101 | 31 | 31 | 0 | 0 | 0.05 | 0.27 | 4.66 | 0.12 | 4.44 | 13.6 | | 35.0 | | | 11 | 0.3 | 7.2 | 16 | 0.0 | 247 | 269 | | 177 | 2.03 |
| 13507 | 3 oz | Pancreas, brsd | 85 | 199 | 60 | 19.4 | 0.0 | 0.0 | 0.0 | 0.0 | 12.8 | 5.8 | 4.6 | 0.6 | 0.25 | 0.38 | 340 | 0 | 0 | 0 | 0 | 0 | 0.02 | 0.18 | 2.18 | 0.04 | 4.71 | 11.1 | 0.72 | 17.0 | 0.3 | | 10 | 0.1 | 1.8 | 16 | 0.0 | 366 | 247 | | 44 | 2.28 |
| 13547 | 4 oz | Pancreas, raw | 113 | 172 | 74 | 16.7 | 0.0 | 0.0 | 0.0 | 0.0 | 11.1 | 5.0 | 4.0 | 0.5 | 0.21 | 0.33 | 294 | 0 | 0 | 0 | 0 | 0 | 0.03 | 0.28 | 4.18 | 0.08 | 6.78 | 14.7 | 1.13 | 20.3 | | | 9 | 0.1 | 2.6 | 24 | 0.0 | 452 | 475 | | 85 | 2.18 |
| 13550 | 3 oz | Spleen, brsd | 85 | 133 | 66 | 22.5 | 0.0 | 0.0 | 0.0 | 0.0 | 4.1 | 1.3 | 1.1 | 0.3 | | | 327 | 0 | 0 | 0 | 0 | 0 | 0.04 | 0.27 | 4.99 | 0.07 | 4.50 | 3.4 | | 22.1 | | | 11 | 0.1 | 32.9 | 18 | 0.1 | 290 | 211 | | 49 | 3.35 |
| 13549 | 4 oz | Spleen, raw | 113 | 114 | 78 | 19.4 | 0.0 | 0.0 | 0.0 | 0.0 | 3.5 | 1.2 | 0.9 | 0.3 | | | 282 | 0 | 0 | 0 | 0 | 0 | 0.05 | 0.39 | 8.93 | 0.12 | 6.03 | 4.5 | | 26.0 | | | 10 | 0.1 | 47.3 | 24 | 0.1 | 316 | 405 | | 95 | 3.21 |
| 13527 | 3 oz | Tongue, brsd | 85 | 234 | 58 | 18.4 | 0.0 | 0.0 | 0.0 | 0.0 | 17.3 | 6.7 | 8.5 | 1.1 | 0.51 | 0.55 | 161 | 0 | 0 | 0 | 0 | 0 | 0.07 | 0.36 | 3.14 | 0.14 | 5.36 | 2.6 | 0.29 | 6.0 | 0.3 | | 9 | 0.2 | 2.2 | 14 | 0.0 | 114 | 134 | | 57 | 2.54 |
| 13551 | 4 oz | Tongue, raw | 113 | 251 | 67 | 17.7 | 0.0 | 0.0 | 0.0 | 0.0 | 19.4 | 7.5 | 9.6 | 1.2 | 0.58 | 0.61 | 176 | 0 | 0 | 0 | 0 | 0 | 0.17 | 0.43 | 5.25 | 0.20 | 8.14 | 4.5 | 1.10 | 6.8 | | | 10 | 0.2 | 3.0 | 24 | 0.1 | 208 | 290 | | 88 | 2.62 |
| | | Pork | | | | | | | | | | | | | | | | | | | | | | | | | | | | | | | | | | | | | | | | |
| 12143 | 3 oz | Brains, brsd | 85 | 117 | 76 | 10.3 | 0.0 | 0.0 | 0.0 | 0.0 | 8.1 | 1.8 | 1.5 | 1.2 | 0.55 | 0.49 | 2169 | 0 | 0 | 0 | 0 | 0 | 0.07 | 0.19 | 2.83 | 0.12 | 1.21 | 3.4 | 1.55 | 11.9 | | | 8 | 0.2 | 1.5 | 10 | 0.1 | 187 | 166 | 15.7 | 77 | 1.26 |
| 12142 | 4 oz | Brains, raw | 113 | 144 | 78 | 11.6 | 0.0 | 0.0 | 0.0 | 0.0 | 10.4 | 2.4 | 1.9 | 1.6 | 0.72 | 0.63 | 2480 | 0 | 0 | 0 | 0 | 0 | 0.18 | 0.31 | 4.84 | 0.21 | 2.47 | 6.8 | 3.16 | 15.3 | | | 11 | 0.3 | 1.8 | 16 | 0.1 | 319 | 292 | 18.0 | 136 | 1.44 |
| 12145 | 3 oz | Chitlings, small intestines, ckd | 85 | 258 | 62 | 8.8 | 0.0 | 0.0 | 0.0 | 0.0 | 24.5 | 8.6 | 8.2 | 6.1 | 0.16 | 3.84 | 122 | 0 | 0 | 0 | 0 | 0 | 0.00 | 0.07 | 0.09 | 0.01 | 0.88 | 2.6 | 0.19 | 0.0 | | | 23 | 0.2 | 3.1 | 9 | 0.0 | 40 | 7 | 33.1 | 33 | 4.30 |
| 12144 | 4 oz | Chitlings, small intestines, raw | 113 | 285 | 66 | 11.4 | 0.4 | 0.0 | 0.4 | 0.0 | 26.1 | 9.0 | 8.9 | 6.6 | 0.17 | 4.70 | 180 | 0 | 0 | 0 | 0 | 0 | 0.01 | 0.08 | 0.09 | 0.01 | 0.92 | 2.3 | 0.22 | 5.0 | | | 23 | 0.2 | 2.2 | 7 | 0.0 | 33 | 131 | 32.1 | 40 | 2.36 |
| 12147 | 1 ea | Ears, ckd | 111 | 184 | 73 | 17.8 | 0.2 | 0.0 | 0.2 | 0.0 | 12.0 | 4.3 | 5.5 | 1.3 | 0.10 | 1.18 | 100 | 0 | 0 | 0 | 0 | 0 | 0.02 | 0.08 | 0.62 | 0.01 | 0.04 | 0.0 | 0.04 | 0.0 | | | 20 | 0.0 | 1.7 | 8 | 0.0 | 27 | 44 | 4.9 | 185 | 0.22 |
| 12146 | 1 ea | Ears, raw | 113 | 264 | 61 | 25.4 | 0.7 | 0.0 | 0.7 | 0.0 | 17.1 | 6.1 | 7.8 | 1.8 | 0.15 | 1.67 | 93 | 0 | 0 | 0 | 0 | 0 | 0.09 | 0.12 | 0.88 | 0.02 | 0.08 | 0.0 | 0.08 | 0.0 | | | 24 | 0.0 | 2.7 | 8 | 0.0 | 46 | 62 | 4.9 | 216 | 0.21 |
| 12178 | 3 oz | Feet, ckd | 85 | 165 | 66 | 16.3 | 0.0 | 0.0 | 0.0 | 0.0 | 10.5 | 3.6 | 4.9 | 1.1 | 0.09 | 1.05 | 85 | 0 | 0 | 0 | 0 | 0 | 0.01 | 0.05 | 0.44 | 0.08 | 0.15 | 0.9 | 0.20 | 0.0 | | | 38 | 0.0 | 0.4 | 4 | 0.0 | 41 | 124 | 4.0 | 26 | 0.92 |
| 12208 | 3 oz | Feet, pickled | 85 | 173 | 69 | 11.5 | 0.0 | 0.0 | 0.0 | 0.0 | 13.7 | 4.7 | 6.4 | 1.5 | 0.12 | 1.37 | 78 | 0 | 0 | 0 | 0 | 0 | 0.01 | 0.04 | 0.31 | 0.32 | 0.53 | 3.4 | 0.27 | 0.0 | 0.3 | | 27 | 0.0 | 0.5 | 3 | 0.0 | 29 | 200 | 6.5 | 785 | 1.05 |
| 12148 | 1 ea | Feet, raw | 190 | 502 | 58 | 42.0 | 0.0 | 0.0 | 0.0 | 0.0 | 35.7 | 12.3 | 16.8 | 3.9 | 0.30 | 3.59 | 201 | 0 | 0 | 0 | 0 | 0 | 0.08 | 0.19 | 2.11 | 0.23 | 0.51 | 3.8 | 0.68 | 0.0 | | | 112 | 0.1 | 0.9 | 13 | 0.0 | 104 | 521 | 8.2 | 118 | 2.45 |
| 12303 | 1 ea | Heart, brsd | 129 | 191 | 68 | 30.4 | 0.5 | 0.0 | | | 6.5 | 1.7 | 1.5 | 1.7 | 0.13 | 1.55 | 285 | 28 | 9 | 9 | 0 | 0 | 0.72 | 2.19 | 7.80 | 0.50 | 4.89 | 5.2 | 3.19 | 2.6 | 0.4 | | 9 | 0.7 | 7.5 | 31 | 0.1 | 230 | 266 | 23.6 | 45 | 3.99 |
| 12149 | 1 ea | Heart, raw | 226 | 267 | 76 | 39.1 | 3.0 | 0.0 | | | 9.9 | 2.6 | 2.3 | 2.5 | 0.18 | 2.35 | 296 | 57 | 18 | 18 | 0 | 0 | 1.39 | 2.69 | 15.30 | 0.88 | 8.57 | 9.0 | 5.70 | 12.0 | | | 11 | 0.9 | 10.6 | 43 | 0.1 | 382 | 664 | 23.5 | 127 | 6.33 |
| 12133 | 1 ea | Hocks, ckd | 51 | 167 | 47 | 14.2 | 0.0 | 0.0 | 0.0 | 0.0 | 11.8 | 4.3 | 5.3 | 1.2 | | | 55 | 5 | 2 | 2 | 0 | 0 | 0.27 | 0.16 | 2.64 | 0.18 | 0.33 | 2.0 | 0.25 | 0.2 | 0.2 | | 9 | 0.1 | 0.8 | 10 | 0.0 | 108 | 187 | | 163 | 2.12 |
| 12150 | 4 oz | Jowl, raw | 113 | 740 | 22 | 7.2 | 0.0 | 0.0 | 0.0 | 0.0 | 78.6 | 28.6 | 37.2 | 9.2 | 0.66 | 8.51 | 102 | 10 | 3 | 3 | 0 | 0 | 0.44 | 0.27 | 5.13 | 0.10 | 0.93 | 1.1 | 0.28 | 0.0 | | | 5 | 0.0 | 0.5 | 3 | 0.0 | 97 | 167 | 1.7 | 28 | 0.95 |
| 12152 | 3 oz | Kidneys, brsd | 85 | 128 | 69 | 21.6 | 0.0 | 0.0 | 0.0 | 0.0 | 4.0 | 1.3 | 1.3 | 0.3 | 0.01 | 0.31 | 408 | 221 | 66 | 66 | 0 | 0 | 0.34 | 1.35 | 4.92 | 0.39 | 6.62 | 34.9 | 2.44 | 9.0 | | | 11 | 0.6 | 4.5 | 15 | 0.1 | 204 | 122 | 265.2 | 68 | 3.53 |
| 12151 | 1 ea | Kidneys, raw | 233 | 233 | 80 | 38.4 | 0.0 | 0.0 | 0.0 | 0.0 | 7.6 | 2.4 | 2.5 | 0.6 | 0.02 | 0.58 | 743 | 461 | 137 | 137 | 0 | 0 | 0.79 | 3.96 | 19.13 | 1.03 | 19.78 | 97.9 | 7.29 | 31.0 | | | 21 | 1.4 | 11.4 | 40 | 0.3 | 475 | 534 | 442.7 | 282 | 6.41 |
| 12013 | 3 pce | Liver, brsd | 54 | 89 | 64 | 14.0 | 2.0 | 0.0 | 0.0 | 2.0 | 2.4 | 0.8 | 0.3 | 0.6 | 0.04 | 0.51 | 192 | 9718 | 2915 | 2915 | 0 | 0 | 0.14 | 1.19 | 4.56 | 0.31 | 10.10 | 88.0 | 2.58 | 12.7 | 0.2 | | 5 | 0.3 | 9.7 | 8 | 0.2 | 130 | 81 | 36.5 | 26 | 3.63 |
| 12154 | 4 oz | Liver, raw | 113 | 151 | 71 | 24.2 | 2.8 | 0.0 | 0.0 | 2.8 | 4.1 | 1.3 | 0.6 | 1.0 | 0.06 | 0.89 | 340 | 24465 | 7339 | 7339 | 0 | 0 | 0.32 | 3.40 | 17.29 | 0.78 | 29.38 | 239.6 | 7.51 | 28.6 | | | 10 | 0.8 | 26.3 | 20 | 0.4 | 325 | 308 | 59.6 | 98 | 6.51 |

| Code | Amount | Description | Basic Components | | | | | | | | | Additional Fats | | | | | | Vit A & Components | | | | | Vitamins | | | | | | | | | | Minerals | | | | | | | | | |
|---|---|---|---|---|---|---|---|---|---|---|---|---|---|---|---|---|---|---|---|---|---|---|---|---|---|---|---|---|---|---|---|---|---|---|---|---|---|---|---|---|---|---|
| | | | Weight (g) | Calories | % Water | Protein (g) | Carbs (g) | Fiber (g) | Sugar (g) | Other Carbs (g) | Fat (g) | Sat Fat (g) | Mono Fat (g) | Poly Fat (g) | Omega 3 (g) | Omega 6 (g) | Choles (mg) | Vit A (IU) | Vit A (RE) | Retinol (RE) | Carotenoids (RE) | Beta Carotene (mcg) | Thiamin (mg) | Riboflavin (mg) | Niacin (NE) | Vit B6 (mg) | Vit B12 (mcg) | Folate (mcg) | Panto (mg) | Vit C (mg) | Vit D (mg) | Vit E (α TE) | Calcium (mg) | Copper (mg) | Iron (mg) | Magnes (mg) | Mang (mg) | Phos (mg) | Potassium (mg) | Selenium (mcg) | Sodium (mg) | Zinc (mg) |
| 12156 | 3 oz | Lungs, brsd | 85 | 84 | 80 | 14.1 | 0.0 | 0.0 | 0.0 | 0.0 | 2.6 | 0.9 | 0.6 | 0.3 | 0.02 | 0.28 | 329 | 0 | • | 0 | 0 | 0 | 0.07 | 0.27 | 1.16 | 0.07 | 1.73 | 1.7 | 0.56 | 6.7 | | | 7 | 0.1 | 13.9 | 10 | 0.0 | 158 | 128 | 19.9 | 69 | 2.08 |
| 12155 | 4 oz | Lungs, raw | 113 | 96 | 80 | 15.9 | 0.0 | 0.0 | 0.0 | 0.0 | 3.1 | 1.1 | 0.7 | 0.4 | 0.02 | 0.33 | 362 | 0 | • | 0 | 0 | 0 | 0.10 | 0.49 | 3.79 | 0.11 | 3.11 | 3.4 | 1.02 | 13.9 | | | 8 | 0.1 | 21.4 | 16 | 0.0 | 221 | 342 | 20.1 | 173 | 2.29 |
| 12159 | 3 oz | Pancreas, brsd | 85 | 186 | 60 | 24.2 | 0.0 | 0.0 | 0.0 | 0.0 | 9.2 | 3.2 | 3.2 | 1.7 | 0.07 | 1.40 | 268 | 0 | • | 0 | 0 | 0 | 0.08 | 0.56 | 2.73 | 0.37 | 14.54 | 4.3 | 4.03 | 4.8 | | | 14 | 0.1 | 2.3 | 20 | 0.2 | 247 | 143 | 61.9 | 36 | 3.65 |
| 12158 | 4 oz | Pancreas, raw | 113 | 225 | 67 | 21.0 | 0.0 | 0.0 | 0.0 | 0.0 | 14.9 | 5.2 | 5.2 | 2.8 | 0.10 | 2.28 | 218 | 0 | • | 0 | 0 | 0 | 0.12 | 0.52 | 3.90 | 0.52 | 18.53 | 3.4 | 5.15 | 17.3 | | | 12 | 0.1 | 2.4 | 19 | 0.2 | 264 | 223 | 46.1 | 50 | 2.96 |
| 12161 | 3 oz | Spleen, brsd | 85 | 127 | 67 | 24.0 | 0.0 | 0.0 | 0.0 | 0.0 | 2.7 | 0.9 | 0.7 | 0.2 | 0.00 | 0.20 | 428 | 0 | • | 0 | 0 | 0 | 0.12 | 0.22 | 5.05 | 0.05 | 2.35 | 3.4 | 0.76 | 9.9 | | | 11 | 0.1 | 13.9 | 13 | 0.0 | 241 | 193 | 42.2 | 91 | 3.01 |
| 12160 | 4 oz | Spleen, raw | 113 | 113 | 78 | 20.2 | 0.0 | 0.0 | 0.0 | 0.0 | 2.9 | 1.0 | 0.8 | 0.2 | 0.00 | 0.21 | 410 | 0 | • | 0 | 0 | 0 | 0.15 | 0.34 | 6.63 | 0.07 | 3.68 | 4.5 | 1.20 | 32.2 | | | 11 | 0.1 | 25.2 | 15 | 0.1 | 294 | 447 | 37.1 | 111 | 2.87 |
| 12162 | 4 oz | Stomach, raw | 113 | 177 | 74 | 18.6 | 0.0 | 0.0 | 0.0 | 0.0 | 10.8 | 3.8 | 4.9 | 1.1 | 0.09 | 1.05 | 218 | 0 | • | 0 | 0 | 0 | 0.10 | 0.13 | 5.03 | 0.05 | 1.12 | 2.3 | 0.72 | 0.0 | | | 11 | 0.4 | 2.5 | 10 | 0.0 | 175 | 227 | 28.9 | 59 | 2.27 |
| 12163 | 4 oz | Tongue, raw | 113 | 254 | 66 | 18.4 | 0.0 | 0.0 | 0.0 | 0.0 | 19.4 | 6.7 | 9.2 | 2.0 | 0.09 | 1.92 | 114 | 0 | • | 0 | 0 | 0 | 0.55 | 0.55 | 5.99 | 0.27 | 3.21 | 4.5 | 0.72 | 5.0 | | | 18 | 0.1 | 3.8 | 20 | 0.0 | 218 | 275 | 11.8 | 124 | 3.40 |
| 12180 | 3 oz | Tail, ckd | 85 | 337 | 47 | 14.5 | 0.0 | 0.0 | 0.0 | 0.0 | 30.4 | 10.6 | 14.4 | 3.3 | 0.26 | 3.09 | 110 | 0 | • | 0 | 0 | 0 | 0.06 | 0.06 | 0.95 | 0.23 | 0.47 | 3.4 | 0.36 | 0.0 | | | 12 | 0.1 | 0.7 | 6 | 0.0 | 40 | 133 | 2.6 | 21 | 1.39 |
| 12179 | 4 oz | Tail, raw | 113 | 427 | 46 | 20.1 | 0.0 | 0.0 | 0.0 | 0.0 | 37.9 | 13.1 | 17.9 | 4.2 | 0.32 | 3.84 | 110 | 0 | • | 0 | 0 | 0 | 0.24 | 0.12 | 2.33 | 0.42 | 0.99 | 5.7 | 0.76 | 0.0 | | | 20 | 0.1 | 1.1 | 9 | 0.0 | 56 | 394 | 3.1 | 71 | 2.61 |
| | | Turkey | | | | | | | | | | | | | | | | | | | | | | | | | | | | | | | | | | | | | | | | |
| 16073 | 3 oz | Giblets, ckd | 85 | 142 | 65 | 22.6 | 1.8 | 0.0 | 0.0 | 1.8 | 4.3 | 1.3 | 1.0 | 1.0 | 0.01 | 0.94 | 355 | 5131 | 1526 | 1526 | 0 | 0 | 0.04 | 0.77 | 3.83 | 0.28 | 20.40 | 293.3 | 2.94 | 1.4 | | | 11 | 0.3 | 5.7 | 14 | 0.1 | 173 | 170 | | 50 | 3.13 |
| 16072 | 4 oz | Giblets, raw | 113 | 146 | 73 | 21.9 | 2.4 | 0.0 | 0.0 | 2.4 | 4.7 | 1.4 | 1.0 | 1.2 | 0.01 | 1.11 | 319 | 8661 | 2587 | 2587 | 0 | 0 | 0.09 | 1.30 | 7.15 | 0.49 | 32.09 | 386.5 | 4.46 | 4.3 | | | 9 | 0.4 | 7.7 | 21 | 0.2 | 249 | 357 | | 98 | 2.70 |
| 16004 | 1 ea | Gizzard, ckd | 67 | 109 | 65 | 19.7 | 0.4 | 0.0 | 0.0 | 0.4 | 2.6 | 0.7 | 0.5 | 0.8 | 0.01 | 0.72 | 155 | 124 | 37 | 37 | 0 | 0 | 0.02 | 0.22 | 2.06 | 0.08 | 1.27 | 34.8 | 0.57 | 1.1 | 0.2 | | 10 | 0.1 | 3.6 | 13 | 0.1 | 86 | 141 | 7.8 | 36 | 2.79 |
| 16074 | 1 ea | Gizzard, raw | 113 | 132 | 76 | 21.6 | 0.7 | 0.0 | 0.0 | 0.7 | 4.2 | 1.2 | 0.8 | 1.2 | 0.01 | 1.15 | 179 | 245 | 73 | 73 | 0 | 0 | 0.06 | 0.26 | 3.89 | 0.16 | 2.40 | 58.8 | 1.03 | 3.6 | | | 10 | 0.2 | 4.3 | 19 | 0.1 | 162 | 388 | | 90 | 2.27 |
| 16005 | 3 ea | Hearts, ckd | 87 | 154 | 64 | 23.3 | 1.8 | 0.0 | 0.0 | 1.8 | 5.3 | 1.5 | 1.0 | 1.5 | 0.02 | 1.47 | 197 | 24 | 7 | 7 | 0 | 0 | 0.06 | 0.77 | 2.83 | 0.28 | 6.22 | 68.7 | 2.37 | 1.5 | 0.3 | | 11 | 0.5 | 6.0 | 19 | 0.1 | 178 | 159 | | 48 | 4.58 |
| 16075 | 4 ea | Heart, raw | 116 | 166 | 73 | 21.0 | 0.8 | 0.0 | 0.0 | 0.8 | 8.1 | 2.3 | 1.6 | 2.3 | 0.03 | 2.25 | 133 | 35 | 10 | 10 | 0 | | 0.23 | 1.26 | 4.74 | 0.42 | 8.46 | 83.5 | 3.10 | 3.7 | | | 10 | 0.4 | 5.6 | 26 | 0.1 | 220 | 321 | | 101 | 4.08 |
| 16007 | 1 ea | Liver, ckd | 75 | 127 | 66 | 18.0 | 2.6 | 0.0 | 0.0 | 2.6 | 4.5 | 1.4 | 1.1 | 0.8 | 0.01 | 0.75 | 470 | 9436 | 2806 | 2806 | 0 | 0 | 0.04 | 1.06 | 4.45 | 0.39 | 35.63 | 499.5 | 4.47 | 1.4 | 0.2 | | 8 | 0.4 | 5.9 | 11 | 0.2 | 204 | 146 | 20.0 | 48 | 2.32 |
| 16076 | 1 ea | Liver, raw | 102 | 140 | 70 | 20.4 | 4.2 | 0.0 | 0.0 | 4.2 | 4.0 | 1.3 | 1.0 | 0.7 | 0.01 | 0.68 | 475 | 18403 | 5495 | 5495 | 0 | 0 | 0.06 | 2.21 | 10.30 | 0.78 | 64.57 | 752.8 | 7.81 | 4.6 | | | 7 | 0.5 | 11.0 | 21 | 0.3 | 319 | 303 | | 98 | 2.53 |
| | | Veal | | | | | | | | | | | | | | | | | | | | | | | | | | | | | | | | | | | | | | | | |
| 11598 | 3 oz | Brain, pan fried | 85 | 181 | 69 | 12.3 | 0.0 | 0.0 | 0.0 | 0.0 | 14.3 | 3.4 | 3.6 | 2.1 | | 0.76 | 1802 | 0 | 0 | 0 | 0 | 0 | 0.13 | 0.31 | 4.78 | 0.28 | 18.10 | 5.1 | 0.96 | 12.8 | 0.3 | | 9 | 0.3 | 0.9 | 15 | 0.0 | 369 | 401 | | 150 | 1.55 |
| 11535 | 4 oz | Brain, raw | 113 | 133 | 80 | 11.6 | 0.0 | 0.0 | 0.0 | 0.0 | 9.3 | 2.2 | 1.9 | 1.1 | 0.00 | 0.32 | 1797 | 0 | 0 | 0 | 0 | 0 | 0.15 | 0.29 | 4.86 | 0.32 | 13.79 | 3.4 | 3.07 | 15.8 | 0.3 | | 11 | 0.2 | 2.4 | 16 | 0.0 | 310 | 356 | | 144 | 1.25 |
| 11501 | 3 oz | Heart, brsd | 85 | 158 | 62 | 24.7 | 0.1 | 0.0 | | | 5.7 | 1.5 | 1.2 | 1.5 | 0.09 | 1.37 | 150 | 0 | 0 | 0 | 0 | 0 | 0.30 | 0.79 | 4.15 | 0.18 | 12.33 | 1.7 | 1.40 | 8.5 | 0.3 | | 7 | 0.4 | 3.7 | 15 | 0.1 | 213 | 169 | 9.5 | 49 | 1.90 |
| 11536 | 4 oz | Heart, raw | 113 | 124 | 78 | 19.4 | 0.1 | 0.0 | | | 4.5 | 1.2 | 0.9 | 1.2 | 0.07 | 1.37 | 118 | 0 | 0 | 0 | 0 | 0 | 0.59 | 1.13 | 7.23 | 0.49 | 15.59 | 2.3 | 3.14 | 9.0 | 0.3 | 0.4 | 6 | 0.4 | 4.8 | 20 | 0.0 | 238 | 295 | | 87 | 1.66 |
| 11538 | 3 oz | Kidneys, brsd | 85 | 139 | 68 | 22.4 | 0.0 | 0.0 | 0.0 | 0.0 | 4.8 | 1.5 | 1.1 | 1.0 | 0.16 | 0.74 | 672 | 569 | 171 | 171 | 0 | 0 | 0.16 | 1.69 | 3.94 | 0.15 | 31.37 | 17.9 | 0.73 | 6.8 | 0.3 | | 25 | 0.3 | 2.6 | 20 | 0.1 | 316 | 135 | | 94 | 3.61 |
| 11537 | 4 oz | Kidneys, raw | 113 | 112 | 79 | 17.9 | 1.0 | 0.0 | | | 3.5 | 1.1 | 0.8 | 0.7 | 0.12 | 0.53 | 411 | 348 | 104 | 104 | 0 | 0 | 0.36 | 2.15 | 7.90 | 0.42 | 31.87 | 23.7 | 3.73 | 5.7 | 0.3 | | 12 | 0.6 | 3.8 | 18 | 0.1 | 272 | 307 | | 201 | 2.23 |
| 11500 | 3 oz | Liver, brsd | 85 | 140 | 67 | 18.4 | 2.3 | 0.0 | 0.0 | 2.3 | 5.9 | 2.2 | 1.3 | 0.9 | 0.07 | 0.36 | 477 | 22851 | 6842 | 6842 | 0 | 0 | 0.11 | 1.65 | 7.21 | 0.42 | 31.03 | 645.2 | 1.94 | 26.4 | 0.3 | | 6 | 6.8 | 2.2 | 16 | 0.1 | 271 | 174 | 48.0 | 45 | 8.09 |
| 11539 | 4 oz | Liver, raw | 113 | 151 | 72 | 20.2 | 5.2 | 0.0 | 0.0 | 5.2 | 4.9 | 1.8 | 1.1 | 0.8 | 0.06 | 0.72 | 349 | 16661 | 5003 | 5003 | 0 | 0 | 0.21 | 1.99 | 13.33 | 0.84 | 52.88 | 725.5 | 3.40 | 24.9 | 0.3 | | 10 | 6.6 | 5.4 | 20 | 0.1 | 303 | 330 | | 70 | 4.55 |
| 11542 | 3 oz | Lungs, brsd | 85 | 88 | 78 | 15.9 | 0.0 | 0.0 | 0.0 | 0.0 | 2.2 | 0.8 | 0.6 | 0.3 | | | 224 | 0 | 0 | 0 | 0 | 0 | 0.03 | 0.11 | 1.95 | 0.05 | 2.02 | 6.8 | | 28.9 | 0.3 | | 6 | 0.2 | 3.1 | 7 | 0.0 | 197 | 121 | | 48 | 1.02 |
| 11541 | 4 oz | Lungs, raw | 113 | 102 | 80 | 18.4 | 0.0 | 0.0 | 0.0 | 0.0 | 2.6 | 0.9 | 0.7 | 0.4 | | | 259 | 0 | 0 | 0 | 0 | 0 | 0.05 | 0.26 | 4.55 | 0.12 | 4.33 | 12.4 | | 44.1 | 0.3 | | 8 | 0.3 | 5.9 | 14 | 0.0 | 325 | 310 | | 122 | 1.31 |
| 11544 | 3 oz | Pancreas, brsd | 85 | 218 | 56 | 24.7 | 0.0 | 0.0 | 0.0 | 0.0 | 12.4 | 4.3 | 4.3 | 2.3 | 0.00 | | 164 | 0 | 0 | 0 | 0 | 0 | 0.16 | 0.43 | 3.53 | 0.16 | 14.70 | 2.6 | | 5.1 | 0.3 | | 15 | 0.1 | 2.0 | 20 | 0.2 | 435 | 236 | | 58 | 4.42 |
| 11543 | 4 oz | Pancreas, raw | 113 | 206 | 71 | 17.0 | 0.0 | 0.0 | 0.0 | 0.0 | 14.8 | 5.1 | 5.1 | 2.8 | 0.00 | | 195 | 0 | 0 | 0 | 0 | 0 | 0.15 | 0.48 | 4.80 | 0.21 | 15.14 | 3.4 | | 18.1 | 0.3 | | 21 | 0.1 | 2.4 | 20 | 0.2 | 372 | 314 | | 76 | 2.94 |
| 11546 | 3 oz | Spleen, brsd | 85 | 110 | 71 | 20.5 | 0.0 | 0.0 | 0.0 | 0.0 | 2.5 | 0.8 | 0.7 | 0.2 | 0.00 | 0.18 | 380 | 0 | 0 | 0 | 0 | 0 | 0.04 | 0.24 | 4.54 | 0.06 | 4.10 | 3.4 | | 34.0 | 0.3 | | 6 | 0.8 | 6.3 | 12 | 0.1 | 265 | 183 | | 49 | 1.62 |
| 11545 | 4 oz | Spleen, raw | 113 | 111 | 78 | 20.7 | 0.0 | 0.0 | 0.0 | 0.0 | 2.5 | 0.8 | 0.7 | 0.2 | 0.00 | 0.18 | 384 | 0 | 0 | 0 | 0 | 0 | 0.05 | 0.39 | 8.93 | 0.12 | 6.03 | 4.5 | | 46.3 | 0.3 | | 7 | 0.2 | 10.5 | 19 | 0.1 | 383 | 409 | | 110 | 1.82 |
| 11548 | 3 oz | Thymus, brsd | 85 | 148 | 64 | 26.9 | 0.0 | 0.0 | 0.0 | 0.0 | 3.6 | 1.3 | 1.3 | 0.7 | 0.00 | 0.40 | 399 | 0 | 0 | 0 | 0 | 0 | 0.05 | 0.14 | 1.73 | 0.08 | 1.85 | 0.9 | | 62.9 | 0.3 | | 3 | 0.0 | 1.7 | 14 | 0.0 | 582 | 291 | | 56 | 2.63 |
| 11547 | 4 oz | Thymus, raw | 113 | 112 | 80 | 20.3 | 0.0 | 0.0 | 0.0 | 0.0 | 2.8 | 0.9 | 1.0 | 0.5 | 0.00 | 0.31 | 303 | 0 | 0 | 0 | 0 | 0 | 0.09 | 0.19 | 2.92 | 0.12 | 3.56 | 3.4 | | 63.3 | 0.3 | | 2 | 0.1 | 2.2 | 18 | 0.2 | 631 | 489 | | 94 | 3.49 |
| 11550 | 3 oz | Tongue, brsd | 85 | 172 | 64 | 22.0 | 0.0 | 0.0 | 0.0 | 0.0 | 8.6 | 3.7 | 3.9 | 0.3 | | 0.24 | 202 | 0 | 0 | 0 | 0 | 0 | 0.06 | 0.30 | 1.25 | 0.13 | 4.51 | 7.7 | 0.63 | 5.1 | 0.3 | | 8 | 0.2 | 1.8 | 15 | 0.0 | 141 | 138 | | 54 | 3.83 |
| 11549 | 4 oz | Tongue, raw | 113 | 148 | 74 | 19.4 | 2.2 | 0.0 | | | 6.2 | 2.7 | 2.8 | 0.4 | | 0.23 | 70 | 1 | 0.3 | 0.3 | 0 | 0 | 0.19 | 0.46 | 2.51 | 0.21 | 6.89 | 5.7 | 1.36 | 5.7 | 0.3 | | 8 | 0.2 | 3.1 | 19 | 0.0 | 180 | 306 | | 93 | 2.97 |
| | | **MEAT SUBSTITUTES, TOFU AND OTHER SOY FOODS** | | | | | | | | | | | | | | | | | | | | | | | | | | | | | | | | | | | | | | | | |
| | | Bacon Substitutes | | | | | | | | | | | | | | | | | | | | | | | | | | | | | | | | | | | | | | | | |
| 7526 | 1/2 cup | Bakon Crumbles, Imagic | 14 | 56 | 16 | 4.0 | 2.0 | 0.2 | | | 3.5 | | | | | | | 0 | 0 | 0 | 0 | 0 | 0.11 | 0.04 | 0.24 | 0.04 | 0.01 | 14.0 | 0.17 | 0.0 | | | 16 | 0.1 | 0.9 | 22 | 0.3 | 50 | 240 | | 343 | 0.50 |
| 7752 | 2 pce | Breakfast Strips, fzn, Morningstar Farms | 16 | 56 | 43 | 1.8 | 2.1 | 0.5 | 0.1 | 1.5 | 4.4 | 0.7 | 1.1 | 2.6 | | | 0 | 0 | 0 | 0 | 0 | 0 | 0.75 | 0.04 | 0.60 | 0.07 | 0.39 | | | 0.0 | | | 7 | | 0.3 | | | 48 | 15 | | 220 | 0.05 |
| 7737 | 2 pce | Stripples, Frozen, Worthington Foods | 16 | 56 | 43 | 1.8 | 2.1 | 0.5 | 0.1 | 1.5 | 4.4 | 0.7 | 1.1 | 2.6 | | | 0 | 0 | 0 | 0 | 0 | 0 | 0.75 | 0.04 | 0.60 | 0.07 | 0.39 | | | 0.0 | | | 7 | | 0.3 | | | 48 | 15 | | 220 | 0.05 |
| | | Beef Substitute | | | | | | | | | | | | | | | | | | | | | | | | | | | | | | | | | | | | | | | | |
| 7634 | 5 pce | Beef Style, fzn, Worthington Foods | 92 | 189 | 58 | 14.4 | 7.3 | 5.6 | 1.0 | 0.7 | 11.3 | 2.1 | 4.6 | 4.4 | | | 0 | 0 | 0 | 0 | 0 | 0 | 1.48 | 0.56 | 10.80 | 0.93 | 6.74 | | | 0.0 | | | 6 | | 4.4 | | | 154 | 75 | | 1043 | 0.37 |
| 7610 | 2 pce | Choplets, cnd, Worthington Foods | 92 | 94 | 72 | 16.7 | 3.1 | 2.3 | 0.4 | 0.3 | 1.6 | 0.9 | 0.3 | 0.3 | | | 0 | 0 | 0 | 0 | 0 | 0 | 0.05 | 0.06 | 0.00 | 0.06 | 0.00 | | | 0.0 | | | 6 | | 0.4 | | | 75 | 40 | | 500 | 0.65 |
| 7608 | 6 pce | Corned Beef, fzn, Worthington Foods | 81 | 197 | 55 | 13.6 | 6.6 | 2.8 | 1.2 | 2.6 | 12.9 | 2.6 | 5.8 | 4.4 | | | 2 | 0 | 0 | 0 | 0 | 0 | 15.08 | 0.10 | 1.94 | 0.43 | 2.45 | | | 0.0 | | | 9 | | 1.7 | | | 130 | 83 | | 745 | 0.37 |
| 7639 | 1 pce | Cutlets, cnd, Worthington Foods | 61 | 66 | 70 | 10.9 | 3.2 | 2.2 | 0.5 | 0.5 | 1.1 | 0.5 | 0.4 | 0.2 | | | 0 | 0 | 0 | 0 | 0 | 0 | 0.03 | 0.04 | 0.00 | 0.04 | 0.00 | | | 0.0 | | | 4 | | 0.2 | | | 50 | 29 | | 340 | 0.43 |
| 7645 | 2 pce | Cutlets, multigrain, cnd, Worthington Foods | 92 | 98 | 71 | 15.4 | 5.3 | 4.3 | 0.3 | 0.7 | 1.7 | 0.7 | 0.3 | 0.8 | | | 0 | 0 | 0 | 0 | 0 | 0 | 0.03 | 0.03 | 0.00 | 0.04 | 0.00 | | | 0.0 | | | 6 | | 0.9 | | | 88 | 31 | | 385 | 0.80 |
| 57432 | 1 ea | Dinner Cuts, cnd, svg, Loma Linda | 67 | 78 | 72 | 12.4 | 3.5 | 3.2 | 0.4 | | 1.6 | 0.4 | 0.5 | 0.7 | | | 0 | 0 | 0 | 0 | 0 | 0 | 0.05 | 0.11 | 0.00 | 0.03 | 0.00 | 14.6 | 0.05 | 0.0 | 0.0 | | 7 | | 0.7 | 13 | | 55 | 19 | | 352 | 0.72 |
| 7606 | 1 ea | Dinner Roast, fzn, Worthington Foods | 85 | 179 | 63 | 12.2 | 4.6 | 2.6 | 1.4 | 0.6 | 12.5 | 2.2 | 5.0 | 5.2 | | | 2 | 0 | 0 | 0 | 0 | 0 | 2.13 | 0.26 | 6.02 | 0.60 | 1.48 | | | 0.0 | | | 36 | | 2.9 | | | 112 | 38 | | 566 | 0.64 |
| 7558 | 2 ea | Fillets, avg | 94 | 273 | 45 | 21.6 | 8.5 | 5.7 | | | 16.9 | 2.7 | 4.1 | 8.8 | | | 0 | 0 | 0 | 0 | 0 | 0 | 1.03 | 0.85 | 11.28 | 1.41 | 3.95 | 95.9 | | 0.0 | | | 89 | 0.9 | 1.9 | 22 | | 423 | 564 | | 461 | 1.32 |
| 7642 | 2 pce | Fillets, fzn, Worthington Foods | 85 | 183 | 56 | 15.6 | 7.9 | 3.9 | 0.5 | 3.5 | 9.8 | 1.9 | 3.5 | 4.3 | | | 2 | 0 | 0 | 0 | 0 | 0 | 0.65 | 0.14 | 0.96 | 0.36 | 2.75 | | | 0.0 | | | 14 | | 2.1 | | | 183 | 133 | | 750 | 0.92 |
| 7552 | 8 ea | Meatballs, avg | 80 | 160 | 58 | 16.8 | 6.4 | 3.7 | | | 7.2 | 1.1 | 1.7 | 3.8 | | | 0 | 0 | 0 | 0 | 0 | 0 | 0.72 | 0.48 | 8.00 | 0.96 | 1.92 | 62.4 | | 0.0 | | | 23 | 0.6 | 1.7 | 14 | | 275 | 144 | | 440 | 1.44 |
| 7613 | 1 pce | Prime Stakes, cnd, Worthington Foods | 92 | 136 | 71 | 9.1 | 4.1 | 3.7 | 0.3 | 0.0 | 9.3 | 1.4 | 2.9 | 4.9 | | | 2 | 0 | 0 | 0 | 0 | 0 | 0.12 | 0.13 | 1.98 | 0.38 | 1.03 | | | 0.0 | | | 12 | | 0.4 | | | 86 | 82 | | 445 | 0.38 |
| 7648 | 1 ea | Roast Beef, svg, Gorilla Foods | 113 | 177 | | 31.9 | 8.0 | | | | 2.0 | | | | | | 0 | | | | | | | | | | | | | | | | | | | | | | | | 789 | |
| 7650 | 1 ea | Roast Beef, w/barbecue sce, svg, Gorilla Foods | 113 | 165 | | 26.1 | 11.0 | | | | 1.9 | | | | | | 0 | | | | | | | | | | | | | | | | | | | | | | | | 692 | |
| 7619 | 2 pce | Saucettes, cnd, Worthington Foods | 76 | 172 | 62 | 11.1 | 2.7 | | | | 13.0 | 2.2 | 3.2 | 7.5 | | | 2 | 0 | 0 | 0 | 0 | 0 | 1.19 | 0.15 | 0.19 | 0.26 | 0.71 | | | 0.0 | | | 17 | | 2.3 | | | 121 | 50 | | 410 | 0.52 |
| 7620 | 3 pce | Savory Slices, cnd, Worthington Foods | 84 | 144 | 66 | 10.1 | 5.2 | 3.3 | 0.6 | 1.3 | 9.3 | 3.6 | 3.8 | 1.7 | | | 2 | 0 | 0 | 0 | 0 | 0 | 0.24 | 0.17 | 1.44 | 0.31 | 1.53 | | | 0.0 | | | 1 | | 1.4 | | | 89 | 40 | | 536 | 0.25 |
| 7735 | 1 pce | Stakelets, fzn, Worthington Foods | 71 | 145 | 58 | 12.3 | 5.7 | 1.7 | 0.2 | 3.8 | 8.0 | 1.4 | 2.7 | 3.9 | | | 2 | 0 | 0 | 0 | 0 | 0 | 1.51 | 0.12 | 3.10 | 0.26 | 1.58 | | | 0.0 | | | 50 | | 1.0 | | | 148 | 95 | | 484 | 0.50 |
| 7628 | 1 ea | Steak, cnd, Worthington Foods | 72 | 83 | 71 | 14.7 | 3.1 | 2.9 | 0.4 | | 1.3 | 0.5 | 0.3 | 0.4 | | | 0 | 0 | 0 | 0 | 0 | 0 | 0.53 | 0.12 | 4.47 | 0.23 | 3.27 | | | 0.0 | | | 5 | | 3.2 | | | 43 | 17 | | 304 | 0.65 |
| 7506 | 1 ea | Steak, Garden, Whole Foods | 142 | 369 | 81 | 22.7 | 51.1 | 14.2 | 2.8 | 34.1 | 8.3 | 2.8 | 4.3 | 1.2 | | | 31 | 142 | 28 | | | | 0.30 | 0.43 | 3.05 | 0.21 | 0.31 | 28.6 | 1.59 | 0.0 | 0.9 | | 239 | 0.4 | 0.0 | 87 | 1.7 | 375 | 550 | 20.9 | 824 | 2.51 |
| 7755 | 1 pce | Swiss Stake, w/gravy, cnd, Loma Linda | 92 | 120 | 71 | 9.0 | 8.4 | 4.1 | 0.6 | 3.7 | 5.6 | 0.8 | 1.5 | 3.3 | | | 2 | 0 | 0 | 0 | 0 | 0 | 1.25 | 0.65 | 5.41 | 1.00 | 5.26 | | 4.66 | 0.0 | | | 24 | | 0.3 | | | 133 | 225 | | 433 | 0.41 |
| 7756 | 6 pce | Tender Bits, cnd, Loma Linda | 85 | 111 | 69 | 10.8 | 6.8 | 3.1 | 0.4 | 3.3 | 4.5 | 0.7 | 1.1 | 2.6 | | | 0 | 0 | 0 | 0 | 0 | 0 | 0.33 | 0.40 | 1.38 | 0.12 | 0.11 | | 1.55 | 0.0 | | | 10 | | 0.7 | | | 89 | 54 | | 436 | 0.34 |
| 7754 | 1 ea | Tender Rounds, cnd, svg, Loma Linda | 80 | 118 | 67 | 13.8 | 4.6 | 3.1 | 0.7 | 0.9 | 5.0 | 0.9 | 1.4 | 2.7 | | | 2 | 0 | 0 | 0 | 0 | 0 | 1.14 | 0.10 | 0.34 | 0.14 | 0.82 | | 0.44 | 0.0 | | | 15 | | 0.6 | | | 78 | 73 | | 326 | 0.66 |
| 7626 | 1 ea | Veelets, fzn, Worthington Foods | 85 | 171 | 52 | 14.5 | 10.4 | 5.2 | 0.6 | 4.6 | 7.9 | 1.5 | 2.5 | 3.9 | | | 1 | 0 | 0 | 0 | 0 | 0 | 1.79 | 0.17 | 1.60 | 0.33 | 2.98 | | | 0.0 | | | 36 | | 0.5 | | | | 121 | | 388 | 0.58 |
| | | Chicken Substitutes | | | | | | | | | | | | | | | | | | | | | | | | | | | | | | | | | | | | | | | | |
| 7548 | 1 pce | Chicken, breaded, fried, avg | 57 | 97 | 70 | 6.3 | 2.8 | 2.5 | | | 6.8 | 1.0 | 2.9 | 2.5 | | | 0 | 0 | 0 | 0 | 0 | 0 | 0.40 | 0.27 | 2.68 | 0.28 | 1.20 | 31.9 | | 0.0 | | | 13 | 0.3 | 1.0 | 7 | | 140 | 171 | | 228 | 0.37 |
| 7649 | 1 ea | Chicken, svg, Gorilla Foods | 57 | 93 | | 18.1 | 3.0 | | | | 1.0 | | | | | | 0 | | | | | | | | | | | | | | | | | | | | | | | | 393 | |
| 7547 | 3 ea | Chicken Slices, avg | 90 | 198 | 59 | 15.3 | 6.3 | 4.0 | | | 12.6 | 2.0 | 3.0 | 6.6 | | | 0 | 0 | 0 | 0 | 0 | 0 | 0.99 | 0.36 | 4.77 | 0.63 | 1.39 | 58.4 | | 0.0 | | | 31 | 0.6 | 1.2 | 15 | | 301 | 297 | | 711 | 0.63 |

| Code | Amount | Description | Basic Components | | | | | | | | | Additional Fats | | | | | | Vit A & Components | | | | | Vitamins | | | | | | | | | | Minerals | | | | | | | | | |
|---|---|---|---|---|---|---|---|---|---|---|---|---|---|---|---|---|---|---|---|---|---|---|---|---|---|---|---|---|---|---|---|---|---|---|---|---|---|---|---|---|---|---|
| | | | Weight (g) | Calories | % Water | Protein (g) | Carbs (g) | Fiber (g) | Sugar (g) | Other Carbs (g) | Fat (g) | Sat Fat (g) | Mono Fat (g) | Poly Fat (g) | Omega 3 (g) | Omega 6 (g) | Choles (mg) | Vit A (IU) | Vit A (RE) | Retinol (RE) | Carotenoids (RE) | Beta Carotene (mcg) | Thiamin (mg) | Riboflavin (mg) | Niacin (NE) | Vit B6 (mg) | Vit B12 (mcg) | Folate (mcg) | Panto (mg) | Vit C (mg) | Vit D (mg) | Vit E (α TE) | Calcium (mg) | Copper (mg) | Iron (mg) | Magnes (mg) | Mang (mg) | Phos (mg) | Potassium (mg) | Selenium (mcg) | Sodium (mg) | Zinc (mg) |
| 7761 | 1 oz | Chicken Supreme, dry, Loma Linda | 28 | 96 | 6 | 15.9 | 6.1 | 4.3 | 0.3 | 1.5 | 0.9 | 0.3 | 0.3 | 0.2 | | | 1 | 0 | 0 | 0 | 0 | 0 | 0.59 | 0.45 | 2.64 | 0.32 | 1.88 | | 1.69 | 0.0 | 0.0 | | 30 | | 1.5 | | | 166 | 482 | | 779 | 0.52 |
| 7640 | 1 ea | Chik-Diced, cnd, svg, Worthington Foods | 55 | 57 | 78 | 5.5 | 0.8 | 0.8 | 0.1 | 0.0 | 3.5 | 0.5 | 0.8 | 2.1 | | | 1 | 0 | 0 | 0 | 0 | 0 | 0.06 | 0.05 | 0.34 | 0.08 | 0.27 | | | 0.0 | | | 8 | | 0.7 | | | 51 | 102 | | 235 | 0.24 |
| 7641 | 1 ea | Chik-Diced, fzn, svg, Worthington Foods | 55 | 83 | 68 | 9.4 | 1.3 | 0.6 | 0.2 | 0.6 | 4.4 | 0.8 | 1.1 | 2.5 | | | 1 | 0 | 0 | 0 | 0 | 0 | 0.31 | 0.13 | 1.18 | 0.20 | 0.87 | | | 0.0 | | | 12 | | 2.0 | | | 107 | 266 | | 360 | 0.25 |
| 7635 | 1 ea | Chik-Ketts, fzn, svg, Worthington Foods | 55 | 121 | 59 | 13.5 | 2.0 | 1.7 | 0.2 | 0.1 | 6.6 | 1.0 | 1.6 | 3.9 | | | 1 | 0 | 0 | 0 | 0 | 0 | 0.36 | 0.12 | 0.75 | 0.12 | 1.26 | | | 0.0 | | | 17 | | 1.7 | | | 82 | 31 | | 389 | 0.54 |
| 7727 | 5 pce | Chik-Nuggets, fzn, Loma Linda | 85 | 245 | 47 | 12.1 | 13.3 | 4.5 | 0.8 | 7.9 | 15.9 | 2.5 | 4.0 | 8.8 | | | 2 | 0 | 0 | 0 | 0 | 0 | 0.67 | 0.30 | 2.89 | 0.45 | 4.50 | | 1.62 | 0.0 | | | 41 | | 1.4 | | | 172 | 153 | | 709 | 0.43 |
| 7665 | 1 ea | Chik-Patties, fzn, Morningstar Farms | 71 | 177 | 51 | 7.3 | 14.9 | 2.5 | 1.6 | 10.8 | 9.8 | 1.3 | 2.6 | 5.9 | | | 1 | 0 | 0 | 0 | 0 | 0 | 2.15 | 0.16 | 1.51 | 0.14 | 0.95 | | | 0.0 | | | 11 | | 1.0 | | | 106 | 163 | | 536 | 0.31 |
| 7637 | 2 pce | Chik-Stiks, fzn, Worthington Foods | 94 | 222 | 57 | 17.4 | 5.1 | 4.1 | 1.0 | | 14.6 | 2.4 | 4.9 | 7.3 | | | 2 | 0 | 0 | 0 | 0 | 0 | 0.65 | 0.07 | 4.93 | 0.68 | 4.13 | | | 0.0 | | | 21 | | 1.7 | | | 178 | 117 | | 711 | 0.62 |
| 7638 | 1 ea | Crispy Chik Patties, fzn, Worthington Foods | 71 | 175 | 51 | 7.8 | 14.8 | 3.8 | 1.1 | 9.8 | 9.4 | 1.4 | 2.4 | 5.7 | | | 1 | 0 | 0 | 0 | 0 | 0 | 1.14 | 0.13 | 0.57 | 0.18 | 0.74 | | | 0.0 | | | 10 | | 1.3 | | | 102 | 200 | | 596 | 0.33 |
| 7729 | 2 pce | Fri-Chik, cnd, Worthington Foods | 90 | 116 | 76 | 9.9 | 1.1 | 1.1 | 0.2 | | 8.0 | 1.1 | 2.1 | 4.8 | | | 2 | 0 | 0 | 0 | 0 | 0 | 0.08 | 0.14 | 0.61 | 0.15 | 2.16 | | | 0.0 | | | 14 | | 1.0 | | | 98 | 146 | | 428 | 0.38 |
| 7753 | 1 pce | Fried Chik'n, fzn, Loma Linda | 57 | 178 | 51 | 10.8 | 0.9 | 0.9 | 0.6 | 0.0 | 14.6 | 1.9 | 3.7 | 8.7 | | | 5 | 0 | 0 | 0 | 0 | 0 | 0.98 | 0.46 | 2.10 | 0.35 | 0.82 | | 2.47 | 0.0 | | | 2 | | 0.6 | | | | 76 | | 503 | 0.20 |
| 7750 | 1 ea | Fried Chik'n, w/gravy, cnd, svg, Loma Linda | 147 | 385 | 57 | 21.2 | 5.8 | 3.1 | 1.0 | 1.8 | 30.9 | 4.4 | 8.1 | 17.7 | | | 6 | 0 | 0 | 0 | 0 | 0 | 1.47 | 0.69 | 3.06 | 0.35 | 2.93 | | 1.91 | 0.0 | | | 15 | | 0.9 | | | 141 | 62 | | 814 | 0.62 |
| | | Chili | | | | | | | | | | | | | | | | | | | | | | | | | | | | | | | | | | | | | | | | |
| 7557 | 1 cup | Vegetarian, avg | 212 | 280 | 64 | 37.5 | 29.9 | 7.8 | | | 4.1 | 0.6 | 1.2 | 1.8 | | | 0 | 1541 | 154 | 0 | 154 | | 0.24 | 0.13 | 2.40 | 0.30 | 0.00 | 162.6 | 0.42 | 30.9 | 0.0 | | 106 | 0.9 | 8.4 | 70 | 1.1 | 430 | 719 | | 1043 | 2.50 |
| 7760 | 1 cup | Vegetarian, cnd, Natural Touch | 307 | 358 | 75 | 23.9 | 28.6 | 14.5 | 2.6 | 11.5 | 16.5 | 2.8 | 4.1 | 9.4 | | | 3 | 627 | 63 | 0 | 63 | | 0.85 | 0.28 | 0.00 | 0.40 | 0.00 | | | 0.0 | | | 49 | | 3.3 | | | 262 | 650 | | 1774 | 1.82 |
| 7609 | 1 ea | Vegetarian, cnd, svg, Worthington Foods | 230 | 294 | 73 | 18.9 | 20.9 | 9.1 | 2.3 | 9.5 | 15.0 | 2.4 | 3.7 | 8.9 | | | 0 | 0 | 0 | 0 | 0 | 0 | 0.05 | 0.07 | 2.25 | 0.67 | 1.61 | | | 0.0 | | | 44 | | 3.2 | | | 241 | 423 | | 1134 | 1.24 |
| 7762 | 1 ea | Corn Dog, fzn, Loma Linda | 71 | 204 | 43 | 10.4 | 19.2 | 2.9 | 1.1 | 15.1 | 9.5 | 1.6 | 2.9 | 5.0 | | | 2 | 0 | 0 | 0 | 0 | 0 | 0.72 | 0.61 | 1.47 | 0.87 | 2.19 | | 4.98 | 0.0 | 0.0 | | 12 | | 0.9 | | | 139 | 39 | | 237 | 0.43 |
| 7644 | 1 pce | Croquettes, fzn, Worthington Foods | 85 | 207 | 52 | 14.3 | 14.2 | 5.7 | 1.4 | 7.1 | 10.3 | 1.7 | 3.7 | 4.8 | | | 2 | 0 | 0 | 0 | 0 | 0 | 0.48 | 0.07 | 2.01 | 0.27 | 2.69 | | | 0.0 | | | 34 | | 1.3 | | | 134 | 191 | | 604 | 0.57 |
| 7632 | 1 ea | Egg Rolls, fzn, Worthington Foods | 85 | 181 | 53 | 6.4 | 19.7 | 2.3 | 0.6 | 16.7 | 8.5 | 1.7 | 4.5 | 2.3 | | | 1 | 0 | 0 | 0 | 0 | 0 | 1.22 | 0.19 | 0.00 | 0.03 | 0.12 | | | 0.0 | | | 15 | | 0.6 | | | 93 | 96 | | 384 | 0.31 |
| | | Fish Substitutes | | | | | | | | | | | | | | | | | | | | | | | | | | | | | | | | | | | | | | | | |
| 7549 | 3 ea | Fish Sticks, avg | 86 | 249 | 45 | 19.8 | 7.7 | 5.2 | | | 15.5 | 2.4 | 3.7 | 8.1 | | | 0 | 0 | 0 | 0 | 0 | 0 | 0.95 | 0.77 | 10.32 | 1.29 | 3.61 | 87.7 | | 0.0 | | | 82 | 0.8 | 1.7 | 20 | | 387 | 516 | | 421 | 1.20 |
| 7763 | 1 oz | Ocean Platter, dry, Loma Linda | 28 | 102 | 5 | 14.7 | 8.2 | 4.8 | 0.4 | 3.0 | 1.1 | 0.3 | 0.3 | 0.5 | | | 1 | 0 | 0 | 0 | 0 | 0 | 1.90 | 0.47 | 1.00 | 0.42 | 1.73 | | 1.55 | 0.0 | 0.0 | | 5 | | 1.4 | | | 160 | 482 | | 484 | 0.51 |
| 7553 | 1/2 cup | Scallops, breaded, fried, avg | 85 | 257 | 43 | 20.4 | 8.0 | 5.4 | | | 15.9 | 2.5 | 3.8 | 8.3 | | | 0 | 0 | 0 | 0 | 0 | 0 | 0.97 | 0.80 | 10.63 | 1.33 | 3.72 | 90.4 | | 0.0 | | | 84 | 0.8 | 1.8 | 20 | | 399 | 531 | | 434 | 1.24 |
| 7731 | 1/2 cup | Skallops, cnd, Worthington Foods | 85 | 86 | 74 | 15.2 | 3.2 | 2.5 | 0.2 | 0.5 | 1.4 | 0.5 | 0.5 | 0.3 | | | 0 | 0 | 0 | 0 | 0 | 0 | 0.03 | 0.03 | 0.00 | 0.01 | 0.00 | | | 0.0 | | | 5 | | 0.6 | | | 60 | 9 | | 411 | 0.67 |
| 7624 | 3 oz | Tuno, fzn, Worthington Foods | 85 | 128 | 70 | 10.0 | 3.2 | 2.1 | 0.1 | 0.9 | 8.5 | 1.4 | 2.0 | 4.9 | | | 1 | 0 | 0 | 0 | 0 | 0 | 0.21 | 0.06 | 1.90 | 0.49 | 3.09 | | | 0.0 | | | 31 | | 1.9 | | | 136 | 53 | | 445 | 0.62 |
| | | Franks/Links | | | | | | | | | | | | | | | | | | | | | | | | | | | | | | | | | | | | | | | | |
| 7744 | 1 ea | Big Franks, cnd, Loma Linda | 51 | 110 | 59 | 10.2 | 2.3 | 2.4 | 0.1 | 0.0 | 6.7 | 1.1 | 1.8 | 3.8 | | | 2 | 0 | 0 | 0 | 0 | 0 | 0.26 | 0.46 | 1.98 | 0.14 | 1.14 | | 1.36 | 0.0 | | | 8 | | 0.8 | | | 74 | 51 | | 243 | 0.89 |
| 7724 | 1 ea | Deli Franks, Morningstar Farms | 45 | 112 | 52 | 10.4 | 3.7 | 2.7 | 0.9 | 0.0 | 6.2 | 0.9 | 2.0 | 3.3 | 0.08 | 3.24 | 0 | 0 | 0 | 0 | 0 | 0 | 0.14 | 0.02 | 0.00 | 0.01 | 0.01 | | 0.02 | 0.0 | | | 17 | 0.0 | 0.6 | 4 | 0.0 | 42 | 50 | | 431 | 0.38 |
| 7550 | 1 ea | Frankfurter, avg | 51 | 102 | 58 | 10.2 | 4.1 | 2.3 | | | 5.1 | 0.8 | 1.2 | 2.7 | | | 0 | 0 | 0 | 0 | 0 | 0 | 0.56 | 0.61 | 8.16 | 0.50 | 1.22 | 39.8 | | 0.0 | | | 17 | 0.4 | 0.9 | 9 | | 175 | 76 | | 219 | 0.61 |
| 7653 | 2 oz | Garden Dog Hotdog, Whole Foods | 57 | 121 | 53 | 19.1 | 4.0 | 1.0 | 1.0 | 2.0 | 2.5 | | | | | | 0 | 0 | 0 | 0 | 0 | 0 | | | | | | | | 3.6 | | | 20 | | 1.4 | | | | 503 | | 312 | |
| 7734 | 1 pce | Leanies Links, fzn, Worthington Foods | 40 | 106 | 54 | 7.3 | 1.7 | 1.4 | 0.6 | | 7.8 | 1.3 | 2.9 | 3.5 | | | 1 | 0 | 0 | 0 | 0 | 0 | 0.20 | 0.12 | 1.00 | 0.18 | 0.84 | | | 0.0 | | | 25 | | 0.9 | | | 93 | 43 | | 425 | 0.23 |
| 7747 | 1 ea | Linketts, cnd, Loma Linda | 35 | 72 | 60 | 6.9 | 1.1 | | | | 4.4 | 0.7 | 1.2 | 2.5 | | | 1 | 0 | 0 | 0 | 0 | 0 | 0.13 | 0.22 | 0.64 | 0.29 | 1.04 | | 0.58 | 0.0 | | | 5 | | 0.4 | | | 41 | 29 | | 160 | 0.46 |
| 7748 | 1 pce | Little Links, cnd, Loma Linda | 23 | 47 | 62 | 4.1 | 1.3 | 0.7 | 0.1 | 0.4 | 2.8 | 0.4 | 0.7 | 1.6 | | | 1 | 0 | 0 | 0 | 0 | 0 | 0.17 | 0.22 | 0.66 | 0.23 | 0.85 | | 0.50 | 0.0 | | | 3 | | 0.2 | | | 28 | 10 | | 113 | 0.28 |
| 7614 | 1 pce | Prosage Links, fzn, Worthington Foods | 22 | 31 | 60 | 4.1 | 0.9 | 0.9 | 0.2 | | 1.2 | 0.2 | 0.3 | 0.6 | | | 0 | 0 | 0 | 0 | 0 | 0 | 3.40 | 0.11 | 2.54 | 0.16 | 1.67 | | | 0.0 | | | 7 | | 1.0 | | | 29 | 29 | | 165 | 0.18 |
| 7730 | 1 pce | Super Links, cnd, Worthington Foods | 48 | 106 | 62 | 6.5 | 2.3 | 1.0 | 0.3 | 1.0 | 7.8 | 1.2 | 1.9 | 4.6 | | | 1 | 0 | 0 | 0 | 0 | 0 | 0.09 | 0.11 | 0.82 | 0.13 | 1.08 | | | 0.0 | | | 9 | | 0.1 | | | 51 | 29 | | 350 | 0.20 |
| 7671 | 1 ea | Vege Frank, Natural Touch | 45 | 99 | 54 | 10.4 | 2.0 | | | | 5.5 | 0.9 | 1.6 | 3.0 | | | 1 | 7 | 1 | 0 | 1 | | 0.03 | 0.07 | 0.00 | | | | | 0.0 | | | 13 | | 0.5 | | | 47 | 53 | | 471 | 0.58 |
| 7733 | 1 pce | Veja Links, cnd, Worthington Foods | 31 | 49 | 69 | 4.6 | 1.0 | 0.4 | 0.2 | 0.4 | 3.0 | 0.6 | 1.5 | 1.0 | | | 1 | 0 | 0 | 0 | 0 | 0 | 0.12 | 0.11 | 1.47 | 0.15 | 0.48 | | | 0.0 | | | 4 | | 0.7 | | | 22 | 18 | | 192 | 0.10 |
| | | Loafs | | | | | | | | | | | | | | | | | | | | | | | | | | | | | | | | | | | | | | | | |
| 7759 | 1 oz | Dry Mix, Natural Touch | 28 | 94 | 6 | 12.7 | 9.4 | 6.1 | 0.6 | 2.7 | 0.6 | 0.1 | 0.3 | 0.2 | | | 1 | 0 | 0 | 0 | 0 | 0 | 0.09 | 0.14 | 0.00 | 0.01 | 0.52 | | | 0.0 | | | 38 | | 1.6 | | | 143 | 380 | | 655 | 0.50 |
| 7738 | 1 oz | Dry Mix, savory dinner, Loma Linda | 28 | 101 | 6 | 14.7 | 7.5 | 4.9 | 0.2 | 2.3 | 1.4 | 0.3 | 0.4 | 0.6 | | | 1 | 0 | 0 | 0 | 0 | 0 | 0.49 | 0.06 | 2.48 | 0.42 | 2.51 | | 2.02 | 0.0 | | | 25 | | 1.4 | | | 148 | 446 | | 604 | 0.41 |
| 7758 | 1 pce | Lentil Rice, Natural Touch | 90 | 166 | 64 | 7.7 | 14.5 | 3.9 | 0.8 | 9.8 | 8.6 | 2.6 | 1.7 | 4.3 | | | 2 | 775 | 78 | 0 | 78 | | 0.05 | 0.12 | 0.00 | 0.03 | 0.07 | | | 0.0 | | | 21 | | 1.2 | | | 202 | 161 | | 366 | 1.04 |
| 7669 | 1 ea | Nine Bean, svg, Natural Touch | 85 | 147 | 65 | 7.7 | 13.2 | 5.6 | 0.9 | 6.8 | 7.0 | 1.2 | 2.4 | 3.4 | | | 3 | 1510 | 151 | 0 | 151 | | 0.06 | 0.11 | 0.00 | | | | | 1.4 | | | 27 | | 0.6 | | | 180 | 187 | | 319 | 0.88 |
| 7560 | 1 ea | Vegetarian Meat, slice, avg | 71 | 142 | 58 | 14.9 | 5.7 | 3.3 | | | 6.4 | 1.0 | 1.5 | 3.3 | | | 0 | 0 | 0 | 0 | 0 | 0 | 0.64 | 0.43 | 7.10 | 0.85 | 1.70 | 55.4 | | 0.0 | | | 21 | 0.5 | 1.5 | 13 | | 244 | 128 | | 390 | 1.28 |
| | | Lunch Meat Substitutes | | | | | | | | | | | | | | | | | | | | | | | | | | | | | | | | | | | | | | | | |
| 7745 | 1 ea | Bolono, fzn, svg, Worthington Foods | 57 | 79 | 66 | 10.1 | 2.2 | 1.7 | 0.4 | 0.0 | 3.3 | 0.8 | 1.0 | 1.6 | | | 2 | 0 | 0 | 0 | 0 | 0 | 0.58 | 0.13 | 0.34 | 0.36 | 0.86 | | | 0.0 | | | 40 | | 2.1 | | | 104 | 125 | | 716 | 0.39 |
| 7551 | 1 pce | Luncheon Slices, avg | 67 | 188 | 46 | 16.8 | 6.0 | 3.4 | | | 10.7 | 1.7 | 2.6 | 5.6 | | | 0 | 0 | 0 | 0 | 0 | 0 | 0.64 | 0.37 | 7.37 | 0.74 | 1.74 | 67.0 | | 0.0 | | | 27 | 0.6 | 1.5 | 15 | | 296 | 188 | | 576 | 1.07 |
| 7651 | 2 ea | Pepperoni, svg, Gorilla Foods | 57 | 121 | | 20.1 | 4.0 | | | | 2.0 | | | | | | 0 | | | | | | | | | | | | | | | | | | | | | | | | 705 | |
| 7618 | 3 pce | Salami, fzn, Worthington Foods | 57 | 129 | 57 | 12.3 | 1.9 | 1.7 | 0.4 | | 8.1 | 0.9 | 1.4 | 5.8 | | | 2 | 0 | 0 | 0 | 0 | 0 | 0.76 | 0.15 | 1.13 | 0.27 | 0.65 | | | 0.0 | | | 26 | | 1.4 | | | 67 | 92 | | 930 | 0.30 |
| 7555 | 3 Tbs | Sandwich Spread, avg | 48 | 72 | 70 | 3.8 | 4.3 | 1.6 | | | 4.3 | 0.7 | 1.0 | 2.3 | | | 0 | 0 | 0 | 0 | 0 | 0 | 0.29 | 0.34 | 6.24 | 0.53 | 1.49 | 49.4 | | 0.0 | | | 21 | 0.3 | 0.7 | 61 | | 106 | 163 | | 302 | 0.62 |
| 7666 | 1 ea | Sandwich Spread, cnd, svg, Loma Linda | 55 | 85 | 69 | 3.9 | 7.2 | 3.1 | 0.5 | 3.6 | 4.5 | 0.9 | 2.1 | 1.4 | | | 1 | 104 | 10 | 0 | 10 | | 0.28 | 0.32 | 1.78 | 0.46 | 3.61 | | 1.08 | 0.0 | | | 20 | | 1.3 | | | 73 | 139 | | 255 | 0.41 |
| 7743 | 1 ea | Smoked Beef Slices, fzn, svg, Worthington Foods | 57 | 123 | 56 | 10.8 | 5.5 | 3.2 | 1.0 | 1.3 | 6.4 | 1.2 | 2.6 | 2.5 | | | 1 | 0 | 0 | 0 | 0 | 0 | 2.12 | 0.14 | 3.15 | 0.30 | 1.73 | | | 0.0 | | | 5 | | 1.3 | | | 112 | 153 | | 727 | 0.14 |
| 7612 | 1 pce | Numete, cnd, Worthington Foods | 55 | 133 | 58 | 6.5 | 5.1 | 3.1 | 0.6 | 1.4 | 9.6 | 2.4 | 4.4 | 2.7 | | | 0 | 0 | 0 | 0 | 0 | 0 | 0.08 | 0.06 | 0.54 | 0.20 | 0.26 | | | 0.0 | | | 10 | | 1.1 | | | 116 | 155 | | 272 | 0.56 |
| 57433 | 1 ea | Nuteena, cnd, svg, Worthington Foods | 55 | 162 | 58 | 5.5 | 5.8 | 1.5 | 0.5 | 3.7 | 13.0 | 5.2 | 5.8 | 1.7 | | | 0 | 0 | 0 | 0 | 0 | 0 | 0.10 | 0.35 | 1.04 | 0.45 | 2.09 | 49.3 | 1.69 | 0.0 | | | 9 | | 0.3 | 33 | | 94 | 166 | | 119 | 0.46 |
| | | Patties/Burgers | | | | | | | | | | | | | | | | | | | | | | | | | | | | | | | | | | | | | | | | |
| 7670 | 1 ea | Better 'N Burgers, Morningstar Farms | 78 | 83 | 71 | 12.8 | 6.9 | 3.9 | 0.4 | 2.6 | 0.5 | 0.1 | 0.3 | 0.1 | 0.02 | 0.13 | 0 | 0 | 0 | 0 | 0 | 0 | 0.23 | 0.51 | 3.78 | 0.18 | 0.00 | 225.4 | 1.03 | 0.0 | | | 80 | 0.2 | 2.7 | 15 | 0.2 | 166 | 398 | | 351 | 0.69 |
| 7725 | 1 ea | Burger Crumbles, Morningstar Farms | 55 | 116 | 60 | 11.1 | 3.3 | 2.5 | 0.6 | 0.2 | 6.5 | 1.6 | 2.3 | 2.5 | 0.26 | 2.20 | 0 | 0 | 0 | 0 | 0 | 0 | 4.96 | 0.18 | 1.49 | 0.27 | 2.18 | | 0.00 | 0.0 | | | 40 | 0.1 | 3.2 | 1 | 0.0 | 87 | 89 | | 238 | 0.82 |
| 7643 | 1 pce | Fri-Pats, fzn, Worthington Foods | 64 | 132 | 57 | 14.5 | 4.2 | 3.5 | 0.2 | 0.5 | 6.3 | 0.9 | 1.6 | 3.8 | | | 2 | 0 | 0 | 0 | 0 | 0 | 2.70 | 0.15 | 3.39 | 0.65 | 1.08 | | | 0.0 | | | 63 | | 1.0 | | | 119 | 127 | | 323 | 0.61 |
| 7722 | 1 ea | Garden Burger, Morningstar Farms | 67 | 119 | 60 | 11.2 | 10.2 | 4.0 | 0.8 | 5.4 | 3.8 | 0.5 | 1.1 | 2.2 | 0.04 | 2.12 | 1 | 766 | 76 | 0 | 76 | | 6.47 | 0.10 | 0.00 | 0.00 | 0.00 | 28.8 | 1.20 | 0.0 | | | 48 | 0.4 | 1.2 | 29 | 0.3 | 124 | 180 | | 382 | 0.58 |
| 7504 | 1 ea | Garden Burger, Whole Foods | 45 | 82 | 58 | 5.1 | 11.4 | 3.2 | 0.6 | 7.6 | 1.9 | 0.6 | 0.9 | 0.3 | | | 7 | 32 | 6 | 0 | | | 0.07 | 0.09 | 0.68 | 0.05 | 0.07 | 6.4 | 0.36 | 0.0 | 0.2 | | 54 | 0.1 | 0.0 | 19 | 0.4 | 84 | 122 | 4.7 | 184 | 0.56 |
| 7728 | 2 Tbs | Gran-Burger, dry, Worthington Foods | 17 | 62 | 2 | 10.2 | 3.5 | 2.5 | 0.1 | 0.9 | 0.8 | 0.2 | 0.3 | 0.3 | | | 0 | 0 | 0 | 0 | 0 | 0 | 0.10 | 0.14 | 2.97 | 0.09 | 0.38 | | 0.17 | 0.0 | | | 35 | | 2.9 | | | 114 | 219 | | 411 | 0.46 |
| 7667 | 1 ea | Ground Meatless Burger, Worthington Foods | 55 | 80 | 68 | 10.9 | 2.9 | 2.8 | 0.1 | 0.0 | 2.7 | 0.5 | 0.7 | 1.5 | | | 0 | 0 | 0 | 0 | 0 | 0 | 0.42 | 0.13 | 3.41 | 0.30 | 3.40 | | | 0.0 | | | 23 | | 2.2 | | | 96 | 96 | | 267 | 0.66 |
| 7673 | 1 ea | Harvest Burger, italian, Green Giant | 90 | 139 | 65 | 17.3 | 7.7 | 4.6 | 0.8 | 2.3 | 4.5 | 1.4 | 0.3 | 0.4 | | | 0 | 30 | 3 | 0 | 3 | | 0.28 | 0.14 | 4.05 | 0.28 | 1.35 | | 0.54 | 0.0 | | | 74 | 0.3 | 2.6 | | | | | | 373 | 6.93 |
| 7674 | 1 ea | Harvest Burger, original, Green Giant | 90 | 137 | 65 | 17.9 | 7.6 | 5.2 | 0.7 | 1.6 | 4.0 | 1.3 | 0.1 | 0.4 | | | 0 | 0 | 0 | 0 | 0 | 0 | 0.29 | 0.14 | 4.32 | 0.29 | 1.44 | | 0.54 | 0.0 | | | 76 | 0.3 | 2.7 | | | | | | 378 | 7.20 |
| 7675 | 1 ea | Harvest Burger, southwestern, Green Giant | 90 | 135 | 65 | 16.2 | 8.6 | 5.4 | 1.0 | 2.3 | 4.0 | 1.4 | 0.2 | 0.4 | | | 0 | 32 | 3 | 0 | 3 | | 0.27 | 0.14 | 4.05 | 0.27 | 1.35 | | 0.54 | 0.0 | | | 71 | 0.3 | 2.5 | | | | | | 371 | 6.66 |
| 7662 | 1 ea | Okra Patty, fzn, Natural Touch | 64 | 105 | 54 | 10.5 | 3.5 | 3.4 | 0.4 | | 5.4 | 1.0 | 1.2 | 3.2 | | | 1 | 0 | 0 | 0 | 0 | 0 | 0.04 | 0.15 | 0.00 | 0.03 | 0.00 | | | 0.0 | | | 33 | | 0.9 | | | 92 | 175 | | 364 | 0.50 |
| 7764 | 1 ea | Patty, dry mix, Loma Linda | 26 | 90 | 6 | 13.9 | 6.5 | 4.9 | 0.4 | 1.2 | 0.9 | 0.2 | 0.3 | 0.4 | | | 1 | 0 | 0 | 0 | 0 | 0 | 0.43 | 0.38 | 2.52 | 0.31 | 1.55 | | 1.65 | 0.0 | | | 22 | | 1.4 | | | 160 | 405 | | 477 | 0.12 |
| 7664 | 1 ea | Prime Patties, fzn, Morningstar Farms | 78 | 115 | 64 | 19.5 | 4.7 | 3.3 | 1.0 | 0.4 | 2.0 | 0.3 | 0.4 | 0.8 | | | 1 | 0 | 0 | 0 | 0 | 0 | 0.62 | 0.30 | 1.12 | 0.50 | 4.42 | | | 1.9 | | | 56 | | 2.6 | | | 153 | 172 | | 301 | 0.90 |
| 7615 | 2 ea | Prosage Patties, Frozen, Worthington Foods | 76 | 160 | 55 | 19.2 | 6.3 | 4.0 | 0.2 | 2.1 | 6.5 | 1.0 | 1.6 | 4.0 | | | 2 | 0 | 0 | 0 | 0 | 0 | 0.96 | 0.17 | 1.04 | 0.55 | 3.02 | | | 0.0 | | | 30 | | 2.4 | | | 192 | 157 | | 591 | 0.68 |
| 57434 | 1 ea | Redi-Burger, cnd, svg, Loma Linda | 85 | 172 | 59 | 16.4 | 4.8 | | | | 9.7 | 1.5 | 2.4 | 5.8 | | | 1 | 0 | 0 | 0 | 0 | 0 | 0.14 | 0.30 | 1.90 | 0.51 | 1.51 | 21.3 | 1.58 | 0.0 | | | 12 | | 1.1 | 16 | | 139 | 122 | | 456 | 1.11 |
| 7554 | 1 ea | Soyburger, avg | 71 | 142 | 58 | 14.9 | 5.7 | 3.3 | | | 6.4 | 1.0 | 1.5 | 3.3 | | | 0 | 0 | 0 | 0 | 0 | 0 | 0.64 | 0.43 | 7.10 | 0.85 | 1.70 | 55.4 | | 0.0 | | | 21 | 0.5 | 1.5 | 13 | | 244 | 128 | | 390 | 1.28 |
| 7562 | 1 ea | Soyburger, w/cheese, avg | 135 | 316 | 50 | 20.7 | 29.5 | 4.1 | | | 12.7 | 4.2 | 3.9 | 3.7 | | | 12 | 220 | 45 | 34 | 11 | | 0.77 | 0.55 | 8.14 | 0.86 | 1.71 | 69.5 | | 0.8 | | | 146 | 0.6 | 2.7 | 27 | | 371 | 211 | | 932 | 1.97 |

| Code | Amount | Description | Weight (g) | Calories | % Water | Protein (g) | Carbs (g) | Fiber (g) | Sugar (g) | Other Carbs (g) | Fat (g) |
|---|---|---|---|---|---|---|---|---|---|---|---|
| 7726 | 1 ea | Spicy Black Bean Burger, Morningstar Farms | 78 | 115 | 60 | 11.8 | 15.2 | 4.8 | 1.4 | 9.0 | 0.8 |
| 57435 | 1 ea | Vege-Burger, cnd, Loma Linda | 55 | 66 | 71 | 10.5 | 2.4 | 2.0 | 0.4 | | 1.6 |
| 7732 | 1/2 cup | Vegetarian Burger, Worthington Foods | 110 | 121 | 71 | 17.4 | 4.3 | 2.3 | 0.3 | 1.7 | 3.8 |
| 7765 | 2 Tbs | Vita-Burger, dry granules, Loma Linda | 10 | 36 | 6 | 4.7 | 3.0 | 1.8 | 0.7 | 0.5 | 0.5 |
| 7556 | 1 ea | Pot Pie, avg | 227 | 524 | 59 | 14.6 | 41.2 | 4.8 | | | 33.8 |
| 7616 | 1 pce | Prosage Roll, fzn, Worthington Foods | 55 | 142 | 54 | 10.0 | 2.0 | | | | 10.4 |
| 7617 | 1 pce | Protose, cnd, Worthington Foods | 55 | 131 | 53 | 12.8 | 4.8 | 2.9 | 0.6 | 1.3 | 6.7 |
| | | Sausage Substitutes | | | | | | | | | |
| 7677 | 1 ea | Breakfast Links, fzn, Green Giant | 23 | 38 | 65 | 4.0 | 1.8 | 1.2 | 0.2 | 0.4 | 1.7 |
| 57436 | 1 pce | Breakfast Links, fzn, Morningstar Farms | 22 | 31 | 60 | 4.1 | 0.9 | 0.9 | 0.2 | | 1.2 |
| 7676 | 1 ea | Breakfast Pattie, fzn, Green Giant | 29 | 48 | 65 | 5.0 | 2.3 | 1.5 | 0.2 | 0.6 | 2.1 |
| 62359 | 1 ea | Breakfast Pattie, Morningstar Fams | 38 | 79 | 54 | 9.9 | 3.7 | 2.0 | 0.6 | 1.2 | 2.3 |
| 7505 | 1 ea | Garden Patty, Whole Foods | 36 | 66 | 59 | 3.6 | 9.1 | 2.0 | 1.0 | 6.1 | 1.6 |
| 7746 | 1 ea | Grillers, fzn, Morningstar Farms | 64 | 140 | 55 | 14.3 | 5.0 | 3.2 | 0.6 | 1.2 | 6.9 |
| 7668 | 1 ea | Ground, svg, Worthington Foods | 55 | 113 | 60 | 11.3 | 3.4 | 2.8 | 0.7 | | 6.0 |
| 7511 | 1 ea | Pattie, avg | 25 | 64 | 50 | 4.6 | 2.5 | 0.7 | | | 4.6 |
| | | Soybeans | | | | | | | | | |
| 90028 | 1/2 cup | Cooked, w/salt, avg | 86 | 149 | 63 | 14.3 | 8.5 | 5.2 | 2.6 | 0.3 | 7.7 |
| 7063 | 1/2 cup | Roasted, dry, avg | 86 | 387 | 1 | 34.1 | 28.1 | 7.0 | 7.1 | 14.0 | 18.6 |
| 7719 | 1/2 cup | Roasted, mature seeds, unsalted, avg | 86 | 405 | 2 | 30.3 | 28.9 | 15.2 | | | 21.8 |
| 7559 | 1 ea | Stew, svg, avg | 270 | 324 | 70 | 45.9 | 18.9 | 3.0 | | | 8.1 |
| 7607 | 1 cup | Stew, Country, cnd, Worthington Foods | 240 | 209 | 81 | 12.7 | 19.6 | 5.4 | 2.2 | 12.0 | 8.8 |
| 7663 | 1 ea | Stroganoff, dry mix, Natural Touch | 23 | 94 | 8 | 5.2 | 9.8 | 3.4 | 1.3 | 5.0 | 3.8 |
| 7507 | 1 ea | Taco Garden, Whole Foods | 35 | 106 | 27 | 6.2 | 17.6 | 4.8 | 0.8 | 12.0 | 1.2 |
| | | Tofu | | | | | | | | | |
| 7540 | 1/2 cup | Silken Extra Firm, Morinaga Nutritional Foods | 126 | 69 | 88 | 9.3 | 2.5 | 0.1 | 1.3 | 1.1 | 2.4 |
| 7542 | 1/2 cup | Silken Firm, Morinaga Nutritional Foods | 126 | 78 | 87 | 8.7 | 3.0 | 0.1 | 1.6 | 1.3 | 3.4 |
| 7541 | 1/2 cup | Silken Soft, Morinaga Nutritional Foods | 124 | 68 | 89 | 6.0 | 3.6 | 0.1 | 1.6 | 1.3 | 3.3 |
| 7625 | 3 pce | Turkee Slices, cnd, Worthington Foods | 94 | 193 | 64 | 13.2 | 3.5 | 1.7 | 0.5 | 1.3 | 14.0 |
| 7622 | 4 pce | Turkey Style, smkd, fzn, Worthington Foods | 76 | 190 | 55 | 13.2 | 4.7 | 3.4 | 1.0 | 0.3 | 13.2 |
| 7633 | 4 pce | Wham, fzn, Worthington Foods | 90 | 163 | 64 | 14.7 | 2.9 | 0.3 | 1.9 | 0.7 | 10.3 |
| | | **NUTS, SEEDS AND PRODUCTS** | | | | | | | | | |
| | | Acorns | | | | | | | | | |
| 4639 | 1 oz | Dried, avg | 28 | 143 | 5 | 2.3 | 15.0 | 1.2 | | | 8.8 |
| 4679 | 1 oz | Flour, full fat, avg | 28 | 140 | 6 | 2.1 | 15.3 | 0.6 | | | 8.5 |
| 4704 | 1 oz | Raw, avg | 28 | 108 | 28 | 1.7 | 11.4 | 0.9 | | | 6.7 |
| | | Almonds | | | | | | | | | |
| 4547 | 1 oz | Blanched, whole, avg | 28 | 164 | 5 | 5.7 | 5.2 | 1.9 | 1.6 | 1.7 | 14.7 |
| 4721 | 1 oz | Blanched, slivered, Blue Diamond | 28 | 170 | 4 | 5.9 | 5.5 | 2.6 | 1.1 | 1.7 | 14.3 |
| 4572 | 2 Tbs | Butter, plain, salted, avg | 32 | 203 | 1 | 4.8 | 6.8 | 1.2 | 3.4 | 2.2 | 18.9 |
| 4534 | 2 Tbs | Butter, plain, unsalted, avg | 32 | 203 | 1 | 4.8 | 6.8 | 1.2 | 3.4 | 2.2 | 18.9 |
| 4691 | 2 Tbs | Butter, w/honey & cinnamon, salted, avg | 32 | 193 | 2 | 5.1 | 8.6 | 1.2 | | | 16.7 |
| 4567 | 2 Tbs | Butter, w/honey & cinnamon, unsalted, avg | 32 | 193 | 2 | 5.1 | 8.6 | 1.2 | 5.3 | 2.2 | 16.7 |
| 4500 | 1 oz | Dried, avg | 28 | 165 | 4 | 5.6 | 5.7 | 3.1 | 1.6 | 1.1 | 14.6 |
| 4571 | 1 oz | Dry Roasted, salted, avg | 28 | 164 | 3 | 4.6 | 6.8 | 3.8 | 1.5 | 1.5 | 14.4 |
| 4549 | 1 oz | Dry Roasted, unsalted, avg | 28 | 164 | 3 | 4.6 | 6.8 | 3.8 | 1.5 | 1.5 | 14.4 |
| 4687 | 1 oz | Honey Roasted, avg | 28 | 166 | 2 | 5.1 | 7.8 | 3.8 | | | 14.0 |
| 4692 | 1 oz | Meal, salted, avg | 28 | 114 | 7 | 11.1 | 8.1 | 3.8 | | | 5.1 |
| 4657 | 1 oz | Nut Meal, avg | 28 | 114 | 7 | 11.1 | 8.1 | 1.0 | 3.2 | 3.9 | 5.1 |
| 4620 | 1 oz | Oil Roasted, salted, avg | 28 | 173 | 3 | 5.7 | 4.5 | 3.1 | 1.3 | 0.0 | 16.2 |
| 4505 | 1 oz | Oil Roasted, unsalted, avg | 28 | 173 | 3 | 5.7 | 4.5 | 3.1 | 1.3 | 0.0 | 16.2 |
| 4553 | 2 Tbs | Paste, packed, avg | 29 | 133 | 14 | 2.6 | 13.9 | 1.4 | 5.0 | 7.4 | 8.0 |
| 4566 | 1 oz | Toasted, whole, avg | 28 | 165 | 3 | 5.7 | 6.4 | 3.1 | 1.8 | 1.5 | 14.2 |
| 4725 | 1 oz | Whole Natural, Blue Diamond | 28 | 168 | 4 | 5.8 | 5.6 | 3.4 | 1.6 | 0.6 | 14.1 |
| 4771 | 1 oz | Amaranth Seeds, Arrowhead Mills | 28 | 101 | 10 | 4.2 | 17.3 | 1.8 | 0.0 | 15.5 | 1.2 |
| 4642 | 1 oz | Beechnuts, dried, avg | 28 | 161 | 7 | 1.7 | 9.4 | 1.0 | | | 14.0 |
| 4643 | 1 oz | Butternuts, dried, avg | 28 | 171 | 3 | 7.0 | 3.4 | 1.3 | | | 16.0 |
| 4535 | 1 oz | Brazil Nuts, dried, avg | 28 | 184 | 3 | 4.0 | 3.6 | 1.5 | 0.7 | 1.3 | 18.5 |
| | | Breadfruit Seeds | | | | | | | | | |
| 4606 | 1 oz | Boiled, avg | 28 | 47 | 59 | 1.5 | 9.0 | 0.6 | | | 0.6 |
| 4605 | 1 oz | Raw, avg | 28 | 53 | 56 | 2.1 | 8.2 | 0.7 | | | 1.6 |
| 4607 | 1 oz | Roasted, avg | 28 | 58 | 50 | 1.7 | 11.2 | 0.7 | | | 0.8 |
| | | Cashews | | | | | | | | | |
| 4662 | 2 Tbs | Butter, salted | 32 | 188 | 3 | 5.6 | 8.8 | 0.6 | 2.1 | 6.1 | 15.8 |
| 4537 | 2 Tbs | Butter, unsalted, avg | 32 | 188 | 3 | 5.6 | 8.8 | 0.6 | 2.1 | 6.1 | 15.8 |

| Code | Sat Fat (g) | Mono Fat (g) | Poly Fat (g) | Omega 3 (g) | Omega 6 (g) | Choles (mg) | Vit A (IU) | Vit A (RE) | Retinol (RE) | Carotenoids (RE) | Beta Carotene (mcg) |
|---|---|---|---|---|---|---|---|---|---|---|---|
| 7726 | 0.3 | 0.2 | 0.4 | 0.04 | 0.31 | 1 | 139 | 14 | 0 | 14 | |
| 57435 | 0.3 | 0.6 | 0.[illegible] | | | 0 | 0 | 0 | 0 | 0 | 0 |
| 7732 | 0.7 | 1.0 | 2.[illegible] | | | 0 | 0 | 0 | 0 | 0 | 0 |
| 7765 | 0.1 | 0.1 | 0.[illegible] | | | 0 | 0 | 0 | 0 | 0 | 0 |
| 7556 | 9.5 | 12.6 | 9.[illegible] | | | 20 | 6267 | 729 | 157 | 572 | |
| 7616 | 2.0 | 3.5 | 4.[illegible] | | | 1 | 0 | 0 | 0 | 0 | 0 |
| 7617 | 1.0 | 3.0 | 2.4 | | | 1 | 0 | 0 | 0 | 0 | 0 |
| 7677 | 0.2 | 0.4 | 1.[illegible] | | | 0 | 0 | 0 | 0 | 0 | 0 |
| 57436 | 0.2 | 0.3 | 0.[illegible] | | | 1 | 0 | 0 | 0 | 0 | 0 |
| 7676 | 0.3 | 0.5 | 1.[illegible] | | | 0 | 0 | 0 | 0 | 0 | 0 |
| 62359 | 0.5 | 0.7 | 1.[illegible] | 0.05 | .25 | 1 | 0 | 0 | 0 | 0 | 0 |
| 7505 | 1.0 | 0.4 | 0.[illegible] | | | 5 | 61 | 12 | | | |
| 7746 | 1.7 | 2.2 | 3.[illegible] | | | 2 | 0 | 0 | 0 | 0 | 0 |
| 7668 | 1.5 | 2.4 | 2.[illegible] | | | 1 | 0 | 0 | 0 | 0 | 0 |
| 7511 | 0.7 | 1.1 | 2.[illegible] | 0.27 | 2.05 | 0 | 160 | 16 | 0 | 16 | |
| 90028 | 1.1 | 1.7 | 4.4 | 0.51 | 3.34 | 0 | 8 | 1 | 0 | 1 | 5 |
| 7063 | 2.7 | 4.1 | 10.[illegible] | 1.23 | 9.25 | 0 | 20 | 2 | 0 | 2 | |
| 7719 | 3.2 | 4.8 | 12.[illegible] | 1.45 | 10.34 | 0 | 172 | 17 | 0 | 17 | |
| 7559 | 1.2 | 3.5 | 3.[illegible] | | | 0 | 0 | 0 | 0 | 0 | 0 |
| 7607 | 1.6 | 2.3 | 4.[illegible] | | | 2 | 2158 | 216 | 0 | 216 | |
| 7663 | 1.8 | 1.1 | 0.[illegible] | | | 11 | 0 | 0 | 0 | 0 | 0 |
| 7507 | 0.6 | 0.4 | 0.[illegible] | | | 0 | 91 | 18 | | | |
| 7540 | 0.4 | 0.4 | 1.[illegible] | | | 0 | 0 | 0 | 0 | 0 | 0 |
| 7542 | 0.5 | 0.7 | 1.9 | | | 0 | 0 | 0 | 0 | 0 | 0 |
| 7541 | 0.4 | 0.6 | 1.9 | | | 0 | 0 | 0 | 0 | 0 | 0 |
| 7625 | 2.3 | 5.4 | 6.[illegible] | | | 2 | 0 | 0 | 0 | 0 | 0 |
| 7622 | 2.6 | 4.9 | 5.4 | | | 2 | 0 | 0 | 0 | 0 | 0 |
| 7633 | 1.6 | 2.7 | 5.9 | | | 2 | 0 | 0 | 0 | 0 | 0 |
| 4639 | 1.1 | 5.6 | 1.7 | 0.00 | 1.69 | 0 | 0 | 0 | 0 | 0 | 0 |
| 4679 | 1.1 | 5.3 | 1.6 | 0.00 | 1.63 | 0 | 14 | 1 | 0 | 1 | 8 |
| 4704 | 0.9 | 4.2 | 1.3 | 0.00 | 1.29 | 0 | 11 | 1 | 0 | 1 | 7 |
| 4547 | 1.4 | 9.5 | 3.1 | 0.11 | 2.97 | 0 | 0 | 0 | 0 | 0 | 0 |
| 4721 | 1.0 | 9.2 | 3.1 | 0.07 | 3.06 | 0 | 0 | 0 | 0 | 0 | 0 |
| 4572 | 1.8 | 12.3 | 4.0 | 0.14 | 3.81 | 0 | 0 | 0 | 0 | 0 | 0 |
| 4534 | 1.8 | 12.3 | 4.0 | 0.14 | 3.81 | 0 | 0 | 0 | 0 | 0 | 0 |
| 4691 | 1.6 | 10.8 | 3.5 | 0.12 | 3.36 | 0 | 0 | 0 | 0 | 0 | 0 |
| 4567 | 1.6 | 10.8 | 3.5 | 0.12 | 3.36 | 0 | 0 | 0 | 0 | 0 | 0 |
| 4500 | 1.4 | 9.5 | 3.1 | 0.10 | 2.94 | 0 | 0 | 0 | 0 | 0 | 0 |
| 4571 | 1.4 | 9.4 | 3.0 | 0.10 | 2.91 | 0 | 0 | 0 | 0 | 0 | 0 |
| 4549 | 1.4 | 9.4 | 3.0 | 0.10 | 2.91 | 0 | 0 | 0 | 0 | 0 | 0 |
| 4687 | 1.3 | 9.1 | 2.9 | 0.10 | 2.83 | 0 | 0 | 0 | 0 | 0 | 0 |
| 4692 | 0.5 | 3.3 | 1.1 | 0.04 | 1.03 | 0 | 0 | 0 | 0 | 0 | 0 |
| 4657 | 0.5 | 3.3 | 1.1 | 0.04 | 1.03 | 0 | 0 | 0 | 0 | 0 | 0 |
| 4620 | 1.5 | 10.5 | 3.4 | 0.12 | 3.25 | 0 | 0 | 0 | 0 | 0 | 0 |
| 4505 | 1.5 | 10.5 | 3.4 | 0.12 | 3.25 | 0 | 0 | 0 | 0 | 0 | 0 |
| 4553 | 0.8 | 5.2 | 1.7 | 0.06 | 1.62 | 0 | 1 | 0 | 0 | 0 | 0 |
| 4566 | 1.3 | 9.2 | 3.0 | 0.10 | 2.86 | 0 | 0 | 0 | 0 | 0 | 0 |
| 4725 | 1.0 | 8.8 | 3.2 | 0.00 | 3.25 | 0 | 0 | 0 | 0 | 0 | 0 |
| 4771 | 0.3 | | | | | 0 | 0 | 0 | 0 | 0 | 0 |
| 4642 | 1.6 | 6.1 | 5.6 | 0.48 | 5.15 | 0 | 0 | 0 | 0 | 0 | 0 |
| 4643 | 0.4 | 2.9 | 12.0 | 2.44 | 9.44 | 0 | 35 | 3 | 0 | 3 | 20 |
| 4535 | 4.5 | 6.4 | 6.7 | 0.02 | 6.66 | 0 | 0 | 0 | 0 | 0 | 0 |
| 4606 | 0.2 | 0.1 | 0.3 | 0.08 | 0.26 | 0 | 67 | 7 | 0 | 7 | 40 |
| 4605 | 0.4 | 0.2 | 0.8 | 0.19 | 0.64 | 0 | 72 | 7 | 0 | 7 | 44 |
| 4607 | 0.2 | 0.1 | 0.4 | 0.09 | 0.31 | 0 | 82 | 8 | 0 | 8 | 49 |
| 4662 | 3.1 | 9.3 | 2.7 | 0.05 | 2.61 | 0 | 0 | 0 | 0 | 0 | 0 |
| 4537 | 3.1 | 9.3 | 2.7 | 0.05 | 2.61 | 0 | 0 | 0 | 0 | 0 | 0 |

| Code | Thiamin (mg) | Riboflavin (mg) | Niacin (NE) | Vit B6 (mg) | Vit B12 (mcg) | Folate (mcg) | Panto (mg) | Vit C (mg) | Vit D (mg) | Vit E (α TE) | Calcium (mg) | Copper (mg) | Iron (mg) | Magnes (mg) | Mang (mg) | Phos (mg) | Potassium (mg) | Selenium (mcg) | Sodium (mg) | Zinc (mg) |
|---|---|---|---|---|---|---|---|---|---|---|---|---|---|---|---|---|---|---|---|---|
| 7726 | 8.03 | 0.14 | 0.00 | 0.21 | 0.07 | | 0.41 | 0.0 | | | 56 | 0.2 | 1.8 | 44 | 0.9 | 150 | 269 | | 499 | 0.93 |
| 57435 | 0.20 | 0.25 | 0.78 | 0.31 | 0.87 | 14.9 | 0.95 | 0.0 | | | 8 | | 0.5 | 12 | | 58 | 30 | | 114 | 0.58 |
| 7732 | 0.25 | 0.20 | 3.92 | 0.47 | 2.28 | | | 0.0 | | | 9 | | 3.5 | | | 112 | 50 | | 538 | 0.77 |
| 7765 | 0.53 | 0.08 | 1.46 | 0.06 | 0.17 | | 0.17 | 0.0 | | | 13 | | 0.9 | | | 74 | 238 | | 168 | 2.28 |
| 7556 | 0.65 | 0.40 | 4.47 | 0.31 | 1.02 | 40.2 | 0.34 | 9.7 | 0.2 | | 66 | 0.3 | 2.9 | 32 | 0.5 | 247 | 331 | | 538 | 1.05 |
| 7616 | 1.03 | 0.19 | 1.55 | 0.24 | 0.75 | | | 0.0 | | | 11 | | 1.9 | | | 74 | 83 | | 392 | 0.38 |
| 7617 | 0.13 | 0.13 | 1.34 | 0.24 | 1.26 | | | 0.0 | | | 1 | | 1.8 | | | 94 | 50 | | 283 | 0.70 |
| 7677 | 0.06 | 0.03 | 0.09 | 0.06 | 0.30 | | 0.12 | 0.0 | | | 22 | 0.1 | 0.6 | | | | | | 115 | 1.54 |
| 57436 | 3.40 | 0.11 | 2.54 | 0.16 | 1.67 | 5.8 | | 0.0 | | | 7 | | 1.0 | 8 | | 26 | 29 | | 165 | 0.17 |
| 7676 | 0.03 | 0.04 | 1.16 | 0.08 | 0.38 | | 0.14 | 0.0 | | | 28 | 0.1 | 1.0 | | | | | | 145 | 1.94 |
| 62359 | 5.40 | 0.13 | 1.84 | 0.19 | 1.50 | | 0.07 | 0.0 | | | 18 | 0.0 | 1.9 | 1 | 0.0 | 106 | 102 | | 259 | 0.37 |
| 7505 | 0.05 | 0.08 | 0.51 | 0.04 | 0.06 | 5.1 | 0.27 | 0.3 | 0.1 | | 41 | 0.1 | 0.3 | 14 | 0.3 | 69 | 72 | 3.8 | 152 | 0.42 |
| 7746 | 11.74 | 0.24 | 2.99 | 0.37 | 4.85 | | | 0.0 | | | 43 | | 1.2 | | | 111 | 127 | | 256 | 0.49 |
| 7668 | 7.76 | 0.08 | 1.05 | 0.37 | 1.72 | | | 0.0 | | | 27 | | 1.6 | | | 104 | 122 | | 331 | 0.48 |
| 7511 | 0.58 | 0.10 | 2.80 | 0.21 | 0.00 | 6.5 | 0.08 | 0.0 | 0.0 | | 16 | 0.1 | 0.9 | 9 | 0.2 | 56 | 58 | 1.9 | 222 | 0.37 |
| 90028 | 0.13 | 0.25 | 0.34 | 0.20 | 0.00 | 46.3 | 0.15 | 1.5 | 0.0 | | 88 | 0.4 | 4.4 | 74 | 0.7 | 211 | 443 | 6.3 | 204 | 0.99 |
| 7063 | 0.37 | 0.65 | 0.91 | 0.19 | 0.00 | 176.3 | 0.41 | 4.0 | 0.0 | | 120 | 0.9 | 3.4 | 196 | 1.9 | 558 | 1173 | 16.6 | 2 | 4.10 |
| 7719 | 0.09 | 0.12 | 1.21 | 0.18 | 0.00 | 181.5 | 0.39 | 1.9 | | | 119 | 0.7 | 3.4 | 125 | 1.9 | 312 | 1264 | 16.4 | 3 | 2.70 |
| 7559 | 1.89 | 1.62 | 32.40 | 2.97 | 5.94 | 278.1 | | 0.0 | | | 84 | 1.8 | 3.5 | 343 | | 594 | 324 | | 1080 | 2.97 |
| 7607 | 1.85 | 0.29 | 4.22 | 0.86 | 3.67 | | | 0.0 | | | 50 | | 5.1 | | | 187 | 269 | | 826 | 1.03 |
| 7663 | 0.14 | 0.17 | 0.38 | 0.12 | 0.54 | | | 0.0 | | | 53 | | 0.5 | | | 104 | 229 | | 607 | 0.51 |
| 7507 | | | | | 0.00 | | | 0.6 | | | 117 | | 0.4 | | | | 150 | | 79 | |
| 7540 | 0.10 | 0.04 | 0.30 | 0.01 | 0.00 | | | 0.0 | | | 39 | 0.3 | 1.5 | 34 | | 126 | 194 | | 79 | 0.76 |
| 7542 | 0.13 | 0.05 | 0.31 | 0.01 | 0.00 | | | 0.0 | | | 40 | 0.3 | 1.3 | 34 | | 113 | 244 | | 45 | 0.77 |
| 7541 | 0.12 | 0.05 | 0.37 | 0.01 | 0.00 | | | 0.0 | | | 38 | 0.3 | 1.0 | 36 | | 77 | 223 | | 6 | 0.64 |
| 7625 | 3.21 | 0.14 | 1.10 | 0.24 | 1.67 | | | 0.0 | | | 8 | | 1.4 | | | 86 | 46 | | 579 | 0.32 |
| 7622 | 13.57 | 0.21 | 2.66 | 0.39 | 2.80 | | | 0.0 | | | 7 | | 2.4 | | | 117 | 93 | | 823 | 0.31 |
| 7633 | 5.58 | 0.30 | 2.86 | 0.37 | 2.36 | | | 0.0 | | | 11 | | 2.2 | | | | 165 | | 853 | 0.28 |
| 4639 | 0.04 | 0.04 | 0.67 | 0.19 | 0.00 | 32.2 | 0.26 | 0.0 | | | 15 | 0.2 | 0.3 | 23 | 0.4 | 29 | 199 | | 0 | 0.19 |
| 4679 | 0.04 | 0.04 | 0.67 | 0.19 | 0.00 | 31.9 | 0.26 | 0.0 | 0.0 | | 12 | 0.2 | 0.3 | 31 | 0.5 | 29 | 199 | | 0 | 0.18 |
| 4704 | 0.03 | 0.03 | 0.51 | 0.15 | 0.00 | 24.4 | 0.20 | 0.0 | 0.0 | | 11 | 0.2 | 0.2 | 17 | 0.4 | 22 | 151 | | 0 | 0.14 |
| 4547 | 0.05 | 0.19 | 0.89 | 0.03 | 0.00 | 10.8 | 0.13 | 0.2 | 0.0 | | 69 | 0.3 | 1.0 | 80 | 0.4 | 149 | 210 | 1.3 | 3 | 0.88 |
| 4721 | 0.04 | 0.19 | 0.88 | 0.03 | 0.00 | 10.9 | | | | | 71 | 0.3 | 1.0 | 85 | | 149 | 176 | | 3 | 0.97 |
| 4572 | 0.04 | 0.20 | 0.92 | 0.02 | 0.00 | 20.9 | 0.08 | 0.2 | 0.0 | | 86 | 0.3 | 1.2 | 97 | 0.8 | 167 | 243 | 1.6 | 144 | 0.98 |
| 4534 | 0.04 | 0.20 | 0.92 | 0.02 | 0.00 | 20.9 | 0.08 | 0.2 | 0.0 | | 86 | 0.3 | 1.2 | 97 | 0.8 | 167 | 243 | 1.5 | 4 | 0.98 |
| 4691 | 0.04 | 0.19 | 0.91 | 0.02 | 0.00 | 20.6 | 0.08 | 0.2 | 0.0 | | 85 | 0.3 | 1.2 | 96 | 0.7 | 166 | 240 | | 54 | 0.96 |
| 4567 | 0.04 | 0.19 | 0.91 | 0.02 | 0.00 | 20.6 | 0.08 | 0.2 | 0.0 | | 85 | 0.3 | 1.2 | 96 | 0.7 | 166 | 240 | 1.0 | 4 | 0.96 |
| 4500 | 0.06 | 0.22 | 0.94 | 0.03 | 0.00 | 16.4 | 0.13 | 0.2 | 0.0 | 6.7 | 74 | 0.3 | 1.0 | 83 | 0.6 | 146 | 205 | 1.3 | 3 | 0.82 |
| 4571 | 0.04 | 0.17 | 0.79 | 0.02 | 0.00 | 17.9 | 0.07 | 0.2 | 0.0 | | 79 | 0.3 | 1.1 | 85 | 0.6 | 153 | 216 | 1.3 | 218 | 1.37 |
| 4549 | 0.04 | 0.17 | 0.79 | 0.02 | 0.00 | 17.9 | 0.07 | 0.2 | 0.0 | | 79 | 0.3 | 1.1 | 85 | 0.6 | 153 | 216 | 1.3 | 3 | 1.37 |
| 4687 | 0.03 | 0.27 | 0.79 | 0.02 | 0.00 | 9.0 | 0.07 | 0.2 | 0.0 | | 74 | 0.3 | 0.8 | 67 | 0.6 | 112 | 157 | | 36 | 0.73 |
| 4692 | 0.09 | 0.47 | 1.76 | 0.03 | 0.00 | 16.0 | 0.13 | 0.2 | 0.0 | | 119 | 0.3 | 2.4 | 81 | 0.6 | 256 | 392 | | 209 | 0.79 |
| 4657 | 0.09 | 0.47 | 1.76 | 0.03 | 0.00 | 16.0 | 0.13 | 0.2 | 0.0 | | 119 | 0.3 | 2.4 | 81 | 0.6 | 256 | 392 | | 2 | 0.79 |
| 4620 | 0.04 | 0.28 | 0.98 | 0.02 | 0.00 | 17.9 | 0.07 | 0.2 | 0.0 | | 66 | 0.3 | 1.1 | 85 | 0.6 | 153 | 191 | 1.3 | 218 | 1.37 |
| 4505 | 0.04 | 0.28 | 0.98 | 0.02 | 0.00 | 17.9 | 0.07 | 0.2 | 0.0 | | 66 | 0.3 | 1.1 | 85 | 0.6 | 153 | 191 | 1.3 | 3 | 1.37 |
| 4553 | 0.02 | 0.12 | 0.41 | 0.01 | 0.00 | 21.2 | 0.03 | 0.0 | 0.0 | | 50 | 0.1 | 0.5 | 38 | 0.2 | 75 | 91 | 1.2 | 3 | 0.43 |
| 4566 | 0.04 | 0.17 | 0.79 | 0.02 | 0.00 | 17.9 | 0.07 | 0.2 | 0.0 | | 79 | 0.3 | 1.4 | 85 | 0.6 | 154 | 216 | 1.3 | 3 | 1.38 |
| 4725 | 0.05 | 0.25 | 0.88 | 0.03 | 0.00 | 12.3 | 0.12 | | | | | | | | | | | | | |
| 4771 | | 0.06 | 0.48 | | 0.00 | | | 0.0 | | | 48 | | 6.4 | | | | 101 | | 0 | |
| 4642 | 0.09 | 0.10 | 0.25 | 0.19 | 0.00 | 31.6 | 0.26 | 4.3 | 0.0 | | 0 | 0.2 | 0.7 | 0 | 0.4 | 0 | 285 | | 11 | 0.10 |
| 4643 | 0.11 | 0.04 | 0.29 | 0.16 | 0.00 | 18.5 | 0.18 | 0.9 | 0.0 | | 15 | 0.1 | 1.1 | 66 | 1.8 | 125 | 118 | 4.8 | 0 | 0.88 |
| 4535 | 0.28 | 0.03 | 0.45 | 0.07 | 0.00 | 1.1 | 0.07 | 0.2 | | | 49 | 0.5 | 1.0 | 63 | 0.2 | 168 | 168 | 828.8 | 1 | 1.29 |
| 4606 | 0.08 | 0.05 | 1.48 | 0.08 | 0.00 | 13.7 | 0.23 | 1.7 | 0.0 | | 17 | 0.3 | 0.2 | 14 | 0.0 | 35 | 245 | | 5 | 0.23 |
| 4605 | 0.13 | 0.08 | 0.12 | 0.09 | 0.00 | 14.8 | 0.25 | 1.8 | 0.0 | | 10 | 0.3 | 1.0 | 15 | 0.0 | 49 | 263 | | 7 | 0.25 |
| 4607 | 0.11 | 0.07 | 2.07 | 0.12 | 0.00 | 16.6 | 0.28 | 2.1 | 0.0 | | 24 | 0.4 | 0.3 | 17 | 0.0 | 49 | 303 | | 8 | 0.29 |
| 4662 | 0.10 | 0.06 | 0.51 | 0.08 | 0.00 | 21.9 | 0.38 | 0.0 | 0.0 | | 14 | 0.7 | 1.6 | 83 | 0.3 | 146 | 175 | 3.7 | 196 | 1.65 |
| 4537 | 0.10 | 0.06 | 0.51 | 0.08 | 0.00 | 21.9 | 0.38 | 0.0 | 0.0 | | 14 | 0.7 | 1.6 | 83 | 0.3 | 146 | 175 | 3.7 | 5 | 1.65 |

| Code | Amount | Description | Basic Components | | | | | | | | | Additional Fats | | | | | | Vit A & Components | | | | | Vitamins | | | | | | | | | | Minerals | | | | | | | | | |
|---|---|---|---|---|---|---|---|---|---|---|---|---|---|---|---|---|---|---|---|---|---|---|---|---|---|---|---|---|---|---|---|---|---|---|---|---|---|---|---|---|---|---|
| | | | Weight (g) | Calories | % Water | Protein (g) | Carbs (g) | Fiber (g) | Sugar (g) | Other Carbs (g) | Fat (g) | Sat Fat (g) | Mono Fat (g) | Poly Fat (g) | Omega 3 (g) | Omega 6 (g) | Choles (mg) | Vit A (IU) | Vit A (RE) | Retinol (RE) | Carotenoids (RE) | Beta Carotene (mcg) | Thiamin (mg) | Riboflavin (mg) | Niacin (NE) | Vit B6 (mg) | Vit B12 (mcg) | Folate (mcg) | Panto (mg) | Vit C (mg) | Vit D (mg) | Vit E (α TE) | Calcium (mg) | Copper (mg) | Iron (mg) | Magnes (mg) | Mang (mg) | Phos (mg) | Potassium (mg) | Selenium (mcg) | Sodium (mg) | Zinc (mg) |
| 4519 | 1 oz | Dry Roasted, salted, avg | 28 | 161 | 2 | 4.3 | 9.2 | 0.8 | 2.0 | 6.3 | 13.0 | 2.6 | 7.6 | 2.2 | 0.05 | 2.14 | 0 | 0 | 0 | 0 | 0 | 0 | 0.06 | 0.06 | 0.39 | 0.07 | 0.00 | 19.4 | 0.34 | 0.0 | 0.0 | | 13 | 0.6 | 1.7 | 73 | 0.2 | 137 | 158 | 3.3 | 179 | 1.57 |
| 4621 | 1 oz | Dry Roasted, unsalted, avg | 28 | 161 | 2 | 4.3 | 9.2 | 0.8 | 2.0 | 6.3 | 13.0 | 2.6 | 7.6 | 2.2 | 0.05 | 2.14 | 0 | 0 | 0 | 0 | 0 | 0 | 0.06 | 0.06 | 0.39 | 0.07 | 0.00 | 19.4 | 0.34 | 0.0 | 0.0 | | 13 | 0.6 | 1.7 | 73 | 0.2 | 137 | 158 | 3.3 | 4 | 1.57 |
| 4596 | 1 oz | Oil Roasted, salted, avg | 28 | 161 | 4 | 4.5 | 8.0 | 1.1 | 1.7 | 5.2 | 13.5 | 2.7 | 8.0 | 2.3 | 0.05 | 2.23 | 0 | 0 | 0 | 0 | 0 | 0 | 0.12 | 0.05 | 0.50 | 0.07 | 0.00 | 19.0 | 0.33 | 0.0 | 0.0 | | 11 | 0.6 | 1.1 | 71 | 0.2 | 119 | 148 | 3.2 | 175 | 1.33 |
| 4622 | 1 oz | Oil Roasted, unsalted, avg | 28 | 161 | 4 | 4.5 | 8.0 | 1.1 | 1.7 | 5.2 | 13.5 | 2.7 | 8.0 | 2.3 | 0.05 | 2.23 | 0 | 0 | 0 | 0 | 0 | 0 | 0.12 | 0.05 | 0.50 | 0.07 | 0.00 | 19.0 | 0.33 | 0.0 | 0.0 | | 11 | 0.6 | 1.1 | 71 | 0.2 | 119 | 148 | 3.2 | 5 | 1.33 |
| | | Chestnuts | | | | | | | | | | | | | | | | | | | | | | | | | | | | | | | | | | | | | | | | |
| 4648 | 1 oz | Cooked, European, avg | 28 | 37 | 68 | 0.6 | 7.8 | 1.4 | 1.9 | 4.5 | 0.4 | 0.1 | 0.1 | 0.2 | 0.02 | 0.14 | 0 | 5 | 1 | 0 | 1 | 3 | 0.04 | 0.03 | 0.20 | 0.07 | 0.00 | 10.8 | 0.09 | 7.5 | 0.0 | | 13 | 0.1 | 0.5 | 15 | 0.2 | 28 | 200 | | 8 | 0.07 |
| 4531 | 1 oz | Dried, peeled, avg | 28 | 103 | 9 | 1.4 | 22.0 | 3.3 | 5.3 | 13.3 | 1.1 | 0.2 | 0.4 | 0.4 | 0.05 | 0.39 | 0 | 0 | 0 | 0 | 0 | 0 | 0.10 | 0.02 | 0.24 | 0.19 | 0.00 | 30.8 | 0.25 | 4.2 | 0.0 | 0.4 | 18 | 0.2 | 0.7 | 21 | 0.3 | 38 | 277 | 1.5 | 10 | 0.10 |
| 4570 | 1 oz | Dried, unpeeled, avg | 28 | 105 | 9 | 1.8 | 21.6 | 3.3 | 5.0 | 13.3 | 1.2 | 0.2 | 0.4 | 0.5 | 0.05 | 0.44 | 0 | 0 | 0 | 0 | 0 | 0 | 0.08 | 0.10 | 0.24 | 0.19 | 0.00 | 30.5 | 0.25 | 4.2 | 0.0 | | 19 | 0.2 | 0.7 | 21 | 0.4 | 49 | 276 | 0.5 | 10 | 0.10 |
| 4658 | 1 oz | Raw, Japanese, avg | 28 | 43 | 61 | 0.6 | 9.8 | 0.3 | | | 0.1 | 0.0 | 0.1 | 0.0 | 0.00 | 0.03 | 0 | 10 | 1 | 0 | 1 | 7 | 0.10 | 0.05 | 0.42 | 0.08 | 0.00 | 13.0 | 0.06 | 7.4 | 0.0 | | 9 | 0.2 | 0.4 | 14 | 0.4 | 20 | 92 | | 4 | 0.31 |
| 4530 | 1 oz | Raw, peeled, avg | 28 | 55 | 52 | 0.5 | 12.4 | 2.2 | 3.0 | 7.2 | 0.3 | 0.1 | 0.1 | 0.1 | 0.01 | 0.12 | 0 | 7 | 1 | 0 | 1 | 5 | 0.04 | 0.00 | 0.31 | 0.10 | 0.00 | 16.2 | 0.13 | 11.3 | 0.0 | 0.1 | 5 | 0.1 | 0.3 | 8 | 0.1 | 11 | 136 | 0.5 | 1 | 0.14 |
| 4568 | 1 oz | Raw, unpeeled, avg | 28 | 60 | 49 | 0.7 | 12.7 | 2.3 | 3.0 | 7.5 | 0.6 | 0.1 | 0.2 | 0.3 | 0.03 | 0.22 | 0 | 8 | 1 | 0 | 1 | 5 | 0.07 | 0.05 | 0.33 | 0.11 | 0.00 | 17.4 | 0.14 | 12.0 | 0.0 | | 8 | 0.1 | 0.3 | 9 | 0.3 | 26 | 145 | | 1 | 0.15 |
| 4538 | 1 oz | Roasted, avg | 28 | 69 | 40 | 0.9 | 14.8 | 1.4 | 3.6 | 9.9 | 0.6 | 0.1 | 0.2 | 0.2 | 0.03 | 0.22 | 0 | 7 | 1 | 0 | 1 | 3 | 0.07 | 0.05 | 0.38 | 0.14 | 0.00 | 19.6 | 0.16 | 7.3 | 0.0 | 0.1 | 8 | 0.1 | 0.3 | 9 | 0.3 | 30 | 166 | 0.3 | 1 | 0.16 |
| | | Coconut | | | | | | | | | | | | | | | | | | | | | | | | | | | | | | | | | | | | | | | | |
| 4511 | 2 Tbs | Dried, sweetened, shredded, avg | 23 | 115 | 13 | 0.7 | 11.0 | 1.0 | 7.9 | 2.0 | 8.2 | 7.2 | 0.3 | 0.1 | 0.00 | 0.09 | 0 | 0 | 0 | 0 | 0 | 0 | 0.01 | 0.00 | 0.11 | 0.06 | 0.00 | 1.9 | 0.17 | 0.2 | 0.0 | 0.2 | 3 | 0.1 | 0.4 | 12 | 0.6 | 25 | 78 | 3.8 | 60 | 0.42 |
| 4510 | 2 Tbs | Dried, unsweetened, avg | 20 | 132 | 3 | 1.4 | 4.9 | 3.3 | 1.6 | 0.0 | 12.9 | 11.4 | 0.6 | 0.1 | 0.00 | 0.14 | 0 | 0 | 0 | 0 | 0 | 0 | 0.01 | 0.02 | 0.12 | 0.06 | 0.00 | 1.8 | 0.16 | 0.3 | 0.0 | | 5 | 0.2 | 0.7 | 18 | 0.6 | 41 | 109 | 3.7 | 7 | 0.40 |
| 4573 | 2 Tbs | Flaked, sweetened, cnd, avg | 19 | 84 | 23 | 0.6 | 7.8 | 0.9 | | | 6.0 | 5.3 | 0.3 | 0.1 | 0.00 | 0.07 | 0 | 0 | 0 | 0 | 0 | 0 | 0.01 | 0.00 | 0.06 | 0.05 | 0.00 | 1.3 | 0.12 | 0.0 | 0.0 | 0.1 | 3 | 0.1 | 0.3 | 9 | 0.4 | 20 | 62 | 3.7 | 4 | 0.30 |
| 4507 | 2 Tbs | Fresh, shredded, avg | 20 | 71 | 47 | 0.7 | 3.0 | 1.8 | 1.2 | 0.0 | 6.7 | 5.9 | 0.3 | 0.1 | 0.00 | 0.07 | 0 | 0 | 0 | 0 | 0 | 0 | 0.01 | 0.00 | 0.11 | 0.01 | 0.00 | 5.3 | 0.06 | 0.7 | 0.0 | 0.1 | 3 | 0.1 | 0.5 | 6 | 0.3 | 23 | 71 | 2.0 | 4 | 0.22 |
| 4559 | 1/2 cup | Milk, cnd, avg | 113 | 223 | 73 | 2.3 | 3.2 | 1.3 | 1.9 | 0.0 | 24.1 | 21.4 | 1.0 | 0.3 | 0.00 | 0.26 | 0 | 0 | 0 | 0 | 0 | 0 | 0.02 | 0.00 | 0.72 | 0.03 | 0.00 | 15.3 | 0.17 | 1.1 | 0.0 | | 20 | 0.3 | 3.7 | 52 | 0.9 | 108 | 249 | 3.8 | 15 | 0.63 |
| 4560 | 1/2 cup | Milk, f/fzn, avg | 120 | 242 | 71 | 1.9 | 6.7 | 2.7 | 4.0 | 0.0 | 25.0 | 22.1 | 1.1 | 0.3 | 0.00 | 0.27 | 0 | 0 | 0 | 0 | 0 | 0 | 0.03 | 0.00 | 0.81 | 0.04 | 0.00 | 17.0 | 0.19 | 1.3 | 0.0 | | 5 | 0.3 | 1.0 | 38 | 1.0 | 71 | 278 | 3.5 | 14 | 0.71 |
| 4528 | 1/2 cup | Milk, raw, avg | 120 | 276 | 68 | 2.7 | 6.6 | 2.6 | 4.0 | 0.0 | 28.6 | 25.3 | 1.2 | 0.3 | 0.00 | 0.31 | 0 | 0 | 0 | 0 | 0 | 0 | 0.03 | 0.00 | 0.91 | 0.04 | 0.00 | 19.3 | 0.22 | 3.4 | 0.0 | | 19 | 0.3 | 2.0 | 44 | 1.1 | 120 | 316 | 7.4 | 18 | 0.80 |
| 4575 | 1 oz | Toasted, dry, avg | 28 | 166 | 1 | 1.5 | 12.4 | 1.8 | 10.6 | 0.0 | 13.2 | 11.7 | 0.6 | 0.1 | 0.00 | 0.14 | 0 | 0 | 0 | 0 | 0 | 0 | 0.02 | 0.03 | 0.17 | 0.09 | 0.00 | 2.6 | 0.23 | 0.4 | 0.0 | 0.3 | 8 | 0.2 | 0.9 | 26 | 0.8 | 59 | 155 | 4.5 | 10 | 0.57 |
| 4527 | 1/2 cup | Water, raw, avg | 120 | 23 | 95 | 0.9 | 4.5 | 1.3 | 3.1 | 0.0 | 0.2 | 0.2 | 0.0 | 0.0 | 0.00 | 0.00 | 0 | 0 | 0 | 0 | 0 | 0 | 0.04 | 0.07 | 0.10 | 0.04 | 0.00 | 3.0 | 0.05 | 2.9 | 0.0 | 0.0 | 29 | 0.0 | 0.3 | 30 | 0.2 | 24 | 300 | 1.2 | 126 | 0.12 |
| | | Filberts/Hazelnuts | | | | | | | | | | | | | | | | | | | | | | | | | | | | | | | | | | | | | | | | |
| 4513 | 1 oz | Dried, avg | 28 | 177 | 5 | 3.6 | 4.3 | 1.7 | 1.3 | 1.3 | 17.5 | 1.3 | 13.7 | 1.7 | 0.04 | 1.63 | 0 | 19 | 2 | 0 | 2 | 12 | 0.14 | 0.03 | 0.32 | 0.17 | 0.00 | 20.1 | 0.32 | 0.3 | 0.0 | 6.7 | 53 | 0.4 | 0.9 | 80 | 0.6 | 87 | 125 | 1.1 | 1 | 0.67 |
| 4650 | 1 oz | Dried, blanched, avg | 28 | 188 | 2 | 3.6 | 4.5 | 1.8 | 1.3 | 1.4 | 18.8 | 1.4 | 14.8 | 1.8 | 0.05 | 1.76 | 0 | 19 | 2 | 0 | 2 | 12 | 0.15 | 0.03 | 0.33 | 0.18 | 0.00 | 20.9 | 0.33 | 0.3 | 0.0 | 7.1 | 55 | 0.4 | 0.9 | 83 | 0.6 | 90 | 129 | 1.1 | 1 | 0.70 |
| 4663 | 1 oz | Dry Roasted, salted, avg | 28 | 185 | 2 | 2.8 | 5.0 | 2.2 | 0.9 | 2.0 | 18.6 | 1.4 | 14.6 | 1.8 | 0.04 | 1.73 | 0 | 0 | 0 | 0 | 0 | 0 | 0.06 | 0.06 | 0.78 | 0.18 | 0.00 | 20.9 | 0.33 | 0.3 | 0.0 | 7.0 | 55 | 0.4 | 0.9 | 83 | 0.6 | 90 | 129 | 1.1 | 218 | 0.70 |
| 4651 | 1 oz | Dry Roasted, unsalted, avg | 28 | 185 | 2 | 2.8 | 5.0 | 2.0 | 0.9 | 2.1 | 18.6 | 1.4 | 14.6 | 1.8 | 0.04 | 1.73 | 0 | 19 | 2 | 0 | 2 | 12 | 0.06 | 0.06 | 0.78 | 0.18 | 0.00 | 20.9 | 0.33 | 0.3 | 0.0 | | 55 | 0.4 | 0.9 | 83 | 0.6 | 90 | 129 | 1.1 | 1 | 0.70 |
| 4664 | 1 oz | Oil Roasted, salted | 28 | 185 | 1 | 4.0 | 5.4 | 1.8 | 1.3 | 2.2 | 17.8 | 1.3 | 13.9 | 1.7 | 0.04 | 1.66 | 0 | 19 | 2 | 0 | 2 | 12 | 0.06 | 0.06 | 0.78 | 0.18 | 0.00 | 21.0 | 0.33 | 0.3 | 0.0 | 7.0 | 55 | 0.4 | 1.0 | 83 | 0.6 | 91 | 130 | 1.2 | 220 | 0.70 |
| 4652 | 1 oz | Oil Roasted, unsalted, avg | 28 | 185 | 1 | 4.0 | 5.4 | 1.8 | 1.3 | 2.2 | 17.8 | 1.3 | 13.9 | 1.7 | 0.04 | 1.66 | 0 | 20 | 2 | 0 | 2 | 12 | 0.06 | 0.06 | 0.78 | 0.18 | 0.00 | 21.0 | 0.33 | 0.3 | 0.0 | | 55 | 0.4 | 1.0 | 83 | 0.6 | 91 | 130 | 1.2 | 1 | 0.70 |
| 4717 | 1 oz | Whole Natural, Westnut | 28 | 164 | 6 | 4.5 | 4.9 | 3.8 | 0.9 | 0.1 | 15.3 | 1.0 | 12.5 | 1.7 | | | 0 | | | | | | 0.17 | 0.06 | 0.32 | 0.17 | 0.00 | | | 0.3 | | | 39 | 0.4 | 1.2 | 46 | | 84 | 166 | | 1 | 0.56 |
| 4777 | 1 oz | Flax Seeds, avg | 28 | 138 | 9 | 5.5 | 9.6 | 7.8 | | | 9.5 | 0.9 | 1.9 | 6.3 | 5.06 | 1.21 | 0 | 0 | 0 | 0 | 0 | 0 | 0.05 | 0.04 | 0.39 | 0.26 | 0.00 | 77.8 | 0.43 | 0.4 | | | 56 | 0.3 | 1.7 | 101 | 0.9 | 139 | 191 | 1.5 | 10 | 1.17 |
| | | Formed Nuts | | | | | | | | | | | | | | | | | | | | | | | | | | | | | | | | | | | | | | | | |
| 4600 | 1 oz | Macadamia Flavor, unsalted | 28 | 173 | 3 | 3.1 | 7.8 | 1.5 | | | 15.8 | 2.4 | 6.6 | 6.1 | 0.44 | 5.66 | 0 | 0.3 | 0.03 | 0 | 0.03 | 0.2 | 0.06 | 0.06 | 0.28 | 0.07 | 0.00 | 26.3 | 0.09 | 0.0 | 0.0 | | 6 | 0.1 | 0.6 | 16 | 1.4 | 84 | 73 | | 13 | 0.82 |
| 4601 | 1 oz | Other Flavors, unsalted | 28 | 181 | 2 | 3.7 | 5.8 | 1.5 | | | 17.4 | 2.6 | 7.2 | 6.8 | 0.50 | 6.27 | 0 | 0.3 | 0.03 | 0 | 0.03 | 0.2 | 0.11 | 0.08 | 0.42 | 0.10 | 0.00 | 35.0 | 0.09 | 0.0 | 0.0 | | 6 | 0.1 | 0.7 | 17 | 1.9 | 102 | 90 | | 25 | 0.83 |
| 4599 | 1 oz | Unflavored, f/wheat & salt, avg | 28 | 174 | 2 | 3.9 | 6.6 | 1.5 | | | 16.2 | 2.4 | 6.6 | 6.4 | 0.47 | 5.88 | 0 | 0.3 | 0.03 | 0 | 0.03 | 0.2 | 0.08 | 0.08 | 0.42 | 0.11 | 0.00 | 39.8 | 0.09 | 0.0 | 0.0 | | 7 | 0.1 | 0.7 | 16 | 2.2 | 104 | 89 | | 141 | 0.82 |
| 4669 | 1 oz | Wheat Germ Nuts, almond, Ana Con Foods | 28 | 196 | 2 | 3.9 | 4.4 | 1.1 | | | 18.6 | | | | | | 0 | | | | | | 0.11 | 0.08 | 0.42 | | 0.00 | | | | | | 7 | | 0.8 | | | 97 | 83 | | 25 | |
| 4671 | 1 oz | Wheat Germ Nuts, black walnut, Ana Con Foods | 28 | 196 | 2 | 3.9 | 4.4 | 1.1 | | | 18.6 | | | | | | 0 | | | | | | 0.11 | 0.08 | 0.42 | | 0.00 | | | | | | 7 | | 0.8 | | | 97 | 83 | | 25 | |
| 4670 | 1 oz | Wheat Germ Nuts, cashew, Ana Con Foods | 28 | 196 | 2 | 3.9 | 4.4 | 1.1 | | | 18.6 | | | | | | 0 | | | | | | 0.11 | 0.08 | 0.42 | | 0.00 | | | | | | 7 | | 0.8 | | | 97 | 83 | | 25 | |
| 4672 | 1 oz | Wheat Germ Nuts, pecan, Ana Con Foods | 28 | 196 | 2 | 3.9 | 4.4 | 1.1 | | | 18.6 | | | | | | 0 | | | | | | 6.16 | 0.08 | 0.42 | | 0.00 | | | | | | 7 | | 0.8 | | | 97 | 83 | | 25 | |
| | | Macadamia Nuts | | | | | | | | | | | | | | | | | | | | | | | | | | | | | | | | | | | | | | | | |
| 4516 | 1 oz | Dried, avg | 28 | 197 | 3 | 2.3 | 3.8 | 2.6 | 1.2 | 0.0 | 20.6 | 3.1 | 16.3 | 0.4 | 0.00 | 0.36 | 0 | 0 | 0 | 0 | 0 | 0 | 0.10 | 0.03 | 0.60 | 0.05 | 0.00 | 4.4 | 0.12 | 0.0 | 0.0 | | 20 | 0.1 | 0.7 | 32 | 0.2 | 38 | 103 | 1.3 | 1 | 0.48 |
| 4587 | 1 oz | Oil Roasted, salted, avg | 28 | 201 | 2 | 2.0 | 3.6 | 2.6 | 1.0 | 0.0 | 21.4 | 3.2 | 16.9 | 0.4 | 0.00 | 0.37 | 0 | 3 | 0.3 | 0 | 0.3 | 2 | 0.06 | 0.03 | 0.57 | 0.06 | 0.00 | 4.4 | 0.12 | 0.0 | 0.0 | | 13 | 0.1 | 0.5 | 33 | 0.2 | 56 | 92 | 1.3 | 73 | 0.31 |
| 4588 | 1 oz | Oil Roasted, unsalted, avg | 28 | 201 | 2 | 2.0 | 3.6 | 2.6 | 1.0 | 0.0 | 21.4 | 3.2 | 16.9 | 0.4 | 0.00 | 0.37 | 0 | 3 | 0.3 | 0 | 0.3 | 2 | 0.06 | 0.03 | 0.57 | 0.06 | 0.00 | 4.5 | 0.12 | 0.0 | 0.0 | | 13 | 0.1 | 0.5 | 33 | 0.2 | 56 | 92 | 1.3 | 2 | 0.31 |
| 4715 | 1 oz | Raw, World Variety Produce | 28 | 207 | 2 | 2.3 | 5.1 | 2.3 | 2.0 | 0.9 | 19.7 | 1.7 | 18.0 | 0.0 | 0.00 | 0.00 | 0 | 3 | 0.3 | 0 | 0.3 | 2 | | | | | 0.00 | | | 0.5 | | | 17 | | 0.6 | | | | | | 6 | |
| | | Mixed Nuts | | | | | | | | | | | | | | | | | | | | | | | | | | | | | | | | | | | | | | | | |
| 4592 | 1 oz | Dry Roasted, salted, avg | 28 | 166 | 2 | 4.8 | 7.1 | 2.5 | 1.1 | 3.5 | 14.4 | 1.9 | 8.8 | 3.0 | 0.05 | 2.94 | 0 | 4 | 0.3 | 0 | 0.3 | 2 | 0.06 | 0.06 | 1.32 | 0.08 | 0.00 | 14.1 | 0.34 | 0.1 | 0.0 | | 20 | 0.4 | 1.0 | 63 | 0.5 | 122 | 167 | 2.1 | 187 | 1.06 |
| 4591 | 1 oz | Dry Roasted, unsalted, avg | 28 | 166 | 2 | 4.8 | 7.1 | 2.5 | 1.1 | 3.5 | 14.4 | 1.9 | 8.8 | 3.0 | 0.05 | 2.94 | 0 | 4 | 0.3 | 0 | 0.3 | 2 | 0.06 | 0.06 | 1.32 | 0.08 | 0.00 | 14.1 | 0.34 | 0.1 | 0.0 | | 20 | 0.4 | 1.0 | 63 | 0.5 | 122 | 167 | 6.4 | 3 | 1.06 |
| 4593 | 1 oz | Oil Roasted, salted | 28 | 173 | 2 | 4.7 | 6.0 | 2.5 | 1.1 | 2.4 | 15.8 | 2.4 | 8.9 | 3.7 | 0.05 | 3.67 | 0 | 5 | 0.6 | 0 | 0.6 | 3 | 0.14 | 0.06 | 1.42 | 0.07 | 0.00 | 23.2 | 0.35 | 0.1 | 0.0 | | 30 | 0.5 | 0.9 | 66 | 0.5 | 130 | 163 | 117.9 | 183 | 1.42 |
| 4533 | 1 oz | Oil Roasted, unsalted | 28 | 173 | 2 | 4.7 | 6.0 | 2.8 | 1.1 | 2.1 | 15.8 | 2.4 | 8.9 | 3.7 | 0.05 | 3.67 | 0 | 5 | 0.6 | 0 | 0.6 | 3 | 0.14 | 0.06 | 1.42 | 0.07 | 0.00 | 23.2 | 0.35 | 0.1 | 0.0 | | 30 | 0.5 | 0.9 | 66 | 0.5 | 130 | 163 | 2.3 | 3 | 1.42 |
| | | Peanut Butter | | | | | | | | | | | | | | | | | | | | | | | | | | | | | | | | | | | | | | | | |
| 4626 | 2 Tbs | Chunky, salted, avg | 32 | 188 | 1 | 7.7 | 6.9 | 2.1 | 2.6 | 2.2 | 16.0 | 3.1 | 7.6 | 4.5 | 0.02 | 4.51 | 0 | 0 | 0 | 0 | 0 | 0 | 0.04 | 0.04 | 4.38 | 0.14 | 0.00 | 29.4 | 0.31 | 0.0 | 0.0 | | 13 | 0.2 | 0.6 | 51 | 0.6 | 101 | 239 | 2.4 | 156 | 0.89 |
| 4576 | 2 Tbs | Chunky, unsalted, avg | 32 | 188 | 1 | 7.7 | 6.9 | 2.1 | 2.6 | 2.2 | 16.0 | 3.1 | 7.6 | 4.5 | 0.02 | 4.51 | 0 | 0 | 0 | 0 | 0 | 0 | 0.04 | 0.04 | 4.38 | 0.14 | 0.00 | 29.4 | 0.31 | 0.0 | 0.0 | | 13 | 0.2 | 0.6 | 51 | 0.6 | 101 | 239 | 2.4 | 5 | 0.89 |
| 4637 | 2 Tbs | Natural, salted, avg | 32 | 187 | 2 | 7.7 | 6.9 | 2.1 | 2.4 | 2.4 | 15.9 | 2.2 | 7.9 | 5.0 | 0.00 | 5.02 | 0 | 0 | 0 | 0 | 0 | 0 | 0.04 | 0.03 | 4.29 | 0.13 | 0.00 | 46.4 | 0.45 | 0.0 | 0.0 | | 17 | 0.2 | 0.7 | 56 | 0.7 | 114 | 210 | 2.4 | 80 | 1.06 |
| 4668 | 2 Tbs | Natural, unsalted, avg | 32 | 187 | 2 | 7.7 | 6.9 | 2.1 | 2.4 | 2.4 | 15.9 | 2.2 | 7.9 | 5.0 | 0.00 | 5.02 | 0 | 0 | 0 | 0 | 0 | 0 | 0.14 | 0.03 | 4.32 | 0.13 | 0.00 | 46.4 | 0.45 | 0.0 | 0.0 | | 17 | 0.2 | 0.7 | 56 | 0.7 | 115 | 211 | 2.4 | 2 | 1.06 |
| 4627 | 2 Tbs | Smooth, salted, avg | 32 | 190 | 1 | 8.1 | 6.2 | 1.9 | 2.5 | 1.8 | 16.3 | 3.3 | 7.8 | 4.4 | 0.02 | 4.38 | 0 | 0 | 0 | 0 | 0 | 0 | 0.03 | 0.03 | 4.29 | 0.15 | 0.00 | 23.7 | 0.26 | 0.0 | 0.0 | | 12 | 0.0 | 0.6 | 51 | 0.1 | 118 | 214 | 2.4 | 149 | 0.93 |
| 4636 | 2 Tbs | Smooth, unsalted, avg | 32 | 190 | 1 | 8.1 | 6.2 | 1.9 | 2.5 | 1.8 | 16.3 | 3.3 | 7.8 | 4.4 | 0.02 | 4.38 | 0 | 0 | 0 | 0 | 0 | 0 | 0.03 | 0.03 | 4.29 | 0.15 | 0.00 | 23.7 | 0.26 | 0.0 | 0.0 | 1.5 | 12 | 0.0 | 0.6 | 51 | 0.1 | 118 | 214 | 2.4 | 5 | 0.93 |
| | | Peanuts | | | | | | | | | | | | | | | | | | | | | | | | | | | | | | | | | | | | | | | | |
| 4753 | 1 oz | Boiled, avg | 28 | 89 | 42 | 3.8 | 6.0 | 2.5 | 1.3 | 2.2 | 6.2 | 0.9 | 3.1 | 1.9 | 0.00 | 1.95 | 0 | 0 | 0 | 0 | 0 | 0 | 0.07 | 0.02 | 1.47 | 0.04 | 0.00 | 20.9 | 0.23 | 0.0 | 0.0 | | 15 | 0.1 | 0.3 | 29 | 0.3 | 55 | 50 | 1.2 | 210 | 0.51 |
| 4590 | 1 oz | Dry Roasted, all types, salted | 28 | 164 | 2 | 6.6 | 6.0 | 2.2 | 1.3 | 2.5 | 13.9 | 1.9 | 6.9 | 4.4 | 0.00 | 4.40 | 0 | 0 | 0 | 0 | 0 | 0 | 0.12 | 0.03 | 3.78 | 0.07 | 0.00 | 40.6 | 0.39 | 0.0 | 0.0 | | 15 | 0.2 | 0.6 | 49 | 0.6 | 100 | 184 | 2.1 | 228 | 0.93 |
| 4756 | 1 oz | Dry Roasted, all types, unsalted | 28 | 164 | 2 | 6.6 | 6.0 | 2.2 | 1.3 | 2.5 | 13.9 | 1.9 | 6.9 | 4.4 | 0.00 | 4.40 | 0 | 0 | 0 | 0 | 0 | 0 | 0.12 | 0.03 | 3.78 | 0.07 | 0.00 | 40.6 | 0.39 | 0.0 | | | 15 | 0.2 | 0.6 | 49 | 0.6 | 100 | 184 | 2.1 | 2 | 0.93 |
| 4695 | 1 oz | Fried, avg | 28 | 159 | 6 | 5.1 | 7.0 | 0.7 | 1.2 | 5.1 | 13.6 | 1.9 | 6.7 | 4.3 | 0.00 | 4.28 | 0 | 0 | 0 | 0 | 0 | 0 | | | | | 0.00 | | | | 0.0 | | 15 | | 0.6 | | | 30 | 156 | | | |
| 4762 | 1 oz | Oil Roasted, salted, avg | 28 | 163 | 2 | 7.4 | 5.3 | 2.6 | 1.0 | 1.7 | 13.8 | 1.9 | 6.9 | 4.4 | 0.00 | 4.37 | 0 | 0 | 0 | 0 | 0 | 0 | 0.07 | 0.03 | 4.00 | 0.07 | 0.00 | 35.3 | 0.39 | 0.0 | 0.0 | 1.9 | 25 | 0.4 | 0.5 | 52 | 0.6 | 145 | 191 | 2.1 | 121 | 1.86 |
| 4542 | 1 oz | Oil Roasted, unsalted, avg | 28 | 163 | 2 | 7.4 | 5.3 | 1.9 | 1.0 | 2.3 | 13.8 | 1.9 | 6.9 | 4.4 | 0.00 | 4.37 | 0 | 0 | 0 | 0 | 0 | 0 | 0.07 | 0.03 | 4.00 | 0.07 | 0.00 | 35.3 | 0.39 | 0.0 | 0.0 | | 25 | 0.4 | 0.5 | 52 | 0.6 | 145 | 191 | 2.1 | 2 | 1.86 |
| 4696 | 1 oz | Raw, avg | 28 | 159 | 6 | 7.2 | 4.5 | 2.4 | 0.9 | 1.3 | 13.8 | 1.9 | 6.8 | 4.4 | 0.00 | 4.37 | 0 | 0 | 0 | 0 | 0 | 0 | 0.18 | 0.04 | 3.39 | 0.10 | 0.00 | 67.2 | 0.50 | 0.0 | 0.0 | | 26 | 0.3 | 1.3 | 47 | 0.5 | 105 | 197 | 2.0 | 5 | 0.92 |
| | | Peanuts, Spanish | | | | | | | | | | | | | | | | | | | | | | | | | | | | | | | | | | | | | | | | |
| 4699 | 1 oz | Oil Roasted, salted, avg | 28 | 162 | 2 | 7.8 | 4.9 | 2.5 | 1.0 | 1.5 | 13.7 | 2.1 | 6.2 | 4.8 | 0.00 | 4.76 | 0 | 0 | 0 | 0 | 0 | 0 | 0.09 | 0.02 | 4.17 | 0.07 | 0.00 | 35.3 | 0.39 | 0.0 | 0.0 | 2.1 | 28 | 0.2 | 0.6 | 47 | 0.7 | 108 | 217 | 2.1 | 121 | 0.56 |
| 4665 | 1 oz | Oil Roasted, unsalted, avg | 28 | 162 | 2 | 7.8 | 4.9 | 2.5 | 1.0 | 1.5 | 13.7 | 2.1 | 6.2 | 4.8 | 0.00 | 4.76 | 0 | 0 | 0 | 0 | 0 | 0 | 0.09 | 0.02 | 4.17 | 0.07 | 0.00 | 35.3 | 0.39 | 0.0 | 0.0 | 2.1 | 28 | 0.2 | 0.6 | 47 | 0.7 | 108 | 217 | 2.1 | 2 | 0.56 |
| 4517 | 1 oz | Raw, avg | 28 | 160 | 6 | 7.3 | 4.4 | 2.7 | 0.9 | 0.9 | 13.9 | 2.1 | 6.2 | 4.8 | 0.00 | 4.81 | 0 | 0 | 0 | 0 | 0 | 0 | 0.19 | 0.04 | 4.45 | 0.10 | 0.00 | 67.2 | 0.50 | 0.0 | 0.0 | | 30 | 0.3 | 1.1 | 53 | 0.7 | 109 | 208 | 2.0 | 6 | 0.59 |
| | | Peanuts, Valencia | | | | | | | | | | | | | | | | | | | | | | | | | | | | | | | | | | | | | | | | |
| 4623 | 1 oz | Dry Roasted, unsalted, avg | 28 | 166 | 2 | 6.8 | 5.2 | 1.9 | 1.2 | 2.1 | 14.4 | 2.2 | 6.5 | 5.0 | 0.00 | 5.01 | 0 | 0 | 0 | 0 | 0 | 0 | 0.04 | 0.04 | 3.81 | 0.07 | 0.00 | 40.6 | 0.39 | 0.0 | 0.0 | | 9 | 0.1 | 0.6 | 42 | 0.5 | 62 | 165 | 2.0 | 2 | 0.86 |

| Code | Amount | | Description | Basic Components | | | | | | | | | Additional Fats | | | | | | Vit A & Components | | | | | Vitamins | | | | | | | | | | Minerals | | | | | | | | | |
|---|---|---|---|---|---|---|---|---|---|---|---|---|---|---|---|---|---|---|---|---|---|---|---|---|---|---|---|---|---|---|---|---|---|---|---|---|---|---|---|---|---|---|---|
| | | | | Weight (g) | Calories | % Water | Protein (g) | Carbs (g) | Fiber (g) | Sugar (g) | Other Carbs (g) | Fat (g) | Sat Fat (g) | Mono Fat (g) | Poly Fat (g) | Omega 3 (g) | Omega 6 (g) | Choles (mg) | Vit A (IU) | Vit A (RE) | Retinol (RE) | Carotenoids (RE) | Beta Carotene (mcg) | Thiamin (mg) | Riboflavin (mg) | Niacin (NE) | Vit B6 (mg) | Vit B12 (mcg) | Folate (mcg) | Panto (mg) | Vit C (mg) | Vit D (mg) | Vit E (α TE) | Calcium (mg) | Copper (mg) | Iron (mg) | Magnes (mg) | Mang (mg) | Phos (mg) | Potassium (mg) | Selenium (mcg) | Sodium (mg) | Zinc (mg) |
| 4701 | 1 | oz | Oil Roasted, salted, avg | 28 | 165 | 2 | 7.6 | 4.6 | 2.5 | 0.9 | 1.2 | 14.3 | 2.2 | 6.5 | 5.0 | 0.00 | 4.98 | 0 | 0 | 0 | 0 | 0 | 0 | 0.03 | 0.04 | 4.00 | 0.07 | 0.00 | 35.3 | 0.39 | 0.0 | 0.0 | 2.0 | 15 | 0.2 | 0.5 | 45 | 0.5 | 89 | 171 | 2.1 | 216 | 0.86 |
| 4666 | 1 | oz | Oil Roasted, unsalted, avg | 28 | 165 | 2 | 7.6 | 4.6 | 2.5 | 0.9 | 1.2 | 14.3 | 2.2 | 6.5 | 5.0 | 0.00 | 4.98 | 0 | 0 | 0 | 0 | 0 | 0 | 0.03 | 0.04 | 4.00 | 0.07 | 0.00 | 35.3 | 0.39 | 0.0 | 0.0 | 2.0 | 15 | 0.2 | 0.5 | 45 | 0.5 | 89 | 171 | 2.1 | 2 | 0.86 |
| 4700 | 1 | oz | Raw, avg | 28 | 160 | 4 | 7.0 | 5.9 | 2.4 | 0.9 | 2.5 | 13.3 | 2.1 | 6.0 | 4.6 | 0.00 | 4.62 | 0 | 0 | 0 | 0 | 0 | 0 | 0.18 | 0.08 | 3.61 | 0.10 | 0.00 | 68.9 | 0.51 | 0.0 | 0.0 | 2.3 | 17 | 0.3 | 0.6 | 52 | 0.6 | 94 | 93 | 2.0 | 0 | 0.94 |
| | | | Peanuts, Virginia | | | | | | | | | | | | | | | | | | | | | | | | | | | | | | | | | | | | | | | | |
| 4703 | 1 | oz | Oil Roasted, salted, avg | 28 | 162 | 2 | 7.3 | 5.6 | 2.5 | 1.1 | 2.0 | 13.6 | 1.8 | 7.1 | 4.1 | 0.01 | 4.09 | 0 | 0 | 0 | 0 | 0 | 0 | 0.08 | 0.03 | 4.12 | 0.07 | 0.00 | 35.0 | 0.39 | 0.0 | 0.0 | 1.9 | 24 | 0.4 | 0.5 | 53 | 0.6 | 142 | 183 | 2.1 | 121 | 1.85 |
| 4667 | 1 | oz | Oil Roasted, unsalted, avg | 28 | 162 | 2 | 7.3 | 5.6 | 2.5 | 1.1 | 2.0 | 13.6 | 1.8 | 7.1 | 4.1 | 0.01 | 4.09 | 0 | 0 | 0 | 0 | 0 | 0 | 0.08 | 0.03 | 4.12 | 0.07 | 0.00 | 35.0 | 0.39 | 0.0 | 0.0 | 1.9 | 24 | 0.4 | 0.5 | 53 | 0.6 | 142 | 183 | 2.1 | 2 | 1.85 |
| 4702 | 1 | oz | Raw, avg | 28 | 158 | 7 | 7.1 | 4.6 | 2.4 | 1.0 | 1.2 | 13.7 | 1.8 | 7.1 | 4.1 | 0.01 | 4.11 | 0 | 0 | 0 | 0 | 0 | 0 | 0.18 | 0.04 | 3.47 | 0.10 | 0.00 | 66.9 | 0.49 | 0.0 | 0.0 | 2.3 | 25 | 0.3 | 0.7 | 48 | 0.5 | 106 | 193 | 2.0 | 3 | 1.24 |
| | | | Pecans | | | | | | | | | | | | | | | | | | | | | | | | | | | | | | | | | | | | | | | | |
| 4578 | 1 | oz | Dried, halves, avg | 28 | 187 | 5 | 2.2 | 5.1 | 2.1 | 1.2 | 1.3 | 13.9 | 1.5 | 11.8 | 4.7 | 0.13 | 4.48 | 0 | 36 | 4 | 0 | 4 | 22 | 0.24 | 0.04 | 0.25 | 0.05 | 0.00 | 11.0 | 0.48 | 0.6 | 0.0 | | 10 | 0.3 | 0.6 | 36 | 1.3 | 81 | 110 | 1.5 | 0 | 1.53 |
| 4583 | 1 | oz | Dry Roasted, salted, avg | 28 | 185 | 1 | 2.2 | 6.2 | 2.6 | 1.3 | 2.3 | 13.1 | 1.5 | 11.3 | 4.5 | 0.13 | 4.28 | 0 | 37 | 4 | 0 | 4 | 22 | 0.09 | 0.03 | 0.26 | 0.05 | 0.00 | 11.4 | 0.50 | 0.6 | 0.0 | | 10 | 0.3 | 0.6 | 37 | 1.3 | 85 | 104 | 1.5 | 218 | 1.59 |
| 4582 | 1 | oz | Dry Roasted, unsalted, avg | 28 | 185 | 1 | 2.2 | 6.2 | 2.6 | 1.3 | 2.3 | 13.1 | 1.5 | 11.3 | 4.5 | 0.13 | 4.28 | 0 | 37 | 4 | 0 | 4 | 22 | 0.09 | 0.03 | 0.26 | 0.05 | 0.00 | 11.4 | 0.50 | 0.6 | 0.0 | | 10 | 0.3 | 0.6 | 37 | 1.3 | 85 | 104 | 1.5 | 0 | 1.59 |
| 4586 | 1 | oz | Oil Roasted, salted, avg | 28 | 192 | 4 | 1.9 | 4.5 | 1.9 | 1.0 | 1.7 | 19.9 | 1.6 | 12.4 | 4.9 | 0.20 | 4.70 | 0 | 36 | 4 | 0 | 4 | 22 | 0.09 | 0.03 | 0.25 | 0.05 | 0.00 | 11.0 | 0.48 | 0.6 | 0.0 | | 10 | 0.3 | 0.6 | 36 | 1.3 | 82 | 101 | 1.5 | 212 | 1.54 |
| 4584 | 1 | oz | Oil Roasted, unsalted, avg | 28 | 192 | 4 | 1.9 | 4.5 | 1.9 | 1.0 | 1.7 | 19.9 | 1.6 | 12.4 | 4.9 | 0.20 | 4.70 | 0 | 36 | 4 | 0 | 4 | 22 | 0.09 | 0.03 | 0.25 | 0.05 | 0.00 | 11.0 | 0.48 | 0.6 | 0.0 | | 10 | 0.3 | 0.6 | 36 | 1.3 | 82 | 101 | 1.5 | 0 | 1.54 |
| 4764 | 1 | oz | Pine Nuts, pignolia, dried, avg | 28 | 158 | 7 | 6.7 | 4.0 | 1.3 | 0.9 | 1.3 | 14.2 | 2.2 | 5.3 | 6.0 | 0.18 | 5.78 | 0 | 8 | 1 | 0 | 1 | 5 | 0.23 | 0.05 | 1.00 | 0.03 | 0.00 | 16.0 | 0.06 | 0.5 | 0.0 | | 7 | 0.3 | 2.6 | 65 | 1.2 | 142 | 168 | 4.6 | 1 | 1.19 |
| 4624 | 1 | oz | Pine Nuts, raw, World Variety Produce | 28 | 197 | 2 | 4.8 | 4.1 | 2.2 | 0.9 | 1.1 | 17.9 | 4.0 | 5.5 | 8.4 | | | 0 | 1 | 0.1 | 0 | 0.1 | 1 | | | | | 0.00 | | | 0.2 | | | 6 | | 1.8 | | | | | | 14 | |
| 4540 | 1 | oz | Pistachio Nuts, dry roasted, salted, avg | 28 | 170 | 2 | 4.2 | 7.7 | 3.0 | 2.0 | 2.5 | 14.8 | 1.9 | 10.0 | 2.2 | 0.08 | 2.15 | 0 | 67 | 7 | 0 | 7 | 40 | 0.12 | 0.07 | 0.39 | 0.07 | 0.00 | 16.5 | 0.34 | 2.0 | 0.0 | | 20 | 0.3 | 0.9 | 36 | 0.1 | 133 | 272 | 1.8 | 218 | 0.38 |
| 4654 | 1 | oz | Pistachio Nuts, dry roasted, unsalted, avg | 28 | 170 | 2 | 4.2 | 7.7 | 3.0 | 1.8 | 2.3 | 14.8 | 1.9 | 10.0 | 2.2 | 0.08 | 2.15 | 0 | 67 | 7 | 0 | 7 | 40 | 0.12 | 0.07 | 0.39 | 0.07 | 0.00 | 16.5 | 0.34 | 2.0 | 0.0 | | 20 | 0.3 | 0.9 | 36 | 0.1 | 133 | 272 | 1.8 | 2 | 0.38 |
| | | | Pumpkin Seeds | | | | | | | | | | | | | | | | | | | | | | | | | | | | | | | | | | | | | | | | |
| 4522 | 1 | oz | Dry, avg | 28 | 151 | 7 | 6.9 | 5.0 | 1.1 | 0.3 | 3.5 | 12.9 | 2.4 | 4.0 | 5.9 | 0.05 | 5.30 | 0 | 106 | 11 | 0 | 11 | 64 | 0.06 | 0.09 | 0.49 | 0.06 | 0.00 | 16.1 | 0.09 | 0.5 | 0.0 | | 12 | 0.4 | 4.2 | 150 | 0.8 | 329 | 226 | 1.6 | 5 | 2.09 |
| 4564 | 1 | oz | Roasted, salted, avg | 28 | 125 | 4 | 5.2 | 15.1 | 1.5 | | | 5.4 | 1.0 | 1.7 | 2.5 | 0.02 | 2.45 | 0 | 17 | 2 | 0 | 2 | 10 | 0.01 | 0.01 | 0.08 | 0.01 | 0.00 | 2.5 | 0.02 | 0.1 | 0.0 | | 15 | 0.2 | 0.9 | 73 | 0.1 | 26 | 257 | 1.6 | 161 | 2.88 |
| 4563 | 1 | oz | Roasted, unsalted, avg | 28 | 125 | 4 | 5.2 | 15.1 | 1.1 | | | 5.4 | 1.0 | 1.7 | 2.5 | 0.02 | 2.45 | 0 | 17 | 2 | 0 | 2 | 10 | 0.01 | 0.01 | 0.08 | 0.01 | 0.00 | 2.5 | 0.02 | 0.1 | 0.0 | | 15 | 0.2 | 0.9 | 73 | 0.1 | 26 | 257 | 1.6 | 5 | 2.88 |
| 4776 | 1 | oz | Psyllium Seed, dried, avg | 28 | 66 | 0 | 0.4 | 25.9 | 16.9 | | | 1.0 | | | | | | | 1126 | 113 | 0 | 113 | 676 | 0.00 | 0.00 | 0.00 | | 0.00 | | | 0.0 | | | 94 | | 5.6 | 14 | 0.4 | 18 | 227 | 392.0 | 15 | 0.59 |
| | | | Sesame Seeds | | | | | | | | | | | | | | | | | | | | | | | | | | | | | | | | | | | | | | | | |
| 4683 | 2 | Tbs | Butter Paste, avg | 32 | 190 | 2 | 5.8 | 8.2 | 1.8 | | | 16.3 | 2.3 | 6.1 | 7.1 | 0.12 | 7.01 | 0 | 16 | 2 | 0 | 2 | 10 | 0.08 | 0.06 | 2.14 | 0.26 | 0.00 | 31.9 | 0.02 | 0.0 | 0.0 | | 307 | 1.3 | 6.1 | 116 | 0.8 | 211 | 186 | 1.9 | 4 | 2.33 |
| 4523 | 1 | oz | Dried, whole, avg | 28 | 160 | 5 | 5.0 | 6.6 | 3.3 | 0.3 | 3.0 | 13.9 | 1.9 | 5.3 | 6.1 | 0.11 | 5.99 | 0 | 3 | 0.3 | 0 | 0.3 | 2 | 0.22 | 0.07 | 1.27 | 0.22 | 0.00 | 27.1 | 0.01 | 0.0 | 0.0 | | 273 | 1.1 | 4.1 | 98 | 0.7 | 176 | 131 | 1.6 | 3 | 2.17 |
| 4619 | 1 | oz | Meal, part defatted, avg | 28 | 159 | 5 | 4.8 | 7.3 | 1.1 | | | 13.4 | 1.9 | 5.1 | 5.9 | 0.10 | 5.78 | 0 | 18 | 2 | 0 | 2 | 12 | 0.72 | 0.08 | 3.58 | 0.04 | 0.00 | 8.3 | 0.79 | 0.0 | 0.0 | | 43 | 0.4 | 4.1 | 97 | 0.4 | 217 | 114 | | 11 | 2.86 |
| 4630 | 1 | oz | Raw, Arrowhead Mills | 28 | 163 | 5 | 5.4 | 3.9 | 3.9 | 0.0 | 0.0 | 15.6 | 1.9 | | | | | 0 | 0 | 0 | 0 | 0 | 0 | 0.07 | 0.05 | 1.24 | | 0.00 | | | 0.0 | | | 31 | | 0.8 | | | 178 | 109 | | 0 | |
| 4706 | 1 | oz | Toasted, roasted, whole, avg | 28 | 158 | 3 | 4.8 | 7.2 | 3.9 | 0.3 | 3.0 | 13.4 | 1.9 | 5.1 | 5.9 | 0.10 | 5.78 | 0 | 3 | 0.3 | 0 | 0.3 | 2 | 0.22 | 0.07 | 1.28 | 0.22 | 0.00 | 27.5 | 0.01 | 0.0 | | | 277 | 0.7 | 4.1 | 100 | 0.7 | 179 | 133 | 1.6 | 3 | 2.00 |
| 4688 | 1 | oz | Toasted, salted, avg | 28 | 159 | 5 | 4.8 | 7.3 | 4.7 | 0.3 | 2.2 | 13.4 | 1.9 | 5.1 | 5.9 | 0.10 | 5.78 | 0 | 18 | 2 | 0 | 2 | 12 | 0.34 | 0.13 | 1.52 | 0.04 | 0.00 | 26.8 | 0.19 | 0.0 | 0.0 | | 37 | 0.4 | 2.2 | 97 | 0.4 | 217 | 114 | 0.5 | 165 | 2.86 |
| 4748 | 1 | oz | Toasted, unsalted, China Bowl Trading Co | 28 | 200 | 5 | 0.0 | 0.0 | 0.0 | 0.0 | 0.0 | 0.0 | 0.0 | 0.0 | 0.0 | 0.00 | 0.00 | | 0 | 0 | 0 | 0 | 0 | | | | | 0.00 | | | | | | | | 43.2 | | | | | | 0 | |
| | | | Sunflower Seeds | | | | | | | | | | | | | | | | | | | | | | | | | | | | | | | | | | | | | | | | |
| 4661 | 2 | Tbs | Butter, salted, avg | 32 | 185 | 1 | 6.3 | 8.8 | 4.1 | 1.3 | 3.4 | 15.3 | 1.6 | 2.9 | 10.1 | 0.02 | 10.05 | 0 | 17 | 2 | 0 | 2 | 10 | 0.10 | 0.09 | 1.70 | 0.26 | 0.00 | 75.8 | 2.25 | 0.9 | 0.0 | | 39 | 0.6 | 1.5 | 118 | 0.7 | 236 | 23 | | 166 | 1.69 |
| 4550 | 2 | Tbs | Butter, unsalted, avg | 32 | 185 | 1 | 6.3 | 8.8 | 2.0 | 1.3 | 5.4 | 15.3 | 1.6 | 2.9 | 10.1 | 0.02 | 10.05 | 0 | 17 | 2 | 0 | 2 | 10 | 0.10 | 0.09 | 1.70 | 0.26 | 0.00 | 75.8 | 2.25 | 0.9 | 0.0 | | 39 | 0.6 | 1.5 | 118 | 0.7 | 236 | 23 | 25.0 | 1 | 1.69 |
| 4551 | 1 | oz | Dry Roasted, unsalted, avg | 28 | 163 | 1 | 5.4 | 6.7 | 3.1 | 1.0 | 2.6 | 13.9 | 1.5 | 2.7 | 9.2 | 0.02 | 9.18 | 0 | 0 | 0 | 0 | 0 | 0 | 0.03 | 0.07 | 1.97 | 0.23 | 0.00 | 66.4 | 1.97 | 0.4 | 0.0 | | 20 | 0.5 | 1.1 | 36 | 0.6 | 323 | 238 | 22.2 | 1 | 1.48 |
| 4545 | 1 | oz | Kernels, dry, avg | 28 | 160 | 5 | 6.4 | 5.3 | 2.9 | 0.9 | 1.4 | 13.9 | 1.5 | 2.6 | 9.2 | 0.02 | 9.13 | 0 | 14 | 1 | 0 | 1 | 8 | 0.64 | 0.07 | 1.26 | 0.22 | 0.00 | 63.6 | 1.89 | 0.4 | 0.0 | | 32 | 0.5 | 1.9 | 99 | 0.6 | 197 | 193 | 16.7 | 1 | 1.42 |
| 4597 | 1 | oz | Kernels, dry roasted, salted, avg | 28 | 163 | 1 | 5.4 | 6.7 | 2.5 | 1.0 | 3.2 | 13.9 | 1.5 | 2.7 | 9.2 | 0.02 | 9.18 | 0 | 0 | 0 | 0 | 0 | 0 | 0.03 | 0.07 | 1.97 | 0.23 | 0.00 | 66.4 | 1.97 | 0.4 | 0.0 | 13.8 | 20 | 0.5 | 1.1 | 36 | 0.6 | 323 | 238 | 22.2 | 218 | 1.48 |
| 4708 | 1 | oz | Kernels, toasted, salted, avg | 28 | 173 | 1 | 4.8 | 5.8 | 3.2 | 1.0 | 1.5 | 15.9 | 1.7 | 3.0 | 10.5 | 0.02 | 10.47 | 0 | 0 | 0 | 0 | 0 | 0 | 0.09 | 0.08 | 1.18 | 0.23 | 0.00 | 66.6 | 1.98 | 0.4 | 0.0 | | 16 | 0.5 | 1.9 | 36 | 0.6 | 324 | 137 | 17.4 | 172 | 1.48 |
| 4598 | 1 | oz | Kernels, toasted, unsalted, avg | 28 | 173 | 1 | 4.8 | 5.8 | 3.2 | 1.0 | 1.5 | 15.9 | 1.7 | 3.0 | 10.5 | 0.02 | 10.47 | 0 | 0 | 0 | 0 | 0 | 0 | 0.09 | 0.08 | 1.18 | 0.23 | 0.00 | 66.6 | 1.98 | 0.4 | 0.0 | | 16 | 0.5 | 1.9 | 36 | 0.6 | 324 | 137 | 21.9 | 1 | 1.48 |
| 4552 | 1 | oz | Oil Roasted, salted, avg | 28 | 172 | 3 | 6.0 | 4.1 | 1.9 | 1.6 | 0.6 | 16.1 | 1.7 | 3.1 | 10.6 | 0.02 | 10.58 | 0 | 14 | 1 | 0 | 1 | 8 | 0.09 | 0.08 | 1.16 | 0.22 | 0.00 | 65.5 | 1.94 | 0.4 | 0.0 | | 16 | 0.5 | 1.9 | 36 | 0.6 | 319 | 135 | 21.9 | 169 | 1.46 |
| 4546 | 1 | oz | Oil Roasted, unsalted, avg | 28 | 172 | 3 | 6.0 | 4.1 | 1.9 | 1.6 | 0.6 | 16.1 | 1.7 | 3.1 | 10.6 | 0.02 | 10.58 | 0 | 14 | 1 | 0 | 1 | 8 | 0.09 | 0.08 | 1.16 | 0.22 | 0.00 | 65.5 | 1.94 | 0.4 | 0.0 | | 16 | 0.5 | 1.9 | 36 | 0.6 | 319 | 135 | 21.9 | 1 | 1.46 |
| 4768 | 1 | oz | Raw, Arrowhead Mills | 28 | 140 | 5 | 6.2 | 4.7 | 1.6 | 0.8 | 2.3 | 11.7 | 1.2 | | | | | 0 | 0 | 0 | 0 | 0 | 0 | 0.47 | 0.05 | 1.24 | | 0.00 | | | 0.0 | | | 31 | | 2.1 | | | | 226 | | 8 | |
| 4525 | 1 | oz | Walnuts, black, dried, avg | 28 | 170 | 4 | 6.8 | 3.4 | 1.4 | | | 15.8 | 1.0 | 3.6 | 10.5 | 0.93 | 9.38 | 0 | 83 | 8 | 0 | 8 | 50 | 0.06 | 0.03 | 0.19 | 0.16 | 0.00 | 18.3 | 0.18 | 0.9 | 0.0 | | 16 | 0.3 | 0.9 | 57 | 1.2 | 130 | 147 | 4.8 | 0 | 0.96 |
| 4557 | 1 | oz | Walnuts, English/Persian, halves, dried, avg | 28 | 180 | 4 | 4.0 | 5.1 | 1.3 | 0.6 | 3.2 | 17.3 | 1.6 | 4.0 | 10.9 | 1.91 | 8.91 | 0 | 35 | 3 | 0 | 3 | 20 | 0.11 | 0.04 | 0.29 | 0.16 | 0.00 | 18.5 | 0.18 | 0.9 | 0.0 | 0.2 | 26 | 0.4 | 0.7 | 47 | 0.8 | 89 | 141 | 1.3 | 3 | 0.76 |
| | | | **POULTRY—CHICKEN, TURKEY, DUCK, EMU, OSTRICH, OTHERS** | | | | | | | | | | | | | | | | | | | | | | | | | | | | | | | | | | | | | | | | |
| | | | *CHICKEN–BONELESS BROILER/FRYER* | | | | | | | | | | | | | | | | | | | | | | | | | | | | | | | | | | | | | | | | |
| | | | Back | | | | | | | | | | | | | | | | | | | | | | | | | | | | | | | | | | | | | | | | |
| 15116 | 1 | ea | Batter Fried | 240 | 794 | 44 | 52.8 | 24.7 | 0.8 | 1.9 | 22.0 | 52.6 | 14.0 | 21.4 | 12.5 | 0.77 | 11.47 | 211 | 286 | 85 | 86 | 0 | 0 | 0.29 | 0.51 | 14.02 | 0.55 | 0.62 | 48.0 | 2.16 | 0.0 | 0.7 | | 62 | 0.2 | 3.6 | 46 | 0.1 | 329 | 432 | 60.7 | 761 | 4.70 |
| 15014 | 1 | ea | Flour Fried | 144 | 477 | 44 | 40.0 | 9.4 | 0.3 | 0.2 | 8.9 | 29.8 | 8.1 | 11.8 | 6.9 | 0.43 | 6.31 | 28 | 177 | 53 | 53 | 0 | 0 | 0.15 | 0.34 | 10.51 | 0.43 | 0.40 | 21.6 | 1.57 | 0.0 | 0.4 | | 35 | 0.1 | 2.3 | 33 | 0.1 | 239 | 325 | 36.7 | 130 | 3.56 |
| 15115 | 1 | ea | Raw | 198 | 632 | 58 | 27.9 | 0.0 | 0.0 | 0.0 | 0.0 | 56.8 | 16.5 | 24.4 | 12.2 | 0.63 | 11.25 | 56 | 497 | 141 | 141 | 0 | 0 | 0.10 | 0.23 | 9.58 | 0.38 | 0.50 | 11.9 | 1.62 | 3.2 | 0.6 | | 26 | 0.1 | 1.9 | 30 | 0.0 | 224 | 285 | | 127 | 2.49 |
| 15118 | 1 | ea | Raw, w/skin | 102 | 140 | 75 | 20.0 | 0.0 | 0.0 | 0.0 | 0.0 | 6.0 | 1.6 | 1.9 | 1.5 | 0.13 | 1.30 | 83 | 101 | 31 | 31 | 0 | 0 | 0.08 | 0.17 | 6.80 | 0.34 | 0.37 | 9.2 | 1.24 | 3.2 | 0.3 | | 17 | 0.1 | 1.1 | 22 | 0.0 | 154 | 208 | | 84 | 1.89 |
| 15015 | 1 | ea | Roasted | 106 | 318 | 54 | 27.6 | 0.0 | 0.0 | 0.0 | 0.0 | 22.3 | 6.2 | 8.8 | 4.9 | 0.28 | 4.46 | 93 | 369 | 105 | 105 | 0 | 0 | 0.06 | 0.21 | 7.12 | 0.29 | 0.29 | 6.4 | 1.07 | 0.0 | 0.3 | | 22 | 0.1 | 1.5 | 21 | 0.0 | 163 | 223 | 29.0 | 92 | 2.38 |
| 15051 | 1 | ea | Roasted, w/o skin | 80 | 191 | 59 | 22.6 | 0.0 | 0.0 | 0.0 | 0.0 | 10.6 | 2.9 | 3.9 | 2.4 | 0.17 | 2.18 | 72 | 76 | 22 | 22 | 0 | 0 | 0.05 | 0.17 | 5.66 | 0.27 | 0.24 | 5.6 | 0.90 | 0.0 | 0.2 | | 19 | 0.1 | 1.1 | 18 | 0.0 | 132 | 190 | 25.8 | 77 | 2.12 |
| | | | Breast | | | | | | | | | | | | | | | | | | | | | | | | | | | | | | | | | | | | | | | | |
| 15013 | 1 | ea | Batter Fried | 280 | 728 | 52 | 69.4 | 25.2 | 0.8 | 5.6 | 18.7 | 37.0 | 9.9 | 15.3 | 8.6 | 0.50 | 7.95 | 238 | 138 | 55 | 56 | 0 | 0 | 0.32 | 0.41 | 29.40 | 1.20 | 0.84 | 42.0 | 2.30 | 0.0 | 0.8 | | 56 | 0.2 | 3.5 | 67 | 0.2 | 518 | 563 | 61.6 | 770 | 2.66 |
| 15003 | 1 | ea | Flour Fried | 196 | 435 | 57 | 62.3 | 3.2 | 0.2 | 0.1 | 2.9 | 17.4 | 4.8 | 6.9 | 3.8 | 0.24 | 3.45 | 74 | 98 | 29 | 29 | 0 | 0 | 0.16 | 0.26 | 26.85 | 1.14 | 0.67 | 11.8 | 1.96 | 0.0 | 0.6 | | 31 | 0.1 | 2.3 | 59 | 0.1 | 457 | 508 | 38.8 | 149 | 2.16 |
| 15053 | 1 | ea | Raw | 290 | 499 | 70 | 60.6 | 0.0 | 0.0 | 0.0 | 0.0 | 26.8 | 7.7 | 11.1 | 5.7 | 0.32 | 5.19 | 86 | 241 | 70 | 70 | 0 | 0 | 0.18 | 0.25 | 28.74 | 1.54 | 0.99 | 11.6 | 2.33 | 2.9 | 0.9 | | 32 | 0.1 | 2.1 | 73 | 0.1 | 505 | 638 | 58.0 | 183 | 2.32 |
| 15054 | 1 | ea | Raw, w/o skin | 236 | 260 | 75 | 54.5 | 0.0 | 0.0 | 0.0 | 0.0 | 2.9 | 0.8 | 0.7 | 0.6 | 0.07 | 0.50 | 37 | 50 | 14 | 14 | 0 | 0 | 0.17 | 0.22 | 26.43 | 1.30 | 0.90 | 9.4 | 1.93 | 2.8 | 0.7 | | 26 | 0.1 | 1.7 | 66 | 0.0 | 463 | 602 | 47.2 | 153 | 1.89 |
| 15001 | 1 | ea | Roasted | 196 | 386 | 62 | 58.4 | 0.0 | 0.0 | 0.0 | 0.0 | 15.2 | 4.3 | 5.9 | 3.3 | 0.20 | 2.90 | 65 | 132 | 53 | 53 | 0 | 0 | 0.13 | 0.23 | 24.89 | 1.10 | 0.63 | 7.8 | 1.83 | 0.0 | 0.5 | | 27 | 0.1 | 2.1 | 53 | 0.0 | 419 | 480 | 43.5 | 139 | 2.00 |
| 15004 | 1 | ea | Roasted, w/o skin | 172 | 284 | 65 | 53.3 | 0.0 | 0.0 | 0.0 | 0.0 | 6.1 | 1.7 | 2.1 | 1.3 | 0.10 | 1.12 | 46 | 36 | 10 | 10 | 0 | 0 | 0.12 | 0.20 | 23.56 | 1.03 | 0.58 | 6.9 | 1.66 | 0.0 | 0.5 | | 26 | 0.1 | 1.8 | 50 | 0.0 | 392 | 440 | 47.5 | 127 | 1.72 |
| | | | Canned | | | | | | | | | | | | | | | | | | | | | | | | | | | | | | | | | | | | | | | | |
| 15207 | 3 | oz | Premium Chunk, in water, Swanson | 85 | 104 | 74 | 16.4 | 1.5 | 1.5 | 0.0 | 0.0 | 3.0 | 1.5 | | | | | 52 | 0 | 0 | 0 | 0 | 0 | | | | | | | | 0.0 | | | 0 | | 0.0 | | | | | | 343 | |
| 15208 | 3 | oz | Premium Chunk, in water, white, Swanson | 85 | 89 | 75 | 16.4 | 1.5 | 0.0 | 0.0 | 1.5 | 1.5 | 0.7 | | | | | 37 | 0 | 0 | 0 | 0 | 0 | | | | | | | | 0.0 | | | 0 | | 0.0 | | | | | | 343 | |
| 15019 | 3 | oz | With Broth | 82 | 135 | 69 | 17.9 | 0.0 | 0.0 | 0.0 | 0.0 | 6.5 | 1.8 | 2.6 | 1.4 | 0.08 | 1.30 | 51 | 96 | 23 | 28 | 0 | 0 | 0.01 | 0.11 | 5.19 | 0.29 | 0.24 | 3.3 | 0.70 | 1.6 | 0.2 | | 11 | 0.0 | 1.3 | 10 | 0.0 | 91 | 113 | 15.2 | 412 | 1.16 |
| 15197 | 3 | oz | With Skin & Broth, Bryan Foods | 85 | 247 | | 15.3 | 0.0 | 0.0 | 0.0 | 0.0 | 11.9 | | | | | | | | | | | | | | | | | | | | | | | | | | | | | | 463 | |
| | | | Drumstick | | | | | | | | | | | | | | | | | | | | | | | | | | | | | | | | | | | | | | | | |
| 15030 | 1 | ea | Batter Fried | 72 | 193 | 53 | 15.8 | 6.0 | 0.2 | 1.3 | 4.4 | 11.4 | 3.0 | 4.6 | 2.7 | 0.17 | 2.51 | 62 | 62 | 19 | 19 | 0 | 0 | 0.08 | 0.15 | 3.67 | 0.19 | 0.20 | 13.0 | 0.73 | 0.0 | 0.2 | | 12 | 0.1 | 1.0 | 14 | 0.0 | 106 | 134 | 15.5 | 194 | 1.68 |
| 15007 | 1 | ea | Flour Fried | 49 | 120 | 57 | 13.2 | 0.8 | 0.0 | 0.0 | 0.7 | 6.7 | 1.8 | 2.7 | 1.5 | 0.09 | 1.44 | 44 | 41 | 12 | 12 | 0 | 0 | 0.04 | 0.11 | 2.96 | 0.17 | 0.16 | 4.9 | 0.60 | 0.0 | 0.1 | | 6 | 0.0 | 0.7 | 11 | 0.0 | 86 | 112 | 9.7 | 44 | 1.42 |
| 15055 | 1 | ea | Raw | 73 | 118 | 72 | 14.1 | 0.0 | 0.0 | 0.0 | 0.0 | 6.3 | 1.7 | 2.5 | 1.4 | 0.08 | 1.28 | 59 | 69 | 20 | 20 | 0 | 0 | 0.05 | 0.13 | 3.98 | 0.22 | 0.26 | 6.6 | 0.86 | 2.0 | 0.2 | | 8 | 0.0 | 0.8 | 15 | 0.0 | 112 | 150 | 15.3 | 61 | 1.46 |
| 15056 | 1 | ea | Raw, w/o skin | 62 | 74 | 76 | 12.8 | 0.0 | 0.0 | 0.0 | 0.0 | 2.1 | 0.5 | 0.7 | 0.5 | 0.04 | 0.45 | 48 | 35 | 11 | 11 | 0 | 0 | 0.05 | 0.12 | 3.58 | 0.21 | 0.23 | 6.2 | 0.80 | 2.0 | 0.2 | | 7 | 0.0 | 0.6 | 14 | 0.0 | 103 | 140 | 13.0 | 55 | 1.37 |
| 15008 | 1 | ea | Roasted | 52 | 112 | 63 | 14.0 | 0.0 | 0.0 | 0.0 | 0.0 | 5.8 | 1.6 | 2.2 | 1.3 | 0.07 | 1.18 | 47 | 52 | 16 | 16 | 0 | 0 | 0.04 | 0.11 | 3.11 | 0.18 | 0.17 | 4.2 | 0.63 | 0.0 | 0.2 | | 6 | 0.0 | 0.7 | 12 | 0.0 | 91 | 119 | 15.1 | 47 | 1.49 |

| Code | Amount | Description | Basic Components | | | | | | | | | Additional Fats | | | | | | Vit A & Components | | | | | Vitamins | | | | | | | | | | Minerals | | | | | | | | | |
|---|---|---|---|---|---|---|---|---|---|---|---|---|---|---|---|---|---|---|---|---|---|---|---|---|---|---|---|---|---|---|---|---|---|---|---|---|---|---|---|---|---|---|
| | | | Weight (g) | Calories | % Water | Protein (g) | Carbs (g) | Fiber (g) | Sugar (g) | Other Carbs (g) | Fat (g) | Sat Fat (g) | Mono Fat (g) | Poly Fat (g) | Omega 3 (g) | Omega 6 (g) | Choles (mg) | Vit A (IU) | Vit A (RE) | Retinol (RE) | Carotenoids (RE) | Beta Carotene (mcg) | Thiamin (mg) | Riboflavin (mg) | Niacin (NE) | Vit B6 (mg) | Vit B12 (mcg) | Folate (mcg) | Panto (mg) | Vit C (mg) | Vit D (mg) | Vit E (α TE) | Calcium (mg) | Copper (mg) | Iron (mg) | Magnes (mg) | Mang (mg) | Phos (mg) | Potassium (mg) | Selenium (mcg) | Sodium (mg) | Zinc (mg) |
| 15035 | 1 ea | Roasted, w/o skin | 44 | 76 | 67 | 12.5 | 0.0 | 0.0 | 0.0 | 0.0 | 2.5 | 0.7 | 0.8 | 0.6 | 0.05 | 0.53 | 41 | 26 | 8 | 8 | 0 | 0 | 0.03 | 0.10 | 2.68 | 0.17 | 0.15 | 4.0 | 0.58 | 0.0 | 0.1 | | 5 | 0.0 | 0.6 | 11 | 0.0 | 81 | 108 | 11.4 | 42 | 1.40 |
| | | Leg | | | | | | | | | | | | | | | | | | | | | | | | | | | | | | | | | | | | | | | | |
| 15151 | 1 ea | Batter Fried | 158 | 431 | 52 | 34.4 | 13.8 | 0.5 | 1.1 | 12.2 | 25.6 | 6.8 | 10.4 | 6.1 | 0.38 | 5.61 | 142 | 144 | 43 | 43 | 0 | 0 | 0.18 | 0.35 | 8.58 | 0.43 | 0.44 | 28.4 | 1.57 | 0.0 | 0.5 | | 28 | 0.1 | 2.2 | 32 | 0.1 | 240 | 299 | 33.2 | 441 | 3.43 |
| 15155 | 1 ea | Flour Fried | 112 | 284 | 55 | 30.0 | 2.8 | 0.1 | 0.1 | 2.6 | 16.1 | 4.4 | 6.4 | 3.7 | 0.22 | 3.39 | 105 | 103 | 31 | 31 | 0 | 0 | 0.10 | 0.26 | 7.34 | 0.38 | 0.35 | 12.3 | 1.34 | 0.0 | 0.3 | | 15 | 0.1 | 1.6 | 27 | 0.0 | 204 | 261 | 22.8 | 99 | 3.00 |
| 15119 | 1 ea | Raw | 167 | 312 | 70 | 30.4 | 0.0 | 0.0 | 0.0 | 0.0 | 20.2 | 5.7 | 8.2 | 4.4 | 0.25 | 4.04 | 139 | 205 | 60 | 60 | 0 | 0 | 0.11 | 0.27 | 9.08 | 0.48 | 0.53 | 18.4 | 1.85 | 4.2 | 0.5 | | 17 | 0.1 | 1.7 | 35 | 0.0 | 249 | 331 | | 132 | 2.96 |
| 15121 | 1 ea | Raw, w/o skin | 130 | 156 | 76 | 26.1 | 0.0 | 0.0 | 0.0 | 0.0 | 5.0 | 1.3 | 1.5 | 1.2 | 0.10 | 1.07 | 104 | 79 | 23 | 23 | 0 | 0 | 0.10 | 0.25 | 7.89 | 0.43 | 0.47 | 13.0 | 1.53 | 4.2 | 0.4 | | 14 | 0.1 | 1.3 | 30 | 0.0 | 217 | 298 | | 112 | 2.68 |
| 15154 | 1 ea | Roasted | 114 | 264 | 61 | 29.6 | 0.0 | 0.0 | 0.0 | 0.0 | 15.4 | 4.2 | 6.0 | 3.4 | 0.21 | 3.09 | 105 | 154 | 44 | 44 | 0 | 0 | 0.08 | 0.24 | 7.07 | 0.38 | 0.34 | 8.0 | 1.32 | 0.0 | 0.3 | | 14 | 0.1 | 1.5 | 26 | 0.0 | 198 | 256 | 26.3 | 99 | 2.96 |
| 15156 | 1 ea | Roasted, w/o skin | 95 | 181 | 65 | 25.6 | 0.0 | 0.0 | 0.0 | 0.0 | 8.0 | 2.2 | 2.9 | 1.9 | 0.13 | 1.66 | 89 | 60 | 18 | 18 | 0 | 0 | 0.07 | 0.22 | 6.00 | 0.35 | 0.30 | 7.6 | 1.18 | 0.0 | 0.3 | | 11 | 0.1 | 1.2 | 23 | 0.0 | 174 | 230 | 26.2 | 86 | 2.72 |
| | | Neck | | | | | | | | | | | | | | | | | | | | | | | | | | | | | | | | | | | | | | | | |
| 15124 | 1 ea | Batter Fried | 52 | 172 | 47 | 10.3 | 4.5 | 0.1 | 0.4 | 4.0 | 12.2 | 3.2 | 5.1 | 2.9 | 0.16 | 2.67 | 47 | 88 | 27 | 27 | 0 | 0 | 0.05 | 0.12 | 2.36 | 0.11 | 0.12 | 7.8 | 0.44 | 0.0 | 0.2 | | 16 | 0.1 | 1.1 | 8 | 0.0 | 60 | 79 | 12.6 | 144 | 1.30 |
| 15082 | 1 ea | Flour Fried | 36 | 120 | 48 | 8.6 | 1.5 | 0.0 | 0.0 | 1.4 | 8.5 | 2.3 | 3.5 | 2.0 | 0.11 | 1.82 | 34 | 68 | 21 | 21 | 0 | 0 | 0.03 | 0.09 | 1.93 | 0.09 | 0.09 | 4.0 | 0.35 | 0.0 | 0.1 | | 11 | 0.0 | 0.9 | 7 | 0.0 | 48 | 65 | 7.8 | 30 | 1.11 |
| 15123 | 1 ea | Raw | 50 | 148 | 60 | 7.1 | 0.0 | 0.0 | 0.0 | 0.0 | 13.1 | 3.6 | 5.3 | 2.8 | 0.14 | 2.60 | 50 | 108 | 33 | 33 | 0 | 0 | 0.02 | 0.10 | 1.80 | 0.09 | 0.13 | 2.5 | 0.43 | 0.6 | 0.2 | | 9 | 0.0 | 0.9 | 6 | 0.0 | 56 | 68 | | 32 | 0.93 |
| 15125 | 1 ea | Raw, w/o skin | 20 | 31 | 71 | 3.5 | 0.0 | 0.0 | 0.0 | 0.0 | 1.8 | 0.5 | 0.5 | 0.4 | 0.03 | 0.38 | 17 | 29 | 9 | 9 | 0 | 0 | 0.01 | 0.05 | 0.82 | 0.06 | 0.06 | 1.6 | 0.22 | 0.5 | 0.1 | | 5 | 0.0 | 0.4 | 3 | 0.0 | 23 | 35 | | 16 | 0.54 |
| 15083 | 1 ea | Simmered | 38 | 94 | 62 | 7.4 | 0.0 | 0.0 | 0.0 | 0.0 | 6.9 | 1.9 | 2.7 | 1.5 | 0.08 | 1.37 | 27 | 61 | 18 | 18 | 0 | 0 | 0.02 | 0.09 | 1.26 | 0.04 | 0.05 | 1.1 | 0.20 | 0.0 | 0.1 | | 10 | 0.0 | 0.9 | 5 | 0.0 | 46 | 41 | 8.6 | 20 | 1.03 |
| 15085 | 1 ea | Simmered, w/o skin | 18 | 32 | 67 | 4.4 | 0.0 | 0.0 | 0.0 | 0.0 | 1.5 | 0.4 | 0.5 | 0.4 | 0.03 | 0.32 | 14 | 22 | 6 | 6 | 0 | 0 | 0.01 | 0.05 | 0.71 | 0.03 | 0.03 | 1.1 | 0.12 | 0.0 | 0.1 | | 8 | 0.0 | 0.5 | 3 | 0.0 | 23 | 25 | 4.6 | 12 | 0.68 |
| | | Skin | | | | | | | | | | | | | | | | | | | | | | | | | | | | | | | | | | | | | | | | |
| 15100 | 3 oz | Batter Fried | 85 | 335 | 36 | 8.8 | 19.7 | 0.6 | 1.6 | 17.5 | 24.5 | 6.5 | 10.5 | 5.8 | 0.31 | 5.42 | 63 | 117 | 36 | 36 | 0 | 0 | 0.15 | 0.15 | 2.84 | 0.05 | 0.14 | 34.0 | 0.39 | 0.0 | 0.3 | | 22 | 0.1 | 1.2 | 10 | 0.1 | 68 | 64 | | 494 | 0.61 |
| 15101 | 3 oz | Flour Fried | 85 | 427 | 28 | 16.2 | 7.9 | 0.3 | 0.2 | 7.5 | 36.2 | 9.9 | 15.3 | 8.0 | 0.39 | 7.45 | 62 | 197 | 60 | 60 | 0 | 0 | 0.08 | 0.14 | 4.95 | 0.09 | 0.15 | 28.1 | 0.57 | 0.0 | 0.3 | | 12 | 0.1 | 1.3 | 14 | 0.1 | 107 | 106 | | 45 | 0.98 |
| 15099 | 4 oz | Raw | 113 | 394 | 54 | 15.0 | 0.0 | 0.0 | 0.0 | 0.0 | 36.6 | 10.3 | 15.3 | 7.7 | 0.35 | 7.13 | 123 | 296 | 88 | 88 | 0 | 0 | 0.04 | 0.08 | 4.51 | 0.10 | 0.26 | 3.4 | 0.78 | 0.0 | 0.3 | | 12 | 0.0 | 1.2 | 15 | 0.0 | 113 | 116 | | 71 | 1.05 |
| 15102 | 3 oz | Roasted | 85 | 386 | 40 | 17.3 | 0.0 | 0.0 | 0.0 | 0.0 | 34.6 | 9.7 | 14.5 | 7.3 | 0.33 | 6.75 | 71 | 223 | 66 | 66 | 0 | 0 | 0.03 | 0.11 | 4.74 | 0.09 | 0.17 | 1.7 | 0.60 | 0.0 | 0.3 | | 12 | 0.1 | 1.3 | 13 | 0.0 | 106 | 116 | | 55 | 1.05 |
| | | Thigh | | | | | | | | | | | | | | | | | | | | | | | | | | | | | | | | | | | | | | | | |
| 15036 | 1 ea | Batter Fried | 86 | 238 | 52 | 18.6 | 7.8 | 0.3 | 1.7 | 5.8 | 14.2 | 3.8 | 5.8 | 3.4 | 0.21 | 3.09 | 80 | 82 | 25 | 25 | 0 | 0 | 0.10 | 0.20 | 4.92 | 0.22 | 0.24 | 16.3 | 0.84 | 0.0 | 0.3 | | 15 | 0.1 | 1.2 | 18 | 0.0 | 133 | 165 | 19.5 | 248 | 1.75 |
| 15009 | 1 ea | Flour Fried | 62 | 162 | 54 | 16.6 | 2.0 | 0.1 | 0.0 | 1.9 | 9.3 | 2.5 | 3.6 | 2.1 | 0.12 | 1.92 | 60 | 61 | 18 | 18 | 0 | 0 | 0.06 | 0.15 | 4.31 | 0.20 | 0.19 | 7.4 | 0.74 | 0.0 | 0.2 | | 9 | 0.1 | 0.9 | 16 | 0.0 | 116 | 147 | 13.0 | 55 | 1.56 |
| 15060 | 1 ea | Raw | 94 | 198 | 68 | 16.3 | 0.0 | 0.0 | 0.0 | 0.0 | 14.4 | 4.1 | 5.9 | 3.1 | 0.17 | 2.86 | 79 | 136 | 39 | 39 | 0 | 0 | 0.06 | 0.14 | 5.10 | 0.24 | 0.28 | 6.6 | 0.97 | 2.2 | 0.3 | | 9 | 0.1 | 0.9 | 19 | 0.0 | 136 | 180 | 19.7 | 71 | 1.50 |
| 15061 | 1 ea | Raw, w/o skin | 69 | 82 | 76 | 13.6 | 0.0 | 0.0 | 0.0 | 0.0 | 2.7 | 0.7 | 0.8 | 0.7 | 0.06 | 0.58 | 57 | 45 | 14 | 14 | 0 | 0 | 0.05 | 0.13 | 4.37 | 0.23 | 0.24 | 6.9 | 0.85 | 2.1 | 0.2 | | 7 | 0.0 | 0.7 | 17 | 0.0 | 116 | 159 | 14.5 | 59 | 1.32 |
| 15010 | 1 ea | Roasted | 62 | 153 | 59 | 15.6 | 0.0 | 0.0 | 0.0 | 0.0 | 9.6 | 2.7 | 3.8 | 2.1 | 0.12 | 1.93 | 58 | 102 | 30 | 30 | 0 | 0 | 0.04 | 0.13 | 3.95 | 0.19 | 0.18 | 4.3 | 0.69 | 0.0 | 0.2 | | 7 | 0.0 | 0.8 | 14 | 0.0 | 108 | 138 | 14.8 | 52 | 1.46 |
| 15012 | 1 ea | Roasted, w/o skin | 52 | 109 | 63 | 13.5 | 0.0 | 0.0 | 0.0 | 0.0 | 5.7 | 1.6 | 2.2 | 1.3 | 0.08 | 1.16 | 49 | 34 | 10 | 10 | 0 | 0 | 0.04 | 0.12 | 3.40 | 0.18 | 0.16 | 4.2 | 0.61 | 0.0 | 0.2 | | 6 | 0.0 | 0.7 | 12 | 0.0 | 95 | 124 | 15.1 | 46 | 1.34 |
| | | Wing | | | | | | | | | | | | | | | | | | | | | | | | | | | | | | | | | | | | | | | | |
| 15034 | 1 ea | Batter Fried | 49 | 159 | 46 | 9.8 | 5.3 | 0.1 | 1.2 | 4.0 | 10.7 | 2.9 | 4.4 | 2.5 | 0.14 | 2.27 | 39 | 55 | 17 | 17 | 0 | 0 | 0.05 | 0.07 | 2.58 | 0.15 | 0.12 | 8.8 | 0.35 | 0.0 | 0.1 | | 10 | 0.0 | 0.6 | 8 | 0.0 | 59 | 68 | 12.0 | 157 | 0.68 |
| 15029 | 1 ea | Flour Fried | 32 | 103 | 49 | 8.4 | 0.8 | 0.0 | 0.0 | 0.7 | 7.1 | 1.9 | 2.8 | 1.6 | 0.09 | 1.43 | 26 | 40 | 12 | 12 | 0 | 0 | 0.02 | 0.04 | 2.14 | 0.13 | 0.09 | 1.9 | 0.28 | 0.0 | 0.1 | | 5 | 0.0 | 0.4 | 6 | 0.0 | 48 | 57 | 7.5 | 25 | 0.56 |
| 15062 | 1 ea | Raw | 49 | 109 | 66 | 9.0 | 0.0 | 0.0 | 0.0 | 0.0 | 7.8 | 2.2 | 3.1 | 1.7 | 0.09 | 1.50 | 38 | 72 | 22 | 22 | 0 | 0 | 0.02 | 0.04 | 2.91 | 0.17 | 0.16 | 2.0 | 0.38 | 0.3 | 0.1 | | 6 | 0.0 | 0.5 | 9 | 0.0 | 65 | 76 | 9.8 | 36 | 0.65 |
| 15046 | 1 ea | Raw, w/o skin | 29 | 37 | 75 | 6.4 | 0.0 | 0.0 | 0.0 | 0.0 | 1.0 | 0.3 | 0.2 | 0.2 | 0.02 | 0.17 | 17 | 17 | 5 | 5 | 0 | 0 | 0.02 | 0.03 | 2.13 | 0.15 | 0.11 | 1.2 | 0.24 | 0.3 | 0.1 | | 4 | 0.0 | 0.3 | 6 | 0.0 | 45 | 56 | 3.8 | 23 | 0.47 |
| 15002 | 1 ea | Roasted | 34 | 99 | 55 | 9.1 | 0.0 | 0.0 | 0.0 | 0.0 | 6.6 | 1.9 | 2.6 | 1.4 | 0.08 | 1.26 | 29 | 54 | 16 | 16 | 0 | 0 | 0.01 | 0.04 | 2.26 | 0.14 | 0.10 | 1.0 | 0.30 | 0.0 | 0.1 | | 5 | 0.0 | 0.4 | 6 | 0.0 | 51 | 63 | 9.0 | 28 | 0.62 |
| 15059 | 1 ea | Roasted, w/o skin | 21 | 43 | 63 | 6.4 | 0.0 | 0.0 | 0.0 | 0.0 | 1.7 | 0.5 | 0.5 | 0.4 | 0.03 | 0.31 | 18 | 13 | 4 | 4 | 0 | 0 | 0.01 | 0.03 | 1.54 | 0.12 | 0.07 | 0.8 | 0.21 | 0.0 | 0.1 | | 3 | 0.0 | 0.2 | 4 | 0.0 | 35 | 44 | 6.2 | 19 | 0.45 |
| | | Whole, w/o giblets or neck | | | | | | | | | | | | | | | | | | | | | | | | | | | | | | | | | | | | | | | | |
| 15072 | 3 oz | Batter Fried | 85 | 246 | 49 | 19.1 | 8.0 | 0.3 | 1.8 | 6.0 | 14.8 | 3.9 | 6.0 | 3.5 | 0.20 | 3.20 | 74 | 79 | 24 | 24 | 0 | 0 | 0.10 | 0.16 | 5.98 | 0.26 | 0.24 | 15.3 | 0.76 | 0.0 | 0.3 | | 18 | 0.1 | 1.2 | 18 | 0.0 | 132 | 157 | 19.6 | 248 | 1.42 |
| 15113 | 3 oz | Dark Meat, batter fried | 85 | 253 | 49 | 18.6 | 8.0 | 0.3 | 0.6 | 7.1 | 15.8 | 4.2 | 6.4 | 3.8 | 0.22 | 3.46 | 76 | 88 | 26 | 26 | 0 | 0 | 0.10 | 0.19 | 4.77 | 0.21 | 0.23 | 15.3 | 0.81 | 0.0 | 0.3 | | 18 | 0.1 | 1.2 | 17 | 0.0 | 123 | 157 | 19.8 | 251 | 1.77 |
| 15112 | 4 oz | Dark Meat, raw | 113 | 268 | 65 | 18.9 | 0.0 | 0.0 | 0.0 | 0.0 | 20.7 | 5.9 | 8.6 | 4.5 | 0.24 | 4.11 | 92 | 192 | 55 | 55 | 0 | 0 | 0.07 | 0.16 | 5.89 | 0.28 | 0.33 | 7.9 | 1.12 | 2.4 | 0.3 | | 12 | 0.1 | 1.1 | 21 | 0.0 | 154 | 201 | | 82 | 1.79 |
| 15114 | 4 oz | Dark Meat, raw, w/o skin | 113 | 141 | 76 | 22.7 | 0.0 | 0.0 | 0.0 | 0.0 | 4.9 | 1.2 | 1.5 | 1.2 | 0.10 | 1.04 | 90 | 81 | 25 | 25 | 0 | 0 | 0.09 | 0.21 | 7.06 | 0.37 | 0.41 | 11.3 | 1.41 | 3.5 | 0.3 | | 14 | 0.1 | 1.2 | 26 | 0.0 | 183 | 251 | | 96 | 2.26 |
| 15080 | 3 oz | Dark Meat, rstd | 85 | 215 | 59 | 22.1 | 0.0 | 0.0 | 0.0 | 0.0 | 13.4 | 3.7 | 5.3 | 3.0 | 0.18 | 2.70 | 77 | 171 | 49 | 49 | 0 | 0 | 0.06 | 0.18 | 5.41 | 0.26 | 0.25 | 6.0 | 0.94 | 0.0 | 0.3 | | 13 | 0.1 | 1.2 | 19 | 0.0 | 143 | 187 | 20.7 | 74 | 2.12 |
| 15081 | 3 oz | Dark Meat, stwd | 85 | 198 | 63 | 20.0 | 0.0 | 0.0 | 0.0 | 0.0 | 12.5 | 3.5 | 4.9 | 2.8 | 0.16 | 2.51 | 70 | 158 | 46 | 46 | 0 | 0 | 0.04 | 0.15 | 3.83 | 0.14 | 0.17 | 5.1 | 0.66 | 0.0 | 0.3 | | 12 | 0.1 | 1.1 | 15 | 0.0 | 113 | 141 | 18.5 | 60 | 1.92 |
| 15219 | 3 oz | Dark Meat, stwd, w/o skin | 85 | 163 | 66 | 22.1 | 0.0 | 0.0 | 0.0 | 0.0 | 7.6 | 2.1 | 2.8 | 1.8 | 0.12 | 1.58 | 75 | 59 | 18 | 18 | 0 | 0 | 0.05 | 0.17 | 4.03 | 0.18 | 0.19 | 6.0 | 0.76 | 0.0 | 0.3 | | 12 | 0.1 | 1.2 | 17 | 0.0 | 122 | 154 | 22.7 | 63 | 2.26 |
| 15073 | 6 oz | Flour Fried | 85 | 229 | 52 | 24.3 | 2.7 | 0.1 | 0.1 | 2.5 | 12.7 | 3.5 | 5.0 | 2.9 | 0.18 | 2.63 | 77 | 76 | 23 | 23 | 0 | 0 | 0.07 | 0.16 | 7.64 | 0.35 | 0.26 | 7.7 | 0.92 | 0.0 | 0.3 | | 14 | 0.1 | 1.2 | 21 | 0.0 | 162 | 199 | 18.4 | 71 | 1.73 |
| 15214 | 3 oz | Fried, w/o skin | 85 | 186 | 58 | 26.0 | 1.4 | 0.1 | 0.0 | 1.3 | 7.8 | 2.1 | 2.8 | 1.8 | 0.13 | 1.62 | 80 | 50 | 15 | 15 | 0 | 0 | 0.07 | 0.17 | 8.21 | 0.41 | 0.29 | 6.0 | 0.99 | 0.0 | 0.3 | | 14 | 0.1 | 1.1 | 23 | 0.0 | 174 | 218 | 27.5 | 77 | 1.90 |
| 15111 | 3 oz | Light Meat, batter fried | 85 | 235 | 50 | 20.1 | 8.1 | 0.3 | 0.6 | 7.2 | 13.1 | 3.5 | 5.4 | 3.1 | 0.18 | 2.81 | 71 | 67 | 20 | 20 | 0 | 0 | 0.10 | 0.12 | 7.79 | 0.33 | 0.24 | 13.6 | 0.67 | 0.0 | 0.3 | | 17 | 0.1 | 1.1 | 19 | 0.0 | 143 | 157 | 19.3 | 244 | 0.90 |
| 15076 | 3 oz | Light Meat, flour fried | 85 | 209 | 55 | 25.9 | 1.5 | 0.1 | 0.0 | 1.4 | 10.3 | 2.8 | 4.1 | 2.3 | 0.13 | 2.06 | 74 | 58 | 17 | 17 | 0 | 0 | 0.06 | 0.11 | 10.20 | 0.46 | 0.28 | 6.0 | 0.82 | 0.0 | 0.3 | | 14 | 0.0 | 1.0 | 23 | 0.0 | 181 | 203 | 17.6 | 65 | 1.07 |
| 15110 | 4 oz | Light Meat, raw | 113 | 210 | 69 | 22.9 | 0.0 | 0.0 | 0.0 | 0.0 | 12.5 | 3.6 | 5.1 | 2.6 | 0.15 | 2.41 | 76 | 112 | 33 | 33 | 0 | 0 | 0.07 | 0.10 | 10.07 | 0.54 | 0.38 | 4.5 | 0.90 | 1.0 | 0.3 | | 12 | 0.0 | 0.9 | 26 | 0.0 | 184 | 231 | | 73 | 1.05 |
| 15153 | 4 oz | Light Meat, raw, w/o skin | 113 | 129 | 75 | 26.2 | 0.0 | 0.0 | 0.0 | 0.0 | 1.9 | 0.5 | 0.4 | 0.4 | 0.05 | 0.32 | 66 | 32 | 9 | 9 | 0 | 0 | 0.08 | 0.10 | 11.98 | 0.61 | 0.43 | 4.5 | 0.93 | 1.4 | 0.3 | | 14 | 0.0 | 0.8 | 31 | 0.0 | 211 | 270 | | 77 | 1.10 |
| 15077 | 3 oz | Light Meat, rstd | 85 | 189 | 60 | 24.7 | 0.0 | 0.0 | 0.0 | 0.0 | 9.3 | 2.6 | 3.6 | 2.0 | 0.11 | 1.76 | 71 | 94 | 27 | 27 | 0 | 0 | 0.05 | 0.10 | 9.44 | 0.44 | 0.27 | 2.6 | 0.79 | 0.0 | 0.3 | | 13 | 0.0 | 1.0 | 21 | 0.0 | 170 | 193 | 19.8 | 64 | 1.05 |
| 15216 | 3 oz | Light Meat, rstd, w/skin | 85 | 147 | 65 | 26.3 | 0.0 | 0.0 | 0.0 | 0.0 | 3.8 | 1.1 | 1.3 | 0.8 | 0.07 | 0.70 | 72 | 25 | 8 | 8 | 0 | 0 | 0.06 | 0.10 | 10.54 | 0.51 | 0.29 | 3.4 | 0.83 | 0.0 | 0.3 | | 13 | 0.0 | 0.9 | 23 | 0.0 | 184 | 210 | 23.8 | 65 | 1.05 |
| 15078 | 3 oz | Light Meat, stwd | 85 | 171 | 65 | 22.2 | 0.0 | 0.0 | 0.0 | 0.0 | 8.5 | 2.4 | 3.3 | 1.8 | 0.10 | 1.62 | 63 | 82 | 24 | 24 | 0 | 0 | 0.03 | 0.10 | 5.90 | 0.23 | 0.17 | 2.6 | 0.45 | 0.0 | 0.3 | | 11 | 0.0 | 0.8 | 17 | 0.0 | 124 | 142 | 17.5 | 54 | 0.97 |
| 15071 | 4 oz | Raw | 113 | 243 | 66 | 21.0 | 0.0 | 0.0 | 0.0 | 0.0 | 17.1 | 4.9 | 7.1 | 3.6 | 0.20 | 3.34 | 85 | 158 | 46 | 46 | 0 | 0 | 0.07 | 0.14 | 7.68 | 0.40 | 0.35 | 6.8 | 1.03 | 1.8 | 0.3 | | 12 | 0.1 | 1.0 | 23 | 0.0 | 166 | 214 | | 79 | 1.48 |
| 15049 | 4 oz | Raw, w/o skin | 113 | 134 | 76 | 24.2 | 0.0 | 0.0 | 0.0 | 0.0 | 3.5 | 0.9 | 1.0 | 0.8 | 0.07 | 0.71 | 79 | 59 | 18 | 18 | 0 | 0 | 0.08 | 0.16 | 9.31 | 0.49 | 0.42 | 7.9 | 1.20 | 2.6 | 0.3 | | 14 | 0.1 | 1.0 | 28 | 0.0 | 195 | 259 | 14.8 | 87 | 1.74 |
| 15074 | 3 oz | Roasted | 85 | 203 | 60 | 23.2 | 0.0 | 0.0 | 0.0 | 0.0 | 11.6 | 3.2 | 4.5 | 2.5 | 0.14 | 2.28 | 75 | 137 | 40 | 40 | 0 | 0 | 0.05 | 0.14 | 7.22 | 0.34 | 0.26 | 4.3 | 0.88 | 0.0 | 0.3 | | 13 | 0.1 | 1.1 | 20 | 0.0 | 155 | 190 | 20.3 | 70 | 1.65 |
| 15075 | 3 oz | Stewed | 85 | 186 | 64 | 21.0 | 0.0 | 0.0 | 0.0 | 0.0 | 10.7 | 3.0 | 4.2 | 2.3 | 0.14 | 2.11 | 66 | 124 | 36 | 36 | 0 | 0 | 0.04 | 0.13 | 4.75 | 0.19 | 0.17 | 4.3 | 0.57 | 0.0 | 0.3 | | 11 | 0.0 | 1.0 | 16 | 0.0 | 118 | 141 | 14.0 | 57 | 1.50 |
| | | *TURKEY-ALL TYPES, BONELESS* | | | | | | | | | | | | | | | | | | | | | | | | | | | | | | | | | | | | | | | | |
| 16083 | 4 oz | Back, raw | 113 | 221 | 68 | 20.5 | 0.0 | 0.0 | 0.0 | 0.0 | 14.8 | 4.1 | 5.6 | 3.6 | 0.24 | 3.36 | 84 | 11 | 3 | 3 | 0 | 0 | 0.07 | 0.21 | 3.03 | 0.33 | 0.41 | 10.2 | 1.04 | 0.0 | 0.3 | | 19 | 0.1 | 1.8 | 20 | 0.0 | 177 | 267 | | 75 | 3.02 |
| 16084 | 3 oz | Back, rstd | 85 | 207 | 58 | 22.6 | 0.0 | 0.0 | 0.0 | 0.0 | 12.2 | 3.6 | 4.3 | 3.1 | 0.20 | 2.90 | 77 | 0 | 0 | 0 | 0 | 0 | 0.05 | 0.19 | 2.93 | 0.26 | 0.29 | 6.8 | 0.91 | 0.0 | 0.3 | | 28 | 0.1 | 1.9 | 19 | 0.0 | 161 | 221 | | 62 | 3.33 |
| 16085 | 4 oz | Breast, raw | 113 | 177 | 70 | 24.7 | 0.0 | 0.0 | 0.0 | 0.0 | 7.9 | 2.2 | 3.0 | 1.9 | 0.11 | 1.69 | 73 | 7 | 2 | 2 | 0 | 0 | 0.07 | 0.13 | 5.88 | 0.54 | 0.47 | 7.9 | 0.70 | 0.0 | 0.3 | | 15 | 0.1 | 1.4 | 27 | 0.0 | 210 | 311 | 11.3 | 67 | 1.77 |
| 16086 | 3 oz | Breast, rstd | 85 | 161 | 63 | 24.4 | 0.0 | 0.0 | 0.0 | 0.0 | 6.3 | 1.8 | 2.1 | 1.5 | 0.09 | 1.37 | 63 | 0 | 0 | 0 | 0 | 0 | 0.05 | 0.11 | 5.41 | 0.41 | 0.31 | 5.1 | 0.54 | 0.0 | 0.3 | | 18 | 0.0 | 1.2 | 23 | 0.0 | 179 | 245 | | 54 | 1.73 |
| 16050 | 3 oz | Canned, in broth | 85 | 139 | 66 | 20.1 | 0.0 | 0.0 | 0.0 | 0.0 | 5.8 | 1.7 | 1.9 | 1.5 | 0.09 | 1.36 | 56 | 0 | 0 | 0 | 0 | 0 | 0.01 | 0.15 | 5.63 | 0.28 | 0.24 | 5.1 | 0.58 | 1.7 | 0.3 | | 10 | 0.1 | 1.6 | 17 | 0.0 | 138 | 190 | | 397 | 2.01 |
| 16275 | 3 oz | Canned, premium chunk, in water, Swanson | 85 | 137 | 64 | 20.6 | 2.7 | 0.0 | 0.0 | 2.7 | 5.5 | 1.4 | | | | | 69 | 0 | 0 | 0 | 0 | 0 | | | | | | | | 0.0 | | | 0 | | 1.0 | | | | | | 315 | |
| 16003 | 3 oz | Ground, ckd | 85 | 200 | 59 | 23.3 | 0.0 | 0.0 | 0.0 | 0.0 | 11.2 | 2.9 | 4.2 | 2.7 | 0.15 | 2.58 | 87 | 0 | 0 | 0 | 0 | 0 | 0.05 | 0.14 | 4.10 | 0.33 | 0.28 | 6.0 | 0.69 | 0.0 | 0.3 | | 21 | 0.1 | 1.6 | 20 | 0.0 | 167 | 230 | 35.9 | 91 | 2.43 |
| 16157 | 4 oz | Ground, raw | 113 | 168 | 72 | 19.8 | 0.0 | 0.0 | 0.0 | 0.0 | 9.3 | 2.5 | 3.5 | 2.3 | 0.11 | 2.14 | 89 | 6 | 2 | 2 | 0 | 0 | 0.06 | 0.15 | 3.94 | 0.40 | 0.38 | 7.9 | 0.78 | 0.0 | 0.3 | | 15 | 0.1 | 1.4 | 21 | 0.0 | 176 | 263 | | 106 | 2.18 |
| 16087 | 4 oz | Leg, raw | 113 | 163 | 73 | 22.0 | 0.0 | 0.0 | 0.0 | 0.0 | 7.6 | 2.3 | 2.3 | 2.1 | 0.12 | 1.91 | 80 | 3 | 1 | 1 | 0 | 0 | 0.09 | 0.24 | 3.33 | 0.38 | 0.44 | 11.3 | 1.23 | 0.0 | 0.3 | | 19 | 0.2 | 1.9 | 24 | 0.0 | 200 | 308 | 17.0 | 84 | 3.49 |
| 16159 | 3 oz | Leg, rstd | 85 | 177 | 61 | 23.7 | 0.0 | 0.0 | 0.0 | 0.0 | 8.3 | 2.6 | 2.4 | 2.3 | 0.14 | 2.13 | 72 | 0 | 0 | 0 | 0 | 0 | 0.05 | 0.20 | 3.03 | 0.28 | 0.31 | 7.7 | 1.03 | 0.0 | 0.3 | | 27 | 0.1 | 2.0 | 20 | 0.0 | 169 | 238 | 2.9 | 65 | 3.63 |
| 16078 | 3 oz | Neck, ckd, w/o skin | 85 | 153 | 65 | 22.8 | 0.0 | 0.0 | 0.0 | 0.0 | 6.2 | 2.1 | 1.4 | 1.9 | 0.11 | 1.71 | 104 | 0 | 0 | 0 | 0 | 0 | 0.03 | 0.16 | 1.45 | 0.18 | 0.20 | 6.8 | 0.60 | 0.0 | 0.3 | | 31 | 0.1 | 2.0 | 13 | 0.0 | 104 | 127 | 32.8 | 48 | 6.05 |
| 16077 | 4 oz | Neck, raw, w/o skin | 113 | 153 | 73 | 22.7 | 0.0 | 0.0 | 0.0 | 0.0 | 6.1 | 2.1 | 1.4 | 1.8 | 0.10 | 1.71 | 89 | 0 | 0 | 0 | 0 | 0 | 0.10 | 0.26 | 3.58 | 0.42 | 0.46 | 12.4 | 1.20 | 0.0 | 0.3 | | 38 | 0.2 | 2.3 | 21 | 0.0 | 210 | 341 | | 105 | 5.74 |
| | | Whole, w/o giblets or neck | | | | | | | | | | | | | | | | | | | | | | | | | | | | | | | | | | | | | | | | |
| 16080 | 4 oz | Dark Meat, raw | 113 | 181 | 71 | 21.4 | 0.0 | 0.0 | 0.0 | 0.0 | 9.9 | 2.9 | 3.4 | 2.6 | 0.16 | 2.37 | 81 | 6 | 2 | 2 | 0 | 0 | 0.08 | 0.23 | 3.23 | 0.36 | 0.43 | 11.3 | 1.16 | 0.0 | 0.3 | | 19 | 0.2 | 1.9 | 23 | 0.0 | 192 | 295 | 17.0 | 80 | 3.33 |

| Code | Amount | Description | Basic Components | | | | | | | | | Additional Fats | | | | | | Vit A & Components | | | | | Vitamins | | | | | | | | | | Minerals | | | | | | | | | |
|---|---|---|---|---|---|---|---|---|---|---|---|---|---|---|---|---|---|---|---|---|---|---|---|---|---|---|---|---|---|---|---|---|---|---|---|---|---|---|---|---|---|---|
| | | | Weight (g) | Calories | % Water | Protein (g) | Carbs (g) | Fiber (g) | Sugar (g) | Other Carbs (g) | Fat (g) | Sat Fat (g) | Mono Fat (g) | Poly Fat (g) | Omega 3 (g) | Omega 6 (g) | Choles (mg) | Vit A (IU) | Vit A (RE) | Retinol (RE) | Carotenoids (RE) | Beta Carotene (mcg) | Thiamin (mg) | Riboflavin (mg) | Niacin (NE) | Vit B6 (mg) | Vit B12 (mcg) | Folate (mcg) | Panto (mg) | Vit C (mg) | Vit D (mg) | Vit E (α TE) | Calcium (mg) | Copper (mg) | Iron (mg) | Magnes (mg) | Mang (mg) | Phos (mg) | Potassium (mg) | Selenium (mcg) | Sodium (mg) | Zinc (mg) |
| 16082 | 4 oz | Dark Meat, raw, w/o skin | 113 | 141 | 74 | 22.7 | 0.0 | 0.0 | 0.0 | 0.0 | 4.9 | 1.7 | 1.1 | 1.5 | 0.08 | 1.38 | 78 | 0 | 0 | 0 | 0 | 0 | 0.09 | 0.25 | 3.48 | 0.41 | 0.45 | 12.4 | 1.31 | 0.0 | 0.3 | | 19 | 0.2 | 2.0 | 25 | 0.0 | 208 | 323 | 17.0 | 87 | 3.64 |
| 16028 | 3 oz | Dark Meat, rstd | 85 | 188 | 60 | 23.4 | 0.0 | 0.0 | 0.0 | 0.0 | 9.8 | 3.0 | 3.1 | 2.6 | 0.16 | 2.42 | 76 | 0 | 0 | 0 | 0 | 0 | 0.05 | 0.20 | 3.00 | 0.27 | 0.31 | 7.7 | 0.99 | 0.0 | 0.3 | | 28 | 0.1 | 1.9 | 20 | 0.0 | 167 | 233 | | 65 | 3.54 |
| 16002 | 3 oz | Dark Meat, rstd, w/o skin | 85 | 159 | 63 | 24.3 | 0.0 | 0.0 | 0.0 | 0.0 | 6.1 | 2.1 | 1.4 | 1.8 | 0.11 | 1.69 | 72 | 0 | 0 | 0 | 0 | 0 | 0.05 | 0.21 | 3.10 | 0.31 | 0.31 | 7.7 | 1.10 | 0.0 | 0.3 | | 27 | 0.1 | 2.0 | 20 | 0.0 | 173 | 247 | 34.8 | 67 | 3.79 |
| 16079 | 4 oz | Light Meat, raw | 113 | 180 | 70 | 24.4 | 0.0 | 0.0 | 0.0 | 0.0 | 8.3 | 2.3 | 3.2 | 2.0 | 0.12 | 1.77 | 73 | 7 | 2 | 2 | 0 | 0 | 0.06 | 0.13 | 5.81 | 0.54 | 0.47 | 7.9 | 0.69 | 0.0 | 0.3 | | 15 | 0.1 | 1.4 | 27 | 0.0 | 208 | 306 | 11.3 | 67 | 1.77 |
| 16081 | 4 oz | Light Meat, raw, w/o skin | 113 | 130 | 74 | 26.7 | 0.0 | 0.0 | 0.0 | 0.0 | 1.8 | 0.6 | 0.3 | 0.5 | 0.03 | 0.40 | 68 | 0 | 0 | 0 | 0 | 0 | 0.07 | 0.14 | 6.60 | 0.63 | 0.51 | 9.0 | 0.78 | 0.0 | 0.3 | | 14 | 0.1 | 1.3 | 31 | 0.0 | 231 | 345 | 11.3 | 71 | 1.83 |
| 16027 | 3 oz | Light Meat, rstd | 85 | 167 | 63 | 24.3 | 0.0 | 0.0 | 0.0 | 0.0 | 7.1 | 2.0 | 2.4 | 1.7 | 0.11 | 1.53 | 65 | 0 | 0 | 0 | 0 | 0 | 0.05 | 0.11 | 5.35 | 0.40 | 0.30 | 5.1 | 0.53 | 0.0 | 0.3 | | 18 | 0.0 | 1.2 | 22 | 0.0 | 177 | 242 | | 54 | 1.73 |
| 16158 | 3 oz | Light Meat, rstd, w/o skin | 85 | 133 | 66 | 25.4 | 0.0 | 0.0 | 0.0 | 0.0 | 2.7 | 0.9 | 0.5 | 0.7 | 0.03 | 0.63 | 59 | 0 | 0 | 0 | 0 | 0 | 0.05 | 0.11 | 5.81 | 0.46 | 0.31 | 5.1 | 0.58 | 0.0 | 0.3 | | 16 | 0.0 | 1.1 | 24 | 0.0 | 186 | 259 | 27.3 | 54 | 1.73 |
| 16068 | 4 oz | Raw | 113 | 181 | 70 | 23.1 | 0.0 | 0.0 | 0.0 | 0.0 | 9.1 | 2.6 | 3.3 | 2.2 | 0.15 | 2.05 | 77 | 7 | 2 | 2 | 0 | 0 | 0.07 | 0.18 | 4.62 | 0.46 | 0.45 | 9.0 | 0.91 | 0.0 | 0.3 | | 17 | 0.1 | 1.6 | 25 | 0.0 | 201 | 301 | | 73 | 2.49 |
| 16069 | 4 oz | Raw, w/o skin | 113 | 134 | 74 | 24.6 | 0.0 | 0.0 | 0.0 | 0.0 | 3.2 | 1.1 | 0.7 | 0.9 | 0.05 | 0.86 | 73 | 0 | 0 | 0 | 0 | 0 | 0.08 | 0.19 | 5.13 | 0.53 | 0.49 | 10.2 | 1.02 | 0.0 | 0.3 | | 16 | 0.1 | 1.6 | 28 | 0.0 | 220 | 334 | | 79 | 2.68 |
| 16026 | 3 oz | Roasted | 85 | 177 | 62 | 23.9 | 0.0 | 0.0 | 0.0 | 0.0 | 8.3 | 2.4 | 2.7 | 2.1 | 0.13 | 1.92 | 70 | 0 | 0 | 0 | 0 | 0 | 0.05 | 0.15 | 4.33 | 0.35 | 0.30 | 6.0 | 0.73 | 0.0 | 0.3 | | 22 | 0.1 | 1.5 | 21 | 0.0 | 173 | 238 | | 58 | 2.52 |
| 16000 | 3 oz | Roasted, w/o skin | 85 | 145 | 65 | 24.9 | 0.0 | 0.0 | 0.0 | 0.0 | 4.2 | 1.4 | 0.9 | 1.2 | 0.07 | 1.10 | 65 | 0 | 0 | 0 | 0 | 0 | 0.05 | 0.15 | 4.62 | 0.39 | 0.31 | 6.0 | 0.80 | 0.0 | 0.3 | | 21 | 0.1 | 1.5 | 22 | 0.0 | 181 | 253 | 31.0 | 60 | 2.63 |
| 16070 | 4 oz | Skin, raw | 113 | 437 | 50 | 14.4 | 0.0 | 0.0 | 0.0 | 0.0 | 41.7 | 10.3 | 17.7 | 9.5 | 0.64 | 8.75 | 103 | 43 | 14 | 14 | 0 | 0 | 0.02 | 0.09 | 1.67 | 0.08 | 0.27 | 4.5 | 0.29 | 0.0 | 0.3 | | 20 | 0.1 | 1.5 | 9 | 0.0 | 93 | 115 | | 41 | 1.44 |
| 16071 | 3 oz | Skin, rstd | 85 | 376 | 40 | 16.7 | 0.0 | 0.0 | 0.0 | 0.0 | 33.7 | 8.3 | 14.4 | 7.7 | 0.52 | 7.07 | 96 | 0 | 0 | 0 | 0 | 0 | 0.02 | 0.12 | 2.26 | 0.07 | 0.20 | 3.4 | 0.26 | 0.0 | | | 30 | 0.1 | 1.5 | 14 | 0.0 | 116 | 136 | | 45 | 1.76 |
| 16088 | 4 oz | Wing, raw | 113 | 223 | 66 | 22.8 | 0.0 | 0.0 | 0.0 | 0.0 | 13.9 | 3.7 | 5.6 | 3.2 | 0.21 | 2.95 | 79 | 12 | 3 | 3 | 0 | 0 | 0.06 | 0.12 | 5.01 | 0.46 | 0.44 | 7.9 | 0.63 | 0.0 | 0.3 | | 16 | 0.1 | 1.4 | 24 | 0.0 | 186 | 271 | 17.0 | 62 | 1.74 |
| 16089 | 3 oz | Wing, rstd | 85 | 195 | 60 | 23.3 | 0.0 | 0.0 | 0.0 | 0.0 | 10.5 | 2.9 | 4.0 | 2.5 | 0.16 | 2.25 | 69 | 0 | 0 | 0 | 0 | 0 | 0.04 | 0.11 | 4.87 | 0.36 | 0.29 | 5.1 | 0.50 | 0.0 | 0.3 | | 20 | 0.0 | 1.2 | 21 | 0.0 | 167 | 226 | | 52 | 1.78 |
| | | *DUCK, EMU, OSTRICH AND OTHER - BONELESS* | | | | | | | | | | | | | | | | | | | | | | | | | | | | | | | | | | | | | | | | |
| | | Cornish Game Hen | | | | | | | | | | | | | | | | | | | | | | | | | | | | | | | | | | | | | | | | |
| 15241 | 4 oz | Raw | 113 | 131 | 76 | 22.6 | 0.0 | 0.0 | 0.0 | 0.0 | 3.8 | 1.0 | 1.2 | 0.9 | 0.06 | 0.85 | 103 | 85 | 25 | 25 | 0 | 0 | 0.10 | 0.24 | 7.62 | 0.44 | 0.45 | 3.4 | 0.72 | 0.7 | | | 14 | 0.1 | 0.8 | 24 | 0.0 | 181 | 304 | | 77 | 1.48 |
| 15242 | 3 oz | Roasted | 85 | 114 | 72 | 19.8 | 0.0 | 0.0 | 0.0 | 0.0 | 3.3 | 0.8 | 1.1 | 0.8 | 0.05 | 0.73 | 90 | 55 | 17 | 17 | 0 | 0 | 0.06 | 0.19 | 5.33 | 0.30 | 0.26 | 1.7 | 0.47 | 0.5 | | | 11 | 0.1 | 0.7 | 16 | 0.0 | 127 | 213 | | 54 | 1.30 |
| 15070 | 3 oz | Roasted, w/o skin | 85 | 161 | 63 | 24.4 | 0.0 | 0.0 | 0.0 | 0.0 | 6.3 | 1.7 | 2.2 | 1.4 | 0.10 | 1.25 | 75 | 45 | 14 | 14 | 0 | 0 | 0.06 | 0.15 | 7.75 | 0.40 | 0.28 | 5.1 | 0.94 | 0.0 | 0.3 | | 13 | 0.1 | 1.0 | 21 | 0.0 | 165 | 206 | 25.3 | 259 | 1.77 |
| | | Duck | | | | | | | | | | | | | | | | | | | | | | | | | | | | | | | | | | | | | | | | |
| 16061 | 4 oz | Raw | 113 | 457 | 48 | 13.0 | 0.0 | 0.0 | 0.0 | 0.0 | 44.4 | 14.3 | 21.1 | 5.7 | 0.44 | 5.30 | 86 | 190 | 58 | 58 | 0 | 0 | 0.22 | 0.24 | 4.44 | 0.21 | 0.28 | 14.7 | 1.07 | 3.2 | 0.3 | | 12 | 0.3 | 2.7 | 17 | 0.0 | 157 | 236 | | 71 | 1.54 |
| 16062 | 4 oz | Raw, w/o skin | 113 | 149 | 74 | 20.7 | 0.0 | 0.0 | 0.0 | 0.0 | 6.7 | 2.5 | 1.7 | 0.8 | 0.09 | 0.76 | 87 | 89 | 27 | 27 | 0 | 0 | 0.41 | 0.51 | 5.99 | 0.38 | 0.45 | 28.3 | 1.81 | 6.6 | 0.3 | | 12 | 0.3 | 2.7 | 21 | 0.0 | 229 | 306 | | 84 | 2.15 |
| 14001 | 3 oz | Roasted | 85 | 286 | 52 | 16.1 | 0.0 | 0.0 | 0.0 | 0.0 | 24.1 | 8.2 | 11.0 | 3.1 | 0.25 | 2.86 | 71 | 179 | 54 | 54 | 0 | 0 | 0.15 | 0.23 | 4.11 | 0.15 | 0.26 | 5.1 | 0.94 | 0.0 | 0.3 | | 9 | 0.2 | 2.3 | 14 | 0.0 | 133 | 173 | 16.9 | 50 | 1.58 |
| 14000 | 3 oz | Roasted, w/o skin | 85 | 171 | 64 | 20.0 | 0.0 | 0.0 | 0.0 | 0.0 | 9.5 | 3.5 | 3.1 | 1.2 | 0.12 | 1.10 | 76 | 65 | 20 | 20 | 0 | 0 | 0.22 | 0.40 | 4.34 | 0.21 | 0.34 | 8.5 | 1.28 | 0.0 | 0.3 | | 10 | 0.2 | 2.3 | 17 | 0.0 | 173 | 214 | 16.9 | 55 | 2.21 |
| 16289 | 4 oz | Emu, thigh, raw, BK Emu Products | 113 | 105 | | 22.6 | | | | | 1.7 | | | | | | 55 | | | | | | | | | | | | | | | | | | 5.7 | | | | | | | |
| | | Goose | | | | | | | | | | | | | | | | | | | | | | | | | | | | | | | | | | | | | | | | |
| 16064 | 4 oz | Raw | 113 | 419 | 50 | 18.0 | 0.0 | 0.0 | 0.0 | 0.0 | 38.0 | 11.[illegible] | 20.1 | 4.2 | 0.24 | 3.72 | 90 | 62 | 9 | 19 | 0 | 0 | 0.10 | 0.28 | 4.08 | 0.44 | 0.38 | 4.5 | 1.46 | 4.7 | 0.3 | | 14 | 0.3 | 2.8 | 20 | 0.0 | 264 | 348 | | 32 | 1.94 |
| 16065 | 4 oz | Raw, w/o skin | 113 | 182 | 68 | 25.8 | 0.0 | 0.0 | 0.0 | 0.0 | 8.1 | 3.2 | 2.1 | 1.0 | 0.11 | 0.90 | 95 | 45 | 4 | 14 | 0 | 0 | 0.15 | 0.43 | 4.84 | 0.72 | 0.55 | 35.0 | 2.23 | 8.1 | 0.3 | | 15 | 0.3 | 2.9 | 27 | 0.0 | 353 | 475 | | 38 | 2.64 |
| 14003 | 3 oz | Roasted | 85 | 259 | 52 | 21.4 | 0.0 | 0.0 | 0.0 | 0.0 | 18.6 | 5.3 | 8.8 | 2.1 | 0.15 | 1.90 | 77 | 60 | 8 | 18 | 0 | 0 | 0.07 | 0.27 | 3.54 | 0.31 | 0.35 | 1.7 | 1.30 | 0.0 | 0.3 | | 11 | 0.2 | 2.4 | 19 | 0.0 | 230 | 280 | 17.0 | 60 | 2.23 |
| 14002 | 3 oz | Roasted, w/o skin | 85 | 202 | 57 | 24.7 | 0.0 | 0.0 | 0.0 | 0.0 | 10.8 | 3.3 | 3.7 | 1.3 | 0.13 | 1.16 | 82 | 34 | 0 | 10 | 0 | 0 | 0.08 | 0.33 | 3.47 | 0.40 | 0.42 | 10.2 | 1.56 | 0.0 | 0.3 | | 12 | 0.2 | 2.4 | 21 | 0.0 | 263 | 330 | 17.0 | 65 | 2.69 |
| 14034 | 4 oz | Guinea Hen, raw | 113 | 179 | 69 | 26.4 | 0.0 | 0.0 | 0.0 | 0.0 | 7.3 | 2.0 | 2.7 | 1.6 | 0.10 | 1.42 | 84 | 104 | 32 | 32 | 0 | 0 | 0.07 | 0.12 | 8.67 | 0.43 | 0.38 | 5.7 | 0.99 | 1.5 | 0.3 | | 12 | 0.0 | 0.9 | 25 | 0.0 | 173 | 218 | | 76 | 1.28 |
| 14035 | 4 oz | Guinea Hen, raw, w/o skin | 113 | 124 | 74 | 23.3 | 0.0 | 0.0 | 0.0 | 0.0 | 2.8 | 0.7 | 0.8 | 0.7 | 0.07 | 0.53 | 71 | 46 | 4 | 14 | 0 | 0 | 0.08 | 0.13 | 9.92 | 0.53 | 0.42 | 6.8 | 1.06 | 1.9 | 0.3 | | 12 | 0.0 | 0.9 | 27 | 0.0 | 191 | 249 | | 78 | 1.36 |
| | | Ostrich, American Ostrich Assoc. | | | | | | | | | | | | | | | | | | | | | | | | | | | | | | | | | | | | | | | | |
| 16326 | 3 oz | Fan Cut, ckd | 85 | 114 | 68 | 21.7 | 0.0 | 0.0 | 0.0 | 0.0 | 2.3 | 0.7 | 1.0 | 0.6 | 0.03 | 0.51 | 65 | | | | | | | | | | | | | | | | | | 2.4 | | | | | | 53 | |
| 16325 | 4 oz | Fan Cut, raw | 113 | 132 | 76 | 24.7 | 0.0 | 0.0 | 0.0 | 0.0 | 3.0 | 1.0 | 1.2 | 0.8 | 0.05 | 0.66 | 82 | | | | | | | | | | | | | | | | 6 | 0.1 | 4.9 | 25 | 0.1 | 240 | 303 | | 85 | 2.25 |
| 16314 | 3 oz | Inside Leg, ckd | 85 | 120 | 70 | 24.7 | 0.0 | 0.0 | 0.0 | 0.0 | 1.6 | 0.5 | 0.6 | 0.5 | 0.13 | 0.38 | 62 | | | | | | | | | | | | | | | | 5 | | 2.7 | | | | | | 71 | |
| 16313 | 4 oz | Inside Leg, raw | 113 | 125 | 76 | 25.3 | 0.0 | 0.0 | 0.0 | 0.0 | 1.9 | 0.5 | 0.7 | 0.6 | 0.16 | 0.46 | 75 | | | | | | | | | | | | | | | | 6 | 0.1 | 2.6 | 25 | 0.1 | 240 | 303 | | 81 | 2.25 |
| 16330 | 3 oz | Inside Strip, ckd | 85 | 139 | 67 | 25.0 | 0.0 | 0.0 | 0.0 | 0.0 | 3.6 | 1.2 | 1.3 | 1.2 | 0.28 | 0.85 | 82 | | | | | | | | | | | | | | | | 4 | | 4.1 | | | | | | 62 | |
| 16329 | 4 oz | Inside Strip, raw | 113 | 138 | 75 | 24.8 | 0.0 | 0.0 | 0.0 | 0.0 | 3.5 | 1.1 | 1.2 | 1.1 | 0.27 | 0.81 | 86 | | | | | | | | | | | | | | | | 6 | 0.1 | 4.7 | 25 | 0.1 | 236 | 298 | | 86 | 2.21 |
| 16316 | 3 oz | Outside Leg, ckd | 85 | 111 | 68 | 22.4 | 0.0 | 0.0 | 0.0 | 0.0 | 1.8 | 0.5 | 0.7 | 0.6 | 0.02 | 0.46 | 65 | | | | | | | | | | | | | | | | | | 2.6 | | | | | | 72 | |
| 16315 | 4 oz | Outside Leg, raw | 113 | 130 | 76 | 25.8 | 0.0 | 0.0 | 0.0 | 0.0 | 2.2 | 0.7 | 0.8 | 0.8 | 0.03 | 0.60 | 73 | | | | | | | | | | | | | | | | 6 | 0.1 | 3.0 | 25 | 0.1 | 238 | 302 | | 102 | 2.24 |
| 16320 | 3 oz | Outside Strip, ckd | 85 | 133 | 67 | 24.3 | 0.0 | 0.0 | 0.0 | 0.0 | 3.3 | 1.1 | 1.1 | 1.0 | 0.26 | 0.77 | 79 | | | | | | | | | | | | | | | | 4 | | 3.7 | | | | | | 61 | |
| 16319 | 4 oz | Outside Strip, raw | 113 | 142 | 75 | 25.3 | 0.0 | 0.0 | 0.0 | 0.0 | 3.8 | 1.3 | 1.3 | 1.2 | 0.30 | 0.90 | 87 | | | | | | | | | | | | | | | | 6 | 0.1 | 4.2 | 25 | 0.1 | 236 | 298 | | 79 | 2.21 |
| 16324 | 3 oz | Oyster Cut, ckd | 85 | 132 | 68 | 24.5 | 0.0 | 0.0 | 0.0 | 0.0 | 3.0 | 1.0 | 1.1 | 1.0 | 0.24 | 0.70 | 77 | | | | | | | | | | | | | | | | 5 | | 4.2 | | | | | | 69 | |
| 16323 | 4 oz | Oyster Cut, raw | 113 | 141 | 76 | 24.4 | 0.0 | 0.0 | 0.0 | 0.0 | 4.1 | 1.4 | 1.5 | 1.3 | 0.33 | 0.97 | 82 | | | | | | | | | | | | | | | | 7 | 0.1 | 4.4 | 25 | 0.1 | 238 | 302 | | 94 | 2.24 |
| 16318 | 3 oz | Round Cut, ckd | 85 | 108 | 68 | 20.5 | 0.0 | 0.0 | 0.0 | 0.0 | 2.3 | 0.7 | 0.8 | 0.7 | 0.18 | 0.53 | 69 | | | | | | | | | | | | | | | | | | 2.4 | | | | | | 54 | |
| 16317 | 4 oz | Round Cut, raw | 113 | 131 | 76 | 24.8 | 0.0 | 0.0 | 0.0 | 0.0 | 2.7 | 0.9 | 0.9 | 0.9 | 0.22 | 0.63 | 80 | | | | | | | | | | | | | | | | 6 | 0.1 | 4.0 | 25 | 0.1 | 238 | 302 | | 81 | 2.24 |
| 16332 | 3 oz | Tenderloin, ckd | 85 | 113 | 66 | 19.8 | 0.0 | 0.0 | 0.0 | 0.0 | 3.2 | 1.0 | 1.2 | 1.0 | 0.08 | 0.83 | 81 | | | | | | | | | | | | | | | | | | 2.4 | | | | | | 61 | |
| 16331 | 4 oz | Tenderloin, raw | 113 | 139 | 74 | 24.9 | 0.0 | 0.0 | 0.0 | 0.0 | 3.5 | 1.1 | 1.4 | 1.0 | 0.05 | 0.84 | 90 | | | | | | | | | | | | | | | | 7 | 0.1 | 5.5 | 24 | 0.1 | 235 | 297 | | 97 | 2.20 |
| 16322 | 3 oz | Tip, trimmed, ckd | 85 | 123 | 69 | 24.2 | 0.0 | 0.0 | 0.0 | 0.0 | 2.2 | 0.7 | 0.8 | 0.7 | 0.17 | 0.51 | 72 | | | | | | | | | | | | | | | | 5 | | 2.4 | | | | | | 68 | |
| 16321 | 4 oz | Tip, trimmed, raw | 113 | 129 | 76 | 24.7 | 0.0 | 0.0 | 0.0 | 0.0 | 2.5 | 0.8 | 0.9 | 0.8 | 0.20 | 0.61 | 81 | | | | | | | | | | | | | | | | 6 | 0.1 | 3.2 | 25 | 0.1 | 241 | 303 | | 76 | 2.26 |
| 16328 | 3 oz | Top Loin, ckd | 85 | 132 | 68 | 23.9 | 0.0 | 0.0 | 0.0 | 0.0 | 3.3 | 1.1 | 1.2 | 1.0 | 0.25 | 0.76 | 79 | | | | | | | | | | | | | | | | 5 | | 2.8 | | | | | | 65 | |
| 16327 | 4 oz | Top Loin, raw | 113 | 134 | 75 | 24.5 | 0.0 | 0.0 | 0.0 | 0.0 | 3.3 | 1.1 | 1.2 | 1.1 | 0.25 | 0.78 | 85 | | | | | | | | | | | | | | | | 7 | 0.1 | 3.5 | 25 | 0.1 | 237 | 301 | | 92 | 2.24 |
| 16022 | 4 oz | Pheasant, raw | 113 | 205 | 68 | 25.7 | 0.0 | 0.0 | 0.0 | 0.0 | 10.5 | 3.[illegible] | 4.9 | 1.3 | 0.11 | 0.92 | 80 | 200 | 60 | 50 | 0 | 0 | 0.03 | 0.16 | 7.27 | 0.75 | 0.87 | 6.8 | 1.05 | 6.0 | 0.3 | | 14 | 0.1 | 1.3 | 23 | 0.0 | 242 | 275 | 15.8 | 45 | 1.08 |
| 16023 | 4 oz | Pheasant, raw, w/o skin | 113 | 150 | 73 | 26.7 | 0.0 | 0.0 | 0.0 | 0.0 | 4.1 | 1.4 | 1.3 | 0.7 | 0.09 | 0.61 | 75 | 186 | 55 | 55 | 0 | 0 | 0.09 | 0.17 | 7.64 | 0.84 | 0.95 | 6.8 | 1.08 | 6.8 | 0.3 | | 15 | 0.1 | 1.3 | 23 | 0.0 | 260 | 296 | 15.8 | 42 | 1.10 |
| 16013 | 4 oz | Quail, raw | 113 | 217 | 70 | 22.1 | 0.0 | 0.0 | 0.0 | 0.0 | 13.7 | 3.8 | 4.7 | 3.4 | 0.49 | 2.76 | 86 | 275 | 82 | 32 | 0 | 0 | 0.23 | 0.29 | 8.52 | 0.68 | 0.49 | 9.0 | 0.87 | 6.9 | 0.3 | | 15 | 0.6 | 4.5 | 26 | 0.0 | 311 | 244 | | 60 | 2.73 |
| 16014 | 4 oz | Quail, raw, w/o skin | 113 | 151 | 70 | 24.6 | 0.0 | 0.0 | 0.0 | 0.0 | 5.1 | 1.5 | 1.4 | 1.3 | 0.08 | 1.19 | 79 | 64 | 19 | 19 | 0 | 0 | 0.32 | 0.32 | 9.27 | 0.60 | 0.53 | 7.9 | 0.89 | 8.1 | 0.3 | | 15 | 0.7 | 5.1 | 28 | 0.0 | 347 | 268 | | 58 | 3.05 |
| 16016 | 4 oz | Squab/Pigeon, raw | 113 | 332 | 57 | 20.9 | 0.0 | 0.0 | 0.0 | 0.0 | 26.9 | 9.5 | 11.0 | 3.5 | 0.08 | 3.20 | 107 | 275 | 82 | 32 | 0 | 0 | 0.24 | 0.25 | 6.84 | 0.46 | 0.45 | 6.8 | 0.86 | 5.9 | 0.3 | | 14 | 0.5 | 4.0 | 25 | 0.0 | 280 | 225 | | 61 | 2.49 |
| 16017 | 4 oz | Squab/Pigeon, raw, w/o skin | 113 | 160 | 73 | 19.8 | 0.0 | 0.0 | 0.0 | 0.0 | 8.5 | 2.2 | 3.0 | 1.8 | 0.05 | 1.41 | 102 | 106 | 32 | 32 | 0 | 0 | 0.32 | 0.32 | 7.75 | 0.60 | 0.53 | 7.9 | 0.89 | 8.1 | 0.3 | | 15 | 0.7 | 5.1 | 28 | 0.0 | 347 | 268 | | 58 | 3.05 |
| | | **SALAD DRESSINGS, DIPS AND MAYONNAISE** | | | | | | | | | | | | | | | | | | | | | | | | | | | | | | | | | | | | | | | | |
| | | *DIPS* | | | | | | | | | | | | | | | | | | | | | | | | | | | | | | | | | | | | | | | | |
| 27132 | 1 Tbs | Avocado, Kraft | 16 | 30 | 71 | 0.5 | 2.0 | 0.0 | 0.3 | 1.8 | 2.0 | 1.5 | | | | | 0 | 0 | 0 | 0 | 0 | 0 | | | | | | | | 0.0 | | | 0 | | 0.0 | | | | 12 | | 120 | |
| 8512 | 1 Tbs | Bacon & Horseradish, Kraft | 16 | 26 | | 0.5 | 1.0 | 0.0 | 0.3 | 0.8 | 2.6 | 1.5 | | | | | 8 | 52 | 10 | | | | | | | | | | | 0.0 | | | 10 | | 0.0 | | | | 21 | | 103 | |
| 8513 | 1 Tbs | Bacon & Onion, Kraft | 16 | 31 | | 0.5 | 1.0 | 0.0 | 0.3 | 0.8 | 2.6 | 1.5 | | | | | 8 | 52 | 10 | | | | | | | | | | | 0.0 | | | 10 | | 0.0 | | | | 26 | | 83 | |
| 27139 | 1 Tbs | Bacon Ranch, Marie's | 14 | 75 | 17 | 0.5 | 1.5 | 0.0 | 0.5 | 1.0 | 8.0 | 1.0 | | | | | 8 | 0 | 0 | 0 | 0 | 0 | | | | | | | | 0.0 | | | 0 | | 0.0 | | | | | | 100 | |
| 27140 | 1 Tbs | Bean, Marie's | 14 | 70 | 38 | 0.3 | 1.0 | 0.3 | 0.3 | 0.5 | 7.0 | 1.0 | | | | | 5 | 50 | 10 | | | | | | | | | | | 0.0 | | | 0 | | 0.2 | | | | | | 80 | |
| 8514 | 1 Tbs | Blue Cheese, Kraft | 16 | 23 | | 0.5 | 1.0 | 0.0 | 0.3 | 0.8 | 2.1 | 1.3 | | | | | 5 | 52 | 10 | | | | | | | | | | | 0.0 | | | 21 | | 0.0 | | | | 13 | | 103 | |
| 8515 | 1 Tbs | Clam, Kraft | 16 | 23 | | 0.5 | 1.0 | 0.0 | 0.3 | 0.8 | 2.1 | 1.3 | | | | | 5 | 52 | 10 | | | | | | | | | | | 0.0 | | | 10 | | 0.0 | | | | 18 | | 108 | |
| 8516 | 1 Tbs | Cucumber, Kraft | 16 | 26 | | 0.3 | 1.0 | 0.0 | 0.5 | 0.5 | 2.1 | 1.5 | | | | | 8 | 52 | 10 | | | | | | | | | | | 0.0 | | | 10 | | 0.0 | | | | 21 | | 72 | |

| Code | Amount | Description | Basic Components | | | | | | | | | Additional Fats | | | | | | Vit A & Components | | | | | Vitamins | | | | | | | | | | Minerals | | | | | | | | | |
|---|---|---|---|---|---|---|---|---|---|---|---|---|---|---|---|---|---|---|---|---|---|---|---|---|---|---|---|---|---|---|---|---|---|---|---|---|---|---|---|---|---|---|
| | | | Weight (g) | Calories | % Water | Protein (g) | Carbs (g) | Fiber (g) | Sugar (g) | Other Carbs (g) | Fat (g) | Sat Fat (g) | Mono Fat (g) | Poly Fat (g) | Omega 3 (g) | Omega 6 (g) | Choles (mg) | Vit A (IU) | Vit A (RE) | Retinol (RE) | Carotenoids (RE) | Beta Carotene (mcg) | Thiamin (mg) | Riboflavin (mg) | Niacin (NE) | Vit B6 (mg) | Vit B12 (mcg) | Folate (mcg) | Panto (mg) | Vit C (mg) | Vit D (mg) | Vit E (α TE) | Calcium (mg) | Copper (mg) | Iron (mg) | Magnes (mg) | Mang (mg) | Phos (mg) | Potassium (mg) | Selenium (mcg) | Sodium (mg) | Zinc (mg) |
| 8518 | 1 Tbs | French Onion, Kraft | 16 | 26 | 78 | 0.3 | 1.0 | 0.0 | 0.3 | 0.8 | 2.1 | 1.3 | | | | | 5 | 52 | 10 | | | | | | | | | | | 0.0 | | | 10 | | 0.0 | | | | 21 | | 83 | |
| 27136 | 1 Tbs | Green Onion, Kraft | 16 | 31 | 70 | 0.5 | 2.1 | 0.0 | 0.3 | 1.8 | 2.1 | 1.5 | | | | | 0 | 0 | 0 | 0 | 0 | 0 | | | | | | | | 0.0 | | | 0 | | 0.0 | | | | 10 | | 98 | |
| 8519 | 1 Tbs | Jalapeno Cheese, Kraft | 16 | 30 | 72 | 1.0 | 0.5 | 0.0 | 0.0 | 0.5 | 2.5 | 1.5 | | | | | 8 | 100 | 20 | | | | | | | | | | | 0.0 | | | 30 | | 0.0 | | | | 12 | | 125 | |
| 8520 | 1 Tbs | Nacho Cheese, Kraft | 16 | 30 | 68 | 1.0 | 1.0 | 0.0 | 0.3 | 0.8 | 2.5 | 1.5 | | | | | 8 | 100 | 20 | | | | | | | | | | | 0.0 | | | 40 | | 0.0 | | | | 18 | | 135 | |
| 8517 | 1 Tbs | Onion, Kraft | 16 | 23 | 78 | 0.3 | 1.0 | 0.0 | 0.3 | 0.8 | 2.1 | 1.3 | | | | | 5 | 52 | 10 | | | | | | | | | | | 0.0 | | | 10 | | 0.0 | | | | 21 | | 83 | |
| 27142 | 1 Tbs | Parmesan Garlic, Marie's | 14 | 70 | 38 | 0.3 | 1.0 | 0.3 | 0.3 | 0.5 | 7.0 | 1.0 | | | | | 5 | 50 | 10 | | | | | | | | | | | 0.6 | | | 0 | | 0.2 | | | | | | 70 | |
| 27141 | 1 Tbs | Ranch, Marie's | 14 | 75 | 24 | 0.0 | 1.5 | 0.0 | 0.5 | 1.0 | 7.5 | 1.0 | | | | | 8 | 50 | 10 | | | | | | | | | | | 0.0 | | | 0 | | 0.2 | | | | | | 70 | |
| | | Sour Cream | | | | | | | | | | | | | | | | | | | | | | | | | | | | | | | | | | | | | | | | |
| 8136 | 1 Tbs | Average | 15 | 33 | 66 | 0.6 | 1.2 | 0.1 | 0.8 | 0.3 | 3.0 | 1.8 | 0.9 | 0.1 | | | 6 | 109 | 27 | 24 | 3 | | 0.01 | 0.03 | 0.07 | 0.00 | 0.04 | 1.7 | 0.05 | 0.1 | 0.0 | | 18 | 0.0 | 0.0 | 2 | 0.0 | 16 | 28 | | 112 | 0.04 |
| 8522 | 1 Tbs | Bacon, Knudsen | 16 | 31 | 72 | 0.5 | 1.0 | 0.0 | 0.5 | 0.5 | 2.6 | 1.5 | | | | | 10 | 52 | 10 | | | | | | | | | | | 0.0 | | | 10 | | 0.0 | | | | 23 | | 88 | |
| 8507 | 1 Tbs | Bacon & Onion, Breakstone's | 16 | 31 | 72 | 0.5 | 1.0 | 0.0 | 0.5 | 0.5 | 2.6 | 1.5 | | | | | 10 | 52 | 13 | | | | | | | | | | | 0.0 | | | | | 0.0 | | | | 23 | | 88 | |
| 8508 | 1 Tbs | Chesapeake Clam, Breakstone's | 16 | 26 | 75 | 0.5 | 1.0 | 0.0 | 0.5 | 0.5 | 2.1 | 1.3 | | | | | 15 | 52 | 13 | | | | | | | | | | | 0.0 | | | 10 | | 0.0 | | | | 18 | | 98 | |
| 8509 | 1 Tbs | French Onion, Breakstone's | 16 | 26 | 75 | 0.5 | 1.0 | 0.0 | 0.5 | 0.5 | 2.1 | 1.5 | | | | | 10 | 52 | 13 | | | | | | | | | | | 0.0 | | | 10 | | 0.0 | | | | 21 | | 83 | |
| 8523 | 1 Tbs | French Onion, Knudsen | 16 | 26 | 75 | 0.5 | 1.0 | 0.0 | 0.5 | 0.5 | 2.1 | 1.5 | | | | | 10 | 52 | 10 | | | | | | | | | | | 0.0 | | | 10 | | 0.0 | | | | | | 83 | |
| 8521 | 1 Tbs | French Onion, Sealtest | 16 | 26 | 75 | 0.5 | 1.0 | 0.0 | 0.5 | 0.5 | 2.1 | 1.5 | | | | | 10 | 52 | 10 | | | | | | | | | | | 0.0 | | | 10 | | 0.0 | | | | 21 | | 83 | |
| 8510 | 1 Tbs | Jalapeno Cheddar, Breakstone's | 16 | 31 | 75 | 0.5 | 1.0 | 0.0 | 0.5 | 0.5 | 2.1 | 1.5 | | | | | 8 | 52 | 13 | | | | | | | | | | | 0.0 | | | 21 | | 0.0 | | | | 28 | | 88 | |
| 8137 | 1 Tbs | Low Calorie, avg | 15 | 22 | 74 | 0.5 | 1.2 | 0.1 | 0.8 | 0.3 | 1.7 | 1.1 | 0.5 | 0.1 | | | 5 | 63 | 16 | 14 | 2 | | 0.01 | 0.03 | 0.07 | 0.00 | 0.04 | 1.7 | 0.05 | 0.1 | 0.0 | | 16 | 0.0 | 0.0 | 2 | 0.0 | 17 | 25 | | 106 | 0.08 |
| 8524 | 1 Tbs | Nacho Cheese, Knudsen | 16 | 31 | 68 | 1.0 | 1.5 | 0.0 | 1.0 | 0.5 | 2.1 | 1.5 | | | | | 8 | 52 | 10 | | | | | | | | | | | 0.0 | | | 21 | | 0.0 | | | | 31 | | 103 | |
| 8511 | 1 Tbs | Toasted Onion, Breakstone's | 16 | 26 | 75 | 0.5 | 1.0 | 0.0 | 0.5 | 0.5 | 2.1 | 1.5 | | | | | 10 | 52 | 13 | | | | | | | | | | | 0.0 | | | 10 | | 0.0 | | | | 21 | | 93 | |
| 27143 | 1 Tbs | Spinach, Marie's | 14 | 70 | | 0.0 | 1.5 | 0.0 | 0.3 | 1.3 | 7.0 | 1.0 | | | | | 5 | 200 | 40 | | | | | | | | | | | 0.0 | | | 0 | | 0.2 | | | | | | 100 | |
| 27144 | 1 Tbs | Sun Dried Tomato, Marie's | 14 | 70 | | 0.3 | 1.0 | 0.3 | 0.3 | 0.5 | 7.0 | 1.0 | | | | | 8 | 0 | 0 | 0 | 0 | 0 | | | | | | | | 0.0 | | | 0 | | 0.0 | | | | | | 68 | |
| | | *MAYONNAISES* | | | | | | | | | | | | | | | | | | | | | | | | | | | | | | | | | | | | | | | | |
| | | Mayonnaise | | | | | | | | | | | | | | | | | | | | | | | | | | | | | | | | | | | | | | | | |
| 8046 | 1 Tbs | Average | 14 | 100 | 15 | 0.2 | 0.4 | 0.0 | 0.3 | 0.1 | 11.1 | 1.7 | 3.2 | 5.8 | 0.59 | 5.19 | 8 | 39 | 12 | 11 | 1 | | 0.00 | 0.00 | 0.00 | 0.08 | 0.04 | 1.1 | 0.03 | 0.0 | 0.0 | | 3 | 0.0 | 0.1 | 0 | 0.0 | 4 | 5 | 0.2 | 80 | 0.02 |
| 8691 | 1 Tbs | Best Foods | 14 | 100 | 15 | 0.2 | 0.1 | 0.0 | | | 11.2 | 1.7 | 3.1 | 6.1 | | | 7 | 60 | 12 | | | | 0.00 | 0.00 | | 0.08 | | | | 0.0 | | | 2 | | 0.1 | | | | | | 80 | |
| 8069 | 1 Tbs | Fat Free, Kraft | 16 | 10 | 87 | 0.0 | 2.0 | 0.0 | 0.5 | 1.5 | 0.0 | 0.0 | 0.0 | 0.0 | 0.00 | 0.00 | 0 | 0 | 0 | 0 | 0 | 0 | | | | | | | | 0.0 | | | 0 | | 0.0 | | | | 5 | | 105 | |
| 8390 | 1 Tbs | Fat Free, Weight Watchers | 14 | 10 | 78 | 0.0 | 3.0 | 0.0 | 2.0 | 1.0 | 0.0 | 0.0 | 0.0 | 0.0 | 0.00 | 0.00 | 0 | 0 | 0 | 0 | 0 | 0 | | | | | | | | 0.0 | | | 0 | | 0.0 | | | | 10 | | 104 | |
| 8231 | 1 Tbs | Imitation, no choles, avg | 14 | 67 | 35 | 0.0 | 2.2 | 0.0 | | | 6.7 | 1.0 | 1.5 | 3.9 | 0.64 | 3.22 | 0 | 0 | 0 | 0 | 0 | 0 | 0.00 | 0.00 | 0.00 | 0.00 | 0.00 | 0.0 | 0.00 | 0.0 | | | 0 | 0.0 | 0.0 | 0 | | 0 | 1 | 0.2 | 49 | 0.02 |
| 8503 | 1 Tbs | Kraft | 14 | 100 | 6 | 0.0 | 0.0 | 0.0 | 0.0 | 0.0 | 11.0 | 2.0 | | | | | 10 | 0 | 0 | 0 | 0 | 0 | | | | | | | | 0.0 | | | 0 | | 0.0 | | | | 0 | | 75 | |
| 8501 | 1 Tbs | Light, Kraft | 15 | 50 | 59 | 0.0 | 1.0 | 0.0 | 0.0 | 1.0 | 5.0 | 1.0 | | | | | 0 | 0 | 0 | 0 | 0 | 0 | | | | | | | | 0.0 | | | 0 | | 0.0 | | | | 10 | | 110 | |
| 8148 | 1 Tbs | Light, low sod, avg | 14 | 32 | 63 | 0.0 | 2.2 | 0.0 | | | 2.7 | 0.5 | 0.6 | 1.4 | | | 3 | 4 | 1 | 0 | 1 | | 0.00 | 0.00 | 0.00 | 0.00 | 0.01 | 0.3 | | 0.0 | | | 0 | 0.0 | 0.0 | 0 | 0.0 | 0 | 1 | | 15 | 0.02 |
| 8387 | 1 Tbs | Light, low sod, Weight Watchers | 14 | 25 | 78 | 0.0 | 1.0 | 0.0 | 0.0 | 1.0 | 2.0 | 1.0 | | | 0.00 | 0.00 | 5 | 0 | 0 | 0 | 0 | 0 | | | | | | | | 0.0 | | | 0 | | 0.0 | | | | 15 | | 39 | |
| 8258 | 1 Tbs | Unsalted, avg | 14 | 100 | 17 | 0.2 | 0.4 | 0.0 | | | 11.1 | 1.7 | 3.2 | 5.2 | 0.53 | 4.67 | 8 | 39 | 12 | 11 | 1 | | 0.00 | 0.00 | 0.00 | 0.08 | 0.04 | 1.1 | 0.03 | 0.0 | 0.0 | 2.9 | 3 | | 0.1 | | | 4 | 5 | 0.2 | 4 | |
| | | Miracle Whip | | | | | | | | | | | | | | | | | | | | | | | | | | | | | | | | | | | | | | | | |
| 8500 | 1 Tbs | Fat Free, Kraft | 16 | 15 | 80 | 0.0 | 3.0 | 0.0 | 2.0 | 1.0 | 0.0 | 0.0 | 0.0 | 0.0 | 0.00 | 0.00 | 0 | 0 | 0 | 0 | 0 | 0 | | | | | | | | 0.0 | | | 0 | | 0.0 | | | | 5 | | 120 | |
| 8122 | 1 Tbs | Light, avg | 14 | 36 | 54 | 0.1 | 3.3 | 0.0 | | | 2.7 | 0.4 | 0.7 | 1.4 | | | 4 | 31 | 9 | 9 | 0 | 0 | 0.00 | 0.00 | 0.00 | 0.00 | 0.03 | 0.8 | | 0.0 | | | 2 | 0.0 | 0.0 | 0 | 0.0 | 4 | 1 | | 99 | 0.03 |
| 8502 | 1 Tbs | Light, Kraft | 15 | 40 | 59 | 0.0 | 3.0 | 0.0 | 2.0 | 1.0 | 3.0 | 0.0 | | | | | 0 | 0 | 0 | 0 | 0 | 0 | | | | | | | | 0.0 | | | 0 | | 0.0 | | | | 0 | | 120 | |
| 8479 | 1 Tbs | Regular, Kraft | 14 | 70 | 34 | 0.0 | 2.0 | 0.0 | 1.0 | 1.0 | 7.0 | 1.0 | | | | | 5 | 0 | 0 | 0 | 0 | 0 | | | | | | | | 0.0 | | | 0 | | 0.0 | | | 2 | 0 | | 85 | |
| | | *SALAD DRESSINGS – LOWER CALORIE* | | | | | | | | | | | | | | | | | | | | | | | | | | | | | | | | | | | | | | | | |
| 8147 | 1 Tbs | Bacon & Tomato, avg | 16 | 32 | 73 | 0.3 | 0.3 | 0.0 | | | 3.4 | 0.6 | 0.9 | 1.8 | | | 1 | 44 | 4 | 0 | 4 | | 0.01 | 0.00 | 0.11 | 0.01 | 0.01 | 0.0 | | 1.4 | | | 1 | 0.0 | 0.0 | 1 | 0.0 | 4 | 17 | | 173 | 0.03 |
| 8566 | 1 Tbs | Bacon & Tomato, Kraft | 16 | 31 | | 0.5 | 1.5 | 0.0 | 1.5 | 0.0 | 2.6 | 0.5 | | | | | 1 | 0 | 0 | 0 | 0 | 0 | | | | | | | | 0.0 | | | 0 | | 0.0 | | | | 21 | | 155 | |
| | | Blue Cheese/Roquefort | | | | | | | | | | | | | | | | | | | | | | | | | | | | | | | | | | | | | | | | |
| 8128 | 1 Tbs | Average | 15 | 15 | 80 | 0.8 | 0.4 | 0.0 | | | 1.1 | 0.2 | 0.5 | 0.4 | | | 0 | 2 | 0.5 | 0.5 | 0 | 0 | 0.00 | 0.02 | 0.01 | 0.00 | 0.03 | 0.5 | | 0.0 | | | 13 | 0.0 | 0.1 | 1 | 0.0 | 12 | 1 | | 180 | 0.04 |
| 8639 | 1 Tbs | Fat Free, avg | 15 | 18 | 72 | 0.5 | 3.5 | 0.0 | 0.5 | 3.0 | 0.0 | 0.0 | 0.0 | 0.0 | 0.00 | 0.00 | 0 | 0 | 0 | 0 | 0 | 0 | | | | | | | | 0.0 | | | 10 | | 0.0 | | | | | | 155 | |
| 8497 | 1 Tbs | Fat Free, Kraft | 18 | 26 | 61 | 0.3 | 6.2 | 0.5 | 1.5 | 4.1 | 0.0 | 0.0 | 0.0 | 0.0 | 0.00 | 0.00 | 0 | 0 | 0 | 0 | 0 | 0 | | | | | | | | 0.0 | | | 0 | | 0.0 | | | | 21 | | 175 | |
| 8537 | 1 Tbs | Marie's | 16 | 50 | 48 | 0.5 | 3.5 | 0.5 | 1.0 | 2.0 | 3.5 | 0.5 | | | | | 5 | 0 | 0 | 0 | 0 | 0 | | | | | | | | 0.0 | | | 20 | | 0.0 | | | | | | 125 | |
| 8431 | 1 Tbs | Wishbone | 15 | 40 | 65 | 0.5 | 1.0 | 0.0 | 0.5 | 0.5 | 3.5 | 0.8 | | | | | 0 | 0 | 0 | 0 | 0 | 0 | | | | | | | | 0.0 | | | 0 | | 0.0 | | | | | | 190 | |
| | | Caesar | | | | | | | | | | | | | | | | | | | | | | | | | | | | | | | | | | | | | | | | |
| 8138 | 1 Tbs | Average | 15 | 17 | 73 | 0.0 | 2.8 | 0.0 | | | 0.7 | 0.1 | 0.3 | 0.2 | | | 0 | 3 | 0.3 | 0 | 0.3 | | 0.00 | 0.00 | 0.01 | 0.00 | 0.00 | 0.3 | | 0.0 | 0.0 | | 4 | 0.0 | 0.0 | 0 | 0.0 | 3 | 4 | | 162 | 0.02 |
| 8400 | 1 Tbs | Fat free, Weight Watchers | 15 | 5 | 93 | 0.0 | 0.5 | 0.0 | 0.5 | 0.0 | 0.0 | 0.0 | 0.0 | 0.0 | 0.00 | 0.00 | 0 | 0 | 0 | 0 | 0 | 0 | | | | | | | | 0.0 | | | 0 | | 0.0 | | | | 12 | | 195 | |
| 8588 | 1 Tbs | Kraft | 16 | 31 | | 0.5 | 1.0 | 0.0 | 1.0 | 0.0 | 2.6 | 0.5 | | | | | 1 | 0 | 0 | 0 | 0 | 0 | | | | | | | | 0.0 | | | 10 | | 0.0 | | | | 5 | | 289 | |
| | | French | | | | | | | | | | | | | | | | | | | | | | | | | | | | | | | | | | | | | | | | |
| 8014 | 1 Tbs | Average | 16 | 21 | 69 | 0.0 | 3.5 | 0.0 | 3.1 | 0.3 | 0.9 | 0.1 | 0.2 | 0.5 | 0.06 | 0.48 | 0 | 208 | 21 | 0 | 21 | | 0.00 | 0.00 | 0.00 | 0.00 | 0.00 | 0.0 | 0.00 | 0.0 | 0.0 | 0.2 | 2 | 0.0 | 0.1 | 0 | 0.0 | 2 | 13 | 0.3 | 126 | 0.03 |
| 8613 | 1 Tbs | Catalina | 17 | 40 | | 0.0 | 4.5 | 0.0 | 3.5 | 1.0 | 2.0 | 0.3 | | | | | 0 | 250 | 50 | | | | | | | | | | | 0.0 | | | 0 | | 0.0 | | | | 38 | | 200 | |
| 8499 | 1 Tbs | Fat Free, Kraft | 18 | 21 | 65 | 0.0 | 6.2 | 0.3 | 2.6 | 3.3 | 0.0 | 0.0 | 0.0 | 0.0 | 0.00 | 0.00 | 0 | 257 | 77 | | | | | | | | | | | 0.0 | | | 0 | | 0.0 | | | | 21 | | 154 | |
| 8401 | 1 Tbs | Fat Free, Weight Watchers | 16 | 20 | 71 | 0.0 | 4.5 | 0.0 | 3.0 | 1.5 | 0.0 | 0.0 | 0.0 | 0.0 | 0.00 | 0.00 | 0 | 0 | 0 | 0 | 0 | 0 | | | | | | | | 0.0 | | | 0 | | 0.0 | | | | 25 | | 100 | |
| | | Honey Dijon | | | | | | | | | | | | | | | | | | | | | | | | | | | | | | | | | | | | | | | | |
| 8504 | 1 Tbs | Fat Free, Kraft | 18 | 26 | 65 | 0.3 | 5.7 | 0.5 | 2.6 | 2.6 | 0.0 | 0.0 | 0.0 | 0.0 | 0.00 | 0.00 | 0 | 0 | 0 | 0 | 0 | 0 | | | | | | | | 0.0 | | | 0 | | 0.2 | | | | 26 | | 170 | |
| 8642 | 1 Tbs | Fat Free, Lipton | 15 | 22 | 62 | 0.5 | 5.0 | 0.0 | 4.5 | 0.5 | 0.0 | 0.0 | 0.0 | 0.0 | 0.00 | 0.00 | 0 | 0 | 0 | 0 | 0 | 0 | | | | | | | | 0.0 | | | 0 | | 0.0 | | | | | | 135 | |
| 8402 | 1 Tbs | Fat Free, Weight Watchers | 15 | 22 | 61 | 0.0 | 5.5 | 0.0 | 2.5 | 3.0 | 0.0 | 0.0 | 0.0 | 0.0 | 0.00 | 0.00 | 0 | 0 | 0 | 0 | 0 | 0 | | | | | | | | 0.0 | | | 0 | | 0.0 | | | | 12 | | 75 | |
| | | Italian | | | | | | | | | | | | | | | | | | | | | | | | | | | | | | | | | | | | | | | | |
| 8016 | 1 Tbs | Average | 15 | 16 | 82 | 0.0 | 0.7 | 0.0 | 0.7 | 0.0 | 1.5 | 0.2 | 0.3 | 0.9 | 0.12 | 0.78 | 1 | 0 | 0 | 0 | 0 | 0 | 0.00 | 0.00 | 0.00 | 0.00 | 0.00 | 0.0 | 0.00 | 0.0 | 0.0 | 0.2 | 0 | 0.0 | 0.0 | 0 | 0.0 | 1 | 2 | 0.2 | 118 | 0.02 |
| 8637 | 1 Tbs | Creamy, fat free, Lipton | 15 | 18 | 73 | 0.0 | 4.0 | 0.5 | 1.5 | 2.0 | 0.0 | 0.0 | 0.0 | 0.0 | 0.00 | 0.00 | 0 | 0 | 0 | 0 | 0 | 0 | | | | | | | | 0.0 | | | 0 | | 0.0 | | | | | | 85 | |
| 8399 | 1 Tbs | Creamy, fat free, Weight Watchers | 15 | 15 | 73 | 0.0 | 3.5 | 0.0 | 1.0 | 2.5 | 0.0 | 0.0 | 0.0 | 0.0 | 0.00 | 0.00 | 0 | 0 | 0 | 0 | 0 | 0 | | | | | | | | 0.0 | | | 0 | | 0.0 | | | | 12 | | 180 | |
| 8615 | 1 Tbs | Creamy, Kraft | 16 | 26 | 72 | 0.0 | 1.5 | 0.0 | 1.0 | 0.5 | 2.6 | 0.5 | | | | | 0 | 0 | 0 | 0 | 0 | 0 | | | | | | | | 0.0 | | | 0 | | 0.0 | | | | 13 | | 129 | |
| 8531 | 1 Tbs | Creamy, Marie's | 16 | 19 | 72 | 0.0 | 2.9 | 0.0 | 1.5 | 1.5 | 1.0 | 0.0 | | | | | 0 | 0 | 0 | 0 | 0 | 0 | | | | | | | | 0.0 | | | 0 | | 0.0 | | | | | | 141 | |
| 8442 | 1 Tbs | Creamy, Wishbone | 15 | 26 | 72 | 0.1 | 2.0 | | | | 2.0 | 0.4 | 0.9 | 0.7 | | | 0 | 0 | 0 | 0 | 0 | 0 | 0.00 | 0.00 | 0.00 | | | | | 0.0 | | | 0 | | 0.0 | | | | | | 148 | |
| 8491 | 1 Tbs | Fat free, Kraft | 16 | 5 | 90 | 0.0 | 1.0 | 0.0 | 1.0 | 0.0 | 0.0 | 0.0 | 0.0 | 0.0 | 0.00 | 0.00 | 0 | 0 | 0 | 0 | 0 | 0 | | | | | | | | 0.0 | | | 0 | | 0.0 | | | | 21 | | 150 | |
| 8505 | 1 Tbs | Fat free, Seven Seas | 16 | 5 | 90 | 0.0 | 1.0 | 0.0 | 1.0 | 0.0 | 0.0 | 0.0 | 0.0 | 0.0 | 0.00 | 0.00 | 0 | 0 | 0 | 0 | 0 | 0 | | | | | | | | 0.0 | | | 0 | | 0.0 | | | | 22 | | 240 | |
| 8403 | 1 Tbs | Fat free, Weight Watchers | 15 | 5 | 90 | 0.0 | 1.0 | 0.0 | 0.5 | 0.5 | 0.0 | 0.0 | 0.0 | 0.0 | 0.00 | 0.00 | 0 | 0 | 0 | 0 | 0 | 0 | | | | | | | | 0.0 | | | 0 | | 0.0 | | | | 12 | | 180 | |

| Code | Amount | Description | Weight (g) | Calories | % Water | Protein (g) | Carbs (g) | Fiber (g) | Sugar (g) | Other Carbs (g) | Fat (g) | Sat Fat (g) | Mono Fat (g) | Poly Fat (g) | Omega 3 (g) | Omega 6 (g) | Choles (mg) | Vit A (IU) | Vit A (RE) | Retinol (RE) | Carotenoids (RE) | Beta Carotene (mcg) | Thiamin (mg) | Riboflavin (mg) | Niacin (NE) | Vit B6 (mg) | Vit B12 (mcg) | Folate (mcg) | Panto (mg) | Vit C (mg) | Vit D (mg) | Vit E (α TE) | Calcium (mg) | Copper (mg) | Iron (mg) | Magnes (mg) | Mang (mg) | Phos (mg) | Potassium (mg) | Selenium (mcg) | Sodium (mg) | Zinc (mg) |
|---|---|---|---|---|---|---|---|---|---|---|---|---|---|---|---|---|---|---|---|---|---|---|---|---|---|---|---|---|---|---|---|---|---|---|---|---|---|---|---|---|---|---|
| | | **Basic Components** | | | | | | | | | | **Additional Fats** | | | | | | **Vit A & Components** | | | | | **Vitamins** | | | | | | | | | | **Minerals** | | | | | | | | | |
| 8560 | 1 Tbs | Kraft | 16 | 36 | | 0.0 | 1.5 | 0.0 | 1.0 | 0.5 | 3.6 | 0.5 | | | | | 0 | 0 | 0 | 0 | 0 | 0 | | | | | | | | 0.0 | | | 0 | | 0.0 | | | | 13 | | 124 | |
| 8257 | 1 Tbs | Unsalted, avg | 15 | 16 | 84 | 0.0 | 0.7 | 0.0 | | | 1.5 | 0.2 | 0.3 | 0.9 | 0.12 | 0.73 | - | 0 | 0 | 0 | 0 | 0 | 0.00 | 0.00 | 0.00 | 0.00 | 0.00 | | 0.00 | 0.0 | 0.0 | 0.2 | 0 | | 0.0 | | | 1 | 2 | 0.2 | 5 | |
| 8413 | 1 Tbs | Wishbone | 16 | 6 | 90 | 0.0 | 1.0 | | | | 0.3 | 0.0 | 0.2 | 0.1 | | | 0 | 9 | 2 | | | | 0.00 | 0.00 | 0.00 | | | | | 0.2 | | | 1 | | 0.0 | | | | | | 255 | |
| | | Ranch | | | | | | | | | | | | | | | | | | | | | | | | | | | | | | | | | | | | | | | | |
| 8493 | 1 Tbs | Fat Free, Kraft | 18 | 26 | 66 | 0.3 | 5.7 | 0.3 | 1.0 | 4.4 | 0.0 | 0.0 | 0.0 | 0.0 | 0.00 | 0.00 | 0 | 0 | 0 | 0 | 0 | 0 | | | | | | | | 0.0 | | | 0 | | 0.0 | | | | 26 | | 159 | |
| 8640 | 1 Tbs | Fat Free, Lipton | 15 | 20 | 69 | 0.0 | 4.5 | 0.0 | 1.0 | 3.5 | 0.0 | 0.0 | 0.0 | 0.0 | 0.00 | 0.00 | 0 | 0 | 0 | 0 | 0 | 0 | | | | | | | | 0.0 | | | 0 | | 0.0 | | | | | | 135 | |
| 8492 | 1 Tbs | Fat Free, peppercorn, Kraft | 18 | 26 | 66 | 0.3 | 5.7 | 0.5 | 1.0 | 4.1 | 0.0 | 0.0 | 0.0 | 0.0 | 0.00 | 0.00 | 0 | 0 | 0 | 0 | 0 | 0 | | | | | | | | 0.0 | | | 0 | | 0.0 | | | | 31 | | 185 | |
| 8506 | 1 Tbs | Fat Free, Seven Seas | 18 | 26 | 63 | 0.3 | 6.2 | 0.5 | 1.5 | 4.1 | 0.0 | 0.0 | 0.0 | 0.0 | 0.00 | 0.00 | 0 | 0 | 0 | 0 | 0 | 0 | | | | | | | | 0.0 | | | 10 | | 0.0 | | | | 28 | | 170 | |
| 8614 | 1 Tbs | Kraft | 15 | 55 | | 0.0 | 1.0 | 0.0 | 0.5 | 0.5 | 5.5 | 1.0 | | | | | 5 | 0 | 0 | 0 | 0 | 0 | | | | | | | | 0.0 | | | 0 | | 0.0 | | | | 20 | | 155 | |
| 8539 | 1 Tbs | Marie's | 15 | 50 | 38 | 0.5 | 3.5 | 0.0 | 1.5 | 2.0 | 3.5 | 0.3 | | | | | 2 | 0 | 0 | 0 | 0 | 0 | | | | | | | | 0.0 | | | 0 | | 0.2 | | | | | | 120 | |
| 8427 | 1 Tbs | Wishbone | 15 | 50 | 56 | 0.0 | 2.5 | 0.0 | 0.5 | 2.0 | 4.0 | 0.8 | | | | | 2 | 0 | 0 | 0 | 0 | 0 | | | | | | | | 0.0 | | | 0 | | 0.0 | | | | | | 120 | |
| 8534 | 1 Tbs | Zesty, Marie's | 16 | 22 | 74 | 0.0 | 3.4 | 0.0 | 1.5 | 1.9 | 0.7 | 0.0 | | | | | 0 | 0 | 0 | 0 | 0 | 0 | | | | | | | | 0.0 | | | 0 | | 0.0 | | | | | | 160 | |
| 8494 | 1 Tbs | Red Wine Vinegar, fat free, Catalina | 16 | 8 | | 0.0 | 1.5 | 0.0 | 1.5 | 0.0 | 0.0 | 0.0 | 0.0 | 0.0 | 0.00 | 0.00 | 0 | 0 | 0 | 0 | 0 | 0 | | | | | | | | 0.0 | | | 0 | | 0.0 | | | | 8 | | 200 | |
| 8643 | 1 Tbs | Roasted Garlic, fat free, Lipton | 15 | 20 | 69 | 0.0 | 4.5 | 0.0 | 2.0 | 2.5 | 0.0 | 0.0 | 0.0 | 0.0 | 0.00 | 0.00 | 0 | 0 | 0 | 0 | 0 | 0 | | | | | | | | 0.0 | | | 0 | | 0.0 | | | | | | 140 | |
| | | Thousand Island | | | | | | | | | | | | | | | | | | | | | | | | | | | | | | | | | | | | | | | | |
| 8023 | 1 Tbs | Average | 15 | 24 | 69 | 0.1 | 2.4 | 0.2 | 2.2 | 0.1 | 1.6 | 0.2 | 0.4 | 0.9 | 0.14 | 0.83 | 2 | 48 | 14 | 14 | 0 | 0 | 0.00 | 0.00 | 0.00 | 0.00 | 0.03 | 0.8 | 0.03 | 0.0 | 0.0 | | 2 | 0.0 | 0.1 | 0 | 0.0 | 3 | 17 | 0.2 | 150 | 0.02 |
| 8495 | 1 Tbs | Fat Free, avg | 18 | 23 | 68 | 0.0 | 5.7 | 0.5 | 3.1 | 2.1 | 0.0 | 0.0 | 0.0 | 0.0 | 0.00 | 0.00 | 0 | 0 | 0 | 0 | 0 | 0 | | | | | | | | 0.0 | | | 0 | | 0.0 | | | | 28 | | 154 | |
| 8638 | 1 Tbs | Fat Free, Lipton | 15 | 18 | 72 | 0.0 | 4.0 | 0.0 | 2.5 | 1.5 | 0.0 | 0.0 | 0.0 | 0.0 | 0.00 | 0.00 | 0 | 0 | 0 | 0 | 0 | 0 | | | | | | | | 0.0 | | | 0 | | 0.0 | | | | | | 145 | |
| 8563 | 1 Tbs | Kraft | 16 | 35 | | 0.0 | 4.0 | 0.0 | 2.5 | 1.5 | 2.0 | 0.5 | | | | | 2 | 0 | 0 | 0 | 0 | 0 | | | | | | | | 0.0 | | | 0 | | 0.0 | | | | 28 | | 160 | |
| 8646 | 1 Tbs | Lipton | 15 | 40 | 59 | 0.0 | 3.5 | 0.0 | 3.0 | 0.5 | 2.5 | 0.5 | | | | | 5 | 0 | 0 | 0 | 0 | 0 | | | | | | | | 0.0 | | | 0 | | 0.0 | | | | | | 125 | |
| | | Vinaigrette | | | | | | | | | | | | | | | | | | | | | | | | | | | | | | | | | | | | | | | | |
| 8543 | 1 Tbs | Classic Herb, fat free, Marie's | 18 | 15 | 77 | 0.0 | 3.6 | 0.0 | 1.5 | 2.1 | 0.0 | 0.0 | 0.0 | 0.0 | 0.00 | 0.00 | 0 | 0 | 0 | 0 | 0 | 0 | | | | | | | | 0.0 | | | 0 | | 0.0 | | | | | | 129 | |
| 8544 | 1 Tbs | Honey Dijon, fat free, Marie's | 18 | 26 | 66 | 0.0 | 5.7 | 0.0 | 4.1 | 1.5 | 0.0 | 0.0 | 0.0 | 0.0 | 0.00 | 0.00 | 0 | 0 | 0 | 0 | 0 | 0 | | | | | | | | 0.0 | | | 0 | | 0.0 | | | | | | 64 | |
| 8545 | 1 Tbs | Italian, fat free, Marie's | 18 | 18 | 75 | 0.0 | 4.1 | 0.0 | 2.1 | 2.1 | 0.0 | 0.0 | 0.0 | 0.0 | 0.00 | 0.00 | 0 | 0 | 0 | 0 | 0 | 0 | | | | | | | | 0.0 | | | 0 | | 0.0 | | | | | | 144 | |
| 8546 | 1 Tbs | Raspberry, fat free, Marie's | 18 | 18 | 75 | 0.0 | 4.1 | 0.0 | 2.6 | 1.5 | 0.0 | 0.0 | 0.0 | 0.0 | 0.00 | 0.00 | 0 | 0 | 0 | 0 | 0 | 0 | | | | | | | | 0.0 | | | 0 | | 0.0 | | | | | | 18 | |
| 8547 | 1 Tbs | Red Wine, fat free, Marie's | 18 | 21 | 69 | 0.0 | 5.1 | 0.0 | 3.1 | 2.1 | 0.0 | 0.0 | 0.0 | 0.0 | 0.00 | 0.00 | 0 | 0 | 0 | 0 | 0 | 0 | | | | | | | | 0.0 | | | 0 | | 0.0 | | | | | | 154 | |
| 8548 | 1 Tbs | White Wine, fat free, Marie's | 18 | 21 | 69 | 0.0 | 5.1 | 0.0 | 3.1 | 2.1 | 0.0 | 0.0 | 0.0 | 0.0 | 0.00 | 0.00 | 0 | 0 | 0 | 0 | 0 | 0 | | | | | | | | 0.0 | | | 0 | | 0.0 | | | | | | 159 | |
| | | *SALAD DRESSINGS - REGULAR* | | | | | | | | | | | | | | | | | | | | | | | | | | | | | | | | | | | | | | | | |
| | | Blue Cheese/Roquefort | | | | | | | | | | | | | | | | | | | | | | | | | | | | | | | | | | | | | | | | |
| 8013 | 1 Tbs | Average | 15 | 76 | 32 | 0.7 | 1.1 | 0.0 | 1.1 | 0.1 | 7.8 | 1.5 | 1.8 | 4.2 | 0.56 | 3.53 | 3 | 32 | 10 | | | | 0.00 | 0.02 | 0.02 | 0.01 | 0.04 | 1.2 | 0.06 | 0.3 | 0.0 | 0.9 | 12 | 0.0 | 0.0 | 0 | 0.0 | 11 | 6 | 0.2 | 164 | 0.04 |
| 8526 | 1 Tbs | Chunky, Marie's | 15 | 90 | 20 | 0.5 | 1.5 | 0.0 | 0.0 | 1.5 | 9.5 | 1.8 | | | | | 8 | 0 | 0 | 0 | 0 | 0 | | | | | | | | 0.0 | | | 0 | | 0.2 | | | | | | 85 | |
| 8581 | 1 Tbs | Kraft | 16 | 44 | | 0.5 | 2.4 | 0.0 | 1.5 | 1.0 | 3.4 | 1.9 | | | | | 5 | 0 | 0 | 0 | 0 | 0 | | | | | | | | 0.0 | | | 10 | | 0.0 | | | | 24 | | 228 | |
| 8253 | 1 Tbs | Unsalted, avg | 15 | 76 | 32 | 0.7 | 1.1 | 0.0 | 1.1 | 0.1 | 7.8 | 1.5 | 1.8 | 4.2 | 0.56 | 3.53 | 3 | 32 | 10 | | | | 0.00 | 0.02 | 0.02 | 0.01 | 0.04 | 1.2 | 0.06 | 0.3 | 0.0 | 0.9 | 12 | 0.0 | 0.0 | 0 | 0.0 | 11 | 6 | 0.2 | 5 | |
| 8575 | 1 Tbs | Buttermilk, Kraft | 14 | 72 | | 0.0 | 1.0 | 0.0 | 1.0 | 0.0 | 7.7 | 1.4 | | | | | - | 0 | 0 | 0 | 0 | 0 | | | | | | | | 0.0 | | | 0 | | 0.0 | | | | 10 | | 111 | |
| 8525 | 1 Tbs | Buttermilk Ranch, Marie's | 15 | 90 | 15 | 0.0 | 2.0 | 0.0 | 1.0 | 1.0 | 9.0 | 1.5 | | | | | 8 | 0 | 0 | 0 | 0 | 0 | | | | | | | | 0.0 | | | 0 | | 0.0 | | | | | | 115 | |
| | | Caesar | | | | | | | | | | | | | | | | | | | | | | | | | | | | | | | | | | | | | | | | |
| 8066 | 1 Tbs | Average | 12 | 56 | 36 | 1.5 | 0.3 | 0.0 | 0.2 | 0.1 | 5.5 | 1.0 | 3.7 | 0.5 | 0.09 | 0.42 | 12 | 24 | 7 | 6 | 0 | | 0.00 | 0.02 | 0.50 | 0.01 | 0.06 | 1.6 | 0.06 | 0.7 | 0.1 | 0.6 | 23 | 0.0 | 0.2 | 3 | 0.0 | 19 | 21 | 3.1 | 207 | 0.13 |
| 8528 | 1 Tbs | Creamy, Marie's | 15 | 125 | | 0.3 | 3.0 | 0.5 | 0.3 | 2.3 | 12.5 | 2.0 | | | | | 12 | 0 | 0 | 0 | 0 | 0 | | | | | | | | 0.0 | | | 10 | | 0.2 | | | | | | 115 | |
| 8590 | 1 Tbs | Creamy, Seven Seas | 14 | 68 | | 0.2 | 0.5 | 0.0 | 0.0 | 0.5 | 7.2 | 1.2 | | | | | 5 | 0 | 0 | 0 | 0 | 0 | | | | | | | | 0.0 | | | 10 | | 0.0 | | | | 5 | | 145 | |
| 8576 | 1 Tbs | Kraft | 15 | 65 | | 0.5 | 1.0 | 0.0 | 0.5 | 0.5 | 6.5 | 1.3 | | | | | - | 0 | 0 | 0 | 0 | 0 | | | | | | | | 0.0 | | | 10 | | 0.0 | | | | 5 | | 185 | |
| 8573 | 1 Tbs | Ranch, Kraft | 14 | 68 | | 0.5 | 0.5 | 0.0 | 0.0 | 0.5 | 7.2 | 1.2 | | | | | 5 | 0 | 0 | 0 | 0 | 0 | | | | | | | | 0.0 | | | 10 | | 0.0 | | | | 5 | | 145 | |
| 8395 | 1 Tbs | Three Cheese, Weight Watchers | 15 | 20 | 70 | 0.5 | 2.5 | 0.0 | 2.0 | 0.5 | 1.0 | 0.0 | | | 0.00 | 0.00 | 5 | 0 | 0 | 0 | 0 | 0 | | | | | | | | 0.0 | | | 10 | | 0.0 | | | | 8 | | 95 | |
| 8577 | 1 Tbs | Coleslaw, Kraft | 16 | 75 | | 0.0 | 4.0 | 0.0 | 4.0 | 0.0 | 6.0 | 1.0 | | | | | 12 | 0 | 0 | 0 | 0 | 0 | | | | | | | | 0.0 | | | 0 | | 0.0 | | | | 5 | | 210 | |
| 8527 | 1 Tbs | Coleslaw, Marie's | 15 | 75 | 36 | 0.0 | 3.0 | 0.0 | 3.0 | 0.0 | 6.5 | 1.0 | | | | | 5 | 0 | 0 | 0 | 0 | 0 | | | | | | | | 0.0 | | | 0 | | 0.0 | | | | | | 105 | |
| 8572 | 1 Tbs | Cucumber Ranch, Kraft | 15 | 75 | | 0.0 | 1.0 | 0.0 | 1.0 | 0.0 | 7.5 | 1.3 | | | | | 0 | 0 | 0 | 0 | 0 | 0 | | | | | | | | 0.0 | | | 0 | | 0.0 | | | | 10 | | 110 | |
| | | French | | | | | | | | | | | | | | | | | | | | | | | | | | | | | | | | | | | | | | | | |
| 8259 | 1 Tbs | Average | 14 | 88 | 24 | 0.0 | 0.5 | 0.0 | | | 9.8 | 2.5 | 2.8 | 4.6 | 0.00 | 4.56 | 0 | 0 | 0 | 0 | 0 | 0 | 0.00 | 0.00 | 0.02 | | | | | 0.0 | | | 1 | | 0.0 | | | 0 | 3 | 0.2 | 92 | |
| 8570 | 1 Tbs | Catalina | 16 | 70 | 39 | 0.0 | 4.0 | 0.0 | 4.0 | 0.0 | 5.5 | 1.0 | | | | | 0 | 250 | 50 | | | | | | | | | | | 0.0 | | | 0 | | 0.0 | | | | 20 | | 195 | |
| 8439 | 1 Tbs | Sweet & Spicy, Lipton | 15 | 65 | 39 | 0.0 | 3.0 | 0.0 | 2.5 | 0.5 | 6.0 | 1.0 | | | | | 0 | 0 | 0 | 0 | 0 | 0 | | | | | | | | 0.6 | | | 0 | | 0.0 | | | | | | 165 | |
| 8541 | 1 Tbs | Tangy, Marie's | 15 | 65 | 34 | 0.0 | 4.0 | 0.0 | 3.5 | 0.5 | 5.5 | 0.8 | | | | | 0 | 0 | 0 | 0 | 0 | 0 | | | | | | | | 0.0 | | | 0 | | 0.0 | | | | | | 130 | |
| 8254 | 1 Tbs | Unsalted, avg | 16 | 69 | 38 | 0.1 | 2.8 | 0.0 | 2.7 | 0.1 | 6.6 | 1.5 | 1.3 | 3.5 | 0.00 | 3.25 | 0 | 11 | 3 | 0 | 3 | | 0.00 | 0.00 | 0.00 | 0.00 | 0.02 | 0.7 | 0.03 | 0.0 | 0.0 | 0.8 | 2 | 0.0 | 0.1 | 0 | 0.0 | 2 | 13 | 0.3 | 0 | |
| 8438 | 1 Tbs | Wishbone | 15 | 60 | 46 | 0.0 | 2.5 | 0.0 | 2.0 | 0.5 | 5.5 | 0.8 | | | | | 0 | 50 | 10 | | | | | | | | | | | 0.0 | | | 0 | | 0.0 | | | | | | 85 | |
| 8578 | 1 Tbs | Garlic, Kraft | 15 | 55 | | 0.0 | 1.0 | 0.0 | 1.0 | 0.0 | 5.5 | 1.0 | | | | | 0 | 0 | 0 | 0 | 0 | 0 | | | | | | | | 0.0 | | | 0 | | 0.0 | | | | 12 | | 175 | |
| 8592 | 1 Tbs | Green Goddess, Seven Seas | 14 | 58 | | 0.0 | 0.5 | 0.0 | 0.5 | 0.0 | 6.3 | 1.0 | | | | | 0 | 0 | 0 | 0 | 0 | 0 | | | | | | | | 0.0 | | | 0 | | 0.0 | | | | 7 | | 126 | |
| 8593 | 1 Tbs | Herbs & Spices, Seven Seas | 15 | 60 | | 0.0 | 0.5 | 0.0 | 0.5 | 0.0 | 6.0 | 1.0 | | | | | 0 | 0 | 0 | 0 | 0 | 0 | | | | | | | | 0.0 | | | 0 | | 0.0 | | | | 5 | | 160 | |
| | | Honey Mustard | | | | | | | | | | | | | | | | | | | | | | | | | | | | | | | | | | | | | | | | |
| 8124 | 1 Tbs | Average | 16 | 52 | 35 | 0.2 | 7.1 | 0.1 | 6.9 | 0.0 | 2.9 | 0.4 | 0.7 | 1.6 | | | 0 | 0 | 0 | 0 | 0 | 0 | 0.00 | 0.00 | 0.03 | 0.00 | 0.00 | 0.5 | 0.01 | 0.1 | 0.0 | | 3 | 0.0 | 0.1 | 2 | 0.0 | 3 | 10 | | 93 | 0.06 |
| 8579 | 1 Tbs | Honey Dijon, Kraft | 16 | 77 | | 0.0 | 2.1 | 0.0 | 1.5 | 0.5 | 7.7 | 1.0 | | | | | 0 | 0 | 0 | 0 | 0 | 0 | | | | | | | | 0.0 | | | 0 | | 0.0 | | | | 18 | | 103 | |
| 8530 | 1 Tbs | Marie's | 15 | 80 | 21 | 0.0 | 4.0 | 0.2 | 3.8 | 0.0 | 7.5 | 1.0 | | | | | 2 | 0 | 0 | 0 | 0 | 0 | | | | | | | | 0.0 | | | 0 | | 0.0 | | | | | | 80 | |
| | | Italian | | | | | | | | | | | | | | | | | | | | | | | | | | | | | | | | | | | | | | | | |
| 8561 | 1 Tbs | Creamy, Kraft | 15 | 55 | | 0.0 | 1.5 | 0.0 | 1.0 | 0.5 | 5.5 | 2.0 | | | | | 0 | 0 | 0 | 0 | 0 | 0 | | | | | | | | 0.0 | | | 0 | | 0.0 | | | | 10 | | 115 | |
| 8591 | 1 Tbs | Creamy, Seven Seas | 15 | 55 | | 0.0 | 1.0 | 0.0 | 1.0 | 0.0 | 6.0 | 1.0 | | | | | 0 | 0 | 0 | 0 | 0 | 0 | | | | | | | | 0.0 | | | 0 | | 0.0 | | | | 5 | | 255 | |
| 8435 | 1 Tbs | Creamy, Wishbone | 15 | 50 | 56 | 0.0 | 1.5 | 0.0 | 1.0 | 0.5 | 5.0 | 1.0 | | | | | 0 | 0 | 0 | 0 | 0 | 0 | | | | | | | | 0.0 | | | 0 | | 0.0 | | | | | | 155 | |
| 8557 | 1 Tbs | Kraft | 15 | 60 | | 0.0 | 1.5 | 0.0 | 1.0 | 0.5 | 6.0 | 1.0 | | | | | - | 0 | 0 | 0 | 0 | 0 | | | | | | | | 0.0 | | | 0 | | 0.0 | | | | 12 | | 120 | |
| 8423 | 1 Tbs | Olive Oil, Lipton | 15 | 35 | 65 | 0.0 | 2.0 | 0.0 | 1.0 | 1.0 | 3.0 | 0.5 | | | | | 0 | 0 | 0 | 0 | 0 | 0 | | | | | | | | 0.0 | | | 0 | | 0.0 | | | | | | 200 | |

| Code | Amount | Description | Basic Components | | | | | | | | | | Additional Fats | | | | | Vit A & Components | | | | | Vitamins | | | | | | | | | | Minerals | | | | | | | | | |
|---|---|---|---|---|---|---|---|---|---|---|---|---|---|---|---|---|---|---|---|---|---|---|---|---|---|---|---|---|---|---|---|---|---|---|---|---|---|---|---|---|---|---|
| | | | Weight (g) | Calories | % Water | Protein (g) | Carbs (g) | Fiber (g) | Sugar (g) | Other Carbs (g) | Fat (g) | Sat Fat (g) | Mono Fat (g) | Poly Fat (g) | Omega 3 (g) | Omega 6 (g) | Choles (mg) | Vit A (IU) | Vit A (RE) | Retinol (RE) | Carotenoids (RE) | Beta Carotene (mcg) | Thiamin (mg) | Riboflavin (mg) | Niacin (NE) | Vit B6 (mg) | Vit B12 (mcg) | Folate (mcg) | Panto (mg) | Vit C (mg) | Vit D (mg) | Vit E (α TE) | Calcium (mg) | Copper (mg) | Iron (mg) | Magnes (mg) | Mang (mg) | Phos (mg) | Potassium (mg) | Selenium (mcg) | Sodium (mg) | Zinc (mg) |
| 8596 | 1 Tbs | Two Cheese, Seven Seas | 16 | 36 | | 0.0 | 1.5 | 0.0 | 1.0 | 0.5 | 3.6 | 0.5 | | | | | 0 | 0 | 0 | 0 | 0 | 0 | | | | | | | | 0.0 | | | 0 | | 0.0 | | | | 13 | | 124 | |
| 8256 | 1 Tbs | Unsalted, avg | 15 | 70 | 40 | 0.1 | 1.5 | 0.0 | 1.5 | 0.0 | 7.2 | 1.1 | 1.7 | 4.2 | 0.50 | 3.69 | 10 | 12 | 4 | | | | 0.00 | 0.00 | 0.03 | 0.00 | 0.02 | 0.7 | 0.03 | 0.0 | 0.0 | 0.8 | 2 | 0.0 | 0.0 | | | 1 | 2 | 0.2 | 5 | |
| 8434 | 1 Tbs | Wishbone | 15 | 50 | 58 | 0.0 | 1.5 | 0.0 | 1.0 | 0.5 | 4.5 | 0.8 | | | | | 0 | 0 | 0 | 0 | 0 | 0 | | | | | | | | 0.0 | | | 0 | | 0.0 | | | | | | 295 | |
| 8536 | 1 Tbs | Poppyseed, Marie's | 15 | 75 | 22 | 0.0 | 4.0 | 0.0 | 3.0 | 1.0 | 6.0 | 0.8 | | | | | 5 | 0 | 0 | 0 | 0 | 0 | | | | | | | | 0.0 | | | 0 | | 0.0 | | | | | | 100 | |
| | | Ranch | | | | | | | | | | | | | | | | | | | | | | | | | | | | | | | | | | | | | | | | |
| 8529 | 1 Tbs | Creamy, Marie's | 15 | 95 | 10 | 0.3 | 1.5 | 0.0 | 0.3 | 1.3 | 10.0 | 1.5 | | | | | 8 | 0 | 0 | 0 | 0 | 0 | | | | | | | | 0.0 | | | 0 | | 0.0 | | | | | | 85 | |
| 8555 | 1 Tbs | Kraft | 14 | 82 | 30 | 0.0 | 1.0 | 0.0 | 0.5 | 0.5 | 8.7 | 1.4 | | | | | 2 | 0 | 0 | 0 | 0 | 0 | | | | | | | | 0.0 | | | 0 | | 0.0 | | | | 5 | | 130 | |
| 8580 | 1 Tbs | Peppercorn, Kraft | 14 | 82 | 30 | 0.5 | 0.5 | 0.0 | 0.5 | 0.0 | 8.7 | 1.4 | | | | | 5 | 0 | 0 | 0 | 0 | 0 | | | | | | | | 0.0 | | | 10 | | 0.0 | | | | 10 | | 164 | |
| 8583 | 1 Tbs | Salsa, Kraft | 14 | 63 | 51 | 0.0 | 0.5 | 0.0 | 0.5 | 0.0 | 6.3 | 1.0 | | | | | 5 | 0 | 0 | 0 | 0 | 0 | | | | | | | | 0.0 | | | 0 | | 0.0 | | | | 10 | | 154 | |
| 8594 | 1 Tbs | Seven Seas | 14 | 72 | 30 | 0.0 | 1.0 | 0.0 | 0.5 | 0.5 | 7.7 | 1.2 | | | | | 2 | 0 | 0 | 0 | 0 | 0 | | | | | | | | 0.0 | | | 0 | | 0.0 | | | | 5 | | 121 | |
| 8428 | 1 Tbs | Wishbone | 15 | 80 | 39 | 0.0 | 0.5 | 0.0 | 0.5 | 0.0 | 8.5 | 1.3 | | | | | 5 | 0 | 0 | 0 | 0 | 0 | | | | | | | | 0.0 | | | 0 | | 0.0 | | | | | | 105 | |
| | | Russian | | | | | | | | | | | | | | | | | | | | | | | | | | | | | | | | | | | | | | | | |
| 8022 | 1 Tbs | Average | 15 | 74 | 34 | 0.2 | 1.6 | 0.0 | 1.6 | 0.0 | 7.6 | 1.1 | 1.8 | 4.4 | 0.53 | 3.88 | 3 | 104 | 31 | | | | 0.01 | 0.01 | 0.09 | 0.00 | 0.05 | 1.6 | 0.06 | 0.9 | 0.0 | 0.9 | 3 | 0.0 | 0.1 | 0 | 0.0 | 6 | 24 | 0.2 | 130 | 0.06 |
| 8582 | 1 Tbs | Kraft | 16 | 63 | | 0.0 | 4.8 | 0.0 | 4.4 | 0.5 | 4.8 | 0.7 | | | | | 0 | 194 | 39 | | | | | | | | | | | 0.0 | | | 0 | | 0.0 | | | | 19 | | 136 | |
| 8599 | 1 Tbs | Seven Seas | 15 | 75 | | 0.0 | 1.5 | 0.0 | 1.0 | 0.5 | 8.0 | 1.3 | | | | | 0 | 0 | 0 | 0 | 0 | 0 | | | | | | | | 0.0 | | | 0 | | 0.0 | | | | 10 | | 115 | |
| 8437 | 1 Tbs | Wishbone | 15 | 55 | 29 | 0.0 | 7.5 | 0.0 | 3.5 | 4.0 | 3.0 | 0.5 | | | | | 0 | 50 | 10 | | | | | | | | | | | 0.6 | | | 0 | | 0.0 | | | | | | 175 | 0.00 |
| 8584 | 1 Tbs | Salsa Zesty Garden, Kraft | 16 | 36 | | 0.0 | 1.5 | 0.0 | 1.5 | 0.0 | 3.1 | 0.5 | | | | | 0 | 155 | 31 | | | | | | | | | | | 0.0 | | | 0 | | 0.0 | | | | 15 | | 145 | |
| 8144 | 1 Tbs | Sesame Seed, avg | 15 | 66 | 39 | 0.5 | 1.3 | 0.2 | | | 6.8 | 0.9 | 1.8 | 3.8 | 0.30 | 3.47 | 0 | 104 | 31 | | | | 0.00 | 0.00 | 0.00 | 0.00 | 0.00 | 0.0 | 0.00 | 0.0 | 0.0 | 0.8 | 3 | | 0.1 | 0 | 0.0 | 6 | 24 | 0.2 | 150 | 0.02 |
| 8540 | 1 Tbs | Sour Cream & Dill, Marie's | 15 | 95 | 23 | 0.0 | 1.5 | 0.0 | 0.3 | 1.3 | 10.0 | 1.5 | | | | | 8 | 0 | 0 | 0 | 0 | 0 | | | | | | | | 0.0 | | | 0 | | 0.0 | | | | | | 80 | |
| | | Thousand Island | | | | | | | | | | | | | | | | | | | | | | | | | | | | | | | | | | | | | | | | |
| 8024 | 1 Tbs | Average | 16 | 60 | 46 | 0.1 | 2.4 | 0.0 | 2.0 | 0.4 | 5.7 | 1.0 | 1.3 | 3.2 | 0.40 | 2.64 | 4 | 51 | 15 | 11 | 4 | | 0.00 | 0.00 | 0.00 | 0.00 | 0.03 | 1.0 | 0.04 | 0.0 | 0.0 | | 2 | 0.0 | 0.1 | 0 | 0.0 | 3 | 18 | 0.3 | 112 | 0.02 |
| 8586 | 1 Tbs | Kraft | 16 | 57 | 51 | 0.0 | 2.6 | 0.0 | 2.6 | 0.0 | 5.2 | 0.8 | | | | | 5 | 0 | 0 | 0 | 0 | 0 | | | | | | | | 0.0 | | | 0 | | 0.0 | | | | 18 | | 160 | |
| 8432 | 1 Tbs | Wishbone | 15 | 65 | 36 | 0.0 | 3.5 | 0.0 | 3.0 | 0.5 | 6.0 | 1.0 | | | | | 5 | 0 | 0 | 0 | 0 | 0 | | | | | | | | 0.0 | | | 0 | | 0.0 | | | | | | 170 | |
| 8587 | 1 Tbs | With Bacon, Kraft | 14 | 58 | 40 | 0.0 | 2.4 | 0.0 | 1.9 | 0.5 | 5.8 | 1.0 | | | | | 0 | 0 | 0 | 0 | 0 | 0 | | | | | | | | 0.0 | | | 0 | | 0.0 | | | | 14 | | 92 | |
| | | Vinegar & Oil | | | | | | | | | | | | | | | | | | | | | | | | | | | | | | | | | | | | | | | | |
| 8035 | 1 Tbs | Average | 16 | 72 | 47 | 0.0 | 0.4 | 0.0 | 0.4 | 0.0 | 8.0 | 1.5 | 2.4 | 3.9 | 0.22 | 3.63 | 0 | 0 | 0 | 0 | 0 | 0 | 0.00 | 0.00 | 0.00 | 0.00 | 0.00 | 0.0 | 0.00 | 0.0 | 0.0 | 0.6 | 0 | 0.0 | 0.0 | 0 | 0.0 | 0 | 1 | 0.3 | 0 | 0.00 |
| 8595 | 1 Tbs | Red Wine, Seven Seas | 16 | 57 | | 0.0 | 1.0 | 0.0 | 1.0 | 0.0 | 5.7 | 1.0 | | | | | 0 | 0 | 0 | 0 | 0 | 0 | | | | | | | | 0.0 | | | 0 | | 0.0 | | | | 8 | | 263 | |
| 8429 | 1 Tbs | Wishbone | 15 | 30 | 69 | 0.0 | 2.0 | 0.0 | 1.5 | 0.5 | 2.5 | 0.3 | | | | | 0 | 0 | 0 | 0 | 0 | 0 | | | | | | | | 0.0 | | | 0 | | 0.0 | | | | | | 125 | |
| 8150 | 1 Tbs | Vinegar, Sugar & Water, avg | 16 | 8 | 84 | 0.0 | 2.2 | 0.0 | 2.2 | 0.0 | 0.0 | 0.0 | 0.0 | 0.0 | 0.00 | 0.00 | 0 | 0 | 0 | 0 | 0 | 0 | 0.00 | 0.00 | 0.00 | 0.00 | 0.00 | 0.0 | 0.00 | 0.0 | 0.0 | 0.0 | 1 | 0.0 | 0.0 | 1 | 0.0 | 0 | 5 | | 164 | 0.00 |
| 8123 | 1 Tbs | Yogurt, avg | 15 | 11 | 85 | 0.4 | 1.1 | 0.0 | 1.0 | 0.1 | 0.6 | 0.3 | 0.1 | 0.1 | | | 2 | 15 | 4 | 3 | 0.4 | | 0.00 | 0.02 | 0.01 | 0.00 | 0.04 | 1.0 | 0.05 | 0.4 | 0.0 | | 15 | 0.0 | 0.0 | 2 | 0.0 | 12 | 22 | | 58 | 0.07 |
| | | *SALADS* | | | | | | | | | | | | | | | | | | | | | | | | | | | | | | | | | | | | | | | | |
| 52068 | 1/2 cup | Antipasto Salad, Orval Kent | 100 | 220 | | 6.0 | 2.0 | 1.3 | 0.7 | 0.0 | 21.0 | 5.0 | | | | | 20 | 100 | 20 | | | | | | | | | | | 4.8 | | | 80 | | 0.7 | | | | | | 650 | |
| 52069 | 1/2 cup | Artichoke Salad, marinated, Orval Kent | 100 | 150 | | 1.0 | 5.0 | 2.0 | 2.0 | 1.0 | 14.0 | 2.0 | | | | | 0 | 100 | 20 | | | | | | | | | | | 9.0 | | | 20 | | 0.4 | | | | | | 600 | |
| | | Bean Salads | | | | | | | | | | | | | | | | | | | | | | | | | | | | | | | | | | | | | | | | |
| 52052 | 1/2 cup | Medley, Orval Kent | 151 | 242 | | 7.6 | 31.7 | 7.6 | 7.6 | 16.6 | 10.6 | 1.5 | | | | | 0 | 151 | 30 | | | | | | | | | | | 1.8 | | | 91 | | 1.1 | | | | | | 649 | |
| 56118 | 1/2 cup | String Bean, avg | 75 | 70 | 82 | 1.9 | 6.7 | 1.5 | | | 4.2 | 0.6 | 1.0 | 2.4 | | | 0 | 99 | 11 | 2 | 9 | 54 | 0.03 | 0.05 | 0.20 | 0.02 | 0.01 | 26.4 | | 2.2 | | | 18 | 0.1 | 0.7 | 13 | | 32 | 112 | | 257 | 0.27 |
| 57510 | 1/2 cup | Three Bean, avg | 104 | 83 | 78 | 3.6 | 17.5 | 4.5 | 7.7 | 5.2 | 0.2 | 0.0 | 0.0 | 0.1 | 0.09 | 0.05 | 0 | 104 | 10 | 0 | 10 | 60 | 0.07 | 0.08 | 0.36 | 0.03 | 0.00 | 44.5 | 0.15 | 2.2 | 0.0 | | 12 | 0.1 | 0.5 | 25 | 0.2 | 66 | 59 | 1.1 | 203 | 0.46 |
| 56109 | 1/2 cup | Carrot Raisin Salad, avg | 88 | 203 | 58 | 1.3 | 20.9 | 2.0 | 18.2 | 0.7 | 14.0 | 2.0 | 3.9 | 7.3 | 0.82 | 6.31 | 10 | 14530 | 1453 | 14 | 1439 | 6992 | 0.08 | 0.05 | 0.64 | 0.22 | 0.05 | 9.2 | 0.15 | 5.4 | 0.1 | 3.6 | 26 | 0.1 | 0.7 | 14 | 0.1 | 46 | 317 | 2.1 | 118 | 0.19 |
| 52034 | 1/2 cup | Carrot Raisin Salad, Orval Kent | 100 | 170 | | 1.0 | 17.0 | 2.0 | 14.0 | 1.0 | 11.0 | 2.0 | | | | | 5 | 8000 | 1600 | | | | | | | | | | | 1.2 | | | 40 | | 0.4 | | | | | | 310 | |
| | | Chicken Salads | | | | | | | | | | | | | | | | | | | | | | | | | | | | | | | | | | | | | | | | |
| 52040 | 1/2 cup | Deluxe, Orval Kent | 100 | 250 | | 15.0 | 5.0 | 0.0 | 1.0 | 4.0 | 20.0 | 3.5 | | | | | 55 | 0 | 0 | 0 | 0 | 0 | | | | | | | | 1.2 | | | 20 | | 0.7 | | | | | | 700 | |
| 52061 | 1/2 cup | Orval Kent | 100 | 250 | | 10.0 | 9.0 | 2.0 | 4.0 | 3.0 | 20.0 | 4.0 | | | | | 55 | 100 | 20 | | | | | | | | | | | 1.2 | | | 40 | | 0.4 | | | | | | 600 | |
| 52001 | 1/2 cup | White Meat, Orval Kent | 100 | 250 | | 15.0 | 5.0 | 2.0 | 2.0 | 1.0 | 19.0 | 3.0 | | | | | 55 | 100 | 20 | | | | | | | | | | | 1.2 | | | 20 | | 0.4 | | | | | | 500 | |
| 56002 | 1/2 cup | With Celery, avg | 78 | 268 | 53 | 10.6 | 1.3 | 0.2 | 0.2 | 0.9 | 24.6 | 3.1 | 4.5 | 15.8 | 0.87 | 14.93 | 48 | 155 | 31 | 29 | 2 | | 0.03 | 0.07 | 3.28 | 0.34 | 0.19 | 8.5 | 0.49 | 1.1 | 0.1 | 5.8 | 16 | 0.0 | 0.6 | 11 | 0.0 | 80 | 138 | 10.1 | 201 | 0.80 |
| | | Coleslaw/Cabbage Slaw | | | | | | | | | | | | | | | | | | | | | | | | | | | | | | | | | | | | | | | | |
| 52024 | 1/2 cup | Claremont, Orval Kent | 100 | 110 | | 1.0 | 14.0 | 4.0 | 9.0 | 1.0 | 6.0 | 1.5 | | | | | 0 | 400 | 80 | | | | | | | | | | | 0.0 | | | 40 | | 1.1 | | | | | | 600 | |
| 52021 | 1/2 cup | Creamy, Orval Kent | 100 | 170 | | 1.0 | 12.0 | 2.8 | 9.2 | 0.0 | 13.0 | 2.0 | | | | | 15 | 200 | 40 | | | | | | | | | | | 2.4 | | | 20 | | 0.7 | | | | | | 190 | |
| 52035 | 1/2 cup | Cucumber & Onion, Orval Kent | 100 | 40 | | 1.0 | 10.0 | 1.0 | 8.0 | 1.0 | 0.0 | 0.0 | 0.0 | 0.0 | 0.00 | 0.00 | 0 | 300 | 60 | | | | | | | | | | | 1.2 | | | 20 | | 0.4 | | | | | | 460 | |
| 52022 | 1/2 cup | Dixie Style, Orval Kent | 100 | 180 | | 1.0 | 17.0 | 2.0 | 13.0 | 2.0 | 12.0 | 1.5 | | | | | 0 | 100 | 20 | | | | | | | | | | | 108.0 | | | 40 | | 0.4 | | | | | | 180 | |
| 52004 | 1/2 cup | Orval Kent | 100 | 90 | | 1.0 | 17.0 | 2.0 | 12.0 | 3.0 | 2.0 | 0.0 | 0.0 | 1.0 | | | 0 | 0 | 0 | 0 | 0 | 0 | | | | | 0.00 | | | 1.2 | | | 40 | | 0.4 | | | | | | 230 | |
| 52025 | 1/2 cup | Shredded, Orval Kent | 100 | 100 | | 1.0 | 13.0 | 2.0 | 11.0 | 0.0 | 5.0 | 0.5 | | | | | 5 | 100 | 20 | | | | | | | | | | | 96.0 | | | 400 | | 0.4 | | | | | | 290 | |
| 52042 | 1/2 cup | Sour Cream & Honey, Orval Kent | 100 | 170 | | 1.0 | 16.0 | 2.0 | 10.0 | 4.0 | 11.0 | 2.5 | | | | | 10 | 100 | 20 | | | | | | | | | | | 66.0 | | | 40 | | 0.4 | | | | | | 280 | |
| 52023 | 1/2 cup | Vinegar & Oil, Orval Kent | 100 | 160 | | 1.0 | 15.0 | 2.0 | 10.0 | 3.0 | 11.0 | 1.5 | | | | | 0 | 500 | 100 | | | | | | | | | | | 96.0 | | | 40 | | 0.4 | | | | | | 570 | |
| 56003 | 1/2 cup | Egg Salad, avg | 92 | 294 | 57 | 8.5 | 1.5 | 0.0 | 1.3 | 0.2 | 28.4 | 5.3 | 8.8 | 12.1 | | | 289 | 435 | 131 | 131 | 0 | | 0.04 | 0.33 | 0.04 | 0.23 | 0.79 | 31.2 | 1.09 | 0.0 | 1.0 | | 38 | 0.0 | 0.9 | 6 | 0.0 | 118 | 91 | 19.7 | 335 | 0.72 |
| 52066 | 1/2 cup | Egg Salad, Orval Kent | 100 | 230 | | 9.0 | 8.0 | 0.0 | 4.0 | 4.0 | 18.0 | 4.0 | | | | | 240 | 0 | 0 | 0 | 0 | 0 | | | | | | | | 0.0 | | | 40 | | 1.4 | | | | | | 570 | |
| 52010 | 1/2 cup | Fruit Salad, Orval Kent | 110 | 60 | | 1.0 | 14.0 | 1.8 | 12.3 | 0.0 | 0.0 | 0.0 | 0.0 | 0.0 | 0.00 | 0.00 | 0 | 0 | 0 | 0 | 0 | 0 | | | | | | | | 54.0 | | | 0 | | 18.0 | | | | | | 10 | |
| | | Green Garden/Tossed Salads | | | | | | | | | | | | | | | | | | | | | | | | | | | | | | | | | | | | | | | | |
| 5677 | 1 cup | Average | 139 | 25 | 95 | 1.3 | 5.0 | 1.6 | 3.2 | 0.3 | 0.3 | 0.0 | 0.0 | 0.1 | 0.05 | 0.09 | 0 | 2790 | 279 | 0 | 279 | 1673 | 0.07 | 0.05 | 0.56 | 0.09 | 0.00 | 47.7 | 0.19 | 14.9 | 0.0 | 0.2 | 20 | 0.1 | 0.6 | 14 | 0.2 | 31 | 268 | 1.9 | 15 | 0.24 |
| 56624 | 1 cup | With Cheese & Egg, avg | 145 | 68 | 90 | 5.9 | 3.2 | | | | 3.9 | 2.0 | 1.2 | 0.3 | | | 65 | 550 | 77 | 3 | 73 | | 0.06 | 0.12 | 0.65 | 0.07 | 0.20 | 56.6 | 0.35 | 6.5 | | | 67 | 0.1 | 0.4 | 16 | 0.2 | 88 | 248 | 4.9 | 80 | 0.67 |
| 56625 | 1 cup | With Chicken, avg | 145 | 70 | 87 | 11.6 | 2.5 | | | | 1.5 | 0.4 | 0.5 | 0.4 | | | 48 | 622 | 64 | 1 | 63 | | 0.07 | 0.09 | 3.92 | 0.29 | 0.13 | 45.0 | 0.39 | 11.6 | | | 25 | 0.1 | 0.7 | 22 | 0.2 | 113 | 297 | 10.3 | 139 | 0.59 |
| 56626 | 1 cup | With Pasta & Seafood, avg | 278 | 253 | 80 | 11.0 | 21.3 | | | | 13.9 | 1.7 | 3.2 | 6.1 | | | 33 | 4164 | 425 | 81 | 345 | | 0.19 | 0.14 | 2.36 | 0.22 | 1.14 | 125.1 | 0.25 | 25.6 | | | 47 | 0.2 | 2.1 | 33 | 0.4 | 136 | 400 | 29.7 | 1048 | 1.11 |
| 56627 | 1 cup | With Shrimp, avg | 157 | 71 | 89 | 9.7 | 4.4 | | | | 1.6 | 0.4 | 0.5 | 0.3 | | | 119 | 526 | 52 | 1 | 51 | | 0.08 | 0.11 | 0.77 | 0.09 | 2.51 | 58.1 | 0.33 | 6.1 | | | 39 | 0.1 | 0.6 | 25 | 0.1 | 107 | 268 | 25.4 | 325 | 0.85 |
| 52062 | 1/2 cup | Ham Salad, Orval Kent | 100 | 270 | | 9.0 | 6.0 | 2.0 | 3.0 | 1.0 | 24.0 | 5.0 | | | | | 35 | 100 | 20 | | | | | | | | | | | 6.0 | | | 20 | | 0.7 | | | | | | 1030 | |
| 52002 | 1/2 cup | Mushroom Salad, Orval Kent | 100 | 90 | | 2.0 | 5.0 | 1.0 | 1.0 | 3.0 | 7.0 | 1.0 | | | | | 0 | 0 | 0 | 0 | 0 | 0 | | | | | | | | 2.4 | | | 20 | | 0.4 | | | | | | 620 | |
| 52063 | 1/2 cup | Olive Salad, Orval Kent | 100 | 100 | | 1.0 | 7.0 | 2.0 | 2.0 | 3.0 | 8.0 | 1.0 | | | | | 0 | 500 | 100 | | | | | | | | | | | 2.4 | | | 80 | | 2.7 | | | | | | 1620 | |
| 52084 | 1/2 cup | Olive Salad, Progresso | 96 | 100 | | 0.0 | 4.0 | 2.0 | 2.0 | 0.0 | 10.0 | 0.0 | 6.0 | 0.0 | 0.00 | 0.00 | 0 | 0 | 0 | 0 | 0 | 0 | | | | | | | | 0.0 | | | 0 | | 1.4 | | | | | | 1440 | |
| | | Pasta Salads | | | | | | | | | | | | | | | | | | | | | | | | | | | | | | | | | | | | | | | | |
| 52092 | 1/2 cup | Caesar, prep f/dry, Kraft | 91 | 232 | | 4.6 | 19.9 | 1.3 | 3.3 | 15.3 | 14.6 | 2.7 | | | | | 10 | 66 | 13 | | | | 0.10 | 0.07 | 1.06 | | | | | 0.8 | | | 40 | | 1.2 | 27 | | 100 | 206 | | 432 | |
| 52049 | 1/2 cup | California, Orval Kent | 93 | 133 | | 2.7 | 19.3 | 2.0 | 5.3 | 12.0 | 4.7 | 0.7 | | | | | 0 | 266 | 53 | | | | | | | | | | | 4.0 | | | 13 | | 1.0 | | | | | | 372 | |
| 52067 | 1/2 cup | Cheese Tortellini Vinaigrette, Orval Kent | 100 | 164 | | 4.3 | 17.9 | 2.9 | 2.9 | 12.1 | 7.9 | 1.8 | | | | | 7 | 71 | 14 | | | | | | | | | | | 0.9 | | | 71 | | 1.3 | | | | | | 564 | |

| Code | Amount | Description | Weight (g) | Calories | % Water | Protein (g) | Carbs (g) | Fiber (g) | Sugar (g) | Other Carbs (g) | Fat (g) | Sat Fat (g) | Mono Fat (g) | Poly Fat (g) | Omega 3 (g) | Omega 6 (g) | Choles (mg) | Vit A (IU) | Vit A (RE) | Retinol (RE) | Carotenoids (RE) | Beta Carotene (mcg) | Thiamin (mg) | Riboflavin (mg) | Niacin (NE) | Vit B6 (mg) | Vit B12 (mcg) | Folate (mcg) | Panto (mg) | Vit C (mg) | Vit D (mg) | Vit E (α TE) | Calcium (mg) | Copper (mg) | Iron (mg) | Magnes (mg) | Mang (mg) | Phos (mg) | Potassium (mg) | Selenium (mcg) | Sodium (mg) | Zinc (mg) |
|---|---|---|---|---|---|---|---|---|---|---|---|---|---|---|---|---|---|---|---|---|---|---|---|---|---|---|---|---|---|---|---|---|---|---|---|---|---|---|---|---|---|---|
| | | **Basic Components** | | | | | | | | | | **Additional Fats** | | | | | | **Vit A & Components** | | | | | **Vitamins** | | | | | | | | | | **Minerals** | | | | | | | | | |
| 52050 | 1/2 cup | Cold Rigatoni, Orval Kent | 130 | 170 | | 4.0 | 22.0 | 3.0 | 3.0 | 16.0 | 7.0 | 1.5 | | | | | 0 | 300 | 60 | | | | | | | | | | | 2.4 | | | 60 | | 0.7 | | | | | | 860 | |
| 52044 | 1/2 cup | Cold Vermicelli, Orval Kent | 106 | 129 | | 3.8 | 17.4 | 1.5 | 2.3 | 13.6 | 4.5 | 1.1 | | | | | 0 | 76 | 15 | | | | | | | | | | | 2.7 | | | 45 | | 0.8 | | | | | | 636 | |
| 52006 | 1/2 cup | Creamy, Orval Kent | 106 | 129 | | 3.8 | 24.2 | 1.5 | 5.3 | 17.4 | 1.9 | 0.4 | 0.4 | 1.1 | | | 8 | 76 | 15 | | | | | | | | | | | 2.7 | | | 30 | | 0.5 | | | | | | 424 | |
| 52045 | 1/2 cup | Dill, w/chicken, Orval Kent | 106 | 242 | | 11.4 | 21.2 | 2.3 | 1.5 | 17.4 | 14.4 | 2.3 | | | | | 23 | 76 | 15 | | | | | | | | | | | 1.8 | | | 15 | | 1.1 | | | | | | 545 | |
| 52047 | 1/2 cup | Honey Mustard, Orval Kent | 93 | 206 | | 3.3 | 23.3 | 2.0 | 5.3 | 15.9 | 10.6 | 2.0 | | | | | 3 | 199 | 40 | | | | | | | | | | | 0.0 | | | 13 | | 1.2 | | | | | | 379 | |
| 52036 | 1/2 cup | Italian, Orval Kent | 106 | 174 | | 3.0 | 16.7 | 2.3 | 1.5 | 12.9 | 10.6 | 1.5 | | | | | 0 | 76 | 15 | | | | | | | | | | | 9.1 | | | 30 | | 1.4 | | | | | | 432 | |
| 52097 | 1/2 cup | Italian, light, prep f/dry, Kraft | 95 | 127 | 68 | 5.4 | 22.7 | 1.3 | 3.3 | 18.1 | 1.3 | 0.7 | | | | | 1 | 134 | 27 | | | | 0.10 | | | | | | | 0.8 | | | 54 | | 1.2 | 21 | | 100 | 147 | | 442 | |
| 52054 | 1/2 cup | Italian Ziti, Orval Kent | 93 | 140 | | 6.0 | 10.6 | 1.3 | 1.3 | 8.0 | 8.0 | 3.0 | | | | | 13 | 996 | 199 | | | | | | | | | | | 3.2 | | | 133 | | 0.7 | | | | | | 465 | |
| 52055 | 1/2 cup | Lemon Dill Orzo, Orval Kent | 106 | 121 | | 3.8 | 16.7 | 1.5 | 0.8 | 14.4 | 4.5 | 1.9 | | | | | 8 | 1325 | 265 | | | | | | | | | | | 4.5 | | | 30 | | 0.5 | | | | | | 416 | |
| 56004 | 1/2 cup | Macaroni, avg | 88 | 229 | 60 | 2.3 | 14.1 | 0.9 | 2.3 | 10.9 | 18.5 | 2.0 | 3.0 | 12.7 | 0.69 | 11.95 | 14 | 90 | 22 | 19 | 3 | | 0.09 | 0.05 | 0.71 | 0.17 | 0.06 | 10.2 | 0.15 | 1.8 | 0.0 | 4.9 | 15 | 0.1 | 0.8 | 10 | 0.1 | 34 | 85 | 8.5 | 175 | 0.27 |
| 52005 | 1/2 cup | Macaroni, Orval Kent | 106 | 106 | | 3.8 | 23.5 | 0.8 | 6.8 | 15.9 | 1.9 | 0.0 | 0.0 | 1.1 | | | 8 | 76 | 15 | | | | | | | | | | | 0.9 | | | 30 | | 0.8 | | | | | | 401 | |
| 52031 | 1/2 cup | Macaroni, reduced fat, Orval Kent | 106 | 159 | | 3.8 | 25.0 | 1.5 | 8.3 | 15.1 | 4.5 | 0.8 | | | | | 8 | 0 | 0 | 0 | 0 | 0 | | | | | | | | 1.8 | | | 0 | | 2.7 | | | | | | 568 | |
| 52043 | 1/2 cup | Macaroni, w/sour cream & cheddar, Orval Kent | 106 | 212 | | 3.8 | 18.9 | 2.3 | 3.0 | 13.6 | 13.6 | 3.8 | | | | | 19 | 151 | 30 | | | | | | | | | | | 6.8 | | | 45 | | 4.1 | | | | | | 515 | |
| 52027 | 1/2 cup | Macaroni Country, Orval Kent | 106 | 227 | | 3.0 | 22.7 | 2.3 | 9.1 | 11.4 | 13.6 | 2.3 | | | | | 8 | 76 | 15 | | | | | | | | | | | 1.8 | | | 15 | | 0.8 | | | | | | 856 | |
| 52026 | 1/2 cup | Macaroni Ditalini, Orval Kent | 106 | 197 | | 3.0 | 17.4 | 2.3 | 5.3 | 9.8 | 12.9 | 1.9 | | | | | 8 | 76 | 15 | | | | | | | | | | | 1.8 | | | 15 | | 0.5 | | | | | | 621 | |
| 52028 | 1/2 cup | Macaroni Seashell, Orval Kent | 106 | 204 | | 3.0 | 21.2 | 1.5 | 5.3 | 14.4 | 12.1 | 1.9 | | | | | 8 | 0 | 0 | 0 | 0 | 0 | | | | | | | | 1.8 | | | 15 | | 1.4 | | | | | | 477 | |
| 52037 | 1/2 cup | Mediterranean, Orval Kent | 106 | 182 | | 3.0 | 15.9 | 2.3 | 0.8 | 12.9 | 12.1 | 1.9 | | | | | 0 | 568 | 114 | | | | | | | | | | | 1.8 | | | 30 | | 1.4 | | | | | | 318 | |
| 52051 | 1/2 cup | Oriental, Orval Kent | 106 | 136 | | 2.3 | 20.4 | 1.5 | 8.3 | 10.6 | 5.3 | 0.8 | | | | | 0 | 227 | 45 | | | | | | | | | | | 2.7 | | | 15 | | 0.8 | | | | | | 371 | |
| 52095 | 1/2 cup | Parmesan Pepper, prep f/dry, Kraft | 93 | 239 | | 5.3 | 18.6 | 1.3 | 2.0 | 15.3 | 16.6 | 3.0 | | | | | 13 | 199 | 40 | | | | 0.10 | 0.09 | 1.06 | | | | | 0.0 | | | 53 | | 1.2 | | | 100 | 100 | | 405 | |
| 52053 | 1/2 cup | Prima, Orval Kent | 106 | 204 | | 5.3 | 7.6 | 1.5 | 0.8 | 5.3 | 16.7 | 4.5 | | | | | 15 | 227 | 45 | | | | | | | | | | | 2.7 | | | 30 | | 1.4 | | | | | | 545 | |
| 52046 | 1/2 cup | Primavera, Orval Kent | 93 | 166 | | 4.0 | 16.6 | 1.3 | 2.0 | 13.3 | 9.3 | 1.7 | | | | | 7 | 498 | 100 | | | | | | | | | | | 0.8 | | | 27 | | 1.8 | | | | | | 445 | |
| 52094 | 1/2 cup | Primavera, prep f/dry, Kraft | 95 | 187 | 61 | 5.4 | 22.7 | 1.3 | 2.7 | 18.7 | 8.0 | 1.7 | | | | | 1 | 134 | 27 | | | | 0.10 | 0.11 | 1.34 | | | | | 0.8 | | | 54 | | 1.2 | 21 | | 100 | 134 | | 488 | |
| 52090 | 1/2 cup | Ranch, w/bacon, prep f/dry, Kraft | 90 | 240 | | 4.7 | 20.0 | 1.3 | 2.0 | 16.7 | 15.3 | 2.7 | | | | | 10 | 200 | 40 | | | | 0.15 | 0.09 | 1.33 | | | | | 0.0 | | | 13 | | 1.2 | 21 | | 67 | 113 | | 333 | |
| 52007 | 1/2 cup | Rotelli, Orval Kent | 106 | 129 | | 3.8 | 25.0 | 1.5 | 6.1 | 17.4 | 1.9 | 0.0 | 0.0 | 1.1 | | | 0 | 76 | 15 | | | | | | | | | | | 4.5 | | | 15 | | 0.8 | | | | | | 401 | |
| 52048 | 1/2 cup | Tarragon, w/tuna, Orval Kent | 93 | 159 | | 5.3 | 15.9 | 1.3 | 2.7 | 12.0 | 8.6 | 1.3 | | | | | 10 | 0 | 0 | 0 | 0 | 0 | | | | | | | | 0.8 | | | 13 | | 0.7 | | | | | | 445 | |
| 52038 | 1/2 cup | Vegetable, Orval Kent | 106 | 189 | | 3.8 | 18.9 | 2.3 | 0.8 | 15.9 | 10.6 | 1.9 | | | | | 0 | 151 | 30 | | | | | | | | | | | 0.9 | | | 45 | | 1.4 | | | | | | 386 | |
| | | Potato Salads | | | | | | | | | | | | | | | | | | | | | | | | | | | | | | | | | | | | | | | | |
| 56005 | 1/2 cup | Average | 125 | 179 | 76 | 3.4 | 14.0 | 1.6 | 4.0 | 8.4 | 10.3 | 1.8 | 3.1 | 4.7 | 0.47 | 4.20 | 35 | 261 | 41 | 23 | 18 | | 0.10 | 0.07 | 1.11 | 0.18 | 0.00 | 8.4 | 0.67 | 12.5 | 0.3 | | 24 | 0.1 | 0.8 | 19 | 0.1 | 65 | 318 | 5.1 | 661 | 0.39 |
| 52014 | 1/2 cup | Baked Style, Orval Kent | 106 | 129 | | 3.0 | 12.9 | 1.5 | 1.5 | 9.8 | 7.6 | 3.0 | | | | | 8 | 0 | 0 | 0 | 0 | 0 | | | | | | | | 0.0 | | | 30 | | 0.5 | | | | | | 326 | |
| 52020 | 1/2 cup | Country Style, w/egg, Orval Kent | 106 | 151 | | 1.5 | 18.9 | 2.3 | 6.8 | 9.8 | 8.3 | 1.1 | | | | | 4 | 76 | 15 | | | | | | | | | | | 4.5 | | | 1 | | 0.5 | | | | | | 553 | |
| 52030 | 1/2 cup | Country Style, w/egg, reduced fat, Orval Kent | 106 | 106 | | 2.3 | 16.7 | 1.5 | 4.5 | 10.6 | 3.0 | 0.4 | | | | | 8 | 76 | 15 | | | | | | | | | | | 1.8 | | | 15 | | 0.3 | | | | | | 530 | |
| 52017 | 1/2 cup | Creole, Orval Kent | 106 | 167 | | 2.3 | 15.9 | 2.3 | 0.8 | 12.9 | 10.6 | 1.5 | | | | | 19 | 0 | 0 | 0 | 0 | 0 | | | | | | | | 1.8 | | | 15 | | 0.8 | | | | | | 386 | |
| 52015 | 1/2 cup | German, Orval Kent | 106 | 106 | | 1.5 | 18.2 | 1.5 | 4.5 | 12.1 | 3.0 | 3.0 | | | | | 4 | 0 | 0 | 0 | 0 | 0 | | | | | | | | 0.9 | | | 15 | | 0.8 | | | | | | 318 | |
| 52056 | 1/2 cup | Herb, Orval Kent | 106 | 114 | | 1.5 | 11.4 | 3.0 | 0.8 | 7.6 | 6.8 | 1.1 | | | | | 0 | 76 | 15 | | | | | | | | | | | 0.9 | | | 15 | | 0.8 | | | | | | 371 | |
| 52018 | 1/2 cup | Mustard, Orval Kent | 106 | 144 | | 1.5 | 15.9 | 1.5 | 5.3 | 9.1 | 8.3 | 1.1 | | | | | 4 | 0 | 0 | 0 | 0 | 0 | | | | | | | | 1.8 | | | 15 | | 1.1 | | | | | | 538 | |
| 52033 | 1/2 cup | Mustard, reduced fat, Orval Kent | 106 | 98 | | 2.3 | 15.9 | 2.3 | 3.8 | 9.8 | 3.4 | 0.4 | | | | | 8 | 303 | 61 | | | | | | | | | | | 0.0 | | | 15 | | 0.3 | | | | | | 515 | |
| 52019 | 1/2 cup | Orval Kent | 106 | 151 | | 1.5 | 16.7 | 2.3 | 3.0 | 11.4 | 9.1 | 1.5 | | | | | 0 | 76 | 15 | | | | | | | | | | | 4.5 | | | 0 | | 0.3 | | | | | | 295 | |
| 52003 | 1/2 cup | Red, Orval Kent | 106 | 83 | | 1.5 | 15.1 | 2.3 | 3.8 | 9.1 | 1.9 | 0.0 | 0.4 | 1.1 | | | 11 | 76 | 15 | | | | | | | | | | | 4.5 | | | 15 | | 0.5 | | | | | | 447 | |
| 52013 | 1/2 cup | Red, w/egg, Orval Kent | 106 | 189 | | 2.3 | 21.2 | 1.5 | 4.5 | 15.1 | 11.4 | 1.5 | | | | | 15 | 76 | 15 | | | | | | | | | | | 6.8 | | | 15 | | 0.3 | | | | | | 598 | |
| 52032 | 1/2 cup | Reduced Fat, Orval Kent | 106 | 106 | | 2.3 | 16.7 | 2.3 | 5.3 | 9.1 | 3.8 | 0.4 | | | | | 8 | 76 | 15 | | | | | | | | | | | 2.7 | | | 15 | | 0.0 | | | | | | 485 | |
| 52041 | 1/2 cup | Sour Cream & Dill, Orval Kent | 106 | 159 | | 2.3 | 15.9 | 2.3 | 0.8 | 12.9 | 9.8 | 2.3 | | | | | 19 | 76 | 15 | | | | | | | | | | | 9.1 | | | 15 | | 0.3 | | | | | | 394 | |
| 52065 | 1/2 cup | Seafood Salad, Orval Kent | 100 | 230 | | 6.0 | 13.0 | 7.4 | 5.6 | 0.0 | 17.0 | 2.5 | | | | | 20 | 0 | 0 | 0 | 0 | 0 | | | | | | | | 0.0 | | | 20 | | 0.4 | | | | | | 770 | |
| 52064 | 1/2 cup | Shrimp Salad, Orval Kent | 100 | 170 | | 7.0 | 5.0 | 3.0 | 2.0 | 0.0 | 14.0 | 2.0 | | | | | 35 | 0 | 0 | 0 | 0 | 0 | | | | | | | | 0.0 | | | 40 | | 0.7 | | | | | | 620 | |
| 5537 | 1 cup | Spinach Salad, avg | 74 | 89 | 74 | 4.3 | 9.7 | 1.7 | 0.8 | 7.2 | 3.9 | 0.9 | 1.4 | 0.9 | | | 51 | 2237 | 240 | 24 | 216 | 1281 | 0.11 | 0.25 | 1.41 | 0.10 | 0.16 | 75.9 | 0.60 | 9.6 | 0.2 | | 51 | 0.1 | 1.6 | 33 | 0.4 | 73 | 277 | | 157 | 0.55 |
| 56007 | 1/2 cup | Tuna Salad, avg | 102 | 191 | 63 | 16.3 | 9.6 | 0.0 | 4.9 | 4.7 | 9.4 | 1.6 | 2.9 | 4.2 | 0.41 | 3.79 | 13 | 99 | 28 | | | | 0.03 | 0.07 | 6.83 | 0.08 | 1.22 | 8.2 | 0.27 | 2.2 | 3.3 | | 17 | 0.1 | 1.0 | 19 | 0.0 | 182 | 182 | 42.0 | 410 | 0.57 |
| 52009 | 1/2 cup | Tuna Salad, Orval Kent | 100 | 130 | | 12.0 | 8.0 | 2.0 | 3.0 | 3.0 | 5.0 | 0.9 | 1.4 | 2.7 | | | 25 | 0 | 0 | 0 | 0 | 0 | | | | | | | | 1.2 | | | 20 | | 0.7 | | | | | | 490 | |
| 56006 | 1/2 cup | Waldorf Salad, avg | 68 | 203 | 58 | 1.7 | 6.3 | 1.1 | 3.0 | 2.1 | 19.9 | 2.1 | 3.6 | 13.4 | 1.18 | 12.16 | 10 | 98 | 20 | 15 | 5 | | 0.05 | 0.02 | 0.18 | 0.18 | 0.04 | 13.6 | 0.16 | 2.9 | 0.0 | 3.9 | 21 | 0.1 | 0.4 | 20 | 0.3 | 41 | 134 | 0.5 | 117 | 0.31 |
| | | **SANDWICHES** | | | | | | | | | | | | | | | | | | | | | | | | | | | | | | | | | | | | | | | | |
| 56023 | 1 ea | Avocado & Cheese, on wheat, avg | 214 | 468 | 58 | 16.1 | 40.0 | 7.8 | 4.5 | 27.7 | 29.8 | 8.7 | 11.6 | 7.5 | 0.47 | 6.92 | 31 | 892 | 140 | 72 | 68 | | 0.36 | 0.37 | 4.29 | 0.42 | 0.26 | 91.7 | 1.27 | 11.1 | 0.2 | 3.0 | 281 | 0.4 | 3.5 | 102 | 1.9 | 336 | 679 | 29.3 | 593 | 2.68 |
| 56021 | 1 ea | Avocado & Cheese, on white, avg | 210 | 478 | 58 | 15.3 | 40.9 | 4.9 | 4.2 | 31.9 | 29.3 | 8.8 | 11.3 | 7.3 | 0.47 | 6.75 | 34 | 892 | 140 | 72 | 68 | | 0.37 | 0.39 | 3.77 | 0.32 | 0.26 | 79.7 | 1.16 | 11.1 | 0.3 | 3.0 | 294 | 0.3 | 3.1 | 54 | 0.5 | 241 | 582 | 21.6 | 550 | 1.71 |
| 56010 | 1 ea | Bacon, Lettuce & Tomato, on wheat, avg | 137 | 328 | 53 | 12.1 | 31.7 | 4.5 | 3.8 | 23.4 | 18.1 | 4.4 | 6.4 | 6.3 | 0.42 | 5.80 | 20 | 261 | 31 | 7 | 24 | | 0.37 | 0.20 | 3.96 | 0.24 | 0.33 | 48.3 | 0.64 | 12.0 | 0.2 | 3.0 | 55 | 0.2 | 2.7 | 64 | 1.6 | 219 | 342 | 26.1 | 670 | 1.90 |
| 56008 | 1 ea | Bacon, Lettuce & Tomato, on white, avg | 133 | 336 | 52 | 11.3 | 32.5 | 1.8 | 3.6 | 27.1 | 17.7 | 4.5 | 6.1 | 6.1 | 0.42 | 5.64 | 22 | 260 | 31 | 7 | 24 | | 0.39 | 0.21 | 3.49 | 0.15 | 0.33 | 37.3 | 0.55 | 11.9 | 0.2 | 3.0 | 67 | 0.1 | 2.2 | 22 | 0.4 | 133 | 252 | 19.2 | 630 | 1.02 |
| | | Beef | | | | | | | | | | | | | | | | | | | | | | | | | | | | | | | | | | | | | | | | |
| 56020 | 1 ea | Corned Beef & Swiss, on rye, avg | 156 | 420 | 49 | 27.7 | 21.7 | 0.1 | 1.5 | 20.0 | 25.6 | 9.4 | 7.4 | 6.3 | 0.52 | 5.78 | 32 | 286 | 81 | 79 | 2 | | 0.19 | 0.33 | 2.72 | 0.17 | 1.73 | 19.1 | 0.65 | 1.0 | 0.4 | 2.9 | 268 | 0.1 | 3.1 | 28 | 0.1 | 272 | 225 | 29.1 | 1392 | 3.64 |
| 56983 | 1 ea | Fried Beef Pocket, fzn, Ore Ida | 142 | 371 | 51 | 15.0 | 34.1 | 2.0 | 2.0 | 30.1 | 20.0 | 5.0 | | | | | 45 | 0 | 0 | 0 | 0 | 0 | | | | | | | | 0.0 | | | 40 | | 2.7 | | | | 240 | | 671 | |
| 56263 | 1 ea | Meatball, w/spaghetti sauce, avg | 189 | 435 | 54 | 29.3 | 36.0 | 2.6 | | | 18.5 | 6.9 | 7.9 | 1.2 | | | 37 | 632 | 63 | 0 | 63 | | 0.29 | 0.34 | 8.23 | 0.35 | 2.82 | 30.7 | | 16.4 | | | 68 | 0.3 | 4.4 | 42 | | 231 | 527 | | 418 | 5.45 |
| 69024 | 1 ea | Patty, w/cheese, Kid Cuisine | 177 | 270 | 67 | 10.0 | 40.0 | 5.0 | 22.0 | 13.0 | 7.0 | 4.0 | | | | | 20 | 0 | 0 | 0 | 0 | 0 | | | | | | | | 3.6 | | | 100 | | 1.1 | | | | | | 330 | |
| 56038 | 1 ea | Patty Melt, w/ground beef on rye, avg | 182 | 561 | 46 | 36.8 | 22.0 | 3.0 | 2.2 | 16.8 | 36.8 | 13.2 | 11.7 | 8.4 | 0.39 | 7.87 | 113 | 465 | 123 | 111 | 12 | | 0.25 | 0.46 | 6.14 | 0.35 | 2.43 | 24.8 | 0.60 | 0.1 | 0.5 | 3.4 | 221 | 0.1 | 4.2 | 36 | 0.0 | 327 | 391 | 42.5 | 701 | 7.11 |
| 56043 | 1 ea | Roast Beef, on white, avg | 160 | 418 | 45 | 29.1 | 37.3 | 1.4 | 7.2 | 28.6 | 16.2 | 3.3 | 4.1 | 7.9 | 0.44 | 7.46 | 44 | 37 | 11 | 11 | 0 | | 0.32 | 0.31 | 6.47 | 0.38 | 2.16 | 32.7 | 0.81 | 11.8 | 0.4 | 1.9 | 73 | 0.1 | 4.1 | 29 | 0.3 | 207 | 436 | 40.9 | 1580 | 3.71 |
| 56045 | 1 ea | Roast Beef, on whole wheat, avg | 169 | 422 | 46 | 30.9 | 37.5 | 4.3 | 7.7 | 25.5 | 17.1 | 3.3 | 4.5 | 8.4 | 0.45 | 7.86 | 43 | 39 | 12 | 12 | 0 | | 0.31 | 0.31 | 7.18 | 0.49 | 2.24 | 45.5 | 0.93 | 12.2 | 0.4 | 2.9 | 62 | 0.2 | 4.7 | 77 | 1.7 | 307 | 547 | 49.7 | 1672 | 4.79 |
| 56669 | 1 ea | Roast Beef, w/cheese, avg | 176 | 473 | 44 | 32.2 | 45.4 | | | | 18.0 | 9.0 | 3.7 | 3.5 | | | 77 | 194 | 46 | 41 | 5 | | 0.39 | 0.46 | 5.90 | 0.33 | 2.06 | 63.4 | 0.69 | 0.0 | | | 183 | 0.2 | 5.1 | 40 | 0.3 | 401 | 345 | 34.3 | 1633 | 5.37 |
| 56670 | 1 ea | Steak, avg | 204 | 459 | 51 | 30.4 | 52.0 | | | | 14.1 | 3.8 | 5.3 | 3.3 | | | 73 | 367 | 45 | 45 | 0 | | 0.41 | 0.37 | 7.30 | 0.37 | 1.57 | 89.8 | 0.92 | 5.5 | | | 92 | 0.2 | 5.2 | 49 | 0.4 | 298 | 524 | 42.0 | 798 | 4.53 |
| 56014 | 1 ea | Cheese, grilled, on wheat, avg | 132 | 420 | 38 | 19.7 | 33.3 | 4.3 | 3.8 | 25.1 | 24.5 | 13.1 | 7.8 | 2.2 | 0.15 | 1.78 | 54 | 844 | 212 | 191 | 20 | | 0.26 | 0.35 | 2.74 | 0.17 | 0.41 | 39.6 | 0.66 | 0.0 | 0.3 | 0.5 | 402 | 0.2 | 2.5 | 73 | 1.6 | 585 | 270 | 29.5 | 1227 | 3.08 |
| 56012 | 1 ea | Cheese, grilled, on white, avg | 128 | 429 | 36 | 18.9 | 34.2 | 1.5 | 3.5 | 29.2 | 24.1 | 13.2 | 7.5 | 2.0 | 0.15 | 1.61 | 56 | 844 | 212 | 191 | 20 | | 0.28 | 0.36 | 2.22 | 0.06 | 0.40 | 27.8 | 0.56 | 0.0 | 0.3 | 0.5 | 415 | 0.1 | 2.1 | 27 | 0.3 | 492 | 174 | 22.0 | 1184 | 2.11 |
| | | Chicken | | | | | | | | | | | | | | | | | | | | | | | | | | | | | | | | | | | | | | | | |
| 56278 | 1 ea | BBQ, avg | 119 | 250 | 54 | 20.6 | 26.2 | 1.5 | | | 6.2 | 1.6 | 2.2 | 1.6 | | | 51 | 137 | 20 | 9 | 11 | | 0.28 | 0.27 | 7.29 | 0.30 | 0.19 | 20.8 | | 0.9 | | | 69 | 0.1 | 2.3 | 29 | | 165 | 218 | | 424 | 1.52 |
| 69015 | 1 ea | Broccoli & Cheese Pocket, Weight Watchers | 142 | 250 | 58 | 13.0 | 40.0 | 1.0 | 4.0 | 35.0 | 6.0 | 2.5 | | | | | 25 | 500 | 100 | | | | | | | | | | | 2.4 | | | 60 | | 0.7 | | | | 220 | | 310 | |
| 56000 | 1 ea | Fillet, avg | 182 | 515 | 47 | 24.2 | 38.8 | 1.3 | 6.0 | 31.5 | 29.5 | 8.5 | 10.4 | 8.4 | 0.96 | 7.42 | 50 | 100 | 31 | 31 | 0 | | 0.33 | 0.24 | 6.81 | 0.20 | 0.38 | 100.1 | 0.60 | 8.9 | 0.3 | | 60 | 0.2 | 4.7 | 35 | 0.5 | 233 | 353 | 40.4 | 957 | 1.87 |
| 56656 | 1 ea | Fillet, w/cheese, avg | 228 | 632 | 46 | 29.4 | 41.5 | | | | 38.8 | 12.4 | 13.7 | 9.9 | | | 78 | 620 | 123 | 115 | 13 | | 0.41 | 0.46 | 9.07 | 0.41 | 0.46 | 109.4 | 1.35 | 3.0 | | | 258 | 0.2 | 3.6 | 43 | 0.4 | 406 | 333 | 48.1 | 1238 | 2.90 |
| 69025 | 1 ea | Kid Cuisine | 234 | 440 | 60 | 15.0 | 63.0 | 4.0 | 25.0 | 34.0 | 14.0 | 3.0 | | | | | 20 | 100 | 20 | | | | | | | | | | | 0.0 | | | 60 | | 2.7 | | | | | | 680 | |

| Code | Amount | Description | Weight (g) | Calories | % Water | Protein (g) | Carbs (g) | Fiber (g) | Sugar (g) | Other Carbs (g) | Fat (g) | Sat Fat (g) | Mono Fat (g) | Poly Fat (g) | Omega 3 (g) | Omega 6 (g) | Choles (mg) |
|---|---|---|---|---|---|---|---|---|---|---|---|---|---|---|---|---|---|
| | | **Basic Components** | | | | | | | | | | **Additional Fats** | | | | | |
| 56018 | 1 ea | Salad, on wheat, avg | 123 | 387 | 41 | 12.7 | 34.5 | 4.6 | 3.4 | 26.5 | 23.5 | 3.6 | 6.3 | 12.2 | 0.94 | 11.17 | 30 |
| 56016 | 1 ea | Salad, on white, avg | 119 | 398 | 39 | 11.8 | 35.5 | 1.7 | 3.1 | 30.8 | 23.1 | 3.7 | 6.0 | 12.0 | 0.94 | 11.01 | 33 |
| 56982 | 1 ea | Vegetable & Cheese Pocket, Ore Ida | 142 | 361 | 49 | 13.0 | 44.1 | 3.0 | 7.0 | 34.1 | 14.0 | 4.0 | | | | | 20 |
| 56026 | 1 ea | Egg Salad, on wheat, avg | 130 | 401 | 43 | 11.6 | 34.6 | 4.5 | 3.7 | 26.4 | 25.3 | 4.3 | 7.1 | 12.2 | 0.31 | 5.54 | 155 |
| 56024 | 1 ea | Egg Salad, on white, avg | 126 | 410 | 42 | 10.7 | 35.6 | 1.6 | 3.3 | 30.7 | 24.9 | 4.4 | 6.8 | 12.0 | 0.30 | 5.37 | 157 |
| | | Fish | | | | | | | | | | | | | | | |
| 69066 | 1 ea | With Cheese, Mrs Paul's | 121 | 330 | | 10.0 | 38.0 | 3.0 | 5.0 | 30.0 | 15.0 | 4.0 | | | | | 25 |
| 66011 | 1 ea | With Cheese & Tartar Sauce, avg | 183 | 523 | 45 | 20.7 | 47.6 | 0.4 | | | 28.5 | 8.1 | 8.9 | 9.4 | 0.96 | 8.47 | 68 |
| 66010 | 1 ea | With Tartar Sauce, avg | 158 | 431 | 47 | 16.9 | 41.1 | 0.4 | | | 22.8 | 5.2 | 7.7 | 8.2 | 0.63 | 7.62 | 55 |
| | | Hamburgers/Cheeseburgers | | | | | | | | | | | | | | | |
| 66014 | 1 ea | Cheeseburger, avg | 102 | 319 | 37 | 14.8 | 31.7 | | | | 15.2 | 6.5 | 5.8 | 1.5 | | | 50 |
| 66016 | 1 ea | Cheeseburger, double, avg | 155 | 457 | 42 | 27.7 | 22.0 | | | | 28.5 | 13.0 | 11.0 | 1.9 | | | 110 |
| 66013 | 1 ea | Cheeseburger, double, w/condmnts & vegs, avg | 166 | 417 | 51 | 21.2 | 35.2 | | | | 21.1 | 8.7 | 7.8 | 2.7 | | | 60 |
| 56648 | 1 ea | Cheeseburger, large, avg | 185 | 609 | 39 | 30.2 | 47.4 | | | | 32.9 | 14.8 | 12.7 | 2.4 | | | 96 |
| 66012 | 1 ea | Cheeseburger, large, double, w/cond&vegs, avg | 258 | 704 | 51 | 37.9 | 39.7 | | | | 43.6 | 17.7 | 17.4 | 4.7 | | | 142 |
| 56651 | 1 ea | Cheeseburger, large, w/bacon & condmnts, avg | 195 | 608 | 44 | 32.0 | 37.0 | | | | 36.9 | 16.2 | 14.5 | 2.7 | | | 111 |
| 56649 | 1 ea | Cheeseburger, large, w/condiments & veg, avg | 219 | 563 | 52 | 28.3 | 38.3 | | | | 32.9 | 15.0 | 12.6 | 2.0 | 0.39 | 1.64 | 88 |
| 56650 | 1 ea | Cheeseburger, large, w/ham, cond & vegs, avg | 254 | 744 | 50 | 39.6 | 37.6 | | | | 48.3 | 21.1 | 18.9 | 3.9 | | | 122 |
| 56652 | 1 ea | Cheeseburger, triple, avg | 304 | 796 | 54 | 55.9 | 26.7 | | | | 51.1 | 21.7 | 21.5 | 3.2 | | | 161 |
| 56647 | 1 ea | Cheeseburger, w/condiments, avg | 113 | 295 | 48 | 15.9 | 26.6 | | | | 14.1 | 6.3 | 5.3 | 1.1 | 0.18 | 0.91 | 37 |
| 66015 | 1 ea | Cheeseburger, w/condiments & vegs, avg | 154 | 359 | 55 | 17.9 | 28.2 | | | | 19.9 | 9.2 | 7.2 | 1.5 | 0.55 | 0.92 | 52 |
| 66007 | 1 ea | Hamburger, avg | 90 | 274 | 38 | 12.3 | 30.5 | | | | 11.8 | 4.1 | 5.5 | 0.9 | 0.07 | 0.84 | 35 |
| 66009 | 1 ea | Hamburger, double, avg | 176 | 544 | 41 | 29.9 | 42.9 | | | | 28.0 | 10.4 | 12.1 | 2.3 | | | 99 |
| 66006 | 1 ea | Hamburger, double, w/condiments, avg | 215 | 576 | 50 | 31.8 | 38.7 | | | | 32.5 | 12.0 | 14.1 | 2.8 | | | 103 |
| 56660 | 1 ea | Hamburger, large, avg | 137 | 426 | 42 | 22.6 | 31.8 | | | | 22.9 | 8.4 | 9.9 | 2.1 | | | 71 |
| 56662 | 1 ea | Hamburger, large, dbl, w/condmnts & vegs, avg | 226 | 540 | 54 | 34.4 | 40.2 | | | | 26.7 | 10.5 | 10.3 | 2.8 | | | 122 |
| 56661 | 1 ea | Hamburger, large, w/condiments & vegs, avg | 218 | 512 | 56 | 25.9 | 40.1 | | | | 27.5 | 10.4 | 11.4 | 2.2 | 0.24 | 1.96 | 87 |
| 56663 | 1 ea | Hamburger, triple, w/condiments, avg | 259 | 692 | 52 | 50.0 | 28.5 | | | | 41.4 | 15.9 | 18.2 | 2.7 | | | 142 |
| 56658 | 1 ea | Hamburger, w/condiments, avg | 107 | 275 | 45 | 12.4 | 34.6 | 2.4 | 6.8 | 25.4 | 9.9 | 3.6 | 3.4 | 1.0 | 0.11 | 0.90 | 30 |
| 56659 | 1 ea | Hamburger, w/condiments & vegetables, avg | 110 | 279 | 49 | 12.9 | 27.3 | | | | 13.5 | 4.1 | 5.3 | 2.6 | | | 26 |
| | | Ham | | | | | | | | | | | | | | | |
| 56032 | 1 ea | On rye, avg | 150 | 283 | 60 | 21.7 | 20.7 | 0.1 | 1.0 | 19.5 | 13.5 | 2.4 | 3.8 | 6.0 | 0.35 | 5.65 | 47 |
| 56030 | 1 ea | On wheat, avg | 169 | 352 | 54 | 23.6 | 33.6 | 4.5 | 3.8 | 25.3 | 14.6 | 2.9 | 4.7 | 6.1 | 0.34 | 5.70 | 45 |
| 56028 | 1 ea | On white, avg | 170 | 373 | 54 | 23.4 | 35.6 | 1.7 | 3.7 | 30.2 | 14.6 | 3.0 | 4.5 | 6.1 | 0.34 | 5.69 | 49 |
| 69018 | 1 ea | Pocket, w/cheese, Weight Watchers | 142 | 240 | 62 | 14.0 | 32.0 | 5.0 | 1.0 | 26.0 | 7.0 | 2.5 | | | | | 10 |
| 56065 | 1 ea | Salad, on wheat, avg | 144 | 381 | 47 | 12.5 | 40.3 | 4.5 | 5.0 | 30.8 | 20.2 | 4.7 | 7.0 | 7.6 | 0.51 | 6.98 | 29 |
| 56063 | 1 ea | Salad, on white, avg | 140 | 390 | 46 | 11.7 | 41.3 | 1.5 | 4.7 | 35.0 | 19.8 | 4.8 | 6.7 | 7.4 | 0.51 | 6.82 | 31 |
| 56036 | 1 ea | With Cheese, on wheat, avg | 170 | 424 | 49 | 24.5 | 34.0 | 4.5 | 4.0 | 25.4 | 22.2 | 8.3 | 6.2 | 6.4 | 0.39 | 5.80 | 59 |
| 56034 | 1 ea | With Cheese, on white, avg | 166 | 433 | 48 | 23.7 | 34.9 | 1.6 | 3.8 | 29.5 | 21.8 | 8.4 | 5.9 | 6.1 | 0.39 | 5.63 | 61 |
| 56033 | 1 ea | With Swiss, on rye, avg | 150 | 339 | 54 | 22.4 | 21.7 | 0.1 | 2.0 | 19.5 | 19.1 | 6.5 | 5.1 | 6.0 | 0.41 | 5.62 | 57 |
| | | Hotdog | | | | | | | | | | | | | | | |
| 66004 | 1 ea | Hotdog, avg | 98 | 242 | 54 | 10.4 | 18.0 | | | | 14.5 | 5.1 | 6.9 | 1.7 | 0.42 | 1.28 | 44 |
| 56667 | 1 ea | Hotdog, w/chili, avg | 114 | 296 | 48 | 13.6 | 31.4 | | | | 13.5 | 4.9 | 6.6 | 1.2 | 0.14 | 1.04 | 51 |
| 56284 | 1 ea | Hotdog, w/chili & cheese, avg | 264 | 729 | 50 | 29.6 | 48.2 | 3.6 | | | 46.6 | 21.0 | 19.1 | 3.6 | | | 98 |
| 56041 | 1 ea | Peanut Butter & Jam, on wheat, avg | 114 | 370 | 28 | 13.4 | 50.1 | 6.1 | 18.6 | 25.4 | 15.5 | 3.0 | 7.0 | 4.1 | 0.04 | 3.98 | 0 |
| 56039 | 1 ea | Peanut Butter & Jam, on white, avg | 110 | 379 | 27 | 12.6 | 51.0 | 3.3 | 18.3 | 29.5 | 15.1 | 3.1 | 6.6 | 3.9 | 0.04 | 3.81 | 3 |
| 69016 | 1 ea | Pizza Pocket, Weight Watchers | 142 | 300 | 50 | 17.0 | 46.0 | 4.0 | 2.0 | 40.0 | 7.0 | 2.5 | | | | | 15 |
| 69072 | 1 ea | Reuben, avg | 239 | 462 | 64 | 27.9 | 24.8 | 2.2 | 2.2 | 20.4 | 29.1 | 9.9 | 9.5 | 7.1 | 0.54 | 6.54 | 80 |
| 69021 | 1 ea | Reuben Pocket, Weight Watchers | 142 | 250 | 57 | 12.0 | 42.0 | 5.0 | 6.0 | 31.0 | 6.0 | 2.0 | | | | | 20 |
| | | Submarine | | | | | | | | | | | | | | | |
| 56671 | 1 ea | Cold Cuts, avg | 228 | 456 | 58 | 21.8 | 51.1 | 1.7 | | | 18.6 | 6.8 | 8.2 | 2.3 | | | 36 |
| 56672 | 1 ea | Roast Beef, avg | 216 | 410 | 59 | 28.7 | 44.3 | | | | 13.0 | 7.1 | 1.8 | 2.6 | | | 73 |
| 56673 | 1 ea | Tuna Salad, avg | 256 | 584 | 54 | 29.7 | 55.3 | | | | 27.9 | 5.3 | 13.4 | 7.3 | | | 49 |
| 56047 | 1 ea | Tuna Salad, on white, avg | 131 | 356 | 45 | 14.8 | 39.7 | 1.9 | 5.2 | 32.6 | 15.1 | 2.4 | 3.8 | 7.9 | 0.52 | 7.32 | 15 |
| 56049 | 1 ea | Tuna Salad, on whole wheat, avg | 135 | 346 | 46 | 15.6 | 38.7 | 4.8 | 5.5 | 28.3 | 15.5 | 2.3 | 4.1 | 8.1 | 0.53 | 7.48 | 12 |
| | | Turkey | | | | | | | | | | | | | | | |
| 56055 | 1 ea | Ham & Cheese, on rye, avg | 150 | 353 | 54 | 22.2 | 20.5 | 0.1 | 0.8 | 19.5 | 21.3 | 8.1 | 4.7 | 6.8 | 0.42 | 6.31 | 66 |
| 56058 | 1 ea | Ham & Cheese, on wheat, avg | 170 | 422 | 49 | 24.2 | 33.6 | 4.5 | 3.7 | 25.4 | 22.3 | 8.4 | 5.5 | 7.0 | 0.41 | 6.37 | 64 |
| 56056 | 1 ea | Ham & Cheese, on white, avg | 166 | 431 | 49 | 23.4 | 34.6 | 1.6 | 3.4 | 29.5 | 21.9 | 8.4 | 5.2 | 6.7 | 0.41 | 6.19 | 67 |
| 56103 | 1 ea | Ham, on rye, avg | 150 | 281 | 60 | 21.3 | 20.1 | 0.1 | 0.5 | 19.5 | 13.6 | 2.5 | 2.8 | 6.9 | 0.38 | 6.52 | 55 |
| 56105 | 1 ea | Ham, on wheat, avg | 169 | 350 | 55 | 23.2 | 33.1 | 4.5 | 3.3 | 25.3 | 14.8 | 2.9 | 3.7 | 7.0 | 0.37 | 6.53 | 53 |
| 56107 | 1 ea | Ham, on white, avg | 166 | 361 | 54 | 22.4 | 34.2 | 1.6 | 3.0 | 29.5 | 14.4 | 3.0 | 3.4 | 6.8 | 0.36 | 6.39 | 56 |
| 56053 | 1 ea | On wheat, avg | 169 | 364 | 53 | 26.1 | 32.7 | 4.3 | 2.9 | 25.5 | 15.2 | 2.3 | 3.5 | 8.5 | 0.45 | 7.93 | 43 |
| 56051 | 1 ea | On white, avg | 165 | 326 | 55 | 26.6 | 35.3 | 1.6 | 2.7 | 31.0 | 7.9 | 1.7 | 2.1 | 3.4 | 0.18 | 3.17 | 43 |
| 56989 | 1 ea | Swiss & Broccoli Pocket, Ore Ida | 170 | 380 | 52 | 18.0 | 49.0 | 3.0 | 9.0 | 37.0 | 14.0 | 5.0 | | | | | 35 |

| Code | Vit A (IU) | Vit A (RE) | Retinol (RE) | Carotenoids (RE) | Beta Carotene (mcg) | Thiamin (mg) | Riboflavin (mg) | Niacin (NE) | Vit B6 (mg) | Vit B12 (mcg) | Folate (mcg) | Panto (mg) | Vit C (mg) | Vit D (mg) | Vit E (α TE) | Calcium (mg) | Copper (mg) | Iron (mg) | Magnes (mg) | Mang (mg) | Phos (mg) | Potassium (mg) | Selenium (mcg) | Sodium (mg) | Zinc (mg) |
|---|---|---|---|---|---|---|---|---|---|---|---|---|---|---|---|---|---|---|---|---|---|---|---|---|---|
| | **Vit A & Components** | | | | | **Vitamins** | | | | | | | | | | **Minerals** | | | | | | | | | |
| 56018 | 87 | 24 | 23 | 1 | | 0.27 | 0.19 | 4.50 | 0.36 | 0.12 | 41.6 | 0.68 | 0.6 | 0.3 | 5.8 | 63 | 0.3 | 2.8 | 68 | 1.7 | 212 | 259 | 31.5 | 542 | 1.85 |
| 56016 | 87 | 24 | 23 | 1 | | 0.29 | 0.20 | 3.97 | 0.25 | 0.13 | 29.4 | 0.57 | 0.6 | 0.3 | 5.8 | 76 | 0.1 | 2.3 | 20 | 0.4 | 114 | 158 | 23.7 | 499 | 0.85 |
| 56982 | 501 | 100 | | | | | | | | | | | 2.4 | | | 150 | | 0.7 | | | | 210 | | 631 | |
| 56026 | 252 | 76 | 76 | 0 | 0 | 0.28 | 0.32 | 2.82 | 0.30 | 0.44 | 53.3 | 0.99 | 0.0 | 0.7 | 2.9 | 73 | 0.2 | 2.9 | 66 | 1.7 | 231 | 234 | 36.9 | 611 | 1.80 |
| 56024 | 252 | 76 | 76 | 0 | 0 | 0.29 | 0.33 | 2.29 | 0.20 | 0.44 | 41.1 | 0.89 | 0.0 | 0.7 | 2.9 | 87 | 0.1 | 2.4 | 18 | 0.3 | 134 | 133 | 29.1 | 568 | 0.81 |
| 69066 | 0 | 0 | 0 | 0 | 0 | | | | | | | | 0.0 | | | 150 | | 2.7 | | | | | | 630 | |
| 66011 | 432 | 97 | 87 | 10 | | 0.46 | 0.42 | 4.23 | 0.11 | 1.08 | 91.5 | 0.44 | 2.7 | | | 185 | 0.1 | 3.5 | 37 | 0.4 | 311 | 353 | 88.6 | 939 | 1.17 |
| 66010 | 109 | 30 | 30 | 0 | | 0.33 | 0.22 | 3.40 | 0.11 | 1.07 | 85.3 | 0.58 | 2.8 | | 0.9 | 84 | 0.2 | 2.6 | 33 | 0.4 | 212 | 340 | 79.9 | 615 | 1.00 |
| 66014 | 153 | 37 | 32 | 5 | | 0.40 | 0.40 | 3.70 | 0.09 | 0.97 | 54.1 | 0.43 | 0.0 | | | 141 | 0.1 | 2.4 | 21 | 0.2 | 196 | 164 | 22.6 | 500 | 2.37 |
| 66016 | 332 | 79 | 69 | 10 | | 0.25 | 0.37 | 6.01 | 0.25 | 2.31 | 68.2 | 0.62 | 0.0 | | 1.2 | 232 | 0.1 | 3.4 | 33 | 0.2 | 374 | 308 | 32.1 | 635 | 4.96 |
| 66013 | 398 | 65 | 43 | 22 | | 0.35 | 0.28 | 8.05 | 0.18 | 1.93 | 61.4 | 0.43 | 1.7 | | | 171 | 0.1 | 3.4 | 30 | 0.3 | 242 | 335 | 23.6 | 1051 | 3.49 |
| 56648 | 616 | 148 | 129 | 19 | | 0.48 | 0.57 | 11.17 | 0.28 | 2.53 | 74.0 | 0.74 | 0.0 | | | 91 | 0.2 | 5.5 | 39 | 0.3 | 422 | 644 | 38.9 | 1589 | 5.55 |
| 66012 | 348 | 54 | 36 | 18 | | 0.36 | 0.49 | 7.25 | 0.41 | 3.41 | 74.8 | 0.85 | 1.0 | | | 240 | 0.2 | 5.9 | 52 | 0.3 | 395 | 596 | 28.9 | 1148 | 6.68 |
| 56651 | 406 | 80 | 53 | 27 | | 0.31 | 0.41 | 6.63 | 0.31 | 2.34 | 85.8 | 0.35 | 2.1 | | | 162 | 0.2 | 4.7 | 45 | 0.3 | 400 | 332 | 33.0 | 1043 | 6.83 |
| 56649 | 613 | 129 | 95 | 34 | | 0.39 | 0.46 | 7.38 | 0.28 | 2.56 | 81.0 | 0.72 | 7.9 | | 1.2 | 206 | 0.2 | 4.7 | 44 | 0.3 | 311 | 445 | 37.4 | 1108 | 4.60 |
| 56650 | 505 | 104 | 65 | 40 | | 0.53 | 0.56 | 9.17 | 0.38 | 2.87 | 78.7 | 1.04 | 7.4 | | | 302 | 0.2 | 5.0 | 51 | 0.4 | 531 | 538 | 32.5 | 1712 | 6.63 |
| 56652 | 359 | 85 | 74 | 11 | | 0.61 | 0.64 | 11.46 | 0.61 | 5.90 | 69.9 | 1.16 | 2.7 | | | 283 | 0.3 | 8.3 | 61 | 0.4 | 541 | 821 | 25.5 | 1213 | 10.88 |
| 56647 | 462 | 94 | 82 | 12 | | 0.25 | 0.23 | 3.72 | 0.11 | 0.94 | 54.2 | 0.32 | 1.9 | | 0.5 | 111 | 0.1 | 2.4 | 20 | 0.2 | 176 | 223 | 19.8 | 616 | 2.09 |
| 66015 | 431 | 71 | 52 | 18 | | 0.32 | 0.23 | 6.38 | 0.15 | 1.23 | 64.7 | 0.34 | 2.3 | | | 182 | 0.1 | 2.6 | 26 | 0.3 | 216 | 229 | 20.5 | 976 | 2.62 |
| 66007 | 0 | 0 | 0 | 0 | 0 | 0.33 | 0.27 | 3.72 | 0.06 | 0.89 | 53.1 | 0.37 | 0.0 | | 0.5 | 63 | 0.1 | 2.4 | 19 | 0.2 | 103 | 145 | 21.7 | 387 | 2.00 |
| 66009 | 0 | 0 | 0 | 0 | 0 | 0.33 | 0.37 | 8.25 | 0.32 | 2.92 | 77.4 | 0.67 | 0.0 | | 1.3 | 86 | 0.2 | 4.6 | 37 | 0.3 | 234 | 363 | 39.6 | 554 | 5.72 |
| 66006 | 54 | 4 | 0 | 4 | | 0.34 | 0.41 | 6.73 | 0.37 | 3.33 | 83.9 | 0.77 | 1.1 | | | 92 | 0.2 | 5.5 | 45 | 0.3 | 284 | 527 | 44.9 | 742 | 5.81 |
| 56660 | 0 | 0 | 0 | 0 | 0 | 0.29 | 0.29 | 6.25 | 0.23 | 2.06 | 60.3 | 0.53 | 0.0 | | 0.7 | 74 | 0.1 | 3.6 | 27 | 0.2 | 175 | 267 | 27.1 | 474 | 4.11 |
| 56662 | 102 | 11 | 0 | 11 | | 0.36 | 0.38 | 7.57 | 0.54 | 4.07 | 76.8 | 0.54 | 1.1 | | | 102 | 0.2 | 5.9 | 50 | 0.2 | 314 | 570 | 25.5 | 791 | 5.67 |
| 56661 | 312 | 33 | 0 | 33 | | 0.41 | 0.37 | 7.28 | 0.33 | 2.38 | 82.8 | 0.72 | 2.6 | | 1.2 | 96 | 0.2 | 4.9 | 44 | 0.3 | 233 | 480 | 33.6 | 824 | 4.88 |
| 56663 | 158 | 16 | 0 | 16 | | 0.31 | 0.54 | 10.96 | 0.62 | 4.92 | 75.1 | 0.67 | 1.3 | | | 65 | 0.2 | 8.3 | 54 | 0.2 | 394 | 785 | 55.7 | 712 | 10.75 |
| 56658 | 75 | 10 | 0 | 10 | 58 | 0.29 | 0.24 | 3.95 | 0.12 | 1.10 | 52.4 | 0.28 | 2.2 | | 0.4 | 127 | 0.2 | 2.7 | 24 | 0.4 | 116 | 254 | 20.9 | 539 | 2.27 |
| 56659 | 83 | 9 | 0 | 9 | | 0.23 | 0.20 | 3.68 | 0.12 | 0.88 | 51.7 | 0.30 | 1.7 | | | 63 | 0.1 | 2.6 | 22 | 0.3 | 124 | 227 | 20.6 | 504 | 2.06 |
| 56032 | 28 | 8 | 8 | 0.1 | | 0.99 | 0.31 | 5.45 | 0.47 | 0.71 | 15.2 | 0.54 | 22.9 | 0.6 | 1.9 | 48 | 0.1 | 2.3 | 26 | 0.1 | 238 | 363 | 25.9 | 1566 | 2.11 |
| 56030 | 26 | 8 | 8 | 0 | 0 | 1.04 | 0.33 | 6.78 | 0.57 | 0.67 | 39.0 | 0.81 | 22.1 | 0.7 | 1.9 | 62 | 0.3 | 3.1 | 77 | 1.7 | 351 | 483 | 38.4 | 1697 | 3.05 |
| 56028 | 26 | 8 | 8 | 0 | 0 | 1.08 | 0.36 | 6.46 | 0.48 | 0.68 | 28.1 | 0.73 | 22.7 | 0.8 | | 78 | 0.2 | 2.7 | 32 | 0.4 | 266 | 398 | 31.9 | 1704 | 2.16 |
| 69018 | 200 | 40 | | | | | | | | | | | 3.6 | | | 100 | | 1.1 | | | | 250 | | 480 | |
| 56065 | 27 | 8 | 8 | 0 | 0 | 0.53 | 0.23 | 4.09 | 0.28 | 0.51 | 37.6 | 0.62 | 3.7 | 0.2 | 2.9 | 59 | 0.2 | 2.8 | 68 | 1.7 | 243 | 279 | 34.3 | 1002 | 2.11 |
| 56063 | 27 | 8 | 8 | 0 | 0 | 0.54 | 0.24 | 3.56 | 0.17 | 0.50 | 25.4 | 0.52 | 3.7 | 0.3 | 2.9 | 72 | 0.1 | 2.3 | 21 | 0.3 | 147 | 179 | 26.6 | 958 | 1.13 |
| 56036 | 370 | 90 | 80 | 10 | | 0.78 | 0.37 | 5.47 | 0.46 | 0.65 | 40.3 | 0.82 | 14.8 | 0.6 | 1.9 | 236 | 0.3 | 3.0 | 79 | 1.7 | 503 | 432 | 36.6 | 1707 | 3.37 |
| 56034 | 370 | 90 | 80 | 10 | | 0.80 | 0.39 | 4.96 | 0.36 | 0.65 | 28.5 | 0.71 | 14.8 | 0.6 | 1.9 | 249 | 0.2 | 2.5 | 32 | 0.4 | 410 | 335 | 29.1 | 1664 | 2.41 |
| 56033 | 278 | 79 | 77 | 2 | | 0.72 | 0.36 | 4.06 | 0.35 | 1.17 | 15.7 | 0.55 | 15.3 | 0.6 | 1.9 | 258 | 0.1 | 2.2 | 29 | 0.1 | 328 | 344 | 25.4 | 1602 | 2.59 |
| 66004 | 0 | 0 | 0 | 0 | 0 | 0.24 | 0.27 | 3.65 | 0.05 | 0.51 | 48.0 | 0.51 | 0.1 | | | 24 | 0.1 | 2.3 | 13 | 0.1 | 97 | 143 | 26.0 | 670 | 1.98 |
| 56667 | 58 | 6 | 0 | 6 | | 0.22 | 0.40 | 3.74 | 0.05 | 0.30 | 73.0 | 0.55 | 2.7 | | | 19 | 0.1 | 3.3 | 10 | 0.1 | 192 | 166 | 13.0 | 480 | 0.78 |
| 56284 | 814 | 167 | 128 | 39 | | 0.49 | 0.51 | 4.76 | 0.26 | 1.40 | 48.3 | | 22.0 | | | 420 | 0.2 | 5.2 | 61 | | 599 | 507 | | 2307 | 4.73 |
| 56041 | 2 | 0.2 | 0 | 0.2 | | 0.29 | 0.17 | 6.14 | 0.24 | 0.01 | 55.8 | 0.61 | 0.4 | 0.1 | | 63 | 0.4 | 3.0 | 104 | 2.0 | 246 | 361 | 26.0 | 376 | 2.09 |
| 56039 | 2 | 0.2 | 0 | 0.2 | | 0.30 | 0.19 | 5.63 | 0.13 | 0.00 | 44.0 | 0.51 | 0.4 | 0.2 | | 76 | 0.3 | 2.5 | 58 | 0.7 | 153 | 265 | 18.5 | 332 | 1.14 |
| 69016 | 500 | 100 | | | | | | | | | | | 3.6 | | | 150 | | 1.4 | | | | 250 | | 490 | |
| 69072 | 457 | 130 | 126 | 4 | | 0.21 | 0.34 | 2.79 | 0.27 | 1.70 | 38.1 | 0.72 | 12.9 | 0.4 | 3.0 | 288 | 0.1 | 4.2 | 38 | 0.2 | 284 | 361 | 30.2 | 1949 | 3.72 |
| 69021 | 400 | 80 | | | | | | | | | | | 9.0 | | | 80 | | 1.8 | | | | 380 | | 400 | |
| 56671 | 424 | 80 | 80 | 0 | 0 | 1.00 | 0.80 | 5.49 | 0.14 | 1.09 | 86.6 | 0.89 | 12.3 | | | 189 | 0.3 | 2.5 | 68 | 0.5 | 287 | 394 | 30.8 | 1651 | 2.58 |
| 56672 | 413 | 50 | 50 | 0 | 0 | 0.41 | 0.41 | 5.96 | 0.32 | 1.81 | 71.3 | 0.78 | 5.6 | | | 41 | 0.4 | 2.8 | 67 | 0.4 | 192 | 330 | 25.7 | 845 | 4.38 |
| 56673 | 187 | 41 | 41 | 0 | 0 | 0.46 | 0.33 | 11.34 | 0.23 | 1.61 | 102.4 | 1.87 | 3.6 | | | 74 | 0.4 | 2.6 | 79 | 0.5 | 220 | 335 | 60.2 | 1293 | 1.87 |
| 56047 | 78 | 22 | 21 | 1 | | 0.29 | 0.21 | 5.81 | 0.12 | 0.66 | 28.7 | 0.46 | 1.2 | 1.9 | 2.9 | 76 | 0.2 | 2.5 | 25 | 0.4 | 167 | 180 | 55.1 | 605 | 0.74 |
| 56049 | 78 | 22 | 21 | 1 | | 0.27 | 0.19 | 6.34 | 0.23 | 0.67 | 40.8 | 0.57 | 1.2 | 1.9 | | 63 | 0.3 | 3.0 | 72 | 1.7 | 263 | 280 | 62.8 | 649 | 1.72 |
| 56055 | 381 | 93 | 82 | 11 | | 0.22 | 0.36 | 3.29 | 0.24 | 0.40 | 17.4 | 0.76 | 0.1 | 0.2 | 1.9 | 229 | 0.1 | 3.4 | 27 | 0.1 | 376 | 294 | 20.4 | 1313 | 3.02 |
| 56058 | 370 | 90 | 80 | 10 | | 0.28 | 0.38 | 4.73 | 0.34 | 0.36 | 41.5 | 1.03 | 0.0 | 0.4 | 1.9 | 238 | 0.3 | 4.2 | 78 | 1.7 | 487 | 418 | 33.3 | 1460 | 3.94 |
| 56056 | 370 | 90 | 80 | 10 | | 0.30 | 0.40 | 4.21 | 0.23 | 0.36 | 29.6 | 0.93 | 0.0 | 0.4 | 1.9 | 251 | 0.2 | 3.7 | 32 | 0.4 | 394 | 321 | 25.8 | 1418 | 2.99 |
| 56103 | 28 | 8 | 8 | 0.1 | | 0.22 | 0.33 | 4.30 | 0.29 | 0.27 | 16.9 | 0.87 | 0.1 | 0.3 | 1.9 | 51 | 0.1 | 4.1 | 25 | 0.1 | 214 | 342 | 20.8 | 1186 | 3.00 |
| 56105 | 26 | 8 | 8 | 0 | 0 | 0.29 | 0.35 | 5.68 | 0.39 | 0.23 | 40.7 | 1.14 | 0.0 | 0.4 | 1.9 | 65 | 0.3 | 4.8 | 76 | 1.7 | 328 | 462 | 33.5 | 1330 | 3.91 |
| 56107 | 26 | 8 | 8 | 0 | 0 | 0.31 | 0.37 | 5.20 | 0.28 | 0.23 | 29.1 | 1.03 | 0.0 | 0.5 | 1.9 | 78 | 0.2 | 4.4 | 30 | 0.4 | 237 | 367 | 26.2 | 1294 | 2.97 |
| 56053 | 39 | 12 | 12 | 0 | 0 | 0.28 | 0.23 | 9.77 | 0.51 | 1.77 | 39.5 | 0.93 | 0.0 | 0.4 | 2.9 | 59 | 0.2 | 2.7 | 77 | 1.6 | 359 | 418 | 51.9 | 1666 | 2.35 |
| 56051 | 14 | 4 | 4 | 0 | 0 | 0.32 | 0.27 | 9.81 | 0.37 | 1.85 | 28.6 | 0.85 | 0.0 | 0.5 | | 74 | 0.1 | 2.3 | 33 | 0.4 | 279 | 337 | 47.0 | 1663 | 1.46 |
| 56989 | 500 | 100 | | | | | | | | | | | 0.0 | | | 200 | | 1.1 | | | | 250 | | 690 | |

| Code | Amount | Description | Basic Components | | | | | | | | | Additional Fats | | | | | | Vit A & Components | | | | | Vitamins | | | | | | | | | | Minerals | | | | | | | | | |
|---|---|---|---|---|---|---|---|---|---|---|---|---|---|---|---|---|---|---|---|---|---|---|---|---|---|---|---|---|---|---|---|---|---|---|---|---|---|---|---|---|---|---|
| | | | Weight (g) | Calories | % Water | Protein (g) | Carbs (g) | Fiber (g) | Sugar (g) | Other Carbs (g) | Fat (g) | Sat Fat (g) | Mono Fat (g) | Poly Fat (g) | Omega 3 (g) | Omega 6 (g) | Choles (mg) | Vit A (IU) | Vit A (RE) | Retinol (RE) | Carotenoids (RE) | Beta Carotene (mcg) | Thiamin (mg) | Riboflavin (mg) | Niacin (NE) | Vit B6 (mg) | Vit B12 (mcg) | Folate (mcg) | Panto (mg) | Vit C (mg) | Vit D (mg) | Vit E (α TE) | Calcium (mg) | Copper (mg) | Iron (mg) | Magnes (mg) | Mang (mg) | Phos (mg) | Potassium (mg) | Selenium (mcg) | Sodium (mg) | Zinc (mg) |
| | | **SAUCES AND GRAVIES** | | | | | | | | | | | | | | | | | | | | | | | | | | | | | | | | | | | | | | | | |
| | | *GRAVIES* | | | | | | | | | | | | | | | | | | | | | | | | | | | | | | | | | | | | | | | | |
| | | Au Jus Gravy | | | | | | | | | | | | | | | | | | | | | | | | | | | | | | | | | | | | | | | | |
| 53034 | 1/2 cup | Canned, avg | 119 | 19 | 94 | 1.4 | 3.0 | 0.0 | 0.1 | 2.9 | 0.2 | 0.1 | 0.1 | 0.0 | 0.00 | 0.01 | 0 | 0 | 0 | 0 | 0 | 0 | 0.02 | 0.07 | 1.07 | 0.01 | 0.12 | 2.4 | 0.02 | 1.2 | 0.0 | 0.0 | 5 | 0.1 | 0.7 | 2 | 0.2 | 36 | 96 | 0.5 | 60 | 1.19 |
| 53107 | 1 ea | Dry Mix, pkt, avg | 24 | 75 | 3 | 2.2 | 11.4 | | | | 2.3 | 0.5 | 1.1 | 0.1 | 0.01 | 0.05 | 1 | 2 | 0.2 | | | | 0.11 | 0.08 | 0.98 | 0.04 | 0.03 | 19.4 | 0.04 | 0.2 | 0.0 | | 34 | 0.0 | 2.2 | 13 | 0.1 | 37 | 67 | 1.5 | 2781 | 0.17 |
| 53035 | 1/2 cup | Dry Mix, prep, avg | 123 | 16 | 96 | 0.6 | 2.0 | 0.0 | 0.1 | 1.9 | 0.7 | 0.3 | 0.3 | 0.0 | 0.00 | 0.02 | 1 | 0 | 0 | 0 | 0 | 0 | 0.00 | 0.00 | 0.00 | 0.00 | 0.00 | 0.0 | 0.00 | 0.0 | 0.0 | 0.0 | 11 | 0.0 | 0.0 | 4 | 0.0 | 0 | 0 | | 482 | 0.07 |
| 53032 | 1/2 cup | Beef Gravy, cnd, avg | 116 | | | | | | | | | | | | | | | | | | | | | | | | | | | | | | | | | | | | | | | |
| | | Brown Gravy | | | | | | | | | | | | | | | | | | | | | | | | | | | | | | | | | | | | | | | | |
| 53036 | 1 ea | Dry Mix, pkt, avg | 22 | 81 | 5 | 2.4 | 13.1 | 0.4 | 0.3 | 12.4 | 2.1 | 0.7 | 1.0 | 0.1 | 0.01 | 0.08 | 1 | 5 | 1 | | | | 0.04 | 0.09 | 0.81 | 0.02 | 0.15 | 6.8 | 0.02 | 0.1 | 0.0 | | 29 | 0.0 | 0.4 | 7 | 0.1 | 45 | 58 | 1.3 | 1065 | 0.24 |
| 53027 | 1/2 cup | Dry Mix, prep, avg | 129 | 37 | 92 | 1.2 | 6.5 | 0.1 | 0.1 | 6.3 | 0.9 | 0.4 | 0.4 | 0.0 | 0.01 | 0.03 | 1 | 0 | 0 | 0 | 0 | 0 | 0.02 | 0.04 | 0.40 | 0.00 | 0.00 | 0.0 | 0.00 | 0.0 | 0.0 | | 34 | 0.0 | 0.1 | 5 | 0.0 | 22 | 28 | 0.0 | 538 | 0.15 |
| 53150 | 1 oz | Light, dry mix, Pioneer Food Service | 28 | 81 | 18 | 2.4 | 15.4 | 0.4 | 1.0 | 13.9 | 1.1 | 0.2 | | | | | 0 | 0 | 0 | 0 | 0 | 0 | 0.05 | 0.01 | 0.12 | | | 3.1 | | 0.1 | | | 4 | | 0.7 | | | | 144 | | 1880 | |
| 53399 | 1 ea | Quick, dry mix, pkt, Loma Linda | 6 | 19 | 8 | 0.8 | 3.8 | 0.4 | 0.1 | 3.3 | 0.2 | 0.0 | 0.0 | 0.1 | | | 0 | 0 | 0 | 0 | 0 | 0 | 0.42 | 0.00 | 0.00 | 0.00 | 0.00 | | | 0.0 | | | 4 | | 0.1 | | | 10 | 7 | | 352 | 0.02 |
| 53307 | 1/2 cup | With Onions, Franco American | 158 | 67 | 90 | 0.0 | 10.7 | 0.0 | 5.4 | 5.4 | 2.7 | 0.0 | | | | | 13 | 0 | 0 | 0 | 0 | 0 | | | | | | | | 0.0 | | | 0 | | 0.0 | | | | | | 911 | |
| | | Chicken Gravy | | | | | | | | | | | | | | | | | | | | | | | | | | | | | | | | | | | | | | | | |
| 53400 | 1 ea | Dry Mix, pkt, Loma Linda | 6 | 18 | 8 | 1.2 | 3.0 | 0.4 | 0.1 | 2.5 | 0.1 | 0.0 | 0.0 | 0.0 | | | 0 | 0 | 0 | 0 | 0 | 0 | 0.31 | 0.01 | 0.00 | 0.01 | 0.00 | | | 0.0 | | | 3 | | 0.2 | | | 23 | 30 | | 392 | 0.06 |
| 53309 | 1/2 cup | Franco American | 118 | 80 | 88 | 0.0 | 6.0 | 0.0 | 0.0 | 6.0 | 6.0 | 2.0 | | | | | 10 | 0 | 0 | 0 | 0 | 0 | | | | | | | | 0.0 | | | 0 | | 0.0 | | | | | | 480 | |
| 53005 | 1/2 cup | Giblet, avg | 130 | 97 | 85 | 6.1 | 6.4 | 0.5 | 0.1 | 5.7 | 5.2 | 1.4 | 2.2 | 1.0 | | | 55 | 1091 | 327 | 327 | 0 | 0 | 0.03 | 0.19 | 1.58 | 0.05 | 2.34 | 49.2 | 0.03 | 0.6 | 0.0 | | 16 | 0.2 | 1.5 | 5 | 0.2 | 62 | 151 | 1.8 | 682 | 1.47 |
| 53375 | 1/2 cup | Libby's | 122 | 120 | 85 | 2.0 | 6.0 | 0.0 | 0.0 | 6.0 | 8.5 | 1.2 | | | | | 10 | 0 | 0 | 0 | 0 | 0 | | | | | | | | 0.0 | | | 0 | | 0.0 | | | | | | 660 | |
| | | Country Gravy | | | | | | | | | | | | | | | | | | | | | | | | | | | | | | | | | | | | | | | | |
| 53091 | 1 oz | Dry Mix, Lawry's | 28 | 106 | 5 | 3.0 | 18.5 | 0.0 | | | 2.2 | | | | | | | | | | | | | | | | | | | | | | | | | | | | 192 | | 1288 | |
| 53401 | 1 ea | Dry Mix, pkt, Loma Linda | 6 | 22 | 7 | 0.6 | 3.7 | 0.4 | 0.0 | 3.2 | 0.6 | 0.1 | 0.4 | 0.0 | | | 0 | 0 | 0 | 0 | 0 | 0 | 0.00 | 0.01 | 0.00 | 0.01 | 0.01 | | | 0.0 | | | 1 | | 0.0 | | | 7 | 7 | | 249 | 0.02 |
| 53194 | 1 oz | Dry Mix, Trio | 28 | 121 | 4 | 2.5 | 18.2 | 2.5 | 8.0 | 7.7 | 4.3 | 1.1 | 0.5 | 1.9 | 0.21 | 1.63 | 2 | 0 | 0 | 0 | 0 | 0 | 0.03 | 0.05 | 0.35 | 0.01 | 0.03 | 2.8 | 0.09 | 0.0 | | | 18 | 0.0 | 0.4 | 4 | 0.0 | 31 | 39 | | 717 | 0.18 |
| | | Mushroom Gravy | | | | | | | | | | | | | | | | | | | | | | | | | | | | | | | | | | | | | | | | |
| 53026 | 1/2 cup | Canned, avg | 119 | 60 | 89 | 1.5 | 6.5 | 0.5 | 0.1 | 5.9 | 3.2 | 0.5 | 1.4 | 1.2 | 0.08 | 1.13 | 0 | 0 | 0 | 0 | 0 | 0 | 0.04 | 0.07 | 0.80 | 0.02 | 0.00 | 14.3 | 1.31 | 0.0 | 0.0 | | 8 | 0.1 | 0.8 | 2 | 0.4 | 18 | 126 | 2.3 | 678 | 0.83 |
| 53038 | 1 ea | Dry Mix, avg | 21 | 69 | 3 | 2.1 | 13.6 | 1.0 | 0.3 | 12.3 | 0.8 | 0.5 | 0.3 | 0.0 | 0.00 | 0.02 | 1 | 0 | 0 | 0 | 0 | 0 | 0.04 | 0.08 | 0.78 | 0.02 | 0.15 | 6.5 | 0.02 | 1.5 | 0.1 | | 48 | 0.1 | 0.2 | 7 | 0.1 | 43 | 55 | 1.1 | 1382 | 0.32 |
| 53402 | 1 ea | Dry Mix, pkt, Loma Linda | 5 | 16 | 8 | 0.8 | 2.6 | 0.7 | 0.1 | 1.8 | 0.2 | 0.1 | 0.1 | 0.0 | | | 0 | 0 | 0 | 0 | 0 | 0 | 0.00 | 0.01 | 0.00 | 0.01 | 0.00 | | | 0.0 | | | 1 | | 0.3 | | | 15 | 31 | | 304 | 0.05 |
| 53039 | 1/2 cup | Dry Mix, prep, avg | 129 | 35 | 92 | 1.1 | 6.9 | 0.5 | 0.1 | 6.2 | 0.4 | 0.3 | 0.1 | 0.0 | 0.00 | 0.01 | 0 | 0 | 0 | 0 | 0 | 0 | 0.03 | 0.04 | 0.39 | 0.01 | 0.08 | 1.3 | 0.01 | 0.8 | 0.0 | | 25 | 0.1 | 0.1 | 4 | 0.0 | 22 | 28 | | 700 | 0.16 |
| 53312 | 1/2 cup | Franco American | 118 | 40 | 90 | 2.0 | 6.0 | 0.0 | 0.0 | 6.0 | 2.0 | 0.0 | | | | | 10 | 0 | 0 | 0 | 0 | 0 | | | | | | | | 0.0 | | | 0 | | 0.0 | | | | | | 600 | |
| | | Onion Gravy | | | | | | | | | | | | | | | | | | | | | | | | | | | | | | | | | | | | | | | | |
| 53040 | 1 ea | Dry Mix, pkt, avg | 24 | 77 | 4 | 2.2 | 16.2 | 1.4 | 0.3 | 14.5 | 0.7 | 0.4 | 0.2 | 0.0 | 0.00 | 0.02 | 0 | 0 | 0 | 0 | 0 | 0 | 0.05 | 0.10 | 0.89 | 0.02 | 0.17 | 7.4 | 0.02 | 1.7 | 0.0 | | 67 | 0.0 | 0.2 | 8 | 0.1 | 49 | 63 | 1.5 | 1005 | 0.21 |
| 53403 | 1 ea | Dry Mix, pkt, Loma Linda | 5 | 18 | 8 | 0.5 | 3.2 | 0.6 | 0.1 | 2.5 | 0.3 | 0.1 | 0.2 | 0.0 | | | 0 | 0 | 0 | 0 | 0 | 0 | 0.03 | 0.02 | 0.00 | 0.02 | 0.00 | | | 0.0 | | | 1 | | 0.1 | | | 10 | 25 | | 229 | 0.04 |
| 53041 | 1/2 cup | Dry Mix, prep, avg | 130 | 39 | 91 | 1.1 | 8.1 | 0.7 | 0.2 | 7.2 | 0.4 | 0.2 | 0.1 | 0.0 | 0.00 | 0.01 | 0 | 0 | 0 | 0 | 0 | 0 | 0.00 | 0.00 | 0.00 | 0.00 | 0.00 | 0.0 | 0.00 | 0.0 | 0.0 | | 36 | 0.0 | 0.0 | 1 | 0.0 | 0 | 0 | | 504 | 0.14 |
| 53167 | 1 oz | Pepper Gravy, dry mix, Miller's Pride | 28 | 124 | 8 | 1.4 | 16.4 | 0.1 | 5.0 | 11.3 | 5.9 | 1.4 | | | | | 0 | 2 | 0.4 | | | | 0.25 | 0.58 | 0.72 | | | 16.0 | | 0.0 | | | 3 | | 0.5 | | | | 112 | | 1061 | |
| 53144 | 1 oz | Pepper Gravy, dry mix, RediMix | 28 | 130 | 7 | 1.7 | 17.2 | 0.4 | | | 6.0 | 0.9 | 3.4 | 1.6 | | | 0 | 2 | 0.4 | 0.3 | 0.1 | | 0.08 | 0.06 | 0.69 | 0.01 | 0.03 | 3.0 | 0.07 | 0.0 | | | 11 | 0.0 | 0.6 | 3 | | 18 | 26 | 1.2 | 437 | 0.11 |
| | | Pork Gravy | | | | | | | | | | | | | | | | | | | | | | | | | | | | | | | | | | | | | | | | |
| 53042 | 1 ea | Dry Mix, pkt, avg | 21 | 77 | 4 | 1.8 | 13.4 | 0.5 | 0.3 | 12.6 | 1.8 | 0.9 | 0.8 | 0.1 | 0.01 | 0.09 | 2 | 25 | 6 | | | | 0.03 | 0.06 | 0.48 | 0.02 | 0.11 | 6.5 | 0.07 | 0.3 | 0.0 | | 29 | 0.0 | 0.8 | 7 | 0.1 | 39 | 49 | 1.3 | 1125 | 0.22 |
| 53043 | 1/2 cup | Dry Mix, prep, avg | 129 | 39 | 92 | 1.0 | 6.7 | 0.5 | 0.1 | 6.1 | 1.0 | 0.4 | 0.4 | 0.1 | 0.01 | 0.10 | 1 | 0 | 0 | 0 | 0 | 0 | 0.03 | 0.03 | 0.39 | 0.01 | 0.08 | 1.5 | 0.01 | 0.8 | 0.0 | | 15 | 0.0 | 0.1 | 5 | 0.0 | 22 | 28 | | 618 | 0.13 |
| 53311 | 1/2 cup | Franco American | 118 | 90 | 85 | 2.0 | 6.0 | 2.0 | 0.0 | 4.0 | 8.0 | 3.0 | | | | | 8 | 0 | 0 | 0 | 0 | 0 | | | | | | | | 0.0 | | | 0 | | 0.0 | | | | | | 680 | |
| | | Sausage Gravy | | | | | | | | | | | | | | | | | | | | | | | | | | | | | | | | | | | | | | | | |
| 53119 | 1/2 cup | Average | 120 | 206 | 72 | 8.4 | 8.6 | 0.1 | | | 15.3 | 5.5 | 6.3 | 2.5 | | | 34 | 366 | 93 | 85 | 8 | | 0.24 | 0.24 | 1.40 | 0.12 | 0.70 | 5.6 | | 1.3 | | | 128 | 0.1 | 0.6 | 19 | | 143 | 244 | | 408 | 1.00 |
| 53376 | 1/2 cup | Libby's | 128 | 180 | 81 | 2.0 | 6.0 | 0.0 | 0.0 | 6.0 | 14.1 | 2.6 | | | | | 10 | 0 | 0 | 0 | 0 | 0 | | | | | | | | 0.0 | | | 0 | | 0.0 | | | | | | 561 | |
| 53191 | 1/2 cup | RTS, Chef Mate | 124 | 192 | 75 | 5.7 | 7.8 | 0.9 | 1.0 | 6.0 | 15.4 | 4.0 | 5.8 | 4.3 | 0.34 | 3.93 | 26 | 0 | 0 | 0 | 0 | 0 | 0.20 | 0.08 | 1.30 | 0.08 | 0.42 | 1.2 | 0.20 | 0.1 | | | 7 | 0.0 | 0.7 | 6 | 0.0 | 51 | 95 | | 471 | 0.68 |
| | | Turkey Gravy | | | | | | | | | | | | | | | | | | | | | | | | | | | | | | | | | | | | | | | | |
| 53033 | 1/2 cup | Canned, avg | 119 | 61 | 89 | 3.1 | 6.1 | 0.5 | 0.1 | 5.5 | 2.5 | 0.7 | 1.1 | 0.6 | 0.04 | 0.55 | 2 | 0 | 0 | 0 | 0 | 0 | 0.02 | 0.10 | 1.55 | 0.01 | 0.12 | 2.4 | 0.02 | 0.0 | 0.0 | | 5 | 0.1 | 0.8 | 2 | 0.2 | 35 | 130 | 0.7 | 687 | 0.95 |
| 53044 | 1 ea | Dry Mix, avg | 25 | 92 | 5 | 2.6 | 16.3 | 1.0 | 0.3 | 14.9 | 1.8 | 0.5 | 0.6 | 0.6 | 0.05 | 0.49 | 4 | 9 | 2 | | | | 0.05 | 0.11 | 0.69 | 0.05 | 0.14 | 20.5 | 0.25 | 0.1 | 0.1 | | 36 | 0.0 | 0.8 | 11 | 0.1 | 64 | 107 | 1.3 | 1098 | 0.31 |
| 53045 | 1/2 cup | Dry Mix, prep, avg | 130 | 43 | 91 | 1.5 | 7.5 | 0.5 | 0.2 | 6.8 | 0.9 | 0.3 | 0.4 | 0.2 | 0.01 | 0.20 | 1 | 0 | 0 | 0 | 0 | 0 | 0.03 | 0.06 | 0.52 | 0.01 | 0.13 | 1.7 | 0.01 | 0.9 | 0.0 | | 25 | 0.0 | 0.1 | 5 | 0.1 | 25 | 32 | | 745 | 0.13 |
| 53313 | 1/2 cup | Franco American | 118 | 50 | 90 | 2.0 | 6.0 | 0.0 | 0.0 | 6.0 | 2.0 | 0.0 | | | | | 10 | 0 | 0 | 0 | 0 | 0 | | | | | | | | 0.0 | | | 0 | | 0.0 | | | | | | 580 | |
| 53046 | 1 ea | Unspecified Gravy, dry mix, avg | 25 | 86 | 4 | 3.3 | 14.5 | 1.0 | 0.3 | 13.1 | 2.0 | 0.7 | 0.8 | 0.4 | 0.03 | 0.33 | 1 | 0 | 0 | 0 | 0 | 0 | 0.05 | 0.11 | 0.93 | 0.03 | 0.17 | 7.8 | 0.03 | 1.8 | 0.0 | | 38 | 0.0 | 0.3 | 11 | 0.1 | 51 | 66 | 1.5 | 1432 | 0.35 |
| 53047 | 1/2 cup | Unspecified Gravy, dry mix, prep, avg | 130 | 43 | 91 | 1.6 | 7.2 | 0.5 | 0.2 | 6.5 | 1.0 | 0.4 | 0.4 | 0.2 | 0.01 | 0.13 | 0 | 0 | 0 | 0 | 0 | 0 | 0.03 | 0.05 | 0.39 | 0.01 | 0.09 | 1.7 | 0.01 | 0.9 | 0.0 | | 18 | 0.0 | 0.1 | 5 | 0.1 | 25 | 32 | | 707 | 0.13 |
| | | *SAUCES* | | | | | | | | | | | | | | | | | | | | | | | | | | | | | | | | | | | | | | | | |
| | | Alfredo Sauce | | | | | | | | | | | | | | | | | | | | | | | | | | | | | | | | | | | | | | | | |
| 53431 | 1/2 cup | Alfredo Sauce, Bernardi's | 126 | 180 | 76 | 6.0 | 10.0 | 0.5 | 4.0 | 5.5 | 13.0 | 9.0 | | | | | 35 | 200 | 40 | | | | | | | | | | | 0.0 | | | 150 | | 0.0 | | | | | | 500 | |
| 53212 | 1 oz | Alfredo Sauce, dry mix, Nestle | 28 | 150 | 2 | 4.3 | 10.2 | 0.6 | 1.5 | 8.1 | 10.2 | 3.7 | 3.8 | 2.4 | 0.21 | 2.20 | 16 | 159 | 48 | | | | 0.04 | 0.02 | 0.58 | 0.04 | 0.11 | 33.0 | 0.29 | 0.0 | | | 131 | 0.0 | 0.3 | 9 | 0.0 | 116 | 71 | 2.6 | 725 | 0.42 |
| 53396 | 1/2 cup | Alfredo Sauce, reduced fat, DiGiorno | 138 | 340 | | 10.0 | 32.0 | 0.0 | 6.0 | 26.0 | 20.0 | 2.0 | | | | | 60 | 800 | 160 | | | | 0.00 | 0.20 | 0.00 | | | | | 0.0 | | | 300 | | 0.0 | 16 | | 200 | 160 | | 1200 | |
| | | Barbeque Sauce | | | | | | | | | | | | | | | | | | | | | | | | | | | | | | | | | | | | | | | | |
| 53000 | 1 Tbs | Average | 16 | 12 | 81 | 0.3 | 2.0 | 0.2 | 1.9 | 0.0 | 0.3 | 0.0 | 0.1 | 0.1 | 0.01 | 0.10 | 0 | 139 | 14 | | | | 0.00 | 0.00 | 0.14 | 0.01 | 0.00 | 0.6 | 0.05 | 1.1 | 0.0 | | 3 | 0.0 | 0.1 | 3 | 0.0 | 3 | 28 | 0.2 | 130 | 0.03 |
| 53536 | 1 Tbs | Low sodium, avg | 16 | 12 | 81 | 0.3 | 2.0 | 0.5 | | | 0.3 | 0.0 | 0.1 | 0.1 | | | 0 | 139 | 14 | 0 | 14 | | 0.00 | 0.00 | 0.14 | 0.01 | 0.00 | 1.9 | | 1.1 | | | 3 | 0.0 | 0.1 | 3 | | 3 | 97 | | 21 | 0.04 |
| 53418 | 1 Tbs | Honey, Kraft | 17 | 30 | 58 | 0.0 | 6.5 | 0.0 | 5.5 | 1.0 | 0.0 | 0.0 | 0.0 | 0.0 | 0.00 | 0.00 | 0 | 100 | 20 | | | | | | | | | | | 0.0 | | | 0 | | 0.0 | | | | 48 | | 175 | |
| 53416 | 1 Tbs | Original, Kraft | 17 | 25 | 62 | 0.0 | 6.0 | 0.0 | 5.0 | 1.0 | 0.0 | 0.0 | 0.0 | 0.0 | 0.00 | 0.00 | 0 | 100 | 20 | | | | | | | | | | | 0.0 | | | 0 | | 0.2 | | | | 38 | | 220 | |
| 53417 | 1 Tbs | Mesquite, Kraft | 17 | 25 | 62 | 0.0 | 6.0 | 0.0 | 5.0 | 1.0 | 0.0 | 0.0 | 0.0 | 0.0 | 0.00 | 0.00 | 0 | 100 | 20 | | | | | | | | | | | 0.0 | | | 0 | | | | | | 32 | | 220 | |
| | | Bearnaise Sauce | | | | | | | | | | | | | | | | | | | | | | | | | | | | | | | | | | | | | | | | |
| 53021 | 1/2 cup | Average | 73 | 322 | 46 | 2.4 | 1.0 | 0.1 | 1.0 | 0.0 | 33.9 | 20.0 | 10.5 | 1.6 | 0.47 | 1.17 | 237 | 1391 | 353 | 320 | 33 | | 0.02 | 0.09 | 0.04 | 0.05 | 0.43 | 19.8 | 0.47 | 0.6 | 1.0 | 0.6 | 29 | 0.0 | 0.6 | 6 | 0.1 | 72 | 47 | 5.3 | 444 | 0.42 |
| 53048 | 1 ea | Dry Mix, pkt, avg | 25 | 90 | 6 | 3.5 | 14.9 | 0.2 | | | 2.3 | 0.3 | 1.0 | 0.8 | 0.06 | 0.79 | 0 | 1 | 0.3 | | | | 0.03 | 0.05 | 0.15 | 0.01 | 0.10 | 3.3 | 0.10 | 0.5 | | | 41 | 0.0 | 0.1 | 7 | 0.0 | 37 | 73 | | 848 | 0.17 |
| 53111 | 1/2 cup | Dry Mix, prep w/milk, avg | 127 | 349 | 61 | 4.2 | 8.7 | | | | 34.0 | 20.8 | 9.9 | 1.5 | 0.51 | 1.02 | 94 | 1255 | 377 | 377 | 0 | | 0.04 | 0.13 | 0.13 | 0.04 | 0.25 | 5.1 | 0.25 | 0.9 | | | 114 | 0.1 | 0.1 | 13 | 0.0 | 93 | 149 | | 630 | 0.38 |
| 53018 | 1/2 cup | Bechamel Sauce, avg | 145 | 142 | 84 | 1.6 | 6.9 | 0.3 | 0.9 | 5.6 | 12.1 | 7.3 | 3.7 | 0.6 | 0.17 | 0.47 | 31 | 454 | 113 | 101 | 12 | | 0.07 | 0.06 | 0.57 | 0.01 | 0.03 | 3.7 | 0.06 | 0.0 | 0.2 | 0.2 | 13 | 0.0 | 0.5 | 5 | 0.1 | 18 | 28 | 2.3 | 1126 | 0.07 |
| 53100 | 1/2 cup | Black Bean Sauce, avg | 138 | 128 | 79 | 3.4 | 14.3 | 1.9 | | | 6.1 | 1.1 | 2.7 | 2.0 | | | 0 | 60 | 9 | 3 | 6 | | 0.08 | 0.05 | 0.49 | 0.07 | 0.01 | 35.2 | | 2.6 | 0.0 | | 32 | 0.1 | 0.8 | 22 | | 52 | 190 | | 1326 | 0.43 |
| 53019 | 1/2 cup | Bordelaise Sauce, avg | 233 | 207 | 86 | 2.8 | 10.1 | 0.7 | 3.0 | 6.4 | 12.6 | 7.8 | 3.8 | 0.5 | 0.19 | 0.34 | 33 | 579 | 125 | 101 | 24 | | 0.08 | 0.10 | 1.57 | 0.06 | 0.11 | 12.5 | 0.12 | 7.1 | 0.2 | 0.2 | 32 | 0.0 | 1.6 | 18 | 0.5 | 45 | 204 | 3.3 | 522 | 0.21 |
| | | Clam Sauce | | | | | | | | | | | | | | | | | | | | | | | | | | | | | | | | | | | | | | | | |
| 53278 | 1/2 cup | Red, Progresso | 125 | 80 | | 6.0 | 8.0 | 1.0 | 5.0 | 2.0 | 3.0 | 0.5 | 1.5 | 1.0 | | | 5 | 200 | 40 | | | | | | | | | | | 0.0 | | | 20 | | 0.7 | | | | | | 620 | |
| 53101 | 1/2 cup | White, avg | 120 | 299 | 57 | 21.2 | 4.8 | 0.1 | 2.2 | 2.6 | 21.3 | 2.8 | 14.7 | 2.1 | | | 55 | 498 | 144 | 142 | 2 | | 0.13 | 0.35 | 2.79 | 0.11 | 81.60 | 24.3 | | 18.8 | | | 83 | 0.6 | 23.4 | 17 | | 282 | 530 | | 490 | 2.30 |

| Code | Amount | Description | Basic Components | | | | | | | | | Additional Fats | | | | | |
|---|---|---|---|---|---|---|---|---|---|---|---|---|---|---|---|---|---|
| | | | Weight (g) | Calories | % Water | Protein (g) | Carbs (g) | Fiber (g) | Sugar (g) | Other Carbs (g) | Fat (g) | Sat Fat (g) | Mono Fat (g) | Poly Fat (g) | Omega 3 (g) | Omega 6 (g) | Choles (mg) |
| 53282 | 1/2 cup | White, Progresso | 124 | 90 | 85 | 5.0 | 2.0 | 0.0 | 0.0 | 2.0 | 7.0 | 1.5 | 5.0 | 0.5 | | | 10 |
| 53355 | 1/2 cup | Creole Sauce, RTS, Chef Mate | 124 | 50 | 89 | 1.8 | 7.4 | 1.6 | 5.8 | 0.0 | 1.4 | 0.1 | 0.5 | 0.6 | 0.03 | 0.55 | 0 |
| | | Curry Sauce | | | | | | | | | | | | | | | |
| 53016 | 1/2 cup | Average | 115 | 75 | 89 | 2.6 | 3.3 | 0.3 | 0.3 | 2.7 | 5.6 | 1.0 | 2.6 | 1.7 | 0.13 | 1.60 | 0 |
| 53031 | 1 ea | Dry Mix, pkt, avg | 35 | 149 | 4 | 3.3 | 17.7 | 0.5 | | | 8.1 | 1.2 | 3.5 | 3.0 | 0.21 | 2.82 | 0 |
| 53108 | 1/2 cup | Dry Mix, prep w/milk, avg | 136 | 135 | 79 | 5.3 | 12.9 | 1.0 | 1.0 | 10.9 | 7.4 | 3.0 | 2.6 | 1.4 | 0.15 | 1.24 | 18 |
| | | Enchilada Sauce | | | | | | | | | | | | | | | |
| 53103 | 1/2 cup | Green, avg | 125 | 89 | 87 | 1.9 | 7.3 | 1.3 | | | 6.4 | 3.6 | 1.8 | 0.5 | | | 19 |
| 53102 | 1/2 cup | Red, avg | 125 | 165 | 80 | 1.7 | 6.5 | 1.2 | | | 15.5 | 8.1 | 4.9 | 1.5 | | | 45 |
| 53208 | 1/2 cup | RTS, Nestle | 120 | 60 | 88 | 1.7 | 8.1 | 1.2 | 0.7 | 6.2 | 2.4 | 0.3 | 0.7 | 1.1 | 0.06 | 1.05 | 0 |
| 53347 | 1/2 cup | Santiago | 124 | 42 | 93 | 1.0 | 8.0 | 1.4 | 3.8 | 2.8 | 0.4 | 0.0 | 0.0 | 0.4 | | | 0 |
| 53474 | 1/2 cup | Fish Sauce, RTS, avg | 144 | 50 | 71 | 7.3 | 5.2 | 0.0 | | | 0.0 | 0.0 | 0.0 | 0.0 | 0.00 | 0.00 | 0 |
| 53389 | 1/2 cup | Four Cheese Sauce, DiGior no | 126 | 400 | 56 | 10.0 | 4.0 | 0.0 | 4.0 | 0.0 | 38.0 | 22.0 | | | | | 90 |
| | | Hollandaise Sauce | | | | | | | | | | | | | | | |
| 53020 | 1/2 cup | Average | 80 | 342 | 47 | 4.0 | 1.0 | 0.0 | 0.5 | 0.5 | 36.4 | 20.5 | 11.1 | 2.0 | | | 360 |
| 53112 | 1/2 cup | Dry Mix, prep w/milk, avg | 128 | 353 | 61 | 4.2 | 9.0 | | | | 34.3 | 21.0 | 10.0 | 1.5 | 0.50 | 0.97 | 95 |
| 53110 | 1/2 cup | Dry Mix, prep w/water, avg | 130 | 120 | 84 | 2.4 | 6.9 | 0.4 | | | 9.9 | 5.8 | 3.0 | 0.5 | 0.13 | 0.34 | 26 |
| 53472 | 1/2 cup | Hoisin Sauce, RTS, avg | 128 | 282 | 44 | 4.2 | 56.4 | 3.6 | | | 4.3 | 0.7 | 1.2 | 2.2 | 0.22 | 1.95 | 4 |
| 27162 | 1/2 cup | Lemon Sauce, RTS, Chef Mate | 128 | 172 | 67 | 0.3 | 40.8 | 0.0 | 31.4 | 9.5 | 0.8 | 0.1 | 0.2 | 0.4 | 0.03 | 0.33 | 0 |
| 53279 | 1/2 cup | Lobster Sauce, Progresso | 123 | 100 | 86 | 3.0 | 6.0 | 2.0 | 3.0 | 1.0 | 7.0 | 1.0 | 2.5 | 3.5 | | | 5 |
| 53125 | 1/2 cup | Mole Poblana Sauce, avg | 131 | 215 | 72 | 4.6 | 16.9 | 5.5 | | | 14.4 | 4.4 | 6.3 | 3.7 | | | 1 |
| 53126 | 1/2 cup | Mole Verde Sauce, avg | 132 | 78 | 86 | 4.5 | 7.8 | 2.2 | | | 3.9 | 0.8 | 1.2 | 1.6 | | | 0 |
| 53017 | 1/2 cup | Mornay Sauce, avg | 172 | 366 | 67 | 11.6 | 12.0 | 0.4 | 6.5 | 5.2 | 30.8 | 14.0 | 9.9 | 5.2 | 0.41 | 4.79 | 159 |
| 53473 | 1/2 cup | Oyster Sauce, RTS, avg | 32 | 16 | 80 | 0.4 | 3.5 | 0.1 | | | 0.1 | 0.0 | 0.0 | 0.0 | 0.00 | 0.02 | 0 |
| | | Pasta Sauce, Tomato Based | | | | | | | | | | | | | | | |
| 7474 | 1/2 cup | Chunky, Prego | 130 | 120 | 79 | 2.0 | 20.0 | 3.0 | 14.0 | 3.0 | 3.0 | 0.5 | | | | | 0 |
| 7473 | 1/2 cup | Chunky, garlic, Prego | 130 | 130 | 76 | 3.0 | 23.0 | 3.0 | 15.0 | 5.0 | 3.0 | 0.5 | | | | | 0 |
| 53539 | 1/2 cup | Low sodium | 125 | 136 | 75 | 2.3 | 19.9 | 3.8 | | | 6.0 | 0.9 | 3.1 | 1.6 | | | 0 |
| 53008 | 1/2 cup | Marinara | 125 | 94 | 82 | 2.2 | 13.2 | 2.5 | 6.8 | 3.9 | 4.7 | 0.7 | 1.1 | 2.7 | | | 0 |
| 53342 | 1/2 cup | Three cheese, Prego | 130 | 100 | 81 | 3.0 | 18.0 | 3.0 | 14.0 | 1.0 | 2.0 | 1.0 | | | | | 5 |
| 53011 | 1/2 cup | With meat | 125 | 150 | 74 | 4.2 | 18.7 | 4.0 | 9.9 | 4.8 | 7.1 | 1.4 | 3.5 | 1.6 | | | 8 |
| 53014 | 1/2 cup | With mushrooms, cnd, avg | 123 | 108 | 84 | 1.6 | 12.7 | 1.2 | 7.6 | 3.9 | 3.0 | 0.4 | 1.5 | 0.8 | | | 0 |
| 53288 | 1/2 cup | With mushrooms, Weight Watchers | 113 | 60 | | 2.0 | 11.0 | 4.0 | 6.0 | 1.0 | 0.0 | 0.0 | 0.0 | 0.0 | 0.00 | 0.00 | 0 |
| 53540 | 1/2 cup | Peanut Sauce, avg | 120 | 372 | 47 | 15.3 | 15.4 | 3.8 | | | 31.0 | 5.9 | 14.6 | 8.9 | | | 0 |
| 53106 | 1/2 cup | Pesto Sauce, avg | 116 | 622 | 21 | 20.2 | 9.0 | 1.8 | | | 57.8 | 14.5 | 36.3 | 4.2 | | | 35 |
| 53392 | 1/2 cup | Pesto Sauce, DiGiorno | 124 | 640 | | 16.0 | 6.0 | 0.0 | 0.0 | 6.0 | 62.0 | 14.0 | 41.9 | 5.1 | | | 30 |
| | | Pizza Sauce | | | | | | | | | | | | | | | |
| 53366 | 1/4 cup | Chunky, Contadina | 63 | 30 | 88 | 0.9 | 6.0 | 1.0 | 2.0 | 3.0 | 0.0 | 0.0 | 0.0 | 0.0 | 0.00 | 0.00 | 0 |
| 53215 | 1/4 cup | Original, Contadina | 61 | 24 | 90 | 1.0 | 3.9 | 1.0 | 2.9 | 0.0 | 0.6 | 0.0 | | | 0.00 | 0.00 | 0 |
| 53277 | 1/4 cup | Progresso | 63 | 35 | 87 | 1.0 | 5.0 | 1.0 | 2.0 | 2.0 | 1.0 | 0.0 | | | | | 0 |
| 53214 | 1/4 cup | With Cheese, Contadina | 63 | 30 | 87 | 1.0 | 4.0 | 1.0 | 3.0 | 0.0 | 1.3 | 0.0 | | | 0.00 | 0.00 | 0 |
| 53378 | 1/2 cup | Sloppy Joe Sauce, Libby's | 118 | 68 | 85 | 1.5 | 15.1 | 1.5 | 6.1 | 7.6 | 0.0 | 0.0 | 0.0 | 0.0 | 0.00 | 0.00 | 0 |
| | | Stir Fry Sauce | | | | | | | | | | | | | | | |
| 53447 | 2 Tbs | Hunan, avg | 30 | 56 | 60 | 0.0 | 6.6 | | 4.6 | | 3.1 | | | | | | |
| 53448 | 2 Tbs | Mandarin, China Bowl Trading Co | 29 | 30 | 84 | 0.0 | 1.5 | | | | 2.5 | | | | | | |
| 53352 | 2 Tbs | RTS, Chef Mate | 30 | 32 | 74 | 0.5 | 4.7 | 0.0 | 1.9 | 2.8 | 1.3 | 0.2 | 0.4 | 0.6 | 0.04 | 0.59 | 0 |
| 53262 | 1 oz | Sweet & Sour, La Choy | 28 | 30 | 72 | 0.5 | 7.2 | 0.3 | 5.6 | 1.3 | 0.0 | 0.0 | | | | | 0 |
| 53269 | 1 oz | Szechwan, La Choy | 28 | 16 | 84 | 0.6 | 3.5 | 0.4 | 2.9 | 0.1 | 0.0 | 0.0 | | | | | 0 |
| 53260 | 1 oz | Teriyaki, La Choy | 28 | 22 | 77 | 0.5 | 5.2 | 0.3 | 4.1 | 0.8 | 0.0 | 0.0 | | | | | 0 |
| 53057 | 1 ea | Stroganoff Sauce, dry mix, pkt, avg | 46 | 161 | 5 | 5.6 | 26.5 | 0.5 | | | 4.4 | 2.8 | 1.2 | 0.1 | 0.04 | 0.08 | 12 |
| 53058 | 1/2 cup | Stroganoff Sauce, prep f/dry mix, w/mlk & wtr, avg | 123 | 113 | 78 | 4.9 | 14.1 | 0.2 | | | 4.5 | 2.8 | 1.3 | 0.2 | 0.06 | 0.10 | 16 |
| | | Sweet & Sour Sauce | | | | | | | | | | | | | | | |
| 53059 | 1 ea | Dry, pkt, avg | 57 | 222 | 1 | 0.6 | 54.8 | 1.1 | 50.8 | 2.8 | 0.1 | 0.0 | 0.0 | 0.0 | 0.01 | 0.03 | 0 |
| 53261 | 1 oz | Duck, La Choy | 28 | 46 | 56 | 0.0 | 11.4 | 0.0 | 11.2 | 0.3 | 0.0 | 0.0 | | | | | 0 |
| 53264 | 1 oz | La Choy | 28 | 48 | 57 | 0.0 | 11.8 | 0.0 | 11.3 | 0.5 | 0.0 | 0.0 | | | | | 0 |
| 53357 | 2 Tbs | RTS, Chef Mate | 33 | 40 | 71 | 0.2 | 8.2 | 0.3 | 6.9 | 1.1 | 0.8 | 0.1 | 0.2 | 0.4 | 0.02 | 0.35 | 0 |
| 53001 | 2 Tbs | Szechuan Sauce | 31 | 23 | 81 | 0.6 | 4.0 | 0.4 | 3.6 | 0.0 | 0.6 | 0.1 | 0.2 | 0.2 | 0.02 | 0.20 | 0 |
| 53003 | 1 Tbs | Tartar Sauce, avg | 14 | 74 | 34 | 0.2 | 0.6 | 0.0 | 0.4 | 0.2 | 8.2 | 1.5 | 2.6 | 4.1 | 0.00 | 4.06 | 7 |
| 53122 | 1 Tbs | Tartar Sauce, low calorie | 14 | 31 | 63 | 0.1 | 2.3 | 0.0 | | | 2.5 | 0.4 | 0.6 | 1.3 | | | 3 |
| | | Teriyaki Sauce | | | | | | | | | | | | | | | |
| 53109 | 2 Tbs | Dry Mix, prep w/water, avg | 35 | 16 | 84 | 0.5 | 3.4 | | | | 0.1 | 0.0 | 0.0 | 0.1 | 0.01 | 0.06 | 0 |
| 53268 | 2 Tbs | Light, La Choy | 36 | 37 | 68 | 2.1 | 7.0 | 0.0 | 5.2 | 1.8 | 0.0 | 0.0 | | | | | 0 |
| 27161 | 2 Tbs | RTS, Chef Mate | 32 | 42 | 69 | 0.3 | 7.5 | 0.0 | 5.6 | 1.9 | 1.2 | 0.1 | 0.3 | 0.6 | 0.03 | 0.52 | 0 |
| | | White Sauce | | | | | | | | | | | | | | | |
| 53468 | 1/4 cup | Medium, prep f/recipe, avg | 62 | 91 | 75 | 2.4 | 5.7 | 0.1 | | | 6.6 | 1.8 | 2.7 | 1.8 | 0.09 | 1.68 | 4 |

| Code | Description | Vit A & Components | | | | | Vitamins | | | | | | | | | | Minerals | | | | | | | | | |
|---|---|---|---|---|---|---|---|---|---|---|---|---|---|---|---|---|---|---|---|---|---|---|---|---|---|---|
| | | Vit A (IU) | Vit A (RE) | Retinol (RE) | Carotenoids (RE) | Beta Carotene (mcg) | Thiamin (mg) | Riboflavin (mg) | Niacin (NE) | Vit B6 (mg) | Vit B12 (mcg) | Folate (mcg) | Panto (mg) | Vit C (mg) | Vit D (mg) | Vit E (α TE) | Calcium (mg) | Copper (mg) | Iron (mg) | Magnes (mg) | Mang (mg) | Phos (mg) | Potassium (mg) | Selenium (mcg) | Sodium (mg) | Zinc (mg) |
| 53282 | White, Progresso | 0 | 0 | 0 | 0 | 0 | | | | | | | | 1.2 | | | 0 | | 0.7 | | | | | | 470 | |
| 53355 | Creole Sauce, RTS, Chef Mate | 467 | 47 | | | | 0.07 | 0.05 | 1.05 | 0.14 | 0.00 | 17.4 | 0.33 | 0.0 | | | 69 | 0.1 | 0.6 | 17 | 0.2 | 35 | 374 | | 678 | 0.20 |
| | Curry Sauce | | | | | | | | | | | | | | | | | | | | | | | | | |
| 53016 | Average | 207 | 61 | 56 | 5 | | 0.03 | 0.05 | 1.63 | 0.01 | 0.11 | 2.8 | 0.04 | 0.1 | 0.0 | | 9 | 0.1 | 0.5 | 3 | 0.1 | 38 | 104 | 1.1 | 392 | 0.15 |
| 53031 | Dry Mix, pkt, avg | 36 | 4 | | | | 0.04 | 0.07 | 0.28 | 0.02 | 0.14 | 3.1 | 0.14 | 0.7 | 0.0 | | 62 | 0.0 | 1.1 | 14 | 0.0 | 52 | 123 | | 1428 | 0.31 |
| 53108 | Dry Mix, prep w/milk, avg | 171 | 20 | | | | 0.05 | 0.27 | 0.27 | 0.05 | 0.54 | 8.2 | 0.14 | 1.4 | | | 242 | 0.5 | 0.5 | 23 | 0.0 | 140 | 248 | | 638 | 0.54 |
| | Enchilada Sauce | | | | | | | | | | | | | | | | | | | | | | | | | |
| 53103 | Green, avg | 2441 | 276 | 52 | 224 | | 0.05 | 0.09 | 1.38 | 0.10 | 0.06 | 8.8 | | 54.1 | 0.0 | | 39 | 0.1 | 0.7 | 22 | | 59 | 292 | | 184 | 0.30 |
| 53102 | Red, avg | 3038 | 389 | 128 | 262 | | 0.05 | 0.10 | 0.65 | 0.12 | 0.05 | 11.2 | | 10.1 | 0.0 | | 31 | 0.1 | 0.5 | 15 | | 45 | 196 | | 168 | 0.23 |
| 53208 | RTS, Nestle | 493 | 49 | | | | 0.07 | 0.04 | 1.27 | 0.17 | 0.00 | 9.6 | 0.32 | 8.5 | | 0.0 | 29 | 0.1 | 1.2 | 20 | 0.2 | 42 | 334 | | 310 | 0.23 |
| 53347 | Santiago | | | | | | 0.02 | 0.02 | 0.00 | | | | | 0.0 | | | 16 | | 0.4 | | | 20 | 162 | | 552 | |
| 53474 | Fish Sauce, RTS, avg | 3 | 0 | | | | 0.02 | 0.08 | 3.33 | 0.57 | 0.69 | 73.4 | 0.17 | 0.7 | | | 62 | 0.1 | 1.1 | 252 | 0.3 | 10 | 415 | 13.1 | 11117 | 0.29 |
| 53389 | Four Cheese Sauce, DiGior no | 1500 | 300 | | | | 0.06 | 0.20 | 0.00 | | | | | 0.0 | | | 300 | | 0.0 | 0 | | 200 | 150 | | 820 | |
| | Hollandaise Sauce | | | | | | | | | | | | | | | | | | | | | | | | | |
| 53020 | Average | 1543 | 403 | 373 | 30 | | 0.04 | 0.15 | 0.03 | 0.09 | 0.73 | 33.9 | 1.25 | 3.4 | 1.2 | | 39 | 0.0 | 0.8 | 3 | | 115 | 39 | 16.3 | 312 | 0.71 |
| 53112 | Dry Mix, prep w/milk, avg | 1164 | 349 | 349 | 0 | 0 | 0.04 | 0.17 | 0.12 | 0.04 | 0.26 | 5.1 | 0.26 | 0.8 | | | 120 | 0.1 | 0.1 | 13 | 0.0 | 97 | 155 | | 570 | 0.38 |
| 53110 | Dry Mix, prep w/water, avg | 368 | 110 | 110 | 0 | 0 | 0.03 | 0.09 | 0.03 | 0.26 | 0.39 | 10.4 | 0.39 | 0.1 | | | 62 | 0.1 | 0.5 | 4 | 0.0 | 64 | 62 | | 785 | 0.39 |
| 53472 | Hoisin Sauce, RTS, avg | 13 | 1 | | | | 0.01 | 0.28 | 1.50 | 0.08 | 0.00 | 29.4 | 0.09 | 0.5 | | 0.0 | 41 | 0.2 | 1.3 | 31 | 0.3 | 49 | 152 | 2.3 | 2067 | 0.41 |
| 27162 | Lemon Sauce, RTS, Chef Mate | 0 | 0 | 0 | 0 | 0 | 0.01 | 0.01 | 0.04 | 0.01 | 0.00 | 1.3 | 0.03 | 11.0 | | | 5 | 0.0 | 0.5 | 3 | 0.0 | 5 | 26 | | 10 | 0.05 |
| 53279 | Lobster Sauce, Progresso | 300 | 60 | | | | | | | | | | | 0.0 | | | 20 | | 1.1 | | | | | | 430 | |
| 53125 | Mole Poblana Sauce, avg | 5019 | 502 | 0 | 502 | | 0.03 | 0.00 | 2.15 | 0.33 | 0.06 | 36.7 | 0.31 | 0.0 | 0.0 | | 31 | 0.2 | 2.4 | 42 | 0.3 | 107 | 427 | | 176 | 0.60 |
| 53126 | Mole Verde Sauce, avg | 816 | 81 | 0 | 81 | | 0.06 | 0.08 | 2.53 | 0.11 | 0.09 | 17.4 | | 23.5 | 0.0 | | 22 | 0.2 | 1.8 | 50 | | 133 | 380 | | 467 | 0.75 |
| 53017 | Mornay Sauce, avg | 1204 | 327 | 298 | 29 | | 0.12 | 0.31 | 0.55 | 0.11 | 0.79 | 19.3 | 0.72 | 1.7 | 1.6 | 1.0 | 315 | 0.1 | 0.8 | 24 | 0.1 | 253 | 215 | 8.5 | 805 | 1.15 |
| 53473 | Oyster Sauce, RTS, avg | 7 | 2 | | | | 0.00 | 0.04 | 0.47 | 0.01 | 0.13 | 4.8 | 0.01 | 0.0 | | | 10 | 0.0 | 0.1 | 1 | 0.0 | 7 | 17 | 1.4 | 875 | 0.03 |
| | Pasta Sauce, Tomato Based | | | | | | | | | | | | | | | | | | | | | | | | | |
| 7474 | Chunky, Prego | 1000 | 100 | 0 | 100 | 586 | | | | | 0.00 | | | 9.0 | | | 60 | | 1.1 | | | | | | 580 | |
| 7473 | Chunky, garlic, Prego | 1000 | 100 | 0 | 100 | 586 | | | | | 0.00 | | | 4.8 | | | 60 | | 1.4 | | | | | | 570 | |
| 53539 | Low sodium | 1534 | 154 | 0 | 154 | 901 | 0.07 | 0.07 | 1.88 | 0.44 | 0.00 | 26.3 | | 14.0 | | | 35 | 0.1 | 0.8 | 30 | | 45 | 480 | | 38 | 0.26 |
| 53008 | Marinara | 1380 | 138 | 0 | 138 | 809 | 0.09 | 0.09 | 1.71 | 0.23 | 0.00 | 11.6 | 0.31 | 21.1 | 0.0 | | 31 | 0.3 | 1.6 | 31 | | 51 | 565 | 1.7 | 656 | 0.46 |
| 53342 | Three cheese, Prego | 750 | 150 | | | | | | | | 0.00 | | | 15.0 | | | 60 | | 0.7 | | | | | | 460 | |
| 53011 | With meat | 1441 | 288 | | | | 0.07 | 0.09 | 2.25 | 0.44 | 0.25 | 26.1 | 0.21 | 13.2 | 0.0 | | 34 | 0.1 | 1.0 | 30 | | 56 | 476 | 2.6 | 590 | 0.68 |
| 53014 | With mushrooms, cnd, avg | 2408 | 241 | 0 | 241 | 1412 | 0.08 | 0.08 | 0.93 | 0.16 | 0.00 | 12.5 | 0.42 | 9.3 | 0.0 | | 15 | 0.4 | 1.0 | 15 | | 30 | 332 | 2.2 | 494 | 0.34 |
| 53288 | With mushrooms, Weight Watchers | 498 | 50 | 0 | 50 | 292 | | | | | | | | 14.9 | | | 0 | | 1.1 | | | | 194 | | 419 | |
| 53540 | Peanut Sauce, avg | 6 | 0.6 | 0 | 0.6 | | 0.09 | 0.06 | 8.14 | 0.25 | 0.00 | 52.2 | | 13.5 | | | 24 | 0.4 | 1.0 | 100 | | 202 | 482 | | 298 | 1.58 |
| 53106 | Pesto Sauce, avg | 1266 | 173 | 64 | 109 | | 0.04 | 0.21 | 0.88 | 0.18 | 0.63 | 33.0 | | 10.4 | 0.0 | | 834 | 0.2 | 4.9 | 67 | | 414 | 413 | | 844 | 2.06 |
| 53392 | Pesto Sauce, DiGiorno | 1500 | 300 | | | | 0.06 | 0.20 | 0.00 | 0.17 | | 3.4 | | 0.0 | | | 500 | | 0.7 | 48 | | 300 | 120 | | 1000 | 2.22 |
| | Pizza Sauce | | | | | | | | | | | | | | | | | | | | | | | | | |
| 53366 | Chunky, Contadina | 200 | 40 | | | | | | | | | | | 9.0 | | | 20 | | 0.4 | | | | | | 280 | |
| 53215 | Original, Contadina | 290 | 29 | | | | | | | | | | | 5.8 | | | 20 | | 0.7 | | | | | | 290 | |
| 53277 | Progresso | 400 | 80 | | | | | | | | | | | 6.0 | | | 20 | | 0.7 | | | | | | 140 | |
| 53214 | With Cheese, Contadina | 300 | 30 | | | | | | | | | | | 6.0 | | | 20 | | 0.4 | | | | | | 350 | |
| 53378 | Sloppy Joe Sauce, Libby's | 454 | 91 | | | | | | | | | | | 9.1 | | | 31 | | 0.5 | | | | | | 650 | |
| | Stir Fry Sauce | | | | | | | | | | | | | | | | | | | | | | | | | |
| 53447 | Hunan, avg | | | | | | | | | | | | | | | | | | | | | | | | 280 | |
| 53448 | Mandarin, China Bowl Trading Co | | | | | | | | | | | | | | | | | | | | | | | | 80 | |
| 53352 | RTS, Chef Mate | 8 | 1 | | | | 0.00 | 0.01 | 0.27 | 0.01 | 0.00 | 1.2 | 0.03 | 1.4 | | | 3 | 0.0 | 0.2 | 3 | 0.0 | 9 | 16 | | 467 | 0.04 |
| 53262 | Sweet & Sour, La Choy | 46 | 9 | | | | | | | | | | | 3.0 | | | 0 | | 0.2 | | | | | | 169 | |
| 53269 | Szechwan, La Choy | 17 | 3 | | | | | | | | | | | 1.2 | | | 0 | | 1.2 | | | | | | 133 | |
| 53260 | Teriyaki, La Choy | 25 | 5 | | | | | | | | | | | 1.6 | | | 0 | | 3.5 | | | | | | 246 | |
| 53057 | Stroganoff Sauce, dry mix, pkt, avg | 222 | 67 | 59 | 7 | | 0.84 | 0.48 | 0.63 | 0.05 | 0.28 | 3.7 | 0.60 | 0.4 | 0.0 | | 307 | 0.1 | 1.3 | 19 | 0.2 | 126 | 398 | | 1863 | 1.10 |
| 53058 | Stroganoff Sauce, prep f/dry mix, w/mlk & wtr, avg | 175 | 53 | 46 | 6 | | 0.36 | 0.32 | 0.31 | 0.05 | 0.25 | 3.7 | 0.37 | 0.6 | 0.0 | | 216 | 0.0 | 0.6 | 16 | 0.1 | 125 | 279 | | 760 | 0.46 |
| | Sweet & Sour Sauce | | | | | | | | | | | | | | | | | | | | | | | | | |
| 53059 | Dry, pkt, avg | 0 | 0 | 0 | 0 | 0 | 0.01 | 0.07 | 0.63 | 0.28 | 0.00 | 1.7 | 0.51 | 0.0 | 0.0 | 0.0 | 31 | 0.0 | 1.2 | 7 | 0.0 | 34 | 50 | | 587 | 0.07 |
| 53261 | Duck, La Choy | 0 | 0 | 0 | 0 | 0 | | | | | | | | 0.0 | | | 0 | | 0.2 | | | | | | 96 | |
| 53264 | La Choy | 0 | 0 | 0 | 0 | 0 | | | | | | | | 0.0 | | | 2 | | 0.0 | | | | | | 99 | |
| 53357 | RTS, Chef Mate | 25 | 3 | | | | 0.01 | 0.00 | 0.07 | 0.01 | 0.00 | 0.7 | 0.02 | 0.0 | | | 6 | 0.0 | 0.3 | 2 | 0.1 | 3 | 22 | | 116 | 0.03 |
| 53001 | Szechuan Sauce | 269 | 27 | | | | 0.01 | 0.01 | 0.28 | 0.02 | 0.00 | 1.2 | 0.09 | 2.2 | 0.0 | | 6 | 0.1 | 0.3 | 6 | 0.1 | 6 | 54 | 0.4 | 253 | 0.06 |
| 53003 | Tartar Sauce, avg | 31 | 9 | 9 | 0 | | 0.00 | 0.00 | 0.00 | 0.01 | 0.00 | 0.6 | 0.04 | 0.1 | 0.0 | | 3 | 0.0 | 0.1 | 0 | 0.0 | 4 | 11 | 0.6 | 99 | 0.02 |
| 53122 | Tartar Sauce, low calorie | 20 | 2 | 0 | 2 | | 0.00 | 0.00 | 0.01 | 0.00 | 0.00 | 0.2 | | 0.1 | | | 2 | 0.0 | 0.1 | 0 | | 1 | 5 | | 83 | 0.02 |
| | Teriyaki Sauce | | | | | | | | | | | | | | | | | | | | | | | | | |
| 53109 | Dry Mix, prep w/water, avg | 0 | 0 | 0 | 0 | 0 | 0.00 | 0.01 | 0.16 | 0.02 | 0.00 | 3.5 | 0.04 | 0.0 | 0.0 | 0.0 | 14 | 0.2 | 0.3 | 10 | 0.0 | 27 | 27 | | 593 | 0.02 |
| 53268 | Light, La Choy | 0 | 0 | 0 | 0 | 0 | | | | | | | | 0.0 | | | 1 | | 0.9 | | | | | | 878 | |
| 27161 | RTS, Chef Mate | 0 | 0 | 0 | 0 | 0 | 0.00 | 0.01 | 0.19 | 0.01 | 0.00 | 1.0 | 0.02 | 0.0 | | | 3 | 0.0 | 0.2 | 3 | 0.0 | 7 | 16 | | 319 | 0.03 |
| | White Sauce | | | | | | | | | | | | | | | | | | | | | | | | | |
| 53468 | Medium, prep f/recipe, avg | 343 | 34 | | | | 0.04 | 0.11 | 0.25 | 0.02 | 0.17 | 5.0 | 0.20 | 0.5 | | | 73 | 0.0 | 0.2 | 9 | 0.0 | 61 | 97 | 2.5 | 219 | 0.25 |

| Code | Amount | Description | Basic Components | | | | | | | | | Additional Fats | | | | | | Vit A & Components | | | | | Vitamins | | | | | | | | | | Minerals | | | | | | | | | |
|---|---|---|---|---|---|---|---|---|---|---|---|---|---|---|---|---|---|---|---|---|---|---|---|---|---|---|---|---|---|---|---|---|---|---|---|---|---|---|---|---|---|---|
| | | | Weight (g) | Calories | % Water | Protein (g) | Carbs (g) | Fiber (g) | Sugar (g) | Other Carbs (g) | Fat (g) | Sat Fat (g) | Mono Fat (g) | Poly Fat (g) | Omega 3 (g) | Omega 6 (g) | Choles (mg) | Vit A (IU) | Vit A (RE) | Retinol (RE) | Carotenoids (RE) | Beta Carotene (mcg) | Thiamin (mg) | Riboflavin (mg) | Niacin (NE) | Vit B6 (mg) | Vit B12 (mcg) | Folate (mcg) | Panto (mg) | Vit C (mg) | Vit D (mg) | Vit E (α TE) | Calcium (mg) | Copper (mg) | Iron (mg) | Magnes (mg) | Mang (mg) | Phos (mg) | Potassium (mg) | Selenium (mcg) | Sodium (mg) | Zinc (mg) |
| 53469 | 1/4 cup | Thick, prep f/recipe, avg | 62 | 115 | 69 | 2.5 | 7.2 | 0.2 | | | 8.6 | 2.1 | 3.6 | 2.4 | 0.12 | 2.31 | 4 | 417 | 42 | | | | 0.05 | 0.12 | 0.37 | 0.02 | 0.16 | 6.8 | 0.20 | 0.4 | | | 69 | 0.0 | 0.3 | 9 | 0.0 | 60 | 92 | 3.2 | 231 | 0.25 |
| 53467 | 1/4 cup | Thin, prep f/recipe, avg | 62 | 65 | 81 | 2.3 | 4.6 | 0.1 | | | 4.2 | 1.3 | 1.7 | 1.0 | 0.06 | 0.92 | 5 | 250 | 25 | | | | 0.03 | 0.11 | 0.16 | 0.03 | 0.19 | 3.7 | 0.21 | 0.5 | | | 78 | 0.0 | 0.1 | 9 | 0.0 | 63 | 101 | 2.0 | 203 | 0.26 |
| | | **SNACK FOODS–CHIPS, PRETZELS, POPCORN** | | | | | | | | | | | | | | | | | | | | | | | | | | | | | | | | | | | | | | | | |
| 44061 | 1 pce | Bagel Chips, avg | 18 | 77 | 3 | 1.6 | 13.5 | 1.4 | | | 1.9 | 0.3 | 0.5 | 0.9 | | | 0 | 0 | 0 | 0 | 0 | 0 | 0.03 | 0.03 | 0.40 | 0.05 | 0.00 | 14.9 | | 0.0 | | | 2 | 0.1 | 0.4 | 11 | | 37 | 43 | | 108 | 0.23 |
| 44188 | 1 oz | Bagel Chips, onion, multigrain, Pepperidge Farm | 28 | 120 | 7 | 3.0 | 19.0 | 1.0 | 1.0 | 17.0 | 3.5 | 0.0 | | | | | 0 | 0 | 0 | 0 | 0 | 0 | 0.09 | 0.03 | 0.80 | | | | | 0.0 | | | | | 1.1 | | | | | | 200 | |
| 44029 | 1 oz | Bugles, avg | 28 | 143 | 2 | 1.6 | 17.6 | 0.3 | 2.8 | 14.5 | 7.5 | 6.4 | 0.5 | 0.2 | 0.00 | 0.22 | 0 | 89 | 9 | 0 | 9 | | 0.09 | 0.07 | 0.39 | 0.01 | 0.00 | 0.8 | 0.06 | 0.0 | 0.0 | | 1 | 0.0 | 0.7 | 3 | 0.0 | 12 | 23 | 1.1 | 286 | 0.06 |
| 44030 | 1 oz | Bugles, nacho, avg | 28 | 150 | 2 | 1.8 | 16.0 | 0.3 | 0.0 | 15.7 | 8.9 | 7.5 | 0.6 | 0.2 | 0.01 | 0.23 | 1 | 88 | 11 | 0 | 11 | 64 | 0.06 | 0.03 | 0.39 | 0.03 | 0.00 | 1.4 | 0.11 | 0.0 | 0.0 | | 10 | 0.0 | 0.4 | 7 | 0.0 | 21 | 34 | 1.1 | 267 | 0.13 |
| | | Cheese Curls | | | | | | | | | | | | | | | | | | | | | | | | | | | | | | | | | | | | | | | | |
| 44115 | 1 ea | Barbecue, bag, Weight Watchers | 14 | 59 | 4 | 1.0 | 10.8 | 1.0 | 0.0 | 9.9 | 1.5 | 0.0 | | | 0.00 | 0.00 | 0 | 0 | 0 | 0 | 0 | 0 | | | | | | | | 0.0 | | | 0 | | 0.0 | | | | 44 | | 108 | |
| 44246 | 8 pce | Cheetos | 15 | 80 | 2 | 1.1 | 8.6 | 0.5 | 0.5 | 7.5 | 4.8 | 1.3 | | | | | 0 | | | | | | | | | | | | | | | | | | | | | | | | 150 | |
| 44114 | 1 ea | Original, bag, Weight Watchers | 14 | 69 | 2 | 1.0 | 9.9 | 0.0 | 0.0 | 9.9 | 2.5 | 1.0 | | | | | 0 | 0 | 0 | 0 | 0 | 0 | | | | | | | | 0.0 | | | 0 | | 0.0 | | | | 108 | | 84 | |
| 44108 | 1 ea | Pizza, bag, Weight Watchers | 14 | 59 | 1 | 1.0 | 10.8 | 1.0 | 0.0 | 9.9 | 2.0 | 0.0 | | | 0.00 | 0.00 | 0 | 0 | 0 | 0 | 0 | 0 | | | | | | | | 0.0 | | | 0 | | 0.0 | | | | 35 | | 123 | |
| 44107 | 1 ea | Ranch, bag, Weight Watchers | 14 | 59 | 5 | 1.0 | 9.9 | 1.0 | 0.0 | 8.9 | 2.0 | 0.0 | | | 0.00 | 0.00 | 0 | 0 | 0 | 0 | 0 | 0 | | | | | | | | 0.0 | | | 0 | | 0.0 | | | | 35 | | 168 | |
| | | Cheese Puffs | | | | | | | | | | | | | | | | | | | | | | | | | | | | | | | | | | | | | | | | |
| 44001 | 1 cup | Average | 20 | 111 | 2 | 1.5 | 10.8 | 0.2 | 0.3 | 10.3 | 6.9 | 1.3 | 4.1 | 1.0 | 0.04 | 0.91 | 1 | 53 | 7 | 7 | 0.1 | | 0.05 | 0.07 | 0.65 | 0.03 | 0.03 | 24.0 | 0.07 | 0.0 | 0.0 | | 12 | 0.0 | 0.5 | 4 | 0.0 | 22 | 33 | 0.6 | 210 | 0.08 |
| 44176 | 1 cup | Caramel, fat free, Health Valley | 30 | 110 | 11 | 2.0 | 24.0 | 2.0 | 2.0 | 20.0 | 0.0 | 0.0 | 0.0 | 0.0 | 0.00 | 0.00 | 0 | 0 | 0 | 0 | 0 | 0 | | | | | | | | 0.0 | | | 0 | | 0.7 | | | | | | 60 | |
| 44245 | 21 pce | Cheetos | 28 | 150 | 2 | 2.0 | 16.0 | 1.0 | 1.0 | 14.0 | 9.0 | 2.0 | | | | | 0 | | | | | | | | | | | | | | | | | | | | | | | | 300 | |
| 44251 | 21 pce | Cheetos, Flamin' Hot | 28 | 160 | 2 | 2.0 | 16.0 | 1.0 | 1.0 | 14.0 | 9.0 | 2.0 | | | | | 0 | | | | | | | | | | | | | | | | | | | | | | | | 240 | |
| 44249 | 13 pce | Cheetos, Jumbo | 28 | 160 | 2 | 2.0 | 15.0 | 1.0 | 1.0 | 13.0 | 10.0 | 2.5 | | | | | 5 | | | | | | | | | | | | | | | | | | | | | | | | 330 | |
| 44174 | 1 cup | Fat Free, Health Valley | 20 | 73 | 11 | 2.0 | 15.3 | 1.3 | 1.3 | 12.7 | 0.0 | 0.0 | 0.0 | 0.0 | 0.00 | 0.00 | 0 | 67 | 13 | | | | | | | | | | | 0.0 | | | 0 | | 0.2 | | | | | | 173 | |
| 44172 | 1 cup | Green Onion, fat free, Health Valley | 20 | 73 | 12 | 2.0 | 15.3 | 1.3 | 1.3 | 12.7 | 0.0 | 0.0 | 0.0 | 0.0 | 0.00 | 0.00 | 0 | 67 | 13 | | | | | | | | | | | 0.0 | | | 0 | | 0.2 | | | | | | 173 | |
| 44171 | 1 cup | Zesty Chili, fat free, Health Valley | 20 | 73 | 12 | 2.0 | 15.3 | 1.3 | 1.3 | 12.7 | 0.0 | 0.0 | 0.0 | 0.0 | 0.00 | 0.00 | 0 | 67 | 13 | | | | | | | | | | | 0.0 | | | 0 | | 0.2 | | | | | | 173 | |
| | | Chex Snack Mix | | | | | | | | | | | | | | | | | | | | | | | | | | | | | | | | | | | | | | | | |
| 44032 | 1/2 cup | Average | 21 | 89 | 4 | 2.3 | 13.7 | 1.2 | 1.4 | 11.1 | 3.6 | 1.1 | 1.9 | 0.6 | 0.01 | 0.41 | 0 | 30 | 3 | | | | 0.33 | 0.10 | 3.53 | 0.33 | 2.60 | 0.0 | 0.09 | 10.0 | 0.0 | | 7 | 0.1 | 5.2 | 13 | 0.3 | 39 | 56 | | 214 | 0.44 |
| 44205 | 1/2 cup | Bold & Zesty, Ralston Purina | 34 | 160 | 19 | 3.0 | 17.0 | 5.0 | 4.0 | 8.0 | 7.0 | 1.5 | | | | | 0 | 400 | 40 | | | | 0.15 | 0.07 | 2.00 | 0.02 | 0.60 | 40.0 | | 12.0 | | | 0 | | 5.4 | | | | | | 390 | |
| 44206 | 1/2 cup | Cheese, Ralston Purina | 25 | 106 | 4 | 2.3 | 18.2 | 1.5 | 1.5 | 15.2 | 3.4 | 0.8 | | | | | 0 | 0 | 0 | 0 | 0 | 0 | 0.23 | 0.05 | 3.03 | 0.23 | 0.63 | 45.5 | | 1.8 | | | 0 | | 2.7 | | | | | | 189 | |
| 44207 | 1/2 cup | Traditional, Ralston Purina | 23 | 100 | 4 | 2.3 | 16.9 | 0.8 | 1.5 | 14.6 | 2.7 | 0.8 | | | | | 0 | 0 | 0 | 0 | 0 | 0 | 0.23 | 0.03 | 2.30 | 0.23 | 0.63 | 46.0 | | 0.5 | | | 0 | | 3.4 | | | | | | 215 | |
| | | Corn Chips | | | | | | | | | | | | | | | | | | | | | | | | | | | | | | | | | | | | | | | | |
| 44026 | 16 pce | Barbecue, avg | 29 | 152 | 1 | 2.0 | 16.3 | 1.5 | 0.0 | 14.8 | 9.5 | 1.3 | 2.7 | 4.7 | 0.36 | 4.32 | 0 | 177 | 18 | 0 | 18 | | 0.02 | 0.06 | 0.48 | 0.07 | 0.00 | 11.3 | 0.04 | 0.5 | 0.0 | | 38 | 0.0 | 0.4 | 22 | 0.2 | 60 | 68 | 1.2 | 221 | 0.31 |
| 44280 | 29 pce | Cheddar/Sour Cream, Fritos | 28 | 160 | 2 | 2.0 | 15.0 | 1.0 | 1.0 | 13.0 | 10.0 | 1.5 | | | | | 0 | | | | | | | | | | | | | | | | | | | | | | | | 260 | |
| 44002 | 1 cup | Plain, avg | 26 | 140 | 1 | 1.7 | 14.8 | 1.3 | 0.0 | 13.5 | 8.7 | 1.2 | 2.5 | 4.3 | 0.33 | 3.95 | 0 | 24 | 2 | 0 | 2 | | 0.01 | 0.04 | 0.31 | 0.06 | 0.00 | 5.2 | 0.10 | 0.0 | 0.0 | | 33 | 0.0 | 0.3 | 20 | 0.1 | 48 | 37 | 1.7 | 164 | 0.33 |
| 44278 | 32 pce | Plain, Fritos | 28 | 160 | 2 | 2.0 | 15.0 | 1.0 | 0.0 | 14.0 | 10.0 | 1.5 | | | | | 0 | | | | | | | | | | | | | | | | | | | | | | | | 160 | |
| 44283 | 10 pce | Ranch, Fritos | 28 | 150 | 2 | 2.0 | 16.0 | 1.0 | 0.0 | 15.0 | 9.0 | 1.5 | | | | | 0 | | | | | | | | | | | | | | | | | | | | | | | | 135 | |
| 44284 | 28 pce | Sour Cream/Onion, Fritos | 28 | 160 | 2 | 2.0 | 15.0 | 1.0 | 1.0 | 13.0 | 10.0 | 1.5 | | | | | 0 | | | | | | | | | | | | | | | | | | | | | | | | 170 | |
| | | Corn Nuts | | | | | | | | | | | | | | | | | | | | | | | | | | | | | | | | | | | | | | | | |
| 44034 | 16 pce | Barbecue, avg | 29 | 126 | 2 | 2.6 | 20.8 | 2.4 | 0.0 | 18.4 | 4.1 | 0.7 | 2.1 | 0.9 | 0.01 | 0.92 | 0 | 98 | 10 | 0 | 10 | | 0.10 | 0.04 | 0.44 | 0.05 | 0.00 | 0.0 | 0.11 | 0.1 | 0.0 | | 5 | 0.0 | 0.5 | 32 | 0.1 | 82 | 83 | | 283 | 0.55 |
| 44069 | 16 pce | Nacho, avg | 29 | 127 | 2 | 2.7 | 20.8 | 2.3 | 0.0 | 18.4 | 4.1 | 0.7 | 2.1 | 0.9 | 0.01 | 0.91 | 1 | 11 | 1 | 0 | 1 | | 0.11 | 0.02 | 0.35 | 0.06 | 0.00 | 4.3 | 0.16 | 4.5 | 0.0 | | 10 | 0.0 | 0.5 | 32 | 0.1 | 90 | 90 | | 184 | 0.52 |
| 44031 | 16 pce | Plain, avg | 29 | 127 | 1 | 2.5 | 21.3 | 2.0 | 0.0 | 19.3 | 4.1 | 0.7 | 2.1 | 0.9 | 0.01 | 0.91 | 0 | 0 | 0 | 0 | 0 | 0 | 0.01 | 0.04 | 0.49 | 0.07 | 0.00 | 0.0 | 0.11 | 0.0 | 0.0 | | 3 | 0.0 | 0.5 | 33 | 0.1 | 80 | 81 | 4.3 | 159 | 0.52 |
| | | Crackers, see page 145 | | | | | | | | | | | | | | | | | | | | | | | | | | | | | | | | | | | | | | | | |
| 44035 | 1/2 cup | Doo Dads Snack Mix, avg | 28 | 128 | 3 | 2.9 | 18.0 | 1.9 | | | 5.2 | 1.0 | 3.1 | 0.9 | 0.01 | 0.60 | 0 | 42 | 12 | | | | 0.10 | 0.07 | 1.50 | 0.06 | 0.00 | 11.2 | 0.16 | 0.0 | | | 21 | 0.1 | 0.7 | 17 | 0.5 | 83 | 78 | | 356 | 0.63 |
| | | Fruit Snacks | | | | | | | | | | | | | | | | | | | | | | | | | | | | | | | | | | | | | | | | |
| 44113 | 1 ea | Apple, pouch, Weight Watchers | 14 | 49 | 5 | 0.0 | 12.8 | 2.0 | 8.9 | 2.0 | 0.0 | 0.0 | 0.0 | 0.0 | 0.00 | 0.00 | 0 | 0 | 0 | 0 | 0 | 0 | | | | | | | | 0.0 | | | 0 | | 0.0 | | | | 59 | | 123 | |
| 44116 | 1 ea | Apple Chips, bag, Weight Watchers | 21 | 69 | | 0.0 | 17.7 | 3.0 | 12.8 | 2.0 | 0.0 | 0.0 | 0.0 | 0.0 | 0.00 | 0.00 | 0 | 0 | 0 | 0 | 0 | 0 | | | | | | | | 0.0 | | | 0 | | 0.0 | | | | | | 123 | |
| 44112 | 1 ea | Cinnamon, pouch, Weight Watchers | 14 | 49 | 5 | 0.0 | 12.8 | 2.0 | 8.9 | 2.0 | 0.0 | 0.0 | 0.0 | 0.0 | 0.00 | 0.00 | 0 | 0 | 0 | 0 | 0 | 0 | | | | | | | | 0.0 | | | 0 | | 0.0 | | | | 59 | | 123 | |
| 44212 | 1 ea | Leather, bars, avg | 23 | 81 | 14 | 0.4 | 18.1 | 0.8 | | | 1.2 | 0.9 | 0.1 | 0.0 | 0.00 | 0.04 | 0 | 27 | 3 | 0 | 3 | | 0.01 | 0.01 | 0.02 | 0.07 | 0.00 | 0.9 | 0.02 | 16.1 | | | 7 | 0.0 | 0.2 | 5 | 0.0 | 13 | 32 | 0.6 | 18 | 0.04 |
| 44213 | 1 ea | Leather, bars, w/cream, avg | 24 | 89 | 12 | 0.2 | 18.7 | 0.9 | | | 2.0 | 0.6 | 1.0 | 0.2 | 0.01 | 0.21 | 1 | 13 | 3 | | | | 0.01 | 0.01 | 0.02 | 0.07 | 0.01 | 0.7 | 0.02 | 14.9 | | | 5 | 0.0 | 0.2 | 3 | 0.0 | 7 | 51 | 0.6 | 23 | 0.04 |
| 44214 | 1 ea | Leather, pces, avg | 21 | 72 | 12 | 0.2 | 16.4 | 0.7 | 10.5 | 5.2 | 1.5 | 0.2 | 0.6 | 0.6 | 0.04 | 0.52 | 0 | 24 | 3 | 0 | 3 | | 0.01 | 0.02 | 0.02 | 0.06 | 0.00 | 2.9 | 0.07 | 11.8 | 0.0 | | 4 | 0.0 | 0.2 | 3 | 0.0 | 5 | 34 | 0.6 | 85 | 0.04 |
| 44111 | 1 ea | Peach, pouch, Weight Watchers | 14 | 49 | 5 | 0.0 | 12.8 | 2.0 | 8.9 | 2.0 | 0.0 | 0.0 | 0.0 | 0.0 | 0.00 | 0.00 | 0 | 0 | 0 | 0 | 0 | 0 | | | | | | | | 0.0 | | | 0 | | 0.0 | | | | 59 | | 123 | |
| 44110 | 1 ea | Strawberry, pouch, Weight Watchers | 14 | 49 | 5 | 0.0 | 12.8 | 2.0 | 10.8 | 0.0 | 0.0 | 0.0 | 0.0 | 0.0 | 0.00 | 0.00 | 0 | 0 | 0 | 0 | 0 | 0 | | | | | | | | 0.0 | | | 0 | | 0.0 | | | | 69 | | 123 | |
| 44260 | 13 pce | Funyuns, Frito-Lay | 28 | 140 | 2 | 2.0 | 18.0 | 1.0 | 1.0 | 16.0 | 7.0 | 1.5 | | | | | 0 | | | | | | | | | | | | | | | | | | | | | | | | 250 | |
| | | Handi-Snacks | | | | | | | | | | | | | | | | | | | | | | | | | | | | | | | | | | | | | | | | |
| 57095 | 1 ea | Cheese N Breadstick, pkg, Kraft | 32 | 130 | | 4.0 | 11.0 | 0.0 | 3.0 | 8.0 | 7.0 | 4.0 | | | | | 15 | 400 | 114 | | | | | 0.07 | | | 0.12 | | | 0.0 | | | 80 | | 0.0 | 0 | | 150 | 60 | | 340 | 0.30 |
| 57096 | 1 ea | Cheese N Crackers, pkg, Kraft | 31 | 130 | | 4.0 | 10.0 | 0.0 | 2.0 | 8.0 | 8.0 | 4.5 | | | | | 15 | 300 | 36 | | | | | 0.14 | | | 0.12 | | | 0.0 | | | 80 | | 0.4 | 0 | | 150 | 55 | | 340 | 0.30 |
| 57097 | 1 ea | Cheese N Pretzels, pkg, Kraft | 30 | 110 | | 4.0 | 11.0 | 0.5 | 2.0 | 8.5 | 6.0 | 4.0 | | | | | 15 | 300 | 36 | | | | | 0.07 | | | 0.12 | | | 0.0 | | | 80 | | 0.0 | 0 | | 150 | 55 | | 420 | 0.30 |
| 57099 | 1 ea | Peanut Butter N Cracker, pkg, Kraft | 31 | 180 | | 5.0 | 12.0 | 1.0 | 3.0 | 8.0 | 12.0 | 3.0 | | | | | 0 | 0 | 0 | 0 | 0 | 0 | | 0.10 | | | 0.00 | | | 0.0 | | | 0 | | 0.7 | 32 | | 80 | 150 | | 150 | 0.30 |
| 57100 | 1 ea | Peanut Butter N Graham, pkg, Kraft | 32 | 170 | | 5.0 | 14.0 | 1.0 | 4.0 | 9.0 | 10.0 | 2.5 | | | | | 0 | 0 | 0 | 0 | 0 | 0 | | 0.07 | | | 0.00 | | | 0.0 | | | 0 | | 0.7 | 24 | | 60 | 150 | | 130 | 0.30 |
| 44261 | 16 pce | Munchos, Frito-Lay | 28 | 150 | | 1.0 | 18.0 | 1.0 | 0.0 | 17.0 | 10.0 | 2.5 | | | | | 0 | | | | | | | | | | | | | | | | | | | | | | | | 270 | |
| | | Popcorn | | | | | | | | | | | | | | | | | | | | | | | | | | | | | | | | | | | | | | | | |
| 44104 | 1 ea | Butter, bag, Weight Watchers | 19 | 91 | | 2.0 | 14.2 | 3.0 | 0.0 | 11.2 | 2.5 | 0.0 | | | 0.00 | 0.00 | 0 | 0 | 0 | 0 | 0 | 0 | | | | | | | | 0.0 | | | 0 | | 0.4 | | | | 51 | | 102 | |
| 44106 | 1 ea | Butter Toffee, bag, Weight Watchers | 26 | 112 | 3 | 1.0 | 21.4 | 1.0 | 11.2 | 9.2 | 2.5 | 1.0 | | | | | 0 | 0 | 0 | 0 | 0 | 0 | | | | | | | | 0.0 | | | 0 | | 0.7 | | | | 46 | | 92 | |
| 44014 | 1 cup | Caramel, avg | 35 | 151 | 3 | 1.3 | 27.7 | 1.8 | 13.6 | 12.3 | 4.5 | 1.3 | 1.0 | 1.6 | 0.14 | 1.42 | 2 | 18 | 4 | 3 | 1 | | 0.02 | 0.02 | 0.77 | 0.01 | 0.00 | 0.7 | 0.03 | 0.0 | 0.0 | | 15 | 0.0 | 0.6 | 12 | 0.1 | 29 | 38 | 1.3 | 72 | 0.20 |
| 44105 | 1 ea | Caramel, bag, Weight Watchers | 26 | 102 | 3 | 1.0 | 22.4 | 1.0 | 11.2 | 10.2 | 1.0 | 0.0 | | | 0.00 | 0.00 | 0 | 0 | 0 | 0 | 0 | 0 | | | | | | | | 0.0 | | | 0 | | 0.7 | | | | 61 | | 46 | |
| 44037 | 1 cup | Caramel, w/peanuts, avg | 42 | 168 | 3 | 2.7 | 33.9 | 1.6 | 17.2 | 15.1 | 3.3 | 0.4 | 1.1 | 1.4 | 0.03 | 1.35 | 0 | 27 | 3 | 0 | 3 | | 0.02 | 0.05 | 0.84 | 0.08 | 0.00 | 6.7 | 0.10 | 0.0 | 0.0 | | 28 | 0.1 | 1.6 | 34 | 0.3 | 53 | 149 | 1.6 | 124 | 0.52 |
| 44038 | 1 cup | Cheese, avg | 11 | 58 | 2 | 1.0 | 5.7 | 1.1 | 0.1 | 4.5 | 3.7 | 0.7 | 1.1 | 1.7 | 0.10 | 1.60 | 1 | 27 | 5 | | | | 0.01 | 0.03 | 0.16 | 0.03 | 0.06 | 1.2 | 0.05 | 0.1 | 0.0 | | 12 | 0.0 | 0.2 | 10 | 0.1 | 40 | 29 | 1.3 | 98 | 0.22 |
| 44072 | 1 cup | Plain, air popped, avg | 8 | 31 | 4 | 1.0 | 6.2 | 1.2 | 0.0 | 5.0 | 0.3 | 0.0 | 0.1 | 0.2 | 0.00 | 0.15 | 0 | 0.2 | 0 | 0 | 0.2 | | 0.02 | 0.02 | 0.16 | 0.02 | 0.00 | 1.8 | 0.03 | 0.0 | 0.0 | | 1 | 0.0 | 0.2 | 10 | 0.1 | 24 | 24 | 0.8 | 0 | 0.28 |

| Code | Amount | | Description | Weight (g) | Calories | % Water | Protein (g) | Carbs (g) | Fiber (g) | Sugar (g) | Other Carbs (g) | Fat (g) | Sat Fat (g) | Mono Fat (g) | Poly Fat (g) | Omega 3 (g) | Omega 6 (g) | Choles (mg) |
|---|---|---|---|---|---|---|---|---|---|---|---|---|---|---|---|---|---|---|
| | | | **Basic Components** | | | | | | | | | | **Additional Fats** | | | | | |
| 44066 | 1 | cup | Plain, microwave, low fat, low sod, avg | 6 | 25 | 3 | 0.8 | 4.3 | 0.9 | 0.1 | 3.4 | 0.6 | 0.1 | 0.2 | 0.3 | | | 0 |
| 44292 | 1 | cup | Plain, popped in oil, avg | 11 | 55 | 3 | 1.0 | 6.3 | 1.1 | 0.1 | 5.1 | 3.1 | 0.5 | 0.9 | 1.5 | | | 0 |
| 44013 | 1 | cup | Plain, popped in oil, salted, avg | 11 | 55 | 3 | 1.0 | 6.3 | 1.1 | 0.1 | 5.1 | 3.1 | 0.5 | 0.9 | 1.5 | 0.08 | 1.39 | 0 |
| 44103 | 1 | ea | White Cheddar, bag, Weight Watchers | 19 | 91 | 2 | 2.0 | 12.2 | 2.0 | 0.0 | 10.2 | 4.1 | 1.0 | | | | | 0 |
| | | | Popcorn Cakes | | | | | | | | | | | | | | | |
| 44022 | 1 | ea | Average | 10 | 38 | 5 | 1.0 | 8.0 | 0.3 | 0.1 | 7.6 | 0.3 | 0.0 | 0.1 | 0.1 | 0.00 | 0.13 | 0 |
| 44287 | 1 | ea | Cheddar Cheese, Chico San | 9 | 48 | | 1.0 | 9.7 | | | | 1.9 | | | | | | 0 |
| 44070 | 1 | ea | Low Sodium, avg | 9 | 35 | 5 | 0.7 | 7.5 | | 0.0 | | 0.2 | 0.0 | 0.1 | 0.1 | 0.00 | 0.08 | 0 |
| 44039 | 1 | cup | Pork Skins, barbecue | 32 | 172 | 2 | 18.5 | 0.5 | | 0.0 | | 10.2 | 3.7 | 4.8 | 1.1 | 0.00 | 1.10 | 37 |
| | | | Potato Chips | | | | | | | | | | | | | | | |
| 44046 | 20 | pce | Barbecue, avg | 26 | 142 | 2 | 1.7 | 13.3 | 0.3 | 0.3 | 12.8 | 9.6 | 2.5 | 1.9 | 4.9 | 0.09 | 4.78 | 1 |
| 44042 | 1 | cup | Cheese, avg | 20 | 99 | 2 | 1.7 | 11.5 | 1.0 | 0.2 | 10.3 | 5.4 | 1.7 | 1.5 | 1.9 | 0.03 | 1.88 | 1 |
| 44045 | 1 | oz | Cheese, Pringles | 28 | 154 | 2 | 2.0 | 14.2 | 0.9 | 0.3 | 12.9 | 10.4 | 2.7 | 2.0 | 5.2 | 0.10 | 5.12 | 1 |
| 44006 | 15 | ea | Plain, avg | 30 | 161 | 2 | 2.1 | 15.9 | 1.4 | 0.3 | 14.2 | 10.4 | 3.3 | 3.0 | 3.7 | 0.06 | 3.60 | 0 |
| 44043 | 20 | pce | Plain, light, avg | 40 | 188 | 1 | 2.8 | 26.8 | 2.3 | 0.4 | 24.0 | 8.3 | 1.7 | 1.9 | 4.4 | 0.08 | 4.28 | 0 |
| 44024 | 1 | oz | Plain, light, Pringles | 28 | 140 | 1 | 1.6 | 18.2 | 1.0 | 2.8 | 14.4 | 7.2 | 1.4 | 1.7 | 3.8 | 0.07 | 3.71 | 0 |
| 44044 | 1 | oz | Plain, Pringles | 28 | 156 | 1 | 1.7 | 14.3 | 1.0 | 0.3 | 13.0 | 10.8 | 2.6 | 2.0 | 5.6 | 0.10 | 5.49 | 0 |
| 44076 | 1 | oz | Plain, unsalted, avg | 28 | 150 | 2 | 2.0 | 14.8 | 1.3 | 0.0 | 13.5 | 9.7 | 3.1 | 2.8 | 3.4 | 0.05 | 3.36 | 0 |
| 5437 | 1 | oz | Sour Cream & Onion, avg | 28 | 149 | 2 | 2.3 | 14.4 | 1.5 | 2.3 | 10.7 | 9.5 | 2.5 | 1.7 | 4.9 | 0.02 | 4.84 | 2 |
| 44046 | 1 | oz | Sour Cream & Onion, Pringles | 28 | 153 | 2 | 1.8 | 14.4 | 0.3 | 0.3 | 13.7 | 10.4 | 2.7 | 2.0 | 5.3 | 0.10 | 5.15 | 1 |
| 44025 | 10 | pce | White Potato Skins, avg | 20 | 112 | 1 | 1.2 | 10.2 | 0.7 | 1.3 | 8.2 | 7.3 | 1.9 | 1.2 | 3.9 | 0.01 | 3.84 | 0 |
| 44047 | 1 | cup | Potato Sticks | 36 | 188 | 2 | 2.4 | 19.2 | 1.2 | 0.4 | 17.6 | 12.4 | 3.2 | 2.2 | 6.4 | 0.03 | 6.42 | 0 |
| | | | Pretzels | | | | | | | | | | | | | | | |
| 44270 | 3 | pce | Bavarian, Rold Gold | 28 | 110 | 3 | 3.0 | 21.0 | 1.0 | 1.0 | 19.0 | 2.0 | 0.5 | | | | | 0 |
| 44033 | 10 | pce | Cheddar Cheese, Mars Snacks | 30 | 139 | 2 | 3.0 | 20.0 | | | | 5.1 | | | | | | 2 |
| 44015 | 5 | pce | Hard, avg | 30 | 114 | 3 | 2.7 | 23.8 | 1.0 | 0.5 | 22.3 | 1.1 | 0.2 | 0.4 | 0.4 | 0.02 | 0.34 | 0 |
| 44215 | 3 | ea | Hard, chocolate coated, avg | 33 | 151 | 2 | 2.5 | 23.4 | 1.1 | | | 5.5 | 2.5 | 1.8 | 0.7 | 0.05 | 0.66 | 0 |
| 44079 | 5 | ea | Hard, unsalted, avg | 30 | 114 | 3 | 2.7 | 23.8 | 0.8 | 0.0 | 22.9 | 1.1 | 0.2 | 0.4 | 0.4 | 0.02 | 0.34 | 0 |
| 44109 | 1 | ea | Oat Bran Nuggets, bag, Weight Watchers | 42 | 168 | 4 | 4.0 | 32.6 | 3.0 | 0.0 | 29.6 | 2.5 | 0.0 | | | 0.00 | 0.00 | 0 |
| 42093 | 1 | ea | Soft, avg | 55 | 190 | 15 | 4.5 | 38.4 | 0.9 | | | 1.7 | 0.7 | 0.8 | 0.2 | | | 2 |
| 42453 | 1 | ea | Soft, dipped in butter, Auntie Anne's | 140 | 410 | | 12.0 | 82.0 | 4.0 | 11.0 | 67.0 | 4.5 | 2.0 | | | | | 10 |
| 42458 | 1 | ea | Soft, raisin, Auntie Anne's | 165 | 500 | | 11.0 | 111.0 | 4.0 | 40.0 | 67.0 | 0.5 | 0.0 | | | | | 0 |
| 42456 | 1 | ea | Soft, whole wheat, Auntie Anne's | 140 | 390 | | 13.0 | 82.0 | 8.0 | 13.0 | 61.0 | 1.5 | 0.0 | | | | | 0 |
| 44274 | 1 | ea | Sourdough, fat free, Rold Gold | 28 | 80 | 15 | 2.0 | 17.0 | 1.0 | 1.0 | 15.0 | 0.0 | 0.0 | 0.0 | 0.0 | 0.00 | 0.00 | 0 |
| 44275 | 48 | pce | Sticks, fat free, Rold Gold | 28 | 110 | 3 | 3.0 | 23.0 | 1.0 | 1.0 | 21.0 | 0.0 | 0.0 | 0.0 | 0.0 | 0.00 | 0.00 | 0 |
| 44269 | 48 | pce | Sticks, Rold Gold | 28 | 110 | 3 | 3.0 | 23.0 | 1.0 | 1.0 | 21.0 | 1.0 | 0.0 | | | 0.00 | 0.00 | 0 |
| 44137 | 5 | ea | Twist, lightly salted, Michael Seasons | 30 | 116 | | 2.1 | 23.3 | | | | 1.1 | | | | | | |
| 44119 | 7 | ea | Twist, Mr Salty | 30 | 120 | | 3.0 | 23.0 | 1.0 | 1.0 | 21.0 | 1.5 | 0.0 | 0.5 | 0.0 | 0.00 | 0.00 | 0 |
| 44136 | 5 | ea | Twist, unsalted, Michael Seasons | 30 | 116 | | 2.1 | 23.3 | | | | 1.1 | | | | | | |
| 44135 | 5 | ea | Wheat Mini, lightly salted, Michael Seasons | 30 | 116 | | 4.2 | 21.2 | | | | 0.0 | 0.0 | 0.0 | 0.0 | 0.00 | 0.00 | |
| 44134 | 5 | ea | Wheat Mini, unsalted, Michael Seasons | 30 | 116 | | 4.2 | 21.2 | | | | 0.0 | 0.0 | 0.0 | 0.0 | 0.00 | 0.00 | |
| 44048 | 1 | oz | Whole Wheat, avg | 28 | 101 | 4 | 3.1 | 22.7 | 2.2 | 0.0 | 20.6 | 0.7 | 0.2 | 0.3 | 0.2 | 0.01 | 0.22 | 0 |
| 44067 | 2 | ea | Yogurt Covered, avg | 8 | 37 | 5 | 0.7 | 5.4 | 0.1 | | | 1.5 | 1.2 | 0.2 | 0.0 | | | 0 |
| 44140 | 1 | oz | Rice Bites, all flavors, American Grains, avg | 28 | 119 | | 2.0 | 21.7 | | | | 3.0 | | | | | | |
| | | | Rice Cakes | | | | | | | | | | | | | | | |
| 44080 | 1 | ea | Brown, avg | 9 | 35 | 6 | 0.7 | 7.3 | 0.4 | 0.0 | 7.0 | 0.3 | 0.1 | 0.1 | 0.1 | 0.00 | 0.09 | 0 |
| 44021 | 1 | ea | Brown, salted, avg | 9 | 35 | 6 | 0.7 | 7.3 | 0.4 | 0.0 | 7.0 | 0.3 | 0.1 | 0.1 | 0.1 | 0.00 | 0.09 | 0 |
| 44049 | 1 | ea | Brown/Buckwheat, avg | 9 | 34 | 6 | 0.8 | 7.2 | 0.3 | 0.0 | 6.9 | 0.3 | 0.1 | 0.1 | 0.1 | 0.01 | 0.09 | 0 |
| 44050 | 1 | ea | Brown/Corn, avg | 9 | 35 | 6 | 0.8 | 7.3 | 0.3 | 0.0 | 7.0 | 0.3 | 0.1 | 0.1 | 0.1 | 0.00 | 0.10 | 0 |
| 44051 | 1 | ea | Brown/Multi-Grain, avg | 9 | 35 | 6 | 0.8 | 7.2 | 0.3 | 0.0 | 6.9 | 0.3 | 0.1 | 0.1 | 0.1 | 0.04 | 0.09 | 0 |
| 44052 | 1 | ea | Brown/Rye, avg | 9 | 35 | 7 | 0.7 | 7.2 | 0.4 | 0.0 | 6.8 | 0.3 | 0.1 | 0.1 | 0.1 | 0.01 | 0.13 | 0 |
| 44053 | 1 | ea | Brown/Sesame Seed, avg | 9 | 35 | 6 | 0.7 | 7.3 | 0.5 | 0.0 | 6.8 | 0.3 | 0.0 | 0.1 | 0.1 | 0.00 | 0.10 | 0 |
| | | | Snack Mix | | | | | | | | | | | | | | | |
| 44197 | 1/2 | cup | Goldfish, cheddar, Pepperidge Farm | 36 | 180 | 14 | 1.0 | 19.0 | 1.0 | 3.0 | 15.0 | 10.0 | 1.5 | | | | | 5 |
| 44194 | 1/2 | cup | Goldfish, Pepperidge Farm | 36 | 170 | 2 | 5.0 | 21.0 | 2.0 | 3.0 | 16.0 | 8.0 | 1.5 | | | | | 5 |
| 44195 | 1/2 | cup | Nutty, Pepperidge Farm | 36 | 180 | 2 | 5.0 | 20.0 | 2.0 | 2.0 | 16.0 | 9.0 | 1.5 | | | | | 25 |
| | | | Snack Sticks | | | | | | | | | | | | | | | |
| 44189 | 9 | pce | Pumpernickel, Pepperidge Farm | 31 | 150 | 4 | 3.0 | 20.0 | 1.0 | 1.0 | 18.0 | 6.0 | 0.5 | | | | | 0 |
| 44217 | 1 | oz | Sesame, avg | 28 | 151 | 2 | 3.1 | 13.0 | 0.8 | | | 10.3 | 1.8 | 3.1 | 4.9 | 0.27 | 4.59 | 0 |
| 44084 | 1 | oz | Sesame, unsalted, avg | 28 | 151 | 2 | 3.1 | 13.0 | | | | 10.3 | 1.8 | 3.1 | 4.9 | 0.27 | 4.59 | 0 |
| 44191 | 9 | pce | Three Cheese, Pepperidge Farm | 31 | 140 | 3 | 4.0 | 20.0 | 1.0 | 1.0 | 18.0 | 5.0 | 2.0 | | | | | 5 |
| | | | Sun Chips | | | | | | | | | | | | | | | |
| 44257 | 13 | pce | French Onion | 28 | 140 | 2 | 2.0 | 19.0 | 2.0 | 2.0 | 15.0 | 6.0 | 1.0 | | | | | 0 |
| 44258 | 13 | pce | Harvest Cheddar | 28 | 140 | 2 | 2.0 | 18.0 | 2.0 | 2.0 | 14.0 | 6.0 | 1.0 | | | | | 0 |
| 44256 | 14 | pce | Original | 28 | 140 | 2 | 2.0 | 18.0 | 2.0 | 2.0 | 14.0 | 7.0 | 1.0 | | | | | 0 |
| 44020 | 10 | ea | Taro Chips, avg | 23 | 115 | 2 | 0.5 | 15.7 | 1.7 | 0.6 | 13.4 | 5.7 | 1.5 | 1.0 | 3.0 | 0.01 | 2.94 | 0 |
| | | | Tortilla Chips | | | | | | | | | | | | | | | |
| 44302 | 1 | oz | Lime N Chili, baked, Guiltless Gourmet | 28 | 110 | 4 | 2.0 | 22.0 | 2.0 | 2.0 | 18.0 | 2.0 | 0.0 | | | 0.00 | 0.00 | 0 |
| 44263 | 6 | pce | Lime N Chili, Tostitos | 28 | 150 | 2 | 2.0 | 17.0 | 1.0 | 0.0 | 16.0 | 7.0 | 1.0 | | | | | 0 |
| 44303 | 1 | oz | Nacho, baked, Guiltless Gourmet | 28 | 110 | 4 | 2.0 | 22.0 | 2.0 | 2.0 | 18.0 | 2.0 | 0.0 | | | 0.00 | 0.00 | 0 |

| Code | Vit A (IU) | Vit A (RE) | Retinol (RE) | Carotenoids (RE) | Beta Carotene (mcg) | Thiamin (mg) | Riboflavin (mg) | Niacin (NE) | Vit B6 (mg) | Vit B12 (mcg) | Folate (mcg) | Panto (mg) | Vit C (mg) | Vit D (mg) | Vit E (α TE) | Calcium (mg) | Copper (mg) | Iron (mg) | Magnes (mg) | Mang (mg) | Phos (mg) | Potassium (mg) | Selenium (mcg) | Sodium (mg) | Zinc (mg) |
|---|---|---|---|---|---|---|---|---|---|---|---|---|---|---|---|---|---|---|---|---|---|---|---|---|---|
| | **Vit A & Components** | | | | | **Vitamins** | | | | | | | | | | **Minerals** | | | | | | | | | |
| 44066 | 6 | 1 | 0 | 1 | | 0.02 | 0.01 | 0.12 | 0.01 | 0.00 | 1.0 | | 0.0 | | | 1 | 0.0 | 0.1 | 9 | | 16 | 14 | | 29 | 0.23 |
| 44292 | 17 | 2 | 0 | 2 | | 0.01 | 0.01 | 0.17 | 0.02 | 0.00 | 1.9 | | 0.0 | | | 1 | 0.0 | 0.3 | 12 | | 27 | 25 | 0.8 | 97 | 0.29 |
| 44013 | 17 | 2 | 0 | 2 | 10 | 0.01 | 0.01 | 0.17 | 0.02 | 0.00 | 1.9 | 0.03 | 0.0 | 0.0 | | 1 | 0.0 | 0.3 | 12 | 0.1 | 27 | 25 | 0.8 | 97 | 0.29 |
| 44103 | 0 | 0 | 0 | 0 | 0 | | | | | | | | 0.0 | | | 0 | | 0.4 | | | | 61 | | 127 | |
| 44022 | 7 | 1 | 0 | 1 | | 0.01 | 0.02 | 0.60 | 0.02 | 0.00 | 1.8 | 0.04 | 0.0 | 0.0 | | 1 | 0.1 | 0.2 | 16 | 0.1 | 28 | 33 | 1.0 | 29 | 0.40 |
| 44287 | | | | | | | | | | | | | | | | | | | | | | 34 | | | |
| 44070 | 22 | 2 | | | | 0.02 | 0.00 | 0.46 | 0.01 | 0.00 | 1.7 | 0.07 | 0.0 | 0.0 | 0.0 | 2 | 0.0 | 0.1 | 10 | 0.2 | 14 | 14 | 0.9 | 3 | 0.18 |
| 44039 | 483 | 58 | | | | 0.03 | 0.14 | 1.08 | 0.05 | 0.04 | 9.9 | 0.14 | 0.5 | 0.0 | | 14 | 0.1 | 0.3 | 0 | 0.0 | 70 | 58 | | 853 | 0.23 |
| 44046 | 196 | 25 | 0 | 25 | 153 | 0.05 | 0.03 | 0.65 | 0.12 | 0.00 | 6.0 | 0.22 | 2.5 | 0.0 | | 17 | 0.0 | 0.4 | 14 | 0.1 | 44 | 129 | 2.1 | 187 | 0.18 |
| 44042 | 7 | 2 | | | | 0.03 | 0.03 | 1.00 | 0.07 | 0.00 | 0.0 | 0.16 | 10.8 | 0.0 | | 14 | 0.1 | 0.4 | 15 | 0.1 | 60 | 306 | 1.6 | 159 | 0.18 |
| 44045 | 0.3 | 0.03 | 0 | 0.03 | | 0.05 | 0.03 | 0.73 | 0.15 | 0.00 | 5.0 | 0.09 | 2.4 | 0.0 | | 31 | 0.0 | 0.4 | 15 | 0.0 | 46 | 107 | 2.3 | 211 | 0.18 |
| 44006 | 0 | 0 | 0 | 0 | 0 | 0.05 | 0.06 | 1.15 | 0.20 | 0.00 | 13.5 | 0.12 | 9.3 | 0.0 | | 7 | 0.1 | 0.5 | 20 | 0.1 | 50 | 383 | 2.4 | 178 | 0.33 |
| 44043 | 0 | 0 | 0 | 0 | 0 | 0.08 | 0.11 | 2.80 | 0.27 | 0.00 | 10.8 | 0.11 | 10.3 | 0.0 | | 8 | 0.2 | 0.5 | 36 | 0.2 | 77 | 698 | 3.2 | 197 | 0.03 |
| 44024 | 0 | 0 | 0 | 0 | 0 | 0.05 | 0.02 | 1.18 | 0.22 | 0.00 | 6.4 | 0.07 | 3.4 | 0.0 | | 10 | 0.0 | 0.4 | 18 | 0.1 | 43 | 281 | 2.3 | 120 | 0.17 |
| 44044 | 0 | 0 | 0 | 0 | 0 | 0.06 | 0.03 | 0.88 | 0.04 | 0.00 | 2.0 | 0.06 | 2.3 | 0.0 | | 7 | 0.0 | 0.4 | 16 | 0.1 | 44 | 282 | 2.3 | 184 | 0.17 |
| 44076 | 0 | 0 | 0 | 0 | 0 | 0.05 | 0.06 | 1.07 | 0.18 | 0.00 | 12.6 | 0.11 | 8.7 | 0.0 | | 7 | 0.1 | 0.5 | 19 | 0.1 | 46 | 357 | 2.3 | 2 | 0.31 |
| 5437 | 48 | 6 | | | | 0.05 | 0.06 | 1.13 | 0.19 | 0.28 | 17.4 | 0.23 | 10.4 | 0.1 | | 20 | 0.1 | 0.4 | 21 | 0.1 | 49 | 373 | 2.3 | 175 | 0.27 |
| 44046 | 211 | 27 | 0 | 27 | 165 | 0.05 | 0.03 | 0.70 | 0.13 | 0.00 | 6.4 | 0.23 | 2.7 | 0.0 | | 18 | 0.0 | 0.4 | 15 | 0.1 | 47 | 139 | 2.3 | 202 | 0.20 |
| 44025 | 0 | 0 | 0 | 0 | 0 | 0.04 | 0.02 | 0.63 | 0.03 | 0.00 | 1.4 | | 1.6 | | | 5 | 0.0 | 0.3 | 12 | | 31 | 202 | 1.6 | 131 | 0.12 |
| 44047 | 0 | 0 | 0 | 0 | 0 | 0.03 | 0.04 | 1.72 | 0.12 | 0.00 | 14.4 | 0.15 | 17.0 | 0.0 | | 6 | 0.1 | 0.8 | 23 | 0.2 | 62 | 445 | 2.9 | 90 | 0.36 |
| 44270 | | | | | | | | | | | | | | | | | | | | | | | | 440 | |
| 44033 | 20 | 2 | | | | 0.09 | 0.17 | 0.95 | 0.01 | 0.04 | 2.4 | 0.14 | 0.0 | | | 59 | 0.0 | 0.3 | 7 | 0.1 | 43 | 39 | | 335 | 0.22 |
| 44015 | 0 | 0 | 0 | 0 | 0 | 0.14 | 0.19 | 1.58 | 0.03 | 0.00 | 51.3 | 0.09 | 0.0 | 0.0 | | 11 | 0.1 | 1.3 | 11 | 0.5 | 34 | 44 | 1.7 | 515 | 0.26 |
| 44215 | 3 | 1 | | | | 0.03 | 0.07 | 0.26 | 0.06 | 0.00 | 3.0 | 0.25 | 0.2 | 0.0 | | 24 | 0.1 | 0.7 | 14 | 0.2 | 48 | 74 | 1.9 | 188 | 0.30 |
| 44079 | 0 | 0 | 0 | 0 | 0 | 0.14 | 0.19 | 1.58 | 0.03 | 0.00 | 24.9 | 0.09 | 0.0 | 0.0 | | 11 | 0.1 | 1.3 | 11 | 0.5 | 34 | 44 | 1.7 | 87 | 0.26 |
| 44109 | 0 | 0 | 0 | 0 | 0 | | | | | | | | 0.0 | | | 0 | | 0.7 | | | | 74 | | 247 | |
| 42093 | 0 | 0 | 0 | 0 | 0 | 0.23 | 0.16 | 2.35 | 0.01 | 0.00 | 7.7 | | 0.0 | 0.0 | | 13 | 0.1 | 2.2 | 12 | | 43 | 48 | | 772 | 0.52 |
| 42453 | 100 | 20 | | | | | | | | | | | | | | 40 | | 2.7 | | | | | | 1050 | |
| 42458 | 0 | 0 | 0 | 0 | 0 | | | | | | | | | | | 40 | | 2.7 | | | | | | 490 | |
| 42456 | 0 | 0 | 0 | 0 | 0 | | | | | | | | | | | 40 | | 2.7 | | | | | | 1290 | |
| 44274 | | | | | | | | | | | | | | | | | | | | | | | | 300 | |
| 44275 | | | | | | | | | | | | | | | | | | | | | | | | 530 | |
| 44269 | | | | | | | | | | | | | | | | | | | | | | | | 430 | |
| 44137 | | | | | | | | | | | | | | | | | | | | | | | | 360 | |
| 44119 | | | | | | | | | | | | | | | | | | 1.4 | | | | 35 | | 810 | |
| 44136 | | | | | | | | | | | | | | | | | | | | | | | | 63 | |
| 44135 | | | | | | | | | | | | | | | | | | | | | | | | 270 | |
| 44134 | | | | | | | | | | | | | | | | | | | | | | | | 32 | |
| 44048 | 0 | 0 | 0 | 0 | 0 | 0.12 | 0.08 | 1.83 | 0.08 | 0.00 | 15.1 | 0.23 | 0.3 | 0.0 | | 8 | 0.1 | 0.8 | 8 | 0.7 | 35 | 120 | | 57 | 0.17 |
| 44067 | 20 | 6 | 6 | 0.02 | | 0.03 | 0.03 | 0.22 | 0.00 | 0.04 | 1.3 | | 0.1 | | | 12 | 0.0 | 0.1 | 2 | | 12 | 19 | | 5 | 0.06 |
| 44140 | | | | | | | | | | | | | | | | | | | | | | | | 178 | |
| 44080 | 4 | 0.5 | 0 | 0.5 | | 0.01 | 0.01 | 0.70 | 0.01 | 0.00 | 1.9 | 0.09 | 0.0 | 0.0 | | 1 | 0.0 | 0.1 | 12 | 0.3 | 32 | 26 | 2.2 | 2 | 0.27 |
| 44021 | 4 | 0.5 | 0 | 0.5 | | 0.01 | 0.01 | 0.70 | 0.01 | 0.00 | 1.9 | 0.09 | 0.0 | 0.0 | | 1 | 0.0 | 0.1 | 12 | 0.3 | 32 | 26 | 2.2 | 29 | 0.27 |
| 44049 | 0 | 0 | 0 | 0 | 0 | 0.01 | 0.01 | 0.73 | 0.01 | 0.00 | 1.9 | 0.10 | 0.0 | 0.0 | | 1 | 0.0 | 0.1 | 14 | 0.6 | 34 | 27 | 1.5 | 10 | 0.23 |
| 44050 | 0 | 0 | 0 | 0 | 0 | 0.01 | 0.01 | 0.58 | 0.01 | 0.00 | 1.7 | 0.08 | 0.0 | 0.0 | | 1 | 0.0 | 0.1 | 10 | 0.5 | 29 | 25 | | 26 | 0.20 |
| 44051 | 0 | 0 | 0 | 0 | 0 | 0.01 | 0.02 | 0.59 | 0.01 | 0.00 | 1.8 | 0.09 | 0.0 | 0.0 | | 2 | 0.0 | 0.2 | 12 | 0.5 | 33 | 26 | | 23 | 0.23 |
| 44052 | 0.3 | 0.03 | 0 | 0.03 | 0.2 | 0.01 | 0.01 | 0.63 | 0.01 | 0.00 | 0.5 | 0.10 | 0.0 | 0.0 | | 2 | 0.0 | 0.2 | 13 | 0.3 | 34 | 28 | | 10 | 0.27 |
| 44053 | 0 | 0 | 0 | 0 | 0 | 0.00 | 0.01 | 0.65 | 0.01 | 0.00 | 1.6 | 0.13 | 0.3 | 0.0 | | 1 | 0.0 | 0.1 | 12 | 0.4 | 34 | 26 | 2.2 | 20 | 0.27 |
| 44197 | 0 | 0 | 0 | 0 | 0 | 0.22 | 0.14 | 1.60 | | | | | 0.0 | | | 20 | | 0.7 | | | | | | 390 | |
| 44194 | 0 | 0 | 0 | 0 | 0 | 0.22 | 0.14 | 1.60 | | | | | 0.0 | | | 40 | | 1.8 | | | | | | 360 | |
| 44195 | 0 | 0 | 0 | 0 | 0 | 0.22 | 0.14 | 1.60 | | | | | 0.0 | | | 40 | | 0.7 | | | | | | 330 | |
| 44189 | 0 | 0 | 0 | 0 | 0 | 0.09 | 0.07 | 0.80 | | | | | 0.0 | | | 0 | | 0.7 | | | | | | 340 | |
| 44217 | 25 | 3 | 0 | 3 | | 0.03 | 0.02 | 0.43 | 0.02 | 0.00 | 6.2 | 0.07 | 0.0 | | | 48 | 0.1 | 0.2 | 13 | 0.3 | 39 | 50 | 4.8 | 417 | 0.33 |
| 44084 | 25 | 3 | 0 | 3 | | 0.03 | 0.02 | 0.43 | 0.02 | 0.00 | 6.2 | 0.07 | 0.0 | | | 48 | 0.1 | 0.2 | 13 | 0.3 | 39 | 50 | 4.8 | 8 | 0.33 |
| 44191 | 0 | 0 | 0 | 0 | 0 | 0.09 | 0.07 | 0.80 | | | | | 0.0 | | | 40 | | 0.7 | | | | | | 410 | |
| 44257 | | | | | | | | | | | | | | | | | | | | | | | | 115 | |
| 44258 | | | | | | | | | | | | | | | | | | | | | | | | 115 | |
| 44256 | | | | | | | | | | | | | | | | | | | | | | | | 115 | |
| 44020 | 0 | 0 | 0 | 0 | 0 | 0.04 | 0.01 | 0.12 | 0.10 | 0.00 | 4.6 | 0.15 | 1.1 | 0.0 | | 14 | 0.1 | 0.3 | 19 | 0.0 | 30 | 174 | 0.4 | 79 | 0.09 |
| 44302 | 0 | 0 | 0 | 0 | 0 | | | | | | | | 0.0 | | | 60 | | 3.6 | | | | | | 200 | |
| 44263 | | | | | | | | | | | | | | | | | | | | | | | | 180 | |
| 44303 | 0 | 0 | 0 | 0 | 0 | | | | | | | | 0.0 | | | 60 | | 0.4 | | | | | | 200 | |

| Code | Amount | Description | Weight (g) | Calories | % Water | Protein (g) | Carbs (g) | Fiber (g) | Sugar (g) | Other Carbs (g) | Fat (g) | Sat Fat (g) | Mono Fat (g) | Poly Fat (g) | Omega 3 (g) | Omega 6 (g) | Choles (mg) |
|---|---|---|---|---|---|---|---|---|---|---|---|---|---|---|---|---|---|
| | | | Basic Components | | | | | | | | | Additional Fats | | | | | |
| 44054 | 20 ea | Nacho, light, avg | 32 | 142 | 1 | 2.8 | 22.9 | 1.5 | 0.4 | 21.0 | 4.9 | 0.9 | 2.9 | 0.7 | 0.03 | 0.64 | 1 |
| 44004 | 1 cup | Nacho, Doritos | 26 | 129 | 2 | 2.0 | 16.2 | 1.4 | 0.3 | 14.6 | 6.7 | 1.3 | 3.9 | 0.9 | 0.04 | 0.88 | 1 |
| 44131 | 11 ea | Nacho, Michael Seasons | 28 | 138 | | 2.0 | 18.8 | | | | 4.9 | | | | | | |
| 44018 | 16 pce | Plain, avg | 29 | 145 | 2 | 2.0 | 18.2 | 1.9 | 0.3 | 16.0 | 7.6 | 1.5 | 4.5 | 1.1 | 0.04 | 1.01 | 0 |
| 44301 | 1 oz | Plain, baked, blue corn, Guiltless Gourmet | 28 | 110 | 4 | 3.0 | 22.0 | 2.0 | 0.0 | 20.0 | 2.0 | 0.0 | | | 0.00 | 0.00 | 0 |
| 44298 | 1 oz | Plain, baked, Guiltless Gourmet | 28 | 110 | 0 | 3.0 | 22.0 | 2.0 | 0.0 | 20.0 | 2.0 | 0.0 | | | 0.00 | 0.00 | 0 |
| 44266 | 13 pce | Plain, baked, Tostitos | 28 | 110 | | 3.0 | 24.0 | 2.0 | 0.0 | 22.0 | 1.0 | 0.0 | | | 0.00 | 0.00 | 0 |
| 44267 | 13 pce | Plain, baked, unsalted, Tostitos | 28 | 110 | | 3.0 | 24.0 | 2.0 | 0.0 | 22.0 | 1.0 | 0.0 | | | 0.00 | 0.00 | 0 |
| 44223 | 18 pce | Plain, Doritos | 28 | 140 | 2 | 2.0 | 19.0 | 1.0 | 0.0 | 18.0 | 6.0 | 1.0 | | | | | 0 |
| 44130 | 11 ea | Plain, lightly salted, Michael Seasons | 28 | 138 | | 2.0 | 18.8 | | | | 4.9 | | | | | | |
| 44127 | 11 ea | Plain, unsalted, Michael Seasons | 28 | 138 | | 2.0 | 18.8 | | | | 4.9 | | | | | | |
| 44133 | 11 ea | Plain, white, lightly salted, Michael Seasons | 28 | 138 | | 2.0 | 18.8 | | | | 4.9 | | | | | | |
| 44255 | 6 pce | Plain, white, Santitas | 28 | 140 | 2 | 2.0 | 19.0 | 1.0 | 1.0 | 17.0 | 6.0 | 1.0 | | | | | 0 |
| 44055 | 16 pce | Ranch, avg | 28 | 137 | 2 | 2.1 | 18.1 | 1.1 | 0.3 | 16.7 | 6.7 | 1.3 | 3.9 | 0.9 | 0.04 | 0.88 | 0 |
| 44268 | 11 pce | Ranch, baked, lowfat, Tostitos | 28 | 120 | 2 | 2.0 | 21.0 | 1.0 | 0.0 | 20.0 | 3.0 | 0.5 | | | | | 0 |
| 44128 | 11 ea | Ranch, Michael Seasons | 28 | 138 | | 2.0 | 18.8 | | | | 4.9 | | | | | | |
| 44129 | 11 ea | Salsa, Michael Seasons | 28 | 138 | | 2.0 | 18.8 | | | | 4.9 | | | | | | |
| 44057 | 16 pce | Taco, avg | 28 | 134 | 2 | 2.2 | 17.7 | 1.5 | 0.3 | 15.9 | 6.8 | 1.3 | 4.0 | 0.9 | 0.04 | 0.90 | 1 |
| 44227 | 15 pce | Taco, Doritos | 28 | 140 | 2 | 2.0 | 18.0 | 1.0 | 1.0 | 16.0 | 7.0 | 1.5 | | | | | 0 |
| 44151 | 1 oz | Tortilla Bites, all flavors, American Grains | 28 | 109 | | 4.0 | 21.7 | | | | 1.0 | | | | | | |
| | | Trail Mix | | | | | | | | | | | | | | | |
| 44058 | 1/2 cup | Average | 75 | 346 | 9 | 10.4 | 33.7 | 3.8 | | | 22.0 | 4.2 | 9.4 | 7.2 | 0.05 | 7.18 | 0 |
| 44060 | 1/2 cup | Tropical, avg | 70 | 285 | 9 | 4.4 | 45.9 | 4.5 | | | 12.0 | 5.9 | 1.7 | 3.6 | 0.03 | 3.58 | 0 |
| 44085 | 1/2 cup | Unsalted, avg | 75 | 346 | 9 | 10.4 | 33.7 | 3.8 | | | 22.0 | 4.2 | 9.4 | 7.2 | 0.05 | 7.18 | 0 |
| 44059 | 1/2 cup | With Chocolate Chips, avg | 73 | 353 | 7 | 10.4 | 32.8 | 4.1 | | | 23.3 | 4.5 | 9.9 | 8.2 | 0.06 | 8.18 | 3 |
| 44086 | 1/2 cup | With Chocolate Chips, unsalted, avg | 73 | 353 | 7 | 10.4 | 32.8 | 4.1 | | | 23.3 | 4.5 | 9.9 | 8.2 | 0.06 | 8.18 | 3 |
| | | Wheat Snacks | | | | | | | | | | | | | | | |
| 44179 | 1/2 cup | Apple Cinnamon, Spicer's | 30 | 100 | | 4.0 | 14.0 | 6.0 | 5.3 | 2.7 | 3.3 | 0.0 | | | | | 0 |
| 44180 | 1/2 cup | Barbecue, Spicer's | 30 | 100 | | 4.0 | 12.0 | 6.0 | 0.0 | 6.0 | 4.0 | 0.0 | | | | | 0 |
| 44181 | 1/2 cup | Cheddar Cheese, Spicer's | 30 | 100 | | 4.0 | 12.0 | 6.0 | 0.0 | 6.0 | 4.0 | 0.0 | | | | | 0 |
| 44182 | 1/2 cup | Chocolate, Spicer's | 30 | 100 | | 4.0 | 14.0 | 6.0 | 5.3 | 2.7 | 3.3 | 0.0 | | | | | 0 |
| 44183 | 1/2 cup | Maple Walnut, Spicer's | 30 | 100 | | 4.0 | 14.0 | 6.0 | 5.3 | 2.7 | 3.3 | 0.0 | | | | | 0 |
| 44184 | 1/2 cup | Ranch, Spicer's | 30 | 100 | | 4.0 | 12.0 | 6.0 | 0.0 | 6.0 | 4.0 | 0.0 | | | | | 0 |
| 44185 | 1/2 cup | Sour Cream & Onion, Spicer's | 30 | 100 | | 4.0 | 12.0 | 6.0 | 0.0 | 6.0 | 4.0 | 0.0 | | | | | 0 |
| 44186 | 1/2 cup | Vanilla Malt, Spicer's | 30 | 100 | | 4.0 | 14.0 | 6.0 | 5.3 | 2.7 | 3.3 | 0.0 | | | | | 0 |
| | | **SOUPS AND STEWS** | | | | | | | | | | | | | | | |
| | | *CANNED SOUPS AND STEWS* | | | | | | | | | | | | | | | |
| | | Asparagus Cream Soup | | | | | | | | | | | | | | | |
| 50056 | 1/2 cup | Condensed, avg | 152 | 105 | 84 | 2.8 | 13.0 | 0.6 | 2.7 | 9.6 | 5.0 | 1.2 | 1.1 | 2.2 | 0.06 | 2.16 | 6 |
| 50057 | 1 cup | Prep, w/milk, avg | 248 | 161 | 86 | 6.3 | 16.4 | 0.7 | 8.4 | 7.3 | 8.2 | 3.3 | 2.1 | 2.2 | 0.10 | 2.13 | 22 |
| 50058 | 1 cup | Prep, w/water, avg | 244 | 85 | 92 | 2.3 | 10.7 | 0.5 | 2.3 | 7.9 | 4.1 | 1.0 | 1.0 | 1.9 | 0.05 | 1.78 | 5 |
| 50188 | 1 cup | Bacon Cream Soup, prep w/water, avg | 244 | 117 | 91 | 3.4 | 9.3 | 0.2 | | | 7.4 | 2.1 | 3.3 | 1.5 | | | 10 |
| | | Bean Soup | | | | | | | | | | | | | | | |
| 50648 | 1/2 cup | Bean & Frank, cond, avg | 132 | 187 | 68 | 10.0 | 22.2 | 6.1 | 7.9 | 8.2 | 7.0 | 2.1 | 2.7 | 1.7 | 0.36 | 1.25 | 12 |
| 50063 | 1 cup | Bean & Frank, prep w/water, avg | 250 | 188 | 83 | 10.0 | 22.0 | 5.7 | 7.9 | 8.4 | 7.0 | 2.1 | 2.7 | 1.7 | 0.35 | 1.25 | 12 |
| 50647 | 1/2 cup | Bean w/Bacon, cond, avg | 134 | 173 | 70 | 7.9 | 22.8 | 7.9 | 2.5 | 12.3 | 5.9 | 1.5 | 2.2 | 1.8 | 0.44 | 1.37 | 3 |
| 50510 | 1 cup | Bean w/Bacon, cond, Healthy Request | 256 | 300 | 70 | 14.0 | 52.0 | 14.0 | 12.0 | 26.0 | 4.0 | 2.0 | | | | | 10 |
| 50000 | 1 cup | Bean w/Bacon, prep w/water, avg | 253 | 172 | 84 | 7.9 | 22.8 | 8.6 | 2.5 | 11.7 | 5.9 | 1.5 | 2.2 | 1.8 | 0.43 | 1.37 | 3 |
| 50064 | 1 cup | Bean w/Ham, chunky, RTS, avg | 243 | 231 | 79 | 12.6 | 27.2 | 11.2 | 2.4 | 13.6 | 8.5 | 3.3 | 3.8 | 0.9 | 0.09 | 0.85 | 22 |
| 50411 | 1 cup | Bean w/Ham, RTS, Progresso | 238 | 160 | 83 | 10.0 | 25.0 | 8.0 | 2.0 | 15.0 | 2.0 | 0.5 | 1.0 | 0.5 | | | 10 |
| 50646 | 1/2 cup | Black Bean, cond, avg | 128 | 116 | 75 | 6.2 | 19.7 | 8.7 | 4.2 | 6.8 | 1.7 | 0.4 | 0.6 | 0.5 | 0.13 | 0.40 | 0 |
| 50050 | 1 cup | Black Bean, prep w/water, avg | 247 | 116 | 87 | 5.6 | 19.8 | 4.4 | 4.3 | 11.0 | 1.5 | 0.4 | 0.5 | 0.5 | 0.10 | 0.35 | 0 |
| 50425 | 1 cup | Black Bean, RTS, Progresso | 242 | 170 | 82 | 8.0 | 30.0 | 10.0 | 0.0 | 20.0 | 1.5 | 0.0 | 0.0 | 0.5 | | | 2 |
| 50325 | 1 cup | Black Bean, Taste Adventure | 242 | 139 | 85 | 6.4 | 27.7 | 6.4 | | | 0.5 | | | | | | |
| 50353 | 1 cup | Black Bean & Vegetable, fat free, Health Valley | 240 | 110 | 85 | 11.0 | 24.0 | 12.0 | 8.0 | 4.0 | 0.0 | 0.0 | 0.0 | 0.0 | 0.00 | 0.00 | 0 |
| 50438 | 1 cup | Black Bean w/Bacon, prep, Old El Paso | 245 | 160 | 83 | 11.0 | 26.0 | 7.0 | 2.0 | 17.0 | 1.5 | 0.5 | 0.5 | 0.5 | | | 5 |
| 50359 | 1 cup | Five Bean, fat free, Health Valley | 240 | 140 | 82 | 10.0 | 32.0 | 13.0 | 9.0 | 10.0 | 0.0 | 0.0 | 0.0 | 0.0 | 0.00 | 0.00 | 0 |
| 50433 | 1 cup | Macaroni & Bean, RTS, Progresso | 246 | 160 | | 7.0 | 23.0 | 6.0 | 1.0 | 16.0 | 4.0 | 1.0 | 1.0 | 1.5 | | | 2 |
| 50327 | 1 cup | Navy Bean, Taste Adventure | 234 | 155 | | 9.3 | 12.4 | 3.1 | | | 0.5 | | | | | | |
| 50640 | 8 oz | 16 Bean, Bascom's | 226 | 788 | 10 | 54.8 | 143.8 | | | | 3.4 | | | | | | |
| | | Beef Broth/Bouillon/Consomme | | | | | | | | | | | | | | | |
| 50470 | 1/2 cup | Condensed, Campbell's | 124 | 25 | 94 | 4.0 | 2.0 | 0.0 | 2.0 | 0.0 | 0.0 | 0.0 | 0.0 | 0.0 | 0.00 | 0.00 | 5 |
| 50220 | 1/2 cup | Double Strength, cond, Campbell's | 124 | 15 | 96 | 3.0 | 1.0 | 0.0 | 0.0 | 1.0 | 0.0 | 0.0 | 0.0 | 0.0 | 0.00 | 0.00 | 5 |
| 50183 | 1 cup | Low Sodium, avg | 240 | 38 | 96 | 4.8 | 1.0 | 0.0 | 1.0 | 0.0 | 1.4 | 0.4 | 0.6 | 0.3 | | | 0 |
| 50001 | 1 cup | RTS, avg | 240 | 17 | 98 | 2.7 | 0.1 | 0.0 | 0.1 | 0.0 | 0.5 | 0.3 | 0.2 | 0.0 | 0.00 | 0.02 | 0 |
| 50595 | 1 cup | RTS, Swanson | 235 | 20 | 97 | 2.0 | 1.0 | 0.0 | 1.0 | 0.0 | 1.0 | 0.5 | | | | | 0 |
| 50366 | 1 cup | Soup, fat free, Health Valley | 240 | 30 | 98 | 5.0 | 2.0 | 0.0 | 2.0 | 0.0 | 0.0 | 0.0 | 0.0 | 0.0 | 0.00 | 0.00 | 0 |
| 50355 | 1 cup | Soup, fat free, unsltd, Health Valley | 240 | 18 | 98 | 4.9 | 0.0 | 0.0 | 0.0 | 0.0 | 0.0 | 0.0 | 0.0 | 0.0 | 0.00 | 0.00 | 0 |
| 50663 | 1/2 cup | With Gelatin, cond, avg | 123 | 30 | 93 | 5.4 | 1.8 | 0.0 | 1.3 | 0.5 | 0.0 | 0.0 | 0.0 | 0.0 | 0.00 | 0.00 | 0 |
| 50098 | 1 cup | With Gelatin, prep w/water, avg | 241 | 29 | 96 | 5.4 | 1.8 | 0.0 | 1.3 | 0.5 | 0.0 | 0.0 | 0.0 | 0.0 | 0.00 | 0.00 | 0 |

| Code | Description | Vit A (IU) | Vit A (RE) | Retinol (RE) | Carotenoids (RE) | Beta Carotene (mcg) | Thiamin (mg) | Riboflavin (mg) | Niacin (NE) | Vit B6 (mg) | Vit B12 (mcg) | Folate (mcg) | Panto (mg) | Vit C (mg) | Vit D (mg) | Vit E (α TE) | Calcium (mg) | Copper (mg) | Iron (mg) | Magnes (mg) | Mang (mg) | Phos (mg) | Potassium (mg) | Selenium (mcg) | Sodium (mg) | Zinc (mg) |
|---|---|---|---|---|---|---|---|---|---|---|---|---|---|---|---|---|---|---|---|---|---|---|---|---|---|---|
| | | Vit A & Components | | | | | Vitamins | | | | | | | | | | Minerals | | | | | | | | | |
| 44054 | Nacho, light, avg | 122 | 13 | 0 | 13 | | 0.07 | 0.09 | 0.13 | 0.07 | 0.00 | 8.3 | 0.09 | 0.1 | 0.0 | | 51 | 0.0 | 0.5 | 31 | 0.1 | 102 | 87 | 2.1 | 321 | |
| 44004 | Nacho, Doritos | 96 | 11 | 0 | 11 | | 0.03 | 0.05 | 0.37 | 0.07 | 0.01 | 3.6 | 0.08 | 0.5 | 0.0 | | 38 | 0.0 | 0.4 | 21 | 0.1 | 63 | 56 | 1.7 | 184 | 0.31 |
| 44131 | Nacho, Michael Seasons | | | | | | | | | | | | | | | | | | | | | | | | 119 | |
| 44018 | Plain, avg | 57 | 6 | 0 | 6 | | 0.02 | 0.05 | 0.37 | 0.08 | 0.00 | 2.9 | 0.23 | 0.0 | 0.0 | | 45 | 0.0 | 0.4 | 26 | 0.1 | 59 | 57 | 1.9 | 153 | 0.44 |
| 44301 | Plain, baked, blue corn, Guiltless Gourmet | 0 | 0 | 0 | 0 | 0 | | | | | | | | 0.0 | | | 60 | | 0.7 | | | | | | 140 | |
| 44298 | Plain, baked, Guiltless Gourmet | 0 | 0 | 0 | 0 | 0 | | | | | | | | 0.0 | | | 60 | | 0.4 | | | | | | 160 | |
| 44266 | Plain, baked, Tostitos | | | | | | | | | | | | | | | | | | | | | | | | 140 | |
| 44267 | Plain, baked, unsalted, Tostitos | | | | | | | | | | | | | | | | | | | | | | | | 0 | |
| 44223 | Plain, Doritos | | | | | | | | | | | | | | | | | | | | | | | | 65 | |
| 44130 | Plain, lightly salted, Michael Seasons | | | | | | | | | | | | | | | | | | | | | | | | 114 | |
| 44127 | Plain, unsalted, Michael Seasons | | | | | | | | | | | | | | | | | | | | | | | | 10 | |
| 44133 | Plain, white, lightly salted, Michael Seasons | | | | | | | | | | | | | | | | | | | | | | | | 119 | |
| 44255 | Plain, white, Santitas | | | | | | | | | | | | | | | | | | | | | | | | 75 | |
| 44055 | Ranch, avg | 72 | 8 | 0 | 8 | | 0.03 | 0.07 | 0.41 | 0.06 | 0.00 | 4.8 | 0.17 | 0.3 | 0.0 | | 39 | 0.0 | 0.4 | 25 | 0.1 | 67 | 68 | 1.9 | 171 | 0.35 |
| 44268 | Ranch, baked, lowfat, Tostitos | | | | | | | | | | | | | | | | | | | | | | | | 170 | |
| 44128 | Ranch, Michael Seasons | | | | | | | | | | | | | | | | | | | | | | | | 40 | |
| 44129 | Salsa, Michael Seasons | | | | | | | | | | | | | | | | | | | | | | | | 79 | |
| 44057 | Taco, avg | 253 | 25 | 0 | 25 | | 0.07 | 0.06 | 0.56 | 0.08 | 0.00 | 5.9 | 0.08 | 0.3 | 0.0 | | 43 | 0.1 | 0.6 | 25 | 0.1 | 67 | 61 | 1.9 | 220 | 0.36 |
| 44227 | Taco, Doritos | | | | | | | | | | | | | | | | | | | | | | | | 200 | |
| 44151 | Tortilla Bites, all flavors, American Grains | | | | | | | | | | | | | | | | | | | | | | | | 198 | |
| | Trail Mix | | | | | | | | | | | | | | | | | | | | | | | | | |
| 44058 | Average | 14 | 2 | 0 | 2 | | 0.35 | 0.15 | 3.53 | 0.22 | 0.00 | 53.3 | 0.67 | 1.0 | | | 58 | 0.7 | 2.3 | 118 | 0.8 | 259 | 514 | | 172 | 2.41 |
| 44060 | Tropical, avg | 34 | 4 | 0 | 4 | | 0.31 | 0.08 | 1.04 | 0.23 | 0.00 | 29.4 | 0.85 | 5.3 | | | 40 | 0.4 | 1.8 | 67 | 0.7 | 130 | 496 | | 7 | 0.82 |
| 44085 | Unsalted, avg | 14 | 2 | 0 | 2 | | 0.35 | 0.15 | 3.53 | 0.22 | 0.00 | 53.3 | 0.67 | 1.0 | | | 58 | 0.7 | 2.3 | 118 | 0.8 | 259 | 514 | | 8 | 2.41 |
| 44059 | With Chocolate Chips, avg | 32 | 4 | | | | 0.30 | 0.16 | 3.22 | 0.19 | 0.00 | 47.5 | 0.70 | 0.9 | | | 80 | 0.6 | 2.5 | 118 | 0.8 | 283 | 473 | | 88 | 2.29 |
| 44086 | With Chocolate Chips, unsalted, avg | 32 | 4 | | | | 0.30 | 0.16 | 3.22 | 0.19 | 0.00 | 47.5 | 0.70 | 0.9 | | | 80 | 0.6 | 2.5 | 118 | 0.8 | 283 | 473 | | 20 | 2.29 |
| | Wheat Snacks | | | | | | | | | | | | | | | | | | | | | | | | | |
| 44179 | Apple Cinnamon, Spicer's | 0 | 0 | 0 | 0 | 0 | | | | | | | | 0.0 | | | 0 | | 1.2 | | | | | | 70 | |
| 44180 | Barbecue, Spicer's | 0 | 0 | 0 | 0 | 0 | | | | | | | | 0.0 | | | 40 | | 1.4 | | | | | | 180 | |
| 44181 | Cheddar Cheese, Spicer's | 0 | 0 | 0 | 0 | 0 | | | | | | | | 0.0 | | | 40 | | 1.4 | | | | | | 180 | |
| 44182 | Chocolate, Spicer's | 0 | 0 | 0 | 0 | 0 | | | | | | | | 0.0 | | | 27 | | 1.2 | | | | | | 80 | |
| 44183 | Maple Walnut, Spicer's | 0 | 0 | 0 | 0 | 0 | | | | | | | | 0.0 | | | 0 | | 1.2 | | | | | | 70 | |
| 44184 | Ranch, Spicer's | 0 | 0 | 0 | 0 | 0 | | | | | | | | 0.0 | | | 40 | | 1.4 | | | | | | 180 | |
| 44185 | Sour Cream & Onion, Spicer's | 0 | 0 | 0 | 0 | 0 | | | | | | | | 0.0 | | | 40 | | 1.4 | | | | | | 180 | |
| 44186 | Vanilla Malt, Spicer's | 0 | 0 | 0 | 0 | 0 | | | | | | | | 0.0 | | | 0 | | 1.2 | | | | | | 70 | |
| | **SOUPS AND STEWS** | | | | | | | | | | | | | | | | | | | | | | | | | |
| | *CANNED SOUPS AND STEWS* | | | | | | | | | | | | | | | | | | | | | | | | | |
| | Asparagus Cream Soup | | | | | | | | | | | | | | | | | | | | | | | | | |
| 50056 | Condensed, avg | 540 | 55 | | | | 0.07 | 0.09 | 0.94 | 0.02 | 0.05 | 28.9 | 0.17 | 3.3 | | | 35 | 0.2 | 1.0 | 5 | 0.5 | 47 | 210 | 2.9 | 1189 | 1.06 |
| 50057 | Prep, w/milk, avg | 600 | 34 | 40 | 45 | | 0.10 | 0.28 | 0.88 | 0.06 | 0.50 | 29.8 | 0.52 | 4.0 | | | 174 | 0.1 | 0.9 | 20 | 0.4 | 154 | 360 | | 1042 | 0.93 |
| 50058 | Prep, w/water, avg | 444 | 44 | | | | 0.05 | 0.08 | 0.78 | 0.01 | 0.05 | 22.0 | 0.12 | 2.7 | | | 29 | 0.1 | 0.8 | 5 | 0.4 | 39 | 173 | | 981 | 0.88 |
| 50188 | Bacon Cream Soup, prep w/water, avg | 561 | 56 | 0 | 56 | | 0.03 | 0.06 | 0.82 | 0.02 | 0.10 | 1.7 | | 0.2 | | | 34 | 0.1 | 0.6 | 2 | | 37 | 88 | | 986 | 0.63 |
| | Bean Soup | | | | | | | | | | | | | | | | | | | | | | | | | |
| 50648 | Bean & Frank, cond, avg | 874 | 87 | | | | 0.11 | 0.06 | 1.03 | 0.13 | 0.03 | 31.7 | 0.09 | 0.9 | 0.0 | | 87 | 0.4 | 2.3 | 49 | 0.8 | 166 | 479 | 9.1 | 1097 | 1.19 |
| 50063 | Bean & Frank, prep w/water, avg | 870 | 88 | | | | 0.11 | 0.06 | 1.02 | 0.13 | 0.07 | 30.0 | 0.10 | 1.0 | 0.0 | | 88 | 0.4 | 2.3 | 48 | 0.8 | 165 | 478 | 8.5 | 1092 | 1.18 |
| 50647 | Bean w/Bacon, cond, avg | 887 | 88 | | | | 0.09 | 0.03 | 0.56 | 0.04 | 0.04 | 31.8 | 0.09 | 1.6 | 0.0 | | 80 | 0.4 | 2.1 | 44 | 0.7 | 131 | 402 | 8.6 | 950 | 1.03 |
| 50510 | Bean w/Bacon, cond, Healthy Request | 1000 | 200 | | | | | | | | | | | 0.0 | | | 120 | | 3.6 | | | | | | 960 | |
| 50000 | Bean w/Bacon, prep w/water, avg | 888 | 89 | 0 | 89 | | 0.09 | 0.03 | 0.57 | 0.04 | 0.05 | 31.9 | 0.10 | 1.5 | 0.0 | | 81 | 0.4 | 2.0 | 46 | 0.7 | 132 | 402 | 8.1 | 951 | 1.03 |
| 50064 | Bean w/Ham, chunky, RTS, avg | 3951 | 396 | | | | 0.15 | 0.15 | 1.70 | 0.12 | 0.07 | 29.2 | 0.10 | 4.4 | 0.0 | | 78 | 0.4 | 3.2 | 46 | 0.7 | 143 | 425 | 16.8 | 972 | 1.07 |
| 50411 | Bean w/Ham, RTS, Progresso | 1500 | 300 | | | | | | | | | | | 0.0 | | | 80 | | 2.7 | | | | | | 870 | |
| 50646 | Black Bean, cond, avg | 570 | 58 | 0 | 58 | | 0.05 | 0.05 | 0.52 | 0.09 | 0.00 | 25.6 | 0.20 | 0.3 | 0.0 | | 45 | 0.4 | 1.9 | 42 | 0.6 | 96 | 320 | | 1242 | 1.41 |
| 50050 | Black Bean, prep w/water, avg | 506 | 49 | 0 | 49 | | 0.08 | 0.05 | 0.53 | 0.09 | 0.02 | 24.7 | 0.20 | 0.7 | 0.0 | | 44 | 0.4 | 2.1 | 42 | 0.6 | 106 | 274 | 1.0 | 1198 | 1.41 |
| 50425 | Black Bean, RTS, Progresso | 200 | 40 | | | | | | | | | | | 0.0 | | | 60 | | 3.6 | | | | | | 730 | |
| 50325 | Black Bean, Taste Adventure | | | | | | | | | | | | | | | | | | | | | | 650 | | 565 | |
| 50353 | Black Bean & Vegetable, fat free, Health Valley | 10000 | 2000 | | | | 0.34 | 0.11 | 1.35 | 0.22 | | 135.0 | | 9.0 | | | 40 | | 3.6 | | | | 676 | | 280 | |
| 50438 | Black Bean w/Bacon, prep, Old El Paso | 0 | 0 | 0 | 0 | 0 | | | | | | | | 0.0 | | | 60 | | 7.2 | | | | | | 960 | |
| 50359 | Five Bean, fat free, Health Valley | 10000 | 2000 | | | | | | | | | | | 12.0 | | | 80 | | 5.4 | | | | | | 250 | |
| 50433 | Macaroni & Bean, RTS, Progresso | 200 | 40 | | | | | | | | | | | 0.0 | | | 40 | | 1.8 | | | | | | 800 | |
| 50327 | Navy Bean, Taste Adventure | | | | | | | | | | | | | | | | | | | | | | 763 | | 350 | |
| 50640 | 16 Bean, Bascom's | | | | | | 3.60 | 0.68 | 8.22 | | | | | | | | 137 | | 18.5 | | | | | | 34 | |
| | Beef Broth/Bouillon/Consomme | | | | | | | | | | | | | | | | | | | | | | | | | |
| 50470 | Condensed, Campbell's | 0 | 0 | 0 | 0 | 0 | | | | | | | | 0.0 | | | 0 | | 0.4 | | | | | | 820 | |
| 50220 | Double Strength, cond, Campbell's | 0 | 0 | 0 | 0 | 0 | 0.00 | 0.02 | 0.93 | 0.01 | 0.09 | 2.5 | | 0.0 | 0.0 | 0.0 | 0 | 0.0 | 0.4 | 2 | | 16 | 67 | | 900 | 0.00 |
| 50183 | Low Sodium, avg | 0 | 0 | 0 | 0 | 0 | 0.00 | 0.07 | 3.29 | 0.02 | 0.24 | 4.8 | | 0.0 | 0.0 | | 10 | 0.1 | 0.5 | 2 | | 72 | 206 | | 72 | 0.24 |
| 50001 | RTS, avg | 0 | 0 | 0 | 0 | 0 | 0.00 | 0.05 | 1.87 | 0.02 | 0.17 | 4.8 | 0.05 | 0.0 | 0.0 | 0.0 | 14 | 0.0 | 0.4 | 5 | 0.0 | 31 | 130 | 1.7 | 782 | 0.00 |
| 50595 | RTS, Swanson | 0 | 0 | 0 | 0 | 0 | | | | | | | | 0.0 | | | 0 | | 0.4 | | | | | | 820 | |
| 50366 | Soup, fat free, Health Valley | 0 | 0 | 0 | 0 | 0 | | | 0.98 | | | | | 4.8 | | | 0 | | 0.0 | | | | 196 | | 160 | |
| 50355 | Soup, fat free, unsltd, Health Valley | | | | | | | | 0.98 | | | | | | | | | | | | | | 196 | | 74 | |
| 50663 | With Gelatin, cond, avg | 0 | 0 | 0 | 0 | 0 | 0.02 | 0.03 | 0.77 | 0.02 | 0.00 | 3.0 | 0.05 | 0.9 | 0.0 | | 9 | 0.2 | 0.5 | 0 | 0.4 | 32 | 154 | 2.5 | 640 | 0.37 |
| 50098 | With Gelatin, prep w/water, avg | 0 | 0 | 0 | 0 | 0 | 0.02 | 0.03 | 0.77 | 0.02 | 0.00 | 2.9 | 0.05 | 1.0 | 0.0 | | 10 | 0.2 | 0.5 | 0 | 0.4 | 31 | 154 | | 636 | 0.37 |

| Code | Amount | Description | Basic Components | | | | | | | | | Additional Fats | | | | | | Vit A & Components | | | | | Vitamins | | | | | | | | | | Minerals | | | | | | | | | |
|---|---|---|---|---|---|---|---|---|---|---|---|---|---|---|---|---|---|---|---|---|---|---|---|---|---|---|---|---|---|---|---|---|---|---|---|---|---|---|---|---|---|---|
| | | | Weight (g) | Calories | % Water | Protein (g) | Carbs (g) | Fiber (g) | Sugar (g) | Other Carbs (g) | Fat (g) | Sat Fat (g) | Mono Fat (g) | Poly Fat (g) | Omega 3 (g) | Omega 6 (g) | Choles (mg) | Vit A (IU) | Vit A (RE) | Retinol (RE) | Carotenoids (RE) | Beta Carotene (mcg) | Thiamin (mg) | Riboflavin (mg) | Niacin (NE) | Vit B6 (mg) | Vit B12 (mcg) | Folate (mcg) | Panto (mg) | Vit C (mg) | Vit D (mg) | Vit E (α TE) | Calcium (mg) | Copper (mg) | Iron (mg) | Magnes (mg) | Mang (mg) | Phos (mg) | Potassium (mg) | Selenium (mcg) | Sodium (mg) | Zinc (mg) |
| | | Beef Soup | | | | | | | | | | | | | | | | | | | | | | | | | | | | | | | | | | | | | | | | |
| 50275 | 8 oz | Barley, prep w/water, Corn Products Company | 227 | 67 | 92 | 4.0 | 10.7 | | | | 1.3 | | | | | | | | | | | | | | | | | | | | | | | | 1.0 | | | | 120 | | 895 | |
| 50412 | 1 cup | Barley, RTS, Progresso | 242 | 130 | 88 | 10.0 | 13.0 | 3.0 | 0.0 | 10.0 | 4.0 | 1.5 | 1.5 | 0.0 | 0.00 | 0.00 | 25 | 1500 | 300 | | | | | | | | | | | 0.0 | | | 40 | | 1.8 | | | | | | 780 | |
| 50452 | 1/2 cup | Barley w/Vegetables, cond, Campbell's | 126 | 80 | 83 | 5.0 | 11.0 | 2.0 | 1.0 | 8.0 | 2.0 | 1.0 | | | | | 15 | 1250 | 250 | | | | | | | | | | | 1.2 | | | 20 | | 0.7 | | | | | | 920 | |
| 50066 | 1 cup | Chunky, RTS, avg | 240 | 170 | 83 | 11.7 | 19.6 | 1.4 | 2.2 | 16.0 | 5.1 | 2.5 | 2.1 | 0.2 | 0.02 | 0.17 | 14 | 2611 | 262 | | | | 0.06 | 0.15 | 2.71 | 0.13 | 0.62 | 13.4 | 0.43 | 7.0 | 0.0 | | 31 | 0.2 | 2.3 | 5 | 0.2 | 120 | 336 | 6.0 | 866 | 2.64 |
| 50685 | 1/2 cup | Mushroom, cond, avg | 126 | 77 | 86 | 5.8 | 6.6 | 0.0 | 0.5 | 6.0 | 3.0 | 1.5 | 1.3 | 0.1 | 0.01 | 0.09 | 6 | 0 | 0 | 0 | 0 | 0 | 0.03 | 0.08 | 1.13 | 0.05 | 0.20 | 8.8 | 0.24 | 0.0 | 0.0 | | 5 | 0.3 | 0.9 | 9 | 0.4 | 37 | 159 | | 974 | 1.39 |
| 50453 | 1/2 cup | Mushroom, cond, Campbell's | 126 | 70 | 87 | 5.0 | 6.0 | 1.0 | 1.0 | 4.0 | 3.0 | 1.0 | | | | | 10 | 0 | 0 | 0 | 0 | 0 | | | | | | | | 0.0 | | | 0 | | 0.7 | | | | | | 1000 | |
| 50708 | 1 cup | Mushroom, low sod, avg | 251 | 173 | 83 | 10.8 | 18.8 | 0.5 | | | 5.8 | 2.7 | 2.2 | 0.2 | | | 15 | 4937 | 494 | 0 | 494 | | 0.10 | 0.28 | 2.84 | 0.15 | 0.65 | 17.6 | | 7.5 | | | 33 | 0.3 | 2.4 | 5 | | 125 | 351 | | 63 | 2.76 |
| 50198 | 1 cup | Mushroom, prep w/water, avg | 244 | 73 | 93 | 5.8 | 6.3 | 0.2 | 0.5 | 5.6 | 3.0 | 1.5 | 1.2 | 0.1 | 0.02 | 0.10 | 7 | 0 | 0 | 0 | 0 | 0 | 0.04 | 0.06 | 0.95 | 0.05 | 0.20 | 9.8 | 0.22 | 4.6 | | | 5 | 0.2 | 0.9 | 10 | 0.5 | 34 | 154 | | 942 | 1.46 |
| 50649 | 1/2 cup | Noodle, cond, avg | 126 | 84 | 84 | 4.9 | 9.0 | 0.8 | 0.6 | 7.6 | 3.1 | 1.1 | 1.2 | 0.5 | 0.06 | 0.42 | 5 | 633 | 63 | | | | 0.07 | 0.06 | 1.07 | 0.04 | 0.20 | 18.9 | 0.20 | 0.4 | 0.0 | | 15 | 0.1 | 1.1 | 6 | 0.3 | 47 | 100 | 7.4 | 956 | 1.55 |
| 50003 | 1 cup | Noodle, prep w/water, avg | 244 | 83 | 92 | 4.8 | 9.0 | 0.7 | 0.7 | 7.6 | 3.1 | 1.1 | 1.2 | 0.5 | 0.05 | 0.41 | 5 | 630 | 63 | | | | 0.07 | 0.06 | 1.07 | 0.04 | 0.20 | 19.5 | 0.20 | 0.2 | 0.0 | | 15 | 0.1 | 1.1 | 5 | 0.3 | 46 | 100 | 7.3 | 952 | 1.54 |
| 50413 | 1 cup | Noodle, RTS, Progresso | 241 | 140 | 86 | 13.0 | 15.0 | 1.0 | 2.0 | 12.0 | 3.5 | 1.5 | 1.5 | 0.0 | 0.00 | 0.00 | 30 | 750 | 150 | | | | | | | | | | | 0.0 | | | 20 | | 1.8 | | | | | | 950 | |
| 50442 | 1 cup | Old El Paso | 240 | 120 | 88 | 10.0 | 14.0 | 0.0 | 2.0 | 12.0 | 2.5 | 1.5 | 0.5 | 0.5 | | | 25 | 2000 | 400 | | | | | | | | | | | 9.0 | | | 40 | | 1.4 | | | | | | 690 | |
| 50529 | 1 cup | Pasta, chunky, RTS, Campbell's | 245 | 150 | 85 | 13.0 | 18.0 | 2.0 | 5.0 | 11.0 | 3.0 | 1.0 | | | | | 20 | 3000 | 600 | | | | | | | | | | | 1.2 | | | 40 | | 1.8 | | | | | | 970 | |
| 50385 | 1 cup | Pasta w/Vegetables, Progresso | 239 | 120 | 89 | 11.0 | 10.0 | 3.0 | 0.5 | 6.5 | 3.5 | 1.5 | 1.5 | 0.0 | 0.00 | 0.00 | 20 | 1250 | 250 | | | | | | | | | | | 2.4 | | | 20 | | 1.8 | | | | | | 830 | |
| 50550 | 1 cup | Pepper Steak, chunky, RTS, Campbell's | 245 | 140 | 86 | 11.0 | 18.0 | 3.0 | 4.0 | 11.0 | 2.5 | 1.0 | | | | | 20 | 2500 | 500 | | | | | | | | | | | 4.8 | | | 40 | | 1.8 | | | | | | 830 | |
| 50552 | 1 cup | Steak 'N Potato, chunky, RTS, Campbell's | 245 | 160 | 84 | 12.0 | 20.0 | 3.0 | 1.0 | 16.0 | 4.0 | 1.0 | | | | | 20 | 0 | 0 | 0 | 0 | 0 | | | | | | | | 3.6 | | | 20 | | 1.4 | | | | | | 890 | |
| 50206 | 1 cup | Stroganoff, chunky, avg | 240 | 235 | 80 | 12.2 | 21.6 | 1.4 | | | 11.7 | 5.1 | 4.2 | 2.4 | | | 50 | 1968 | 197 | 0 | 197 | | 0.10 | 0.22 | 0.24 | 0.14 | 0.62 | 14.4 | | 0.0 | | | 48 | 0.2 | 2.1 | 5 | | 120 | 336 | | 1044 | 2.64 |
| 50553 | 8 oz | Stroganoff, chunky, RTS, Campbell's | 227 | 231 | 79 | 11.9 | 20.8 | 3.0 | 3.0 | 14.9 | 11.9 | 4.5 | | | | | 33 | 1861 | 372 | | | | | | | | | | | 0.0 | | | 60 | | 2.0 | | | | | | 878 | |
| 50683 | 1/2 cup | Vegetable Beef, cond, avg | 126 | 79 | 84 | 5.6 | 10.2 | 2.0 | 1.0 | 7.2 | 1.9 | 0.9 | 0.8 | 0.1 | 0.01 | 0.10 | 5 | 1900 | 190 | | | | 0.04 | 0.05 | 1.04 | 0.08 | 0.31 | 10.6 | 0.35 | 2.4 | 0.0 | 0.0 | 16 | 0.2 | 1.1 | 6 | 0.3 | 40 | 174 | 2.8 | 795 | 1.55 |
| 50014 | 1 cup | Vegetable Beef, prep w/water, avg | 244 | 78 | 92 | 5.6 | 10.2 | 0.5 | 1.1 | 8.6 | 1.9 | 0.9 | 0.8 | 0.1 | 0.02 | 0.10 | 5 | 1891 | 190 | 0 | 190 | | 0.04 | 0.05 | 1.03 | 0.08 | 0.32 | 10.5 | 0.34 | 2.4 | 0.0 | | 17 | 0.2 | 1.1 | 5 | 0.3 | 41 | 173 | 4.4 | 791 | 1.54 |
| 50530 | 1 cup | Vegetable Beef, RTS, chunky, Campbell's | 245 | 160 | 83 | 13.0 | 18.0 | 3.0 | 4.0 | 11.0 | 4.0 | 1.0 | | | | | 25 | 7500 | 1500 | | | | | | | | | | | 1.2 | | | 40 | | 1.8 | | | | | | 900 | |
| 50561 | 1 cup | Vegetable Beef, RTS, Healthy Request | 245 | 140 | 85 | 9.0 | 20.0 | 3.0 | 4.0 | 13.0 | 2.5 | 1.0 | | | | | 20 | 5000 | 1000 | | | | | | | | | | | 2.4 | | | 40 | | 1.1 | | | | | | 480 | |
| 50047 | 1 cup | Vegetable Stew, avg | 245 | 194 | 82 | 14.2 | 17.4 | 2.5 | 6.4 | 8.6 | 7.6 | 2.5 | 3.1 | 0.4 | | 0.00 | 34 | 2377 | 262 | 0 | 262 | | 0.07 | 0.12 | 2.45 | 0.20 | 1.59 | 31.1 | 0.29 | 7.4 | 0.1 | | 29 | 0.1 | 2.2 | 39 | 0.2 | 110 | 426 | 13.5 | 1007 | 4.24 |
| 50210 | 1 cup | Birds Nest Soup, avg | 244 | 110 | 89 | 14.0 | 6.1 | 0.0 | | | 2.7 | 0.8 | 1.1 | 0.5 | | | 27 | 7 | 2 | 2 | 0 | 0 | 0.10 | 0.11 | 5.12 | 0.17 | 0.31 | 5.3 | | 0.0 | | | 15 | 0.1 | 0.8 | 10 | | 124 | 244 | | 1508 | 0.92 |
| 50180 | 1 cup | Borscht Soup, avg | 245 | 74 | 93 | 3.1 | 6.5 | 1.7 | | | 4.1 | 2.5 | 1.2 | 0.2 | | | 7 | 170 | 38 | 31 | 7 | | 0.04 | 0.08 | 1.32 | 0.07 | 0.15 | 34.8 | | 11.0 | | | 47 | 0.0 | 0.7 | 27 | | 59 | 314 | | 497 | 0.23 |
| 50204 | 1 cup | Bouillabaisse Soup, avg | 227 | 241 | 78 | 33.7 | 4.8 | 0.6 | | | 9.0 | 2.0 | 4.0 | 1.5 | | | 91 | 474 | 89 | 62 | 27 | | 0.24 | 0.19 | 5.05 | 0.38 | 10.42 | 28.0 | | 11.9 | | | 84 | 0.4 | 4.0 | 73 | | 340 | 733 | | 418 | 1.86 |
| | | Broccoli Soup | | | | | | | | | | | | | | | | | | | | | | | | | | | | | | | | | | | | | | | | |
| 50455 | 1/2 cup | Cheese, cond, Campbell's | 124 | 110 | 84 | 3.0 | 9.0 | 2.0 | 2.0 | 5.0 | 7.0 | 3.0 | | | | | 10 | 1500 | 300 | | | | | | | | | | | 1.2 | | | 40 | | 0.4 | | | | | | 860 | |
| 50259 | 1 cup | Cheese, prep, Corn Products Company | 248 | 365 | 78 | 8.8 | 13.1 | | | | 30.6 | | | | | | | | | | | | | 0.50 | | | | | | | | | 219 | | | | | | 204 | | 1225 | |
| 50531 | 1 cup | Chicken & Cheese, RTS, Campbell's | 245 | 200 | 85 | 9.0 | 14.0 | 1.0 | 1.0 | 12.0 | 12.0 | 5.0 | | | | | 25 | 1000 | 200 | | | | | | | | | | | 0.0 | | | 40 | | 0.4 | | | | | | 1120 | |
| 50189 | 1 cup | Cream, avg | 237 | 235 | 81 | 8.7 | 15.8 | 1.8 | | | 15.9 | 6.0 | 5.9 | 3.4 | | | 24 | 1358 | 208 | 117 | 91 | | 0.10 | 0.39 | 0.68 | 0.15 | 0.61 | 37.2 | | 43.3 | | | 246 | 0.1 | 0.7 | 38 | | 209 | 427 | | 787 | 0.90 |
| 50472 | 1/2 cup | Cream, cond, Campbell's | 124 | 100 | 85 | 2.0 | 9.0 | 1.0 | 2.0 | 6.0 | 6.0 | 2.5 | | | | | 5 | 300 | 60 | | | | | | | | | | | 2.4 | | | 20 | | 0.4 | | | | | | 770 | |
| 50514 | 1/2 cup | Cream, cond, Healthy Request | 124 | 70 | 88 | 2.0 | 9.0 | 1.0 | 3.0 | 5.0 | 2.0 | 1.0 | | | | | 5 | 500 | 100 | | | | | | | | | | | 3.6 | | | 20 | | 0.0 | | | | | | 480 | |
| 50264 | 1 cup | Cream, prep w/milk, Corn Products Company | 248 | 175 | 86 | 11.7 | 10.2 | | | | 10.2 | | | | | | | 146 | 29 | | | | 0.22 | 0.25 | | | | | | | | | 146 | | 3.9 | | | | 379 | | 744 | |
| 50402 | 1 cup | Cream, RTS, Progresso | 244 | 88 | 92 | 2.4 | 13.3 | 2.4 | | | 2.8 | 0.7 | 0.9 | 0.6 | 0.13 | 0.45 | 5 | 293 | 32 | | | | 0.03 | 0.06 | 0.32 | 0.07 | 0.00 | 29.3 | 0.27 | 5.9 | | | 41 | 0.0 | 1.2 | 15 | 0.1 | 39 | 161 | | 578 | 0.27 |
| 50386 | 1 cup | Pasta, RTS, Progresso | 243 | 70 | | 3.0 | 14.0 | 3.0 | 2.0 | 9.0 | 1.0 | 0.0 | 0.0 | 0.5 | | | 2 | 3000 | 600 | | | | | | | | | | | 6.0 | | | 40 | | 1.4 | | | | | | 720 | |
| 50048 | 1 cup | Brunswick Stew, avg | 250 | 174 | 83 | 15.6 | 20.7 | 3.2 | 4.2 | 13.3 | 3.9 | 1.0 | 1.3 | 1.0 | 0.08 | 0.94 | 34 | 465 | 51 | 6 | 44 | | 0.12 | 0.16 | 5.77 | 0.37 | 0.18 | 43.7 | 1.03 | 17.5 | 0.1 | | 37 | 0.2 | 1.7 | 46 | 0.5 | 168 | 538 | 12.1 | 451 | 1.37 |
| | | Celery Soup | | | | | | | | | | | | | | | | | | | | | | | | | | | | | | | | | | | | | | | | |
| 50650 | 1/2 cup | Cream of Celery, cond, avg | 126 | 91 | 85 | 1.7 | 8.9 | 0.8 | 0.7 | 7.4 | 5.6 | 1.4 | 1.3 | 2.5 | 0.08 | 2.44 | 14 | 307 | 30 | | | | 0.03 | 0.05 | 0.33 | 0.01 | 0.05 | 2.4 | 1.16 | 0.3 | 0.1 | | 40 | 0.1 | 0.6 | 6 | 0.3 | 38 | 123 | 2.3 | 954 | 0.15 |
| 50515 | 1/2 cup | Cream of Celery, cond, Healthy Request | 124 | 70 | 86 | 2.0 | 11.0 | 1.0 | 3.0 | 7.0 | 2.0 | 0.5 | | | | | 5 | 0 | 0 | 0 | 0 | 0 | | | | | | | | 0.0 | | | 150 | | 0.0 | | | | | | 480 | |
| 50015 | 1 cup | Cream of Celery, prep w/milk, avg | 248 | 164 | 86 | 5.7 | 14.5 | 0.7 | 6.7 | 7.1 | 9.7 | 3.9 | 2.5 | 2.7 | 0.12 | 2.53 | 32 | 461 | 67 | 37 | 30 | | 0.07 | 0.25 | 0.44 | 0.06 | 0.50 | 8.4 | 1.51 | 1.5 | 1.4 | | 186 | 0.2 | 0.7 | 22 | 0.3 | 151 | 310 | 4.7 | 1009 | 0.20 |
| 50016 | 1 cup | Cream of Celery, prep w/water, avg | 244 | 90 | 92 | 1.7 | 8.8 | 0.7 | 0.7 | 7.4 | 5.6 | 1.4 | 1.3 | 2.5 | 0.07 | 2.44 | 15 | 307 | 32 | | | | 0.03 | 0.05 | 0.33 | 0.01 | 0.24 | 2.4 | 1.12 | 0.2 | 0.1 | | 39 | 0.1 | 0.6 | 7 | 0.3 | 37 | 122 | 2.2 | 949 | 0.15 |
| | | Cheese Soup | | | | | | | | | | | | | | | | | | | | | | | | | | | | | | | | | | | | | | | | |
| 50651 | 1/2 cup | Condensed, avg | 128 | 155 | 77 | 5.4 | 10.5 | 1.0 | 1.3 | 8.2 | 10.4 | 6.6 | 3.0 | 0.3 | 0.12 | 0.18 | 29 | 1084 | 109 | | | | 0.02 | 0.13 | 0.40 | 0.03 | 0.00 | 3.8 | 0.09 | 0.0 | 0.1 | | 142 | 0.1 | 0.7 | 4 | 0.3 | 136 | 154 | 4.6 | 956 | 0.64 |
| 50495 | 1/2 cup | Nacho, cond, Campbell's | 124 | 140 | 78 | 5.0 | 11.0 | 2.0 | 2.0 | 7.0 | 8.0 | 4.0 | | | | | 15 | 1250 | 250 | | | | | | | | | | | 1.2 | | | 100 | | 0.4 | | | | | | 810 | |
| 50071 | 1 cup | Prepared, w/milk, avg | 251 | 231 | 82 | 9.5 | 16.2 | 1.0 | 7.5 | 7.7 | 14.6 | 9.1 | 4.1 | 0.5 | 0.18 | 0.28 | 48 | 1242 | 148 | 43 | 105 | | 0.06 | 0.33 | 0.50 | 0.08 | 0.43 | 10.0 | 0.48 | 1.3 | 1.3 | | 289 | 0.1 | 0.8 | 20 | 0.3 | 251 | 341 | 7.0 | 1019 | 0.69 |
| 50072 | 1 cup | Prepared, w/water, avg | 247 | 156 | 88 | 5.4 | 10.5 | 1.0 | 1.4 | 8.2 | 10.5 | 6.7 | 3.0 | 0.3 | 0.12 | 0.17 | 30 | 1087 | 109 | | | | 0.02 | 0.14 | 0.40 | 0.02 | 0.00 | 4.9 | 0.10 | 0.0 | 0.1 | | 141 | 0.1 | 0.7 | 5 | 0.3 | 136 | 153 | 4.4 | 958 | 0.64 |
| | | Chicken Broth/Bouillon/Consomme | | | | | | | | | | | | | | | | | | | | | | | | | | | | | | | | | | | | | | | | |
| 50653 | 1/2 cup | Condensed, avg | 126 | 39 | 92 | 5.6 | 0.9 | 0.0 | 0.3 | 0.6 | 1.3 | 0.4 | 0.6 | 0.3 | 0.01 | 0.25 | 1 | 0 | 0 | 0 | 0 | 0 | 0.01 | 0.06 | 2.81 | 0.03 | 0.25 | 5.0 | 0.05 | 0.0 | 0.0 | | 8 | 0.1 | 0.5 | 3 | 0.3 | 76 | 214 | 2.9 | 789 | 0.25 |
| 50364 | 1 cup | Fat Free, Health Valley | 240 | 30 | 97 | 6.0 | 0.0 | 0.0 | 0.0 | 0.0 | 0.0 | 0.0 | 0.0 | 0.0 | 0.00 | 0.00 | 0 | 0 | 0 | 0 | 0 | 0 | | 0.03 | 2.44 | | | | | 1.2 | | | 20 | | 1.8 | | | | 146 | | 170 | |
| 50004 | 1 cup | Prepared, w/water, avg | 244 | 39 | 96 | 4.9 | 0.9 | 0.0 | 0.3 | 0.6 | 1.4 | 0.4 | 0.6 | 0.3 | 0.02 | 0.24 | 0 | 0 | 0 | 0 | 0 | 0 | 0.01 | 0.07 | 3.34 | 0.02 | 0.24 | 4.9 | 0.05 | 0.0 | 0.0 | | 10 | 0.1 | 0.5 | 2 | 0.2 | 73 | 210 | 0.0 | 776 | 0.25 |
| 50555 | 1 cup | RTS, Healthy Request | 245 | 20 | 96 | 3.0 | 1.0 | 0.0 | 1.0 | 0.0 | 0.0 | 0.0 | 0.0 | 0.0 | 0.00 | 0.00 | 0 | 0 | 0 | 0 | 0 | 0 | | | | | | | | 9.0 | | | 0 | | 0.0 | | | | | | 450 | |
| 50583 | 1 cup | RTS, low sod, Campbell's | 188 | 31 | 96 | 3.1 | 1.5 | 0.0 | 0.8 | 0.8 | 1.5 | 0.8 | | | | | 4 | 0 | 0 | 0 | 0 | 0 | | | | | | | | 0.0 | | | 15 | | 0.0 | | | | | | 107 | |
| 50416 | 1 cup | RTS, Progresso | 233 | 20 | 97 | 2.0 | 1.0 | 0.0 | | | 0.5 | | | | | | 5 | 0 | 0 | 0 | 0 | 0 | | | | | | | | 0.0 | | | 0 | | 0.0 | | | | | | 860 | |
| 50280 | 8 oz | Soup, prep w/water, Corn Products Company | 227 | 20 | 98 | 1.3 | 1.3 | | | | | | | | | | | | | | | | | | 0.53 | | | | | | | | | | | | | | 93 | | 935 | |
| | | Chicken Soup | | | | | | | | | | | | | | | | | | | | | | | | | | | | | | | | | | | | | | | | |
| 50415 | 1 cup | Barley, RTS, Progresso | 241 | 110 | 88 | 10.0 | 14.0 | 3.0 | 0.0 | 11.0 | 2.5 | 0.5 | 1.0 | 0.5 | | | 15 | 1750 | 350 | | | | | | | | | | | 0.0 | | | 20 | | 1.4 | | | | | | 720 | |
| 50483 | 1/2 cup | Broth w/Noodles, cond, Campbell's | 126 | 80 | 84 | 3.0 | 12.0 | 1.0 | 1.0 | 10.0 | 2.5 | 1.0 | | | | | 15 | 750 | 150 | | | | | | | | | | | 0.0 | | | 20 | | 1.1 | | | | | | 840 | |
| 50458 | 1/2 cup | Chicken & Stars, cond, Campbell's | 126 | 70 | 87 | 3.0 | 9.0 | 1.0 | 1.0 | 7.0 | 2.0 | 0.5 | | | | | 1 | 750 | 150 | | | | | | | | | | | 1.2 | | | 20 | | 0.7 | | | | | | 1010 | |
| 50654 | 1/2 cup | Cream of Chicken, cond, avg | 126 | 117 | 82 | 3.4 | 9.3 | 0.3 | 0.6 | 8.4 | 7.4 | 2.1 | 3.3 | 1.5 | 0.06 | 1.41 | 10 | 562 | 57 | | | | 0.03 | 0.06 | 0.82 | 0.02 | 0.09 | 1.6 | 0.21 | 0.1 | 0.1 | | 34 | 0.1 | 0.6 | 3 | 0.4 | 38 | 88 | 7.9 | 990 | 0.63 |
| 50516 | 1/2 cup | Cream of Chicken, cond, Healthy Request | 124 | 80 | 85 | 2.0 | 12.0 | 0.0 | 2.0 | 10.0 | 2.0 | 1.0 | | | | | 10 | 500 | 100 | | | | | | | | | | | 24.0 | | | 0 | | 0.0 | | | | | | 480 | |
| 50006 | 1 cup | Cream of Chicken, prep w/milk, avg | 248 | 191 | 85 | 7.5 | 15.0 | 0.2 | 6.7 | 8.0 | 11.5 | 4.6 | 4.5 | 1.6 | 0.12 | 1.51 | 27 | 714 | 94 | 34 | 60 | | 0.07 | 0.26 | 0.92 | 0.07 | 0.55 | 7.7 | 0.57 | 1.2 | 1.2 | | 181 | 0.1 | 0.7 | 17 | 0.4 | 151 | 273 | 8.5 | 1047 | 0.67 |
| 50018 | 1 cup | Cream of Chicken, prep w/water, avg | 244 | 117 | 91 | 3.4 | 9.3 | 0.2 | 0.6 | 8.4 | 7.4 | 2.1 | 3.3 | 1.5 | 0.07 | 1.42 | 10 | 561 | 56 | | | | 0.03 | 0.06 | 0.82 | 0.02 | 0.10 | 1.7 | 0.20 | 0.2 | 0.1 | | 34 | 0.1 | 0.6 | 2 | 0.4 | 37 | 88 | | 986 | 0.63 |
| 50420 | 1 cup | Cream of Chicken, RTS, Progresso | 239 | 170 | 83 | 8.0 | 11.0 | 0.0 | 0.0 | 11.0 | 10.0 | 3.5 | 3.5 | 1.0 | | | 35 | 300 | 60 | | | | | | | | | | | 0.0 | | | 20 | | 1.4 | | | | | | 880 | |
| 50652 | 1/2 cup | Dumpling, cond, avg | 123 | 97 | 84 | 5.6 | 6.1 | 0.5 | 0.4 | 5.2 | 5.5 | 1.3 | 2.5 | 1.3 | 0.04 | 1.23 | 33 | 520 | 52 | | | | 0.02 | 0.07 | 1.76 | 0.04 | 0.16 | 2.5 | 0.15 | 0.0 | 0.0 | | 15 | 0.1 | 0.6 | 4 | 0.5 | 62 | 117 | 12.1 | 865 | 0.37 |
| 50074 | 1 cup | Dumpling, prep, avg | 241 | 96 | 92 | 5.6 | 6.0 | 0.5 | 0.4 | 5.2 | 5.5 | 1.3 | 2.5 | 1.3 | 0.02 | 1.23 | 34 | 518 | 53 | | | | 0.02 | 0.07 | 1.75 | 0.04 | 0.17 | 2.4 | 0.14 | 0.0 | 0.0 | | 14 | 0.1 | 0.6 | 5 | 0.5 | 60 | 116 | 11.8 | 860 | 0.37 |
| 50600 | 8 oz | Grilled Chicken, Nestle Foods | 227 | 191 | 82 | 8.6 | 22.2 | 3.4 | 6.4 | 12.5 | 7.5 | 1.8 | 3.0 | 1.4 | | | 30 | 1362 | 272 | | | | | | | | | | | 5.7 | | | 45 | | 0.7 | | | | 375 | | 1090 | |
| 50076 | 1/2 cup | Gumbo, cond, avg | 126 | 57 | 88 | 2.6 | 8.4 | 2.0 | 1.5 | 4.9 | 1.4 | 0.3 | 0.7 | 0.4 | 0.01 | 0.31 | 4 | 136 | 14 | | | | 0.25 | 0.38 | 0.67 | 0.06 | 0.03 | 6.3 | 0.20 | 5.0 | 0.0 | | 24 | 0.1 | 0.9 | 4 | 0.3 | 25 | 76 | 8.4 | 959 | 0.38 |
| 50077 | 1 cup | Gumbo, prep, avg | 244 | 56 | 94 | 2.6 | 8.4 | 2.0 | 1.5 | 5.0 | 1.4 | 0.3 | 0.7 | 0.3 | 0.00 | 0.32 | 5 | 137 | 15 | | | | 0.02 | 0.05 | 0.66 | 0.06 | 0.02 | 4.9 | 0.20 | 4.9 | 0.0 | | 24 | 0.1 | 0.9 | 5 | 0.3 | 24 | 76 | 8.1 | 954 | 0.38 |

| Code | Amount | Description | Weight (g) | Calories | % Water | Protein (g) | Carbs (g) | Fiber (g) | Sugar (g) | Other Carbs (g) | Fat (g) | Sat Fat (g) | Mono Fat (g) | Poly Fat (g) | Omega 3 (g) | Omega 6 (g) | Choles (mg) | Vit A (IU) | Vit A (RE) | Retinol (RE) | Carotenoids (RE) | Beta Carotene (mcg) |
|---|---|---|---|---|---|---|---|---|---|---|---|---|---|---|---|---|---|---|---|---|---|---|
| | | | Basic Components | | | | | | | | | Additional Fats | | | | | | Vit A & Components | | | | |
| 50079 | 1/2 cup | Mushroom, cond, avg | 152 | 166 | 80 | 5.3 | 11.6 | 0.3 | 0.9 | 10.4 | 11.1 | 2.9 | 4.9 | 2.8 | 0.14 | 2.66 | 12 | 1376 | 137 | | | |
| 50080 | 1 cup | Mushroom, prep w/water, avg | 244 | 132 | 90 | 4.4 | 9.3 | 0.2 | 0.7 | 8.3 | 9.2 | 2.4 | 4.0 | 2.3 | 0.10 | 2.20 | 10 | 1135 | 112 | | | |
| 50656 | 1/2 cup | Noodle, cond, avg | 123 | 75 | 85 | 4.0 | 9.4 | 0.7 | 0.6 | 8.0 | 2.3 | 0.6 | 1.0 | 0.5 | 0.02 | 0.44 | 6 | 654 | 55 | | | |
| 50511 | 1/2 cup | Noodle, cond, Healthy Request | 126 | 70 | 87 | 3.0 | 9.0 | 0.0 | 1.0 | 8.0 | 2.0 | 0.5 | | | | | 15 | 500 | 130 | | | |
| 50443 | 1 cup | Noodle, Old El Paso | 239 | 110 | 90 | 9.0 | 10.0 | 0.0 | 0.0 | 10.0 | 3.0 | 1.0 | 1.0 | 1.0 | | | 25 | 3500 | 700 | | | |
| 50005 | 1 cup | Noodle, prep w/water, avg | 241 | 75 | 92 | 4.0 | 9.4 | 0.7 | 0.6 | 8.0 | 2.5 | 0.7 | 1.1 | 0.6 | 0.02 | 0.51 | 7 | 711 | 72 | | | |
| 50081 | 1 cup | Noodle, RTS, chunky, avg | 240 | 175 | 84 | 12.7 | 17.0 | 3.8 | 1.4 | 11.8 | 6.0 | 1.4 | 2.7 | 1.5 | 0.00 | 1.51 | 19 | 1222 | 122 | | | |
| 50540 | 1 cup | Noodle, RTS, chunky, Campbell's | 245 | 130 | 87 | 9.0 | 16.0 | 2.0 | 3.0 | 11.0 | 3.0 | 1.0 | | | | | 20 | 2500 | 500 | | | |
| 50585 | 1 cup | Noodle, RTS, low sod, Campbell's | 245 | 95 | 92 | 4.8 | 11.9 | 1.2 | 1.2 | 9.5 | 3.6 | 1.2 | | | | | 18 | 1189 | 238 | | | |
| 50427 | 1 cup | Noodle, RTS, Progresso | 238 | 80 | 91 | 9.0 | 8.0 | 1.0 | 0.0 | 7.0 | 2.0 | 0.5 | 1.0 | 0.5 | | | 20 | 3000 | 600 | | | |
| 50330 | 1 cup | Noodle, Weight Watchers | 241 | 121 | 87 | 7.3 | 20.2 | 3.2 | 12.1 | 4.9 | 1.6 | 0.4 | | | | | 24 | 809 | 152 | | | |
| 50048 | 1 cup | Noodle & Meatball, RTS, avg | 248 | 173 | 83 | 15.5 | 20.5 | 3.2 | 4.2 | 13.2 | 3.9 | 1.0 | 1.3 | 1.0 | 0.08 | 0.93 | 34 | 461 | 50 | 6 | 44 | |
| 50462 | 1/2 cup | Noodle O'S, cond, Campbell's | 126 | 80 | 84 | 4.0 | 10.0 | 1.0 | 1.0 | 8.0 | 3.0 | 1.0 | | | | | 15 | 1000 | 200 | | | |
| 50658 | 1/2 cup | Rice, cond, avg | 123 | 60 | 88 | 3.6 | 7.2 | 0.6 | 0.4 | 6.2 | 1.9 | 0.5 | 0.9 | 0.4 | 0.01 | 0.39 | 6 | 663 | 66 | | | |
| 50513 | 1/2 cup | Rice, cond, Healthy Request | 126 | 60 | 87 | 2.0 | 10.0 | 1.0 | 1.0 | 8.0 | 2.5 | 1.0 | | | | | 15 | 1000 | 200 | | | |
| 50439 | 1 cup | Rice, Old El Paso | 238 | 90 | 91 | 8.0 | 10.0 | 0.0 | 1.0 | 9.0 | 2.5 | 0.5 | 1.0 | 0.5 | | | 15 | 3500 | 700 | | | |
| 50020 | 1 cup | Rice, prep w/water, avg | 241 | 60 | 94 | 3.5 | 7.2 | 0.7 | 0.2 | 6.2 | 1.9 | 0.5 | 0.9 | 0.4 | 0.02 | 0.39 | 7 | 660 | 55 | | | |
| 50085 | 1 cup | Rice, RTS, chunky, avg | 240 | 127 | 87 | 12.3 | 13.0 | 1.0 | 2.1 | 9.9 | 3.2 | 1.0 | 1.4 | 0.7 | 0.02 | 0.62 | 12 | 5858 | 586 | | | |
| 50444 | 8 oz | Rice, Weight Watchers | 302 | 112 | 91 | 6.1 | 17.2 | 4.1 | 11.2 | 2.0 | 1.5 | 0.0 | | | | | 10 | 1014 | 203 | | | |
| 50466 | 1/2 cup | Rice, wild, cond, Campbell's | 126 | 70 | 87 | 3.0 | 9.0 | 1.0 | 1.0 | 7.0 | 2.0 | 0.5 | | | | | 10 | 400 | 80 | | | |
| 50428 | 1 cup | Rice Vegetable, RTS, Progresso | 238 | 110 | 89 | 7.0 | 12.0 | 0.5 | 0.0 | 11.5 | 3.0 | 1.0 | 1.5 | 0.5 | | | 15 | 1250 | 250 | | | |
| 50389 | 1 cup | Rotini Pasta, Progresso | 238 | 90 | 90 | 10.0 | 8.0 | 0.0 | 0.0 | 8.0 | 2.0 | 0.5 | 1.0 | 0.5 | | | 20 | 2250 | 450 | | | |
| 50203 | 1 cup | Stew, avg | 252 | 287 | 78 | 24.1 | 15.2 | 2.1 | | | 14.1 | 4.0 | 5.6 | 3.1 | | | 86 | 7673 | 793 | 39 | 754 | |
| 50382 | 1 cup | Tortellini in Chicken Broth, RTS, Progresso | 236 | 80 | | 4.0 | 10.0 | 2.0 | 1.0 | 7.0 | 2.0 | 0.5 | 1.0 | 0.5 | | | 5 | 3000 | 600 | | | |
| 50088 | 1 cup | Vegetable, chunky, RTS, avg | 240 | 166 | 83 | 12.3 | 18.9 | 0.2 | 9.7 | 9.0 | 4.8 | 1.4 | 2.2 | 1.0 | 0.05 | 0.94 | 17 | 5990 | 600 | | | |
| 50659 | 1/2 cup | Vegetable, cond, avg | 123 | 75 | 86 | 3.6 | 8.6 | 0.9 | 1.0 | 6.7 | 2.9 | 0.8 | 1.3 | 0.6 | 0.02 | 0.55 | 9 | 2667 | 267 | | | |
| 50512 | 1/2 cup | Vegetable, cond, Healthy Request | 126 | 80 | 84 | 3.0 | 12.0 | 1.0 | 4.0 | 7.0 | 2.0 | 0.5 | | | | | 5 | 2000 | 400 | | | |
| 50219 | 1 cup | Vegetable, low sod, prep, avg | 241 | 166 | 83 | 12.3 | 19.0 | 1.0 | 2.2 | 15.8 | 4.8 | 1.4 | 2.2 | 1.0 | | | 17 | 6013 | 603 | 0 | 603 | |
| 50441 | 1 cup | Vegetable, Old El Paso | 240 | 110 | 89 | 9.0 | 13.0 | 0.0 | 4.0 | 9.0 | 2.5 | 0.5 | 1.0 | 1.0 | | | 15 | 3000 | 600 | | | |
| 50091 | 1 cup | Vegetable, prep, avg | 241 | 75 | 93 | 3.6 | 8.6 | 1.0 | 1.0 | 6.6 | 2.8 | 0.8 | 1.3 | 0.6 | 0.02 | 0.55 | 10 | 2656 | 265 | | | |
| 50426 | 1 cup | Vegetable, Progresso | 240 | 100 | 90 | 9.0 | 10.0 | 1.0 | 0.0 | 9.0 | 2.5 | 0.5 | 1.0 | 0.5 | | | 15 | 1750 | 350 | | | |
| 50559 | 1 cup | Vegetable, RTS, Healthy Request | 245 | 110 | 87 | 6.0 | 18.0 | 2.0 | 5.0 | 11.0 | 2.0 | 1.0 | | | | | 10 | 4500 | 900 | | | |
| 50457 | 1/2 cup | Vegetable Alphabet, cond, Campbell's | 126 | 80 | 84 | 4.0 | 11.0 | 1.0 | 1.0 | 9.0 | 2.0 | 1.0 | | | | | 10 | 750 | 150 | | | |
| 50535 | 1 cup | Vegetable w/Chicken Nuggets, RTS, Campbell's | 245 | 90 | 90 | 6.0 | 12.0 | 2.0 | 2.0 | 8.0 | 2.0 | 0.5 | | | | | 10 | 1500 | 300 | | | |
| | | Chili Soup | | | | | | | | | | | | | | | | | | | | |
| 50660 | 1/2 cup | Beef, cond, avg | 132 | 170 | 71 | 6.7 | 21.5 | 9.6 | 2.0 | 9.8 | 6.6 | 3.3 | 2.8 | 0.3 | 0.04 | 0.21 | 13 | 1517 | 152 | | | |
| 50007 | 1 cup | Beef, prep w/water, avg | 250 | 170 | 85 | 6.7 | 21.5 | 9.5 | 1.3 | 10.7 | 6.6 | 3.4 | 2.8 | 0.3 | 0.05 | 0.20 | 12 | 1510 | 150 | | | |
| 50468 | 1/2 cup | Beef w/Beans, cond, Campbell's | 128 | 170 | 69 | 7.0 | 24.0 | 4.0 | 4.0 | 16.0 | 5.0 | 2.5 | | | | | 15 | 750 | 150 | | | |
| 50538 | 8 oz | Beef w/Beans, RTS, chunky, Campbell's | 227 | 218 | 76 | 15.3 | 27.6 | 6.5 | 2.9 | 18.2 | 5.1 | 1.5 | | | | | 15 | 1091 | 218 | | | |
| 50368 | 1 cup | Chili w/Beans Soup, Old El Paso | 228 | 200 | 80 | 19.0 | 15.0 | 6.0 | 0.0 | 9.0 | 7.0 | 1.5 | 2.5 | 1.5 | | | 30 | | | | | |
| | | Clam Chowder | | | | | | | | | | | | | | | | | | | | |
| 50661 | 1/2 cup | Manhattan, cond, avg | 126 | 77 | 84 | 2.2 | 12.3 | 1.5 | 1.9 | 8.9 | 2.2 | 0.4 | 0.4 | 1.3 | 0.09 | 1.20 | 3 | 966 | 97 | | | |
| 50021 | 1 cup | Manhattan, prep w/water, avg | 244 | 78 | 92 | 2.2 | 12.2 | 1.5 | 1.9 | 8.9 | 2.2 | 0.4 | 0.4 | 1.3 | 0.09 | 1.20 | 2 | 964 | 98 | | | |
| 50093 | 1 cup | Manhattan, RTS, chunky, avg | 240 | 134 | 86 | 7.2 | 18.8 | 2.9 | 2.4 | 13.5 | 3.4 | 2.1 | 1.0 | 0.1 | 0.05 | 0.07 | 14 | 3293 | 329 | | | |
| 50432 | 1 cup | Manhattan, RTS, Progresso | 239 | 110 | 88 | 12.0 | 11.0 | 3.0 | 3.0 | 5.0 | 2.0 | 0.0 | 0.5 | 1.5 | | | 10 | 2250 | 450 | | | |
| 50662 | 1/2 cup | New England, cond, avg | 126 | 88 | 82 | 5.5 | 10.9 | 0.8 | 3.4 | 6.8 | 2.5 | 0.4 | 1.1 | 0.9 | 0.06 | 0.88 | 5 | 10 | 1 | 1 | 0.1 | |
| 50008 | 1 cup | New England, prep w/milk, avg | 248 | 164 | 85 | 9.5 | 16.6 | 1.5 | 6.5 | 8.6 | 6.6 | 3.0 | 2.3 | 1.1 | 0.12 | 0.97 | 22 | 164 | 40 | 36 | 4 | |
| 50195 | 1 cup | New England, prep w/water, avg | 244 | 95 | 90 | 4.8 | 12.4 | 1.5 | | | 2.9 | 0.4 | 1.2 | 1.1 | 0.07 | 1.00 | 5 | 7 | 1 | 0 | 1 | |
| 50545 | 1 cup | New England, RTS, chunky, Campbell's | 245 | 240 | 80 | 7.0 | 21.0 | 2.0 | 1.0 | 18.0 | 15.0 | 5.0 | | | | | 10 | 0 | 0 | 0 | 0 | 0 |
| 50563 | 1 cup | New England, RTS, Healthy Request | 245 | 120 | 87 | 5.0 | 17.0 | 1.0 | 2.0 | 14.0 | 3.0 | 0.5 | | | | | 15 | 0 | 0 | 0 | 0 | 0 |
| | | Corn Soup | | | | | | | | | | | | | | | | | | | | |
| 50532 | 1 cup | Chicken Chowder, RTS, chunky, Campbell's | 245 | 250 | 82 | 10.0 | 18.0 | 3.0 | 4.0 | 11.0 | 15.0 | 7.0 | | | | | 25 | 4000 | 800 | | | |
| 50271 | 1 cup | Chowder, prep w/milk, Corn Products Company | 248 | 175 | 86 | 7.3 | 19.0 | | | | 7.3 | | | | | | | 146 | 29 | | | |
| 50419 | 1 cup | Chowder, RTS, Progresso | 244 | 180 | 85 | 5.0 | 20.0 | 2.0 | 4.0 | 14.0 | 10.0 | 4.0 | 4.0 | 1.0 | | | 10 | 300 | 60 | | | |
| 50487 | 1/2 cup | Condensed, Campbell's | 124 | 120 | 78 | 2.0 | 20.0 | 2.0 | 7.0 | 11.0 | 3.5 | 1.0 | | | | | 5 | 500 | 50 | 0 | 50 | 300 |
| 50358 | 1 cup | Vegetable, fat free, Health Valley | 240 | 80 | 90 | 6.0 | 17.0 | 5.0 | 9.0 | 3.0 | 0.0 | 0.0 | 0.0 | 0.0 | 0.00 | 0.00 | 0 | 10000 | 2000 | | | |
| 50213 | 1 cup | Crab Soup, prep w/milk, avg | 248 | 253 | 81 | 20.5 | 11.8 | 0.3 | | | 13.6 | 4.6 | 4.9 | 3.1 | | | 92 | 600 | 148 | 132 | 16 | |
| 50099 | 1 cup | Crab Soup, RTS, avg | 244 | 76 | 92 | 5.5 | 10.3 | 0.7 | | | 1.5 | 0.4 | 0.7 | 0.4 | 0.02 | 0.37 | 10 | 505 | 51 | | | |
| 50190 | 1 cup | Egg Drop Soup, avg | 244 | 73 | 94 | 7.5 | 1.1 | 0.0 | | | 3.8 | 1.2 | 1.5 | 0.6 | | | 102 | 135 | 41 | 41 | 0 | 0 |
| 50101 | 1 cup | Escarole Soup, avg | 248 | 27 | 97 | 1.5 | 1.8 | | | | 1.8 | 0.5 | 0.8 | 0.4 | 0.02 | 0.35 | 2 | 2170 | 218 | | | |
| 50710 | 1 cup | Fish Broth, avg | 237 | 38 | 96 | 4.7 | 0.9 | 0.0 | | | 1.4 | 0.4 | 0.6 | 0.3 | | | 0 | 0 | 0 | 0 | 0 | 0 |
| 50103 | 1 cup | Gazpacho Soup, avg | 244 | 46 | 94 | 7.1 | 4.4 | 0.5 | | | 0.2 | 0.0 | 0.0 | 0.1 | 0.01 | 0.05 | 0 | 2603 | 261 | | | |
| 50208 | 1 cup | Ham, Pasta & Vegetable Soup, avg | 244 | 63 | 93 | 5.3 | 8.3 | 1.7 | | | 1.0 | 0.3 | 0.4 | 0.2 | | | 7 | 2572 | 257 | 0 | 257 | |
| 50182 | 1 cup | Hot & Sour Soup, avg | 244 | 132 | 88 | 12.1 | 5.4 | 0.5 | | | 6.1 | 2.0 | 2.5 | 1.0 | | | 22 | 14 | 2 | 1 | 1 | |
| 50200 | 1 cup | Lamb Stew, avg | 252 | 272 | 76 | 18.4 | 28.0 | 5.8 | | | 10.0 | 4.4 | 3.8 | 0.7 | | | 53 | 3142 | 315 | 0 | 315 | |
| | | Lentil Soup | | | | | | | | | | | | | | | | | | | | |
| 50324 | 1 cup | Curry, Taste Adventure | 241 | 138 | | 6.4 | 29.7 | 5.3 | | | 0.5 | | | | | | | | | | | |
| 50105 | 1 cup | Ham, RTS, avg | 248 | 139 | 86 | 9.3 | 20.2 | 1.9 | | | 2.8 | 1.1 | 1.3 | 0.3 | 0.02 | 0.30 | 7 | 360 | 35 | | | |
| 50575 | 1 cup | RTS, Campbell's | 245 | 130 | 86 | 7.0 | 24.0 | 5.0 | 3.0 | 16.0 | 0.5 | 0.5 | 0.0 | 0.0 | 0.00 | 0.00 | 0 | 2000 | 400 | | | |
| 50430 | 1 cup | RTS, Progresso | 241 | 140 | 85 | 9.0 | 22.0 | 7.0 | 0.0 | 15.0 | 2.0 | 0.0 | 1.0 | 1.0 | | | 0 | 750 | 150 | | | |

| Code | Thiamin (mg) | Riboflavin (mg) | Niacin (NE) | Vit B6 (mg) | Vit B12 (mcg) | Folate (mcg) | Panto (mg) | Vit C (mg) | Vit D (mg) | Vit E (α TE) | Calcium (mg) | Copper (mg) | Iron (mg) | Magnes (mg) | Mang (mg) | Phos (mg) | Potassium (mg) | Selenium (mcg) | Sodium (mg) | Zinc (mg) |
|---|---|---|---|---|---|---|---|---|---|---|---|---|---|---|---|---|---|---|---|---|
| | Vitamins | | | | | | | | | | Minerals | | | | | | | | | |
| 50079 | 0.03 | 0.14 | 1.98 | 0.06 | 0.08 | 3.0 | 0.30 | 0.0 | 0.0 | | 35 | 0.1 | 1.1 | 11 | 0.2 | 33 | 192 | 4.4 | 1175 | 1.22 |
| 50080 | 0.02 | 0.11 | 1.63 | 0.05 | 0.05 | 0.2 | 0.24 | 0.0 | 0.0 | | 29 | 0.2 | 0.9 | 10 | 0.2 | 27 | 154 | | 942 | 0.98 |
| 50656 | 0.06 | 0.07 | 1.51 | 0.03 | 0.16 | 19.7 | 0.17 | 0.0 | 0.0 | | 14 | 0.2 | 0.8 | 5 | 0.3 | 37 | 55 | 12.1 | 981 | 0.29 |
| 50511 | | | | | | | | 0.0 | | | 0 | | 0.7 | | | | | | 430 | |
| 50443 | | | | | | | | 4.8 | | | 40 | | 1.1 | | | | | | | |
| 50005 | 0.05 | 0.06 | 1.39 | 0.03 | 0.14 | 21.7 | 0.17 | 0.2 | 0.0 | | 17 | 0.2 | 0.8 | 5 | 0.3 | 36 | 55 | 6.3 | 1136 | 0.40 |
| 50081 | 0.07 | 0.17 | 4.32 | 0.05 | 0.31 | 38.4 | 0.36 | 0.0 | 0.0 | | 24 | 0.2 | 1.4 | 10 | 0.2 | 72 | 108 | 25.2 | 850 | 0.96 |
| 50540 | | | | | | | | 2.4 | | | 40 | | 1.1 | | | | | | 1050 | |
| 50585 | | | | | | | | 0.0 | | | 24 | | 0.9 | | | | | | 137 | |
| 50427 | | | | | | | | 0.0 | | | 20 | | 1.1 | | | | | | 730 | |
| 50330 | | | | | | | | 0.0 | | | 49 | | 1.2 | | | | 364 | | 598 | |
| 50048 | 0.12 | 0.16 | 5.72 | 0.37 | 0.18 | 43.3 | 1.02 | 17.3 | 0.1 | | 37 | 0.2 | 1.7 | 46 | 0.5 | 167 | 534 | 12.0 | 448 | 1.36 |
| 50462 | | | | | | | | 1.2 | | | 20 | | 1.1 | | | | | | 980 | |
| 50658 | 0.02 | 0.02 | 1.13 | 0.02 | 0.16 | 1.1 | 0.17 | 0.1 | 0.0 | | 17 | 0.1 | 0.8 | 0 | 0.4 | 21 | 101 | 5.0 | 813 | 0.26 |
| 50513 | | | | | | | | 12.0 | | | 0 | | 0.0 | | | | | | 480 | |
| 50439 | | | | | | | | 6.0 | | | 40 | | 0.7 | | | | | | 630 | |
| 50020 | 0.02 | 0.02 | 1.13 | 0.02 | 0.14 | 1.0 | 0.17 | 0.2 | 0.0 | | 17 | 0.1 | 0.7 | 0 | 0.4 | 22 | 101 | 4.8 | 815 | 0.26 |
| 50085 | 0.02 | 0.10 | 4.10 | 0.05 | 0.31 | 3.8 | 0.36 | 3.8 | 0.0 | | 34 | 0.2 | 1.9 | 10 | 0.2 | 72 | 108 | 10.8 | 838 | 0.96 |
| 50444 | | | | | | | | 0.0 | | | 61 | | 1.1 | | | | 436 | | 730 | |
| 50466 | | | | | | | | 15.0 | | | 20 | | 0.4 | | | | | | 900 | |
| 50428 | | | | | | | | 0.0 | | | 20 | | 1.1 | | | | | | 750 | |
| 50389 | | | | | | | | 3.6 | | | 0 | | 0.7 | | | | | | 850 | |
| 50203 | 0.14 | 0.20 | 8.93 | 0.45 | 0.24 | 18.1 | | 12.3 | | | 33 | 0.2 | 1.9 | 43 | | 219 | 633 | | 469 | 1.89 |
| 50382 | | | | | | | | 0.0 | | | 40 | | 1.8 | | | | | | 750 | |
| 50088 | 0.04 | 0.17 | 3.29 | 0.10 | 0.24 | 12.0 | 0.34 | 5.5 | 0.0 | | 26 | 0.2 | 1.5 | 10 | 0.2 | 106 | 367 | 12.2 | 1038 | 2.16 |
| 50659 | 0.04 | 0.06 | 1.23 | 0.05 | 0.12 | 4.9 | 0.17 | 1.0 | 0.0 | | 17 | 0.1 | 0.9 | 6 | 0.4 | 41 | 155 | 5.5 | 948 | 0.37 |
| 50512 | | | | | | | | 1.2 | | | 20 | | 0.4 | | | | | | 480 | |
| 50219 | 0.05 | 0.17 | 3.30 | 0.10 | 0.24 | 12.1 | | 5.5 | 0.0 | | 27 | 0.2 | 1.5 | 10 | | 106 | 369 | | 34 | 2.17 |
| 50441 | | | | | | | | | | | 60 | | 1.1 | | | | | | 620 | |
| 50091 | 0.04 | 0.06 | 1.23 | 0.05 | 0.12 | 4.8 | 0.17 | 1.0 | 0.0 | | 17 | 0.1 | 0.9 | 7 | 0.4 | 41 | 154 | 5.3 | 945 | 0.37 |
| 50426 | | | | | | | | 0.0 | | | 0 | | 1.4 | | | | | | 680 | |
| 50559 | | | | | | | | 3.6 | | | 20 | | 0.7 | | | | | | 480 | |
| 50457 | | | | | | | | 0.0 | | | 20 | | 0.7 | | | | | | 880 | |
| 50535 | | | | | | | | 0.0 | | | 20 | | 0.7 | | | | | | 800 | |
| 50660 | 0.06 | 0.08 | 1.07 | 0.16 | 0.32 | 18.5 | 0.66 | 4.1 | 0.0 | | 44 | 0.4 | 2.1 | 30 | 1.1 | 149 | 528 | 25.6 | 1040 | 1.40 |
| 50007 | 0.06 | 0.07 | 1.07 | 0.16 | 0.32 | 17.5 | 0.50 | 4.0 | 0.0 | | 42 | 0.4 | 2.1 | 30 | 1.0 | 148 | 525 | 6.0 | 1035 | 1.40 |
| 50468 | | | | | | | | 1.2 | | | 40 | | 1.8 | | | | | | 910 | |
| 50538 | | | | | | | | 6.5 | | | 58 | | 3.3 | | | | | | 756 | |
| 50368 | | | | | | | | | | | 60 | | 3.6 | | | | | | 420 | |
| 50661 | 0.03 | 0.04 | 0.82 | 0.10 | 4.07 | 10.1 | 0.19 | 4.0 | 0.0 | | 24 | 0.1 | 1.6 | 10 | 0.4 | 42 | 189 | 9.4 | 576 | 0.93 |
| 50021 | 0.03 | 0.04 | 0.82 | 0.10 | 4.05 | 9.8 | 0.00 | 3.9 | 0.0 | | 27 | 0.1 | 1.6 | 12 | 0.4 | 41 | 188 | 9.3 | 578 | 0.98 |
| 50093 | 0.06 | 0.06 | 1.85 | 0.26 | 7.92 | 9.4 | 0.24 | 12.2 | 0.0 | | 67 | 0.2 | 2.6 | 19 | 0.2 | 84 | 384 | 16.1 | 1001 | 1.68 |
| 50432 | | | | | | | | 3.6 | | | 40 | | 1.8 | | | | | | 710 | |
| 50662 | 0.02 | 0.04 | 0.93 | 0.08 | 9.85 | 3.7 | 0.33 | 2.4 | 0.6 | | 42 | 0.1 | 1.4 | 8 | 0.3 | 43 | 115 | 10.6 | 936 | 0.76 |
| 50008 | 0.07 | 0.24 | 1.03 | 0.13 | 10.24 | 9.7 | 0.69 | 3.5 | 1.2 | | 186 | 0.1 | 1.5 | 22 | 0.3 | 156 | 300 | 12.9 | 992 | 0.80 |
| 50195 | 0.02 | 0.04 | 0.96 | 0.08 | 8.00 | 3.7 | 0.32 | 2.0 | | | 44 | 0.1 | 1.5 | 7 | 0.3 | 54 | 146 | 10.2 | 915 | 0.75 |
| 50545 | | | | | | | | 0.0 | | | 40 | | 1.4 | | | | | | 980 | |
| 50563 | | | | | | | | 0.0 | | | 100 | | 1.4 | | | | | | 480 | |
| 50532 | | | | | | | | 2.4 | | | 20 | | 0.7 | | | | | | 870 | |
| 50271 | 0.22 | 1.24 | | | | | | | | | 146 | | 1.6 | | | | 306 | | 830 | |
| 50419 | | | | | | | | 6.0 | | | 0 | | 0.7 | | | | | | 780 | |
| 50487 | | | | | | | | 0.0 | | | 20 | | 0.4 | | | | | | 730 | |
| 50358 | | | | | | | | 9.0 | | | 40 | | 5.4 | | | | | | 240 | |
| 50213 | 0.16 | 0.30 | 2.93 | 0.20 | 5.80 | 46.7 | | 4.5 | | | 250 | 0.5 | 1.1 | 47 | | 298 | 486 | | 530 | 3.72 |
| 50099 | 0.20 | 0.07 | 1.34 | 0.12 | 0.20 | 14.6 | 0.29 | 0.0 | 0.0 | | 66 | 0.5 | 1.2 | 15 | 0.5 | 88 | 327 | 6.3 | 1235 | 1.46 |
| 50190 | 0.02 | 0.19 | 3.03 | 0.05 | 0.49 | 15.4 | | 0.0 | | | 22 | 0.1 | 0.8 | 5 | | 107 | 220 | | 730 | 0.48 |
| 50101 | 0.07 | 0.05 | 2.31 | 0.22 | 0.50 | 34.7 | 0.17 | 4.5 | | | 32 | 0.4 | 0.7 | 5 | 1.2 | 79 | 265 | | 3864 | 2.23 |
| 50710 | 0.00 | 0.07 | 3.25 | 0.02 | 0.24 | 9.5 | | 0.0 | | 0.0 | 71 | 0.1 | 0.5 | 2 | | 71 | 204 | | 754 | 0.24 |
| 50103 | 0.05 | 0.02 | 0.93 | 0.15 | 0.00 | 9.8 | 0.17 | 7.1 | 0.0 | | 24 | 0.1 | 1.0 | 7 | 0.7 | 37 | 224 | 3.7 | 739 | 0.24 |
| 50208 | 0.15 | 0.08 | 1.54 | 0.12 | 0.07 | 15.2 | | 10.9 | | | 27 | 0.1 | 0.9 | 20 | | 63 | 227 | | 532 | 0.68 |
| 50182 | 0.19 | 0.22 | 4.58 | 0.15 | 0.35 | 11.8 | | 0.7 | | | 29 | 0.2 | 1.8 | 27 | | 161 | 351 | | 1522 | 1.17 |
| 50200 | 0.24 | 0.27 | 5.31 | 0.41 | 1.49 | 33.7 | | 14.3 | | | 35 | 0.4 | 2.3 | 53 | | 202 | 723 | | 1023 | 3.19 |
| 50324 | | | | | | | | | | | | | | | | | 467 | | 554 | |
| 50105 | 0.17 | 0.11 | 1.35 | 0.22 | 0.30 | 49.6 | 0.35 | 4.2 | 0.3 | | 42 | 0.2 | 2.7 | 22 | 0.3 | 184 | 357 | 0.7 | 1319 | 0.74 |
| 50575 | | | | | | | | 0.0 | | | 40 | | 3.6 | | | | | | 880 | |
| 50430 | | | | | | | | 0.0 | | | 40 | | 3.6 | | | | | | 750 | |

| Code | Amount | Description | Basic Components | | | | | | | | | Additional Fats | | | | | | Vit A & Components | | | | | Vitamins | | | | | | | | | | Minerals | | | | | | | | | |
|---|---|---|---|---|---|---|---|---|---|---|---|---|---|---|---|---|---|---|---|---|---|---|---|---|---|---|---|---|---|---|---|---|---|---|---|---|---|---|---|---|---|---|
| | | | Weight (g) | Calories | % Water | Protein (g) | Carbs (g) | Fiber (g) | Sugar (g) | Other Carbs (g) | Fat (g) | Sat Fat (g) | Mono Fat (g) | Poly Fat (g) | Omega 3 (g) | Omega 6 (g) | Choles (mg) | Vit A (IU) | Vit A (RE) | Retinol (RE) | Carotenoids (RE) | Beta Carotene (mcg) | Thiamin (mg) | Riboflavin (mg) | Niacin (NE) | Vit B6 (mg) | Vit B12 (mcg) | Folate (mcg) | Panto (mg) | Vit C (mg) | Vit D (mg) | Vit E (α TE) | Calcium (mg) | Copper (mg) | Iron (mg) | Magnes (mg) | Mang (mg) | Phos (mg) | Potassium (mg) | Selenium (mcg) | Sodium (mg) | Zinc (mg) |
| 50395 | 1 cup | Shells, RTS, Progresso | 242 | 130 | 87 | 7.0 | 22.0 | 4.0 | 0.0 | 18.0 | 1.5 | 0.0 | 0.5 | 0.5 | | | 0 | 200 | 40 | | | | | | | | | | | 0.0 | | | 20 | | 2.7 | | | | | | 840 | |
| 50273 | 8 oz | With Bacon, prep w/water CPC | 227 | 93 | 91 | 5.3 | 9.3 | | | | 4.0 | | | | | | | | | | | | 0.08 | 0.14 | | | | | | | | | 27 | | 1.9 | | | | 120 | | 921 | |
| 50362 | 1 cup | With Carrots, fat free, Health Valley | 240 | 90 | 85 | 10.0 | 25.0 | 14.0 | 7.0 | 4.0 | 0.0 | 0.0 | 0.0 | 0.0 | 0.00 | 0.00 | 0 | 10000 | 2000 | | | | 0.10 | 0.16 | 5.63 | 0.45 | | 27.0 | | 2.4 | | | 60 | | 5.4 | | | | 439 | | 220 | |
| 50431 | 1 cup | With Sausage, RTS, Progresso | 241 | 170 | 85 | 8.0 | 19.0 | 5.0 | 0.0 | 14.0 | 7.0 | 2.0 | 2.5 | 1.0 | | | 15 | 2000 | 400 | | | | | | | | | | | 3.6 | | | 20 | | 1.8 | | | | | | 780 | |
| 50214 | 1 cup | Lobster Bisque Soup, avg | 248 | 273 | 79 | 20.1 | 12.7 | 0.2 | | | 15.5 | 5.7 | 5.8 | 3.1 | | | 72 | 757 | 194 | 179 | 16 | | 0.09 | 0.37 | 1.05 | 0.13 | 2.59 | 17.2 | | 1.9 | | | 270 | 1.3 | 0.5 | 50 | | 305 | 538 | | 858 | 2.67 |
| 50215 | 1 cup | Lobster Gumbo Soup, avg | 244 | 178 | 84 | 9.8 | 19.7 | 4.0 | | | 7.3 | 1.4 | 3.1 | 2.3 | | | 24 | 1481 | 206 | 89 | 118 | | 0.20 | 0.12 | 2.25 | 0.20 | 1.01 | 68.0 | | 28.5 | | | 110 | 0.9 | 1.8 | 54 | | 129 | 610 | | 669 | 1.55 |
| 50394 | 1 cup | Meatballs & Pasta Soup, RTS, Progresso | 237 | 140 | 88 | 7.0 | 13.0 | 0.0 | 0.0 | 13.0 | 7.0 | 3.0 | 3.0 | 0.5 | | | 15 | 750 | 150 | | | | | | | | | | | 0.0 | | | 40 | | 1.1 | | | | | | 700 | |
| | | Minestrone Soup | | | | | | | | | | | | | | | | | | | | | | | | | | | | | | | | | | | | | | | | |
| 50410 | 1 cup | Beef, RTS, Progresso | 241 | 140 | 86 | 12.0 | 14.0 | 3.0 | 0.0 | 11.0 | 4.0 | 1.5 | 2.5 | 0.0 | 0.00 | 0.00 | 25 | 2000 | 400 | | | | | | | | | | | 2.4 | | | 40 | | 2.7 | | | | | | 850 | |
| 50417 | 1 cup | Chicken, RTS, Progresso | 239 | 120 | 88 | 10.0 | 12.0 | 2.0 | 0.0 | 10.0 | 3.5 | 1.0 | 1.5 | 1.0 | | | 20 | 2500 | 500 | | | | | | | | | | | 0.0 | | | 40 | | 1.4 | | | | | | 790 | |
| 50107 | 1 cup | Chunky, RTS, avg | 240 | 127 | 87 | 5.1 | 20.7 | 5.8 | 2.4 | 12.6 | 2.8 | 1.5 | 0.9 | 0.3 | 0.05 | 0.22 | 5 | 4351 | 434 | | | | 0.06 | 0.12 | 1.18 | 0.24 | 0.00 | 52.8 | 0.72 | 4.8 | 0.0 | | 60 | 0.2 | 1.8 | 14 | 0.7 | 110 | 612 | 5.3 | 864 | 1.44 |
| 50664 | 1/2 cup | Condensed, avg | 123 | 84 | 83 | 4.3 | 11.3 | 1.0 | 1.5 | 8.8 | 2.5 | 0.5 | 0.7 | 1.1 | 0.14 | 0.97 | 1 | 2347 | 235 | | | | 0.05 | 0.04 | 0.95 | 0.10 | 0.00 | 35.7 | 0.34 | 1.1 | 0.0 | | 34 | 0.1 | 0.9 | 7 | 0.4 | 57 | 314 | 3.4 | 915 | 0.74 |
| 50519 | 1/2 cup | Condensed, Healthy Request | 126 | 90 | 80 | 4.0 | 17.0 | 2.0 | 2.0 | 13.0 | 1.0 | 0.5 | | | | | 0 | 2250 | 225 | 0 | 225 | 1350 | | | | | | | | 0.0 | | | 20 | | 1.1 | | | | | | 480 | |
| 50328 | 1 cup | Condensed, Taste Adventure | 234 | 124 | | 7.2 | 24.7 | 3.1 | | | 0.5 | | | | | | | | | | | | | | | | | | | | | | | | | | | | 526 | | 320 | |
| 50356 | 1 cup | Fat Free, Health Valley | 240 | 80 | 88 | 8.0 | 21.0 | 11.0 | 6.0 | 4.0 | 0.0 | 0.0 | 0.0 | 0.0 | 0.00 | 0.00 | 0 | 10000 | 2000 | | | | | | | | | | | 4.8 | | | 40 | | 3.6 | | | | | | 210 | |
| 50009 | 1 cup | Prepared, w/water, avg | 241 | 82 | 91 | 4.3 | 11.2 | 1.0 | 1.5 | 8.7 | 2.5 | 0.6 | 0.7 | 1.1 | 0.14 | 0.96 | 2 | 2338 | 234 | 0 | 234 | | 0.05 | 0.04 | 0.94 | 0.10 | 0.00 | 36.2 | 0.34 | 1.2 | 0.0 | | 34 | 0.1 | 0.9 | 7 | 0.4 | 55 | 313 | | 911 | 0.74 |
| 50577 | 1 ea | RTS, can, Campbell's | 305 | 140 | 88 | 5.0 | 24.0 | 3.0 | 5.0 | 16.0 | 3.0 | 1.5 | | | | | 5 | 4500 | 900 | | | | | | | | | | | 1.2 | | | 80 | | 1.1 | | | | | | 1220 | |
| 50445 | 8 oz | Weight Watchers | 227 | 99 | 89 | 3.8 | 17.5 | 4.6 | 5.3 | 7.6 | 1.5 | 0.4 | | | | | 4 | 2288 | 458 | | | | | | | | | | | 0.9 | | | 76 | | 1.4 | | | | 381 | | 580 | |
| 50391 | 1 cup | With Shells, RTS, Progresso | 240 | 120 | 88 | 5.0 | 20.0 | 4.0 | 2.0 | 14.0 | 1.5 | 0.0 | 1.0 | 0.0 | 0.00 | 0.00 | 0 | 2000 | 400 | | | | | | | | | | | 4.8 | | | 20 | | 1.1 | | | | | | 700 | |
| | | Mushroom Soup | | | | | | | | | | | | | | | | | | | | | | | | | | | | | | | | | | | | | | | | |
| 50665 | 1/2 cup | Barley, cond, avg | 126 | 77 | 85 | 1.9 | 12.1 | 0.8 | | | 2.3 | 0.4 | 1.0 | 0.7 | 0.04 | 0.68 | 0 | 199 | 20 | | | | 0.03 | 0.09 | 0.88 | 0.18 | 0.00 | 6.3 | 0.13 | 0.0 | 0.0 | | 13 | 0.2 | 0.5 | 9 | 0.1 | 63 | 96 | | 920 | 0.50 |
| 50111 | 1 cup | Barley, prep w/water, avg | 244 | 73 | 92 | 1.9 | 11.7 | 0.7 | | | 2.3 | 0.4 | 1.0 | 0.7 | 0.02 | 0.68 | 0 | 198 | 20 | | | | 0.02 | 0.09 | 0.88 | 0.17 | 0.00 | 4.9 | 0.12 | 0.0 | 0.0 | | 12 | 0.2 | 0.5 | 10 | 0.1 | 61 | 93 | | 891 | 0.49 |
| 50667 | 1/2 cup | Beef Stock, cond, avg | 126 | 86 | 85 | 3.2 | 9.3 | 0.1 | 0.7 | 8.5 | 4.0 | 1.6 | 1.4 | 0.8 | 0.10 | 0.68 | 8 | 1260 | 126 | | | | 0.04 | 0.10 | 1.21 | 0.04 | 0.00 | 9.2 | 0.24 | 1.0 | 0.0 | 0.0 | 10 | 0.3 | 0.8 | 9 | 0.4 | 37 | 159 | 4.7 | 974 | 1.39 |
| 50113 | 1 cup | Beef Stock, prep w/water, avg | 244 | 85 | 92 | 3.1 | 9.3 | 0.7 | 0.7 | 7.9 | 4.0 | 1.6 | 1.4 | 0.8 | 0.10 | 0.68 | 7 | 1254 | 124 | | | | 0.03 | 0.10 | 1.21 | 0.04 | 0.00 | 9.3 | 0.24 | 1.0 | 0.0 | | 10 | 0.3 | 0.8 | 10 | 0.4 | 37 | 159 | | 969 | 1.38 |
| 50666 | 1/2 cup | Cream of Mushroom, cond, avg | 126 | 130 | 81 | 2.0 | 9.3 | 0.4 | 0.6 | 8.3 | 9.5 | 2.6 | 1.8 | 4.5 | 0.04 | 4.44 | 1 | 0 | 0 | 0 | 0 | 0 | 0.03 | 0.08 | 0.81 | 0.01 | 0.13 | 3.8 | 0.25 | 1.1 | 0.0 | | 33 | 0.1 | 0.5 | 5 | 0.3 | 43 | 84 | 1.5 | 872 | 0.60 |
| 50517 | 1/2 cup | Cream of Mushroom, cond, Healthy Request | 124 | 70 | 87 | 1.0 | 10.0 | 0.0 | 2.0 | 8.0 | 2.5 | 1.0 | | | | | 10 | 0 | 0 | 0 | 0 | 0 | | | | | | | | 0.0 | | | 100 | | 0.0 | | | | | | 480 | |
| 50587 | 8 oz | Cream of Mushroom, low sod, RTS, Campbell's | 227 | 152 | 88 | 2.3 | 13.7 | 2.3 | 3.8 | 7.6 | 10.7 | 3.0 | | | | | 15 | 0 | 0 | 0 | 0 | 0 | | | | | | | | 0.0 | | | 46 | | 0.8 | | | | | | 50 | |
| 50011 | 1 cup | Cream of Mushroom, prep w/milk, avg | 248 | 203 | 85 | 6.1 | 15.0 | 0.5 | 6.7 | 7.8 | 13.6 | 5.1 | 3.0 | 4.6 | 0.10 | 4.51 | 20 | 154 | 37 | 33 | 4 | | 0.08 | 0.28 | 0.91 | 0.06 | 0.50 | 9.9 | 0.62 | 2.2 | 1.2 | | 179 | 0.1 | 0.6 | 20 | 0.3 | 156 | 270 | 4.0 | 918 | 0.64 |
| 50049 | 1 cup | Cream of Mushroom, prep w/water, avg | 244 | 129 | 90 | 2.3 | 9.3 | 0.5 | 0.6 | 8.2 | 9.0 | 2.4 | 1.7 | 4.2 | 0.02 | 4.17 | 2 | 0 | 0 | 0 | 0 | 0 | 0.05 | 0.09 | 0.72 | 0.01 | 0.05 | 4.9 | 0.29 | 1.0 | | | 46 | 0.1 | 0.5 | 5 | 0.3 | 49 | 100 | 1.5 | 881 | 0.59 |
| 50574 | 1 cup | Cream of Mushroom, RTS, Campbell's | 245 | 170 | 89 | 3.0 | 9.0 | 3.0 | 1.0 | 5.0 | 13.0 | 4.0 | | | | | 15 | 0 | 0 | 0 | 0 | 0 | | | | | | | | 0.0 | | | 0 | | 0.0 | | | | | | 970 | |
| 50421 | 1 cup | Cream of Mushroom, RTS, Progresso | 238 | 140 | 90 | 3.0 | 12.0 | 1.0 | 0.0 | 11.0 | 8.0 | 3.5 | 3.5 | 0.0 | 0.00 | 0.00 | 20 | 0 | 0 | 0 | 0 | 0 | | | | | | | | 0.0 | | | 20 | | 0.7 | | | | | | 920 | |
| 50488 | 1/2 cup | Golden, cond, Campbell's | 124 | 80 | 86 | 2.0 | 10.0 | 1.0 | 1.0 | 8.0 | 3.0 | 1.0 | | | | | 5 | 750 | 75 | 0 | 75 | 450 | | | | | | | | 0.0 | | | 0 | | 0.4 | | | | | | 930 | |
| | | Onion Soup | | | | | | | | | | | | | | | | | | | | | | | | | | | | | | | | | | | | | | | | |
| 50022 | 1 cup | Average | 241 | 58 | 93 | 3.8 | 8.2 | 1.0 | 2.4 | 4.8 | 1.7 | 0.3 | 0.7 | 0.7 | 0.05 | 0.60 | 0 | 0 | 0 | 0 | 0 | 0 | 0.03 | 0.02 | 0.60 | 0.05 | 0.00 | 15.2 | 0.00 | 1.2 | 0.0 | | 27 | 0.1 | 0.7 | 2 | 0.2 | 12 | 67 | 4.3 | 1053 | 0.61 |
| 50668 | 1/2 cup | Condensed, avg | 123 | 57 | 86 | 3.8 | 8.2 | 0.9 | 2.7 | 4.6 | 1.7 | 0.3 | 0.8 | 0.7 | 0.05 | 0.60 | 0 | 0 | 0 | 0 | 0 | 0 | 0.03 | 0.02 | 0.60 | 0.05 | 0.00 | 15.3 | 0.00 | 1.2 | 0.0 | | 27 | 0.1 | 0.7 | 2 | 0.2 | 11 | 69 | 4.3 | 1058 | 0.62 |
| 50669 | 1/2 cup | Creamy, cond, avg | 126 | 111 | 81 | 2.8 | 13.1 | 0.5 | | | 5.3 | 1.5 | 2.1 | 1.5 | 0.10 | 1.35 | 15 | 297 | 30 | | | | 0.05 | 0.08 | 0.50 | 0.03 | 0.05 | 7.2 | 0.30 | 1.3 | | | 34 | 0.1 | 0.6 | 6 | 0.3 | 38 | 123 | 2.9 | 958 | 0.15 |
| 50194 | 1 cup | Creamy, prep w/milk, avg | 248 | 186 | 84 | 6.8 | 18.4 | 0.7 | | | 9.4 | 4.0 | 3.3 | 1.6 | 0.17 | 1.42 | 32 | 451 | 69 | | | | 0.10 | 0.27 | 0.61 | 0.07 | 0.50 | 22.3 | 0.69 | 2.5 | | | 179 | 0.1 | 0.7 | 22 | 0.2 | 154 | 310 | | 1004 | 0.62 |
| 50196 | 1 cup | Creamy, prep w/water, avg | 244 | 107 | 90 | 2.8 | 12.7 | 1.0 | | | 5.3 | 1.5 | 2.1 | 1.5 | 0.10 | 1.34 | 15 | 295 | 29 | | | | 0.05 | 0.08 | 0.50 | 0.02 | 0.05 | 6.8 | 0.29 | 1.2 | | | 34 | 0.1 | 0.6 | 5 | 0.2 | 37 | 120 | | 927 | 0.15 |
| 50486 | 1/2 cup | French, cond, Campbell's | 126 | 70 | 86 | 2.0 | 10.0 | 1.0 | 5.0 | 4.0 | 2.5 | 0.0 | | | | | 5 | 0 | 0 | 0 | 0 | 0 | | | | | | | | 2.4 | | | 20 | | 0.4 | | | | | | 980 | |
| 50294 | 8 oz | French, prep w/water, Corn Products Company | 227 | 67 | 92 | 2.7 | 12.0 | | | | 1.3 | | | | | | | | | | | | | | | | | | | | | | | | 0.5 | | | | 187 | | 868 | |
| | | Oyster Stew | | | | | | | | | | | | | | | | | | | | | | | | | | | | | | | | | | | | | | | | |
| 50670 | 1/2 cup | Condensed, avg | 123 | 59 | 90 | 2.1 | 4.1 | 0.0 | 0.4 | 3.7 | 3.8 | 2.5 | 0.9 | 0.2 | 0.02 | 0.12 | 14 | 71 | 7 | | | | 0.02 | 0.04 | 0.23 | 0.01 | 2.20 | 2.5 | 0.12 | 3.2 | 2.0 | | 22 | 1.6 | 1.0 | 5 | 0.4 | 48 | 49 | 8.4 | 984 | 10.33 |
| 50024 | 1 cup | Prepared, w/milk, avg | 245 | 135 | 89 | 6.1 | 9.8 | 0.0 | 6.4 | 3.3 | 7.9 | 5.0 | 2.1 | 0.3 | 0.07 | 0.22 | 32 | 225 | 44 | 34 | 10 | | 0.07 | 0.23 | 0.34 | 0.06 | 2.62 | 9.8 | 0.49 | 4.4 | 3.5 | | 167 | 1.6 | 1.1 | 20 | 0.4 | 162 | 235 | 33.1 | 1041 | 10.34 |
| 50115 | 1 cup | Prepared, w/water, avg | 241 | 58 | 95 | 2.1 | 4.1 | 0.0 | 0.4 | 3.7 | 3.8 | 2.5 | 0.9 | 0.2 | 0.02 | 0.12 | 14 | 70 | 7 | | | | 0.02 | 0.04 | 0.23 | 0.01 | 2.19 | 2.4 | 0.12 | 3.1 | 1.9 | | 22 | 1.6 | 1.0 | 5 | 0.4 | 48 | 48 | | 981 | 10.29 |
| | | Pasta Soups | | | | | | | | | | | | | | | | | | | | | | | | | | | | | | | | | | | | | | | | |
| 50627 | 1 cup | Bolognese, fat free, Health Valley | 240 | 70 | 90 | 5.0 | 17.0 | 7.0 | 8.0 | 2.0 | 0.0 | 0.0 | 0.0 | 0.0 | 0.00 | 0.00 | 0 | 2000 | 400 | | | | | | | | | | | 6.0 | | | 40 | | 0.2 | | | | | | 135 | |
| 50626 | 1 cup | Cacciatore, fat free, Health Valley | 240 | 90 | 88 | 6.0 | 19.0 | 4.0 | 4.0 | 11.0 | 0.0 | 0.0 | 0.0 | 0.0 | 0.00 | 0.00 | 0 | 2000 | 400 | | | | | | | | | | | 15.0 | | | 40 | | 2.7 | | | | | | 210 | |
| 50624 | 1 cup | Fagioli, fat free, Health Valley | 240 | 80 | 90 | 6.0 | 17.0 | 4.0 | 8.0 | 5.0 | 0.0 | 0.0 | 0.0 | 0.0 | 0.00 | 0.00 | 0 | 2000 | 400 | | | | | | | | | | | 15.0 | | | 40 | | 0.2 | | | | | | 250 | |
| 50625 | 1 cup | Primavera, fat free, Health Valley | 240 | 80 | 87 | 8.0 | 21.0 | 11.0 | 6.0 | 4.0 | 0.0 | 0.0 | 0.0 | 0.0 | 0.00 | 0.00 | 0 | 2000 | 400 | | | | | | | | | | | 4.8 | | | 40 | | 0.4 | | | | | | 210 | |
| 50628 | 1 cup | Romano, fat free, Health Valley | 240 | 140 | 81 | 10.0 | 32.0 | 13.0 | 9.0 | 10.0 | 0.0 | 0.0 | 0.0 | 0.0 | 0.00 | 0.00 | 0 | 2000 | 400 | | | | | | | | | | | 12.0 | | | 80 | | 5.4 | | | | | | 250 | |
| 50623 | 1 cup | Rotini Vegetable, fat free, Health Valley | 240 | 100 | 89 | 4.0 | 20.0 | 4.0 | 4.0 | 12.0 | 0.0 | 0.0 | 0.0 | 0.0 | 0.00 | 0.00 | 0 | 1000 | 200 | | | | | | | | | | | 12.0 | | | 4 | | 2.7 | | | | | | 290 | |
| 50490 | 1/2 cup | Vegetable, cond, Campbell's | 126 | 90 | 82 | 2.0 | 18.0 | 2.0 | 8.0 | 8.0 | 1.0 | 0.0 | | | | | 0 | 2250 | 225 | 0 | 225 | 1350 | | | | | | | | 0.0 | | | 20 | | 0.7 | | | | | | 830 | |
| | | Pea Soup | | | | | | | | | | | | | | | | | | | | | | | | | | | | | | | | | | | | | | | | |
| 50671 | 1/2 cup | Green, cond, avg | 132 | 165 | 68 | 8.6 | 26.7 | 2.9 | 4.1 | 19.7 | 2.9 | 1.4 | 1.0 | 0.4 | 0.04 | 0.34 | 0 | 202 | 20 | 0 | 20 | | 0.11 | 0.07 | 1.24 | 0.05 | 0.00 | 1.8 | 0.13 | 1.7 | 0.0 | | 28 | 0.4 | 2.0 | 40 | 0.7 | 125 | 191 | 9.8 | 921 | 1.72 |
| 50185 | 1 cup | Green, low sod, prep w/water, avg | 250 | 165 | 84 | 8.5 | 26.5 | 0.8 | 4.0 | 21.8 | 3.0 | 1.4 | 1.0 | 0.4 | | | 0 | 203 | 20 | 0 | 20 | | 0.10 | 0.07 | 1.25 | 0.05 | 0.00 | 2.5 | | 1.8 | 0.0 | | 28 | 0.4 | 1.9 | 40 | | 125 | 190 | | 25 | 1.70 |
| 50117 | 1 cup | Green, prep w/milk, avg | 254 | 239 | 78 | 12.6 | 32.3 | 2.8 | 10.2 | 19.3 | 7.0 | 4.0 | 2.2 | 0.5 | 0.10 | 0.43 | 18 | 356 | 58 | 38 | 20 | | 0.15 | 0.27 | 1.34 | 0.10 | 0.43 | 7.9 | 0.56 | 2.8 | 1.2 | | 173 | 0.4 | 2.0 | 56 | 0.7 | 239 | 376 | 3.2 | 970 | 1.76 |
| 50050 | 1 cup | Green, prep w/water, avg | 250 | 165 | 84 | 8.6 | 26.5 | 2.8 | 4.0 | 19.8 | 2.9 | 1.4 | 1.0 | 0.4 | 0.05 | 0.33 | 0 | 203 | 20 | 0 | 20 | | 0.11 | 0.07 | 1.24 | 0.05 | 0.00 | 1.8 | 0.13 | 1.8 | 0.0 | | 28 | 0.4 | 1.9 | 40 | 0.7 | 125 | 190 | 9.3 | 918 | 1.71 |
| 50122 | 1 cup | Pepper Pot Soup, avg | 241 | 104 | 90 | 6.4 | 9.4 | 0.5 | 1.2 | 7.7 | 4.6 | 2.0 | 2.0 | 0.4 | 0.05 | 0.31 | 10 | 865 | 87 | | | | 0.05 | 0.05 | 1.22 | 0.06 | 0.17 | 9.6 | 0.34 | 1.4 | 0.0 | | 24 | 0.1 | 0.9 | 5 | 0.6 | 41 | 152 | 4.3 | 971 | 1.22 |
| 50673 | 1/2 cup | Pepper Pot Soup, cond, avg | 123 | 103 | 81 | 6.4 | 9.4 | 0.5 | 1.1 | 7.8 | 4.6 | 2.1 | 2.0 | 0.4 | 0.04 | 0.31 | 10 | 868 | 87 | | | | 0.05 | 0.05 | 1.23 | 0.06 | 0.17 | 9.8 | 0.34 | 1.4 | 0.0 | | 23 | 0.1 | 0.9 | 5 | 0.6 | 42 | 153 | | 974 | 1.23 |
| 50207 | 1 cup | Pork, Rice & Vegetable Soup, avg | 244 | 122 | 89 | 11.8 | 8.5 | 0.9 | | | 4.3 | 1.4 | 2.0 | 0.4 | | | 39 | 4934 | 494 | 1 | 493 | | 0.25 | 0.14 | 2.44 | 0.22 | 0.24 | 7.5 | | 1.3 | | | 20 | 0.1 | 1.1 | 15 | | 95 | 220 | | 603 | 1.91 |
| | | Potato Soup | | | | | | | | | | | | | | | | | | | | | | | | | | | | | | | | | | | | | | | | |
| 50674 | 1/2 cup | Cream of Potato, cond, avg | 126 | 74 | 85 | 1.8 | 11.5 | 0.5 | 0.8 | 10.2 | 2.4 | 1.2 | 0.6 | 0.4 | 0.04 | 0.38 | 6 | 290 | 29 | | | | 0.04 | 0.04 | 0.54 | 0.04 | 0.05 | 3.0 | 0.88 | 0.0 | 0.1 | | 20 | 0.3 | 0.5 | 1 | 0.4 | 47 | 137 | 2.4 | 1004 | 0.63 |
| 50266 | 1 cup | Cream of Potato, prep w/milk, Corn Products Co | 248 | 175 | 86 | 7.3 | 19.0 | | | | 7.3 | | | | | | | 146 | 29 | | | | 0.04 | 1.24 | | | | | | | | | 146 | | 1.6 | | | | 365 | | 963 | |
| 50197 | 1 cup | Cream of Potato, prep w/water, avg | 244 | 73 | 92 | 1.8 | 11.5 | 0.5 | 0.8 | 10.2 | 2.4 | 1.2 | 0.6 | 0.4 | 0.02 | 0.39 | 5 | 288 | 29 | | | | 0.03 | 0.04 | 0.54 | 0.04 | 0.05 | 2.9 | 0.83 | 0.0 | 0.1 | | 20 | 0.3 | 0.5 | 2 | 0.4 | 46 | 137 | | 1000 | 0.63 |
| 50548 | 1 cup | Ham Chowder, RTS, chunky, Campbell's | 245 | 220 | 83 | 6.0 | 16.0 | 3.0 | 1.0 | 12.0 | 14.0 | 8.0 | | | | | 20 | 0 | 0 | 0 | 0 | 0 | | | | | | | | 0.0 | | | 20 | | 1.1 | | | | | | 840 | |
| 50027 | 1 cup | Vichyssoise, avg | 248 | 149 | 87 | 5.8 | 17.2 | 0.5 | 1.8 | 14.9 | 6.4 | 3.8 | 1.7 | 0.6 | 0.10 | 0.47 | 22 | 444 | 67 | 33 | 34 | | 0.08 | 0.24 | 0.64 | 0.09 | 0.50 | 9.2 | 1.69 | 1.2 | 1.2 | | 166 | 0.3 | 0.5 | 17 | 0.4 | 161 | 322 | 2.2 | 1061 | 0.67 |
| 50216 | 1 cup | Salmon Soup, cream style, avg | 248 | 258 | 77 | 28.0 | 6.5 | 0.2 | | | 12.6 | 3.3 | 4.5 | 3.6 | | | 74 | 464 | 61 | 19 | 42 | | 0.05 | 0.29 | 9.52 | 0.39 | 5.54 | 22.6 | | 0.7 | | | 288 | 0.2 | 1.6 | 45 | | 451 | 523 | | 1535 | 1.61 |
| | | Scotch Broth Soup | | | | | | | | | | | | | | | | | | | | | | | | | | | | | | | | | | | | | | | | |
| 50675 | 1/2 cup | Condensed, avg | 123 | 81 | 84 | 5.0 | 9.5 | 1.2 | 0.9 | 7.4 | 2.6 | 1.1 | 0.8 | 0.6 | 0.09 | 0.46 | 5 | 2188 | 219 | | | | 0.02 | 0.05 | 1.17 | 0.07 | 0.27 | 9.8 | 0.34 | 0.9 | 0.0 | | 15 | 0.2 | 0.8 | 4 | 0.4 | 55 | 160 | 2.7 | 1016 | 1.60 |
| 50500 | 1/2 cup | Condensed, Campbell's | 124 | 80 | 85 | 4.0 | 9.0 | 1.0 | 0.0 | 8.0 | 3.0 | 1.5 | | | | | 5 | 2500 | 500 | | | | | | | | | | | 1.2 | | | 20 | | 1.4 | | | | | | 900 | |

| Code | Amount | Description | Basic Components | | | | | | | | | Additional Fats | | | | | | Vit A & Components | | | | |
|---|---|---|---|---|---|---|---|---|---|---|---|---|---|---|---|---|---|---|---|---|---|---|
| | | | Weight (g) | Calories | % Water | Protein (g) | Carbs (g) | Fiber (g) | Sugar (g) | Other Carbs (g) | Fat (g) | Sat Fat (g) | Mono Fat (g) | Poly Fat (g) | Omega 3 (g) | Omega 6 (g) | Choles (mg) | Vit A (IU) | Vit A (RE) | Retinol (RE) | Carotenoids (RE) | Beta Carotene (mcg) |
| 50124 | 1 cup | Prepared, w/water, avg | 241 | 80 | 92 | 5.0 | 9.5 | 1.2 | 0.9 | 7.4 | 2.6 | 1.1 | 0.8 | 0.6 | 0.10 | 0.46 | 5 | 2179 | 217 | | | |
| 50205 | 1 cup | Seafood Stew, avg | 252 | 169 | 83 | 20.3 | 15.3 | 2.4 | | | 2.9 | 0.3 | 1.0 | 0.6 | | | 96 | 4904 | 532 | 62 | 470 | |
| | | Shrimp Soup | | | | | | | | | | | | | | | | | | | | |
| 50676 | 1/2 cup | Cream of Shrimp, cond, avg | 126 | 91 | 85 | 2.8 | 8.2 | 0.3 | 0.6 | 7.3 | 5.2 | 3.3 | 1.5 | 0.2 | 0.07 | 0.12 | 16 | 159 | 16 | | | |
| 50127 | 1 cup | Cream of Shrimp, prep w/milk, avg | 248 | 164 | 86 | 6.8 | 13.9 | 0.2 | 6.7 | 6.9 | 9.3 | 5.3 | 2.7 | 0.3 | 0.14 | 0.27 | 35 | 312 | 55 | 50 | 5 | |
| 50128 | 1 cup | Cream of Shrimp, prep w/water, avg | 244 | 90 | 92 | 2.8 | 8.2 | 0.2 | | | 5.2 | 3.2 | 1.5 | 0.2 | 0.07 | 0.12 | 17 | 159 | 15 | | | |
| 50217 | 1 cup | Gumbo, avg | 244 | 151 | 85 | 9.6 | 18.2 | 3.7 | | | 4.9 | 1.0 | 1.9 | 0.6 | | | 49 | 1171 | 151 | 52 | 99 | |
| | | Split Pea Soup | | | | | | | | | | | | | | | | | | | | |
| 50590 | 8 oz | RTS, low sod, Campbell's | 227 | 179 | 82 | 8.9 | 28.3 | 3.7 | 4.5 | 20.1 | 3.0 | 2.2 | | | | | 4 | 930 | 136 | | | |
| 50424 | 1 cup | RTS, Progresso | 244 | 170 | 83 | 10.0 | 25.0 | 5.0 | 4.0 | 16.0 | 3.0 | 1.0 | 1.5 | 0.5 | | | 5 | 100 | 20 | | | |
| 50361 | 1 cup | With Carrots, fat free, Health Valley | 240 | 110 | 89 | 8.0 | 17.0 | 4.0 | 7.0 | 6.0 | 0.0 | 0.0 | 0.0 | 0.0 | 0.00 | 0.00 | 0 | 10000 | 2000 | | | |
| 50672 | 1/2 cup | With Ham, cond, avg | 134 | 189 | 66 | 10.3 | 27.9 | 2.3 | 3.4 | 22.2 | 4.4 | 1.3 | 1.8 | 0.6 | 0.05 | 0.58 | 8 | 444 | 44 | | | |
| 50025 | 1 cup | With Ham, prep w/water, avg | 253 | 190 | 82 | 10.3 | 28.1 | 2.3 | 3.4 | 22.4 | 4.4 | 1.3 | 1.8 | 0.6 | 0.05 | 0.58 | 8 | 445 | 46 | | | |
| 50118 | 1 cup | With Ham, RTS, chunky, avg | 240 | 185 | 81 | 11.1 | 26.9 | 4.1 | 3.2 | 19.6 | 4.0 | 1.5 | 1.6 | 0.6 | 0.05 | 0.53 | 7 | 4872 | 437 | | | |
| 50565 | 1 cup | With Ham, RTS, Healthy Request | 245 | 170 | 81 | 10.0 | 29.0 | 4.0 | 7.0 | 18.0 | 1.5 | 0.5 | | | | | 10 | 2250 | 450 | | | |
| 50436 | 1 cup | With Ham, RTS, Progresso | 243 | 160 | 85 | 9.0 | 20.0 | 5.0 | 1.0 | 14.0 | 4.0 | 1.5 | 2.0 | 0.5 | | | 15 | 1250 | 250 | | | |
| 50501 | 1/2 cup | With Ham & Bacon, cond, Campbell's | 128 | 180 | 65 | 10.0 | 28.0 | 5.0 | 4.0 | 19.0 | 3.5 | 2.0 | | | | | 5 | 500 | 100 | | | |
| 50677 | 1/2 cup | Stock Pot Soup, cond, avg | 128 | 100 | 82 | 4.9 | 11.5 | 0.5 | | | 3.9 | 0.9 | 1.0 | 1.8 | 0.13 | 1.60 | 4 | 3968 | 397 | | | |
| 50130 | 1 cup | Stock Pot Soup, prep w/water, avg | 248 | 99 | 91 | 4.9 | 11.5 | 0.5 | | | 3.9 | 0.9 | 1.0 | 1.8 | 0.12 | 1.61 | 5 | 3995 | 399 | | | |
| 50209 | 1 cup | Sweet & Sour Soup, avg | 244 | 73 | 91 | 3.3 | 15.1 | 1.9 | | | 0.8 | 0.3 | 0.3 | 0.1 | | | 5 | 309 | 31 | 0 | 31 | |
| | | Tomato Soup | | | | | | | | | | | | | | | | | | | | |
| 50678 | 1/2 cup | Beef Noodle, cond, avg | 126 | 141 | 74 | 4.5 | 21.3 | 1.5 | | | 4.3 | 1.6 | 1.7 | 0.7 | 0.09 | 0.58 | 4 | 536 | 53 | | | |
| 50132 | 1 cup | Beef Noodle, prep w/water, avg | 244 | 139 | 87 | 4.5 | 21.2 | 1.5 | | | 4.3 | 1.6 | 1.7 | 0.7 | 0.10 | 0.59 | 5 | 534 | 54 | | | |
| 50687 | 1/2 cup | Bisque, cond, avg | 128 | 123 | 75 | 2.3 | 23.7 | 1.0 | 14.8 | 7.8 | 2.5 | 0.5 | 0.7 | 1.1 | 0.14 | 0.96 | 5 | 719 | 72 | 0 | 72 | |
| 50134 | 1 cup | Bisque, prep w/milk, avg | 251 | 198 | 82 | 6.3 | 29.4 | 0.5 | 21.0 | 7.9 | 6.6 | 3.1 | 1.9 | 1.2 | 0.20 | 1.03 | 23 | 879 | 110 | 34 | 76 | |
| 50135 | 1 cup | Bisque, prep w/water, avg | 247 | 124 | 87 | 2.3 | 23.7 | 0.5 | 14.8 | 8.4 | 2.5 | 0.5 | 0.7 | 1.1 | 0.15 | 0.96 | 5 | 721 | 72 | 0 | 72 | |
| 50688 | 1/2 cup | Condensed, avg | 126 | 86 | 81 | 2.1 | 16.6 | 0.5 | 8.8 | 7.4 | 1.9 | 0.4 | 0.4 | 1.0 | 0.16 | 0.79 | 0 | 699 | 71 | 0 | 71 | |
| 50520 | 1/2 cup | Condensed, Healthy Request | 124 | 90 | 81 | 1.0 | 18.0 | 1.0 | 11.0 | 6.0 | 1.5 | 0.5 | | | | | 0 | 400 | 40 | 0 | 40 | 240 |
| 50485 | 1/2 cup | Fiesta, cond, Campbell's | 126 | 70 | 84 | 1.0 | 16.0 | 1.0 | 8.0 | 7.0 | 0.0 | 0.0 | 0.0 | 0.0 | 0.00 | 0.00 | 0 | 400 | 40 | 0 | 40 | 240 |
| 50580 | 8 oz | Garden, RTS, Campbell's | 227 | 112 | 87 | 3.7 | 20.1 | 3.0 | 9.7 | 7.4 | 3.0 | 1.5 | | | | | 4 | 1861 | 136 | 0 | 186 | 1116 |
| 50408 | 1 cup | Garden, RTS, Progresso | 245 | 98 | 88 | 3.5 | 19.0 | 4.0 | | | 1.0 | 0.2 | 0.5 | 0.3 | 0.02 | 0.32 | 0 | 1348 | 135 | 0 | 135 | |
| 50012 | 1 cup | Prepared, w/milk, avg | 248 | 161 | 85 | 6.1 | 22.3 | 2.7 | 14.9 | 4.7 | 6.0 | 2.9 | 1.6 | 1.1 | 0.22 | 0.89 | 17 | 848 | 109 | 36 | 73 | |
| 50028 | 1 cup | Prepared, w/water, avg | 244 | 85 | 90 | 2.0 | 16.6 | 0.5 | 8.8 | 7.3 | 1.9 | 0.4 | 0.4 | 1.0 | 0.17 | 0.78 | 0 | 688 | 58 | 0 | 68 | |
| 50679 | 1/2 cup | Rice, cond, avg | 128 | 119 | 77 | 2.1 | 21.9 | 1.7 | 9.9 | 10.4 | 2.7 | 0.5 | 0.6 | 1.3 | 0.23 | 1.11 | 1 | 753 | 76 | | | |
| 50137 | 1 cup | Rice, prep w/water, avg | 247 | 119 | 88 | 2.1 | 21.9 | 1.5 | 9.9 | 10.6 | 2.7 | 0.5 | 0.6 | 1.4 | 0.22 | 1.11 | 2 | 756 | 77 | | | |
| 50393 | 1 cup | Rotini, RTS, Progresso | 239 | 90 | 90 | 4.0 | 16.0 | 3.0 | 5.0 | 8.0 | 1.0 | 0.0 | 0.5 | 0.0 | 0.00 | 0.00 | 5 | 500 | 100 | | | |
| 50711 | 1 cup | RTS, low sod, avg | 240 | 84 | 90 | 1.9 | 16.3 | 0.5 | | | 1.9 | 0.4 | 0.4 | 0.9 | | | 0 | 677 | 57 | 0 | 67 | |
| 50591 | 8 oz | RTS, low sod, Campbell's | 227 | 129 | 86 | 3.0 | 21.3 | 1.5 | 12.9 | 6.9 | 4.6 | 1.9 | | | | | 8 | 952 | 95 | 0 | 95 | 571 |
| 50437 | 1 cup | RTS, Progresso | 241 | 90 | 90 | 3.0 | 15.0 | 4.0 | 8.0 | 3.0 | 2.0 | 0.0 | 0.5 | 1.5 | | | 0 | 1500 | 300 | | | |
| 50397 | 1 cup | Tortellini, RTS, Progresso | 239 | 120 | 89 | 5.0 | 13.0 | 2.0 | 5.0 | 6.0 | 5.0 | 1.5 | 2.5 | 1.0 | | | 10 | 1500 | 300 | | | |
| 50360 | 1 cup | Vegetable, fat free, Health Valley | 240 | 80 | 90 | 6.0 | 17.0 | 5.0 | 9.0 | 3.0 | 0.0 | 0.0 | 0.0 | 0.0 | 0.00 | 0.00 | 0 | 10000 | 2000 | | | |
| 50566 | 1 cup | Vegetable, RTS, Healthy Request | 245 | 120 | 87 | 4.0 | 22.0 | 3.0 | 9.0 | 10.0 | 2.0 | 0.5 | | | | | 5 | 4500 | 450 | 0 | 450 | 2700 |
| 50422 | 1 cup | Tortellini Soup, RTS, Progresso | 238 | 210 | 84 | 5.0 | 15.0 | 0.0 | 0.0 | 15.0 | 15.0 | 8.0 | 4.0 | 1.5 | | | 30 | 1000 | 200 | | | |
| | | Turkey Soup | | | | | | | | | | | | | | | | | | | | |
| 50138 | 1 cup | Chunky, RTS, avg | 236 | 135 | 86 | 10.2 | 14.1 | 1.0 | 2.1 | 11.0 | 4.4 | 1.2 | 1.8 | 1.1 | 0.05 | 1.04 | 9 | 7156 | 715 | | | |
| 50680 | 1/2 cup | Noodle, cond, avg | 126 | 69 | 86 | 3.9 | 8.7 | 0.8 | 0.8 | 7.2 | 2.0 | 0.6 | 0.8 | 0.5 | 0.03 | 0.47 | 5 | 294 | 29 | | | |
| 50141 | 1 cup | Noodle, prep w/water, avg | 244 | 68 | 93 | 3.9 | 8.6 | 0.7 | 0.7 | 7.2 | 2.0 | 0.6 | 0.8 | 0.5 | 0.02 | 0.45 | 5 | 293 | 29 | | | |
| 50681 | 1/2 cup | Vegetable, cond, avg | 123 | 74 | 86 | 3.1 | 8.7 | 0.6 | 1.0 | 7.0 | 3.0 | 0.9 | 1.3 | 0.7 | 0.04 | 0.62 | 1 | 2455 | 246 | | | |
| 50143 | 1 cup | Vegetable, prep w/water, avg | 241 | 72 | 93 | 3.1 | 8.6 | 0.5 | 1.1 | 7.1 | 3.0 | 0.9 | 1.3 | 0.7 | 0.05 | 0.63 | 2 | 2444 | 243 | | | |
| 50567 | 1 cup | Vegetable & Wild Rice, RTS, Healthy Request | 245 | 120 | 87 | 7.0 | 17.0 | 2.0 | 3.0 | 12.0 | 2.5 | 1.0 | | | | | 15 | 6000 | 1200 | | | |
| 50212 | 1 cup | Turtle Vegetable Soup, avg | 244 | 117 | 90 | 12.9 | 4.3 | 0.7 | | | 4.2 | 0.9 | 1.1 | 1.7 | | | 59 | 241 | 42 | 26 | 15 | |
| 50201 | 1 cup | Veal Stew, avg | 252 | 192 | 83 | 16.1 | 15.9 | 2.6 | | | 6.8 | 2.8 | 2.6 | 0.6 | | | 55 | 6144 | 615 | 0 | 615 | |
| | | Vegetable Soup | | | | | | | | | | | | | | | | | | | | |
| 50357 | 1 cup | Barley, fat free, Health Valley | 240 | 90 | 89 | 6.0 | 19.0 | 4.0 | 4.0 | 11.0 | 0.0 | 0.0 | 0.0 | 0.0 | 0.00 | 0.00 | 0 | 10000 | 2000 | | | |
| 50709 | 1 cup | Broth, bouillon, avg | 235 | 16 | 95 | 2.0 | 2.0 | 0.0 | | | 0.0 | 0.0 | 0.0 | 0.0 | 0.00 | 0.00 | 0 | 7 | 1 | | | |
| 50599 | 1 cup | Broth, Swanson | 235 | 20 | 95 | 2.0 | 3.0 | 0.0 | 3.0 | 0.0 | 1.0 | 0.0 | | | | | 0 | 200 | 20 | 0 | 20 | 120 |
| 50144 | 1 cup | Chunky, RTS, avg | 240 | 122 | 88 | 3.5 | 19.0 | 1.2 | 6.6 | 11.2 | 3.7 | 0.6 | 1.6 | 1.4 | 0.10 | 1.30 | 0 | 5878 | 588 | 0 | 583 | |
| 50508 | 1/2 cup | Condensed, Campbell's | 126 | 90 | 82 | 3.0 | 16.0 | 2.0 | 5.0 | 9.0 | 1.0 | 0.5 | | | | | 5 | 3000 | 300 | 0 | 300 | 1800 |
| 50518 | 1/2 cup | Condensed, Healthy Request | 126 | 90 | 83 | 3.0 | 16.0 | 2.0 | 4.0 | 10.0 | 1.0 | 0.5 | | | | | 5 | 3000 | 600 | | | |
| 50365 | 1 cup | Fat Free, Health Valley | 240 | 80 | 90 | 6.0 | 17.0 | 4.0 | 8.0 | 5.0 | 0.0 | 0.0 | 0.0 | 0.0 | 0.00 | 0.00 | 0 | 10000 | 2000 | | | |
| 50186 | 1 cup | Low Sodium, avg | 241 | 82 | 92 | 2.4 | 12.8 | 0.8 | | | 2.4 | 0.4 | 1.1 | 0.9 | | | 0 | 3955 | 396 | 0 | 395 | |
| 50562 | 1 cup | RTS, Healthy Request | 245 | 100 | 88 | 3.0 | 20.0 | 2.0 | 6.0 | 12.0 | 1.0 | 0.0 | | | | | 0 | 5000 | 500 | 0 | 500 | 3000 |
| 50383 | 1 cup | RTS, Progresso | 238 | 90 | 90 | 4.0 | 15.0 | 3.0 | 4.0 | 8.0 | 2.0 | 0.5 | 1.0 | 0.5 | | | 2 | 3500 | 700 | | | |
| 50682 | 1/2 cup | Vegetarian, cond, avg | 123 | 73 | 85 | 2.1 | 12.0 | 0.6 | 4.2 | 7.2 | 1.9 | 0.3 | 0.8 | 0.7 | 0.05 | 0.68 | 0 | 3017 | 301 | 0 | 301 | |
| 50013 | 1 cup | Vegetarian, prep w/water, avg | 241 | 72 | 92 | 2.1 | 12.0 | 0.5 | 4.3 | 7.2 | 1.9 | 0.3 | 0.8 | 0.7 | 0.05 | 0.67 | 0 | 3005 | 301 | | | |
| 50446 | 8 oz | Weight Watchers | 227 | 99 | 89 | 3.1 | 20.6 | 4.6 | 8.4 | 7.6 | 0.8 | 0.0 | | | | | 0 | 2669 | 534 | | | |
| 50684 | 1/2 cup | With Beef Broth, cond, avg | 123 | 81 | 83 | 3.0 | 13.2 | 1.6 | 3.0 | 8.6 | 1.9 | 0.4 | 0.6 | 0.8 | 0.11 | 0.68 | 1 | 2100 | 210 | | | |
| 50147 | 1 cup | With Beef Broth, prep w/water, avg | 241 | 82 | 92 | 3.0 | 13.1 | 0.5 | 2.9 | 9.7 | 1.9 | 0.4 | 0.6 | 0.8 | 0.12 | 0.67 | 2 | 2089 | 210 | | | |
| 50202 | 1 cup | Venison Stew, avg | 252 | 164 | 83 | 18.6 | 17.9 | 3.0 | | | 1.9 | 0.7 | 0.5 | 0.4 | | | 58 | 5340 | 534 | 0 | 534 | |
| 50181 | 1 cup | Won Ton Soup, avg | 241 | 188 | 83 | 14.1 | 16.0 | 0.9 | | | 7.0 | 2.2 | 3.0 | 1.0 | | | 53 | 871 | 97 | 14 | 82 | |

| Code | Vitamins | | | | | | | | | | Minerals | | | | | | | | | |
|---|---|---|---|---|---|---|---|---|---|---|---|---|---|---|---|---|---|---|---|---|
| | Thiamin (mg) | Riboflavin (mg) | Niacin (NE) | Vit B6 (mg) | Vit B12 (mcg) | Folate (mcg) | Panto (mg) | Vit C (mg) | Vit D (mg) | Vit E (α TE) | Calcium (mg) | Copper (mg) | Iron (mg) | Magnes (mg) | Mang (mg) | Phos (mg) | Potassium (mg) | Selenium (mcg) | Sodium (mg) | Zinc (mg) |
| 50124 | 0.02 | 0.05 | 1.16 | 0.07 | 0.27 | 9.6 | 0.24 | 1.0 | 0.0 | | 14 | 0.2 | 0.8 | 5 | 0.4 | 55 | 159 | 4.3 | 1012 | 1.59 |
| 50205 | 0.18 | 0.21 | 3.47 | 0.34 | 24.33 | 34.5 | | 31.2 | | | 81 | 0.5 | 9.4 | 45 | | 222 | 811 | | 935 | 1.84 |
| 50676 | 0.02 | 0.03 | 0.43 | 0.04 | 0.59 | 3.8 | 0.14 | 0.0 | 0.3 | | 18 | 0.1 | 0.5 | 9 | 0.4 | 33 | 59 | 5.7 | 930 | 0.76 |
| 50127 | 0.06 | 0.23 | 0.53 | 0.45 | 1.04 | 9.9 | 0.55 | 1.2 | 1.6 | | 164 | 0.1 | 0.6 | 22 | 0.4 | 146 | 248 | 7.9 | 1037 | 0.80 |
| 50128 | 0.02 | 0.03 | 0.43 | 0.05 | 0.59 | 3.7 | 0.15 | 0.0 | | | 17 | 0.1 | 0.5 | 10 | 0.4 | 32 | 59 | 5.6 | 975 | 0.75 |
| 50217 | 0.14 | 0.10 | 2.45 | 0.20 | 0.30 | 58.8 | | 26.2 | | | 98 | 0.3 | 2.8 | 51 | | 129 | 522 | | 530 | 0.95 |
| 50590 | | | | | | | | 0.0 | | | 30 | | 1.3 | | | | | | 37 | |
| 50424 | | | | | | | | 0.0 | | | 0 | | 2.7 | | | | | | 870 | |
| 50361 | 0.10 | 0.16 | 5.63 | 0.45 | | | | 9.0 | | | 40 | | 5.4 | | | | 439 | | 230 | |
| 50672 | 0.15 | 0.08 | 1.47 | 0.07 | 0.27 | 2.5 | 0.27 | 1.5 | 0.0 | | 21 | 0.4 | 2.3 | 48 | 0.7 | 213 | 398 | 9.9 | 1035 | 1.32 |
| 50025 | 0.15 | 0.08 | 1.47 | 0.07 | 0.25 | 2.5 | 0.25 | 1.5 | 0.0 | | 23 | 0.4 | 2.3 | 48 | 0.7 | 213 | 400 | | 1037 | 1.32 |
| 50118 | 0.12 | 0.09 | 2.52 | 0.22 | 0.24 | 4.6 | 0.48 | 7.0 | 0.0 | | 34 | 0.2 | 2.1 | 38 | 0.6 | 178 | 305 | 9.8 | 955 | 3.12 |
| 50565 | | | | | | | | 1.2 | | | 20 | | 1.8 | | | | | | 430 | |
| 50436 | | | | | | | | 2.4 | | | 40 | | 1.8 | | | | | | 880 | |
| 50501 | | | | | | | | 0.0 | | | 20 | | 1.8 | | | | | | 850 | |
| 50677 | 0.04 | 0.05 | 1.22 | 0.09 | 0.00 | 10.2 | 0.36 | 2.0 | 0.0 | | 22 | 0.1 | 0.9 | 4 | 0.3 | 54 | 237 | | 1044 | 1.15 |
| 50130 | 0.04 | 0.05 | 1.23 | 0.09 | 0.00 | 9.9 | 0.35 | 2.0 | 0.0 | | 22 | 0.1 | 0.9 | 5 | 0.3 | 55 | 238 | | 1052 | 1.16 |
| 50209 | 0.09 | 0.07 | 0.92 | 0.11 | 0.03 | 17.2 | | 18.8 | | | 29 | 0.1 | 0.7 | 17 | | 49 | 278 | | 1322 | 0.36 |
| 50678 | 0.08 | 0.09 | 1.88 | 0.09 | 0.19 | 18.9 | 0.19 | 0.0 | 0.0 | | 18 | 0.1 | 1.1 | 8 | 0.3 | 57 | 222 | 5.0 | 921 | 0.76 |
| 50132 | 0.08 | 0.09 | 1.87 | 0.09 | 0.20 | 19.5 | 0.20 | 0.0 | 0.0 | | 17 | 0.1 | 1.1 | 7 | 0.3 | 56 | 220 | 4.9 | 917 | 0.75 |
| 50687 | 0.07 | 0.07 | 1.14 | 0.09 | 0.00 | 15.4 | 0.13 | 5.9 | 0.0 | | 40 | 0.1 | 0.8 | 9 | 0.3 | 60 | 416 | | 1044 | 0.58 |
| 50134 | 0.11 | 0.27 | 1.25 | 0.14 | 0.43 | 21.3 | 0.50 | 7.0 | 1.2 | | 186 | 0.1 | 0.9 | 25 | 0.3 | 173 | 605 | 3.2 | 1109 | 0.63 |
| 50135 | 0.07 | 0.07 | 1.15 | 0.09 | 0.00 | 14.8 | 0.12 | 5.9 | 0.0 | | 40 | 0.1 | 0.8 | 10 | 0.3 | 59 | 417 | | 1047 | 0.59 |
| 50688 | 0.09 | 0.05 | 1.42 | 0.11 | 0.00 | 14.7 | 0.15 | 66.8 | 0.0 | | 14 | 0.3 | 1.8 | 8 | 0.3 | 34 | 265 | 0.5 | 698 | 0.24 |
| 50520 | | | | | | | | 24.0 | | | 0 | | 0.4 | | | | | | 450 | |
| 50485 | | | | | | | | 6.0 | | | 20 | | 0.7 | | | | | | 850 | |
| 50580 | | | | | | | | 0.9 | | | 74 | | 1.1 | | | | | | 670 | |
| 50408 | 0.17 | 0.10 | 1.59 | 0.11 | 0.00 | 24.5 | 0.46 | 4.4 | | | 56 | 0.1 | 1.6 | 29 | 0.2 | 66 | 304 | 4.4 | 480 | 0.47 |
| 50012 | 0.13 | 0.25 | 1.52 | 0.16 | 0.45 | 20.8 | 0.55 | 67.7 | 1.2 | | 159 | 0.3 | 1.8 | 22 | 0.3 | 149 | 449 | 2.2 | 744 | 0.29 |
| 50028 | 0.09 | 0.05 | 1.42 | 0.11 | 0.00 | 14.6 | 0.15 | 66.4 | 0.0 | | 12 | 0.3 | 1.8 | 7 | 0.3 | 34 | 264 | 0.5 | 695 | 0.24 |
| 50679 | 0.06 | 0.05 | 1.05 | 0.08 | 0.00 | 14.1 | 0.13 | 14.7 | 0.0 | | 23 | 0.1 | 0.8 | 5 | 0.4 | 33 | 329 | 2.3 | 813 | 0.51 |
| 50137 | 0.06 | 0.05 | 1.05 | 0.08 | 0.00 | 13.6 | 0.12 | 14.8 | 0.0 | | 22 | 0.1 | 0.8 | 5 | 0.4 | 35 | 331 | 2.2 | 815 | 0.51 |
| 50393 | | | | | | | | 3.6 | | | 60 | | 1.8 | | | | | | 820 | |
| 50711 | 0.10 | 0.05 | 1.39 | 0.12 | 0.00 | 14.4 | | 65.3 | | | 12 | 0.2 | 1.7 | 7 | | 34 | 259 | | 48 | 0.24 |
| 50591 | | | | | | | | 27.4 | | | 30 | | 1.1 | | | | | | 46 | |
| 50437 | | | | | | | | 0.1 | | | 20 | | 1.8 | | | | | | 930 | |
| 50397 | | | | | | | | 1.2 | | | 60 | | 1.8 | | | | | | 910 | |
| 50360 | 0.10 | 0.08 | 2.25 | 0.14 | | 0.4 | | 9.0 | | | 40 | | 5.4 | | | | 608 | | 240 | |
| 50566 | | | | | | | | 4.8 | | | 60 | | 1.1 | | | | | | 480 | |
| 50422 | | | | | | | | 0.0 | | | 150 | | 1.4 | | | | | | 880 | |
| 50138 | 0.04 | 0.11 | 3.59 | 0.31 | 2.12 | 11.1 | 0.92 | 6.4 | 0.0 | | 50 | 0.2 | 1.9 | 24 | 0.2 | 104 | 361 | | 923 | 2.12 |
| 50680 | 0.07 | 0.06 | 1.40 | 0.04 | 0.16 | 18.9 | 0.18 | 0.1 | 0.0 | | 11 | 0.1 | 0.9 | 5 | 0.3 | 48 | 76 | 11.2 | 819 | 0.58 |
| 50141 | 0.07 | 0.06 | 1.40 | 0.04 | 0.15 | 19.5 | 0.17 | 0.2 | 0.0 | | 12 | 0.1 | 1.0 | 5 | 0.3 | 49 | 76 | 10.7 | 815 | 0.58 |
| 50681 | 0.03 | 0.04 | 1.01 | 0.05 | 0.17 | 4.9 | 0.48 | 0.0 | 0.0 | | 17 | 0.1 | 0.8 | 4 | 0.2 | 41 | 176 | 5.3 | 929 | 0.62 |
| 50143 | 0.03 | 0.04 | 1.00 | 0.05 | 0.17 | 4.8 | 0.48 | 0.0 | 0.0 | | 17 | 0.1 | 0.8 | 5 | 0.2 | 41 | 176 | | 906 | 0.61 |
| 50567 | | | | | | | | 2.4 | | | 40 | | 0.7 | | | | | | 480 | |
| 50212 | 0.08 | 0.16 | 1.61 | 0.10 | 0.56 | 17.5 | | 6.8 | | | 68 | 0.1 | 1.2 | 17 | | 117 | 281 | | 473 | 0.59 |
| 50201 | 0.14 | 0.23 | 6.91 | 0.40 | 0.55 | 25.6 | | 11.8 | | | 38 | 0.2 | 1.4 | 35 | | 192 | 547 | | 607 | 2.08 |
| 50357 | | | | | | | | 15.0 | | | 40 | | | | | | | | 210 | |
| 50709 | 0.00 | 0.02 | 0.54 | 0.02 | 0.12 | 3.8 | | 0.0 | | 0.0 | 7 | 0.0 | 0.1 | 7 | | 38 | 54 | | 3114 | 0.00 |
| 50599 | | | | | | | | 0.0 | | | 0 | | 0.0 | | | | | | 1000 | |
| 50144 | 0.07 | 0.06 | 1.20 | 0.19 | 0.00 | 16.6 | 0.34 | 6.0 | 0.0 | | 55 | 0.2 | 1.6 | 7 | 0.5 | 72 | 396 | 7.0 | 1010 | 3.12 |
| 50508 | | | | | | | | 1.2 | | | 20 | | 0.7 | | | | | | 820 | |
| 50518 | | | | | | | | 2.4 | | | 20 | | 0.7 | | | | | | 480 | |
| 50365 | 0.26 | 0.08 | 2.25 | 0.18 | | 27.0 | | 15.0 | | | 40 | | 1.8 | | | | 406 | | 250 | |
| 50186 | 0.05 | 0.05 | 0.81 | 0.13 | 0.00 | 11.3 | | 4.0 | 0.0 | | 39 | 0.2 | 1.1 | 5 | | 22 | 268 | | 43 | 2.12 |
| 50562 | | | | | | | | 0.0 | | | 40 | | 1.1 | | | | | | 470 | |
| 50383 | | | | | | | | 1.2 | | | 40 | | 1.4 | | | | | | 850 | |
| 50682 | 0.05 | 0.05 | 0.92 | 0.06 | 0.00 | 10.6 | 0.34 | 1.5 | 0.0 | | 21 | 0.1 | 1.1 | 7 | 0.5 | 34 | 210 | 4.3 | 827 | 0.46 |
| 50013 | 0.05 | 0.05 | 0.92 | 0.06 | 0.00 | 10.6 | 0.34 | 1.4 | 0.0 | | 22 | 0.1 | 1.1 | 7 | 0.5 | 34 | 210 | 4.3 | 822 | 0.46 |
| 50446 | | | | | | | | 1.8 | | | 61 | | 1.4 | | | | 381 | | 519 | |
| 50684 | 0.05 | 0.05 | 0.97 | 0.06 | 0.00 | 10.5 | 0.34 | 2.3 | 0.0 | | 17 | 0.2 | 1.0 | 6 | 0.3 | 39 | 193 | 2.7 | 813 | 0.80 |
| 50147 | 0.05 | 0.05 | 0.97 | 0.06 | 0.00 | 9.6 | 0.34 | 2.4 | 0.0 | | 17 | 0.2 | 1.0 | 7 | 0.3 | 39 | 193 | 2.7 | 810 | 0.80 |
| 50202 | 0.22 | 0.40 | 5.59 | 0.39 | 3.21 | 30.3 | | 26.8 | | | 30 | 0.4 | 3.5 | 45 | | 207 | 766 | | 678 | 2.03 |
| 50181 | 0.42 | 0.27 | 4.67 | 0.19 | 0.40 | 19.1 | | 3.2 | | | 31 | 0.1 | 1.9 | 22 | | 154 | 313 | | 759 | 1.12 |

| Code | Amount | Description | Basic Components | | | | | | | | | Additional Fats | | | | | |
|---|---|---|---|---|---|---|---|---|---|---|---|---|---|---|---|---|---|
| | | | Weight (g) | Calories | % Water | Protein (g) | Carbs (g) | Fiber (g) | Sugar (g) | Other Carbs (g) | Fat (g) | Sat Fat (g) | Mono Fat (g) | Poly Fat (g) | Omega 3 (g) | Omega 6 (g) | Choles (mg) |
| | | *DEHYDRATED AND PREPARED SOUPS* | | | | | | | | | | | | | | | |
| 50148 | 1 ea | Asparagus Soup, cream of, dry mix, svg, avg | 14 | 51 | 5 | 1.9 | 7.8 | 0.3 | 1.8 | 5.7 | 1.5 | 0.2 | 0.6 | 0.6 | 0.04 | 0.53 | 0 |
| 50149 | 1 cup | Asparagus Soup, cream of, prep f/dry mix, avg | 251 | 58 | 94 | 2.2 | 9.0 | 0.4 | 2.0 | 6.6 | 1.7 | 0.1 | 0.8 | 0.7 | 0.05 | 0.60 | 0 |
| | | Bean Soup | | | | | | | | | | | | | | | |
| 50150 | 1 oz | Bean w/Bacon, dry mix, avg | 28 | 104 | 4 | 5.4 | 16.2 | 8.6 | 1.4 | 6.2 | 2.1 | 0.9 | 0.9 | 0.2 | 0.02 | 0.14 | 3 |
| 50151 | 1 cup | Bean w/Bacon, prep f/dry mix, avg | 265 | 106 | 90 | 5.5 | 16.4 | 9.0 | 1.6 | 5.8 | 2.1 | 1.0 | 0.9 | 0.2 | 0.03 | 0.13 | 3 |
| 50338 | 1 ea | Black Bean, soup in a cup, dry, Nile Spice | 54 | 171 | 7 | 11.3 | 35.1 | 11.5 | 3.3 | 20.3 | 1.5 | 0.2 | 0.2 | 0.9 | | | 0 |
| 50629 | 1/3 cup | Black Bean w/Couscous, fat free, dry, Health Valley | 43 | 130 | 4 | 6.0 | 29.0 | 5.0 | 3.0 | 21.0 | 0.0 | 0.0 | 0.0 | 0.0 | 0.00 | 0.00 | 0 |
| 50630 | 1/3 cup | Black Bean w/Rice, fat free, dry, Health Valley | 33 | 100 | 4 | 5.0 | 22.0 | 4.0 | 2.0 | 16.0 | 0.0 | 0.0 | 0.0 | 0.0 | 0.00 | 0.00 | 0 |
| 56836 | 1 ea | Garbanzo Couscous, dry cup, Nile Spice | 59 | 216 | 9 | 8.8 | 39.5 | 2.4 | 2.1 | 34.9 | 2.6 | 0.3 | 1.0 | 1.2 | | | 0 |
| 56842 | 1 ea | Red Beans & Rice, soup in a cup, dry, Nile Spice | 53 | 166 | 6 | 10.3 | 35.1 | 9.6 | 2.7 | 22.8 | 1.2 | 0.2 | 0.2 | 0.7 | | | 0 |
| | | Beef Soup | | | | | | | | | | | | | | | |
| 50192 | 1 ea | Bouillon, dry cube, avg | 4 | 7 | 3 | 0.7 | 0.6 | 0.0 | | | 0.2 | 0.1 | 0.1 | 0.0 | 0.00 | 0.00 | 0 |
| 50051 | 1 ea | Bouillon, dry pkt, avg | 6 | 14 | 3 | 1.0 | 1.4 | 0.0 | | | 0.5 | 0.3 | 0.2 | 0.0 | 0.00 | 0.02 | 1 |
| 50707 | 1 ea | Bouillon, low sod, dry mix, svg, avg | 6 | 16 | 2 | 1.0 | 1.1 | 0.0 | | | 0.8 | 0.2 | 0.3 | 0.3 | | | 1 |
| 50033 | 1 cup | Bouillon, prep f/dry cube, avg | 241 | 7 | 98 | 0.8 | 0.8 | 0.0 | 0.8 | 0.0 | 0.2 | 0.1 | 0.1 | 0.0 | 0.00 | 0.00 | 0 |
| 50032 | 1 cup | Bouillon, prep f/dry pkt, avg | 244 | 20 | 97 | 1.3 | 1.9 | 0.0 | 1.9 | 0.0 | 0.7 | 0.3 | 0.3 | 0.0 | 0.00 | 0.02 | 0 |
| 50165 | 1 ea | Consomme, w/gelatin, dry mix, svg, avg | 13 | 18 | 1 | 2.2 | 2.1 | 0.0 | | | 0.0 | 0.0 | 0.0 | 0.0 | 0.00 | 0.00 | 0 |
| 50166 | 1 cup | Consomme, w/gelatin, prep f/mix, avg | 249 | 17 | 95 | 2.2 | 2.1 | 0.0 | | | 0.0 | 0.0 | 0.0 | 0.0 | 0.00 | 0.00 | 0 |
| 50152 | 1 ea | Noodle, dry mix, svg, avg | 9 | 30 | 5 | 1.6 | 4.4 | 0.2 | 0.3 | 3.8 | 0.6 | 0.2 | 0.2 | 0.1 | 0.01 | 0.11 | 1 |
| 50153 | 1 cup | Noodle, prep f/mix, avg | 251 | 40 | 95 | 2.2 | 6.0 | 0.8 | 0.5 | 4.8 | 0.8 | 0.3 | 0.4 | 0.2 | 0.03 | 0.15 | 3 |
| 50178 | 1 ea | Vegetable, dry, svg, avg | 16 | 55 | 5 | 3.0 | 8.3 | 0.3 | | | 1.2 | 0.6 | 0.5 | 0.0 | 0.01 | 0.04 | 1 |
| 50044 | 1 cup | Vegetable, prep f/dry mix, avg | 253 | 53 | 94 | 2.9 | 8.0 | 0.5 | 0.9 | 6.6 | 1.1 | 0.6 | 0.5 | 0.1 | 0.00 | 0.03 | 0 |
| 50622 | 1 ea | Broccoli & Cheese Soup, cup a soup, Lipton | 16 | 70 | 15 | 2.0 | 8.0 | 1.0 | 3.0 | 4.0 | 3.0 | 1.5 | | | | | 2 |
| 50380 | 1 ea | Carrot Dill Soup, in a cup, Nile Spice | 28 | 98 | 6 | 3.6 | 18.3 | 3.6 | 5.6 | 9.1 | 2.0 | 1.1 | 0.3 | 0.1 | | | 5 |
| 50154 | 1 ea | Cauliflower Soup, dry mix, svg, avg | 19 | 68 | 4 | 2.9 | 10.8 | 0.2 | | | 1.7 | 0.3 | 0.7 | 0.6 | 0.05 | 0.60 | 0 |
| 50155 | 1 cup | Cauliflower Soup, prep f/dry mix, avg | 256 | 69 | 93 | 2.9 | 10.7 | 0.2 | | | 1.7 | 0.3 | 0.7 | 0.6 | 0.05 | 0.59 | 0 |
| 50156 | 1 ea | Celery Cream Soup, dry, svg, avg | 17 | 61 | 5 | 2.5 | 9.5 | 0.5 | 0.9 | 8.2 | 1.6 | 0.2 | 0.7 | 0.6 | 0.04 | 0.55 | 1 |
| 50157 | 1 cup | Celery Cream Soup, prep f/dry, avg | 254 | 63 | 94 | 2.6 | 9.8 | 0.5 | 0.9 | 8.4 | 1.6 | 0.3 | 0.7 | 0.6 | 0.05 | 0.56 | 0 |
| | | Chicken Soup | | | | | | | | | | | | | | | |
| 50193 | 1 ea | Bouillon, dry cube, avg | 5 | 10 | 2 | 0.7 | 1.2 | 0.0 | | | 0.2 | 0.1 | 0.1 | 0.1 | 0.00 | 0.08 | 1 |
| 50611 | 1 ea | Bouillon, dry, cup a soup, Lipton | 6 | 20 | 24 | 0.0 | 3.0 | 0.0 | 0.0 | 3.0 | 1.0 | 0.0 | | | | | 0 |
| 50034 | 1 cup | Bouillon, prep f/dry mix, avg | 244 | 22 | 97 | 1.3 | 1.4 | 0.0 | 1.4 | 0.0 | 1.1 | 0.3 | 0.4 | 0.4 | 0.00 | 0.34 | 0 |
| 50159 | 1 ea | Noodle, dry mix, svg, avg | 11 | 38 | 4 | 2.1 | 5.3 | 0.3 | 1.1 | 3.9 | 0.8 | 0.2 | 0.4 | 0.2 | 0.02 | 0.23 | 2 |
| 50608 | 1 ea | Noodle, dry, cup a soup, Lipton | 16 | 60 | 9 | 3.0 | 10.0 | 0.0 | 0.0 | 10.0 | 1.0 | 0.5 | | | | | 10 |
| 50631 | 1/3 cup | Noodle, fat free, dry, Health Valley | 32 | 80 | 5 | 3.0 | 18.0 | 2.0 | 1.0 | 15.0 | 0.0 | 0.0 | 0.0 | 0.0 | 0.00 | 0.00 | 0 |
| 50037 | 1 cup | Noodle, prep f/dry mix, avg | 252 | 53 | 94 | 2.9 | 7.4 | 0.8 | 1.2 | 5.5 | 1.2 | 0.3 | 0.5 | 0.4 | 0.03 | 0.33 | 3 |
| 50160 | 1 ea | Rice, dry mix, svg, avg | 16 | 59 | 4 | 2.4 | 9.1 | 0.3 | 1.6 | 7.2 | 1.4 | 0.3 | 0.6 | 0.4 | 0.03 | 0.39 | 3 |
| 50161 | 1 cup | Rice, prep f/dry mix, avg | 253 | 61 | 94 | 2.5 | 9.3 | 0.8 | 1.5 | 7.0 | 1.4 | 0.3 | 0.6 | 0.4 | 0.03 | 0.40 | 3 |
| 50162 | 1 ea | Vegetable, dry mix, svg, avg | 11 | 38 | 5 | 2.1 | 6.1 | 0.3 | 0.7 | 5.0 | 0.6 | 0.1 | 0.2 | 0.1 | 0.00 | 0.12 | 2 |
| 50620 | 1 ea | Vegetable, dry, cup a soup, Lipton | 14 | 50 | 11 | 1.0 | 10.0 | 0.0 | 0.5 | 9.5 | 1.0 | 0.5 | | | | | 10 |
| 50038 | 1 cup | Vegetable, prep f/dry mix, avg | 251 | 50 | 95 | 2.7 | 7.8 | 0.5 | 0.9 | 6.4 | 0.8 | 0.2 | 0.3 | 0.2 | 0.00 | 0.15 | 3 |
| 50158 | 1 ea | Cream of Chicken, dry pkt, avg | 18 | 78 | 4 | 1.3 | 9.8 | 0.3 | 4.1 | 5.3 | 3.9 | 2.5 | 0.9 | 0.3 | 0.00 | 0.30 | 2 |
| 50613 | 1 ea | Cream of Chicken, dry, cup a soup, Lipton | 17 | 70 | 11 | 1.0 | 11.0 | 0.0 | 2.0 | 9.0 | 2.5 | 0.5 | | | | | 0 |
| 50036 | 1 cup | Cream of Chicken, prep f/dry pkt, avg | 261 | 107 | 91 | 1.8 | 13.3 | 0.3 | 5.7 | 7.3 | 5.3 | 3.4 | 1.2 | 0.4 | 0.00 | 0.42 | 3 |
| | | Chili Soup | | | | | | | | | | | | | | | |
| 50317 | 1 cup | With Beans, Chef Mate | 253 | 412 | 70 | 17.7 | 29.1 | 11.1 | 0.2 | 17.7 | 25.0 | 10.9 | 10.8 | 1.4 | 0.25 | 1.11 | 56 |
| 50319 | 1 cup | With Beans, spicy, Chef Mate | 253 | 423 | 68 | 16.9 | 32.9 | 4.3 | 0.2 | 28.4 | 24.7 | 10.7 | 10.8 | 1.1 | 0.20 | 0.90 | 56 |
| 50318 | 1 cup | Without Beans, Chef Mate | 250 | 430 | 70 | 18.5 | 17.6 | 3.0 | 0.2 | 14.4 | 31.5 | 14.4 | 13.6 | 1.8 | 0.23 | 1.40 | 85 |
| 50163 | 1 ea | Clam Chowder, manhattan, dry mix, svg, avg | 19 | 66 | 4 | 2.1 | 10.9 | 0.6 | | | 1.6 | 0.3 | 0.7 | 0.5 | 0.00 | 0.50 | 0 |
| 50164 | 1 ea | Clam Chowder, new england, dry mix, svg, avg | 13 | 54 | 4 | 1.6 | 7.4 | 0.7 | | | 2.1 | 0.4 | 1.0 | 0.7 | 0.00 | 0.67 | 0 |
| 50632 | 1/2 cup | Corn Chowder, fat free, dry, Health Valley | 31 | 90 | 3 | 4.0 | 20.0 | 3.0 | 1.0 | 16.0 | 0.0 | 0.0 | 0.0 | 0.0 | 0.00 | 0.00 | 0 |
| 50335 | 1 ea | Corn Chowder, soup in a cup, dry, Nile Spice | 30 | 110 | 5 | 3.1 | 22.2 | 3.0 | 4.2 | 15.1 | 1.9 | 0.9 | 0.3 | 0.3 | | | 4 |
| 50167 | 1 ea | Leek Soup, dry mix, svg, avg | 17 | 64 | 2 | 1.9 | 10.3 | 0.6 | 2.5 | 7.2 | 1.9 | 0.9 | 0.8 | 0.1 | 0.01 | 0.06 | 2 |
| 50168 | 1 cup | Leek Soup, prep f/dry mix, avg | 254 | 71 | 93 | 2.1 | 11.4 | 3.0 | 2.8 | 5.6 | 2.1 | 1.0 | 0.9 | 0.1 | 0.02 | 0.06 | 3 |
| | | Lentil Soup | | | | | | | | | | | | | | | |
| 50633 | 1/3 cup | Couscous, fat free, dry, Health Valley | 43 | 130 | 3 | 7.0 | 28.0 | 5.0 | 1.0 | 22.0 | 0.0 | 0.0 | 0.0 | 0.0 | 0.00 | 0.00 | 0 |
| 56841 | 1 ea | Curry Couscous, soup in a cup, dry, Nile Spice | 56 | 197 | 9 | 10.2 | 36.2 | 3.6 | 5.2 | 27.5 | 1.3 | 0.2 | 0.6 | 0.4 | | | 0 |
| 50341 | 1 ea | Soup in a cup, dry, Nile Spice | 52 | 166 | 6 | 11.3 | 34.3 | 11.5 | 1.8 | 21.0 | 1.4 | 0.2 | 0.0 | 0.0 | | | 0 |
| | | Minestrone Soup | | | | | | | | | | | | | | | |
| 50169 | 1 ea | Dry, svg, avg | 17 | 61 | 5 | 3.4 | 9.1 | 0.6 | 2.5 | 6.0 | 1.3 | 0.6 | 0.6 | 0.1 | 0.01 | 0.06 | 1 |
| 56840 | 1 ea | Dry, couscous, soup in a cup, Nile Spice | 53 | 178 | 7 | 8.1 | 37.4 | 5.5 | 3.6 | 28.4 | 1.1 | 0.1 | 0.1 | 0.3 | | | 0 |
| 50336 | 1 ea | Dry, soup in a cup, Nile Spice | 45 | 143 | 7 | 8.0 | 29.7 | 6.8 | 3.3 | 19.5 | 1.1 | 0.1 | 0.1 | 0.4 | | | 0 |
| 50170 | 1 cup | Prep f/dry mix, avg | 254 | 79 | 92 | 4.4 | 11.9 | 1.3 | 3.0 | 7.5 | 1.7 | 0.8 | 0.7 | 0.1 | 0.03 | 0.08 | 3 |
| 50351 | 1 cup | Moroccan Stew, meal in a cup, Sahara Moroccan | 248 | 153 | | 4.4 | 32.8 | 2.2 | | | 0.0 | 0.0 | 0.0 | 0.0 | 0.00 | 0.00 | |
| | | Mushroom Soup | | | | | | | | | | | | | | | |
| 50616 | 1 ea | Cream of Mushroom, cup a soup, dry, Lipton | 15 | 60 | 9 | 1.0 | 10.0 | 0.0 | 2.0 | 8.0 | 2.0 | 0.0 | | | | | 0 |
| 50171 | 1 ea | Dry Mix, svg, avg | 17 | 75 | 3 | 1.7 | 8.7 | 0.6 | 1.0 | 7.1 | 3.8 | 0.6 | 1.8 | 1.2 | 0.00 | 1.22 | 0 |
| 50039 | 1 cup | Prep f/dry mix, avg | 253 | 96 | 92 | 2.2 | 11.1 | 0.8 | 1.3 | 9.1 | 4.9 | 0.8 | 2.3 | 1.5 | 0.00 | 1.54 | 0 |
| 50377 | 1 ea | Soup in a cup, dry, Nile Spice | 36 | 137 | 5 | 3.6 | 26.3 | 1.3 | 1.5 | 23.5 | 2.3 | 1.4 | 0.0 | 0.1 | | | 6 |

| Code | Vit A & Components | | | | | Vitamins | | | | | | | | | | Minerals | | | | | | | | | |
|---|---|---|---|---|---|---|---|---|---|---|---|---|---|---|---|---|---|---|---|---|---|---|---|---|---|
| | Vit A (IU) | Vit A (RE) | Retinol (RE) | Carotenoids (RE) | Beta Carotene (mcg) | Thiamin (mg) | Riboflavin (mg) | Niacin (NE) | Vit B6 (mg) | Vit B12 (mcg) | Folate (mcg) | Panto (mg) | Vit C (mg) | Vit D (mg) | Vit E (α TE) | Calcium (mg) | Copper (mg) | Iron (mg) | Magnes (mg) | Mang (mg) | Phos (mg) | Potassium (mg) | Selenium (mcg) | Sodium (mg) | Zinc (mg) |
| 50148 | 236 | 24 | | | | 0.03 | 0.04 | 0.42 | 0.01 | 0.03 | 6.4 | 0.07 | 0.7 | 0.0 | | 19 | 0.1 | 0.5 | 3 | 0.3 | 26 | 115 | | 697 | 0.59 |
| 50149 | 271 | 28 | | | | 0.05 | 0.05 | 0.50 | 0.01 | 0.03 | 7.5 | 0.08 | 0.8 | 0.0 | | 23 | 0.1 | 0.5 | 3 | 0.3 | 30 | 133 | | 801 | 0.68 |
| 50150 | 59 | 6 | | | | 0.06 | 0.03 | 0.39 | 0.03 | 0.03 | 8.4 | 0.06 | 1.1 | 0.0 | | 54 | 0.3 | 1.4 | 30 | 0.4 | 88 | 322 | | 917 | 0.69 |
| 50151 | 53 | 5 | | | | 0.05 | 0.27 | 0.40 | 0.03 | 0.03 | 8.0 | 0.05 | 1.1 | 0.0 | | 56 | 0.3 | 1.3 | 29 | 0.5 | 90 | 326 | 5.8 | 928 | 0.69 |
| 50338 | 676 | 135 | | | 110 | 0.17 | 0.12 | 1.06 | 0.11 | 0.00 | 163.8 | 0.45 | 7.8 | 0.0 | | 72 | 0.3 | 3.3 | 94 | 0.6 | 187 | 680 | 0.0 | 603 | 1.45 |
| 50629 | 100 | 20 | | | | | | | | | | | 3.6 | | | 40 | | 1.8 | | | | | | 280 | |
| 50630 | 100 | 20 | | | | | | | | | | | 3.6 | | | 40 | | 1.8 | | | | | | 280 | |
| 56836 | 50 | 10 | | | | | | | | | | | 3.9 | | | 53 | | 1.9 | | | | 502 | | 504 | |
| 56842 | 24 | 2 | 0 | 2 | 15 | 0.18 | 0.11 | 1.15 | 0.08 | 0.00 | 27.7 | 0.20 | 2.4 | 0.0 | | 90 | 0.1 | 3.0 | 18 | 0.2 | 201 | 587 | 0.0 | 590 | 0.31 |
| 50192 | 2 | 1 | | | | 0.01 | 0.01 | 0.13 | 0.01 | 0.04 | 1.3 | 0.01 | 0.0 | | | 2 | 0.0 | 0.1 | 2 | 0.0 | 9 | 16 | 1.1 | 960 | 0.01 |
| 50051 | 3 | 0 | | | | 0.00 | 0.01 | 0.27 | 0.01 | 0.06 | 1.9 | 0.02 | 0.0 | 0.0 | | 4 | 0.0 | 0.1 | 3 | 0.0 | 19 | 27 | 1.7 | 1019 | 0.00 |
| 50707 | 30 | 9 | 0 | 9 | | 0.01 | 0.03 | 0.15 | 0.01 | 0.02 | 1.9 | | 0.1 | | | 11 | 0.0 | 0.1 | 3 | | 10 | 19 | | 64 | 0.01 |
| 50033 | 2 | 1 | 1 | 0 | | 0.01 | 0.01 | 0.16 | 0.00 | 0.00 | 2.4 | 0.02 | 0.0 | 0.0 | | 2 | 0.0 | 0.1 | 2 | 0.0 | 12 | 19 | 1.7 | 1157 | 0.01 |
| 50032 | 5 | 1 | 1 | 0 | 0 | 0.00 | 0.02 | 0.36 | 0.00 | 0.00 | 0.0 | 0.00 | 0.0 | 0.0 | | 10 | 0.0 | 0.0 | 7 | 0.0 | 24 | 37 | 1.7 | 1362 | 0.07 |
| 50165 | 7 | 2 | | | | 0.01 | 0.03 | 0.58 | 0.03 | 0.13 | 4.2 | 0.04 | 0.0 | 0.0 | | 8 | 0.0 | 0.1 | 7 | 0.1 | 42 | 58 | | 3406 | 0.00 |
| 50166 | 7 | 1 | 0 | 1 | | 0.00 | 0.02 | 0.57 | 0.02 | 0.12 | 4.0 | 0.05 | 0.0 | 0.0 | 0.0 | 7 | 0.0 | 0.1 | 7 | 0.0 | 40 | 57 | 1.7 | 3299 | 0.00 |
| 50152 | 6 | 1 | | | | 0.09 | 0.04 | 0.50 | 0.02 | 0.00 | 11.0 | 0.00 | 0.4 | 0.0 | | 4 | 0.0 | 0.2 | 7 | 0.1 | 29 | 59 | 3.2 | 757 | 0.07 |
| 50153 | 8 | 2 | | | | 0.12 | 0.06 | 0.69 | 0.04 | 0.00 | 15.1 | 0.00 | 0.5 | 0.0 | | 5 | 0.1 | 0.3 | 10 | 0.1 | 40 | 80 | 4.5 | 1042 | 0.10 |
| 50178 | 246 | 25 | | | | 0.03 | 0.04 | 0.48 | 0.06 | 0.32 | 8.2 | 0.27 | 1.4 | 0.0 | | 13 | 0.0 | 0.9 | 24 | 0.3 | 38 | 77 | | 1034 | 0.28 |
| 50044 | 238 | 23 | | | | 0.03 | 0.04 | 0.46 | 0.05 | 0.25 | 7.6 | 0.25 | 1.3 | 0.0 | | 13 | 0.0 | 0.9 | 23 | 0.3 | 35 | 76 | 3.0 | 1002 | 0.27 |
| 50622 | 0 | 0 | 0 | 0 | 0 | | | | | | | | 0.0 | | | 40 | | 0.0 | | | | | | 550 | |
| 50380 | 3444 | 689 | | | | 0.09 | 0.40 | 2.05 | 0.17 | 0.01 | 18.4 | 0.28 | 2.9 | 0.0 | | 56 | 0.1 | 0.7 | 24 | 0.2 | 59 | 417 | 0.0 | 536 | 0.25 |
| 50154 | 6 | 1 | 0 | 1 | | 0.07 | 0.08 | 0.46 | 0.02 | 0.19 | 3.2 | 0.09 | 3.8 | 0.0 | | 9 | 0.0 | 0.4 | 2 | 0.1 | 51 | 105 | | 845 | 0.25 |
| 50155 | 5 | 1 | 0 | 1 | | 0.08 | 0.08 | 0.51 | 0.03 | 0.18 | 2.6 | 0.10 | 2.6 | 0.0 | | 10 | 0.0 | 0.5 | 3 | 0.1 | 51 | 105 | | 842 | 0.26 |
| 50156 | 263 | 26 | | | | 0.02 | 0.04 | 0.29 | 0.01 | 0.04 | 2.0 | 0.99 | 0.2 | 0.0 | | 35 | 0.1 | 0.5 | 5 | 0.2 | 32 | 106 | | 818 | 0.14 |
| 50157 | 269 | 28 | | | | 0.03 | 0.05 | 0.30 | 0.00 | 0.05 | 2.0 | 1.02 | 0.3 | 0.0 | | 36 | 0.1 | 0.5 | 5 | 0.2 | 33 | 109 | | 838 | 0.13 |
| 50193 | 13 | 4 | | | | 0.01 | 0.02 | 0.20 | 0.01 | 0.02 | 1.6 | 0.03 | 0.1 | 0.0 | | 10 | 0.0 | 0.1 | 3 | 0.0 | 10 | 19 | 1.4 | 1200 | 0.01 |
| 50611 | 0 | 0 | 0 | 0 | 0 | | | | | | | | 0.0 | | | 0 | | 0.0 | | | | | | 580 | |
| 50034 | 39 | 12 | | | | 0.01 | 0.03 | 0.20 | 0.00 | 0.02 | 2.4 | 0.05 | 0.0 | 0.0 | | 15 | 0.0 | 0.1 | 5 | 0.0 | 12 | 24 | 0.0 | 1484 | 0.01 |
| 50159 | 45 | 5 | | | | 0.05 | 0.04 | 0.63 | 0.06 | 0.00 | 13.4 | 0.00 | 0.2 | 0.0 | | 23 | 0.0 | 0.4 | 5 | 0.1 | 23 | 23 | 7.0 | 923 | 0.14 |
| 50608 | 0 | 0 | 0 | 0 | 0 | | | | | | | | 0.0 | | | 0 | | 0.7 | | | | | | 540 | |
| 50631 | 100 | 20 | | | | | | | | | | | 6.0 | | | 20 | | 1.4 | | | | | | 360 | |
| 50037 | 63 | 5 | | | | 0.07 | 0.06 | 0.88 | 0.01 | 0.00 | 17.6 | 0.01 | 0.3 | 0.0 | | 33 | 0.0 | 0.5 | 8 | 0.1 | 33 | 30 | 9.6 | 1283 | 0.20 |
| 50160 | 64 | 6 | | | | 0.01 | 0.00 | 0.36 | 0.02 | 0.08 | 0.5 | 0.08 | 0.1 | 0.0 | | 7 | 0.1 | 0.1 | 0 | 0.2 | 11 | 11 | | 968 | 0.13 |
| 50161 | 0 | 0 | 0 | 0 | 0 | 0.00 | 0.00 | 0.36 | 0.03 | 0.08 | 0.5 | 0.08 | 0.0 | 0.0 | | 8 | 0.1 | 0.0 | 0 | 0.2 | 10 | 10 | 5.3 | 982 | 0.13 |
| 50162 | 11 | 1 | | | | 0.05 | 0.04 | 0.53 | 0.07 | 0.08 | 3.1 | 0.11 | 0.9 | 0.0 | | 11 | 0.0 | 0.5 | 17 | 0.2 | 25 | 53 | | 627 | 0.16 |
| 50620 | 0 | 0 | 0 | 0 | 0 | | | | | | | | 0.0 | | | 0 | | 0.4 | | | | | | 520 | |
| 50038 | 15 | 3 | 2 | 1 | | 0.07 | 0.05 | 0.69 | 0.09 | 0.10 | 2.5 | 0.25 | 1.3 | 0.0 | | 15 | 0.0 | 0.6 | 23 | 0.3 | 33 | 68 | 4.3 | 808 | 0.21 |
| 50158 | 297 | 89 | | | | 0.07 | 0.15 | 1.98 | 0.04 | 0.18 | 4.0 | 0.52 | 0.4 | 0.0 | | 56 | 0.2 | 0.3 | 4 | 0.5 | 70 | 158 | | 868 | 1.08 |
| 50613 | 0 | 0 | 0 | 0 | 0 | | | | | | | | 0.0 | | | 20 | | 0.0 | | | | | | 650 | |
| 50036 | 407 | 123 | 110 | 13 | | 0.10 | 0.20 | 2.61 | 0.05 | 0.26 | 5.2 | 0.78 | 0.5 | 0.0 | | 76 | 0.3 | 0.3 | 5 | 0.8 | 97 | 214 | 8.1 | 1185 | 1.57 |
| 50317 | 3013 | 301 | 0 | 301 | | 0.11 | 0.20 | 3.47 | 0.23 | 1.44 | | 0.66 | 0.8 | | | 89 | 0.3 | 4.8 | 46 | 0.4 | 167 | 511 | | 1171 | 3.87 |
| 50319 | 2004 | 210 | 0 | 210 | | 0.15 | 0.15 | 2.99 | 0.26 | 0.86 | | 0.70 | 1.3 | | | 83 | 0.3 | 5.4 | 53 | 0.6 | 177 | 648 | | 1485 | 2.83 |
| 50318 | 2900 | 303 | | | | 0.14 | 0.27 | 4.85 | 0.34 | 1.83 | | 0.78 | 1.8 | | | 68 | 0.4 | 4.4 | 45 | 0.4 | 162 | 530 | | 1588 | 4.50 |
| 50163 | 1020 | 102 | | | | 0.03 | 0.04 | 0.86 | 0.11 | 4.37 | 10.1 | 0.13 | 4.2 | 0.0 | | 25 | 0.1 | 1.7 | 11 | 0.4 | 44 | 199 | | 1343 | 0.99 |
| 50164 | 5 | 1 | | | | 0.01 | 0.09 | 0.48 | 0.04 | 5.07 | 1.9 | 0.17 | 1.2 | 0.0 | | 44 | 0.1 | 0.7 | 4 | 0.1 | 57 | 117 | | 427 | 0.39 |
| 50632 | 100 | 20 | | | | | | | | | | | 9.0 | | | 20 | | 1.4 | | | | | | 360 | |
| 50335 | 617 | 123 | | | 165 | 0.08 | 0.37 | 2.25 | 0.09 | 0.00 | 40.7 | 0.67 | 9.4 | 0.0 | | 19 | 0.1 | 0.7 | 39 | 0.2 | 89 | 289 | 0.0 | 405 | 0.42 |
| 50167 | 5 | 1 | 0 | 1 | | 0.05 | 0.03 | 0.32 | 0.02 | 0.03 | 7.7 | 0.10 | 2.5 | 0.0 | | 28 | 0.0 | 0.4 | 9 | 0.0 | 29 | 81 | | 874 | 0.21 |
| 50168 | 5 | 1 | 0 | 1 | | 0.05 | 0.03 | 0.25 | 0.03 | 0.03 | 7.6 | 0.10 | 2.5 | 0.0 | | 30 | 0.0 | 0.5 | 10 | 0.0 | 30 | 89 | 4.8 | 965 | 0.24 |
| 50633 | 100 | 20 | | | | | | | | | | | 4.8 | | | 40 | | 1.8 | | | | | | 360 | |
| 56841 | 46 | 9 | | | | | | | | | | | 1.9 | | | 51 | | 2.8 | | | | 564 | | 729 | |
| 50341 | 665 | 133 | | | | 0.16 | 0.16 | 1.16 | 0.04 | 0.00 | 15.0 | 0.12 | 46.6 | 0.0 | 0.0 | 54 | 0.0 | 4.5 | 13 | 0.1 | 222 | 714 | 0.0 | 543 | 0.11 |
| 50169 | 225 | 23 | | | | 0.05 | 0.03 | 0.78 | 0.09 | 0.00 | 27.0 | 0.29 | 0.9 | 0.0 | | 29 | 0.1 | 0.8 | 6 | 0.3 | 47 | 260 | | 785 | 0.61 |
| 56840 | 152 | 30 | | | 867 | 0.11 | 0.11 | 1.75 | 0.13 | 0.00 | 53.8 | 0.63 | 13.0 | 0.0 | | 53 | 0.2 | 1.7 | 44 | 0.5 | 132 | 397 | 0.0 | 673 | |
| 50336 | 200 | 40 | | | 60 | 0.09 | 0.10 | 0.90 | 0.05 | 0.00 | 10.0 | 0.22 | 3.6 | 0.0 | 0.0 | 67 | 0.1 | 1.9 | 14 | 0.2 | 136 | 457 | 0.0 | 586 | 0.15 |
| 50170 | 295 | 30 | | | | 0.08 | 0.05 | 1.02 | 0.10 | 0.00 | 35.6 | 0.38 | 1.0 | 0.0 | | 38 | 0.1 | 1.0 | 8 | 0.4 | 61 | 340 | 3.6 | 1026 | 0.76 |
| 50351 | | | | | | | | | | | | | | | | | | | | | | | | 404 | |
| 50616 | 0 | 0 | 0 | 0 | 0 | | | | | | | | 0.0 | | | 0 | | 0.0 | | | | | | 590 | |
| 50171 | 5 | 1 | 0 | 1 | | 0.22 | 0.09 | 0.39 | 0.01 | 0.10 | 3.1 | 0.19 | 0.9 | 0.0 | | 52 | 0.0 | 0.4 | 4 | 0.2 | 60 | 156 | | 796 | 0.07 |
| 50039 | 8 | 1 | 0 | 1 | | 0.28 | 0.11 | 0.50 | 0.03 | 0.25 | 5.1 | 0.24 | 1.0 | 0.3 | | 66 | 0.0 | 0.5 | 5 | 0.3 | 76 | 200 | 5.1 | 1020 | 0.09 |
| 50377 | 24 | 5 | | | | 0.10 | 0.50 | 2.96 | 0.09 | 0.00 | 8.1 | 0.57 | 1.9 | 0.0 | | 23 | 0.1 | 1.0 | 12 | 0.2 | 46 | 192 | 0.0 | 610 | 0.31 |

| Code | Amount | Description | Basic Components | | | | | | | | | Additional Fats | | | | | | Vit A & Components | | | | | Vitamins | | | | | | | | | | Minerals | | | | | | | | | |
|---|---|---|---|---|---|---|---|---|---|---|---|---|---|---|---|---|---|---|---|---|---|---|---|---|---|---|---|---|---|---|---|---|---|---|---|---|---|---|---|---|---|---|
| | | | Weight (g) | Calories | % Water | Protein (g) | Carbs (g) | Fiber (g) | Sugar (g) | Other Carbs (g) | Fat (g) | Sat Fat (g) | Mono Fat (g) | Poly Fat (g) | Omega 3 (g) | Omega 6 (g) | Choles (mg) | Vit A (IU) | Vit A (RE) | Retinol (RE) | Carotenoids (RE) | Beta Carotene (mcg) | Thiamin (mg) | Riboflavin (mg) | Niacin (NE) | Vit B6 (mg) | Vit B12 (mcg) | Folate (mcg) | Panto (mg) | Vit C (mg) | Vit D (ing) | Vit E (α TE) | Calcium (mg) | Copper (mg) | Iron (mg) | Magnes (mg) | Mang (mg) | Phos (mg) | Potassium (mg) | Selenium (mcg) | Sodium (mg) | Zinc (mg) |
| | | Onion Soup ||||||||||||||||||||||||||||||||||||||||
|50054|1 ea|Dry Packet, avg|39|115|4|4.5|20.9|4.1|6.7|10.1|2.3|0.5|1.4|0.3|0.00|0.27|2|8|1|0|1||0.11|0.24|1.99|0.04|0.00|6.3|0.00|0.9|0.0||55|0.1|0.6|25|0.2|126|260|9.6|3493|0.23|
|50526|1/3 cup|Dry Mix, Campbell's|37|106|4|0.0|26.4|0.0|15.9|10.6|0.0|0.0|0.0|0.0|0.00|0.00|0|0|0|0|0|0||||||||0.0|||0||0.0||||||2801||
|50040|1 cup|Prep f/dry pkt, avg|246|27|96|1.1|5.1|1.0|1.5|2.5|0.6|0.1|0.3|0.1|0.00|0.07|0|2|0.3|0|0.3||0.03|0.06|0.48|0.00|0.00|1.5|0.00|0.2|0.0||12|0.0|0.1|5|0.1|30|64|2.5|849|0.06|
|50172|1 ea|Oxtail Soup, dry mix, svg, avg|16|60|5|2.4|7.7|0.1|1.5|6.0|2.2|1.1|0.9|0.1|0.01|0.07|2|8|2||||0.02|0.03|0.72|0.03|0.16|4.8|0.05|0.0|0.0||10|0.0|0.2|8|0.1|51|72||1034|0.00|
|50173|1 cup|Oxtail Soup, prep f/dry mix, avg|253|71|93|2.8|9.0|0.5|1.8|6.7|2.6|1.3|1.1|0.1|0.03|0.08|3|10|3|3|0|0|0.03|0.03|0.76|0.03|0.25|5.1|0.05|0.0|0.0||10|0.0|0.3|10|0.1|61|83|1.8|1209|0.00|
| | | Pasta Soup ||||||||||||||||||||||||||||||||||||||||
|50634|1/3 cup|Italiano, fat free, dry, Health Valley|26|85|2|3.0|18.7|1.8|0.6|16.3|0.0|0.0|0.0|0.0|0.00|0.00|0|60|12|||||||||||7.3|||12||0.9||||||218||
|56835|1 ea|Mediterranean, soup in a cup, dry, Nile Spice|53|207|8|8.5|33.3|1.5|0.8|31.0|4.4|2.6|1.6|0.2|||11|71|14|||||||||||2.5|||93||1.3||||240||636||
|56834|1 ea|Parmesan, soup in a cup, dry, Nile Spice|49|177|10|6.9|32.5|1.7|1.9|28.9|2.7|0.8|0.5|0.1|||7|702|140||||0.01|0.21|0.70|0.22|0.51|3.5|0.06|6.3|0.0||85|0.1|0.4|5|0.1|13|120|0.0|543|2.75|
|56839|1 ea|Primavera, soup in a cup, dry, Nile Spice|50|189|8|7.0|34.7|2.7|2.6|29.4|2.5|1.3|0.5|0.2|||7|2264|453|||||||||||17.1|||59||0.6||||232||348||
|50374|1 ea|Potato Leek Soup, in a cup, dry, Nile Spice|30|112|6|4.1|19.1|3.3|3.9|12.0|2.8|1.6|0.0|0.1|||8|104|10|0|10|62|0.07|0.09|0.83|0.06|0.00|7.2|0.11|5.9|0.0|0.0|62|0.0|0.6|8|0.1|44|396|0.0|571|0.11|
|50635|1/3 cup|Potato w/Broccoli Soup, fat free, dry, Health Valley|27|70|3|4.0|15.0|2.0|2.0|11.0|0.0|0.0|0.0|0.0|0.00|0.00|0|100|20|||||||||||12.0|||60||0.7||||||360||
| | | Pea Soup ||||||||||||||||||||||||||||||||||||||||
|50615|1 ea|Green, cup a soup, dry, Lipton|26|110|7|3.0|17.0|3.0|1.0|13.0|3.5|1.0|||||0|0|0|0|0|0||||||||0.0|||0||0.0||||||620||
|50174|1 ea|Split, dry mix, svg, avg|28|100|4|5.7|17.0|2.8|2.5|11.6|1.2|0.4|0.6|0.2|0.04|0.20|0|36|4|0|4||0.17|0.11|1.01|0.04|0.28|11.3|0.20|0.3|0.0||17|0.1|0.8|35|0.2|100|178||914|0.44|
|50041|1 cup|Split, prep f/dry, avg|255|125|87|7.2|21.3|2.8|3.2|15.4|1.5|0.4|0.7|0.3|0.05|0.23|3|46|5||||0.21|0.14|1.26|0.05|0.25|39.5|0.25|0.0|0.0||20|0.2|0.9|43|0.3|125|224|4.6|1147|0.56|
|50337|1 ea|Split, soup in a cup, dry, Nile Spice|53|196|5|12.8|34.5|8.4|6.7|19.4|1.1|0.1|0.1|0.1|||0|577|116|||336|0.02|0.15|0.65|0.05|0.00|5.1|0.08|2.6|0.0||20|0.0|2.0|7|0.1|15|74|0.0|597|0.08|
|50636|1/2 cup|Split, w/croutons, fat free, dry, Health Valley|37|130|2|8.0|25.0|2.0|2.0|21.0|0.0|0.0|0.0|0.0|0.00|0.00|0|250|50|||||||||||6.0|||40||1.4||||||360||
|50347|1 ea|Splittin, meal in a cup, Fantastic Foods|56|190|13|12.0|35.0|8.0|5.0|22.0|1.0|0.0|||0.00|0.00|0|1250|250|||||||||||9.0|||20||1.8||||||470||
|50610|1 ea|Virginia, cup a soup, dry, Lipton|31|130|11|3.0|19.0|3.0|1.0|15.0|5.0|2.0|||||0|0|0|0|0|0||||||||0.0|||0||0.4||||||630||
| | | Tomato Soup ||||||||||||||||||||||||||||||||||||||||
|50175|1 ea|Dry, svg, avg|21|76|4|1.8|14.3|0.4|7.7|6.3|1.8|0.8|0.7|0.2|0.00|0.17|1|615|62|0|62||0.05|0.03|0.58|0.07|0.06|4.9|0.08|3.4|0.0||40|0.1|0.3|11|0.1|49|218||697|0.15|
|50621|1 ea|Dry, cup a soup, Lipton|26|90|9|2.0|19.0|1.0|12.0|6.0|2.0|1.0|||||2|200|40|||||||||||6.0|||60||0.4||||||490||
|50349|1 cup|Parmesan, Casbah Sahara|248|164||4.4|28.4|2.2|||2.2|||||||||||||||||||||||||||||492||415||
|50042|1 cup|Prep f/dry mix, avg|265|103|90|2.5|19.4|0.5|10.4|8.5|2.4|1.1|0.9|0.2|0.00|0.24|0|832|82|0|82||0.06|0.05|0.78|0.10|0.08|6.6|0.11|4.5|0.0||53|0.1|0.4|13|0.1|66|294|0.5|943|0.21|
|50378|1 ea|Rice, soup in a cup, Nile Spice|36|134|10|4.6|22.7|1.4|4.3|17.0|2.8|1.3|1.2|0.3|||6|1318|330|||0||||||||9.0|||54||0.9||||468||552||
|50176|1/3 cup|Vegetable, dry, avg|6|19|4|0.7|3.6|0.2|1.9|1.5|0.3|0.1|0.1|0.0|0.00|0.03|0|67|7|0|7||0.02|0.02|0.28|0.02|0.00|3.6|0.05|2.1|0.0||3|0.0|0.2|7|0.1|10|36|1.4|403|0.06|
|50043|1 cup|Vegetable, prep f/dry mix, avg|253|56|94|2.0|10.2|0.5|4.0|5.7|0.9|0.4|0.3|0.1|0.00|0.08|0|190|20|0|20||0.06|0.05|0.79|0.05|0.00|10.1|0.14|6.1|0.0||8|0.0|0.6|20|0.2|30|104|4.6|1146|0.17|
| | | Vegetable Soup ||||||||||||||||||||||||||||||||||||||||
|50179|1 ea|Cream of Vegetable, dry mix, svg, avg|18|80|3|1.4|9.4|0.5|0.8|8.0|4.3|1.1|1.9|1.1|0.07|1.06|0|27|3||||0.93|0.08|0.40|0.02|0.09|5.4|0.13|3.0|0.0||24|0.1|0.5|9|0.1|41|73|3.7|892|0.29|
|50045|1 cup|Cream of Vegetable, prep f/dry mix, avg|260|107|91|1.9|12.3|0.5|1.0|10.7|5.7|1.4|2.5|1.5|0.10|1.38|0|36|3||||1.22|0.11|0.52|0.03|0.13|7.8|0.16|3.9|0.0||31|0.1|0.5|10|0.2|55|96|4.9|1170|0.26|
|50617|1 ea|Dry, cup a soup, Lipton|13|50|4|2.0|9.0|1.0|1.0|7.0|1.0|0.0|||||10|0|0|0|0|0||||||||0.0|||0||0.4||||||500||
|50187|1 cup|Low sodium, prep f/dry mix, avg|253|56|94|2.0|10.1|0.5|0.9|8.7|0.8|0.3|0.3|0.1|||0|190|20|0|20||0.05|0.05|0.78|0.05|0.00|10.1||6.1|0.0||8|0.0|0.6|20||30|104||51|0.18|
|56837|1 ea|Parmesan Couscous, dry soup cup, Nile Spice|54|196|11|8.2|34.1|2.0|0.3|31.8|2.9|1.5|1.1|0.3|||8|425|85|||||||||||13.9|||79||1.1||||321||565||
| | | *HOMEMADE SOUPS* ||||||||||||||||||||||||||||||||||||||||
|50689|1 cup|Fish Stock|233|40|97|5.3|0.0|0.0|0.0|0.0|1.9|0.5|0.5|0.3|0.21|0.05|2|0|0|0|0|0|0.08|0.18|2.77|0.09|1.61|46.6|0.77|0.2|||7|0.1|0.0|16|0.1|130|336|2.3|363|0.14|
|50228|1 cup|Ratatouille|214|265|81|2.4|11.8||||24.6|3.3|17.9|2.2|0.18|2.04|0|815|82|0|82||0.13|0.06|1.10|0.25|0.00|34.2|0.22|41.3|||56|0.2|1.3|32|0.3|62|486||330|0.41|
|50690|1 cup|Shark Fin Soup|216|99|90|6.9|8.2|0.0|||4.3|1.1|1.3|0.7|0.48|0.11|4|0|0|0|0|0|0.06|0.08|1.06|0.06|0.41|19.4|0.28|0.2|||22|0.2|2.0|15|0.1|45|114||1082|1.77|
| | | Stew ||||||||||||||||||||||||||||||||||||||||
|50225|1 cup|Beef|252|222|80|22.6|20.1||||5.3|1.9|2.1|0.3|0.03|0.29|60|6625|663|0|663||0.18|0.24|3.58|0.33|1.54|25.2|0.52|14.1|||33|0.3|3.2|40|0.3|224|527||461|5.70|
|50046|1 cup|Beef Vegetable|245|218|82|15.7|15.2|2.0|5.6|7.6|10.5|4.9|4.5|0.5||0.22|64|2401|568|0|568||0.15|0.17|4.66|0.28|1.60|37.0|0.30|17.1|0.1||29|0.2|2.9|39|0.3|184|613|15.2|292|5.29|
|50226|1 cup|Brunswick|243|231|79|26.7|17.4||||6.2|1.6|2.1|1.5|0.11|1.33|70|433|51||||0.13|0.20|6.61|0.39|0.17|21.9|0.90|14.1|||39|0.2|2.0|44|0.3|182|508||437|2.09|
| | | **SPICES, FLAVORS AND SEASONINGS** ||||||||||||||||||||||||||||||||||||||||
|90095|1 tsp|Accent Flavor Enhancer|2|0||0.0|0.0|0.0|0.0|0.0|0.0|0.0|0.0|0.0|0.00|0.00|0|0|0|0|0|0|||||0.00|||0.0|||0||0.0||||||320||
|26000|1 tsp|Allspice, ground, avg|2|5|8|0.1|1.4|0.4|||0.2|0.1|0.0|0.0|0.00|0.05|0|11|1|0|1|6|0.00|0.00|0.06|0.01|0.00|0.7||0.8|0.0||13|0.0|0.1|3|0.1|2|21|0.1|2|0.02|
|26302|1/2 oz|Anchovy Paste, Sokol & Company|14|29|39|2.4|4.1||||0.3||||||7||||||||||0.00|0.0|||||59||7.2||||||1747||
|26106|1 tsp|Anise Seed, avg|2|7|10|0.4|1.0|0.3|||0.3|0.0|0.2|0.1|0.00|0.06|0|6|1|0|1|4|0.01|0.01|0.06|0.01|0.00|0.2|0.02|0.4|||13|0.0|0.7|3|0.0|9|29|0.1|0|0.11|
|26493|1 tsp|Annatto Seed, American Spice & Trade Assoc|2|7|10|0.3|1.4|0.7|||0.1|||||||1|0.1|0|0.1|1|||||0.00|||0.1|||4||0.6||||||0||
|26107|1 tsp|Bay Leaf, dried, avg|1|3|5|0.1|0.8|0.3|||0.1|0.0|0.0|0.0|0.01|0.01|0|62|6|0|6|37|0.00|0.00|0.02|0.01|0.00|1.8||0.5|||8|0.0|0.4|1|0.1|1|5||0|0.04|
| | | Basil ||||||||||||||||||||||||||||||||||||||||
|26001|1 tsp|Ground, avg|2|5|6|0.3|1.2|0.8|||0.1|0.0|0.0|0.0|0.03|0.01|0|188|19|0|19|113|0.00|0.01|0.14|0.02|0.00|5.5||1.2|0.0||42|0.0|0.8|8|0.1|10|69|0.1|1|0.12|
|26054|1 tsp|Leaves, dried, Foran Spice Company|1|3|6|0.1|0.6|0.2|||0.0||||||0|150|15|0|15|90|0.00|0.00|0.07||0.00|||0.6|||21||0.4|||5|37||0||
|26045|1 Tbs|Leaves, fresh, chpd, avg|3|1|91|0.1|0.1|0.1|||0.0|0.0|0.0|0.0|0.01|0.00|0|116|12|0|12|69|0.00|0.00|0.03|0.00|0.00|1.9|0.01|0.5|0.0||5|0.0|0.1|2|0.0|2|14||0|0.03|
|26100|1 tsp|Cajun Seasoning, Lawry's|3|7|5|0.2|1.1|0.2|||0.1|||||||||||||||0.00|||||||||||||29||474||
|26018|1 tsp|Caraway Seed, avg|2|7|10|0.4|1.0|0.8|||0.3|0.0|0.1|0.1|0.00|0.06|0|7|1|0|1|4|0.01|0.01|0.07|0.01|0.00|0.2||0.4|0.0||14|0.0|0.3|5|0.0|11|27|0.2|0|0.11|
|26039|1 tsp|Cardamom, ground, avg|2|6|8|0.2|1.4|0.6|||0.1|0.0|0.0|0.0|0.00|0.01|0|0|0|0|0|0|0.00|0.00|0.02||0.00|||0.4|0.0||8|0.0|0.3|5|0.6|4|22||0|0.15|
|26057|1 tsp|Cardamom Seeds, Foran Spice Company|2|7|8|0.2|1.5|0.2|||0.1||||||0||||||0.00|0.00|0.05||0.00||||||6||0.2|||4|24||0||
|26027|1 tsp|Cayenne/Red Pepper, dried, avg|2|6|8|0.2|1.1|0.5|||0.3|0.1|0.1|0.2|0.01|0.15|0|832|83|0|83|499|0.01|0.02|0.17|0.04|0.00|2.1||1.5|0.0||3|0.0|0.2|3|0.0|6|40|0.2|1|0.05|
|26174|1 tsp|Celery Salt, Heller Seasonings|4|2|1|0.1|0.2|0.0|||0.2|0.0|0.1|0.0|||0|0.3|0.03|0|0.03|0.2|0.00|0.00|0.00|0.00|0.00|0.0|0.00|0.1||0.0|12|0.0|0.3|4||3|9|0.1|1319|0.05|
|26040|1 tsp|Celery Seed, avg|2|8|6|0.4|0.8|0.2|||0.5|0.0|0.3|0.1|0.00|0.07|0|1|0.1|0|0.1|1|0.01|0.01|0.06|0.01|0.00|0.2||0.3|0.0||35|0.0|0.9|9|0.2|11|28|0.2|3|0.14|
|26108|1 tsp|Chervil, dried, avg|1|2|7|0.2|0.5|0.1|||0.0|0.0|0.0|0.0|0.00|0.02|0|59|6|0|6|35|0.00|0.01|0.05|0.01|0.00|2.7||0.5|0.0||13|0.0|0.3|1|0.0|4|47|0.3|1|0.09|
|26171|1 Tbs|Chervil, fresh, avg|4|2|81|0.1|0.5|0.1|||0.0|0.0||||0.00|0|0|0|0|0|0|0.00|0.00|0.00||0.00|||0.4|||0||0.0|||0|0||0||
| | | Chili ||||||||||||||||||||||||||||||||||||||||
|26480|1/4 oz|Dry Mix, Old El Paso|7|22|6|0.4|3.5|0.9|0.0|2.6|0.4||||||0|263|26|||||||||0.00|||0.0|||0||0.3||||||674||
|26524|1 tsp|Pepper, dried, American Spice & Trade Assoc|2|6|14|0.3|1.1|0.7|||0.2|||||||420|42|0|42|252|||||0.00|||0.7|||4||0.2||||||3||
|26076|1 tsp|Pepper, dried, Foren Spice Company|2|8|6|0.3|1.2|0.7|||0.3||||||0|1036|104|0|104|622|0.01|0.03|0.28||0.00|||1.3|||2||0.2|||6|42||0||
|26072|1 tsp|Pepper, dried, red, Foran Spice Company|3|13|6|0.4|1.7|0.5|||0.4||||||0|1554|155|0|155|932|0.02|0.05|0.43||0.00|||1.9|||3||0.3|||10|63||0||
|26002|1 tsp|Powder, avg|2|6|8|0.2|1.1|0.7|||0.3|0.1|0.1|0.1|0.01|0.13|0|699|70|0|70|419|0.01|0.02|0.16|0.04|0.00|2.0||1.3|0.0||6|0.0|0.3|3|0.0|6|38|0.2|20|0.05|
|26096|1 tsp|Seasoning, Lawry's|3|10|5|0.4|1.8|0.0|||0.1|||||||||||||||0.00|||||||||||||||183||

| Code | Amount | Description | Weight (g) | Calories | % Water | Protein (g) | Carbs (g) | Fiber (g) | Sugar (g) | Other Carbs (g) | Fat (g) | Sat Fat (g) | Mono Fat (g) | Poly Fat (g) | Omega 3 (g) | Omega 6 (g) | Choles (mg) | Vit A (IU) | Vit A (RE) | Retinol (RE) | Carotenoids (RE) | Beta Carotene (mcg) | Thiamin (mg) | Riboflavin (mg) | Niacin (NE) | Vit B6 (mg) | Vit B12 (mcg) | Folate (mcg) | Panto (mg) | Vit C (mg) | Vit D (mg) | Vit E (α TE) | Calcium (mg) | Copper (mg) | Iron (mg) | Magnes (mg) | Mang (mg) | Phos (mg) | Potassium (mg) | Selenium (mcg) | Sodium (mg) | Zinc (mg) |
|---|---|---|---|---|---|---|---|---|---|---|---|---|---|---|---|---|---|---|---|---|---|---|---|---|---|---|---|---|---|---|---|---|---|---|---|---|---|---|---|---|---|---|
| | | | **Basic Components** | | | | | | | | | **Additional Fats** | | | | | | **Vit A & Components** | | | | | **Vitamins** | | | | | | | | | | **Minerals** | | | | | | | | | |
| 26003 | 1 tsp | Cinnamon, avg | 2 | 5 | 10 | 0.1 | 1.6 | 1.1 | | | 0.1 | 0.0 | 0.0 | 0.0 | 0.00 | 0.01 | 0 | 5 | 1 | 0 | 1 | 3 | 0.00 | 0.00 | 0.03 | 0.00 | 0.00 | 0.6 | | 0.6 | 0.0 | | 25 | 0.0 | 0.8 | 1 | 0.3 | 1 | 10 | 0.0 | 1 | 0.04 |
| 26019 | 1 tsp | Cloves, ground, avg | 2 | 6 | 7 | 0.1 | 1.2 | 0.7 | | | 0.4 | 0.1 | 0.0 | 0.1 | 0.09 | 0.05 | 0 | 11 | 1 | 0 | 1 | 6 | 0.00 | 0.01 | 0.03 | 0.03 | 0.00 | 1.9 | | 1.6 | 0.0 | | 13 | 0.0 | 0.2 | 5 | 0.6 | 2 | 22 | 0.1 | 5 | 0.02 |
| | | Coriander/Cilantro | | | | | | | | | | | | | | | | | | | | | | | | | | | | | | | | | | | | | | | | |
| 26020 | 1 tsp | Dried, avg | 1 | 3 | 7 | 0.2 | 0.5 | 0.1 | | | 0.0 | 0.0 | 0.0 | 0.0 | 0.00 | 0.00 | 0 | 59 | 6 | 0 | 6 | 33 | 0.01 | 0.01 | 0.11 | 0.01 | 0.00 | 2.7 | | 5.7 | 0.0 | | 12 | 0.0 | 0.4 | 7 | 0.1 | 5 | 45 | 0.3 | 2 | 0.05 |
| 26038 | 1 Tbs | Fresh, avg | 1 | 0 | 93 | 0.0 | 0.0 | 0.0 | 0.0 | 0.0 | 0.0 | 0.0 | 0.0 | 0.0 | 0.00 | 0.00 | 0 | 28 | 3 | 0 | 3 | 16 | 0.00 | 0.00 | 0.01 | 0.00 | 0.00 | 0.1 | 0.00 | 0.1 | 0.0 | | 1 | 0.0 | 0.0 | 0 | 0.0 | 0 | 5 | 0.0 | 0 | 0.00 |
| 26041 | 1 tsp | Seed, avg | 2 | 6 | 9 | 0.2 | 1.1 | 0.8 | | | 0.4 | 0.0 | 0.3 | 0.0 | 0.00 | 0.04 | 0 | 0 | 0 | 0 | 0 | 0 | 0.00 | 0.01 | 0.04 | | 0.00 | 0.0 | | 0.4 | 0.0 | | 14 | 0.0 | 0.3 | 7 | 0.0 | 8 | 25 | 0.5 | 1 | 0.09 |
| 26036 | 1 tsp | Cumin Seed, avg | 2 | 7 | 8 | 0.4 | 0.9 | 0.2 | | | 0.4 | 0.0 | 0.3 | 0.1 | 0.00 | 0.06 | 0 | 25 | 3 | 0 | 3 | 15 | 0.01 | 0.01 | 0.09 | 0.01 | 0.00 | 0.2 | | 0.2 | 0.0 | | 19 | 0.0 | 1.3 | 7 | 0.1 | 10 | 36 | 0.1 | 3 | 0.10 |
| 26004 | 1 tsp | Curry Powder, avg | 2 | 6 | 10 | 0.3 | 1.2 | 0.7 | | | 0.3 | 0.0 | 0.1 | 0.1 | 0.01 | 0.04 | 0 | 20 | 2 | 0 | 2 | 12 | 0.01 | 0.01 | 0.07 | 0.01 | 0.00 | 3.1 | 0.00 | 0.2 | 0.0 | | 10 | 0.0 | 0.6 | 5 | 0.1 | 7 | 31 | 0.3 | 1 | 0.08 |
| | | Dill | | | | | | | | | | | | | | | | | | | | | | | | | | | | | | | | | | | | | | | | |
| 26109 | 1 tsp | Seed, avg | 2 | 6 | 8 | 0.3 | 1.1 | 0.4 | | | 0.3 | 0.0 | 0.2 | 0.0 | 0.00 | 0.02 | 0 | 1 | 0.1 | 0 | 0.1 | 1 | 0.01 | 0.01 | 0.06 | 0.01 | 0.00 | 0.2 | | 0.4 | 0.0 | | 30 | 0.0 | 0.3 | 5 | 0.0 | 6 | 24 | 0.2 | 0 | 0.10 |
| 26021 | 1 tsp | Weed, dried, avg | 1 | 3 | 7 | 0.2 | 0.6 | 0.1 | | | 0.0 | 0.0 | 0.0 | 0.0 | 0.00 | 0.00 | 0 | 59 | 6 | 0 | 6 | 35 | 0.00 | 0.00 | 0.03 | 0.01 | 0.00 | | | 0.5 | 0.0 | | 18 | 0.0 | 0.5 | 5 | 0.0 | 5 | 33 | 0.0 | 2 | 0.03 |
| 26047 | 1 Tbs | Weed, fresh, avg | 1 | 0 | 86 | 0.0 | 0.1 | 0.0 | | | 0.0 | 0.0 | 0.0 | 0.0 | 0.00 | 0.00 | 0 | 77 | 8 | 0 | 8 | 46 | 0.00 | 0.00 | 0.02 | 0.00 | 0.00 | 1.5 | 0.00 | 0.8 | 0.0 | | 2 | 0.0 | 0.1 | 1 | 0.0 | 1 | 7 | | 1 | 0.01 |
| 26105 | 1 tsp | Fennel Seed, avg | 2 | 7 | 9 | 0.3 | 1.0 | 0.8 | | | 0.3 | 0.0 | 0.2 | 0.0 | 0.00 | 0.03 | 0 | 3 | 0.3 | 0 | 0.3 | 2 | 0.01 | 0.01 | 0.12 | | 0.00 | | | 0.4 | 0.0 | | 24 | 0.0 | 0.4 | 8 | 0.1 | 10 | 34 | | 2 | 0.07 |
| 7295 | 1/4 oz | Fenugreek Leaves, fresh, avg | 7 | 2 | 88 | 0.3 | 0.3 | | | | 0.0 | | | | | | | 0 | 0 | 0 | 0 | 0 | 0.00 | 0.02 | 0.06 | | 0.00 | | | 4.3 | | | 11 | 0.0 | 0.9 | 5 | | | 2 | | 5 | |
| 26022 | 1 tsp | Fenugreek Seed, avg | 4 | 13 | 9 | 0.9 | 2.3 | 1.0 | | | 0.3 | 0.1 | | | | | 0 | 2 | 0.2 | 0 | 0.2 | 0 | 0.01 | 0.01 | 0.07 | | 0.00 | 2.3 | | 0.1 | 0.0 | | 7 | 0.0 | 1.3 | 8 | 0.0 | 12 | 31 | 0.3 | 3 | 0.10 |
| 26555 | 1 ea | Fish Seasoning, 1/8 pkt, Shake N Bake | 76 | 280 | | 4.0 | 56.0 | 4.0 | 4.0 | 48.0 | 6.0 | 0.0 | | | | | 0 | 0 | 0 | 0 | 0 | 0 | | | | | 0.00 | | | 0.0 | | | 0 | | 0.0 | | | | 100 | | 1680 | |
| 26246 | 1/4 oz | Garlic, Kalsec | 7 | 60 | 1 | 0.0 | 0.1 | 0.0 | 0.0 | 0.1 | 6.7 | 0.9 | | | | | 0 | 0 | 0 | 0 | 0 | 0 | | | | | 0.00 | | | 0.0 | | | 2 | | 0.1 | | | | | | 12 | |
| | | Ginger | | | | | | | | | | | | | | | | | | | | | | | | | | | | | | | | | | | | | | | | |
| 26023 | 1 tsp | Ground, avg | 2 | 7 | 9 | 0.2 | 1.4 | 0.3 | | | 0.1 | 0.0 | 0.0 | 0.0 | 0.01 | 0.02 | 0 | 3 | 0.3 | 0 | 0.3 | 2 | 0.00 | 0.00 | 0.10 | 0.02 | 0.00 | 0.8 | | 0.1 | 0.0 | | 2 | 0.0 | 0.2 | 4 | 0.5 | 3 | 27 | 0.8 | 1 | 0.09 |
| 3462 | 1/4 oz | Root, crystallized, avg | 7 | 24 | 12 | 0.0 | 6.1 | 0.0 | 2.6 | 3.5 | 0.0 | 0.0 | | | | 0.00 | 0 | 7 | 1 | 0 | 1 | 4 | 0.01 | 0.03 | 0.49 | | 0.00 | | | 2.8 | 0.0 | | 16 | | 1.5 | | | 25 | 185 | | 4 | |
| 26044 | 1 Tbs | Root, fresh, avg | 6 | 4 | 82 | 0.1 | 0.9 | 0.1 | | | 0.0 | 0.0 | 0.0 | 0.0 | 0.00 | 0.01 | 0 | 0 | 0 | 0 | 0 | 0 | 0.00 | 0.00 | 0.04 | 0.01 | 0.00 | 0.7 | 0.01 | 0.3 | 0.0 | | 1 | 0.0 | 0.0 | 3 | 0.0 | 2 | 25 | 0.0 | 1 | 0.02 |
| 26553 | 1 ea | Italian Herb Seasoning, 1/8 pkt, Shake N Bake | 80 | 320 | | 8.0 | 56.0 | 0.0 | 8.0 | 48.0 | 4.0 | 0.0 | | | | | 0 | 0 | 0 | 0 | 0 | 0 | | | | | 0.00 | | | 0.0 | | | 0 | | 2.9 | | | | 200 | | 2400 | |
| 26099 | 1 tsp | Lemon Pepper, Lawry's | 3 | 7 | 5 | 0.2 | 1.4 | 0.1 | | | 0.1 | | | | | | | | | | | | | | | | 0.00 | | | | | | | | | | | | 13 | | 390 | |
| 26645 | 1/4 oz | Licorice Powder, avg | 7 | 15 | 9 | 0.4 | 3.1 | | | | 0.1 | | | | | | | 0 | 0 | 0 | 0 | 0 | | | | | 0.00 | | | | | | 41 | | 3.5 | | | | | | | |
| 26024 | 1 tsp | Mace, ground, avg | 2 | 9 | 8 | 0.1 | 1.0 | 0.4 | | | 0.6 | 0.2 | 0.2 | 0.1 | 0.00 | 0.09 | 0 | 16 | 2 | 0 | 2 | 10 | 0.01 | 0.01 | 0.03 | 0.01 | 0.00 | 1.5 | | 0.4 | 0.0 | | 5 | 0.0 | 0.3 | 3 | 0.0 | 2 | 9 | 0.1 | 2 | 0.05 |
| 26183 | 1 tsp | Mackakscha, ethiopian mixed spice, avg | 4 | 12 | 12 | 0.3 | 2.4 | 0.5 | | | 0.4 | | | | | | | 85 | 9 | 0 | 9 | 51 | 0.00 | 0.00 | 0.18 | | 0.00 | | | | | | 0 | | | | | 9 | | | | |
| 26025 | 1 tsp | Marjoram, dried, avg | 1 | 3 | 8 | 0.1 | 0.6 | 0.4 | | | 0.1 | 0.0 | 0.0 | 0.0 | 0.03 | 0.01 | 0 | 81 | 8 | 0 | 8 | 48 | 0.00 | 0.00 | 0.04 | 0.01 | 0.00 | 2.7 | | 0.5 | 0.0 | | 20 | 0.0 | 0.8 | 3 | 0.1 | 3 | 15 | 0.0 | 1 | 0.04 |
| | | Mexican Seasoning Mixes | | | | | | | | | | | | | | | | | | | | | | | | | | | | | | | | | | | | | | | | |
| 26479 | 1/4 oz | Burrito, dry, Old El Paso | 7 | 23 | 6 | 0.6 | 3.5 | 1.2 | 0.0 | 2.3 | 0.0 | 0.0 | 0.0 | 0.0 | 0.00 | 0.00 | 0 | 117 | 23 | | | | | | | | 0.00 | | | 0.0 | | | 23 | | 0.4 | | | | | | 338 | |
| 26481 | 1/4 oz | Enchilada, dry, Old El Paso | 7 | 18 | 6 | 0.0 | 3.5 | 0.9 | 0.0 | 2.6 | 0.0 | 0.0 | 0.0 | 0.0 | 0.00 | 0.00 | 0 | 525 | 105 | | | | | | | | 0.00 | | | 0.0 | | | 0 | | 0.0 | | | | | | 945 | |
| 26605 | 1 Tbs | Taco, dry, Natural Touch | 9 | 30 | 10 | 4.2 | 2.3 | 1.5 | 0.4 | 0.4 | 0.5 | 0.1 | 0.2 | 0.2 | | | 0 | 61 | 6 | 0 | 6 | | 0.03 | 0.02 | 0.00 | 0.03 | 0.00 | | | 0.0 | | | 15 | | 0.5 | | | 56 | 189 | | 293 | 0.16 |
| 26478 | 1 Tbs | Taco, dry, Pancho Villa | 9 | 30 | 5 | 0.0 | 7.5 | 0.0 | 3.0 | 4.5 | 0.0 | 0.0 | 0.0 | 0.0 | 0.00 | 0.00 | 0 | | | | | | | | | | 0.00 | | | | | | | | | | | | | | 825 | |
| 26647 | 1/4 oz | Mint Leaves, avg | 7 | 2 | 89 | 0.2 | 0.4 | | | | 0.0 | | | | | | 0 | 86 | 9 | 0 | 9 | 52 | 0.01 | 0.01 | 0.05 | | 0.00 | 7.7 | | 4.5 | 0.0 | | 14 | | 0.3 | | 0.1 | 3 | 13 | | 0 | |
| 26051 | 1 tsp | Monosodium Glutamate, msg, Anjinomoto | 4 | 11 | 0 | | | | | | | | | | | | | | | | | | | | | | 0.00 | | | | | | 1 | | 0.0 | | | 0 | 0 | | 496 | |
| 26069 | 1 tsp | Mustard Powder, Foran Spice Company | 3 | 17 | 3 | 1.0 | 0.6 | 0.1 | | | 1.3 | | | | | | 0 | 2 | 0.2 | 0 | 0.2 | 1 | 0.02 | 0.01 | 0.25 | | 0.00 | | | 0.7 | | | 9 | | 0.2 | | | 24 | 21 | | 0 | |
| 26110 | 1 tsp | Mustard Seed, yellow, avg | 4 | 19 | 7 | 1.0 | 1.4 | 0.6 | | | 1.2 | 0.1 | 0.8 | 0.2 | 0.11 | 0.10 | 0 | 2 | 0.3 | 0 | 0.3 | 1 | 0.02 | 0.02 | 0.32 | 0.01 | 0.00 | 3.0 | | 0.1 | | | 21 | 0.0 | 0.4 | 12 | 0.1 | 34 | 27 | 5.4 | 0 | 0.23 |
| 26026 | 1 tsp | Nutmeg, ground, avg | 2 | 10 | 6 | 0.1 | 1.0 | 0.4 | | | 0.7 | 0.5 | 0.1 | 0.0 | 0.00 | 0.01 | 0 | 2 | 0.2 | 0 | 0.2 | 1 | 0.01 | 0.00 | 0.03 | 0.01 | 0.00 | 1.5 | | 0.1 | 0.0 | | 4 | 0.0 | 0.1 | 4 | 0.1 | 4 | 7 | 0.0 | 0 | 0.04 |
| | | Oils | | | | | | | | | | | | | | | | | | | | | | | | | | | | | | | | | | | | | | | | |
| 26240 | 1/4 oz | Cinnamon, Kalsec | 7 | 62 | 1 | 0.0 | 0.0 | 0.0 | 0.0 | 0.0 | 6.9 | 1.0 | | | | | 0 | 0 | 0 | 0 | 0 | 0 | | | | | 0.00 | | | 0.0 | | | 0 | | 0.1 | | | | | | 0 | |
| 26199 | 1/4 oz | Clove, Kalsec | 7 | 62 | 1 | 0.0 | 0.0 | 0.0 | 0.0 | 0.0 | 6.9 | 1.0 | | | | | 0 | 0 | 0 | 0 | 0 | 0 | | | | | 0.00 | | | 0.0 | | | 0 | | 0.1 | | | | | | 0 | |
| 26263 | 1/4 oz | Peppermint, Kalsec | 7 | 62 | 1 | 0.0 | 0.0 | 0.0 | 0.0 | 0.0 | 6.9 | 1.0 | | | | | 0 | 0 | 0 | 0 | 0 | 0 | | | | | 0.00 | | | 0.0 | | | 0 | | 0.1 | | | | | | 0 | |
| 26008 | 1 tsp | Onion Powder, avg | 2 | 7 | 5 | 0.2 | 1.6 | 0.1 | | | 0.0 | 0.0 | 0.0 | 0.0 | 0.00 | 0.01 | 0 | 0 | 0 | 0 | 0 | 0 | 0.01 | 0.00 | 0.01 | 0.03 | 0.00 | 3.3 | 0.03 | 0.3 | 0.0 | | 7 | 0.0 | 0.1 | 2 | 0.0 | 7 | 19 | 0.0 | 1 | 0.05 |
| 26175 | 1 tsp | Onion Salt, Heller Seasonings | 6 | 3 | 1 | 0.1 | 0.7 | 0.1 | | | 0.0 | | | | | | 0 | 0 | 0 | 0 | 0 | 0 | 0.00 | 0.00 | 0.01 | 0.01 | 0.00 | 1.2 | 0.01 | 0.1 | 0.0 | 0.0 | 6 | 0.0 | 0.0 | 3 | | 3 | 9 | 0.2 | 1977 | 0.04 |
| | | Oregano | | | | | | | | | | | | | | | | | | | | | | | | | | | | | | | | | | | | | | | | |
| 26310 | 1 Tbs | Fresh, avg | 6 | 4 | 82 | 0.1 | 0.6 | | | | 0.1 | | | | | | | 81 | 8 | 0 | 8 | 49 | 0.00 | | | | 0.00 | | | 2.7 | 0.0 | | 19 | | | 3 | 0.0 | 2 | 20 | | 0 | 0.05 |
| 26009 | 1 tsp | Ground, avg | 2 | 6 | 7 | 0.2 | 1.3 | 0.9 | | | 0.2 | 0.1 | 0.0 | 0.1 | 0.08 | 0.02 | 0 | 138 | 14 | 0 | 14 | 73 | 0.01 | 0.01 | 0.12 | 0.02 | 0.00 | 5.5 | | 1.0 | 0.0 | | 32 | 0.0 | 0.9 | 5 | 0.1 | 4 | 33 | 0.1 | 0 | 0.09 |
| 26519 | 1 tsp | Mediterranean, dried, Amer Spice & Trade Assoc | 2 | 7 | 10 | 0.3 | 1.3 | 0.8 | | | 0.1 | | | | | | | 112 | 11 | 0 | 11 | 67 | | | | | 0.00 | | | 0.1 | | | 31 | | 1.1 | | | | | | 1 | |
| 26518 | 1 tsp | Mexican, dried, American Spice & Trade Assoc | 2 | 7 | 10 | 0.3 | 1.3 | 0.7 | | | 0.1 | | | | | | | 164 | 16 | 0 | 16 | 99 | | | | | 0.00 | | | 0.1 | | | 24 | | 0.3 | | | | | | 0 | |
| | | Paprika | | | | | | | | | | | | | | | | | | | | | | | | | | | | | | | | | | | | | | | | |
| 26010 | 1 tsp | Average | 2 | 6 | 10 | 0.3 | 1.1 | 0.4 | | | 0.3 | 0.0 | 0.0 | 0.2 | 0.02 | 0.15 | 0 | 1212 | 121 | 0 | 121 | 727 | 0.01 | 0.03 | 0.31 | 0.04 | 0.00 | 2.1 | 0.04 | 1.4 | 0.0 | | 4 | 0.0 | 0.5 | 4 | 0.0 | 7 | 47 | 0.1 | 1 | 0.08 |
| 26616 | 1 tsp | Hot Hungarian, Budapest's | 2 | 0 | | 0.0 | 0.0 | 0.0 | 0.0 | 0.0 | 0.0 | 0.0 | 0.0 | 0.0 | 0.00 | 0.00 | | 1200 | 120 | 0 | 120 | 720 | | | | | 0.00 | | | | | | | | | | | | | | 0 | |
| 26615 | 1 tsp | Sweet Hungarian, Budapest's | 2 | 0 | | 0.0 | 0.0 | 0.0 | 0.0 | 0.0 | 0.0 | 0.0 | 0.0 | 0.0 | 0.00 | 0.00 | | 1200 | 120 | 0 | 120 | 720 | | | | | 0.00 | | | | | | | | | | | | | | 0 | |
| 26016 | 1 tsp | Pepper, black, avg | 2 | 5 | 10 | 0.2 | 1.3 | 0.5 | | | 0.1 | 0.0 | 0.0 | 0.0 | 0.00 | 0.02 | 0 | 4 | 0.4 | 0 | 0.4 | 2 | 0.00 | 0.00 | 0.02 | 0.01 | 0.00 | 0.2 | | 0.4 | 0.0 | | 9 | 0.0 | 0.6 | 4 | 0.1 | 3 | 25 | 0.1 | 1 | 0.03 |
| 26037 | 1 tsp | Pepper, white, avg | 2 | 6 | 11 | 0.2 | 1.4 | 0.5 | | | 0.0 | 0.0 | 0.0 | 0.0 | 0.00 | 0.01 | 0 | 0 | 0 | 0 | 0 | 0 | 0.00 | 0.00 | 0.00 | 0.01 | 0.00 | 0.2 | | 0.4 | 0.0 | | 5 | 0.0 | 0.3 | 2 | 0.1 | 4 | 1 | 0.1 | 0 | 0.02 |
| 26628 | 1 Tbs | Peppermint, fresh, avg | 16 | 11 | 79 | 0.6 | 2.4 | 1.3 | | | 0.2 | 0.0 | 0.0 | 0.1 | 0.07 | 0.01 | 0 | 680 | 68 | 0 | 68 | 408 | 0.01 | 0.04 | 0.27 | 0.02 | 0.00 | 18.2 | 0.05 | 5.1 | | | 39 | 0.1 | 0.8 | 13 | 0.2 | 12 | 91 | | 5 | 0.18 |
| 26015 | 1 tsp | Poppyseed, avg | 3 | 16 | 7 | 0.5 | 0.7 | 0.3 | | | 1.3 | 0.1 | 0.2 | 0.9 | 0.01 | 0.91 | 0 | 0 | 0 | 0 | 0 | 0 | 0.03 | 0.01 | 0.03 | 0.01 | 0.00 | 1.7 | | 0.1 | 0.0 | | 43 | 0.0 | 0.3 | 10 | 0.2 | 25 | 21 | 0.0 | 1 | 0.31 |
| 26558 | 1 ea | Pork Seasoning, bbq, 1/8 pkt, Shake N Bake | 80 | 280 | | 0.0 | 64.0 | 0.0 | 32.0 | 32.0 | 0.0 | 0.0 | 0.0 | 0.0 | 0.00 | 0.00 | 0 | 1600 | 320 | | | | | | | | 0.00 | | | 0.0 | | | 0 | | 0.0 | | | | 320 | | 2000 | |
| 26551 | 1 ea | Pork Seasoning, hot & spicy, 1/8 pkt, Shake N Bake | 64 | 262 | | 5.8 | 46.5 | 0.0 | 5.8 | 40.7 | 2.9 | 0.0 | | | | | 0 | 0 | 0 | 0 | 0 | 0 | | | | | 0.00 | | | 0.0 | | | 0 | | 0.0 | | | | 145 | | 1280 | |
| 26548 | 1 ea | Potato Seasoning, cheddar, 1/6 pkt, Shake N Bake | 42 | 180 | | 12.0 | 12.0 | 0.0 | 6.0 | 6.0 | 12.0 | 9.0 | | | | | 30 | 0 | 0 | 0 | 0 | 0 | | | | | 0.00 | | | 0.0 | | | 240 | | 0.0 | | | | 270 | | 2280 | |
| 26549 | 1 ea | Potato Seasoning, herb & garlic, 1/6 pkt, Shake N Bake | 42 | 120 | | 0.0 | 30.0 | 0.0 | 6.0 | 24.0 | 0.0 | 0.0 | 0.0 | 0.0 | 0.00 | 0.00 | 0 | 0 | 0 | 0 | 0 | 0 | | | | | 0.00 | | | 0.0 | | | 0 | | 0.0 | | | | 120 | | 2220 | |
| | | Poultry Seasoning Mixes | | | | | | | | | | | | | | | | | | | | | | | | | | | | | | | | | | | | | | | | |
| 26028 | 1 tsp | Average | 1 | 3 | 9 | 0.1 | 0.7 | 0.1 | | | 0.1 | 0.0 | 0.0 | 0.0 | 0.01 | 0.01 | 0 | 26 | 3 | 0 | 3 | 16 | 0.00 | 0.00 | 0.03 | 0.01 | 0.00 | 1.4 | | 0.1 | 0.0 | | 10 | 0.0 | 0.4 | 2 | 0.1 | 2 | 7 | 0.1 | 0 | 0.03 |
| 26557 | 1 ea | Barbecue, 1/8 pkt, Shake N Bake | 96 | 360 | | 0.0 | 72.0 | 0.0 | 40.0 | 32.0 | 8.0 | 0.0 | | | | | 0 | 1600 | 320 | | | | | | | | 0.00 | | | 9.6 | | | 0 | | 0.0 | | | | 320 | | 3280 | |
| 26552 | 1 ea | Hot & Spicy, 1/8 pkt, Shake N Bake | 80 | 320 | | 8.0 | 56.0 | 0.0 | 8.0 | 48.0 | 8.0 | 0.0 | | | | | 0 | 0 | 0 | 0 | 0 | 0 | | | | | 0.00 | | | 0.0 | | | 0 | | 2.9 | | | | 160 | | 1520 | |
| 26029 | 1 tsp | Pumpkin Pie, avg | 2 | 7 | 8 | 0.1 | 1.4 | 0.3 | | | 0.3 | 0.1 | 0.0 | 0.0 | 0.00 | 0.01 | 0 | 5 | 1 | 0 | 1 | 3 | 0.00 | 0.00 | 0.04 | 0.01 | 0.00 | 1.0 | | 0.5 | 0.0 | | 14 | 0.0 | 0.4 | 3 | 0.3 | 2 | 13 | 0.2 | 1 | 0.05 |

| Code | Amount | Description | Weight (g) | Calories | % Water | Protein (g) | Carbs (g) | Fiber (g) | Sugar (g) | Other Carbs (g) | Fat (g) | Sat Fat (g) | Mono Fat (g) | Poly Fat (g) | Omega 3 (g) | Omega 6 (g) | Choles (mg) | Vit A (IU) | Vit A (RE) | Retinol (RE) | Carotenoids (RE) | Beta Carotene (mcg) | Thiamin (mg) | Riboflavin (mg) | Niacin (NE) | Vit B6 (mg) | Vit B12 (mcg) | Folate (mcg) | Panto (mg) | Vit C (mg) | Vit D (mg) | Vit E (α TE) | Calcium (mg) | Copper (mg) | Iron (mg) | Magnes (mg) | Mang (mg) | Phos (mg) | Potassium (mg) | Selenium (mcg) | Sodium (mg) | Zinc (mg) |
|---|---|---|---|---|---|---|---|---|---|---|---|---|---|---|---|---|---|---|---|---|---|---|---|---|---|---|---|---|---|---|---|---|---|---|---|---|---|---|---|---|---|---|
| | | **Basic Components** → Weight–Fat; **Additional Fats** → Sat Fat–Choles; **Vit A & Components** → Vit A–Beta Carotene; **Vitamins** → Thiamin–Vit E; **Minerals** → Calcium–Zinc | | | | | | | | | | | | | | | | | | | | | | | | | | | | | | | | | | | | | | | | |
| 26077 | 1 tsp | Red Pepper, Foran Spice Company | 2 | 8 | 6 | 0.3 | 1.1 | 0.5 | | | 0.3 | | | | | | 0 | 628 | 63 | 0 | 63 | 377 | 0.01 | 0.02 | 0.27 | | 0.00 | | | 0.6 | | | 2 | | 0.2 | | | 6 | 42 | | 0 | |
| 26111 | 1 tsp | Saffron, avg | 1 | 3 | 12 | 0.1 | 0.7 | 0.0 | | | 0.1 | 0.0 | 0.0 | 0.0 | 0.01 | 0.01 | 0 | 5 | 1 | 0 | 1 | 3 | 0.00 | 0.00 | 0.01 | 0.01 | 0.00 | 0.9 | | 0.8 | 0.0 | | 1 | 0.0 | 0.1 | 3 | 0.3 | 3 | 17 | 0.1 | 1 | 0.01 |
| 26311 | 1 Tbs | Sage, fresh, avg | 2 | 2 | 66 | 0.1 | 0.3 | | | | 0.1 | | | | | | | 43 | 4 | 0 | 4 | 26 | 0.00 | | | | 0.00 | | | | 0.0 | | 12 | | | 3 | 0.2 | 1 | 8 | | 0 | 0.03 |
| 26031 | 1 tsp | Sage, ground, avg | 1 | 3 | 8 | 0.1 | 0.6 | 0.4 | | | 0.1 | 0.1 | 0.0 | 0.0 | 0.01 | 0.01 | 0 | 59 | 6 | 0 | 6 | 35 | 0.01 | 0.00 | 0.06 | 0.01 | 0.00 | 2.7 | | 0.3 | 0.0 | | 17 | 0.0 | 0.3 | 4 | 0.0 | 1 | 11 | 0.0 | 0 | 0.05 |
| | | Salt | | | | | | | | | | | | | | | | | | | | | | | | | | | | | | | | | | | | | | | | |
| 26048 | 1 tsp | Light, Morton | 6 | | 0 | 0.0 | 0.0 | | | | 0.0 | 0.0 | 0.0 | 0.0 | 0.00 | 0.00 | | | | | | | | | | | 0.00 | | | | | | 2 | | | 4 | | | 1560 | | 1170 | |
| 26280 | 1/4 oz | Rock, Azko Salt Incorporated | 7 | 0 | 0 | 0.0 | 0.0 | 0.0 | 0.0 | 0.0 | 0.0 | 0.0 | 0.0 | 0.0 | 0.00 | 0.00 | 0 | 0 | 0 | 0 | 0 | 0 | 0.00 | 0.00 | 0.00 | 0.00 | 0.00 | 0.0 | 0.00 | 0.0 | 0.0 | 0.0 | 21 | | | 0 | | | | | 2695 | |
| 26273 | 1 tsp | Sea, avg | 6 | 0 | 0 | 0.0 | 0.0 | 0.0 | 0.0 | 0.0 | 0.0 | 0.0 | 0.0 | 0.0 | 0.00 | 0.00 | 0 | 0 | 0 | 0 | 0 | 0 | 0.00 | 0.00 | 0.00 | 0.00 | 0.00 | 0.0 | 0.00 | 0.0 | 0.0 | 0.0 | 2 | 0.0 | 0.0 | 0 | 0.0 | 0 | 1 | 0.2 | 2511 | 0.00 |
| 26098 | 1 tsp | Seasoned, no msg, Lowry's | 4 | 3 | 5 | 0.1 | 0.6 | 0.1 | | | 0.1 | | | | | | | | | | | | | | | | 0.00 | | | | | | | | | | | | 12 | | 1234 | |
| 26014 | 1 tsp | Table, avg | 6 | 0 | 0 | 0.0 | 0.0 | 0.0 | 0.0 | 0.0 | 0.0 | 0.0 | 0.0 | 0.0 | 0.00 | 0.00 | 0 | 0 | 0 | 0 | 0 | 0 | 0.00 | 0.00 | 0.00 | 0.00 | 0.00 | 0.0 | 0.00 | 0.0 | 0.0 | 0.0 | 1 | 0.0 | 0.0 | 0 | 0.0 | 0 | 0 | 0.0 | 2325 | 0.01 |
| | | Salt Substitutes | | | | | | | | | | | | | | | | | | | | | | | | | | | | | | | | | | | | | | | | |
| 26090 | 1 tsp | Morton | 5 | 0 | 0 | 0.0 | 0.1 | | | | 0.0 | 0.0 | 0.0 | 0.0 | 0.00 | 0.00 | | | | | | | | | | | 0.00 | | | | | | 28 | | | | | 23 | 2515 | | 0 | |
| 26632 | 1 tsp | Nu-Salt, Sweet N Low | 5 | 0 | | 0.0 | 0.0 | 0.0 | 0.0 | 0.0 | 0.0 | 0.0 | 0.0 | 0.0 | 0.00 | 0.00 | 0 | 0 | 0 | 0 | 0 | 0 | | | | | 0.00 | | | 0.0 | | 0.0 | 0 | | | 0 | | | 2650 | | 0 | |
| 26091 | 1 tsp | Seasoned, Morton | 4 | 2 | 1 | 0.0 | 0.4 | | | | 0.0 | | | | | | | | | | | | | | | | 0.00 | | | | | | | | | | | | 1732 | | 1 | |
| 26112 | 1 tsp | Savory, ground, avg | 2 | 5 | 9 | 0.1 | 1.4 | 0.9 | | | 0.1 | 0.1 | | | | | 0 | 103 | 10 | 0 | 10 | 62 | 0.01 | | 0.08 | | 0.00 | | | 1.0 | 0.0 | | 43 | 0.0 | 0.8 | 8 | 0.1 | 3 | 21 | 0.1 | 0 | 0.09 |
| 26530 | 1 tsp | Savory Leaves, dried, American Spice & Trade Assoc | 1 | 3 | 11 | 0.1 | 0.7 | 0.4 | | | 0.0 | | | | | | | 42 | 4 | 0 | 4 | 25 | | | | | 0.00 | | | 0.0 | | | 19 | | 0.2 | | | | | | 0 | |
| 26631 | 1 tsp | Spearmint, dried, avg | 0 | 0 | 11 | 0.0 | 0.0 | 0.0 | | | 0.0 | 0.0 | 0.0 | 0.0 | 0.00 | 0.00 | 0 | 0 | 0 | 0 | 0 | 0 | 0.00 | 0.00 | 0.00 | 0.00 | 0.00 | 0.0 | 0.00 | 0.0 | | | 0 | 0.0 | 0.0 | 0 | 0.0 | 0 | 0 | | 0 | 0.00 |
| 26630 | 1 Tbs | Spearmint, fresh, avg | 6 | 3 | 86 | 0.2 | 0.5 | 0.4 | | | 0.0 | 0.0 | 0.0 | 0.0 | 0.02 | 0.00 | 0 | 243 | 24 | 0 | 24 | 146 | 0.00 | 0.01 | 0.06 | 0.01 | 0.00 | 6.3 | 0.01 | 0.8 | | | 12 | 0.0 | 0.7 | 4 | 0.1 | 4 | 27 | | 2 | 0.07 |
| 26320 | 1 Tbs | Tarragon, fresh, avg | 6 | 3 | 86 | 0.2 | 0.4 | | | | 0.1 | | | | | | | 38 | 4 | 0 | 4 | 23 | 0.01 | | | | 0.00 | | | 0.1 | 0.0 | | 10 | | | 3 | | 3 | 27 | | 1 | 0.04 |
| 26032 | 1 tsp | Tarragon, ground, avg | 2 | 6 | 8 | 0.5 | 1.0 | 0.1 | | | 0.1 | 0.0 | 0.0 | 0.1 | 0.06 | 0.01 | 0 | 84 | 8 | 0 | 8 | 50 | 0.01 | 0.03 | 0.18 | 0.02 | 0.00 | 5.5 | | 1.0 | 0.0 | | 23 | 0.0 | 0.6 | 7 | 0.2 | 6 | 60 | 0.1 | 1 | 0.08 |
| 26312 | 1 Tbs | Thyme, fresh, avg | 4 | 4 | 69 | 0.1 | 0.6 | | | | 0.1 | | | | | | | 51 | 5 | 0 | 5 | 30 | 0.01 | | | | 0.00 | | | | | | 25 | | | 3 | 0.1 | 3 | 11 | | 1 | 0.08 |
| 26033 | 1 tsp | Thyme, ground, avg | 1 | 3 | 8 | 0.1 | 0.6 | 0.4 | | | 0.1 | 0.0 | 0.0 | 0.0 | 0.01 | 0.00 | 0 | 38 | 4 | 0 | 4 | 23 | 0.01 | 0.00 | 0.05 | 0.01 | 0.00 | 2.7 | | 0.5 | 0.0 | | 19 | 0.0 | 1.2 | 2 | 0.1 | 2 | 8 | 0.0 | 1 | 0.06 |
| 26034 | 1 tsp | Turmeric, ground, avg | 2 | 7 | 11 | 0.2 | 1.3 | 0.4 | | | 0.2 | 0.1 | 0.0 | 0.0 | 0.01 | 0.03 | 0 | 0 | 0 | 0 | 0 | 0 | 0.00 | 0.00 | 0.10 | 0.04 | 0.00 | 0.8 | | 0.5 | 0.0 | | 4 | 0.0 | 0.8 | 4 | 0.2 | 5 | 50 | 0.1 | 1 | 0.09 |
| 26086 | 1 tsp | Turmeric, ground, Foran Spice Company | 2 | 8 | 6 | 0.2 | 1.4 | 0.5 | | | 0.2 | | | | | | 0 | | | | | | 0.00 | 0.00 | 0.10 | | 0.00 | | | 1.0 | | | 4 | | 0.9 | | | 5 | 50 | | 0 | |
| | | Vanilla Flavorings | | | | | | | | | | | | | | | | | | | | | | | | | | | | | | | | | | | | | | | | |
| 26624 | 1 tsp | Extract, avg | 4 | 12 | 53 | 0.0 | 0.5 | 0.0 | | | 0.0 | 0.0 | 0.0 | 0.0 | 0.00 | 0.00 | 0 | 0 | 0 | 0 | 0 | 0 | 0.00 | 0.00 | 0.02 | 0.00 | 0.00 | 0.0 | 0.00 | 0.0 | | 0.0 | 0 | 0.0 | 0.0 | 0 | 0.0 | 0 | 6 | 0.0 | 0 | 0.00 |
| 26625 | 1 tsp | Extract, imitation, w/alcohol, avg | 4 | 9 | 64 | 0.0 | 0.1 | 0.0 | | | 0.0 | 0.0 | 0.0 | 0.0 | 0.00 | 0.00 | 0 | 0 | 0 | 0 | 0 | 0 | 0.00 | 0.00 | 0.01 | 0.00 | 0.00 | 0.0 | 0.00 | 0.0 | | 0.0 | 0 | 0.0 | 0.0 | 0 | 0.0 | 1 | 4 | | 0 | 0.00 |
| 26626 | 1 tsp | Extract, imitation, w/o alcohol, avg | 4 | 2 | 86 | 0.0 | 0.6 | 0.0 | | | 0.0 | 0.0 | 0.0 | 0.0 | 0.00 | 0.00 | 0 | 0 | 0 | 0 | 0 | 0 | 0.00 | 0.00 | 0.01 | 0.00 | 0.00 | 0.0 | 0.00 | 0.0 | | 0.0 | 0 | 0.0 | 0.0 | 0 | 0.0 | 0 | 0 | 0.0 | 0 | 0.00 |
| 26290 | 1 tsp | Vanillin, Rhone Poulenc | 5 | 22 | 0 | | 5.0 | | | | | | | | | | | | | | | | | | | | 0.00 | | | | | | 0 | | 0.0 | 0 | | 0 | 0 | | 0 | |
| | | **SUPPLEMENTS AND FORMULAS–BARS, LIQUIDS AND MIXES** | | | | | | | | | | | | | | | | | | | | | | | | | | | | | | | | | | | | | | | | |
| | | Carnation Breakfast Bars | | | | | | | | | | | | | | | | | | | | | | | | | | | | | | | | | | | | | | | | |
| 62204 | 1 ea | Chocolate Chip | 36 | 150 | 12 | 2.0 | 22.0 | 0.8 | 10.0 | 11.2 | 6.1 | 2.5 | | | | | 0 | 1250 | 250 | | | | 0.37 | 0.42 | 5.00 | 0.50 | 1.50 | 100.1 | 2.50 | 15.0 | 2.5 | | 500 | 0.5 | 4.5 | 100 | | 250 | 55 | | 80 | 3.74 |
| 62319 | 1 ea | Chocolate Chunk Granola | 36 | 389 | 17 | 5.6 | 61.1 | 2.8 | 27.8 | 30.5 | 14.0 | 6.0 | | | | | 0 | 3472 | 694 | | | | 1.04 | 1.18 | 13.90 | 1.39 | 4.17 | 278.0 | 6.94 | 41.7 | 6.9 | | 1389 | 1.4 | 12.5 | 278 | | 694 | 111 | | 153 | 10.40 |
| 62320 | 1 ea | Honey & Oats Granola | 36 | 130 | 17 | 2.0 | 23.0 | 1.0 | 9.0 | 13.0 | 4.0 | 1.4 | | | | | 0 | 1250 | 250 | | | | 0.37 | 0.42 | 5.00 | 0.50 | 1.50 | 100.1 | 2.50 | 15.0 | 2.5 | | 500 | 0.5 | 4.5 | 100 | | 250 | 40 | | 55 | 3.74 |
| 62203 | 1 ea | Peanut Butter & Chocolate Chip | 36 | 150 | 15 | 3.0 | 21.0 | 0.5 | 10.0 | 10.5 | 5.0 | 2.2 | | | | | 0 | 1250 | 250 | | | | 0.37 | 0.42 | 5.00 | 0.50 | 0.15 | 100.1 | 2.50 | 15.0 | 2.5 | | 500 | 0.5 | 4.5 | 100 | | 250 | 80 | | 90 | 3.74 |
| | | Carnation Instant Breakfast Drinks | | | | | | | | | | | | | | | | | | | | | | | | | | | | | | | | | | | | | | | | |
| 62172 | 1 ea | Cafe Mocha, dry pkt | 37 | 129 | | 4.0 | 27.7 | 0.4 | 22.8 | 4.5 | 0.4 | 0.0 | | | | | 3 | 1731 | 520 | | | | 0.30 | 0.13 | 4.96 | 0.40 | 0.59 | 98.8 | 1.98 | 26.7 | 0.0 | | 346 | 0.5 | 4.4 | 79 | | 99 | 336 | | 99 | 2.96 |
| 62444 | 1 cup | Cafe Mocha, RTS | 251 | 176 | | 10.0 | 28.0 | 0.0 | 26.4 | 1.5 | 2.5 | 0.0 | | | | | 5 | 1800 | 540 | | | | 0.30 | 0.35 | 4.02 | 0.40 | 1.20 | 80.3 | 2.01 | 24.1 | 2.0 | | 399 | 0.4 | 3.5 | 80 | | 279 | 439 | | 168 | 3.01 |
| 62059 | 1 ea | Chocolate, dry pkt | 37 | 130 | | 4.0 | 28.1 | 1.0 | 22.1 | 5.0 | 1.1 | 0.4 | | | | | 3 | 1755 | 527 | | | | 0.30 | 0.14 | 5.03 | 0.40 | 0.60 | 100.3 | 2.01 | 27.1 | 0.0 | | 301 | 0.5 | 4.5 | 80 | | 100 | 361 | | 100 | 3.00 |
| 62170 | 1 ea | Chocolate, dry pkt, sugar free | 21 | 70 | | 4.0 | 12.0 | 1.0 | 6.0 | 5.0 | 1.0 | 0.4 | | | | | 3 | 1750 | 525 | | | | 0.30 | 0.10 | 5.00 | 0.40 | 0.60 | 100.0 | 2.00 | 27.0 | 0.0 | | 300 | 0.5 | 4.5 | 80 | | 100 | 350 | | 90 | 3.00 |
| 62447 | 1 cup | Chocolate, RTS | 251 | 176 | | 10.0 | 29.6 | 0.8 | 27.2 | 1.5 | 2.5 | 0.0 | | | | | 5 | 1800 | 540 | | | | 0.30 | 0.35 | 4.02 | 0.40 | 1.20 | 80.3 | 2.01 | 24.1 | 2.0 | | 399 | 0.4 | 3.5 | 80 | | 279 | 487 | | 183 | 3.01 |
| 62060 | 1 ea | Chocolate Malt, dry pkt | 36 | 132 | | 4.1 | 26.4 | 0.9 | 16.2 | 9.3 | 1.4 | 0.4 | | | | | 3 | 1775 | 533 | | | | 0.31 | 0.07 | 5.08 | 0.41 | 0.61 | 101.5 | 2.03 | 27.4 | 0.0 | | 253 | 0.5 | 4.6 | 81 | | 102 | 253 | | 132 | 3.06 |
| 62171 | 1 ea | Chocolate Malt, dry pkt, sugar free | 20 | 71 | | 4.0 | 11.1 | 1.0 | 6.1 | 4.0 | 1.6 | 1.0 | | | | | 3 | 1768 | 531 | | | | 0.30 | 0.10 | 5.06 | 0.40 | 0.61 | 101.0 | 2.02 | 27.3 | 0.0 | | 253 | 0.5 | 4.5 | 81 | | 101 | 263 | | 121 | 3.04 |
| 62058 | 1 ea | Strawberry Crème, dry pkt | 36 | 130 | | 4.0 | 27.9 | 0.0 | 17.9 | 10.0 | 0.0 | 0.0 | 0.0 | 0.0 | 0.00 | 0.00 | 3 | 1745 | 525 | | | | 0.30 | 0.14 | 5.00 | 0.40 | 0.60 | 99.7 | 1.99 | 26.9 | 0.0 | | 349 | 0.5 | 4.5 | 80 | | 100 | 249 | | 159 | 2.99 |
| 62169 | 1 ea | Strawberry Crème, dry pkt, sugar free | 20 | 70 | | 4.0 | 12.0 | 0.0 | 7.0 | 5.0 | 0.0 | 0.0 | 0.0 | 0.0 | 0.00 | 0.00 | 3 | 1750 | 526 | | | | 0.30 | 0.14 | 5.00 | 0.40 | 0.60 | 100.0 | 2.00 | 27.0 | 0.0 | | 350 | 0.5 | 4.5 | 80 | | 100 | 250 | | 90 | 3.00 |
| 62445 | 1 cup | Strawberry Crème, RTS | 252 | 176 | | 10.0 | 28.0 | 0.0 | 26.4 | 1.5 | 2.5 | 0.0 | | | | | 5 | 1799 | 540 | | | | 0.30 | 0.33 | 4.03 | 0.40 | 1.21 | 80.6 | 1.99 | 23.9 | 2.0 | | 401 | 0.4 | 3.5 | 81 | | 280 | 375 | | 169 | 3.02 |
| 62057 | 1 ea | Vanilla, dry pkt | 36 | 131 | | 4.0 | 27.2 | 0.0 | 17.1 | 10.1 | 0.0 | 0.0 | 0.0 | 0.0 | 0.00 | 0.00 | 3 | 1760 | 528 | | | | 0.30 | 0.14 | 5.04 | 0.40 | 0.60 | 100.4 | 2.01 | 27.1 | 0.0 | | 352 | 0.5 | 4.5 | 80 | | 100 | 251 | | 111 | 3.02 |
| 62168 | 1 ea | Vanilla, dry pkt, sugar free | 20 | 69 | | 4.0 | 11.9 | 0.0 | 6.9 | 5.0 | 0.0 | 0.0 | 0.0 | 0.0 | 0.00 | 0.00 | 3 | 1733 | 520 | | | | 0.30 | 0.13 | 4.96 | 0.40 | 0.59 | 99.0 | 1.98 | 26.7 | 0.0 | | 347 | 0.5 | 4.5 | 79 | | 99 | 248 | | 89 | 2.98 |
| 62222 | 1 cup | Vanilla, prep w/whole milk | 280 | 291 | 77 | 16.0 | 37.0 | 0.0 | 20.0 | 17.0 | 9.0 | 0.0 | | | 0.00 | 0.00 | 34 | 2000 | 400 | | | | 0.60 | 1.19 | 7.00 | 0.80 | 3.00 | 140.0 | 3.50 | 21.0 | 6.0 | | 599 | 0.7 | 6.3 | 81 | | 451 | 711 | | 230 | 6.00 |
| 62446 | 1 cup | Vanilla, RTS | 250 | 160 | | 10.0 | 24.8 | 0.0 | 23.2 | 1.5 | 2.5 | 0.0 | | | | | 2 | 1798 | 540 | | | | 0.30 | 0.35 | 4.00 | 0.40 | 1.20 | 80.0 | 2.00 | 24.0 | 2.0 | | 400 | 0.4 | 3.5 | 80 | | 280 | 288 | | 145 | 3.00 |
| | | Ensure Drinks | | | | | | | | | | | | | | | | | | | | | | | | | | | | | | | | | | | | | | | | |
| 62146 | 1 cup | High Calorie Plus, RTS | 259 | 355 | 70 | 13.0 | 47.3 | | | | 12.6 | | | | | | | 834 | 167 | | | | 0.50 | 0.57 | 6.67 | 0.67 | 2.00 | 134.0 | 3.34 | 50.0 | 1.7 | | 167 | 0.3 | 3.0 | 67 | 0.8 | 167 | 460 | 12.0 | 250 | 3.75 |
| 62039 | 1 cup | High Nitrogen, RTS | 253 | 250 | 79 | 10.5 | 33.4 | | | | 8.4 | | | | | | | 893 | 179 | | | | 0.41 | 0.46 | 5.36 | 0.54 | 1.70 | 108.0 | 2.68 | 53.6 | 1.8 | | 179 | 0.4 | 3.2 | 72 | 0.9 | 179 | 370 | 13.0 | 190 | 4.02 |
| 62044 | 1 cup | High Nitrogen Plus, RTS | 259 | 355 | 70 | 14.8 | 47.3 | | | | 11.8 | | | | | | | 1250 | 250 | | | | 0.75 | 0.85 | 10.00 | 1.00 | 3.00 | 200.0 | 5.00 | 75.0 | 2.5 | | 250 | 0.5 | 4.5 | 100 | 1.3 | 250 | 430 | 18.0 | 280 | 5.63 |
| 62314 | 1 cup | High Protein, RTS | 253 | 225 | 80 | 12.0 | 30.8 | | | | 6.0 | 0.6 | | | | | | 1250 | 250 | | | | 0.38 | 0.43 | 5.00 | 0.50 | 1.50 | 100.0 | 2.50 | 30.0 | 2.5 | | 250 | 0.5 | 4.5 | 100 | 1.3 | 250 | 500 | 18.0 | 290 | 5.63 |
| 62038 | 1 cup | Vanilla, prep f/mix | 252 | 250 | 79 | 8.8 | 34.3 | | | | 8.8 | | | | | | | 625 | 125 | | | | 0.38 | 0.43 | 5.00 | 0.50 | 1.50 | 100.0 | 2.50 | 37.5 | 1.3 | | 125 | 0.3 | 2.3 | 50 | 0.6 | 125 | 370 | 9.0 | 200 | 2.82 |
| 62310 | 1 cup | With Fiber, RTS | 255 | 260 | 77 | 9.4 | 38.3 | 3.4 | | | 8.8 | | | | | | | 850 | 170 | | | | 0.39 | 0.44 | 5.10 | 0.51 | 1.60 | 102.0 | 2.55 | 51.0 | 1.7 | | 170 | 0.3 | 3.1 | 68 | 0.9 | 170 | 400 | 12.0 | 200 | 3.83 |
| | | Menu Magic | | | | | | | | | | | | | | | | | | | | | | | | | | | | | | | | | | | | | | | | |
| 62241 | 1 cup | Bread Pudding, prep f/mix | 298 | 441 | 64 | 8.0 | 90.0 | 2.0 | 74.0 | 14.0 | 6.0 | 2.0 | | | | | 9 | 298 | 60 | | | | 0.24 | 0.14 | 1.60 | | | | | 2.4 | | | 301 | | 2.2 | | | | 212 | | 519 | |
| 62219 | 1 cup | Great Nog, prep f/mix | 287 | 310 | 76 | 17.0 | 40.0 | 0.0 | 25.0 | 15.0 | 9.5 | | | | | | 43 | 2000 | 400 | | | | 0.60 | 1.19 | 7.00 | 0.80 | 3.00 | 140.0 | 3.50 | 21.0 | 6.0 | | 499 | 0.7 | 6.3 | 181 | | 399 | 709 | | 241 | 6.00 |
| 62215 | 1 cup | Lemon Shake, prep f/mix | 260 | 460 | 62 | 16.0 | 66.0 | 0.0 | 36.0 | 30.0 | 14.0 | 4.0 | | | | | 8 | 1500 | 300 | | | | 0.45 | 0.51 | 6.00 | 0.60 | 1.80 | 120.0 | 3.00 | 18.0 | 3.0 | | 400 | 0.6 | 5.4 | 161 | | 400 | 601 | | 320 | 4.50 |
| 62242 | 1 cup | Vanilla Mousse, prep f/mix | 121 | 221 | 65 | 2.0 | 28.1 | | | | 12.1 | | | | | | 0 | 0 | 0 | 0 | 0 | 0 | | | | | | | | 0.0 | | | 40 | 0.1 | | | | 80 | 121 | | 70 | |
| 62239 | 1 cup | Vanilla Pudding, low cal, prep f/mix | 270 | 181 | 85 | 8.0 | 30.0 | 0.0 | 12.0 | 18.0 | 2.6 | 0.0 | | | 0.00 | 0.00 | 0 | 400 | 80 | | | | | | | | | | | | | | 300 | | 0.0 | 32 | | | 421 | | 721 | 1.20 |
| 62216 | 1 cup | Vanilla Shake, prep f/mix | 260 | 400 | 66 | 12.0 | 62.0 | 0.0 | 34.0 | 28.0 | 12.0 | 2.0 | | | | | 8 | 1500 | 300 | | | | 0.45 | 0.51 | 6.00 | 0.60 | 1.80 | 120.0 | 3.00 | 18.0 | 3.0 | | 400 | 0.6 | 5.4 | 161 | | 299 | 460 | | 260 | 4.50 |
| 62073 | 1 cup | Nutra Shake | 260 | 400 | 66 | 12.0 | 62.0 | | | | 12.0 | 7.9 | 3.6 | 0.5 | | | 36 | 400 | 80 | | | | 0.18 | 0.85 | | 0.16 | 1.44 | | 1.60 | | 2.4 | | 500 | | | | | 360 | 444 | | 110 | 2.40 |
| 62074 | 1 cup | Nutra Shake, w/fiber | 260 | 400 | 62 | 14.7 | 80.0 | 5.3 | | | 2.7 | | | | | | 0 | 400 | 80 | | | | 0.18 | 0.85 | | 0.16 | 1.60 | | 1.60 | | 2.1 | | 500 | | | 64 | | 400 | 440 | | 147 | 2.40 |
| | | NutriCare Drinks | | | | | | | | | | | | | | | | | | | | | | | | | | | | | | | | | | | | | | | | |
| 62048 | 1 ea | Vanilla, dry pkt | 32 | 120 | 7 | 7.0 | 21.0 | | | | 1.0 | | | | | | 5 | 1250 | 250 | | | | 0.50 | 0.06 | 7.00 | 0.70 | 1.10 | 0.1 | 3.50 | 20.0 | 0.8 | | 0 | 0.7 | 6.3 | 100 | 1.3 | 0 | 300 | 20.0 | 120 | 5.30 |
| 62282 | 1 cup | Vanilla, prep w/2% lowfat milk | 227 | 209 | 78 | 13.5 | 28.5 | 0.1 | 23.7 | 4.7 | 4.7 | 2.5 | 1.3 | 0.3 | | | 16 | 2 | 0.4 | | | | 0.15 | 0.68 | 0.27 | 0.12 | 0.78 | 11.0 | 1.26 | 2.3 | 2.0 | | 368 | 0.0 | 0.4 | 123 | | 316 | 654 | | 204 | 0.84 |
| 62281 | 1 cup | Vanilla, prep w/whole milk | 276 | 270 | 78 | 14.9 | 32.7 | 0.1 | 26.8 | 5.7 | 9.0 | 5.1 | 2.4 | 0.5 | | | 33 | 309 | 62 | | | | 0.17 | 0.75 | 0.29 | 0.13 | 0.87 | 12.4 | 1.48 | 2.3 | 2.4 | | 386 | 0.0 | 0.4 | 146 | | 339 | 723 | | 226 | 0.94 |

| Code | Amount | | Description | Weight (g) | Calories | % Water | Protein (g) | Carbs (g) | Fiber (g) | Sugar (g) | Other Carbs (g) | Fat (g) | Sat Fat (g) | Mono Fat (g) | Poly Fat (g) | Omega 3 (g) | Omega 6 (g) | Choles (mg) | Vit A (IU) | Vit A (RE) | Retinol (RE) | Carotenoids (RE) | Beta Carotene (mcg) | Thiamin (mg) | Riboflavin (mg) | Niacin (NE) | Vit B6 (mg) | Vit B12 (mcg) | Folate (mcg) | Panto (mg) | Vit C (mg) | Vit D (mg) | Vit E (α TE) | Calcium (mg) | Copper (mg) | Iron (mg) | Magnes (mg) | Mang (mg) | Phos (mg) | Potassium (mg) | Selenium (mcg) | Sodium (mg) | Zinc (mg) |
|---|---|---|---|---|---|---|---|---|---|---|---|---|---|---|---|---|---|---|---|---|---|---|---|---|---|---|---|---|---|---|---|---|---|---|---|---|---|---|---|---|---|---|---|
| | | | | Basic Components | | | | | | | | | Additional Fats | | | | | | Vit A & Components | | | | | Vitamins | | | | | | | | | | Minerals | | | | | | | | | |
| | | | Power Bars | | | | | | | | | | | | | | | | | | | | | | | | | | | | | | | | | | | | | | | | |
| 62275 | 1 | ea | Apple Cinnamon | 65 | 230 | 10 | 10.0 | 45.0 | 3.0 | 20.0 | 22.0 | 2.5 | 0.5 | 1.5 | 0.5 | | | 0 | 0 | 0 | 0 | 0 | 0 | 1.50 | 1.70 | 20.00 | 2.00 | 6.00 | 400.0 | 10.00 | 60.0 | | | 300 | 0.7 | 6.3 | 140 | | 350 | 110 | | 90 | 5.25 |
| 62276 | 1 | ea | Banana | 65 | 230 | 13 | 9.0 | 45.0 | 3.0 | 20.0 | 22.0 | 2.0 | 0.5 | 1.0 | 0.5 | | | 0 | 0 | 0 | 0 | 0 | 0 | 1.50 | 1.70 | 20.00 | 2.00 | 6.00 | 400.0 | 10.00 | 60.0 | | | 300 | 0.7 | 6.3 | 140 | | 350 | 200 | | 90 | 5.25 |
| 62278 | 1 | ea | Chocolate | 65 | 230 | 11 | 10.0 | 45.0 | 3.0 | 14.0 | 28.0 | 2.0 | 0.5 | 0.5 | 1.0 | | | 0 | 0 | 0 | 0 | 0 | 0 | 1.50 | 1.70 | 20.00 | 2.00 | 6.00 | 400.0 | 10.00 | 60.0 | | | 300 | 0.7 | 6.3 | 140 | | 350 | 145 | | 90 | 5.25 |
| 62279 | 1 | ea | Malt Nut | 65 | 230 | 10 | 10.0 | 45.0 | 3.0 | 18.0 | 24.0 | 2.5 | 0.5 | 1.0 | 1.0 | | | 0 | 0 | 0 | 0 | 0 | 0 | 1.50 | 1.70 | 20.00 | 2.00 | 6.00 | 400.0 | 10.00 | 60.0 | | | 300 | 0.7 | 6.3 | 140 | | 350 | 110 | | 90 | 5.25 |
| 62280 | 1 | ea | Mocha | 65 | 230 | 10 | 10.0 | 45.0 | 3.0 | 17.0 | 25.0 | 2.5 | 1.0 | 1.0 | 0.5 | | | 0 | 0 | 0 | 0 | 0 | 0 | 1.50 | 1.70 | 20.00 | 2.00 | 6.00 | 400.0 | 10.00 | 60.0 | | | 300 | 0.7 | 6.3 | 140 | | 350 | 145 | | 90 | 5.25 |
| 62361 | 1 | ea | Oatmeal Raisin | 65 | 230 | 10 | 10.0 | 45.0 | 3.0 | 20.0 | 22.0 | 2.5 | | | | | | 0 | | | | | | 1.50 | 1.70 | 20.00 | 2.00 | 6.00 | 400.0 | | 60.0 | | | 300 | 0.7 | 6.3 | 140 | | 350 | 145 | | 90 | 5.25 |
| 62206 | 1 | ea | Peanut Butter | 65 | 230 | | 10.0 | 45.0 | 3.0 | 20.0 | 22.0 | 2.5 | | | | | | 0 | | | | | | 1.50 | 1.70 | 20.00 | 2.00 | 6.00 | 400.0 | | 60.0 | | | 300 | 0.7 | 5.4 | 140 | | 350 | 150 | | 110 | 5.25 |
| 62277 | 1 | ea | Wild Berry | 65 | 230 | 10 | 10.0 | 45.0 | 3.0 | 14.0 | 28.0 | 2.5 | 0.5 | 1.5 | 0.5 | | | 0 | 0 | 0 | 0 | 0 | 0 | 1.50 | 1.70 | 20.00 | 2.00 | 6.00 | 400.0 | 10.00 | 60.0 | | | 300 | 0.7 | 6.3 | 140 | | 350 | 110 | | 90 | 5.25 |
| | | | Sweet Success Bars | | | | | | | | | | | | | | | | | | | | | | | | | | | | | | | | | | | | | | | | |
| 62180 | 1 | ea | Chocolate Brownie | 33 | 120 | 9 | 2.0 | 23.0 | 3.0 | 13.0 | 7.0 | 4.0 | 2.0 | 0.5 | 0.6 | | | 3 | 750 | 150 | | | | 0.22 | 0.25 | 3.00 | 0.30 | 0.90 | 60.1 | 1.50 | 9.0 | 1.5 | | 150 | | 2.7 | 60 | | 150 | 140 | | 45 | 0.59 |
| 62179 | 1 | ea | Chocolate Chip | 33 | 120 | 9 | 2.0 | 23.0 | 3.0 | 10.0 | 10.0 | 4.0 | 2.0 | 0.4 | 0.5 | | | 3 | 750 | 150 | | | | 0.22 | 0.25 | 3.00 | 0.30 | 0.90 | 60.1 | 1.50 | 9.0 | 1.5 | | 150 | | 2.7 | 60 | | 150 | 110 | | 40 | 0.59 |
| 62178 | 1 | ea | Chocolate Peanut Butter | 33 | 120 | 9 | 2.0 | 23.0 | 3.0 | 12.0 | 8.0 | 4.0 | 2.0 | 0.6 | 0.6 | | | 3 | 750 | 150 | | | | 0.22 | 0.25 | 3.00 | 0.30 | 0.90 | 60.1 | 1.50 | 9.0 | 1.5 | | 150 | | 2.7 | 60 | | 150 | 125 | | 35 | 0.59 |
| 62201 | 1 | ea | Chocolate Raspberry | 33 | 120 | 9 | 2.0 | 23.0 | 0.0 | 10.0 | 13.0 | 4.0 | 2.0 | | | | | 3 | 750 | 150 | | | | 0.22 | 0.25 | 3.00 | 0.30 | 0.90 | 60.1 | 1.50 | 9.0 | 1.5 | | 150 | | 2.7 | 60 | | 150 | | | 35 | 0.59 |
| 62202 | 1 | ea | Oatmeal Raisin | 33 | 120 | 9 | 2.0 | 23.0 | 3.0 | 10.0 | 10.0 | 4.0 | 2.0 | | | | | 3 | 750 | 150 | | | | 0.22 | 0.25 | 3.00 | 0.30 | 0.90 | 60.1 | 1.50 | 9.0 | 1.5 | | 150 | | 2.7 | 60 | | 150 | | | 30 | 0.59 |
| | | | Sweet Success Drinks | | | | | | | | | | | | | | | | | | | | | | | | | | | | | | | | | | | | | | | | |
| 62200 | 1 | oz | Chocolate, dry mix | 28 | 79 | 9 | 6.1 | 16.6 | 5.3 | 10.5 | 0.9 | 1.4 | 0.8 | | | | | 3 | 1094 | 219 | | | | 0.39 | 0.22 | 6.13 | 0.61 | 1.05 | 122.6 | 2.63 | 18.4 | 0.9 | | 175 | 0.6 | 5.5 | 105 | | 88 | 306 | | 184 | 3.95 |
| 62199 | 1 | cup | Chocolate, prep w/skim milk | 265 | 180 | 81 | 15.0 | 30.0 | 6.0 | | | 2.0 | 1.0 | | | | | 6 | 1750 | 350 | | | | 0.52 | 0.60 | 7.00 | 0.70 | 2.10 | 140.0 | 3.50 | 21.0 | 3.5 | | 500 | 0.7 | 6.3 | 140 | | 350 | 750 | | 336 | 5.25 |
| 62185 | 1 | cup | Chocolate, RTS | 250 | 158 | 82 | 9.5 | 30.1 | 4.8 | 23.7 | 1.6 | 2.5 | 0.0 | | | | | 5 | 1385 | 277 | | | | 0.43 | 0.47 | 5.50 | 0.55 | 1.65 | 110.0 | 2.78 | 16.5 | 2.8 | | 395 | 0.6 | 5.0 | 110 | | 278 | 442 | | 190 | 4.25 |
| 62184 | 1 | cup | Chocolate Almond, RTS | 250 | 158 | 82 | 9.5 | 30.1 | 4.8 | 23.7 | 1.6 | 2.5 | 0.0 | 2.2 | 0.2 | | | 5 | 1385 | 277 | | | | 0.43 | 0.47 | 5.50 | 0.55 | 1.65 | 110.0 | 2.78 | 16.5 | 2.8 | | 395 | 0.6 | 5.0 | 110 | | 278 | 442 | | 190 | 4.25 |
| 62196 | 1 | oz | Chocolate Chip, dry mix | 28 | 79 | 9 | 6.1 | 16.6 | 5.3 | 11.4 | 0.0 | 1.7 | 1.4 | | | | | 3 | 1094 | 219 | | | | 0.39 | 0.22 | 6.13 | 0.61 | 1.05 | 122.6 | 2.63 | 18.4 | 0.9 | | 175 | 0.6 | 5.5 | 105 | | 88 | 175 | | 149 | 3.95 |
| 62195 | 1 | cup | Chocolate Chip, prep w/skim milk | 265 | 180 | 81 | 15.0 | 30.0 | 6.0 | | | 2.6 | 1.6 | | | | | 6 | 1750 | 350 | | | | 0.52 | 0.60 | 7.00 | 0.70 | 2.10 | 140.0 | 3.50 | 21.0 | 3.5 | | 500 | 0.7 | 6.3 | 140 | | 350 | 600 | | 288 | 5.25 |
| 62198 | 1 | oz | Chocolate Fudge, dry mix | 28 | 79 | 10 | 6.1 | 16.6 | 5.3 | 9.6 | 1.8 | 1.4 | 0.8 | | | | | 3 | 1094 | 219 | | | | 0.39 | 0.22 | 6.13 | 0.61 | 1.05 | 122.6 | 2.63 | 18.4 | 0.9 | | 175 | 0.6 | 5.5 | 105 | | 88 | 306 | | 184 | 3.95 |
| 62197 | 1 | cup | Chocolate Fudge, prep w/skim milk | 265 | 180 | 81 | 15.0 | 30.0 | 6.0 | | | 2.0 | | | | | | 6 | 1750 | 350 | | | | 0.52 | 0.60 | 7.00 | 0.70 | 2.10 | 140.0 | 3.50 | 21.0 | 3.5 | | 500 | 0.7 | 6.3 | 140 | | 350 | 750 | | 336 | 5.25 |
| 62186 | 1 | cup | Chocolate Fudge, RTS | 250 | 158 | 82 | 9.5 | 30.1 | 4.8 | 23.7 | 1.6 | 2.5 | 0.0 | 2.2 | 0.2 | | | 5 | 1385 | 277 | | | | 0.43 | 0.47 | 5.50 | 0.55 | 1.65 | 110.0 | 2.78 | 16.5 | 2.8 | | 395 | 0.6 | 5.0 | 110 | | 278 | 442 | | 175 | 4.25 |
| 62271 | 1 | cup | Chocolate Mint, RTS | 265 | 167 | 82 | 10.1 | 31.9 | 5.0 | 25.1 | 1.7 | 2.7 | 0.0 | | | | | 5 | 1468 | 294 | | | | 0.45 | 0.50 | 5.83 | 0.58 | 1.75 | 116.6 | 2.94 | 17.5 | 2.9 | | 419 | 0.6 | 5.3 | 117 | | 294 | 469 | | 201 | 4.51 |
| 62188 | 1 | oz | Chocolate Mocha, dry mix | 28 | 79 | 10 | 6.1 | 16.6 | 5.3 | 8.8 | 2.6 | 1.4 | 0.8 | | | | | 3 | 1094 | 219 | | | | 0.39 | 0.22 | 6.13 | 0.61 | 1.05 | 122.6 | 2.63 | 18.4 | 0.9 | | 175 | 0.6 | 5.5 | 105 | | 88 | 350 | | 184 | 3.95 |
| 62187 | 1 | cup | Chocolate Mocha, prep w/skim milk | 265 | 180 | 81 | 15.0 | 30.0 | 6.0 | | | 1.3 | 1.0 | | | | | 6 | 1750 | 350 | | | | 0.52 | 0.60 | 7.00 | 0.70 | 2.10 | 140.0 | 3.50 | 21.0 | 3.5 | | 500 | 0.7 | 6.3 | 140 | | 350 | 800 | | 336 | 5.25 |
| 62181 | 1 | cup | Chocolate Mocha, RTS | 250 | 158 | 82 | 9.5 | 30.1 | 4.8 | 23.7 | 1.6 | 2.5 | 0.0 | 0.6 | 1.8 | | | 5 | 1385 | 277 | | | | 0.43 | 0.47 | 5.50 | 0.55 | 1.65 | 110.0 | 2.78 | 16.5 | 2.8 | | 395 | 0.6 | 5.0 | 110 | | 278 | 402 | | 175 | 4.25 |
| 62182 | 1 | cup | Chocolate Raspberry, RTS | 250 | 158 | 82 | 9.5 | 30.1 | 4.8 | 23.7 | 1.6 | 2.5 | 0.0 | 2.2 | 0.2 | | | 5 | 1385 | 277 | | | | 0.43 | 0.47 | 5.50 | 0.55 | 1.65 | 110.0 | 2.78 | 16.5 | 2.8 | | 382 | 0.6 | 5.0 | 110 | | 278 | 442 | | 175 | 4.25 |
| 62272 | 1 | cup | Strawberry, RTS | 265 | 167 | 82 | 10.1 | 31.9 | 5.0 | 25.1 | 1.7 | 2.7 | 0.0 | | | | | 5 | 1468 | 294 | | | | 0.45 | 0.50 | 5.83 | 0.58 | 1.75 | 116.6 | 2.94 | 17.5 | 2.9 | | 419 | 0.6 | 5.3 | 117 | | 294 | 310 | | 175 | 4.51 |
| 62190 | 1 | oz | Vanilla, dry mix | 28 | 79 | 9 | 6.1 | 17.5 | 5.3 | 7.9 | 4.4 | 0.6 | 0.0 | | | | | 3 | 1094 | 219 | | | | 0.39 | 0.22 | 6.13 | 0.61 | 1.05 | 122.6 | 2.63 | 18.4 | 0.9 | | 175 | 0.6 | 5.5 | 105 | | 88 | 376 | | 158 | 3.95 |
| 62189 | 1 | cup | Vanilla, prep w/skim milk | 265 | 180 | 81 | 15.0 | 33.0 | 6.0 | | | 1.0 | 0.6 | | | | | 6 | 1250 | 250 | | | | 0.52 | 0.60 | 7.00 | 0.70 | 2.10 | 140.0 | 3.50 | 21.0 | 3.5 | | 500 | 0.7 | 6.3 | 140 | | 350 | 830 | | 312 | 5.25 |
| 62183 | 1 | cup | Vanilla, RTS | 250 | 158 | 82 | 9.5 | 30.1 | 4.8 | 23.7 | 1.6 | 2.5 | 0.0 | 2.1 | 0.3 | | | 5 | 1385 | 277 | | | | 0.43 | 0.47 | 5.50 | 0.55 | 1.65 | 110.0 | 2.78 | 16.5 | 2.8 | | 395 | 0.6 | 5.0 | 110 | | 278 | 292 | | 175 | 4.25 |
| 62136 | 5 | oz | Sustacal, pudding | 142 | 240 | 65 | 6.8 | 32.0 | | | | 9.5 | 1.5 | 4.2 | 3.8 | | | 4 | 750 | 225 | 225 | 0 | 0 | 0.23 | 0.26 | 3.00 | 0.30 | 0.90 | 60.0 | 1.50 | 9.0 | | | 220 | 0.3 | 2.7 | 60 | 0.7 | 220 | 320 | | 120 | 2.30 |
| 62134 | 1 | cup | Sustacal, vanilla drink, high cal, RTS | 258 | 360 | | 14.4 | 45.0 | 0.0 | | | 13.6 | 2.1 | 3.4 | 8.1 | | | 4 | 1000 | 300 | 300 | 0 | 0 | 0.45 | 0.51 | 6.00 | 0.60 | 1.80 | 120.0 | 3.00 | 18.0 | | | 200 | 0.4 | 3.6 | 80 | 0.6 | 200 | 350 | | 200 | 3.00 |
| | | | Slim Fast Drinks | | | | | | | | | | | | | | | | | | | | | | | | | | | | | | | | | | | | | | | | |
| 62005 | 1 | ea | Chocolate Malt, dry mix, 1 scoop | 28 | 100 | 4 | 5.0 | 20.0 | 2.0 | 17.0 | 1.0 | 1.0 | 0.5 | | | | | 5 | 750 | 225 | 225 | 0 | 0 | 0.45 | 0.17 | 7.00 | 0.59 | 1.20 | 100.0 | 2.49 | 18.0 | 1.0 | | 150 | 0.2 | 6.3 | 100 | 0.0 | 100 | 260 | 0.0 | 120 | 4.48 |
| 62006 | 1 | ea | Strawberry, dry mix, 1 scoop | 28 | 100 | 4 | 5.0 | 20.0 | 2.0 | 18.0 | 0.0 | 0.5 | | | | | | 5 | 750 | 75 | 0 | 75 | 450 | 0.45 | 0.17 | 7.00 | 0.59 | 1.20 | 100.0 | 2.49 | 18.0 | 1.0 | | 150 | 0.2 | 6.3 | 100 | 0.0 | 100 | 210 | 0.0 | 130 | 4.51 |
| 62004 | 1 | ea | Vanilla, dry mix, 1 scoop | 28 | 100 | 4 | 5.0 | 20.0 | 2.0 | 18.0 | 0.0 | 0.5 | | | | | | 5 | 750 | 225 | 225 | 0 | | 0.45 | 0.17 | 7.00 | 0.59 | 1.20 | 100.0 | 2.49 | 18.0 | 1.0 | | 150 | 0.2 | 6.3 | 100 | | 100 | 210 | | 130 | 4.51 |
| | | | Slim Fast, Ultra Drinks | | | | | | | | | | | | | | | | | | | | | | | | | | | | | | | | | | | | | | | | |
| 62013 | 1 | ea | Chocolate, dry mix, 1 scoop | 33 | 120 | 3 | 5.0 | 24.0 | 5.0 | 17.2 | 1.9 | 1.0 | 0.5 | | | | | 5 | 750 | 225 | 225 | 0 | 0 | 0.46 | 0.17 | 9.90 | 0.59 | 2.11 | 100.0 | 3.99 | 27.0 | 2.5 | | 150 | 0.2 | 6.3 | 100 | 0.7 | 100 | 280 | 17.5 | 130 | 4.49 |
| 62019 | 1 | ea | Fruit, dry mix, 1 scoop | 31 | 100 | 3 | 10.0 | 17.0 | 5.0 | 8.0 | 4.0 | 1.0 | 0.0 | 0.5 | 0.5 | 0.00 | 0.00 | 5 | 750 | 75 | 0 | 75 | 450 | 0.45 | 0.17 | 10.01 | 0.60 | 2.10 | 100.0 | 4.00 | 27.0 | 2.5 | | 150 | 0.2 | 6.3 | 100 | 0.7 | 100 | 300 | 17.5 | 210 | 4.49 |
| 62020 | 1 | cup | Fruit, prep w/orange juice | 279 | 200 | 80 | 11.0 | 44.0 | 6.0 | | | 0.1 | | | | | | | 833 | 250 | | | | 0.52 | 0.60 | 7.00 | 0.70 | 2.10 | 140.0 | 3.50 | 60.0 | | | 400 | 0.7 | 6.3 | 140 | 1.0 | 400 | 590 | | 30 | 5.25 |
| 62012 | 1 | ea | Mocha, dry mix, 1 scoop | 33 | 120 | 3 | 5.0 | 24.0 | 5.0 | 18.0 | 1.0 | 1.0 | 0.5 | | | | | 5 | 750 | 225 | 225 | 0 | 0 | 0.45 | 0.17 | 1.00 | 0.60 | 2.10 | 100.0 | 4.00 | 27.0 | 2.5 | | 150 | 0.2 | 6.3 | 100 | 0.7 | 100 | 210 | 17.5 | 110 | 4.50 |
| 62010 | 1 | ea | Strawberry, dry mix, 1 scoop | 33 | 100 | 10 | 5.0 | 24.1 | 4.0 | | | 0.6 | | | | | | | 835 | 251 | | | | 0.45 | 0.17 | 7.02 | 0.60 | 1.20 | 100.3 | 2.51 | 18.1 | | | 150 | 0.7 | 6.3 | 100 | 1.0 | 150 | 321 | | 120 | 4.51 |
| 62009 | 1 | ea | Vanilla, dry mix, 1 scoop | 33 | 120 | 3 | 5.0 | 25.0 | 5.0 | 19.0 | 1.0 | 0.5 | | | 0.0 | | | 5 | 750 | 225 | 225 | 0 | 0 | 0.45 | 0.17 | 10.00 | 0.60 | 2.11 | 100.0 | 4.00 | 27.0 | 2.5 | | 150 | 0.2 | 6.3 | 100 | 0.7 | 100 | 160 | 17.5 | 130 | 4.49 |
| | | | **SWEETENERS AND SWEET SUBSTITUTES** | | | | | | | | | | | | | | | | | | | | | | | | | | | | | | | | | | | | | | | | |
| | | | *JAMS AND JELLIES* | | | | | | | | | | | | | | | | | | | | | | | | | | | | | | | | | | | | | | | | |
| | | | Apple Butter | | | | | | | | | | | | | | | | | | | | | | | | | | | | | | | | | | | | | | | | |
| 23000 | 1 | Tbs | Average | 18 | 31 | 56 | 0.1 | 7.7 | 0.3 | 6.4 | 1.1 | C.0 | 0.0 | 0.0 | 0.0 | 0.00 | 0.00 | 0 | 21 | 2 | | | | 0.00 | 0.00 | 0.02 | 0.01 | 0.00 | 0.2 | 0.01 | 0.1 | 0.0 | | 3 | 0.0 | 0.1 | 1 | 0.1 | 2 | 16 | 0.1 | 1 | 0.01 |
| 23393 | 1 | Tbs | Apricot, avg | 15 | 22 | 62 | 0.0 | 5.5 | 0.5 | 5.0 | 0.0 | C.0 | 0.0 | 0.0 | 0.0 | 0.00 | 0.00 | 0 | 0 | 0 | 0 | 0 | 0 | | | | | | | | 0.0 | | | 30 | | 0.7 | | | | | | 2 | |
| 23394 | 1 | Tbs | Raspberry, avg | 15 | 22 | 62 | 0.0 | 5.5 | 0.5 | 5.0 | 0.0 | C.0 | 0.0 | 0.0 | 0.0 | 0.00 | 0.00 | 0 | 0 | 0 | 0 | 0 | 0 | | | | | | | | 0.0 | | | 30 | | 0.7 | | | | | | 2 | |
| 23395 | 1 | Tbs | Strawberry, avg | 15 | 22 | 62 | 0.0 | 5.5 | 0.5 | 5.0 | 0.0 | C.0 | 0.0 | 0.0 | 0.0 | 0.00 | 0.00 | 0 | 0 | 0 | 0 | 0 | 0 | | | | | | | | 0.0 | | | 30 | | 0.7 | | | | | | 2 | |
| 23277 | 1 | Tbs | Fruit Spread, grape, red cal, Kraft | 17 | 20 | | 5.0 | 0.0 | 0.0 | 0.0 | 0.0 | C.0 | 0.0 | 0.0 | 0.0 | 0.00 | 0.00 | 0 | 0 | 0 | 0 | 0 | 0 | | | | | | | | 0.0 | | | 0 | | 0.0 | | | | 25 | | 20 | |
| 23278 | 1 | Tbs | Fruit Spread, strawberry, red cal, Kraft | 20 | 20 | | 0.0 | 5.0 | 0.0 | 5.0 | 0.0 | C.0 | 0.0 | 0.0 | 0.0 | 0.00 | 0.00 | 0 | 0 | 0 | 0 | 0 | 0 | | | | | | | | 0.0 | | | 0 | | 0.0 | | | | 25 | | 20 | |
| | | | Jam/Preserves | | | | | | | | | | | | | | | | | | | | | | | | | | | | | | | | | | | | | | | | |
| 23054 | 1 | Tbs | Average | 20 | 48 | 34 | 0.1 | 12.9 | 0.2 | 9.7 | 3.0 | C.0 | 0.0 | 0.0 | 0.0 | 0.00 | 0.00 | 0 | 2 | 0.2 | | | | 0.00 | 0.00 | 0.01 | 0.00 | 0.00 | 6.6 | 0.00 | 1.8 | 0.0 | 0.0 | 4 | 0.0 | 0.1 | 1 | 0.0 | 2 | 15 | 0.4 | 8 | 0.01 |
| 23205 | 1 | Tbs | Apricot, avg | 20 | 48 | 34 | 0.1 | 12.9 | 0.2 | 12.0 | 0.6 | C.0 | 0.0 | 0.0 | 0.0 | 0.00 | 0.00 | 0 | 41 | 4 | 0 | 4 | | 0.00 | 0.00 | 0.01 | 0.00 | 0.00 | 6.6 | 0.00 | 1.8 | 0.0 | 0.0 | 4 | 0.0 | 0.1 | 1 | 0.0 | 2 | 15 | 0.4 | 8 | 0.01 |
| 23299 | 1 | Tbs | Apricot, Kraft | 20 | 50 | 34 | 0.0 | 13.0 | 0.0 | 7.0 | 6.0 | C.0 | 0.0 | 0.0 | 0.0 | 0.00 | 0.00 | 0 | 0 | 0 | 0 | 0 | 0 | | | | | | | | 2.4 | | | 0 | | 0.0 | | | | 25 | | 10 | |
| 23166 | 1 | Tbs | Artificially Sweetened, avg | 20 | 2 | 46 | 0.1 | 10.7 | 0.5 | | | C.1 | 0.0 | 0.0 | 0.0 | | | 0 | 0 | 0 | 0 | 0 | 0 | 0.00 | 0.00 | 0.00 | 0.00 | 0.00 | 1.8 | | 0.0 | | | 2 | 0.0 | 0.1 | 1 | | 2 | 14 | | 0 | 0.01 |
| 23298 | 1 | Tbs | Blackberry, Kraft | 20 | 50 | 34 | 0.0 | 13.0 | 0.5 | 7.0 | 5.5 | C.0 | 0.0 | 0.0 | 0.0 | 0.00 | 0.00 | 0 | 0 | 0 | 0 | 0 | 0 | | | | | | | | 0.0 | | | 0 | | 0.0 | | | | 15 | | 10 | |
| 23288 | 1 | Tbs | Grape, Kraft | 20 | 60 | 34 | 0.0 | 14.0 | 0.0 | 8.0 | 6.0 | C.0 | 0.0 | 0.0 | 0.0 | 0.00 | 0.00 | 0 | 0 | 0 | 0 | 0 | 0 | | | | | | | | 0.0 | | | 0 | | 0.0 | | | | 20 | | 10 | |
| 23295 | 1 | Tbs | Orange Marmalade, Kraft | 20 | 50 | 28 | 0.0 | 14.0 | 0.0 | 7.0 | 7.0 | C.0 | 0.0 | 0.0 | 0.0 | 0.00 | 0.00 | 0 | 0 | 0 | 0 | 0 | 0 | | | | | | | | 1.2 | | | 0 | | 0.0 | | | | 5 | | 10 | |
| 23296 | 1 | Tbs | Peach, Kraft | 20 | 50 | 28 | 0.0 | 14.0 | 0.0 | 8.0 | 6.0 | C.0 | 0.0 | 0.0 | 0.0 | 0.00 | 0.00 | 0 | 0 | 0 | 0 | 0 | 0 | | | | | | | | 1.2 | | | 0 | | 0.0 | | | | 15 | | 10 | |
| 23300 | 1 | Tbs | Pineapple, Kraft | 20 | 50 | 28 | 0.0 | 14.0 | 0.0 | 8.0 | 6.0 | C.0 | 0.0 | 0.0 | 0.0 | 0.00 | 0.00 | 0 | 0 | 0 | 0 | 0 | 0 | | | | | | | | 0.0 | | | 0 | | 0.0 | | | | 10 | | 10 | |
| 23287 | 1 | Tbs | Red Plum, Kraft | 20 | 60 | 34 | 0.0 | 13.0 | 0.0 | 8.0 | 5.0 | C.0 | 0.0 | 0.0 | 0.0 | 0.00 | 0.00 | 0 | 0 | 0 | 0 | 0 | 0 | | | | | | | | 0.0 | | | 0 | | 0.0 | | | | 15 | | 10 | |
| 23167 | 1 | Tbs | Reduced Sugar, avg | 20 | 36 | 52 | 0.2 | 8.9 | 0.6 | 7.3 | 1.0 | C.1 | 0.0 | 0.0 | 0.1 | | | 0 | 4 | 0.4 | 0 | 0.4 | | 0.00 | 0.02 | 0.06 | 0.03 | 0.00 | 1.7 | | 7.6 | | | 1 | 0.0 | 0.2 | 1 | | 1 | 12 | | 5 | 0.05 |
| 23391 | 1 | Tbs | Raspberry, fruit sweetened, Kraft | 15 | 25 | 56 | 0.0 | 6.0 | 0.5 | 5.5 | 0.0 | C.0 | 0.0 | 0.0 | 0.0 | 0.00 | 0.00 | 0 | 0 | 0 | 0 | 0 | 0 | | | | | | | | 0.0 | | | 30 | | 0.9 | | | | | | 2 | |
| 23297 | 1 | Tbs | Raspberry, Kraft | 20 | 50 | 34 | 0.0 | 13.0 | 0.0 | 7.0 | 6.0 | C.0 | 0.0 | 0.0 | 0.0 | 0.00 | 0.00 | 0 | 0 | 0 | 0 | 0 | 0 | | | | | | | | 0.0 | | | 0 | | 0.0 | | | | 20 | | 10 | |

| Code | Amount | Description | Weight (g) | Calories | % Water | Protein (g) | Carbs (g) | Fiber (g) | Sugar (g) | Other Carbs (g) | Fat (g) | Sat Fat (g) | Mono Fat (g) | Poly Fat (g) | Omega 3 (g) | Omega 6 (g) | Chol (mg) | Vit A (IU) | Vit A (RE) | Retinol (RE) | Carotenoids (RE) | Beta Carotene (mcg) | Thiamin (mg) | Riboflavin (mg) | Niacin (NE) | Vit B6 (mg) | Vit B12 (mcg) | Folate (mcg) | Panto (mg) | Vit C (mg) | Vit D (mg) | Vit E (α TE) | Calcium (mg) | Copper (mg) | Iron (mg) | Magnes (mg) | Mang (mg) | Phos (mg) | Potassium (mg) | Selenium (mcg) | Sodium (mg) | Zinc (mg) |
|---|---|---|---|---|---|---|---|---|---|---|---|---|---|---|---|---|---|---|---|---|---|---|---|---|---|---|---|---|---|---|---|---|---|---|---|---|---|---|---|---|---|---|
| | | **Basic Components** | | | | | | | | | | **Additional Fats** | | | | | | **Vit A & Components** | | | | | **Vitamins** | | | | | | | | | | **Minerals** | | | | | | | | | |
| 23175 | 1 Tbs | Strawberry, avg | 20 | 54 | 29 | 0.1 | 14.0 | | | | 0.0 | 0.0 | | | | 0.00 | 0 | 2 | 0.2 | 0 | 0.2 | | 0.00 | 0.01 | 0.04 | | | | | 3.0 | | | 4 | | 0.2 | | | 2 | 18 | | 2 | |
| 23390 | 1 Tbs | Strawberry, fruit sweetened, Kraft | 15 | 25 | 56 | 0.0 | 6.0 | 0.5 | 5.5 | 0.0 | 0.0 | 0.0 | 0.0 | 0.0 | 0.00 | 0.00 | 0 | 0 | 0 | 0 | 0 | 0 | | | | | | | | 0.0 | | | 30 | | 0.9 | | | | | | 2 | |
| 23286 | 1 Tbs | Strawberry, Kraft | 20 | 50 | 34 | 0.0 | 13.0 | 0.0 | 8.0 | 5.0 | 0.0 | 0.0 | 0.0 | 0.0 | 0.00 | 0.00 | 0 | 0 | 0 | 0 | 0 | 0 | | | | | | | | 2.4 | | | 0 | | 0.0 | | | | 15 | | 10 | |
| | | Jelly | | | | | | | | | | | | | | | | | | | | | | | | | | | | | | | | | | | | | | | | |
| 23003 | 1 Tbs | Average | 19 | 51 | 28 | 0.1 | 13.5 | 0.2 | 7.9 | 5.4 | 0.0 | 0.0 | 0.0 | 0.0 | 0.00 | 0.01 | 0 | 3 | 0.4 | 0 | 0.4 | | 0.00 | 0.00 | 0.01 | 0.00 | 0.00 | 0.2 | 0.04 | 0.2 | 0.0 | 0.0 | 2 | 0.0 | 0.0 | 1 | 0.0 | 1 | 12 | 0.4 | 7 | 0.01 |
| 23092 | 1 Tbs | Artificially Sweetened, avg | 19 | 6 | 42 | 0.1 | 10.9 | 0.2 | | | 0.0 | 0.0 | 0.0 | 0.0 | 0.00 | 0.00 | 0 | 0 | 0 | 0 | 0 | 0 | 0.00 | 0.00 | 0.00 | 0.01 | 0.00 | 0.2 | | 0.0 | | | 1 | 0.0 | 0.0 | 1 | | 1 | 13 | | 0 | 0.00 |
| 23291 | 1 Tbs | Blackberry, Kraft | 20 | 50 | 34 | 0.0 | 13.0 | 0.0 | 7.0 | 6.0 | 0.0 | 0.0 | 0.0 | 0.0 | 0.00 | 0.00 | 0 | 0 | 0 | 0 | 0 | 0 | | | | | | | | 0.0 | | | 0 | | 0.0 | | | | 15 | | 10 | |
| 23293 | 1 Tbs | Grape, Kraft | 20 | 50 | 28 | 0.0 | 14.0 | 0.0 | 8.0 | 6.0 | 0.0 | 0.0 | 0.0 | 0.0 | 0.00 | 0.00 | 0 | 0 | 0 | 0 | 0 | 0 | | | | | | | | 0.0 | | | 0 | | 0.0 | | | | 5 | | 10 | |
| 23290 | 1 Tbs | Guava, Kraft | 20 | 50 | 34 | 0.0 | 13.0 | 0.0 | 7.0 | 6.0 | 0.0 | 0.0 | 0.0 | 0.0 | 0.00 | 0.00 | 0 | 0 | 0 | 0 | 0 | 0 | | | | | | | | 3.6 | | | 0 | | 0.0 | | | | 25 | | 10 | |
| 23289 | 1 Tbs | Red Current, Kraft | 20 | 50 | 34 | 0.0 | 13.0 | 0.0 | 7.0 | 6.0 | 0.0 | 0.0 | 0.0 | 0.0 | 0.00 | 0.00 | 0 | 0 | 0 | 0 | 0 | 0 | | | | | | | | 0.0 | | | 0 | | 0.0 | | | | 20 | | 10 | |
| 23165 | 1 Tbs | Reduced Sugar, avg | 19 | 34 | 53 | 0.1 | 8.8 | 0.2 | 8.6 | 0.0 | 0.0 | 0.0 | 0.0 | 0.0 | | | 0 | [illegible] | 0.2 | 0 | 0.2 | | 0.00 | 0.00 | 0.03 | 0.01 | 0.00 | 0.2 | | 0.0 | | | 1 | 0.0 | 0.0 | 1 | | 1 | 13 | | 0 | 0.01 |
| 23294 | 1 Tbs | Strawberry, Kraft | 20 | 60 | 28 | 0.0 | 14.0 | 0.0 | 8.0 | 6.0 | 0.0 | 0.0 | 0.0 | 0.0 | 0.00 | 0.00 | 0 | 0 | 0 | 0 | 0 | 0 | | | | | | | | 0.0 | | | 0 | | 0.0 | | | | 15 | | 10 | |
| | | *SUGARS, SUGAR SUBSTITUTES AND SYRUPS* | | | | | | | | | | | | | | | | | | | | | | | | | | | | | | | | | | | | | | | | |
| | | Artificial Sweeteners | | | | | | | | | | | | | | | | | | | | | | | | | | | | | | | | | | | | | | | | |
| 25038 | 1 ea | Aspartame, pkt, Nutrisweet | 1 | 4 | 12 | 0.0 | 0.9 | 0.0 | 0.0 | 0.9 | 0.0 | 0.0 | 0.0 | 0.0 | 0.00 | 0.00 | 0 | 0 | 0 | 0 | 0 | 0 | 0.00 | 0.00 | 0.00 | 0.00 | 0.00 | 0.0 | 0.00 | 0.0 | 0.0 | 0.0 | 0 | 0.0 | 0.0 | 0 | 0.0 | 0 | 0 | 0.0 | 0 | 0.00 |
| 25037 | 1 tsp | Aspartame, pwd, Nutrisweet | 5 | 19 | 4 | 4.8 | 0.0 | 0.0 | 0.0 | 0.0 | 0.0 | 0.0 | 0.0 | 0.0 | 0.00 | 0.00 | 0 | 0 | 0 | 0 | 0 | 0 | 0.00 | 0.00 | 0.00 | | 0.00 | | | 0.0 | | | 0 | | 0.1 | | | 0 | 1 | | 2 | |
| 25070 | 1 tsp | Saccharin, liquid, avg | 5 | 0 | 98 | 0.0 | 0.1 | 0.0 | 0.1 | 0.0 | 0.0 | 0.0 | 0.0 | 0.0 | 0.00 | 0.00 | 0 | 0 | 0 | 0 | 0 | 0 | 0.00 | 0.00 | 0.00 | 0.00 | 0.00 | 0.0 | | 0.0 | 0.0 | 0.0 | 0 | 0.0 | 0.0 | 0 | | 0 | 5 | | 1 | 0.00 |
| 25041 | 1 ea | Saccharin, pkt, avg | 0 | 0 | 0 | 0.0 | 0.0 | 0.0 | 0.0 | 0.0 | 0.0 | 0.0 | 0.0 | 0.0 | 0.00 | 0.00 | 0 | 0 | 0 | 0 | 0 | 0 | 0.00 | 0.00 | 0.00 | 0.00 | 0.00 | 0.0 | | 0.0 | 0.0 | 0.0 | 0 | 0.0 | 0.0 | 0 | | 0 | 0 | | 0 | 0.00 |
| 25207 | 1 ea | Sweet Magic | 1 | 0 | | 0.0 | 0.0 | 0.0 | 0.0 | 0.0 | 0.0 | 0.0 | 0.0 | 0.0 | 0.00 | 0.00 | 0 | 0 | 0 | 0 | 0 | 0 | | | | | | | | 0.0 | | | 0 | | 0.0 | | | | | | 100 | |
| 25124 | 1 tsp | Weight Watchers | 5 | 25 | | 0.0 | 5.0 | 0.0 | 5.0 | 0.0 | 0.0 | 0.0 | 0.0 | 0.0 | 0.00 | 0.00 | 0 | 0 | 0 | 0 | 0 | 0 | | | | | | | | 0.0 | | | 0 | | 0.0 | | | | 0 | | 150 | |
| | | Cane Sugar | | | | | | | | | | | | | | | | | | | | | | | | | | | | | | | | | | | | | | | | |
| 25067 | 1 tsp | Brown, liquid, avg | 7 | 18 | 32 | 0.0 | 4.7 | 0.0 | 4.7 | 0.0 | 0.0 | 0.0 | 0.0 | 0.0 | 0.00 | 0.00 | 0 | 0 | 0 | 0 | 0 | 0 | 0.00 | 0.00 | 0.00 | 0.00 | 0.00 | 0.0 | | 0.0 | 0.0 | 0.0 | 4 | 0.0 | 0.1 | 1 | | 1 | 17 | | 2 | 0.01 |
| 25005 | 1 tsp | Brown, packed, avg | 5 | 19 | 2 | 0.0 | 4.9 | 0.0 | 4.9 | 0.0 | 0.0 | 0.0 | 0.0 | 0.0 | 0.00 | 0.00 | 0 | 0 | 0 | 0 | 0 | 0 | 0.00 | 0.00 | 0.00 | 0.00 | 0.00 | 0.1 | 0.01 | 0.0 | 0.0 | 0.0 | 4 | 0.0 | 0.1 | 1 | 0.0 | 1 | 17 | 0.1 | 2 | 0.01 |
| 25201 | 1 tsp | Brown, unpacked, avg | 5 | 19 | 2 | 0.0 | 4.9 | 0.0 | 4.9 | 0.0 | 0.0 | 0.0 | 0.0 | 0.0 | 0.00 | 0.00 | 0 | 0 | 0 | 0 | 0 | 0 | 0.00 | 0.00 | 0.00 | 0.00 | 0.00 | 0.1 | 0.01 | 0.0 | 0.0 | 0.0 | 4 | 0.0 | 0.1 | 1 | 0.0 | 1 | 17 | 0.1 | 2 | 0.01 |
| 25068 | 1 tsp | Caramelized, avg | 5 | 19 | 2 | 0.0 | 4.9 | 0.0 | 4.8 | 0.0 | 0.0 | 0.0 | 0.0 | 0.0 | 0.00 | 0.00 | 0 | 0 | 0 | 0 | 0 | 0 | 0.00 | 0.00 | 0.00 | 0.00 | 0.00 | 0.1 | | 0.0 | 0.0 | 0.0 | 4 | 0.0 | 0.1 | 1 | | 1 | 17 | | 2 | 0.01 |
| 25071 | 1 tsp | Raw, avg | 4 | 15 | 2 | 0.0 | 3.9 | 0.0 | 3.8 | 0.0 | 0.0 | 0.0 | 0.0 | 0.0 | 0.00 | 0.00 | 0 | 0 | 0 | 0 | 0 | 0 | 0.00 | 0.00 | 0.00 | 0.00 | 0.00 | 0.0 | | 0.0 | 0.0 | 0.0 | 3 | 0.0 | 0.1 | 1 | | 1 | 14 | | 2 | 0.01 |
| 90065 | 1 tsp | Syrup, avg | 7 | 18 | 26 | 0.0 | 4.8 | 0.0 | 4.8 | 0.0 | 0.0 | 0.0 | 0.0 | 0.0 | 0.00 | 0.00 | 0 | 0 | 0 | 0 | 0 | 0 | 0.01 | 0.00 | 0.01 | | | | | 0.0 | 0.0 | 0.0 | 4 | | 0.3 | | | 2 | 30 | | 0 | |
| 25006 | 1 tsp | White, granulated, avg | 4 | 15 | 0 | 0.0 | 4.0 | 0.0 | 3.9 | 0.1 | 0.0 | 0.0 | 0.0 | 0.0 | 0.00 | 0.00 | 0 | 0 | 0 | 0 | 0 | 0 | 0.00 | 0.00 | 0.00 | 0.00 | 0.00 | 0.0 | 0.00 | 0.0 | 0.0 | 0.0 | 0 | 0.0 | 0.0 | 0 | 0.0 | 0 | 0 | 0.0 | 0 | 0.00 |
| 25008 | 1 tsp | White, powdered, avg | 2 | 8 | 0 | 0.0 | 2.0 | 0.0 | 1.9 | 0.1 | 0.0 | 0.0 | 0.0 | 0.0 | 0.00 | 0.00 | 0 | 0 | 0 | 0 | 0 | 0 | 0.00 | 0.00 | 0.00 | 0.00 | 0.00 | 0.0 | 0.00 | 0.0 | 0.0 | 0.0 | 0 | 0.0 | 0.0 | 0 | 0.0 | 0 | 0 | 0.0 | 0 | 0.00 |
| | | Corn Syrup | | | | | | | | | | | | | | | | | | | | | | | | | | | | | | | | | | | | | | | | |
| 25113 | 1/2 oz | Crystalline Fructose, CornSweet | 14 | 56 | 0 | 0.0 | 14.0 | 0.0 | 14.0 | 0.0 | 0.0 | 0.0 | 0.0 | 0.0 | 0.00 | 0.00 | 0 | 0 | 0 | 0 | 0 | 0 | 0.00 | 0.00 | 0.00 | 0.00 | 0.00 | 0.0 | 0.00 | 0.0 | 0.0 | 0.0 | 0 | 0.0 | 0.0 | 0 | | 0 | 0 | | 0 | 0.00 |
| 25010 | 1 Tbs | Dark, avg | 20 | 56 | 23 | 0.0 | 15.3 | 0.0 | 7.4 | 7.9 | 0.0 | 0.0 | 0.0 | 0.0 | 0.00 | 0.00 | 0 | 0 | 0 | 0 | 0 | 0 | 0.00 | 0.00 | 0.00 | 0.00 | 0.00 | 0.0 | 0.00 | 0.0 | 0.0 | 0.0 | 4 | 0.0 | 0.1 | 2 | 0.0 | 2 | 9 | 0.2 | 31 | 0.01 |
| 25203 | 1 Tbs | Hi-Fructose, avg | 19 | 53 | 24 | 0.0 | 14.4 | 0.0 | 9.5 | 4.9 | 0.0 | 0.0 | 0.0 | 0.0 | 0.00 | 0.00 | 0 | 0 | 0 | 0 | 0 | 0 | 0.00 | 0.00 | 0.00 | 0.00 | 0.00 | 0.0 | 0.00 | 0.0 | 0.0 | 0.0 | 0 | 0.0 | 0.0 | 0 | 0.0 | 0 | 0 | 0.1 | 0 | 0.00 |
| 25000 | 1 Tbs | Light, avg | 20 | 56 | 23 | 0.0 | 15.3 | 0.0 | 10.2 | 5.1 | 0.0 | 0.0 | 0.0 | 0.0 | 0.00 | 0.00 | 0 | 0 | 0 | 0 | 0 | 0 | 0.00 | 0.00 | 0.00 | 0.00 | 0.00 | 0.0 | 0.00 | 0.0 | 0.0 | 0.0 | 1 | 0.0 | 0.0 | 0 | 0.0 | 0 | 1 | 0.1 | 24 | 0.00 |
| 25198 | 1 Tbs | Fruit Sweet, fruit juice sweetener, Wax Orchards | 15 | 30 | 50 | 0.0 | 7.5 | 0.5 | 7.0 | 0.0 | 0.0 | 0.0 | 0.0 | 0.0 | 0.00 | 0.00 | 0 | 0 | 0 | 0 | 0 | 0 | | | | | | | | 0.0 | | | 30 | | 0.7 | | | | | | 2 | |
| | | Fruit Syrups | | | | | | | | | | | | | | | | | | | | | | | | | | | | | | | | | | | | | | | | |
| 23399 | 1 Tbs | Apricot Passion, Wax Orchards | 15 | 30 | 47 | 0.0 | 7.5 | 0.5 | 7.0 | 0.0 | 0.0 | 0.0 | 0.0 | 0.0 | 0.00 | 0.00 | 0 | 0 | 0 | 0 | 0 | 0 | | | | | | | | 0.0 | | | 30 | | 0.7 | | | | | | 2 | |
| 23398 | 1 Tbs | Blueberry, Wax Orchards | 15 | 30 | 47 | 0.0 | 7.5 | 0.5 | 7.0 | 0.0 | 0.0 | 0.0 | 0.0 | 0.0 | 0.00 | 0.00 | 0 | 0 | 0 | 0 | 0 | 0 | | | | | | | | 0.0 | | | 30 | | 0.7 | | | | | | 2 | |
| 23396 | 1 Tbs | Raspberry, Wax Orchards | 15 | 30 | 47 | 0.0 | 7.5 | 0.5 | 7.0 | 0.0 | 0.0 | 0.0 | 0.0 | 0.0 | 0.00 | 0.00 | 0 | 0 | 0 | 0 | 0 | 0 | | | | | | | | 0.0 | | | 30 | | 0.7 | | | | | | 2 | |
| 23397 | 1 Tbs | Strawberry, Wax Orchards | 15 | 30 | 47 | 0.0 | 7.5 | 0.5 | 7.0 | 0.0 | 0.0 | 0.0 | 0.0 | 0.0 | 0.00 | 0.00 | 0 | 0 | 0 | 0 | 0 | 0 | | | | | | | | 0.0 | | | 30 | | 0.7 | | | | | | 2 | |
| 25066 | 1 Tbs | Grenadine Syrup, avg | 20 | 53 | 28 | 0.0 | 14.3 | 0.0 | 13.6 | 0.7 | 0.0 | 0.0 | 0.0 | 0.0 | 0.00 | 0.00 | 0 | 0.4 | 0.04 | 0 | 0.04 | | 0.00 | 0.00 | 0.01 | 0.00 | 0.00 | 0.2 | | 0.6 | 0.0 | | 1 | 0.0 | 0.0 | 1 | | 1 | 6 | | 10 | 0.01 |
| 25001 | 1 Tbs | Honey, avg | 21 | 64 | 17 | 0.1 | 17.3 | 0.0 | 16.4 | 0.8 | 0.0 | 0.0 | 0.0 | 0.0 | 0.00 | 0.00 | 0 | 0 | 0 | 0 | 0 | 0 | 0.00 | 0.01 | 0.03 | 0.01 | 0.00 | 0.4 | 0.01 | 0.1 | 0.0 | 0.0 | 1 | 0.0 | 0.1 | 0 | 0.0 | 1 | 11 | 0.2 | 1 | 0.05 |
| 25204 | 1 Tbs | Malt Syrup, avg | 24 | 76 | 21 | 1.5 | 17.1 | 0.0 | | | 0.0 | 0.0 | 0.0 | 0.0 | 0.00 | 0.00 | 0 | 0 | 0 | 0 | 0 | 0 | 0.00 | 0.09 | 1.95 | 0.12 | 0.00 | 2.9 | 0.04 | 0.0 | 0.0 | 0.0 | 15 | 0.0 | 0.2 | 17 | 0.0 | 57 | 77 | 3.0 | 8 | 0.03 |
| 25202 | 1 Tbs | Maple Sugar, avg | 9 | 32 | 8 | 0.0 | 8.2 | 0.0 | 7.8 | 0.4 | 0.0 | 0.0 | 0.0 | 0.0 | 0.00 | 0.01 | 0 | 2 | 0.2 | 0 | 0.2 | | 0.00 | 0.00 | 0.00 | 0.00 | 0.00 | 0.0 | 0.00 | 0.0 | 0.0 | 0.0 | 8 | 0.0 | 0.1 | 2 | 0.4 | 0 | 25 | 0.1 | 1 | 0.55 |
| 25002 | 1 Tbs | Maple Syrup, avg | 20 | 52 | 32 | 0.0 | 13.4 | 0.0 | 12.7 | 0.7 | 0.0 | 0.0 | 0.0 | 0.0 | 0.00 | 0.02 | 0 | 0 | 0 | 0 | 0 | 0 | 0.00 | 0.00 | 0.01 | 0.00 | 0.00 | 0.0 | 0.01 | 0.0 | 0.0 | 0.0 | 13 | 0.0 | 0.2 | 3 | 0.7 | 0 | 41 | 0.1 | 2 | 0.83 |
| | | Molasses | | | | | | | | | | | | | | | | | | | | | | | | | | | | | | | | | | | | | | | | |
| 25004 | 1 Tbs | Blackstrap Cane, avg | 20 | 47 | 29 | 0.0 | 12.2 | 0.0 | 8.6 | 3.6 | 0.0 | 0.0 | 0.0 | 0.0 | 0.00 | 0.00 | 0 | 0 | 0 | 0 | 0 | 0 | 0.01 | 0.01 | 0.22 | 0.14 | 0.00 | 0.2 | 0.18 | 0.0 | 0.0 | 0.0 | 172 | 0.4 | 3.5 | 43 | 0.5 | 8 | 498 | 3.6 | 11 | 0.20 |
| 90050 | 1 Tbs | Light Cane, avg | 20 | 50 | 24 | 0.0 | 13.0 | 0.0 | 12.0 | 1.0 | 0.0 | 0.0 | 0.0 | 0.0 | 0.00 | 0.00 | 0 | 0 | 0 | 0 | 0 | 0 | 0.01 | 0.01 | 0.04 | 0.13 | | 0.0 | | 0.0 | 0.0 | 0.0 | 33 | | 0.9 | 49 | | 9 | 183 | | 3 | 0.06 |
| 90051 | 1 Tbs | Medium Cane, avg | 20 | 46 | 24 | 0.0 | 12.0 | 0.0 | 11.0 | 1.0 | 0.0 | 0.0 | 0.0 | 0.0 | 0.00 | 0.00 | 0 | 0 | 0 | 0 | 0 | 0 | 0.02 | 0.02 | 0.24 | | | | | 0.0 | 0.0 | 0.0 | 58 | | 1.2 | | | 14 | 213 | | 7 | |
| | | Pancake Syrup | | | | | | | | | | | | | | | | | | | | | | | | | | | | | | | | | | | | | | | | |
| 23090 | 1 Tbs | Butter type, avg | 20 | 59 | 24 | 0.0 | 14.8 | 0.0 | 9.2 | 5.6 | 0.3 | 0.2 | 0.1 | 0.0 | 0.00 | 0.01 | 1 | 12 | 3 | 3 | 0.3 | | 0.00 | 0.00 | 0.00 | 0.00 | 0.00 | 0.0 | 0.01 | 0.0 | 0.0 | | 0 | 0.0 | 0.0 | 0 | 0.0 | 2 | 1 | 0.1 | 20 | 0.01 |
| 25152 | 1 Tbs | Butter, Hungry Jack | 20 | 53 | 34 | 0.0 | 13.1 | 0.0 | 7.1 | 5.9 | 0.0 | 0.0 | 0.0 | 0.0 | 0.00 | 0.00 | 0 | 0 | 0 | 0 | 0 | 0 | | | | | | | | 0.0 | | | 0 | | 0.1 | | | | | | 23 | |
| 23091 | 1 Tbs | Butter, lite, avg | 18 | 29 | 55 | 0.0 | 7.5 | 0.0 | 4.6 | 2.9 | 0.0 | 0.0 | 0.0 | 0.0 | 0.00 | 0.00 | 0 | 0 | 0 | 0 | 0 | 0 | 0.01 | 0.01 | 0.01 | 0.00 | 0.00 | 0.0 | | 0.0 | | 0.0 | 2 | 0.0 | 0.3 | 1 | | 1 | 6 | | 37 | 0.02 |
| 25153 | 1 Tbs | Butter, lite, Hungry Jack | 20 | 28 | 64 | 0.0 | 7.0 | 0.2 | 6.6 | 0.1 | 0.0 | 0.0 | 0.0 | 0.0 | 0.00 | 0.00 | 0 | 0 | 0 | 0 | 0 | 0 | | | | | | | | 0.0 | | | 1 | | 0.0 | | | | | | 53 | |
| 23042 | 1 Tbs | Regular, avg | 20 | 57 | 24 | 0.0 | 15.1 | 0.0 | 9.4 | 5.8 | 0.0 | 0.0 | 0.0 | 0.0 | 0.00 | 0.00 | 0 | 0 | 0 | 0 | 0 | 0 | 0.00 | 0.00 | 0.00 | 0.00 | 0.00 | 0.0 | 0.00 | 0.0 | 0.0 | 0.0 | 0 | 0.0 | 0.0 | 0 | 0.0 | 2 | 0 | 0.1 | 17 | 0.01 |
| 23176 | 1 Tbs | Regular, Hungry Jack | 20 | 53 | 34 | 0.0 | 13.1 | 0.0 | 7.1 | 5.9 | 0.0 | 0.0 | 0.0 | 0.0 | 0.00 | 0.00 | 0 | 0 | 0 | 0 | 0 | 0 | | | | | | | | 0.0 | | | 0 | | 0.1 | | | | | | 23 | |
| 25222 | 1 Tbs | Regular, Log Cabin | 20 | 50 | 35 | 0.0 | 13.0 | 0.0 | 7.8 | 5.3 | 0.0 | 0.0 | 0.0 | 0.0 | 0.00 | 0.00 | 0 | 0 | 0 | 0 | 0 | 0 | | | | | | | | 0.0 | | | 0 | | 0.0 | | | | 0 | | 15 | |
| 23172 | 1 Tbs | Regular, lite, avg | 15 | 25 | 55 | 0.0 | 6.6 | 0.0 | 5.8 | 0.9 | 0.0 | 0.0 | 0.0 | 0.0 | 0.00 | 0.00 | 0 | 0 | 0 | 0 | 0 | 0 | 0.00 | 0.00 | 0.00 | 0.00 | 0.00 | 0.0 | 0.00 | 0.0 | 0.0 | 0.0 | 0 | 0.0 | 0.0 | 0 | 0.0 | 6 | 0 | 0.1 | 30 | 0.00 |
| 23177 | 1 Tbs | Regular, lite, Hungry Jack | 20 | 28 | 64 | 0.0 | 7.0 | 0.2 | 6.6 | 0.1 | 0.0 | 0.0 | 0.0 | 0.0 | 0.00 | 0.00 | 0 | 0 | 0 | 0 | 0 | 0 | | | | | | | | 0.0 | | | 1 | | 0.0 | | | | | | 53 | |
| 25223 | 1 Tbs | Regular, lite, Log Cabin | 15 | 25 | 56 | 0.0 | 6.5 | 0.0 | 6.3 | 0.3 | 0.0 | 0.0 | 0.0 | 0.0 | 0.00 | 0.00 | 0 | 0 | 0 | 0 | 0 | 0 | | | | | | | | 0.0 | | | 0 | | 0.0 | | | | 0 | | 45 | |
| 25111 | 1 Tbs | Sorghum Syrup, avg | 21 | 61 | 20 | 0.0 | 15.7 | 0.0 | 14.4 | 1.3 | 0.0 | 0.0 | 0.0 | 0.0 | 0.00 | 0.00 | 0 | 0 | 0 | 0 | 0 | 0 | 0.02 | 0.03 | 0.02 | 0.14 | 0.00 | 0.0 | 0.17 | 0.0 | 0.0 | 0.0 | 31 | 0.0 | 0.8 | 21 | 0.3 | 12 | 210 | 0.1 | 2 | 0.09 |
| | | **VEGETABLES AND LEGUMES** | | | | | | | | | | | | | | | | | | | | | | | | | | | | | | | | | | | | | | | | |
| 5010 | 1/2 cup | Alfalfa Sprouts, avg | 16 | 5 | 91 | 0.6 | 0.6 | 0.4 | 0.1 | 0.1 | 0.1 | 0.0 | 0.0 | 0.1 | 0.03 | 0.04 | 0 | 25 | 3 | 0 | 3 | 15 | 0.01 | 0.02 | 0.08 | 0.01 | 0.00 | 5.8 | 0.09 | 1.3 | 0.0 | | 5 | 0.0 | 0.2 | 4 | 0.0 | 11 | 13 | 0.1 | 1 | 0.15 |
| | | Amaranth | | | | | | | | | | | | | | | | | | | | | | | | | | | | | | | | | | | | | | | | |
| 5837 | 1/2 cup | Boiled, salted, avg | 66 | 14 | 92 | 1.4 | 2.7 | 1.2 | | | 0.1 | 0.0 | 0.0 | 0.1 | 0.00 | 0.05 | 0 | 1828 | 183 | 0 | 183 | 1008 | 0.01 | 0.09 | 0.37 | 0.12 | 0.00 | 37.5 | 0.04 | 27.1 | 0.0 | | 138 | 0.1 | 1.5 | 36 | 0.6 | 48 | 423 | 0.6 | 170 | 0.58 |

| Code | Amount | Description | Basic Components | | | | | | | | | Additional Fats | | | | | | Vit A & Components | | | | | Vitamins | | | | | | | | | | Minerals | | | | | | | | | |
|---|---|---|---|---|---|---|---|---|---|---|---|---|---|---|---|---|---|---|---|---|---|---|---|---|---|---|---|---|---|---|---|---|---|---|---|---|---|---|---|---|---|---|
| | | | Weight (g) | Calories | % Water | Protein (g) | Carbs (g) | Fiber (g) | Sugar (g) | Other Carbs (g) | Fat (g) | Sat Fat (g) | Mono Fat (g) | Poly Fat (g) | Omega 3 (g) | Omega 6 (g) | Choles (mg) | Vit A (IU) | Vit A (RE) | Retinol (RE) | Carotenoids (RE) | Beta Carotene (mcg) | Thiamin (mg) | Riboflavin (mg) | Niacin (NE) | Vit B6 (mg) | Vit B12 (mcg) | Folate (mcg) | Panto (mg) | Vit C (mg) | Vit D (mg) | Vit E (α TE) | Calcium (mg) | Copper (mg) | Iron (mg) | Magnes (mg) | Mang (mg) | Phos (mg) | Potassium (mg) | Selenium (mcg) | Sodium (mg) | Zinc (mg) |
| 5377 | 1/2 cup | Leaf, boiled, drained, avg | 66 | 14 | 92 | 1.4 | 2.7 | 1.2 | | | 0.1 | 0.0 | 0.0 | 0.1 | 0.00 | 0.05 | 0 | 1828 | 183 | 0 | 183 | 1008 | 0.01 | 0.09 | 0.37 | 0.12 | 0.00 | 37.5 | 0.04 | 27.1 | 0.0 | | 138 | 0.1 | 1.5 | 36 | 0.6 | 48 | 423 | 0.6 | 14 | 0.58 |
| 5375 | 1/2 cup | Raw, chpd, avg | 14 | 3 | 92 | 0.3 | 0.6 | 0.2 | | | 0.0 | 0.0 | 0.0 | 0.0 | 0.00 | 0.02 | 0 | 408 | 41 | 0 | 41 | 225 | 0.00 | 0.02 | 0.09 | 0.03 | 0.00 | 11.9 | 0.01 | 6.1 | 0.0 | | 30 | 0.0 | 0.3 | 8 | 0.1 | 7 | 86 | 0.1 | 3 | 0.13 |
| 5721 | 1 ea | Arrowhead, boiled, avg | 12 | 9 | 77 | 0.5 | 1.9 | | | | 0.0 | | | | | | 0 | 0 | 0 | 0 | 0 | 0 | 0.02 | 0.01 | 0.14 | 0.02 | 0.00 | 1.1 | 0.05 | 0.0 | 0.0 | | 1 | 0.0 | 0.1 | 6 | 0.0 | 24 | 106 | 0.1 | 2 | 0.03 |
| 5719 | 1 ea | Arrowhead, raw, avg | 12 | 12 | 72 | 0.6 | 2.4 | | | | 0.0 | | | | | | 0 | 0 | 0 | 0 | 0 | 0 | 0.02 | 0.01 | 0.20 | 0.03 | 0.00 | 1.7 | 0.07 | 0.1 | 0.0 | | 1 | 0.0 | 0.3 | 6 | 0.0 | 21 | 111 | 0.1 | 3 | 0.03 |
| | | Artichokes | | | | | | | | | | | | | | | | | | | | | | | | | | | | | | | | | | | | | | | | |
| 5192 | 1/2 cup | Frozen, boiled, avg | 84 | 38 | 86 | 2.6 | 7.7 | 3.9 | 0.9 | 2.9 | 0.4 | 0.1 | 0.0 | 0.2 | 0.05 | 0.13 | 0 | 138 | 13 | 0 | 13 | 81 | 0.05 | 0.13 | 0.77 | 0.07 | 0.00 | 100.0 | 0.17 | 4.2 | 0.0 | 0.1 | 18 | 0.1 | 0.5 | 26 | 0.2 | 51 | 222 | 0.2 | 45 | 0.30 |
| 5000 | 1 ea | Globe, boiled, avg | 120 | 60 | 84 | 4.2 | 13.4 | 6.5 | 1.3 | 5.6 | 0.2 | 0.0 | 0.0 | 0.1 | 0.02 | 0.06 | 0 | 212 | 22 | 0 | 22 | 130 | 0.08 | 0.08 | 1.20 | 0.13 | 0.00 | 61.2 | 0.41 | 12.0 | 0.0 | 0.2 | 54 | 0.3 | 1.5 | 72 | 0.3 | 103 | 425 | 0.2 | 114 | 0.59 |
| 6709 | 1 ea | Globe, raw, avg | 128 | 60 | 85 | 4.2 | 13.4 | 6.9 | 2.7 | 3.8 | 0.2 | 0.0 | 0.0 | 0.1 | 0.02 | 0.06 | 0 | 237 | 23 | 0 | 23 | 138 | 0.09 | 0.08 | 1.34 | 0.15 | 0.00 | 87.0 | 0.43 | 15.0 | 0.0 | | 56 | 0.3 | 1.6 | 77 | 0.3 | 115 | 474 | 0.3 | 120 | 0.63 |
| 5191 | 1/2 cup | Hearts, marinated, avg | 65 | 64 | 81 | 1.6 | 5.0 | 2.9 | 0.6 | 1.6 | 5.2 | 0.8 | 1.2 | 2.9 | 0.37 | 2.57 | 0 | 107 | 11 | 0 | 11 | 64 | 0.02 | 0.07 | 0.53 | 0.06 | 0.00 | 56.9 | 0.14 | 19.8 | 0.0 | | 15 | 0.1 | 0.6 | 18 | 0.2 | 39 | 168 | 0.4 | 344 | 0.21 |
| 6464 | 1 pce | Hearts, Progresso | 41 | 18 | | 1.0 | 3.0 | 0.5 | 0.5 | 2.0 | 0.0 | 0.0 | 0.0 | 0.0 | 0.00 | 0.00 | 0 | 0 | 0 | 0 | 0 | 0 | | | | | 0.00 | | | 1.8 | | | 0 | | 0.5 | | | | | | 120 | |
| 5077 | 1/2 cup | Jerusalem, raw, avg | 75 | 57 | 78 | 1.5 | 13.0 | 1.2 | 1.9 | 10.0 | 0.0 | 0.0 | 0.0 | 0.0 | 0.00 | 0.00 | 0 | 15 | 2 | 0 | 2 | 9 | 0.15 | 0.04 | 0.97 | 0.06 | 0.00 | 10.0 | 0.30 | 3.0 | 0.0 | 0.1 | 10 | 0.1 | 2.6 | 13 | 0.0 | 58 | 322 | 0.5 | 3 | 0.09 |
| 6033 | 1/2 cup | Arugula, leaf, raw, avg | 10 | 3 | 92 | 0.3 | 0.4 | 0.2 | | | 0.1 | 0.0 | 0.0 | 0.0 | 0.02 | 0.01 | 0 | 237 | 24 | 0 | 24 | 142 | 0.00 | 0.01 | 0.03 | 0.01 | 0.00 | 9.7 | 0.04 | 1.5 | 0.0 | | 16 | 0.0 | 0.1 | 5 | 0.0 | 5 | 37 | 0.0 | 3 | 0.05 |
| | | Asparagus | | | | | | | | | | | | | | | | | | | | | | | | | | | | | | | | | | | | | | | | |
| 5003 | 1/2 cup | Boiled, avg | 90 | 22 | 92 | 2.3 | 3.8 | 1.4 | 1.4 | 0.9 | 0.3 | 0.1 | 0.0 | 0.1 | 0.01 | 0.12 | 0 | 485 | 49 | 0 | 49 | 288 | 0.11 | 0.11 | 0.97 | 0.11 | 0.00 | 131.4 | 0.14 | 9.7 | 0.0 | 0.3 | 18 | 0.1 | 0.7 | 9 | 0.1 | 49 | 144 | 1.5 | 10 | 0.38 |
| 5842 | 1/2 cup | Canned, unsalted, avg | 122 | 18 | 94 | 2.2 | 3.0 | 1.2 | 0.9 | 0.9 | 0.2 | 0.1 | 0.0 | 0.1 | 0.00 | 0.10 | 0 | 642 | 65 | 0 | 65 | 383 | 0.07 | 0.11 | 1.04 | 0.12 | 0.00 | 104.1 | 0.15 | 20.1 | 0.0 | | 18 | 0.1 | 0.7 | 11 | 0.2 | 46 | 210 | 2.0 | 32 | 0.57 |
| 5245 | 1/2 cup | Canned, w/liquid, avg | 122 | 18 | 94 | 2.2 | 3.0 | 1.2 | 0.7 | 1.1 | 0.2 | 0.1 | 0.0 | 0.1 | 0.00 | 0.10 | 0 | 642 | 65 | 0 | 65 | 383 | 0.07 | 0.11 | 1.04 | 0.12 | 0.00 | 104.1 | 0.15 | 20.1 | 0.0 | | 18 | 0.1 | 0.7 | 11 | 0.2 | 46 | 210 | 2.0 | 346 | 0.57 |
| 6263 | 1/2 cup | Canned, 50% less salt, Green Giant | 120 | 18 | 96 | 1.4 | 3.0 | 1.1 | 0.7 | 1.2 | 0.0 | 0.0 | 0.0 | 0.0 | 0.00 | 0.00 | 0 | 318 | 32 | 0 | 32 | 188 | | | | | 0.00 | | | 10.0 | | | 13 | | 0.5 | | | | | | 212 | |
| 6264 | 3 oz | Canned, white spears, Pillsbury | 85 | 12 | 94 | 1.7 | 2.0 | 0.8 | | | 0.1 | 0.1 | 0.0 | 0.0 | | | 0 | 488 | 49 | 0 | 49 | 289 | 0.06 | 0.06 | 0.61 | | 0.00 | | | 18.0 | | | 12 | | 0.4 | | | 28 | 164 | | 310 | |
| 5005 | 1/2 cup | Frozen, boiled, avg | 90 | 25 | 91 | 2.7 | 4.4 | 1.4 | 1.4 | 1.5 | 0.4 | 0.1 | 0.0 | 0.2 | 0.01 | 0.16 | 0 | 736 | 74 | 0 | 74 | 437 | 0.06 | 0.09 | 0.94 | 0.02 | 0.00 | 121.5 | 0.14 | 22.0 | 0.0 | 0.4 | 21 | 0.2 | 0.6 | 12 | 0.2 | 49 | 196 | 1.5 | 4 | 0.50 |
| 5001 | 1/2 cup | Raw, avg | 67 | 15 | 92 | 1.5 | 3.0 | 1.4 | 1.4 | 0.2 | 0.1 | 0.0 | 0.0 | 0.1 | 0.00 | 0.06 | 0 | 391 | 39 | 0 | 39 | 230 | 0.09 | 0.09 | 0.78 | 0.09 | 0.00 | 85.8 | 0.12 | 8.8 | 0.0 | 1.3 | 14 | 0.1 | 0.6 | 12 | 0.2 | 38 | 183 | 1.5 | 1 | 0.31 |
| | | Balsam Pear | | | | | | | | | | | | | | | | | | | | | | | | | | | | | | | | | | | | | | | | |
| 5403 | 1/2 cup | Leaf tips, ckd, avg | 58 | 20 | 89 | 2.1 | 3.9 | 1.1 | | | 0.1 | 0.0 | 0.0 | 0.0 | 0.04 | 0.01 | 0 | 1005 | 100 | 0 | 100 | 602 | 0.09 | 0.16 | 0.58 | 0.44 | 0.00 | 50.8 | 0.03 | 32.2 | 0.0 | | 24 | 0.1 | 0.6 | 55 | 0.3 | 45 | 349 | 0.5 | 8 | 0.17 |
| 5402 | 1/2 cup | Leaf tips, raw, avg | 48 | 14 | 89 | 2.5 | 1.6 | 1.1 | 0.4 | 0.1 | 0.3 | 0.1 | 0.0 | 0.1 | 0.11 | 0.02 | 0 | 832 | 83 | 0 | 83 | 498 | 0.09 | 0.17 | 0.53 | 0.39 | 0.00 | 61.4 | 0.03 | 42.2 | 0.0 | | 40 | 0.1 | 1.0 | 41 | 0.3 | 48 | 292 | 0.4 | 5 | 0.14 |
| 5405 | 1/2 cup | Pods, ckd, avg | 62 | 12 | 94 | 0.5 | 2.7 | 1.2 | | | 0.1 | 0.0 | 0.0 | 0.0 | 0.00 | 0.05 | 0 | 70 | 7 | 0 | 7 | 41 | 0.03 | 0.03 | 0.17 | 0.03 | 0.00 | 31.7 | 0.12 | 20.5 | 0.0 | | 6 | 0.0 | 0.2 | 10 | 0.1 | 22 | 198 | 0.1 | 4 | 0.48 |
| 5404 | 1/2 cup | Pods, raw, avg | 46 | 8 | 94 | 0.5 | 1.7 | 1.3 | | | 0.1 | 0.0 | 0.0 | 0.0 | 0.00 | 0.04 | 0 | 175 | 17 | 0 | 17 | 105 | 0.02 | 0.02 | 0.18 | 0.02 | 0.00 | 33.1 | 0.10 | 38.6 | 0.0 | | 9 | 0.0 | 0.2 | 8 | 0.0 | 14 | 136 | 0.1 | 2 | 0.37 |
| | | Bamboo Shoots | | | | | | | | | | | | | | | | | | | | | | | | | | | | | | | | | | | | | | | | |
| 5249 | 1/2 cup | Boiled, avg | 60 | 7 | 96 | 0.9 | 1.2 | 0.6 | | | 0.1 | 0.0 | 0.0 | 0.1 | 0.01 | 0.05 | 0 | 0 | 0 | 0 | 0 | 0 | 0.01 | 0.03 | 0.18 | 0.06 | 0.00 | 1.4 | 0.04 | 0.0 | 0.0 | | 7 | 0.0 | 0.1 | 2 | 0.1 | 12 | 320 | 0.2 | 2 | 0.28 |
| 5401 | 1/2 cup | Canned, sliced, avg | 66 | 13 | 94 | 1.1 | 2.1 | 0.9 | | | 0.3 | 0.1 | 0.0 | 0.1 | 0.02 | 0.10 | 0 | 5 | 1 | 0 | 1 | 3 | 0.02 | 0.02 | 0.09 | 0.09 | 0.00 | 2.1 | 0.06 | 0.7 | 0.0 | | 5 | 0.1 | 0.2 | 3 | 0.1 | 17 | 53 | 0.3 | 5 | 0.43 |
| 6463 | 2 oz | Canned, La Choy | 57 | 6 | 96 | 0.4 | 1.7 | 1.0 | 0.7 | 0.0 | 0.1 | 0.0 | | | | | 0 | 0 | 0 | 0 | 0 | 0 | | | | | 0.00 | | | 0.0 | | | 0 | | 0.0 | | | | | | 0 | |
| 5230 | 1/2 cup | Sliced, raw, avg | 76 | 21 | 91 | 2.0 | 4.0 | 1.7 | 0.8 | 1.4 | 0.2 | 0.1 | 0.0 | 0.1 | 0.02 | 0.09 | 0 | 15 | 2 | 0 | 2 | 9 | 0.11 | 0.05 | 0.46 | 0.18 | 0.00 | 5.4 | 0.12 | 3.0 | 0.0 | | 10 | 0.1 | 0.4 | 2 | 0.2 | 45 | 405 | 0.6 | 3 | 0.84 |
| | | Beans—Mature Legumes | | | | | | | | | | | | | | | | | | | | | | | | | | | | | | | | | | | | | | | | |
| 7443 | 1/2 cup | Adzuki, unsalted, Eden | 130 | 110 | 79 | 7.0 | 19.0 | 5.0 | | | 0.0 | 0.0 | 0.0 | 0.0 | 0.00 | 0.00 | 0 | 0 | 0 | 0 | 0 | 0 | 0.06 | 0.07 | 0.80 | | | | | 0.0 | 0.0 | | 40 | | 1.8 | 40 | | 100 | 250 | | 10 | 0.90 |
| 57056 | 1/2 cup | Baked, barbecue, B&M | 133 | 170 | | 7.0 | 32.0 | 6.0 | 8.0 | 18.0 | 2.0 | 0.5 | 0.5 | 0.5 | | | 2 | 0 | 0 | 0 | 0 | 0 | | | | | | | | 0.0 | | | 80 | | 3.6 | | | | | | 360 | |
| 57058 | 1/2 cup | Baked, brick oven, B&M | 131 | 180 | | 8.0 | 32.0 | 7.0 | 10.0 | 15.0 | 2.0 | 0.5 | 0.5 | 0.5 | | | 5 | 0 | 0 | 0 | 0 | 0 | | | | | | | | 0.0 | | | 60 | | 4.5 | | | | | | 390 | |
| 57055 | 1/2 cup | Baked, extra hearty, B&M | 131 | 190 | | 8.0 | 36.0 | 8.0 | 14.0 | 14.0 | 2.0 | 0.5 | 1.0 | 0.5 | | | 2 | 0 | 0 | 0 | 0 | 0 | | | | | | | | 0.0 | | | 60 | | 4.5 | | | | | | 450 | |
| 7163 | 1/2 cup | Baked, fat free, Health Valley | 120 | 110 | 74 | 7.0 | 24.0 | 7.0 | 11.0 | 6.0 | 0.0 | 0.0 | 0.0 | 0.0 | 0.00 | 0.00 | 0 | 4500 | 450 | 0 | 450 | 2595 | | | | | 0.00 | | | 12.0 | | | 40 | | 2.7 | | | | | | 135 | |
| 7162 | 1/2 cup | Baked, fat free, unsalted, Health Valley | 120 | 110 | 74 | 7.0 | 24.0 | 7.0 | 11.0 | 6.0 | 0.0 | 0.0 | 0.0 | 0.0 | 0.00 | 0.00 | 0 | 4500 | 450 | 0 | 450 | 2595 | | | | | 0.00 | | | 12.0 | | | 40 | | 2.7 | | | | | | 25 | |
| 57054 | 1/2 cup | Baked Beans, 99% fat free, B&M | 130 | 160 | | 8.0 | 31.0 | 7.0 | 8.0 | 16.0 | 1.0 | 0.0 | 0.0 | 0.5 | | | 0 | 0 | 0 | 0 | 0 | 0 | | | | | | | | 0.0 | | | 60 | | 3.6 | | | | | | 220 | |
| 57053 | 1/2 cup | Baked, red kidney, B&M | 132 | 170 | | 7.0 | 32.0 | 6.0 | 10.0 | 16.0 | 2.0 | 0.5 | 0.5 | 0.5 | | | 2 | 0 | 0 | 0 | 0 | 0 | | | | | | | | 0.0 | | | 60 | | 3.6 | | | | | | 440 | |
| 57052 | 1/2 cup | Baked, yellow eye, B&M | 130 | 170 | | 8.0 | 28.0 | 7.0 | 7.0 | 14.0 | 2.0 | 0.5 | 1.0 | 0.5 | | | 2 | 0 | 0 | 0 | 0 | 0 | | | | | | | | 0.0 | | | 60 | | 4.5 | | | | | | 460 | |
| 57057 | 1/2 cup | Baked, w/honey, B&M | 134 | 170 | | 8.0 | 30.0 | 8.0 | 7.0 | 15.0 | 1.5 | 0.0 | 0.0 | 1.0 | | | 0 | 0 | 0 | 0 | 0 | 0 | | | | | | | | 0.0 | | | 60 | | 4.5 | | | | | | 450 | |
| 6089 | 1/2 cup | Broadbeans/Fava, boiled, avg | 100 | 62 | 84 | 4.8 | 10.1 | 3.6 | 1.8 | 4.7 | 0.5 | 0.1 | 0.0 | 0.3 | 0.18 | 0.12 | 0 | 270 | 27 | 0 | 27 | 156 | 0.13 | 0.09 | 1.20 | 0.03 | 0.00 | 57.8 | 0.07 | 19.8 | 0.0 | | 18 | 0.1 | 1.5 | 31 | 0.3 | 73 | 193 | 1.0 | 41 | 0.47 |
| 7026 | 1/2 cup | Broadbeans/Fava, raw, avg | 75 | 256 | 11 | 19.6 | 43.7 | 18.8 | 3.2 | 21.8 | 1.1 | 0.2 | 0.2 | 0.5 | 0.03 | 0.44 | 0 | 40 | 4 | 0 | 4 | 22 | 0.42 | 0.25 | 2.12 | 0.27 | 0.00 | 317.3 | 0.73 | 1.0 | 0.0 | | 77 | 0.6 | 5.0 | 144 | 1.2 | 316 | 796 | 6.1 | 10 | 2.36 |
| 7171 | 1/2 cup | Broadbeans/Fava, cnd, Progresso | 130 | 110 | 78 | 6.0 | 20.0 | 5.0 | 0.0 | 15.0 | 0.5 | 0.0 | 0.0 | 0.0 | 0.00 | 0.00 | 0 | 0 | 0 | 0 | 0 | 0 | | | | | 0.00 | | | 0.0 | | | 20 | | 1.4 | | | | | | 250 | |
| 7174 | 1/2 cup | Black, cnd, Old El Paso | 130 | 100 | 80 | 7.0 | 17.0 | 7.0 | 0.0 | 10.0 | 1.0 | 0.0 | 0.0 | 0.5 | | | 0 | 0 | 0 | 0 | 0 | 0 | | | | | 0.00 | | | 0.0 | | | 40 | | 2.7 | | | | | | 400 | |
| 7835 | 1/2 cup | Black, 50% less salt, cnd, S&W | 127 | 70 | 81 | 5.0 | 17.0 | 6.0 | 1.0 | 10.0 | 0.0 | 0.0 | 0.0 | 0.0 | 0.00 | 0.00 | 0 | 0 | 0 | 0 | 0 | 0 | | | | | | | | 2.4 | | | 40 | | 1.8 | | | | 360 | | 260 | |
| 7178 | 1/2 cup | Black, refried, cnd, Old El Paso | 120 | 120 | 76 | 6.0 | 18.0 | 6.0 | 2.0 | 10.0 | 2.0 | 0.0 | 0.0 | 1.0 | | | 0 | 0 | 0 | 0 | 0 | 0 | | | | | 0.00 | | | 0.0 | | | 60 | | 2.7 | | | | | | 340 | |
| 7823 | 1/2 cup | Butter, cnd, S&W | 124 | 70 | 79 | 6.0 | 18.0 | 5.0 | 1.0 | 12.0 | 0.0 | 0.0 | 0.0 | 0.0 | 0.00 | 0.00 | 0 | 0 | 0 | 0 | 0 | 0 | | | | | | | | 2.4 | | | 40 | | 1.8 | | | | 470 | | 440 | |
| 7169 | 1/2 cup | Cannellini, cnd, Progresso | 130 | 100 | 80 | 5.0 | 18.0 | 5.0 | 0.0 | 13.0 | 0.5 | 0.0 | 0.0 | 0.5 | | | 0 | 0 | 0 | 0 | 0 | 0 | | | | | 0.00 | | | 0.0 | | | 40 | | 1.8 | | | | | | 270 | |
| 90099 | 1/2 cup | Chili, cnd, Campbell's | 130 | 130 | 76 | 6.0 | 21.0 | 6.0 | 4.0 | 11.0 | 3.0 | 1.0 | | | | | 5 | 300 | 30 | 0 | 30 | 173 | | | | | | | | 1.2 | | | 60 | | 1.4 | | | | | | 490 | |
| 5764 | 1/2 cup | Hyacinth, boiled, avg | 44 | 22 | 87 | 1.3 | 4.0 | 1.6 | | | 0.1 | 0.1 | 0.1 | 0.0 | 0.00 | 0.00 | 0 | 62 | 6 | 0 | 6 | 36 | 0.02 | 0.04 | 0.21 | 0.01 | 0.00 | 20.5 | 0.02 | 2.2 | 0.0 | | 18 | 0.0 | 0.3 | 18 | 0.1 | 22 | 115 | 0.7 | 1 | 0.17 |
| 5763 | 1/2 cup | Hyacinth, raw, avg | 40 | 18 | 88 | 0.8 | 3.7 | 1.5 | | | 0.1 | 0.0 | 0.0 | 0.0 | 0.00 | 0.00 | 0 | 44 | 4 | 0 | 4 | 25 | 0.03 | 0.04 | 0.21 | 0.01 | 0.00 | 24.6 | 0.02 | 5.2 | 0.0 | | 20 | 0.0 | 0.3 | 16 | 0.1 | 20 | 101 | 0.6 | 1 | 0.15 |
| 7001 | 1/2 cup | Garbanzo/Chickpeas, boiled, avg | 82 | 134 | 60 | 7.3 | 22.5 | 6.2 | 1.0 | 15.3 | 2.1 | 0.2 | 0.5 | 1.0 | 0.04 | 0.91 | 0 | 22 | 2 | 0 | 2 | 14 | 0.10 | 0.05 | 0.43 | 0.11 | 0.00 | 141.0 | 0.23 | 1.1 | 0.0 | | 40 | 0.3 | 2.4 | 39 | 0.8 | 138 | 239 | 3.0 | 6 | 1.25 |
| 7175 | 1/2 cup | Garbanzo/Chickpeas, cnd, Old El Paso | 130 | 120 | 78 | 5.0 | 20.0 | 7.0 | 0.0 | 13.0 | 2.5 | 0.0 | 1.0 | 1.5 | | | 0 | 0 | 0 | 0 | 0 | 0 | | | | | 0.00 | | | 0.0 | | | 40 | | 1.8 | | | | | | 280 | |
| 7000 | 1/2 cup | Garbanzo/Chickpeas, raw, avg | 100 | 364 | 12 | 19.3 | 60.7 | 17.4 | 10.7 | 32.6 | 6.0 | 0.6 | 1.4 | 2.7 | 0.10 | 2.59 | 0 | 67 | 7 | 0 | 7 | 40 | 0.48 | 0.21 | 1.54 | 0.54 | 0.00 | 557.0 | 1.59 | 4.0 | 0.0 | | 105 | 0.8 | 6.2 | 115 | 2.2 | 366 | 875 | 8.2 | 24 | 3.43 |
| 7445 | 1/2 cup | Garbanzo/Chickpeas, unsalted, cnd, Eden | 130 | 120 | 77 | 7.0 | 19.0 | 5.0 | | | 1.5 | | | | | | 0 | | | | | | 0.09 | 0.07 | 0.40 | | 0.00 | | | | 0.0 | | 60 | | 1.4 | 60 | | 100 | 250 | | | 1.50 |
| 7021 | 1/2 cup | Great Northern, boiled, avg | 88 | 104 | 69 | 7.3 | 18.6 | 6.2 | 1.9 | 10.5 | 0.4 | 0.1 | 0.0 | 0.2 | 0.07 | 0.09 | 0 | 1 | 0.1 | 0 | 0.1 | 1 | 0.14 | 0.05 | 0.60 | 0.10 | 0.00 | 89.8 | 0.23 | 1.1 | 0.0 | | 60 | 0.2 | 1.9 | 44 | 0.5 | 145 | 344 | 3.6 | 2 | 0.77 |
| 7837 | 1/2 cup | Great Northern, cnd, S&W | 127 | 70 | 81 | 6.0 | 17.0 | 6.0 | 3.0 | 8.0 | 0.0 | 0.0 | 0.0 | 0.0 | 0.00 | 0.00 | 0 | 0 | 0 | 0 | 0 | 0 | | | | | | | | 1.2 | | | 40 | | 1.4 | | | | 360 | | 490 | |
| 7008 | 1/2 cup | Kidney, all types, boiled, avg | 88 | 112 | 67 | 7.6 | 20.1 | 5.6 | 1.9 | 12.5 | 0.4 | 0.1 | 0.0 | 0.2 | 0.15 | 0.09 | 0 | 0 | 0 | 0 | 0 | 0 | 0.14 | 0.05 | 0.51 | 0.11 | 0.00 | 114.4 | 0.19 | 1.1 | 0.0 | | 25 | 0.2 | 2.6 | 40 | 0.4 | 125 | 355 | 1.1 | 2 | 0.94 |
| 7173 | 1/2 cup | Kidney, cnd, Progresso | 130 | 110 | 77 | 7.0 | 20.0 | 8.0 | 0.0 | 12.0 | 0.5 | 0.0 | 0.0 | 0.0 | 0.00 | 0.00 | 0 | 0 | 0 | 0 | 0 | 0 | | | | | 0.00 | | | 0.0 | | | 40 | | 1.8 | | | | | | 280 | |
| 7446 | 1/2 cup | Kidney, fat free, unsalted, cnd, Eden | 130 | 100 | 78 | 8.0 | 18.0 | 10.0 | | | 0.0 | 0.0 | 0.0 | 0.0 | 0.00 | 0.00 | 0 | 0 | 0 | 0 | 0 | 0 | 0.15 | 0.03 | 0.40 | | 0.00 | | | | 0.0 | | 60 | | 1.4 | 40 | | 150 | 440 | | 15 | 1.20 |
| 5319 | 1/2 cup | Lima, baby, boiled, avg | 85 | 105 | 67 | 5.8 | 20.1 | 4.5 | 2.8 | 12.8 | 0.3 | 0.1 | 0.0 | 0.1 | 0.04 | 0.09 | 0 | 315 | 31 | 0 | 31 | 181 | 0.12 | 0.08 | 0.88 | 0.16 | 0.00 | 22.4 | 0.22 | 8.6 | 0.0 | | 27 | 0.3 | 2.1 | 63 | 1.1 | 111 | 485 | 1.7 | 14 | 0.67 |
| 5527 | 1/2 cup | Lima, baby, cnd, low sod, avg | 87 | 62 | 81 | 3.5 | 11.6 | 3.1 | 1.7 | 6.7 | 0.3 | 0.1 | 0.0 | 0.1 | 0.04 | 0.08 | 0 | 131 | 13 | 0 | 13 | 75 | 0.03 | 0.04 | 0.46 | 0.05 | 0.00 | 13.9 | 0.08 | 7.6 | 0.0 | | 24 | 0.1 | 1.4 | 30 | 0.6 | 62 | 248 | 1.0 | 3 | 0.56 |
| 7009 | 1/2 cup | Lima, baby, dry, avg | 101 | 338 | 12 | 20.8 | 63.4 | 20.8 | 8.6 | 34.0 | 0.9 | 0.2 | 0.1 | 0.4 | 0.13 | 0.29 | 0 | 5 | 1 | 0 | 1 | 3 | 0.58 | 0.22 | 1.73 | 0.33 | 0.00 | 404.0 | 1.28 | 0.0 | 0.0 | | 82 | 0.7 | 6.3 | 190 | 1.7 | 374 | 1417 | 7.1 | 13 | 2.63 |
| 5019 | 1/2 cup | Lima, baby, fzn, ckd | 90 | 94 | 72 | 6.0 | 17.5 | 5.4 | 2.5 | 9.6 | 0.3 | 0.1 | 0.0 | 0.1 | 0.04 | 0.09 | 0 | 150 | 15 | 0 | 15 | 88 | 0.06 | 0.05 | 0.69 | 0.10 | 0.00 | 13.9 | 0.16 | 5.2 | 0.0 | | 25 | 0.2 | 1.8 | 50 | 0.7 | 101 | 370 | 1.5 | 26 | 0.50 |
| 7010 | 1/2 cup | Lima, large, boiled, avg | 94 | 108 | 70 | 7.3 | 19.6 | 6.6 | 2.7 | 10.3 | 0.4 | 0.1 | 0.0 | 0.2 | 0.05 | 0.11 | 0 | 0 | 0 | 0 | 0 | 0 | 0.15 | 0.05 | 0.40 | 0.15 | 0.00 | 78.1 | 0.40 | 0.0 | 0.0 | | 16 | 0.2 | 2.2 | 40 | 0.5 | 104 | 478 | 4.2 | 2 | 0.89 |
| 7011 | 1/2 cup | Lima, large, cnd, avg | 120 | 95 | 77 | 5.9 | 17.9 | 5.8 | 2.5 | 9.6 | 0.2 | 0.0 | 0.0 | 0.1 | 0.03 | 0.06 | 0 | 0 | 0 | 0 | 0 | 0 | 0.07 | 0.04 | 0.31 | 0.11 | 0.00 | 60.5 | 0.31 | 0.0 | 0.0 | | 25 | 0.2 | 2.2 | 47 | 0.4 | 89 | 264 | 5.4 | 403 | 0.78 |
| 5247 | 1/2 cup | Lima, large, fzn, ckd, avg | 85 | 85 | 74 | 5.2 | 16.0 | 4.9 | 2.5 | 8.6 | 0.3 | 0.1 | 0.0 | 0.1 | 0.05 | 0.09 | 0 | 162 | 16 | 0 | 16 | 94 | 0.06 | 0.05 | 0.91 | 0.10 | 0.00 | 18.0 | 0.14 | 10.9 | 0.0 | | 19 | 0.0 | 1.2 | 29 | 0.3 | 54 | 347 | 1.4 | 45 | 0.37 |
| 5680 | 1/2 cup | Lima, large, raw, avg | 78 | 88 | 70 | 5.3 | 15.8 | 3.8 | 2.3 | 9.6 | 0.7 | 0.2 | 0.0 | 0.3 | 0.11 | 0.22 | 0 | 236 | 23 | 0 | 23 | 135 | 0.17 | 0.08 | 1.15 | 0.16 | 0.00 | 26.5 | 0.19 | 18.3 | 0.0 | | 27 | 0.2 | 2.4 | 45 | 1.0 | 106 | 364 | 1.4 | 6 | 0.61 |
| 7176 | 1/2 cup | Mexican, cnd, Old El Paso | 130 | 110 | | 7.0 | 19.0 | 7.0 | 0.0 | 12.0 | 0.5 | 0.0 | 0.0 | 0.5 | | | 0 | 200 | 40 | 0 | 40 | 231 | | | | | 0.00 | | | 0.0 | | | 40 | | 1.8 | | | | | | 630 | |

| Code | Amount | Description | Basic Components | | | | | | | | | Additional Fats | | | | | | Vit A & Components | | | | | Vitamins | | | | | | | | | | Minerals | | | | | | | | | |
|---|---|---|---|---|---|---|---|---|---|---|---|---|---|---|---|---|---|---|---|---|---|---|---|---|---|---|---|---|---|---|---|---|---|---|---|---|---|---|---|---|---|---|
| | | | Weight (g) | Calories | % Water | Protein (g) | Carbs (g) | Fiber (g) | Sugar (g) | Other Carbs (g) | Fat (g) | Sat Fat (g) | Mono Fat (g) | Poly Fat (g) | Omega 3 (g) | Omega 6 (g) | Choles (mg) | Vit A (IU) | Vit A (RE) | Retinol (RE) | Carotenoids (RE) | Beta Carotene (mcg) | Thiamin (mg) | Riboflavin (mg) | Niacin (NE) | Vit B6 (mg) | Vit B12 (mcg) | Folate (mcg) | Panto (mg) | Vit C (mg) | Vit D (mg) | Vit E (α TE) | Calcium (mg) | Copper (mg) | Iron (mg) | Magnes (mg) | Mang (mg) | Phos (mg) | Potassium (mg) | Selenium (mcg) | Sodium (mg) | Zinc (mg) |
| 7022 | 1/2 cup | Navy, ckd, avg | 91 | 129 | 63 | 7.9 | 23.9 | 5.8 | 2.0 | 16.1 | 0.5 | 0.1 | 0.0 | 0.2 | 0.10 | 0.12 | 0 | 2 | 0.2 | 0 | 0.2 | 1 | 0.18 | 0.06 | 0.48 | 0.15 | 0.00 | 127.4 | 0.23 | 0.8 | 0.0 | | 64 | 0.3 | 2.3 | 54 | 0.5 | 143 | 335 | 5.3 | 1 | 0.96 |
| 7447 | 1/2 cup | Navy, unsalted, cnd, Eden | 130 | 110 | 78 | 7.0 | 20.0 | 7.0 | | | 0.5 | | | | | | 0 | | | | | | 0.12 | 0.03 | 0.40 | | 0.00 | | | | 0.0 | | 80 | | 2.7 | 60 | | 150 | 300 | | 15 | 0.90 |
| 7013 | 1/2 cup | Pinto, boiled, avg | 86 | 118 | 64 | 7.1 | 22.1 | 7.4 | 1.9 | 12.8 | 0.4 | 0.1 | 0.1 | 0.2 | 0.09 | 0.07 | 0 | 2 | 0.2 | 0 | 0.2 | 1 | 0.16 | 0.08 | 0.34 | 0.13 | 0.00 | 147.9 | 0.25 | 1.8 | 0.0 | | 41 | 0.2 | 2.2 | 47 | 0.5 | 138 | 402 | 6.1 | 2 | 0.93 |
| 7177 | 1/2 cup | Pinto, cnd, Old El Paso | 130 | 110 | 79 | 6.0 | 19.0 | 7.0 | 0.0 | 12.0 | 0.5 | 0.0 | 0.0 | 0.5 | | | 0 | 0 | 0 | 0 | 0 | 0 | | | | | 0.00 | | | 0.0 | | | 40 | | 1.8 | | | | | | 420 | |
| 7448 | 1/2 cup | Pinto, cnd, unsalted, fat free, Eden | 130 | 100 | 80 | 6.0 | 18.0 | 6.0 | | | 0.0 | 0.0 | 0.0 | 0.0 | 0.00 | 0.00 | 0 | | | | | | 0.03 | 0.03 | 0.40 | | 0.00 | | | | 0.0 | | 60 | | 1.8 | 40 | | 100 | 350 | | 15 | 0.90 |
| 5731 | 3 oz | Pinto, fzn, ckd | 85 | 138 | 58 | 7.9 | 26.3 | 7.3 | 2.2 | 16.7 | 0.4 | 0.0 | 0.0 | 0.2 | 0.15 | 0.08 | 0 | 0 | 0 | 0 | 0 | 0 | 0.23 | 0.09 | 0.54 | 0.16 | 0.00 | 28.5 | 0.22 | 0.6 | 0.0 | | 44 | 0.1 | 2.3 | 46 | 0.4 | 85 | 549 | 1.2 | 71 | 0.59 |
| 7023 | 1/2 cup | Pork & Beans, w/sweet sauce, cnd, avg | 126 | 140 | 71 | 6.7 | 26.5 | 6.6 | 10.5 | 9.4 | 1.8 | 0.7 | 0.8 | 0.2 | 0.04 | 0.20 | 0 | 144 | 14 | 0 | 14 | 80 | 0.06 | 0.08 | 0.44 | 0.11 | 0.00 | 47.1 | 0.13 | 3.8 | 0.0 | | 77 | 0.1 | 2.1 | 43 | 0.5 | 132 | 335 | 5.9 | 423 | 1.89 |
| 7004 | 1/2 cup | Pork & Beans, w/tomato sauce, cnd, avg | 126 | 123 | 73 | 6.5 | 24.4 | 6.0 | 7.2 | 11.2 | 1.3 | 0.5 | 0.6 | 0.2 | 0.03 | 0.14 | 0 | 156 | 15 | 0 | 15 | 87 | 0.07 | 0.06 | 0.63 | 0.09 | 0.00 | 28.4 | 0.67 | 3.9 | 0.0 | | 71 | 0.3 | 4.1 | 44 | 0.6 | 147 | 378 | 5.9 | 554 | 7.38 |
| 7024 | 1/2 cup | Refried, cnd, avg | 126 | 118 | 76 | 6.9 | 19.5 | 6.7 | 2.1 | 10.7 | 1.6 | 0.6 | 0.7 | 0.2 | 0.03 | 0.17 | 1[illegible] | 0 | 0 | 0 | 0 | 0 | 0.03 | 0.02 | 0.40 | 0.18 | 0.00 | 13.9 | 0.12 | 7.6 | 0.0 | | 44 | 0.2 | 2.1 | 42 | 0.2 | 108 | 336 | 1.6 | 377 | 1.47 |
| 7179 | 1/2 cup | Refried, cnd, fat free, Old El Paso | 124 | 110 | 77 | 6.0 | 20.0 | 6.0 | 1.0 | 13.0 | 0.0 | 0.0 | 0.0 | 0.0 | 0.00 | 0.00 | 0 | 0 | 0 | 0 | 0 | 0 | | | | | 0.00 | | | 0.0 | | | 40 | | 1.8 | | | | | | 480 | |
| 7185 | 1/2 cup | Refried, cnd, vegetarian, Old El Paso | 118 | 100 | 79 | 6.0 | 16.0 | 6.0 | 2.0 | 8.0 | 1.0 | 0.0 | 0.0 | 0.5 | | | 0 | 0 | 0 | 0 | 0 | 0 | | | | | 0.00 | | | 0.0 | | | 40 | | 1.4 | | | | | | 490 | |
| 7181 | 1/2 cup | Refried, cnd, w/cheese, Old El Paso | 120 | 130 | | 7.0 | 18.0 | 6.0 | 1.0 | 11.0 | 3.5 | 1.5 | 1.0 | 0.5 | | | [illegible] | 0 | 0 | 0 | 0 | 0 | | | | | 0.00 | | | 0.0 | | | 80 | | 1.8 | | | | | | 500 | |
| 7182 | 1/2 cup | Refried, cnd, w/green chilies, Old El Paso | 122 | 110 | | 6.0 | 19.0 | 6.0 | 1.0 | 12.0 | 0.5 | 0.0 | | | | | [illegible] | 0 | 0 | 0 | 0 | 0 | | | | | 0.00 | | | 0.0 | | | 40 | | 1.8 | | | | | | 720 | |
| 7183 | 1/2 cup | Refried, cnd, w/sausage, Old El Paso | 118 | 200 | | 7.0 | 14.0 | 8.0 | 1.0 | 5.0 | 13.0 | 5.0 | 5.0 | 2.0 | | | 1[illegible] | 0 | 0 | 0 | 0 | 0 | | | | | 0.00 | | | 0.0 | | | 40 | | 1.4 | | | | | | 360 | |
| 5732 | 1/2 cup | Shell, cnd, avg | 122 | 37 | 91 | 2.1 | 7.6 | 4.1 | | | 0.2 | 0.0 | 0.0 | 0.1 | 0.09 | 0.05 | 0 | 273 | 27 | 0 | 28 | 162 | 0.04 | 0.07 | 0.25 | 0.06 | 0.00 | 22.0 | 0.16 | 3.8 | 0.0 | | 35 | 0.1 | 1.2 | 18 | 0.5 | 37 | 133 | 1.0 | 407 | 0.33 |
| 7063 | 1/2 cup | Soybeans, dry roasted, avg | 86 | 387 | 1 | 34.1 | 28.1 | 7.0 | 7.1 | 14.0 | 18.6 | 2.7 | 4.1 | 10.5 | 1.23 | 9.25 | 0 | 20 | 2 | 0 | 2 | | 0.37 | 0.65 | 0.91 | 0.19 | 0.00 | 176.3 | 0.41 | 4.0 | 0.0 | | 120 | 0.9 | 3.4 | 196 | 1.9 | 558 | 1173 | 16.6 | 2 | 4.10 |
| 7003 | 1/2 cup | White, boiled, avg | 90 | 128 | 63 | 8.1 | 23.2 | 9.4 | 2.0 | 11.9 | 0.6 | 0.1 | 0.1 | 0.2 | 0.11 | 0.14 | 0 | 0 | 0 | 0 | 0 | 0 | 0.21 | 0.05 | 0.24 | 0.11 | 0.00 | 123.3 | 0.23 | 0.0 | 0.0 | | 66 | 0.1 | 2.6 | 61 | 0.5 | 152 | 417 | 1.2 | 2 | 0.98 |
| 7838 | 1/2 cup | White, cnd, S&W | 122 | 80 | 78 | 7.0 | 19.0 | 6.0 | 1.0 | 12.0 | 0.5 | 0.0 | | | 0.00 | 0.00 | 0 | 0 | 0 | 0 | 0 | 0 | | | | | | | | 0.0 | | | 60 | | 1.4 | | | | 350 | | 440 | |
| 7002 | 1/2 cup | White, raw, avg | 108 | 363 | 12 | 22.8 | 67.3 | 26.9 | 5.9 | 34.5 | 1.3 | 0.3 | 0.1 | 0.5 | 0.25 | 0.30 | 0 | 0 | 0 | 0 | 0 | 0 | 0.80 | 0.22 | 1.45 | 0.47 | 0.00 | 416.9 | 0.79 | 0.0 | 0.0 | | 187 | 0.7 | 8.3 | 198 | 1.4 | 481 | 1665 | 13.8 | 13 | 3.03 |
| 7031 | 1/2 cup | Winged/Goabean, dry, boiled, avg | 86 | 126 | 67 | 9.1 | 12.8 | 2.1 | 2.2 | 8.6 | 5.0 | 0.7 | 1.8 | 1.3 | 0.08 | 1.25 | 0 | 0 | 0 | 0 | 0 | 0 | 0.25 | 0.11 | 0.71 | 0.04 | 0.00 | 8.9 | 0.13 | 0.0 | 0.0 | | 122 | 0.7 | 3.7 | 46 | 1.0 | 132 | 241 | 2.5 | 11 | 1.24 |
| 7030 | 1/2 cup | Winged/Goabean, mature, dry, avg | 91 | 372 | 8 | 27.0 | 37.9 | 6.2 | 6.4 | 25.3 | 14.8 | 2.1 | 5.5 | 3.9 | 0.24 | 3.70 | 0 | 0 | 0 | 0 | 0 | 0 | 0.94 | 0.41 | 2.81 | 0.16 | 0.00 | 40.6 | 0.72 | 0.0 | 0.0 | | 400 | 2.6 | 12.2 | 163 | 3.4 | 410 | 889 | 7.5 | 35 | 4.08 |
| 7033 | 1/2 cup | Yard Long, boiled, avg | 86 | 101 | 69 | 7.1 | 18.1 | 3.3 | | | 0.4 | 0.1 | 0.0 | 0.2 | 0.08 | 0.09 | 0 | 4 | [illegible] | 0 | 2 | 10 | 0.18 | 0.06 | 0.47 | 0.08 | 0.00 | 125.6 | 0.34 | 0.3 | 0.0 | | 36 | 0.2 | 2.3 | 84 | 0.4 | 156 | 271 | 2.4 | 4 | 0.93 |
| 7032 | 1/2 cup | Yard Long, mature, raw, avg | 84 | 291 | 8 | 20.4 | 52.0 | 9.2 | | | 1.1 | 0.3 | 0.1 | 0.5 | 0.22 | 0.26 | 0 | 44 | [illegible] | 0 | 4 | 24 | 0.75 | 0.20 | 1.81 | 0.31 | 0.00 | 552.7 | 1.31 | 1.3 | 0.0 | | 116 | 0.7 | 7.2 | 284 | 1.3 | 470 | 972 | 6.9 | 14 | 2.94 |
| | | Beets | | | | | | | | | | | | | | | | | | | | | | | | | | | | | | | | | | | | | | | | |
| 5022 | 1/2 cup | Boiled, diced, avg | 85 | 37 | 87 | 1.4 | 8.5 | 1.7 | 6.2 | 0.6 | 0.2 | 0.0 | 0.0 | 0.1 | 0.00 | 0.05 | 0 | 30 | 3 | 0 | 3 | 10 | 0.02 | 0.03 | 0.28 | 0.06 | 0.00 | 68.0 | 0.12 | 3.1 | 0.0 | 0.0 | 14 | 0.1 | 0.7 | 20 | 0.3 | 32 | 259 | 0.6 | 65 | 0.30 |
| 5309 | 1/2 cup | Canned, w/liquid, avg | 123 | 34 | 92 | 1.0 | 8.1 | 1.5 | 6.4 | 0.2 | 0.1 | 0.0 | 0.0 | 0.0 | 0.00 | 0.03 | 0 | 32 | [illegible] | 0 | 4 | 11 | 0.01 | 0.05 | 0.19 | 0.07 | 0.00 | 35.7 | 0.18 | 3.4 | 0.0 | | 16 | 0.1 | 0.8 | 20 | 0.3 | 20 | 162 | 0.6 | 310 | 0.28 |
| 5357 | 1/2 cup | Canned, w/liquid, low sod, avg | 123 | 34 | 92 | 1.0 | 8.1 | 1.5 | 6.4 | 0.2 | 0.1 | 0.0 | 0.0 | 0.0 | 0.00 | 0.03 | 0 | 32 | [illegible] | 0 | 4 | 11 | 0.01 | 0.05 | 0.19 | 0.07 | 0.00 | 35.7 | 0.18 | 3.4 | 0.0 | | 16 | 0.1 | 0.8 | 20 | 0.3 | 20 | 175 | 0.6 | 26 | 0.28 |
| 6610 | 1/2 cup | Canned, harvard, Green Giant | 135 | 97 | 81 | 1.4 | 22.8 | 2.6 | 14.7 | 5.5 | 0.1 | 0.0 | | | | | 0 | 0 | 0 | 0 | 0 | 0 | | | | | 0.00 | | | 0.0 | | | 18 | | 0.5 | | | | | | 404 | |
| 5025 | 1/2 cup | Greens, boiled, avg | 72 | 19 | 89 | 1.9 | 3.9 | 2.1 | 0.7 | 1.1 | 0.1 | 0.0 | 0.0 | 0.1 | 0.00 | 0.05 | 0 | 3672 | 367 | 0 | 367 | 2201 | 0.08 | 0.21 | 0.36 | 0.10 | 0.00 | 10.3 | 0.24 | 17.9 | 0.0 | 0.2 | 82 | 0.2 | 1.4 | 49 | 0.4 | 30 | 654 | 0.6 | 174 | 0.36 |
| 5312 | 1/2 cup | Greens, raw, avg | 38 | 7 | 92 | 0.7 | 1.5 | 1.4 | 0.1 | 0.0 | 0.0 | 0.0 | 0.0 | 0.0 | 0.00 | 0.01 | 0 | 2318 | 232 | 0 | 232 | 1389 | 0.04 | 0.08 | 0.15 | 0.04 | 0.00 | 5.6 | 0.09 | 11.4 | 0.0 | 0.6 | 45 | 0.1 | 1.3 | 27 | 0.1 | 15 | 208 | 0.3 | 76 | 0.14 |
| 5310 | 1/2 cup | Pickled, w/liquid, slices, avg | 114 | 74 | 82 | 0.9 | 18.6 | 2.3 | 16.3 | 0.0 | 0.1 | 0.0 | 0.0 | 0.0 | 0.00 | 0.03 | 0 | 3 | [illegible] | 0 | 1 | 3 | 0.01 | 0.05 | 0.29 | 0.06 | 0.00 | 30.2 | 0.16 | 2.6 | 0.0 | | 13 | 0.1 | 0.5 | 17 | 0.3 | 19 | 169 | 1.1 | 301 | 0.30 |
| 6669 | 1 ea | Raw, avg | 82 | 36 | 87 | 1.2 | 8.2 | 0.7 | | | 0.1 | | | | | | | 6 | [illegible] | 0 | 2 | 5 | 0.04 | 0.02 | 0.33 | 0.04 | 0.00 | 75.9 | 0.12 | 9.0 | | | 13 | | 0.7 | 17 | | 39 | 266 | | 59 | 0.30 |
| 5507 | 1/2 cup | Root Juice, avg | 118 | 41 | 88 | 1.3 | 9.6 | | | | | | | | | | 0 | | | | | | | | | | 0.00 | | | 3.4 | | | | | | | | 34 | 286 | | 236 | |
| 5407 | 2 oz | Borage, boiled, drained, avg | 57 | 14 | 92 | 1.2 | 2.0 | 0.6 | 0.6 | 0.8 | 0.5 | 0.1 | 0.1 | 0.1 | 0.00 | 0.07 | 0 | 2499 | 250 | 0 | 250 | 1498 | 0.03 | 0.09 | 0.54 | 0.05 | 0.00 | 5.7 | 0.03 | 18.5 | 0.0 | | 58 | 0.1 | 2.1 | 32 | 0.2 | 31 | 280 | 0.5 | 50 | 0.13 |
| 5406 | 1/2 cup | Borage, raw | 44 | 9 | 93 | 0.8 | 1.3 | 0.4 | 0.4 | 0.6 | 0.3 | 0.1 | 0.1 | 0.0 | 0.00 | 0.05 | 0 | 1848 | 185 | 0 | 185 | 1109 | 0.03 | 0.07 | 0.40 | 0.04 | 0.00 | 5.8 | 0.02 | 15.4 | 0.0 | | 41 | 0.1 | 1.5 | 23 | 0.2 | 23 | 207 | 0.4 | 35 | 0.09 |
| | | Broccoli | | | | | | | | | | | | | | | | | | | | | | | | | | | | | | | | | | | | | | | | |
| 5513 | 1/2 cup | Batter Dipped, fried, avg | 42 | 60 | 74 | 1.7 | 4.4 | 1.0 | 0.9 | 2.5 | 4.4 | 0.7 | 1.1 | 2.4 | | | [illegible] | 476 | 57 | 4 | 46 | 274 | 0.04 | 0.07 | 0.37 | 0.06 | 0.03 | 21.3 | 0.29 | 26.3 | 0.1 | | 33 | 0.0 | 0.5 | 10 | 0.1 | 35 | 120 | 2.1 | 31 | 0.19 |
| 5456 | 1/2 cup | Cooked Broccoli, w/cheese sauce, avg | 114 | 109 | 81 | 6.1 | 6.3 | 2.1 | 3.9 | 0.3 | 7.3 | 3.5 | 2.4 | 1.0 | | | 1[illegible] | 1294 | 176 | 65 | 111 | 660 | 0.06 | 0.17 | 0.52 | 0.13 | 0.18 | 41.3 | 0.40 | 56.8 | 0.3 | | 148 | 0.1 | 0.8 | 25 | 0.3 | 128 | 269 | 2.3 | 365 | 0.74 |
| 5457 | 1/2 cup | Cooked, w/cream sauce, avg | 114 | 93 | 83 | 3.9 | 7.7 | 1.9 | 3.1 | 2.7 | 5.8 | 1.8 | 2.3 | 1.4 | | | [illegible] | 1492 | 190 | 55 | 134 | 796 | 0.06 | 0.13 | 0.45 | 0.11 | 0.15 | 22.6 | 0.09 | 27.5 | 0.4 | | 88 | 0.1 | 0.5 | 19 | 0.2 | 80 | 186 | 1.1 | 347 | 0.38 |
| 56944 | 1 ea | Cuts in Butter, svg, Green Giant | 127 | 44 | 90 | 2.5 | 7.3 | 2.9 | | | 1.8 | 0.9 | 0.5 | 0.2 | | | [illegible] | 846 | 169 | | | | 0.04 | 0.09 | 0.25 | | 0.00 | | | 57.1 | | | 39 | | 0.3 | | | 51 | 221 | | 475 | |
| 5030 | 1/2 cup | Frozen, boiled, avg | 92 | 26 | 91 | 2.9 | 4.9 | 2.8 | 1.7 | 0.5 | 0.1 | 0.0 | 0.0 | 0.1 | 0.04 | 0.01 | 0 | 1741 | 174 | 0 | 174 | 1036 | 0.05 | 0.07 | 0.42 | 0.12 | 0.00 | 51.9 | 0.25 | 36.9 | 0.0 | | 47 | 0.0 | 0.6 | 18 | 0.3 | 51 | 166 | 2.8 | 22 | 0.28 |
| 5867 | 1/2 cup | Leaves, raw, avg | 44 | 12 | 91 | 1.3 | 2.3 | 0.8 | | | 0.2 | 0.0 | 0.0 | 0.1 | 0.06 | 0.02 | 0 | 7040 | 704 | 0 | 704 | 4224 | 0.03 | 0.05 | 0.28 | 0.07 | 0.00 | 31.2 | 0.24 | 41.0 | 0.0 | | 21 | 0.0 | 0.4 | 11 | 0.1 | 29 | 143 | 1.3 | 12 | 0.18 |
| 5026 | 1/2 cup | Raw, chpd, avg | 44 | 12 | 91 | 1.3 | 2.3 | 1.3 | 0.9 | 0.1 | 0.2 | 0.0 | 0.0 | 0.1 | 0.06 | 0.02 | 0 | 678 | 68 | 0 | 68 | 403 | 0.03 | 0.05 | 0.28 | 0.07 | 0.00 | 31.2 | 0.24 | 41.0 | 0.0 | 0.2 | 21 | 0.0 | 0.4 | 11 | 0.1 | 29 | 143 | 1.3 | 12 | 0.18 |
| 6387 | 3 oz | Spears, Green Giant | 85 | 23 | 93 | 1.8 | 3.7 | 2.1 | 1.3 | 0.3 | 0.2 | 0.0 | | | | | 0 | 349 | 35 | 0 | 35 | 208 | | | | | 0.00 | | | 29.0 | | | 26 | | 0.6 | | | | | | 105 | |
| 5653 | 1/2 cup | Steamed, avg | 78 | 22 | 91 | 2.3 | 4.1 | 2.3 | 1.6 | 0.2 | 0.3 | 0.0 | 0.0 | 0.1 | 0.10 | 0.03 | 0 | 1140 | 114 | 0 | 114 | 679 | 0.05 | 0.09 | 0.47 | 0.11 | 0.00 | 47.0 | 0.40 | 61.7 | 0.0 | 0.4 | 37 | 0.0 | 0.7 | 19 | 0.2 | 51 | 253 | | 21 | 0.31 |
| | | Brussel Sprouts | | | | | | | | | | | | | | | | | | | | | | | | | | | | | | | | | | | | | | | | |
| 5033 | 1/2 cup | Boiled, avg | 78 | 30 | 87 | 2.0 | 6.8 | 2.0 | 3.1 | 1.6 | 0.4 | 0.1 | 0.0 | 0.2 | 0.13 | 0.06 | 0 | 561 | 56 | 0 | 56 | 335 | 0.08 | 0.06 | 0.47 | 0.14 | 0.00 | 46.8 | 0.20 | 48.4 | 0.0 | 0.7 | 28 | 0.1 | 0.9 | 16 | 0.2 | 44 | 247 | 1.2 | 16 | 0.26 |
| 6351 | 3 oz | Butter Sauce, Green Giant | 85 | 54 | 85 | 2.6 | 7.7 | 3.2 | 2.5 | 2.0 | 1.3 | 1.0 | | | | | [illegible] | 181 | 36 | | | | | | | | 0.00 | | | 33.2 | | | 19 | | 0.3 | | | | | | 221 | |
| 5035 | 1/2 cup | Frozen, boiled, avg | 78 | 33 | 87 | 2.8 | 6.5 | 3.2 | 2.7 | 0.6 | 0.3 | 0.1 | 0.0 | 0.2 | 0.10 | 0.05 | 0 | 459 | 46 | 0 | 46 | 275 | 0.08 | 0.09 | 0.42 | 0.23 | 0.00 | 78.8 | 0.27 | 35.6 | 0.0 | 0.5 | 19 | 0.1 | 0.6 | 19 | 0.2 | 42 | 253 | 1.2 | 18 | 0.28 |
| 5031 | 1/2 cup | Raw, avg | 44 | 19 | 86 | 1.5 | 3.9 | 1.7 | 1.0 | 1.3 | 0.1 | 0.0 | 0.0 | 0.1 | 0.04 | 0.02 | 0 | 389 | 39 | 0 | 39 | 231 | 0.06 | 0.04 | 0.33 | 0.10 | 0.00 | 26.9 | 0.14 | 37.4 | 0.0 | 0.4 | 18 | 0.0 | 0.6 | 10 | 0.1 | 30 | 171 | 0.7 | 11 | 0.18 |
| 6760 | 1/2 cup | Burdock Root, boiled, 1" pces, avg | 62 | 55 | 76 | 1.3 | 13.1 | 1.1 | | | 0.1 | 0.0 | 0.0 | 0.0 | 0.00 | 0.03 | 0 | 0 | 0 | 0 | 0 | 0 | 0.02 | 0.04 | 0.20 | 0.17 | 0.00 | 12.1 | 0.22 | 1.6 | 0.0 | | 30 | 0.1 | 0.5 | 24 | 0.2 | 58 | 223 | 0.6 | 2 | 0.24 |
| 6759 | 1/2 cup | Burdock Root, raw, 1" pces, avg | 59 | 42 | 80 | 0.9 | 10.3 | 1.9 | | | 0.1 | 0.0 | 0.0 | 0.0 | 0.00 | 0.03 | 0 | 0 | 0 | 0 | 0 | 0 | 0.01 | 0.02 | 0.18 | 0.14 | 0.00 | 13.5 | 0.19 | 1.8 | 0.0 | | 24 | 0.0 | 0.5 | 22 | 0.1 | 30 | 182 | 0.4 | 3 | 0.19 |
| | | Cabbage | | | | | | | | | | | | | | | | | | | | | | | | | | | | | | | | | | | | | | | | |
| 5038 | 1/2 cup | Common, boiled, shred, avg | 75 | 16 | 94 | 0.8 | 3.3 | 1.7 | 1.3 | 0.4 | 0.3 | 0.0 | 0.0 | 0.1 | 0.08 | 0.06 | 0 | 99 | 10 | 0 | 10 | 59 | 0.04 | 0.04 | 0.21 | 0.08 | 0.00 | 15.0 | 0.10 | 15.1 | 0.0 | 0.1 | 23 | 0.0 | 0.1 | 6 | 0.1 | 11 | 73 | 0.5 | 6 | 0.07 |
| 5608 | 1/2 cup | Common, pickled, avg | 75 | 16 | 91 | 1.2 | 3.3 | 2.3 | | | 0.1 | 0.0 | 0.0 | 0.0 | 0.02 | 0.01 | 0 | 142 | 14 | 0 | 14 | 86 | 0.00 | 0.03 | 0.14 | 0.08 | 0.00 | 31.5 | 0.08 | 0.5 | 0.0 | | 36 | 0.0 | 0.4 | 9 | 0.1 | 32 | 640 | | 208 | 0.15 |
| 5036 | 1 cup | Common, raw, shred, avg | 70 | 17 | 92 | 1.0 | 3.8 | 1.6 | 1.8 | 0.3 | 0.2 | 0.0 | 0.0 | 0.1 | 0.05 | 0.04 | 0 | 93 | 9 | 0 | 9 | 55 | 0.04 | 0.03 | 0.21 | 0.07 | 0.00 | 30.1 | 0.10 | 22.5 | 0.0 | 0.1 | 33 | 0.0 | 0.4 | 10 | 0.1 | 16 | 172 | 0.6 | 13 | 0.13 |
| 5535 | 1/2 cup | Kim Chee, avg | 75 | 16 | 92 | 1.2 | 3.1 | 0.9 | 1.0 | 1.2 | 0.2 | 0.0 | 0.0 | 0.1 | 0.04 | 0.03 | 0 | 2131 | 213 | 0 | 213 | 1279 | 0.04 | 0.05 | 0.38 | 0.17 | 0.00 | 44.0 | 0.08 | 39.8 | 0.0 | | 73 | 0.0 | 0.6 | 14 | 0.2 | 30 | 188 | | 498 | 0.18 |
| 5041 | 1 cup | Pak Choi/Bok Choy, raw, shred, avg | 70 | 9 | 95 | 1.0 | 1.5 | 0.7 | 0.3 | 0.5 | 0.1 | 0.0 | 0.0 | 0.1 | 0.04 | 0.03 | 0 | 2100 | 210 | 0 | 210 | 1250 | 0.03 | 0.05 | 0.35 | 0.14 | 0.00 | 46.0 | 0.06 | 31.5 | 0.0 | 0.1 | 73 | 0.0 | 0.6 | 13 | 0.1 | 26 | 176 | 0.3 | 45 | 0.13 |
| 5671 | 1/2 cup | Pak Choi/Bok Choy, stmd, avg | 85 | 11 | 96 | 1.3 | 1.9 | 0.9 | 0.9 | 0.2 | 0.2 | 0.0 | 0.0 | 0.1 | 0.04 | 0.03 | 0 | 77 | 8 | 0 | 8 | 50 | 0.03 | 0.06 | 0.40 | 0.15 | 0.00 | 47.3 | 0.07 | 2.7 | 0.0 | | 89 | 0.0 | 0.7 | 16 | 0.1 | 31 | 213 | | 55 | 0.16 |
| 5235 | 1/2 cup | Pe Tsai, boiled, shred | 60 | 8 | 95 | 0.9 | 1.4 | 1.6 | | | 0.1 | 0.0 | 0.0 | 0.0 | 0.03 | 0.01 | 0 | 580 | 58 | 0 | 58 | 349 | 0.03 | 0.03 | 0.30 | 0.11 | 0.00 | 32.0 | 0.05 | 9.5 | 0.0 | | 19 | 0.0 | 0.2 | 6 | 0.1 | 23 | 135 | 0.2 | 5 | 0.11 |
| 5040 | 1 cup | Pe Tsai, raw, avg | 76 | 12 | 94 | 0.9 | 2.5 | 2.4 | | | 0.2 | 0.0 | 0.0 | 0.1 | 0.04 | 0.01 | 0 | 912 | 91 | 0 | 91 | 547 | 0.03 | 0.04 | 0.30 | 0.18 | 0.00 | 59.8 | 0.08 | 20.5 | 0.0 | 0.1 | 59 | 0.0 | 0.2 | 10 | 0.1 | 22 | 181 | 0.5 | 7 | 0.17 |
| 5238 | 1/2 cup | Red, boiled, avg | 75 | 16 | 94 | 0.8 | 3.5 | 1.5 | 2.0 | 0.0 | 0.2 | 0.0 | 0.0 | 0.1 | 0.04 | 0.03 | 0 | 20 | [illegible] | 0 | 2 | 13 | 0.03 | 0.01 | 0.15 | 0.11 | 0.00 | 9.5 | 0.16 | 25.8 | 0.0 | | 28 | 0.1 | 0.3 | 8 | 0.1 | 22 | 105 | 0.5 | 6 | 0.11 |
| 5533 | 1/2 cup | Red, pickled, avg | 75 | 110 | 60 | 0.4 | 28.7 | 0.6 | 27.7 | 0.4 | 0.1 | 0.0 | 0.0 | 0.0 | 0.02 | 0.02 | 0 | 10 | [illegible] | 0 | 1 | 6 | 0.01 | 0.01 | 0.11 | 0.06 | 0.00 | 4.1 | 0.08 | 9.3 | 0.0 | | 36 | 0.1 | 0.6 | 13 | 0.1 | 16 | 154 | | 14 | 0.11 |
| 5042 | 1 cup | Red, raw, shred | 70 | 19 | 92 | 1.0 | 4.3 | 1.4 | 2.9 | 0.0 | 0.2 | 0.0 | 0.0 | 0.1 | 0.05 | 0.04 | 0 | 28 | 3 | 0 | 3 | 16 | 0.04 | 0.02 | 0.21 | 0.15 | 0.00 | 14.5 | 0.23 | 39.9 | 0.0 | 0.1 | 36 | 0.1 | 0.3 | 10 | 0.1 | 29 | 144 | 0.6 | 8 | 0.15 |
| 5145 | 1/2 cup | Sauerkraut, cnd, avg | 118 | 22 | 92 | 1.1 | 5.1 | 2.9 | 0.9 | 1.2 | 0.2 | 0.0 | 0.0 | 0.1 | 0.03 | 0.03 | 0 | 21 | 2 | 0 | 2 | 14 | 0.02 | 0.03 | 0.17 | 0.15 | 0.00 | 28.0 | 0.11 | 17.3 | 0.0 | | 35 | 0.1 | 1.7 | 15 | 0.2 | 24 | 201 | 0.7 | 780 | 0.22 |
| 5531 | 1/2 cup | Sauerkraut, cnd, low sod, avg | 71 | 13 | 92 | 0.6 | 3.1 | 1.8 | | | 0.1 | 0.0 | 0.0 | 0.0 | 0.02 | 0.02 | 0 | 3 | [illegible] | 0 | 1 | 9 | 0.01 | 0.01 | 0.10 | 0.06 | 0.00 | 17.0 | 0.07 | 10.4 | 0.0 | | 21 | 0.1 | 1.0 | 9 | 0.1 | 14 | 121 | | 219 | 0.13 |
| 5044 | 1/2 cup | Savoy, boiled, avg | 72 | 17 | 92 | 1.3 | 3.9 | 2.0 | 1.5 | 0.4 | 0.1 | 0.0 | 0.0 | 0.0 | 0.02 | 0.01 | 0 | 640 | 64 | 0 | 64 | 384 | 0.04 | 0.01 | 0.02 | 0.11 | 0.00 | 33.3 | 0.11 | 12.2 | 0.0 | | 22 | 0.0 | 0.3 | 17 | 0.1 | 24 | 132 | 0.5 | 17 | 0.17 |
| 5043 | 1 cup | Savoy, raw, avg | 70 | 19 | 91 | 1.4 | 4.3 | 2.2 | 2.0 | 0.1 | 0.1 | 0.0 | 0.0 | 0.0 | 0.02 | 0.01 | 0 | 700 | 70 | 0 | 70 | 420 | 0.05 | 0.02 | 0.21 | 0.13 | 0.00 | 56.1 | 0.13 | 21.7 | 0.0 | 0.1 | 24 | 0.0 | 0.3 | 20 | 0.1 | 29 | 161 | 0.6 | 20 | 0.19 |
| 7263 | 1/2 cup | Cactus/Nopales, ckd, unsalted, avg | 74 | 11 | 94 | 1.0 | 2.4 | 1.5 | | | 0.0 | 0.0 | 0.0 | 0.0 | 0.00 | 0.01 | 0 | 340 | 34 | 0 | 34 | 204 | 0.01 | 0.03 | 0.22 | 0.05 | 0.00 | 2.2 | 0.11 | 3.9 | | | 121 | 0.0 | 0.4 | 35 | 0.3 | 12 | 144 | 0.5 | 15 | 0.16 |
| 7262 | 1/2 cup | Cactus/Nopales, raw, avg | 43 | 7 | 94 | 0.6 | 1.5 | 1.0 | | | 0.1 | 0.0 | 0.0 | 0.0 | 0.00 | 0.02 | 0 | 178 | 18 | 0 | 18 | 106 | 0.01 | 0.02 | 0.23 | 0.03 | 0.00 | 1.3 | 0.08 | 5.8 | | | 70 | 0.0 | 0.3 | 25 | 0.2 | 7 | 137 | 0.3 | 9 | 0.12 |

| Code | Amount | Description | Basic Components | | | | | | | | | Additional Fats | | | | | | Vit A & Components | | | | | Vitamins | | | | | | | | | | Minerals | | | | | | | | | |
|---|---|---|---|---|---|---|---|---|---|---|---|---|---|---|---|---|---|---|---|---|---|---|---|---|---|---|---|---|---|---|---|---|---|---|---|---|---|---|---|---|---|---|
| | | | Weight (g) | Calories | % Water | Protein (g) | Carbs (g) | Fiber (g) | Sugar (g) | Other Carbs (g) | Fat (g) | Sat Fat (g) | Mono Fat (g) | Poly Fat (g) | Omega 3 (g) | Omega 6 (g) | Choles (mg) | Vit A (IU) | Vit A (RE) | Retinol (RE) | Carotenoids (RE) | Beta Carotene (mcg) | Thiamin (mg) | Riboflavin (mg) | Niacin (NE) | Vit B6 (mg) | Vit B12 (mcg) | Folate (mcg) | Panto (mg) | Vit C (mg) | Vit D (mg) | Vit E (α TE) | Calcium (mg) | Copper (mg) | Iron (mg) | Magnes (mg) | Mang (mg) | Phos (mg) | Potassium (mg) | Selenium (mcg) | Sodium (mg) | Zinc (mg) |
| 5511 | 1 tsp | Capers, avg | 5 | 0 | 86 | 0.2 | 0.1 | 0.2 | 0.0 | | 0.0 | | | | | | 0 | 12 | 1 | 0 | 1 | 7 | | | | | 0.00 | | | 0.0 | | | 2 | | 0.1 | | | | | | 105 | |
| | | Carrots | | | | | | | | | | | | | | | | | | | | | | | | | | | | | | | | | | | | | | | | |
| 5439 | 1 ea | Baby, raw, avg | 10 | 4 | 90 | 0.1 | 0.8 | 0.2 | 0.5 | 0.1 | 0.1 | 0.0 | 0.0 | 0.0 | 0.00 | 0.02 | 0 | 1501 | 150 | 0 | 150 | 730 | 0.00 | 0.01 | 0.09 | 0.01 | 0.00 | 3.3 | 0.02 | 0.8 | 0.0 | | 2 | 0.0 | 0.1 | 1 | 0.0 | 4 | 28 | 0.1 | 4 | 0.02 |
| 5198 | 1/2 cup | Canned, w/liquid, avg | 123 | 28 | 93 | 0.7 | 6.6 | 2.2 | 3.8 | 0.6 | 0.2 | 0.0 | 0.0 | 0.1 | 0.01 | 0.07 | 0 | 11894 | 1189 | 0 | 1189 | 5781 | 0.02 | 0.03 | 0.52 | 0.14 | 0.00 | 10.0 | 0.17 | 2.5 | 0.0 | | 38 | 0.1 | 0.6 | 11 | 0.6 | 25 | 213 | 0.5 | 295 | 0.36 |
| 5888 | 1/2 cup | Canned, w/liquid, unsalted, avg | 123 | 28 | 93 | 0.7 | 6.6 | 2.2 | 3.8 | 0.6 | 0.2 | 0.0 | 0.0 | 0.1 | 0.01 | 0.07 | 0 | 11894 | 1189 | 0 | 1189 | 5781 | 0.02 | 0.03 | 0.52 | 0.14 | 0.00 | 10.0 | 0.17 | 2.5 | 0.0 | | 38 | 0.1 | 0.6 | 11 | 0.6 | 25 | 194 | 0.5 | 42 | 0.36 |
| 5517 | 1/4 cup | Chips, dried, avg | 18 | 66 | 4 | 1.6 | 13.1 | 3.6 | 9.3 | 0.2 | 0.3 | 0.1 | 0.0 | 0.1 | 0.02 | 0.11 | 0 | 17999 | 1800 | 0 | 1800 | 8920 | 0.13 | 0.09 | 1.29 | 0.22 | 0.00 | 15.1 | 0.22 | 10.0 | 0.0 | | 39 | 0.1 | 0.7 | 22 | 0.2 | 61 | 448 | | 54 | 0.31 |
| 5633 | 1/2 cup | Cooked, glzd, avg | 80 | 116 | 70 | 0.8 | 16.7 | 2.1 | 12.4 | 2.2 | 5.6 | 1.1 | 2.4 | 1.8 | | | 0 | 16626 | 1707 | 68 | 1639 | 7966 | 0.02 | 0.04 | 0.35 | 0.17 | 0.01 | 9.4 | 0.21 | 1.5 | 0.1 | | 31 | 0.1 | 0.6 | 12 | 0.5 | 24 | 188 | 0.8 | 130 | 0.22 |
| 5634 | 1/2 cup | Cooked, w/cheese sauce, avg | 114 | 88 | 82 | 3.8 | 10.7 | 2.0 | | | 3.5 | 1.9 | 1.1 | 0.4 | | | 10 | 14293 | 1444 | 24 | 1420 | 6904 | 0.05 | 0.14 | 0.36 | 0.17 | 0.22 | 10.6 | 0.40 | 1.8 | 0.0 | | 132 | 0.1 | 0.4 | 17 | 0.5 | 105 | 242 | 1.3 | 490 | 0.37 |
| 5358 | 1/2 cup | Frozen, boiled, drained, avg | 73 | 26 | 90 | 0.9 | 6.0 | 2.6 | 3.3 | 0.2 | 0.1 | 0.0 | 0.0 | 0.0 | 0.01 | 0.03 | 0 | 12922 | 1292 | 0 | 1292 | 6279 | 0.02 | 0.03 | 0.32 | 0.09 | 0.00 | 7.9 | 0.12 | 2.0 | 0.0 | | 20 | 0.1 | 0.3 | 7 | 0.3 | 19 | 115 | 0.4 | 43 | 0.18 |
| 5226 | 1/2 cup | Juice, cnd, avg | 118 | 47 | 89 | 1.1 | 11.0 | 0.9 | 7.1 | 2.9 | 0.2 | 0.0 | 0.0 | 0.1 | 0.01 | 0.07 | 0 | 12916 | 1292 | 0 | 1292 | 6280 | 0.11 | 0.06 | 0.46 | 0.26 | 0.00 | 4.5 | 0.27 | 10.0 | 0.0 | | 28 | 0.1 | 0.5 | 17 | 0.2 | 50 | 345 | 0.7 | 34 | 0.21 |
| 5045 | 1 ea | Raw, 7 1/2", avg | 72 | 31 | 88 | 0.7 | 7.3 | 2.2 | 4.8 | 0.4 | 0.1 | 0.0 | 0.0 | 0.1 | 0.01 | 0.05 | 0 | 20253 | 2025 | 0 | 2025 | 9843 | 0.07 | 0.04 | 0.67 | 0.11 | 0.00 | 10.1 | 0.14 | 6.7 | 0.0 | | 19 | 0.0 | 0.4 | 11 | 0.1 | 32 | 233 | 0.8 | 25 | 0.14 |
| 6772 | 1/2 cup | Raw, chpd, avg | 64 | 28 | 88 | 0.7 | 6.5 | 1.9 | 4.2 | 0.3 | 0.1 | 0.0 | 0.0 | 0.0 | 0.01 | 0.04 | 0 | 18003 | 1800 | 0 | 1800 | 8749 | 0.06 | 0.04 | 0.59 | 0.09 | 0.00 | 9.0 | 0.13 | 6.0 | 0.0 | | 17 | 0.0 | 0.3 | 10 | 0.1 | 28 | 207 | 0.7 | 22 | 0.13 |
| 5655 | 1/2 cup | Steamed, avg | 78 | 34 | 88 | 0.8 | 7.9 | 2.3 | 5.1 | 0.4 | 0.1 | 0.0 | 0.0 | 0.1 | 0.01 | 0.05 | 0 | 19780 | 1977 | 0 | 1977 | 9610 | 0.07 | 0.04 | 0.69 | 0.11 | 0.00 | 10.4 | 0.12 | 5.5 | 0.0 | | 21 | 0.0 | 0.4 | 12 | 0.1 | 34 | 252 | | 27 | 0.16 |
| 5625 | 1/2 cup | Cassava, ckd, avg | 68 | 82 | 68 | 2.1 | 18.4 | 0.1 | | | 0.3 | 0.1 | 0.1 | 0.1 | 0.02 | 0.04 | 0 | 6 | 1 | 0 | 1 | 4 | 0.12 | 0.06 | 0.86 | 0.19 | 0.00 | 9.8 | 0.20 | 21.4 | 0.1 | | 59 | 0.1 | 2.3 | 43 | 0.3 | 43 | 469 | 0.1 | 164 | 0.16 |
| 5356 | 1/2 cup | Cassava, raw, avg | 103 | 165 | 60 | 1.4 | 39.2 | 1.9 | | | 0.3 | 0.1 | 0.1 | 0.0 | 0.02 | 0.03 | 0 | 26 | 2 | 0 | 3 | 15 | 0.09 | 0.05 | 0.88 | 0.09 | 0.00 | 27.8 | 0.11 | 21.2 | 0.0 | | 16 | 0.1 | 0.3 | 22 | 0.4 | 28 | 279 | 0.7 | 14 | 0.35 |
| | | Cauliflower | | | | | | | | | | | | | | | | | | | | | | | | | | | | | | | | | | | | | | | | |
| 5539 | 5 pce | Batter Dipped, fried, avg | 130 | 251 | 69 | 6.0 | 12.8 | 2.1 | 3.8 | 6.9 | 20.1 | 4.8 | 5.2 | 9.1 | 0.00 | 0.00 | 30 | 165 | 45 | 41 | 4 | 23 | 0.10 | 0.16 | 0.74 | 0.19 | 0.17 | 40.1 | 0.27 | 46.7 | 0.3 | | 166 | 0.0 | 0.9 | 19 | 0.3 | 173 | 333 | 4.5 | 239 | 0.64 |
| 5051 | 1/2 cup | Boiled, avg | 62 | 14 | 93 | 1.1 | 2.5 | 1.7 | 0.8 | 0.1 | 0.3 | 0.0 | 0.0 | 0.1 | 0.10 | 0.03 | 0 | 11 | 1 | 0 | 1 | 7 | 0.03 | 0.03 | 0.25 | 0.11 | 0.00 | 27.3 | 0.31 | 27.5 | 0.0 | 0.0 | 10 | 0.0 | 0.2 | 6 | 0.1 | 20 | 88 | 0.3 | 9 | 0.11 |
| 5053 | 1/2 cup | Frozen, boiled, avg | 90 | 17 | 94 | 1.4 | 3.4 | 2.4 | 0.9 | 0.0 | 0.2 | 0.0 | 0.0 | 0.1 | 0.07 | 0.02 | 0 | 20 | 2 | 0 | 2 | 11 | 0.03 | 0.05 | 0.28 | 0.08 | 0.00 | 36.9 | 0.09 | 28.2 | 0.0 | 0.0 | 15 | 0.0 | 0.4 | 8 | 0.1 | 22 | 125 | 0.5 | 16 | 0.12 |
| 7266 | 1/2 cup | Green, ckd, unsalted, avg | 62 | 20 | 90 | 1.9 | 3.9 | 2.0 | | | 0.2 | 0.0 | 0.0 | 0.1 | 0.07 | 0.02 | 0 | 87 | 9 | 0 | 9 | 52 | 0.04 | 0.06 | 0.42 | 0.13 | 0.00 | 25.4 | 0.42 | 45.0 | | | 20 | 0.0 | 0.4 | 12 | 0.2 | 35 | 172 | 0.5 | 14 | 0.39 |
| 7265 | 1/2 cup | Green, raw, avg | 32 | 10 | 90 | 0.9 | 1.9 | 1.0 | | | 0.1 | 0.0 | 0.0 | 0.0 | 0.03 | 0.01 | 0 | 49 | 5 | 0 | 5 | 29 | 0.03 | 0.03 | 0.23 | 0.07 | 0.00 | 18.2 | 0.22 | 28.2 | | | 11 | 0.0 | 0.2 | 6 | 0.1 | 20 | 96 | 0.2 | 7 | 0.20 |
| 5607 | 1/2 ea | Pickled, avg | 14 | 6 | 88 | 0.2 | 1.4 | 0.3 | 1.0 | 0.1 | 0.0 | 0.0 | 0.0 | 0.0 | 0.01 | 0.00 | 0 | 52 | 5 | 0 | 5 | 32 | 0.01 | 0.01 | 0.06 | 0.02 | 0.00 | 4.1 | 0.01 | 6.1 | 0.0 | | 4 | 0.0 | 0.1 | 2 | 0.0 | 5 | 33 | 0.1 | 22 | 0.02 |
| 5049 | 1/2 cup | Raw, avg | 50 | 12 | 92 | 1.0 | 2.6 | 1.3 | 1.2 | 0.2 | 0.1 | 0.0 | 0.0 | 0.0 | 0.04 | 0.01 | 0 | 10 | 1 | 0 | 1 | 6 | 0.03 | 0.03 | 0.26 | 0.11 | 0.00 | 28.5 | 0.33 | 23.2 | 0.0 | 0.0 | 11 | 0.0 | 0.2 | 8 | 0.1 | 22 | 152 | 0.3 | 15 | 0.14 |
| 5641 | 1/2 cup | With Cheese/Cream Sauce, avg | 81 | 73 | 83 | 3.3 | 4.6 | 0.9 | 2.1 | 1.6 | 4.8 | 2.2 | 1.7 | 0.8 | | | 10 | 174 | 41 | 37 | 4 | 23 | 0.04 | 0.11 | 0.29 | 0.10 | 0.17 | 22.2 | 0.18 | 21.4 | 0.3 | | 88 | 0.1 | 0.2 | 11 | 0.1 | 73 | 183 | | 258 | 0.37 |
| 56957 | 1/2 cup | With Cheese Sauce, fzn, Green Giant | 99 | 60 | 86 | 2.2 | 7.8 | 2.1 | 4.0 | 1.8 | 2.3 | 0.7 | | | | | 4 | 1112 | 111 | | | | | | | | 0.00 | | | 19.3 | | | 51 | | 0.3 | | | | | | 510 | |
| | | Celery | | | | | | | | | | | | | | | | | | | | | | | | | | | | | | | | | | | | | | | | |
| 5606 | 1/2 cup | Pickled, avg | 75 | 11 | 94 | 0.5 | 2.8 | 1.1 | 0.9 | 0.9 | 0.1 | 0.0 | 0.0 | 0.0 | | | 0 | 80 | 8 | 0 | 8 | 46 | 0.02 | 0.03 | 0.18 | 0.05 | 0.00 | 12.0 | 0.12 | 3.5 | 0.0 | | 26 | 0.0 | 0.3 | 8 | 0.1 | 16 | 177 | | 183 | 0.08 |
| 5054 | 1/2 cup | Raw, avg | 60 | 10 | 95 | 0.5 | 2.2 | 1.0 | 0.6 | 0.6 | 0.1 | 0.0 | 0.0 | 0.0 | 0.00 | 0.04 | 0 | 80 | 8 | 0 | 8 | 47 | 0.03 | 0.03 | 0.19 | 0.05 | 0.00 | 16.8 | 0.11 | 4.2 | 0.0 | 0.2 | 24 | 0.0 | 0.2 | 7 | 0.1 | 15 | 172 | 0.5 | 52 | 0.08 |
| 5200 | 1/2 cup | Root/Celeriac, ckd, avg | 78 | 21 | 92 | 0.7 | 4.6 | 0.9 | 1.2 | 2.5 | 0.1 | 0.0 | 0.0 | 0.1 | 0.01 | 0.07 | 0 | 0 | 0 | 0 | 0 | 0 | 0.02 | 0.03 | 0.33 | 0.08 | 0.00 | 2.7 | 0.16 | 2.8 | 0.0 | | 20 | 0.0 | 0.3 | 9 | 0.1 | 51 | 135 | 0.3 | 48 | 0.16 |
| 5742 | 1/2 cup | Root/Celeriac, raw, avg | 78 | 33 | 88 | 1.2 | 7.2 | 1.4 | 1.6 | 4.2 | 0.2 | 0.1 | 0.0 | 0.1 | 0.00 | 0.12 | 0 | 0 | 0 | 0 | 0 | 0 | 0.04 | 0.05 | 0.55 | 0.13 | 0.00 | 5.9 | 0.27 | 6.2 | 0.0 | | 34 | 0.1 | 0.5 | 16 | 0.1 | 90 | 234 | 0.5 | 78 | 0.26 |
| 5659 | 1/2 cup | Steamed, avg | 75 | 12 | 95 | 0.6 | 2.7 | 1.3 | 0.8 | 0.7 | 0.1 | 0.0 | 0.0 | 0.1 | 0.00 | 0.05 | 0 | 96 | 10 | 0 | 10 | 58 | 0.10 | 0.03 | 0.23 | 0.06 | 0.00 | 17.9 | 0.14 | 4.5 | 0.0 | 0.3 | 30 | 0.0 | 0.3 | 8 | 0.1 | 19 | 216 | | 65 | 0.10 |
| 5414 | 1/2 cup | Chayote, boiled, chpd, avg | 80 | 19 | 93 | 0.5 | 4.1 | 2.2 | | | 0.4 | 0.1 | 0.0 | 0.2 | 0.10 | 0.06 | 0 | 38 | 4 | 0 | 4 | 24 | 0.02 | 0.03 | 0.34 | 0.09 | 0.00 | 14.5 | 0.33 | 6.4 | 0.0 | | 10 | 0.1 | 0.2 | 10 | 0.1 | 23 | 138 | 0.2 | 1 | 0.25 |
| 6781 | 1/2 cup | Chayote, raw, avg | 66 | 13 | 94 | 0.5 | 3.0 | 1.1 | | | 0.1 | 0.0 | 0.0 | 0.0 | 0.02 | 0.01 | 0 | 37 | 4 | 0 | 4 | 24 | 0.02 | 0.02 | 0.31 | 0.05 | 0.00 | 61.4 | 0.16 | 5.1 | 0.0 | | 11 | 0.1 | 0.2 | 8 | 0.1 | 12 | 83 | 0.1 | 1 | 0.49 |
| 5415 | 1/2 cup | Chicory, greens, raw, chpd, avg | 90 | 21 | 92 | 1.5 | 4.2 | 3.6 | 0.6 | 0.0 | 0.3 | 0.1 | 0.0 | 0.1 | 0.02 | 0.10 | 0 | 3600 | 360 | 0 | 360 | 2160 | 0.05 | 0.09 | 0.45 | 0.09 | 0.00 | 99.0 | 1.04 | 21.6 | 0.0 | | 90 | 0.3 | 0.8 | 27 | 0.4 | 42 | 378 | 0.3 | 40 | 0.38 |
| 5416 | 1/2 cup | Chicory, root, raw pces, avg | 45 | 33 | 80 | 0.6 | 7.9 | 0.9 | 1.1 | 5.9 | 0.1 | 0.0 | 0.0 | 0.0 | 0.01 | 0.03 | 0 | 3 | 0 | 0 | 0 | 3 | 0.02 | 0.01 | 0.18 | 0.11 | 0.00 | 10.3 | 0.15 | 2.3 | 0.0 | | 18 | 0.0 | 0.4 | 10 | 0.1 | 27 | 130 | 0.3 | 22 | 0.15 |
| | | Collards | | | | | | | | | | | | | | | | | | | | | | | | | | | | | | | | | | | | | | | | |
| 5061 | 1/2 cup | Boiled, unsalted, avg | 95 | 25 | 92 | 2.0 | 4.7 | 2.7 | 0.1 | 1.9 | 0.3 | 0.0 | 0.0 | 0.2 | 0.09 | 0.07 | 0 | 2973 | 297 | 0 | 297 | 1784 | 0.04 | 0.10 | 0.55 | 0.12 | 0.00 | 88.3 | 0.21 | 17.3 | 0.0 | | 113 | 0.0 | 0.4 | 16 | 0.5 | 25 | 247 | 1.0 | 9 | 0.40 |
| 5062 | 1/2 cup | Frozen Collards, boiled, avg | 85 | 31 | 88 | 2.5 | 6.0 | 2.4 | 0.1 | 3.6 | 0.3 | 0.1 | 0.0 | 0.2 | 0.11 | 0.05 | 0 | 5084 | 508 | 0 | 508 | 3050 | 0.04 | 0.10 | 0.54 | 0.10 | 0.00 | 64.7 | 0.10 | 22.4 | 0.0 | | 179 | 0.0 | 1.0 | 26 | 0.6 | 23 | 213 | 1.3 | 43 | 0.23 |
| 5898 | 1/2 cup | Frozen, boiled, salted, avg | 85 | 31 | 88 | 2.5 | 6.0 | 2.4 | 0.1 | 3.6 | 0.3 | 0.0 | 0.0 | 0.2 | 0.11 | 0.05 | 0 | 5084 | 508 | 0 | 508 | 3050 | 0.04 | 0.10 | 0.54 | 0.10 | 0.00 | 64.7 | 0.10 | 22.4 | 0.0 | | 179 | 0.0 | 1.0 | 26 | 0.6 | 23 | 213 | 1.3 | 243 | 0.23 |
| 5060 | 1/2 cup | Raw, avg | 18 | 5 | 91 | 0.4 | 1.0 | 0.6 | 0.1 | 0.3 | 0.1 | 0.0 | 0.0 | 0.0 | 0.02 | 0.02 | 0 | 688 | 69 | 0 | 69 | 413 | 0.01 | 0.02 | 0.13 | 0.03 | 0.00 | 29.9 | 0.05 | 6.4 | 0.0 | | 26 | 0.0 | 0.0 | 2 | 0.0 | 2 | 30 | 0.2 | 4 | 0.02 |
| | | Corn | | | | | | | | | | | | | | | | | | | | | | | | | | | | | | | | | | | | | | | | |
| 5252 | 1/2 cup | White, cnd, avg | 105 | 83 | 77 | 2.5 | 20.4 | 2.1 | 3.0 | 15.3 | 0.5 | 0.1 | 0.2 | 0.2 | 0.01 | 0.24 | 0 | 0 | 0 | 0 | 0 | 0 | 0.04 | 0.08 | 1.23 | 0.06 | 0.00 | 51.8 | 0.71 | 8.5 | 0.0 | 0.0 | 5 | 0.1 | 0.4 | 24 | 0.1 | 67 | 195 | 0.7 | 286 | 0.48 |
| 5564 | 1/2 cup | White, cnd, creamed, avg | 128 | 92 | 79 | 2.2 | 23.2 | 1.5 | 4.2 | 17.4 | 0.5 | 0.1 | 0.2 | 0.3 | 0.01 | 0.25 | 0 | 0 | 0 | 0 | 0 | 0 | 0.03 | 0.07 | 1.23 | 0.08 | 0.00 | 57.3 | 0.23 | 5.9 | 0.0 | | 4 | 0.1 | 0.5 | 22 | 0.0 | 65 | 172 | 0.8 | 365 | 0.68 |
| 7207 | 1/2 cup | White, cnd, creamed, low sod, avg | 128 | 92 | 79 | 2.2 | 23.2 | 1.5 | 4.2 | 17.4 | 0.5 | 0.1 | 0.2 | 0.3 | 0.01 | 0.25 | 0 | 0 | 0 | 0 | 0 | 0 | 0.03 | 0.07 | 1.23 | 0.08 | 0.00 | 57.3 | 0.23 | 5.9 | 0.0 | | 4 | 0.1 | 0.5 | 22 | 0.0 | 65 | 172 | 0.8 | 4 | 0.68 |
| 6017 | 1/2 cup | White, cnd, unsalted, avg | 105 | 83 | 77 | 2.5 | 20.4 | 2.1 | 3.0 | 15.3 | 0.5 | 0.1 | 0.2 | 0.2 | 0.01 | 0.24 | 0 | 0 | 0 | 0 | 0 | 0 | 0.04 | 0.08 | 1.23 | 0.06 | 0.00 | 51.8 | 0.71 | 8.5 | 0.0 | | 5 | 0.1 | 0.4 | 24 | 0.1 | 67 | 195 | 0.7 | 3 | 0.48 |
| 7203 | 1/2 cup | White, fresh, boiled, avg | 82 | 89 | 70 | 2.7 | 20.6 | 2.2 | 1.6 | 16.7 | 1.0 | 0.2 | 0.3 | 0.5 | 0.01 | 0.48 | 0 | 0 | 0 | 0 | 0 | 0 | 0.18 | 0.06 | 1.32 | 0.05 | 0.00 | 38.0 | 0.72 | 5.1 | 0.0 | | 2 | 0.0 | 0.5 | 26 | 0.2 | 84 | 204 | 0.7 | 14 | 0.39 |
| 5393 | 1/2 cup | White, fzn, boiled, avg | 82 | 66 | 77 | 2.3 | 16.1 | 2.0 | 1.5 | 12.6 | 0.4 | 0.1 | 0.1 | 0.2 | 0.00 | 0.16 | 0 | 0 | 0 | 0 | 0 | 0 | 0.07 | 0.06 | 1.07 | 0.11 | 0.00 | 25.4 | 0.15 | 2.5 | 0.0 | | 3 | 0.0 | 0.3 | 16 | 0.1 | 47 | 121 | 0.6 | 4 | 0.33 |
| 5567 | 1 ea | White, on the cob, fzn, boiled, unsalted, avg | 63 | 59 | 73 | 2.0 | 14.0 | 1.3 | 1.6 | 11.1 | 0.5 | 0.1 | 0.1 | 0.2 | 0.01 | 0.21 | 0 | 0 | 0 | 0 | 0 | 0 | 0.11 | 0.04 | 0.96 | 0.14 | 0.00 | 19.2 | 0.16 | 3.0 | 0.0 | 0.0 | 2 | 0.0 | 0.4 | 18 | 0.1 | 47 | 158 | 0.4 | 3 | 0.40 |
| 6015 | 1/2 cup | White, raw, avg | 77 | 66 | 76 | 2.5 | 14.6 | 2.1 | | | 0.9 | 0.1 | 0.3 | 0.4 | 0.01 | 0.42 | 0 | 0 | 0 | 0 | 0 | 0 | 0.15 | 0.05 | 1.31 | 0.04 | 0.00 | 35.3 | 0.59 | 5.2 | 0.0 | | 2 | 0.0 | 0.4 | 28 | 0.1 | 69 | 208 | 0.5 | 12 | 0.35 |
| 6342 | 1/2 cup | White, w/butter sauce, Green Giant | 75 | 80 | 75 | 1.9 | 14.1 | 2.3 | 3.1 | 8.6 | 1.8 | 0.9 | | | | | 2 | 116 | 23 | | | | | | | | 0.00 | | | 1.1 | | | 6 | | 0.2 | | | | | | 212 | |
| 5067 | 1/2 cup | Yellow, cnd, avg | 105 | 83 | 77 | 2.5 | 20.4 | 2.1 | 2.9 | 15.3 | 0.5 | 0.1 | 0.2 | 0.2 | 0.01 | 0.24 | 0 | 253 | 25 | 0 | 25 | 101 | 0.04 | 0.08 | 1.23 | 0.06 | 0.00 | 51.8 | 0.71 | 8.5 | 0.0 | 0.0 | 5 | 0.1 | 0.4 | 24 | 0.1 | 67 | 195 | 0.7 | 286 | 0.48 |
| 5068 | 1/2 cup | Yellow, cnd, creamed, avg | 128 | 92 | 79 | 2.2 | 23.2 | 1.5 | 4.2 | 17.4 | 0.5 | 0.1 | 0.2 | 0.3 | 0.01 | 0.25 | 0 | 124 | 13 | 0 | 13 | 51 | 0.03 | 0.07 | 1.23 | 0.08 | 0.00 | 57.3 | 0.23 | 5.9 | 0.0 | 0.0 | 4 | 0.1 | 0.5 | 22 | 0.0 | 65 | 172 | 0.8 | 365 | 0.68 |
| 5243 | 1/2 cup | Yellow, cnd, unsalted, avg | 105 | 83 | 77 | 2.5 | 20.4 | 2.1 | 2.9 | 15.3 | 0.5 | 0.1 | 0.2 | 0.2 | 0.01 | 0.24 | 0 | 253 | 25 | 0 | 25 | 101 | 0.04 | 0.08 | 1.23 | 0.06 | 0.00 | 51.8 | 0.71 | 8.5 | 0.0 | | 5 | 0.1 | 0.4 | 24 | 0.1 | 67 | 195 | 0.7 | 3 | 0.48 |
| 5379 | 1/2 cup | Yellow, fresh, boiled, avg | 82 | 89 | 70 | 2.7 | 20.6 | 2.3 | 2.1 | 16.2 | 1.0 | 0.2 | 0.3 | 0.5 | 0.01 | 0.48 | 0 | 178 | 18 | 0 | 18 | 72 | 0.18 | 0.06 | 1.32 | 0.05 | 0.00 | 38.0 | 0.72 | 5.1 | 0.0 | | 2 | 0.0 | 0.5 | 26 | 0.2 | 84 | 204 | 0.7 | 14 | 0.39 |
| 5378 | 1/2 cup | Yellow, fresh, raw, avg | 77 | 66 | 76 | 2.5 | 14.6 | 2.1 | 4.5 | 8.1 | 0.9 | 0.1 | 0.3 | 0.4 | 0.01 | 0.42 | 0 | 216 | 22 | 0 | 22 | 87 | 0.15 | 0.05 | 1.31 | 0.04 | 0.00 | 35.3 | 0.59 | 5.2 | 0.0 | | 2 | 0.0 | 0.4 | 28 | 0.1 | 69 | 208 | 0.5 | 12 | 0.35 |
| 5065 | 1/2 cup | Yellow, fzn, boiled, avg | 82 | 66 | 77 | 2.3 | 16.1 | 2.0 | 1.5 | 12.6 | 0.4 | 0.1 | 0.1 | 0.2 | 0.00 | 0.16 | 0 | 180 | 18 | 0 | 18 | 72 | 0.07 | 0.06 | 1.07 | 0.11 | 0.00 | 25.4 | 0.15 | 2.5 | 0.0 | 0.0 | 3 | 0.0 | 0.3 | 16 | 0.1 | 47 | 121 | 0.6 | 4 | 0.33 |
| 5364 | 1 ea | Yellow, on the cob, fzn, boiled, avg | 63 | 59 | 73 | 2.0 | 14.0 | 1.8 | 1.3 | 11.0 | 0.5 | 0.1 | 0.1 | 0.2 | 0.01 | 0.21 | 0 | 133 | 13 | 0 | 13 | 53 | 0.11 | 0.04 | 0.96 | 0.14 | 0.00 | 19.2 | 0.16 | 3.0 | 0.0 | | 2 | 0.0 | 0.4 | 18 | 0.1 | 47 | 158 | 0.4 | 3 | 0.40 |
| 6343 | 3 oz | Yellow, w/butter sauce, Green Giant | 85 | 89 | 75 | 2.0 | 16.1 | 1.8 | 3.6 | 10.7 | 2.0 | 0.9 | | | | | 3 | 79 | 16 | | | | | | | | 0.00 | | | 2.2 | | | 3 | | 0.3 | | | | | | 240 | |
| 5470 | 1/2 cup | Yellow Hominy, cnd, avg | 80 | 58 | 82 | 1.2 | 11.4 | 2.0 | 0.1 | 9.4 | 0.7 | 0.1 | 0.2 | 0.3 | 0.01 | 0.31 | 0 | 88 | 9 | 0 | 9 | 35 | 0.00 | 0.00 | 0.03 | 0.00 | 0.00 | 0.8 | 0.12 | 0.0 | 0.0 | | 8 | 0.0 | 0.5 | 13 | 0.1 | 28 | 7 | 2.4 | 168 | 0.84 |
| 5640 | 1/2 cup | Yellow Hominy, boiled, avg | 82 | 72 | 76 | 1.7 | 16.7 | 4.7 | | | 1.0 | 0.1 | 0.2 | 0.5 | | | 0 | 0 | 0 | 0 | 0 | 0 | 0.00 | 0.00 | 0.00 | 0.01 | 0.00 | 0.8 | 0.04 | 0.0 | 0.0 | | 8 | 0.0 | 0.8 | 14 | 0.0 | 34 | 8 | | 145 | 0.85 |
| | | Cowpeas/Blackeyed Peas | | | | | | | | | | | | | | | | | | | | | | | | | | | | | | | | | | | | | | | | |
| 7018 | 1/2 cup | Boiled, avg | 86 | 100 | 70 | 6.6 | 17.9 | 5.6 | 2.8 | 9.5 | 0.5 | 0.1 | 0.0 | 0.2 | 0.07 | 0.12 | 0 | 13 | 2 | 0 | 2 | 10 | 0.17 | 0.05 | 0.43 | 0.09 | 0.00 | 178.9 | 0.35 | 0.3 | 0.0 | | 21 | 0.2 | 2.2 | 46 | 0.4 | 134 | 239 | 2.2 | 3 | 1.11 |
| 7016 | 1/2 cup | Canned, avg | 120 | 92 | 80 | 5.7 | 16.3 | 4.0 | 2.6 | 9.7 | 0.7 | 0.2 | 0.1 | 0.3 | 0.10 | 0.18 | 0 | 16 | 1 | 0 | 1 | 7 | 0.09 | 0.09 | 0.42 | 0.05 | 0.00 | 61.4 | 0.23 | 3.2 | 0.0 | | 24 | 0.1 | 1.2 | 34 | 0.3 | 84 | 206 | 2.8 | 359 | 0.84 |
| 5115 | 1/2 cup | Frozen, boiled, drained, avg | 85 | 112 | 66 | 7.2 | 20.2 | 5.4 | 3.2 | 11.6 | 0.6 | 0.1 | 0.1 | 0.2 | 0.10 | 0.14 | 0 | 64 | 7 | 0 | 7 | 39 | 0.22 | 0.05 | 0.62 | 0.08 | 0.00 | 119.9 | 0.18 | 2.2 | 0.0 | | 20 | 0.2 | 1.8 | 43 | 0.7 | 104 | 319 | 2.9 | 4 | 1.21 |
| 7017 | 1/2 cup | Raw, avg | 84 | 282 | 12 | 19.7 | 50.4 | 8.9 | 5.8 | 35.7 | 1.1 | 0.3 | 0.1 | 0.5 | 0.17 | 0.29 | 0 | 42 | 4 | 0 | 4 | 24 | 0.72 | 0.19 | 1.75 | 0.30 | 0.00 | 531.7 | 1.26 | 1.3 | 0.0 | | 92 | 0.7 | 6.9 | 155 | 1.3 | 356 | 934 | 7.6 | 13 | 2.83 |
| 5374 | 1/2 cup | Cress, garden, boiled, drained, avg | 68 | 16 | 92 | 1.3 | 2.6 | 0.5 | 0.3 | 1.8 | 0.4 | 0.0 | 0.1 | 0.1 | 0.04 | 0.09 | 0 | 5236 | 524 | 0 | 524 | 3142 | 0.04 | 0.11 | 0.54 | 0.11 | 0.00 | 25.2 | 0.11 | 15.6 | 0.0 | | 41 | 0.1 | 0.5 | 18 | 0.3 | 33 | 240 | 0.6 | 5 | 0.10 |
| 5372 | 1/2 cup | Cress, garden, raw, avg | 25 | 8 | 89 | 0.6 | 1.4 | 0.3 | 0.4 | 0.7 | 0.2 | 0.0 | 0.1 | 0.1 | 0.02 | 0.04 | 0 | 2325 | 233 | 0 | 233 | 1395 | 0.02 | 0.06 | 0.25 | 0.06 | 0.00 | 20.1 | 0.06 | 17.3 | 0.0 | | 20 | 0.0 | 0.3 | 10 | 0.1 | 19 | 152 | 0.2 | 4 | 0.06 |
| 5639 | 1/2 cup | Cucumber, ckd, avg | 90 | 14 | 94 | 0.6 | 3.2 | 1.1 | 2.1 | 0.0 | 0.1 | 0.0 | 0.0 | 0.1 | | | 0 | 45 | 4 | 0 | 4 | 27 | 0.03 | 0.02 | 0.30 | 0.05 | 0.00 | 10.7 | 0.14 | 4.2 | 0.0 | | 15 | 0.0 | 0.3 | 12 | 0.1 | 17 | 148 | 9.9 | 247 | 0.24 |
| 5071 | 1/2 cup | Cucumber, w/peel, raw, avg | 52 | 7 | 96 | 0.4 | 1.4 | 0.4 | 1.0 | 0.0 | 0.1 | 0.0 | 0.0 | 0.0 | 0.02 | 0.01 | 0 | 112 | 11 | 0 | 11 | 66 | 0.01 | 0.01 | 0.11 | 0.02 | 0.00 | 6.8 | 0.09 | 2.8 | 0.0 | 0.0 | 7 | 0.0 | 0.1 | 6 | 0.0 | 10 | 75 | 0.0 | 1 | 0.10 |
| 5242 | 1/2 cup | Dandelion, greens, boiled, avg | 53 | 17 | 90 | 1.1 | 3.4 | 1.5 | 0.5 | 1.3 | 0.3 | 0.1 | 0.0 | 0.1 | 0.02 | 0.12 | 0 | 6201 | 620 | 0 | 620 | 3721 | 0.07 | 0.09 | 0.27 | 0.08 | 0.00 | 6.6 | 0.03 | 9.5 | 0.0 | | 74 | 0.1 | 1.0 | 13 | 0.1 | 22 | 123 | 0.2 | 23 | 0.15 |

| Code | Amount | Description | Basic Components | | | | | | | | | Additional Fats | | | | | | Vit A & Components | | | | | Vitamins | | | | | | | | | | Minerals | | | | | | | | | |
|---|---|---|---|---|---|---|---|---|---|---|---|---|---|---|---|---|---|---|---|---|---|---|---|---|---|---|---|---|---|---|---|---|---|---|---|---|---|---|---|---|---|---|
| | | | Weight (g) | Calories | % Water | Protein (g) | Carbs (g) | Fiber (g) | Sugar (g) | Other Carbs (g) | Fat (g) | Sat Fat (g) | Mono Fat (g) | Poly Fat (g) | Omega 3 (g) | Omega 6 (g) | Choles (mg) | Vit A (IU) | Vit A (RE) | Retinol (RE) | Carotenoids (RE) | Beta Carotene (mcg) | Thiamin (mg) | Riboflavin (mg) | Niacin (NE) | Vit B6 (mg) | Vit B12 (mcg) | Folate (mcg) | Panto (mg) | Vit C (mg) | Vit D (mg) | Vit E (α TE) | Calcium (mg) | Copper (mg) | Iron (mg) | Magnes (mg) | Mang (mg) | Phos (mg) | Potassium (mg) | Selenium (mcg) | Sodium (mg) | Zinc (mg) |
| 5509 | 1/2 cup | Dandelion, leaves, avg | 28 | 13 | 86 | 0.7 | 3.1 | 0.6 | | | 0.2 | | | | | | 0 | 2453 | 246 | 0 | 246 | 1475 | 0.05 | 0.05 | 0.22 | | 0.00 | | | 8.4 | | | 44 | 0.0 | 0.9 | 10 | 0.1 | 20 | 123 | | 21 | 0.34 |
| 6910 | 1/2 cup | Dock/Sorrel, geens, raw, avg | 66 | 15 | 93 | 1.3 | 2.1 | 1.9 | | | 0.5 | | | | | | 0 | 2640 | 264 | 0 | 264 | 1584 | 0.03 | 0.07 | 0.33 | 0.08 | 0.00 | 8.7 | 0.03 | 31.7 | 0.0 | | 29 | 0.1 | 1.6 | 68 | 0.2 | 42 | 257 | 0.6 | 3 | 0.13 |
| 5418 | 1/2 cup | Dock/Sorrel, greens, ckd, avg | 50 | 10 | 94 | 0.9 | 1.5 | 1.3 | | | 0.3 | | | | | | 0 | 1737 | 174 | 0 | 174 | 1041 | 0.02 | 0.04 | 0.21 | 0.05 | 0.00 | 3.9 | 0.02 | 13.1 | 0.0 | | 19 | 0.1 | 1.0 | 44 | 0.2 | 26 | 160 | 0.4 | 2 | 0.09 |
| | | Eggplant | | | | | | | | | | | | | | | | | | | | | | | | | | | | | | | | | | | | | | | | |
| 5642 | 1 pce | Batter Dipped, fried, avg | 50 | 75 | 74 | 1.2 | 6.0 | 1.2 | 1.7 | 3.1 | 5.3 | 1.3 | 2.3 | 1.5 | | | 9 | 35 | 5 | 0 | 3 | 15 | 0.06 | 0.04 | 0.45 | 0.04 | 0.06 | 7.1 | | 0.6 | | | 27 | 0.1 | 0.5 | 6 | 0.1 | 26 | 106 | | 32 | 0.14 |
| 5072 | 1/2 cup | Boiled, avg | 50 | 14 | 92 | 0.4 | 3.3 | 1.3 | 2.1 | 0.0 | 0.1 | 0.0 | 0.0 | 0.0 | 0.01 | 0.04 | 0 | 32 | 3 | 0 | 3 | 18 | 0.04 | 0.01 | 0.30 | 0.04 | 0.00 | 7.2 | 0.04 | 0.6 | 0.0 | 0.0 | 3 | 0.1 | 0.2 | 6 | 0.1 | 11 | 124 | 0.2 | 2 | 0.08 |
| 5611 | 1/2 cup | Pickled, avg | 68 | 23 | 87 | 0.6 | 5.0 | 1.7 | 2.7 | 0.5 | 0.5 | 0.1 | 0.0 | 0.3 | 0.04 | 0.23 | 0 | 34 | 3 | 0 | 3 | 20 | 0.03 | 0.05 | 0.45 | 0.10 | 0.00 | 13.6 | 0.05 | 0.0 | 0.0 | | 17 | 0.1 | 0.5 | 4 | 0.1 | 6 | 8 | | 1138 | 0.16 |
| 5371 | 1/2 cup | Raw, cubes, avg | 41 | 11 | 92 | 0.4 | 2.5 | 1.0 | 1.4 | 0.1 | 0.1 | 0.0 | 0.0 | 0.0 | 0.01 | 0.03 | 0 | 34 | 3 | 0 | 3 | 20 | 0.02 | 0.01 | 0.25 | 0.03 | 0.00 | 7.8 | 0.10 | 0.7 | 0.0 | | 3 | 0.0 | 0.1 | 6 | 0.1 | 9 | 89 | 0.1 | 1 | 0.06 |
| 47614 | 1/2 cup | Endive, raw, Freida's Specialty Produce | 22 | 4 | 94 | 0.3 | 0.8 | 0.6 | 0.2 | 0.0 | 0.0 | 0.0 | 0.0 | 0.0 | 0.00 | 0.00 | 0 | 453 | 45 | 0 | 45 | 272 | | | | | 0.00 | | | 1.6 | | | 10 | | 0.2 | | | | | | 5 | |
| 5450 | 1/2 cup | Fennel, bulb, raw, slices, avg | 44 | 14 | 90 | 0.5 | 3.2 | 1.4 | 0.1 | 1.8 | 0.1 | | | | | | 0 | 59 | 6 | 0 | 6 | 34 | 0.00 | 0.01 | 0.28 | 0.02 | 0.00 | 11.9 | 0.10 | 5.3 | 0.0 | | 22 | 0.0 | 0.3 | 7 | 0.1 | 22 | 182 | 0.3 | 23 | 0.09 |
| 5508 | 1/2 cup | Fennel, leaves, avg | 24 | 5 | 86 | 0.6 | 1.5 | 0.8 | | | 0.1 | | | | | | 0 | 1253 | 125 | 0 | 125 | 752 | 0.06 | 0.03 | 0.05 | 0.02 | 0.00 | 24.0 | 0.06 | 22.3 | | | 26 | 0.0 | 0.6 | 12 | | 12 | 119 | | 21 | 0.06 |
| 5541 | 1/2 cup | Grape Leaves, avg | 28 | 19 | 79 | 1.3 | 3.8 | | | | 0.3 | | | | | | 0 | 7557 | 756 | 0 | 756 | 4534 | 0.06 | 0.02 | 0.34 | | 0.00 | | | 3.1 | 0.0 | | 200 | | 1.9 | | | 11 | 71 | | 6 | |
| | | Green Beans | | | | | | | | | | | | | | | | | | | | | | | | | | | | | | | | | | | | | | | | |
| 5011 | 1/2 cup | Snap/String, boiled, avg | 62 | 22 | 89 | 1.2 | 4.9 | 2.0 | 1.2 | 1.7 | 0.2 | 0.0 | 0.0 | 0.1 | 0.06 | 0.03 | 0 | 413 | 42 | 0 | 42 | 240 | 0.05 | 0.06 | 0.38 | 0.03 | 0.00 | 20.6 | 0.05 | 6.0 | 0.0 | | 29 | 0.1 | 0.8 | 16 | 0.2 | 24 | 185 | 0.2 | 2 | 0.22 |
| 5017 | 1/2 cup | Snap/String, cnd w/liquid, avg | 120 | 18 | 95 | 1.0 | 4.2 | 1.8 | 1.4 | 1.0 | 0.1 | 0.0 | 0.0 | 0.1 | 0.04 | 0.02 | 0 | 335 | 38 | 0 | 38 | 221 | 0.03 | 0.06 | 0.24 | 0.04 | 0.00 | 21.8 | 0.13 | 4.1 | 0.0 | | 29 | 0.1 | 1.1 | 16 | 0.4 | 23 | 110 | 0.2 | 311 | 0.24 |
| 5013 | 1/2 cup | Snap/String, fzn, boiled, avg | 68 | 19 | 91 | 1.0 | 4.4 | 2.0 | 1.8 | 0.6 | 0.1 | 0.0 | 0.0 | 0.1 | 0.03 | 0.02 | 0 | 273 | 27 | 0 | 27 | 157 | 0.02 | 0.06 | 0.26 | 0.04 | 0.00 | 15.6 | 0.03 | 2.8 | 0.0 | | 33 | 0.0 | 0.6 | 16 | 0.2 | 21 | 86 | 0.3 | 6 | 0.33 |
| 5009 | 1/2 cup | Snap/String, raw, avg | 55 | 17 | 90 | 1.0 | 3.9 | 1.9 | 1.4 | 0.6 | 0.1 | 0.0 | 0.0 | 0.0 | 0.02 | 0.01 | 0 | 367 | 37 | 0 | 37 | 212 | 0.05 | 0.06 | 0.41 | 0.04 | 0.00 | 20.1 | 0.05 | 9.0 | 0.0 | | 20 | 0.0 | 0.6 | 14 | 0.1 | 21 | 115 | 0.3 | 3 | 0.13 |
| 5231 | 1/2 cup | String, cnd w/liquid, low sod, avg | 120 | 18 | 95 | 1.0 | 4.2 | 1.8 | 1.4 | 1.0 | 0.1 | 0.0 | 0.0 | 0.1 | 0.04 | 0.02 | 0 | 385 | 38 | 0 | 38 | 221 | 0.03 | 0.06 | 0.24 | 0.04 | 0.00 | 21.8 | 0.13 | 4.1 | 0.0 | | 29 | 0.1 | 1.1 | 16 | 0.4 | 23 | 110 | 0.2 | 17 | 0.24 |
| 6250 | 1/2 cup | String, 50% less salt, cnd, Green Giant | 120 | 22 | 95 | 0.8 | 4.3 | 1.4 | 1.7 | 1.2 | 0.1 | 0.0 | | | | | 0 | 414 | 41 | 0 | 41 | 239 | | | | | 0.00 | | | 1.4 | | | 25 | | 0.7 | | | | | | 200 | |
| 5603 | 1/2 cup | String, pickled, avg | 68 | 19 | 91 | 1.1 | 4.5 | 1.1 | 1.8 | 1.6 | 0.1 | 0.0 | 0.0 | 0.0 | 0.02 | 0.01 | 0 | 377 | 38 | 0 | 38 | 218 | 0.04 | 0.06 | 0.42 | 0.04 | 0.00 | 18.4 | | 8.2 | 0.0 | | 22 | 0.0 | 0.6 | 16 | | 23 | 129 | | 149 | 0.14 |
| 6348 | 3 oz | String, w/butter sauce, Green Giant | 85 | 28 | 91 | 1.0 | 4.4 | 1.6 | | | 1.4 | 0.8 | 0.4 | 0.0 | | | 3 | 226 | 23 | 0 | 23 | 130 | 0.03 | 0.06 | 0.48 | | 0.00 | | | 3.3 | | | 25 | | 0.4 | | | 20 | 105 | | 227 | |
| 5504 | 1 Tbs | Horseradish, fresh, raw, avg | 15 | 9 | 77 | 0.4 | 1.9 | | | | 0.0 | 0.0 | 0.0 | 0.0 | | | 0 | 2 | 0.2 | 0 | 0.2 | 1 | 0.02 | 0.02 | 0.09 | 0.03 | 0.00 | | | 17.1 | | | 16 | 0.0 | 0.2 | 5 | 0.1 | 10 | 83 | 0.0 | 1 | 0.21 |
| 5765 | 1/2 cup | Jew's Ear, raw, avg | 50 | 12 | 93 | 0.2 | 3.4 | | | | 0.0 | | | | | | 0 | 0 | 0 | 0 | 0 | 0 | 0.04 | 0.10 | 0.04 | 0.04 | 0.00 | 9.6 | 1.00 | 0.3 | 0.0 | | 8 | 0.2 | 0.3 | 12 | 0.1 | 7 | 22 | 5.6 | 4 | 0.33 |
| 5420 | 1/2 cup | Jute/Potherb, boiled, avg | 44 | 16 | 87 | 1.6 | 3.2 | 0.9 | | | 0.1 | 0.0 | 0.0 | 0.0 | 0.00 | 0.04 | 0 | 2281 | 228 | 0 | 228 | 1370 | 0.04 | 0.08 | 0.39 | 0.25 | 0.00 | 45.8 | 0.03 | 14.5 | 0.0 | | 93 | 0.1 | 1.4 | 27 | 0.1 | 32 | 242 | 0.4 | 5 | 0.35 |
| 5419 | 1/2 cup | Jute/Potherb, raw, avg | 14 | 5 | 88 | 0.7 | 0.8 | 0.2 | | | 0.0 | 0.0 | 0.0 | 0.0 | 0.00 | 0.02 | 0 | 778 | 78 | 0 | 78 | 467 | 0.02 | 0.08 | 0.18 | 0.08 | 0.00 | 17.2 | 0.01 | 5.2 | 0.0 | | 29 | 0.0 | 0.7 | 9 | 0.0 | 12 | 78 | 0.1 | 1 | 0.11 |
| | | Kale | | | | | | | | | | | | | | | | | | | | | | | | | | | | | | | | | | | | | | | | |
| 5075 | 1/2 cup | Boiled, drained, unsalted, avg | 65 | 18 | 91 | 1.2 | 3.7 | 1.3 | 0.8 | 1.6 | 0.3 | 0.0 | 0.0 | 0.1 | 0.07 | 0.05 | 0 | 4810 | 481 | 0 | 481 | 2886 | 0.03 | 0.05 | 0.32 | 0.09 | 0.00 | 8.6 | 0.03 | 26.6 | 0.0 | 0.6 | 47 | 0.1 | 0.6 | 12 | 0.3 | 18 | 148 | 0.6 | 15 | 0.16 |
| 5076 | 1/2 cup | Frozen, boiled, avg | 65 | 19 | 90 | 1.8 | 3.4 | 1.3 | 0.7 | 1.4 | 0.3 | 0.0 | 0.0 | 0.2 | 0.08 | 0.05 | 0 | 4130 | 413 | 0 | 413 | 2477 | 0.03 | 0.07 | 0.44 | 0.06 | 0.00 | 9.3 | 0.03 | 16.4 | 0.0 | 0.1 | 90 | 0.0 | 0.6 | 12 | 0.3 | 18 | 209 | 0.6 | 10 | 0.12 |
| 5208 | 1 cup | Raw, chpd, avg | 67 | 34 | 84 | 2.2 | 6.7 | 1.3 | 1.5 | 3.9 | 0.5 | 0.1 | 0.0 | 0.2 | 0.12 | 0.09 | 0 | 5963 | 596 | 0 | 596 | 3578 | 0.07 | 0.09 | 0.67 | 0.18 | 0.00 | 19.6 | 0.06 | 80.4 | 0.0 | | 90 | 0.2 | 1.1 | 23 | 0.5 | 38 | 299 | 0.6 | 29 | 0.29 |
| 5079 | 1/2 cup | Kohlrabi, boiled, drained, unsalted, avg | 82 | 24 | 90 | 1.5 | 5.5 | 0.9 | 3.9 | 0.6 | 0.1 | 0.0 | 0.0 | 0.0 | 0.02 | 0.02 | 0 | 29 | 3 | 0 | 3 | 20 | 0.03 | 0.02 | 0.32 | 0.13 | 0.00 | 9.9 | 0.13 | 44.3 | 0.0 | | 20 | 0.1 | 0.3 | 16 | 0.1 | 37 | 279 | 0.7 | 17 | 0.25 |
| 5078 | 1/2 cup | Kohlrabi, raw, avg | 68 | 18 | 91 | 1.2 | 4.2 | 2.4 | 1.8 | 0.0 | 0.1 | 0.0 | 0.0 | 0.0 | 0.02 | 0.01 | 0 | 24 | 3 | 0 | 3 | 16 | 0.03 | 0.01 | 0.27 | 0.10 | 0.00 | 10.9 | 0.11 | 42.2 | 0.0 | | 16 | 0.1 | 0.3 | 13 | 0.1 | 31 | 238 | 0.5 | 14 | 0.02 |
| 5203 | 1/2 cup | Leeks, boiled, drained, unsalted, avg | 52 | 16 | 91 | 0.4 | 4.0 | 0.5 | 0.5 | 2.9 | 0.1 | 0.0 | 0.0 | 0.1 | 0.03 | 0.02 | 0 | 24 | 3 | 0 | 3 | 16 | 0.01 | 0.01 | 0.10 | 0.06 | 0.00 | 12.6 | 0.04 | 2.2 | 0.0 | | 16 | 0.0 | 0.6 | 7 | 0.1 | 9 | 45 | 0.3 | 5 | 0.03 |
| 5205 | 1/2 cup | Leeks, raw, chpd, avg | 44 | 27 | 83 | 0.7 | 6.2 | 0.8 | 1.7 | 3.7 | 0.1 | 0.0 | 0.0 | 0.1 | 0.04 | 0.03 | 0 | 42 | 4 | 0 | 4 | 26 | 0.03 | 0.01 | 0.18 | 0.10 | 0.00 | 28.2 | 0.06 | 5.3 | 0.0 | | 26 | 0.1 | 0.9 | 12 | 0.2 | 15 | 79 | 0.4 | 9 | 0.05 |
| 6130 | 1 oz | Lemon Grass, leaves, avg | 28 | 18 | 72 | 0.4 | 4.0 | | | | 0.4 | | | | | | | 11295 | 1130 | 0 | 1130 | 6777 | 0.01 | 0.03 | 0.14 | | 0.00 | | | 6.7 | | | 45 | | 1.5 | | | 12 | | | | |
| 7006 | 1/2 cup | Lentils, boiled, avg | 99 | 115 | 70 | 8.9 | 19.9 | 7.8 | 1.8 | 10.3 | 0.4 | 0.1 | 0.1 | 0.2 | 0.04 | 0.14 | 0 | 8 | 1 | 0 | 1 | 6 | 0.17 | 0.07 | 1.05 | 0.18 | 0.00 | 179.2 | 0.63 | 1.5 | 0.0 | | 19 | 0.2 | 3.3 | 36 | 0.5 | 178 | 365 | 2.8 | 2 | 1.26 |
| 7005 | 1/2 cup | Lentils, raw, avg | 96 | 324 | 11 | 27.0 | 54.8 | 29.3 | 5.2 | 20.4 | 0.9 | 0.1 | 0.2 | 0.4 | 0.09 | 0.34 | 0 | 37 | 4 | 0 | 4 | 22 | 0.46 | 0.24 | 2.52 | 0.51 | 0.00 | 415.7 | 1.78 | 6.0 | 0.0 | | 49 | 0.8 | 8.7 | 103 | 1.4 | 436 | 869 | 7.9 | 10 | 3.47 |
| | | Lettuce | | | | | | | | | | | | | | | | | | | | | | | | | | | | | | | | | | | | | | | | |
| 5080 | 1 cup | Butterhead, avg | 56 | 7 | 96 | 0.7 | 1.3 | 0.6 | 0.7 | 0.0 | 0.1 | 0.0 | 0.0 | 0.1 | 0.05 | 0.02 | 0 | 543 | 54 | 0 | 54 | 326 | 0.03 | 0.03 | 0.17 | 0.03 | 0.00 | 41.0 | 0.10 | 4.5 | 0.0 | 0.2 | 18 | 0.0 | 0.2 | 7 | 0.1 | 13 | 144 | 0.1 | 3 | 0.10 |
| 5083 | 1 cup | Iceberg, avg | 55 | 7 | 96 | 0.6 | 1.1 | 0.8 | 0.4 | 0.0 | 0.1 | 0.0 | 0.0 | 0.1 | 0.04 | 0.02 | 0 | 182 | 18 | 0 | 18 | 109 | 0.03 | 0.02 | 0.10 | 0.02 | 0.00 | 30.8 | 0.03 | 2.1 | 0.0 | 0.2 | 10 | 0.0 | 0.3 | 5 | 0.1 | 11 | 87 | 0.1 | 5 | 0.12 |
| 5086 | 1 cup | Looseleaf, avg | 56 | 10 | 94 | 0.7 | 2.0 | 1.1 | 0.9 | 0.0 | 0.2 | 0.0 | 0.0 | 0.1 | 0.06 | 0.03 | 0 | 1064 | 106 | 0 | 106 | 638 | 0.03 | 0.04 | 0.22 | 0.03 | 0.00 | 27.9 | 0.11 | 10.1 | 0.0 | | 38 | 0.0 | 0.8 | 6 | 0.4 | 14 | 148 | 0.1 | 5 | 0.16 |
| 5637 | 1 cup | Mixed Salad Greens, raw, avg | 55 | 9 | 94 | 0.9 | 1.6 | 0.9 | 0.4 | 0.3 | 0.1 | 0.0 | 0.0 | 0.1 | | | 0 | 1495 | 150 | 0 | 150 | 896 | 0.04 | 0.05 | 0.24 | 0.04 | 0.00 | 63.6 | 0.15 | 8.9 | 0.0 | | 30 | 0.0 | 0.7 | 13 | 0.3 | 18 | 174 | | 14 | 0.23 |
| 5088 | 1 cup | Romaine, avg | 56 | 8 | 95 | 0.9 | 1.3 | 1.0 | 0.3 | 0.1 | 0.1 | 0.0 | 0.0 | 0.1 | 0.04 | 0.02 | 0 | 1456 | 146 | 0 | 146 | 874 | 0.06 | 0.06 | 0.28 | 0.03 | 0.00 | 76.2 | 0.10 | 13.4 | 0.0 | 0.2 | 20 | 0.0 | 0.6 | 3 | 0.4 | 25 | 162 | 0.1 | 4 | 0.14 |
| 5392 | 1/2 cup | Lotus Root, boiled, drained, sliced, avg | 60 | 40 | 81 | 0.9 | 9.6 | 1.9 | | | 0.0 | 0.0 | 0.0 | 0.0 | 0.00 | 0.01 | 0 | 0 | 0 | 0 | 0 | 0 | 0.08 | 0.01 | 0.18 | 0.13 | 0.00 | 4.7 | 0.18 | 16.4 | 0.0 | | 16 | 0.1 | 0.5 | 13 | 0.1 | 47 | 218 | 0.4 | 27 | 0.20 |
| 5391 | 10 ea | Lotus Root, raw, slices, avg | 81 | 60 | 79 | 2.1 | 13.9 | 4.0 | | | 0.1 | 0.0 | 0.0 | 0.0 | 0.00 | 0.01 | 0 | 0 | 0 | 0 | 0 | 0 | 0.13 | 0.18 | 0.32 | 0.21 | 0.00 | 10.3 | 0.31 | 35.6 | 0.0 | | 36 | 0.2 | 0.9 | 19 | 0.2 | 81 | 450 | 0.6 | 32 | 0.32 |
| | | Mixed Vegetables | | | | | | | | | | | | | | | | | | | | | | | | | | | | | | | | | | | | | | | | |
| 6644 | 1/2 cup | Broccoli & Cauliflower, Birds Eye | 91 | 22 | 93 | 1.9 | 4.4 | 2.3 | 2.4 | | 0.2 | 0.1 | | | | | 0 | 407 | 41 | 0 | 41 | 242 | | | | | 0.00 | | | | 1.4 | | 29 | | 0.4 | | | | | | 23 | |
| 56942 | 3 oz | Brocc, Cauliflower & Carrots, Green Giant | 85 | 23 | 90 | 2.0 | 5.6 | 2.1 | | | 0.1 | 0.0 | 0.0 | 0.0 | 0.00 | 0.00 | 0 | 2652 | 265 | 0 | 265 | 1591 | 0.01 | 0.06 | 0.49 | | 0.00 | | | 25.1 | | | 31 | | 0.7 | | | 39 | 188 | | 29 | |
| 57533 | 1 ea | Brocc, Caulif & Carrots, w/cheese, svg, Green | 141 | 75 | 85 | 3.2 | 12.9 | 1.9 | | | 2.0 | 0.5 | 0.9 | 0.1 | | | 4 | 3745 | 749 | | | | 0.01 | 0.18 | 0.41 | | 0.00 | | | 16.2 | | | 76 | | 0.6 | | | 214 | 296 | | 650 | |
| 6234 | 1/2 cup | Broccoli, Corn & Red Peppers, Birds Eye | 102 | 54 | 84 | 2.5 | 12.4 | 2.6 | 2.9 | 6.8 | 0.5 | 0.1 | | | | | 0 | 844 | 84 | 0 | 84 | 507 | 0.07 | 0.08 | 1.12 | 0.14 | 0.00 | 58.9 | 0.20 | 38.2 | | | 21 | 0.0 | 0.5 | 18 | | 60 | 204 | | 15 | |
| 6636 | 1/2 cup | Broccoli, Grn Beans, Prl Onions & Ppprs, Birds Eye | 43 | 12 | 92 | 0.7 | 2.7 | 0.9 | 1.4 | 0.3 | 0.1 | 0.0 | | | | | 0 | 354 | 35 | 0 | 35 | 212 | | | | | 0.00 | | | 14.6 | | | 17 | | 0.3 | | | | | | 6 | |
| 6645 | 1/2 cup | Broccoli, Rd Peppers, Onions & Mushrms, Birds Eye | 99 | 25 | 93 | 1.8 | 4.8 | 2.2 | 3.0 | | 0.3 | 0.1 | | | | | 0 | 1098 | 110 | 0 | 110 | 658 | | | | | 0.00 | | | 51.6 | | | 30 | | 0.5 | | | | | | 21 | |
| 6236 | 1/2 cup | Brussel Sprouts, Caulif & Carrots, Birds Eye | 89 | 31 | 89 | 2.2 | 6.6 | 2.6 | 2.6 | 1.4 | 0.2 | 0.0 | | | | | 0 | 4151 | 415 | 0 | 415 | 2488 | 0.06 | 0.07 | 0.53 | 0.16 | 0.00 | 62.3 | 0.22 | 41.7 | | | 24 | 0.0 | 0.6 | 13 | | 39 | 235 | | 22 | |
| 5548 | 1/2 cup | Canned, avg | 122 | 44 | 90 | 1.7 | 8.7 | 4.6 | | | 0.3 | 0.1 | 0.0 | 0.1 | 0.04 | [illegible] | 0 | 6199 | 620 | 0 | 620 | 3221 | 0.04 | 0.05 | 0.59 | 0.09 | 0.00 | 22.0 | 0.14 | 4.6 | 0.0 | | 26 | 0.1 | 0.8 | 18 | 0.5 | 45 | 168 | 0.2 | 273 | 0.62 |
| 5516 | 1/2 cup | Canned, low sod, avg | 91 | 33 | 90 | 1.3 | 6.5 | 2.8 | | | 0.2 | 0.0 | 0.0 | 0.1 | 0.03 | 0.08 | 0 | 4623 | 462 | 0 | 462 | 2402 | 0.03 | 0.04 | 0.44 | 0.07 | 0.00 | 16.4 | 0.14 | 3.5 | 0.0 | | 19 | 0.1 | 0.6 | 14 | 0.3 | 34 | 126 | 0.3 | 24 | 0.46 |
| 6238 | 1/2 cup | Cauliflower, Carrots & Snow Pea Pods, Birds Eye | 90 | 28 | 91 | 1.6 | 6.1 | 2.5 | 3.0 | 0.6 | 0.2 | 0.0 | | | | | 0 | 8086 | 808 | 0 | 808 | 4349 | 0.04 | 0.05 | 0.54 | 0.14 | 0.00 | 26.5 | 0.20 | 27.5 | | | 26 | 0.0 | 0.6 | 12 | | 29 | 182 | | 26 | |
| 6267 | 1/2 cup | Corn, Mexicorn, cnd, Green Giant | 78 | 68 | 77 | 1.7 | 14.4 | 1.5 | 4.4 | 8.4 | 0.5 | 0.1 | | | | | 0 | 51 | 5 | 0 | 5 | 30 | | | | | 0.00 | | | 1.2 | | | 6 | | 0.2 | | | | | | 434 | |
| 5515 | 1/2 cup | Corn w/Red & Green Peppers, cnd w/liquid, avg | 114 | 85 | 78 | 2.7 | 20.7 | 2.3 | 3.9 | 14.6 | 0.6 | 0.1 | 0.2 | 0.3 | 0.01 | 0.29 | 0 | 264 | 26 | 0 | 26 | 157 | 0.03 | 0.09 | 1.08 | 0.11 | 0.00 | 38.6 | 0.51 | 10.0 | 0.0 | | 6 | 0.1 | 0.9 | 28 | 0.0 | 71 | 174 | 0.7 | 396 | 0.42 |
| 6590 | 1/2 cup | French Style, Green Giant | 112 | 52 | 89 | 1.8 | 5.3 | 1.9 | 1.9 | 1.5 | 2.7 | 1.8 | | | | | 8 | 869 | 87 | 0 | 87 | 521 | | | | | 0.00 | | | 18.1 | | | 34 | | 0.5 | | | | | | 342 | |
| 5549 | 3 oz | Frozen, avg | 85 | 54 | 82 | 2.8 | 11.5 | 3.4 | | | 0.4 | 0.1 | 0.0 | 0.2 | 0.05 | [illegible] | 0 | 4316 | 432 | 0 | 432 | 2215 | 0.10 | 0.07 | 1.06 | 0.03 | 0.00 | 24.7 | 0.14 | 8.8 | 0.0 | | 21 | 0.1 | 0.8 | 20 | 0.2 | 50 | 180 | 0.3 | 40 | 0.38 |
| 5187 | 1/2 cup | Frozen, boiled, avg | 91 | 54 | 83 | 2.6 | 11.9 | 4.0 | 2.9 | 5.0 | 0.1 | 0.0 | 0.0 | 0.1 | 0.02 | 0.05 | 0 | 3892 | 389 | 0 | 389 | 1998 | 0.06 | 0.11 | 0.77 | 0.07 | 0.00 | 17.3 | 0.14 | 2.9 | 0.0 | | 23 | 0.1 | 0.7 | 20 | 0.3 | 46 | 154 | 0.3 | 32 | 0.45 |
| 6358 | 1/2 cup | Heartland Style, Green Giant | 46 | 16 | 91 | 0.9 | 2.9 | 1.3 | 0.9 | 0.7 | 0.1 | 0.0 | | | | | 0 | 1084 | 108 | 0 | 108 | 650 | | | | | 0.00 | | | 13.0 | | | 16 | | 0.2 | | | | | | 17 | |
| 6591 | 1/2 cup | Italian Style Parmesan, Green Giant | 112 | 66 | 85 | 3.9 | 7.3 | 2.7 | 1.9 | 2.7 | 2.3 | 1.4 | | | | | 6 | 2062 | 412 | | | | | | | | 0.00 | | | 13.7 | | | 75 | | 0.5 | | | | | | 226 | |
| 6206 | 1/2 cup | Japanese Style, Birds Eye | 127 | 79 | 88 | 2.3 | 8.1 | 2.2 | 4.3 | 1.6 | 4.7 | 2.3 | | | | | 1 | 955 | 96 | 0 | 96 | 573 | 0.05 | 0.09 | 0.38 | 0.11 | 0.00 | 35.4 | 0.15 | 44.4 | | | 39 | 0.1 | 0.7 | 22 | | 50 | 179 | | 320 | |
| 6357 | 1/2 cup | Manhattan Style, Green Giant | 40 | 13 | 91 | 0.9 | 2.2 | 0.9 | 1.0 | 0.4 | 0.1 | 0.0 | | | | | 0 | 150 | 15 | 0 | 15 | 90 | | | | | 0.00 | | | 9.3 | | | 14 | | 0.2 | | | | | | 7 | |
| 6356 | 1/2 cup | New England, Green Giant | 57 | 50 | 80 | 1.5 | 8.7 | 2.1 | 1.3 | 5.4 | 1.0 | 0.2 | | | | | 0 | 1345 | 135 | 0 | 135 | 807 | | | | | 0.00 | | | 5.1 | | | 11 | | 0.5 | | | | | | 48 | |
| 6593 | 1/2 cup | Normandy Style, Green Giant | 112 | 77 | 85 | 1.8 | 10.6 | 1.7 | 2.0 | 6.9 | 2.9 | 1.9 | | | | | 9 | 218 | 22 | 0 | 22 | 131 | | | | | 0.00 | | | 10.0 | | | 27 | | 0.9 | | | | | | 270 | |
| 57151 | 3 oz | Oriental Style, Nestle | 85 | 61 | | 1.0 | 9.1 | 1.0 | 2.7 | 5.4 | 2.4 | 0.3 | | | | | 0 | 1349 | 135 | 0 | 135 | 810 | | | | | 0.00 | | | 2.0 | | | 7 | | 0.4 | | | | | | 476 | |
| 5281 | 1/2 cup | Peas & Carrots, cnd, avg | 128 | 49 | 88 | 2.8 | 10.9 | 2.6 | 4.9 | 3.4 | 0.3 | 0.1 | 0.0 | 0.2 | 0.03 | 0.13 | 0 | 7386 | 739 | 0 | 739 | 3935 | 0.09 | 0.07 | 0.74 | 0.11 | 0.00 | 23.4 | 0.15 | 8.4 | 0.0 | | 29 | 0.1 | 1.0 | 18 | 0.5 | 59 | 128 | 1.2 | 333 | 0.74 |
| 5123 | 1/2 cup | Peas & Carrots, fzn, ckd, avg | 80 | 38 | 86 | 2.5 | 8.1 | 2.5 | 2.6 | 3.0 | 0.3 | 0.1 | 0.0 | 0.2 | 0.03 | 0.13 | 0 | 6209 | 621 | 0 | 621 | 3308 | 0.18 | 0.05 | 0.92 | 0.07 | 0.00 | 20.8 | 0.13 | 6.5 | 0.0 | | 18 | 0.1 | 0.8 | 13 | 0.2 | 39 | 126 | 0.9 | 54 | 0.36 |
| 7494 | 1/2 cup | Peas & Mushrooms, ckd, avg | 95 | 65 | 81 | 4.3 | 11.8 | 2.8 | | | 0.3 | 0.0 | 0.0 | 0.1 | | | 0 | 512 | 51 | 0 | 51 | 298 | 0.23 | 0.16 | 1.86 | 0.10 | 0.00 | 48.7 | 0.11 | 8.2 | 0.0 | | 20 | 0.2 | 1.4 | 24 | | 87 | 195 | 3.8 | 291 | 0.85 |

| Code | Amount | Description | Basic Components: Weight (g) | Calories | % Water | Protein (g) | Carbs (g) | Fiber (g) | Sugar (g) | Other Carbs (g) | Fat (g) | Additional Fats: Sat Fat (g) | Mono Fat (g) | Poly Fat (g) | Omega 3 (g) | Omega 6 (g) | Choles (mg) | Vit A & Components: Vit A (IU) | Vit A (RE) | Retinol (RE) | Carotenoids (RE) | Beta Carotene (mcg) | Vitamins: Thiamin (mg) | Riboflavin (mg) | Niacin (NE) | Vit B6 (mg) | Vit B12 (mcg) | Folate (mcg) | Panto (mg) | Vit C (mg) | Vit D (mg) | Vit E (α TE) | Minerals: Calcium (mg) | Copper (mg) | Iron (mg) | Magnes (mg) | Mang (mg) | Phos (mg) | Potassium (mg) | Selenium (mcg) | Sodium (mg) | Zinc (mg) |
|---|---|---|---|---|---|---|---|---|---|---|---|---|---|---|---|---|---|---|---|---|---|---|---|---|---|---|---|---|---|---|---|---|---|---|---|---|---|---|---|---|---|---|
| 5577 | 1/2 cup | Peas & Onions, cnd, avg | 60 | 31 | 86 | 2.0 | 5.1 | 1.4 | | | 0.2 | 0.0 | 0.0 | 0.1 | 0.02 | 0.09 | 0 | 97 | 10 | 0 | 10 | 57 | 0.06 | 0.04 | 0.77 | 0.12 | 0.00 | 16.0 | 0.10 | 1.8 | 0.0 | | 10 | 0.1 | 0.5 | 10 | 0.2 | 31 | 58 | 0.2 | 265 | 0.35 |
| 6090 | 1/2 cup | Peas & Onions, fzn, ckd, avg | 90 | 40 | 88 | 2.3 | 7.8 | 2.0 | 3.2 | 2.6 | 0.2 | 0.0 | 0.0 | 0.1 | 0.01 | 0.07 | 0 | 312 | 32 | 0 | 32 | 186 | 0.14 | 0.06 | 0.94 | 0.08 | 0.00 | 17.9 | 0.08 | 6.2 | 0.0 | | 13 | 0.1 | 0.8 | 12 | 0.1 | 31 | 105 | 0.4 | 33 | 0.26 |
| 56729 | 1/2 cup | Peas & Potatoes, w/cream sauce, Birds Eye | 114 | 75 | 85 | 3.6 | 11.8 | 2.7 | 4.5 | 4.6 | 1.8 | 0.8 | 0.5 | 0.5 | | | 3 | 302 | 60 | | | | 0.14 | 0.11 | 0.80 | 0.11 | 0.23 | 24.1 | 0.31 | 8.6 | | | 50 | 0.1 | 0.7 | 19 | | 70 | 196 | | 378 | |
| 6354 | 1/2 cup | Santa Fe Style, Green Giant | 59 | 42 | 82 | 1.5 | 8.4 | 1.4 | 1.9 | 5.1 | 0.3 | 0.1 | | | | | 0 | 192 | 19 | 0 | 19 | 115 | | | | | 0.00 | | | 10.9 | | | 9 | | 0.3 | | | | | | 8 | |
| 6353 | 1/2 cup | Seattle Style, Green Giant | 51 | 19 | 90 | 1.0 | 3.6 | 1.5 | 0.7 | 1.4 | 0.1 | 0.0 | | | | | 0 | 860 | 86 | 0 | 86 | 516 | | | | | 0.00 | | | 6.9 | | | 18 | | 0.4 | | | | | | 10 | |
| 7419 | 1/2 cup | Soup Vegetables, Birds Eye | 63 | 33 | 87 | 1.1 | 6.9 | 1.3 | 2.0 | 3.6 | 0.2 | 0.0 | | | | | 0 | 1383 | 138 | 0 | 138 | 830 | | | | | 0.00 | | | 1.6 | | | 9 | | 0.2 | | | | | | 33 | |
| 70616 | 3 oz | Stew Vegetables, Ore Ida | 85 | 49 | 85 | 1.0 | 10.9 | 0.5 | 1.0 | 9.4 | 0.0 | 0.0 | 0.0 | 0.0 | 0.00 | 0.00 | 0 | 638 | 64 | 0 | 64 | 383 | 0.07 | 0.03 | 1.39 | | 0.00 | | | 3.1 | | | 0 | | 0.0 | | | | 198 | | 49 | |
| 5251 | 1/2 cup | Succotash, boiled, avg | 96 | 110 | 68 | 4.9 | 23.4 | 4.3 | 4.3 | 14.8 | 0.8 | 0.1 | 0.1 | 0.4 | 0.06 | 0.31 | 0 | 282 | 28 | 0 | 28 | 167 | 0.16 | 0.09 | 1.28 | 0.11 | 0.00 | 31.5 | 0.54 | 7.9 | 0.0 | | 16 | 0.2 | 1.5 | 51 | 0.7 | 112 | 394 | 0.6 | 16 | 0.60 |
| 5601 | 1/2 cup | Succotash, cnd, avg | 128 | 81 | 82 | 3.3 | 17.9 | 3.3 | 2.9 | 11.6 | 0.6 | 0.1 | 0.1 | 0.3 | 0.05 | 0.25 | 0 | 187 | 19 | 0 | 19 | 115 | 0.04 | 0.07 | 0.82 | 0.06 | 0.00 | 40.6 | 0.40 | 5.9 | 0.0 | | 14 | 0.1 | 0.7 | 24 | 0.5 | 70 | 209 | 0.8 | 283 | 0.64 |
| 5154 | 1/2 cup | Succotash, fzn, ckd, avg | 85 | 79 | 74 | 3.7 | 17.0 | 3.5 | 2.9 | 10.6 | 0.8 | 0.1 | 0.1 | 0.4 | 0.06 | 0.31 | 0 | 196 | 20 | 0 | 20 | 117 | 0.06 | 0.06 | 1.11 | 0.08 | 0.00 | 28.2 | 0.20 | 5.0 | 0.0 | | 13 | 0.1 | 0.8 | 20 | 0.2 | 60 | 225 | 0.5 | 38 | 0.38 |
| 5805 | 3 oz | Succotash, raw, avg | 85 | 84 | 73 | 4.3 | 16.7 | 3.2 | 3.2 | 10.2 | 0.9 | 0.2 | 0.2 | 0.4 | 0.06 | 0.35 | 0 | 248 | 25 | 0 | 25 | 148 | 0.18 | 0.07 | 1.35 | 0.11 | 0.00 | 33.9 | 0.11 | 12.8 | 0.0 | | 15 | 0.2 | 1.6 | 41 | 0.6 | 96 | 314 | 0.5 | 3 | 0.52 |
| 5600 | 1/2 cup | Succotash, w/creamed corn, cnd, avg | 133 | 102 | 78 | 3.5 | 23.4 | 4.0 | 4.0 | 15.4 | 0.7 | 0.1 | 0.1 | 0.3 | 0.05 | 0.29 | 0 | 188 | 19 | 0 | 19 | 112 | 0.04 | 0.09 | 0.81 | 0.17 | 0.00 | 58.9 | 0.29 | 8.5 | 0.0 | | 15 | 0.2 | 0.7 | 1 | 0.9 | 78 | 243 | 0.8 | 326 | 0.57 |
| 6352 | 3 oz | Western Style, Green Giant | 85 | 62 | 83 | 1.5 | 10.6 | 2.5 | 1.1 | 7.1 | 1.5 | 0.3 | | | | | 0 | 151 | 15 | 0 | 15 | 91 | | | | | 0.00 | | | 3.7 | | | 20 | | 0.4 | | | | | | 13 | |
| 6344 | 3 oz | With Butter Sauce, Green Giant | 85 | 54 | 84 | 2.0 | 9.5 | 2.6 | 2.7 | 4.3 | 1.5 | 1.0 | | | | | 3 | 1673 | 335 | | | | | | | | 0.00 | | | 2.2 | | | 19 | | 0.5 | | | | | | 196 | |
| | | Mung Bean Sprouts | | | | | | | | | | | | | | | | | | | | | | | | | | | | | | | | | | | | | | | | |
| 5197 | 1/2 cup | Canned, drained, avg | 62 | 7 | 96 | 0.9 | 1.3 | 0.5 | 0.4 | 0.4 | 0.0 | 0.0 | 0.0 | 0.0 | 0.00 | 0.01 | 0 | 14 | 1 | 0 | 1 | 7 | 0.02 | 0.04 | 0.14 | 0.02 | 0.00 | 6.0 | 0.09 | 0.2 | 0.0 | | 9 | 0.1 | 0.3 | 6 | 0.0 | 20 | 17 | 0.4 | 87 | 0.17 |
| 6459 | 2 oz | Canned, La Choy | 57 | 9 | 96 | 0.7 | 1.5 | 0.7 | 0.0 | 0.8 | 0.0 | 0.0 | | | | | 0 | 0 | 0 | 0 | 0 | 0 | | | | | 0.00 | | | 9.7 | | | 7 | | 0.2 | | | | | | 14 | |
| 5020 | 1/2 cup | Raw, avg | 52 | 16 | 90 | 1.6 | 3.1 | 0.9 | 1.1 | 1.1 | 0.1 | 0.0 | 0.0 | 0.0 | 0.01 | 0.02 | 0 | 11 | 1 | 0 | 1 | 6 | 0.04 | 0.06 | 0.39 | 0.05 | 0.00 | 31.6 | 0.20 | 6.9 | 0.0 | | 7 | 0.1 | 0.5 | 11 | 0.1 | 28 | 77 | 0.3 | 3 | 0.21 |
| 5246 | 1/2 cup | Stir Fried, avg | 62 | 31 | 84 | 2.7 | 6.6 | 1.2 | 2.5 | 2.9 | 0.1 | 0.0 | 0.0 | 0.0 | 0.01 | 0.04 | 0 | 19 | 2 | 0 | 2 | 11 | 0.09 | 0.11 | 0.74 | 0.08 | 0.00 | 43.2 | 0.35 | 9.9 | 0.0 | | 8 | 0.2 | 1.2 | 20 | 0.2 | 49 | 136 | 0.4 | 6 | 0.56 |
| 6828 | 1/2 cup | Mountain Yam, ckd, avg | 72 | 59 | 77 | 1.2 | 14.4 | 2.2 | | | 0.1 | 0.0 | 0.0 | 0.0 | 0.00 | 0.02 | 0 | 0 | 0 | 0 | 0 | 0 | 0.06 | 0.01 | 0.09 | 0.15 | 0.00 | 8.7 | 0.35 | 0.0 | | | 6 | 0.1 | 0.3 | 7 | 0.2 | 29 | 356 | 0.6 | 9 | 0.23 |
| 6827 | 1/2 cup | Mountain Yam, raw, avg | 68 | 46 | 81 | 0.9 | 11.1 | 2.0 | | | 0.1 | 0.0 | 0.0 | 0.0 | 0.00 | 0.03 | 0 | 0 | 0 | 0 | 0 | 0 | 0.07 | 0.01 | 0.33 | 0.12 | 0.00 | 9.5 | 0.29 | 1.8 | 0.0 | | 18 | 0.1 | 0.3 | 8 | 0.2 | 23 | 284 | 0.5 | 9 | 0.18 |
| | | Mushrooms | | | | | | | | | | | | | | | | | | | | | | | | | | | | | | | | | | | | | | | | |
| 5514 | 5 ea | Batter Dipped, fried, avg | 70 | 148 | 66 | 2.3 | 8.2 | 0.7 | 1.9 | 5.6 | 12.2 | 2.1 | 3.0 | 6.4 | | | 14 | 35 | 10 | 9 | 0.4 | 2 | 0.07 | 0.22 | 1.64 | 0.05 | 0.06 | 7.8 | 0.91 | 1.3 | | | 54 | 0.2 | 0.8 | 8 | 0.1 | 103 | 180 | | 120 | 0.42 |
| 6274 | 1 ea | Broiled in Butter, svg, cnd, B&B | 120 | 30 | 93 | 2.8 | 4.0 | 2.0 | 1.4 | 0.5 | 0.4 | 0.2 | | | | | 0 | 0 | 0 | 0 | 0 | 0 | | | | | 0.00 | | | 0.0 | | | 7 | | 0.5 | | | | | | 462 | |
| 5094 | 1/2 cup | Canned, drained, avg | 78 | 19 | 91 | 1.5 | 3.9 | 1.9 | 0.1 | 1.9 | 0.2 | 0.0 | 0.0 | 0.1 | 0.00 | 0.09 | 0 | 0 | 0 | 0 | 0 | 0 | 0.07 | 0.02 | 1.24 | 0.05 | 0.00 | 9.6 | 0.63 | 0.0 | 0.8 | 0.0 | 9 | 0.2 | 0.6 | 12 | 0.1 | 51 | 101 | 3.2 | 331 | 0.56 |
| 6616 | 1/2 cup | Canned, Green Giant | 120 | 28 | 93 | 2.5 | 4.0 | 1.8 | 1.0 | 1.2 | 0.2 | 0.0 | | | | | 0 | 0 | 0 | 0 | 0 | 0 | | | | | 0.00 | | | 0.0 | | | 6 | | 0.4 | | | | | | 438 | |
| 6113 | 1/4 cup | Chanterelle, dried, avg | 36 | 122 | 12 | 6.5 | 18.6 | 7.1 | 0.0 | 11.6 | 2.4 | 0.3 | 1.1 | 1.0 | | | 0 | 8 | 1 | 0 | 1 | 5 | | | | | 0.00 | | | 0.4 | | | 17 | | 4.1 | | | | | | 12 | |
| 7350 | 3 oz | Enoki, raw, Freida's Specialty Produce | 85 | 34 | 89 | 1.7 | 6.0 | 2.6 | 1.7 | 1.7 | 0.0 | 0.0 | 0.0 | 0.0 | 0.00 | 0.00 | 0 | 0 | 0 | 0 | 0 | 0 | | | | | 0.00 | | | 0.0 | | | 0 | | 0.9 | | | | | | 0 | |
| 7338 | 10 pce | Morel, dried, Freida's Specialty Produce | 13 | 49 | 14 | 3.3 | 6.5 | 0.0 | 0.0 | 6.5 | 0.0 | 0.0 | 0.0 | 0.0 | 0.00 | 0.00 | 0 | 0 | 0 | 0 | 0 | 0 | | | | | 0.00 | | | 0.0 | | | 0 | | 2.3 | | | | | | 0 | |
| 6110 | 1/4 cup | Oyster, dried, World Variety Produce | 36 | 130 | 7 | 9.7 | 19.5 | 3.7 | | | 1.5 | 0.2 | 0.3 | 1.0 | | | 0 | 4 | 0.4 | 0 | 0.4 | 2 | | | | | 0.00 | | | 2.3 | | | 4 | | 3.4 | | | | | | 35 | |
| 7309 | 3 oz | Oyster, raw, American Mushroom Institute | 85 | 28 | 91 | 3.7 | 2.8 | 0.9 | 0.9 | 0.9 | 0.0 | 0.0 | 0.0 | 0.0 | 0.00 | 0.00 | 0 | 0 | 0 | 0 | 0 | 0 | | | | | 0.00 | | | 0.0 | | | 0 | | 1.3 | | | | | | 28 | |
| 5614 | 1/2 cup | Pickled, avg | 78 | 18 | 92 | 1.4 | 3.6 | 0.9 | 1.3 | 1.4 | 0.3 | 0.0 | 0.0 | 0.1 | 0.00 | 0.11 | 0 | 0 | 0 | 0 | 0 | 0 | 0.05 | 0.27 | 2.35 | 0.06 | 0.00 | 9.2 | 1.48 | 1.8 | 0.8 | | 4 | 0.3 | 0.8 | 8 | 0.1 | 64 | 232 | | 158 | 0.47 |
| 6111 | 1/4 cup | Porcini, dried, World Variety Produce | 36 | 127 | 9 | 11.1 | 17.7 | 5.8 | 0.8 | 11.1 | 1.4 | 0.2 | 0.7 | 0.6 | | | | 4 | 0.4 | 0 | 0.4 | 2 | | | | | 0.00 | | | 0.2 | | | 10 | | 7.5 | | | | | | 14 | |
| 7346 | 10 pce | Portabella, dried, Freida's Specialty Produce | 6 | 0 | | 1.5 | 1.5 | 0.0 | 0.0 | 1.5 | 0.0 | 0.0 | 0.0 | 0.0 | 0.00 | 0.00 | 0 | 0 | 0 | 0 | 0 | 0 | | | | | 0.00 | | | 0.0 | | | 0 | | 0.0 | | | | | | 0 | |
| 7310 | 3 oz | Portabella, raw, American Mushroom Institute | 85 | 20 | 91 | 3.0 | 4.0 | 3.0 | 1.0 | 0.0 | 0.0 | 0.0 | 0.0 | 0.0 | 0.00 | 0.00 | 0 | 0 | 0 | 0 | 0 | 0 | | | | | 0.00 | | | | | | 40 | | 0.4 | | | | | | 10 | |
| 5090 | 1/2 cup | Raw, sliced, avg | 35 | 9 | 92 | 0.7 | 1.6 | 0.4 | 0.5 | 0.7 | 0.1 | 0.0 | 0.0 | 0.1 | 0.00 | 0.06 | 0 | 0 | 0 | 0 | 0 | 0 | 0.04 | 0.16 | 1.44 | 0.03 | 0.00 | 7.4 | 0.77 | 1.2 | 0.7 | 0.0 | 2 | 0.2 | 0.4 | 3 | 0.0 | 36 | 129 | 4.3 | 1 | 0.26 |
| 5385 | 1/2 cup | Shiitake, ckd, pces, avg | 72 | 40 | 84 | 1.1 | 10.3 | 1.5 | | | 0.2 | 0.0 | 0.0 | 0.0 | 0.00 | 0.02 | 0 | 0 | 0 | 0 | 0 | 0 | 0.03 | 0.12 | 1.08 | 0.11 | 0.00 | 15.0 | 2.58 | 0.2 | 5.0 | | 2 | 0.6 | 0.3 | 10 | 0.1 | 21 | 84 | 17.9 | 3 | 0.96 |
| 5383 | 4 ea | Shiitake, dried, avg | 15 | 44 | 10 | 1.4 | 11.3 | 1.7 | | | 0.1 | 0.0 | 0.0 | 0.0 | 0.00 | 0.02 | 0 | 0 | 0 | 0 | 0 | 0 | 0.05 | 0.19 | 2.12 | 0.14 | 0.00 | 24.5 | 3.29 | 0.5 | 6.2 | | 2 | 0.8 | 0.3 | 20 | 0.2 | 44 | 230 | 20.4 | 2 | 1.15 |
| 7308 | 3 oz | Shiitake, raw, American Mushroom Institute | 85 | 33 | 91 | 1.9 | 4.7 | 0.9 | 0.9 | 2.8 | 0.0 | 0.0 | 0.0 | 0.0 | 0.00 | 0.00 | 0 | 0 | 0 | 0 | 0 | 0 | | | | | 0.00 | | | 2.2 | | | 0 | | 1.3 | | | | | | 19 | |
| 5657 | 1/2 cup | Steamed, sliced, avg | 78 | 19 | 92 | 1.6 | 3.6 | 0.9 | 1.1 | 1.6 | 0.3 | 0.0 | 0.0 | 0.1 | 0.00 | 0.13 | 0 | 0 | 0 | 0 | 0 | 0 | 0.07 | 0.33 | 3.07 | 0.07 | 0.00 | 14.0 | 1.57 | 2.3 | 0.0 | 0.1 | 4 | 0.4 | 1.0 | 8 | 0.1 | 81 | 289 | | 3 | 0.57 |
| 5643 | 3 ea | Stuffed, avg | 72 | 169 | 56 | 6.4 | 11.8 | 1.4 | 2.6 | 7.8 | 11.0 | 3.2 | 4.4 | 2.7 | | | 9 | 426 | 105 | 91 | 14 | 82 | 0.13 | 0.36 | 3.38 | 0.10 | 0.14 | 17.7 | 1.87 | 4.7 | 0.9 | | 104 | 0.4 | 1.4 | 16 | 0.1 | 147 | 312 | | 418 | 0.90 |
| | | Mustard Greens | | | | | | | | | | | | | | | | | | | | | | | | | | | | | | | | | | | | | | | | |
| 5096 | 1/2 cup | Boiled, avg | 70 | 10 | 94 | 1.6 | 1.5 | 1.4 | 0.0 | 0.1 | 0.2 | 0.0 | 0.1 | 0.0 | 0.02 | 0.02 | 0 | 2122 | 212 | 0 | 212 | 1273 | 0.03 | 0.04 | 0.30 | 0.07 | 0.00 | 51.4 | 0.08 | 17.7 | 0.0 | 1.4 | 52 | 0.1 | 0.5 | 10 | 0.2 | 29 | 141 | 0.4 | 11 | 0.08 |
| 5097 | 1/2 cup | Frozen, boiled, avg | 75 | 14 | 94 | 1.7 | 2.3 | 2.1 | 0.1 | 0.2 | 0.2 | 0.0 | 0.1 | 0.0 | 0.02 | 0.02 | 0 | 3353 | 335 | 0 | 335 | 2012 | 0.03 | 0.04 | 0.19 | 0.08 | 0.00 | 52.1 | 0.01 | 10.4 | 0.0 | 1.3 | 76 | 0.0 | 0.8 | 10 | 0.2 | 18 | 104 | 0.5 | 19 | 0.15 |
| 7298 | 1 oz | Leaves, raw, avg | 28 | 10 | 90 | 1.1 | 0.9 | | | | 0.2 | | | | | | | 0 | 0 | 0 | 0 | 0 | 0.01 | | | | 0.00 | | | 9.2 | | | 43 | | 0.4 | | | | | | | |
| | | Okra | | | | | | | | | | | | | | | | | | | | | | | | | | | | | | | | | | | | | | | | |
| 5644 | 1/2 cup | Batter Dipped, fried, avg | 46 | 87 | 69 | 1.4 | 5.8 | 1.0 | | | 6.7 | 1.1 | 1.7 | 3.6 | | | 8 | 180 | 21 | 5 | 16 | 94 | 0.07 | 0.05 | 0.38 | 0.06 | 0.03 | 18.7 | 0.09 | 5.2 | 0.1 | | 52 | 0.0 | 0.4 | 18 | 0.3 | 53 | 107 | | 69 | 0.25 |
| 5100 | 1/2 cup | Frozen, boiled, avg | 92 | 26 | 91 | 1.9 | 5.3 | 2.6 | 1.8 | 0.9 | 0.3 | 0.1 | 0.0 | 0.1 | 0.00 | 0.07 | 0 | 473 | 47 | 0 | 47 | 270 | 0.09 | 0.11 | 0.72 | 0.04 | 0.00 | 134.3 | 0.22 | 11.2 | 0.0 | | 88 | 0.1 | 0.6 | 47 | 0.9 | 42 | 215 | 0.6 | 3 | 0.57 |
| 5775 | 1/2 cup | Raw, avg | 50 | 16 | 90 | 1.0 | 3.8 | 1.6 | 1.2 | 1.0 | 0.1 | 0.0 | 0.0 | 0.0 | 0.00 | 0.01 | 0 | 330 | 33 | 0 | 33 | 190 | 0.10 | 0.03 | 0.50 | 0.11 | 0.00 | 43.9 | 0.12 | 10.6 | 0.0 | | 40 | 0.0 | 0.4 | 28 | 0.5 | 32 | 152 | 0.3 | 4 | 0.30 |
| 5099 | 1/2 cup | Raw, boiled, avg | 80 | 26 | 90 | 1.5 | 5.8 | 2.0 | 1.6 | 2.2 | 0.1 | 0.0 | 0.0 | 0.0 | 0.00 | 0.04 | 0 | 460 | 46 | 0 | 46 | 266 | 0.11 | 0.04 | 0.70 | 0.15 | 0.00 | 36.6 | 0.17 | 13.0 | 0.0 | | 50 | 0.1 | 0.4 | 46 | 0.7 | 45 | 258 | 0.6 | 4 | 0.44 |
| | | Onions | | | | | | | | | | | | | | | | | | | | | | | | | | | | | | | | | | | | | | | | |
| 5108 | 1/2 cup | Boiled, avg | 105 | 46 | 88 | 1.4 | 10.7 | 1.5 | 6.5 | 2.7 | 0.2 | 0.0 | 0.0 | 0.1 | 0.00 | 0.07 | 0 | 0 | 0 | 0 | 0 | 0 | 0.04 | 0.02 | 0.17 | 0.14 | 0.00 | 15.7 | 0.12 | 5.5 | 0.0 | 0.1 | 23 | 0.1 | 0.3 | 12 | 0.2 | 37 | 174 | 0.6 | 3 | 0.22 |
| 7367 | 3 ea | Boiler, raw, Freida's Specialty Produce | 85 | 30 | 90 | 1.0 | 7.0 | 2.0 | 5.0 | 0.0 | 0.0 | 0.0 | 0.0 | 0.0 | 0.00 | 0.00 | 0 | 0 | 0 | 0 | 0 | 0 | | | | | 0.00 | | | 6.0 | | | 0 | | 0.0 | | | | | | 0 | |
| 5574 | 1/2 cup | Canned, avg | 112 | 21 | 94 | 1.0 | 4.5 | 1.3 | | | 0.1 | 0.0 | 0.0 | 0.0 | 0.00 | 0.04 | 0 | 0 | 0 | 0 | 0 | 0 | 0.04 | 0.01 | 0.07 | 0.15 | 0.00 | 10.9 | 0.11 | 4.8 | 0.0 | | 50 | 0.1 | 0.1 | 7 | 0.1 | 31 | 124 | 0.3 | 416 | 0.32 |
| 6621 | 1/2 cup | Canned, whole, Green Giant | 122 | 38 | 91 | 0.9 | 8.4 | 1.1 | 4.9 | 2.4 | 0.1 | 0.0 | | | | | 0 | 0 | 0 | 0 | 0 | 0 | | | | | 0.00 | | | 0.5 | | | 18 | | 0.5 | | | | | | 407 | |
| 5532 | 1/2 cup | Creamed, avg | 114 | 100 | 82 | 2.6 | 11.0 | 1.3 | 5.7 | 4.0 | 5.5 | 1.7 | 2.2 | 1.3 | 0.00 | | 5 | 196 | 57 | 52 | 5 | 31 | 0.05 | 0.09 | 0.25 | 0.11 | 0.14 | 12.8 | 0.21 | 4.0 | 0.4 | | 65 | 0.1 | 0.3 | 13 | 0.1 | 65 | 177 | | 334 | 0.31 |
| 5113 | 1 Tbs | Flakes, dehydrated, avg | 4 | 14 | 4 | 0.4 | 3.3 | 0.4 | 2.7 | 0.3 | 0.0 | 0.0 | 0.0 | 0.0 | 0.00 | 0.01 | 0 | 0 | 0 | 0 | 0 | 0 | 0.02 | 0.00 | 0.04 | 0.06 | 0.00 | 6.6 | 0.06 | 3.0 | 0.0 | 0.0 | 10 | 0.0 | 0.1 | 4 | 0.1 | 12 | 65 | 0.2 | 1 | 0.08 |
| 5300 | 1/2 cup | Frozen, chpd, boiled, avg | 105 | 29 | 92 | 0.8 | 6.9 | 1.9 | 4.3 | 0.7 | 0.1 | 0.0 | 0.0 | 0.0 | 0.00 | 0.04 | 0 | 36 | 3 | 0 | 3 | 19 | 0.02 | 0.03 | 0.15 | 0.07 | 0.00 | 14.1 | 0.10 | 2.7 | 0.0 | | 17 | 0.0 | 0.3 | 6 | 0.1 | 20 | 113 | 0.4 | 13 | 0.07 |
| 5530 | 1/2 cup | Pearl, pickled, avg | 92 | 40 | 87 | 1.2 | 9.3 | 1.5 | 3.6 | 4.2 | 0.2 | 0.0 | 0.0 | 0.1 | 0.00 | 0.06 | 0 | 0 | 0 | 0 | 0 | 0 | 0.04 | 0.02 | 0.15 | 0.12 | 0.00 | 13.7 | 0.07 | 4.8 | 0.0 | 0.2 | 20 | 0.1 | 0.2 | 10 | 0.1 | 32 | 152 | 0.4 | 215 | 0.19 |
| 5101 | 1/2 cup | Raw, chpd, avg | 80 | 30 | 90 | 0.9 | 6.9 | 1.4 | 5.0 | 0.5 | 0.1 | 0.0 | 0.0 | 0.0 | 0.00 | 0.05 | 0 | 0 | 0 | 0 | 0 | 0 | 0.03 | 0.02 | 0.12 | 0.09 | 0.00 | 15.2 | 0.08 | 5.1 | 0.0 | 0.1 | 16 | 0.0 | 0.2 | 8 | 0.1 | 26 | 126 | 0.5 | 2 | 0.15 |
| 5190 | 2 ea | Rings, fzn, ckd, avg | 20 | 81 | 28 | 1.1 | 7.6 | 0.3 | 1.9 | 5.5 | 5.3 | 1.7 | 2.2 | 1.0 | 0.06 | 0.96 | 0 | 45 | 5 | 0 | 5 | 28 | 0.06 | 0.03 | 0.72 | 0.02 | 0.00 | 13.2 | 0.05 | 0.3 | 0.0 | 0.1 | 6 | 0.0 | 0.3 | 4 | 0.1 | 16 | 26 | 0.7 | 75 | 0.08 |
| 56725 | 1/2 cup | Small, w/cream sauce, Birds Eye | 126 | 58 | 89 | 1.8 | 9.8 | 1.5 | 5.2 | 3.2 | 1.6 | 0.7 | 0.5 | 0.4 | | | 4 | 51 | 10 | | | | 0.03 | 0.09 | 0.13 | 0.08 | 0.25 | 15.1 | 0.23 | 5.8 | | | 66 | 0.0 | 3.4 | 11 | | 43 | 164 | | 325 | |
| 5114 | 1/2 cup | Spring/Green, avg | 50 | 16 | 90 | 0.9 | 3.7 | 1.3 | 1.6 | 0.8 | 0.1 | 0.0 | 0.0 | 0.0 | 0.00 | 0.04 | 0 | 193 | 20 | 0 | 20 | 117 | 0.03 | 0.04 | 0.26 | 0.03 | 0.00 | 32.0 | 0.04 | 9.4 | 0.0 | 0.1 | 36 | 0.0 | 0.7 | 10 | 0.1 | 18 | 138 | 0.3 | 8 | 0.19 |
| 5649 | 1/2 cup | Steamed, avg | 105 | 40 | 90 | 1.2 | 9.1 | 1.9 | 6.5 | 0.7 | 0.2 | 0.0 | 0.0 | 0.1 | 0.00 | 0.06 | 0 | 0 | 0 | 0 | 0 | 0 | 0.04 | 0.02 | 0.15 | 0.12 | 0.00 | 16.2 | 0.11 | 5.1 | 0.0 | 0.3 | 21 | 0.1 | 0.2 | 10 | 0.1 | 35 | 165 | | 3 | 0.20 |
| 5650 | 1/2 cup | Stir Fried, avg | 105 | 40 | 90 | 1.2 | 9.1 | 1.9 | 6.5 | 0.7 | 0.2 | 0.0 | 0.0 | 0.1 | 0.00 | 0.06 | 0 | 0 | 0 | 0 | 0 | 0 | 0.04 | 0.02 | 0.15 | 0.12 | 0.00 | 16.2 | 0.11 | 5.4 | 0.0 | 0.3 | 21 | 0.1 | 0.2 | 10 | 0.1 | 35 | 165 | | 3 | 0.20 |

| Code | Amount | Description | Weight (g) | Calories | % Water | Protein (g) | Carbs (g) | Fiber (g) | Sugar (g) | Other Carbs (g) | Fat (g) | Sat Fat (g) | Mono Fat (g) | Poly Fat (g) | Omega 3 (g) | Omega 6 (g) | Choles (mg) | Vit A (IU) | Vit A (RE) | Retinol (RE) | Carotenoids (RE) | Beta Carotene (mcg) | Thiamin (mg) | Riboflavin (mg) | Niacin (NE) | Vit B6 (mg) | Vit B12 (mcg) | Folate (mcg) | Panto (mg) | Vit C (mg) | Vit D (mg) | Vit E (α TE) | Calcium (mg) | Copper (mg) | Iron (mg) | Magnes (mg) | Mang (mg) | Phos (mg) | Potassium (mg) | Selenium (mcg) | Sodium (mg) | Zinc (mg) |
|---|---|---|---|---|---|---|---|---|---|---|---|---|---|---|---|---|---|---|---|---|---|---|---|---|---|---|---|---|---|---|---|---|---|---|---|---|---|---|---|---|---|---|
| | | | Basic Components | | | | | | | | | Additional Fats | | | | | | Vit A & Components | | | | | Vitamins | | | | | | | | | | Minerals | | | | | | | | | |
| 7270 | 1/2 cup | Palm Hearts, cnd, avg | 73 | 20 | 90 | 1.8 | 3.4 | 1.8 | | | 0.5 | 0.1 | 0.1 | 0.1 | 0.01 | 0.13 | 0 | 0 | [illegible] | 0 | 0 | 0 | 0.01 | 0.04 | 0.32 | 0.02 | 0.00 | 28.5 | 0.09 | 5.8 | | | 42 | 0.1 | 2.3 | 28 | 1.0 | 47 | 129 | 0.5 | 311 | 0.84 |
| 5522 | 1/2 cup | Palm Hearts, ckd, avg | 73 | 75 | 70 | 2.0 | 19.4 | 1.1 | | | 0.1 | 0.1 | 0.0 | [illegible] | | | 0 | 47 | 5 | 0 | 5 | 29 | 0.03 | 0.12 | 0.62 | 0.53 | 0.00 | 14.9 | | 5.0 | 0.0 | | 13 | 0.5 | 1.2 | 7 | | 102 | 1318 | | 10 | 2.72 |
| 5212 | 1/2 cup | Parsnips, raw, boiled, avg | 78 | 63 | 78 | 1.0 | 15.2 | 3.1 | 4.3 | 7.8 | 0.2 | 0.0 | 0.1 | 0.0 | 0.00 | 0.03 | 0 | 0 | [illegible] | 0 | 0 | 0 | 0.06 | 0.04 | 0.56 | 0.07 | 0.00 | 45.4 | 0.46 | 10.1 | 0.0 | 0.8 | 29 | 0.1 | 0.5 | 23 | 0.2 | 54 | 286 | 1.3 | 8 | 0.20 |
| 5211 | 1/2 cup | Parsnips, raw, sliced, avg | 66 | 50 | 80 | 0.8 | 11.9 | 3.2 | 3.2 | 5.5 | 0.2 | 0.0 | 0.1 | 0.0 | 0.00 | 0.03 | 0 | 0 | [illegible] | 0 | 0 | 0 | 0.06 | 0.03 | 0.46 | 0.06 | 0.00 | 44.1 | 0.40 | 11.2 | 0.0 | 0.7 | 24 | 0.1 | 0.4 | 19 | 0.4 | 47 | 248 | 1.2 | 7 | 0.39 |
| | | Peas | | | | | | | | | | | | | | | | | | | | | | | | | | | | | | | | | | | | | | | | |
| 5117 | 1/2 cup | Green, boiled, avg | 80 | 67 | 78 | 4.3 | 12.5 | 4.4 | 4.6 | 3.4 | 0.2 | 0.0 | 0.0 | 0.1 | 0.02 | 0.07 | 0 | 473 | 48 | 0 | 48 | 278 | 0.21 | 0.12 | 1.62 | 0.17 | 0.00 | 50.6 | 0.12 | 11.4 | 0.0 | | 22 | 0.1 | 1.2 | 31 | 0.4 | 94 | 217 | 1.5 | 2 | 0.95 |
| 5214 | 1/2 cup | Green, cnd w/liquid, avg | 124 | 66 | 86 | 4.0 | 12.1 | 4.0 | 3.1 | 5.0 | 0.4 | 0.1 | 0.0 | 0.2 | 0.03 | 0.13 | 0 | 477 | 47 | 0 | 47 | 273 | 0.14 | 0.09 | 1.04 | 0.08 | 0.00 | 35.3 | 0.11 | 12.2 | 0.0 | | 22 | 0.1 | 1.3 | 21 | 0.3 | 66 | 124 | 1.6 | 310 | 0.87 |
| 5267 | 1/2 cup | Green, cnd w/liquid, unsalted, avg | 124 | 66 | 86 | 4.0 | 12.1 | 4.0 | 3.1 | 5.0 | 0.4 | 0.1 | 0.0 | 0.2 | 0.03 | 0.14 | 0 | 477 | 47 | 0 | 47 | 273 | 0.14 | 0.09 | 1.04 | 0.08 | 0.00 | 35.3 | 0.11 | 12.2 | 0.0 | | 22 | 0.1 | 1.3 | 21 | 0.3 | 66 | 124 | 1.6 | 11 | 0.87 |
| 6624 | 1/2 cup | Green, cnd, 50% less sod, Green Giant | 120 | 61 | 87 | 4.1 | 10.6 | 4.1 | 3.1 | 3.4 | 0.2 | 0.0 | | | | | 0 | 367 | 37 | 0 | 37 | 213 | | | | | 0.00 | | | 6.6 | | | 22 | | 1.0 | | | | | | 188 | |
| 5118 | 1/2 cup | Green, fzn, boiled, avg | 80 | 62 | 80 | 4.1 | 11.4 | 4.4 | 4.4 | 2.6 | 0.2 | 0.0 | 0.0 | 0.1 | 0.02 | 0.08 | 0 | 534 | 54 | 0 | 54 | 311 | 0.23 | 0.08 | 1.18 | 0.09 | 0.00 | 46.9 | 0.11 | 7.9 | 0.0 | | 19 | 0.1 | 1.3 | 23 | 0.3 | 72 | 134 | 0.8 | 70 | 0.75 |
| 5116 | 1/2 cup | Green, raw, avg | 72 | 58 | 79 | 3.9 | 10.4 | 3.7 | 4.0 | 2.7 | 0.3 | 0.1 | 0.0 | 0.1 | 0.03 | 0.11 | 0 | 461 | 46 | 0 | 46 | 267 | 0.19 | 0.10 | 1.50 | 0.12 | 0.00 | 46.8 | 0.07 | 28.8 | 0.0 | 0.1 | 18 | 0.1 | 1.1 | 24 | 0.3 | 78 | 176 | 1.3 | 4 | 0.89 |
| 6360 | 1/2 cup | Green, w/butter sauce, Green Giant | 57 | 48 | 80 | 1.9 | 7.8 | 2.3 | 2.1 | 3.4 | 1.1 | 0.8 | | | | | 2 | 285 | 57 | | | | | | | | 0.00 | | | 2.2 | | | 10 | | 0.8 | | | | | | 198 | |
| 5783 | 1/2 cup | Pigeon, boiled, avg | 76 | 84 | 72 | 4.5 | 14.8 | 4.7 | | | 1.0 | 0.3 | 0.0 | 0.7 | 0.03 | 0.65 | 0 | 99 | 10 | 0 | 10 | 57 | 0.27 | 0.13 | 1.63 | 0.04 | 0.00 | 76.0 | 0.48 | 21.4 | 0.0 | | 31 | 0.1 | 1.2 | 30 | 0.3 | 90 | 347 | 0.9 | 4 | 0.62 |
| 5781 | 1/2 cup | Pigeon, raw, avg | 77 | 105 | 66 | 5.5 | 18.4 | 3.9 | | | 1.3 | 0.3 | 0.0 | 0.7 | 0.03 | 0.64 | 0 | 108 | 11 | 0 | 11 | 62 | 0.31 | 0.13 | 1.69 | 0.05 | 0.00 | 133.2 | 0.52 | 30.0 | 0.0 | | 32 | 0.1 | 1.2 | 52 | 0.4 | 98 | 425 | 1.2 | 4 | 0.80 |
| 7020 | 1/2 cup | Split, boiled, avg | 98 | 116 | 70 | 8.2 | 20.7 | 8.1 | 2.8 | 9.7 | 0.4 | 0.1 | 0.1 | 0.2 | 0.03 | 0.13 | 0 | 7 | [illegible] | 0 | 1 | 6 | 0.19 | 0.05 | 0.87 | 0.05 | 0.00 | 63.6 | 0.58 | 0.4 | 0.0 | | 14 | 0.2 | 1.3 | 35 | 0.4 | 97 | 355 | 0.6 | 2 | 0.98 |
| 7019 | 1/2 cup | Split, raw, avg | 98 | 334 | 11 | 24.1 | 59.2 | 25.0 | 7.8 | 26.4 | 1.1 | 0.2 | 0.2 | 0.5 | 0.08 | 0.40 | 0 | 146 | 15 | 0 | 15 | 85 | 0.71 | 0.21 | 2.83 | 0.17 | 0.00 | 268.5 | 1.72 | 1.8 | 0.0 | | 54 | 0.8 | 4.3 | 113 | 1.4 | 359 | 961 | 1.6 | 15 | 2.95 |
| | | Peas, Edible Pods | | | | | | | | | | | | | | | | | | | | | | | | | | | | | | | | | | | | | | | | |
| 5296 | 1/2 cup | Frozen, boiled, avg | 80 | 42 | 87 | 2.8 | 7.2 | 2.5 | 3.7 | 1.1 | 0.3 | 0.1 | 0.0 | 0.1 | 0.02 | 0.11 | 0 | 134 | 14 | 0 | 14 | 79 | 0.05 | 0.10 | 0.45 | 0.14 | 0.00 | 28.2 | 0.69 | 17.6 | 0.0 | | 47 | 0.1 | 1.9 | 22 | 0.2 | 46 | 174 | 0.6 | 4 | 0.39 |
| 5122 | 1/2 cup | Snow, boiled, avg | 80 | 34 | 89 | 2.6 | 5.6 | 2.2 | 2.8 | 0.6 | 0.2 | 0.0 | 0.0 | 0.1 | 0.01 | 0.07 | 0 | 105 | 10 | 0 | 10 | 60 | 0.10 | 0.06 | 0.43 | 0.12 | 0.00 | 23.3 | 0.54 | 38.3 | 0.0 | | 34 | 0.1 | 1.6 | 21 | 0.1 | 44 | 192 | 0.6 | 3 | 0.30 |
| 6836 | 1/2 cup | Snow, raw, chpd, avg | 49 | 21 | 89 | 1.4 | 3.7 | 1.3 | 2.0 | 0.5 | 0.1 | 0.0 | 0.0 | 0.0 | 0.01 | 0.04 | 0 | 71 | 7 | 0 | 7 | 40 | 0.07 | 0.04 | 0.29 | 0.08 | 0.00 | 20.4 | 0.37 | 29.4 | 0.0 | | 21 | 0.0 | 1.0 | 12 | 0.1 | 26 | 98 | 0.3 | 2 | 0.13 |
| 5665 | 1/2 cup | Steamed, avg | 82 | 34 | 89 | 2.3 | 6.2 | 2.1 | 3.3 | 0.8 | 0.2 | 0.0 | 0.0 | 0.1 | 0.01 | 0.06 | 0 | 113 | 11 | 0 | 11 | 66 | 0.11 | 0.06 | 0.47 | 0.12 | 0.00 | 29.0 | 0.57 | 41.8 | 0.0 | | 35 | 0.1 | 1.7 | 20 | 0.2 | 43 | 164 | | 3 | 0.22 |
| | | Peppers, Hot | | | | | | | | | | | | | | | | | | | | | | | | | | | | | | | | | | | | | | | | |
| 6469 | 1 Tbs | Cherry, cnd, Progresso | 14 | 16 | | 0.0 | 1.0 | 0.5 | 0.5 | 0.0 | 1.0 | 0.0 | | | | | 0 | 259 | 26 | 0 | 26 | 140 | | | | | 0.00 | | | 9.3 | | | 0 | | 0.0 | | | | | | 16 | |
| 7260 | 1 Tbs | Chile, sun dried, avg | 2 | 6 | 7 | 0.2 | 1.4 | 0.6 | | | 0.1 | 0.0 | 0.0 | 0.1 | 0.00 | 0.06 | 0 | 530 | 53 | 0 | 53 | 311 | 0.00 | 0.02 | 0.17 | 0.02 | 0.00 | 1.0 | 0.02 | 0.6 | | | 1 | 0.0 | 0.1 | 2 | 0.0 | 3 | 37 | 0.1 | 2 | 0.02 |
| 6470 | 1 Tbs | Fried, cnd, Progresso | 14 | 31 | | 0.0 | 1.6 | 0.5 | 1.0 | 0.0 | 2.6 | 0.3 | | | | | 0 | 0 | 0 | 0 | 0 | 0 | | | | | 0.00 | | | 7.8 | | | 0 | | 0.0 | | | | | | 31 | |
| 6301 | 1/4 cup | Green Chiles, cnd, Ortega | 34 | 15 | | 1.0 | 3.0 | 0.0 | 0.0 | 3.0 | 0.0 | 0.0 | 0.0 | 0.0 | 0.00 | 0.00 | 0 | 100 | 10 | 0 | 10 | 59 | | | | | 0.00 | | | 27.0 | | | | | 0.7 | | | | 115 | | 30 | |
| 5399 | 1/4 cup | Green Chili, raw, chpd, avg | 38 | 15 | 88 | 0.8 | 3.6 | 0.6 | 1.9 | 1.1 | 0.1 | 0.0 | 0.0 | 0.0 | 0.00 | 0.04 | 0 | 293 | 29 | 0 | 29 | 172 | 0.03 | 0.03 | 0.36 | 0.11 | 0.00 | 8.9 | 0.02 | 92.3 | 0.0 | | 7 | 0.1 | 0.5 | 9 | 0.1 | 17 | 129 | 0.2 | 3 | 0.11 |
| 5063 | 1/4 cup | Green Chili, cnd, chpd, avg | 34 | 7 | 92 | 0.3 | 1.7 | 0.4 | 1.1 | 0.2 | 0.0 | 0.0 | 0.0 | 0.0 | 0.00 | 0.02 | 0 | 207 | 21 | 0 | 21 | 122 | 0.01 | 0.02 | 0.27 | 0.05 | 0.00 | 3.4 | 0.01 | 23.1 | 0.0 | | 2 | 0.0 | 0.2 | 5 | 0.0 | 6 | 64 | 0.1 | 399 | 0.06 |
| 5293 | 1/4 cup | Jalapenos, cnd, avg | 34 | 9 | 89 | 0.3 | 1.6 | 0.9 | 0.6 | 0.2 | 0.3 | 0.0 | 0.0 | 0.2 | 0.01 | 0.17 | 0 | 578 | 58 | 0 | 58 | 339 | 0.01 | 0.01 | 0.14 | 0.06 | 0.00 | 4.8 | 0.14 | 3.4 | 0.0 | | 8 | 0.0 | 0.6 | 5 | 0.0 | 6 | 66 | 0.1 | 568 | 0.12 |
| 6306 | 1/4 cup | Jalapenos, cnd, Ortega | 34 | 15 | | 1.0 | 3.0 | 1.0 | 1.0 | 1.0 | 0.0 | 0.0 | 0.0 | 0.0 | 0.00 | 0.00 | 0 | 100 | 10 | 0 | 10 | 59 | | | | | 0.00 | | | 27.0 | | | | | 0.7 | | | | 115 | | 30 | |
| 6417 | 1 ea | Jalapenos, pickled, Old El Paso | 13 | 2 | 92 | 0.0 | 0.5 | 0.0 | 0.0 | 0.5 | 0.0 | 0.0 | 0.0 | 0.0 | 0.00 | 0.00 | 0 | | | | | | | | | | 0.00 | | | | | | | | | | | | | | 190 | |
| 6099 | 1 ea | Jalapenos, raw, avg | 45 | 11 | 90 | 0.4 | 2.2 | | | | 0.3 | | | | | | | 304 | 30 | 0 | 30 | 178 | | | | | 0.00 | | | 52.6 | | | | | | | | | 2 | | 2 | |
| 5291 | 1/4 cup | Red Chili, cnd, avg | 34 | 7 | 92 | 0.3 | 1.7 | 0.4 | 0.4 | 0.9 | 0.0 | 0.0 | 0.0 | 0.0 | 0.00 | 0.02 | 0 | 4043 | 404 | 0 | 404 | 2190 | 0.01 | 0.02 | 0.27 | 0.05 | 0.00 | 3.4 | 0.01 | 23.1 | 0.0 | | 2 | 0.0 | 0.2 | 5 | 0.0 | 6 | 64 | 0.1 | 399 | 0.06 |
| 5288 | 1/4 cup | Red Chili, raw, avg | 38 | 15 | 88 | 0.8 | 3.6 | 0.6 | 2.0 | 1.0 | 0.1 | 0.0 | 0.0 | 0.0 | 0.00 | 0.04 | 0 | 4085 | 409 | 0 | 409 | 2213 | 0.03 | 0.03 | 0.36 | 0.11 | 0.00 | 8.9 | 0.02 | 92.3 | 0.0 | | 7 | 0.1 | 0.5 | 9 | 0.1 | 17 | 129 | 0.2 | 3 | 0.11 |
| 6468 | 1/4 ea | Roasted, cnd, Progresso | 14 | 5 | | 0.0 | 0.5 | 0.0 | 0.5 | 0.0 | 0.0 | 0.0 | 0.0 | 0.0 | 0.00 | 0.00 | 0 | 500 | 50 | 0 | 50 | 293 | | | | | 0.00 | | | 10.5 | | | 0 | | 0.4 | | | | | | 30 | |
| 6100 | 1 ea | Serrano, raw, avg | 45 | 20 | 90 | | | | | | | | | | | | | 633 | 63 | 0 | 63 | 372 | | | | | 0.00 | | | 36.8 | | | | | | | | | 2 | | 2 | |
| 6471 | 1 ea | Tuscan, cnd, Progresso | 9 | 3 | | 0.0 | 0.3 | 0.3 | 0.0 | 0.0 | 0.0 | 0.0 | 0.0 | 0.0 | 0.00 | 0.00 | 0 | 0 | 0 | 0 | 0 | 0 | | | | | 0.00 | | | 0.0 | | | 0 | | 0.0 | | | | | | 106 | |
| | | Peppers, Sweet | | | | | | | | | | | | | | | | | | | | | | | | | | | | | | | | | | | | | | | | |
| 5126 | 1/2 cup | Green, boiled, chpd, avg | 68 | 19 | 92 | 0.6 | 4.6 | 0.8 | 2.4 | 1.3 | 0.1 | 0.0 | 0.0 | 0.1 | 0.01 | 0.07 | 0 | 403 | 40 | 0 | 40 | 235 | 0.04 | 0.02 | 0.32 | 0.16 | 0.00 | 10.9 | 0.05 | 50.6 | 0.0 | 0.5 | 6 | 0.0 | 0.3 | 7 | 0.1 | 12 | 113 | 0.2 | 1 | 0.08 |
| 5578 | 1/2 cup | Green, cnd, avg | 70 | 13 | 91 | 0.6 | 2.7 | 0.8 | 1.5 | 0.3 | 0.2 | 0.0 | 0.0 | 0.1 | 0.01 | 0.10 | 0 | 109 | 11 | 0 | 11 | 66 | 0.02 | 0.02 | 0.38 | 0.12 | 0.00 | 11.4 | 0.03 | 32.5 | 0.0 | | 29 | 0.1 | 0.6 | 8 | 0.1 | 14 | 102 | 0.2 | 958 | 0.13 |
| 5284 | 1/2 cup | Green, fzn, boiled, avg | 68 | 12 | 95 | 0.6 | 2.7 | 0.6 | 1.3 | 0.7 | 0.1 | 0.0 | 0.0 | 0.1 | 0.01 | 0.06 | 0 | 197 | 20 | 0 | 20 | 116 | 0.03 | 0.02 | 0.73 | 0.07 | 0.00 | 6.7 | 0.02 | 28.0 | 0.0 | | 5 | 0.0 | 0.4 | 5 | 0.1 | 9 | 49 | 0.1 | 3 | 0.03 |
| 5214 | 1/2 cup | Green, raw, chpd, avg | 74 | 39 | 86 | 2.4 | 7.2 | 2.4 | 1.8 | 3.0 | 0.2 | 0.0 | 0.0 | 0.1 | 0.02 | 0.08 | 0 | 285 | 28 | 0 | 28 | 163 | 0.08 | 0.05 | 0.62 | 0.05 | 0.00 | 21.1 | 0.07 | 7.3 | 0.0 | | 13 | 0.1 | 0.8 | 13 | 0.2 | 39 | 74 | 1.0 | 185 | 0.52 |
| 5661 | 1/2 cup | Green, stmd, avg | 68 | 18 | 92 | 0.6 | 4.4 | 1.2 | 1.7 | 1.5 | 0.1 | 0.0 | 0.0 | 0.1 | 0.01 | 0.06 | 0 | 409 | 41 | 0 | 41 | 240 | 0.04 | 0.02 | 0.33 | 0.15 | 0.00 | 12.7 | 0.05 | 51.7 | 0.0 | 0.5 | 6 | 0.0 | 0.3 | 7 | 0.1 | 13 | 120 | | 1 | 0.08 |
| 5568 | 1/2 cup | Red, cnd, avg | 70 | 13 | 91 | 0.6 | 2.7 | 0.8 | 1.5 | 0.3 | 0.2 | 0.0 | 0.0 | 0.1 | 0.01 | 0.10 | 0 | 364 | 36 | 0 | 36 | 197 | 0.02 | 0.02 | 0.38 | 0.12 | 0.00 | 11.4 | 0.03 | 32.5 | 0.0 | | 29 | 0.1 | 0.6 | 8 | 0.1 | 14 | 102 | 0.2 | 958 | 0.13 |
| 5278 | 1/2 cup | Red, ckd, avg | 68 | 19 | 92 | 0.6 | 4.6 | 0.8 | 2.2 | 1.5 | 0.1 | 0.0 | 0.0 | 0.1 | 0.01 | 0.07 | 0 | 2557 | 256 | 0 | 256 | 1385 | 0.04 | 0.02 | 0.32 | 0.16 | 0.00 | 10.9 | 0.05 | 116.3 | 0.0 | | 6 | 0.0 | 0.3 | 7 | 0.1 | 12 | 113 | 0.2 | 1 | 0.08 |
| 5286 | 1/2 cup | Red, fzn, boiled, avg | 68 | 12 | 95 | 0.6 | 2.7 | 1.1 | 1.3 | 0.2 | 0.1 | 0.0 | 0.0 | 0.1 | 0.01 | 0.06 | 0 | 2273 | 227 | 0 | 227 | 1231 | 0.03 | 0.02 | 0.73 | 0.07 | 0.00 | 6.7 | 0.02 | 28.0 | 0.0 | | 5 | 0.0 | 0.4 | 5 | 0.1 | 9 | 49 | 0.1 | 3 | 0.03 |
| 5218 | 1/2 cup | Red, raw, avg | 74 | 13 | 95 | 0.7 | 2.9 | 1.2 | 1.4 | 0.3 | 0.1 | 0.0 | 0.0 | 0.1 | 0.01 | 0.07 | 0 | 2474 | 247 | 0 | 247 | 1339 | 0.04 | 0.02 | 0.80 | 0.08 | 0.00 | 7.3 | 0.02 | 30.5 | 0.0 | | 6 | 0.0 | 0.4 | 5 | 0.1 | 10 | 53 | 0.1 | 3 | 0.04 |
| 5663 | 1/2 cup | Red, stmd, avg | 68 | 18 | 92 | 0.6 | 4.4 | 1.2 | 1.8 | 1.4 | 0.1 | 0.0 | 0.0 | 0.1 | 0.01 | 0.06 | 0 | 3682 | 368 | 0 | 368 | 1995 | 0.04 | 0.02 | 0.33 | 0.15 | 0.00 | 12.7 | 0.05 | 110.2 | 0.0 | 0.5 | 6 | 0.0 | 0.3 | 7 | 0.1 | 13 | 120 | | 1 | 0.08 |
| 5441 | 1 ea | Yellow, raw, large, avg | 180 | 49 | 92 | 1.8 | 11.4 | 1.6 | 4.5 | 5.3 | 0.4 | 0.1 | 0.0 | 0.2 | 0.02 | 0.18 | 0 | 428 | 43 | 0 | 43 | 189 | 0.05 | 0.04 | 1.60 | 0.30 | 0.00 | 46.8 | 0.30 | 331.2 | 0.0 | | 20 | 0.2 | 0.8 | 22 | 0.2 | 43 | 382 | 0.5 | 4 | 0.31 |
| 5229 | 1/2 cup | Poi, avg | 120 | 134 | 72 | 0.5 | 32.6 | 0.5 | | | 0.2 | 0.0 | 0.0 | 0.1 | 0.02 | 0.05 | 0 | 24 | 2 | 0 | 2 | 14 | 0.16 | 0.05 | 1.32 | 0.33 | 0.00 | 25.7 | 0.35 | 4.8 | 0.0 | | 19 | 0.2 | 1.1 | 29 | 0.4 | 47 | 220 | 0.8 | 14 | 0.26 |
| 5580 | 1/2 cup | Pokeberry Shoots, boiled, avg | 82 | 16 | 93 | 1.9 | 2.5 | 1.2 | | | 0.3 | 0.1 | 0.0 | 0.1 | 0.01 | 0.14 | 0 | 7134 | 713 | 0 | 713 | 4280 | 0.06 | 0.20 | 0.90 | 0.09 | 0.00 | 7.1 | 0.03 | 67.2 | 0.0 | | 43 | 0.1 | 1.0 | 11 | 0.3 | 27 | 151 | 0.7 | 15 | 0.16 |
| 5579 | 1/2 cup | Pokeberry Shoots, raw, avg | 80 | 18 | 92 | 2.1 | 3.0 | 1.4 | | | 0.3 | 0.1 | 0.0 | 0.1 | 0.01 | 0.13 | 0 | 6960 | 696 | 0 | 696 | 4176 | 0.06 | 0.26 | 0.96 | 0.12 | 0.00 | 12.6 | 0.04 | 108.8 | 0.0 | | 42 | 0.1 | 1.4 | 14 | 0.3 | 35 | 194 | 0.7 | 18 | 0.19 |
| | | Potatoes, Plain | | | | | | | | | | | | | | | | | | | | | | | | | | | | | | | | | | | | | | | | |
| 5334 | 1 ea | Baked, long, avg | 202 | 220 | 71 | 4.6 | 50.9 | 4.8 | 3.2 | 42.8 | 0.2 | 0.1 | 0.0 | 0.1 | 0.02 | 0.06 | 0 | 0 | 0 | 0 | 0 | 0 | 0.22 | 0.07 | 3.33 | 0.70 | 0.00 | 22.2 | 1.12 | 26.1 | 0.0 | | 20 | 0.6 | 2.7 | 55 | 0.5 | 115 | 844 | 1.6 | 16 | 0.65 |
| 5328 | 1 ea | Boiled, f/fzn, avg | 70 | 45 | 83 | 1.4 | 10.1 | 1.0 | 0.6 | 8.6 | 0.1 | 0.0 | 0.0 | 0.0 | 0.01 | 0.03 | 0 | 0 | 0 | 0 | 0 | 0 | 0.07 | 0.02 | 0.93 | 0.14 | 0.00 | 5.9 | 0.20 | 6.6 | 0.0 | | 5 | 0.1 | 0.6 | 8 | 0.1 | 18 | 201 | 0.1 | 14 | 0.17 |
| 5586 | 1/2 cup | Canned, w/liquid, avg | 150 | 537 | 6 | 16.3 | 116.5 | 3.0 | | | 1.7 | 0.7 | 0.2 | 0.4 | 0.11 | 0.31 | 3 | 90 | 14 | 12 | 2 | 11 | 0.28 | 0.45 | 6.30 | 1.33 | 0.00 | 44.8 | 2.79 | 24.0 | | | 213 | 0.9 | 5.3 | 111 | 0.7 | 356 | 2772 | 39.4 | 123 | 1.80 |
| 5129 | 1 ea | Flesh, baked, avg | 156 | 145 | 75 | 3.1 | 33.7 | 2.3 | 2.7 | 28.7 | 0.2 | 0.0 | 0.0 | 0.1 | 0.02 | 0.05 | 0 | 0 | 0 | 0 | 0 | 0 | 0.16 | 0.03 | 2.18 | 0.47 | 0.00 | 14.2 | 0.87 | 20.0 | 0.0 | 0.0 | 8 | 0.3 | 0.5 | 39 | 0.3 | 78 | 610 | 0.5 | 8 | 0.45 |
| 5136 | 1/2 cup | Flesh, boiled, avg | 78 | 67 | 78 | 1.3 | 15.6 | 1.4 | 0.8 | 13.4 | 0.1 | 0.0 | 0.0 | 0.0 | 0.01 | 0.02 | 0 | 0 | 0 | 0 | 0 | 0 | 0.08 | 0.01 | 1.02 | 0.21 | 0.00 | 6.9 | 0.40 | 5.8 | 0.0 | 0.0 | 6 | 0.1 | 0.2 | 16 | 0.1 | 31 | 256 | 0.2 | 4 | 0.21 |
| 6120 | 3 oz | Flesh, boiled, new potato, avg | 85 | 54 | 80 | 2.1 | 10.9 | 1.6 | 0.3 | 8.9 | 0.1 | | | | | | 0 | 0 | 0 | 0 | 0 | 0 | 0.07 | 0.02 | 0.76 | | 0.00 | | | 17.9 | | | 3 | | 0.4 | 16 | | | 366 | | 3 | 0.34 |
| 5345 | 1 ea | Flesh, microwaved, avg | 156 | 156 | 74 | 3.3 | 36.3 | 2.5 | 2.8 | 31.1 | 0.2 | 0.0 | 0.0 | 0.1 | 0.02 | 0.05 | 0 | 0 | 0 | 0 | 0 | 0 | 0.20 | 0.04 | 2.54 | 0.50 | 0.00 | 19.3 | 0.93 | 23.6 | 0.0 | | 8 | 0.4 | 0.6 | 39 | 0.3 | 170 | 641 | 0.6 | 11 | 0.51 |
| 5582 | 1/2 cup | Flesh, raw, diced, avg | 75 | 59 | 79 | 1.6 | 13.5 | 1.2 | 1.1 | 11.2 | 0.1 | 0.0 | 0.0 | 0.0 | 0.01 | 0.02 | 0 | 0 | 0 | 0 | 0 | 0 | 0.07 | 0.03 | 1.11 | 0.19 | 0.00 | 9.6 | 0.28 | 14.8 | 0.0 | | 5 | 0.2 | 0.6 | 16 | 0.2 | 34 | 407 | 0.2 | 4 | 0.29 |
| 6121 | 3 oz | Flesh, raw, new potato, avg | 85 | 54 | 82 | 2.0 | 10.9 | 1.4 | 0.5 | 8.9 | 0.1 | | | | | | 0 | 0 | 0 | 0 | 0 | 0 | 0.08 | 0.03 | 1.11 | | 0.00 | | | 20.4 | | | 4 | | 0.5 | 17 | | | 438 | | 3 | 0.34 |
| 5340 | 1 ea | Microwaved, avg | 202 | 212 | 72 | 4.9 | 48.7 | 4.6 | 3.1 | 40.9 | 0.2 | 0.1 | 0.0 | 0.1 | 0.02 | 0.06 | 0 | 0 | 0 | 0 | 0 | 0 | 0.24 | 0.06 | 3.45 | 0.69 | 0.00 | 24.2 | 0.92 | 30.5 | 0.0 | | 22 | 0.7 | 2.5 | 55 | 0.6 | 212 | 903 | 0.8 | 16 | 0.73 |
| 5715 | 1 ea | Raw, Produce Marketing Association | 127 | 93 | 79 | 3.1 | 21.9 | 2.3 | 1.5 | 18.1 | 0.2 | | | | | | | 0 | 0 | 0 | 0 | 0 | 0.12 | 0.03 | 1.50 | 0.22 | 0.00 | 26.7 | 0.36 | 23.1 | 0.0 | | 11 | 0.1 | 1.0 | 27 | 0.2 | 58 | 617 | | 4 | 0.36 |
| 5339 | 1 ea | Skin, baked, avg | 58 | 115 | 47 | 2.5 | 26.7 | 4.6 | 0.8 | 21.3 | 0.1 | 0.0 | 0.0 | 0.0 | 0.01 | 0.02 | 0 | 0 | 0 | 0 | 0 | 0 | 0.07 | 0.06 | 1.78 | 0.36 | 0.00 | 12.5 | 0.50 | 7.8 | 0.0 | | 20 | 0.5 | 4.1 | 25 | 0.4 | 59 | 332 | 0.4 | 12 | 0.28 |
| 5368 | 1 ea | Skin, boiled, avg | 34 | 27 | 78 | 1.0 | 5.8 | 1.1 | 0.2 | 4.5 | 0.0 | 0.0 | 0.0 | 0.0 | 0.00 | 0.01 | 0 | 0 | 0 | 0 | 0 | 0 | 0.01 | 0.01 | 0.41 | 0.08 | 0.00 | 3.3 | 0.12 | 1.8 | 0.0 | | 15 | 0.3 | 2.1 | 10 | 0.5 | 18 | 138 | 0.1 | 5 | 0.15 |
| 5350 | 1 ea | Skin, microwaved, avg | 58 | 77 | 64 | 2.5 | 17.2 | 3.2 | 0.8 | 13.2 | 0.1 | 0.0 | 0.0 | 0.0 | 0.01 | 0.02 | 0 | 0 | 0 | 0 | 0 | 0 | 0.04 | 0.04 | 1.29 | 0.29 | 0.00 | 9.6 | 0.34 | 8.9 | 0.0 | | 27 | 0.5 | 3.4 | 21 | 0.6 | 48 | 377 | 0.3 | 9 | 0.30 |
| 5784 | 1 ea | Skin, raw, avg | 38 | 22 | 83 | 1.0 | 4.7 | 0.9 | | | 0.0 | 0.0 | 0.0 | 0.0 | 0.00 | 0.01 | 0 | 0 | 0 | 0 | 0 | 0 | 0.01 | 0.01 | 0.39 | 0.09 | 0.00 | 6.6 | 0.11 | 4.3 | 0.0 | | 11 | 0.2 | 1.2 | 9 | 0.2 | 14 | 157 | 0.1 | 4 | 0.13 |
| | | Potato Dishes | | | | | | | | | | | | | | | | | | | | | | | | | | | | | | | | | | | | | | | | |
| 6528 | 3 oz | Au Gratin, baked, Basic American Foods | 85 | 81 | 74 | 1.8 | 13.0 | 0.9 | 2.2 | 9.9 | 2.6 | 0.7 | | | | | 1 | | | | | | | 0.01 | 0.70 | | 0.00 | | | 3.7 | | | 38 | | 0.2 | | | 71 | 185 | | 355 | |

| Code | Amount | Description | Basic Components | | | | | | | | | Additional Fats | | | | | | Vit A & Components | | | | | Vitamins | | | | | | | | | | Minerals | | | | | | | | | |
|---|---|---|---|---|---|---|---|---|---|---|---|---|---|---|---|---|---|---|---|---|---|---|---|---|---|---|---|---|---|---|---|---|---|---|---|---|---|---|---|---|---|---|
| | | | Weight (g) | Calories | % Water | Protein (g) | Carbs (g) | Fiber (g) | Sugar (g) | Other Carbs (g) | Fat (g) | Sat Fat (g) | Mono Fat (g) | Poly Fat (g) | Omega 3 (g) | Omega 6 (g) | Choles (mg) | Vit A (IU) | Vit A (RE) | Retinol (RE) | Carotenoids (RE) | Beta Carotene (mcg) | Thiamin (mg) | Riboflavin (mg) | Niacin (NE) | Vit B6 (mg) | Vit B12 (mcg) | Folate (mcg) | Panto (mg) | Vit C (mg) | Vit D (mg) | Vit E (α TE) | Calcium (mg) | Copper (mg) | Iron (mg) | Magnes (mg) | Mang (mg) | Phos (mg) | Potassium (mg) | Selenium (mcg) | Sodium (mg) | Zinc (mg) |
| 6527 | 1 oz | Au Gratin, dry, Basic American Foods | 28 | 102 | 7 | 2.7 | 19.6 | 1.5 | 3.4 | 14.7 | 1.4 | 0.6 | 0.6 | 0.2 | | | 2 | | | | | | | 0.01 | 1.01 | | 0.00 | | | 5.8 | | | 59 | | 0.4 | | | 110 | 286 | | 522 | |
| 5786 | 1/2 cup | Au Gratin, prep f/recipe, w/butter, avg | 122 | 161 | 74 | 6.2 | 13.8 | 2.2 | | | 9.3 | 5.8 | 2.6 | 0.3 | 0.12 | 0.21 | 28 | 322 | 46 | | | | 0.08 | 0.14 | 1.21 | 0.21 | 0.00 | 13.4 | 0.47 | 12.1 | 0.5 | | 145 | 0.2 | 0.8 | 24 | 0.2 | 138 | 483 | 3.3 | 528 | 0.84 |
| 57362 | 3 oz | Au Gratin, prep, Idahoan | 85 | 90 | 74 | 3.0 | 14.0 | | | | 2.0 | | | | | | | | | | | | 0.03 | 0.07 | 0.80 | | 0.00 | | | 2.4 | | | 40 | | 0.4 | 16 | | 60 | 265 | | 340 | |
| 6427 | 1 ea | Baked, w/butter & sour cream, avg | 312 | 463 | 70 | 7.7 | 52.7 | | | | 25.2 | 12.1 | 8.0 | 3.4 | | | 40 | 200 | 40 | | | | 0.09 | 0.14 | 3.00 | | 0.00 | | | 33.0 | | | 650 | | 2.7 | | | | 1420 | | 203 | |
| 70612 | 1 ea | Baked, w/butter, Ore Ida | 143 | 204 | 70 | 4.1 | 27.2 | 4.1 | 0.5 | 22.6 | 9.2 | 3.1 | 3.1 | 0.5 | | | 0 | 429 | 86 | | | | 0.09 | 0.10 | 3.05 | | 0.00 | | | 21.4 | | | 57 | | 1.0 | | | | 602 | | 357 | |
| 70613 | 1 ea | Baked, w/cheese, Ore Ida | 143 | 194 | 71 | 4.1 | 27.6 | 3.1 | 0.5 | 24.0 | 8.2 | 2.6 | 3.6 | 0.0 | 0.00 | 0.00 | 0 | 0 | 0 | 0 | 0 | 0 | 0.11 | 0.16 | 2.36 | | 0.00 | | | 3.4 | | | 80 | | 2.1 | | | | 643 | | 470 | |
| 6177 | 1 ea | Baked, w/cheese sauce, avg | 296 | 474 | 66 | 14.6 | 46.5 | | | | 28.7 | 10.6 | 10.7 | 6.0 | | | 18 | 835 | 228 | 205 | 23 | 137 | 0.24 | 0.21 | 3.34 | 0.71 | 0.18 | 26.6 | 1.30 | 26.0 | | | 311 | 0.6 | 3.0 | 65 | 0.5 | 320 | 1166 | 7.7 | 382 | 1.89 |
| 6178 | 1 ea | Baked, w/cheese sauce & bacon, avg | 299 | 451 | 65 | 18.4 | 44.6 | | | | 25.9 | 10.1 | 9.7 | 4.8 | | | 30 | 628 | 173 | 156 | 17 | 104 | 0.27 | 0.24 | 3.98 | 0.75 | 0.33 | 29.9 | 1.29 | 28.7 | | | 308 | 0.6 | 3.1 | 69 | 0.5 | 347 | 1178 | 9.6 | 972 | 2.15 |
| 6179 | 1 ea | Baked, w/cheese sauce & broccoli, avg | 339 | 403 | 70 | 13.7 | 46.4 | | | | 21.4 | 8.5 | 7.7 | 4.2 | | | 20 | 1695 | 278 | 200 | 78 | 467 | 0.27 | 0.27 | 3.59 | 0.78 | 0.34 | 61.0 | 1.42 | 48.5 | | | 336 | 0.6 | 3.3 | 78 | 0.8 | 346 | 1441 | 5.8 | 485 | 2.03 |
| 6180 | 1 ea | Baked, w/cheese sauce & chili, avg | 395 | 482 | 70 | 23.2 | 55.7 | | | | 21.8 | 13.0 | 6.8 | 0.9 | | | 32 | 766 | 174 | 137 | 36 | 218 | 0.28 | 0.36 | 4.19 | 0.95 | 0.24 | 47.4 | 2.57 | 31.6 | | | 411 | 0.8 | 6.1 | 111 | 0.7 | 498 | 1572 | 5.5 | 699 | 3.79 |
| 6400 | 1 ea | Baked, w/ranch flavor, Ore Ida | 140 | 180 | | 5.0 | 27.0 | 3.0 | 3.0 | 21.0 | 6.0 | 2.0 | 2.0 | 0.0 | 0.00 | 0.00 | 0 | 200 | 20 | | | | | | | | 0.00 | | | 12.0 | | | 60 | | 0.4 | | | | 420 | | 400 | |
| 70614 | 1 ea | Baked, w/sour cream & chives, Ore Ida | 143 | 184 | 70 | 4.1 | 28.6 | 3.1 | 0.5 | 25.0 | 6.1 | 1.5 | 4.6 | 0.0 | 0.00 | 0.00 | 0 | 0 | 0 | 0 | 0 | 0 | 0.13 | 0.10 | 2.37 | | 0.00 | | | 5.1 | | | 57 | | 1.9 | | | | 633 | | 378 | |
| 6325 | 3 oz | Dices, w/peel, fzn, Nestle | 85 | 120 | 71 | 2.0 | 19.0 | 2.0 | 0.0 | 17.0 | 3.5 | 1.0 | | | | | 5 | 0 | 0 | 0 | 0 | 0 | | | | | 0.00 | | | 6.0 | | | 0 | | 0.7 | | | | | | 50 | |
| 5790 | 10 ea | French Fries, fzn, avg | 65 | 101 | 67 | 1.6 | 15.8 | 1.9 | | | 3.8 | 0.6 | 2.4 | 0.4 | 0.02 | 0.37 | 0 | 0 | 0 | 0 | 0 | 0 | 0.07 | 0.01 | 1.11 | 0.16 | 0.00 | 7.8 | 0.19 | 6.4 | 0.0 | | 4 | 0.1 | 0.6 | 11 | 0.1 | 42 | 212 | 0.2 | 15 | 0.21 |
| 5332 | 10 ea | French Fries, fzn, cottage, oven htd, avg | 50 | 109 | 53 | 1.7 | 17.0 | 1.6 | 0.5 | 14.9 | 4.1 | 1.9 | 1.7 | 0.3 | 0.02 | 0.29 | 0 | 0 | 0 | 0 | 0 | 0 | 0.06 | 0.02 | 1.21 | 0.12 | 0.00 | 8.3 | 0.34 | 4.8 | 0.0 | | 5 | 0.1 | 0.7 | 11 | 0.2 | 32 | 240 | 0.2 | 22 | 0.20 |
| 7408 | 3 oz | French Fries, fzn, crinkle cut 1/8", Nestle | 85 | 140 | 62 | 2.0 | 23.0 | 1.0 | 0.0 | 22.0 | 4.0 | 1.0 | | | | | 0 | 0 | 0 | 0 | 0 | 0 | | | | | 0.00 | | | 0.0 | | | 0 | | 0.4 | | | | | | 35 | |
| 7404 | 3 oz | French Fries, fzn, crinkle cut 3/8", Nestle | 85 | 110 | 72 | 2.0 | 17.0 | 2.0 | 0.0 | 15.0 | 4.0 | 2.0 | | | | | 5 | 0 | 0 | 0 | 0 | 0 | | | | | 0.00 | | | 0.0 | | | 0 | | 0.4 | | | | | | 40 | |
| 6317 | 3 oz | French Fries, fzn, crinkle cut 1/2", Nestle | 85 | 110 | 72 | 2.0 | 18.0 | 2.0 | 0.0 | 16.0 | 3.5 | 1.5 | | | | | 5 | 0 | 0 | 0 | 0 | 0 | | | | | 0.00 | | | 0.0 | | | 0 | | 0.4 | | | | | | 40 | |
| 5961 | 10 ea | French Fries, fzn, prep, salted, avg | 50 | 100 | 57 | 1.6 | 15.6 | 1.6 | 0.4 | 13.6 | 3.8 | 0.6 | 2.4 | 0.4 | 0.02 | 0.37 | 0 | 0 | 0 | 0 | 0 | 0 | 0.06 | 0.01 | 1.04 | 0.15 | 0.00 | 6.0 | 0.17 | 5.1 | 0.0 | | 4 | 0.1 | 0.6 | 11 | 0.1 | 41 | 209 | 0.2 | 133 | 0.20 |
| 5330 | 1 cup | French Fries, fzn, prep in veg oil, avg | 57 | 180 | 38 | 2.3 | 22.6 | 1.8 | 0.3 | 20.5 | 9.5 | 2.2 | 5.4 | 0.8 | 0.03 | 0.58 | 0 | 0 | 0 | 0 | 0 | 0 | 0.10 | 0.02 | 1.85 | 0.13 | 0.00 | 16.5 | 0.37 | 5.9 | 0.0 | | 11 | 0.1 | 0.4 | 19 | 0.1 | 53 | 417 | 0.5 | 123 | 0.22 |
| 6314 | 3 oz | French Fries, fzn, shoestring 1/4", Nestle | 85 | 130 | 68 | 2.0 | 20.0 | 2.0 | 0.0 | 18.0 | 5.0 | 1.5 | | | | | 5 | 0 | 0 | 0 | 0 | 0 | | | | | 0.00 | | | 1.2 | | | 0 | | 0.0 | | | | | | 55 | |
| 6323 | 3 oz | French Fries, fzn, steak cut 7/8", w/peel, Nestle | 85 | 100 | 71 | 2.0 | 18.0 | 2.0 | 0.0 | 16.0 | 3.0 | 1.5 | | | | | 5 | 0 | 0 | 0 | 0 | 0 | | | | | 0.00 | | | 3.6 | | | 0 | | 0.4 | | | | | | 50 | |
| 7403 | 3 oz | French Fries, fzn, steak cut, thin, Nestle | 85 | 130 | 65 | 2.0 | 20.0 | 2.0 | 0.0 | 18.0 | 5.0 | 2.0 | | | | | 5 | 0 | 0 | 0 | 0 | 0 | | | | | 0.00 | | | 1.2 | | | 0 | | 0.4 | | | | 70 | | | |
| 6315 | 3 oz | French Fries, fzn, straight cut /516", Nestle | 85 | 120 | 67 | 2.0 | 19.0 | 2.0 | 0.0 | 17.0 | 4.0 | 1.5 | | | | | 5 | 0 | 0 | 0 | 0 | 0 | | | | | 0.00 | | | 0.0 | | | 0 | | 0.4 | | | | | | 40 | |
| 6321 | 3 oz | French Fries, fzn, 5/16" w/peel, Nestle | 85 | 120 | 69 | 2.0 | 19.0 | 2.0 | 0.0 | 17.0 | 4.5 | 1.5 | | | | | 5 | 0 | 0 | 0 | 0 | 0 | | | | | 0.00 | | | 2.4 | | | 0 | | 0.4 | | | | | | 55 | |
| 5589 | 1/2 cup | Hash Browns, fzn, avg | 105 | 86 | 79 | 2.2 | 18.6 | 1.5 | 0.1 | 17.0 | 0.7 | 0.2 | 0.0 | 0.3 | 0.07 | 0.21 | 0 | 0 | 0 | 0 | 0 | 0 | 0.10 | 0.01 | 1.74 | 0.09 | 0.00 | 4.4 | 0.34 | 8.6 | 0.0 | | 10 | 0.1 | 1.0 | 12 | 0.2 | 49 | 299 | 0.3 | 23 | 0.22 |
| 6335 | 1 ea | Hash Browns, patty, fzn, Nestle | 63 | 120 | 65 | 1.0 | 15.0 | 2.0 | 0.0 | 13.0 | 6.0 | 2.5 | | | | | 10 | 0 | 0 | 0 | 0 | 0 | | | | | 0.00 | | | 1.2 | | | 0 | | 0.0 | | | | | | 300 | |
| 5140 | 1/2 cup | Hash Browns, prep f/fzn, avg | 78 | 170 | 56 | 2.5 | 21.9 | 1.6 | 0.1 | 20.3 | 9.0 | 3.5 | 4.0 | 1.0 | 0.10 | 0.94 | 0 | 0 | 0 | 0 | 0 | 0 | 0.09 | 0.02 | 1.89 | 0.10 | 0.00 | 5.1 | 0.35 | 4.9 | 0.0 | 0.1 | 12 | 0.1 | 1.2 | 13 | 0.2 | 56 | 340 | 0.2 | 27 | 0.25 |
| 5273 | 1 cup | Hash Browns, prep f/recipe, avg | 156 | 326 | 62 | 3.8 | 33.2 | 3.1 | 0.2 | 30.0 | 21.7 | 8.5 | 9.7 | 2.5 | 0.24 | 2.26 | 0 | 0 | 0 | 0 | 0 | 0 | 0.12 | 0.03 | 3.12 | 0.43 | 0.00 | 12.0 | 0.78 | 8.9 | 0.0 | | 12 | 0.3 | 1.3 | 31 | 0.2 | 66 | 501 | 0.5 | 37 | 0.47 |
| 6643 | 3 oz | Hash Browns, prep, Idahoan | 85 | 142 | 66 | 1.5 | 18.0 | 1.5 | 0.0 | 16.5 | 7.5 | 1.1 | 2.2 | 3.4 | | | 0 | 0 | 0 | 0 | 0 | 0 | 0.02 | | 1.20 | | 0.00 | | | | | | 15 | | | 12 | | 45 | 202 | | 75 | |
| 70608 | 2 ea | Hash Browns, toaster, Ore Ida | 100 | 192 | 60 | 2.0 | 24.2 | 1.0 | 0.5 | 22.7 | 12.0 | 2.0 | 3.0 | 0.5 | | | 0 | 0 | 0 | 0 | 0 | 0 | 0.08 | 0.03 | 2.07 | 0.18 | 0.00 | | | 0.0 | | | 0 | | 0.4 | | | | 182 | | 556 | |
| 6642 | 3 oz | Hash Browns, unprep, Idahoan | 85 | 318 | 8 | 6.4 | 66.9 | 3.2 | 0.0 | 63.7 | 1.6 | 0.0 | 0.0 | 0.0 | 0.00 | 0.00 | 0 | 0 | 0 | 0 | 0 | 0 | 0.10 | | 5.09 | | 0.00 | | | 19.1 | | | 64 | | 1.1 | 51 | | 191 | 1051 | | 382 | |
| 5590 | 1 ea | Hash Browns, w/butter sauce, fzn, avg | 170 | 230 | 72 | 3.2 | 31.1 | 4.9 | | | 11.3 | 4.4 | 4.1 | 2.3 | 0.23 | 2.10 | 29 | 143 | 20 | 19 | 2 | 10 | 0.09 | 0.04 | 1.92 | 0.36 | 0.00 | 20.4 | 0.53 | 9.7 | | | 43 | 0.1 | 1.3 | 19 | 0.3 | 49 | 422 | 0.5 | 131 | 0.43 |
| 5591 | 1/2 cup | Hash Browns, w/butter sauce, prep f/fzn, avg | 72 | 128 | 64 | 1.8 | 17.4 | 2.7 | | | 6.3 | 2.4 | 2.3 | 1.3 | 0.13 | 1.17 | 17 | 80 | 12 | 11 | 1 | 6 | 0.04 | 0.02 | 1.02 | 0.19 | 0.00 | 9.5 | 0.26 | 2.7 | | | 24 | 0.1 | 0.7 | 11 | 0.2 | 27 | 235 | 0.2 | 73 | 0.24 |
| 6397 | 1/2 cup | Mashed, dry, w/natural butter flavor, Ore Ida | 59 | 80 | | 2.0 | 14.0 | 0.5 | 0.5 | 13.0 | 2.0 | 0.5 | 0.5 | 0.0 | 0.00 | 0.00 | 2 | 100 | 20 | | | | | | | | 0.00 | | | 3.6 | | | 0 | | 0.0 | | | | 210 | | 140 | |
| 6639 | 1/2 cup | Mashed, dry flakes, Idahoan | 90 | 56 | 8 | 1.1 | 12.4 | | | | 0.0 | 0.0 | 0.0 | 0.0 | 0.00 | 0.00 | | 0 | 0 | 0 | 0 | 0 | | | 0.45 | | 0.00 | | | 2.7 | | | | | | 22 | | 22 | 208 | | 14 | |
| 57367 | 1/2 cup | Mashed, prep f/flakes, Idahoan | 105 | 112 | 78 | 2.5 | 16.2 | | | | 3.7 | | | | | | | 125 | 12 | | | | 0.04 | 0.04 | 1.00 | | 0.00 | | | 3.0 | | | 25 | | 0.4 | 20 | | 50 | 262 | | 281 | |
| 5464 | 1/2 cup | Mashed, prep f/flakes, w/whole milk & butter, | 105 | 119 | 76 | 2.0 | 15.7 | 2.4 | 0.9 | 12.4 | 5.9 | 3.6 | 1.7 | 0.3 | 0.10 | 0.16 | 15 | 189 | 22 | 19 | 3 | 17 | 0.12 | 0.05 | 0.70 | 0.01 | 0.08 | 7.8 | 0.13 | 10.2 | 0.2 | | 51 | 0.0 | 0.2 | 19 | 0.1 | 59 | 245 | 1.5 | 349 | 0.19 |
| 5138 | 1/2 cup | Mashed, prep f/flakes, w/whole milk & marg, avg | 105 | 119 | 76 | 2.0 | 15.7 | 2.4 | 1.0 | 12.3 | 5.9 | 1.5 | 2.4 | 1.6 | 0.09 | 1.53 | 4 | 189 | 22 | | | | 0.12 | 0.05 | 0.70 | 0.01 | 0.00 | 7.8 | 0.13 | 10.2 | 0.2 | | 51 | 0.0 | 0.2 | 19 | 0.1 | 59 | 245 | 0.5 | 349 | 0.19 |
| 5585 | 1/2 cup | Mashed, prep f/granules, w/milk & butter, avg | 105 | 113 | 78 | 2.2 | 15.1 | 2.3 | | | 5.2 | 3.2 | 1.5 | 0.2 | 0.09 | 0.15 | 15 | 194 | 20 | 18 | 2 | 10 | 0.08 | 0.08 | 0.80 | 0.01 | 0.00 | 8.4 | 0.13 | 6.3 | 0.2 | | 37 | 0.0 | 0.2 | 20 | 0.0 | 63 | 151 | 1.4 | 270 | 0.26 |
| 5469 | 1/2 cup | Mashed, prep f/granules, w/milk & marg, avg | 105 | 113 | 78 | 2.2 | 15.1 | 2.3 | | | 5.2 | 1.3 | 2.1 | 1.4 | 0.08 | 1.35 | 3 | 208 | 21 | | | | 0.08 | 0.08 | 0.80 | 0.01 | 0.00 | 7.3 | 0.13 | 6.3 | 0.2 | | 37 | 0.0 | 0.2 | 20 | 0.0 | 63 | 152 | 0.5 | 276 | 0.25 |
| 6545 | 1/2 cup | Mashed, prep f/granules, w/vit C, avg | 105 | 92 | 84 | 2.4 | 16.5 | 1.7 | 1.2 | 13.7 | 2.0 | 0.7 | | | | | 2 | | | | | | 0.00 | 0.05 | 1.18 | | 0.00 | | | 25.7 | | | 27 | | 0.4 | | | 63 | 296 | | 227 | |
| 5137 | 1/2 cup | Mashed, w/whole milk, avg | 105 | 81 | 78 | 2.0 | 18.5 | 2.1 | 1.1 | 15.3 | 0.6 | 0.3 | 0.2 | 0.1 | 0.02 | 0.04 | 2 | 20 | 6 | 5 | 1 | 5 | 0.09 | 0.04 | 1.18 | 0.24 | 0.00 | 8.6 | 0.50 | 7.0 | 0.2 | | 27 | 0.1 | 0.3 | 19 | 0.1 | 50 | 314 | 0.6 | 318 | 0.30 |
| 5569 | 1/2 cup | Mashed, w/whole milk & butter, avg | 105 | 111 | 76 | 2.0 | 17.5 | 2.1 | 1.2 | 14.2 | 4.4 | 2.9 | 1.2 | 0.2 | 0.06 | 0.10 | 13 | 177 | 21 | 19 | 2 | 14 | 0.09 | 0.04 | 1.13 | 0.24 | 0.00 | 8.3 | 0.60 | 6.4 | 0.2 | | 27 | 0.1 | 0.3 | 19 | 0.1 | 48 | 303 | 0.5 | 310 | 0.28 |
| 5787 | 1/2 cup | O'Brien, fzn, avg | 97 | 74 | 80 | 1.8 | 17.0 | 1.8 | | | 0.1 | 0.0 | 0.0 | 0.1 | 0.01 | 0.05 | | 144 | 15 | 13 | 1 | 7 | 0.05 | 0.04 | 1.10 | 0.20 | 0.00 | 7.9 | 0.42 | 11.0 | 0.0 | | 13 | 0.1 | 1.0 | 17 | 0.1 | 48 | 242 | 1.2 | 32 | 0.28 |
| 5269 | 1/2 cup | O'Brien, prep f/fzn, avg | 97 | 198 | 62 | 2.2 | 21.2 | 1.6 | 3.9 | 15.7 | 12.8 | 3.2 | 5.6 | 3.4 | 0.21 | 3.15 | 0 | 182 | 18 | 17 | 1 | 9 | 0.05 | 0.13 | 1.41 | 0.37 | 0.00 | 11.9 | 0.71 | 10.1 | 0.0 | | 19 | 0.2 | 0.9 | 33 | 0.2 | 90 | 459 | 1.2 | 42 | 0.53 |
| 70605 | 1/2 cup | O'Brien, prep f/dry mix, Ore Ida | 78 | 55 | 82 | 0.9 | 12.1 | 1.9 | 0.9 | 9.3 | 0.0 | 0.0 | 0.0 | 0.0 | 0.00 | 0.00 | 0 | 0 | 0 | 0 | 0 | 0 | 0.07 | 0.02 | 1.19 | | 0.00 | | | 3.7 | | | 0 | | 0.0 | | | | 148 | | 14 | |
| 5268 | 1/2 cup | O'Brien, prep f/recipe, avg | 97 | 79 | 80 | 2.3 | 15.0 | 1.0 | 2.1 | 11.9 | 1.2 | 0.8 | 0.3 | 0.1 | 0.02 | 0.04 | 4 | 467 | 55 | 51 | 4 | 27 | 0.07 | 0.05 | 0.98 | 0.21 | 0.00 | 8.1 | 0.42 | 16.2 | 0.0 | | 35 | 0.1 | 0.5 | 17 | 0.1 | 49 | 258 | 1.2 | 210 | 0.29 |
| 5263 | 1 ea | Pancakes, prep f/recipe, avg | 76 | 207 | 47 | 4.7 | 21.7 | 1.5 | 1.0 | 19.2 | 11.6 | 2.3 | 3.5 | 5.0 | 0.30 | 4.67 | 73 | 109 | 11 | 10 | 1 | 5 | 0.10 | 0.13 | 1.63 | 0.29 | 0.14 | 12.2 | 0.56 | 16.7 | 0.2 | | 18 | 0.3 | 1.2 | 25 | 0.3 | 84 | 597 | 3.5 | 386 | 0.63 |
| 6521 | 1 oz | Pearls, w/ched cheese, dry mix, Basic American Foods | 28 | 111 | 8 | 2.2 | 21.0 | 1.8 | 1.2 | 18.1 | 2.0 | 0.6 | | | | | 0 | | | | | | 0.00 | 0.22 | 1.26 | | 0.00 | | | 3.9 | | | 18 | | 0.4 | | | 58 | 313 | | 410 | |
| 6540 | 3 oz | Pearls, w/ched cheese, prep, Basic American Foods | 85 | 88 | 76 | 1.7 | 16.2 | 1.3 | 1.0 | 13.9 | 1.6 | 0.5 | | | | | 0 | | | | | | 0.00 | 0.17 | 0.96 | | 0.00 | | | 3.1 | | | 14 | | 0.3 | | | 46 | 246 | | 322 | |
| 6520 | 1 oz | Pearls, w/sour cream&chives, dry mix, Basic Am. Foods | 28 | 112 | 8 | 2.2 | 20.7 | 1.8 | 0.4 | 18.5 | 2.2 | 0.6 | | | | | 0 | | | | | | 0.00 | 0.03 | 1.32 | | 0.00 | | | 4.7 | | | 15 | | 0.4 | | | 61 | 330 | | 447 | |
| 6539 | 3 oz | Pearls, w/sour cream&chives, prep, Basic Am. Foods | 85 | 85 | 76 | 1.7 | 16.2 | 1.4 | 0.3 | 14.5 | 1.6 | 0.5 | 1.1 | 0.1 | | | 0 | | | | | | 0.00 | 0.03 | 0.96 | | 0.00 | | | 3.5 | | | 11 | | 0.3 | | | 47 | 251 | | 340 | |
| 5788 | 1/2 cup | Puffs, fzn, avg | 64 | 113 | 62 | 1.7 | 15.6 | 1.5 | | | 5.5 | 2.6 | 2.2 | 0.4 | 0.00 | 0.41 | 0 | 8 | 1 | 0 | 1 | 4 | 0.12 | 0.04 | 1.16 | 0.12 | 0.00 | 10.6 | 0.37 | 4.4 | 0.0 | | 15 | 0.0 | 0.8 | 10 | 0.1 | 24 | 194 | 0.2 | 381 | 0.15 |
| 6332 | 12 ea | Rounds, fzn, Nestle | 85 | 160 | 64 | 2.0 | 20.0 | 2.0 | 0.0 | 18.0 | 8.0 | 2.0 | | | | | 0 | 0 | 0 | 0 | 0 | 0 | | | | | 0.00 | | | 1.2 | | | 0 | | 0.4 | | | | | | 390 | |
| 5588 | 1 ea | Scalloped, dry mix, avg | 156 | 558 | 6 | 12.1 | 115.3 | 13.4 | 6.9 | 95.0 | 7.2 | 1.9 | 0.2 | 3.1 | 0.73 | 2.31 | 8 | 0 | 0 | 0 | 0 | 0 | 0.09 | 0.19 | 7.07 | 0.28 | 0.00 | 49.5 | 2.18 | 25.7 | 0.5 | | 97 | 0.4 | 3.1 | 92 | 1.0 | 307 | 1412 | 12.3 | 2462 | 1.44 |
| 6525 | 1 oz | Scalloped, dry mix, Basic American Foods | 28 | 102 | 7 | 2.7 | 20.4 | 1.5 | 1.8 | 17.1 | 1.1 | 0.4 | 0.5 | 0.1 | | | 2 | | | | | | | 0.06 | 0.98 | | 0.00 | | | 6.4 | | | 47 | | 0.3 | | | 76 | 258 | | 410 | |
| 6526 | 3 oz | Scalloped, prep f/dry mix, Basic American Foods | 85 | 81 | 74 | 1.8 | 13.0 | 1.0 | 1.2 | 10.8 | 2.3 | 0.6 | 1.1 | 0.6 | | | 1 | | | | | | | 0.04 | 0.60 | | 0.00 | | | 4.1 | | | 31 | | 0.2 | | | 49 | 167 | | 283 | |
| 57368 | 3 oz | Scalloped, prep f/dry mix, Idahoan | 85 | 90 | 75 | 2.0 | 16.0 | | | | 2.0 | | | | | | | | | | | | 0.03 | 0.07 | 0.80 | | 0.00 | | | 2.4 | | | 40 | | 0.4 | 16 | | 60 | 245 | | 300 | |
| 5785 | 1/2 cup | Scalloped, prep f/recipe, w/butter, avg | 122 | 105 | 81 | 3.5 | 13.2 | 2.3 | | | 4.5 | 2.8 | 1.3 | 0.2 | 0.07 | 0.13 | 15 | 165 | 23 | | | | 0.08 | 0.11 | 1.28 | 0.22 | 0.00 | 13.4 | 0.63 | 12.9 | 0.5 | | 70 | 0.2 | 0.7 | 23 | 0.2 | 77 | 461 | 2.0 | 409 | 0.49 |
| 5270 | 1/2 cup | Scalloped, prep f/recipe, w/marg, avg | 122 | 105 | 81 | 3.5 | 13.2 | 2.3 | 0.7 | 10.1 | 4.5 | 1.7 | 1.6 | 0.9 | 0.07 | 0.84 | 7 | 165 | 23 | | | | 0.08 | 0.11 | 1.28 | 0.22 | 0.00 | 13.4 | 0.63 | 12.9 | 0.5 | | 70 | 0.2 | 0.7 | 23 | 0.2 | 77 | 461 | 2.0 | 409 | 0.49 |
| 56317 | 1/2 cup | Scalloped, w/ham, avg | 116 | 117 | 77 | 5.8 | 13.0 | 1.1 | | | 5.2 | 2.9 | 1.6 | 0.3 | | | 19 | 150 | 21 | 21 | 0 | | 0.12 | 0.09 | 1.77 | 0.11 | 0.10 | 10.2 | | 3.3 | | | 37 | 0.1 | 0.5 | 17 | | 89 | 252 | | 538 | 0.63 |
| 57363 | 3 oz | Slices, dry, Idahoan | 85 | 70 | | 1.0 | 15.0 | | | | 0.0 | 0.0 | 0.0 | 0.0 | 0.00 | 0.00 | | 0 | 0 | 0 | 0 | 0 | | | 0.40 | | 0.00 | | | 2.4 | | | | | 0.4 | 8 | | 20 | 115 | | 12 | |
| 57364 | 3 oz | Slices, prep, Idahoan | 85 | 70 | 78 | 1.0 | 15.0 | | | | 0.0 | 0.0 | 0.0 | 0.0 | 0.00 | 0.00 | | 0 | 0 | 0 | 0 | 0 | 0.03 | 0.03 | 0.40 | | 0.00 | | | 2.4 | | | 10 | | 0.4 | 8 | | 20 | 115 | | 230 | |
| 70600 | 1/2 cup | Tater Tots, bacon flavor, Ore Ida | 62 | 111 | 63 | 1.5 | 14.8 | 0.7 | 0.4 | 13.6 | 5.2 | 1.1 | 1.9 | 0.4 | | | 0 | 0 | 0 | 0 | 0 | 0 | 0.33 | 0.02 | 1.12 | | 0.00 | | | 0.0 | | | 0 | | 0.2 | | | | 162 | | 361 | |

| Code | Amount | Description | Weight (g) | Calories | % Water | Protein (g) | Carbs (g) | Fiber (g) | Sugar (g) | Other Carbs (g) | Fat (g) | Sat Fat (g) | Mono Fat (g) | Poly Fat (g) | Omega 3 (g) | Omega 6 (g) | Choles (mg) |
|---|---|---|---|---|---|---|---|---|---|---|---|---|---|---|---|---|---|
| | | | Basic Components | | | | | | | | | Additional Fats | | | | | |
| 70599 | 1/2 cup | Tater Tots, onion flavor, Ore Ida | 62 | 111 | 64 | 1.5 | 14.8 | 1.5 | 0.4 | 12.9 | 5.2 | 1.1 | 2.2 | 0.4 | | | 0 |
| 70598 | 1/2 cup | Tater Tots, Ore Ida | 62 | 107 | 61 | 1.5 | 15.5 | 1.5 | 0.4 | 13.7 | 5.9 | 1.1 | 1.8 | 0.0 | 0.00 | 0.00 | 0 |
| 6324 | 3 oz | Wedges, w/peel, fzn, Nestle | 85 | 110 | 72 | 2.0 | 19.0 | 2.0 | 0.0 | 17.0 | 2.5 | 1.0 | | | | | 5 |
| | | Pumpkin | | | | | | | | | | | | | | | |
| 5396 | 1/2 cup | Boiled, avg | 122 | 24 | 94 | 0.9 | 6.0 | 1.3 | 3.9 | 0.7 | 0.1 | 0.0 | 0.0 | 0.0 | 0.00 | 0.00 | 0 |
| 5142 | 1/2 cup | Canned, avg | 122 | 41 | 90 | 1.3 | 9.9 | 3.5 | 4.0 | 2.3 | 0.3 | 0.2 | 0.0 | 0.0 | 0.01 | 0.01 | 0 |
| 5793 | 1/2 cup | Raw, avg | 58 | 15 | 92 | 0.6 | 3.8 | 0.3 | 2.6 | 0.9 | 0.1 | 0.0 | 0.0 | 0.0 | 0.00 | 0.00 | 0 |
| 5426 | 1/2 cup | Purslane, boiled, avg | 58 | 10 | 94 | 0.9 | 2.1 | 0.5 | | | 0.1 | 0.0 | 0.0 | 0.0 | | | 0 |
| 5425 | 1/2 cup | Purslane, raw, avg | 22 | 4 | 94 | 0.3 | 0.8 | 0.2 | | | 0.0 | 0.0 | 0.0 | 0.0 | | | 0 |
| 5451 | 1/2 cup | Radicchio, raw, avg | 20 | 5 | 93 | 0.3 | 0.9 | 0.2 | | | 0.1 | 0.0 | 0.0 | 0.0 | 0.00 | 0.02 | 0 |
| | | Radishes | | | | | | | | | | | | | | | |
| 5593 | 1/2 cup | Oriental, boiled, avg | 74 | 13 | 95 | 0.5 | 2.5 | 1.2 | | | 0.2 | 0.1 | 0.0 | 0.1 | 0.05 | 0.03 | 0 |
| 5594 | 1/2 cup | Oriental, dried, avg | 58 | 157 | 20 | 4.6 | 36.8 | 17.2 | | | 0.4 | 0.1 | 0.1 | 0.2 | 0.12 | 0.07 | 0 |
| 5144 | 1/2 cup | Red, slices, avg | 58 | 12 | 95 | 0.3 | 2.1 | 0.9 | 1.2 | 0.0 | 0.3 | 0.0 | 0.0 | 0.0 | 0.02 | 0.01 | 0 |
| 5550 | 1/2 cup | White Icicle, raw, avg | 50 | 7 | 95 | 0.6 | 1.3 | 0.7 | 0.6 | 0.0 | 0.1 | 0.0 | 0.0 | 0.0 | 0.01 | 0.01 | 0 |
| 7225 | 1/2 cup | Rutabaga, boiled, cubes, avg | 85 | 33 | 89 | 1.1 | 7.4 | 1.5 | 3.0 | 2.9 | 0.2 | 0.0 | 0.0 | 0.1 | 0.05 | 0.03 | 0 |
| 7214 | 1/2 cup | Rutabaga, raw, avg | 70 | 25 | 90 | 0.8 | 5.7 | 1.8 | 3.9 | 0.0 | 0.1 | 0.0 | 0.0 | 0.1 | 0.04 | 0.02 | 0 |
| 5221 | 1/2 cup | Salsify, boiled, avg | 68 | 46 | 81 | 1.9 | 10.5 | 2.1 | 8.4 | 0.0 | 0.1 | 0.0 | 0.0 | 0.1 | 0.01 | 0.04 | 0 |
| 5794 | 1/2 cup | Salsify, raw, avg | 66 | 54 | 77 | 2.2 | 12.3 | 2.2 | 1.9 | 8.2 | 0.1 | 0.0 | 0.0 | 0.1 | 0.01 | 0.05 | 0 |
| | | Seaweed | | | | | | | | | | | | | | | |
| 5254 | 1/4 cup | Agar, dried, avg | 4 | 12 | 9 | 0.2 | 3.2 | 0.3 | | | 0.0 | 0.0 | 0.0 | 0.0 | 0.00 | 0.00 | 0 |
| 5253 | 1/2 cup | Agar, raw, avg | 40 | 10 | 91 | 0.2 | 2.7 | 0.2 | | | 0.0 | 0.0 | 0.0 | 0.0 | 0.00 | 0.00 | 0 |
| 5255 | 1/2 cup | Irish Moss, raw, avg | 40 | 20 | 81 | 0.6 | 4.9 | 0.5 | | | 0.1 | 0.0 | 0.0 | 0.0 | 0.02 | 0.00 | 0 |
| 5256 | 1/2 cup | Kelp, raw, avg | 40 | 17 | 82 | 0.7 | 3.8 | 0.5 | | | 0.2 | 0.1 | 0.0 | 0.0 | 0.00 | 0.01 | 0 |
| 5257 | 1/2 cup | Laver, raw, avg | 40 | 14 | 85 | 2.3 | 2.0 | 0.1 | | | 0.1 | 0.0 | 0.0 | 0.0 | 0.03 | 0.01 | 0 |
| 5620 | 1/2 cup | Pickled, avg | 75 | 114 | 57 | 1.0 | 29.2 | 0.2 | | | 0.1 | 0.0 | 0.0 | 0.0 | 0.00 | 0.00 | 0 |
| 5260 | 1/4 cup | Spirulina, dried, avg | 4 | 12 | 5 | 2.3 | 1.0 | 0.1 | | | 0.3 | 0.1 | 0.0 | 0.1 | 0.03 | 0.05 | 0 |
| 5836 | 3 oz | Spirulina, raw, avg | 85 | 22 | 91 | 5.0 | 2.1 | 0.3 | | | 0.3 | 0.1 | 0.0 | 0.1 | 0.04 | 0.05 | 0 |
| 5261 | 1/2 cup | Wakame, raw, avg | 40 | 18 | 80 | 1.2 | 3.7 | 0.2 | | | 0.3 | 0.1 | 0.0 | 0.1 | 0.07 | 0.01 | 0 |
| 5428 | 1 Tbs | Shallots, freeze dried, chpd, avg | 1 | 3 | 2 | 0.1 | 0.8 | 0.0 | 0.1 | 0.6 | 0.0 | 0.0 | 0.0 | 0.0 | 0.00 | 0.00 | 0 |
| 5427 | 1 Tbs | Shallots, raw, chpd, avg | 10 | 7 | 80 | 0.3 | 1.7 | 0.1 | 0.3 | 1.3 | 0.0 | 0.0 | 0.0 | 0.0 | 0.00 | 0.00 | 0 |
| 5259 | 1/2 cup | Soybeans, green, boiled, avg | 90 | 127 | 69 | 11.2 | 10.0 | 3.8 | 2.7 | 3.5 | 5.8 | 0.7 | 1.1 | 2.7 | 0.32 | 2.39 | 0 |
| 5258 | 1/2 cup | Soybeans, green, raw, avg | 128 | 188 | 68 | 16.6 | 14.2 | 5.4 | 3.8 | 5.0 | 8.7 | 1.0 | 1.6 | 4.1 | 0.48 | 3.61 | 0 |
| | | Spinach | | | | | | | | | | | | | | | |
| 5147 | 1/2 cup | Boiled, avg | 90 | 21 | 91 | 2.7 | 3.4 | 2.2 | 0.0 | 1.2 | 0.2 | 0.0 | 0.0 | 0.1 | 0.08 | 0.01 | 0 |
| 5595 | 1/2 cup | Canned, w/liquid, avg | 117 | 22 | 93 | 2.5 | 3.4 | 1.9 | 0.0 | 1.5 | 0.4 | 0.1 | 0.0 | 0.2 | 0.14 | 0.03 | 0 |
| 5973 | 1/2 cup | Canned, w/liquid, unsalted, avg | 117 | 22 | 93 | 2.5 | 3.4 | 2.6 | 0.0 | 0.8 | 0.4 | 0.1 | 0.0 | 0.2 | 0.14 | 0.03 | 0 |
| 5498 | 1 oz | Dehydrated, Basic Vegetable Products | 28 | 69 | 5 | 9.0 | 11.1 | 2.8 | 0.1 | 8.1 | 1.1 | | | | | | 0 |
| 5148 | 1/2 cup | Frozen, boiled, drained, unsalted, avg | 95 | 27 | 90 | 3.0 | 5.1 | 2.8 | 0.0 | 2.2 | 0.2 | 0.0 | 0.0 | 0.1 | 0.06 | 0.01 | 0 |
| 56959 | 1/2 cup | Frozen, creamed, Green Giant | 109 | 84 | 82 | 3.7 | 10.1 | 2.0 | 3.9 | 4.3 | 3.2 | 1.6 | | | | | 0 |
| 5510 | 1/2 cup | Juice, avg | 118 | 7 | 95 | 1.7 | 0.6 | | | | | | | | | | 0 |
| 5146 | 1 cup | Raw, chpd, avg | 30 | 7 | 92 | 0.9 | 1.1 | 0.8 | 0.1 | 0.1 | 0.1 | 0.0 | 0.0 | 0.0 | 0.03 | 0.01 | 0 |
| 5670 | 1/2 cup | Steamed, avg | 95 | 21 | 92 | 2.7 | 3.3 | 2.6 | 0.0 | 0.8 | 0.3 | 0.1 | 0.0 | 0.1 | 0.11 | 0.02 | 0 |
| 5669 | 1/2 cup | Stir Fried, avg | 90 | 20 | 92 | 2.6 | 3.2 | 2.4 | 0.0 | 0.7 | 0.3 | 0.1 | 0.0 | 0.1 | 0.10 | 0.02 | 0 |
| 6347 | 3 oz | With Butter Sauce, fzn, Green Giant | 85 | 37 | 90 | 2.1 | 3.9 | 1.3 | 0.6 | 2.0 | 1.4 | 0.9 | | | | | 2 |
| | | Sprouts | | | | | | | | | | | | | | | |
| 5725 | 1/2 cup | Kidney Bean, boiled, avg | 64 | 21 | 89 | 3.1 | 3.0 | 0.8 | | | 0.4 | 0.1 | 0.0 | 0.2 | 0.12 | 0.08 | 0 |
| 5724 | 1/2 cup | Kidney Bean, raw, avg | 92 | 27 | 91 | 3.9 | 3.8 | 1.0 | | | 0.5 | 0.1 | 0.0 | 0.3 | 0.16 | 0.10 | 0 |
| 5458 | 1/2 cup | Soybeans, raw, avg | 35 | 43 | 69 | 4.6 | 3.3 | 0.4 | 1.0 | 2.0 | 2.3 | 0.3 | 0.5 | 1.3 | 0.16 | 1.17 | 0 |
| 5459 | 1/2 cup | Steamed, avg | 47 | 38 | 80 | 4.0 | 3.1 | 0.4 | | | 2.1 | 0.3 | 0.5 | 1.2 | 0.14 | 1.04 | 0 |
| 5795 | 1/2 cup | Stir Fried, avg | 62 | 78 | 67 | 8.1 | 5.8 | 0.5 | | | 4.4 | 0.6 | 1.0 | 2.5 | 0.29 | 2.19 | 0 |
| | | Squash | | | | | | | | | | | | | | | |
| 5314 | 1/2 cup | Acorn, baked, avg | 102 | 57 | 83 | 1.1 | 14.9 | 4.5 | 3.6 | 6.8 | 0.1 | 0.0 | 0.0 | 0.1 | 0.04 | 0.02 | 0 |
| 5800 | 1/2 cup | Acorn, raw, cubes, avg | 70 | 28 | 88 | 0.6 | 7.3 | 1.0 | 1.7 | 4.5 | 0.1 | 0.0 | 0.0 | 0.0 | 0.02 | 0.01 | 0 |
| 7369 | 1/2 cup | Banana, raw, Freida's Specialty Produce | 57 | 20 | 90 | 0.7 | 4.7 | 0.7 | 2.0 | 2.0 | 0.0 | 0.0 | 0.0 | 0.0 | 0.00 | 0.00 | 0 |
| 5318 | 1/2 cup | Butternut, bkd, mshd, avg | 122 | 49 | 88 | 1.1 | 12.8 | 3.4 | 3.1 | 6.3 | 0.1 | 0.0 | 0.0 | 0.0 | 0.03 | 0.02 | 0 |
| 5274 | 1/2 cup | Butternut, ckd f/fzn, avg | 120 | 47 | 88 | 1.5 | 12.1 | 3.4 | 4.9 | 3.8 | 0.1 | 0.0 | 0.0 | 0.0 | 0.02 | 0.01 | 0 |
| 5801 | 1/2 cup | Butternut, raw, avg | 70 | 31 | 86 | 0.7 | 8.2 | 2.4 | 1.9 | 3.9 | 0.1 | 0.0 | 0.0 | 0.0 | 0.02 | 0.01 | 0 |
| 5322 | 1/2 cup | Crookneck, ckd, avg | 90 | 18 | 94 | 0.8 | 3.9 | 1.3 | 2.0 | 0.6 | 0.3 | 0.1 | 0.0 | 0.1 | 0.07 | 0.04 | 0 |
| 5321 | 1/2 cup | Crookneck, raw, avg | 65 | 12 | 94 | 0.6 | 2.6 | 1.2 | 1.4 | 0.0 | 0.2 | 0.0 | 0.0 | 0.1 | 0.04 | 0.02 | 0 |
| 5453 | 1/2 cup | Hubbard, bkd, avg | 120 | 60 | 85 | 3.0 | 13.0 | 3.2 | 3.1 | 6.7 | 0.7 | 0.2 | 0.1 | 0.3 | 0.19 | 0.12 | 0 |
| 5803 | 1/2 cup | Hubbard, raw, avg | 58 | 23 | 88 | 1.2 | 5.0 | 1.7 | 1.4 | 1.9 | 0.3 | 0.1 | 0.0 | 0.1 | 0.08 | 0.05 | 0 |
| 5325 | 1/2 cup | Scallop, boiled, mshd, unsalted, avg | 120 | 19 | 95 | 1.2 | 4.0 | 2.3 | 2.2 | 0.1 | 0.2 | 0.0 | 0.0 | 0.1 | 0.05 | 0.03 | 0 |
| 5323 | 1/2 cup | Scallop, raw, avg | 65 | 12 | 94 | 0.8 | 2.5 | 1.1 | 1.3 | 0.1 | 0.1 | 0.0 | 0.0 | 0.1 | 0.03 | 0.02 | 0 |
| 5455 | 1/2 cup | Spaghetti, boiled, avg | 78 | 21 | 92 | 0.5 | 5.0 | 1.1 | | | 0.2 | 0.0 | 0.0 | 0.1 | 0.06 | 0.04 | 0 |
| 5804 | 1/2 cup | Spaghetti, raw, avg | 50 | 16 | 92 | 0.3 | 3.5 | 0.8 | | | 0.3 | 0.1 | 0.0 | 0.1 | 0.07 | 0.05 | 0 |
| 5152 | 1/2 cup | Summer, boiled, unsalted, avg | 90 | 18 | 94 | 0.8 | 3.9 | 1.3 | 1.8 | 0.8 | 0.3 | 0.1 | 0.0 | 0.1 | 0.07 | 0.04 | 0 |
| 5597 | 1/2 cup | Summer, cnd, drained, unsalted, avg | 108 | 14 | 96 | 0.7 | 3.2 | 1.5 | 1.7 | 0.0 | 0.1 | 0.0 | 0.0 | 0.0 | 0.02 | 0.01 | 0 |
| 5797 | 1/2 cup | Summer, ckd f/fzn, avg | 96 | 24 | 92 | 1.2 | 5.3 | 1.3 | 2.4 | 1.6 | 0.2 | 0.0 | 0.0 | 0.1 | 0.05 | 0.03 | 0 |
| 5151 | 1/2 cup | Summer, raw, avg | 56 | 11 | 94 | 0.7 | 2.4 | 1.1 | 1.2 | 0.2 | 0.1 | 0.0 | 0.0 | 0.0 | 0.03 | 0.02 | 0 |

| Code | Vit A (IU) | Vit A (RE) | Retinol (RE) | Carotenoids (RE) | Beta Carotene (mcg) | Thiamin (mg) | Riboflavin (mg) | Niacin (NE) | Vit B6 (mg) | Vit B12 (mcg) | Folate (mcg) | Panto (mg) | Vit C (mg) | Vit D (mg) | Vit E (α TE) | Calcium (mg) | Copper (mg) | Iron (mg) | Magnes (mg) | Mang (mg) | Phos (mg) | Potassium (mg) | Selenium (mcg) | Sodium (mg) | Zinc (mg) |
|---|---|---|---|---|---|---|---|---|---|---|---|---|---|---|---|---|---|---|---|---|---|---|---|---|---|
| | Vit A & Components | | | | | Vitamins | | | | | | | | | | Minerals | | | | | | | | | |
| 70599 | 0 | 0 | 0 | 0 | 0 | 0.05 | | 1.13 | | 0.00 | | | 0.0 | | | 0 | | 0.2 | | | | 185 | | 273 | |
| 70598 | 0 | 0 | 0 | 0 | 0 | 0.04 | 0.01 | 1.05 | 0.14 | 0.00 | | | 0.7 | | | 0 | | 0.0 | | | | 162 | | 251 | |
| 6324 | 0 | 0 | 0 | 0 | 0 | | | | | 0.00 | | | 9.0 | | | 0 | | 0.7 | | | | | | 35 | |
| | | | | | | | | | | | | | | | | | | | | | | | | | |
| 5396 | 1320 | 132 | 0 | 132 | 7779 | 0.04 | 0.10 | 0.50 | 0.05 | 0.00 | 10.4 | 0.25 | 5.7 | 0.0 | | 18 | 0.1 | 0.7 | 11 | 0.1 | 37 | 281 | 0.2 | 1 | 0.28 |
| 5142 | 26908 | 259 | 0 | 2691 | 15889 | 0.03 | 0.07 | 0.45 | 0.07 | 0.00 | 15.0 | 0.49 | 5.1 | 0.0 | 1.2 | 32 | 0.1 | 1.7 | 28 | 0.2 | 43 | 251 | 0.5 | 5 | 0.21 |
| 5793 | 928 | 93 | 0 | 93 | 548 | 0.03 | 0.06 | 0.35 | 0.04 | 0.00 | 9.4 | 0.17 | 5.2 | 0.0 | | 12 | 0.1 | 0.5 | 7 | 0.1 | 26 | 197 | 0.2 | 1 | 0.19 |
| 5426 | 1074 | 107 | 0 | 107 | 644 | 0.02 | 0.05 | 0.27 | 0.04 | 0.00 | 4.9 | 0.02 | 6.1 | 0.0 | | 45 | 0.1 | 0.4 | 39 | 0.2 | 21 | 283 | 0.5 | 25 | 0.10 |
| 5425 | 230 | 29 | 0 | 29 | 174 | 0.01 | 0.02 | 0.11 | 0.02 | 0.00 | 2.5 | 0.01 | 4.6 | 0.0 | | 14 | 0.0 | 0.4 | 15 | 0.1 | 10 | 109 | 0.2 | 10 | 0.04 |
| 5451 | 5 | | 0 | 1 | 4 | 0.00 | 0.01 | 0.05 | 0.01 | 0.00 | 12.0 | 0.05 | 1.6 | 0.0 | | 4 | 0.1 | 0.1 | 3 | 0.0 | 8 | 60 | 0.2 | 4 | 0.12 |
| | | | | | | | | | | | | | | | | | | | | | | | | | |
| 5593 | 0 | 0 | 0 | 0 | 0 | 0.00 | 0.02 | 0.11 | 0.03 | 0.00 | 12.9 | 0.08 | 11.2 | 0.0 | 0.0 | 13 | 0.1 | 0.1 | 7 | 0.0 | 18 | 211 | 0.5 | 10 | 0.10 |
| 5594 | 0 | 0 | 0 | 0 | 0 | 0.16 | 0.39 | 1.97 | 0.36 | 0.00 | 171.1 | 1.07 | 0.0 | 0.0 | 0.0 | 365 | 0.9 | 3.9 | 99 | 0.3 | 118 | 2027 | 0.4 | 161 | 1.24 |
| 5144 | 5 | | 0 | 1 | 3 | 0.00 | 0.03 | 0.17 | 0.04 | 0.00 | 15.7 | 0.05 | 13.2 | 0.0 | | 12 | 0.0 | 0.2 | 5 | 0.0 | 10 | 135 | 0.4 | 14 | 0.17 |
| 5550 | 0 | 0 | 0 | 0 | 0 | 0.01 | 0.01 | 0.15 | 0.04 | 0.00 | 7.0 | 0.09 | 14.5 | 0.0 | 0.0 | 14 | 0.0 | 0.4 | 4 | 0.0 | 14 | 140 | 0.3 | 3 | 0.06 |
| 7225 | 477 | 48 | 0 | 48 | 286 | 0.07 | 0.03 | 0.61 | 0.09 | 0.00 | 12.8 | 0.13 | 16.0 | 0.0 | 0.1 | 41 | 0.0 | 0.5 | 20 | 0.1 | 48 | 277 | 0.6 | 17 | 0.30 |
| 7214 | 435 | 4 | 0 | 41 | 244 | 0.06 | 0.03 | 0.49 | 0.07 | 0.00 | 14.7 | 0.11 | 17.5 | 0.0 | 0.0 | 33 | 0.0 | 0.4 | 16 | 0.1 | 41 | 236 | 0.5 | 14 | 0.24 |
| 5221 | 0 | 0 | 0 | 0 | 0 | 0.04 | 0.12 | 0.27 | 0.15 | 0.00 | 10.3 | 0.19 | 3.1 | 0.0 | | 32 | 0.0 | 0.4 | 12 | 0.1 | 38 | 192 | 0.4 | 11 | 0.20 |
| 5794 | 0 | 0 | 0 | 0 | 0 | 0.05 | 0.15 | 0.33 | 0.18 | 0.00 | 17.4 | 0.24 | 5.3 | 0.0 | | 40 | 0.1 | 0.5 | 15 | 0.2 | 50 | 251 | 0.5 | 13 | 0.25 |
| | | | | | | | | | | | | | | | | | | | | | | | | | |
| 5254 | 0 | 0 | 0 | 0 | 0 | 0.00 | 0.01 | 0.01 | 0.01 | 0.00 | 23.2 | 0.12 | 0.0 | 0.0 | | 25 | 0.0 | 0.9 | 31 | 0.2 | 2 | 45 | 0.3 | 4 | 0.23 |
| 5253 | 0 | 0 | 0 | 0 | 0 | 0.00 | 0.01 | 0.02 | 0.01 | 0.00 | 33.9 | 0.12 | 0.0 | 0.0 | | 22 | 0.0 | 0.7 | 27 | 0.1 | 2 | 90 | 0.3 | 4 | 0.23 |
| 5255 | 47 | 5 | 0 | 5 | 29 | 0.01 | 0.19 | 0.24 | 0.03 | 0.00 | 72.8 | 0.07 | 1.2 | 0.0 | | 29 | 0.1 | 3.6 | 58 | 0.1 | 63 | 25 | 0.3 | 27 | 0.78 |
| 5256 | 46 | 5 | 0 | 5 | 29 | 0.02 | 0.06 | 0.19 | 0.00 | 0.00 | 72.0 | 0.26 | 1.2 | 0.0 | | 67 | 0.1 | 1.1 | 48 | 0.1 | 17 | 36 | 0.3 | 93 | 0.49 |
| 5257 | 2081 | 208 | 0 | 208 | 1248 | 0.04 | 0.18 | 0.59 | 0.06 | 0.00 | 58.4 | 0.21 | 15.6 | 0.0 | | 28 | 0.1 | 0.7 | 1 | 0.4 | 23 | 142 | 0.3 | 19 | 0.42 |
| 5620 | 434 | 48 | 0 | 48 | 291 | 0.02 | 0.07 | 0.32 | 0.02 | 0.00 | 30.9 | 0.15 | 2.5 | 0.0 | | 56 | 0.2 | 1.1 | 28 | 0.3 | 21 | 143 | | 109 | 0.28 |
| 5260 | 23 | 2 | 0 | 2 | 14 | 0.10 | 0.15 | 0.51 | 0.01 | 0.00 | 3.8 | 0.14 | 0.4 | 0.0 | | 5 | 0.2 | 1.1 | 8 | 0.1 | 5 | 55 | 0.3 | 42 | 0.08 |
| 5836 | 48 | 5 | 0 | 5 | 31 | 0.19 | 0.29 | 1.02 | 0.03 | 0.00 | 7.8 | 0.28 | 0.8 | 0.0 | | 10 | 0.5 | 2.4 | 16 | 0.2 | 9 | 108 | 0.6 | 83 | 0.17 |
| 5261 | 144 | 14 | 0 | 14 | 86 | 0.02 | 0.09 | 0.64 | 0.00 | 0.00 | 78.4 | 0.28 | 1.2 | 0.0 | | 60 | 0.1 | 0.9 | 43 | 0.6 | 32 | 20 | 0.3 | 349 | 0.15 |
| 5428 | 561 | 56 | 0 | 56 | 337 | 0.00 | 0.00 | 0.01 | 0.02 | 0.00 | 1.2 | 0.01 | 0.4 | 0.0 | | 2 | 0.0 | 0.1 | 1 | 0.0 | 3 | 16 | 0.1 | 1 | 0.02 |
| 5427 | 119 | 12 | 0 | 12 | 71 | 0.01 | 0.00 | 0.02 | 0.03 | 0.00 | 3.4 | 0.03 | 0.8 | 0.0 | | 4 | 0.0 | 0.1 | 2 | 0.0 | 6 | 33 | 0.1 | 1 | 0.04 |
| 5259 | 140 | 14 | 0 | 14 | 83 | 0.23 | 0.14 | 1.13 | 0.05 | 0.00 | 99.9 | 0.12 | 15.3 | 0.0 | | 130 | 0.1 | 2.3 | 54 | 0.5 | 142 | 485 | 1.3 | 13 | 0.82 |
| 5258 | 230 | 23 | 0 | 23 | 133 | 0.56 | 0.22 | 2.11 | 0.08 | 0.00 | 211.2 | 0.19 | 37.1 | 0.0 | | 252 | 0.2 | 4.5 | 83 | 0.7 | 248 | 794 | 1.9 | 19 | 1.27 |
| | | | | | | | | | | | | | | | | | | | | | | | | | |
| 5147 | 7371 | 737 | 0 | 737 | 4374 | 0.09 | 0.21 | 0.44 | 0.22 | 0.00 | 131.4 | 0.13 | 8.8 | 0.0 | | 122 | 0.2 | 3.2 | 78 | 0.8 | 50 | 419 | 1.3 | 63 | 0.68 |
| 5595 | 7525 | 752 | 0 | 752 | 4465 | 0.02 | 0.12 | 0.32 | 0.09 | 0.00 | 67.9 | 0.04 | 15.8 | 0.0 | | 97 | 0.1 | 1.8 | 66 | 0.6 | 37 | 269 | 1.4 | 373 | 0.49 |
| 5973 | 7525 | 752 | 0 | 752 | 4465 | 0.02 | 0.12 | 0.32 | 0.09 | 0.00 | 67.9 | 0.04 | 15.8 | 0.0 | | 97 | 0.1 | 1.8 | 66 | 0.6 | 37 | 269 | 1.4 | 88 | 0.49 |
| 5498 | 21209 | 2121 | 0 | 2121 | 1259 | 0.25 | 0.60 | 2.29 | 0.62 | 0.00 | 514.0 | 0.20 | 88.8 | | | 313 | | 3.6 | 249 | | 155 | 1762 | | 249 | 1.67 |
| 5148 | 7395 | 739 | 0 | 739 | 4386 | 0.06 | 0.16 | 0.40 | 0.14 | 0.00 | 102.6 | 0.08 | 11.7 | 0.0 | | 139 | 0.1 | 1.4 | 66 | 0.9 | 46 | 283 | 1.6 | 82 | 0.66 |
| 56959 | 1483 | 297 | | | | | | | | 0.00 | | | 13.8 | | | 118 | | 0.7 | | | | | | 524 | |
| 5510 | | | | | | | | | | 0.00 | | | 34.2 | | | 1 | | | | | 52 | 486 | | 86 | |
| 5146 | 2015 | 202 | 0 | 202 | 1196 | 0.02 | 0.06 | 0.22 | 0.06 | 0.00 | 58.2 | 0.02 | 8.4 | 0.0 | 0.5 | 30 | 0.0 | 0.8 | 24 | 0.3 | 15 | 167 | 0.3 | 24 | 0.16 |
| 5670 | 6070 | 607 | 0 | 607 | 3601 | 0.06 | 0.17 | 0.62 | 0.17 | 0.00 | 120.7 | 0.06 | 16.1 | 0.0 | | 89 | 0.1 | 2.4 | 75 | 0.8 | 40 | 494 | | 75 | 0.50 |
| 5669 | 5448 | 545 | 0 | 545 | 3233 | 0.06 | 0.16 | 0.62 | 0.17 | 0.00 | 148.5 | 0.04 | 21.5 | 0.0 | | 89 | 0.1 | 2.4 | 71 | 0.8 | 44 | 502 | | 71 | 0.48 |
| 6347 | 2009 | 201 | 0 | 201 | 1192 | | | | | 0.00 | | | 16.1 | | | 81 | | 0.9 | | | | | | 239 | |
| | | | | | | | | | | | | | | | | | | | | | | | | | |
| 5725 | 1 | 0.1 | 0 | 0.1 | 1 | 0.23 | 0.17 | 1.93 | 0.06 | 0.00 | 30.3 | 0.24 | 22.8 | 0.0 | | 12 | 0.1 | 0.6 | 15 | 0.1 | 24 | 124 | 0.4 | 4 | 0.28 |
| 5724 | 2 | 0.2 | 0 | 0.2 | 1 | 0.34 | 0.23 | 2.69 | 0.08 | 0.00 | 54.2 | 0.34 | 35.6 | 0.0 | | 16 | 0.1 | 0.7 | 19 | 0.2 | 34 | 172 | 0.6 | 6 | 0.37 |
| 5458 | 4 | 0.4 | 0 | 0.4 | 2 | 0.12 | 0.04 | 0.40 | 0.06 | 0.00 | 60.2 | 0.33 | 5.4 | 0.0 | | 23 | 0.1 | 0.7 | 25 | 0.2 | 57 | 169 | 0.2 | 5 | 0.41 |
| 5459 | 5 | 0.5 | 0 | 0.5 | 3 | 0.10 | 0.02 | 0.51 | 0.05 | 0.00 | 37.6 | 0.35 | 3.9 | 0.0 | | 28 | 0.2 | 0.6 | 28 | 0.3 | 63 | 167 | 0.3 | 5 | 0.49 |
| 5795 | 11 | 1 | 0 | 1 | 7 | 0.26 | 0.12 | 0.68 | 0.10 | 0.00 | 78.7 | 0.74 | 7.4 | 0.0 | | 51 | 0.3 | 0.2 | 60 | 0.7 | 134 | 352 | 0.4 | 9 | 1.30 |
| | | | | | | | | | | | | | | | | | | | | | | | | | |
| 5314 | 437 | 44 | 0 | 44 | 261 | 0.17 | 0.01 | 0.90 | 0.20 | 0.00 | 19.1 | 0.51 | 11.0 | 0.0 | | 45 | 0.1 | 0.9 | 44 | 0.2 | 46 | 446 | 0.7 | 4 | 0.17 |
| 5800 | 238 | 24 | 0 | 24 | 142 | 0.10 | 0.01 | 0.49 | 0.11 | 0.00 | 11.7 | 0.28 | 7.7 | 0.0 | | 23 | 0.0 | 0.5 | 22 | 0.1 | 25 | 243 | 0.3 | 2 | 0.09 |
| 7369 | 2347 | 235 | 0 | 235 | 1397 | | | | | 0.00 | | | 6.0 | | | 13 | | 0.2 | | | | | | 0 | |
| 5318 | 8541 | 854 | 0 | 854 | 5083 | 0.09 | 0.02 | 1.18 | 0.15 | 0.00 | 23.4 | 0.44 | 18.4 | 0.0 | | 50 | 0.1 | 0.7 | 35 | 0.2 | 33 | 346 | 0.6 | 5 | 0.16 |
| 5274 | 4007 | 401 | 0 | 401 | 2386 | 0.06 | 0.05 | 0.56 | 0.08 | 0.00 | 19.7 | 0.18 | 4.2 | 0.0 | | 23 | 0.0 | 0.7 | 11 | 0.2 | 17 | 160 | 0.6 | 2 | 0.14 |
| 5801 | 5460 | 546 | 0 | 546 | 3250 | 0.07 | 0.01 | 0.84 | 0.11 | 0.00 | 18.7 | 0.28 | 14.7 | 0.0 | | 34 | 0.1 | 0.5 | 24 | 0.1 | 23 | 246 | 0.3 | 3 | 0.11 |
| 5322 | 258 | 26 | 0 | 26 | 155 | 0.04 | 0.04 | 0.46 | 0.08 | 0.00 | 18.1 | 0.12 | 4.9 | 0.0 | | 24 | 0.1 | 0.3 | 22 | 0.2 | 35 | 173 | 0.2 | 1 | 0.35 |
| 5321 | 220 | 22 | 0 | 22 | 131 | 0.03 | 0.03 | 0.30 | 0.07 | 0.00 | 14.9 | 0.07 | 5.5 | 0.0 | | 14 | 0.1 | 0.3 | 14 | 0.1 | 21 | 138 | 0.1 | 1 | 0.19 |
| 5453 | 7242 | 725 | 0 | 725 | 4314 | 0.09 | 0.06 | 0.67 | 0.21 | 0.00 | 19.4 | 0.54 | 11.4 | 0.0 | | 20 | 0.1 | 0.6 | 26 | 0.2 | 28 | 430 | 0.7 | 10 | 0.18 |
| 5803 | 3132 | 313 | 0 | 313 | 1364 | 0.04 | 0.02 | 0.29 | 0.09 | 0.00 | 9.5 | 0.23 | 6.4 | 0.0 | | 8 | 0.0 | 0.2 | 11 | 0.1 | 12 | 186 | 0.3 | 4 | 0.08 |
| 5325 | 102 | 11 | 0 | 11 | 64 | 0.06 | 0.03 | 0.56 | 0.10 | 0.00 | 24.8 | 0.09 | 13.0 | 0.0 | | 18 | 0.1 | 0.4 | 23 | 0.2 | 34 | 168 | 0.2 | 1 | 0.29 |
| 5323 | 72 | 7 | 0 | 7 | 43 | 0.05 | 0.02 | 0.39 | 0.07 | 0.00 | 19.6 | 0.07 | 11.7 | 0.0 | | 12 | 0.1 | 0.3 | 15 | 0.1 | 23 | 118 | 0.1 | 1 | 0.19 |
| 5455 | 86 | 9 | 0 | 9 | 51 | 0.03 | 0.02 | 0.63 | 0.08 | 0.00 | 6.2 | 0.28 | 2.7 | 0.0 | | 16 | 0.0 | 0.3 | 9 | 0.1 | 11 | 91 | 0.2 | 14 | 0.16 |
| 5804 | 25 | 3 | 0 | 3 | 15 | 0.02 | 0.01 | 0.47 | 0.05 | 0.00 | 6.0 | 0.18 | 1.0 | 0.0 | | 12 | 0.0 | 0.2 | 6 | 0.1 | 6 | 54 | 0.2 | 8 | 0.09 |
| 5152 | 258 | 26 | 0 | 26 | 155 | 0.04 | 0.04 | 0.46 | 0.06 | 0.00 | 18.1 | 0.12 | 4.9 | 0.0 | | 24 | 0.1 | 0.3 | 22 | 0.2 | 35 | 173 | 0.2 | 1 | 0.35 |
| 5597 | 131 | 13 | 0 | 13 | 77 | 0.02 | 0.03 | 0.45 | 0.05 | 0.00 | 11.2 | 0.05 | 2.9 | 0.0 | | 13 | 0.1 | 0.8 | 14 | 0.1 | 23 | 104 | 0.2 | 5 | 0.31 |
| 5797 | 187 | 19 | 0 | 19 | 114 | 0.03 | 0.05 | 0.42 | 0.10 | 0.00 | 12.2 | 0.10 | 6.5 | 0.0 | | 19 | 0.1 | 0.5 | 26 | 0.3 | 39 | 243 | 0.3 | 6 | 0.33 |
| 5151 | 110 | 11 | 0 | 11 | 67 | 0.04 | 0.02 | 0.31 | 0.06 | 0.00 | 14.3 | 0.06 | 8.3 | 0.0 | | 11 | 0.0 | 0.3 | 13 | 0.1 | 20 | 109 | 0.1 | 1 | 0.15 |

| Code | Amount | Description | Basic Components: Weight (g) | Calories | % Water | Protein (g) | Carbs (g) | Fiber (g) | Sugar (g) | Other Carbs (g) | Fat (g) | Additional Fats: Sat Fat (g) | Mono Fat (g) | Poly Fat (g) | Omega 3 (g) | Omega 6 (g) | Choles (mg) |
|---|---|---|---|---|---|---|---|---|---|---|---|---|---|---|---|---|---|
| 5599 | 1/2 cup | Zucchini, cnd, italian style, avg | 114 | 33 | 91 | 1.2 | 7.8 | 2.3 | 4.4 | 1.0 | 0.1 | 0.0 | 0.0 | 0.1 | 0.03 | 0.02 | 0 |
| 5598 | 1/2 cup | Zucchini, ckd f/fzn, avg | 112 | 19 | 95 | 1.3 | 4.0 | 1.5 | 1.9 | 0.6 | 0.1 | 0.0 | 0.0 | 0.1 | 0.04 | 0.02 | 0 |
| 5624 | 1/2 cup | Zucchini, pickled, avg | 85 | 26 | 91 | 0.9 | 6.0 | 1.0 | 4.7 | 0.4 | 0.2 | 0.0 | 0.1 | 0.1 | 0.04 | 0.03 | 0 |
| 5667 | 1/2 cup | Zucchini, stmd, avg | 90 | 13 | 95 | 1.1 | 2.6 | 1.1 | 1.5 | 0.1 | 0.1 | 0.0 | 0.0 | 0.1 | 0.03 | 0.02 | 0 |
| 5668 | 1/2 cup | Zucchini, stir fried, avg | 90 | 13 | 95 | 1.1 | 2.6 | 1.1 | 1.5 | 0.1 | 0.1 | 0.0 | 0.0 | 0.1 | 0.03 | 0.02 | 0 |
| 5326 | 1/2 cup | Zucchini, raw, avg | 65 | 9 | 95 | 0.8 | 1.9 | 0.8 | 1.1 | 0.0 | 0.1 | 0.0 | 0.0 | 0.0 | 0.02 | 0.01 | 0 |
| 5304 | 1/2 cup | Winter, bkd, mshd, avg | 122 | 48 | 89 | 1.1 | 10.7 | 3.4 | 2.6 | 4.7 | 0.8 | 0.2 | 0.1 | 0.3 | 0.20 | 0.12 | 0 |
| 5833 | 1/2 cup | Winter, raw, avg | 58 | 21 | 89 | 0.8 | 5.1 | 0.9 | 1.3 | 2.9 | 0.1 | 0.0 | 0.0 | 0.1 | 0.03 | 0.02 | 0 |
| | | Sweet Potatoes/Yams | | | | | | | | | | | | | | | |
| 5158 | 1/2 cup | Baked, avg | 100 | 103 | 73 | 1.7 | 24.3 | 3.0 | 10.0 | 11.3 | 0.1 | 0.0 | 0.0 | 0.0 | 0.01 | 0.04 | 0 |
| 5161 | 1/2 cup | Boiled, avg | 164 | 172 | 73 | 2.7 | 39.9 | 3.0 | 19.0 | 17.9 | 0.5 | 0.1 | 0.0 | 0.2 | 0.03 | 0.18 | 0 |
| 5162 | 1/2 cup | Canned, mshd, avg | 128 | 129 | 74 | 2.5 | 29.7 | 2.2 | 20.5 | 7.0 | 0.3 | 0.1 | 0.0 | 0.1 | 0.02 | 0.10 | 0 |
| 5552 | 1/2 cup | Canned, w/syrup, avg | 114 | 101 | 77 | 1.1 | 23.8 | 2.8 | 15.4 | 5.6 | 0.2 | 0.0 | 0.0 | 0.1 | 0.02 | 0.09 | 0 |
| 5542 | 1/2 cup | Frozen, bkd, avg | 88 | 88 | 74 | 1.5 | 20.6 | 1.6 | 15.0 | 4.0 | 0.1 | 0.0 | 0.0 | 0.0 | 0.01 | 0.04 | 0 |
| 6880 | 1/2 cup | Raw, avg | 66 | 69 | 73 | 1.1 | 16.0 | 2.0 | 3.8 | 10.3 | 0.2 | 0.0 | 0.0 | 0.1 | 0.01 | 0.07 | 0 |
| 5059 | 1/2 cup | Swiss Chard, boiled, avg | 88 | 18 | 93 | 1.7 | 3.6 | 1.8 | 0.4 | 1.4 | 0.1 | 0.0 | 0.0 | 0.0 | 0.00 | 0.02 | 0 |
| 5057 | 1/2 cup | Swiss Chard, raw, avg | 18 | 3 | 93 | 0.3 | 0.7 | 0.3 | 0.2 | 0.2 | 0.0 | 0.0 | 0.0 | 0.0 | 0.00 | 0.01 | 0 |
| | | Taro | | | | | | | | | | | | | | | |
| 7237 | 1/2 cup | Baked, avg | 66 | 91 | 61 | 1.3 | 22.6 | 3.5 | | | 0.2 | 0.0 | 0.0 | 0.1 | | | 0 |
| 6069 | 10 ea | Dried, avg | 23 | 65 | 27 | 0.9 | 15.3 | 0.2 | | | 0.1 | | | | | | |
| 5369 | 1/2 cup | Raw, slices, avg | 52 | 58 | 71 | 0.8 | 13.8 | 2.1 | 0.4 | 11.2 | 0.1 | 0.0 | 0.0 | 0.0 | 0.01 | 0.03 | 0 |
| 5444 | 1/2 cup | Tomatillos, raw, chpd, avg | 66 | 21 | 92 | 0.6 | 3.8 | 1.3 | | | 0.7 | 0.1 | 0.1 | 0.3 | 0.01 | 0.26 | 0 |
| | | Tomatoes | | | | | | | | | | | | | | | |
| 6927 | 1/2 cup | Canned, crushed, avg | 55 | 18 | 89 | 0.9 | 4.0 | 1.0 | | | 0.2 | 0.0 | 0.0 | 0.1 | 0.00 | 0.06 | 0 |
| 5474 | 1/2 cup | Canned, stewed, avg | 128 | 36 | 91 | 1.2 | 8.7 | 1.3 | | | 0.2 | 0.0 | 0.0 | 0.1 | 0.00 | 0.07 | 0 |
| 6542 | 1/2 cup | Canned, tidbits, Contadina | 124 | 40 | 93 | 0.0 | 8.0 | 2.0 | 6.0 | 0.0 | 0.0 | 0.0 | 0.0 | 0.0 | 0.00 | 0.00 | 0 |
| 5179 | 1/2 cup | Canned, unsalted, avg | 120 | 23 | 94 | 1.1 | 5.2 | 1.2 | 3.0 | 1.0 | 0.2 | 0.0 | 0.0 | 0.1 | 0.00 | 0.06 | 0 |
| 5545 | 1/2 cup | Canned, wedges in tomato juice, avg | 130 | 34 | 92 | 1.0 | 8.2 | 1.3 | 5.1 | 1.8 | 0.2 | 0.0 | 0.0 | 0.1 | 0.00 | 0.08 | 0 |
| 6477 | 1/2 cup | Canned, whole, peeled, Progresso | 121 | 25 | 95 | 1.0 | 4.0 | 1.0 | 3.0 | 0.0 | 0.0 | 0.0 | 0.0 | 0.0 | 0.00 | 0.00 | 0 |
| 5471 | 1/2 cup | Canned, whole, unsalted, avg | 120 | 23 | 94 | 1.1 | 5.2 | 1.2 | 2.9 | 1.2 | 0.2 | 0.0 | 0.0 | 0.1 | 0.00 | 0.06 | 0 |
| 5546 | 1/2 cup | Canned, w/green chilies, avg | 120 | 18 | 94 | 0.8 | 4.3 | 1.2 | 0.8 | 2.3 | 0.1 | 0.0 | 0.0 | 0.0 | 0.00 | 0.03 | 0 |
| 5536 | 1 ea | Green, ckd, avg | 144 | 238 | 72 | 4.1 | 16.4 | 2.0 | 3.9 | 10.6 | 17.8 | 4.7 | 7.7 | 4.5 | 0.16 | 4.32 | 32 |
| 5630 | 1/2 cup | Green, pickled, avg | 71 | 26 | 90 | 0.8 | 6.0 | 1.0 | 4.3 | 0.7 | 0.2 | 0.0 | 0.1 | 0.1 | | | 0 |
| 5519 | 1/2 cup | Green, raw, chpd, avg | 90 | 22 | 93 | 1.1 | 4.6 | 1.0 | 2.3 | 1.3 | 0.2 | 0.0 | 0.0 | 0.1 | 0.00 | 0.07 | 0 |
| 5473 | 1/2 cup | Paste, avg | 131 | 107 | 74 | 4.8 | 25.3 | 5.4 | 3.1 | 16.8 | 0.7 | 0.1 | 0.1 | 0.3 | 0.01 | 0.28 | 0 |
| 5181 | 1/2 cup | Paste, unsalted, avg | 131 | 107 | 74 | 4.8 | 25.3 | 5.4 | 3.1 | 16.8 | 0.7 | 0.1 | 0.1 | 0.3 | 0.01 | 0.28 | 0 |
| 5476 | 1/2 cup | Puree, avg | 125 | 50 | 88 | 2.1 | 12.0 | 2.5 | 7.9 | 1.6 | 0.2 | 0.0 | 0.0 | 0.1 | 0.00 | 0.07 | 0 |
| 6479 | 1/2 cup | Puree, thick style, Progresso | 126 | 50 | 89 | 2.0 | 10.0 | 2.0 | 6.0 | 2.0 | 0.0 | 0.0 | 0.0 | 0.0 | 0.00 | 0.00 | 0 |
| 5225 | 1/2 cup | Puree, unsalted, avg | 125 | 50 | 88 | 2.1 | 12.0 | 2.5 | 7.9 | 1.6 | 0.2 | 0.0 | 0.0 | 0.1 | 0.00 | 0.07 | 0 |
| 5178 | 1/2 cup | Raw, boiled, unsalted, avg | 120 | 32 | 92 | 1.3 | 7.0 | 1.2 | 3.8 | 2.0 | 0.5 | 0.1 | 0.1 | 0.2 | 0.01 | 0.20 | 0 |
| 5627 | 1 ea | Raw, brld, avg | 123 | 32 | 92 | 1.3 | 7.1 | 2.0 | 4.6 | 0.6 | 0.5 | 0.1 | 0.1 | 0.2 | 0.00 | 0.13 | 0 |
| 5170 | 1/2 cup | Raw, chpd, avg | 90 | 19 | 94 | 0.8 | 4.2 | 1.0 | 2.5 | 0.7 | 0.3 | 0.0 | 0.0 | 0.1 | 0.00 | 0.12 | 0 |
| 5628 | 1 ea | Raw, fried, avg | 101 | 165 | 73 | 2.6 | 11.2 | 1.2 | 8.2 | 1.7 | 12.6 | 3.3 | 5.4 | 3.2 | 0.00 | 0.00 | 22 |
| 5468 | 1/2 cup | Raw, stewed, avg | 50 | 40 | 81 | 1.0 | 6.6 | 0.9 | 3.7 | 2.0 | 1.3 | 0.3 | 0.5 | 0.4 | 0.02 | 0.42 | 0 |
| 5180 | 1/2 cup | Sauce, cnd, avg | 122 | 37 | 89 | 1.6 | 8.8 | 1.7 | 4.6 | 2.4 | 0.2 | 0.0 | 0.0 | 0.1 | 0.00 | 0.08 | 0 |
| 7232 | 1/2 cup | Sauce, cnd, low sod, avg | 122 | 37 | 89 | 1.6 | 8.8 | 1.8 | | | 0.2 | 0.0 | 0.0 | 0.1 | | | 0 |
| 6294 | 1/2 cup | Sauce, cnd, thick & zesty, Contadina | 124 | 40 | 91 | 2.0 | 6.0 | 2.0 | 4.0 | 0.0 | 0.0 | 0.0 | 0.0 | 0.0 | 0.00 | 0.00 | 0 |
| 5446 | 1/2 cup | Sun Dried, avg | 27 | 70 | 15 | 3.8 | 15.1 | 3.3 | 5.7 | 6.1 | 0.8 | 0.1 | 0.1 | 0.3 | 0.00 | 0.30 | 0 |
| 7482 | 1/2 cup | Sun Dried, packed in oil, drained, avg | 55 | 117 | 54 | 2.8 | 12.8 | 3.2 | | | 7.8 | 1.0 | 4.8 | 1.1 | 0.04 | 1.09 | 0 |
| 6116 | 1/2 cup | Sun Dried, yellow, World Variety Produce | 27 | 79 | 23 | 3.4 | 15.1 | 3.2 | 5.7 | 6.2 | 0.6 | 0.3 | 0.4 | 0.0 | | | 0 |
| | | Turnips | | | | | | | | | | | | | | | |
| 5184 | 1/2 cup | Boiled, mshd, unsalted, avg | 58 | 12 | 94 | 0.4 | 2.8 | 1.2 | 1.1 | 0.6 | 0.0 | 0.0 | 0.0 | 0.0 | 0.02 | 0.01 | 0 |
| 5819 | 1/2 cup | Frozen, boiled, avg | 78 | 18 | 94 | 1.2 | 3.4 | 1.6 | 1.6 | 0.3 | 0.2 | 0.0 | 0.0 | 0.1 | 0.07 | 0.02 | 0 |
| 5820 | 1/2 cup | Greens, cnd, w/liquid, avg | 117 | 16 | 95 | 1.6 | 2.8 | 2.0 | | | 0.4 | 0.1 | 0.0 | 0.1 | 0.10 | 0.04 | 0 |
| 5186 | 1/2 cup | Greens, fzn, boiled, avg | 82 | 25 | 90 | 2.7 | 4.1 | 2.8 | 0.1 | 1.2 | 0.3 | 0.1 | 0.0 | 0.1 | 0.10 | 0.04 | 0 |
| 5185 | 1/2 cup | Greens, raw, boiled, avg | 72 | 14 | 93 | 0.8 | 3.1 | 2.5 | 0.1 | 0.5 | 0.2 | 0.0 | 0.0 | 0.1 | 0.05 | 0.02 | 0 |
| 5547 | 1/2 cup | Greens, raw, chpd, avg | 27 | 7 | 91 | 0.4 | 1.5 | 0.9 | 0.3 | 0.4 | 0.1 | 0.0 | 0.0 | 0.0 | 0.02 | 0.01 | 0 |
| 5623 | 10 ea | Pickled, avg | 70 | 29 | 88 | 0.6 | 7.0 | 1.1 | 5.6 | 0.3 | 0.1 | 0.0 | 0.0 | 0.0 | 0.04 | 0.01 | 0 |
| 5182 | 1/2 cup | Raw, avg | 65 | 18 | 92 | 0.6 | 4.0 | 1.2 | 2.5 | 0.4 | 0.1 | 0.0 | 0.0 | 0.0 | 0.03 | 0.01 | 0 |
| 5823 | 1/2 cup | With Greens, fzn, boiled, avg | 86 | 15 | 94 | 1.8 | 2.5 | 1.5 | | | 0.1 | 0.0 | 0.0 | 0.1 | 0.05 | 0.02 | 0 |
| 5629 | 1/2 cup | Vegetable Tempura, avg | 32 | 51 | 71 | 1.3 | 4.6 | 0.4 | 0.6 | 3.5 | 3.1 | 0.6 | 1.0 | 1.3 | | | 21 |
| 5387 | 1/2 cup | Waterchestnuts, cnd, w/liquid, avg | 70 | 35 | 86 | 0.6 | 8.7 | 1.8 | 1.8 | 5.2 | 0.0 | 0.0 | 0.0 | 0.0 | 0.00 | 0.01 | 0 |
| 5386 | 1/2 oz | Waterchestnuts, raw, avg | 62 | 60 | 74 | 0.9 | 14.8 | 1.9 | 3.0 | 10.0 | 0.1 | 0.0 | 0.0 | 0.0 | 0.01 | 0.02 | 0 |
| 5222 | 1/2 cup | Watercress, fresh, avg | 17 | 2 | 95 | 0.4 | 0.2 | 0.3 | 0.0 | 0.0 | 0.0 | 0.0 | 0.0 | 0.0 | 0.00 | 0.00 | 0 |
| 5432 | 1/2 cup | Waxgourd, boiled, cubes, avg | 88 | 11 | 96 | 0.4 | 2.7 | 0.9 | 0.9 | 0.9 | 0.2 | 0.0 | 0.0 | 0.1 | 0.00 | 0.08 | 0 |

| Code | Vit A & Components: Vit A (IU) | Vit A (RE) | Retinol (RE) | Carotenoids (RE) | Beta Carotene (mcg) | Vitamins: Thiamin (mg) | Riboflavin (mg) | Niacin (NE) | Vit B6 (mg) | Vit B12 (mcg) | Folate (mcg) | Panto (mg) | Vit C (mg) | Vit D (mg) | Vit E (α TE) | Minerals: Calcium (mg) | Copper (mg) | Iron (mg) | Magnes (mg) | Mang (mg) | Phos (mg) | Potassium (mg) | Selenium (mcg) | Sodium (mg) | Zinc (mg) |
|---|---|---|---|---|---|---|---|---|---|---|---|---|---|---|---|---|---|---|---|---|---|---|---|---|---|
| 5599 | 614 | 62 | 0 | 62 | 366 | 0.05 | 0.05 | 0.60 | 0.17 | 0.00 | 34.4 | 0.31 | 2.6 | 0.0 | | 19 | 0.1 | 0.8 | 16 | 0.3 | 33 | 312 | 0.5 | 426 | 0.30 |
| 5598 | 484 | 48 | 0 | 48 | 287 | 0.05 | 0.04 | 0.43 | 0.05 | 0.00 | 8.7 | 0.30 | 4.1 | 0.0 | | 19 | 0.1 | 0.5 | 15 | 0.3 | 28 | 217 | 0.2 | 2 | 0.22 |
| 5624 | 418 | 42 | 0 | 42 | 249 | 0.04 | 0.02 | 0.25 | 0.07 | 0.00 | 10.7 | 0.07 | 11.0 | 0.0 | | 14 | 0.0 | 0.4 | 15 | 0.1 | 23 | 161 | | 73 | 0.16 |
| 5667 | 292 | 29 | 0 | 29 | 174 | 0.06 | 0.03 | 0.34 | 0.07 | 0.00 | 16.9 | 0.07 | 6.9 | 0.0 | | 13 | 0.1 | 0.4 | 20 | 0.1 | 29 | 223 | | 3 | 0.18 |
| 5668 | 276 | 28 | 0 | 28 | 164 | 0.06 | 0.03 | 0.34 | 0.07 | 0.00 | 15.9 | 0.07 | 6.9 | 0.0 | | 13 | 0.1 | 0.4 | 20 | 0.1 | 29 | 223 | | 3 | 0.18 |
| 5326 | 221 | 22 | 0 | 22 | 131 | 0.05 | 0.02 | 0.26 | 0.06 | 0.00 | 14.4 | 0.05 | 5.8 | 0.0 | | 10 | 0.0 | 0.3 | 14 | 0.1 | 21 | 161 | 0.1 | 2 | 0.13 |
| 5304 | 4340 | 434 | 0 | 434 | 2585 | 0.10 | 0.03 | 0.86 | 0.09 | 0.00 | 34.2 | 0.43 | 11.7 | 0.0 | | 17 | 0.1 | 0.4 | 10 | 0.3 | 24 | 533 | 0.5 | 1 | 0.32 |
| 5833 | 2355 | 235 | 0 | 235 | 1402 | 0.06 | 0.02 | 0.46 | 0.05 | 0.00 | 12.6 | 0.23 | 7.1 | 0.0 | 0.1 | 18 | 0.0 | 0.3 | 12 | 0.1 | 19 | 203 | 0.2 | 2 | 0.08 |
| 5158 | 21822 | 2182 | 0 | 2182 | 13092 | 0.07 | 0.13 | 0.60 | 0.24 | 0.00 | 22.6 | 0.65 | 24.6 | 0.0 | | 28 | 0.2 | 0.4 | 20 | 0.6 | 55 | 348 | 0.7 | 10 | 0.29 |
| 5161 | 27969 | 2796 | 0 | 2796 | 16777 | 0.09 | 0.23 | 1.05 | 0.40 | 0.00 | 18.2 | 0.87 | 28.0 | 0.0 | | 34 | 0.3 | 0.9 | 16 | 0.6 | 44 | 302 | 1.1 | 21 | 0.44 |
| 5162 | 19361 | 1937 | 0 | 1937 | 11620 | 0.03 | 0.12 | 1.22 | 0.30 | 0.00 | 13.7 | 0.66 | 6.7 | 0.0 | | 38 | 0.4 | 1.7 | 31 | 1.3 | 67 | 269 | 1.0 | 96 | 0.27 |
| 5552 | 6520 | 652 | 0 | 652 | 3912 | 0.03 | 0.05 | 0.52 | 0.06 | 0.00 | 7.4 | 0.38 | 12.0 | 0.0 | | 17 | 0.1 | 0.9 | 15 | 0.6 | 31 | 211 | 0.8 | 50 | 0.22 |
| 5542 | 14441 | 1444 | 0 | 1444 | 8664 | 0.06 | 0.05 | 0.49 | 0.16 | 0.00 | 19.6 | 0.49 | 8.0 | 0.0 | | 31 | 0.2 | 0.5 | 18 | 0.6 | 39 | 332 | 0.5 | 7 | 0.26 |
| 6880 | 13242 | 1324 | 0 | 1324 | 7944 | 0.04 | 0.10 | 0.44 | 0.17 | 0.00 | 9.1 | 0.39 | 15.0 | 0.0 | | 15 | 0.1 | 0.4 | 7 | 0.2 | 18 | 135 | 0.4 | 9 | 0.18 |
| 5059 | 2762 | 276 | 0 | 276 | 1646 | 0.03 | 0.08 | 0.32 | 0.07 | 0.00 | 7.6 | 0.14 | 15.8 | 0.0 | 0.6 | 51 | 0.1 | 2.0 | 76 | 0.3 | 29 | 483 | 0.8 | 158 | 0.29 |
| 5057 | 594 | 59 | 0 | 59 | 354 | 0.01 | 0.02 | 0.07 | 0.02 | 0.00 | 2.5 | 0.03 | 5.4 | 0.0 | 0.3 | 9 | 0.0 | 0.3 | 15 | 0.1 | 8 | 68 | 0.2 | 38 | 0.06 |
| 7237 | 0 | 0 | 0 | 0 | 0 | 0.07 | 0.02 | 0.49 | 0.23 | 0.00 | 15.2 | | 2.9 | | | 37 | 0.1 | 0.5 | 28 | | 72 | 504 | | 208 | 0.20 |
| 6069 | | | | | | | | | | 0.00 | | | | 0.0 | | 8 | | 1.3 | | | 38 | | | | |
| 5369 | 0 | 0 | 0 | 0 | 0 | 0.05 | 0.01 | 0.31 | 0.15 | 0.00 | 11.5 | 0.16 | 2.3 | 0.0 | | 22 | 0.1 | 0.3 | 17 | 0.2 | 44 | 307 | 0.4 | 6 | 0.12 |
| 5444 | 75 | 7 | 0 | 7 | 44 | 0.03 | 0.02 | 1.22 | 0.04 | 0.00 | 4.6 | 0.10 | 7.7 | 0.0 | | 5 | 0.1 | 0.4 | 13 | 0.1 | 26 | 177 | 0.3 | 1 | 0.15 |
| 6927 | 384 | 39 | 0 | 39 | 226 | 0.04 | 0.03 | 0.67 | 0.08 | 0.00 | 7.2 | 0.15 | 5.1 | 0.0 | | 19 | 0.1 | 0.7 | 11 | 0.1 | 18 | 161 | 0.3 | 73 | 0.15 |
| 5474 | 692 | 69 | 0 | 69 | 405 | 0.06 | 0.04 | 0.91 | 0.02 | 0.00 | 6.9 | 0.15 | 14.6 | 0.0 | | 42 | 0.1 | 0.9 | 15 | 0.1 | 26 | 305 | 0.8 | 283 | 0.22 |
| 6542 | 800 | 80 | 0 | 80 | 469 | | | | | 0.00 | | | 12.0 | | | 0 | | 0.7 | | | | | | 20 | |
| 5179 | 714 | 72 | 0 | 72 | 422 | 0.05 | 0.04 | 0.88 | 0.11 | 0.00 | 9.4 | 0.20 | 17.0 | 0.0 | | 36 | 0.1 | 0.7 | 14 | 0.2 | 23 | 265 | 0.8 | 178 | 0.19 |
| 5545 | 751 | 75 | 0 | 75 | 442 | 0.07 | 0.04 | 0.88 | 0.15 | 0.00 | 13.1 | 0.28 | 19.2 | 0.0 | | 34 | 0.1 | 0.6 | 14 | 0.2 | 30 | 326 | 0.6 | 282 | 0.21 |
| 6477 | 500 | 50 | 0 | 50 | 293 | | | | | 0.00 | | | 12.0 | | | 20 | | 0.7 | | | | | | 220 | |
| 5471 | 714 | 72 | 0 | 72 | 422 | 0.05 | 0.04 | 0.88 | 0.11 | 0.00 | 9.4 | 0.20 | 17.0 | 0.0 | | 36 | 0.1 | 0.7 | 14 | 0.2 | 23 | 272 | 0.8 | 12 | 0.19 |
| 5546 | 468 | 47 | 0 | 47 | 281 | 0.04 | 0.02 | 0.77 | 0.12 | 0.00 | 10.9 | 0.18 | 7.4 | 0.0 | | 24 | 0.1 | 0.3 | 13 | 0.2 | 17 | 128 | 0.5 | 481 | 0.16 |
| 5536 | 688 | 81 | 18 | 63 | 366 | 0.15 | 0.16 | 1.22 | 0.10 | 0.11 | 12.0 | 0.58 | 24.1 | 0.2 | | 85 | 0.1 | 1.3 | 17 | 0.2 | 84 | 269 | | 242 | 0.31 |
| 5630 | 507 | 51 | 0 | 51 | 296 | 0.04 | 0.02 | 0.28 | 0.06 | 0.00 | 5.2 | 0.28 | 17.6 | 0.0 | | 11 | 0.1 | 0.4 | 8 | 0.1 | 19 | 128 | | 82 | 0.07 |
| 5519 | 578 | 58 | 0 | 58 | 338 | 0.05 | 0.04 | 0.45 | 0.07 | 0.00 | 7.9 | 0.45 | 21.1 | 0.0 | | 12 | 0.1 | 0.5 | 9 | 0.1 | 25 | 184 | 0.4 | 12 | 0.06 |
| 5473 | 3203 | 320 | 0 | 320 | 1873 | 0.20 | 0.25 | 4.22 | 0.50 | 0.00 | 29.3 | 0.99 | 55.5 | 0.0 | | 46 | 0.8 | 2.5 | 67 | 0.7 | 103 | 1227 | 1.8 | 1035 | 1.05 |
| 5181 | 3203 | 320 | 0 | 320 | 1873 | 0.20 | 0.25 | 4.22 | 0.50 | 0.00 | 29.3 | 0.99 | 55.5 | 0.0 | 2.8 | 46 | 0.8 | 2.5 | 67 | 0.7 | 103 | 1227 | 1.8 | 115 | 1.05 |
| 5476 | 1594 | 160 | 0 | 160 | 938 | 0.09 | 0.07 | 2.15 | 0.19 | 0.00 | 13.8 | 0.55 | 13.0 | 0.0 | | 21 | 0.2 | 1.5 | 30 | 0.3 | 50 | 532 | 0.9 | 499 | 0.28 |
| 6479 | 1500 | 150 | 0 | 150 | 879 | | | | | 0.00 | | | 18.0 | | | 0 | | 1.4 | | | | | | 30 | |
| 5225 | 1594 | 160 | 0 | 160 | 938 | 0.09 | 0.07 | 2.15 | 0.19 | 0.00 | 13.8 | 0.55 | 13.0 | 0.0 | | 21 | 0.2 | 1.5 | 30 | 0.3 | 50 | 532 | 0.9 | 42 | 0.28 |
| 5178 | 892 | 89 | 0 | 89 | 521 | 0.08 | 0.07 | 0.90 | 0.11 | 0.00 | 15.6 | 0.35 | 27.4 | 0.0 | | 7 | 0.1 | 0.7 | 17 | 0.2 | 37 | 335 | 0.6 | 13 | 0.13 |
| 5627 | 862 | 86 | 0 | 86 | 503 | 0.09 | 0.07 | 0.92 | 0.12 | 0.00 | 16.1 | 0.25 | 27.9 | 0.0 | | 7 | 0.1 | 0.7 | 17 | 0.2 | 37 | 342 | | 14 | 0.14 |
| 5170 | 561 | 56 | 0 | 56 | 327 | 0.05 | 0.04 | 0.57 | 0.07 | 0.00 | 13.5 | 0.22 | 17.2 | 0.0 | | 4 | 0.1 | 0.4 | 10 | 0.1 | 22 | 200 | 0.4 | 8 | 0.08 |
| 5628 | 493 | 58 | 13 | 45 | 263 | 0.10 | 0.12 | 0.95 | 0.07 | 0.08 | 11.7 | 0.20 | 13.8 | 0.2 | | 54 | 0.1 | 0.8 | 12 | 0.1 | 56 | 202 | | 167 | 0.23 |
| 5468 | 333 | 34 | 0 | 34 | 196 | 0.05 | 0.04 | 0.56 | 0.04 | 0.00 | 5.5 | 0.13 | 9.1 | 0.0 | | 13 | 0.0 | 0.5 | 8 | 0.1 | 19 | 124 | 0.6 | 228 | 0.09 |
| 5180 | 1194 | 120 | 0 | 120 | 701 | 0.08 | 0.07 | 1.40 | 0.19 | 0.00 | 11.5 | 0.38 | 16.0 | 0.0 | 0.5 | 17 | 0.2 | 0.9 | 23 | 0.3 | 39 | 453 | 0.7 | 738 | 0.31 |
| 7232 | 1194 | 120 | 0 | 120 | 701 | 0.09 | 0.07 | 1.40 | 0.20 | 0.00 | 11.0 | | 16.0 | | | 17 | 0.2 | 0.9 | 23 | | 39 | 453 | | 13 | 0.31 |
| 6294 | 800 | 80 | 0 | 80 | 469 | | | | | 0.00 | | | 9.5 | | | 0 | | 1.4 | | | | | | 680 | |
| 5446 | 236 | 23 | 0 | 23 | 138 | 0.14 | 0.13 | 2.44 | 0.09 | 0.00 | 18.4 | 0.56 | 10.6 | 0.0 | | 30 | 0.4 | 2.5 | 52 | 0.5 | 96 | 925 | 1.5 | 566 | 0.54 |
| 7482 | 707 | 71 | 0 | 71 | 416 | 0.11 | 0.21 | 2.00 | 0.18 | 0.00 | 12.7 | 0.26 | 56.1 | 0.0 | | 26 | 0.3 | 1.5 | 45 | 0.3 | 76 | 861 | 1.7 | 146 | 0.43 |
| 6116 | 486 | 49 | 0 | 49 | 285 | | | | | 0.00 | | | 4.5 | | | 32 | | 2.3 | | | | | | 23 | |
| 5184 | 0 | 0 | 0 | 0 | 0 | 0.02 | 0.01 | 0.17 | 0.04 | 0.00 | 5.3 | 0.08 | 6.7 | 0.0 | 0.0 | 13 | 0.0 | 0.1 | 5 | 0.1 | 11 | 78 | 0.3 | 29 | 0.12 |
| 5819 | 20 | 2 | 0 | 2 | 9 | 0.03 | 0.02 | 0.44 | 0.05 | 0.00 | 6.2 | 0.11 | 3.0 | 0.0 | 0.0 | 25 | 0.0 | 0.8 | 11 | 0.1 | 20 | 142 | 0.5 | 28 | 0.16 |
| 5820 | 4196 | 420 | 0 | 420 | 2520 | 0.01 | 0.07 | 0.42 | 0.04 | 0.00 | 48.2 | 0.05 | 18.1 | 0.0 | 0.0 | 138 | 0.1 | 1.8 | 23 | 0.3 | 25 | 165 | 0.8 | 324 | 0.27 |
| 5186 | 6540 | 654 | 0 | 654 | 3926 | 0.04 | 0.06 | 0.38 | 0.05 | 0.00 | 32.3 | 0.06 | 17.9 | 0.0 | 1.4 | 125 | 0.1 | 1.6 | 21 | 0.4 | 28 | 184 | 1.0 | 12 | 0.34 |
| 5185 | 3959 | 396 | 0 | 396 | 2376 | 0.03 | 0.05 | 0.30 | 0.13 | 0.00 | 85.0 | 0.20 | 19.7 | 0.0 | 1.2 | 99 | 0.2 | 0.6 | 16 | 0.2 | 21 | 146 | 0.6 | 21 | 0.10 |
| 5547 | 2052 | 205 | 0 | 205 | 1231 | 0.02 | 0.03 | 0.16 | 0.07 | 0.00 | 52.4 | 0.10 | 16.2 | 0.0 | 0.6 | 51 | 0.1 | 0.3 | 8 | 0.1 | 11 | 80 | 0.3 | 11 | 0.05 |
| 5623 | 229 | 23 | 0 | 23 | 137 | 0.02 | 0.02 | 0.21 | 0.06 | 0.00 | 6.3 | 0.07 | 13.0 | 0.0 | | 17 | 0.0 | 0.2 | 7 | 0.1 | 16 | 104 | | 99 | 0.15 |
| 5182 | 0 | 0 | 0 | 0 | 0 | 0.03 | 0.02 | 0.26 | 0.06 | 0.00 | 9.4 | 0.13 | 13.6 | 0.0 | 0.0 | 19 | 0.1 | 0.2 | 7 | 0.1 | 18 | 124 | 0.5 | 44 | 0.18 |
| 5823 | 4438 | 444 | 0 | 444 | 2663 | 0.03 | 0.06 | 0.25 | 0.05 | 0.00 | 18.5 | 0.08 | 8.1 | 0.0 | | 78 | 0.0 | 1.1 | 10 | 0.2 | 15 | 53 | 0.8 | 13 | 0.11 |
| 5629 | 681 | 74 | 9 | 66 | 394 | 0.04 | 0.06 | 0.43 | 0.02 | 0.04 | 7.2 | 0.10 | 1.3 | 0.1 | | 8 | 0.0 | 0.4 | 4 | 0.1 | 22 | 56 | | 10 | 0.14 |
| 5387 | 3 | 0 | 0 | 0 | 0 | 0.01 | 0.02 | 0.25 | 0.11 | 0.00 | 4.1 | 0.15 | 0.9 | 0.0 | | 3 | 0.1 | 0.6 | 3 | 0.1 | 13 | 83 | 0.5 | 6 | 0.27 |
| 5386 | 0 | 0 | 0 | 0 | 0 | 0.09 | 0.12 | 0.62 | 0.20 | 0.00 | 10.0 | 0.30 | 2.5 | 0.0 | | 7 | 0.2 | 0.0 | 14 | 0.2 | 39 | 362 | 0.4 | 9 | 0.31 |
| 5222 | 799 | 80 | 0 | 80 | 479 | 0.02 | 0.02 | 0.03 | 0.02 | 0.00 | 1.6 | 0.05 | 7.3 | 0.0 | 0.2 | 20 | 0.0 | 0.0 | 4 | 0.0 | 10 | 56 | 0.2 | 7 | 0.02 |
| 5432 | 0 | 0 | 0 | 0 | 0 | 0.03 | 0.00 | 0.34 | 0.03 | 0.00 | 3.3 | 0.11 | 9.2 | 0.0 | | 16 | 0.0 | 0.3 | 9 | 0.0 | 15 | 4 | 0.2 | 94 | 0.52 |

| Code | Amount | Description | Basic Components | | | | | | | | | Additional Fats | | | | | | Vit A & Components | | | | | Vitamins | | | | | | | | | | | Minerals | | | | | | | | | |
|---|---|---|---|---|---|---|---|---|---|---|---|---|---|---|---|---|---|---|---|---|---|---|---|---|---|---|---|---|---|---|---|---|---|---|---|---|---|---|---|---|---|---|
| | | | Weight (g) | Calories | % Water | Protein (g) | Carbs (g) | Fiber (g) | Sugar (g) | Other Carbs (g) | Fat (g) | Sat Fat (g) | Mono Fat (g) | Poly Fat (g) | Omega 3 (g) | Omega 6 (g) | Choles (mg) | Vit A (IU) | Vit A (RE) | Retinol (RE) | Carotenoids (RE) | Beta Carotene (mcg) | Thiamin (mg) | Riboflavin (mg) | Niacin (NE) | Vit B6 (mg) | Vit B12 (mcg) | Folate (mcg) | Panto (mg) | Vit C (mg) | Vit D (mg) | Vit E (α TE) | Calcium (mg) | Copper (mg) | Iron (mg) | Magnes (mg) | Mang (mg) | Phos (mg) | Potassium (mg) | Selenium (mcg) | Sodium (mg) | Zinc (mg) |
| 5431 | 1/2 cup | Waxgourd, raw, cubes, avg | 66 | 9 | 96 | 0.3 | 2.0 | 1.9 | | | 0.1 | 0.0 | 0.0 | 0.1 | 0.00 | 0.06 | 0 | 0 | 0 | 0 | 0 | 0 | 0.03 | 0.07 | 0.26 | 0.02 | 0.00 | 3.4 | 0.09 | 8.6 | 0.0 | | 13 | 0.0 | 0.3 | 7 | 0.0 | 13 | 4 | 0.1 | 73 | 0.40 |
| 5436 | 1/2 cup | Yambean/Jicama, boiled, avg | 50 | 19 | 90 | 0.4 | 4.4 | 2.5 | 1.0 | 0.9 | 0.0 | 0.0 | 0.0 | 0.0 | 0.01 | 0.01 | 0 | 10 | | 0 | 1 | 6 | 0.01 | 0.01 | 0.09 | 0.02 | 0.00 | 4.0 | 0.06 | 7.1 | 0.0 | | 6 | 0.0 | 0.3 | 6 | 0.0 | 8 | 68 | 0.3 | 2 | 0.08 |
| 5224 | 1/2 cup | Yambean/Jicama, raw, avg | 60 | 23 | 90 | 0.6 | 5.3 | 2.9 | 1.4 | 1.0 | 0.1 | 0.0 | 0.0 | 0.0 | | | 0 | 13 | | 0 | 1 | 7 | 0.01 | 0.02 | 0.12 | 0.03 | 0.00 | 7.2 | 0.03 | 12.1 | 0.0 | | 7 | 0.0 | 0.4 | 7 | 0.0 | 11 | 90 | | 2 | 0.10 |
| | | Yellow Wax Beans | | | | | | | | | | | | | | | | | | | | | | | | | | | | | | | | | | | | | | | | |
| 5194 | 1/2 cup | Boiled, avg | 62 | 22 | 89 | 1.2 | 4.9 | 2.0 | 1.2 | 1.7 | 0.2 | 0.0 | 0.0 | 0.1 | 0.06 | 0.03 | 0 | 50 | 5 | 0 | 5 | 29 | 0.05 | 0.06 | 0.38 | 0.03 | 0.00 | 20.6 | 0.05 | 6.0 | 0.0 | | 29 | 0.1 | 0.8 | 16 | 0.2 | 24 | 185 | 0.2 | 2 | 0.22 |
| 5195 | 1/2 cup | Frozen, boiled, avg | 68 | 19 | 91 | 1.0 | 4.4 | 2.0 | 1.8 | 0.6 | 0.1 | 0.0 | 0.0 | 0.1 | 0.03 | 0.02 | 0 | 76 | [illegible] | 0 | 7 | 43 | 0.02 | 0.06 | 0.26 | 0.04 | 0.00 | 15.6 | 0.03 | 2.8 | 0.0 | | 33 | 0.0 | 0.6 | 16 | 0.2 | 21 | 86 | 0.3 | 6 | 0.33 |
| 6095 | 1/2 cup | Snap, cnd, avg | 120 | 18 | 95 | 1.0 | 4.2 | 1.8 | 1.6 | 0.8 | 0.1 | 0.0 | 0.0 | 0.1 | 0.04 | 0.02 | 0 | 76 | [illegible] | 0 | 7 | 42 | 0.03 | 0.06 | 0.24 | 0.04 | 0.00 | 21.8 | 0.13 | 4.1 | 0.0 | | 29 | 0.1 | 1.1 | 16 | 0.4 | 23 | 118 | 0.2 | 311 | 0.24 |
| 6094 | 1/2 cup | Snap, cnd, low sod, avg | 120 | 18 | 95 | 1.0 | 4.2 | 1.8 | 1.6 | 0.8 | 0.1 | 0.0 | 0.0 | 0.1 | 0.04 | 0.02 | 0 | 76 | [illegible] | 0 | 7 | 42 | 0.03 | 0.06 | 0.24 | 0.04 | 0.00 | 21.8 | 0.13 | 4.8 | 0.0 | | 29 | 0.1 | 1.1 | 16 | 0.4 | 23 | 118 | 0.2 | 17 | 0.24 |
| 5320 | 1/2 cup | Snap, raw, avg | 55 | 17 | 90 | 1.0 | 3.9 | 1.9 | 1.4 | 0.6 | 0.1 | 0.0 | 0.0 | 0.0 | 0.02 | 0.01 | 0 | 59 | 6 | 0 | 6 | 35 | 0.05 | 0.06 | 0.41 | 0.04 | 0.00 | 20.1 | 0.05 | 9.0 | 0.0 | | 20 | 0.0 | 0.6 | 14 | 0.1 | 21 | 115 | 0.3 | 3 | 0.13 |
| | | **MISCELLANEOUS INGREDIENTS, CONDIMENTS, SALSAS** | | | | | | | | | | | | | | | | | | | | | | | | | | | | | | | | | | | | | | | | |
| | | *BAKING INGREDIENTS* | | | | | | | | | | | | | | | | | | | | | | | | | | | | | | | | | | | | | | | | |
| | | Baking Powder | | | | | | | | | | | | | | | | | | | | | | | | | | | | | | | | | | | | | | | | |
| 28029 | 1 tsp | Average | 4 | 3 | 1 | 0.0 | 0.8 | 0.0 | 0.0 | 0.7 | 0.0 | 0.0 | 0.0 | 0.0 | 0.00 | 0.00 | 0 | 0 | 0 | 0 | 0 | 0 | 0.00 | 0.00 | 0.00 | | | | | 0.0 | | | 231 | | 0.1 | | | 58 | 6 | | 465 | |
| 28050 | 1 tsp | Double Acting, Fleischmann's | 4 | 0 | | 0.0 | 0.0 | 0.0 | 0.0 | 0.0 | 0.0 | 0.0 | 0.0 | 0.0 | 0.00 | 0.00 | 0 | | | | | | | | | | | | | | | | | | | | | | 0 | | 640 | |
| 28006 | 1 tsp | Low Sodium, avg | 5 | 5 | 6 | 0.0 | 2.3 | 0.1 | 0.0 | 2.2 | 0.0 | 0.0 | 0.0 | 0.0 | 0.00 | 0.00 | 0 | 0 | 0 | 0 | 0 | 0 | 0.00 | 0.00 | 0.00 | 0.00 | 0.00 | 0.0 | 0.00 | 0.0 | 0.0 | | 217 | 0.0 | 0.4 | 1 | 0.0 | 343 | 505 | 0.0 | 5 | 0.04 |
| 28003 | 1 tsp | Baking Soda, Ashland Chemical | 5 | 0 | 0 | 0.0 | 0.0 | 0.0 | 0.0 | 0.0 | 0.0 | 0.0 | 0.0 | 0.0 | 0.00 | 0.00 | 0 | 0 | 0 | 0 | 0 | 0 | 0.00 | 0.00 | 0.00 | 0.00 | 0.00 | 0.0 | 0.00 | 0.0 | 0.0 | 0.0 | 0 | 0.0 | 0.0 | 0 | 0.0 | 0 | 0 | 0.0 | 1368 | 0.00 |
| 28052 | 1/4 oz | Baking Soda, low sodium, Ashland Chemical | 7 | 0 | 0 | 0.0 | 0.0 | 0.0 | 0.0 | 0.0 | 0.0 | 0.0 | 0.0 | 0.0 | 0.00 | 0.00 | | | | | | | | | | | | | | | | | 1 | | 0.1 | 0 | | | 2734 | | 19 | |
| | | Candied Fruit | | | | | | | | | | | | | | | | | | | | | | | | | | | | | | | | | | | | | | | | |
| 23001 | 2 Tbs | Fruit Citron, chpd, avg | 28 | 88 | 18 | 0.1 | 22.5 | 0.4 | 22.1 | 0.0 | 0.1 | 0.0 | 0.0 | 0.0 | | 0.00 | 0 | 0 | 0 | 0 | 0 | 0 | 0.00 | 0.00 | 0.00 | 0.00 | 0.00 | | | 0.0 | 0.0 | | 23 | | 0.2 | | | 7 | 34 | | 81 | |
| 23462 | 1 oz | Lemon Peel, avg | 28 | 75 | 22 | 0.0 | 21.5 | 1.9 | 16.8 | 2.8 | 0.0 | 0.0 | 0.0 | 0.0 | 0.00 | 0.00 | 0 | 0 | 0 | 0 | 0 | 0 | | | | | | | | 0.0 | | | 37 | | 0.0 | | | | 103 | | 23 | |
| 23463 | 1 oz | Orange Peel, avg | 28 | 75 | 22 | 0.0 | 21.5 | 1.9 | 16.8 | 2.8 | 0.0 | 0.0 | 0.0 | 0.0 | 0.00 | 0.00 | 0 | 0 | 0 | 0 | 0 | 0 | | | | | | | | 0.0 | | | 37 | | 0.0 | | | | 0 | | 33 | |
| 23238 | 1 oz | Pears, avg | 28 | 85 | 21 | 0.4 | 21.3 | | | | 0.2 | 0.0 | | | | 0.00 | 0 | 20 | 2 | 0 | 2 | | 0.00 | 0.05 | 0.17 | | | | | 2.0 | | | 10 | | 0.4 | | | 13 | 160 | | 2 | |
| 30000 | 1 Tbs | Cornstarch, avg | 8 | 30 | 8 | 0.0 | 7.3 | 0.1 | 0.0 | 7.2 | 0.0 | 0.0 | 0.0 | 0.0 | 0.00 | 0.00 | 0 | 0 | 0 | 0 | 0 | 0 | 0.00 | 0.00 | 0.00 | 0.00 | 0.00 | 0.0 | 0.00 | 0.0 | 0.0 | 0.0 | 0 | 0.0 | 0.0 | 0 | 0.0 | 1 | 0 | 0.2 | 1 | 0.00 |
| 26017 | 1 tsp | Cream Of Tartar, avg | 3 | 8 | 2 | 0.0 | 1.8 | 0.0 | 0.0 | 1.8 | 0.0 | 0.0 | 0.0 | 0.0 | 0.00 | 0.00 | 0 | 0 | 0 | 0 | 0 | 0 | 0.00 | 0.00 | 0.00 | 0.00 | 0.00 | 0.0 | 0.00 | 0.0 | 0.0 | 0.0 | 0 | 0.0 | 0.1 | 0 | 0.0 | 0 | 495 | 0.0 | 2 | 0.01 |
| | | Pectin | | | | | | | | | | | | | | | | | | | | | | | | | | | | | | | | | | | | | | | | |
| 30108 | 1 tsp | Dry, light, Sure-Jell | 4 | 22 | | 0.0 | 4.4 | 0.0 | 4.4 | 0.0 | 0.0 | 0.0 | 0.0 | 0.0 | 0.00 | 0.00 | 0 | 0 | 0 | 0 | 0 | 0 | | | | | 0.00 | | | | | | 0 | | 0.0 | | | | 0 | | 0 | |
| 30107 | 1 tsp | Dry, Sure-Jell | 4 | 22 | | 0.0 | 4.4 | 0.0 | 4.4 | 0.0 | 0.0 | 0.0 | 0.0 | 0.0 | 0.00 | 0.00 | 0 | 0 | 0 | 0 | 0 | 0 | | | | | 0.00 | | | | | | 0 | | 0.0 | | | | 0 | | 0 | |
| 27057 | 1 Tbs | Liquid, Certo | 14 | 2 | 94 | 0.0 | 0.6 | 0.4 | 0.2 | 0.0 | 0.0 | 0.0 | 0.0 | 0.0 | 0.00 | 0.00 | 0 | 0 | 0 | 0 | 0 | 0 | 0.00 | 0.00 | 0.00 | 0.00 | 0.00 | 0.0 | 0.00 | 0.0 | 0.0 | | 0 | 0.0 | | 0 | | 0 | 33 | | 1 | 0.00 |
| 27021 | 1 ea | Unsweetened, dry pkg, avg | 50 | 162 | 9 | 0.2 | 45.2 | 4.3 | 0.0 | 40.9 | 0.2 | 0.0 | 0.0 | 0.0 | 0.01 | 0.04 | 0 | 2 | 0.2 | 0 | 0.2 | 1 | 0.00 | 0.03 | 0.00 | 0.00 | 0.00 | 0.5 | 0.05 | 0.0 | 0.0 | 0.0 | 4 | 0.2 | 1.4 | 0 | 0.0 | 1 | 4 | 0.0 | 100 | 0.23 |
| | | Yeast | | | | | | | | | | | | | | | | | | | | | | | | | | | | | | | | | | | | | | | | |
| 28007 | 1 ea | Bakers, compressed cake, avg | 17 | 18 | 69 | 1.4 | 3.1 | 1.4 | 0.0 | 1.7 | 0.3 | 0.0 | 0.2 | 0.0 | 0.00 | 0.00 | 0 | 0 | 0 | 0 | 0 | 0 | 0.32 | 0.19 | 2.09 | 0.07 | 0.00 | 133.4 | 0.83 | 0.0 | 0.0 | | 3 | 0.0 | 0.6 | 7 | 0.0 | 57 | 102 | 1.4 | 5 | 1.69 |
| 28001 | 1 ea | Bakers, dry active, pkt, avg | 7 | 21 | 8 | 2.7 | 2.7 | 1.5 | 0.0 | 1.2 | 0.3 | 0.0 | 0.2 | 0.0 | 0.00 | 0.00 | 0 | 0.1 | 0.01 | 0 | 0.01 | | 0.17 | 0.38 | 2.79 | 0.11 | 0.00 | 163.8 | 0.79 | 0.0 | 0.0 | | 4 | 0.0 | 1.2 | 7 | 0.0 | 90 | 140 | 1.7 | 4 | 0.45 |
| 28002 | 1 Tbs | Brewers, avg unfortified | 8 | 23 | 5 | 3.0 | 3.1 | 2.5 | 0.1 | 0.4 | 0.1 | 0.0 | 0.0 | 0.0 | 0.00 | 0.00 | 0 | 0 | 0 | 0 | 0 | 0 | 1.25 | 0.34 | 3.03 | 0.40 | 0.00 | 313.0 | 0.68 | 0.0 | 0.0 | | 17 | 0.3 | 1.4 | 18 | | 140 | 151 | 3.4 | 10 | 0.63 |
| 40072 | 1/2 oz | Torula, avg | 7 | 4 | 86 | 0.2 | 0.7 | 0.1 | 0.0 | 0.6 | 0.1 | 0.0 | 0.0 | 0.0 | 0.00 | 0.02 | 0 | 60 | 18 | | | | 0.02 | 0.01 | 0.22 | 0.03 | 0.00 | 5.9 | 0.01 | 0.0 | 0.0 | | 6 | 0.0 | 0.2 | 2 | 0.0 | 5 | 4 | 0.6 | 11 | 0.03 |
| | | *CONDIMENTS* | | | | | | | | | | | | | | | | | | | | | | | | | | | | | | | | | | | | | | | | |
| | | Bacon Bits | | | | | | | | | | | | | | | | | | | | | | | | | | | | | | | | | | | | | | | | |
| 27050 | 1 Tbs | Bac-O-Bits, General Mills | 16 | 67 | 11 | 6.6 | 4.3 | | | | 2.6 | | | | | | 0 | | | | | | 1.38 | 0.05 | 0.29 | | | | | | | | 35 | | 1.1 | | | | 437 | | 274 | |
| 27044 | 1/4 oz | Meatless, avg | 7 | 31 | 8 | 2.2 | 2.0 | 0.7 | | | 1.8 | 0.3 | 0.4 | 0.9 | | | 0 | 0 | 0 | 0 | 0 | 0 | 0.04 | 0.00 | 0.11 | 0.01 | 0.08 | 8.9 | | 0.1 | 0.0 | | 7 | 0.0 | 0.1 | 7 | | 15 | 10 | | 124 | 0.13 |
| 27096 | 1 Tbs | Oscar Mayer | 7 | 24 | 30 | 2.7 | 0.2 | 0.0 | 0.2 | 0.0 | 1.3 | 0.5 | 0.7 | 0.2 | 0.01 | 0.15 | 5 | 0 | 0 | 0 | 0 | 0 | | | | | | | | 0.0 | | | 2 | 0.0 | 0.2 | 5 | | 43 | 39 | | 224 | 0.35 |
| 27000 | 1 Tbs | Catsup, avg | 15 | 16 | 67 | 0.2 | 4.1 | 0.2 | 1.7 | 2.2 | 0.1 | 0.0 | 0.0 | 0.0 | 0.00 | 0.02 | 0 | 152 | 15 | 0 | 15 | 92 | 0.01 | 0.01 | 0.21 | 0.03 | 0.00 | 2.3 | 0.02 | 2.3 | 0.0 | | 3 | 0.0 | 0.1 | 3 | 0.0 | 6 | 72 | 0.1 | 178 | 0.03 |
| 27032 | 1 Tbs | Catsup, low salt, avg | 15 | 16 | 67 | 0.2 | 4.1 | 0.2 | 1.8 | 2.1 | 0.1 | 0.0 | 0.0 | 0.0 | 0.00 | 0.02 | 0 | 152 | 15 | 0 | 15 | 92 | 0.01 | 0.01 | 0.21 | 0.03 | 0.00 | 2.3 | 0.02 | 2.3 | 0.0 | | 3 | 0.0 | 0.1 | 3 | 0.0 | 6 | 72 | 0.1 | 3 | 0.03 |
| 53015 | 1 Tbs | Cheese Sauce, avg | 13 | 28 | 63 | 1.3 | 1.1 | 0.0 | 0.4 | 0.7 | 2.1 | 1.2 | 0.6 | 0.3 | 0.02 | 0.24 | 5 | 75 | 22 | 20 | 2 | | 0.01 | 0.03 | 0.06 | 0.01 | 0.06 | 1.2 | 0.04 | 0.1 | 0.1 | 0.1 | 34 | 0.0 | 0.1 | 2 | 0.0 | 26 | 16 | 0.9 | 66 | 0.14 |
| 53097 | 1 Tbs | Cheese Sauce, lowfat, avg | 15 | 21 | 73 | 1.4 | 1.0 | 0.0 | 0.4 | 0.6 | 1.3 | 0.5 | 0.5 | 0.2 | | | 3 | 57 | 14 | 13 | 1 | | 0.01 | 0.03 | 0.04 | 0.01 | 0.07 | 1.0 | 0.05 | 0.1 | 0.0 | | 41 | 0.0 | 0.1 | 2 | 0.0 | 45 | 24 | 0.6 | 96 | 0.18 |
| 27003 | 1 Tbs | Chili Sauce, avg | 17 | 18 | 68 | 0.4 | 4.2 | 0.2 | 1.9 | 2.1 | 0.1 | 0.0 | 0.0 | 0.0 | | 0.00 | 0 | 238 | 24 | 0 | 24 | | 0.02 | 0.01 | 0.27 | 0.02 | 0.00 | 1.2 | 0.03 | 2.7 | 0.0 | | 3 | 0.1 | 0.1 | 2 | | 9 | 63 | | 227 | 0.05 |
| 27002 | 1 Tbs | Chili Sauce, hot, red pepper, avg | 16 | 3 | 94 | 0.1 | 0.6 | 0.1 | 0.4 | 0.2 | 0.1 | 0.0 | 0.0 | 0.1 | | 0.00 | 0 | 1534 | 153 | 0 | 153 | | 0.00 | 0.01 | 0.10 | 0.02 | 0.00 | 1.6 | 0.04 | 4.8 | 0.0 | | 1 | 0.0 | 0.1 | 2 | | 3 | 90 | 0.1 | 4 | 0.03 |
| 27036 | 1 Tbs | Chutney, avg | 17 | 26 | 57 | 0.2 | 6.7 | 0.4 | 6.0 | 0.3 | 0.1 | 0.0 | 0.0 | 0.0 | | | 0 | 84 | 8 | 0 | 8 | | 0.01 | 0.01 | 0.12 | 0.02 | 0.00 | 1.6 | | 2.9 | | | 5 | 0.0 | 0.2 | 4 | | 7 | 65 | | 38 | 0.03 |
| 27045 | 1 Tbs | Corn Relish, avg | 15 | 13 | 75 | 0.3 | 3.2 | 0.4 | 2.1 | 0.8 | 0.1 | 0.0 | 0.0 | 0.0 | | | 0 | 89 | 9 | 0 | 9 | | 0.01 | 0.01 | 0.15 | 0.02 | 0.00 | 3.5 | | 4.0 | 0.0 | | 2 | 0.0 | 0.1 | 3 | | 7 | 28 | | 54 | 0.04 |
| 27019 | 1 Tbs | Cranberry Orange Relish, avg | 17 | 30 | 53 | 0.1 | 7.9 | 0.0 | 7.3 | 0.5 | 0.0 | 0.0 | 0.0 | 0.0 | 0.00 | 0.00 | 0 | 12 | 1 | 0 | 1 | | 0.01 | 0.00 | 0.02 | 0.00 | 0.00 | 0.5 | 0.01 | 3.1 | 0.0 | | 2 | 0.0 | 0.0 | 1 | 0.0 | 1 | 6 | | 5 | 0.01 |
| | | Croutons | | | | | | | | | | | | | | | | | | | | | | | | | | | | | | | | | | | | | | | | |
| 49098 | 1 Tbs | Bacon Cheddar Toppers, Pepperidge Farm | 7 | 35 | | 1.0 | 4.0 | 0.0 | 0.0 | 4.0 | 2.0 | 0.0 | | | | | 0 | 0 | 0 | 0 | 0 | 0 | 0.00 | 0.00 | 0.00 | | | | | 0.0 | | | 80 | | 0.0 | | | | | | 85 | |
| 49100 | 1 Tbs | Caesar Toppers, Pepperidge Farm | 7 | 35 | | 1.0 | 4.0 | 0.0 | 0.0 | 4.0 | 2.0 | 0.0 | | | | | 0 | 0 | 0 | 0 | 0 | 0 | 0.00 | 0.00 | 0.00 | | | | | 0.0 | | | 40 | | 0.0 | | | | | | 85 | |
| 49099 | 1 Tbs | Cinnamon Raisin Toppers, Pepperidge Farm | 7 | 35 | | 1.0 | 4.0 | 0.0 | 2.0 | 2.0 | 2.0 | 0.0 | | | | | 0 | 0 | 0 | 0 | 0 | 0 | 0.00 | 0.00 | 0.00 | | | | | 0.0 | | | 40 | | 0.0 | | | | | | 15 | |
| 49058 | 1 Tbs | Garlic Italian Toppers, Pepperidge Farm | 7 | 35 | 5 | 1.0 | 4.0 | 0.0 | 0.0 | 4.0 | 1.5 | 0.0 | | | | | 0 | 0 | 0 | 0 | 0 | 0 | 0.03 | 0.00 | 0.00 | | | | | 0.0 | | | 0 | | 0.0 | | | | | | 70 | |
| 27004 | 1 Tbs | Horseradish, avg | 15 | 7 | 85 | 0.2 | 1.7 | 0.5 | 0.7 | 0.5 | 0.1 | 0.0 | 0.0 | 0.1 | 0.01 | 0.04 | 0 | 0 | 0 | | | | 0.00 | 0.00 | 0.06 | 0.01 | 0.00 | 8.6 | 0.01 | 3.7 | 0.0 | | 8 | 0.0 | 0.1 | 4 | 0.0 | 5 | 37 | 0.4 | 47 | 0.12 |
| 53098 | 1 Tbs | Horseradish Sauce, avg | 14 | 29 | 71 | 0.4 | 0.6 | 0.0 | | | 2.9 | 1.8 | 0.8 | 0.1 | | | 6 | 108 | 27 | 24 | 3 | | 0.00 | 0.02 | 0.01 | 0.00 | 0.04 | 1.5 | 0.05 | 0.1 | 0.0 | | 16 | 0.0 | 0.0 | 2 | 0.0 | 12 | 20 | | 41 | 0.04 |
| 27106 | 1 Tbs | Jalapeno Relish, Old El Paso | 15 | 5 | 90 | 0.0 | 1.0 | 1.0 | 0.0 | 0.0 | 0.0 | 0.0 | 0.0 | 0.0 | 0.00 | 0.00 | 0 | | | | | | | | | | | | | | | | | | | | | | | | 110 | |
| | | Mustard | | | | | | | | | | | | | | | | | | | | | | | | | | | | | | | | | | | | | | | | |
| 90054 | 1 Tbs | Brown, avg | 15 | 14 | 78 | 0.9 | 0.8 | 0.3 | 0.4 | 0.1 | 0.9 | 0.2 | 0.2 | 0.6 | 0.00 | 0.60 | 0 | 0 | 0 | 0 | 0 | 0 | 0.00 | 0.00 | 0.00 | | | | | 0.0 | | | 19 | | 0.3 | | | 20 | 20 | | 196 | |
| 27058 | 1 Tbs | Dijon, Nabisco | 16 | 19 | 70 | 1.0 | 1.7 | 0.2 | | 1.0 | 1.4 | 0.1 | 0.5 | 0.4 | | | 0 | 8 | 1 | | | | 0.02 | 0.02 | 0.33 | 0.01 | 0.00 | 0.0 | | 0.1 | | | 22 | 0.0 | 0.4 | | | 35 | 28 | | 388 | 0.24 |
| 27115 | 1 Tbs | Stoneground, Beaverton Foods | 15 | 26 | 58 | 1.0 | 3.4 | 1.8 | 1.2 | 0.4 | 0.2 | | | | | | 0 | 14 | 1 | | | | | | | | | | | 0.0 | | | 19 | | 0.3 | 13 | | 21 | 12 | | 238 | |
| 27005 | 1 Tbs | Yellow, avg | 16 | 12 | 80 | 0.8 | 1.0 | 0.4 | 0.5 | 0.1 | 0.7 | 0.0 | 0.6 | 0.1 | 0.00 | 0.06 | 0 | 0 | 0 | 0 | 0 | 0 | 0.00 | 0.00 | 0.00 | 0.01 | 0.00 | 0.0 | | 0.0 | 0.0 | | 13 | 0.1 | 0.3 | 8 | 0.1 | 12 | 21 | 3.7 | 200 | 0.10 |
| | | Olives | | | | | | | | | | | | | | | | | | | | | | | | | | | | | | | | | | | | | | | | |
| 6499 | 1 ea | Calamata, w/o pits, GL Mezzetta | 4 | 11 | 58 | 0.1 | 0.4 | 0.0 | 0.0 | 0.3 | 1.1 | 0.1 | 0.8 | 0.1 | | | 0 | 2 | 0 | | | | | | | | | | | 0.0 | | | 1 | | 0.0 | | | | | | 65 | |
| 27008 | 1 ea | Green, w/o pits, avg | 4 | 5 | 78 | 0.1 | 0.1 | 0.0 | 0.0 | 0.0 | 0.5 | 0.1 | 0.4 | 0.0 | 0.00 | 0.04 | 0 | 12 | 1 | 0 | 1 | | 0.00 | 0.00 | 0.00 | 0.00 | 0.00 | 0.0 | 0.00 | 0.0 | 0.0 | | 2 | 0.0 | 0.1 | 1 | | 1 | 2 | 0.0 | 96 | 0.00 |
| 27112 | 1 ea | Jumbo, super colossal, California Olive Industry | 10 | 12 | 80 | 0.1 | 0.7 | 0.3 | 0.1 | 0.2 | 1.0 | 0.2 | 0.7 | 0.1 | | | | 308 | 31 | 0 | 31 | | 0.00 | 0.00 | 0.01 | | 0.00 | | | 0.1 | | | 8 | | 0.2 | | | | 1 | | 65 | |
| 27170 | 1 ea | Large, California Olive Industry | 4 | 6 | 76 | 0.0 | 0.3 | 0.1 | 0.0 | 0.1 | 0.5 | 0.1 | 0.4 | 0.0 | | | | 140 | 14 | | | | 0.00 | 0.00 | 0.00 | | 0.00 | | | 0.0 | | | 4 | | 0.1 | | | | 0 | | 25 | |
| 27114 | 1 ea | Medium, California Olive Industry | 3 | 5 | 76 | 0.0 | 0.2 | 0.1 | 0.0 | 0.1 | 0.4 | 0.1 | 0.3 | 0.0 | | | | 105 | 11 | | | | 0.00 | 0.00 | 0.00 | | 0.00 | | | 0.0 | | | 3 | | 0.1 | | | | 0 | | 19 | |
| 27113 | 1 ea | Small, California Olive Industry | 2 | 3 | 76 | 0.0 | 0.2 | 0.1 | 0.0 | 0.1 | 0.3 | 0.0 | 0.2 | 0.0 | | | | 70 | 7 | | | | 0.00 | 0.00 | 0.00 | | 0.00 | | | 0.0 | | | 2 | | 0.1 | | | | 0 | | 12 | |
| 26328 | 1 Tbs | Feppercorns, in brine, Gourmet Club Company | 10 | 6 | 75 | 0.2 | 1.0 | 0.7 | 0.0 | 0.3 | 0.1 | | | | | | 0 | 12 | 1 | 0 | 1 | | | | | | | | | 0.2 | | | 24 | | 0.1 | | | | | | 430 | |
| 6498 | 1/4 oz | Fepperoncini, GL Mezzetta | 7 | 2 | 90 | 0.1 | 0.3 | 0.1 | 0.0 | 0.3 | 0.0 | 0.0 | 0.0 | 0.0 | | | 0 | 17 | 2 | | | | | | | | | | | 0.5 | | | 3 | | 0.0 | | | | | | 91 | |

| Code | Amount | Description | Weight (g) | Calories | % Water | Protein (g) | Carbs (g) | Fiber (g) | Sugar (g) | Other Carbs (g) | Fat (g) | Sat Fat (g) | Mono Fat (g) | Poly Fat (g) | Omega 3 (g) | Omega 6 (g) | Choles (mg) | Vit A (IU) | Vit A (RE) | Retinol (RE) | Carotenoids (RE) | Beta Carotene (mcg) | Thiamin (mg) | Riboflavin (mg) | Niacin (NE) | Vit B6 (mg) | Vit B12 (mcg) | Folate (mcg) | Panto (mg) | Vit C (mg) | Vit D (mg) | Vit E (α TE) | Calcium (mg) | Copper (mg) | Iron (mg) | Magnes (mg) | Mang (mg) | Phos (mg) | Potassium (mg) | Selenium (mcg) | Sodium (mg) | Zinc (mg) |
|---|---|---|---|---|---|---|---|---|---|---|---|---|---|---|---|---|---|---|---|---|---|---|---|---|---|---|---|---|---|---|---|---|---|---|---|---|---|---|---|---|---|---|
| | | Basic Components | | | | | | | | | | Additional Fats | | | | | | Vit A & Components | | | | | Vitamins | | | | | | | | | | Minerals | | | | | | | | | |
| 27043 | 1 ea | Peppers, hot, pickled, avg | 8 | 4 | 84 | 0.1 | 1.0 | 0.1 | 0.7 | 0.2 | 0.0 | 0.0 | 0.0 | 0.0 | | | 0 | 618 | 62 | 0 | 62 | | 0.01 | 0.01 | 0.06 | 0.02 | 0.00 | 1.6 | | 14.0 | 0.0 | | 1 | 0.0 | 0.1 | 2 | | 3 | 22 | | 61 | 0.02 |
| | | Pickles | | | | | | | | | | | | | | | | | | | | | | | | | | | | | | | | | | | | | | | | |
| 27012 | 1 ea | Dill, avg | 65 | 12 | 92 | 0.4 | 2.7 | 0.8 | 0.8 | 1.1 | 0.1 | 0.0 | 0.0 | 0.1 | 0.03 | 0.02 | 0 | 214 | 21 | 0 | 21 | | 0.01 | 0.02 | 0.04 | 0.01 | 0.00 | 0.6 | 0.04 | 1.2 | 0.0 | | 6 | 0.1 | 0.3 | 7 | 0.0 | 14 | 75 | 0.0 | 833 | 0.09 |
| 27099 | 1 pce | Dill, chips, hamburger, Claussen | 3 | 0 | 94 | 0.0 | 0.0 | 0.0 | 0.0 | 0.0 | 0.0 | 0.0 | 0.0 | 0.0 | 0.00 | 0.00 | 0 | 0 | 0 | 0 | 0 | 0 | | | | | | | | 0.0 | | | 4 | 0.0 | 0.0 | 0 | | 0 | 3 | | 41 | 0.01 |
| 27102 | 1 ea | Dill, kosher, Claussen | 33 | 4 | 94 | 0.3 | 0.6 | 0.3 | 0.3 | 0.0 | 0.1 | 0.0 | 0.0 | 0.0 | 0.00 | 0.01 | 0 | 0 | 0 | 0 | 0 | 0 | 0.01 | 0.01 | 0.05 | | | | | 1.0 | | | 17 | 0.1 | 0.2 | 4 | | 14 | 37 | | 312 | 0.10 |
| 27039 | 1 ea | Dill, low salt, avg | 65 | 7 | 94 | 0.3 | 1.5 | 0.8 | 0.7 | 0.0 | 0.1 | 0.0 | 0.0 | 0.1 | | | 0 | 94 | 10 | 0 | 10 | | 0.00 | 0.01 | 0.00 | 0.01 | 0.00 | 0.5 | | 0.6 | 0.0 | | 0 | 0.1 | 0.3 | 3 | | 9 | 15 | | 12 | 0.01 |
| 27023 | 1 ea | Sour, medium, avg | 35 | 4 | 94 | 0.1 | 0.8 | 0.4 | 0.2 | 0.2 | 0.1 | 0.0 | 0.0 | 0.0 | 0.02 | 0.01 | 0 | 51 | 5 | 0 | 5 | | 0.00 | 0.00 | 0.00 | 0.00 | 0.00 | 0.2 | 0.01 | 0.3 | 0.0 | | 0 | 0.0 | 0.1 | 1 | 0.0 | 5 | 8 | 0.0 | 423 | 0.01 |
| 27026 | 1 ea | Sour, medium, low salt, avg | 35 | 4 | 94 | 0.1 | 0.8 | 0.4 | 0.2 | 0.2 | 0.1 | 0.0 | 0.0 | 0.0 | 0.02 | 0.01 | 0 | 51 | 5 | 0 | 5 | | 0.00 | 0.00 | 0.00 | 0.00 | 0.00 | 0.2 | 0.01 | 0.3 | 0.0 | | 0 | 0.0 | 0.1 | 1 | 0.0 | 5 | 8 | 0.0 | 6 | 0.01 |
| 27016 | 1 ea | Sweet, medium, avg | 35 | 41 | 65 | 0.1 | 11.1 | 0.4 | 10.1 | 0.6 | 0.1 | 0.0 | 0.0 | 0.0 | 0.02 | 0.02 | 0 | 44 | 5 | 0 | 5 | | 0.00 | 0.01 | 0.06 | 0.01 | 0.00 | 0.3 | 0.04 | 0.4 | 0.0 | | 1 | 0.0 | 0.2 | 1 | 0.0 | 4 | 11 | 0.0 | 329 | 0.03 |
| 27030 | 1 ea | Sweet, medium, low salt, avg | 35 | 41 | 65 | 0.1 | 11.1 | 0.4 | 10.1 | 0.6 | 0.1 | 0.0 | 0.0 | 0.0 | 0.02 | 0.02 | 0 | 44 | 5 | 0 | 5 | | 0.00 | 0.01 | 0.06 | 0.01 | 0.00 | 0.3 | 0.04 | 0.4 | 0.0 | | 1 | 0.0 | 0.2 | 1 | 0.0 | 4 | 11 | 0.0 | 6 | 0.03 |
| | | Pickles, Relish | | | | | | | | | | | | | | | | | | | | | | | | | | | | | | | | | | | | | | | | |
| 27103 | 1 Tbs | Claussen | 15 | 13 | 78 | 0.1 | 2.8 | 0.2 | 2.2 | 0.4 | 0.1 | 0.0 | 0.0 | 0.0 | 0.00 | 0.02 | 0 | 0 | 0 | 0 | 0 | 0 | 0.00 | 0.00 | 0.02 | | | | | 0.0 | | | 14 | 0.0 | 0.1 | 3 | | 7 | 23 | | 85 | 0.03 |
| 27053 | 1 Tbs | Hamburger, avg | 15 | 19 | 61 | 0.1 | 5.2 | 0.5 | 4.6 | 0.1 | 0.1 | 0.0 | 0.0 | 0.0 | 0.01 | 0.01 | 0 | 40 | 4 | 0 | 4 | | 0.00 | 0.01 | 0.09 | 0.00 | 0.00 | 0.2 | 0.00 | 0.3 | | | 1 | 0.0 | 0.2 | 1 | 0.0 | 3 | 11 | 0.0 | 164 | 0.02 |
| 27051 | 1 Tbs | Hot Dog, avg | 15 | 14 | 72 | 0.2 | 3.5 | 0.2 | 3.1 | 0.2 | 0.1 | 0.0 | 0.0 | 0.0 | 0.01 | 0.01 | 0 | 25 | 3 | 0 | 3 | | 0.01 | 0.01 | 0.08 | 0.00 | 0.00 | 0.2 | 0.00 | 0.2 | | | 1 | 0.0 | 0.2 | 3 | 0.0 | 6 | 12 | 0.0 | 164 | 0.03 |
| 27062 | 1 Tbs | Sweet, avg | 15 | 21 | 63 | 0.1 | 5.1 | 0.3 | 4.6 | 0.3 | 0.1 | 0.0 | 0.0 | 0.0 | | 0.00 | 0 | 15 | 2 | 0 | 2 | | 0.00 | 0.00 | 0.00 | 0.00 | 0.00 | 0.0 | 0.01 | 0.9 | 0.0 | | 3 | 0.1 | 0.1 | 1 | 0.0 | 2 | 30 | 0.2 | 107 | 0.01 |
| | | Soy Sauce | | | | | | | | | | | | | | | | | | | | | | | | | | | | | | | | | | | | | | | | |
| 7523 | 1 Tbs | Dark, China Bowl Trading Company | 18 | 0 | 71 | 0.0 | 0.0 | 0.0 | 0.0 | 0.0 | 0.0 | 0.0 | 0.0 | 0.0 | 0.00 | 0.00 | 0 | 0 | 0 | 0 | 0 | 0 | | | | | | | | 0.0 | | | 0 | | 0.0 | | | | | | 900 | |
| 7524 | 1 Tbs | Light, China Bowl Trading Company | 18 | 0 | 71 | 0.0 | 0.0 | 0.0 | 0.0 | 0.0 | 0.0 | 0.0 | 0.0 | 0.0 | 0.00 | 0.00 | 0 | 0 | 0 | 0 | 0 | 0 | | | | | | | | 0.0 | | | 0 | | | | | | | | 900 | |
| 90035 | 1 Tbs | Low Sodium, avg | 18 | 10 | 71 | 0.9 | 1.5 | 0.1 | | | 0.0 | 0.0 | 0.0 | 0.0 | 0.00 | 0.01 | 0 | 0 | 0 | 0 | 0 | 0 | 0.01 | 0.02 | 0.60 | 0.03 | 0.00 | 2.8 | 0.06 | 0.0 | | 0.0 | 3 | 0.0 | 0.4 | 6 | 0.1 | 20 | 32 | 0.1 | 600 | 0.07 |
| 53124 | 1 Tbs | Steak Sauce, avg | 16 | 10 | 79 | 0.3 | 2.4 | 0.3 | | | 0.1 | 0.0 | 0.0 | 0.0 | | | 0 | 150 | 15 | 0 | 15 | | 0.01 | 0.01 | 0.20 | 0.02 | 0.00 | 1.0 | | 2.6 | 0.0 | | 3 | 0.0 | 0.2 | 4 | | 6 | 64 | | 233 | 0.05 |
| 53085 | 1 Tbs | Tabasco Sauce, avg | 16 | 2 | 95 | 0.1 | 0.3 | 0.1 | 0.0 | 0.2 | 0.1 | 0.0 | 0.0 | 0.0 | 0.01 | 0.03 | 0 | 669 | 67 | | | | 0.01 | 0.01 | 0.05 | 0.03 | 9.60 | 0.2 | 0.02 | 0.1 | 0.0 | | 4 | 0.0 | 0.4 | 1 | | 3 | 21 | | 95 | 0.02 |
| 53004 | 1 Tbs | Teriyaki Sauce, RTS, avg | 18 | 15 | 68 | 1.1 | 2.9 | 0.0 | 1.5 | 1.4 | 0.0 | 0.0 | 0.0 | 0.0 | 0.00 | 0.00 | 0 | 0 | 0 | 0 | 0 | 0 | 0.01 | 0.01 | 0.23 | 0.02 | 0.00 | 3.6 | 0.04 | 0.0 | 0.0 | 0.0 | 5 | 0.0 | 0.3 | 11 | 0.0 | 28 | 41 | 0.2 | 690 | 0.02 |
| 27035 | 1 Tbs | Tomato Relish, avg | 20 | 30 | 52 | 0.3 | 7.8 | 0.4 | 6.5 | 1.0 | 0.0 | 0.0 | 0.0 | 0.0 | | | 0 | 253 | 25 | 0 | 25 | 148 | 0.01 | 0.01 | 0.12 | 0.03 | 0.00 | 2.5 | 0.10 | 9.8 | 0.0 | | 9 | 0.0 | 0.3 | 6 | 0.0 | 9 | 79 | | 452 | 0.03 |
| 27048 | 1 Tbs | Vegetable Relish, avg | 9 | 4 | 88 | 0.1 | 0.9 | 0.1 | 0.7 | 0.1 | 0.0 | 0.0 | 0.0 | 0.0 | | | 0 | 17 | 2 | 0 | 2 | | 0.00 | 0.00 | 0.03 | 0.01 | 0.00 | 1.2 | 0.02 | 0.7 | 0.0 | | 2 | 0.0 | 0.0 | 1 | 0.0 | 2 | 17 | | 42 | 0.02 |
| | | Vinegar | | | | | | | | | | | | | | | | | | | | | | | | | | | | | | | | | | | | | | | | |
| 27061 | 1 Tbs | Apple Cider, Nakano | 15 | 1 | 99 | 0.0 | 0.1 | 0.0 | 0.0 | 0.1 | 0.0 | | | | | | 0 | 0 | 0 | 0 | 0 | 0 | | | | | | | | 0.1 | | | 1 | | 0.1 | | | | | | 3 | |
| 27130 | 1 Tbs | Balsamic, Nakano | 15 | 10 | 84 | 0.1 | 2.3 | 0.0 | 2.2 | 0.1 | 0.0 | | | | | | 0 | 0 | 0 | 0 | 0 | 0 | | | | | | | | 0.1 | | | 5 | | 0.1 | | | | 12 | | 4 | |
| 27007 | 1 Tbs | Cider, avg | 15 | 2 | 94 | 0.0 | 0.9 | 0.0 | 0.9 | 0.0 | 0.0 | 0.0 | 0.0 | 0.0 | 0.00 | 0.00 | 0 | 0 | 0 | 0 | 0 | 0 | 0.00 | 0.00 | 0.00 | 0.00 | 0.00 | 0.0 | 0.00 | 0.0 | 0.0 | 0.0 | 1 | 0.0 | 0.1 | 3 | 0.0 | 1 | 15 | 0.0 | 0 | 0.00 |
| 27159 | 1 Tbs | Malt, w/tarragon flavoring, Fleischmann's | 15 | 3 | 95 | 0.0 | 0.1 | 0.0 | 0.1 | 0.0 | 0.0 | 0.0 | 0.0 | 0.0 | 0.00 | 0.00 | | 0.15 | 0.03 | | | | 0.08 | 0.08 | 0.08 | | | | | 0.3 | | | 0 | | 0.1 | | | 0 | 2 | | 1 | |
| 27059 | 1 Tbs | Red Wine, Nakano | 15 | 0 | 99 | 0.0 | 0.1 | 0.0 | 0.0 | 0.1 | 0.0 | | | | | | 0 | 0 | 0 | 0 | 0 | 0 | | | | | | | | 0.1 | | | 1 | | 0.1 | | | | | | 2 | |
| 27147 | 1 Tbs | Rice, Fleischmann's | 15 | 7 | 87 | 0.0 | 0.5 | 0.0 | 0.5 | 0.0 | 0.0 | 0.0 | 0.0 | 0.0 | 0.00 | 0.00 | | 0.15 | 0.03 | | | | 0.08 | 0.08 | 0.08 | | | | | 0.1 | | | 0 | | 0.1 | | | 0 | 1 | | 1 | |
| 27060 | 1 Tbs | White Wine, Nakano | 15 | 0 | 100 | 0.0 | 0.0 | 0.0 | 0.0 | 0.0 | 0.0 | 0.0 | 0.0 | 0.0 | 0.00 | 0.00 | 0 | 0 | 0 | 0 | 0 | 0 | | | | | | | | 0.2 | | | 1 | | 0.1 | | | | | | 2 | |
| 53084 | 1 Tbs | Worcestershire Sauce, Lea & Perrins | 14 | 17 | 75 | 0.2 | 3.0 | | | | 0.0 | | | | | | | 13 | 1 | 0 | 1 | | 0.00 | 0.02 | 0.15 | | | | | 0.1 | | | 18 | | 1.0 | | | | | | 133 | |
| | | SALSAS | | | | | | | | | | | | | | | | | | | | | | | | | | | | | | | | | | | | | | | | |
| 27125 | 1 Tbs | Cheese 'N Salsa Dip, medium, Old El Paso | 14 | 19 | 74 | 0.2 | 1.4 | 0.0 | 0.0 | 1.4 | 1.4 | 0.5 | | | | | 1 | 0 | 0 | 0 | 0 | 0 | | | | | | | | 0.0 | | | 10 | | 0.0 | | | | | | 145 | |
| 27124 | 1 Tbs | Cheese 'N Salsa Dip, mild, Old El Paso | 14 | 19 | 74 | 0.2 | 1.4 | 0.0 | 0.0 | 1.4 | 1.4 | 0.5 | | | | | 1 | 0 | 0 | 0 | 0 | 0 | | | | | | | | 0.0 | | | 10 | | 0.0 | | | | | | 145 | |
| 27127 | 1 Tbs | Chunky Salsa Dip, medium, Old El Paso | 15 | 8 | 83 | 0.5 | 1.5 | 0.5 | 1.0 | 0.0 | 0.0 | 0.0 | 0.0 | 0.0 | 0.00 | 0.00 | 0 | 50 | 10 | | | | | | | | | | | 0.0 | | | 0 | | 0.0 | | | | | | 115 | |
| 27126 | 1 Tbs | Chunky Salsa Dip, mild, Old El Paso | 15 | 8 | 83 | 0.5 | 1.5 | 0.5 | 1.0 | 0.0 | 0.0 | 0.0 | 0.0 | 0.0 | 0.00 | 0.00 | 0 | 50 | 10 | | | | | | | | | | | 0.0 | | | 0 | | 0.0 | | | | | | 115 | |
| 27086 | 1 Tbs | Green Chile, mild, Ortega | 16 | 5 | 93 | 0.0 | 1.0 | 0.0 | 0.5 | 0.5 | 0.0 | 0.0 | 0.0 | 0.0 | 0.00 | 0.00 | 0 | | | | | | | | | | | | | 0.6 | | | | | | | | | 40 | | 105 | |
| 53121 | 1 Tbs | Guacamole, w/tomatoes, avg | 15 | 18 | 79 | 0.3 | 1.1 | 0.3 | | | 1.6 | 0.3 | 1.0 | 0.2 | | | 0 | 84 | 8 | 0 | 8 | 50 | 0.01 | 0.01 | 0.22 | 0.03 | 0.00 | 7.1 | | 1.8 | 0.0 | | 2 | 0.0 | 0.1 | 5 | | 5 | 71 | | 28 | 0.05 |
| 27083 | 1 Tbs | Medium, Ortega | 16 | 5 | 92 | 0.0 | 1.0 | 0.5 | 0.5 | 0.0 | 0.0 | 0.0 | 0.0 | 0.0 | 0.00 | 0.00 | 0 | 103 | 10 | 0 | 10 | | | | | | | | | 10.8 | | | | | 0.2 | | | | 46 | | 165 | |
| 27084 | 1 Tbs | Mild, Ortega | 16 | 5 | 92 | 0.0 | 1.0 | 0.5 | 0.5 | 0.0 | 0.0 | 0.0 | 0.0 | 0.0 | 0.00 | 0.00 | 0 | 103 | 10 | 0 | 10 | | | | | | | | | 10.8 | | | | | 0.2 | | | | 46 | | 165 | |
| 27123 | 1 Tbs | Thick 'N Chunky, medium, Old El Paso | 15 | 5 | 93 | 0.0 | 1.0 | 0.0 | 0.5 | 0.5 | 0.0 | 0.0 | 0.0 | 0.0 | 0.00 | 0.00 | 0 | 50 | 10 | | | | | | | | | | | 2.4 | | | 0 | | 0.0 | | | | | | 70 | |
| 27122 | 1 Tbs | Thick 'N Chunky, mild, Old El Paso | 15 | 5 | 93 | 0.0 | 1.0 | 0.0 | 0.5 | 0.5 | 0.0 | 0.0 | 0.0 | 0.0 | 0.00 | 0.00 | 0 | 50 | 10 | | | | | | | | | | | 2.4 | | | 0 | | 0.0 | | | | | | 70 | |
| 27121 | 1 Tbs | Italian, hot, Progresso | 15 | 5 | 93 | 0.0 | 1.0 | 0.3 | 0.5 | 0.3 | 0.0 | 0.0 | 0.0 | 0.0 | 0.00 | 0.00 | 0 | 50 | 5 | | | | | | | | | | | 1.8 | | | 0 | | 0.0 | | | | | | 85 | |
| 27120 | 1 Tbs | Italian, medium, Progresso | 15 | 5 | 93 | 0.0 | 1.0 | 0.3 | 0.5 | 0.3 | 0.0 | 0.0 | 0.0 | 0.0 | 0.00 | 0.00 | 0 | 50 | 5 | | | | | | | | | | | 1.8 | | | 0 | | 0.0 | | | | | | 85 | |
| 27119 | 1 Tbs | Italian, mild, Progresso | 15 | 5 | 93 | 0.0 | 1.0 | 0.3 | 0.5 | 0.3 | 0.0 | 0.0 | 0.0 | 0.0 | 0.00 | 0.00 | 0 | 50 | 5 | | | | | | | | | | | 1.8 | | | 0 | | 0.0 | | | | | | 85 | |

SECTION 8

# SUPPLEMENTARY TABLES

# TABLE A Amino Acid Content for Selected Foods

| Code | Amount | Description | Weight (g) | Alanine (g) | Arginine (g) | Aspartic acid (g) | Cystine (g) | Glutamic acid (g) | Glycine (g) | Histidine (g) | Isoleucine (g) | Leucine (g) | Lysine (g) | Methionine (g) | Phenylalanine (g) | Proline (g) | Serine (g) | Threonine (g) | Tryptophan (g) | Tyrosine (g) | Valine (g) |
|---|---|---|---|---|---|---|---|---|---|---|---|---|---|---|---|---|---|---|---|---|---|
| | | **BEVERAGES** | | | | | | | | | | | | | | | | | | | |
| | | Alcoholic | | | | | | | | | | | | | | | | | | | |
| 22738 | 1 ea | Beer, 12 fl oz, avg | 356 | 0.04 | 0.03 | 0.04 | 0.01 | 0.11 | 0.03 | 0.02 | 0.02 | 0.02 | 0.02 | 0.00 | 0.02 | 0.11 | 0.02 | 0.02 | 0.01 | 0.05 | 0.03 |
| 22742 | 1 ea | Beer, 12 fl oz, light, avg | 354 | 0.03 | 0.02 | 0.04 | 0.01 | 0.08 | 0.02 | 0.01 | 0.01 | 0.02 | 0.02 | 0.00 | 0.02 | 0.08 | 0.01 | 0.01 | 0.01 | 0.04 | 0.02 |
| 22734 | 1 ea | Coffee Liqueur | 52 | 0.00 | 0.00 | 0.00 | 0.00 | 0.00 | 0.00 | 0.00 | 0.00 | 0.00 | 0.00 | 0.00 | 0.00 | 0.00 | 0.00 | 0.00 | 0.00 | 0.00 | 0.00 |
| 22736 | 1 ea | Coffee Liqueur, w/cream | 47 | 0.04 | 0.05 | 0.09 | 0.01 | 0.26 | 0.03 | 0.03 | 0.08 | 0.12 | 0.10 | 0.03 | 0.06 | 0.12 | 0.07 | 0.06 | 0.02 | 0.06 | 0.08 |
| 22795 | 1 ea | Mixed Drink, Bloody Mary | 238 | 0.02 | 0.01 | 0.07 | 0.00 | 0.22 | 0.01 | 0.01 | 0.01 | 0.01 | 0.02 | 0.00 | 0.01 | 0.01 | 0.01 | 0.01 | 0.00 | 0.01 | 0.01 |
| 22809 | 1 ea | Mixed Drink, Screwdriver | 243 | 0.03 | 0.09 | 0.14 | 0.01 | 0.06 | 0.02 | 0.00 | 0.01 | 0.02 | 0.02 | 0.01 | 0.02 | 0.08 | 0.02 | 0.01 | 0.00 | 0.01 | 0.02 |
| 22810 | 1 ea | Mixed Drink, Tequila Sunrise | 250 | 0.02 | 0.04 | 0.07 | 0.01 | 0.03 | 0.01 | 0.00 | 0.01 | 0.01 | 0.01 | 0.00 | 0.01 | 0.04 | 0.01 | 0.01 | 0.00 | 0.00 | 0.01 |
| | | Coffee | | | | | | | | | | | | | | | | | | | |
| 20012 | 1 cup | Coffee, brewed, avg | 237 | 0.01 | 0.00 | 0.01 | 0.00 | 0.05 | 0.01 | 0.00 | 0.00 | 0.01 | 0.00 | 0.00 | 0.01 | 0.01 | 0.00 | 0.00 | 0.00 | 0.00 | 0.01 |
| 20109 | 1 cup | Coffee, mocha, w/sugar, prep f/pwd, avg | 250 | 0.02 | 0.02 | 0.05 | 0.01 | 0.09 | 0.02 | 0.01 | 0.02 | 0.03 | 0.02 | 0.01 | 0.02 | 0.02 | 0.02 | 0.02 | 0.01 | 0.02 | 0.03 |
| 20023 | 1 cup | Coffee, prep f/pwd, avg | 238 | 0.01 | 0.00 | 0.01 | 0.00 | 0.05 | 0.01 | 0.00 | 0.00 | 0.01 | 0.00 | 0.00 | 0.01 | 0.01 | 0.00 | 0.00 | 0.00 | 0.00 | 0.01 |
| 20091 | 1 cup | Coffee, prep f/pwd, decaf, avg | 179 | 0.01 | 0.00 | 0.01 | 0.00 | 0.03 | 0.01 | 0.00 | 0.00 | 0.01 | 0.00 | 0.00 | 0.01 | 0.01 | 0.00 | 0.00 | 0.00 | 0.00 | 0.01 |
| 20048 | 1 cup | Coffee Substitute, cereal grain, prep f/pwd, avg | 240 | 0.01 | 0.01 | 0.01 | 0.00 | 0.04 | 0.01 | 0.00 | 0.01 | 0.01 | 0.01 | 0.00 | 0.01 | 0.02 | 0.01 | 0.00 | 0.00 | 0.00 | 0.01 |
| | | Dairy Mixed Drinks | | | | | | | | | | | | | | | | | | | |
| 44 | 1 cup | Carob Beverage, prep f/mix, avg | 256 | 0.27 | 0.28 | 0.59 | 0.07 | 1.63 | 0.17 | 0.21 | 0.47 | 0.76 | 0.62 | 0.20 | 0.38 | 0.76 | 0.42 | 0.35 | 0.11 | 0.38 | 0.52 |
| 39 | 1 cup | Chocolate Drink, prep w/water, avg | 266 | 0.30 | 0.32 | 0.66 | 0.08 | 1.73 | 0.20 | 0.22 | 0.50 | 0.81 | 0.65 | 0.20 | 0.41 | 0.79 | 0.45 | 0.38 | 0.12 | 0.40 | 0.56 |
| 151 | 1 cup | Chocolate Drink, prep w/water, sugar free, avg | 272 | 0.26 | 0.29 | 0.57 | 0.07 | 1.37 | 0.19 | 0.17 | 0.39 | 0.63 | 0.51 | 0.15 | 0.34 | 0.59 | 0.36 | 0.31 | 0.10 | 0.32 | 0.46 |
| 38 | 1 cup | Chocolate Malt, prep f/mix, avg | 265 | 0.28 | 0.29 | 0.61 | 0.07 | 1.68 | 0.17 | 0.22 | 0.48 | 0.78 | 0.64 | 0.20 | 0.39 | 0.78 | 0.44 | 0.36 | 0.11 | 0.39 | 0.54 |
| 70 | 1 cup | Chocolate Milk, prep w/whole milk & syrup, avg | 263 | 0.28 | 0.30 | 0.62 | 0.07 | 1.67 | 0.18 | 0.22 | 0.48 | 0.78 | 0.63 | 0.20 | 0.39 | 0.77 | 0.44 | 0.36 | 0.11 | 0.39 | 0.54 |
| | | Cocoa | | | | | | | | | | | | | | | | | | | |
| 48 | 1 cup | Hot, prep w/water, avg | 275 | 0.14 | 0.16 | 0.32 | 0.04 | 0.76 | 0.10 | 0.10 | 0.22 | 0.35 | 0.28 | 0.08 | 0.19 | 0.33 | 0.20 | 0.17 | 0.06 | 0.18 | 0.26 |
| 21 | 1 cup | Hot, prep w/whole milk, avg | 250 | 0.34 | 0.37 | 0.75 | 0.09 | 1.88 | 0.23 | 0.24 | 0.54 | 0.86 | 0.70 | 0.22 | 0.45 | 0.83 | 0.50 | 0.41 | 0.13 | 0.44 | 0.62 |
| 61 | 1 ea | Hot Mix, dry pkt, avg | 31 | 0.07 | 0.07 | 0.15 | 0.02 | 0.35 | 0.05 | 0.04 | 0.10 | 0.16 | 0.13 | 0.04 | 0.09 | 0.15 | 0.09 | 0.08 | 0.03 | 0.08 | 0.12 |
| 75 | 1 ea | Hot Mix, low cal, dry pkt, avg | 19 | 0.04 | 0.04 | 0.09 | 0.01 | 0.21 | 0.03 | 0.03 | 0.06 | 0.10 | 0.08 | 0.02 | 0.05 | 0.09 | 0.06 | 0.05 | 0.02 | 0.05 | 0.07 |
| 166 | 1 ea | Hot Mix, w/marsh, dry pkt, Carnation | 28 | 0.05 | 0.05 | 0.11 | 0.01 | 0.25 | 0.03 | 0.04 | 0.07 | 0.12 | 0.09 | 0.03 | 0.06 | 0.11 | 0.07 | 0.06 | 0.02 | 0.06 | 0.08 |
| 172 | 1 ea | Hot Mix, Rich Chocolate, dry pkt, Carnation | 28 | 0.05 | 0.05 | 0.10 | 0.01 | 0.24 | 0.03 | 0.03 | 0.07 | 0.11 | 0.09 | 0.03 | 0.06 | 0.10 | 0.06 | 0.05 | 0.02 | 0.06 | 0.08 |
| 73 | 1 cup | Prep w/water, avg | 279 | 0.09 | 0.10 | 0.20 | 0.03 | 0.47 | 0.06 | 0.06 | 0.13 | 0.21 | 0.18 | 0.05 | 0.12 | 0.20 | 0.12 | 0.11 | 0.04 | 0.11 | 0.16 |
| 17 | 1 cup | Eggnog, avg | 254 | 0.33 | 0.36 | 0.71 | 0.09 | 1.88 | 0.21 | 0.23 | 0.56 | 0.90 | 0.73 | 0.21 | 0.45 | 0.86 | 0.53 | 0.43 | 0.13 | 0.45 | 0.62 |
| 45 | 1 Tbs | Eggnog Mix, avg | 14 | 0.00 | 0.00 | 0.00 | 0.00 | 0.01 | 0.00 | 0.00 | 0.00 | 0.00 | 0.00 | 0.00 | 0.00 | 0.00 | 0.00 | 0.00 | 0.00 | 0.00 | 0.00 |
| 20026 | 1 cup | Grape Juice Drink, avg | 250 | 0.03 | 0.02 | 0.01 | 0.00 | 0.04 | 0.01 | 0.00 | 0.00 | 0.01 | 0.01 | 0.00 | 0.01 | 0.01 | 0.01 | 0.01 | 0.00 | 0.00 | 0.01 |
| 20039 | 1 tsp | Iced Tea, instant, lemon, diet, dry mix, avg | 1 | 0.00 | 0.00 | 0.00 | 0.00 | 0.00 | 0.00 | 0.00 | 0.00 | 0.00 | 0.00 | 0.00 | 0.00 | 0.00 | 0.00 | 0.00 | 0.00 | 0.00 | 0.00 |
| 20120 | 1 cup | Iced Tea, instant, lemon, w/sugar, vit C, prep, avg | 182 | 0.01 | 0.01 | 0.03 | 0.01 | 0.06 | 0.01 | 0.00 | 0.01 | 0.01 | 0.01 | 0.00 | 0.00 | 0.01 | 0.01 | 0.01 | 0.01 | 0.01 | 0.01 |
| | | Instant Breakfast | | | | | | | | | | | | | | | | | | | |
| 101 | 1 cup | Prep w/1% milk, avg | 281 | 0.28 | 0.29 | 0.61 | 0.07 | 1.68 | 0.17 | 0.22 | 0.49 | 0.79 | 0.64 | 0.20 | 0.39 | 0.78 | 0.44 | 0.36 | 0.11 | 0.39 | 0.54 |
| 26 | 1 cup | Prep w/2% milk, avg | 281 | 0.28 | 0.30 | 0.62 | 0.08 | 1.70 | 0.17 | 0.22 | 0.49 | 0.80 | 0.64 | 0.20 | 0.39 | 0.79 | 0.44 | 0.37 | 0.11 | 0.39 | 0.54 |
| 27 | 1 cup | Prep w/nonfat milk, avg | 282 | 0.29 | 0.30 | 0.63 | 0.08 | 1.75 | 0.18 | 0.23 | 0.50 | 0.82 | 0.66 | 0.21 | 0.40 | 0.81 | 0.45 | 0.38 | 0.12 | 0.40 | 0.56 |
| 25 | 1 cup | Prep w/whole milk, avg | 281 | 0.28 | 0.29 | 0.61 | 0.07 | 1.68 | 0.17 | 0.22 | 0.49 | 0.79 | 0.64 | 0.20 | 0.39 | 0.78 | 0.44 | 0.36 | 0.11 | 0.39 | 0.54 |
| 20000 | 1 cup | Lemonade, prep f/conc, avg | 248 | 0.01 | 0.01 | 0.03 | 0.00 | 0.03 | 0.02 | 0.00 | 0.01 | 0.01 | 0.01 | 0.00 | 0.01 | 0.01 | 0.01 | 0.00 | 0.00 | 0.00 | 0.01 |
| 197 | 1 cup | Milkshake, chocolate, avg | 227 | 0.23 | 0.24 | 0.50 | 0.06 | 1.38 | 0.14 | 0.18 | 0.40 | 0.65 | 0.52 | 0.16 | 0.32 | 0.64 | 0.36 | 0.30 | 0.09 | 0.32 | 0.44 |
| 199 | 1 cup | Milkshake, vanilla, avg | 227 | 0.29 | 0.30 | 0.63 | 0.08 | 1.75 | 0.18 | 0.23 | 0.51 | 0.82 | 0.66 | 0.21 | 0.40 | 0.81 | 0.45 | 0.38 | 0.12 | 0.40 | 0.56 |
| 20058 | 1 cup | Orange Apricot, juice drink, cnd, avg | 250 | 0.03 | 0.05 | 0.13 | 0.01 | 0.06 | 0.02 | 0.01 | 0.02 | 0.03 | 0.03 | 0.01 | 0.02 | 0.05 | 0.03 | 0.02 | 0.01 | 0.01 | 0.02 |
| 20059 | 1 cup | Pineapple Grapefruit, juice drink, cnd, avg | 250 | 0.02 | 0.04 | 0.08 | 0.01 | 0.05 | 0.02 | 0.01 | 0.02 | 0.02 | 0.02 | 0.01 | 0.01 | 0.03 | 0.03 | 0.01 | 0.01 | 0.01 | 0.02 |
| 20025 | 1 cup | Pineapple Orange Drink, cnd, avg | 250 | 0.03 | 0.06 | 0.12 | 0.01 | 0.06 | 0.02 | 0.01 | 0.02 | 0.02 | 0.02 | 0.01 | 0.02 | 0.06 | 0.03 | 0.02 | 0.01 | 0.01 | 0.02 |
| 41 | 1 cup | Strawberry Milk, prep f/mix, avg | 266 | 0.26 | 0.27 | 0.58 | 0.07 | 1.59 | 0.16 | 0.21 | 0.46 | 0.74 | 0.60 | 0.19 | 0.37 | 0.74 | 0.41 | 0.34 | 0.11 | 0.37 | 0.51 |
| | | **CANDIES AND CONFECTIONS** | | | | | | | | | | | | | | | | | | | |
| | | Baking Chocolate and Coating | | | | | | | | | | | | | | | | | | | |
| 23200 | 1/2 cup | Semi-Sweet Chocolate, w/butter, avg | 85 | 0.17 | 0.20 | 0.36 | 0.04 | 0.54 | 0.16 | 0.06 | 0.14 | 0.22 | 0.18 | 0.04 | 0.17 | 0.15 | 0.16 | 0.14 | 0.05 | 0.14 | 0.22 |
| 23010 | 1 ea | Unsweetened Square, avg | 28 | 0.13 | 0.16 | 0.29 | 0.04 | 0.43 | 0.13 | 0.05 | 0.11 | 0.17 | 0.14 | 0.03 | 0.14 | 0.12 | 0.12 | 0.11 | 0.04 | 0.11 | 0.17 |

TABLE A **Amino Acid Content for Selected Foods *(continued)***

| Code | Amount | Description | Weight (g) | Alanine (g) | Arginine (g) | Aspartic acid (g) | Cystine (g) | Glutamic acid (g) | Glycine (g) | Histidine (g) | Isoleucine (g) | Leucine (g) | Lysine (g) | Methionine (g) | Phenylalanine (g) | Proline (g) | Serine (g) | Threonine (g) | Tryptophan (g) | Tyrosine (g) | Valine (g) |
|---|---|---|---|---|---|---|---|---|---|---|---|---|---|---|---|---|---|---|---|---|---|
| 23011 | 1/2 cup | Unsweetened Square, grated, avg | 66 | 0.31 | 0.38 | 0.67 | 0.08 | 1.02 | 0.30 | 0.12 | 0.26 | 0.41 | 0.34 | 0.07 | 0.33 | 0.29 | 0.29 | 0.27 | 0.10 | 0.25 | 0.41 |
| | | Baking Chips and Morsels | | | | | | | | | | | | | | | | | | | |
| 23119 | 1/2 cup | Butterscotch Chips, avg | 85 | 0.06 | 0.06 | 0.13 | 0.02 | 0.37 | 0.04 | 0.05 | 0.11 | 0.17 | 0.14 | 0.04 | 0.09 | 0.17 | 0.10 | 0.08 | 0.03 | 0.09 | 0.12 |
| 23243 | 1/2 cup | Carob Chips, avg | 85 | 0.50 | 0.11 | 0.43 | 0.02 | 0.31 | 0.23 | 0.10 | 0.18 | 0.38 | 0.17 | 0.07 | 0.13 | 0.30 | 0.26 | 0.23 | 0.04 | 0.10 | 0.38 |
| 23423 | 1 Tbs | Milk Chocolate, M&M's mini bits | 14 | 0.02 | 0.02 | 0.06 | 0.00 | 0.14 | 0.02 | 0.01 | 0.04 | 0.06 | 0.04 | 0.01 | 0.04 | 0.06 | 0.03 | 0.03 | 0.01 | 0.03 | 0.04 |
| 23012 | 1/2 cup | Semi-Sweet Chocolate Chips, avg | 84 | 0.16 | 0.20 | 0.35 | 0.04 | 0.54 | 0.16 | 0.06 | 0.14 | 0.22 | 0.18 | 0.04 | 0.17 | 0.15 | 0.15 | 0.14 | 0.05 | 0.13 | 0.21 |
| 23421 | 1 Tbs | Semi-Sweet Chocolate Mini Bits, M&M's | 14 | 0.03 | 0.04 | 0.06 | 0.01 | 0.09 | 0.03 | 0.01 | 0.02 | 0.04 | 0.03 | 0.01 | 0.03 | 0.03 | 0.03 | 0.02 | 0.01 | 0.02 | 0.04 |
| 23121 | 1/2 cup | White Chips, avg | 85 | 0.14 | 0.15 | 0.31 | 0.04 | 0.86 | 0.09 | 0.11 | 0.25 | 0.40 | 0.33 | 0.10 | 0.20 | 0.40 | 0.22 | 0.18 | 0.06 | 0.20 | 0.28 |
| | | Candy and Candy Bars | | | | | | | | | | | | | | | | | | | |
| 23115 | 5 pce | Butterscotch candy, avg | 30 | 0.00 | 0.00 | 0.00 | 0.00 | 0.00 | 0.00 | 0.00 | 0.00 | 0.00 | 0.00 | 0.00 | 0.00 | 0.00 | 0.00 | 0.00 | 0.00 | 0.00 | 0.00 |
| 23015 | 5 pce | Caramels, avg | 50 | 0.07 | 0.08 | 0.16 | 0.02 | 0.45 | 0.05 | 0.06 | 0.13 | 0.21 | 0.17 | 0.05 | 0.10 | 0.21 | 0.12 | 0.10 | 0.03 | 0.10 | 0.14 |
| 23117 | 5 ea | Caramels, chocolate flvd roll, avg | 25 | 0.02 | 0.02 | 0.04 | 0.01 | 0.08 | 0.02 | 0.01 | 0.02 | 0.04 | 0.03 | 0.01 | 0.02 | 0.03 | 0.02 | 0.02 | 0.01 | 0.02 | 0.03 |
| 23118 | 1 ea | Carob, avg, 3.1 oz. bar | 87 | 0.51 | 0.11 | 0.44 | 0.03 | 0.31 | 0.23 | 0.11 | 0.18 | 0.38 | 0.17 | 0.07 | 0.13 | 0.31 | 0.26 | 0.23 | 0.04 | 0.10 | 0.39 |
| 23023 | 5 ea | Chocolate Covered Fondant/Mints, avg | 55 | 0.05 | 0.06 | 0.11 | 0.01 | 0.16 | 0.05 | 0.02 | 0.04 | 0.07 | 0.05 | 0.01 | 0.05 | 0.05 | 0.05 | 0.04 | 0.02 | 0.04 | 0.06 |
| 23098 | 1 ea | Crisped Rice Almond bar, 1 oz, avg | 28 | 0.09 | 0.17 | 0.18 | 0.04 | 0.44 | 0.10 | 0.05 | 0.08 | 0.14 | 0.07 | 0.03 | 0.10 | 0.10 | 0.08 | 0.06 | 0.03 | 0.07 | 0.10 |
| 23099 | 1 ea | Crisped Rice Chocolate Chip bar, 1 oz, avg | 28 | 0.07 | 0.11 | 0.13 | 0.03 | 0.27 | 0.07 | 0.03 | 0.06 | 0.11 | 0.06 | 0.03 | 0.07 | 0.07 | 0.07 | 0.05 | 0.02 | 0.06 | 0.08 |
| 23053 | 1 pce | Divinity Candy, w/o nuts, recipe, avg | 11 | 0.01 | 0.01 | 0.01 | 0.00 | 0.02 | 0.00 | 0.00 | 0.01 | 0.01 | 0.01 | 0.00 | 0.01 | 0.01 | 0.01 | 0.01 | 0.00 | 0.01 | 0.01 |
| 23404 | 1 ea | Fruit Leather, avg, .74 oz | 21 | 0.01 | 0.01 | 0.04 | 0.00 | 0.03 | 0.01 | 0.00 | 0.01 | 0.01 | 0.01 | 0.00 | 0.01 | 0.01 | 0.01 | 0.01 | 0.00 | 0.01 | 0.01 |
| 23025 | 1 pce | Fudge, chocolate, recipe, avg | 17 | 0.01 | 0.01 | 0.02 | 0.00 | 0.05 | 0.01 | 0.01 | 0.01 | 0.02 | 0.02 | 0.01 | 0.01 | 0.02 | 0.01 | 0.01 | 0.00 | 0.01 | 0.02 |
| 23026 | 1 pce | Fudge, chocolate w/nuts, recipe, avg | 19 | 0.02 | 0.06 | 0.06 | 0.01 | 0.11 | 0.02 | 0.01 | 0.03 | 0.04 | 0.03 | 0.01 | 0.03 | 0.03 | 0.03 | 0.02 | 0.01 | 0.02 | 0.03 |
| 23126 | 1 pce | Fudge chocolate marshmallow, recipe, avg | 20 | 0.02 | 0.02 | 0.04 | 0.00 | 0.08 | 0.03 | 0.01 | 0.02 | 0.03 | 0.03 | 0.01 | 0.02 | 0.04 | 0.02 | 0.02 | 0.01 | 0.02 | 0.03 |
| 23127 | 1 pce | Fudge chocolate marsh w/nuts recipe, avg | 22 | 0.03 | 0.05 | 0.06 | 0.01 | 0.12 | 0.04 | 0.01 | 0.03 | 0.05 | 0.03 | 0.01 | 0.03 | 0.04 | 0.03 | 0.03 | 0.01 | 0.02 | 0.04 |
| 23128 | 1 pce | Fudge, peanut butter, recipe, avg | 16 | 0.02 | 0.06 | 0.06 | 0.01 | 0.12 | 0.03 | 0.01 | 0.02 | 0.04 | 0.03 | 0.01 | 0.03 | 0.03 | 0.03 | 0.02 | 0.01 | 0.02 | 0.03 |
| 23124 | 1 pce | Fudge, penuche w/brn sugar & nuts, avg | 14 | 0.01 | 0.04 | 0.03 | 0.01 | 0.07 | 0.01 | 0.01 | 0.02 | 0.03 | 0.02 | 0.01 | 0.02 | 0.02 | 0.02 | 0.01 | 0.00 | 0.01 | 0.02 |
| 23027 | 1 pce | Fudge, vanilla, recipe, avg | 16 | 0.01 | 0.01 | 0.01 | 0.00 | 0.03 | 0.00 | 0.00 | 0.01 | 0.02 | 0.01 | 0.00 | 0.01 | 0.02 | 0.01 | 0.01 | 0.00 | 0.01 | 0.01 |
| 23028 | 1 pce | Fudge, vanilla w/nuts, recipe, avg | 15 | 0.02 | 0.04 | 0.04 | 0.01 | 0.08 | 0.02 | 0.01 | 0.02 | 0.03 | 0.02 | 0.01 | 0.02 | 0.02 | 0.02 | 0.01 | 0.01 | 0.01 | 0.02 |
| 23016 | 1 ea | Kisses, milk chocolate, 1.6 oz pkg, Hershey's | 44 | 0.11 | 0.09 | 0.26 | 0.02 | 0.64 | 0.07 | 0.05 | 0.16 | 0.28 | 0.18 | 0.07 | 0.17 | 0.26 | 0.14 | 0.13 | 0.04 | 0.14 | 0.20 |
| 23058 | 1 ea | Milk Chocolate candy bar w/crsp rice, 1.4 oz, avg | 40 | 0.10 | 0.09 | 0.21 | 0.02 | 0.52 | 0.07 | 0.04 | 0.13 | 0.23 | 0.14 | 0.05 | 0.14 | 0.20 | 0.12 | 0.11 | 0.03 | 0.11 | 0.16 |
| 23019 | 1 ea | Milk Chocolate candy bar w/peanuts, 1 oz, avg | 28 | 0.18 | 0.46 | 0.52 | 0.05 | 0.94 | 0.24 | 0.11 | 0.17 | 0.32 | 0.18 | 0.06 | 0.24 | 0.23 | 0.22 | 0.12 | 0.05 | 0.19 | 0.21 |
| 23022 | 1/2 cup | Milk Chocolate Covered Raisins, avg | 95 | 0.14 | 0.16 | 0.37 | 0.03 | 0.82 | 0.10 | 0.08 | 0.16 | 0.28 | 0.19 | 0.10 | 0.18 | 0.27 | 0.18 | 0.15 | 0.04 | 0.15 | 0.21 |
| 23419 | 5 pce | Milk Chocolate Coated Peanuts, 5 pces | 20 | 0.10 | 0.20 | 0.27 | 0.03 | 0.54 | 0.11 | 0.05 | 0.11 | 0.20 | 0.12 | 0.04 | 0.14 | 0.16 | 0.12 | 0.10 | 0.03 | 0.11 | 0.14 |
| 23018 | 1 ea | Milk chocolate w/almonds, 1.45 oz bar, avg | 41 | 0.13 | 0.19 | 0.32 | 0.03 | 0.81 | 0.12 | 0.07 | 0.18 | 0.31 | 0.18 | 0.07 | 0.19 | 0.27 | 0.16 | 0.14 | 0.05 | 0.15 | 0.22 |
| 23137 | 1 ea | Peanut Bar, 1.4 oz, avg | 40 | 0.24 | 0.73 | 0.74 | 0.08 | 1.27 | 0.37 | 0.15 | 0.21 | 0.39 | 0.22 | 0.07 | 0.31 | 0.27 | 0.30 | 0.21 | 0.06 | 0.25 | 0.26 |
| 23081 | 1/2 cup | Peanut Brittle, recipe, avg | 74 | 0.22 | 0.65 | 0.67 | 0.07 | 1.15 | 0.33 | 0.14 | 0.19 | 0.36 | 0.20 | 0.07 | 0.29 | 0.24 | 0.27 | 0.19 | 0.05 | 0.22 | 0.23 |
| 23120 | 1/2 cup | Peanut Butter candy, avg | 84 | 0.61 | 1.80 | 1.85 | 0.20 | 3.20 | 0.91 | 0.39 | 0.54 | 1.00 | 0.56 | 0.14 | 0.79 | 0.69 | 0.75 | 0.53 | 0.15 | 0.62 | 0.65 |
| 23138 | 1 pce | Praline Candy, recipe, avg | 39 | 0.04 | 0.13 | 0.08 | 0.02 | 0.18 | 0.04 | 0.03 | 0.04 | 0.06 | 0.03 | 0.02 | 0.05 | 0.04 | 0.04 | 0.03 | 0.02 | 0.03 | 0.05 |
| 23142 | 20 pce | Sesame Crunch candy, avg | 35 | 0.19 | 0.53 | 0.33 | 0.07 | 0.80 | 0.24 | 0.11 | 0.15 | 0.27 | 0.11 | 0.12 | 0.19 | 0.16 | 0.20 | 0.15 | 0.08 | 0.15 | 0.20 |
| 23145 | 1 ea | Sweet Chocolate bar, 1.45 oz, avg | 41 | 0.07 | 0.09 | 0.16 | 0.02 | 0.24 | 0.07 | 0.03 | 0.06 | 0.10 | 0.08 | 0.02 | 0.08 | 0.07 | 0.07 | 0.06 | 0.02 | 0.06 | 0.10 |
| 23147 | 1 pce | Taffy candy, homemade, avg | 15 | 0.00 | 0.00 | 0.00 | 0.00 | 0.00 | 0.00 | 0.00 | 0.00 | 0.00 | 0.00 | 0.00 | 0.00 | 0.00 | 0.00 | 0.00 | 0.00 | 0.00 | 0.00 |
| 23173 | 1 pce | Toffee candy, homemade, avg | 12 | 0.00 | 0.00 | 0.01 | 0.00 | 0.03 | 0.00 | 0.00 | 0.01 | 0.01 | 0.01 | 0.00 | 0.01 | 0.01 | 0.01 | 0.01 | 0.00 | 0.01 | 0.01 |
| 23148 | 1 pce | Truffles candy, homemade, avg | 12 | 0.02 | 0.02 | 0.06 | 0.00 | 0.14 | 0.02 | 0.01 | 0.04 | 0.06 | 0.04 | 0.01 | 0.04 | 0.06 | 0.03 | 0.03 | 0.01 | 0.03 | 0.04 |
| 23008 | 1 cup | Marshmallows, miniature, avg | 46 | 0.08 | 0.07 | 0.06 | 0.00 | 0.10 | 0.19 | 0.01 | 0.01 | 0.03 | 0.04 | 0.01 | 0.02 | 0.13 | 0.03 | 0.02 | 0.00 | 0.00 | 0.02 |
| | | **CEREALS, DRY AND COOKED** | | | | | | | | | | | | | | | | | | | |
| | | Corn Grits | | | | | | | | | | | | | | | | | | | |
| 40093 | 1 cup | Enriched, white, ckd, avg | 242 | 0.25 | 0.17 | 0.23 | 0.06 | 0.64 | 0.14 | 0.10 | 0.12 | 0.42 | 0.09 | 0.07 | 0.17 | 0.30 | 0.16 | 0.13 | 0.02 | 0.14 | 0.17 |
| 40150 | 1/4 cup | Enriched, white, dry, avg | 39 | 0.26 | 0.17 | 0.24 | 0.06 | 0.64 | 0.14 | 0.10 | 0.12 | 0.42 | 0.10 | 0.07 | 0.17 | 0.30 | 0.16 | 0.13 | 0.02 | 0.14 | 0.17 |
| 38007 | 1 cup | Enriched, yellow, ckd, avg | 242 | 0.25 | 0.17 | 0.23 | 0.06 | 0.64 | 0.14 | 0.10 | 0.12 | 0.42 | 0.09 | 0.07 | 0.17 | 0.30 | 0.16 | 0.13 | 0.02 | 0.14 | 0.17 |
| 38006 | 1/4 cup | Enriched, yellow, dry, avg | 39 | 0.26 | 0.17 | 0.24 | 0.06 | 0.64 | 0.14 | 0.10 | 0.12 | 0.42 | 0.10 | 0.07 | 0.17 | 0.30 | 0.16 | 0.13 | 0.02 | 0.14 | 0.17 |
| 40152 | 1 ea | Instant Cheese flvr, dry pkt, Quaker | 28 | 0.17 | 0.12 | 0.16 | 0.04 | 0.45 | 0.09 | 0.07 | 0.09 | 0.29 | 0.07 | 0.05 | 0.11 | 0.21 | 0.11 | 0.09 | 0.02 | 0.10 | 0.12 |
| 40233 | 1 cup | Instant Cheese flvr, prep, Quaker | 178 | 0.21 | 0.14 | 0.20 | 0.05 | 0.54 | 0.11 | 0.09 | 0.11 | 0.34 | 0.09 | 0.06 | 0.14 | 0.25 | 0.14 | 0.11 | 0.02 | 0.12 | 0.15 |

TABLE A **Amino Acid Content for Selected Foods *(continued)***

| Code | Amount | Description | Weight (g) | Alanine (g) | Arginine (g) | Aspartic acid (g) | Cystine (g) | Glutamic acid (g) | Glycine (g) | Histidine (g) | Isoleucine (g) | Leucine (g) | Lysine (g) | Methionine (g) | Phenylalanine (g) | Proline (g) | Serine (g) | Threonine (g) | Tryptophan (g) | Tyrosine (g) | Valine (g) |
|---|---|---|---|---|---|---|---|---|---|---|---|---|---|---|---|---|---|---|---|---|---|
| 40153 | 1 ea | Instant Imit Bacon, dry pkt, Quaker | 28 | 0.19 | 0.13 | 0.18 | 0.05 | 0.48 | 0.11 | 0.08 | 0.09 | 0.32 | 0.07 | 0.05 | 0.13 | 0.22 | 0.12 | 0.10 | 0.02 | 0.10 | 0.13 |
| 40243 | 1 ea | Instant Imit Bacon, prep f/dry pkt, Quaker | 141 | 0.18 | 0.12 | 0.17 | 0.04 | 0.47 | 0.10 | 0.08 | 0.09 | 0.30 | 0.07 | 0.05 | 0.12 | 0.22 | 0.12 | 0.09 | 0.02 | 0.10 | 0.13 |
| 40154 | 1 ea | Instant Imit Ham Bits, dry pkt, Quaker | 28 | 0.19 | 0.13 | 0.18 | 0.05 | 0.49 | 0.11 | 0.08 | 0.09 | 0.32 | 0.08 | 0.05 | 0.13 | 0.23 | 0.12 | 0.10 | 0.02 | 0.11 | 0.13 |
| 40234 | 1 cup | Instant Ham Bits prep, Quaker | 176 | 0.23 | 0.15 | 0.22 | 0.06 | 0.59 | 0.13 | 0.10 | 0.11 | 0.38 | 0.09 | 0.07 | 0.15 | 0.27 | 0.15 | 0.12 | 0.02 | 0.13 | 0.16 |
| 40094 | 1 cup | Unenriched, white, ckd, avg | 242 | 0.25 | 0.17 | 0.23 | 0.06 | 0.64 | 0.14 | 0.10 | 0.12 | 0.42 | 0.09 | 0.07 | 0.17 | 0.30 | 0.16 | 0.13 | 0.02 | 0.14 | 0.17 |
| 40173 | 1/4 cup | Unenriched, white, dry, avg | 39 | 0.26 | 0.17 | 0.24 | 0.06 | 0.64 | 0.14 | 0.10 | 0.12 | 0.42 | 0.10 | 0.07 | 0.17 | 0.30 | 0.16 | 0.13 | 0.02 | 0.14 | 0.17 |
| 40081 | 1 cup | Unenriched, yellow, ckd, avg | 242 | 0.25 | 0.17 | 0.23 | 0.06 | 0.64 | 0.14 | 0.10 | 0.12 | 0.42 | 0.09 | 0.07 | 0.17 | 0.30 | 0.16 | 0.13 | 0.02 | 0.14 | 0.17 |
| 40174 | 1/4 cup | Unenriched, yellow, dry, avg | 39 | 0.26 | 0.17 | 0.24 | 0.06 | 0.64 | 0.14 | 0.10 | 0.12 | 0.42 | 0.10 | 0.07 | 0.17 | 0.30 | 0.16 | 0.13 | 0.02 | 0.14 | 0.17 |
| 40078 | 1 cup | Cream of Rice, ckd, avg | 244 | 0.09 | 0.18 | 0.20 | 0.04 | 0.34 | 0.12 | 0.06 | 0.04 | 0.18 | 0.09 | 0.06 | 0.09 | 0.09 | 0.10 | 0.11 | 0.03 | 0.12 | 0.14 |
| 40155 | 1/4 cup | Cream of Rice, dry, avg | 43 | 0.11 | 0.22 | 0.25 | 0.05 | 0.43 | 0.16 | 0.08 | 0.14 | 0.22 | 0.11 | 0.08 | 0.11 | 0.11 | 0.12 | 0.14 | 0.04 | 0.15 | 0.18 |
| | | Cream of Wheat | | | | | | | | | | | | | | | | | | | |
| 40162 | 1 ea | Apple, Banana & Maple, dry pkt, avg | 35 | 0.08 | 0.10 | 0.11 | 0.05 | 0.80 | 0.09 | 0.05 | 0.10 | 0.17 | 0.06 | 0.04 | 0.12 | 0.26 | 0.12 | 0.07 | 0.03 | 0.07 | 0.11 |
| 40163 | 1 ea | Apple, Banana & Maple, prep f/dry pkt, avg | 150 | 0.08 | 0.10 | 0.11 | 0.05 | 0.80 | 0.09 | 0.05 | 0.09 | 0.17 | 0.06 | 0.04 | 0.12 | 0.26 | 0.12 | 0.07 | 0.03 | 0.07 | 0.11 |
| 40157 | 1 cup | Cooked, avg | 251 | 0.12 | 0.15 | 0.16 | 0.08 | 1.27 | 0.13 | 0.08 | 0.15 | 0.26 | 0.09 | 0.06 | 0.18 | 0.42 | 0.19 | 0.11 | 0.05 | 0.11 | 0.16 |
| 40156 | 1/4 cup | Dry, avg | 43 | 0.14 | 0.18 | 0.19 | 0.09 | 1.52 | 0.16 | 0.09 | 0.18 | 0.31 | 0.11 | 0.08 | 0.22 | 0.50 | 0.23 | 0.13 | 0.06 | 0.13 | 0.20 |
| 40159 | 1/4 cup | Instant, dry, avg | 44 | 0.15 | 0.18 | 0.20 | 0.10 | 1.57 | 0.16 | 0.10 | 0.18 | 0.32 | 0.11 | 0.08 | 0.23 | 0.52 | 0.24 | 0.13 | 0.06 | 0.13 | 0.21 |
| 40160 | 1 cup | Prep f/instant, avg | 241 | 0.14 | 0.17 | 0.19 | 0.09 | 1.46 | 0.15 | 0.09 | 0.17 | 0.30 | 0.10 | 0.07 | 0.21 | 0.48 | 0.22 | 0.12 | 0.05 | 0.12 | 0.19 |
| 40158 | 1/4 cup | Quick, dry, avg | 44 | 0.14 | 0.18 | 0.19 | 0.09 | 1.51 | 0.16 | 0.09 | 0.18 | 0.31 | 0.11 | 0.08 | 0.22 | 0.50 | 0.23 | 0.13 | 0.06 | 0.13 | 0.20 |
| 40079 | 1 cup | Quick, prep, avg | 239 | 0.11 | 0.14 | 0.15 | 0.07 | 1.21 | 0.13 | 0.07 | 0.14 | 0.25 | 0.08 | 0.06 | 0.18 | 0.40 | 0.18 | 0.10 | 0.04 | 0.10 | 0.16 |
| | | Farina | | | | | | | | | | | | | | | | | | | |
| 40006 | 1 cup | Enriched, ckd, avg | 233 | 0.09 | 0.12 | 0.13 | 0.09 | 1.17 | 0.10 | 0.07 | 0.13 | 0.22 | 0.06 | 0.05 | 0.16 | 0.36 | 0.15 | 0.09 | 0.04 | 0.09 | 0.14 |
| 40077 | 1 cup | Unenriched, ckd, avg | 233 | 0.09 | 0.12 | 0.13 | 0.09 | 1.17 | 0.10 | 0.07 | 0.13 | 0.22 | 0.06 | 0.05 | 0.16 | 0.36 | 0.15 | 0.09 | 0.04 | 0.09 | 0.14 |
| 40183 | 1/4 cup | Unenriched, dry, avg | 44 | 0.14 | 0.17 | 0.19 | 0.13 | 1.68 | 0.15 | 0.09 | 0.18 | 0.32 | 0.09 | 0.07 | 0.23 | 0.51 | 0.22 | 0.12 | 0.06 | 0.12 | 0.20 |
| | | Malt-o-Meal | | | | | | | | | | | | | | | | | | | |
| 40188 | 1 cup | Chocolate, ckd w/salt, avg | 240 | 0.10 | 0.13 | 0.14 | 0.10 | 1.26 | 0.11 | 0.07 | 0.14 | 0.24 | 0.07 | 0.05 | 0.17 | 0.38 | 0.16 | 0.09 | 0.04 | 0.09 | 0.15 |
| 40187 | 1/4 cup | Chocolate, dry, avg | 41 | 0.13 | 0.16 | 0.18 | 0.12 | 1.55 | 0.14 | 0.09 | 0.17 | 0.29 | 0.08 | 0.07 | 0.21 | 0.47 | 0.20 | 0.11 | 0.06 | 0.11 | 0.18 |
| 40014 | 1 cup | Plain, ckd, avg | 240 | 0.10 | 0.13 | 0.14 | 0.10 | 1.26 | 0.11 | 0.07 | 0.14 | 0.24 | 0.07 | 0.05 | 0.17 | 0.38 | 0.16 | 0.09 | 0.04 | 0.09 | 0.15 |
| 40165 | 1/4 cup | Plain, dry, avg | 41 | 0.13 | 0.16 | 0.18 | 0.12 | 1.55 | 0.14 | 0.09 | 0.17 | 0.29 | 0.08 | 0.07 | 0.21 | 0.47 | 0.20 | 0.11 | 0.06 | 0.11 | 0.18 |
| 40235 | 1 cup | Maltex, wheat cereal, ckd, avg | 249 | 0.16 | 0.20 | 0.22 | 0.15 | 1.94 | 0.17 | 0.11 | 0.21 | 0.37 | 0.10 | 0.08 | 0.26 | 0.59 | 0.25 | 0.14 | 0.07 | 0.14 | 0.23 |
| 40164 | 1/4 cup | Maltex, wheat cereal, dry, avg | 38 | 0.12 | 0.16 | 0.17 | 0.12 | 1.53 | 0.13 | 0.09 | 0.16 | 0.29 | 0.08 | 0.06 | 0.21 | 0.47 | 0.20 | 0.11 | 0.05 | 0.11 | 0.18 |
| | | Oatmeal | | | | | | | | | | | | | | | | | | | |
| 90076 | 1 ea | Apple Cinnamon, dry pkt, Quaker | 35 | 0.17 | 0.23 | 0.28 | 0.08 | 0.72 | 0.16 | 0.08 | 0.14 | 0.25 | 0.14 | 0.06 | 0.17 | 0.18 | 0.15 | 0.11 | 0.05 | 0.11 | 0.18 |
| 40073 | 1 ea | Apple Cinnamon, prep f/dry pkt, Quaker | 149 | 0.17 | 0.23 | 0.27 | 0.08 | 0.71 | 0.16 | 0.08 | 0.13 | 0.24 | 0.13 | 0.06 | 0.17 | 0.18 | 0.14 | 0.11 | 0.04 | 0.11 | 0.18 |
| 90077 | 1 ea | Brown Sugar & Raisins, dry pkt, Quaker | 42 | 0.25 | 0.34 | 0.41 | 0.12 | 1.05 | 0.24 | 0.11 | 0.20 | 0.36 | 0.20 | 0.09 | 0.25 | 0.26 | 0.21 | 0.16 | 0.07 | 0.16 | 0.27 |
| 38317 | 1 ea | Brown Sugar & Raisins, prep f/dry pkt, Quaker | 195 | 0.25 | 0.34 | 0.41 | 0.12 | 1.06 | 0.24 | 0.12 | 0.20 | 0.37 | 0.20 | 0.09 | 0.26 | 0.27 | 0.22 | 0.17 | 0.07 | 0.17 | 0.27 |
| 90079 | 1 ea | Cinnamon Spice, dry pkt, Quaker | 46 | 0.20 | 0.28 | 0.33 | 0.09 | 0.86 | 0.19 | 0.09 | 0.16 | 0.30 | 0.16 | 0.07 | 0.21 | 0.22 | 0.17 | 0.13 | 0.05 | 0.13 | 0.22 |
| 40074 | 1 ea | Cinnamon Spice, prep f/dry pkt, Quaker | 161 | 0.25 | 0.34 | 0.41 | 0.12 | 1.05 | 0.24 | 0.12 | 0.20 | 0.36 | 0.20 | 0.09 | 0.25 | 0.27 | 0.21 | 0.16 | 0.07 | 0.16 | 0.27 |
| 40000 | 1 cup | Cooked, avg | 234 | 0.32 | 0.43 | 0.52 | 0.15 | 1.33 | 0.30 | 0.15 | 0.25 | 0.46 | 0.25 | 0.11 | 0.32 | 0.33 | 0.27 | 0.21 | 0.08 | 0.21 | 0.33 |
| 40167 | 1 ea | Maple & Brown Sugar, dry pkt, Quaker | 42 | 0.22 | 0.30 | 0.36 | 0.10 | 0.93 | 0.21 | 0.10 | 0.17 | 0.32 | 0.18 | 0.08 | 0.22 | 0.23 | 0.19 | 0.14 | 0.06 | 0.14 | 0.24 |
| 40075 | 1 ea | Maple & Brown Sugar, prep f/dry pkt, Quaker | 155 | 0.23 | 0.31 | 0.37 | 0.10 | 0.95 | 0.22 | 0.10 | 0.03 | 0.33 | 0.18 | 0.08 | 0.23 | 0.24 | 0.19 | 0.15 | 0.06 | 0.15 | 0.24 |
| 90080 | 1 ea | Raisin Spice, dry pkt, Quaker | 42 | 0.23 | 0.31 | 0.38 | 0.11 | 0.97 | 0.22 | 0.11 | 0.18 | 0.34 | 0.18 | 0.08 | 0.23 | 0.24 | 0.20 | 0.15 | 0.06 | 0.15 | 0.24 |
| 40076 | 1 ea | Raisin Spice, prep f/dry pkt, Quaker | 158 | 0.22 | 0.30 | 0.36 | 0.10 | 0.93 | 0.21 | 0.10 | 0.17 | 0.32 | 0.18 | 0.08 | 0.22 | 0.23 | 0.19 | 0.14 | 0.06 | 0.14 | 0.23 |
| 38008 | 1/4 cup | Rolled Oats, dry, avg | 20 | 0.17 | 0.23 | 0.27 | 0.08 | 0.70 | 0.16 | 0.08 | 0.13 | 0.24 | 0.13 | 0.06 | 0.17 | 0.18 | 0.14 | 0.11 | 0.04 | 0.11 | 0.18 |
| 40080 | 1 cup | Wheatena, whole wheat cereal, ckd | 243 | 0.17 | 0.23 | 0.25 | 0.11 | 1.53 | 0.20 | 0.11 | 0.18 | 0.33 | 0.13 | 0.08 | 0.23 | 0.50 | 0.23 | 0.14 | 0.08 | 0.14 | 0.22 |
| 40169 | 1/4 cup | Wheatena, whole wheat cereal, dry | 35 | 0.16 | 0.21 | 0.23 | 0.10 | 1.43 | 0.18 | 0.10 | 0.17 | 0.31 | 0.12 | 0.07 | 0.21 | 0.47 | 0.21 | 0.13 | 0.07 | 0.13 | 0.21 |
| 40002 | 1 cup | Whole Wheat Natural Cereal, ckd, avg | 240 | 0.17 | 0.22 | 0.25 | 0.11 | 1.52 | 0.19 | 0.11 | 0.18 | 0.33 | 0.13 | 0.07 | 0.23 | 0.50 | 0.23 | 0.14 | 0.07 | 0.14 | 0.22 |
| 40001 | 1/4 cup | Whole Wheat Natural Cereal, dry, avg | 21 | 0.08 | 0.11 | 0.12 | 0.05 | 0.74 | 0.09 | 0.05 | 0.09 | 0.16 | 0.06 | 0.04 | 0.11 | 0.24 | 0.11 | 0.07 | 0.04 | 0.07 | 0.11 |
| | | **CEREALS, READY TO EAT** | | | | | | | | | | | | | | | | | | | |
| 40258 | 1 cup | Alpha Bits, Post | 28 | 0.13 | 0.14 | 0.18 | 0.05 | 0.49 | 0.11 | 0.05 | 0.10 | 0.20 | 0.08 | 0.04 | 0.12 | 0.14 | 0.10 | 0.07 | 0.03 | 0.08 | 0.12 |
| 40281 | 1 cup | Bran Flakes, 100% Bran, Nabisco | 66 | 0.40 | 0.58 | 0.60 | 0.16 | 1.60 | 0.48 | 0.23 | 0.26 | 0.49 | 0.32 | 0.12 | 0.32 | 0.51 | 0.37 | 0.27 | 0.13 | 0.23 | 0.39 |

TABLE A **Amino Acid Content for Selected Foods *(continued)***

| Code | Amount | | Description | Weight (g) | Alanine (g) | Arginine (g) | Aspartic acid (g) | Cystine (g) | Glutamic acid (g) | Glycine (g) | Histidine (g) | Isoleucine (g) | Leucine (g) | Lysine (g) | Methionine (g) | Phenylalanine (g) | Proline (g) | Serine (g) | Threonine (g) | Tryptophan (g) | Tyrosine (g) | Valine (g) |
|---|---|---|---|---|---|---|---|---|---|---|---|---|---|---|---|---|---|---|---|---|---|---|
| 40259 | 1 | cup | Bran Flakes, Post | 47 | 0.23 | 0.31 | 0.33 | 0.11 | 1.46 | 0.26 | 0.14 | 0.20 | 0.35 | 0.18 | 0.08 | 0.24 | 0.47 | 0.27 | 0.17 | 0.09 | 0.16 | 0.26 |
| | | | Cap'n Crunch | | | | | | | | | | | | | | | | | | | |
| 40032 | 1 | cup | Original, Quaker | 37 | 0.13 | 0.08 | 0.12 | 0.04 | 0.40 | 0.07 | 0.05 | 0.07 | 0.22 | 0.05 | 0.04 | 0.09 | 0.15 | 0.09 | 0.06 | 0.01 | 0.07 | 0.10 |
| 40034 | 1 | cup | Peanut Butter, Quaker | 35 | 0.15 | 0.19 | 0.23 | 0.05 | 0.51 | 0.12 | 0.06 | 0.10 | 0.25 | 0.08 | 0.04 | 0.13 | 0.17 | 0.12 | 0.08 | 0.02 | 0.10 | 0.12 |
| 40033 | 1 | cup | Crunchberries, Quaker | 35 | 0.12 | 0.07 | 0.11 | 0.04 | 0.36 | 0.06 | 0.04 | 0.07 | 0.20 | 0.05 | 0.04 | 0.08 | 0.14 | 0.08 | 0.06 | 0.01 | 0.07 | 0.09 |
| 40297 | 1 | cup | Cheerios, General Mills | 23 | 0.13 | 0.18 | 0.21 | 0.06 | 0.54 | 0.13 | 0.05 | 0.11 | 0.18 | 0.10 | 0.04 | 0.13 | 0.13 | 0.11 | 0.08 | 0.03 | 0.08 | 0.14 |
| 40051 | 1 | cup | Cheerios, Honey Nut, General Mills | 33 | 0.16 | 0.22 | 0.25 | 0.07 | 0.61 | 0.16 | 0.07 | 0.12 | 0.34 | 0.13 | 0.05 | 0.15 | 0.16 | 0.13 | 0.10 | 0.07 | 0.10 | 0.16 |
| | | | Chex | | | | | | | | | | | | | | | | | | | |
| 40323 | 1 | cup | Bran, Ralston Purina | 49 | 0.25 | 0.35 | 0.37 | 0.10 | 0.98 | 0.29 | 0.14 | 0.16 | 0.30 | 0.20 | 0.07 | 0.19 | 0.31 | 0.23 | 0.16 | 0.08 | 0.14 | 0.24 |
| 40325 | 1 | cup | Corn, Ralston Purina | 28 | 0.16 | 0.06 | 0.11 | 0.04 | 0.42 | 0.06 | 0.05 | 0.07 | 0.28 | 0.04 | 0.05 | 0.10 | 0.19 | 0.09 | 0.07 | 0.01 | 0.08 | 0.10 |
| 40333 | 1 | cup | Rice, Ralston Purina | 33 | 0.07 | 0.14 | 0.16 | 0.03 | 0.32 | 0.10 | 0.05 | 0.09 | 0.14 | 0.07 | 0.05 | 0.07 | 0.07 | 0.08 | 0.08 | 0.02 | 0.09 | 0.11 |
| 40335 | 1 | cup | Wheat, Ralston Purina | 46 | 0.17 | 0.23 | 0.25 | 0.09 | 1.31 | 0.19 | 0.10 | 0.18 | 0.31 | 0.14 | 0.08 | 0.22 | 0.45 | 0.25 | 0.15 | 0.09 | 0.13 | 0.22 |
| 40257 | 1 | cup | Cocoa Pebbles, Post | 32 | 0.06 | 0.12 | 0.14 | 0.02 | 0.24 | 0.09 | 0.04 | 0.08 | 0.12 | 0.06 | 0.04 | 0.06 | 0.06 | 0.07 | 0.07 | 0.02 | 0.08 | 0.10 |
| | | | Corn Flakes | | | | | | | | | | | | | | | | | | | |
| 40195 | 1 | cup | Corn Flakes, Kellogg's | 28 | 0.15 | 0.06 | 0.11 | 0.04 | 0.39 | 0.05 | 0.05 | 0.07 | 0.26 | 0.03 | 0.04 | 0.09 | 0.18 | 0.09 | 0.06 | 0.01 | 0.07 | 0.09 |
| 40145 | 1 | cup | Corn Flakes, low sodium, avg | 25 | 0.16 | 0.06 | 0.11 | 0.04 | 0.41 | 0.05 | 0.05 | 0.07 | 0.28 | 0.04 | 0.04 | 0.09 | 0.19 | 0.09 | 0.06 | 0.01 | 0.08 | 0.09 |
| 40017 | 1 | cup | Crispy Rice, avg | 28 | 0.07 | 0.13 | 0.15 | 0.03 | 0.27 | 0.10 | 0.05 | 0.09 | 0.14 | 0.07 | 0.05 | 0.07 | 0.07 | 0.07 | 0.08 | 0.02 | 0.09 | 0.11 |
| 40240 | 1 | cup | Crispy Rice, low sod, avg | 28 | 0.06 | 0.12 | 0.01 | 0.02 | 0.23 | 0.08 | 0.04 | 0.08 | 0.12 | 0.06 | 0.04 | 0.06 | 0.06 | 0.06 | 0.07 | 0.02 | 0.08 | 0.09 |
| 40040 | 1 | cup | Crispy Wheat 'N Raisins, General Mills | 43 | 0.10 | 0.14 | 0.15 | 0.06 | 0.90 | 0.12 | 0.07 | 0.11 | 0.20 | 0.08 | 0.05 | 0.14 | 0.29 | 0.15 | 0.09 | 0.05 | 0.08 | 0.14 |
| 40030 | 1 | cup | C.W. Post, Post | 97 | 0.44 | 0.64 | 0.75 | 0.20 | 2.05 | 0.47 | 0.21 | 0.41 | 0.68 | 0.35 | 0.16 | 0.46 | 0.53 | 0.42 | 0.33 | 0.13 | 0.33 | 0.52 |
| 40031 | 1 | cup | C.W. Post w/raisins, Post | 103 | 0.44 | 0.63 | 0.74 | 0.20 | 2.02 | 0.46 | 0.21 | 0.41 | 0.67 | 0.35 | 0.16 | 0.45 | 0.53 | 0.42 | 0.32 | 0.12 | 0.33 | 0.51 |
| 40217 | 1 | cup | Frosted Flakes, Kellogg's | 41 | 0.13 | 0.05 | 0.09 | 0.03 | 0.34 | 0.05 | 0.04 | 0.06 | 0.23 | 0.03 | 0.04 | 0.08 | 0.16 | 0.08 | 0.05 | 0.01 | 0.07 | 0.08 |
| 40043 | 1 | cup | Frosted Mini-Wheats, Kellogg's | 51 | 0.18 | 0.25 | 0.27 | 0.09 | 1.38 | 0.20 | 0.11 | 0.19 | 0.33 | 0.15 | 0.08 | 0.23 | 0.47 | 0.26 | 0.16 | 0.09 | 0.14 | 0.23 |
| 40146 | 1 | cup | Frosted Rice Krinkles, avg | 45 | 0.09 | 0.18 | 0.20 | 0.04 | 0.34 | 0.12 | 0.06 | 0.11 | 0.18 | 0.09 | 0.06 | 0.09 | 0.09 | 0.10 | 0.11 | 0.03 | 0.12 | 0.14 |
| 40266 | 1 | cup | Fruity Pebbles, Post | 32 | 0.05 | 0.11 | 0.12 | 0.02 | 0.21 | 0.07 | 0.04 | 0.07 | 0.11 | 0.05 | 0.04 | 0.05 | 0.05 | 0.06 | 0.06 | 0.02 | 0.07 | 0.08 |
| 40299 | 1 | cup | Golden Grahams, General Mills | 39 | 0.13 | 0.08 | 0.12 | 0.04 | 0.50 | 0.07 | 0.05 | 0.08 | 0.24 | 0.06 | 0.04 | 0.10 | 0.20 | 0.10 | 0.07 | 0.02 | 0.08 | 0.10 |
| | | | Granola | | | | | | | | | | | | | | | | | | | |
| 40064 | 1 | cup | Apple Cinnamon, 100% Nat, Quaker | 104 | 0.49 | 0.65 | 0.86 | 0.20 | 2.53 | 0.46 | 0.26 | 0.54 | 0.87 | 0.53 | 0.20 | 0.55 | 0.80 | 0.54 | 0.40 | 0.15 | 0.40 | 0.63 |
| 40048 | 1 | cup | Lowfat, oat & wheat germ, homemade, avg | 122 | 0.72 | 1.34 | 1.04 | 0.31 | 2.37 | 0.65 | 0.37 | 0.66 | 1.07 | 0.65 | 0.26 | 0.72 | 0.63 | 0.52 | 0.55 | 0.18 | 0.47 | 0.81 |
| 40008 | 1 | cup | Lowfat, NatureValley, General Mills | 113 | 0.62 | 0.87 | 1.02 | 0.29 | 2.64 | 0.63 | 0.26 | 0.53 | 0.88 | 0.47 | 0.19 | 0.63 | 0.65 | 0.54 | 0.40 | 0.16 | 0.41 | 0.68 |
| 40063 | 1 | cup | Lowfat, 100%Natural Oats & Honey, Quaker | 104 | 0.48 | 0.71 | 0.87 | 0.20 | 2.52 | 0.47 | 0.26 | 0.52 | 0.85 | 0.50 | 0.19 | 0.54 | 0.77 | 0.52 | 0.38 | 0.14 | 0.39 | 0.61 |
| 40065 | 1 | cup | Lowfat, 100% Natural Raisin & Dates, Quaker | 110 | 0.52 | 0.75 | 0.94 | 0.21 | 2.66 | 0.50 | 0.27 | 0.55 | 0.91 | 0.54 | 0.21 | 0.58 | 0.83 | 0.55 | 0.41 | 0.15 | 0.41 | 0.65 |
| 40277 | 1 | cup | Grape Nuts, Post | 109 | 0.49 | 0.65 | 0.73 | 0.25 | 4.06 | 0.55 | 0.31 | 0.52 | 0.90 | 0.39 | 0.21 | 0.65 | 1.35 | 0.69 | 0.41 | 0.23 | 0.39 | 0.64 |
| 40265 | 1 | cup | Grape Nuts Flakes, Post | 39 | 0.16 | 0.21 | 0.24 | 0.08 | 1.33 | 0.18 | 0.10 | 0.17 | 0.30 | 0.13 | 0.07 | 0.21 | 0.44 | 0.23 | 0.13 | 0.08 | 0.13 | 0.21 |
| 40264 | 1 | cup | Honey Comb, Post | 22 | 0.10 | 0.06 | 0.09 | 0.03 | 0.28 | 0.05 | 0.03 | 0.05 | 0.16 | 0.03 | 0.03 | 0.07 | 0.11 | 0.06 | 0.04 | 0.01 | 0.05 | 0.07 |
| 40054 | 1 | cup | King Vitaman, Quaker | 21 | 0.08 | 0.05 | 0.07 | 0.03 | 0.24 | 0.04 | 0.03 | 0.05 | 0.14 | 0.03 | 0.02 | 0.06 | 0.10 | 0.05 | 0.04 | 0.01 | 0.04 | 0.06 |
| 40010 | 1 | cup | Kix , General Mills | 19 | 0.09 | 0.05 | 0.08 | 0.03 | 0.27 | 0.04 | 0.03 | 0.05 | 0.15 | 0.03 | 0.03 | 0.06 | 0.11 | 0.06 | 0.04 | 0.01 | 0.05 | 0.06 |
| 40011 | 1 | cup | Life, Quaker | 44 | 0.20 | 0.28 | 0.40 | 0.08 | 0.89 | 0.19 | 0.10 | 0.21 | 0.34 | 0.23 | 0.07 | 0.22 | 0.26 | 0.21 | 0.16 | 0.06 | 0.16 | 0.24 |
| 40300 | 1 | cup | Lucky Charms, General Mills | 32 | 0.12 | 0.17 | 0.20 | 0.06 | 0.51 | 0.12 | 0.05 | 0.10 | 0.17 | 0.09 | 0.04 | 0.12 | 0.13 | 0.10 | 0.08 | 0.03 | 0.08 | 0.13 |
| 40041 | 1 | cup | Oat Flakes, Post | 48 | 0.38 | 0.46 | 0.77 | 0.13 | 1.56 | 0.32 | 0.18 | 0.40 | 0.66 | 0.47 | 0.13 | 0.37 | 0.44 | 0.38 | 0.34 | 0.12 | 0.27 | 0.43 |
| 40018 | 1 | cup | Puffed rice, Quaker | 14 | 0.04 | 0.07 | 0.08 | 0.02 | 0.14 | 0.05 | 0.03 | 0.05 | 0.07 | 0.04 | 0.03 | 0.04 | 0.04 | 0.04 | 0.04 | 0.01 | 0.05 | 0.06 |
| 40023 | 1 | cup | Puffed Wheat, Quaker | 12 | 0.07 | 0.09 | 0.10 | 0.03 | 0.60 | 0.07 | 0.05 | 0.08 | 0.13 | 0.05 | 0.03 | 0.09 | 0.18 | 0.10 | 0.05 | 0.03 | 0.05 | 0.08 |
| 40066 | 1 | cup | Quisp, Quaker | 30 | 0.11 | 0.07 | 0.10 | 0.03 | 0.32 | 0.05 | 0.04 | 0.06 | 0.18 | 0.04 | 0.03 | 0.08 | 0.13 | 0.07 | 0.05 | 0.01 | 0.06 | 0.08 |
| 40209 | 1 | cup | Raisin Bran, Kellogg's | 61 | 0.24 | 0.33 | 0.35 | 0.11 | 1.54 | 0.28 | 0.14 | 0.21 | 0.37 | 0.19 | 0.09 | 0.26 | 0.50 | 0.29 | 0.18 | 0.10 | 0.17 | 0.27 |
| 40260 | 1 | cup | Raisin Bran, Post | 56 | 0.19 | 0.26 | 0.28 | 0.09 | 1.24 | 0.23 | 0.11 | 0.17 | 0.30 | 0.15 | 0.07 | 0.21 | 0.40 | 0.23 | 0.15 | 0.08 | 0.13 | 0.22 |
| 40105 | 1 | cup | Rice Krispies, Frosted, Kelloggs | 35 | 0.07 | 0.13 | 0.15 | 0.03 | 0.26 | 0.09 | 0.05 | 0.08 | 0.13 | 0.07 | 0.05 | 0.07 | 0.07 | 0.07 | 0.08 | 0.02 | 0.09 | 0.10 |
| 40210 | 1 | cup | Rice Krispies, Kelloggs | 26 | 0.06 | 0.12 | 0.14 | 0.03 | 0.24 | 0.09 | 0.05 | 0.08 | 0.12 | 0.06 | 0.04 | 0.06 | 0.06 | 0.07 | 0.08 | 0.02 | 0.08 | 0.10 |
| 40062 | 1 | ea | Shredded Wheat, large biscuit, 1.7 oz, avg | 47 | 0.20 | 0.26 | 0.28 | 0.10 | 1.48 | 0.22 | 0.12 | 0.20 | 0.35 | 0.16 | 0.09 | 0.24 | 0.50 | 0.28 | 0.17 | 0.10 | 0.15 | 0.25 |
| 40022 | 1 | cup | Shredded Wheat, small biscuit, avg | 43 | 0.18 | 0.24 | 0.26 | 0.09 | 1.36 | 0.20 | 0.11 | 0.18 | 0.32 | 0.14 | 0.08 | 0.22 | 0.46 | 0.26 | 0.16 | 0.09 | 0.14 | 0.23 |
| 40149 | 1 | cup | Sugar Frosted Flakes, Ralston | 38 | 0.16 | 0.06 | 0.12 | 0.04 | 0.43 | 0.06 | 0.05 | 0.07 | 0.29 | 0.04 | 0.05 | 0.10 | 0.20 | 0.09 | 0.07 | 0.01 | 0.08 | 0.10 |

TABLE A **Amino Acid Content for Selected Foods *(continued)***

| Code | Amount | Description | Weight (g) | Alanine (g) | Arginine (g) | Aspartic acid (g) | Cystine (g) | Glutamic acid (g) | Glycine (g) | Histidine (g) | Isoleucine (g) | Leucine (g) | Lysine (g) | Methionine (g) | Phenylalanine (g) | Proline (g) | Serine (g) | Threonine (g) | Tryptophan (g) | Tyrosine (g) | Valine (g) |
|---|---|---|---|---|---|---|---|---|---|---|---|---|---|---|---|---|---|---|---|---|---|
| 40339 | 1 cup | Sugar Sparkled Flakes, avg | 38 | 0.16 | 0.06 | 0.11 | 0.04 | 0.42 | 0.06 | 0.05 | 0.07 | 0.28 | 0.04 | 0.04 | 0.10 | 0.19 | 0.09 | 0.07 | 0.01 | 0.08 | 0.10 |
| 40261 | 1 cup | Super Golden Crisp, Post | 33 | 0.08 | 0.10 | 0.12 | 0.04 | 0.72 | 0.08 | 0.06 | 0.09 | 0.15 | 0.06 | 0.04 | 0.11 | 0.22 | 0.12 | 0.07 | 0.03 | 0.06 | 0.10 |
| 40070 | 1 cup | Tasteeos, avg | 24 | 0.16 | 0.22 | 0.26 | 0.07 | 0.68 | 0.16 | 0.07 | 0.14 | 0.23 | 0.12 | 0.05 | 0.16 | 0.17 | 0.14 | 0.10 | 0.04 | 0.11 | 0.18 |
| 40071 | 1 cup | Team Rice, Nabisco | 42 | 0.13 | 0.19 | 0.22 | 0.05 | 0.58 | 0.14 | 0.07 | 0.13 | 0.23 | 0.10 | 0.07 | 0.13 | 0.18 | 0.13 | 0.11 | 0.04 | 0.12 | 0.16 |
| 40263 | 1 cup | Toasties, Post | 24 | 0.16 | 0.06 | 0.12 | 0.04 | 0.43 | 0.06 | 0.05 | 0.08 | 0.29 | 0.04 | 0.05 | 0.10 | 0.20 | 0.10 | 0.07 | 0.01 | 0.08 | 0.10 |
| 40021 | 1 cup | Total Wheat w/calcium, General Mills | 40 | 0.15 | 0.20 | 0.22 | 0.07 | 1.15 | 0.17 | 0.09 | 0.15 | 0.27 | 0.12 | 0.07 | 0.19 | 0.39 | 0.22 | 0.13 | 0.07 | 0.11 | 0.19 |
| 40306 | 1 cup | Trix, General Mills | 28 | 0.07 | 0.04 | 0.06 | 0.02 | 0.19 | 0.03 | 0.02 | 0.03 | 0.12 | 0.02 | 0.02 | 0.04 | 0.08 | 0.04 | 0.03 | 0.01 | 0.04 | 0.04 |
| 40307 | 1 cup | Wheaties, General Mills | 29 | 0.11 | 0.14 | 0.15 | 0.05 | 0.81 | 0.12 | 0.06 | 0.11 | 0.19 | 0.08 | 0.05 | 0.13 | 0.27 | 0.15 | 0.09 | 0.05 | 0.08 | 0.14 |
| | | CHEESE | | | | | | | | | | | | | | | | | | | |
| | | American Process Cheese & Cheese Food | | | | | | | | | | | | | | | | | | | |
| 1001 | 1 oz | Cold Pack, avg | 28 | 0.14 | 0.23 | 0.33 | 0.03 | 1.12 | 0.09 | 0.22 | 0.25 | 0.48 | 0.54 | 0.14 | 0.27 | 0.55 | 0.26 | 0.18 | 0.08 | 0.30 | 0.32 |
| 1096 | 1/4 cup | Lowfat, avg | 28 | 0.17 | 0.29 | 0.42 | 0.04 | 1.43 | 0.11 | 0.28 | 0.32 | 0.61 | 0.69 | 0.18 | 0.35 | 0.70 | 0.33 | 0.22 | 0.10 | 0.38 | 0.41 |
| 1072 | 1 pce | Slice, avg | 21 | 0.10 | 0.17 | 0.25 | 0.03 | 0.84 | 0.07 | 0.16 | 0.19 | 0.36 | 0.40 | 0.10 | 0.20 | 0.41 | 0.19 | 0.13 | 0.06 | 0.22 | 0.24 |
| 1027 | 1/4 cup | Asiago, avg | 27 | 0.23 | 0.23 | 0.39 | 0.07 | 1.40 | 0.13 | 0.26 | 0.38 | 0.73 | 0.64 | 0.19 | 0.41 | 0.91 | 0.40 | 0.26 | 0.10 | 0.42 | 0.53 |
| 1003 | 1/4 cup | Blue, avg | 34 | 0.20 | 0.23 | 0.46 | 0.03 | 1.64 | 0.13 | 0.24 | 0.35 | 0.61 | 0.59 | 0.18 | 0.35 | 0.66 | 0.35 | 0.25 | 0.10 | 0.41 | 0.49 |
| 1004 | 1/4 cup | Brie, avg | 36 | 0.29 | 0.25 | 0.45 | 0.04 | 1.47 | 0.13 | 0.24 | 0.34 | 0.65 | 0.62 | 0.20 | 0.39 | 0.82 | 0.39 | 0.25 | 0.11 | 0.40 | 0.45 |
| 1037 | 1/4 cup | Brick, avg | 28 | 0.17 | 0.23 | 0.41 | 0.03 | 1.43 | 0.11 | 0.21 | 0.30 | 0.58 | 0.55 | 0.15 | 0.32 | 0.67 | 0.34 | 0.23 | 0.08 | 0.29 | 0.38 |
| 1109 | 1/4 cup | Brick, w/salami, avg | 28 | 0.18 | 0.23 | 0.41 | 0.04 | 1.35 | 0.13 | 0.20 | 0.29 | 0.55 | 0.53 | 0.14 | 0.30 | 0.63 | 0.32 | 0.22 | 0.08 | 0.28 | 0.36 |
| 1006 | 1/4 cup | Camembert, avg | 62 | 0.47 | 0.40 | 0.74 | 0.06 | 2.41 | 0.22 | 0.39 | 0.56 | 1.06 | 1.02 | 0.33 | 0.64 | 1.35 | 0.64 | 0.41 | 0.18 | 0.66 | 0.74 |
| | | Cheddar Cheese | | | | | | | | | | | | | | | | | | | |
| 1008 | 1/4 cup | Avg | 28 | 0.18 | 0.24 | 0.41 | 0.03 | 1.57 | 0.11 | 0.23 | 0.40 | 0.62 | 0.53 | 0.17 | 0.34 | 0.72 | 0.38 | 0.23 | 0.08 | 0.31 | 0.43 |
| 1089 | 1/4 cup | Low Fat, low sod, avg | 28 | 0.18 | 0.24 | 0.40 | 0.03 | 1.53 | 0.11 | 0.22 | 0.39 | 0.60 | 0.52 | 0.16 | 0.33 | 0.71 | 0.37 | 0.22 | 0.08 | 0.30 | 0.42 |
| 1451 | 1/4 cup | Low Sod, avg | 28 | 0.18 | 0.24 | 0.40 | 0.03 | 1.53 | 0.11 | 0.22 | 0.39 | 0.60 | 0.52 | 0.16 | 0.33 | 0.71 | 0.37 | 0.22 | 0.08 | 0.30 | 0.42 |
| 1010 | 1/4 cup | Colby, avg | 28 | 0.17 | 0.23 | 0.39 | 0.03 | 1.50 | 0.11 | 0.22 | 0.38 | 0.59 | 0.51 | 0.16 | 0.32 | 0.69 | 0.36 | 0.22 | 0.08 | 0.30 | 0.41 |
| | | Cottage Cheese | | | | | | | | | | | | | | | | | | | |
| 1047 | 1/2 cup | 1% Fat, avg | 113 | 0.65 | 0.57 | 0.85 | 0.12 | 2.72 | 0.27 | 0.42 | 0.74 | 1.29 | 1.01 | 0.38 | 0.68 | 1.46 | 0.71 | 0.56 | 0.14 | 0.67 | 0.78 |
| 1012 | 1/2 cup | 1% Fat, small curd, avg | 105 | 0.61 | 0.54 | 0.80 | 0.11 | 2.55 | 0.26 | 0.39 | 0.69 | 1.21 | 0.95 | 0.35 | 0.63 | 1.37 | 0.66 | 0.52 | 0.13 | 0.63 | 0.73 |
| 1013 | 1/2 cup | 1% Fat, large curd, avg | 112 | 0.65 | 0.57 | 0.85 | 0.12 | 2.72 | 0.27 | 0.42 | 0.74 | 1.29 | 1.01 | 0.38 | 0.68 | 1.46 | 0.70 | 0.56 | 0.14 | 0.67 | 0.78 |
| 1099 | 1/2 cup | 1% Fat, low sod, avg | 112 | 0.65 | 0.57 | 0.84 | 0.12 | 2.70 | 0.27 | 0.41 | 0.73 | 1.28 | 1.01 | 0.38 | 0.67 | 1.43 | 0.70 | 0.55 | 0.14 | 0.66 | 0.77 |
| 1049 | 1/2 cup | 2% Fat, creamed w/fruit, avg | 113 | 0.52 | 0.46 | 0.68 | 0.09 | 2.17 | 0.22 | 0.33 | 0.59 | 1.03 | 0.81 | 0.30 | 0.54 | 1.17 | 0.56 | 0.44 | 0.11 | 0.53 | 0.62 |
| 1046 | 1 oz | Chesire Cheese, avg | 28 | 0.17 | 0.23 | 0.39 | 0.03 | 1.48 | 0.10 | 0.21 | 0.37 | 0.58 | 0.50 | 0.16 | 0.32 | 0.68 | 0.35 | 0.21 | 0.08 | 0.29 | 0.40 |
| 1045 | 1 oz | Caraway Cheese, avg | 28 | 0.18 | 0.25 | 0.42 | 0.03 | 1.59 | 0.11 | 0.23 | 0.40 | 0.62 | 0.54 | 0.17 | 0.34 | 0.73 | 0.38 | 0.23 | 0.08 | 0.31 | 0.43 |
| | | Cream Cheese | | | | | | | | | | | | | | | | | | | |
| 1015 | 1 Tbs | Avg | 14 | 0.03 | 0.04 | 0.07 | 0.01 | 0.23 | 0.02 | 0.04 | 0.05 | 0.10 | 0.09 | 0.02 | 0.06 | 0.09 | 0.05 | 0.04 | 0.01 | 0.05 | 0.06 |
| 1452 | 1 Tbs | Fat Free, avg | 14 | 0.06 | 0.07 | 0.14 | 0.02 | 0.44 | 0.04 | 0.07 | 0.10 | 0.18 | 0.17 | 0.05 | 0.11 | 0.17 | 0.10 | 0.08 | 0.02 | 0.09 | 0.11 |
| 1098 | 1 Tbs | Light, avg | 15 | 0.05 | 0.06 | 0.11 | 0.01 | 0.36 | 0.03 | 0.06 | 0.08 | 0.15 | 0.14 | 0.04 | 0.09 | 0.15 | 0.08 | 0.07 | 0.01 | 0.08 | 0.09 |
| 1453 | 1 Tbs | Whipped, avg | 10 | 0.02 | 0.03 | 0.05 | 0.01 | 0.16 | 0.01 | 0.03 | 0.04 | 0.07 | 0.06 | 0.02 | 0.04 | 0.07 | 0.04 | 0.03 | 0.01 | 0.03 | 0.04 |
| 1050 | 1/4 cup | Edam, avg | 33 | 0.21 | 0.27 | 0.49 | 0.07 | 1.72 | 0.14 | 0.29 | 0.37 | 0.72 | 0.75 | 0.20 | 0.40 | 0.91 | 0.43 | 0.26 | 0.10 | 0.41 | 0.51 |
| 1016 | 1/4 cup | Feta Cheese, avg | 38 | 0.24 | 0.18 | 0.29 | 0.03 | 0.90 | 0.04 | 0.15 | 0.30 | 0.52 | 0.45 | 0.14 | 0.25 | 0.51 | 0.44 | 0.24 | 0.07 | 0.25 | 0.40 |
| 1052 | 1/4 cup | Fontina Cheese, avg | 27 | 0.20 | 0.21 | 0.35 | 0.06 | 1.27 | 0.11 | 0.24 | 0.34 | 0.66 | 0.58 | 0.17 | 0.37 | 0.82 | 0.37 | 0.23 | 0.09 | 0.38 | 0.48 |
| 1132 | 1 oz | Gjetost, avg | 28 | 0.08 | 0.08 | 0.18 | 0.01 | 0.51 | 0.05 | 0.07 | 0.13 | 0.25 | 0.21 | 0.08 | 0.14 | 0.30 | 0.12 | 0.10 | 0.03 | 0.14 | 0.20 |
| | | Goat Cheese | | | | | | | | | | | | | | | | | | | |
| 1078 | 1 oz | Hard, avg | 28 | 0.15 | 0.25 | 0.43 | 0.04 | 1.59 | 0.10 | 0.23 | 0.35 | 0.74 | 0.61 | 0.23 | 0.34 | 1.03 | 0.33 | 0.32 | 0.09 | 0.33 | 0.59 |
| 1079 | 1 oz | Semi-soft, avg | 28 | 0.10 | 0.18 | 0.30 | 0.03 | 1.13 | 0.07 | 0.16 | 0.25 | 0.52 | 0.43 | 0.16 | 0.24 | 0.73 | 0.23 | 0.23 | 0.06 | 0.24 | 0.42 |
| 1080 | 1/4 cup | Soft, avg | 62 | 0.20 | 0.34 | 0.57 | 0.05 | 2.14 | 0.13 | 0.31 | 0.47 | 0.99 | 0.82 | 0.31 | 0.46 | 1.39 | 0.44 | 0.43 | 0.12 | 0.45 | 0.79 |

TABLE A **Amino Acid Content for Selected Foods *(continued)***

| Code | Amount | Description | Weight (g) | Alanine (g) | Arginine (g) | Aspartic acid (g) | Cystine (g) | Glutamic acid (g) | Glycine (g) | Histidine (g) | Isoleucine (g) | Leucine (g) | Lysine (g) | Methionine (g) | Phenylalanine (g) | Proline (g) | Serine (g) | Threonine (g) | Tryptophan (g) | Tyrosine (g) | Valine (g) |
|---|---|---|---|---|---|---|---|---|---|---|---|---|---|---|---|---|---|---|---|---|---|
| 1054 | 1/4 cup | Gouda, avg | 33 | 0.21 | 0.27 | 0.49 | 0.07 | 1.72 | 0.14 | 0.29 | 0.37 | 0.72 | 0.74 | 0.20 | 0.40 | 0.91 | 0.43 | 0.26 | 0.10 | 0.41 | 0.51 |
| 1074 | 1/4 cup | Gruyere, avg | 27 | 0.24 | 0.24 | 0.41 | 0.07 | 1.48 | 0.13 | 0.28 | 0.40 | 0.76 | 0.67 | 0.20 | 0.43 | 0.95 | 0.42 | 0.27 | 0.10 | 0.44 | 0.55 |
| 1055 | 1/4 cup | Limburger, avg | 34 | 0.20 | 0.21 | 0.45 | 0.03 | 1.37 | 0.12 | 0.18 | 0.37 | 0.64 | 0.51 | 0.19 | 0.34 | 0.74 | 0.35 | 0.23 | 0.09 | 0.37 | 0.44 |
| 1017 | 1/4 cup | Monterey Jack, avg | 28 | 0.18 | 0.24 | 0.40 | 0.03 | 1.54 | 0.11 | 0.22 | 0.39 | 0.60 | 0.53 | 0.17 | 0.33 | 0.71 | 0.37 | 0.22 | 0.08 | 0.30 | 0.42 |
| | | Mozzarella Cheese | | | | | | | | | | | | | | | | | | | |
| 1100 | 1/4 cup | Low Sod, Lifeline | 28 | 0.20 | 0.29 | 0.48 | 0.39 | 1.56 | 0.13 | 0.25 | 0.32 | 0.65 | 0.67 | 0.19 | 0.35 | 0.69 | 0.39 | 0.25 | 0.09 | 0.38 | 0.42 |
| 1058 | 1/4 cup | Part Skim, avg | 28 | 0.19 | 0.26 | 0.45 | 0.04 | 1.44 | 0.12 | 0.23 | 0.29 | 0.60 | 0.62 | 0.17 | 0.32 | 0.64 | 0.36 | 0.23 | 0.09 | 0.36 | 0.39 |
| 1056 | 1/4 cup | Whole Milk, avg | 28 | 0.15 | 0.21 | 0.36 | 0.03 | 1.15 | 0.09 | 0.19 | 0.24 | 0.48 | 0.50 | 0.14 | 0.26 | 0.51 | 0.29 | 0.19 | 0.07 | 0.28 | 0.31 |
| 1021 | 1/4 cup | Muenster, avg | 29 | 0.18 | 0.24 | 0.43 | 0.04 | 1.50 | 0.12 | 0.22 | 0.31 | 0.61 | 0.58 | 0.15 | 0.33 | 0.70 | 0.35 | 0.24 | 0.09 | 0.30 | 0.40 |
| 1102 | 1/4 cup | Muenster, low sod, avg | 33 | 0.21 | 0.27 | 0.49 | 0.04 | 1.70 | 0.13 | 0.25 | 0.35 | 0.69 | 0.66 | 0.17 | 0.38 | 0.79 | 0.40 | 0.27 | 0.10 | 0.34 | 0.46 |
| 1060 | 1/4 cup | Neufchatel, avg | 58 | 0.17 | 0.21 | 0.39 | 0.05 | 1.25 | 0.11 | 0.20 | 0.29 | 0.53 | 0.49 | 0.13 | 0.31 | 0.50 | 0.29 | 0.23 | 0.05 | 0.26 | 0.32 |
| | | Parmesan Cheese | | | | | | | | | | | | | | | | | | | |
| 1075 | 1 Tbs | Grated, avg | 6 | 0.07 | 0.08 | 0.14 | 0.02 | 0.52 | 0.04 | 0.09 | 0.12 | 0.22 | 0.21 | 0.06 | 0.12 | 0.27 | 0.13 | 0.08 | 0.03 | 0.13 | 0.16 |
| 1061 | 1 ea | Hard, cube, avg | 10 | 0.10 | 0.12 | 0.21 | 0.02 | 0.75 | 0.06 | 0.13 | 0.17 | 0.32 | 0.30 | 0.09 | 0.18 | 0.38 | 0.19 | 0.12 | 0.04 | 0.18 | 0.22 |
| 1103 | 1 Tbs | Low Sod, avg | 6 | 0.07 | 0.08 | 0.14 | 0.02 | 0.52 | 0.04 | 0.09 | 0.12 | 0.22 | 0.21 | 0.06 | 0.12 | 0.27 | 0.13 | 0.08 | 0.03 | 0.13 | 0.16 |
| 1112 | 1 Tbs | Shredded, avg | 5 | 0.05 | 0.06 | 0.11 | 0.01 | 0.40 | 0.03 | 0.07 | 0.09 | 0.17 | 0.16 | 0.05 | 0.09 | 0.20 | 0.10 | 0.06 | 0.02 | 0.10 | 0.12 |
| 1062 | 1/4 cup | Port Du Salut, avg | 28 | 0.20 | 0.21 | 0.44 | 0.03 | 1.34 | 0.12 | 0.17 | 0.36 | 0.62 | 0.50 | 0.18 | 0.33 | 0.72 | 0.34 | 0.22 | 0.09 | 0.36 | 0.43 |
| 1023 | 1/4 cup | Provolone, avg | 33 | 0.21 | 0.31 | 0.52 | 0.03 | 1.87 | 0.13 | 0.34 | 0.33 | 0.69 | 0.80 | 0.21 | 0.39 | 0.83 | 0.44 | 0.30 | 0.10 | 0.46 | 0.49 |
| 1024 | 1/4 cup | Ricotta, part skim , avg | 62 | 0.27 | 0.34 | 0.54 | 0.05 | 1.33 | 0.16 | 0.25 | 0.32 | 0.67 | 0.73 | 0.15 | 0.30 | 0.58 | 0.31 | 0.28 | 0.07 | 0.32 | 0.38 |
| 1064 | 1/4 cup | Ricotta, whole milk, avg | 62 | 0.27 | 0.34 | 0.54 | 0.05 | 1.32 | 0.16 | 0.25 | 0.32 | 0.66 | 0.72 | 0.15 | 0.30 | 0.58 | 0.31 | 0.28 | 0.07 | 0.32 | 0.37 |
| 1066 | 1 Tbs | Romano, avg | 6 | 0.05 | 0.06 | 0.11 | 0.01 | 0.40 | 0.03 | 0.07 | 0.09 | 0.17 | 0.16 | 0.05 | 0.09 | 0.20 | 0.10 | 0.06 | 0.02 | 0.10 | 0.12 |
| 1026 | 1 Tbs | Roquefort, avg | 8 | 0.08 | 0.06 | 0.09 | 0.01 | 0.29 | 0.01 | 0.05 | 0.10 | 0.17 | 0.15 | 0.04 | 0.08 | 0.16 | 0.14 | 0.08 | 0.02 | 0.08 | 0.13 |
| | | Swiss Cheese | | | | | | | | | | | | | | | | | | | |
| 1027 | 1/4 cup | Avg | 27 | 0.23 | 0.23 | 0.39 | 0.07 | 1.40 | 0.13 | 0.26 | 0.38 | 0.73 | 0.64 | 0.19 | 0.41 | 0.91 | 0.40 | 0.26 | 0.10 | 0.42 | 0.53 |
| 1093 | 1/4 cup | Lowfat, avg | 33 | 0.28 | 0.28 | 0.47 | 0.09 | 1.72 | 0.15 | 0.32 | 0.46 | 0.89 | 0.78 | 0.24 | 0.50 | 1.11 | 0.50 | 0.31 | 0.12 | 0.51 | 0.64 |
| 1104 | 1/4 cup | Low Sod, avg | 33 | 0.28 | 0.28 | 0.47 | 0.09 | 1.72 | 0.15 | 0.32 | 0.46 | 0.89 | 0.78 | 0.24 | 0.50 | 1.11 | 0.50 | 0.31 | 0.12 | 0.51 | 0.64 |
| 1067 | 1/4 cup | Tilsit, whole milk, avg | 28 | 0.20 | 0.21 | 0.45 | 0.03 | 1.37 | 0.12 | 0.18 | 0.37 | 0.64 | 0.51 | 0.19 | 0.34 | 0.74 | 0.35 | 0.23 | 0.09 | 0.37 | 0.44 |
| | | **DAIRY PRODUCTS** | | | | | | | | | | | | | | | | | | | |
| | | Cream | | | | | | | | | | | | | | | | | | | |
| 500 | 1 Tbs | Half & half, avg | 15 | 0.01 | 0.02 | 0.03 | 0.00 | 0.09 | 0.01 | 0.01 | 0.03 | 0.04 | 0.03 | 0.01 | 0.02 | 0.04 | 0.02 | 0.02 | 0.01 | 0.02 | 0.03 |
| 501 | 1 Tbs | Light, avg | 15 | 0.01 | 0.01 | 0.03 | 0.00 | 0.08 | 0.01 | 0.01 | 0.02 | 0.04 | 0.03 | 0.01 | 0.02 | 0.04 | 0.02 | 0.02 | 0.01 | 0.02 | 0.03 |
| 527 | 1 Tbs | Medium, 25% fat, avg | 15 | 0.01 | 0.01 | 0.03 | 0.00 | 0.07 | 0.01 | 0.01 | 0.02 | 0.03 | 0.03 | 0.01 | 0.02 | 0.03 | 0.02 | 0.02 | 0.00 | 0.02 | 0.02 |
| 587 | 1 Tbs | Whipping, heavy, avg | 15 | 0.01 | 0.01 | 0.02 | 0.00 | 0.06 | 0.01 | 0.01 | 0.02 | 0.03 | 0.02 | 0.01 | 0.01 | 0.03 | 0.02 | 0.01 | 0.00 | 0.01 | 0.02 |
| 503 | 1 Tbs | Whipping, heavy, whipped, avg | 15 | 0.01 | 0.01 | 0.02 | 0.00 | 0.06 | 0.01 | 0.01 | 0.02 | 0.03 | 0.02 | 0.01 | 0.01 | 0.03 | 0.02 | 0.01 | 0.00 | 0.01 | 0.02 |
| 586 | 1 Tbs | Whipping, light, avg | 15 | 0.01 | 0.01 | 0.02 | 0.00 | 0.06 | 0.01 | 0.01 | 0.02 | 0.03 | 0.02 | 0.01 | 0.01 | 0.03 | 0.02 | 0.01 | 0.00 | 0.01 | 0.02 |
| 515 | 1 Tbs | Whipping, light, whipped, avg | 15 | 0.03 | 0.03 | 0.06 | 0.01 | 0.18 | 0.02 | 0.02 | 0.05 | 0.08 | 0.07 | 0.02 | 0.04 | 0.08 | 0.05 | 0.04 | 0.01 | 0.04 | 0.06 |
| 534 | 1 Tbs | Creamer, coffee whitener, avg | 15 | 0.01 | 0.01 | 0.02 | 0.00 | 0.03 | 0.01 | 0.00 | 0.01 | 0.01 | 0.01 | 0.00 | 0.01 | 0.01 | 0.01 | 0.01 | 0.00 | 0.01 | 0.01 |
| 506 | 1 Tbs | Creamer, powder, avg | 6 | 0.01 | 0.01 | 0.02 | 0.00 | 0.06 | 0.01 | 0.01 | 0.02 | 0.03 | 0.02 | 0.01 | 0.01 | 0.03 | 0.02 | 0.01 | 0.00 | 0.01 | 0.02 |
| | | Dessert Toppings | | | | | | | | | | | | | | | | | | | |
| 513 | 2 Tbs | Dry Mix, avg | 3 | 0.00 | 0.01 | 0.01 | 0.00 | 0.03 | 0.00 | 0.00 | 0.01 | 0.01 | 0.01 | 0.00 | 0.01 | 0.01 | 0.01 | 0.01 | 0.00 | 0.01 | 0.01 |
| 508 | 2 Tbs | Frozen, semi solid, avg | 9 | 0.00 | 0.00 | 0.01 | 0.00 | 0.02 | 0.00 | 0.00 | 0.01 | 0.01 | 0.01 | 0.00 | 0.01 | 0.01 | 0.01 | 0.00 | 0.00 | 0.01 | 0.01 |
| 509 | 2 Tbs | Prep w/milk, avg | 10 | 0.01 | 0.01 | 0.02 | 0.00 | 0.07 | 0.01 | 0.01 | 0.02 | 0.03 | 0.03 | 0.01 | 0.02 | 0.03 | 0.02 | 0.01 | 0.00 | 0.02 | 0.02 |
| 514 | 2 Tbs | Pressurized, avg | 9 | 0.00 | 0.00 | 0.01 | 0.00 | 0.02 | 0.00 | 0.00 | 0.00 | 0.01 | 0.01 | 0.00 | 0.00 | 0.01 | 0.00 | 0.00 | 0.00 | 0.00 | 0.01 |
| 526 | 2 Tbs | Whipped Cream Substitute, non dairy, prep, avg | 10 | 0.00 | 0.00 | 0.01 | 0.00 | 0.02 | 0.00 | 0.03 | 0.01 | 0.01 | 0.01 | 0.00 | 0.00 | 0.01 | 0.05 | 0.00 | 0.00 | 0.00 | 0.01 |
| 510 | 2 Tbs | Whipped Cream Topping, pressurized, avg | 8 | 0.01 | 0.01 | 0.02 | 0.00 | 0.05 | 0.01 | 0.01 | 0.01 | 0.02 | 0.02 | 0.01 | 0.01 | 0.02 | 0.01 | 0.01 | 0.00 | 0.01 | 0.02 |
| | | Milk, Cow | | | | | | | | | | | | | | | | | | | |
| 32 | 1/3 cup | Buttermilk, dried, avg | 40 | 0.45 | 0.47 | 0.99 | 0.12 | 2.73 | 0.28 | 0.35 | 0.79 | 1.28 | 1.04 | 0.33 | 0.63 | 1.26 | 0.71 | 0.59 | 0.18 | 0.63 | 0.88 |
| 58 | 1 cup | Buttermilk, reconstd f/dry, avg | 245 | 0.30 | 0.32 | 0.66 | 0.08 | 1.61 | 0.18 | 0.24 | 0.51 | 0.82 | 0.69 | 0.20 | 0.44 | 0.84 | 0.43 | 0.39 | 0.09 | 0.35 | 0.61 |
| 7 | 1 cup | Buttermilk, skim, cultured, avg | 245 | 0.28 | 0.29 | 0.61 | 0.07 | 1.49 | 0.17 | 0.22 | 0.47 | 0.76 | 0.64 | 0.19 | 0.40 | 0.77 | 0.40 | 0.37 | 0.08 | 0.32 | 0.56 |
| 11 | 1/4 cup | Condensed milk, sweet, cnd, avg | 76 | 0.20 | 0.21 | 0.43 | 0.05 | 1.20 | 0.12 | 0.15 | 0.35 | 0.56 | 0.45 | 0.14 | 0.28 | 0.55 | 0.31 | 0.26 | 0.08 | 0.28 | 0.38 |

TABLE A **Amino Acid Content for Selected Foods *(continued)***

| Code | Amount | | Description | Weight (g) | Alanine (g) | Arginine (g) | Aspartic acid (g) | Cystine (g) | Glutamic acid (g) | Glycine (g) | Histidine (g) | Isoleucine (g) | Leucine (g) | Lysine (g) | Methionine (g) | Phenylalanine (g) | Proline (g) | Serine (g) | Threonine (g) | Tryptophan (g) | Tyrosine (g) | Valine (g) |
|---|---|---|---|---|---|---|---|---|---|---|---|---|---|---|---|---|---|---|---|---|---|---|
| 80 | 1 | cup | Evaporated, 2% fat, avg | 252 | 0.61 | 0.65 | 1.35 | 0.17 | 3.73 | 0.38 | 0.48 | 1.08 | 1.74 | 1.41 | 0.45 | 0.86 | 1.73 | 0.97 | 0.80 | 0.25 | 0.86 | 1.19 |
| 10 | 1 | cup | Evaporated, skim milk, cnd, avg | 256 | 0.63 | 0.67 | 1.40 | 0.17 | 3.85 | 0.39 | 0.50 | 1.11 | 1.80 | 1.46 | 0.46 | 0.89 | 1.78 | 1.00 | 0.83 | 0.26 | 0.89 | 1.23 |
| 15 | 1 | cup | Evaporated, whole milk, cnd, avg | 252 | 0.56 | 0.59 | 1.24 | 0.15 | 3.43 | 0.35 | 0.44 | 0.99 | 1.60 | 1.29 | 0.41 | 0.79 | 1.58 | 0.89 | 0.74 | 0.23 | 0.79 | 1.09 |
| 196 | 1 | cup | Filled Milk, fluid w/blend of hydro veg oil, avg | 244 | 0.27 | 0.28 | 0.59 | 0.07 | 1.62 | 0.16 | 0.21 | 0.47 | 0.76 | 0.61 | 0.20 | 0.37 | 0.75 | 0.42 | 0.35 | 0.11 | 0.37 | 0.52 |
| 4 | 1 | cup | Lowfat milk, 1%, acidophilus w/added vit A, avg | 244 | 0.26 | 0.28 | 0.58 | 0.07 | 1.60 | 0.16 | 0.21 | 0.46 | 0.75 | 0.61 | 0.19 | 0.37 | 0.74 | 0.42 | 0.35 | 0.11 | 0.37 | 0.51 |
| 53 | 1 | cup | Lowfat milk, 1%, avg | 247 | 0.28 | 0.29 | 0.62 | 0.07 | 1.70 | 0.17 | 0.22 | 0.49 | 0.80 | 0.64 | 0.21 | 0.39 | 0.79 | 0.44 | 0.37 | 0.11 | 0.39 | 0.54 |
| 19 | 1 | cup | Lowfat milk, 1%, chocolate, avg | 250 | 0.27 | 0.28 | 0.59 | 0.07 | 1.61 | 0.16 | 0.21 | 0.47 | 0.75 | 0.61 | 0.19 | 0.37 | 0.75 | 0.42 | 0.35 | 0.11 | 0.37 | 0.52 |
| 54 | 1 | cup | Lowfat milk, 1%, low lactose, avg | 246 | 0.28 | 0.29 | 0.62 | 0.07 | 1.69 | 0.17 | 0.22 | 0.49 | 0.79 | 0.64 | 0.20 | 0.39 | 0.78 | 0.44 | 0.37 | 0.11 | 0.39 | 0.54 |
| 55 | 1 | cup | Lowfat milk, 1%, low lactose, fort w/calc, avg | 247 | 0.28 | 0.29 | 0.62 | 0.07 | 1.70 | 0.17 | 0.22 | 0.49 | 0.80 | 0.64 | 0.21 | 0.39 | 0.79 | 0.44 | 0.37 | 0.11 | 0.39 | 0.54 |
| 64 | 1 | cup | Lowfat milk, 1%, protein fort w/added vit A, avg | 246 | 0.32 | 0.33 | 0.70 | 0.08 | 1.93 | 0.19 | 0.25 | 0.56 | 0.90 | 0.73 | 0.23 | 0.44 | 0.89 | 0.50 | 0.41 | 0.13 | 0.44 | 0.62 |
| 79 | 1 | cup | Lowfat milk, 1%, reconstd f/dry, avg | 245 | 0.26 | 0.27 | 0.58 | 0.07 | 1.59 | 0.16 | 0.21 | 0.46 | 0.74 | 0.60 | 0.19 | 0.37 | 0.74 | 0.41 | 0.35 | 0.11 | 0.37 | 0.51 |
| 2 | 1 | cup | Lowfat milk, 2%, acidophilus w/added vit A, avg | 244 | 0.27 | 0.28 | 0.59 | 0.07 | 1.62 | 0.16 | 0.21 | 0.47 | 0.76 | 0.61 | 0.20 | 0.37 | 0.75 | 0.42 | 0.35 | 0.11 | 0.37 | 0.52 |
| 18 | 1 | cup | Lowfat milk, 2%, chocolate, avg | 250 | 0.26 | 0.28 | 0.58 | 0.07 | 1.60 | 0.16 | 0.21 | 0.46 | 0.75 | 0.61 | 0.19 | 0.37 | 0.74 | 0.42 | 0.34 | 0.11 | 0.37 | 0.51 |
| 63 | 1 | cup | Lowfat milk, 2%, protein fort w/added vit A, avg | 246 | 0.32 | 0.33 | 0.70 | 0.09 | 1.94 | 0.20 | 0.25 | 0.56 | 0.91 | 0.73 | 0.23 | 0.45 | 0.90 | 0.50 | 0.42 | 0.13 | 0.45 | 0.62 |
| 132 | 1 | cup | Nonfat/Skim milk, avg | 245 | 0.28 | 0.29 | 0.60 | 0.07 | 1.67 | 0.17 | 0.21 | 0.48 | 0.78 | 0.63 | 0.20 | 0.38 | 0.77 | 0.43 | 0.36 | 0.11 | 0.38 | 0.53 |
| 59 | 1 | cup | Nonfat/Skim milk, chocolate, avg | 250 | 0.30 | 0.31 | 0.65 | 0.08 | 1.80 | 0.18 | 0.23 | 0.52 | 0.84 | 0.68 | 0.22 | 0.41 | 0.83 | 0.47 | 0.39 | 0.12 | 0.41 | 0.58 |
| 131 | 1/3 | cup | Nonfat/Skim milk, dry pwd, avg | 23 | 0.27 | 0.28 | 0.59 | 0.07 | 1.63 | 0.16 | 0.21 | 0.47 | 0.76 | 0.62 | 0.19 | 0.37 | 0.75 | 0.42 | 0.35 | 0.11 | 0.37 | 0.52 |
| 69 | 1/3 | cup | Nonfat/Skim milk, instant, dry, avg | 23 | 0.27 | 0.28 | 0.58 | 0.07 | 1.61 | 0.16 | 0.21 | 0.46 | 0.75 | 0.61 | 0.19 | 0.37 | 0.74 | 0.42 | 0.35 | 0.11 | 0.37 | 0.51 |
| 57 | 1 | cup | Nonfat/Skim milk, instant, reconstd, avg | 245 | 0.27 | 0.29 | 0.61 | 0.07 | 1.67 | 0.17 | 0.22 | 0.48 | 0.78 | 0.63 | 0.20 | 0.38 | 0.77 | 0.43 | 0.36 | 0.11 | 0.38 | 0.53 |
| 56 | 1 | cup | Nonfat/Skim milk, low lactose, avg | 245 | 0.29 | 0.30 | 0.63 | 0.08 | 1.75 | 0.18 | 0.23 | 0.50 | 0.82 | 0.66 | 0.21 | 0.40 | 0.81 | 0.45 | 0.38 | 0.12 | 0.40 | 0.56 |
| 65 | 1 | cup | Nonfat/Skim milk, protein fort w/added vit A, avg | 246 | 0.32 | 0.34 | 0.70 | 0.09 | 1.94 | 0.20 | 0.25 | 0.56 | 0.91 | 0.74 | 0.23 | 0.45 | 0.90 | 0.50 | 0.42 | 0.13 | 0.45 | 0.62 |
| 20 | 1 | cup | Whole milk, chocolate, avg | 250 | 0.26 | 0.27 | 0.57 | 0.07 | 1.58 | 0.16 | 0.20 | 0.46 | 0.74 | 0.60 | 0.19 | 0.36 | 0.73 | 0.41 | 0.34 | 0.11 | 0.36 | 0.50 |
| 66 | 1/3 | cup | Whole milk, dry pwd, avg | 43 | 0.37 | 0.39 | 0.82 | 0.10 | 2.25 | 0.23 | 0.29 | 0.65 | 1.06 | 0.85 | 0.27 | 0.52 | 1.04 | 0.58 | 0.49 | 0.15 | 0.52 | 0.72 |
| 52 | 1 | cup | Whole milk, low sod, avg | 244 | 0.25 | 0.26 | 0.55 | 0.07 | 1.51 | 0.15 | 0.19 | 0.44 | 0.71 | 0.57 | 0.18 | 0.35 | 0.70 | 0.39 | 0.33 | 0.10 | 0.35 | 0.48 |
| 78 | 1 | cup | Whole milk, reconstd f/dry pwd, avg | 244 | 0.26 | 0.27 | 0.57 | 0.07 | 1.57 | 0.16 | 0.20 | 0.46 | 0.74 | 0.60 | 0.19 | 0.36 | 0.73 | 0.41 | 0.34 | 0.11 | 0.36 | 0.50 |
| 1 | 1 | cup | Whole milk, 3.3% fat, avg | 244 | 0.26 | 0.28 | 0.58 | 0.07 | 1.60 | 0.16 | 0.21 | 0.46 | 0.75 | 0.61 | 0.19 | 0.37 | 0.74 | 0.42 | 0.35 | 0.11 | 0.37 | 0.51 |
| 62 | 1 | cup | Whole milk, 3.7% fat, avg | 244 | 0.26 | 0.28 | 0.58 | 0.07 | 1.60 | 0.16 | 0.21 | 0.46 | 0.75 | 0.60 | 0.19 | 0.37 | 0.74 | 0.41 | 0.34 | 0.11 | 0.37 | 0.51 |
| 23 | 1 | cup | Milk, goat, avg | 244 | 0.29 | 0.29 | 0.51 | 0.11 | 1.53 | 0.12 | 0.22 | 0.51 | 0.77 | 0.71 | 0.20 | 0.38 | 0.90 | 0.44 | 0.40 | 0.11 | 0.44 | 0.59 |
| 22 | 1 | cup | Milk, human breast milk, avg | 246 | 0.09 | 0.11 | 0.20 | 0.05 | 0.41 | 0.06 | 0.06 | 0.14 | 0.23 | 0.17 | 0.05 | 0.11 | 0.20 | 0.11 | 0.11 | 0.04 | 0.13 | 0.15 |
| 150 | 1 | cup | Milk, Indian Buffalo, avg | 244 | 0.32 | 0.28 | 0.75 | 0.12 | 1.16 | 0.20 | 0.19 | 0.50 | 0.89 | 0.68 | 0.24 | 0.40 | 0.89 | 0.55 | 0.44 | 0.13 | 0.45 | 0.53 |
| 42 | 1 | cup | Milk, Sheep, avg | 245 | 0.65 | 0.48 | 0.79 | 0.08 | 2.45 | 0.10 | 0.40 | 0.81 | 1.41 | 1.23 | 0.37 | 0.68 | 1.40 | 1.18 | 0.64 | 0.20 | 0.68 | 1.08 |
| | | | Sour Cream | | | | | | | | | | | | | | | | | | | |
| 504 | 2 | Tbs | Avg | 29 | 0.03 | 0.03 | 0.07 | 0.01 | 0.18 | 0.02 | 0.02 | 0.05 | 0.09 | 0.07 | 0.02 | 0.04 | 0.08 | 0.05 | 0.04 | 0.01 | 0.04 | 0.06 |
| 515 | 2 | Tbs | Half & Half, avg | 30 | 0.03 | 0.03 | 0.06 | 0.01 | 0.18 | 0.02 | 0.02 | 0.05 | 0.08 | 0.07 | 0.02 | 0.04 | 0.08 | 0.05 | 0.04 | 0.01 | 0.04 | 0.06 |
| 505 | 2 | Tbs | Imitation, avg | 29 | 0.02 | 0.02 | 0.04 | 0.00 | 0.14 | 0.01 | 0.02 | 0.04 | 0.06 | 0.05 | 0.02 | 0.03 | 0.07 | 0.04 | 0.03 | 0.01 | 0.04 | 0.05 |
| 143 | 1 | Tbs | Whey, acid, dried, avg | 3 | 0.02 | 0.01 | 0.03 | 0.01 | 0.06 | 0.01 | 0.01 | 0.02 | 0.03 | 0.03 | 0.01 | 0.01 | 0.02 | 0.02 | 0.02 | 0.01 | 0.01 | 0.02 |
| 144 | 1 | cup | Whey, acid, fluid, avg | 246 | 0.08 | 0.05 | 0.18 | 0.03 | 0.33 | 0.03 | 0.04 | 0.09 | 0.18 | 0.16 | 0.03 | 0.06 | 0.11 | 0.09 | 0.09 | 0.04 | 0.05 | 0.09 |
| 145 | 1 | Tbs | Whey, sweet, dried, avg | 8 | 0.05 | 0.03 | 0.10 | 0.02 | 0.18 | 0.02 | 0.02 | 0.06 | 0.10 | 0.08 | 0.02 | 0.03 | 0.06 | 0.05 | 0.07 | 0.02 | 0.03 | 0.06 |
| 146 | 1 | cup | Whey, sweet, fluid, avg | 246 | 0.10 | 0.06 | 0.20 | 0.04 | 0.36 | 0.04 | 0.04 | 0.12 | 0.19 | 0.17 | 0.04 | 0.07 | 0.13 | 0.10 | 0.13 | 0.03 | 0.06 | 0.11 |
| | | | Yogurt | | | | | | | | | | | | | | | | | | | |
| 2579 | 1 | ea | Coffee, lowfat, 8 oz, avg | 245 | 0.47 | 0.33 | 0.87 | 0.10 | 2.16 | 0.27 | 0.27 | 0.60 | 1.11 | 0.99 | 0.32 | 0.60 | 1.31 | 0.68 | 0.45 | 0.06 | 0.56 | 0.91 |
| 2574 | 1 | ea | Coffee, nonfat, 8 oz, avg | 227 | 0.45 | 0.32 | 0.84 | 0.10 | 2.07 | 0.25 | 0.26 | 0.58 | 1.07 | 0.95 | 0.31 | 0.58 | 1.26 | 0.66 | 0.44 | 0.06 | 0.54 | 0.88 |
| 2575 | 1 | ea | Coffee, whole milk, 8 oz, avg | 227 | 0.43 | 0.30 | 0.79 | 0.09 | 1.96 | 0.24 | 0.25 | 0.55 | 1.01 | 0.90 | 0.30 | 0.55 | 1.19 | 0.62 | 0.41 | 0.06 | 0.51 | 0.83 |
| 2493 | 1 | ea | Fruit, lowfat, 8 oz, avg | 245 | 0.42 | 0.30 | 0.78 | 0.09 | 1.91 | 0.23 | 0.24 | 0.53 | 0.98 | 0.88 | 0.29 | 0.53 | 1.16 | 0.61 | 0.40 | 0.06 | 0.49 | 0.81 |
| 2102 | 1 | ea | Fruit, lowfat, w/nuts, 8 oz, avg | 227 | 0.39 | 0.28 | 0.74 | 0.08 | 1.81 | 0.22 | 0.23 | 0.50 | 0.93 | 0.83 | 0.27 | 0.50 | 1.10 | 0.57 | 0.38 | 0.05 | 0.47 | 0.77 |
| 2511 | 1 | ea | Fruit, nonfat, 8 oz, avg | 241 | 0.45 | 0.32 | 0.84 | 0.10 | 2.08 | 0.26 | 0.26 | 0.58 | 1.07 | 0.95 | 0.31 | 0.58 | 1.26 | 0.66 | 0.43 | 0.06 | 0.54 | 0.88 |
| 2492 | 1 | ea | Maple, lowfat, 8 oz, avg | 245 | 0.47 | 0.33 | 0.87 | 0.10 | 2.16 | 0.27 | 0.27 | 0.60 | 1.11 | 0.99 | 0.32 | 0.60 | 1.31 | 0.68 | 0.45 | 0.06 | 0.56 | 0.91 |
| 2494 | 1 | ea | Plain, lowfat, 8 oz, avg | 245 | 0.50 | 0.35 | 0.93 | 0.11 | 2.30 | 0.28 | 0.29 | 0.64 | 1.18 | 1.05 | 0.35 | 0.64 | 1.39 | 0.73 | 0.48 | 0.07 | 0.59 | 0.97 |
| 2510 | 1 | ea | Plain, nonfat, 8 oz, avg | 245 | 0.55 | 0.38 | 1.02 | 0.12 | 2.51 | 0.31 | 0.32 | 0.70 | 1.29 | 1.15 | 0.38 | 0.70 | 1.52 | 0.79 | 0.53 | 0.07 | 0.65 | 1.06 |
| 2565 | 1 | ea | Plain, whole milk, 8 oz, avg | 245 | 0.33 | 0.23 | 0.62 | 0.07 | 1.52 | 0.19 | 0.19 | 0.42 | 0.78 | 0.70 | 0.23 | 0.42 | 0.92 | 0.48 | 0.32 | 0.04 | 0.39 | 0.64 |

TABLE A **Amino Acid Content for Selected Foods *(continued)***

| Code | Amount | Description | Weight (g) | Alanine (g) | Arginine (g) | Aspartic acid (g) | Cystine (g) | Glutamic acid (g) | Glycine (g) | Histidine (g) | Isoleucine (g) | Leucine (g) | Lysine (g) | Methionine (g) | Phenylalanine (g) | Proline (g) | Serine (g) | Threonine (g) | Tryptophan (g) | Tyrosine (g) | Valine (g) |
|---|---|---|---|---|---|---|---|---|---|---|---|---|---|---|---|---|---|---|---|---|---|
| 2577 | 1 ea | Vanilla, lowfat, 8 oz, avg | 245 | 0.47 | 0.33 | 0.87 | 0.10 | 2.16 | 0.27 | 0.27 | 0.60 | 1.11 | 0.99 | 0.32 | 0.60 | 1.31 | 0.68 | 0.45 | 0.06 | 0.56 | 0.91 |
| 2098 | 1 ea | Vanilla, nonfat, 8 oz, avg | 227 | 0.45 | 0.32 | 0.84 | 0.10 | 2.07 | 0.25 | 0.26 | 0.58 | 1.07 | 0.95 | 0.31 | 0.58 | 1.26 | 0.66 | 0.44 | 0.06 | 0.54 | 0.88 |
| 2564 | 1 ea | Vanilla, whole milk, 8 oz, avg | 227 | 0.43 | 0.30 | 0.79 | 0.09 | 1.96 | 0.24 | 0.25 | 0.55 | 1.01 | 0.90 | 0.30 | 0.55 | 1.19 | 0.62 | 0.41 | 0.06 | 0.51 | 0.83 |
| | | **DESSERTS** | | | | | | | | | | | | | | | | | | | |
| | | Brownies | | | | | | | | | | | | | | | | | | | |
| 47030 | 1 ea | Low Calorie, low sod, avg | 22 | 0.04 | 0.04 | 0.06 | 0.02 | 0.20 | 0.03 | 0.02 | 0.04 | 0.06 | 0.04 | 0.02 | 0.04 | 0.06 | 0.05 | 0.03 | 0.01 | 0.03 | 0.04 |
| 47683 | 1 oz | Low Calorie, low sod, dry mix, avg | 28 | 0.03 | 0.03 | 0.04 | 0.02 | 0.23 | 0.03 | 0.02 | 0.03 | 0.05 | 0.03 | 0.01 | 0.04 | 0.08 | 0.04 | 0.02 | 0.01 | 0.02 | 0.04 |
| 47000 | 1 ea | With Nuts, avg | 61 | 0.13 | 0.16 | 0.24 | 0.06 | 0.58 | 0.10 | 0.06 | 0.14 | 0.22 | 0.16 | 0.07 | 0.15 | 0.18 | 0.17 | 0.12 | 0.04 | 0.10 | 0.16 |
| 47028 | 1 ea | Without Nuts, avg | 33 | 0.06 | 0.08 | 0.11 | 0.03 | 0.29 | 0.05 | 0.03 | 0.06 | 0.09 | 0.06 | 0.02 | 0.07 | 0.09 | 0.07 | 0.05 | 0.02 | 0.05 | 0.07 |
| 47027 | 1 oz | Without Nuts, dry mix, avg | 28 | 0.04 | 0.06 | 0.08 | 0.02 | 0.27 | 0.05 | 0.02 | 0.04 | 0.07 | 0.05 | 0.02 | 0.05 | 0.08 | 0.05 | 0.04 | 0.02 | 0.04 | 0.06 |
| 47019 | 1 ea | With Walnuts, prep f/rec, avg | 24 | 0.07 | 0.10 | 0.12 | 0.03 | 0.29 | 0.06 | 0.03 | 0.06 | 0.11 | 0.07 | 0.03 | 0.07 | 0.09 | 0.08 | 0.05 | 0.02 | 0.05 | 0.08 |
| | | Cakes | | | | | | | | | | | | | | | | | | | |
| 46004 | 1 pce | Angel Food Cake, prep, avg | 28 | 0.09 | 0.08 | 0.15 | 0.04 | 0.29 | 0.06 | 0.04 | 0.09 | 0.13 | 0.10 | 0.05 | 0.09 | 0.09 | 0.11 | 0.07 | 0.02 | 0.06 | 0.10 |
| 46002 | 1 pce | Boston Cream Pie cake, coml prep, avg | 92 | 0.09 | 0.10 | 0.16 | 0.04 | 0.50 | 0.07 | 0.05 | 0.11 | 0.17 | 0.12 | 0.05 | 0.11 | 0.18 | 0.13 | 0.09 | 0.03 | 0.08 | 0.12 |
| 46010 | 1 pce | Carrot Cake w/cream cheese frosting, prep f/rec, avg | 111 | 0.20 | 0.32 | 0.38 | 0.10 | 1.12 | 0.17 | 0.12 | 0.21 | 0.37 | 0.23 | 0.11 | 0.24 | 0.35 | 0.28 | 0.18 | 0.06 | 0.17 | 0.25 |
| 46054 | 1 pce | Carrot Cake w/o frosting, prep f/mix, avg | 70 | 0.16 | 0.17 | 0.27 | 0.07 | 0.83 | 0.12 | 0.08 | 0.16 | 0.27 | 0.17 | 0.08 | 0.18 | 0.27 | 0.21 | 0.13 | 0.04 | 0.12 | 0.18 |
| 46013 | 1 pce | Chocolate Cake, coml prep, w/frosting, avg | 64 | 0.12 | 0.13 | 0.22 | 0.05 | 0.51 | 0.09 | 0.06 | 0.12 | 0.20 | 0.15 | 0.05 | 0.13 | 0.17 | 0.15 | 0.11 | 0.04 | 0.10 | 0.15 |
| 46066 | 1 pce | Chocolate Cake, German, w/icing, avg | 11 | 0.02 | 0.02 | 0.03 | 0.01 | 0.08 | 0.01 | 0.01 | 0.02 | 0.03 | 0.02 | 0.01 | 0.02 | 0.02 | 0.02 | 0.01 | 0.01 | 0.01 | 0.02 |
| 46059 | 1 pce | Chocolate Cake, prep f/mix, avg | 65 | 0.16 | 0.20 | 0.30 | 0.07 | 0.79 | 0.14 | 0.08 | 0.16 | 0.26 | 0.17 | 0.07 | 0.18 | 0.25 | 0.20 | 0.13 | 0.05 | 0.13 | 0.19 |
| 46118 | 1 pce | Chocolate Cake w/vanilla icing, avg | 103 | 0.16 | 0.20 | 0.30 | 0.07 | 0.80 | 0.14 | 0.08 | 0.16 | 0.27 | 0.18 | 0.07 | 0.19 | 0.26 | 0.20 | 0.13 | 0.05 | 0.13 | 0.19 |
| 46092 | 1 pce | Coffee Cake, cheese, avg | 76 | 0.19 | 0.23 | 0.36 | 0.08 | 1.32 | 0.16 | 0.14 | 0.25 | 0.43 | 0.30 | 0.11 | 0.27 | 0.47 | 0.28 | 0.20 | 0.06 | 0.20 | 0.27 |
| 46492 | 1 oz | Coffee Cake, cinnamon, w/crumb top, dry mix, avg | 28 | 0.04 | 0.05 | 0.05 | 0.03 | 0.47 | 0.05 | 0.03 | 0.05 | 0.09 | 0.03 | 0.02 | 0.07 | 0.16 | 0.07 | 0.04 | 0.02 | 0.04 | 0.06 |
| 46093 | 1 pce | Coffee Cake, cinnamon, w/crumb top, prep f/mix, avg | 63 | 0.16 | 0.20 | 0.26 | 0.08 | 1.20 | 0.15 | 0.10 | 0.18 | 0.31 | 0.16 | 0.08 | 0.20 | 0.40 | 0.22 | 0.14 | 0.05 | 0.14 | 0.20 |
| 46096 | 1 pce | Coffee Cake, crème filled, w/chocolate frosting, avg | 90 | 0.16 | 0.19 | 0.25 | 0.09 | 1.35 | 0.16 | 0.10 | 0.18 | 0.33 | 0.15 | 0.08 | 0.22 | 0.45 | 0.23 | 0.14 | 0.05 | 0.14 | 0.21 |
| 46097 | 1 pce | Coffee Cake, fruit, avg | 50 | 0.11 | 0.13 | 0.16 | 0.05 | 0.72 | 0.14 | 0.06 | 0.10 | 0.18 | 0.09 | 0.05 | 0.12 | 0.26 | 0.13 | 0.08 | 0.03 | 0.08 | 0.12 |
| 46206 | 1 pce | Coffee Cake, plain, avg | 63 | 0.16 | 0.20 | 0.26 | 0.08 | 1.20 | 0.15 | 0.10 | 0.18 | 0.31 | 0.16 | 0.08 | 0.20 | 0.40 | 0.22 | 0.14 | 0.05 | 0.14 | 0.20 |
| 46205 | 1 pce | Fruit cake, avg | 43 | 0.05 | 0.11 | 0.12 | 0.03 | 0.27 | 0.05 | 0.03 | 0.05 | 0.09 | 0.05 | 0.03 | 0.06 | 0.07 | 0.07 | 0.04 | 0.02 | 0.04 | 0.06 |
| 46006 | 1 pce | Gingerbread, prep f/mix, avg | 67 | 0.11 | 0.14 | 0.20 | 0.06 | 0.66 | 0.10 | 0.06 | 0.12 | 0.20 | 0.13 | 0.05 | 0.13 | 0.22 | 0.16 | 0.10 | 0.04 | 0.09 | 0.13 |
| 46119 | 1 pce | Marble Cake, prep w/chocolate icing, avg | 111 | 0.16 | 0.18 | 0.29 | 0.07 | 0.66 | 0.13 | 0.07 | 0.16 | 0.25 | 0.19 | 0.07 | 0.17 | 0.21 | 0.21 | 0.14 | 0.05 | 0.13 | 0.19 |
| 46070 | 1 pce | Pineapple cake, upside down, prep f/rec, avg | 115 | 0.15 | 0.17 | 0.25 | 0.08 | 1.09 | 0.13 | 0.09 | 0.17 | 0.30 | 0.16 | 0.09 | 0.20 | 0.39 | 0.22 | 0.13 | 0.05 | 0.14 | 0.19 |
| 46495 | 1 pce | Pound Cake, fat free, avg | 80 | 0.20 | 0.20 | 0.35 | 0.10 | 0.86 | 0.14 | 0.10 | 0.22 | 0.35 | 0.25 | 0.12 | 0.23 | 0.29 | 0.27 | 0.17 | 0.06 | 0.16 | 0.25 |
| 46073 | 1 pce | Pound Cake, prep w/butter, avg | 54 | 0.13 | 0.15 | 0.22 | 0.07 | 0.79 | 0.11 | 0.08 | 0.14 | 0.25 | 0.15 | 0.08 | 0.16 | 0.27 | 0.19 | 0.12 | 0.04 | 0.12 | 0.16 |
| 46011 | 1 ea | Snack Cake, chocolate creme filled, w/icing, avg | 50 | 0.06 | 0.07 | 0.10 | 0.03 | 0.45 | 0.06 | 0.03 | 0.07 | 0.12 | 0.07 | 0.03 | 0.08 | 0.15 | 0.09 | 0.06 | 0.02 | 0.05 | 0.08 |
| 46426 | 1 ea | Snack Cake, chocolate w/frosting, low fat, avg | 43 | 0.08 | 0.09 | 0.14 | 0.04 | 0.41 | 0.07 | 0.04 | 0.09 | 0.14 | 0.10 | 0.04 | 0.10 | 0.14 | 0.11 | 0.07 | 0.03 | 0.07 | 0.10 |
| 46105 | 1 ea | Snack Cake, chocolate w/fruit & cream, avg | 43 | 0.07 | 0.08 | 0.11 | 0.04 | 0.52 | 0.06 | 0.04 | 0.09 | 0.15 | 0.10 | 0.04 | 0.09 | 0.19 | 0.10 | 0.07 | 0.03 | 0.07 | 0.10 |
| 46001 | 1 pce | Sponge Cake, coml prep, avg | 38 | 0.09 | 0.10 | 0.15 | 0.05 | 0.46 | 0.07 | 0.05 | 0.10 | 0.16 | 0.11 | 0.05 | 0.10 | 0.15 | 0.13 | 0.08 | 0.03 | 0.07 | 0.11 |
| 46082 | 1 pce | White Cake, avg | 62 | 0.09 | 0.11 | 0.15 | 0.05 | 0.69 | 0.08 | 0.06 | 0.11 | 0.19 | 0.11 | 0.06 | 0.13 | 0.24 | 0.14 | 0.08 | 0.03 | 0.09 | 0.13 |
| 46007 | 1 pce | White Cake w/choc icing, prep f/rec, avg | 100 | 0.08 | 0.10 | 0.14 | 0.05 | 0.62 | 0.07 | 0.05 | 0.10 | 0.18 | 0.10 | 0.05 | 0.12 | 0.22 | 0.13 | 0.08 | 0.03 | 0.08 | 0.12 |
| 46003 | 1 pce | White Cake w/coconut icing, prep f/rec, avg | 112 | 0.20 | 0.24 | 0.34 | 0.10 | 1.16 | 0.16 | 0.11 | 0.22 | 0.38 | 0.23 | 0.12 | 0.26 | 0.40 | 0.28 | 0.18 | 0.06 | 0.17 | 0.26 |
| 46017 | 1 pce | White Cake w/white frosting, prep f/rec, avg | 71 | 0.09 | 0.10 | 0.14 | 0.05 | 0.63 | 0.08 | 0.05 | 0.10 | 0.18 | 0.10 | 0.05 | 0.12 | 0.22 | 0.13 | 0.08 | 0.03 | 0.08 | 0.12 |
| 46012 | 1 pce | Yellow Cake w/chocolate frosting, avg | 64 | 0.10 | 0.12 | 0.19 | 0.05 | 0.50 | 0.08 | 0.05 | 0.11 | 0.18 | 0.13 | 0.05 | 0.12 | 0.17 | 0.14 | 0.09 | 0.03 | 0.09 | 0.13 |
| 46015 | 1 pce | Yellow Cake w/vanilla frosting, avg | 64 | 0.09 | 0.10 | 0.17 | 0.04 | 0.48 | 0.07 | 0.05 | 0.11 | 0.18 | 0.14 | 0.06 | 0.11 | 0.17 | 0.14 | 0.09 | 0.03 | 0.09 | 0.13 |
| 46091 | 1 pce | Yellow Cake w/o frosting, prep f/recipe, avg | 80 | 0.16 | 0.19 | 0.27 | 0.08 | 1.06 | 0.14 | 0.10 | 0.19 | 0.33 | 0.20 | 0.10 | 0.21 | 0.38 | 0.24 | 0.15 | 0.05 | 0.15 | 0.21 |
| | | Cookies | | | | | | | | | | | | | | | | | | | |
| 47026 | 1 ea | Animal Cookie, avg | 1 | 0.00 | 0.00 | 0.00 | 0.00 | 0.02 | 0.00 | 0.00 | 0.00 | 0.00 | 0.00 | 0.00 | 0.00 | 0.01 | 0.00 | 0.00 | 0.00 | 0.00 | 0.00 |
| 47036 | 1 ea | Chocolate Chip cookie, baked f/refrig dough, avg | 12 | 0.02 | 0.02 | 0.03 | 0.01 | 0.16 | 0.02 | 0.01 | 0.03 | 0.04 | 0.03 | 0.01 | 0.03 | 0.05 | 0.03 | 0.02 | 0.01 | 0.02 | 0.03 |
| 47032 | 1 ea | Chocolate Chip Cookie, low fat, avg | 10 | 0.02 | 0.02 | 0.03 | 0.01 | 0.18 | 0.02 | 0.01 | 0.02 | 0.04 | 0.02 | 0.01 | 0.03 | 0.06 | 0.03 | 0.02 | 0.01 | 0.02 | 0.03 |
| 47001 | 1 ea | Chocolate Chip cookie, soft, avg | 15 | 0.02 | 0.02 | 0.03 | 0.01 | 0.15 | 0.02 | 0.01 | 0.02 | 0.04 | 0.02 | 0.01 | 0.03 | 0.05 | 0.03 | 0.02 | 0.01 | 0.02 | 0.03 |
| 47044 | 1 ea | Chocolate Fudge Cookie, avg | 21 | 0.06 | 0.06 | 0.07 | 0.01 | 0.24 | 0.09 | 0.02 | 0.04 | 0.06 | 0.05 | 0.01 | 0.04 | 0.12 | 0.05 | 0.03 | 0.01 | 0.03 | 0.05 |
| 47039 | 1 ea | Chocolate Sandwich Cookie, low sod, w/fructose, avg | 10 | 0.02 | 0.02 | 0.03 | 0.01 | 0.12 | 0.02 | 0.01 | 0.02 | 0.03 | 0.02 | 0.01 | 0.02 | 0.04 | 0.02 | 0.02 | 0.01 | 0.01 | 0.02 |

## TABLE A Amino Acid Content for Selected Foods *(continued)*

| Code | Amount | Description | Weight (g) | Alanine (g) | Arginine (g) | Aspartic acid (g) | Cystine (g) | Glutamic acid (g) | Glycine (g) | Histidine (g) | Isoleucine (g) | Leucine (g) | Lysine (g) | Methionine (g) | Phenylalanine (g) | Proline (g) | Serine (g) | Threonine (g) | Tryptophan (g) | Tyrosine (g) | Valine (g) |
|---|---|---|---|---|---|---|---|---|---|---|---|---|---|---|---|---|---|---|---|---|---|
| 47038 | 1 ea | Chocolate Sandwich Cookie, chocolate icing, avg | 17 | 0.03 | 0.03 | 0.05 | 0.01 | 0.13 | 0.03 | 0.01 | 0.03 | 0.04 | 0.03 | 0.01 | 0.03 | 0.04 | 0.03 | 0.03 | 0.01 | 0.02 | 0.04 |
| 47040 | 1 ea | Chocolate Sandwich Cookie, extra crème, avg | 13 | 0.02 | 0.02 | 0.03 | 0.01 | 0.13 | 0.02 | 0.01 | 0.02 | 0.03 | 0.02 | 0.01 | 0.02 | 0.04 | 0.02 | 0.01 | 0.01 | 0.01 | 0.02 |
| 47041 | 1 ea | Chocolate Wafer cookie, avg | 6 | 0.01 | 0.02 | 0.02 | 0.01 | 0.10 | 0.01 | 0.01 | 0.02 | 0.03 | 0.02 | 0.01 | 0.02 | 0.03 | 0.02 | 0.01 | 0.01 | 0.01 | 0.02 |
| 49014 | 1 ea | Cone, sugar, rolled type, avg | 10 | 0.02 | 0.03 | 0.03 | 0.02 | 0.28 | 0.03 | 0.02 | 0.03 | 0.05 | 0.02 | 0.01 | 0.04 | 0.09 | 0.04 | 0.02 | 0.01 | 0.02 | 0.03 |
| 49111 | 1 ea | Cone, wafer type, cake cone, avg | 29 | 0.07 | 0.08 | 0.09 | 0.05 | 0.82 | 0.08 | 0.05 | 0.09 | 0.16 | 0.05 | 0.04 | 0.12 | 0.28 | 0.11 | 0.06 | 0.03 | 0.06 | 0.10 |
| 47012 | 1 ea | Fig Cookie, avg | 16 | 0.02 | 0.02 | 0.06 | 0.01 | 0.15 | 0.02 | 0.01 | 0.02 | 0.04 | 0.02 | 0.01 | 0.02 | 0.06 | 0.03 | 0.02 | 0.01 | 0.02 | 0.02 |
| 47043 | 1 ea | Fortune cookie, avg | 8 | 0.01 | 0.01 | 0.02 | 0.01 | 0.11 | 0.01 | 0.01 | 0.01 | 0.02 | 0.01 | 0.01 | 0.02 | 0.04 | 0.02 | 0.01 | 0.00 | 0.01 | 0.02 |
| 47045 | 1 ea | Gingersnap Cookie, avg | 7 | 0.01 | 0.01 | 0.02 | 0.01 | 0.13 | 0.01 | 0.01 | 0.01 | 0.03 | 0.01 | 0.01 | 0.02 | 0.04 | 0.02 | 0.01 | 0.01 | 0.01 | 0.02 |
| 47009 | 1 ea | Ladyfinger cookie, w/lemon juice, avg | 11 | 0.06 | 0.07 | 0.10 | 0.02 | 0.21 | 0.04 | 0.03 | 0.06 | 0.09 | 0.07 | 0.03 | 0.06 | 0.07 | 0.08 | 0.05 | 0.01 | 0.04 | 0.06 |
| 47042 | 1 ea | Macaroon Coconut cookie, avg | 24 | 0.04 | 0.07 | 0.08 | 0.02 | 0.13 | 0.03 | 0.02 | 0.04 | 0.07 | 0.05 | 0.02 | 0.05 | 0.03 | 0.05 | 0.03 | 0.01 | 0.03 | 0.05 |
| 47046 | 1 ea | Marshmallow cookie, w/choc coating, avg | 13 | 0.03 | 0.03 | 0.04 | 0.01 | 0.10 | 0.06 | 0.01 | 0.02 | 0.03 | 0.03 | 0.01 | 0.02 | 0.06 | 0.02 | 0.02 | 0.00 | 0.01 | 0.02 |
| 47109 | 1 ea | Molasses Cookie, avg | 15 | 0.03 | 0.03 | 0.04 | 0.02 | 0.27 | 0.03 | 0.02 | 0.03 | 0.06 | 0.03 | 0.01 | 0.04 | 0.09 | 0.04 | 0.02 | 0.01 | 0.02 | 0.04 |
| 47047 | 1 ea | Oatmeal cookie, avg | 18 | 0.05 | 0.07 | 0.08 | 0.03 | 0.29 | 0.05 | 0.03 | 0.04 | 0.08 | 0.04 | 0.02 | 0.05 | 0.09 | 0.06 | 0.03 | 0.02 | 0.04 | 0.05 |
| 47612 | 1 oz | Oatmeal cookie, fat free, avg | 28 | 0.06 | 0.08 | 0.10 | 0.04 | 0.47 | 0.06 | 0.04 | 0.06 | 0.11 | 0.06 | 0.03 | 0.08 | 0.15 | 0.08 | 0.05 | 0.02 | 0.05 | 0.08 |
| 47048 | 1 ea | Oatmeal cookie, soft type, avg | 15 | 0.04 | 0.06 | 0.07 | 0.03 | 0.21 | 0.04 | 0.02 | 0.04 | 0.07 | 0.04 | 0.02 | 0.05 | 0.06 | 0.05 | 0.03 | 0.01 | 0.03 | 0.05 |
| 47003 | 1 ea | Oatmeal Raisin Cookie, prep f/recipe, avg | 15 | 0.04 | 0.06 | 0.07 | 0.02 | 0.23 | 0.04 | 0.02 | 0.04 | 0.07 | 0.04 | 0.02 | 0.05 | 0.07 | 0.05 | 0.03 | 0.01 | 0.03 | 0.05 |
| 49102 | 1 ea | Peanut Butter cookie, avg | 15 | 0.06 | 0.13 | 0.14 | 0.02 | 0.34 | 0.07 | 0.03 | 0.05 | 0.10 | 0.06 | 0.02 | 0.07 | 0.09 | 0.08 | 0.05 | 0.02 | 0.05 | 0.06 |
| 47056 | 1 ea | Peanut Butter cookie, soft type, avg | 15 | 0.03 | 0.07 | 0.07 | 0.01 | 0.20 | 0.04 | 0.02 | 0.03 | 0.05 | 0.03 | 0.01 | 0.04 | 0.05 | 0.04 | 0.03 | 0.01 | 0.03 | 0.03 |
| 47059 | 1 ea | Peanut Butter Sandwich Cookie, avg | 14 | 0.05 | 0.10 | 0.11 | 0.02 | 0.30 | 0.06 | 0.03 | 0.05 | 0.09 | 0.05 | 0.02 | 0.06 | 0.09 | 0.06 | 0.04 | 0.02 | 0.04 | 0.06 |
| 47060 | 1 ea | Peanut Butter Sandwich Cookie, low sod, w/fructose, av | 10 | 0.04 | 0.10 | 0.10 | 0.01 | 0.24 | 0.05 | 0.02 | 0.04 | 0.07 | 0.04 | 0.01 | 0.05 | 0.06 | 0.05 | 0.03 | 0.01 | 0.04 | 0.04 |
| 47062 | 1 ea | Pecan Cookie, shortbread, avg | 14 | 0.02 | 0.04 | 0.03 | 0.02 | 0.21 | 0.02 | 0.02 | 0.03 | 0.05 | 0.02 | 0.01 | 0.03 | 0.07 | 0.04 | 0.02 | 0.01 | 0.02 | 0.03 |
| 48091 | 1 ea | Raisin Cookie, Bakes, fat free, Health Valley | 27 | 0.02 | 0.02 | 0.02 | 0.01 | 0.16 | 0.02 | 0.01 | 0.02 | 0.03 | 0.02 | 0.01 | 0.02 | 0.05 | 0.03 | 0.01 | 0.01 | 0.01 | 0.02 |
| 47061 | 1 ea | Raisin Cookie, soft type, avg | 15 | 0.02 | 0.03 | 0.04 | 0.01 | 0.17 | 0.02 | 0.01 | 0.02 | 0.04 | 0.03 | 0.01 | 0.03 | 0.05 | 0.03 | 0.02 | 0.01 | 0.02 | 0.03 |
| 47011 | 1 ea | Snickerdoodle cookie, avg | 20 | 0.03 | 0.04 | 0.05 | 0.02 | 0.27 | 0.03 | 0.02 | 0.04 | 0.07 | 0.03 | 0.02 | 0.04 | 0.09 | 0.05 | 0.03 | 0.01 | 0.03 | 0.04 |
| 47064 | 1 ea | Sugar Cookie, avg | 15 | 0.03 | 0.03 | 0.05 | 0.02 | 0.20 | 0.02 | 0.02 | 0.03 | 0.06 | 0.04 | 0.02 | 0.04 | 0.07 | 0.04 | 0.03 | 0.01 | 0.03 | 0.04 |
| 47069 | 1 ea | Sugar Cookie, creme filled wafer, avg | 9 | 0.01 | 0.01 | 0.02 | 0.01 | 0.12 | 0.01 | 0.01 | 0.01 | 0.03 | 0.01 | 0.01 | 0.02 | 0.04 | 0.02 | 0.01 | 0.01 | 0.01 | 0.02 |
| 47070 | 1 ea | Sugar Cookie, w/o sod, w/fructose, avg | 4 | 0.00 | 0.00 | 0.01 | 0.00 | 0.04 | 0.00 | 0.00 | 0.00 | 0.01 | 0.00 | 0.00 | 0.01 | 0.01 | 0.01 | 0.00 | 0.00 | 0.00 | 0.01 |
| 47071 | 1 ea | Vanilla Sandwich Cookie | 10 | 0.01 | 0.02 | 0.02 | 0.01 | 0.15 | 0.02 | 0.01 | 0.02 | 0.03 | 0.02 | 0.01 | 0.02 | 0.05 | 0.02 | 0.01 | 0.01 | 0.01 | 0.02 |
| 47008 | 1 ea | Vanilla Wafer Cookie | 4 | 0.01 | 0.01 | 0.01 | 0.00 | 0.05 | 0.01 | 0.00 | 0.01 | 0.01 | 0.01 | 0.00 | 0.01 | 0.02 | 0.01 | 0.01 | 0.00 | 0.01 | 0.01 |
| | | Doughnuts | | | | | | | | | | | | | | | | | | | |
| 45518 | 1 ea | Cake Doughnut, chocolate, glazed or sugared, avg | 42 | 0.08 | 0.10 | 0.15 | 0.04 | 0.42 | 0.07 | 0.04 | 0.09 | 0.14 | 0.10 | 0.04 | 0.09 | 0.14 | 0.11 | 0.07 | 0.02 | 0.07 | 0.10 |
| 45524 | 1 ea | Cake Doughnut, chocolate, iced, avg | 43 | 0.08 | 0.11 | 0.16 | 0.04 | 0.49 | 0.08 | 0.05 | 0.09 | 0.16 | 0.11 | 0.04 | 0.10 | 0.17 | 0.12 | 0.08 | 0.03 | 0.08 | 0.11 |
| 45563 | 1 ea | Raised/Yeast Doughnut, creme filled, avg | 85 | 0.20 | 0.23 | 0.32 | 0.11 | 1.58 | 0.19 | 0.12 | 0.23 | 0.41 | 0.20 | 0.10 | 0.26 | 0.53 | 0.28 | 0.18 | 0.07 | 0.17 | 0.25 |
| 45506 | 1 ea | Raised/Yeast Doughnut, glazed, avg | 60 | 0.14 | 0.16 | 0.23 | 0.08 | 1.12 | 0.14 | 0.09 | 0.16 | 0.28 | 0.14 | 0.07 | 0.19 | 0.38 | 0.20 | 0.13 | 0.05 | 0.12 | 0.18 |
| 49109 | 1 ea | Raised/Yeast Doughnut, glazed, donut hole, avg | 13 | 0.03 | 0.04 | 0.05 | 0.02 | 0.24 | 0.03 | 0.02 | 0.03 | 0.06 | 0.03 | 0.01 | 0.04 | 0.08 | 0.04 | 0.03 | 0.01 | 0.03 | 0.04 |
| 45507 | 1 ea | Raised/Yeast Doughnut, jelly filled, avg | 85 | 0.19 | 0.21 | 0.29 | 0.10 | 1.47 | 0.18 | 0.11 | 0.21 | 0.37 | 0.18 | 0.09 | 0.24 | 0.50 | 0.26 | 0.16 | 0.06 | 0.16 | 0.23 |
| | | Frozen Desserts | | | | | | | | | | | | | | | | | | | |
| 2004 | 1/2 cup | Ice Cream, vanilla, avg | 66 | 0.08 | 0.08 | 0.17 | 0.02 | 0.45 | 0.06 | 0.06 | 0.13 | 0.21 | 0.17 | 0.05 | 0.10 | 0.22 | 0.12 | 0.10 | 0.03 | 0.10 | 0.14 |
| 2008 | 1/2 cup | Ice Cream, vanilla, french, soft serve, avg | 86 | 0.14 | 0.15 | 0.26 | 0.03 | 0.64 | 0.14 | 0.09 | 0.18 | 0.30 | 0.25 | 0.08 | 0.15 | 0.32 | 0.19 | 0.15 | 0.04 | 0.15 | 0.21 |
| 2006 | 1/2 cup | Ice Cream, vanilla, rich, 16% fat, avg | 74 | 0.10 | 0.10 | 0.18 | 0.02 | 0.48 | 0.11 | 0.06 | 0.13 | 0.22 | 0.18 | 0.06 | 0.11 | 0.25 | 0.13 | 0.10 | 0.03 | 0.11 | 0.15 |
| 2009 | 1/2 cup | Ice Milk, vanilla, avg | 66 | 0.10 | 0.10 | 0.18 | 0.02 | 0.48 | 0.10 | 0.06 | 0.13 | 0.22 | 0.18 | 0.06 | 0.11 | 0.24 | 0.12 | 0.10 | 0.03 | 0.10 | 0.15 |
| 2011 | 1/2 cup | Sherbet, orange, avg | 99 | 0.03 | 0.04 | 0.08 | 0.01 | 0.20 | 0.02 | 0.03 | 0.06 | 0.10 | 0.08 | 0.02 | 0.05 | 0.10 | 0.05 | 0.04 | 0.01 | 0.05 | 0.07 |
| | | Fruit Desserts | | | | | | | | | | | | | | | | | | | |
| 49005 | 1/2 cup | Brown Betty, apple, avg | 103 | 0.09 | 0.10 | 0.15 | 0.04 | 0.73 | 0.10 | 0.05 | 0.10 | 0.17 | 0.07 | 0.04 | 0.12 | 0.25 | 0.12 | 0.07 | 0.03 | 0.06 | 0.12 |
| 49003 | 1 pce | Cobbler, apple, avg | 104 | 0.06 | 0.07 | 0.11 | 0.03 | 0.55 | 0.06 | 0.04 | 0.08 | 0.14 | 0.07 | 0.04 | 0.09 | 0.20 | 0.09 | 0.06 | 0.02 | 0.06 | 0.09 |

TABLE A **Amino Acid Content for Selected Foods *(continued)***

| Code | Amount | | Description | Weight (g) | Alanine (g) | Arginine (g) | Aspartic acid (g) | Cystine (g) | Glutamic acid (g) | Glycine (g) | Histidine (g) | Isoleucine (g) | Leucine (g) | Lysine (g) | Methionine (g) | Phenylalanine (g) | Proline (g) | Serine (g) | Threonine (g) | Tryptophan (g) | Tyrosine (g) | Valine (g) |
|---|---|---|---|---|---|---|---|---|---|---|---|---|---|---|---|---|---|---|---|---|---|---|
| 49008 | 1 | pce | Cobbler, peach, avg | 130 | 0.09 | 0.08 | 0.17 | 0.04 | 0.62 | 0.07 | 0.05 | 0.09 | 0.16 | 0.08 | 0.05 | 0.10 | 0.22 | 0.11 | 0.08 | 0.02 | 0.07 | 0.11 |
| 49036 | 1 | pce | Crisp, apple, avg | 78 | 0.05 | 0.05 | 0.08 | 0.03 | 0.43 | 0.05 | 0.03 | 0.05 | 0.10 | 0.04 | 0.02 | 0.07 | 0.14 | 0.07 | 0.04 | 0.02 | 0.04 | 0.06 |
| 49135 | 1 | pce | Crisp, apricot, avg | 139 | 0.06 | 0.06 | 0.20 | 0.02 | 0.33 | 0.05 | 0.03 | 0.05 | 0.10 | 0.07 | 0.02 | 0.07 | 0.13 | 0.08 | 0.05 | 0.02 | 0.04 | 0.06 |
| 49009 | 1 | pce | Crisp, peach, avg | 139 | 0.07 | 0.05 | 0.15 | 0.02 | 0.37 | 0.05 | 0.03 | 0.05 | 0.09 | 0.04 | 0.03 | 0.06 | 0.12 | 0.07 | 0.05 | 0.01 | 0.04 | 0.07 |
| 49006 | 1 | ea | Dumpling, apple, avg | 151 | 0.07 | 0.07 | 0.11 | 0.05 | 0.70 | 0.07 | 0.04 | 0.08 | 0.15 | 0.05 | 0.04 | 0.10 | 0.24 | 0.10 | 0.06 | 0.02 | 0.06 | 0.09 |
| 49015 | 1 | pce | Strudel, apple, avg | 71 | 0.08 | 0.10 | 0.15 | 0.04 | 0.60 | 0.07 | 0.05 | 0.10 | 0.18 | 0.11 | 0.05 | 0.11 | 0.22 | 0.13 | 0.08 | 0.03 | 0.08 | 0.12 |
| | | | Gelatin Dessert | | | | | | | | | | | | | | | | | | | |
| 23155 | 2 1/2 | g | Dry Mix, per 1/2 c svg, avg | 2 | 0.02 | 0.01 | 0.01 | 0.00 | 0.02 | 0.04 | 0.00 | 0.00 | 0.01 | 0.01 | 0.00 | 0.00 | 0.03 | 0.01 | 0.00 | 0.00 | 0.00 | 0.00 |
| 23157 | 1 | ea | Dry Mix, sugar free, env, avg | 10 | 0.58 | 0.48 | 0.38 | 0.00 | 0.63 | 1.38 | 0.05 | 0.08 | 0.18 | 0.25 | 0.04 | 0.13 | 0.89 | 0.19 | 0.11 | 0.00 | 0.02 | 0.15 |
| 23009 | 1 | ea | Dry Mix, unswtnd, env, avg | 7 | 0.56 | 0.46 | 0.37 | 0.00 | 0.61 | 1.33 | 0.05 | 0.08 | 0.17 | 0.24 | 0.04 | 0.12 | 0.86 | 0.18 | 0.10 | 0.00 | 0.02 | 0.15 |
| 23093 | 1/2 | cup | Prep, sugar free, avg | 117 | 0.13 | 0.11 | 0.09 | 0.00 | 0.15 | 0.32 | 0.01 | 0.02 | 0.04 | 0.06 | 0.01 | 0.03 | 0.21 | 0.04 | 0.02 | 0.00 | 0.01 | 0.03 |
| 23156 | 1/2 | cup | Prep, w/added fruit, avg | 106 | 0.10 | 0.09 | 0.10 | 0.01 | 0.15 | 0.22 | 0.03 | 0.02 | 0.04 | 0.05 | 0.01 | 0.03 | 0.15 | 0.04 | 0.03 | 0.00 | 0.01 | 0.03 |
| | | | Pastries and Sweet Rolls | | | | | | | | | | | | | | | | | | | |
| 45522 | 1 | ea | Croissant, apple, avg | 57 | 0.17 | 0.18 | 0.26 | 0.08 | 1.12 | 0.17 | 0.09 | 0.19 | 0.32 | 0.18 | 0.09 | 0.20 | 0.41 | 0.22 | 0.15 | 0.05 | 0.14 | 0.21 |
| 42015 | 1 | ea | Croissant, butter, avg | 57 | 0.18 | 0.19 | 0.28 | 0.10 | 1.30 | 0.16 | 0.11 | 0.21 | 0.35 | 0.19 | 0.10 | 0.23 | 0.44 | 0.25 | 0.16 | 0.06 | 0.15 | 0.23 |
| 45523 | 1 | ea | Croissant, cheese, avg | 57 | 0.19 | 0.21 | 0.30 | 0.10 | 1.48 | 0.17 | 0.12 | 0.23 | 0.39 | 0.21 | 0.11 | 0.26 | 0.51 | 0.27 | 0.17 | 0.06 | 0.17 | 0.26 |
| 45572 | 1 | ea | Danish Pastry, cheese, avg | 71 | 0.21 | 0.23 | 0.36 | 0.10 | 1.43 | 0.17 | 0.15 | 0.26 | 0.46 | 0.31 | 0.12 | 0.29 | 0.51 | 0.30 | 0.21 | 0.06 | 0.21 | 0.29 |
| 45571 | 1 | ea | Danish Pastry, cinnamon, avg | 65 | 0.18 | 0.20 | 0.30 | 0.09 | 1.22 | 0.16 | 0.10 | 0.20 | 0.34 | 0.19 | 0.09 | 0.23 | 0.41 | 0.24 | 0.16 | 0.05 | 0.15 | 0.22 |
| 45569 | 1 | ea | Danish Pastry, fruit, avg | 71 | 0.14 | 0.15 | 0.21 | 0.08 | 1.14 | 0.13 | 0.08 | 0.16 | 0.28 | 0.13 | 0.08 | 0.19 | 0.39 | 0.20 | 0.12 | 0.05 | 0.12 | 0.18 |
| 45573 | 1 | ea | Danish Pastry, nut, avg | 65 | 0.17 | 0.28 | 0.31 | 0.09 | 1.23 | 0.17 | 0.11 | 0.20 | 0.34 | 0.18 | 0.09 | 0.22 | 0.40 | 0.24 | 0.15 | 0.06 | 0.15 | 0.23 |
| 45590 | 1 | ea | Fruit burritos, apple or cherry, avg | 155 | 0.17 | 0.21 | 0.26 | 0.11 | 1.72 | 0.19 | 0.12 | 0.18 | 0.35 | 0.12 | 0.09 | 0.26 | 0.59 | 0.26 | 0.14 | 0.06 | 0.16 | 0.21 |
| 49041 | 7 | pce | Nacho chips w/cinnamon & sugar, avg | 109 | 0.54 | 0.36 | 0.50 | 0.13 | 1.35 | 0.30 | 0.22 | 0.26 | 0.88 | 0.20 | 0.15 | 0.35 | 0.63 | 0.34 | 0.27 | 0.05 | 0.29 | 0.37 |
| 42164 | 1 | ea | Sweet Rolls, cheese, avg | 66 | 0.18 | 0.21 | 0.32 | 0.07 | 1.14 | 0.15 | 0.12 | 0.21 | 0.37 | 0.26 | 0.09 | 0.23 | 0.40 | 0.25 | 0.17 | 0.05 | 0.17 | 0.23 |
| 42166 | 1 | ea | Sweet Rolls, cinnamon, prep f/refrig dough, w/frosting, | 30 | 0.05 | 0.07 | 0.08 | 0.03 | 0.53 | 0.06 | 0.04 | 0.06 | 0.11 | 0.04 | 0.03 | 0.08 | 0.18 | 0.08 | 0.05 | 0.02 | 0.05 | 0.07 |
| 42165 | 1 | ea | Sweet Rolls, cinnamon, refrig dough, w/frosting, avg | 30 | 0.05 | 0.06 | 0.07 | 0.03 | 0.48 | 0.05 | 0.03 | 0.05 | 0.11 | 0.04 | 0.03 | 0.07 | 0.17 | 0.07 | 0.04 | 0.02 | 0.05 | 0.06 |
| 42033 | 1 | ea | Sweet Rolls, cinnamon Raisin, avg | 60 | 0.14 | 0.17 | 0.24 | 0.07 | 1.04 | 0.13 | 0.09 | 0.16 | 0.27 | 0.15 | 0.07 | 0.18 | 0.35 | 0.20 | 0.13 | 0.04 | 0.12 | 0.17 |
| 42167 | 1 | ea | Sweet Rolls, cinnamon Raisin nut, avg | 57 | 0.14 | 0.20 | 0.23 | 0.07 | 1.00 | 0.13 | 0.09 | 0.15 | 0.27 | 0.14 | 0.08 | 0.18 | 0.33 | 0.19 | 0.12 | 0.05 | 0.12 | 0.17 |
| 45683 | 1 | ea | Toaster Pastry, brown sugar cinnamon, avg | 50 | 0.08 | 0.09 | 0.11 | 0.05 | 0.70 | 0.08 | 0.05 | 0.08 | 0.16 | 0.07 | 0.04 | 0.11 | 0.24 | 0.11 | 0.07 | 0.03 | 0.07 | 0.09 |
| 45679 | 1 | ea | Toaster Pastry, strawberry, w/frosting, lowfat, Pop Tart | 52 | 0.10 | 0.11 | 0.17 | 0.05 | 0.70 | 0.09 | 0.05 | 0.11 | 0.18 | 0.12 | 0.04 | 0.12 | 0.24 | 0.14 | 0.09 | 0.04 | 0.08 | 0.13 |
| | | | Pastry, Pie and Dessert Crusts | | | | | | | | | | | | | | | | | | | |
| 45530 | 1 | ea | Cookie Crust, chocolate, bkd, whl, avg | 219 | 0.41 | 0.49 | 0.72 | 0.22 | 3.02 | 0.40 | 0.23 | 0.46 | 0.79 | 0.51 | 0.19 | 0.54 | 1.01 | 0.58 | 0.39 | 0.17 | 0.37 | 0.57 |
| 45676 | 1 | pce | Cookie Crust, plain, bkd, avg | 22 | 0.03 | 0.04 | 0.05 | 0.02 | 0.22 | 0.03 | 0.02 | 0.04 | 0.06 | 0.04 | 0.02 | 0.04 | 0.07 | 0.05 | 0.03 | 0.01 | 0.03 | 0.04 |
| 45500 | 1 | pce | Graham Cracker Crust, bkd, avg | 30 | 0.04 | 0.05 | 0.06 | 0.03 | 0.41 | 0.05 | 0.03 | 0.05 | 0.09 | 0.03 | 0.02 | 0.06 | 0.14 | 0.06 | 0.04 | 0.02 | 0.04 | 0.05 |
| 45521 | 1 | ea | Pastry Crust, cream puff shell, 3 1/2 ", avg | 66 | 0.28 | 0.31 | 0.48 | 0.13 | 1.19 | 0.20 | 0.14 | 0.28 | 0.47 | 0.33 | 0.16 | 0.31 | 0.39 | 0.39 | 0.24 | 0.07 | 0.22 | 0.32 |
| 45528 | 1 | ea | Pastry Crust, phyllo dough, avg | 19 | 0.04 | 0.05 | 0.06 | 0.03 | 0.45 | 0.05 | 0.03 | 0.05 | 0.09 | 0.03 | 0.02 | 0.07 | 0.16 | 0.07 | 0.04 | 0.02 | 0.04 | 0.05 |
| 49114 | 1 | pce | Pie Crust, prep f/mix | 20 | 0.04 | 0.05 | 0.05 | 0.03 | 0.47 | 0.05 | 0.03 | 0.05 | 0.09 | 0.03 | 0.02 | 0.07 | 0.16 | 0.06 | 0.04 | 0.02 | 0.04 | 0.06 |
| 45503 | 1 | ea | Pie Crust, prep f/mix, whl, avg | 160 | 0.32 | 0.37 | 0.43 | 0.24 | 3.73 | 0.36 | 0.23 | 0.40 | 0.74 | 0.21 | 0.19 | 0.52 | 1.25 | 0.52 | 0.28 | 0.12 | 0.29 | 0.45 |
| 49115 | 1 | pce | Pie Crust, prep f/recipe, avg | 23 | 0.05 | 0.06 | 0.06 | 0.03 | 0.50 | 0.05 | 0.03 | 0.05 | 0.10 | 0.03 | 0.03 | 0.07 | 0.17 | 0.07 | 0.04 | 0.02 | 0.04 | 0.06 |
| 45501 | 1 | ea | Pie Crust, prep f/recipe, whl, avg | 180 | 0.37 | 0.46 | 0.49 | 0.24 | 3.89 | 0.41 | 0.26 | 0.40 | 0.79 | 0.25 | 0.20 | 0.58 | 1.33 | 0.57 | 0.31 | 0.14 | 0.35 | 0.46 |
| 45540 | 1 | ea | Popover Crust, prep f/mix, whl, avg | 33 | 0.11 | 0.12 | 0.17 | 0.06 | 0.66 | 0.09 | 0.06 | 0.12 | 0.20 | 0.11 | 0.06 | 0.13 | 0.22 | 0.15 | 0.09 | 0.03 | 0.09 | 0.13 |
| | | | Pies | | | | | | | | | | | | | | | | | | | |
| 48061 | 1 | pce | Apple Pie, 1/8 of 9" pie, avg | 125 | 0.07 | 0.09 | 0.12 | 0.05 | 0.73 | 0.08 | 0.05 | 0.09 | 0.16 | 0.09 | 0.04 | 0.11 | 0.25 | 0.12 | 0.07 | 0.03 | 0.07 | 0.10 |
| 48013 | 1 | ea | Apple Pie, fried, avg | 85 | 0.08 | 0.10 | 0.12 | 0.05 | 0.79 | 0.09 | 0.05 | 0.08 | 0.16 | 0.06 | 0.04 | 0.12 | 0.27 | 0.12 | 0.07 | 0.03 | 0.07 | 0.10 |
| 48076 | 1 | pce | Apple Pie, frozen, bkd, 1/8 of 9" pie, avg | 125 | 0.07 | 0.09 | 0.12 | 0.05 | 0.73 | 0.08 | 0.05 | 0.09 | 0.16 | 0.09 | 0.04 | 0.11 | 0.25 | 0.12 | 0.07 | 0.03 | 0.07 | 0.10 |
| 48089 | 1 | pce | Apple Pie, prep f/recipe, 1/8 of 9" pie, avg | 155 | 0.12 | 0.15 | 0.17 | 0.08 | 1.22 | 0.13 | 0.08 | 0.13 | 0.25 | 0.09 | 0.07 | 0.18 | 0.42 | 0.18 | 0.10 | 0.04 | 0.11 | 0.15 |
| 48090 | 1 | pce | Banana Cream Pie, prep f/mix, 1/8 of 9" pie, avg | 92 | 0.11 | 0.14 | 0.24 | 0.05 | 0.72 | 0.09 | 0.08 | 0.15 | 0.26 | 0.18 | 0.06 | 0.15 | 0.27 | 0.16 | 0.12 | 0.04 | 0.12 | 0.16 |
| 48069 | 1 | pce | Banana Cream Pie, prep f/recipe, 1/8 of 9" pie, avg | 144 | 0.22 | 0.27 | 0.41 | 0.10 | 1.53 | 0.18 | 0.17 | 0.29 | 0.52 | 0.33 | 0.13 | 0.30 | 0.59 | 0.35 | 0.24 | 0.08 | 0.24 | 0.33 |
| 48091 | 1 | pce | Blueberry Pie, prep f/frozen, avg | 125 | 0.02 | 0.02 | 0.02 | 0.01 | 0.16 | 0.02 | 0.01 | 0.02 | 0.03 | 0.02 | 0.01 | 0.02 | 0.05 | 0.03 | 0.01 | 0.01 | 0.01 | 0.02 |
| 48092 | 1 | pce | Blueberry Pie, prep f/recipe, avg | 147 | 0.13 | 0.17 | 0.19 | 0.07 | 1.17 | 0.15 | 0.08 | 0.13 | 0.26 | 0.08 | 0.07 | 0.19 | 0.40 | 0.18 | 0.11 | 0.04 | 0.11 | 0.16 |
| 48093 | 1 | pce | Butterscotch Pie, prep f/rec, 1/8 of 9" pie, avg | 127 | 0.21 | 0.26 | 0.39 | 0.09 | 1.45 | 0.17 | 0.15 | 0.29 | 0.50 | 0.33 | 0.13 | 0.28 | 0.56 | 0.34 | 0.23 | 0.08 | 0.24 | 0.32 |

TABLE A **Amino Acid Content for Selected Foods *(continued)***

| Code | Amount | | Description | Weight (g) | Alanine (g) | Arginine (g) | Aspartic acid (g) | Cystine (g) | Glutamic acid (g) | Glycine (g) | Histidine (g) | Isoleucine (g) | Leucine (g) | Lysine (g) | Methionine (g) | Phenylalanine (g) | Proline (g) | Serine (g) | Threonine (g) | Tryptophan (g) | Tyrosine (g) | Valine (g) |
|---|---|---|---|---|---|---|---|---|---|---|---|---|---|---|---|---|---|---|---|---|---|---|
| 49004 | 1 | pce | Cheesecake, avg | 80 | 0.20 | 0.20 | 0.32 | 0.06 | 0.82 | 0.18 | 0.11 | 0.22 | 0.37 | 0.30 | 0.11 | 0.21 | 0.38 | 0.25 | 0.18 | 0.05 | 0.18 | 0.25 |
| 49011 | 1 | pce | Cheesecake w/cherry topping, avg | 142 | 0.25 | 0.29 | 0.63 | 0.09 | 1.43 | 0.17 | 0.21 | 0.35 | 0.61 | 0.53 | 0.17 | 0.36 | 0.55 | 0.39 | 0.29 | 0.07 | 0.30 | 0.39 |
| 49119 | 1 | ea | Cherry Pie, fried, avg | 85 | 0.08 | 0.10 | 0.12 | 0.05 | 0.79 | 0.09 | 0.05 | 0.08 | 0.16 | 0.06 | 0.04 | 0.12 | 0.27 | 0.12 | 0.07 | 0.03 | 0.07 | 0.10 |
| 48077 | 1 | pce | Cherry Pie, prep f/frozen, 1/8 of 9" pie, avg | 125 | 0.09 | 0.12 | 0.16 | 0.04 | 0.61 | 0.07 | 0.06 | 0.12 | 0.20 | 0.14 | 0.05 | 0.12 | 0.23 | 0.13 | 0.09 | 0.03 | 0.09 | 0.14 |
| 48094 | 1 | pce | Cherry Pie, prep f/recipe, 1/8 pie, avg | 180 | 0.15 | 0.18 | 0.61 | 0.09 | 1.42 | 0.17 | 0.10 | 0.16 | 0.31 | 0.12 | 0.08 | 0.22 | 0.50 | 0.23 | 0.13 | 0.06 | 0.14 | 0.19 |
| 48096 | 1 | pce | Chocolate Cream Pie, RTS, 1/8 of 8" pie, avg | 113 | 0.14 | 0.15 | 0.21 | 0.05 | 0.68 | 0.20 | 0.05 | 0.11 | 0.19 | 0.13 | 0.04 | 0.13 | 0.28 | 0.14 | 0.10 | 0.04 | 0.08 | 0.14 |
| 48071 | 1 | pce | Chocolate Cream Pie, prep f/rec, 1/8 of 9", avg | 142 | 0.25 | 0.30 | 0.46 | 0.10 | 1.62 | 0.20 | 0.16 | 0.32 | 0.55 | 0.36 | 0.14 | 0.32 | 0.61 | 0.37 | 0.26 | 0.09 | 0.27 | 0.36 |
| 48072 | 1 | pce | Coconut Cream Pie, RTS, 1/6 of 7" pie, avg | 64 | 0.05 | 0.07 | 0.09 | 0.02 | 0.32 | 0.04 | 0.03 | 0.07 | 0.11 | 0.08 | 0.03 | 0.06 | 0.12 | 0.07 | 0.05 | 0.02 | 0.05 | 0.08 |
| 48084 | 1 | pce | Coconut Custard Pie, avg | 104 | 1.24 | 1.77 | 2.36 | 0.53 | 8.99 | 1.02 | 0.87 | 1.78 | 3.01 | 2.09 | 0.76 | 1.71 | 3.41 | 1.88 | 1.35 | 0.49 | 1.40 | 2.06 |
| 48081 | 1 | pce | Egg Custard Pie, RTS, 1/6 of 8" pie, avg | 105 | 0.24 | 0.26 | 0.44 | 0.10 | 1.14 | 0.17 | 0.13 | 0.30 | 0.48 | 0.37 | 0.14 | 0.28 | 0.42 | 0.35 | 0.24 | 0.07 | 0.22 | 0.33 |
| 49118 | 1 | ea | Fruit pie, fried, avg | 128 | 0.12 | 0.14 | 0.20 | 0.08 | 1.16 | 0.13 | 0.08 | 0.15 | 0.27 | 0.15 | 0.07 | 0.18 | 0.40 | 0.20 | 0.11 | 0.05 | 0.12 | 0.18 |
| 49120 | 1 | ea | Lemon Pie, fried, avg | 85 | 0.08 | 0.10 | 0.12 | 0.05 | 0.79 | 0.09 | 0.05 | 0.08 | 0.16 | 0.06 | 0.04 | 0.12 | 0.27 | 0.12 | 0.07 | 0.03 | 0.07 | 0.10 |
| 48101 | 1 | pce | Lemon Meringue Pie, prep f/rec, 1/8 of 9", avg | 127 | 0.21 | 0.24 | 0.35 | 0.11 | 1.10 | 0.17 | 0.11 | 0.21 | 0.37 | 0.23 | 0.12 | 0.25 | 0.37 | 0.30 | 0.18 | 0.06 | 0.17 | 0.24 |
| 48083 | 1 | pce | Mince Pie, prep f/rec, 1/8 of 9", avg | 165 | 0.14 | 0.20 | 0.26 | 0.08 | 1.29 | 0.12 | 0.11 | 0.12 | 0.25 | 0.10 | 0.09 | 0.18 | 0.38 | 0.17 | 0.12 | 0.04 | 0.12 | 0.16 |
| 48073 | 1 | pce | Peach Pie, baked f/frozen, 1/6 of 8" pie, avg | 117 | 0.08 | 0.08 | 0.15 | 0.04 | 0.63 | 0.07 | 0.04 | 0.08 | 0.14 | 0.07 | 0.04 | 0.09 | 0.21 | 0.11 | 0.07 | 0.03 | 0.06 | 0.10 |
| 48087 | 1 | pce | Peach Pie, prep f/recipe, 1/8 of 9 " pie, avg | 139 | 0.12 | 0.12 | 0.20 | 0.06 | 0.99 | 0.11 | 0.07 | 0.11 | 0.22 | 0.08 | 0.06 | 0.15 | 0.34 | 0.16 | 0.09 | 0.04 | 0.10 | 0.14 |
| 48086 | 1 | pce | Pecan Pie, RTS, 1/6 of 8" pie, avg | 113 | 0.19 | 0.32 | 0.35 | 0.11 | 0.98 | 0.17 | 0.11 | 0.20 | 0.34 | 0.23 | 0.11 | 0.23 | 0.30 | 0.27 | 0.17 | 0.07 | 0.16 | 0.23 |
| 48075 | 1 | pce | Pumpkin Pie, RTS, 1/6 of 8" pie, avg | 109 | 0.16 | 0.18 | 0.32 | 0.06 | 0.90 | 0.11 | 0.10 | 0.22 | 0.37 | 0.28 | 0.10 | 0.20 | 0.36 | 0.24 | 0.17 | 0.06 | 0.18 | 0.25 |
| 48011 | 1 | pce | Strawberryb Chiffon Pie, 1/8 of 9" pie, avg | 139 | 0.24 | 0.22 | 0.28 | 0.04 | 0.93 | 0.46 | 0.07 | 0.13 | 0.23 | 0.15 | 0.06 | 0.15 | 0.51 | 0.17 | 0.11 | 0.03 | 0.09 | 0.15 |
| 48104 | 1 | pce | Vanilla Pie, cream, prep f/rec, 1/8 of 9" pie, avg | 126 | 0.21 | 0.26 | 0.39 | 0.09 | 1.44 | 0.17 | 0.15 | 0.29 | 0.50 | 0.34 | 0.13 | 0.28 | 0.56 | 0.34 | 0.23 | 0.08 | 0.24 | 0.32 |
| | | | Pudding | | | | | | | | | | | | | | | | | | | |
| 2628 | 1/2 | cup | Banana, prep f/mix, inst, w/2% milk, avg | 147 | 0.13 | 0.14 | 0.29 | 0.04 | 0.81 | 0.08 | 0.10 | 0.23 | 0.38 | 0.31 | 0.10 | 0.19 | 0.37 | 0.21 | 0.17 | 0.05 | 0.19 | 0.26 |
| 2631 | 1/2 | cup | Banana, prep f/mix, w/2% milk, avg | 140 | 0.13 | 0.14 | 0.29 | 0.04 | 0.81 | 0.08 | 0.11 | 0.23 | 0.38 | 0.31 | 0.10 | 0.19 | 0.37 | 0.21 | 0.17 | 0.05 | 0.19 | 0.26 |
| 2632 | 1 | ea | Banana, RTE, 5 oz pkg, avg | 142 | 0.11 | 0.12 | 0.24 | 0.03 | 0.67 | 0.07 | 0.09 | 0.19 | 0.32 | 0.25 | 0.08 | 0.15 | 0.31 | 0.17 | 0.14 | 0.04 | 0.15 | 0.21 |
| 2617 | 1/2 | cup | Bread w/Raisins, avg | 126 | 0.27 | 0.30 | 0.52 | 0.11 | 1.35 | 0.17 | 0.17 | 0.33 | 0.54 | 0.40 | 0.17 | 0.31 | 0.48 | 0.36 | 0.27 | 0.08 | 0.26 | 0.37 |
| 2635 | 1 | oz | Chocolate, mix, avg | 28 | 0.03 | 0.04 | 0.07 | 0.01 | 0.11 | 0.03 | 0.01 | 0.03 | 0.04 | 0.04 | 0.01 | 0.03 | 0.03 | 0.03 | 0.03 | 0.01 | 0.03 | 0.04 |
| 2634 | 1/2 | cup | Chocolate, prep f/mix w/2% milk, avg | 147 | 0.16 | 0.17 | 0.35 | 0.04 | 0.90 | 0.11 | 0.11 | 0.26 | 0.41 | 0.34 | 0.10 | 0.21 | 0.40 | 0.23 | 0.20 | 0.06 | 0.21 | 0.29 |
| 2605 | 1/2 | cup | Chocolate, prep f/mix, w/whl milk, avg | 147 | 0.16 | 0.17 | 0.34 | 0.04 | 0.89 | 0.10 | 0.11 | 0.25 | 0.41 | 0.33 | 0.10 | 0.21 | 0.40 | 0.23 | 0.19 | 0.06 | 0.21 | 0.29 |
| 2637 | 1/2 | cup | Chocolate, prep f/rec, w/2% milk, avg | 157 | 0.17 | 0.19 | 0.38 | 0.05 | 0.95 | 0.12 | 0.12 | 0.27 | 0.43 | 0.35 | 0.11 | 0.23 | 0.41 | 0.25 | 0.21 | 0.07 | 0.22 | 0.31 |
| 2601 | 1/2 | cup | Chocolate, prep f/rec, w/whl milk, avg | 157 | 0.17 | 0.19 | 0.38 | 0.05 | 0.94 | 0.12 | 0.12 | 0.27 | 0.43 | 0.35 | 0.11 | 0.23 | 0.41 | 0.25 | 0.21 | 0.07 | 0.22 | 0.31 |
| 2610 | 1 | ea | Chocolate, RTE, cnd, avg | 142 | 0.13 | 0.15 | 0.30 | 0.04 | 0.74 | 0.10 | 0.09 | 0.21 | 0.34 | 0.27 | 0.08 | 0.18 | 0.32 | 0.19 | 0.16 | 0.05 | 0.17 | 0.24 |
| 2658 | 1 | oz | Chocolate, rennin, dry mix, avg | 28 | 0.04 | 0.04 | 0.06 | 0.01 | 0.10 | 0.05 | 0.01 | 0.02 | 0.04 | 0.03 | 0.01 | 0.03 | 0.04 | 0.03 | 0.02 | 0.01 | 0.02 | 0.04 |
| 2659 | 1/2 | cup | Chocolate, rennin, prep f/mix, w/2%milk, avg | 136 | 0.15 | 0.16 | 0.33 | 0.04 | 0.86 | 0.11 | 0.11 | 0.25 | 0.40 | 0.32 | 0.10 | 0.20 | 0.39 | 0.22 | 0.19 | 0.06 | 0.20 | 0.28 |
| 2660 | 1/2 | cup | Chocolate, rennin, prep f/mix, w/whl milk, avg | 136 | 0.15 | 0.16 | 0.32 | 0.04 | 0.85 | 0.11 | 0.11 | 0.24 | 0.39 | 0.32 | 0.10 | 0.20 | 0.39 | 0.22 | 0.18 | 0.06 | 0.20 | 0.28 |
| 2638 | 1 | oz | Coconut Cream, dry mix, avg | 28 | 0.01 | 0.03 | 0.02 | 0.00 | 0.05 | 0.01 | 0.01 | 0.01 | 0.02 | 0.01 | 0.00 | 0.01 | 0.01 | 0.01 | 0.01 | 0.00 | 0.01 | 0.01 |
| 2639 | 1/2 | cup | Coconut Cream, prep f/mix, w/2%milk, avg | 147 | 0.14 | 0.17 | 0.31 | 0.04 | 0.85 | 0.09 | 0.11 | 0.24 | 0.39 | 0.32 | 0.10 | 0.20 | 0.38 | 0.22 | 0.18 | 0.06 | 0.19 | 0.27 |
| 2615 | 1/2 | cup | Coconut Cream, prep f/mix w/whl mlk, avg | 147 | 0.14 | 0.17 | 0.31 | 0.04 | 0.85 | 0.09 | 0.11 | 0.24 | 0.39 | 0.31 | 0.10 | 0.20 | 0.38 | 0.22 | 0.18 | 0.06 | 0.19 | 0.27 |
| 2644 | 1/2 | cup | Lemon, prep f/mix, w/2% milk, avg | 147 | 0.13 | 0.14 | 0.29 | 0.04 | 0.81 | 0.08 | 0.10 | 0.23 | 0.38 | 0.31 | 0.10 | 0.19 | 0.37 | 0.21 | 0.17 | 0.05 | 0.19 | 0.26 |
| 2616 | 1/2 | cup | Lemon, prep f/mix, w/whl milk, avg | 147 | 0.13 | 0.14 | 0.29 | 0.03 | 0.79 | 0.08 | 0.10 | 0.23 | 0.37 | 0.30 | 0.09 | 0.18 | 0.37 | 0.20 | 0.17 | 0.05 | 0.18 | 0.25 |
| 2647 | 1 | ea | Lemon, RTE, cnd, avg | 142 | 0.01 | 0.01 | 0.01 | 0.00 | 0.02 | 0.00 | 0.00 | 0.00 | 0.01 | 0.00 | 0.00 | 0.01 | 0.01 | 0.00 | 0.00 | 0.00 | 0.00 | 0.01 |
| 2649 | 1/2 | cup | Rice, prep f/mix, w/whl milk, avg | 144 | 0.13 | 0.14 | 0.29 | 0.04 | 0.81 | 0.08 | 0.11 | 0.23 | 0.38 | 0.31 | 0.10 | 0.19 | 0.37 | 0.21 | 0.17 | 0.05 | 0.19 | 0.26 |
| 2650 | 1/2 | cup | Rice, prep f/rec, avg | 152 | 0.21 | 0.26 | 0.44 | 0.07 | 1.10 | 0.14 | 0.14 | 0.29 | 0.48 | 0.35 | 0.13 | 0.26 | 0.43 | 0.27 | 0.22 | 0.07 | 0.23 | 0.34 |
| 2651 | 1 | ea | Rice, RTE, cnd, avg | 142 | 0.10 | 0.11 | 0.21 | 0.03 | 0.56 | 0.07 | 0.07 | 0.16 | 0.26 | 0.20 | 0.07 | 0.13 | 0.25 | 0.15 | 0.12 | 0.04 | 0.13 | 0.18 |
| 2652 | 1 | oz | Tapioca, dry mix, avg | 92 | 0.01 | 0.01 | 0.01 | 0.00 | 0.02 | 0.00 | 0.00 | 0.00 | 0.01 | 0.00 | 0.00 | 0.00 | 0.01 | 0.00 | 0.00 | 0.00 | 0.00 | 0.00 |
| 2653 | 1/2 | cup | Tapioca, prep f/mix, w/2% milk, avg | 141 | 0.13 | 0.14 | 0.30 | 0.04 | 0.82 | 0.08 | 0.11 | 0.24 | 0.38 | 0.31 | 0.10 | 0.19 | 0.38 | 0.21 | 0.17 | 0.05 | 0.19 | 0.26 |
| 2603 | 1/2 | cup | Tapioca, prep f/rec, w/whl milk, avg | 152 | 0.31 | 0.33 | 0.61 | 0.11 | 1.21 | 0.19 | 0.18 | 0.40 | 0.64 | 0.53 | 0.19 | 0.35 | 0.50 | 0.44 | 0.32 | 0.09 | 0.31 | 0.45 |
| 2611 | 1 | ea | Tapioca, RTE, cnd, avg | 142 | 0.10 | 0.10 | 0.21 | 0.03 | 0.57 | 0.06 | 0.07 | 0.16 | 0.26 | 0.21 | 0.07 | 0.13 | 0.26 | 0.15 | 0.12 | 0.04 | 0.13 | 0.18 |
| 2656 | 1 | oz | Vanilla, dry mix, avg | 28 | 0.01 | 0.00 | 0.01 | 0.00 | 0.01 | 0.00 | 0.00 | 0.00 | 0.01 | 0.00 | 0.00 | 0.00 | 0.01 | 0.00 | 0.00 | 0.00 | 0.00 | 0.00 |
| 2655 | 1/2 | cup | Vanilla, prep f/mix, w/2% milk, avg | 142 | 0.13 | 0.13 | 0.28 | 0.03 | 0.78 | 0.08 | 0.10 | 0.23 | 0.37 | 0.30 | 0.09 | 0.18 | 0.36 | 0.20 | 0.17 | 0.05 | 0.18 | 0.25 |
| 2608 | 1/2 | cup | Vanilla, prep f/mix, w/whl milk, avg | 142 | 0.13 | 0.13 | 0.28 | 0.03 | 0.76 | 0.08 | 0.10 | 0.22 | 0.36 | 0.29 | 0.09 | 0.18 | 0.35 | 0.20 | 0.16 | 0.05 | 0.18 | 0.24 |

TABLE A **Amino Acid Content for Selected Foods *(continued)***

| Code | Amount | | Description | Weight (g) | Alanine (g) | Arginine (g) | Aspartic acid (g) | Cystine (g) | Glutamic acid (g) | Glycine (g) | Histidine (g) | Isoleucine (g) | Leucine (g) | Lysine (g) | Methionine (g) | Phenylalanine (g) | Proline (g) | Serine (g) | Threonine (g) | Tryptophan (g) | Tyrosine (g) | Valine (g) |
|---|---|---|---|---|---|---|---|---|---|---|---|---|---|---|---|---|---|---|---|---|---|---|
| 2602 | 1/2 | cup | Vanilla, prep f/rec, w/whl milk, avg | 123 | 0.13 | 0.14 | 0.29 | 0.04 | 0.80 | 0.08 | 0.11 | 0.23 | 0.38 | 0.30 | 0.10 | 0.18 | 0.37 | 0.21 | 0.17 | 0.05 | 0.18 | 0.26 |
| 2612 | 1 | ea | Vanilla, RTS, cnd, avg | 142 | 0.11 | 0.11 | 0.24 | 0.03 | 0.65 | 0.07 | 0.09 | 0.19 | 0.31 | 0.25 | 0.08 | 0.15 | 0.30 | 0.17 | 0.14 | 0.04 | 0.15 | 0.21 |
| 2662 | 1/2 | cup | Vanilla, rennin, prep f/mix, w/2%milk, avg | 133 | 0.13 | 0.14 | 0.29 | 0.04 | 0.81 | 0.08 | 0.11 | 0.24 | 0.38 | 0.31 | 0.10 | 0.19 | 0.38 | 0.21 | 0.18 | 0.05 | 0.19 | 0.26 |
| 2663 | 1/2 | cup | Vanilla, rennin, prep f/mix, w/whl milk, avg | 133 | 0.13 | 0.14 | 0.29 | 0.04 | 0.80 | 0.08 | 0.11 | 0.23 | 0.37 | 0.30 | 0.09 | 0.18 | 0.37 | 0.21 | 0.17 | 0.05 | 0.18 | 0.25 |
| 2664 | 1/2 | cup | Vanilla, rennin, prep f/rec, avg | 137 | 0.13 | 0.14 | 0.29 | 0.04 | 0.80 | 0.08 | 0.11 | 0.23 | 0.38 | 0.30 | 0.10 | 0.18 | 0.37 | 0.21 | 0.17 | 0.05 | 0.18 | 0.26 |
| | | | **DESSERT TOPPINGS** | | | | | | | | | | | | | | | | | | | |
| 23069 | 2 | Tbs | Butterscotch Topping, avg | 41 | 0.02 | 0.02 | 0.04 | 0.01 | 0.12 | 0.01 | 0.02 | 0.04 | 0.06 | 0.05 | 0.01 | 0.03 | 0.06 | 0.03 | 0.03 | 0.01 | 0.03 | 0.04 |
| 23070 | 2 | Tbs | Caramel Topping, avg | 41 | 0.02 | 0.02 | 0.04 | 0.01 | 0.12 | 0.01 | 0.02 | 0.04 | 0.06 | 0.05 | 0.01 | 0.03 | 0.06 | 0.03 | 0.03 | 0.01 | 0.03 | 0.04 |
| 46037 | 2 | Tbs | Chocolate Frosting, RTE, avg | 29 | 0.01 | 0.02 | 0.03 | 0.00 | 0.05 | 0.01 | 0.01 | 0.01 | 0.02 | 0.02 | 0.00 | 0.02 | 0.01 | 0.01 | 0.01 | 0.00 | 0.01 | 0.02 |
| 23056 | 2 | Tbs | Chocolate Topping, avg | 38 | 0.03 | 0.03 | 0.06 | 0.01 | 0.09 | 0.03 | 0.01 | 0.02 | 0.04 | 0.03 | 0.01 | 0.03 | 0.02 | 0.02 | 0.02 | 0.01 | 0.02 | 0.03 |
| 23014 | 2 | Tbs | Chocolate fudge Topping, avg | 42 | 0.09 | 0.09 | 0.19 | 0.03 | 0.32 | 0.06 | 0.04 | 0.09 | 0.15 | 0.12 | 0.03 | 0.08 | 0.11 | 0.09 | 0.09 | 0.03 | 0.07 | 0.11 |
| 46211 | 1 | ea | Coconut Frosting, RTE, can, avg | 462 | 0.29 | 0.95 | 0.60 | 0.16 | 1.33 | 0.31 | 0.13 | 0.26 | 0.44 | 0.25 | 0.14 | 0.33 | 0.29 | 0.31 | 0.22 | 0.14 | 0.23 | 0.34 |
| 46212 | 1 | ea | Cream Cheese Frosting, RTE, can, avg | 462 | 0.01 | 0.01 | 0.01 | 0.00 | 0.08 | 0.01 | 0.00 | 0.01 | 0.02 | 0.01 | 0.00 | 0.01 | 0.03 | 0.01 | 0.01 | 0.00 | 0.01 | 0.01 |
| 23071 | 2 | Tbs | Marshmallow Crème Topping, avg | 38 | 0.03 | 0.03 | 0.02 | 0.00 | 0.04 | 0.07 | 0.00 | 0.00 | 0.01 | 0.01 | 0.00 | 0.01 | 0.05 | 0.01 | 0.01 | 0.00 | 0.00 | 0.01 |
| 46042 | 1 | ea | Sour Cream Frosting, RTE, can, avg | 462 | 0.02 | 0.02 | 0.02 | 0.01 | 0.14 | 0.01 | 0.01 | 0.02 | 0.03 | 0.02 | 0.01 | 0.02 | 0.05 | 0.03 | 0.01 | 0.01 | 0.02 | 0.02 |
| | | | Vanilla Frosting | | | | | | | | | | | | | | | | | | | |
| 46043 | 1 | ea | Dry Mix pkg, avg | 411 | 0.08 | 0.05 | 0.08 | 0.02 | 0.21 | 0.04 | 0.03 | 0.04 | 0.14 | 0.02 | 0.02 | 0.05 | 0.10 | 0.05 | 0.04 | 0.00 | 0.04 | 0.05 |
| 46044 | 2 | Tbs | Prep f/mix, w/butter, avg | 40 | 0.00 | 0.00 | 0.01 | 0.00 | 0.02 | 0.00 | 0.00 | 0.00 | 0.01 | 0.00 | 0.00 | 0.00 | 0.01 | 0.00 | 0.00 | 0.00 | 0.00 | 0.00 |
| 46045 | 2 | Tbs | Prep f/recipe, w/butter, avg | 40 | 0.01 | 0.01 | 0.02 | 0.00 | 0.05 | 0.00 | 0.01 | 0.01 | 0.02 | 0.02 | 0.01 | 0.01 | 0.02 | 0.01 | 0.01 | 0.00 | 0.01 | 0.02 |
| 46046 | 2 | Tbs | Prep f/recipe, w/marg, avg | 40 | 0.00 | 0.00 | 0.01 | 0.00 | 0.03 | 0.00 | 0.00 | 0.01 | 0.01 | 0.01 | 0.00 | 0.01 | 0.01 | 0.01 | 0.01 | 0.00 | 0.01 | 0.01 |
| 46009 | 2 | Tbs | RTE, avg | 31 | 0.00 | 0.00 | 0.00 | 0.00 | 0.01 | 0.00 | 0.00 | 0.00 | 0.00 | 0.00 | 0.00 | 0.00 | 0.00 | 0.00 | 0.00 | 0.00 | 0.00 | 0.00 |
| | | | White Frosting | | | | | | | | | | | | | | | | | | | |
| 46047 | 1 | ea | Dry Mix pkg, avg | 207 | 0.31 | 0.28 | 0.46 | 0.10 | 0.62 | 0.31 | 0.11 | 0.24 | 0.37 | 0.31 | 0.15 | 0.25 | 0.27 | 0.30 | 0.20 | 0.05 | 0.16 | 0.28 |
| 46048 | 2 | Tbs | Prep f/Mix, avg | 40 | 0.04 | 0.04 | 0.06 | 0.01 | 0.08 | 0.04 | 0.01 | 0.03 | 0.05 | 0.04 | 0.02 | 0.03 | 0.03 | 0.04 | 0.03 | 0.01 | 0.02 | 0.04 |
| 46041 | 2 | Tbs | Prep f/Recipe, avg | 40 | 0.04 | 0.04 | 0.07 | 0.02 | 0.09 | 0.02 | 0.01 | 0.04 | 0.06 | 0.04 | 0.02 | 0.04 | 0.03 | 0.05 | 0.03 | 0.01 | 0.03 | 0.04 |
| | | | **EGGS, SUBSTITUTES, EGG DISHES** | | | | | | | | | | | | | | | | | | | |
| | | | Chicken Egg Whites | | | | | | | | | | | | | | | | | | | |
| 19522 | 1 | ea | Cooked, avg | 33 | 0.20 | 0.19 | 0.35 | 0.09 | 0.46 | 0.12 | 0.08 | 0.20 | 0.29 | 0.24 | 0.12 | 0.20 | 0.14 | 0.24 | 0.16 | 0.04 | 0.14 | 0.22 |
| 19609 | 1/4 | cup | Dried, avg | 27 | 1.26 | 1.19 | 2.23 | 0.57 | 2.92 | 0.77 | 0.43 | 1.24 | 1.85 | 1.49 | 0.75 | 1.28 | 0.85 | 1.51 | 1.00 | 0.27 | 0.85 | 1.39 |
| 19506 | 1 | ea | Raw, avg | 33 | 0.20 | 0.19 | 0.35 | 0.09 | 0.46 | 0.12 | 0.08 | 0.20 | 0.29 | 0.24 | 0.12 | 0.20 | 0.13 | 0.24 | 0.16 | 0.04 | 0.13 | 0.22 |
| 19608 | 1 | ea | Raw, fzn, avg | 33 | 0.19 | 0.18 | 0.33 | 0.08 | 0.43 | 0.11 | 0.07 | 0.18 | 0.27 | 0.22 | 0.11 | 0.19 | 0.13 | 0.22 | 0.15 | 0.04 | 0.13 | 0.21 |
| | | | Chicken Egg Yolks | | | | | | | | | | | | | | | | | | | |
| 19523 | 1 | ea | Cooked, avg | 17 | 0.15 | 0.20 | 0.28 | 0.05 | 0.36 | 0.09 | 0.07 | 0.14 | 0.25 | 0.23 | 0.07 | 0.12 | 0.12 | 0.24 | 0.15 | 0.03 | 0.13 | 0.16 |
| 19571 | 1/4 | cup | Dried, avg | 17 | 0.30 | 0.41 | 0.57 | 0.10 | 0.74 | 0.18 | 0.15 | 0.29 | 0.51 | 0.46 | 0.14 | 0.25 | 0.24 | 0.50 | 0.31 | 0.07 | 0.26 | 0.32 |
| 19572 | 1 | oz | Frozen, avg | 28 | 0.22 | 0.31 | 0.43 | 0.08 | 0.55 | 0.13 | 0.11 | 0.22 | 0.38 | 0.34 | 0.11 | 0.19 | 0.18 | 0.37 | 0.23 | 0.05 | 0.19 | 0.24 |
| 19532 | 1/4 | cup | Frozen, salted, avg | 61 | 0.44 | 0.61 | 0.84 | 0.15 | 1.08 | 0.26 | 0.22 | 0.43 | 0.75 | 0.68 | 0.21 | 0.36 | 0.36 | 0.73 | 0.45 | 0.10 | 0.38 | 0.48 |
| 19566 | 1 | oz | Frozen, sugared, avg | 28 | 0.20 | 0.28 | 0.38 | 0.07 | 0.49 | 0.12 | 0.11 | 0.20 | 0.34 | 0.31 | 0.10 | 0.17 | 0.16 | 0.33 | 0.21 | 0.05 | 0.17 | 0.22 |
| 19508 | 1/4 | cup | Raw, avg | 61 | 0.53 | 0.73 | 1.00 | 0.18 | 1.29 | 0.32 | 0.25 | 0.52 | 0.90 | 0.81 | 0.25 | 0.44 | 0.43 | 0.87 | 0.54 | 0.12 | 0.46 | 0.57 |
| | | | Chicken Whole Eggs | | | | | | | | | | | | | | | | | | | |
| 19538 | 1/4 | cup | Creamed, avg | 60 | 0.23 | 0.25 | 0.13 | 0.09 | 0.73 | 0.14 | 0.11 | 0.25 | 0.41 | 0.33 | 0.14 | 0.24 | 0.26 | 0.32 | 0.21 | 0.06 | 0.19 | 0.28 |
| 19539 | 1 | ea | Deviled, avg | 31 | 0.20 | 0.22 | 0.36 | 0.08 | 0.47 | 0.12 | 0.08 | 0.20 | 0.31 | 0.26 | 0.11 | 0.19 | 0.14 | 0.27 | 0.17 | 0.04 | 0.15 | 0.22 |
| 19527 | 1/4 | cup | Dried, avg | 21 | 0.55 | 0.60 | 1.00 | 0.23 | 1.30 | 0.33 | 0.24 | 0.54 | 0.85 | 0.71 | 0.31 | 0.53 | 0.40 | 0.74 | 0.48 | 0.12 | 0.41 | 0.61 |
| 19509 | 1 | ea | Fried, avg | 46 | 0.35 | 0.37 | 0.62 | 0.14 | 0.81 | 0.21 | 0.15 | 0.34 | 0.53 | 0.45 | 0.19 | 0.33 | 0.25 | 0.46 | 0.30 | 0.08 | 0.25 | 0.38 |
| 19604 | 1 | ea | Frozen, avg | 50 | 0.33 | 0.36 | 0.60 | 0.14 | 0.78 | 0.20 | 0.14 | 0.33 | 0.51 | 0.43 | 0.19 | 0.32 | 0.24 | 0.44 | 0.29 | 0.07 | 0.24 | 0.36 |
| 19510 | 1 | ea | Hard Cooked/Boiled, avg | 50 | 0.35 | 0.38 | 0.63 | 0.15 | 0.82 | 0.21 | 0.15 | 0.34 | 0.54 | 0.45 | 0.20 | 0.33 | 0.25 | 0.47 | 0.30 | 0.08 | 0.26 | 0.38 |
| 19534 | 1 | ea | Omelet, plain, w/milk & butter, avg | 61 | 0.35 | 0.38 | 0.63 | 0.15 | 0.82 | 0.21 | 0.15 | 0.34 | 0.54 | 0.45 | 0.20 | 0.33 | 0.25 | 0.47 | 0.30 | 0.08 | 0.26 | 0.38 |
| 19614 | 1 | ea | Omelet, w/chicken, avg | 95 | 0.65 | 0.71 | 1.14 | 0.22 | 1.73 | 0.47 | 0.32 | 0.66 | 1.00 | 0.94 | 0.36 | 0.58 | 0.53 | 0.70 | 0.55 | 0.15 | 0.47 | 0.69 |
| 19611 | 1 | ea | Omelet, w/dark green vegs, avg | 84 | 0.36 | 0.39 | 0.66 | 0.14 | 0.93 | 0.23 | 0.15 | 0.37 | 0.59 | 0.49 | 0.20 | 0.35 | 0.31 | 0.48 | 0.32 | 0.09 | 0.28 | 0.37 |
| 19610 | 1 | ea | Omelet, w/fish, avg | 88 | 0.55 | 0.59 | 0.95 | 0.18 | 1.35 | 0.35 | 0.25 | 0.56 | 0.88 | 0.73 | 0.30 | 0.49 | 0.41 | 0.62 | 0.46 | 0.14 | 0.38 | 0.63 |
| 19612 | 1 | ea | Omelet, w/mushrooms, avg | 69 | 0.32 | 0.33 | 0.57 | 0.12 | 0.81 | 0.19 | 0.14 | 0.32 | 0.50 | 0.43 | 0.17 | 0.30 | 0.27 | 0.41 | 0.28 | 0.07 | 0.24 | 0.35 |

TABLE A **Amino Acid Content for Selected Foods *(continued)***

| Code | Amount | Description | Weight (g) | Alanine (g) | Arginine (g) | Aspartic acid (g) | Cystine (g) | Glutamic acid (g) | Glycine (g) | Histidine (g) | Isoleucine (g) | Leucine (g) | Lysine (g) | Methionine (g) | Phenylalanine (g) | Proline (g) | Serine (g) | Threonine (g) | Tryptophan (g) | Tyrosine (g) | Valine (g) |
|---|---|---|---|---|---|---|---|---|---|---|---|---|---|---|---|---|---|---|---|---|---|
| 19613 | 1 ea | Omelet, w/sausage, avg | 95 | 0.56 | 0.59 | 0.95 | 0.18 | 1.42 | 0.43 | 0.26 | 0.50 | 0.82 | 0.76 | 0.29 | 0.47 | 0.47 | 0.62 | 0.46 | 0.11 | 0.38 | 0.55 |
| 19517 | 1 ea | Poached, avg | 50 | 0.35 | 0.37 | 0.62 | 0.14 | 0.81 | 0.21 | 0.15 | 0.34 | 0.53 | 0.45 | 0.19 | 0.33 | 0.25 | 0.46 | 0.30 | 0.08 | 0.25 | 0.38 |
| 19501 | 1 ea | Raw, avg | 50 | 0.35 | 0.37 | 0.63 | 0.14 | 0.81 | 0.21 | 0.15 | 0.34 | 0.54 | 0.45 | 0.19 | 0.33 | 0.25 | 0.46 | 0.30 | 0.08 | 0.25 | 0.38 |
| 19516 | 1 ea | Scrambled, avg | 61 | 0.36 | 0.39 | 0.66 | 0.15 | 0.92 | 0.22 | 0.16 | 0.37 | 0.58 | 0.49 | 0.21 | 0.36 | 0.30 | 0.49 | 0.32 | 0.08 | 0.28 | 0.41 |
| 19620 | 1/2 cup | Scrambled, no choles, avg | 70 | 0.50 | 0.46 | 0.73 | 0.18 | 1.34 | 0.29 | 0.20 | 0.52 | 0.77 | 0.57 | 0.31 | 0.51 | 0.44 | 0.60 | 0.38 | 0.13 | 0.36 | 0.63 |
| 19621 | 1/2 cup | Scrambled, no choles, w/cheese, avg | 70 | 0.50 | 0.46 | 0.73 | 0.18 | 1.34 | 0.29 | 0.20 | 0.52 | 0.77 | 0.57 | 0.31 | 0.51 | 0.44 | 0.60 | 0.38 | 0.13 | 0.36 | 0.63 |
| 19540 | 1/2 cup | Scrambled, prep f/dry, avg | 107 | 0.56 | 0.61 | 0.95 | 0.23 | 1.24 | 0.32 | 0.23 | 0.60 | 0.85 | 0.65 | 0.31 | 0.54 | 0.39 | 0.73 | 0.47 | 0.15 | 0.40 | 0.69 |
| 19551 | 1/2 cup | Scrambled, prep f/fzn, avg | 70 | 0.51 | 0.47 | 0.76 | 0.19 | 1.38 | 0.30 | 0.21 | 0.54 | 0.79 | 0.58 | 0.31 | 0.53 | 0.46 | 0.61 | 0.39 | 0.13 | 0.37 | 0.65 |
| 19552 | 1/2 cup | Scrambled, prep f/liquid, avg | 105 | 0.83 | 0.86 | 1.31 | 0.32 | 2.08 | 0.54 | 0.32 | 0.82 | 1.19 | 0.86 | 0.47 | 0.84 | 0.58 | 0.97 | 0.61 | 0.21 | 0.54 | 0.97 |
| | | Other Eggs | | | | | | | | | | | | | | | | | | | |
| 19528 | 1 ea | Duck, raw, avg | 70 | 0.44 | 0.53 | 0.54 | 0.20 | 1.23 | 0.29 | 0.22 | 0.41 | 0.76 | 0.66 | 0.40 | 0.58 | 0.33 | 0.66 | 0.51 | 0.18 | 0.42 | 0.61 |
| 19529 | 1 ea | Goose,raw, avg | 144 | 0.97 | 1.18 | 1.20 | 0.44 | 2.76 | 0.65 | 0.49 | 0.92 | 1.69 | 1.47 | 0.89 | 1.29 | 0.74 | 1.48 | 1.13 | 0.40 | 0.94 | 1.36 |
| 19530 | 1 ea | Quail, raw, avg | 9 | 0.07 | 0.07 | 0.11 | 0.03 | 0.15 | 0.04 | 0.03 | 0.07 | 0.10 | 0.08 | 0.04 | 0.06 | 0.05 | 0.09 | 0.06 | 0.02 | 0.05 | 0.08 |
| 19531 | 1 ea | Turkey, raw, avg | 79 | 0.61 | 0.67 | 1.04 | 0.25 | 1.34 | 0.35 | 0.25 | 0.66 | 0.92 | 0.71 | 0.34 | 0.59 | 0.42 | 0.80 | 0.52 | 0.17 | 0.44 | 0.76 |
| | | Substitutes | | | | | | | | | | | | | | | | | | | |
| 19524 | 1/4 cup | Frozen, avg | 60 | 0.37 | 0.35 | 0.56 | 0.14 | 1.01 | 0.22 | 0.15 | 0.40 | 0.58 | 0.43 | 0.23 | 0.39 | 0.33 | 0.45 | 0.29 | 0.10 | 0.27 | 0.48 |
| 19525 | 1/4 cup | Liquid, avg | 63 | 0.44 | 0.45 | 0.69 | 0.17 | 1.10 | 0.28 | 0.17 | 0.43 | 0.62 | 0.46 | 0.25 | 0.44 | 0.30 | 0.51 | 0.32 | 0.11 | 0.29 | 0.51 |
| 19526 | 1 oz | Powder, avg | 28 | 0.95 | 0.90 | 1.36 | 0.37 | 2.06 | 0.55 | 0.35 | 0.92 | 1.31 | 0.94 | 0.57 | 0.93 | 0.57 | 1.11 | 0.68 | 0.23 | 0.61 | 1.12 |
| | | **FAST FOODS, GENERIC** | | | | | | | | | | | | | | | | | | | |
| | | Breakfast Items | | | | | | | | | | | | | | | | | | | |
| 56600 | 1 ea | Biscuit w/Egg | 136 | 0.51 | 0.58 | 0.85 | 0.23 | 2.22 | 0.36 | 0.26 | 0.58 | 0.90 | 0.59 | 0.29 | 0.58 | 0.77 | 0.71 | 0.45 | 0.16 | 0.42 | 0.66 |
| 56601 | 1 ea | Biscuit w/Egg & Bacon | 150 | 0.84 | 0.94 | 1.34 | 0.29 | 3.06 | 0.77 | 0.43 | 0.82 | 1.31 | 1.02 | 0.42 | 0.81 | 1.09 | 0.94 | 0.68 | 0.22 | 0.59 | 0.95 |
| 56602 | 1 ea | Biscuit w/Egg & Ham | 192 | 1.06 | 1.19 | 1.73 | 0.37 | 3.77 | 0.84 | 0.59 | 1.00 | 1.65 | 1.38 | 0.54 | 0.99 | 1.19 | 1.10 | 0.87 | 0.27 | 0.73 | 1.08 |
| 66028 | 1 ea | Biscuit w/Egg & Sausage | 180 | 0.97 | 1.07 | 1.54 | 0.33 | 3.53 | 0.83 | 0.50 | 0.92 | 1.50 | 1.20 | 0.49 | 0.90 | 1.21 | 1.07 | 0.79 | 0.25 | 0.68 | 1.05 |
| 56603 | 1 ea | Biscuit w/Egg & Steak | 148 | 0.93 | 1.01 | 1.48 | 0.30 | 3.18 | 0.74 | 0.50 | 0.87 | 1.43 | 1.18 | 0.46 | 0.83 | 1.04 | 0.94 | 0.75 | 0.23 | 0.64 | 0.98 |
| 66029 | 1 ea | Biscuit w/Egg, Cheese & Bacon | 144 | 0.71 | 0.84 | 1.21 | 0.24 | 3.01 | 0.63 | 0.46 | 0.77 | 1.29 | 1.11 | 0.40 | 0.78 | 1.17 | 0.86 | 0.62 | 0.21 | 0.64 | 0.92 |
| 56604 | 1 ea | Biscuit w/Ham | 113 | 0.68 | 0.77 | 1.08 | 0.22 | 2.89 | 0.62 | 0.43 | 0.58 | 1.06 | 0.92 | 0.33 | 0.62 | 0.90 | 0.60 | 0.54 | 0.17 | 0.45 | 0.60 |
| 66030 | 1 ea | Biscuit w/Sausage | 124 | 0.53 | 0.60 | 0.79 | 0.19 | 2.98 | 0.57 | 0.32 | 0.48 | 0.90 | 0.65 | 0.26 | 0.53 | 1.05 | 0.56 | 0.43 | 0.14 | 0.39 | 0.55 |
| 56605 | 1 ea | Biscuit w/Steak | 141 | 0.62 | 0.68 | 0.94 | 0.19 | 2.92 | 0.58 | 0.38 | 0.56 | 1.01 | 0.79 | 0.30 | 0.57 | 0.98 | 0.57 | 0.49 | 0.16 | 0.44 | 0.62 |
| 56606 | 1 ea | Croissant w/Egg & Cheese | 127 | 0.47 | 0.60 | 0.89 | 0.19 | 2.60 | 0.33 | 0.39 | 0.63 | 1.06 | 0.92 | 0.33 | 0.66 | 1.06 | 0.72 | 0.47 | 0.18 | 0.57 | 0.76 |
| 56607 | 1 ea | Croissant w/Egg, Cheese & Bacon | 129 | 0.64 | 0.80 | 1.16 | 0.23 | 3.21 | 0.50 | 0.50 | 0.79 | 1.34 | 1.18 | 0.42 | 0.81 | 1.30 | 0.89 | 0.61 | 0.22 | 0.70 | 0.95 |
| 56608 | 1 ea | Croissant w/Egg, Cheese & Ham | 152 | 0.90 | 1.04 | 1.52 | 0.31 | 3.57 | 0.70 | 0.59 | 0.90 | 1.54 | 1.37 | 0.49 | 0.92 | 1.23 | 0.99 | 0.77 | 0.26 | 0.73 | 1.01 |
| 56609 | 1 ea | Croissant w/Egg, Cheese & Sausage | 160 | 0.93 | 1.08 | 1.54 | 0.30 | 3.78 | 0.80 | 0.58 | 0.95 | 1.60 | 1.41 | 0.51 | 0.95 | 1.40 | 1.07 | 0.79 | 0.26 | 0.78 | 1.11 |
| 66031 | 1 ea | English Muffins w/Cheese & Sausage | 115 | 0.61 | 0.74 | 1.02 | 0.17 | 3.27 | 0.59 | 0.49 | 0.63 | 1.18 | 1.12 | 0.35 | 0.69 | 1.29 | 0.69 | 0.53 | 0.19 | 0.61 | 0.76 |
| 66033 | 1 ea | English Muffins w/Egg, Cheese & Sausage | 165 | 0.92 | 1.10 | 1.57 | 0.30 | 4.19 | 0.79 | 0.66 | 0.98 | 1.72 | 1.56 | 0.53 | 1.01 | 1.62 | 1.10 | 0.81 | 0.28 | 0.87 | 1.16 |
| 66032 | 1 ea | English Muffins w/Egg, Cheese & Canadian Bacon | 146 | 0.78 | 0.93 | 1.37 | 0.28 | 3.41 | 0.58 | 0.57 | 0.86 | 1.46 | 1.30 | 0.48 | 0.87 | 1.25 | 0.98 | 0.70 | 0.24 | 0.73 | 1.00 |
| 19533 | 1 ea | Scrambled Eggs | 47 | 0.36 | 0.39 | 0.61 | 0.14 | 0.83 | 0.21 | 0.15 | 0.39 | 0.56 | 0.43 | 0.20 | 0.35 | 0.27 | 0.47 | 0.31 | 0.10 | 0.26 | 0.45 |
| | | Chicken | | | | | | | | | | | | | | | | | | | |
| 15065 | 1 pce | Pieces, breaded, fried | 17 | 0.14 | 0.16 | 0.23 | 0.04 | 0.49 | 0.13 | 0.08 | 0.14 | 0.21 | 0.21 | 0.07 | 0.12 | 0.15 | 0.11 | 0.11 | 0.03 | 0.09 | 0.14 |
| 15066 | 6 pce | Pieces, breaded, fried w/barbeque sauce | 130 | 0.86 | 0.97 | 1.39 | 0.25 | 2.94 | 0.78 | 0.49 | 0.85 | 1.25 | 1.26 | 0.44 | 0.70 | 0.87 | 0.65 | 0.68 | 0.20 | 0.56 | 0.83 |
| 15180 | 6 pce | Pieces, breaded, fried w/honey | 115 | 0.86 | 0.96 | 1.39 | 0.24 | 2.93 | 0.78 | 0.49 | 0.85 | 1.25 | 1.25 | 0.44 | 0.70 | 0.88 | 0.65 | 0.68 | 0.20 | 0.56 | 0.83 |
| 15067 | 6 pce | Pieces, breaded, fried w/mustard sauce | 130 | 0.86 | 0.97 | 1.39 | 0.25 | 2.94 | 0.78 | 0.49 | 0.85 | 1.25 | 1.26 | 0.44 | 0.70 | 0.87 | 0.65 | 0.68 | 0.20 | 0.56 | 0.83 |
| 15068 | 6 pce | Pieces, breaded, fried w/sweet & sour sauce | 130 | 0.86 | 0.97 | 1.39 | 0.25 | 2.94 | 0.78 | 0.49 | 0.85 | 1.25 | 1.26 | 0.44 | 0.70 | 0.87 | 0.65 | 0.68 | 0.20 | 0.56 | 0.83 |
| | | Desserts | | | | | | | | | | | | | | | | | | | |
| 47150 | 1 ea | Brownie, w/out nuts | 60 | 0.09 | 0.11 | 0.17 | 0.04 | 0.62 | 0.08 | 0.06 | 0.12 | 0.20 | 0.13 | 0.05 | 0.12 | 0.24 | 0.13 | 0.09 | 0.03 | 0.10 | 0.14 |
| 66034 | 1 ea | Caramel Sundae | 155 | 0.24 | 0.25 | 0.53 | 0.06 | 1.46 | 0.15 | 0.19 | 0.42 | 0.68 | 0.55 | 0.17 | 0.34 | 0.67 | 0.38 | 0.31 | 0.10 | 0.34 | 0.47 |
| 45588 | 1 ea | Danish Pastry, cheese | 91 | 0.24 | 0.28 | 0.37 | 0.10 | 1.41 | 0.18 | 0.14 | 0.26 | 0.46 | 0.28 | 0.13 | 0.29 | 0.53 | 0.31 | 0.21 | 0.07 | 0.22 | 0.30 |
| 45512 | 1 ea | Danish Pastry, cinnamon | 88 | 0.19 | 0.22 | 0.29 | 0.10 | 1.26 | 0.16 | 0.11 | 0.21 | 0.36 | 0.20 | 0.11 | 0.24 | 0.44 | 0.27 | 0.17 | 0.06 | 0.17 | 0.24 |
| 45513 | 1 ea | Danish Pastry, fruit | 94 | 0.19 | 0.22 | 0.29 | 0.09 | 1.25 | 0.16 | 0.11 | 0.21 | 0.36 | 0.19 | 0.10 | 0.24 | 0.43 | 0.27 | 0.17 | 0.06 | 0.17 | 0.24 |
| 2035 | 1/2 cup | Frozen Yogurt, chocolate, soft serve | 72 | 0.11 | 0.12 | 0.23 | 0.03 | 0.55 | 0.08 | 0.07 | 0.15 | 0.25 | 0.20 | 0.06 | 0.14 | 0.23 | 0.14 | 0.12 | 0.04 | 0.13 | 0.18 |

TABLE A **Amino Acid Content for Selected Foods *(continued)***

| Code | Amount | Description | Weight (g) | Alanine (g) | Arginine (g) | Aspartic acid (g) | Cystine (g) | Glutamic acid (g) | Glycine (g) | Histidine (g) | Isoleucine (g) | Leucine (g) | Lysine (g) | Methionine (g) | Phenylalanine (g) | Proline (g) | Serine (g) | Threonine (g) | Tryptophan (g) | Tyrosine (g) | Valine (g) |
|---|---|---|---|---|---|---|---|---|---|---|---|---|---|---|---|---|---|---|---|---|---|
| 2064 | 1/2 cup | Frozen Yogurt, vanilla, soft serve | 72 | 0.09 | 0.10 | 0.21 | 0.03 | 0.57 | 0.06 | 0.07 | 0.16 | 0.26 | 0.21 | 0.07 | 0.13 | 0.26 | 0.15 | 0.12 | 0.04 | 0.13 | 0.18 |
| 2032 | 1 ea | Hot Fudge Sundae | 158 | 0.19 | 0.21 | 0.41 | 0.05 | 0.96 | 0.14 | 0.12 | 0.27 | 0.44 | 0.35 | 0.10 | 0.24 | 0.41 | 0.26 | 0.22 | 0.07 | 0.23 | 0.32 |
| 2031 | 1 ea | Ice Milk Cone, soft serve, svg | 103 | 0.13 | 0.14 | 0.27 | 0.04 | 0.84 | 0.09 | 0.10 | 0.21 | 0.35 | 0.27 | 0.09 | 0.18 | 0.37 | 0.20 | 0.16 | 0.05 | 0.17 | 0.24 |
| 49117 | 1 ea | Lemon Pie | 128 | 0.12 | 0.14 | 0.20 | 0.03 | 1.16 | 0.13 | 0.08 | 0.15 | 0.27 | 0.15 | 0.07 | 0.18 | 0.40 | 0.20 | 0.11 | 0.05 | 0.12 | 0.18 |
| 2033 | 1 ea | Strawberry sundae | 153 | 0.21 | 0.22 | 0.49 | 0.05 | 1.23 | 0.13 | 0.16 | 0.35 | 0.57 | 0.46 | 0.14 | 0.28 | 0.56 | 0.32 | 0.27 | 0.08 | 0.28 | 0.39 |
| 7208 | 1 ea | French Fries, medium svg | 76 | 0.10 | 0.14 | 0.70 | 0.02 | 0.47 | 0.11 | 0.05 | 0.13 | 0.18 | 0.16 | 0.03 | 0.13 | 0.10 | 0.11 | 0.14 | 0.04 | 0.08 | 0.15 |
| 56666 | 5 pce | Hushpuppies | 78 | 0.31 | 0.26 | 0.38 | 0.09 | 0.83 | 0.17 | 0.13 | 0.23 | 0.52 | 0.23 | 0.12 | 0.24 | 0.35 | 0.27 | 0.20 | 0.05 | 0.20 | 0.28 |
| | | Milkshakes | | | | | | | | | | | | | | | | | | | |
| 2020 | 1 cup | Chocolate | 166 | 0.18 | 0.19 | 0.41 | 0.05 | 1.13 | 0.11 | 0.15 | 0.33 | 0.53 | 0.43 | 0.13 | 0.26 | 0.52 | 0.29 | 0.24 | 0.08 | 0.26 | 0.36 |
| 2022 | 1 cup | Strawberry | 226 | 0.25 | 0.26 | 0.55 | 0.07 | 1.53 | 0.16 | 0.20 | 0.44 | 0.72 | 0.58 | 0.18 | 0.35 | 0.71 | 0.40 | 0.33 | 0.10 | 0.35 | 0.49 |
| 2024 | 1 cup | Vanilla | 166 | 0.19 | 0.20 | 0.42 | 0.05 | 1.16 | 0.12 | 0.15 | 0.34 | 0.54 | 0.44 | 0.14 | 0.27 | 0.53 | 0.30 | 0.25 | 0.08 | 0.27 | 0.37 |
| 6176 | 8 1/2 pce | Onion Rings | 83 | 0.12 | 0.22 | 0.17 | 0.07 | 1.15 | 0.14 | 0.08 | 0.15 | 0.24 | 0.10 | 0.06 | 0.17 | 0.36 | 0.18 | 0.10 | 0.05 | 0.11 | 0.15 |
| | | Potatoes | | | | | | | | | | | | | | | | | | | |
| 6177 | 1 ea | Baked w/Cheese Sauce | 296 | 0.40 | 0.56 | 1.71 | 0.10 | 3.02 | 0.30 | 0.42 | 0.76 | 1.16 | 1.04 | 0.31 | 0.69 | 1.20 | 0.74 | 0.49 | 0.19 | 0.62 | 0.87 |
| 6178 | 1 ea | Baked w/Cheese Sauce & Bacon | 299 | 0.59 | 0.78 | 2.10 | 0.14 | 3.68 | 0.52 | 0.54 | 0.94 | 1.45 | 1.35 | 0.40 | 0.86 | 1.46 | 0.91 | 0.65 | 0.23 | 0.75 | 1.09 |
| 6179 | 1 ea | Baked w/Cheese sauce & Broccoli | 339 | 0.40 | 0.54 | 1.55 | 0.10 | 2.72 | 0.29 | 0.38 | 0.69 | 1.03 | 0.95 | 0.28 | 0.62 | 1.06 | 0.67 | 0.46 | 0.17 | 0.55 | 0.80 |
| 6180 | 1 ea | Baked w/Cheese Sauce & Chili | 395 | 0.76 | 1.00 | 2.62 | 0.18 | 4.66 | 0.64 | 0.67 | 1.15 | 1.82 | 1.67 | 0.49 | 1.06 | 1.75 | 1.13 | 0.81 | 0.29 | 0.91 | 1.33 |
| 5463 | 1/2 cup | Hash Browns | 72 | 0.07 | 0.09 | 0.45 | 0.01 | 0.30 | 0.07 | 0.03 | 0.08 | 0.12 | 0.10 | 0.02 | 0.08 | 0.06 | 0.07 | 0.09 | 0.03 | 0.05 | 0.10 |
| 6185 | 1/3 cup | Mashed | 80 | 0.06 | 0.08 | 0.37 | 0.02 | 0.33 | 0.05 | 0.04 | 0.08 | 0.13 | 0.12 | 0.03 | 0.08 | 0.09 | 0.08 | 0.07 | 0.03 | 0.07 | 0.11 |
| | | Salads | | | | | | | | | | | | | | | | | | | |
| 56628 | 1 1/2 cup | Chef Style, w/turkey, ham & cheese | 326 | 1.29 | 1.49 | 2.28 | 0.29 | 4.63 | 1.02 | 0.81 | 1.34 | 2.09 | 2.14 | 0.67 | 1.13 | 1.49 | 1.22 | 1.07 | 0.30 | 0.99 | 1.39 |
| 5461 | 3/4 cup | Coleslaw | 99 | 0.06 | 0.09 | 0.14 | 0.02 | 0.27 | 0.04 | 0.03 | 0.07 | 0.08 | 0.07 | 0.02 | 0.05 | 0.19 | 0.08 | 0.05 | 0.02 | 0.03 | 0.06 |
| 6173 | 1/3 cup | Potato | 95 | 0.07 | 0.08 | 0.22 | 0.02 | 0.19 | 0.05 | 0.03 | 0.08 | 0.13 | 0.09 | 0.03 | 0.10 | 0.06 | 0.07 | 0.07 | 0.02 | 0.06 | 0.08 |
| 56623 | 1 1/2 cup | Tossed Vegetable, w/o dressing | 207 | 0.10 | 0.13 | 0.28 | 0.03 | 0.47 | 0.10 | 0.05 | 0.14 | 0.14 | 0.14 | 0.03 | 0.10 | 0.15 | 0.09 | 0.10 | 0.02 | 0.06 | 0.12 |
| | | Sandwiches, Cheeseburger | | | | | | | | | | | | | | | | | | | |
| 66016 | 1 ea | Double, plain | 155 | 1.43 | 1.60 | 2.19 | 0.28 | 5.29 | 1.55 | 0.89 | 1.19 | 2.22 | 2.15 | 0.63 | 1.17 | 1.94 | 1.06 | 1.05 | 0.35 | 0.97 | 1.41 |
| 66013 | 1 ea | Double, w/condiments & vegetables | 166 | 1.09 | 1.21 | 1.69 | 0.21 | 4.12 | 1.18 | 0.68 | 0.91 | 1.68 | 1.64 | 0.48 | 0.89 | 1.47 | 0.81 | 0.80 | 0.27 | 0.74 | 1.08 |
| 66012 | 1 ea | Double, w/condiments & vegetables, large | 258 | 2.10 | 2.27 | 3.12 | 0.39 | 7.12 | 2.32 | 1.18 | 1.62 | 2.99 | 2.92 | 0.85 | 1.55 | 2.45 | 1.39 | 1.47 | 0.47 | 1.24 | 1.89 |
| 56654 | 1 ea | Double, w/double deck bun, condiments & vegs | 228 | 1.49 | 1.66 | 2.25 | 0.32 | 5.97 | 1.61 | 0.92 | 1.27 | 2.33 | 2.16 | 0.65 | 1.27 | 2.16 | 1.17 | 1.10 | 0.37 | 1.00 | 1.51 |
| 56653 | 1 ea | Double, w/double deck bun, plain | 160 | 1.11 | 1.23 | 1.68 | 0.24 | 4.45 | 1.20 | 0.68 | 0.94 | 1.74 | 1.62 | 0.48 | 0.95 | 1.62 | 0.87 | 0.81 | 0.28 | 0.75 | 1.12 |
| 66014 | 1 ea | Plain | 102 | 0.72 | 0.80 | 1.08 | 0.17 | 3.16 | 0.77 | 0.45 | 0.63 | 1.16 | 1.02 | 0.32 | 0.65 | 1.15 | 0.60 | 0.53 | 0.19 | 0.49 | 0.75 |
| 56648 | 1 ea | Plain, large | 185 | 1.54 | 1.71 | 2.33 | 0.31 | 5.86 | 1.67 | 0.95 | 1.29 | 2.40 | 2.29 | 0.68 | 1.28 | 2.15 | 1.16 | 1.13 | 0.38 | 1.05 | 1.53 |
| 56651 | 1 ea | With Bacon & Condiments, large | 195 | 1.66 | 1.85 | 2.52 | 0.33 | 5.91 | 1.86 | 0.99 | 1.36 | 2.48 | 2.42 | 0.71 | 1.33 | 2.16 | 1.23 | 1.20 | 0.39 | 1.07 | 1.61 |
| 56647 | 1 ea | With Condiments | 113 | 0.77 | 0.86 | 1.18 | 0.18 | 3.42 | 0.83 | 0.48 | 0.68 | 1.24 | 1.10 | 0.34 | 0.70 | 1.24 | 0.65 | 0.58 | 0.20 | 0.53 | 0.81 |
| 66015 | 1 ea | With Condiments & Vegetables | 154 | 0.86 | 0.96 | 1.33 | 0.20 | 3.85 | 0.93 | 0.54 | 0.76 | 1.39 | 1.22 | 0.38 | 0.78 | 1.37 | 0.73 | 0.65 | 0.22 | 0.59 | 0.91 |
| 56649 | 1 ea | With condiments & Vegetables, large | 219 | 1.43 | 1.59 | 2.21 | 0.29 | 5.58 | 1.54 | 0.88 | 1.20 | 2.21 | 2.12 | 0.62 | 1.19 | 1.97 | 1.08 | 1.05 | 0.35 | 0.96 | 1.42 |
| 56650 | 1 ea | With Ham, Condiments & Vegetables, large | 254 | 2.06 | 2.29 | 3.15 | 0.43 | 7.57 | 2.16 | 1.27 | 1.70 | 3.12 | 3.05 | 0.90 | 1.68 | 2.67 | 1.67 | 1.52 | 0.50 | 1.35 | 1.96 |
| 56652 | 1 ea | With Triple Meat, plain | 304 | 3.28 | 3.50 | 4.74 | 0.57 | 10.00 | 3.65 | 1.76 | 2.40 | 4.47 | 4.41 | 1.27 | 2.26 | 3.44 | 2.29 | 2.23 | 0.70 | 1.83 | 2.78 |
| 56000 | 1 ea | Sandwiches, Chicken fillet | 182 | 1.22 | 1.35 | 1.97 | 0.33 | 4.44 | 1.13 | 0.70 | 1.21 | 1.78 | 1.74 | 0.61 | 1.01 | 1.33 | 0.92 | 0.95 | 0.28 | 0.76 | 1.20 |
| 56656 | 1 ea | Sandwiches, Chicken fillet w/cheese | 228 | 1.38 | 1.58 | 2.23 | 0.38 | 5.63 | 1.48 | 0.86 | 1.37 | 2.18 | 2.11 | 0.70 | 1.26 | 2.06 | 1.20 | 1.08 | 0.35 | 1.01 | 1.48 |
| 56657 | 1 ea | Sandwiches, Egg & cheese | 146 | 0.65 | 0.78 | 1.13 | 0.27 | 3.18 | 0.48 | 0.41 | 0.78 | 1.24 | 0.93 | 0.38 | 0.80 | 1.18 | 0.93 | 0.59 | 0.22 | 0.59 | 0.94 |
| 56665 | 1 ea | Sandwiches, Egg, ham, & cheese | 143 | 0.85 | 1.01 | 1.49 | 0.29 | 3.70 | 0.65 | 0.60 | 0.94 | 1.57 | 1.40 | 0.49 | 0.96 | 1.36 | 1.04 | 0.75 | 0.26 | 0.76 | 1.09 |
| | | Sandwiches, Hamburger | | | | | | | | | | | | | | | | | | | |
| 66007 | 1 ea | Plain | 90 | 0.67 | 0.71 | 0.95 | 0.16 | 2.68 | 0.76 | 0.35 | 0.52 | 0.94 | 0.77 | 0.25 | 0.52 | 0.90 | 0.49 | 0.46 | 0.15 | 0.35 | 0.61 |
| 56660 | 1 ea | Plain, large | 137 | 1.31 | 1.37 | 1.85 | 0.25 | 4.32 | 1.48 | 0.66 | 0.95 | 1.74 | 1.58 | 0.48 | 0.91 | 1.42 | 0.93 | 0.88 | 0.27 | 0.66 | 1.09 |
| 56658 | 1 ea | With Condiments | 107 | 0.67 | 0.72 | 0.96 | 0.16 | 2.73 | 0.76 | 0.35 | 0.53 | 0.95 | 0.77 | 0.26 | 0.53 | 0.90 | 0.54 | 0.47 | 0.15 | 0.35 | 0.61 |
| 56659 | 1 ea | With Condiment & Vegetables | 110 | 0.70 | 0.74 | 1.01 | 0.16 | 2.84 | 0.78 | 0.36 | 0.54 | 0.98 | 0.80 | 0.26 | 0.55 | 0.93 | 0.56 | 0.48 | 0.16 | 0.37 | 0.63 |
| 56661 | 1 ea | With Condiments & Vegetables, large | 218 | 1.47 | 1.55 | 2.14 | 0.29 | 5.06 | 1.56 | 0.74 | 1.07 | 1.95 | 1.77 | 0.54 | 1.03 | 1.60 | 1.05 | 0.99 | 0.31 | 0.74 | 1.23 |
| 66009 | 1 ea | Double, plain | 176 | 1.78 | 1.85 | 2.50 | 0.33 | 5.56 | 2.01 | 0.89 | 1.26 | 2.32 | 2.16 | 0.65 | 1.19 | 1.83 | 1.22 | 1.17 | 0.36 | 0.88 | 1.45 |
| 66006 | 1 ea | Double, w/condiments | 215 | 1.88 | 1.97 | 2.64 | 0.35 | 5.93 | 2.12 | 0.94 | 1.34 | 2.45 | 2.28 | 0.69 | 1.27 | 1.94 | 1.29 | 1.25 | 0.38 | 0.94 | 1.54 |

TABLE A **Amino Acid Content for Selected Foods *(continued)***

| Code | Amount | | Description | Weight (g) | Alanine (g) | Arginine (g) | Aspartic acid (g) | Cystine (g) | Glutamic acid (g) | Glycine (g) | Histidine (g) | Isoleucine (g) | Leucine (g) | Lysine (g) | Methionine (g) | Phenylalanine (g) | Proline (g) | Serine (g) | Threonine (g) | Tryptophan (g) | Tyrosine (g) | Valine (g) |
|---|---|---|---|---|---|---|---|---|---|---|---|---|---|---|---|---|---|---|---|---|---|---|
| 56662 | 1 | ea | Double, w/condiments & vegetables, large | 226 | 2.04 | 2.13 | 2.92 | 0.37 | 6.33 | 2.31 | 1.02 | 1.44 | 2.64 | 2.51 | 0.75 | 1.35 | 2.03 | 1.38 | 1.35 | 0.41 | 1.01 | 1.65 |
| 56663 | 1 | ea | With Triple Meat & Condiments | 259 | 3.08 | 3.21 | 4.33 | 0.52 | 8.75 | 3.50 | 1.52 | 2.13 | 3.94 | 3.83 | 1.12 | 1.96 | 2.87 | 2.01 | 2.02 | 0.61 | 1.52 | 2.43 |
| 66004 | 1 | ea | Sandwiches, Hotdog, plain | 98 | 0.59 | 0.65 | 0.85 | 0.14 | 2.34 | 0.63 | 0.29 | 0.44 | 0.75 | 0.63 | 0.20 | 0.41 | 0.75 | 0.47 | 0.35 | 0.10 | 0.28 | 0.47 |
| 56667 | 1 | ea | Sandwiches, Hotdog w/chili | 114 | 0.75 | 0.84 | 1.13 | 0.18 | 2.90 | 0.81 | 0.37 | 0.57 | 0.97 | 0.83 | 0.25 | 0.53 | 0.91 | 0.60 | 0.47 | 0.13 | 0.36 | 0.61 |
| | | | **FATS, OILS, AND MARGARINE** | | | | | | | | | | | | | | | | | | | |
| | | | Beef Fat | | | | | | | | | | | | | | | | | | | |
| 8340 | 1 | oz | Beef Fat, all cuts, raw, avg | 28 | 0.14 | 0.15 | 0.21 | 0.03 | 0.34 | 0.13 | 0.08 | 0.10 | 0.18 | 0.19 | 0.06 | 0.09 | 0.10 | 0.09 | 0.10 | 0.03 | 0.08 | 0.11 |
| 8688 | 1 | Tbs | Beef Fat, drippings, avg | 13 | 0.01 | 0.01 | 0.01 | 0.00 | 0.05 | 0.01 | 0.00 | 0.01 | 0.01 | 0.00 | 0.00 | 0.01 | 0.02 | 0.01 | 0.00 | 0.00 | 0.01 | 0.01 |
| | | | Butter | | | | | | | | | | | | | | | | | | | |
| 8000 | 1 | tsp | Salted, avg | 5 | 0.00 | 0.00 | 0.00 | 0.00 | 0.01 | 0.00 | 0.00 | 0.00 | 0.00 | 0.00 | 0.00 | 0.00 | 0.00 | 0.00 | 0.00 | 0.00 | 0.00 | 0.00 |
| 8160 | 1 | tsp | Salted, lightly, avg | 5 | 0.00 | 0.00 | 0.00 | 0.00 | 0.01 | 0.00 | 0.00 | 0.00 | 0.00 | 0.00 | 0.00 | 0.00 | 0.00 | 0.00 | 0.00 | 0.00 | 0.00 | 0.00 |
| 8025 | 1 | tsp | Unsalted, avg | 5 | 0.00 | 0.00 | 0.00 | 0.00 | 0.01 | 0.00 | 0.00 | 0.00 | 0.00 | 0.00 | 0.00 | 0.00 | 0.00 | 0.00 | 0.00 | 0.00 | 0.00 | 0.00 |
| 8142 | 1 | tsp | Whipped, salted, avg | 5 | 0.00 | 0.00 | 0.00 | 0.00 | 0.01 | 0.00 | 0.00 | 0.00 | 0.00 | 0.00 | 0.00 | 0.00 | 0.00 | 0.00 | 0.00 | 0.00 | 0.00 | 0.00 |
| 8341 | 1 | oz | Pork Fat, fresh, raw, avg | 28 | 0.12 | 0.16 | 0.12 | 0.01 | 0.16 | 0.30 | 0.02 | 0.05 | 0.11 | 0.14 | 0.02 | 0.06 | 0.19 | 0.07 | 0.06 | 0.01 | 0.03 | 0.08 |
| | | | Margarines | | | | | | | | | | | | | | | | | | | |
| 8052 | 1 | tsp | Corn Oil, hard, avg | 5 | 0.00 | 0.00 | 0.00 | 0.00 | 0.01 | 0.00 | 0.00 | 0.00 | 0.00 | 0.00 | 0.00 | 0.00 | 0.00 | 0.00 | 0.00 | 0.00 | 0.00 | 0.00 |
| 8061 | 1 | tsp | Corn Oil, soft, avg | 5 | 0.00 | 0.00 | 0.00 | 0.00 | 0.01 | 0.00 | 0.00 | 0.00 | 0.00 | 0.00 | 0.00 | 0.00 | 0.00 | 0.00 | 0.00 | 0.00 | 0.00 | 0.00 |
| 8263 | 1 | tsp | Coconut/safflower/palm oils, hard, avg | 5 | 0.00 | 0.00 | 0.00 | 0.00 | 0.01 | 0.00 | 0.00 | 0.00 | 0.00 | 0.00 | 0.00 | 0.00 | 0.00 | 0.00 | 0.00 | 0.00 | 0.00 | 0.00 |
| 8241 | 1 | tsp | Lard, hard, avg | 5 | 0.00 | 0.00 | 0.00 | 0.00 | 0.01 | 0.00 | 0.00 | 0.00 | 0.00 | 0.00 | 0.00 | 0.00 | 0.00 | 0.00 | 0.00 | 0.00 | 0.00 | 0.00 |
| 8165 | 1 | tsp | Liquid, Parkay | 5 | 0.00 | 0.00 | 0.01 | 0.00 | 0.02 | 0.00 | 0.00 | 0.01 | 0.01 | 0.01 | 0.00 | 0.00 | 0.01 | 0.00 | 0.00 | 0.00 | 0.00 | 0.01 |
| 8155 | 1 | tsp | Light, tub, Fleishmann's | 5 | 0.00 | 0.00 | 0.00 | 0.00 | 0.00 | 0.00 | 0.00 | 0.00 | 0.00 | 0.00 | 0.00 | 0.00 | 0.00 | 0.00 | 0.00 | 0.00 | 0.00 | 0.00 |
| 8249 | 1 | tsp | Palm oil, hard, imitation, avg | 5 | 0.00 | 0.00 | 0.00 | 0.00 | 0.00 | 0.00 | 0.00 | 0.00 | 0.00 | 0.00 | 0.00 | 0.00 | 0.00 | 0.00 | 0.00 | 0.00 | 0.00 | 0.00 |
| 8058 | 1 | tsp | Safflower Oil, soft, avg | 5 | 0.00 | 0.00 | 0.00 | 0.00 | 0.01 | 0.00 | 0.00 | 0.00 | 0.00 | 0.00 | 0.00 | 0.00 | 0.00 | 0.00 | 0.00 | 0.00 | 0.00 | 0.00 |
| 8054 | 1 | tsp | Safflower Oil w/Soybean oil, hard, avg | 5 | 0.00 | 0.00 | 0.00 | 0.00 | 0.01 | 0.00 | 0.00 | 0.00 | 0.00 | 0.00 | 0.00 | 0.00 | 0.00 | 0.00 | 0.00 | 0.00 | 0.00 | 0.00 |
| 8179 | 1 | tsp | Soybean Oil, hard, avg | 5 | 0.00 | 0.00 | 0.00 | 0.00 | 0.01 | 0.00 | 0.00 | 0.00 | 0.00 | 0.00 | 0.00 | 0.00 | 0.00 | 0.00 | 0.00 | 0.00 | 0.00 | 0.00 |
| 8247 | 1 | tsp | Soybean Oil, soft, avg | 5 | 0.00 | 0.00 | 0.00 | 0.00 | 0.01 | 0.00 | 0.00 | 0.00 | 0.00 | 0.00 | 0.00 | 0.00 | 0.00 | 0.00 | 0.00 | 0.00 | 0.00 | 0.00 |
| 8262 | 1 | tsp | Sunflower oil, hard, avg | 5 | 0.00 | 0.00 | 0.00 | 0.00 | 0.01 | 0.00 | 0.00 | 0.00 | 0.00 | 0.00 | 0.00 | 0.00 | 0.00 | 0.00 | 0.00 | 0.00 | 0.00 | 0.00 |
| 8042 | 1 | tsp | Unspecified Oils, hard, avg | 5 | 0.00 | 0.00 | 0.00 | 0.00 | 0.01 | 0.00 | 0.00 | 0.00 | 0.00 | 0.00 | 0.00 | 0.00 | 0.00 | 0.00 | 0.00 | 0.00 | 0.00 | 0.00 |
| 8244 | 1 | tsp | Unspecified Oils, soft, avg | 5 | 0.00 | 0.00 | 0.00 | 0.00 | 0.01 | 0.00 | 0.00 | 0.00 | 0.00 | 0.00 | 0.00 | 0.00 | 0.00 | 0.00 | 0.00 | 0.00 | 0.00 | 0.00 |
| | | | **FISH—FINFISH** | | | | | | | | | | | | | | | | | | | |
| 17288 | 1 | ea | Anchovy, canned in oil, drained, avg | 45 | 0.79 | 0.78 | 1.33 | 0.14 | 1.94 | 0.63 | 0.38 | 0.60 | 1.06 | 1.19 | 0.38 | 0.51 | 0.46 | 0.53 | 0.57 | 0.15 | 0.44 | 0.67 |
| 17188 | 3 | oz | Anchovy, European, raw, avg | 85 | 1.05 | 1.04 | 1.77 | 0.19 | 2.58 | 0.83 | 0.51 | 0.80 | 1.40 | 1.59 | 0.51 | 0.67 | 0.61 | 0.71 | 0.76 | 0.19 | 0.58 | 0.89 |
| | | | Bass | | | | | | | | | | | | | | | | | | | |
| 17029 | 1 | ea | Freshwater, mixed species, bkd/brld, fillet, avg | 62 | 0.91 | 0.90 | 1.54 | 0.16 | 2.24 | 0.72 | 0.44 | 0.69 | 1.22 | 1.38 | 0.44 | 0.59 | 0.53 | 0.61 | 0.66 | 0.17 | 0.51 | 0.77 |
| 17028 | 1 | ea | Freshwater, raw, fillet, avg | 79 | 0.90 | 0.89 | 1.52 | 0.16 | 2.23 | 0.71 | 0.44 | 0.69 | 1.21 | 1.37 | 0.44 | 0.58 | 0.53 | 0.61 | 0.65 | 0.17 | 0.50 | 0.77 |
| 17086 | 1 | ea | Sea bass, mixed species, bkd/brld, fillet, avg | 101 | 1.44 | 1.42 | 2.44 | 0.26 | 3.57 | 1.14 | 0.70 | 1.10 | 1.94 | 2.19 | 0.71 | 0.93 | 0.84 | 0.97 | 1.05 | 0.27 | 0.81 | 1.23 |
| 17225 | 1 | ea | Sea bass, mixed species, raw, fillet, avg | 129 | 1.44 | 1.42 | 2.44 | 0.26 | 3.55 | 1.14 | 0.70 | 1.10 | 1.93 | 2.18 | 0.70 | 0.93 | 0.84 | 0.97 | 1.04 | 0.27 | 0.80 | 1.23 |
| 17104 | 1 | ea | Striped, baked/broiled, fillet, avg | 124 | 1.71 | 1.69 | 2.89 | 0.30 | 4.20 | 1.35 | 0.83 | 1.30 | 2.29 | 2.59 | 0.83 | 1.10 | 1.00 | 1.15 | 1.24 | 0.32 | 0.95 | 1.45 |
| 17226 | 1 | ea | Striped, raw, fillet, avg | 159 | 1.70 | 1.69 | 2.89 | 0.30 | 4.21 | 1.35 | 0.83 | 1.30 | 2.29 | 2.59 | 0.83 | 1.10 | 1.00 | 1.15 | 1.24 | 0.32 | 0.95 | 1.45 |
| 17031 | 1 | ea | Bluefish, baked/broiled, fillet, avg | 117 | 1.81 | 1.80 | 3.08 | 0.32 | 4.49 | 1.44 | 0.88 | 1.38 | 2.45 | 2.76 | 0.89 | 1.17 | 1.06 | 1.23 | 1.32 | 0.34 | 1.01 | 1.54 |
| 17030 | 1 | ea | Bluefish, raw, fillet, avg | 150 | 1.82 | 1.80 | 3.07 | 0.32 | 4.49 | 1.44 | 0.88 | 1.38 | 2.44 | 2.76 | 0.89 | 1.17 | 1.06 | 1.23 | 1.32 | 0.34 | 1.01 | 1.54 |
| 17105 | 1 | ea | Burbot, baked/broiled, fillet, avg | 90 | 1.35 | 1.33 | 2.29 | 0.24 | 3.33 | 1.07 | 0.66 | 1.03 | 1.81 | 2.04 | 0.66 | 0.87 | 0.79 | 0.91 | 0.98 | 0.25 | 0.75 | 1.15 |
| 17191 | 1 | ea | Burbot, raw, fillet, avg | 116 | 1.36 | 1.35 | 2.30 | 0.24 | 3.34 | 1.08 | 0.66 | 1.03 | 1.82 | 2.05 | 0.66 | 0.87 | 0.79 | 0.91 | 0.98 | 0.25 | 0.76 | 1.15 |
| 17106 | 1 | ea | Butterfish, baked/broiled, fillet, avg | 25 | 0.34 | 0.33 | 0.57 | 0.06 | 0.83 | 0.26 | 0.16 | 0.25 | 0.45 | 0.51 | 0.16 | 0.22 | 0.20 | 0.23 | 0.24 | 0.06 | 0.19 | 0.28 |
| 17192 | 1 | ea | Butterfish, raw, fillet, avg | 32 | 0.34 | 0.33 | 0.57 | 0.06 | 0.83 | 0.27 | 0.16 | 0.25 | 0.45 | 0.51 | 0.16 | 0.22 | 0.20 | 0.23 | 0.24 | 0.06 | 0.19 | 0.28 |
| 17087 | 1 | ea | Carp, baked/broiled, avg | 170 | 2.35 | 2.33 | 3.98 | 0.42 | 5.80 | 1.87 | 1.14 | 1.78 | 3.16 | 3.57 | 1.15 | 1.52 | 1.37 | 1.59 | 1.70 | 0.44 | 1.31 | 2.01 |
| 17032 | 1 | ea | Carp, raw, fillet, avg | 218 | 2.35 | 2.33 | 3.99 | 0.42 | 5.80 | 1.87 | 1.14 | 1.79 | 3.16 | 3.58 | 1.15 | 1.52 | 1.38 | 1.59 | 1.70 | 0.44 | 1.31 | 2.00 |
| | | | Catfish | | | | | | | | | | | | | | | | | | | |
| 17179 | 1 | ea | Channel, farmed, baked/broiled, fillet, avg | 143 | 1.62 | 1.60 | 2.75 | 0.29 | 3.99 | 1.28 | 0.79 | 1.23 | 2.17 | 2.46 | 0.79 | 1.05 | 0.95 | 1.09 | 1.17 | 0.30 | 0.90 | 1.38 |
| 17178 | 1 | ea | Channel, farmed, raw, fillet, avg | 159 | 1.50 | 1.48 | 2.53 | 0.27 | 3.69 | 1.19 | 0.73 | 1.14 | 2.00 | 2.27 | 0.73 | 0.97 | 0.87 | 1.01 | 1.08 | 0.28 | 0.83 | 1.27 |

## TABLE A Amino Acid Content for Selected Foods *(continued)*

| Code | Amount | | Description | Weight (g) | Alanine (g) | Arginine (g) | Aspartic acid (g) | Cystine (g) | Glutamic acid (g) | Glycine (g) | Histidine (g) | Isoleucine (g) | Leucine (g) | Lysine (g) | Methionine (g) | Phenylalanine (g) | Proline (g) | Serine (g) | Threonine (g) | Tryptophan (g) | Tyrosine (g) | Valine (g) |
|---|---|---|---|---|---|---|---|---|---|---|---|---|---|---|---|---|---|---|---|---|---|---|
| 17305 | 1 | ea | Channel, wild, baked/broiled, fillet, avg | 143 | 1.60 | 1.59 | 2.70 | 0.28 | 3.95 | 1.27 | 0.78 | 1.22 | 2.14 | 2.43 | 0.78 | 1.03 | 0.93 | 1.08 | 1.16 | 0.30 | 0.89 | 1.36 |
| 17088 | 1 | ea | Channel, wild, breaded, fried, fillet, avg | 87 | 0.96 | 0.94 | 1.58 | 0.18 | 2.37 | 0.74 | 0.46 | 0.73 | 1.31 | 1.39 | 0.46 | 0.63 | 0.60 | 0.66 | 0.69 | 0.17 | 0.54 | 0.82 |
| 17033 | 1 | ea | Channel, wild, raw, steamed/poached, fillet, avg | 159 | 1.58 | 1.56 | 2.67 | 0.28 | 3.93 | 1.25 | 0.77 | 1.20 | 2.11 | 2.38 | 0.77 | 1.02 | 0.92 | 1.06 | 1.14 | 0.29 | 0.88 | 1.34 |
| 17128 | 3 | oz | Steamed/poached, avg | 85 | 1.04 | 1.03 | 1.76 | 0.18 | 2.57 | 0.82 | 0.50 | 0.79 | 1.38 | 1.57 | 0.51 | 0.67 | 0.60 | 0.70 | 0.75 | 0.19 | 0.58 | 0.88 |
| 17034 | 1 | Tbs | Caviar, black/red, sturgeon roe, granular, avg | 16 | 0.26 | 0.25 | 0.38 | 0.07 | 0.53 | 0.12 | 0.10 | 0.17 | 0.34 | 0.29 | 0.10 | 0.17 | 0.19 | 0.30 | 0.20 | 0.05 | 0.15 | 0.20 |
| | | | Cod | | | | | | | | | | | | | | | | | | | |
| 17037 | 1 | ea | Atlantic, baked/broiled, fillet, avg | 180 | 2.48 | 2.47 | 4.21 | 0.44 | 6.14 | 1.98 | 1.21 | 1.89 | 3.35 | 3.78 | 1.22 | 1.60 | 1.45 | 1.68 | 1.80 | 0.46 | 1.39 | 2.12 |
| 17089 | 1 | ea | Atlantic, canned w/liquid, avg | 312 | 4.31 | 4.24 | 7.27 | 0.76 | 10.61 | 3.40 | 2.09 | 3.28 | 5.77 | 6.52 | 2.10 | 2.77 | 2.51 | 2.90 | 3.11 | 0.80 | 2.40 | 3.65 |
| 17038 | 1 | pce | Atlantic, dried & salted, avg | 80 | 3.04 | 3.01 | 5.14 | 0.54 | 7.53 | 2.42 | 1.48 | 2.32 | 4.09 | 4.62 | 1.49 | 1.96 | 1.78 | 2.05 | 2.20 | 0.56 | 1.70 | 2.59 |
| 17036 | 1 | ea | Atlantic, raw, fillet, avg | 231 | 2.49 | 2.47 | 4.20 | 0.44 | 6.14 | 1.98 | 1.21 | 1.90 | 3.35 | 3.79 | 1.22 | 1.61 | 1.46 | 1.68 | 1.80 | 0.46 | 1.39 | 2.12 |
| 17107 | 1 | ea | Pacific, baked/broiled, fillet, avg | 90 | 1.25 | 1.23 | 2.11 | 0.22 | 3.03 | 0.99 | 0.61 | 0.95 | 1.68 | 1.90 | 0.61 | 0.81 | 0.73 | 0.84 | 0.91 | 0.23 | 0.70 | 1.06 |
| 17166 | 1 | ea | Pacific, raw, fillet, avg | 116 | 1.25 | 1.24 | 2.12 | 0.22 | 3.10 | 1.00 | 0.61 | 0.95 | 1.69 | 1.90 | 0.61 | 0.81 | 0.73 | 0.85 | 0.91 | 0.23 | 0.70 | 1.07 |
| 17001 | 3 | oz | Steamed/poached, avg | 85 | 1.15 | 1.14 | 1.94 | 0.20 | 2.83 | 0.91 | 0.56 | 0.88 | 1.54 | 1.74 | 0.56 | 0.74 | 0.67 | 0.77 | 0.83 | 0.21 | 0.64 | 0.98 |
| 17070 | 1 | ea | Croaker, Atlantic, breaded, fried, fillet, avg | 87 | 0.93 | 0.92 | 1.56 | 0.19 | 2.53 | 0.74 | 0.46 | 0.74 | 1.29 | 1.37 | 0.46 | 0.65 | 0.66 | 0.69 | 0.69 | 0.18 | 0.54 | 0.82 |
| 17194 | 1 | ea | Croaker, Atlantic, raw, fillet, avg | 79 | 0.85 | 0.84 | 1.44 | 0.15 | 2.03 | 0.67 | 0.41 | 0.65 | 1.15 | 1.29 | 0.42 | 0.55 | 0.50 | 0.57 | 0.62 | 0.16 | 0.47 | 0.72 |
| 17108 | 1 | ea | Cusk, baked/broiled, fillet, avg | 95 | 1.40 | 1.39 | 2.37 | 0.25 | 3.45 | 1.11 | 0.68 | 1.05 | 1.88 | 2.13 | 0.68 | 0.90 | 0.82 | 0.94 | 1.02 | 0.26 | 0.78 | 1.19 |
| 17195 | 1 | ea | Cusk, raw, fillet, avg | 122 | 1.40 | 1.39 | 2.38 | 0.25 | 3.46 | 1.11 | 0.68 | 1.07 | 1.88 | 2.12 | 0.69 | 0.91 | 0.82 | 0.95 | 1.02 | 0.26 | 0.78 | 1.19 |
| 19099 | 3 | oz | Cuttlefish, mixed species, raw, avg | 85 | 0.83 | 1.01 | 1.33 | 0.18 | 1.83 | 0.87 | 0.27 | 0.60 | 0.97 | 1.03 | 0.31 | 0.49 | 0.56 | 0.62 | 0.59 | 0.15 | 0.44 | 0.60 |
| 19085 | 3 | oz | Cuttlefish, steamed/boiled, avg | 85 | 1.67 | 2.01 | 2.66 | 0.36 | 3.75 | 1.73 | 0.53 | 1.20 | 1.95 | 2.07 | 0.62 | 0.99 | 1.13 | 1.24 | 1.19 | 0.31 | 0.88 | 1.21 |
| 17110 | 1 | ea | Drumfish, baked/broiled, fillet, avg | 154 | 2.09 | 2.08 | 3.54 | 0.37 | 5.17 | 1.66 | 1.02 | 1.60 | 2.82 | 3.19 | 1.03 | 1.35 | 1.22 | 1.41 | 1.52 | 0.39 | 1.17 | 1.79 |
| 17231 | 1 | ea | Drumfish, freshwater, raw, fillet, avg | 198 | 2.10 | 2.08 | 3.56 | 0.37 | 5.19 | 1.67 | 1.02 | 1.60 | 2.83 | 3.19 | 1.03 | 1.36 | 1.23 | 1.42 | 1.52 | 0.39 | 1.17 | 1.79 |
| 17002 | 1 | ea | Fish Sticks/Portions, breaded, fzn, baked, avg | 28 | 0.23 | 0.24 | 0.38 | 0.06 | 0.89 | 0.19 | 0.12 | 0.21 | 0.36 | 0.31 | 0.12 | 0.20 | 0.26 | 0.21 | 0.18 | 0.05 | 0.15 | 0.23 |
| 17103 | 3 | oz | Gefilte, sweet, avg | 85 | 0.44 | 0.48 | 0.62 | 0.09 | 1.40 | 0.32 | 0.21 | 0.39 | 0.65 | 0.67 | 0.20 | 0.39 | 0.27 | 0.38 | 0.39 | 0.07 | 0.30 | 0.44 |
| 17071 | 1 | ea | Grouper, baked/broiled, fillet, avg | 202 | 3.03 | 3.01 | 5.13 | 0.54 | 7.49 | 2.40 | 1.48 | 2.32 | 4.08 | 4.61 | 1.48 | 1.96 | 1.77 | 2.04 | 2.20 | 0.56 | 1.69 | 2.59 |
| 17196 | 1 | ea | Grouper, raw, fillet, avg | 202 | 2.36 | 2.34 | 4.00 | 0.42 | 5.84 | 1.88 | 1.15 | 1.80 | 3.19 | 3.60 | 1.16 | 1.53 | 1.38 | 1.60 | 1.71 | 0.44 | 1.32 | 2.02 |
| | | | Haddock | | | | | | | | | | | | | | | | | | | |
| 17090 | 1 | ea | Baked/broiled, fillet, avg | 150 | 2.20 | 2.18 | 3.72 | 0.39 | 5.43 | 1.74 | 1.07 | 1.63 | 2.95 | 3.35 | 1.08 | 1.42 | 1.29 | 1.48 | 1.59 | 0.41 | 1.23 | 1.88 |
| 17043 | 1 | ea | Raw, fillet, avg | 193 | 2.20 | 2.18 | 3.74 | 0.39 | 5.44 | 1.75 | 1.08 | 1.63 | 2.97 | 3.36 | 1.08 | 1.42 | 1.29 | 1.49 | 1.60 | 0.41 | 1.23 | 1.88 |
| 17010 | 3 | oz | Smoked, avg | 85 | 1.30 | 1.28 | 2.19 | 0.23 | 3.20 | 1.03 | 0.63 | 0.99 | 1.74 | 1.97 | 0.63 | 0.84 | 0.76 | 0.88 | 0.94 | 0.24 | 0.72 | 1.11 |
| 17008 | 3 | oz | Steamed/poached, avg | 85 | 1.22 | 1.20 | 2.06 | 0.22 | 2.99 | 0.96 | 0.59 | 0.92 | 1.63 | 1.84 | 0.60 | 0.78 | 0.71 | 0.82 | 0.88 | 0.23 | 0.68 | 1.04 |
| | | | Halibut | | | | | | | | | | | | | | | | | | | |
| 17291 | 1 | ea | Atlantic/Pacific, baked/broiled, fillet, avg | 318 | 5.12 | 5.09 | 8.68 | 0.91 | 12.65 | 4.07 | 2.50 | 3.91 | 6.90 | 7.79 | 2.51 | 3.31 | 3.00 | 3.47 | 3.72 | 0.95 | 2.87 | 4.39 |
| 17044 | 1 | ea | Atlantic/Pacific, raw, fillet, avg | 408 | 5.14 | 5.10 | 8.69 | 0.91 | 12.69 | 4.08 | 2.50 | 3.91 | 6.90 | 7.79 | 2.51 | 3.32 | 3.00 | 3.46 | 3.72 | 0.95 | 2.87 | 4.37 |
| 17111 | 1 | ea | Greenland, baked/broiled, fillet, avg | 318 | 3.53 | 3.50 | 6.01 | 0.63 | 8.74 | 2.81 | 1.72 | 2.70 | 4.77 | 5.37 | 1.73 | 2.29 | 2.07 | 2.39 | 2.57 | 0.66 | 1.98 | 3.02 |
| 17227 | 1 | ea | Greenland, raw, fillet, avg | 408 | 3.55 | 3.51 | 6.00 | 0.63 | 8.77 | 2.82 | 1.73 | 2.70 | 4.77 | 5.39 | 1.73 | 2.29 | 2.07 | 2.39 | 2.57 | 0.66 | 1.98 | 3.02 |
| | | | Herring | | | | | | | | | | | | | | | | | | | |
| 17047 | 1 | ea | Atlantic, baked/broiled, fillet, avg | 143 | 1.99 | 1.97 | 3.37 | 0.35 | 4.92 | 1.53 | 0.97 | 1.52 | 2.67 | 3.03 | 0.98 | 1.29 | 1.16 | 1.34 | 1.44 | 0.37 | 1.11 | 1.70 |
| 17012 | 3 | oz | Atlantic, pickled, avg | 85 | 0.73 | 0.72 | 1.23 | 0.13 | 1.80 | 0.58 | 0.36 | 0.56 | 0.98 | 1.11 | 0.36 | 0.47 | 0.43 | 0.49 | 0.53 | 0.14 | 0.41 | 0.62 |
| 17045 | 1 | ea | Atlantic, raw, fillet, avg | 184 | 2.01 | 1.99 | 3.39 | 0.36 | 4.93 | 1.53 | 0.97 | 1.52 | 2.69 | 3.04 | 0.98 | 1.29 | 1.17 | 1.35 | 1.45 | 0.37 | 1.12 | 1.70 |
| 17014 | 1 | ea | Atlantic, smoked, kippered, fillet, avg | 65 | 0.97 | 0.96 | 1.64 | 0.17 | 2.39 | 0.77 | 0.47 | 0.73 | 1.30 | 1.47 | 0.47 | 0.62 | 0.56 | 0.65 | 0.70 | 0.18 | 0.54 | 0.83 |
| 17112 | 1 | ea | Pacific, baked/broiled, fillet, avg | 144 | 1.83 | 1.81 | 3.10 | 0.32 | 4.52 | 1.45 | 0.89 | 1.39 | 2.46 | 2.78 | 0.90 | 1.18 | 1.07 | 1.23 | 1.33 | 0.34 | 1.02 | 1.56 |
| 17046 | 1 | ea | Pacific, raw, fillet, avg | 184 | 1.82 | 1.81 | 3.09 | 0.32 | 4.51 | 1.45 | 0.89 | 1.39 | 2.45 | 2.78 | 0.89 | 1.18 | 1.07 | 1.23 | 1.32 | 0.34 | 1.02 | 1.55 |
| 17113 | 1 | ea | Ling, baked/broiled, fillet, avg | 151 | 2.22 | 2.20 | 3.76 | 0.39 | 5.48 | 1.77 | 1.08 | 1.69 | 2.99 | 3.38 | 1.09 | 1.43 | 1.30 | 1.50 | 1.62 | 0.41 | 1.24 | 1.89 |
| 17197 | 1 | ea | Ling, raw, fillet, avg | 193 | 2.22 | 2.20 | 3.74 | 0.39 | 5.46 | 1.75 | 1.08 | 1.69 | 2.97 | 3.36 | 1.08 | 1.43 | 1.30 | 1.50 | 1.61 | 0.41 | 1.24 | 1.89 |
| 17114 | 1 | ea | Lingcod, baked/broiled, fillet, avg | 302 | 4.14 | 4.11 | 7.01 | 0.73 | 10.21 | 3.23 | 2.01 | 3.14 | 5.56 | 6.28 | 2.02 | 2.67 | 2.42 | 2.79 | 3.00 | 0.77 | 2.31 | 3.53 |
| 17198 | 1 | ea | Lingcod, raw, fillet, avg | 386 | 4.13 | 4.09 | 6.99 | 0.73 | 10.19 | 3.27 | 2.01 | 3.14 | 5.56 | 6.25 | 2.02 | 2.66 | 2.41 | 2.78 | 2.99 | 0.76 | 2.30 | 3.51 |
| | | | Mackerel | | | | | | | | | | | | | | | | | | | |
| 17049 | 1 | ea | Atlantic, baked/broiled, fillet, avg | 88 | 1.27 | 1.26 | 2.15 | 0.23 | 3.13 | 1.01 | 0.62 | 0.97 | 1.71 | 1.93 | 0.62 | 0.82 | 0.74 | 0.86 | 0.92 | 0.23 | 0.71 | 1.08 |
| 17048 | 1 | ea | Atlantic, raw, fillet, avg | 112 | 1.27 | 1.24 | 2.14 | 0.22 | 3.11 | 1.00 | 0.61 | 0.96 | 1.69 | 1.92 | 0.62 | 0.81 | 0.74 | 0.85 | 0.91 | 0.23 | 0.70 | 1.07 |
| 17293 | 1 | ea | Jack, canned, drained, avg | 361 | 5.05 | 5.02 | 8.59 | 0.90 | 12.49 | 4.01 | 2.47 | 3.86 | 6.82 | 7.69 | 2.48 | 3.27 | 2.96 | 3.42 | 3.68 | 0.94 | 2.83 | 4.33 |

TABLE A **Amino Acid Content for Selected Foods *(continued)***

| Code | Amount | | Description | Weight (g) | Alanine (g) | Arginine (g) | Aspartic acid (g) | Cystine (g) | Glutamic acid (g) | Glycine (g) | Histidine (g) | Isoleucine (g) | Leucine (g) | Lysine (g) | Methionine (g) | Phenylalanine (g) | Proline (g) | Serine (g) | Threonine (g) | Tryptophan (g) | Tyrosine (g) | Valine (g) |
|---|---|---|---|---|---|---|---|---|---|---|---|---|---|---|---|---|---|---|---|---|---|---|
| 17115 | 1 | ea | King, baked/broiled, fillet, avg | 308 | 4.84 | 4.80 | 8.19 | 0.86 | 11.95 | 3.85 | 2.36 | 3.70 | 6.50 | 7.36 | 2.37 | 3.14 | 2.83 | 3.26 | 3.51 | 0.90 | 2.70 | 4.13 |
| 17228 | 1 | ea | King, raw, fillet, avg | 396 | 4.87 | 4.79 | 8.24 | 0.86 | 12.00 | 3.86 | 2.36 | 3.70 | 6.53 | 7.37 | 2.38 | 3.14 | 2.84 | 3.27 | 3.52 | 0.90 | 2.71 | 4.16 |
| 17092 | 1 | ea | Spanish, baked/broiled, fillet, avg | 146 | 2.09 | 2.06 | 3.53 | 0.37 | 5.14 | 1.65 | 1.01 | 1.59 | 2.80 | 3.17 | 1.02 | 1.34 | 1.22 | 1.40 | 1.50 | 0.39 | 1.16 | 1.78 |
| 17229 | 1 | ea | Spanish, raw, fillet, avg | 187 | 2.19 | 2.15 | 3.70 | 0.39 | 5.39 | 1.73 | 1.06 | 1.66 | 2.94 | 3.31 | 1.07 | 1.41 | 1.28 | 1.47 | 1.58 | 0.40 | 1.22 | 1.86 |
| 17131 | 1 | ea | Pacific/Jack, mixed species, bkd/brld, fillet, avg | 176 | 2.75 | 2.71 | 4.65 | 0.49 | 6.76 | 2.18 | 1.33 | 2.09 | 3.68 | 4.15 | 1.34 | 1.78 | 1.60 | 1.85 | 1.99 | 0.51 | 1.53 | 2.34 |
| 17051 | 1 | ea | Pacific/Jack, raw, fillet, avg | 225 | 2.72 | 2.70 | 4.63 | 0.48 | 6.75 | 2.17 | 1.33 | 2.08 | 3.67 | 4.14 | 1.34 | 1.76 | 1.60 | 1.84 | 1.98 | 0.51 | 1.53 | 2.32 |
| 17109 | 1 | ea | Mahi Mahi, dolphin fish, baked/broiled, fillet, avg | 159 | 2.27 | 2.26 | 3.86 | 0.40 | 5.63 | 1.81 | 1.11 | 1.73 | 3.07 | 3.47 | 1.12 | 1.47 | 1.33 | 1.54 | 1.65 | 0.42 | 1.27 | 1.94 |
| 17240 | 1 | ea | Mahi Mahi, dolphin fish, raw, fillet, avg | 204 | 2.28 | 2.26 | 3.86 | 0.40 | 5.63 | 1.81 | 1.11 | 1.74 | 3.06 | 3.47 | 1.12 | 1.47 | 1.33 | 1.54 | 1.65 | 0.42 | 1.27 | 1.94 |
| 17116 | 3 | oz | Milkfish, baked/broiled, avg | 85 | 1.35 | 1.34 | 2.30 | 0.24 | 3.34 | 1.07 | 0.66 | 1.03 | 1.82 | 2.06 | 0.66 | 0.88 | 0.79 | 0.91 | 0.98 | 0.25 | 0.76 | 1.16 |
| 17199 | 3 | oz | Milkfish, raw, avg | 85 | 1.05 | 1.05 | 1.78 | 0.19 | 2.61 | 0.84 | 0.51 | 0.80 | 1.42 | 1.61 | 0.52 | 0.68 | 0.62 | 0.71 | 0.76 | 0.20 | 0.59 | 0.90 |
| 17117 | 3 | oz | Monkfish, baked/broiled, avg | 85 | 0.95 | 0.94 | 1.62 | 0.17 | 2.35 | 0.76 | 0.46 | 0.73 | 1.28 | 1.45 | 0.47 | 0.62 | 0.56 | 0.64 | 0.69 | 0.18 | 0.53 | 0.81 |
| 17200 | 3 | oz | Monkfish, raw, avg | 85 | 0.74 | 0.74 | 1.26 | 0.13 | 1.84 | 0.59 | 0.36 | 0.57 | 1.00 | 1.13 | 0.36 | 0.48 | 0.44 | 0.50 | 0.54 | 0.14 | 0.42 | 0.63 |
| 17072 | 1 | ea | Mullet, striped, baked/broiled, fillet, avg | 93 | 1.39 | 1.38 | 2.36 | 0.25 | 3.44 | 1.11 | 0.68 | 1.06 | 1.88 | 2.12 | 0.68 | 0.90 | 0.82 | 0.94 | 1.01 | 0.26 | 0.78 | 1.19 |
| 17201 | 1 | ea | Mullet, striped, raw, fillet, avg | 119 | 1.39 | 1.38 | 2.36 | 0.25 | 3.44 | 1.11 | 0.68 | 1.06 | 1.87 | 2.12 | 0.68 | 0.90 | 0.81 | 0.94 | 1.01 | 0.26 | 0.78 | 1.19 |
| 17121 | 3 | oz | Orange Roughy, baked/broiled, avg | 85 | 0.97 | 0.96 | 1.64 | 0.17 | 2.39 | 0.77 | 0.47 | 0.74 | 1.30 | 1.47 | 0.47 | 0.63 | 0.57 | 0.65 | 0.70 | 0.18 | 0.54 | 0.83 |
| 17207 | 3 | oz | Orange Roughy, raw, avg | 85 | 0.76 | 0.75 | 1.28 | 0.13 | 1.86 | 0.60 | 0.37 | 0.58 | 1.02 | 1.15 | 0.37 | 0.49 | 0.44 | 0.51 | 0.55 | 0.14 | 0.42 | 0.64 |
| | | | Perch | | | | | | | | | | | | | | | | | | | |
| 17093 | 1 | ea | Atlantic Ocean, baked/broiled, fillet, avg | 50 | 0.72 | 0.71 | 1.23 | 0.13 | 1.78 | 0.57 | 0.35 | 0.55 | 0.97 | 1.10 | 0.35 | 0.47 | 0.42 | 0.49 | 0.52 | 0.13 | 0.40 | 0.62 |
| 17052 | 1 | ea | Atlantic Ocean, redfish, raw, fillet, avg | 64 | 0.72 | 0.72 | 1.22 | 0.13 | 1.78 | 0.57 | 0.35 | 0.55 | 0.97 | 1.09 | 0.35 | 0.47 | 0.42 | 0.49 | 0.52 | 0.13 | 0.40 | 0.61 |
| 17094 | 1 | ea | Mixed species, baked/broiled, fillet, avg | 46 | 0.69 | 0.69 | 1.17 | 0.12 | 1.71 | 0.55 | 0.34 | 0.53 | 0.93 | 1.05 | 0.34 | 0.45 | 0.40 | 0.46 | 0.50 | 0.13 | 0.39 | 0.59 |
| 17239 | 1 | ea | Mixed species, raw, fillet, avg | 60 | 0.70 | 0.70 | 1.19 | 0.12 | 1.73 | 0.56 | 0.34 | 0.54 | 0.95 | 1.07 | 0.34 | 0.45 | 0.41 | 0.47 | 0.51 | 0.13 | 0.39 | 0.60 |
| | | | Pike | | | | | | | | | | | | | | | | | | | |
| 17095 | 1 | ea | Northern, baked/broiled, fillet, avg | 310 | 4.62 | 4.59 | 7.84 | 0.82 | 11.44 | 3.69 | 2.25 | 3.53 | 6.23 | 7.04 | 2.27 | 2.99 | 2.71 | 3.13 | 3.35 | 0.86 | 2.58 | 3.94 |
| 17160 | 1 | ea | Northern, raw, fillet, avg | 396 | 4.63 | 4.55 | 7.80 | 0.82 | 11.40 | 3.66 | 2.25 | 3.51 | 6.22 | 7.01 | 2.26 | 2.98 | 2.70 | 3.11 | 3.34 | 0.86 | 2.57 | 3.93 |
| 17118 | 1 | ea | Walleye, baked/broiled, fillet, avg | 124 | 1.84 | 1.82 | 3.11 | 0.33 | 4.54 | 1.46 | 0.90 | 1.40 | 2.47 | 2.79 | 0.90 | 1.19 | 1.08 | 1.24 | 1.34 | 0.34 | 1.03 | 1.56 |
| 17202 | 1 | ea | Walleye, raw, fillet, avg | 159 | 1.84 | 1.83 | 3.12 | 0.33 | 4.55 | 1.46 | 0.90 | 1.40 | 2.48 | 2.80 | 0.90 | 1.19 | 1.08 | 1.24 | 1.33 | 0.34 | 1.03 | 1.57 |
| | | | Pollock | | | | | | | | | | | | | | | | | | | |
| 17168 | 1 | ea | Atlantic, baked/broiled, fillet, avg | 302 | 4.56 | 4.50 | 7.70 | 0.81 | 11.23 | 3.62 | 2.22 | 3.47 | 6.13 | 6.92 | 2.23 | 2.94 | 2.66 | 3.08 | 3.29 | 0.84 | 2.54 | 3.87 |
| 17053 | 1 | ea | Atlantic, raw, fillet, avg | 386 | 4.55 | 4.48 | 7.68 | 0.80 | 11.19 | 3.60 | 2.21 | 3.46 | 6.10 | 6.91 | 2.22 | 2.93 | 2.66 | 3.06 | 3.29 | 0.84 | 2.53 | 3.86 |
| 17096 | 1 | ea | Walleye, baked/broiled, fillet, avg | 60 | 0.85 | 0.85 | 1.45 | 0.15 | 2.11 | 0.68 | 0.42 | 0.65 | 1.15 | 1.30 | 0.42 | 0.55 | 0.50 | 0.58 | 0.62 | 0.16 | 0.48 | 0.73 |
| 17167 | 1 | ea | Walleye, raw, fillet, avg | 77 | 0.80 | 0.79 | 1.36 | 0.14 | 1.98 | 0.64 | 0.39 | 0.61 | 1.08 | 1.22 | 0.39 | 0.52 | 0.47 | 0.54 | 0.58 | 0.15 | 0.45 | 0.68 |
| 17073 | 1 | ea | Pompano, baked/broiled, fillet, avg | 88 | 1.26 | 1.25 | 2.14 | 0.22 | 3.12 | 1.00 | 0.61 | 0.96 | 1.70 | 1.92 | 0.62 | 0.81 | 0.74 | 0.85 | 0.92 | 0.23 | 0.70 | 1.07 |
| 17203 | 1 | ea | Pompano, raw, fillet, avg | 112 | 1.25 | 1.24 | 2.12 | 0.22 | 3.09 | 0.99 | 0.61 | 0.95 | 1.68 | 1.90 | 0.61 | 0.81 | 0.73 | 0.84 | 0.91 | 0.23 | 0.70 | 1.07 |
| 17119 | 1 | ea | Pout, ocean, baked/broiled, fillet, avg | 274 | 3.53 | 3.51 | 6.00 | 0.63 | 8.74 | 2.79 | 1.72 | 2.69 | 4.74 | 5.37 | 1.73 | 2.28 | 2.07 | 2.38 | 2.56 | 0.65 | 1.97 | 3.01 |
| 17204 | 1 | ea | Pout, ocean, raw, fillet, avg | 352 | 3.56 | 3.51 | 5.98 | 0.63 | 8.73 | 2.81 | 1.72 | 2.70 | 4.75 | 5.39 | 1.73 | 2.29 | 2.07 | 2.39 | 2.57 | 0.65 | 1.98 | 3.02 |
| 17174 | 1 | ea | Pumpkinseed Sunfish, baked/broiled, fillet, avg | 37 | 0.56 | 0.55 | 0.94 | 0.10 | 1.37 | 0.44 | 0.27 | 0.43 | 0.75 | 0.84 | 0.27 | 0.36 | 0.33 | 0.38 | 0.40 | 0.10 | 0.31 | 0.47 |
| 17216 | 1 | ea | Pumpkinseed Sunfish, raw, fillet, avg | 48 | 0.56 | 0.56 | 0.96 | 0.10 | 1.39 | 0.45 | 0.27 | 0.43 | 0.76 | 0.85 | 0.28 | 0.36 | 0.33 | 0.38 | 0.41 | 0.10 | 0.31 | 0.48 |
| 17074 | 1 | ea | Rockfish, Pacific, mixed species, bkd/brld, avg | 149 | 2.16 | 2.15 | 3.67 | 0.38 | 5.35 | 1.71 | 1.05 | 1.65 | 2.91 | 3.29 | 1.06 | 1.40 | 1.27 | 1.46 | 1.56 | 0.40 | 1.21 | 1.85 |
| 17205 | 1 | ea | Rockfish, Pacific, mixed species, raw, fillet, avg | 191 | 2.16 | 2.14 | 3.67 | 0.38 | 5.35 | 1.72 | 1.05 | 1.65 | 2.90 | 3.29 | 1.06 | 1.40 | 1.27 | 1.46 | 1.57 | 0.40 | 1.21 | 1.85 |
| | | | Roe | | | | | | | | | | | | | | | | | | | |
| 17148 | 1 | Tbs | Herring, avg | 14 | 0.20 | 0.18 | 0.25 | 0.05 | 0.04 | 0.09 | 0.08 | 0.16 | 0.27 | 0.24 | 0.08 | 0.15 | 0.17 | 0.14 | 0.14 | 0.04 | 0.16 | 0.18 |
| 17120 | 1/2 | oz | Mixed species, baked/broiled, avg | 14 | 0.26 | 0.23 | 0.32 | 0.07 | 0.48 | 0.12 | 0.11 | 0.21 | 0.35 | 0.31 | 0.10 | 0.20 | 0.21 | 0.17 | 0.18 | 0.05 | 0.20 | 0.24 |
| 17206 | 1 | Tbs | Mixed species, raw, avg | 14 | 0.20 | 0.18 | 0.25 | 0.05 | 0.37 | 0.09 | 0.08 | 0.16 | 0.27 | 0.24 | 0.08 | 0.15 | 0.17 | 0.14 | 0.14 | 0.04 | 0.16 | 0.18 |
| | | | Sablefish | | | | | | | | | | | | | | | | | | | |
| 17122 | 1 | ea | Baked/broiled, fillet, avg | 302 | 3.14 | 3.11 | 5.32 | 0.56 | 7.76 | 2.49 | 1.53 | 2.39 | 4.23 | 4.77 | 1.54 | 2.03 | 1.84 | 2.12 | 2.28 | 0.58 | 1.75 | 2.68 |
| 17208 | 1 | ea | Raw, fillet, avg | 386 | 3.13 | 3.10 | 5.29 | 0.56 | 7.72 | 2.49 | 1.52 | 2.39 | 4.21 | 4.75 | 1.53 | 2.02 | 1.83 | 2.11 | 2.27 | 0.58 | 1.75 | 2.67 |
| 17075 | 3 | oz | Smoked, avg | 85 | 0.91 | 0.90 | 1.54 | 0.16 | 2.24 | 0.72 | 0.44 | 0.69 | 1.22 | 1.38 | 0.44 | 0.59 | 0.53 | 0.61 | 0.66 | 0.17 | 0.51 | 0.77 |
| | | | Salmon | | | | | | | | | | | | | | | | | | | |
| 17152 | 3 | oz | Chinook, smoked, avg | 85 | 0.94 | 0.93 | 1.59 | 0.17 | 2.32 | 0.75 | 0.46 | 0.72 | 1.27 | 1.43 | 0.46 | 0.61 | 0.55 | 0.63 | 0.68 | 0.17 | 0.52 | 0.80 |
| 17016 | 1 | ea | Coho, wild, steamed/poached, fillet, avg | 310 | 5.15 | 5.08 | 8.68 | 0.91 | 12.68 | 4.06 | 2.50 | 3.91 | 6.88 | 7.78 | 2.51 | 3.32 | 3.00 | 3.47 | 3.72 | 0.95 | 2.86 | 4.37 |

TABLE A **Amino Acid Content for Selected Foods *(continued)***

| Code | Amount | | Description | Weight (g) | Alanine (g) | Arginine (g) | Aspartic acid (g) | Cystine (g) | Glutamic acid (g) | Glycine (g) | Histidine (g) | Isoleucine (g) | Leucine (g) | Lysine (g) | Methionine (g) | Phenylalanine (g) | Proline (g) | Serine (g) | Threonine (g) | Tryptophan (g) | Tyrosine (g) | Valine (g) |
|---|---|---|---|---|---|---|---|---|---|---|---|---|---|---|---|---|---|---|---|---|---|---|
| 17306 | 3 | oz | Nuggets, breaded, fzn, heated, avg | 85 | 0.62 | 0.61 | 1.04 | 0.11 | 1.52 | 0.49 | 0.30 | 0.47 | 0.83 | 0.94 | 0.30 | 0.40 | 0.36 | 0.41 | 0.45 | 0.11 | 0.34 | 0.53 |
| 17171 | 1 | ea | Pink, baked/broiled, fillet, avg | 248 | 3.84 | 3.79 | 6.50 | 0.68 | 3.47 | 3.05 | 1.87 | 2.93 | 5.16 | 5.83 | 1.88 | 2.48 | 2.24 | 2.58 | 2.78 | 0.71 | 2.14 | 3.27 |
| 17056 | 1 | ea | Pink, raw, fillet, avg | 318 | 3.85 | 3.78 | 6.49 | 0.68 | 3.48 | 3.04 | 1.87 | 2.92 | 5.15 | 5.82 | 1.88 | 2.47 | 2.24 | 2.59 | 2.78 | 0.71 | 2.14 | 3.28 |
| 17154 | 3 | oz | Pink, unsalted, canned w/liquid, avg | 85 | 1.02 | 1.00 | 1.73 | 0.18 | 2.51 | 0.81 | 0.49 | 0.78 | 1.37 | 1.55 | 0.50 | 0.66 | 0.59 | 0.69 | 0.74 | 0.19 | 0.57 | 0.87 |
| 17017 | 3 | oz | Pink, w/bone, canned w/liquid, avg | 85 | 1.02 | 1.00 | 1.73 | 0.18 | 2.51 | 0.81 | 0.49 | 0.78 | 1.37 | 1.55 | 0.50 | 0.66 | 0.59 | 0.69 | 0.74 | 0.19 | 0.57 | 0.87 |
| 17058 | 3 | oz | Sockeye, w/bone, canned, drained, avg | 85 | 1.05 | 1.05 | 1.78 | 0.19 | 2.60 | 0.84 | 0.51 | 0.80 | 1.41 | 1.60 | 0.52 | 0.68 | 0.62 | 0.71 | 0.76 | 0.19 | 0.59 | 0.90 |
| 17155 | 3 | oz | Sockeye, w/bone, unsalted, cnd, drained, avg | 85 | 1.05 | 1.05 | 1.78 | 0.19 | 2.60 | 0.84 | 0.51 | 0.80 | 1.41 | 1.60 | 0.52 | 0.68 | 0.62 | 0.71 | 0.76 | 0.19 | 0.59 | 0.90 |
| | | | Sardines | | | | | | | | | | | | | | | | | | | |
| 17297 | 1 | ea | Atlantic, w/bones in oil, canned, drained, avg | 12 | 0.18 | 0.18 | 0.30 | 0.03 | 0.44 | 0.14 | 0.09 | 0.14 | 0.24 | 0.27 | 0.09 | 0.12 | 0.10 | 0.12 | 0.13 | 0.03 | 0.10 | 0.15 |
| 17298 | 1 | ea | Pacific, w/bone in tomato sce, cnd, drained, avg | 38 | 0.38 | 0.40 | 0.63 | 0.05 | 0.88 | 0.31 | 0.26 | 0.30 | 0.52 | 0.53 | 0.18 | 0.30 | 0.25 | 0.28 | 0.30 | 0.06 | 0.24 | 0.35 |
| 17133 | 1 | ea | Skinless, w/o bones in water, avg | 21 | 0.31 | 0.31 | 0.52 | 0.06 | 0.76 | 0.25 | 0.15 | 0.24 | 0.42 | 0.47 | 0.15 | 0.20 | 0.18 | 0.21 | 0.22 | 0.06 | 0.17 | 0.26 |
| 17021 | 3 | oz | With mustard, canned, avg | 85 | 0.99 | 1.03 | 1.63 | 0.14 | 2.26 | 0.81 | 0.67 | 0.78 | 1.33 | 1.37 | 0.47 | 0.78 | 0.64 | 0.71 | 0.78 | 0.15 | 0.61 | 0.91 |
| 17172 | 1 | ea | Scup fish, baked/broiled, fillet, avg | 50 | 0.73 | 0.73 | 1.24 | 0.13 | 1.80 | 0.58 | 0.36 | 0.56 | 0.99 | 1.11 | 0.36 | 0.47 | 0.43 | 0.49 | 0.53 | 0.14 | 0.41 | 0.63 |
| 17210 | 1 | ea | Scup fish, raw, fillet, avg | 64 | 0.73 | 0.72 | 1.24 | 0.13 | 1.80 | 0.58 | 0.36 | 0.56 | 0.98 | 1.11 | 0.36 | 0.47 | 0.43 | 0.49 | 0.53 | 0.14 | 0.41 | 0.62 |
| 17211 | 1 | ea | Shad, American, raw, fillet, avg | 184 | 1.88 | 1.86 | 3.18 | 0.33 | 4.66 | 1.50 | 0.92 | 1.44 | 2.54 | 2.87 | 0.92 | 1.22 | 1.10 | 1.27 | 1.37 | 0.35 | 1.05 | 1.60 |
| 17062 | 1 | ea | Shad, baked/broiled, fillet, avg | 144 | 1.89 | 1.87 | 3.20 | 0.34 | 4.67 | 1.50 | 0.92 | 1.44 | 2.53 | 2.87 | 0.92 | 1.22 | 1.10 | 1.28 | 1.37 | 0.35 | 1.06 | 1.61 |
| 17076 | 3 | oz | Shark, batter fried, mixed species, avg | 85 | 0.94 | 0.93 | 1.57 | 0.18 | 2.52 | 0.74 | 0.46 | 0.74 | 1.29 | 1.39 | 0.46 | 0.64 | 0.63 | 0.67 | 0.72 | 0.18 | 0.54 | 0.82 |
| 17212 | 3 | oz | Shark, raw, mixed species, avg | 85 | 1.08 | 1.07 | 1.83 | 0.19 | 2.66 | 0.86 | 0.53 | 0.82 | 1.45 | 1.64 | 0.53 | 0.70 | 0.63 | 0.73 | 0.78 | 0.20 | 0.60 | 0.92 |
| 17077 | 1 | ea | Sheepshead fish, baked/broiled, fillet, avg | 186 | 2.92 | 2.90 | 4.95 | 0.52 | 7.22 | 2.33 | 1.42 | 2.23 | 3.94 | 4.45 | 1.43 | 1.90 | 1.71 | 1.97 | 2.12 | 0.54 | 1.63 | 2.49 |
| 17213 | 1 | ea | Sheepshead fish, raw, fillet, avg | 238 | 2.90 | 2.88 | 4.93 | 0.52 | 7.19 | 2.31 | 1.42 | 2.22 | 3.90 | 4.43 | 1.42 | 1.88 | 1.70 | 1.96 | 2.11 | 0.54 | 1.62 | 2.48 |
| 17100 | 3 | oz | Smelt, rainbow, baked/broiled, avg | 85 | 1.16 | 1.15 | 1.96 | 0.21 | 2.86 | 0.93 | 0.57 | 0.88 | 1.56 | 1.77 | 0.57 | 0.75 | 0.68 | 0.78 | 0.84 | 0.22 | 0.65 | 0.99 |
| 17063 | 3 | oz | Smelt, rainbow, raw, avg | 85 | 0.91 | 0.90 | 1.54 | 0.16 | 2.24 | 0.72 | 0.44 | 0.69 | 1.22 | 1.38 | 0.44 | 0.58 | 0.53 | 0.61 | 0.66 | 0.17 | 0.51 | 0.77 |
| 17022 | 1 | ea | Snapper, mixed species, baked/broiled, fillet, avg | 170 | 2.70 | 2.67 | 4.57 | 0.48 | 5.68 | 2.14 | 1.32 | 2.06 | 3.64 | 4.11 | 1.32 | 1.75 | 1.58 | 1.82 | 1.96 | 0.50 | 1.51 | 2.31 |
| 17064 | 1 | ea | Snapper, mixed species, raw, fillet, avg | 218 | 2.70 | 2.68 | 4.58 | 0.48 | 5.67 | 2.15 | 1.32 | 2.06 | 3.64 | 4.10 | 1.32 | 1.75 | 1.58 | 1.82 | 1.96 | 0.50 | 1.51 | 2.31 |
| | | | Sole/Flounder | | | | | | | | | | | | | | | | | | | |
| 17068 | 1 | ea | Baked/broiled, fillet, avg | 127 | 1.85 | 1.84 | 3.14 | 0.33 | 4.58 | 1.47 | 0.90 | 1.41 | 2.49 | 2.82 | 0.91 | 1.20 | 1.08 | 1.25 | 1.35 | 0.34 | 1.04 | 1.59 |
| 17042 | 1 | ea | Raw, fillet, avg | 163 | 1.86 | 1.84 | 3.15 | 0.33 | 4.58 | 1.48 | 0.90 | 1.41 | 2.49 | 2.82 | 0.91 | 1.20 | 1.09 | 1.25 | 1.35 | 0.34 | 1.04 | 1.58 |
| 17006 | 3 | oz | Steamed/poached, fillet, avg | 85 | 1.22 | 1.20 | 2.06 | 0.22 | 3.00 | 0.97 | 0.59 | 0.93 | 1.63 | 1.84 | 0.60 | 0.79 | 0.71 | 0.82 | 0.88 | 0.23 | 0.68 | 1.03 |
| 17190 | 1 | ea | Spot fish, baked/broiled, fillet, avg | 50 | 0.72 | 0.71 | 1.22 | 0.13 | 1.77 | 0.57 | 0.35 | 0.55 | 0.96 | 1.09 | 0.35 | 0.46 | 0.42 | 0.48 | 0.52 | 0.13 | 0.40 | 0.61 |
| 17189 | 1 | ea | Spot fish, raw, fillet, avg | 64 | 0.72 | 0.71 | 1.22 | 0.13 | 1.77 | 0.57 | 0.35 | 0.55 | 0.97 | 1.09 | 0.35 | 0.46 | 0.42 | 0.48 | 0.52 | 0.13 | 0.40 | 0.61 |
| 17023 | 1 | ea | Steelhead, sea trout, mixed species, baked/broiled, avg | 186 | 2.42 | 2.38 | 4.09 | 0.43 | 5.95 | 1.92 | 1.18 | 1.84 | 3.24 | 3.66 | 1.18 | 1.56 | 1.41 | 1.63 | 1.75 | 0.45 | 1.35 | 2.06 |
| 17067 | 1 | ea | Steelhead, sea trout, mixed species, raw, fillet, avg | 238 | 2.40 | 2.38 | 4.09 | 0.43 | 5.95 | 1.91 | 1.17 | 1.84 | 3.24 | 3.67 | 1.18 | 1.56 | 1.41 | 1.63 | 1.75 | 0.45 | 1.34 | 2.05 |
| | | | Sturgeon | | | | | | | | | | | | | | | | | | | |
| 17078 | 1 | cup | Baked/broiled, avg | 136 | 1.70 | 1.69 | 2.88 | 0.30 | 4.20 | 1.35 | 0.83 | 1.30 | 2.28 | 2.58 | 0.83 | 1.10 | 1.00 | 1.15 | 1.23 | 0.32 | 0.95 | 1.46 |
| 17214 | 3 | oz | Raw, mixed species, avg | 85 | 0.83 | 0.82 | 1.40 | 0.15 | 2.05 | 0.66 | 0.40 | 0.63 | 1.11 | 1.26 | 0.41 | 0.54 | 0.49 | 0.56 | 0.60 | 0.15 | 0.46 | 0.71 |
| 17079 | 3 | oz | Smoked, mixed species, avg | 85 | 1.61 | 1.59 | 2.72 | 0.28 | 3.96 | 1.28 | 0.78 | 1.22 | 2.16 | 2.44 | 0.79 | 1.04 | 0.94 | 1.08 | 1.16 | 0.30 | 0.89 | 1.37 |
| 17173 | 1 | ea | Sucker fish, white, baked/broiled, fillet, avg | 124 | 1.61 | 1.60 | 2.73 | 0.29 | 3.98 | 1.28 | 0.78 | 1.23 | 2.17 | 2.44 | 0.79 | 1.04 | 0.94 | 1.09 | 1.17 | 0.30 | 0.90 | 1.38 |
| 17215 | 1 | ea | Sucker fish, white, raw, fillet, avg | 159 | 1.61 | 1.59 | 2.73 | 0.29 | 3.98 | 1.28 | 0.78 | 1.23 | 2.16 | 2.45 | 0.79 | 1.04 | 0.94 | 1.09 | 1.17 | 0.30 | 0.90 | 1.37 |
| | | | Swordfish | | | | | | | | | | | | | | | | | | | |
| 17066 | 1 | pce | Baked/broiled, avg | 106 | 1.63 | 1.61 | 2.76 | 0.29 | 4.02 | 1.29 | 0.79 | 1.24 | 2.18 | 2.47 | 0.80 | 1.05 | 0.95 | 1.10 | 1.18 | 0.30 | 0.91 | 1.39 |
| 17065 | 1 | pce | Raw, avg | 136 | 1.63 | 1.62 | 2.76 | 0.29 | 4.03 | 1.29 | 0.79 | 1.24 | 2.19 | 2.48 | 0.80 | 1.05 | 0.95 | 1.10 | 1.18 | 0.30 | 0.91 | 1.39 |
| 17136 | 3 | oz | Steamed/poached, avg | 85 | 1.29 | 1.28 | 2.19 | 0.23 | 0.32 | 1.03 | 0.63 | 0.99 | 1.73 | 1.96 | 0.63 | 0.83 | 0.76 | 0.87 | 0.94 | 0.24 | 0.72 | 1.11 |
| 17081 | 1 | ea | Tilefish, baked/broiled, fillet, avg | 300 | 4.44 | 4.41 | 7.53 | 0.79 | 10.98 | 3.54 | 2.16 | 3.39 | 5.97 | 6.75 | 2.18 | 2.87 | 2.60 | 3.00 | 3.21 | 0.82 | 2.48 | 3.78 |
| 17217 | 1 | ea | Tilefish, raw, fillet, avg | 386 | 4.09 | 4.05 | 6.91 | 0.73 | 10.07 | 3.24 | 1.99 | 3.11 | 5.48 | 6.21 | 2.00 | 2.64 | 2.39 | 2.76 | 2.96 | 0.76 | 2.28 | 3.48 |
| 17218 | 1 | ea | Trout, mixed species, raw, fillet, avg | 79 | 1.00 | 0.98 | 1.68 | 0.18 | 2.45 | 0.79 | 0.48 | 0.76 | 1.34 | 1.51 | 0.49 | 0.64 | 0.58 | 0.67 | 0.72 | 0.18 | 0.55 | 0.85 |
| 17175 | 1 | ea | Trout, mixed species, baked/broiled, fillet, avg | 62 | 1.00 | 0.99 | 1.69 | 0.18 | 2.47 | 0.79 | 0.49 | 0.76 | 1.34 | 1.52 | 0.49 | 0.64 | 0.58 | 0.68 | 0.73 | 0.18 | 0.56 | 0.85 |
| | | | Tuna | | | | | | | | | | | | | | | | | | | |
| 17024 | 1 | ea | Light, canned in oil, drained, avg | 171 | 3.01 | 2.98 | 5.10 | 0.53 | 7.44 | 2.39 | 1.47 | 2.29 | 4.05 | 4.58 | 1.47 | 1.95 | 1.76 | 2.03 | 2.19 | 0.56 | 1.68 | 2.57 |
| 17156 | 1 | ea | Light, canned in oil, drained, unsalted, avg | 171 | 3.01 | 2.98 | 5.10 | 0.53 | 7.44 | 2.39 | 1.47 | 2.29 | 4.05 | 4.58 | 1.47 | 1.95 | 1.76 | 2.03 | 2.19 | 0.56 | 1.68 | 2.57 |
| 17027 | 1 | cup | Light, canned in water, drained, avg | 154 | 2.37 | 2.36 | 4.02 | 0.42 | 5.87 | 1.88 | 1.16 | 1.82 | 3.19 | 3.60 | 1.16 | 1.53 | 1.39 | 1.60 | 1.72 | 0.44 | 1.33 | 2.02 |

TABLE A **Amino Acid Content for Selected Foods *(continued)***

| Code | Amount | | Description | Weight (g) | Alanine (g) | Arginine (g) | Aspartic acid (g) | Cystine (g) | Glutamic acid (g) | Glycine (g) | Histidine (g) | Isoleucine (g) | Leucine (g) | Lysine (g) | Methionine (g) | Phenylalanine (g) | Proline (g) | Serine (g) | Threonine (g) | Tryptophan (g) | Tyrosine (g) | Valine (g) |
|---|---|---|---|---|---|---|---|---|---|---|---|---|---|---|---|---|---|---|---|---|---|---|
| 17157 | 1 | ea | Light, canned in water, drained, unsalted, avg | 165 | 2.54 | 2.52 | 4.31 | 0.45 | 6.29 | 2.01 | 1.24 | 1.95 | 3.42 | 3.86 | 1.25 | 1.64 | 1.49 | 1.72 | 1.85 | 0.47 | 1.42 | 2.16 |
| 17141 | 3 | oz | Smoked, fresh, avg | 85 | 1.22 | 1.21 | 2.07 | 0.22 | 2.15 | 0.97 | 0.60 | 0.94 | 1.65 | 1.86 | 0.60 | 0.79 | 0.72 | 0.83 | 0.89 | 0.23 | 0.68 | 1.05 |
| 17083 | 1 | ea | White, canned in oil, drained, avg | 178 | 2.87 | 2.83 | 4.84 | 0.51 | 7.05 | 2.26 | 1.39 | 2.17 | 3.84 | 4.34 | 1.40 | 1.85 | 1.67 | 1.92 | 2.06 | 0.53 | 1.59 | 2.44 |
| 17158 | 1 | ea | White, canned in oil, drained, unsalted, avg | 178 | 2.87 | 2.83 | 4.84 | 0.51 | 7.05 | 2.26 | 1.39 | 2.17 | 3.84 | 4.34 | 1.40 | 1.85 | 1.67 | 1.92 | 2.06 | 0.53 | 1.59 | 2.44 |
| 17151 | 1 | ea | White, canned in water, drained, avg | 172 | 2.46 | 2.43 | 4.16 | 0.44 | 6.07 | 1.94 | 1.20 | 1.87 | 3.30 | 3.73 | 1.20 | 1.59 | 1.44 | 1.66 | 1.79 | 0.46 | 1.37 | 2.10 |
| 17159 | 1 | ea | White, canned in water, drained, unsalted, avg | 172 | 2.46 | 2.43 | 4.16 | 0.44 | 6.07 | 1.94 | 1.20 | 1.87 | 3.30 | 3.73 | 1.20 | 1.59 | 1.44 | 1.66 | 1.79 | 0.46 | 1.37 | 2.10 |
| 17177 | 3 | oz | Yellowfin, fresh, baked/broiled, avg | 85 | 1.54 | 1.52 | 2.61 | 0.27 | 3.81 | 1.22 | 0.75 | 1.17 | 2.07 | 2.34 | 0.75 | 0.99 | 0.90 | 1.04 | 1.11 | 0.29 | 0.86 | 1.31 |
| 17233 | 3 | oz | Yellowfin, fresh, boneless, raw, avg | 85 | 1.20 | 1.19 | 2.03 | 0.21 | 2.97 | 0.95 | 0.58 | 0.92 | 1.62 | 1.83 | 0.59 | 0.78 | 0.70 | 0.81 | 0.88 | 0.22 | 0.67 | 1.02 |
| 17161 | 1 | ea | Turbot, baked/broiled, fillet, avg | 318 | 3.94 | 3.91 | 6.71 | 0.70 | 9.76 | 3.14 | 1.93 | 3.01 | 5.31 | 6.01 | 1.94 | 2.55 | 2.32 | 2.67 | 2.87 | 0.73 | 2.21 | 3.37 |
| 17220 | 1 | ea | Turbot, raw, fillet, avg | 408 | 3.96 | 3.92 | 6.69 | 0.70 | 9.79 | 3.14 | 1.93 | 3.02 | 5.34 | 6.00 | 1.94 | 2.56 | 2.32 | 2.67 | 2.87 | 0.73 | 2.21 | 3.37 |
| | | | Whitefish | | | | | | | | | | | | | | | | | | | |
| 17162 | 1 | ea | Baked/broiled, fillet, avg | 154 | 2.28 | 2.26 | 3.87 | 0.40 | 5.62 | 1.82 | 1.11 | 1.74 | 3.06 | 3.46 | 1.11 | 1.47 | 1.33 | 1.54 | 1.65 | 0.42 | 1.27 | 1.94 |
| 17221 | 1 | ea | Mixed species, raw, fillet, avg | 198 | 2.28 | 2.26 | 3.88 | 0.41 | 5.64 | 1.81 | 1.11 | 1.74 | 3.07 | 3.47 | 1.12 | 1.48 | 1.34 | 1.54 | 1.66 | 0.42 | 1.28 | 1.95 |
| 17084 | 1 | cup | Smoked, avg | 136 | 1.93 | 1.90 | 3.26 | 0.34 | 4.75 | 1.52 | 0.94 | 1.47 | 2.58 | 2.92 | 0.94 | 1.24 | 1.12 | 1.30 | 1.40 | 0.36 | 1.07 | 1.65 |
| 17144 | 1 | ea | Whiting, baked/broiled, mixed species, fillet, avg | 72 | 1.02 | 1.02 | 1.73 | 0.18 | 2.53 | 0.81 | 0.50 | 0.78 | 1.38 | 1.56 | 0.50 | 0.66 | 0.60 | 0.69 | 0.74 | 0.19 | 0.57 | 0.87 |
| 17222 | 1 | ea | Whiting, raw, mixed species, fillet, avg | 92 | 1.02 | 1.01 | 1.73 | 0.18 | 2.51 | 0.81 | 0.50 | 0.78 | 1.37 | 1.55 | 0.50 | 0.66 | 0.60 | 0.69 | 0.74 | 0.19 | 0.57 | 0.87 |
| 17163 | 1 | ea | Wolfish, Atlantic, baked/broiled, fillet, avg | 238 | 3.24 | 3.19 | 5.47 | 0.57 | 7.97 | 2.57 | 1.57 | 2.45 | 4.33 | 4.90 | 1.58 | 2.08 | 1.89 | 2.18 | 2.34 | 0.60 | 1.80 | 2.76 |
| 17223 | 1 | ea | Wolfish, Atlantic, raw, fillet, avg | 306 | 3.24 | 3.21 | 5.48 | 0.58 | 7.99 | 2.57 | 1.58 | 2.47 | 4.35 | 4.93 | 1.59 | 2.09 | 1.89 | 2.18 | 2.35 | 0.60 | 1.81 | 2.76 |
| 17164 | 1 | ea | Yellowtail fish, baked/broiled, fillet, avg | 292 | 5.23 | 5.20 | 8.88 | 0.93 | 12.94 | 4.15 | 2.55 | 4.00 | 7.04 | 7.97 | 2.56 | 3.39 | 3.07 | 3.53 | 3.80 | 0.97 | 2.92 | 4.47 |
| 17224 | 1 | ea | Yellowtail fish, raw, fillet, avg | 374 | 5.24 | 5.20 | 8.86 | 0.93 | 12.94 | 4.15 | 2.55 | 4.00 | 7.03 | 7.97 | 2.56 | 3.38 | 3.06 | 3.53 | 3.81 | 0.97 | 2.92 | 4.45 |
| | | | **FISH—SHELLFISH AND OTHER FISH** | | | | | | | | | | | | | | | | | | | |
| | | | Abalone | | | | | | | | | | | | | | | | | | | |
| 19041 | 3 | oz | Fried, avg | 85 | 0.99 | 1.20 | 1.58 | 0.22 | 2.40 | 1.03 | 0.32 | 0.73 | 1.18 | 1.22 | 0.37 | 0.61 | 0.72 | 0.75 | 0.71 | 0.19 | 0.53 | 0.73 |
| 19018 | 3 | oz | Raw, avg | 85 | 0.88 | 1.06 | 1.40 | 0.19 | 1.98 | 0.91 | 0.28 | 0.63 | 1.02 | 1.09 | 0.33 | 0.52 | 0.59 | 0.65 | 0.63 | 0.16 | 0.46 | 0.63 |
| 19086 | 3 | oz | Steamed/poached, avg | 85 | 1.76 | 2.13 | 2.81 | 0.38 | 3.95 | 1.82 | 0.56 | 1.27 | 2.05 | 2.18 | 0.66 | 1.05 | 1.19 | 1.30 | 1.25 | 0.33 | 0.93 | 1.27 |
| | | | Clams | | | | | | | | | | | | | | | | | | | |
| 19049 | 15 | ea | Baked/broiled, avg | 150 | 1.36 | 1.63 | 2.16 | 0.30 | 3.06 | 1.40 | 0.43 | 0.98 | 1.57 | 1.68 | 0.51 | 0.81 | 0.92 | 1.00 | 0.97 | 0.25 | 0.72 | 0.98 |
| 19081 | 1 | cup | Breaded, fried, avg | 150 | 1.24 | 1.48 | 1.96 | 0.31 | 3.36 | 1.25 | 0.42 | 0.95 | 1.53 | 1.49 | 0.49 | 0.82 | 1.04 | 1.01 | 0.90 | 0.25 | 0.70 | 0.97 |
| 19002 | 1 | cup | Canned, drained, avg | 160 | 2.48 | 2.98 | 3.94 | 0.54 | 5.55 | 2.56 | 0.78 | 1.78 | 2.88 | 3.06 | 0.92 | 1.46 | 1.66 | 1.82 | 1.76 | 0.46 | 1.31 | 1.79 |
| 19110 | 1 | cup | Fried in crumbs, avg | 153 | 0.78 | 0.93 | 1.21 | 0.29 | 3.67 | 0.77 | 0.35 | 0.71 | 1.19 | 0.82 | 0.35 | 0.74 | 1.22 | 0.85 | 0.61 | 0.20 | 0.51 | 0.79 |
| 19051 | 10 | ea | Smoked, in oil, avg | 100 | 0.86 | 1.03 | 1.36 | 0.19 | 1.92 | 0.89 | 0.27 | 0.62 | 1.00 | 1.06 | 0.32 | 0.51 | 0.58 | 0.63 | 0.61 | 0.16 | 0.45 | 0.62 |
| 19000 | 10 | ea | Steamed, avg | 95 | 1.47 | 1.77 | 2.34 | 0.32 | 3.30 | 1.52 | 0.47 | 1.05 | 1.71 | 1.81 | 0.55 | 0.87 | 0.99 | 1.08 | 1.04 | 0.27 | 0.78 | 1.06 |
| | | | Crab | | | | | | | | | | | | | | | | | | | |
| 19094 | 1 | ea | Alaskan king, leg, raw, avg | 172 | 1.79 | 2.75 | 3.25 | 0.35 | 5.36 | 1.89 | 0.64 | 1.52 | 2.49 | 2.73 | 0.88 | 1.33 | 1.04 | 1.24 | 1.27 | 0.44 | 1.05 | 1.48 |
| 19036 | 1 | ea | Alaskan king, leg, steamed/boiled, avg | 134 | 1.47 | 2.26 | 2.68 | 0.29 | 4.42 | 1.57 | 0.53 | 1.26 | 2.06 | 2.25 | 0.73 | 1.10 | 0.86 | 1.02 | 1.05 | 0.36 | 0.86 | 1.22 |
| 19052 | 1 | cup | Baked/broiled, sauteed, avg | 118 | 1.27 | 1.96 | 2.31 | 0.25 | 3.82 | 1.36 | 0.46 | 1.09 | 1.78 | 1.95 | 0.63 | 0.95 | 0.74 | 0.88 | 0.91 | 0.31 | 0.75 | 1.05 |
| 19124 | 1 | cup | Blue, canned, drained, avg | 135 | 1.56 | 2.41 | 2.85 | 0.31 | 4.71 | 1.67 | 0.56 | 1.34 | 2.19 | 2.41 | 0.78 | 1.17 | 0.91 | 1.09 | 1.12 | 0.38 | 0.92 | 1.30 |
| 19095 | 1 | ea | Blue, raw, avg | 21 | 0.21 | 0.33 | 0.39 | 0.04 | 0.65 | 0.23 | 0.08 | 0.18 | 0.30 | 0.33 | 0.11 | 0.16 | 0.12 | 0.15 | 0.15 | 0.05 | 0.13 | 0.18 |
| 19033 | 1 | cup | Blue, steamed/boiled, avg | 118 | 1.34 | 2.08 | 2.46 | 0.27 | 4.06 | 1.44 | 0.48 | 1.15 | 1.88 | 2.07 | 0.67 | 1.00 | 0.78 | 0.94 | 0.96 | 0.33 | 0.79 | 1.12 |
| 19096 | 1 | ea | Dungeness, raw, avg | 163 | 1.60 | 2.47 | 2.93 | 0.32 | 4.83 | 1.71 | 0.58 | 1.37 | 2.24 | 2.47 | 0.80 | 1.19 | 0.93 | 1.11 | 1.15 | 0.39 | 0.94 | 1.33 |
| 19004 | 1 | ea | Dungeness, steamed/boiled, avg | 127 | 1.60 | 2.47 | 2.92 | 0.32 | 4.82 | 1.70 | 0.58 | 1.37 | 2.25 | 2.46 | 0.80 | 1.19 | 0.93 | 1.11 | 1.14 | 0.39 | 0.94 | 1.33 |
| 19097 | 3 | oz | Queen, raw, avg | 85 | 0.89 | 1.37 | 1.62 | 0.18 | 2.68 | 0.95 | 0.32 | 0.76 | 1.25 | 1.36 | 0.44 | 0.66 | 0.52 | 0.62 | 0.63 | 0.22 | 0.52 | 0.74 |
| 19083 | 3 | oz | Queen, steamed/boiled, avg | 85 | 1.14 | 1.76 | 2.08 | 0.23 | 3.43 | 1.21 | 0.41 | 0.98 | 1.60 | 1.75 | 0.57 | 0.85 | 0.66 | 0.79 | 0.81 | 0.28 | 0.67 | 0.94 |
| 19055 | 1 | ea | Soft shell, floured/breaded, fried, avg | 65 | 0.74 | 1.15 | 1.36 | 0.15 | 2.24 | 0.79 | 0.27 | 0.64 | 1.04 | 1.14 | 0.37 | 0.55 | 0.43 | 0.52 | 0.53 | 0.18 | 0.44 | 0.62 |
| 19087 | 10 | ea | Crayfish, mixed species, raw, avg | 34 | 0.29 | 0.44 | 0.52 | 0.06 | 0.86 | 0.30 | 0.10 | 0.24 | 0.40 | 0.44 | 0.14 | 0.21 | 0.17 | 0.20 | 0.20 | 0.07 | 0.17 | 0.24 |
| 19088 | 3 | oz | Crayfish, mixed species, steamed/boiled, avg | 85 | 0.84 | 1.30 | 1.54 | 0.17 | 2.53 | 0.89 | 0.30 | 0.72 | 1.18 | 1.29 | 0.42 | 0.63 | 0.49 | 0.59 | 0.60 | 0.21 | 0.49 | 0.70 |
| | | | Eel | | | | | | | | | | | | | | | | | | | |
| 17102 | 1 | ea | Baked/broiled, fillet, avg | 159 | 2.27 | 2.26 | 3.85 | 0.40 | 5.61 | 1.81 | 1.11 | 1.73 | 3.05 | 3.45 | 1.11 | 1.47 | 1.33 | 1.53 | 1.65 | 0.42 | 1.27 | 1.94 |
| 17232 | 1 | ea | Raw, fillet, avg | 204 | 2.28 | 2.24 | 3.86 | 0.40 | 5.61 | 1.81 | 1.11 | 1.73 | 3.06 | 3.45 | 1.11 | 1.47 | 1.33 | 1.54 | 1.65 | 0.42 | 1.27 | 1.94 |
| 17041 | 3 | oz | Smoked, avg | 85 | 0.96 | 0.95 | 1.50 | 0.17 | 2.36 | 0.76 | 0.47 | 0.73 | 1.29 | 1.45 | 0.47 | 0.62 | 0.56 | 0.65 | 0.69 | 0.18 | 0.53 | 0.82 |

TABLE A **Amino Acid Content for Selected Foods *(continued)***

| Code | Amount | | Description | Weight (g) | Alanine (g) | Arginine (g) | Aspartic acid (g) | Cystine (g) | Glutamic acid (g) | Glycine (g) | Histidine (g) | Isoleucine (g) | Leucine (g) | Lysine (g) | Methionine (g) | Phenylalanine (g) | Proline (g) | Serine (g) | Threonine (g) | Tryptophan (g) | Tyrosine (g) | Valine (g) |
|---|---|---|---|---|---|---|---|---|---|---|---|---|---|---|---|---|---|---|---|---|---|---|
| 17130 | 1 | cup | Steamed/poached, avg | 123 | 1.80 | 1.78 | 3.05 | 0.32 | 0.44 | 1.43 | 0.88 | 1.38 | 2.42 | 2.73 | 0.83 | 1.16 | 1.05 | 1.22 | 1.30 | 0.33 | 1.00 | 1.54 |
| | | | Lobster | | | | | | | | | | | | | | | | | | | |
| 19057 | 1 | cup | Baked/broiled, avg | 145 | 1.62 | 2.51 | 2.97 | 0.32 | 4.90 | 1.74 | 0.58 | 1.39 | 2.28 | 2.49 | 0.81 | 1.21 | 0.95 | 1.13 | 1.16 | 0.40 | 0.95 | 1.35 |
| 19023 | 1 | ea | Northern, raw, avg | 150 | 1.60 | 2.46 | 2.90 | 0.32 | 4.80 | 1.69 | 0.57 | 1.36 | 2.23 | 2.46 | 0.79 | 1.19 | 0.93 | 1.11 | 1.14 | 0.39 | 0.94 | 1.32 |
| 19006 | 1 | cup | Northern, steamed/boiled, avg | 145 | 1.68 | 2.59 | 3.07 | 0.33 | 5.06 | 1.79 | 0.60 | 1.44 | 2.36 | 2.58 | 0.83 | 1.25 | 0.98 | 1.17 | 1.20 | 0.41 | 0.99 | 1.39 |
| 19098 | 1 | ea | Spiny, raw, avg | 209 | 2.44 | 3.76 | 4.45 | 0.48 | 7.33 | 2.59 | 0.87 | 2.08 | 3.40 | 3.73 | 1.21 | 1.82 | 1.42 | 1.69 | 1.74 | 0.60 | 1.43 | 2.02 |
| 19084 | 1 | ea | Spiny, steamed/boiled, avg | 163 | 2.43 | 3.74 | 4.44 | 0.48 | 7.33 | 2.59 | 0.87 | 2.08 | 3.40 | 3.74 | 1.21 | 1.81 | 1.42 | 1.69 | 1.74 | 0.60 | 1.43 | 2.02 |
| 19024 | 1 | cup | Mussels, Blue, raw, avg | 150 | 1.08 | 1.30 | 1.72 | 0.23 | 2.43 | 1.12 | 0.34 | 0.78 | 1.26 | 1.33 | 0.40 | 0.64 | 0.73 | 0.80 | 0.77 | 0.20 | 0.57 | 0.78 |
| 19044 | 3 | oz | Mussels, Blue, steamed/boiled, avg | 85 | 1.22 | 1.48 | 1.96 | 0.27 | 2.75 | 1.27 | 0.39 | 0.88 | 1.43 | 1.57 | 0.45 | 0.73 | 0.83 | 0.91 | 0.88 | 0.23 | 0.65 | 0.88 |
| | | | Octopus | | | | | | | | | | | | | | | | | | | |
| 19072 | 1 | cup | Dried, avg | 53 | 1.84 | 2.22 | 2.93 | 0.40 | 4.13 | 1.93 | 0.58 | 1.32 | 2.14 | 2.27 | 0.63 | 1.09 | 1.24 | 1.36 | 1.31 | 0.34 | 0.97 | 1.32 |
| 19058 | 1 | cup | Dried, boiled, avg | 107 | 2.01 | 2.42 | 3.20 | 0.44 | 0.45 | 2.03 | 0.64 | 1.44 | 2.33 | 2.48 | 0.75 | 1.19 | 1.35 | 1.49 | 1.42 | 0.37 | 1.06 | 1.44 |
| 19025 | 3 | oz | Raw, avg | 85 | 0.77 | 0.93 | 1.22 | 0.17 | 1.73 | 0.73 | 0.24 | 0.55 | 0.89 | 0.94 | 0.29 | 0.45 | 0.52 | 0.57 | 0.55 | 0.14 | 0.41 | 0.55 |
| 19059 | 3 | oz | Smoked, avg | 85 | 1.31 | 1.57 | 2.08 | 0.28 | 2.94 | 1.35 | 0.41 | 0.94 | 1.52 | 1.62 | 0.49 | 0.77 | 0.88 | 0.97 | 0.93 | 0.24 | 0.69 | 0.94 |
| 19048 | 3 | oz | Steamed/boiled, avg | 85 | 1.53 | 1.85 | 2.45 | 0.33 | 3.45 | 1.53 | 0.49 | 1.11 | 1.78 | 1.90 | 0.57 | 0.91 | 1.04 | 1.14 | 1.09 | 0.28 | 0.81 | 1.11 |
| | | | Oysters | | | | | | | | | | | | | | | | | | | |
| 19027 | 10 | ea | Eastern, boiled/steamed, avg | 70 | 0.60 | 0.72 | 0.95 | 0.13 | 1.34 | 0.62 | 0.19 | 0.43 | 0.70 | 0.73 | 0.22 | 0.35 | 0.40 | 0.44 | 0.42 | 0.11 | 0.32 | 0.43 |
| 19135 | 1 | ea | Eastern, canned w/liquid, avg | 272 | 1.16 | 1.40 | 1.85 | 0.25 | 2.61 | 1.23 | 0.37 | 0.84 | 1.35 | 1.44 | 0.43 | 0.69 | 0.78 | 0.86 | 0.83 | 0.21 | 0.61 | 0.84 |
| 19090 | 10 | ea | Eastern, medium, baked/broiled, avg | 98 | 0.41 | 0.50 | 0.66 | 0.09 | 0.93 | 0.43 | 0.13 | 0.30 | 0.48 | 0.57 | 0.15 | 0.25 | 0.28 | 0.31 | 0.29 | 0.08 | 0.22 | 0.30 |
| 19009 | 10 | ea | Eastern, medium, breaded, fried, avg | 147 | 0.72 | 0.86 | 1.15 | 0.19 | 2.20 | 0.72 | 0.26 | 0.58 | 0.94 | 0.86 | 0.29 | 0.52 | 0.69 | 0.63 | 0.54 | 0.15 | 0.43 | 0.60 |
| 19089 | 10 | ea | Eastern, medium, raw, avg | 142 | 0.45 | 0.54 | 0.72 | 0.10 | 1.01 | 0.45 | 0.14 | 0.32 | 0.52 | 0.55 | 0.17 | 0.27 | 0.30 | 0.33 | 0.32 | 0.08 | 0.24 | 0.32 |
| 19045 | 1 | ea | Pacific, raw, avg | 50 | 0.29 | 0.34 | 0.46 | 0.06 | 0.64 | 0.33 | 0.09 | 0.21 | 0.33 | 0.35 | 0.11 | 0.17 | 0.19 | 0.21 | 0.20 | 0.05 | 0.15 | 0.21 |
| 19008 | 1 | ea | Pacific, steamed/boiled, avg | 25 | 0.28 | 0.34 | 0.46 | 0.06 | 0.64 | 0.23 | 0.09 | 0.21 | 0.33 | 0.35 | 0.11 | 0.17 | 0.19 | 0.21 | 0.20 | 0.05 | 0.15 | 0.21 |
| | | | Scallops | | | | | | | | | | | | | | | | | | | |
| 19061 | 4 | ea | Baked/broiled, avg | 100 | 1.23 | 1.48 | 1.96 | 2.67 | 2.77 | 1.27 | 0.39 | 0.88 | 1.43 | 1.52 | 0.46 | 0.73 | 0.83 | 0.91 | 0.88 | 0.23 | 0.65 | 0.89 |
| 19030 | 4 | ea | Breaded, fried, avg | 62 | 0.66 | 0.79 | 1.04 | 0.16 | 1.72 | 0.66 | 0.22 | 0.50 | 0.81 | 0.79 | 0.25 | 0.43 | 0.53 | 0.53 | 0.48 | 0.13 | 0.36 | 0.51 |
| 19137 | 4 | ea | Raw, avg | 60 | 0.61 | 0.73 | 0.97 | 0.13 | 1.37 | 0.63 | 0.19 | 0.44 | 0.71 | 0.75 | 0.23 | 0.36 | 0.41 | 0.45 | 0.43 | 0.11 | 0.32 | 0.44 |
| 19011 | 1 | cup | Steamed/boiled, avg | 120 | 1.18 | 1.42 | 1.88 | 0.26 | 2.66 | 1.22 | 0.37 | 0.85 | 1.38 | 1.46 | 0.44 | 0.70 | 0.80 | 0.87 | 0.84 | 0.22 | 0.63 | 0.85 |
| | | | Shrimp | | | | | | | | | | | | | | | | | | | |
| 19065 | 4 | ea | Baked/broiled, sauteed, avg | 20 | 0.27 | 0.43 | 0.51 | 0.05 | 0.84 | 0.30 | 0.10 | 0.24 | 0.39 | 0.43 | 0.14 | 0.21 | 0.16 | 0.19 | 0.20 | 0.07 | 0.16 | 0.23 |
| 19012 | 4 | ea | Boiled, avg | 22 | 0.26 | 0.40 | 0.47 | 0.05 | 0.78 | 0.28 | 0.09 | 0.22 | 0.36 | 0.40 | 0.13 | 0.19 | 0.15 | 0.18 | 0.19 | 0.06 | 0.15 | 0.22 |
| 19014 | 4 | ea | Breaded, fried, avg | 30 | 0.35 | 0.53 | 0.63 | 0.08 | 1.16 | 0.37 | 0.13 | 0.31 | 0.51 | 0.52 | 0.18 | 0.28 | 0.25 | 0.27 | 0.26 | 0.09 | 0.21 | 0.31 |
| 19127 | 1 | ea | Canned, drained, avg | 128 | 1.67 | 2.58 | 3.05 | 0.33 | 5.03 | 1.78 | 0.60 | 1.43 | 2.34 | 2.57 | 0.83 | 1.25 | 0.97 | 1.16 | 1.19 | 0.41 | 0.98 | 1.39 |
| 19077 | 20 | ea | Dried, avg | 10 | 0.33 | 0.51 | 0.60 | 0.07 | 0.99 | 0.35 | 0.12 | 0.28 | 0.46 | 0.57 | 0.17 | 0.25 | 0.19 | 0.23 | 0.24 | 0.08 | 0.19 | 0.27 |
| 19125 | 4 | ea | Raw, avg | 24 | 0.28 | 0.43 | 0.50 | 0.05 | 0.83 | 0.29 | 0.10 | 0.24 | 0.38 | 0.42 | 0.14 | 0.21 | 0.16 | 0.19 | 0.20 | 0.07 | 0.16 | 0.23 |
| | | | Squid | | | | | | | | | | | | | | | | | | | |
| 19068 | 1 | cup | Baked/broiled, avg | 140 | 1.57 | 1.90 | 2.51 | 0.36 | 3.81 | 1.63 | 0.51 | 1.15 | 1.86 | 1.93 | 0.59 | 0.96 | 1.15 | 1.19 | 1.12 | 0.30 | 0.85 | 1.16 |
| 19074 | 1 | cup | Canned, avg | 187 | 2.00 | 2.41 | 3.18 | 0.45 | 4.84 | 2.08 | 0.65 | 1.46 | 2.37 | 2.45 | 0.75 | 1.23 | 1.46 | 1.52 | 1.43 | 0.38 | 1.08 | 1.47 |
| 19073 | 3 | oz | Dried, avg | 85 | 2.92 | 3.51 | 4.62 | 0.66 | 7.05 | 3.02 | 0.94 | 2.13 | 3.46 | 3.56 | 1.10 | 1.78 | 2.13 | 2.21 | 2.07 | 0.55 | 1.56 | 2.14 |
| 19047 | 1 | cup | Fried in flour, avg | 105 | 1.12 | 1.35 | 1.78 | 0.25 | 2.72 | 1.17 | 0.37 | 0.82 | 1.33 | 1.38 | 0.42 | 0.69 | 0.82 | 0.85 | 0.80 | 0.21 | 0.60 | 0.83 |
| 19069 | 3 | oz | Pickled, avg | 85 | 0.76 | 0.92 | 1.21 | 0.17 | 1.84 | 0.79 | 0.25 | 0.56 | 0.90 | 0.94 | 0.29 | 0.47 | 0.56 | 0.58 | 0.54 | 0.14 | 0.41 | 0.56 |
| 19093 | 3 | oz | Raw, avg | 85 | 0.80 | 0.97 | 1.28 | 0.17 | 1.80 | 0.83 | 0.25 | 0.58 | 0.94 | 0.99 | 0.30 | 0.47 | 0.54 | 0.59 | 0.57 | 0.15 | 0.42 | 0.58 |
| | | | Surimi | | | | | | | | | | | | | | | | | | | |
| 19037 | 3 | oz | Imitation crab, Alaskan king, avg | 85 | 0.60 | 0.68 | 1.02 | 0.11 | 1.62 | 0.40 | 0.24 | 0.48 | 0.81 | 0.94 | 0.35 | 0.40 | 0.38 | 0.45 | 0.49 | 0.06 | 0.41 | 0.52 |
| 17080 | 3 | oz | Imitation pollock, avg | 85 | 0.76 | 0.86 | 1.29 | 0.14 | 2.04 | 0.50 | 0.30 | 0.60 | 1.02 | 1.18 | 0.44 | 0.51 | 0.48 | 0.56 | 0.62 | 0.08 | 0.52 | 0.65 |

TABLE A **Amino Acid Content for Selected Foods *(continued)***

| Code | Amount | Description | Weight (g) | Alanine (g) | Arginine (g) | Aspartic acid (g) | Cystine (g) | Glutamic acid (g) | Glycine (g) | Histidine (g) | Isoleucine (g) | Leucine (g) | Lysine (g) | Methionine (g) | Phenylalanine (g) | Proline (g) | Serine (g) | Threonine (g) | Tryptophan (g) | Tyrosine (g) | Valine (g) |
|---|---|---|---|---|---|---|---|---|---|---|---|---|---|---|---|---|---|---|---|---|---|
| 19046 | 3 oz | Imitation scallop, avg | 85 | 0.64 | 0.72 | 1.09 | 0.12 | 1.72 | 0.42 | 0.25 | 0.51 | 0.86 | 0.99 | 0.37 | 0.43 | 0.40 | 0.47 | 0.52 | 0.07 | 0.44 | 0.55 |
| 19039 | 3 oz | Imitation shrimp, avg | 85 | 0.62 | 0.70 | 1.05 | 0.11 | 1.67 | 0.41 | 0.24 | 0.49 | 0.83 | 0.96 | 0.36 | 0.41 | 0.39 | 0.46 | 0.51 | 0.06 | 0.42 | 0.53 |
| 19100 | 3 oz | Whelk, mollusks, raw, avg | 85 | 1.33 | 2.10 | 2.18 | 0.16 | 3.12 | 1.28 | 0.41 | 0.70 | 1.62 | 1.25 | 0.51 | 0.70 | 1.00 | 0.94 | 0.91 | 0.26 | 0.65 | 0.88 |
| 19040 | 3 oz | Whelk, mollusks, steamed/boiled, avg | 85 | 2.64 | 4.20 | 4.36 | 0.32 | 6.24 | 2.54 | 0.83 | 1.41 | 3.24 | 2.49 | 1.03 | 1.40 | 2.01 | 1.89 | 1.82 | 0.53 | 1.29 | 1.77 |
| | | **FRUIT, VEGETABLE AND BLENDED JUICES** | | | | | | | | | | | | | | | | | | | |
| | | Apple | | | | | | | | | | | | | | | | | | | |
| 3008 | 1/2 cup | Canned/bottled, avg | 124 | 0.00 | 0.00 | 0.03 | 0.00 | 0.01 | 0.00 | 0.00 | 0.00 | 0.00 | 0.01 | 0.00 | 0.00 | 0.00 | 0.00 | 0.00 | 0.00 | 0.00 | 0.00 |
| 3328 | 1/2 cup | Canned/bottled, w/vit C, avg | 124 | 0.00 | 0.00 | 0.03 | 0.00 | 0.01 | 0.00 | 0.00 | 0.00 | 0.00 | 0.01 | 0.00 | 0.00 | 0.00 | 0.00 | 0.00 | 0.00 | 0.00 | 0.00 |
| 3150 | 1/4 cup | Concentrate, avg | 70 | 0.02 | 0.01 | 0.12 | 0.00 | 0.04 | 0.01 | 0.01 | 0.01 | 0.02 | 0.03 | 0.01 | 0.01 | 0.01 | 0.02 | 0.01 | 0.01 | 0.01 | 0.02 |
| 3010 | 1/2 cup | Concentrate, prep w/water, avg | 120 | 0.01 | 0.00 | 0.06 | 0.00 | 0.02 | 0.00 | 0.00 | 0.00 | 0.01 | 0.01 | 0.00 | 0.00 | 0.00 | 0.01 | 0.00 | 0.00 | 0.00 | 0.01 |
| 3329 | 1/4 cup | Concentrate, w/vit C, avg | 70 | 0.02 | 0.01 | 0.12 | 0.00 | 0.04 | 0.01 | 0.01 | 0.01 | 0.02 | 0.03 | 0.01 | 0.01 | 0.01 | 0.02 | 0.01 | 0.01 | 0.01 | 0.02 |
| 3015 | 1/2 cup | Apricot nectar, canned, avg | 126 | 0.02 | 0.02 | 0.11 | 0.00 | 0.05 | 0.01 | 0.01 | 0.01 | 0.03 | 0.03 | 0.00 | 0.02 | 0.03 | 0.03 | 0.02 | 0.01 | 0.01 | 0.02 |
| 3218 | 1/2 cup | Apricot nectar, w/vit C, canned, avg | 126 | 0.02 | 0.02 | 0.11 | 0.00 | 0.05 | 0.01 | 0.01 | 0.01 | 0.03 | 0.03 | 0.00 | 0.02 | 0.03 | 0.03 | 0.02 | 0.01 | 0.01 | 0.02 |
| 3325 | 1/2 cup | Banana nectar, avg | 125 | 0.02 | 0.02 | 0.05 | 0.01 | 0.05 | 0.02 | 0.04 | 0.02 | 0.03 | 0.02 | 0.01 | 0.02 | 0.02 | 0.02 | 0.02 | 0.01 | 0.01 | 0.02 |
| 3223 | 1/2 cup | Cranberry-apple drink, w/vit C, bottled, avg | 122 | 0.00 | 0.00 | 0.01 | 0.00 | 0.00 | 0.00 | 0.00 | 0.00 | 0.00 | 0.00 | 0.00 | 0.00 | 0.00 | 0.00 | 0.00 | 0.00 | 0.00 | 0.00 |
| 3274 | 1/2 cup | Cranberry-apricot, avg | 122 | 0.01 | 0.01 | 0.04 | 0.00 | 0.02 | 0.00 | 0.00 | 0.00 | 0.01 | 0.01 | 0.00 | 0.01 | 0.01 | 0.01 | 0.01 | 0.00 | 0.00 | 0.01 |
| 3275 | 1/2 cup | Cranberry-grape, avg | 122 | 0.04 | 0.02 | 0.01 | 0.00 | 0.05 | 0.00 | 0.00 | 0.00 | 0.00 | 0.00 | 0.00 | 0.00 | 0.01 | 0.01 | 0.01 | 0.00 | 0.00 | 0.00 |
| | | Grape | | | | | | | | | | | | | | | | | | | |
| 3062 | 1/2 cup | Canned/bottled, avg | 126 | 0.11 | 0.06 | 0.03 | 0.00 | 0.14 | 0.02 | 0.01 | 0.01 | 0.02 | 0.01 | 0.00 | 0.02 | 0.02 | 0.02 | 0.02 | 0.00 | 0.00 | 0.01 |
| 3233 | 1/4 cup | Concentrate, sweetened, w/vit C, avg | 71 | 0.07 | 0.04 | 0.02 | 0.00 | 0.09 | 0.01 | 0.01 | 0.01 | 0.01 | 0.01 | 0.00 | 0.01 | 0.01 | 0.01 | 0.01 | 0.00 | 0.00 | 0.01 |
| 3064 | 1/2 cup | Concentrate, sweetened, w/vit C, prep w/water, avg | 125 | 0.04 | 0.02 | 0.01 | 0.00 | 0.05 | 0.01 | 0.00 | 0.00 | 0.01 | 0.00 | 0.00 | 0.01 | 0.01 | 0.01 | 0.01 | 0.00 | 0.00 | 0.00 |
| | | Grapefruit | | | | | | | | | | | | | | | | | | | |
| 3052 | 1/2 cup | Canned, avg | 124 | 0.03 | 0.05 | 0.13 | 0.00 | 0.05 | 0.01 | 0.01 | 0.01 | 0.02 | 0.02 | 0.00 | 0.01 | 0.06 | 0.03 | 0.01 | 0.00 | 0.01 | 0.02 |
| 3219 | 1/4 cup | Concentrate, avg | 68 | 0.06 | 0.11 | 0.27 | 0.00 | 0.11 | 0.03 | 0.01 | 0.03 | 0.04 | 0.05 | 0.01 | 0.03 | 0.12 | 0.07 | 0.03 | 0.01 | 0.19 | 0.04 |
| 3053 | 1/2 cup | Concentrate, prep w/water, avg | 124 | 0.03 | 0.05 | 0.14 | 0.00 | 0.06 | 0.01 | 0.01 | 0.01 | 0.02 | 0.02 | 0.00 | 0.01 | 0.06 | 0.03 | 0.01 | 0.00 | 0.10 | 0.02 |
| 3051 | 1/2 cup | Fresh, avg | 124 | 0.03 | 0.05 | 0.13 | 0.00 | 0.05 | 0.01 | 0.01 | 0.01 | 0.02 | 0.02 | 0.00 | 0.01 | 0.06 | 0.03 | 0.01 | 0.00 | 0.01 | 0.02 |
| 3165 | 1/2 cup | Sweetened, canned, avg | 125 | 0.03 | 0.05 | 0.13 | 0.00 | 0.05 | 0.01 | 0.01 | 0.01 | 0.02 | 0.02 | 0.00 | 0.01 | 0.06 | 0.03 | 0.01 | 0.01 | 0.01 | 0.02 |
| 3305 | 1/2 cup | Guava drink, w/vit C, avg | 126 | 0.01 | 0.00 | 0.01 | 0.00 | 0.02 | 0.01 | 0.00 | 0.01 | 0.01 | 0.00 | 0.00 | 0.00 | 0.01 | 0.01 | 0.01 | 0.00 | 0.00 | 0.01 |
| 3304 | 1/2 cup | Guava nectar, avg | 125 | 0.01 | 0.00 | 0.01 | 0.00 | 0.02 | 0.01 | 0.00 | 0.01 | 0.01 | 0.00 | 0.00 | 0.00 | 0.01 | 0.01 | 0.01 | 0.00 | 0.00 | 0.01 |
| | | Lemon | | | | | | | | | | | | | | | | | | | |
| 3069 | 1/2 cup | Bottled, avg | 122 | 0.03 | 0.03 | 0.06 | 0.01 | 0.05 | 0.04 | 0.01 | 0.01 | 0.01 | 0.02 | 0.01 | 0.02 | 0.02 | 0.01 | 0.01 | 0.00 | 0.01 | 0.02 |
| 3068 | 1/2 cup | Fresh, avg | 122 | 0.03 | 0.03 | 0.06 | 0.01 | 0.05 | 0.04 | 0.01 | 0.01 | 0.01 | 0.02 | 0.01 | 0.02 | 0.02 | 0.01 | 0.01 | 0.00 | 0.01 | 0.02 |
| 3070 | 1/2 cup | Frozen, avg | 122 | 0.03 | 0.03 | 0.08 | 0.01 | 0.06 | 0.05 | 0.01 | 0.01 | 0.01 | 0.03 | 0.01 | 0.02 | 0.03 | 0.01 | 0.01 | 0.00 | 0.01 | 0.02 |
| 3303 | 1/2 cup | Mango nectar, avg | 125 | 0.02 | 0.01 | 0.02 | 0.00 | 0.03 | 0.01 | 0.01 | 0.01 | 0.02 | 0.02 | 0.00 | 0.01 | 0.01 | 0.01 | 0.01 | 0.00 | 0.01 | 0.01 |
| | | Orange | | | | | | | | | | | | | | | | | | | |
| 3093 | 1/2 cup | Canned, avg | 124 | 0.02 | 0.05 | 0.08 | 0.00 | 0.03 | 0.01 | 0.00 | 0.01 | 0.01 | 0.01 | 0.00 | 0.01 | 0.05 | 0.01 | 0.01 | 0.00 | 0.00 | 0.01 |
| 3092 | 1/2 cup | Chilled, avg | 124 | 0.01 | 0.04 | 0.06 | 0.00 | 0.03 | 0.01 | 0.00 | 0.01 | 0.01 | 0.01 | 0.00 | 0.01 | 0.04 | 0.01 | 0.01 | 0.00 | 0.00 | 0.01 |
| 3094 | 1/4 cup | Concentrate, avg | 70 | 0.04 | 0.11 | 0.18 | 0.01 | 0.08 | 0.02 | 0.01 | 0.02 | 0.03 | 0.02 | 0.01 | 0.02 | 0.10 | 0.03 | 0.02 | 0.00 | 0.01 | 0.03 |
| 3091 | 1/2 cup | Concentrate, prep w/water, avg | 124 | 0.02 | 0.06 | 0.09 | 0.01 | 0.04 | 0.01 | 0.00 | 0.01 | 0.02 | 0.01 | 0.00 | 0.01 | 0.05 | 0.02 | 0.01 | 0.00 | 0.00 | 0.01 |
| 3090 | 1/2 cup | Fresh, avg | 124 | 0.02 | 0.06 | 0.09 | 0.01 | 0.04 | 0.01 | 0.00 | 0.01 | 0.02 | 0.01 | 0.00 | 0.01 | 0.05 | 0.02 | 0.01 | 0.00 | 0.00 | 0.01 |
| 3317 | 1/2 cup | Orange-banana, avg | 125 | 0.02 | 0.06 | 0.10 | 0.01 | 0.06 | 0.02 | 0.03 | 0.02 | 0.03 | 0.02 | 0.01 | 0.02 | 0.05 | 0.03 | 0.02 | 0.01 | 0.01 | 0.02 |
| 3170 | 1/2 cup | Orange-grapefruit, canned, avg | 124 | 0.02 | 0.05 | 0.09 | 0.00 | 0.04 | 0.01 | 0.00 | 0.01 | 0.01 | 0.01 | 0.00 | 0.01 | 0.05 | 0.02 | 0.01 | 0.00 | 0.00 | 0.01 |
| 3095 | 1/2 cup | Papaya nectar, canned, avg | 125 | 0.01 | 0.00 | 0.02 | 0.00 | 0.01 | 0.01 | 0.00 | 0.00 | 0.01 | 0.01 | 0.00 | 0.00 | 0.00 | 0.01 | 0.00 | 0.00 | 0.00 | 0.00 |
| 3200 | 1/2 cup | Passion Fruit, purple, fresh, avg | 124 | 0.04 | 0.00 | 0.19 | 0.00 | 0.12 | 0.00 | 0.01 | 0.01 | 0.01 | 0.01 | 0.00 | 0.01 | 0.00 | 0.07 | 0.00 | 0.00 | 0.00 | 0.01 |
| 3201 | 1/2 cup | Passion Fruit, yellow, avg | 124 | 0.07 | 0.00 | 0.32 | 0.00 | 0.21 | 0.01 | 0.02 | 0.01 | 0.01 | 0.02 | 0.00 | 0.02 | 0.00 | 0.12 | 0.01 | 0.00 | 0.00 | 0.02 |

TABLE A **Amino Acid Content for Selected Foods *(continued)***

| Code | Amount | Description | Weight (g) | Alanine (g) | Arginine (g) | Aspartic acid (g) | Cystine (g) | Glutamic acid (g) | Glycine (g) | Histidine (g) | Isoleucine (g) | Leucine (g) | Lysine (g) | Methionine (g) | Phenylalanine (g) | Proline (g) | Serine (g) | Threonine (g) | Tryptophan (g) | Tyrosine (g) | Valine (g) |
|---|---|---|---|---|---|---|---|---|---|---|---|---|---|---|---|---|---|---|---|---|---|
| 3101 | 1/2 cup | Peach nectar, canned, avg | 124 | 0.02 | 0.01 | 0.06 | 0.00 | 0.05 | 0.01 | 0.01 | 0.01 | 0.02 | 0.0[illegible] | 0.01 | 0.01 | 0.01 | 0.01 | 0.01 | 0.00 | 0.01 | 0.02 |
| 3110 | 1/2 cup | Pear nectar, canned, avg | 125 | 0.00 | 0.00 | 0.03 | 0.00 | 0.0[illegible] | 0.00 | 0.00 | 0.00 | 0.01 | 0.0[illegible] | 0.00 | 0.00 | 0.00 | 0.01 | 0.00 | 0.00 | 0.00 | 0.01 |
| | | Pineapple | | | | | | | | | | | | | | | | | | | |
| 3120 | 1/2 cup | Canned, avg | 125 | 0.02 | 0.02 | 0.06 | 0.00 | 0.05 | 0.02 | 0.01 | 0.01 | 0.02 | 0.03 | 0.01 | 0.01 | 0.01 | 0.03 | 0.01 | 0.01 | 0.01 | 0.02 |
| 3189 | 1/4 cup | Concentrate, avg | 71 | 0.04 | 0.04 | 0.14 | 0.00 | 0.1[illegible] | 0.04 | 0.02 | 0.03 | 0.05 | 0.06 | 0.03 | 0.03 | 0.03 | 0.06 | 0.03 | 0.01 | 0.03 | 0.04 |
| 3119 | 1/2 cup | Concentrate, prep w/water, avg | 125 | 0.02 | 0.02 | 0.07 | 0.00 | 0.06 | 0.02 | 0.01 | 0.02 | 0.02 | 0.03 | 0.01 | 0.02 | 0.02 | 0.03 | 0.02 | 0.01 | 0.02 | 0.02 |
| 3302 | 1/2 cup | Pineapple-orange-banana, avg | 125 | 0.01 | 0.03 | 0.05 | 0.00 | 0.02 | 0.01 | 0.01 | 0.01 | 0.01 | 0.0[illegible] | 0.00 | 0.01 | 0.03 | 0.01 | 0.01 | 0.00 | 0.00 | 0.01 |
| 3128 | 1/2 cup | Prune, Bottled, avg | 128 | 0.03 | 0.01 | 0.25 | 0.00 | 0.04 | 0.01 | 0.01 | 0.02 | 0.02 | 0.02 | 0.01 | 0.02 | 0.03 | 0.02 | 0.02 | 0.00 | 0.01 | 0.02 |
| 3324 | 1/2 cup | Strawberry, avg | 118 | 0.04 | 0.03 | 0.16 | 0.01 | 0.1[illegible] | 0.03 | 0.01 | 0.02 | 0.04 | 0.03 | 0.00 | 0.02 | 0.02 | 0.03 | 0.02 | 0.01 | 0.02 | 0.02 |
| | | Tangerine | | | | | | | | | | | | | | | | | | | |
| 3347 | 1/2 cup | Fresh, avg | 124 | 0.01 | 0.04 | 0.07 | 0.00 | 0.03 | 0.01 | 0.00 | 0.01 | 0.01 | 0.0[illegible] | 0.00 | 0.01 | 0.04 | 0.01 | 0.01 | 0.00 | 0.00 | 0.01 |
| 3141 | 1/2 cup | Concentrate, prep w/water, sweetened, avg | 124 | 0.01 | 0.04 | 0.06 | 0.00 | 0.02 | 0.01 | 0.00 | 0.01 | 0.01 | 0.0[illegible] | 0.00 | 0.01 | 0.03 | 0.01 | 0.01 | 0.00 | 0.00 | 0.01 |
| 3421 | 1/4 cup | Concentrate, sweetened, avg | 71 | 0.02 | 0.07 | 0.11 | 0.01 | 0.05 | 0.01 | 0.00 | 0.01 | 0.02 | 0.0[illegible] | 0.00 | 0.01 | 0.07 | 0.02 | 0.01 | 0.00 | 0.01 | 0.02 |
| 3140 | 1/2 cup | Canned, sweetened, avg | 124 | 0.01 | 0.04 | 0.07 | 0.00 | 0.03 | 0.01 | 0.00 | 0.01 | 0.01 | 0.0[illegible] | 0.00 | 0.01 | 0.04 | 0.01 | 0.01 | 0.00 | 0.00 | 0.01 |
| | | Tomato | | | | | | | | | | | | | | | | | | | |
| 20057 | 1/2 cup | & beef broth, canned, avg | 122 | 0.06 | 0.05 | 0.05 | 0.00 | 0.1[illegible] | 0.16 | 0.01 | 0.01 | 0.02 | 0.03 | 0.00 | 0.02 | 0.09 | 0.02 | 0.01 | 0.00 | 0.00 | 0.02 |
| 20042 | 1/2 cup | & clam juice, canned, avg | 122 | 0.02 | 0.02 | 0.10 | 0.00 | 0.3[illegible] | 0.01 | 0.01 | 0.01 | 0.02 | 0.02 | 0.00 | 0.02 | 0.02 | 0.02 | 0.02 | 0.00 | 0.01 | 0.02 |
| 5397 | 1/2 cup | Canned, unsalted, avg | 122 | 0.03 | 0.02 | 0.12 | 0.00 | 0.37 | 0.01 | 0.01 | 0.02 | 0.03 | 0.03 | 0.00 | 0.02 | 0.02 | 0.02 | 0.02 | 0.01 | 0.01 | 0.02 |
| 5188 | 1/2 cup | Canned, w/salt, avg | 122 | 0.03 | 0.02 | 0.12 | 0.00 | 0.37 | 0.01 | 0.01 | 0.02 | 0.03 | 0.03 | 0.00 | 0.02 | 0.02 | 0.02 | 0.02 | 0.01 | 0.01 | 0.02 |
| | | **FRUITS** | | | | | | | | | | | | | | | | | | | |
| | | Apples | | | | | | | | | | | | | | | | | | | |
| 3308 | 1 ea | Baked, unsweetened, avg | 161 | 0.01 | 0.01 | 0.06 | 0.00 | 0.04 | 0.01 | 0.00 | 0.01 | 0.02 | 0.02 | 0.00 | 0.01 | 0.01 | 0.01 | 0.01 | 0.00 | 0.01 | 0.01 |
| 3388 | 1/2 cup | Boiled, avg | 86 | 0.01 | 0.01 | 0.04 | 0.00 | 0.02 | 0.01 | 0.00 | 0.01 | 0.01 | 0.0[illegible] | 0.00 | 0.01 | 0.01 | 0.01 | 0.01 | 0.00 | 0.00 | 0.01 |
| 3318 | 1 ea | Candied, avg | 184 | 0.08 | 0.08 | 0.19 | 0.02 | 0.43 | 0.05 | 0.06 | 0.13 | 0.21 | 0.1[illegible] | 0.05 | 0.10 | 0.20 | 0.12 | 0.01 | 0.03 | 0.10 | 0.14 |
| 3389 | 1/2 cup | Canned, avg | 102 | 0.01 | 0.01 | 0.03 | 0.00 | 0.02 | 0.01 | 0.00 | 0.01 | 0.01 | 0.0[illegible] | 0.00 | 0.01 | 0.01 | 0.01 | 0.01 | 0.00 | 0.00 | 0.01 |
| 3148 | 1/2 cup | Canned, slices, sweetened, avg | 102 | 0.01 | 0.01 | 0.03 | 0.00 | 0.02 | 0.01 | 0.00 | 0.01 | 0.01 | 0.0[illegible] | 0.00 | 0.01 | 0.01 | 0.01 | 0.01 | 0.00 | 0.00 | 0.01 |
| 3009 | 1/2 cup | Cooked, slices, peeled, avg | 85 | 0.01 | 0.01 | 0.04 | 0.00 | 0.02 | 0.01 | 0.00 | 0.01 | 0.01 | 0.02 | 0.00 | 0.01 | 0.01 | 0.01 | 0.01 | 0.00 | 0.00 | 0.01 |
| 3656 | 1/2 cup | Dried, rings, avg | 43 | 0.01 | 0.01 | 0.07 | 0.01 | 0.04 | 0.02 | 0.01 | 0.02 | 0.02 | 0.02 | 0.00 | 0.01 | 0.01 | 0.02 | 0.01 | 0.00 | 0.01 | 0.02 |
| 3145 | 1/2 cup | Dried, w/o sugar, avg | 128 | 0.01 | 0.01 | 0.05 | 0.00 | 0.03 | 0.01 | 0.00 | 0.01 | 0.02 | 0.02 | 0.00 | 0.01 | 0.01 | 0.01 | 0.01 | 0.00 | 0.01 | 0.01 |
| 3146 | 1/2 cup | Dried, w/sugar, avg | 140 | 0.01 | 0.01 | 0.05 | 0.00 | 0.03 | 0.01 | 0.00 | 0.01 | 0.02 | 0.02 | 0.00 | 0.01 | 0.01 | 0.01 | 0.01 | 0.00 | 0.01 | 0.01 |
| 3392 | 1/2 cup | Frozen, unsweetened, avg | 86 | 0.01 | 0.01 | 0.04 | 0.00 | 0.02 | 0.01 | 0.00 | 0.01 | 0.01 | 0.0[illegible] | 0.00 | 0.01 | 0.01 | 0.01 | 0.01 | 0.00 | 0.00 | 0.01 |
| 3315 | 1 ea | Pickled, avg | 19 | 0.00 | 0.00 | 0.00 | 0.00 | 0.00 | 0.00 | 0.00 | 0.00 | 0.00 | 0.00 | 0.00 | 0.00 | 0.00 | 0.00 | 0.00 | 0.00 | 0.00 | 0.00 |
| 3003 | 1 ea | Raw, w/o peel, avg | 128 | 0.01 | 0.01 | 0.03 | 0.00 | 0.02 | 0.01 | 0.00 | 0.01 | 0.01 | 0.0[illegible] | 0.00 | 0.01 | 0.01 | 0.01 | 0.01 | 0.00 | 0.00 | 0.01 |
| 3000 | 1 ea | Raw, w/peel, avg | 138 | 0.01 | 0.01 | 0.05 | 0.00 | 0.03 | 0.01 | 0.00 | 0.01 | 0.02 | 0.02 | 0.00 | 0.01 | 0.01 | 0.01 | 0.01 | 0.00 | 0.01 | 0.01 |
| | | Applesauce | | | | | | | | | | | | | | | | | | | |
| 3006 | 1/2 cup | Canned, avg | 122 | 0.01 | 0.01 | 0.03 | 0.00 | 0.02 | 0.01 | 0.00 | 0.01 | 0.01 | 0.0[illegible] | 0.00 | 0.01 | 0.01 | 0.01 | 0.01 | 0.00 | 0.00 | 0.01 |
| 3330 | 1/2 cup | Canned, w/vit C, avg | 122 | 0.01 | 0.01 | 0.03 | 0.00 | 0.02 | 0.01 | 0.00 | 0.01 | 0.01 | 0.0[illegible] | 0.00 | 0.01 | 0.01 | 0.01 | 0.01 | 0.00 | 0.00 | 0.01 |
| 3331 | 1/2 cup | Sweetened, avg | 128 | 0.01 | 0.01 | 0.04 | 0.00 | 0.02 | 0.01 | 0.00 | 0.01 | 0.01 | 0.0[illegible] | 0.00 | 0.01 | 0.01 | 0.01 | 0.01 | 0.00 | 0.00 | 0.01 |
| 3147 | 1/2 cup | Sweetened, w/o salt, avg | 128 | 0.01 | 0.01 | 0.04 | 0.00 | 0.02 | 0.01 | 0.00 | 0.01 | 0.01 | 0.0[illegible] | 0.00 | 0.01 | 0.01 | 0.01 | 0.01 | 0.00 | 0.00 | 0.01 |
| | | Apricots | | | | | | | | | | | | | | | | | | | |
| 3398 | 1/2 cup | Canned in extra heavy syrup, w/o skin & pit, avg | 123 | 0.03 | 0.03 | 0.15 | 0.00 | 0.07 | 0.02 | 0.01 | 0.02 | 0.04 | 0.05 | 0.00 | 0.03 | 0.04 | 0.04 | 0.02 | 0.01 | 0.02 | 0.02 |
| 3396 | 1/2 cup | Canned in heavy syrup, w/o skin & pit, avg | 129 | 0.03 | 0.03 | 0.15 | 0.00 | 0.07 | 0.02 | 0.01 | 0.02 | 0.04 | 0.05 | 0.00 | 0.03 | 0.04 | 0.04 | 0.02 | 0.01 | 0.02 | 0.02 |
| 3011 | 1/2 cup | Canned in heavy syrup, w/skin, avg | 120 | 0.03 | 0.03 | 0.15 | 0.00 | 0.06 | 0.02 | 0.01 | 0.02 | 0.04 | 0.04 | 0.00 | 0.03 | 0.04 | 0.04 | 0.02 | 0.01 | 0.01 | 0.02 |
| 3151 | 1/2 cup | Canned in juice, w/skin, halves, avg | 122 | 0.04 | 0.03 | 0.18 | 0.00 | 0.08 | 0.02 | 0.01 | 0.02 | 0.05 | 0.05 | 0.00 | 0.03 | 0.05 | 0.04 | 0.03 | 0.01 | 0.02 | 0.03 |
| 3153 | 1/2 cup | Canned in light syrup, w/skin, avg | 126 | 0.03 | 0.03 | 0.15 | 0.00 | 0.07 | 0.02 | 0.01 | 0.02 | 0.04 | 0.05 | 0.00 | 0.03 | 0.04 | 0.04 | 0.02 | 0.01 | 0.02 | 0.02 |
| 3333 | 1/2 cup | Canned in water, w/o skin, avg | 114 | 0.04 | 0.03 | 0.18 | 0.00 | 0.08 | 0.02 | 0.01 | 0.02 | 0.05 | 0.05 | 0.00 | 0.03 | 0.05 | 0.04 | 0.03 | 0.01 | 0.02 | 0.03 |
| 3632 | 1/2 cup | Canned in water, w/skin, avg | 122 | 0.04 | 0.03 | 0.20 | 0.00 | 0.09 | 0.03 | 0.01 | 0.03 | 0.05 | 0.06 | 0.00 | 0.04 | 0.05 | 0.05 | 0.03 | 0.02 | 0.02 | 0.03 |
| 3014 | 1/2 cup | Dried, sulfured, uncooked, avg | 65 | 0.12 | 0.09 | 0.54 | 0.01 | 0.24 | 0.07 | 0.04 | 0.07 | 0.14 | 0.16 | 0.01 | 0.10 | 0.14 | 0.14 | 0.09 | 0.04 | 0.06 | 0.09 |
| 3155 | 1/2 cup | Frozen, sweetened, avg | 121 | 0.04 | 0.03 | 0.19 | 0.00 | 0.10 | 0.02 | 0.02 | 0.02 | 0.05 | 0.06 | 0.00 | 0.03 | 0.06 | 0.05 | 0.03 | 0.01 | 0.02 | 0.03 |
| 3657 | 1/2 cup | Raw, pitted, fresh, sliced, avg | 82 | 0.06 | 0.04 | 0.26 | 0.00 | 0.13 | 0.03 | 0.02 | 0.03 | 0.06 | 0.08 | 0.00 | 0.04 | 0.08 | 0.07 | 0.04 | 0.01 | 0.02 | 0.04 |

# TABLE A Amino Acid Content for Selected Foods *(continued)*

| Code | Amount | Description | Weight (g) | Alanine (g) | Arginine (g) | Aspartic acid (g) | Cystine (g) | Glutamic acid (g) | Glycine (g) | Histidine (g) | Isoleucine (g) | Leucine (g) | Lysine (g) | Methionine (g) | Phenylalanine (g) | Proline (g) | Serine (g) | Threonine (g) | Tryptophan (g) | Tyrosine (g) | Valine (g) |
|---|---|---|---|---|---|---|---|---|---|---|---|---|---|---|---|---|---|---|---|---|---|
| 3401 | 1/2 cup | Stewed, dried, halves, sulfured, w/sugar, avg | 135 | 0.08 | 0.06 | 0.36 | 0.01 | 0.16 | 0.05 | 0.03 | 0.05 | 0.09 | 0.11 | 0.01 | 0.07 | 0.09 | 0.09 | 0.06 | 0.03 | 0.04 | 0.06 |
| 3217 | 1/2 cup | Stewed, dried, sulfured, stewed, avg | 125 | 0.08 | 0.06 | 0.37 | 0.01 | 0.16 | 0.05 | 0.03 | 0.05 | 0.09 | 0.11 | 0.01 | 0.07 | 0.10 | 0.09 | 0.06 | 0.03 | 0.04 | 0.06 |
| | | Avocado | | | | | | | | | | | | | | | | | | | |
| 3213 | 1/2 cup | Average | 115 | 0.11 | 0.05 | 0.26 | 0.02 | 0.19 | 0.08 | 0.03 | 0.07 | 0.11 | 0.09 | 0.03 | 0.06 | 0.07 | 0.07 | 0.06 | 0.02 | 0.04 | 0.09 |
| 3211 | 1/2 cup | California, pureed, avg | 115 | 0.15 | 0.07 | 0.35 | 0.03 | 0.25 | 0.10 | 0.03 | 0.09 | 0.15 | 0.12 | 0.04 | 0.08 | 0.09 | 0.10 | 0.08 | 0.03 | 0.06 | 0.12 |
| 3658 | 1/2 cup | Sliced, avg | 73 | 0.09 | 0.04 | 0.21 | 0.02 | 0.15 | 0.06 | 0.02 | 0.05 | 0.09 | 0.07 | 0.03 | 0.05 | 0.06 | 0.06 | 0.05 | 0.02 | 0.04 | 0.07 |
| | | Bananas | | | | | | | | | | | | | | | | | | | |
| 3307 | 1/2 cup | Dried, chips, avg | 46 | 0.04 | 0.05 | 0.12 | 0.02 | 0.11 | 0.04 | 0.08 | 0.03 | 0.07 | 0.05 | 0.01 | 0.04 | 0.04 | 0.05 | 0.03 | 0.01 | 0.02 | 0.05 |
| 3361 | 1 ea | Fried, green, avg | 90 | 0.04 | 0.04 | 0.10 | 0.02 | 0.10 | 0.03 | 0.07 | 0.03 | 0.06 | 0.04 | 0.01 | 0.03 | 0.04 | 0.04 | 0.03 | 0.01 | 0.02 | 0.04 |
| 3306 | 1 ea | Fried, ripe, avg | 91 | 0.04 | 0.05 | 0.12 | 0.02 | 0.14 | 0.04 | 0.08 | 0.04 | 0.08 | 0.06 | 0.01 | 0.04 | 0.05 | 0.05 | 0.04 | 0.01 | 0.03 | 0.06 |
| 3021 | 1/2 cup | Raw, slices, avg | 75 | 0.03 | 0.04 | 0.08 | 0.01 | 0.08 | 0.03 | 0.06 | 0.02 | 0.05 | 0.04 | 0.01 | 0.03 | 0.03 | 0.04 | 0.03 | 0.01 | 0.02 | 0.04 |
| | | Blueberries | | | | | | | | | | | | | | | | | | | |
| 3030 | 1/2 cup | Canned in heavy syrup, avg | 128 | 0.04 | 0.04 | 0.07 | 0.01 | 0.10 | 0.03 | 0.01 | 0.03 | 0.05 | 0.02 | 0.01 | 0.03 | 0.03 | 0.03 | 0.02 | 0.00 | 0.01 | 0.03 |
| 3029 | 1/2 cup | Fresh, avg | 72 | 0.02 | 0.02 | 0.04 | 0.01 | 0.06 | 0.02 | 0.01 | 0.02 | 0.03 | 0.01 | 0.01 | 0.02 | 0.02 | 0.01 | 0.01 | 0.00 | 0.01 | 0.02 |
| 3031 | 1/2 cup | Frozen, avg | 78 | 0.01 | 0.02 | 0.03 | 0.00 | 0.04 | 0.01 | 0.00 | 0.01 | 0.02 | 0.01 | 0.01 | 0.01 | 0.01 | 0.01 | 0.01 | 0.00 | 0.00 | 0.01 |
| 3231 | 1/2 cup | Frozen, sweetened, thawed, avg | 115 | 0.02 | 0.02 | 0.04 | 0.00 | 0.06 | 0.02 | 0.01 | 0.01 | 0.03 | 0.01 | 0.01 | 0.02 | 0.02 | 0.01 | 0.01 | 0.00 | 0.01 | 0.02 |
| 3239 | 1/2 cup | Breadfruit, raw, avg | 110 | 0.00 | 0.00 | 0.00 | 0.01 | 0.00 | 0.00 | 0.00 | 0.07 | 0.07 | 0.04 | 0.01 | 0.03 | 0.00 | 0.00 | 0.06 | 0.00 | 0.02 | 0.05 |
| 3665 | 1/2 cup | Carambola/Starfruit, raw, slices, avg | 54 | 0.02 | 0.01 | 0.03 | 0.00 | 0.04 | 0.01 | 0.00 | 0.01 | 0.02 | 0.02 | 0.01 | 0.01 | 0.01 | 0.02 | 0.01 | 0.00 | 0.01 | 0.01 |
| 5414 | 1/2 cup | Chayote, chopped, boiled, avg | 80 | 0.03 | 0.02 | 0.06 | 0.00 | 0.08 | 0.02 | 0.01 | 0.03 | 0.05 | 0.02 | 0.00 | 0.03 | 0.03 | 0.03 | 0.02 | 0.01 | 0.02 | 0.04 |
| 5413 | 1 ea | Chayote, raw, avg | 203 | 0.10 | 0.07 | 0.19 | 0.00 | 0.25 | 0.08 | 0.03 | 0.09 | 0.16 | 0.08 | 0.00 | 0.10 | 0.09 | 0.10 | 0.08 | 0.02 | 0.06 | 0.13 |
| | | Cherries, Sour | | | | | | | | | | | | | | | | | | | |
| 3335 | 1/2 cup | Canned, in extra heavy syrup, avg | 131 | 0.02 | 0.01 | 0.50 | 0.00 | 0.03 | 0.02 | 0.01 | 0.02 | 0.02 | 0.03 | 0.00 | 0.02 | 0.03 | 0.03 | 0.02 | 0.01 | 0.01 | 0.02 |
| 3403 | 1/2 cup | Canned in heavy syrup, avg | 128 | 0.02 | 0.01 | 0.50 | 0.00 | 0.03 | 0.02 | 0.01 | 0.02 | 0.02 | 0.03 | 0.00 | 0.02 | 0.03 | 0.03 | 0.02 | 0.01 | 0.01 | 0.02 |
| 3402 | 1/2 cup | Canned in light syrup, avg | 126 | 0.03 | 0.01 | 0.50 | 0.00 | 0.03 | 0.02 | 0.01 | 0.02 | 0.02 | 0.03 | 0.00 | 0.02 | 0.03 | 0.03 | 0.02 | 0.01 | 0.01 | 0.02 |
| 3035 | 1/2 cup | Canned in water, avg | 122 | 0.03 | 0.01 | 0.50 | 0.00 | 0.03 | 0.02 | 0.01 | 0.02 | 0.02 | 0.03 | 0.00 | 0.02 | 0.03 | 0.03 | 0.02 | 0.01 | 0.01 | 0.02 |
| 3159 | 1/2 cup | Frozen, unsweetened, avg | 78 | 0.02 | 0.01 | 0.38 | 0.00 | 0.02 | 0.01 | 0.01 | 0.01 | 0.02 | 0.02 | 0.00 | 0.01 | 0.02 | 0.02 | 0.01 | 0.01 | 0.01 | 0.02 |
| | | Cherries, Sweet | | | | | | | | | | | | | | | | | | | |
| 3406 | 1/2 cup | Canned in extra heavy syrup, avg | 131 | 0.02 | 0.01 | 0.41 | 0.00 | 0.03 | 0.02 | 0.01 | 0.01 | 0.02 | 0.03 | 0.00 | 0.01 | 0.02 | 0.02 | 0.02 | 0.01 | 0.01 | 0.02 |
| 3336 | 1/2 cup | Canned in juice, avg | 125 | 0.03 | 0.02 | 0.60 | 0.00 | 0.04 | 0.02 | 0.01 | 0.02 | 0.03 | 0.04 | 0.01 | 0.02 | 0.03 | 0.03 | 0.02 | 0.01 | 0.01 | 0.03 |
| 3405 | 1/2 cup | Canned in light syrup, avg | 126 | 0.02 | 0.01 | 0.41 | 0.00 | 0.03 | 0.02 | 0.01 | 0.01 | 0.02 | 0.03 | 0.00 | 0.01 | 0.02 | 0.02 | 0.02 | 0.01 | 0.01 | 0.02 |
| 3038 | 1/2 cup | Canned in heavy syrup, avg | 127 | 0.02 | 0.01 | 0.41 | 0.00 | 0.03 | 0.02 | 0.01 | 0.01 | 0.02 | 0.03 | 0.00 | 0.01 | 0.02 | 0.02 | 0.02 | 0.01 | 0.01 | 0.02 |
| 3404 | 1/2 cup | Canned in water, avg | 124 | 0.03 | 0.01 | 0.51 | 0.00 | 0.03 | 0.02 | 0.01 | 0.02 | 0.02 | 0.03 | 0.00 | 0.02 | 0.03 | 0.03 | 0.02 | 0.01 | 0.01 | 0.02 |
| 3158 | 1/2 cup | Frozen, sweetened, avg | 130 | 0.01 | 0.05 | 0.17 | 1.02 | 0.11 | 0.06 | 0.00 | 0.01 | 0.01 | 0.01 | 0.00 | 0.01 | 0.01 | 0.01 | 0.01 | 0.00 | 0.00 | 0.01 |
| 3037 | 1/2 cup | Raw, w/o pits, avg | 72 | 0.02 | 0.01 | 0.46 | 0.00 | 0.03 | 0.02 | 0.01 | 0.02 | 0.02 | 0.03 | 0.00 | 0.02 | 0.02 | 0.02 | 0.02 | 0.01 | 0.01 | 0.02 |
| 3043 | 1/2 cup | Dates, chopped, pitted, avg | 89 | 0.09 | 0.06 | 0.11 | 0.04 | 0.19 | 0.08 | 0.03 | 0.04 | 0.08 | 0.05 | 0.02 | 0.05 | 0.09 | 0.06 | 0.05 | 0.04 | 0.03 | 0.06 |
| 3310 | 1/2 cup | Elderberries, cooked/canned, avg | 128 | 0.03 | 0.04 | 0.05 | 0.01 | 0.09 | 0.03 | 0.01 | 0.03 | 0.06 | 0.02 | 0.01 | 0.04 | 0.02 | 0.03 | 0.03 | 0.01 | 0.05 | 0.03 |
| 3245 | 1/2 cup | Elderberries, raw, avg | 72 | 0.02 | 0.03 | 0.04 | 0.01 | 0.07 | 0.03 | 0.01 | 0.02 | 0.04 | 0.02 | 0.01 | 0.03 | 0.02 | 0.02 | 0.02 | 0.01 | 0.04 | 0.02 |
| | | Figs | | | | | | | | | | | | | | | | | | | |
| 3410 | 1/2 cup | Canned in extra heavy syrup, avg | 130 | 0.03 | 0.01 | 0.11 | 0.01 | 0.05 | 0.02 | 0.01 | 0.01 | 0.02 | 0.02 | 0.00 | 0.01 | 0.03 | 0.02 | 0.02 | 0.00 | 0.02 | 0.02 |
| 57486 | 1/2 cup | Canned in heavy syrup, avg | 130 | 0.03 | 0.01 | 0.12 | 0.01 | 0.05 | 0.02 | 0.01 | 0.02 | 0.02 | 0.02 | 0.00 | 0.01 | 0.03 | 0.02 | 0.02 | 0.00 | 0.02 | 0.02 |
| 3408 | 1/2 cup | Canned in light syrup, avg | 126 | 0.03 | 0.01 | 0.12 | 0.01 | 0.05 | 0.02 | 0.01 | 0.02 | 0.02 | 0.02 | 0.00 | 0.01 | 0.03 | 0.02 | 0.02 | 0.00 | 0.02 | 0.02 |
| 3678 | 1/2 cup | Canned in water, avg | 124 | 0.03 | 0.01 | 0.12 | 0.01 | 0.05 | 0.02 | 0.01 | 0.01 | 0.02 | 0.02 | 0.00 | 0.01 | 0.03 | 0.02 | 0.02 | 0.00 | 0.02 | 0.02 |
| 3314 | 1/2 cup | Dried, cooked, unsweetened, avg | 130 | 0.10 | 0.04 | 0.39 | 0.03 | 0.16 | 0.06 | 0.02 | 0.05 | 0.07 | 0.07 | 0.01 | 0.04 | 0.11 | 0.08 | 0.05 | 0.01 | 0.07 | 0.06 |
| 3679 | 1/2 cup | Dried, uncooked, avg | 100 | 0.18 | 0.07 | 0.72 | 0.05 | 0.29 | 0.10 | 0.04 | 0.09 | 0.13 | 0.12 | 0.03 | 0.07 | 0.20 | 0.15 | 0.10 | 0.03 | 0.13 | 0.12 |
| 3160 | 1 ea | Raw, medium, avg | 50 | 0.02 | 0.01 | 0.09 | 0.01 | 0.04 | 0.01 | 0.01 | 0.01 | 0.02 | 0.01 | 0.00 | 0.01 | 0.02 | 0.02 | 0.01 | 0.00 | 0.02 | 0.01 |
| | | Fruit Cocktail | | | | | | | | | | | | | | | | | | | |
| 3412 | 1/2 cup | Canned in extra heavy syrup, avg | 130 | 0.03 | 0.02 | 0.10 | 0.01 | 0.07 | 0.02 | 0.01 | 0.01 | 0.02 | 0.02 | 0.01 | 0.01 | 0.02 | 0.02 | 0.02 | 0.00 | 0.01 | 0.02 |
| 3411 | 1/2 cup | Canned in extra light syrup, avg | 123 | 0.02 | 0.02 | 0.09 | 0.00 | 0.07 | 0.02 | 0.01 | 0.01 | 0.02 | 0.01 | 0.01 | 0.01 | 0.02 | 0.02 | 0.02 | 0.00 | 0.01 | 0.02 |
| 3045 | 1/2 cup | Canned in heavy syrup, avg | 124 | 0.02 | 0.02 | 0.09 | 0.00 | 0.07 | 0.02 | 0.01 | 0.01 | 0.02 | 0.01 | 0.01 | 0.01 | 0.02 | 0.02 | 0.02 | 0.00 | 0.01 | 0.02 |
| 3164 | 1/2 cup | Canned in juice, avg | 118 | 0.03 | 0.02 | 0.10 | 0.01 | 0.07 | 0.02 | 0.01 | 0.01 | 0.02 | 0.02 | 0.01 | 0.01 | 0.02 | 0.02 | 0.02 | 0.00 | 0.01 | 0.02 |

TABLE A **Amino Acid Content for Selected Foods *(continued)***

| Code | Amount | Description | Weight (g) | Alanine (g) | Arginine (g) | Aspartic acid (g) | Cystine (g) | Glutamic acid (g) | Glycine (g) | Histidine (g) | Isoleucine (g) | Leucine (g) | Lysine (g) | Methionine (g) | Phenylalanine (g) | Proline (g) | Serine (g) | Threonine (g) | Tryptophan (g) | Tyrosine (g) | Valine (g) |
|---|---|---|---|---|---|---|---|---|---|---|---|---|---|---|---|---|---|---|---|---|---|
| 3163 | 1/2 cup | Canned in light syrup, avg | 121 | 0.02 | 0.02 | 0.09 | 0.00 | 0.07 | 0.02 | 0.01 | 0.01 | 0.02 | 0.01 | 0.01 | 0.01 | 0.02 | 0.02 | 0.02 | 0.00 | 0.01 | 0.02 |
| 3313 | 1/2 cup | Canned in water, w/o sugar, avg | 118 | 0.02 | 0.02 | 0.09 | 0.00 | 0.07 | 0.02 | 0.01 | 0.01 | 0.02 | 0.01 | 0.01 | 0.01 | 0.02 | 0.02 | 0.02 | 0.00 | 0.01 | 0.02 |
| | | Fruit Salad | | | | | | | | | | | | | | | | | | | |
| 3415 | 1/2 cup | Canned in extra heavy syrup, avg | 130 | 0.02 | 0.01 | 0.06 | 0.00 | 0.04 | 0.02 | 0.01 | 0.01 | 0.02 | 0.02 | 0.01 | 0.01 | 0.01 | 0.02 | 0.01 | 0.01 | 0.01 | 0.01 |
| 3414 | 1/2 cup | Canned in heavy syrup, avg | 128 | 0.02 | 0.01 | 0.06 | 0.00 | 0.04 | 0.02 | 0.01 | 0.01 | 0.02 | 0.02 | 0.01 | 0.01 | 0.01 | 0.02 | 0.01 | 0.01 | 0.01 | 0.01 |
| 3355 | 1/2 cup | Canned in heavy syrup, tropical, avg | 129 | 0.02 | 0.01 | 0.07 | 0.00 | 0.00 | 0.02 | 0.01 | 0.01 | 0.02 | 0.02 | 0.01 | 0.01 | 0.01 | 0.02 | 0.01 | 0.01 | 0.01 | 0.02 |
| 3413 | 1/2 cup | Canned in water, avg | 123 | 0.02 | 0.01 | 0.06 | 0.00 | 0.04 | 0.02 | 0.01 | 0.01 | 0.02 | 0.02 | 0.01 | 0.01 | 0.01 | 0.02 | 0.01 | 0.01 | 0.01 | 0.01 |
| | | Grapes | | | | | | | | | | | | | | | | | | | |
| 3059 | 1/2 cup | American type/slip skin, w/o seeds, avg | 46 | 0.01 | 0.02 | 0.04 | 0.00 | 0.06 | 0.01 | 0.01 | 0.00 | 0.01 | 0.01 | 0.01 | 0.01 | 0.01 | 0.01 | 0.01 | 0.00 | 0.01 | 0.01 |
| 3058 | 1/2 cup | European type/adherent skin, avg | 80 | 0.02 | 0.04 | 0.06 | 0.01 | 0.11 | 0.02 | 0.02 | 0.00 | 0.01 | 0.01 | 0.02 | 0.01 | 0.02 | 0.03 | 0.01 | 0.00 | 0.01 | 0.01 |
| 3206 | 1/2 cup | Thompson, seedless, canned in heavy syrup, avg | 128 | 0.03 | 0.04 | 0.08 | 0.01 | 0.13 | 0.02 | 0.02 | 0.01 | 0.01 | 0.01 | 0.02 | 0.01 | 0.02 | 0.03 | 0.02 | 0.00 | 0.01 | 0.02 |
| 3417 | 1/2 cup | Thompson, seedless, canned in water, avg | 123 | 0.03 | 0.05 | 0.08 | 0.01 | 0.13 | 0.02 | 0.02 | 0.00 | 0.01 | 0.01 | 0.02 | 0.01 | 0.02 | 0.03 | 0.02 | 0.00 | 0.01 | 0.02 |
| | | Grapefruit | | | | | | | | | | | | | | | | | | | |
| 3342 | 1/2 cup | Canned in juice, avg | 124 | 0.03 | 0.06 | 0.17 | 0.00 | 0.07 | 0.02 | 0.01 | 0.02 | 0.02 | 0.02 | 0.00 | 0.02 | 0.07 | 0.04 | 0.02 | 0.00 | 0.01 | 0.02 |
| 3050 | 1/2 cup | Canned in light syrup, avg | 127 | 0.03 | 0.05 | 0.14 | 0.00 | 0.05 | 0.01 | 0.01 | 0.01 | 0.02 | 0.02 | 0.00 | 0.01 | 0.06 | 0.03 | 0.01 | 0.00 | 0.01 | 0.02 |
| 3416 | 1/2 cup | Canned in water, avg | 122 | 0.03 | 0.05 | 0.13 | 0.00 | 0.05 | 0.01 | 0.01 | 0.01 | 0.02 | 0.02 | 0.00 | 0.01 | 0.06 | 0.03 | 0.01 | 0.00 | 0.01 | 0.02 |
| 3048 | 1/2 cup | Fresh, sections, avg | 115 | 0.03 | 0.05 | 0.14 | 0.00 | 0.06 | 0.01 | 0.01 | 0.01 | 0.02 | 0.02 | 0.00 | 0.01 | 0.06 | 0.03 | 0.01 | 0.00 | 0.01 | 0.02 |
| 3817 | 1/2 cup | Pink/red, sections, avg | 115 | 0.02 | 0.05 | 0.12 | 0.00 | 0.05 | 0.01 | 0.01 | 0.01 | 0.02 | 0.02 | 0.00 | 0.01 | 0.05 | 0.03 | 0.01 | 0.00 | 0.01 | 0.02 |
| 3686 | 1/2 cup | White, avg | 115 | 0.03 | 0.06 | 0.15 | 0.00 | 0.06 | 0.01 | 0.01 | 0.01 | 0.02 | 0.02 | 0.00 | 0.01 | 0.07 | 0.04 | 0.02 | 0.00 | 0.01 | 0.02 |
| 3634 | 1/2 cup | Guava, raw, avg | 82 | 0.03 | 0.02 | 0.04 | 0.00 | 0.09 | 0.03 | 0.01 | 0.02 | 0.05 | 0.02 | 0.00 | 0.00 | 0.02 | 0.02 | 0.03 | 0.01 | 0.01 | 0.02 |
| 3208 | 1/2 cup | Guava, sauce, cooked, avg | 119 | 0.02 | 0.01 | 0.02 | 0.00 | 0.05 | 0.02 | 0.00 | 0.01 | 0.02 | 0.01 | 0.00 | 0.00 | 0.01 | 0.01 | 0.01 | 0.00 | 0.00 | 0.01 |
| 3066 | 1 ea | Lemon, fresh, w/o peel, avg | 58 | 0.03 | 0.03 | 0.08 | 0.01 | 0.07 | 0.06 | 0.01 | 0.02 | 0.02 | 0.03 | 0.01 | 0.02 | 0.03 | 0.02 | 0.01 | 0.00 | 0.01 | 0.02 |
| 3418 | 1 ea | Lemon, fresh, w/peel, avg | 108 | 0.06 | 0.06 | 0.15 | 0.01 | 0.12 | 0.10 | 0.02 | 0.03 | 0.03 | 0.05 | 0.02 | 0.04 | 0.06 | 0.03 | 0.02 | 0.01 | 0.02 | 0.04 |
| 3255 | 10 ea | Longans, dried, avg | 30 | 0.18 | 0.04 | 0.14 | 0.00 | 0.23 | 0.05 | 0.01 | 0.03 | 0.06 | 0.05 | 0.01 | 0.03 | 0.05 | 0.05 | 0.04 | 0.00 | 0.03 | 0.07 |
| 3254 | 10 ea | Longans, raw, avg | 30 | 0.05 | 0.01 | 0.04 | 0.00 | 0.06 | 0.01 | 0.00 | 0.01 | 0.02 | 0.01 | 0.00 | 0.01 | 0.01 | 0.01 | 0.01 | 0.00 | 0.01 | 0.02 |
| 3639 | 1 ea | Loquats, raw, medium, avg | 16 | 0.00 | 0.00 | 0.01 | 0.00 | 0.01 | 0.00 | 0.00 | 0.00 | 0.00 | 0.00 | 0.00 | 0.00 | 0.00 | 0.00 | 0.00 | 0.00 | 0.00 | 0.00 |
| 3089 | 1/2 cup | Mandarine Orange, canned, avg | 125 | 0.04 | 0.05 | 0.09 | 0.01 | 0.08 | 0.08 | 0.01 | 0.02 | 0.02 | 0.04 | 0.02 | 0.02 | 0.04 | 0.03 | 0.01 | 0.01 | 0.01 | 0.03 |
| 3221 | 1 ea | Mango, fresh, whole, avg | 207 | 0.11 | 0.04 | 0.09 | 0.00 | 0.12 | 0.04 | 0.02 | 0.04 | 0.06 | 0.08 | 0.01 | 0.04 | 0.04 | 0.05 | 0.04 | 0.02 | 0.02 | 0.05 |
| 3216 | 1/2 cup | Nectarines, fresh, avg | 69 | 0.04 | 0.02 | 0.11 | 0.01 | 0.10 | 0.02 | 0.01 | 0.02 | 0.04 | 0.02 | 0.02 | 0.02 | 0.03 | 0.03 | 0.02 | 0.00 | 0.02 | 0.04 |
| | | Oranges | | | | | | | | | | | | | | | | | | | |
| 3715 | 1/2 cup | California navel, avg | 82 | 0.05 | 0.06 | 0.10 | 0.01 | 0.09 | 0.09 | 0.02 | 0.02 | 0.02 | 0.04 | 0.02 | 0.03 | 0.04 | 0.03 | 0.01 | 0.01 | 0.01 | 0.04 |
| 3714 | 1/2 cup | California valencia, avg | 90 | 0.05 | 0.07 | 0.11 | 0.01 | 0.09 | 0.09 | 0.02 | 0.03 | 0.02 | 0.05 | 0.02 | 0.03 | 0.05 | 0.03 | 0.02 | 0.01 | 0.02 | 0.04 |
| 3420 | 1/2 cup | With peel, avg | 85 | 0.06 | 0.08 | 0.13 | 0.01 | 0.11 | 0.11 | 0.02 | 0.03 | 0.03 | 0.06 | 0.02 | 0.04 | 0.05 | 0.04 | 0.02 | 0.01 | 0.02 | 0.05 |
| 3171 | 1 ea | Papaya, fresh, whole, medium, avg | 304 | 0.04 | 0.03 | 0.15 | 0.00 | 0.10 | 0.05 | 0.02 | 0.02 | 0.05 | 0.08 | 0.01 | 0.03 | 0.03 | 0.05 | 0.03 | 0.02 | 0.02 | 0.03 |
| 3722 | 1/2 cup | Passion Fruit, purple, fresh, avg | 118 | 0.21 | 0.00 | 1.00 | 0.00 | 0.65 | 0.02 | 0.06 | 0.03 | 0.04 | 0.05 | 0.00 | 0.08 | 0.01 | 0.37 | 0.02 | 0.00 | 0.01 | 0.06 |
| | | Peaches | | | | | | | | | | | | | | | | | | | |
| 3427 | 1/2 cup | Canned in extra heavy syrup, halves, avg | 131 | 0.04 | 0.02 | 0.10 | 0.01 | 0.09 | 0.02 | 0.01 | 0.02 | 0.04 | 0.02 | 0.01 | 0.02 | 0.03 | 0.03 | 0.02 | 0.00 | 0.02 | 0.03 |
| 3728 | 1/2 cup | Canned in extra light syrup, halves, avg | 124 | 0.03 | 0.01 | 0.08 | 0.00 | 0.08 | 0.02 | 0.01 | 0.01 | 0.03 | 0.02 | 0.01 | 0.02 | 0.02 | 0.02 | 0.02 | 0.00 | 0.01 | 0.03 |
| 3098 | 1/2 cup | Canned in heavy syrup, avg | 131 | 0.04 | 0.02 | 0.10 | 0.01 | 0.09 | 0.02 | 0.01 | 0.02 | 0.03 | 0.02 | 0.01 | 0.02 | 0.02 | 0.03 | 0.02 | 0.00 | 0.02 | 0.03 |
| 3348 | 1/2 cup | Canned in heavy syrup, spiced, avg | 121 | 0.03 | 0.01 | 0.08 | 0.00 | 0.08 | 0.02 | 0.01 | 0.01 | 0.03 | 0.02 | 0.01 | 0.02 | 0.02 | 0.02 | 0.02 | 0.00 | 0.01 | 0.03 |
| 3727 | 1/2 cup | Canned in juices, halves, avg | 124 | 0.05 | 0.02 | 0.13 | 0.01 | 0.12 | 0.03 | 0.01 | 0.02 | 0.04 | 0.02 | 0.02 | 0.02 | 0.03 | 0.04 | 0.03 | 0.00 | 0.02 | 0.04 |
| 3173 | 1/2 cup | Canned in light syrup, halves, avg | 126 | 0.03 | 0.01 | 0.09 | 0.01 | 0.09 | 0.02 | 0.01 | 0.02 | 0.03 | 0.02 | 0.01 | 0.02 | 0.02 | 0.03 | 0.02 | 0.00 | 0.02 | 0.03 |
| 3423 | 1/2 cup | Canned in water, halves, avg | 122 | 0.03 | 0.01 | 0.09 | 0.00 | 0.08 | 0.02 | 0.01 | 0.02 | 0.03 | 0.02 | 0.01 | 0.02 | 0.02 | 0.02 | 0.02 | 0.00 | 0.01 | 0.03 |
| 3729 | 1/2 cup | Dried, cooked, dehydrated, sulfured, stewed, avg | 121 | 0.17 | 0.07 | 0.48 | 0.02 | 0.44 | 0.10 | 0.05 | 0.08 | 0.16 | 0.09 | 0.07 | 0.09 | 0.12 | 0.13 | 0.11 | 0.01 | 0.08 | 0.16 |
| 3430 | 1/2 cup | Dried, cooked, stewed w/sugar, avg | 135 | 0.09 | 0.04 | 0.24 | 0.01 | 0.22 | 0.05 | 0.03 | 0.04 | 0.08 | 0.05 | 0.04 | 0.04 | 0.06 | 0.07 | 0.06 | 0.00 | 0.04 | 0.08 |

TABLE A **Amino Acid Content for Selected Foods *(continued)***

| Code | Amount | Description | Weight (g) | Alanine (g) | Arginine (g) | Aspartic acid (g) | Cystine (g) | Glutamic acid (g) | Glycine (g) | Histidine (g) | Isoleucine (g) | Leucine (g) | Lysine (g) | Methionine (g) | Phenylalanine (g) | Proline (g) | Serine (g) | Threonine (g) | Tryptophan (g) | Tyrosine (g) | Valine (g) |
|---|---|---|---|---|---|---|---|---|---|---|---|---|---|---|---|---|---|---|---|---|---|
| 3428 | 1/2 cup | Dried, dehydrated, sulfured, uncooked, avg | 58 | 0.17 | 0.07 | 0.47 | 0.02 | 0.43 | 0.10 | 0.05 | 0.08 | 0.16 | 0.09 | 0.07 | 0.09 | 0.12 | 0.13 | 0.11 | 0.01 | 0.07 | 0.15 |
| 3729 | 1/2 cup | Dried, halves, avg | 80 | 0.26 | 0.11 | 0.73 | 0.04 | 0.66 | 0.15 | 0.08 | 0.13 | 0.25 | 0.14 | 0.11 | 0.14 | 0.18 | 0.20 | 0.17 | 0.01 | 0.11 | 0.24 |
| 3096 | 1 ea | Fresh, whole, medium, avg | 98 | 0.04 | 0.02 | 0.11 | 0.01 | 0.10 | 0.02 | 0.01 | 0.02 | 0.04 | 0.02 | 0.02 | 0.02 | 0.03 | 0.03 | 0.03 | 0.00 | 0.02 | 0.04 |
| 57481 | 1/2 cup | Frozen, slices, sweetened, thawed, avg | 125 | 0.05 | 0.02 | 0.13 | 0.01 | 0.12 | 0.03 | 0.02 | 0.02 | 0.04 | 0.02 | 0.02 | 0.02 | 0.03 | 0.04 | 0.03 | 0.00 | 0.02 | 0.04 |
| | | Pears | | | | | | | | | | | | | | | | | | | |
| 3107 | 1/2 cup | Canned in heavy syrup, avg | 133 | 0.01 | 0.00 | 0.05 | 0.00 | 0.02 | 0.01 | 0.00 | 0.01 | 0.01 | 0.01 | 0.00 | 0.01 | 0.01 | 0.01 | 0.01 | 0.00 | 0.00 | 0.01 |
| 3179 | 1/2 cup | Canned in juice, avg | 124 | 0.01 | 0.01 | 0.08 | 0.00 | 0.03 | 0.01 | 0.00 | 0.01 | 0.02 | 0.01 | 0.00 | 0.01 | 0.01 | 0.01 | 0.01 | 0.00 | 0.00 | 0.01 |
| 3177 | 1/2 cup | Canned in light syrup, avg | 126 | 0.01 | 0.00 | 0.05 | 0.00 | 0.02 | 0.01 | 0.00 | 0.01 | 0.01 | 0.01 | 0.00 | 0.01 | 0.01 | 0.01 | 0.01 | 0.00 | 0.00 | 0.01 |
| 3645 | 1/2 cup | Canned in water, halves, avg | 122 | 0.01 | 0.00 | 0.05 | 0.00 | 0.02 | 0.01 | 0.00 | 0.01 | 0.01 | 0.01 | 0.00 | 0.01 | 0.01 | 0.01 | 0.01 | 0.00 | 0.00 | 0.01 |
| 3730 | 1/2 cup | Dried, halves, avg | 90 | 0.06 | 0.03 | 0.33 | 0.02 | 0.12 | 0.05 | 0.02 | 0.05 | 0.08 | 0.06 | 0.02 | 0.04 | 0.05 | 0.06 | 0.04 | 0.00 | 0.01 | 0.06 |
| 3104 | 1/2 cup | Fresh, avg | 82 | 0.01 | 0.01 | 0.06 | 0.00 | 0.02 | 0.01 | 0.00 | 0.01 | 0.02 | 0.01 | 0.00 | 0.01 | 0.01 | 0.01 | 0.01 | 0.00 | 0.00 | 0.01 |
| 3272 | 1 ea | Fresh, Asian, avg | 122 | 0.02 | 0.01 | 0.12 | 0.01 | 0.04 | 0.02 | 0.01 | 0.02 | 0.03 | 0.02 | 0.01 | 0.02 | 0.02 | 0.02 | 0.02 | 0.01 | 0.00 | 0.02 |
| | | Persimmons | | | | | | | | | | | | | | | | | | | |
| 3351 | 1 ea | Dried, Japanese, avg | 34 | 0.02 | 0.02 | 0.05 | 0.01 | 0.06 | 0.02 | 0.01 | 0.02 | 0.03 | 0.03 | 0.00 | 0.02 | 0.02 | 0.02 | 0.02 | 0.01 | 0.01 | 0.02 |
| 3193 | 1 ea | Fresh, Japanese, large, avg | 168 | 0.05 | 0.04 | 0.10 | 0.02 | 0.13 | 0.04 | 0.02 | 0.04 | 0.07 | 0.06 | 0.01 | 0.04 | 0.04 | 0.04 | 0.05 | 0.02 | 0.03 | 0.05 |
| 3194 | 1 ea | Fresh, native, small, avg | 25 | 0.01 | 0.01 | 0.02 | 0.00 | 0.03 | 0.01 | 0.00 | 0.01 | 0.01 | 0.01 | 0.00 | 0.01 | 0.01 | 0.01 | 0.01 | 0.00 | 0.01 | 0.01 |
| | | Pineapple | | | | | | | | | | | | | | | | | | | |
| 3440 | 1/2 cup | Canned in extra heavy syrup, chunks, avg | 130 | 0.02 | 0.02 | 0.10 | 0.00 | 0.05 | 0.02 | 0.01 | 0.01 | 0.02 | 0.02 | 0.01 | 0.01 | 0.01 | 0.02 | 0.01 | 0.01 | 0.01 | 0.01 |
| 3114 | 1/2 cup | Canned in heavy syrup, pieces, avg | 127 | 0.02 | 0.02 | 0.10 | 0.00 | 0.05 | 0.02 | 0.01 | 0.01 | 0.02 | 0.02 | 0.01 | 0.01 | 0.01 | 0.02 | 0.01 | 0.01 | 0.01 | 0.01 |
| 3183 | 1/2 cup | Canned in juice, avg | 125 | 0.03 | 0.02 | 0.12 | 0.00 | 0.06 | 0.02 | 0.01 | 0.01 | 0.02 | 0.02 | 0.01 | 0.01 | 0.01 | 0.03 | 0.01 | 0.01 | 0.01 | 0.02 |
| 3181 | 1/2 cup | Canned in light syrup, avg | 126 | 0.02 | 0.02 | 0.10 | 0.00 | 0.05 | 0.02 | 0.01 | 0.01 | 0.02 | 0.02 | 0.01 | 0.01 | 0.01 | 0.02 | 0.01 | 0.01 | 0.01 | 0.02 |
| 3738 | 1/2 cup | Canned in water, slices, avg | 123 | 0.03 | 0.02 | 0.12 | 0.00 | 0.06 | 0.02 | 0.01 | 0.01 | 0.02 | 0.02 | 0.01 | 0.01 | 0.01 | 0.03 | 0.01 | 0.01 | 0.01 | 0.02 |
| 3111 | 1/2 cup | Fresh, chunks, avg | 78 | 0.01 | 0.01 | 0.04 | 0.00 | 0.04 | 0.01 | 0.01 | 0.01 | 0.01 | 0.02 | 0.01 | 0.01 | 0.01 | 0.02 | 0.01 | 0.00 | 0.01 | 0.01 |
| 3118 | 1/2 cup | Frozen, sweetened, avg | 123 | 0.02 | 0.02 | 0.07 | 0.00 | 0.06 | 0.02 | 0.01 | 0.02 | 0.02 | 0.03 | 0.01 | 0.01 | 0.02 | 0.03 | 0.02 | 0.01 | 0.02 | 0.02 |
| 3196 | 1/2 cup | Plantain, cooked, slices, avg | 77 | 0.02 | 0.05 | 0.05 | 0.01 | 0.05 | 0.02 | 0.03 | 0.02 | 0.03 | 0.03 | 0.01 | 0.02 | 0.02 | 0.02 | 0.02 | 0.01 | 0.02 | 0.02 |
| 3195 | 1/2 cup | Plantain, raw, slices, avg | 74 | 0.04 | 0.08 | 0.08 | 0.01 | 0.09 | 0.03 | 0.05 | 0.03 | 0.04 | 0.04 | 0.01 | 0.03 | 0.04 | 0.03 | 0.03 | 0.01 | 0.02 | 0.03 |
| | | Plum | | | | | | | | | | | | | | | | | | | |
| 3124 | 1/2 cup | Canned in heavy syrup, avg | 129 | 0.02 | 0.01 | 0.15 | 0.00 | 0.02 | 0.01 | 0.01 | 0.01 | 0.01 | 0.01 | 0.00 | 0.01 | 0.02 | 0.01 | 0.01 | 0.00 | 0.00 | 0.01 |
| 3185 | 1/2 cup | Canned in juice, avg | 126 | 0.02 | 0.01 | 0.20 | 0.00 | 0.03 | 0.01 | 0.01 | 0.01 | 0.02 | 0.01 | 0.01 | 0.01 | 0.03 | 0.02 | 0.01 | 0.00 | 0.01 | 0.02 |
| 3187 | 1/2 cup | Canned in light syrup, avg | 126 | 0.02 | 0.01 | 0.15 | 0.00 | 0.02 | 0.01 | 0.01 | 0.01 | 0.01 | 0.01 | 0.00 | 0.01 | 0.02 | 0.01 | 0.01 | 0.00 | 0.00 | 0.01 |
| 3123 | 1/2 cup | Fresh, slices, avg | 82 | 0.02 | 0.01 | 0.20 | 0.00 | 0.03 | 0.01 | 0.01 | 0.01 | 0.02 | 0.01 | 0.00 | 0.01 | 0.03 | 0.02 | 0.01 | 0.00 | 0.00 | 0.02 |
| | | Prunes | | | | | | | | | | | | | | | | | | | |
| 3352 | 1/2 cup | Canned in heavy syrup, avg | 117 | 0.04 | 0.02 | 0.32 | 0.01 | 0.05 | 0.02 | 0.02 | 0.02 | 0.03 | 0.02 | 0.01 | 0.02 | 0.04 | 0.03 | 0.02 | 0.00 | 0.01 | 0.02 |
| 3449 | 1/2 cup | Cooked, f/dry, w/sugar, avg | 124 | 0.04 | 0.02 | 0.39 | 0.01 | 0.06 | 0.02 | 0.02 | 0.02 | 0.03 | 0.03 | 0.01 | 0.03 | 0.05 | 0.03 | 0.02 | 0.00 | 0.01 | 0.03 |
| 3448 | 1/2 cup | Cooked, f/dehydrated, avg | 140 | 0.06 | 0.03 | 0.54 | 0.01 | 0.08 | 0.03 | 0.03 | 0.33 | 0.05 | 0.04 | 0.01 | 0.04 | 0.07 | 0.04 | 0.04 | 0.00 | 0.01 | 0.04 |
| 3127 | 1/2 cup | Cooked, stewed f/dry, w/o sugar, avg | 124 | 0.05 | 0.02 | 0.41 | 0.01 | 0.06 | 0.02 | 0.02 | 0.03 | 0.03 | 0.03 | 0.01 | 0.03 | 0.06 | 0.03 | 0.03 | 0.00 | 0.01 | 0.03 |
| 3647 | 1/2 cup | Dried, avg | 85 | 0.07 | 0.03 | 0.63 | 0.01 | 0.09 | 0.03 | 0.03 | 0.04 | 0.05 | 0.04 | 0.02 | 0.04 | 0.09 | 0.05 | 0.04 | 0.00 | 0.02 | 0.05 |
| 3447 | 1/2 cup | Dried, dehydrated, uncooked, avg | 66 | 0.08 | 0.04 | 0.70 | 0.01 | 0.10 | 0.03 | 0.04 | 0.04 | 0.06 | 0.05 | 0.02 | 0.05 | 0.10 | 0.06 | 0.04 | 0.00 | 0.02 | 0.05 |
| | | Raisins | | | | | | | | | | | | | | | | | | | |
| 3450 | 1/2 cup | Seeded, avg | 72 | 0.08 | 0.13 | 0.22 | 0.03 | 0.38 | 0.05 | 0.07 | 0.01 | 0.04 | 0.04 | 0.06 | 0.04 | 0.06 | 0.09 | 0.05 | 0.01 | 0.03 | 0.05 |
| 3202 | 1/2 cup | Seedless, golden, packed, avg | 82 | 0.12 | 0.21 | 0.34 | 0.04 | 0.58 | 0.08 | 0.10 | 0.02 | 0.06 | 0.06 | 0.09 | 0.06 | 0.09 | 0.13 | 0.08 | 0.01 | 0.05 | 0.08 |
| 3546 | 1/2 cup | Seedless, plumped, avg | 80 | 0.11 | 0.51 | 0.11 | 0.08 | 0.17 | 0.07 | 0.07 | 0.06 | 0.10 | 0.08 | 0.02 | 0.07 | 0.28 | 0.07 | 0.07 | 0.00 | 0.05 | 0.08 |
| 3130 | 1/2 cup | Seedless, unpacked, avg | 72 | 0.10 | 0.17 | 0.28 | 0.04 | 0.48 | 0.07 | 0.08 | 0.02 | 0.05 | 0.05 | 0.08 | 0.05 | 0.08 | 0.11 | 0.06 | 0.01 | 0.04 | 0.06 |
| 3133 | 1/2 cup | Rhubarb, Cooked from frozen, w/sugar, avg | 120 | 0.00 | 0.00 | 0.01 | 0.00 | 0.01 | 0.00 | 0.00 | 0.00 | 0.00 | 0.00 | 0.00 | 0.00 | 0.00 | 0.00 | 0.00 | 0.00 | 0.00 | 0.00 |
| 3209 | 1/2 cup | Rhubarb, Raw, diced, avg | 61 | 0.02 | 0.02 | 0.03 | 0.00 | 0.04 | 0.02 | 0.01 | 0.02 | 0.02 | 0.02 | 0.01 | 0.02 | 0.01 | 0.02 | 0.01 | 0.01 | 0.01 | 0.02 |
| 3649 | 1/2 ea | Sapodillas, raw, avg | 120 | 0.02 | 0.02 | 0.04 | 0.00 | 0.05 | 0.02 | 0.02 | 0.02 | 0.03 | 0.05 | 0.00 | 0.02 | 0.04 | 0.02 | 0.01 | 0.01 | 0.02 | 0.02 |
| 3267 | 1 ea | Sapotes, raw, avg | 225 | 0.26 | 0.12 | 1.20 | 0.00 | 0.49 | 0.13 | 0.09 | 0.10 | 0.19 | 0.22 | 0.04 | 0.12 | 0.13 | 0.51 | 0.13 | 0.05 | 0.12 | 0.17 |
| | | Strawberries | | | | | | | | | | | | | | | | | | | |
| 3135 | 1/2 cup | Fresh, slices, avg | 83 | 0.03 | 0.02 | 0.11 | 0.00 | 0.07 | 0.02 | 0.01 | 0.01 | 0.03 | 0.02 | 0.00 | 0.01 | 0.02 | 0.02 | 0.02 | 0.01 | 0.02 | 0.01 |
| 3236 | 1/2 cup | Frozen, sliced, sweetened, avg | 128 | 0.03 | 0.03 | 0.15 | 0.01 | 0.10 | 0.03 | 0.01 | 0.02 | 0.03 | 0.03 | 0.00 | 0.02 | 0.02 | 0.03 | 0.02 | 0.01 | 0.02 | 0.02 |

TABLE A **Amino Acid Content for Selected Foods *(continued)***

| Code | Amount | Description | Weight (g) | Alanine (g) | Arginine (g) | Aspartic acid (g) | Cystine (g) | Glutamic acid (g) | Glycine (g) | Histidine (g) | Isoleucine (g) | Leucine (g) | Lysine (g) | Methionine (g) | Phenylalanine (g) | Proline (g) | Serine (g) | Threonine (g) | Tryptophan (g) | Tyrosine (g) | Valine (g) |
|---|---|---|---|---|---|---|---|---|---|---|---|---|---|---|---|---|---|---|---|---|---|
| 3783 | 1/2 cup | Frozen, thawed, unsweetened, avg | 110 | 0.02 | 0.02 | 0.11 | 0.00 | 0.07 | 0.02 | 0.01 | 0.01 | 0.02 | 0.02 | 0.00 | 0.01 | 0.01 | 0.02 | 0.01 | 0.01 | 0.02 | 0.01 |
| 3453 | 1/2 cup | In heavy syrup, avg | 127 | 0.04 | 0.03 | 0.16 | 0.01 | 0.11 | 0.03 | 0.01 | 0.02 | 0.04 | 0.03 | 0.00 | 0.02 | 0.02 | 0.03 | 0.02 | 0.01 | 0.02 | 0.02 |
| 3237 | 1/2 cup | Tangerines, canned in light syrup, avg | 126 | 0.03 | 0.04 | 0.07 | 0.01 | 0.06 | 0.06 | 0.01 | 0.02 | 0.01 | 0.03 | 0.01 | 0.02 | 0.03 | 0.02 | 0.01 | 0.01 | 0.01 | 0.02 |
| 3139 | 1/2 cup | Tangerines, fresh, sections, avg | 98 | 0.03 | 0.04 | 0.08 | 0.01 | 0.06 | 0.06 | 0.01 | 0.02 | 0.02 | 0.03 | 0.01 | 0.02 | 0.03 | 0.02 | 0.01 | 0.01 | 0.01 | 0.03 |
| 3142 | 1/2 cup | Watermelon, fresh, diced, avg | 76 | 0.01 | 0.04 | 0.03 | 0.00 | 0.05 | 0.01 | 0.00 | 0.01 | 0.01 | 0.05 | 0.00 | 0.01 | 0.02 | 0.01 | 0.02 | 0.01 | 0.01 | 0.01 |
| | | **GRAINS, FLOURS AND FRACTIONS** | | | | | | | | | | | | | | | | | | | |
| 38070 | 1/4 cup | Amaranth, grain, avg | 49 | 0.39 | 0.52 | 0.62 | 0.09 | 1.11 | 0.30 | 0.19 | 0.29 | 0.43 | 0.37 | 0.11 | 0.27 | 0.34 | 0.56 | 0.27 | 0.09 | 0.16 | 0.33 |
| 38242 | 1/4 cup | Amaranth, grain, whole, American Amaranth | 31 | 0.17 | 0.42 | 0.39 | 0.11 | 0.75 | 0.36 | 0.13 | 0.18 | 0.27 | 0.27 | 0.11 | 0.20 | 0.19 | 0.28 | 0.17 | 0.08 | 0.16 | 0.20 |
| 38071 | 1/4 cup | Arrowroot Flour, avg | 32 | 0.00 | 0.00 | 0.02 | 0.00 | 0.02 | 0.00 | 0.00 | 0.00 | 0.01 | 0.00 | 0.00 | 0.00 | 0.00 | 0.00 | 0.00 | 0.00 | 0.00 | 0.00 |
| | | Barley | | | | | | | | | | | | | | | | | | | |
| 38003 | 1/4 cup | Pearled, cooked, avg | 39 | 0.03 | 0.04 | 0.05 | 0.02 | 0.23 | 0.03 | 0.02 | 0.03 | 0.06 | 0.03 | 0.02 | 0.05 | 0.10 | 0.04 | 0.03 | 0.01 | 0.03 | 0.04 |
| 38002 | 1/4 cup | Pearled, dry, avg | 50 | 0.19 | 0.25 | 0.31 | 0.11 | 1.29 | 0.18 | 0.11 | 0.18 | 0.34 | 0.18 | 0.09 | 0.28 | 0.59 | 0.21 | 0.17 | 0.08 | 0.14 | 0.24 |
| 38001 | 1/4 cup | Whole, cooked, avg | 50 | 0.07 | 0.09 | 0.12 | 0.04 | 0.48 | 0.07 | 0.04 | 0.07 | 0.13 | 0.07 | 0.04 | 0.10 | 0.22 | 0.08 | 0.06 | 0.03 | 0.05 | 0.09 |
| 38000 | 1/4 cup | Whole, dry, avg | 46 | 0.22 | 0.29 | 0.36 | 0.13 | 1.50 | 0.21 | 0.13 | 0.21 | 0.39 | 0.21 | 0.11 | 0.32 | 0.68 | 0.24 | 0.20 | 0.10 | 0.16 | 0.28 |
| | | Buckwheat | | | | | | | | | | | | | | | | | | | |
| 38053 | 1/4 cup | Flour, whole, avg | 30 | 0.21 | 0.28 | 0.32 | 0.07 | 0.59 | 0.29 | 0.09 | 0.14 | 0.24 | 0.19 | 0.05 | 0.15 | 0.14 | 0.20 | 0.14 | 0.05 | 0.07 | 0.19 |
| 38278 | 1/4 cup | Groats, dry roasted, avg | 41 | 0.27 | 0.36 | 0.41 | 0.08 | 0.74 | 0.37 | 0.11 | 0.18 | 0.30 | 0.24 | 0.05 | 0.19 | 0.18 | 0.25 | 0.18 | 0.07 | 0.09 | 0.25 |
| 38073 | 1/4 cup | Groats, dry roasted, cooked, avg | 42 | 0.08 | 0.10 | 0.12 | 0.02 | 0.22 | 0.11 | 0.03 | 0.05 | 0.09 | 0.07 | 0.02 | 0.06 | 0.05 | 0.07 | 0.05 | 0.02 | 0.03 | 0.07 |
| 38100 | 1/4 cup | Kasha, cooked, avg | 50 | 0.33 | 0.43 | 0.50 | 0.10 | 0.50 | 0.46 | 0.14 | 0.22 | 0.37 | 0.30 | 0.03 | 0.23 | 0.22 | 0.30 | 0.22 | 0.09 | 0.11 | 0.30 |
| 38101 | 1/4 cup | Kasha, raw, avg | 82 | 0.16 | 0.20 | 0.24 | 0.05 | 0.43 | 0.22 | 0.06 | 0.10 | 0.17 | 0.14 | 0.04 | 0.11 | 0.11 | 0.14 | 0.11 | 0.04 | 0.05 | 0.14 |
| | | Corn | | | | | | | | | | | | | | | | | | | |
| 38005 | 1/4 cup | Flour, masa, enriched, avg | 28 | 0.20 | 0.13 | 0.18 | 0.05 | 0.49 | 0.11 | 0.08 | 0.09 | 0.32 | 0.07 | 0.05 | 0.13 | 0.23 | 0.12 | 0.10 | 0.02 | 0.11 | 0.13 |
| 38161 | 1/4 cup | Flour, masa, enriched, yellow, avg | 28 | 0.20 | 0.13 | 0.18 | 0.05 | 0.49 | 0.11 | 0.08 | 0.09 | 0.32 | 0.07 | 0.05 | 0.13 | 0.23 | 0.12 | 0.10 | 0.02 | 0.11 | 0.13 |
| 38096 | 1/4 cup | Flour, white, whole grain, avg | 29 | 0.15 | 0.10 | 0.14 | 0.04 | 0.38 | 0.08 | 0.06 | 0.07 | 0.25 | 0.06 | 0.04 | 0.10 | 0.18 | 0.10 | 0.08 | 0.01 | 0.08 | 0.10 |
| 38049 | 1/4 cup | Flour, yellow, whole grain, avg | 29 | 0.15 | 0.10 | 0.14 | 0.04 | 0.38 | 0.08 | 0.06 | 0.07 | 0.25 | 0.06 | 0.04 | 0.10 | 0.18 | 0.10 | 0.08 | 0.01 | 0.08 | 0.10 |
| 38253 | 1/4 cup | Meal, white, self rising, enriched, avg | 30 | 0.19 | 0.12 | 0.17 | 0.04 | 0.47 | 0.10 | 0.08 | 0.09 | 0.31 | 0.07 | 0.05 | 0.12 | 0.22 | 0.12 | 0.09 | 0.02 | 0.10 | 0.13 |
| 38059 | 1/4 cup | Meal, yellow, whole grain, avg | 30 | 0.18 | 0.12 | 0.17 | 0.04 | 0.46 | 0.10 | 0.07 | 0.09 | 0.30 | 0.07 | 0.05 | 0.12 | 0.21 | 0.12 | 0.09 | 0.02 | 0.10 | 0.12 |
| 38280 | 1/4 cup | Meal, yellow, self rising, enriched, avg | 30 | 0.19 | 0.12 | 0.17 | 0.04 | 0.47 | 0.10 | 0.08 | 0.09 | 0.31 | 0.07 | 0.05 | 0.12 | 0.22 | 0.12 | 0.09 | 0.02 | 0.10 | 0.13 |
| 38252 | 1/4 cup | White, dry, avg | 42 | 0.30 | 0.20 | 0.28 | 0.07 | 0.74 | 0.15 | 0.12 | 0.14 | 0.49 | 0.11 | 0.03 | 0.19 | 0.35 | 0.19 | 0.15 | 0.03 | 0.16 | 0.20 |
| 38279 | 1/4 cup | Yellow, dry, avg | 42 | 0.30 | 0.20 | 0.28 | 0.07 | 0.74 | 0.15 | 0.12 | 0.14 | 0.49 | 0.11 | 0.03 | 0.19 | 0.35 | 0.19 | 0.15 | 0.03 | 0.16 | 0.20 |
| 38052 | 1/4 cup | Millet, cooked, avg | 60 | 0.19 | 0.07 | 0.14 | 0.04 | 0.46 | 0.05 | 0.05 | 0.09 | 0.27 | 0.04 | 0.04 | 0.11 | 0.17 | 0.12 | 0.07 | 0.02 | 0.06 | 0.11 |
| 38282 | 1/4 cup | Millet, dry, avg | 50 | 0.49 | 0.19 | 0.36 | 0.11 | 1.20 | 0.14 | 0.12 | 0.23 | 0.70 | 0.11 | 0.11 | 0.29 | 0.44 | 0.32 | 0.18 | 0.06 | 0.17 | 0.29 |
| | | Oat | | | | | | | | | | | | | | | | | | | |
| 38078 | 1/4 cup | Bran, cooked, avg | 55 | 0.08 | 0.12 | 0.15 | 0.05 | 0.35 | 0.09 | 0.04 | 0.06 | 0.13 | 0.07 | 0.03 | 0.09 | 0.09 | 0.08 | 0.05 | 0.03 | 0.06 | 0.09 |
| 38064 | 1/4 cup | Bran, dry, avg | 24 | 0.20 | 0.30 | 0.37 | 0.13 | 0.87 | 0.22 | 0.10 | 0.16 | 0.32 | 0.18 | 0.08 | 0.21 | 0.23 | 0.21 | 0.12 | 0.08 | 0.16 | 0.22 |
| 38080 | 1/4 cup | Grain, dry, avg | 39 | 0.34 | 0.46 | 0.57 | 0.16 | 1.45 | 0.33 | 0.16 | 0.27 | 0.50 | 0.27 | 0.12 | 0.35 | 0.36 | 0.29 | 0.22 | 0.09 | 0.22 | 0.37 |
| 38008 | 1/4 cup | Rolled, dry, avg | 20 | 0.17 | 0.23 | 0.27 | 0.08 | 0.70 | 0.16 | 0.08 | 0.13 | 0.24 | 0.13 | 0.06 | 0.17 | 0.18 | 0.14 | 0.11 | 0.04 | 0.11 | 0.18 |
| 38079 | 1/4 cup | Quinoa, grain, dry, avg | 42 | 0.26 | 0.39 | 0.40 | 0.15 | 0.66 | 0.29 | 0.13 | 0.20 | 0.33 | 0.31 | 0.11 | 0.23 | 0.17 | 0.20 | 0.19 | 0.06 | 0.15 | 0.25 |
| 38050 | 1/4 cup | Rice, bran, crude, avg | 30 | 0.29 | 0.32 | 0.39 | 0.10 | 0.56 | 0.26 | 0.11 | 0.17 | 0.31 | 0.20 | 0.09 | 0.19 | 0.20 | 0.20 | 0.17 | 0.03 | 0.12 | 0.26 |
| 38158 | 1/4 cup | Rice, flour, white, avg | 40 | 0.13 | 0.21 | 0.22 | 0.04 | 0.44 | 0.11 | 0.06 | 0.10 | 0.20 | 0.08 | 0.06 | 0.13 | 0.11 | 0.12 | 0.08 | 0.03 | 0.13 | 0.14 |
| | | Rye | | | | | | | | | | | | | | | | | | | |
| 38022 | 1/4 cup | Flour, dark, avg | 32 | 0.19 | 0.20 | 0.31 | 0.09 | 1.25 | 0.17 | 0.10 | 0.17 | 0.31 | 0.16 | 0.07 | 0.23 | 0.48 | 0.24 | 0.16 | 0.05 | 0.09 | 0.22 |
| 38023 | 1/4 cup | Flour, light, avg | 26 | 0.09 | 0.10 | 0.15 | 0.04 | 0.61 | 0.08 | 0.05 | 0.08 | 0.15 | 0.08 | 0.03 | 0.11 | 0.23 | 0.12 | 0.08 | 0.02 | 0.04 | 0.11 |
| 38056 | 1/4 cup | Flour, medium, avg | 26 | 0.10 | 0.11 | 0.17 | 0.05 | 0.68 | 0.09 | 0.05 | 0.09 | 0.17 | 0.08 | 0.04 | 0.12 | 0.26 | 0.13 | 0.08 | 0.03 | 0.05 | 0.12 |
| 38084 | 1/4 cup | Grain, avg | 42 | 0.30 | 0.34 | 0.50 | 0.14 | 1.54 | 0.29 | 0.15 | 0.23 | 0.41 | 0.25 | 0.10 | 0.28 | 0.63 | 0.29 | 0.22 | 0.06 | 0.14 | 0.31 |

## TABLE A Amino Acid Content for Selected Foods *(continued)*

| Code | Amount | Description | Weight (g) | Alanine (g) | Arginine (g) | Aspartic acid (g) | Cystine (g) | Glutamic acid (g) | Glycine (g) | Histidine (g) | Isoleucine (g) | Leucine (g) | Lysine (g) | Methionine (g) | Phenylalanine (g) | Proline (g) | Serine (g) | Threonine (g) | Tryptophan (g) | Tyrosine (g) | Valine (g) |
|---|---|---|---|---|---|---|---|---|---|---|---|---|---|---|---|---|---|---|---|---|---|
| 38085 | 1/4 cup | Sorghum, grain, whole, avg | 48 | 0.49 | 0.17 | 0.36 | 0.06 | 1.17 | 0.17 | 0.12 | 0.21 | 0.72 | 0.11 | 0.08 | 0.26 | 0.41 | 0.22 | 0.17 | 0.06 | 0.15 | 0.27 |
| 38087 | 1/4 cup | Triticale, flour, avg | 32 | 0.16 | 0.22 | 0.25 | 0.09 | 1.30 | 0.18 | 0.10 | 0.15 | 0.29 | 0.12 | 0.07 | 0.21 | 0.38 | 0.19 | 0.13 | 0.05 | 0.12 | 0.20 |
| 38086 | 1/4 cup | Triticale, grain, dry, avg | 48 | 0.23 | 0.32 | 0.38 | 0.13 | 1.92 | 0.27 | 0.15 | 0.23 | 0.44 | 0.18 | 0.10 | 0.31 | 0.57 | 0.28 | 0.19 | 0.08 | 0.18 | 0.29 |
| | | Wheat | | | | | | | | | | | | | | | | | | | |
| 38024 | 1/4 cup | Bran, crude, avg | 14 | 0.11 | 0.15 | 0.16 | 0.05 | 0.40 | 0.13 | 0.06 | 0.07 | 0.13 | 0.08 | 0.03 | 0.08 | 0.12 | 0.10 | 0.07 | 0.04 | 0.06 | 0.10 |
| 38028 | 1/4 cup | Bulgur, cooked, avg | 46 | 0.05 | 0.07 | 0.07 | 0.03 | 0.45 | 0.06 | 0.03 | 0.05 | 0.10 | 0.04 | 0.02 | 0.07 | 0.15 | 0.07 | 0.04 | 0.02 | 0.04 | 0.06 |
| 38027 | 1/4 cup | Bulgur, dry, avg | 35 | 0.15 | 0.20 | 0.22 | 0.10 | 1.36 | 0.17 | 0.10 | 0.16 | 0.29 | 0.12 | 0.07 | 0.20 | 0.45 | 0.20 | 0.12 | 0.07 | 0.13 | 0.19 |
| 38329 | 1/4 cup | Cracked, dry, avg | 30 | 0.15 | 0.19 | 0.21 | 0.10 | 1.30 | 0.17 | 0.10 | 0.15 | 0.28 | 0.11 | 0.06 | 0.19 | 0.43 | 0.19 | 0.12 | 0.06 | 0.12 | 0.19 |
| 38030 | 1/4 cup | Flour, all purpose, white, enr, bleached, avg | 31 | 0.10 | 0.13 | 0.13 | 0.07 | 1.08 | 0.11 | 0.07 | 0.11 | 0.22 | 0.07 | 0.06 | 0.16 | 0.37 | 0.16 | 0.09 | 0.04 | 0.10 | 0.13 |
| 38271 | 1/4 cup | Flour, all purpose, white, unenriched, avg | 31 | 0.10 | 0.13 | 0.13 | 0.07 | 1.08 | 0.11 | 0.07 | 0.11 | 0.22 | 0.07 | 0.06 | 0.16 | 0.37 | 0.16 | 0.09 | 0.04 | 0.10 | 0.13 |
| 46086 | 1/4 cup | Flour, cake, white, enriched, avg | 34 | 0.08 | 0.11 | 0.12 | 0.06 | 0.92 | 0.09 | 0.06 | 0.11 | 0.19 | 0.10 | 0.05 | 0.13 | 0.31 | 0.15 | 0.08 | 0.04 | 0.08 | 0.12 |
| 38065 | 1/4 cup | Flour, gluten, avg | 35 | 0.47 | 0.58 | 0.61 | 0.31 | 4.90 | 0.52 | 0.32 | 0.50 | 0.99 | 0.32 | 0.26 | 0.73 | 1.68 | 0.72 | 0.40 | 0.18 | 0.44 | 0.58 |
| 38054 | 1/4 cup | Flour, semolina, enriched, avg | 42 | 0.16 | 0.20 | 0.22 | 0.15 | 1.92 | 0.17 | 0.11 | 0.21 | 0.36 | 0.10 | 0.08 | 0.26 | 0.59 | 0.25 | 0.14 | 0.07 | 0.14 | 0.23 |
| 38270 | 1/4 cup | Flour, semolina, unenriched, avg | 42 | 0.16 | 0.20 | 0.22 | 0.15 | 1.92 | 0.17 | 0.11 | 0.21 | 0.36 | 0.10 | 0.08 | 0.26 | 0.59 | 0.25 | 0.14 | 0.07 | 0.14 | 0.23 |
| 38098 | 1/4 cup | Flour tortilla mix, white, enriched, avg | 28 | 0.09 | 0.11 | 0.11 | 0.06 | 0.91 | 0.10 | 0.06 | 0.09 | 0.19 | 0.06 | 0.05 | 0.14 | 0.31 | 0.14 | 0.07 | 0.03 | 0.08 | 0.11 |
| 38025 | 1/4 cup | Germ, crude, avg | 29 | 0.43 | 0.54 | 0.60 | 0.13 | 1.16 | 0.41 | 0.19 | 0.25 | 0.46 | 0.43 | 0.13 | 0.27 | 0.36 | 0.32 | 0.28 | 0.09 | 0.20 | 0.35 |
| 38026 | 1/4 cup | Germ, toasted, avg | 28 | 0.52 | 0.66 | 0.73 | 0.16 | 1.41 | 0.50 | 0.23 | 0.30 | 0.55 | 0.52 | 0.16 | 0.33 | 0.43 | 0.39 | 0.34 | 0.11 | 0.25 | 0.42 |
| 38068 | 1/4 cup | Sprouted, avg | 27 | 0.08 | 0.11 | 0.12 | 0.04 | 0.50 | 0.08 | 0.05 | 0.08 | 0.14 | 0.07 | 0.03 | 0.09 | 0.18 | 0.09 | 0.07 | 0.03 | 0.07 | 0.10 |
| | | Wheat, Whole | | | | | | | | | | | | | | | | | | | |
| 38032 | 1/4 cup | Flour, whole, avg | 30 | 0.15 | 0.19 | 0.21 | 0.10 | 1.30 | 0.17 | 0.10 | 0.15 | 0.28 | 0.11 | 0.06 | 0.19 | 0.43 | 0.19 | 0.12 | 0.06 | 0.12 | 0.19 |
| 38090 | 1/4 cup | Grain, durum, avg | 48 | 0.20 | 0.23 | 0.30 | 0.14 | 2.28 | 0.24 | 0.15 | 0.26 | 0.45 | 0.15 | 0.11 | 0.33 | 0.70 | 0.32 | 0.18 | 0.08 | 0.17 | 0.29 |
| 38287 | 1/4 cup | Grain, hard, red, spring, dry, avg | 48 | 0.27 | 0.34 | 0.39 | 0.19 | 2.38 | 0.30 | 0.16 | 0.26 | 0.50 | 0.19 | 0.11 | 0.35 | 0.81 | 0.32 | 0.21 | 0.09 | 0.21 | 0.33 |
| 38029 | 1/4 cup | Grain, hard, red, winter, dry, avg | 48 | 0.22 | 0.29 | 0.31 | 0.15 | 1.92 | 0.25 | 0.14 | 0.22 | 0.41 | 0.16 | 0.10 | 0.28 | 0.62 | 0.28 | 0.18 | 0.08 | 0.19 | 0.27 |
| 38088 | 1/4 cup | Grain, hard, white, dry, avg | 48 | 0.19 | 0.26 | 0.28 | 0.14 | 1.72 | 0.23 | 0.12 | 0.20 | 0.37 | 0.14 | 0.09 | 0.25 | 0.55 | 0.25 | 0.16 | 0.07 | 0.17 | 0.24 |
| 38288 | 1/4 cup | Grain, soft, red, winter, dry, avg | 42 | 0.16 | 0.20 | 0.22 | 0.12 | 1.43 | 0.18 | 0.10 | 0.15 | 0.30 | 0.12 | 0.07 | 0.20 | 0.46 | 0.21 | 0.13 | 0.00 | 0.13 | 0.19 |
| 38089 | 1/4 cup | Grain, soft, white, dry, avg | 42 | 0.17 | 0.21 | 0.22 | 0.12 | 1.47 | 0.18 | 0.10 | 0.16 | 0.31 | 0.13 | 0.07 | 0.20 | 0.47 | 0.22 | 0.14 | 0.00 | 0.13 | 0.20 |
| | | **GRAIN PRODUCTS—BAGELS** | | | | | | | | | | | | | | | | | | | |
| 42594 | 1 ea | Cinnamon Raisin, large, avg | 118 | 0.39 | 0.45 | 0.57 | 0.25 | 3.82 | 0.40 | 0.26 | 0.43 | 0.79 | 0.28 | 0.21 | 0.56 | 1.27 | 0.57 | 0.34 | 0.13 | 0.32 | 0.50 |
| 42592 | 1 ea | Egg, large, avg | 110 | 0.39 | 0.43 | 0.53 | 0.25 | 3.88 | 0.40 | 0.25 | 0.45 | 0.82 | 0.29 | 0.21 | 0.57 | 1.30 | 0.58 | 0.33 | 0.14 | 0.34 | 0.50 |
| | | **GRAIN PRODUCTS—BISCUITS** | | | | | | | | | | | | | | | | | | | |
| | | Dough | | | | | | | | | | | | | | | | | | | |
| 42107 | 1 ea | Chilled, avg | 30 | 0.05 | 0.07 | 0.07 | 0.04 | 0.64 | 0.06 | 0.04 | 0.07 | 0.13 | 0.04 | 0.03 | 0.10 | 0.23 | 0.09 | 0.05 | 0.02 | 0.06 | 0.07 |
| 42109 | 1 ea | Chilled, low fat, avg | 23 | 0.05 | 0.06 | 0.06 | 0.03 | 0.52 | 0.06 | 0.03 | 0.05 | 0.11 | 0.03 | 0.03 | 0.08 | 0.18 | 0.08 | 0.04 | 0.02 | 0.05 | 0.06 |
| 42111 | 1 ea | Chilled, mixed grain, avg | 44 | 0.09 | 0.11 | 0.12 | 0.06 | 0.89 | 0.10 | 0.06 | 0.09 | 0.19 | 0.06 | 0.05 | 0.13 | 0.30 | 0.13 | 0.07 | 0.03 | 0.08 | 0.11 |
| | | Prepared | | | | | | | | | | | | | | | | | | | |
| 42598 | 1 ea | Buttermilk, f/mix, avg | 77 | 0.15 | 0.19 | 0.21 | 0.09 | 1.52 | 0.16 | 0.11 | 0.17 | 0.34 | 0.13 | 0.09 | 0.24 | 0.54 | 0.24 | 0.14 | 0.06 | 0.15 | 0.20 |
| 42001 | 1 ea | Homemade, avg | 60 | 0.14 | 0.16 | 0.20 | 0.08 | 1.31 | 0.14 | 0.10 | 0.16 | 0.31 | 0.14 | 0.08 | 0.21 | 0.47 | 0.21 | 0.13 | 0.05 | 0.14 | 0.19 |
| 42108 | 1 ea | Plain, f/chilled dough, avg | 27 | 0.05 | 0.07 | 0.07 | 0.04 | 0.62 | 0.06 | 0.04 | 0.06 | 0.12 | 0.04 | 0.03 | 0.09 | 0.22 | 0.09 | 0.05 | 0.02 | 0.06 | 0.07 |
| 42110 | 1 ea | Plain, f/chilled dough, low fat, avg | 21 | 0.05 | 0.07 | 0.07 | 0.03 | 0.55 | 0.06 | 0.04 | 0.06 | 0.11 | 0.04 | 0.03 | 0.08 | 0.19 | 0.08 | 0.04 | 0.02 | 0.05 | 0.07 |
| 42112 | 1 ea | Plain, f/chilled dough, mixed grains, avg | 41 | 0.10 | 0.12 | 0.13 | 0.06 | 0.96 | 0.11 | 0.07 | 0.10 | 0.20 | 0.07 | 0.05 | 0.15 | 0.33 | 0.14 | 0.08 | 0.04 | 0.09 | 0.12 |
| | | **GRAIN PRODUCTS—BREADS** | | | | | | | | | | | | | | | | | | | |
| 42039 | 1 pce | Banana Bread, prep f/recipe, w/marg, avg | 60 | 0.10 | 0.12 | 0.17 | 0.05 | 0.67 | 0.09 | 0.07 | 0.11 | 0.20 | 0.11 | 0.06 | 0.13 | 0.23 | 0.15 | 0.09 | 0.03 | 0.09 | 0.13 |
| 42004 | 1/4 cup | Bread Crumbs, plain, dry, grated, avg | 27 | 0.12 | 0.14 | 0.18 | 0.06 | 1.06 | 0.13 | 0.07 | 0.14 | 0.24 | 0.09 | 0.05 | 0.17 | 0.36 | 0.17 | 0.10 | 0.04 | 0.08 | 0.17 |
| 42144 | 1/4 cup | Bread Crumbs, seasoned, dry, grated, avg | 27 | 0.13 | 0.16 | 0.21 | 0.06 | 1.16 | 0.15 | 0.09 | 0.16 | 0.27 | 0.12 | 0.06 | 0.19 | 0.41 | 0.19 | 0.11 | 0.05 | 0.10 | 0.20 |
| 42036 | 1 ea | Bread Sticks, Plain, w/o salt coating, avg | 10 | 0.04 | 0.04 | 0.05 | 0.03 | 0.40 | 0.04 | 0.03 | 0.05 | 0.08 | 0.03 | 0.02 | 0.06 | 0.14 | 0.06 | 0.03 | 0.01 | 0.03 | 0.05 |
| 42052 | 1 pce | Brown Bread, Boston, canned, avg | 45 | 0.09 | 0.11 | 0.15 | 0.05 | 0.69 | 0.09 | 0.06 | 0.08 | 0.16 | 0.07 | 0.04 | 0.10 | 0.22 | 0.11 | 0.07 | 0.03 | 0.07 | 0.10 |
| | | Cornbread | | | | | | | | | | | | | | | | | | | |
| 49012 | 1 ea | Hush Puppies, avg | 22 | 0.08 | 0.08 | 0.11 | 0.03 | 0.39 | 0.06 | 0.04 | 0.07 | 0.16 | 0.07 | 0.04 | 0.08 | 0.15 | 0.09 | 0.06 | 0.02 | 0.06 | 0.09 |
| 42116 | 1 pce | Prepared f/recipe w/2% milk, avg | 65 | 0.24 | 0.20 | 0.31 | 0.08 | 0.90 | 0.15 | 0.12 | 0.19 | 0.44 | 0.19 | 0.10 | 0.21 | 0.37 | 0.23 | 0.17 | 0.04 | 0.17 | 0.23 |
| 42117 | 1 pce | Prepared f/recipe w/whole milk, avg | 65 | 0.24 | 0.20 | 0.31 | 0.08 | 0.89 | 0.15 | 0.12 | 0.19 | 0.44 | 0.19 | 0.10 | 0.21 | 0.37 | 0.23 | 0.17 | 0.04 | 0.17 | 0.23 |

TABLE A **Amino Acid Content for Selected Foods *(continued)***

| Code | Amount | | Description | Weight (g) | Alanine (g) | Arginine (g) | Aspartic acid (g) | Cystine (g) | Glutamic acid (g) | Glycine (g) | Histidine (g) | Isoleucine (g) | Leucine (g) | Lysine (g) | Methionine (g) | Phenylalanine (g) | Proline (g) | Serine (g) | Threonine (g) | Tryptophan (g) | Tyrosine (g) | Valine (g) |
|---|---|---|---|---|---|---|---|---|---|---|---|---|---|---|---|---|---|---|---|---|---|---|
| 42042 | 1 | pce | Cracked Wheat Bread, avg | 25 | 0.08 | 0.09 | 0.11 | 0.05 | 0.59 | 0.08 | 0.05 | 0.08 | 0.15 | 0.06 | 0.04 | 0.10 | 0.23 | 0.10 | 0.07 | 0.03 | 0.06 | 0.10 |
| 42016 | 1/4 | cup | Croutons, plain, avg | 8 | 0.03 | 0.03 | 0.04 | 0.02 | 0.32 | 0.03 | 0.02 | 0.04 | 0.07 | 0.02 | 0.02 | 0.05 | 0.11 | 0.05 | 0.03 | 0.01 | 0.03 | 0.04 |
| 42148 | 1/4 | cup | Croutons, seasoned, avg | 10 | 0.04 | 0.04 | 0.05 | 0.02 | 0.34 | 0.04 | 0.02 | 0.04 | 0.08 | 0.03 | 0.02 | 0.05 | 0.12 | 0.05 | 0.03 | 0.01 | 0.03 | 0.05 |
| | | | Dinner Rolls | | | | | | | | | | | | | | | | | | | |
| 42159 | 1 | ea | Egg, avg | 35 | 0.13 | 0.13 | 0.19 | 0.07 | 0.37 | 0.12 | 0.07 | 0.14 | 0.24 | 0.11 | 0.07 | 0.16 | 0.32 | 0.17 | 0.11 | 0.04 | 0.10 | 0.16 |
| 42022 | 1 | ea | Hard, white, enriched, avg | 57 | 0.19 | 0.20 | 0.26 | 0.12 | 1.38 | 0.20 | 0.12 | 0.22 | 0.39 | 0.14 | 0.10 | 0.28 | 0.63 | 0.27 | 0.16 | 0.07 | 0.16 | 0.25 |
| 42158 | 1 | ea | Prepared f/recipe, w/2% milk, avg | 35 | 0.11 | 0.13 | 0.17 | 0.06 | 0.35 | 0.10 | 0.07 | 0.12 | 0.22 | 0.11 | 0.06 | 0.15 | 0.30 | 0.16 | 0.10 | 0.04 | 0.10 | 0.14 |
| 42019 | 1 | ea | Prepared f/recipe w/whole milk, avg | 35 | 0.11 | 0.13 | 0.17 | 0.06 | 0.35 | 0.10 | 0.07 | 0.12 | 0.22 | 0.12 | 0.06 | 0.15 | 0.30 | 0.16 | 0.10 | 0.04 | 0.10 | 0.14 |
| 42160 | 1 | ea | Wheat, avg | 36 | 0.10 | 0.13 | 0.14 | 0.07 | 1.03 | 0.12 | 0.07 | 0.11 | 0.21 | 0.07 | 0.05 | 0.15 | 0.34 | 0.15 | 0.09 | 0.04 | 0.09 | 0.13 |
| 42057 | 1 | ea | Whole wheat, avg | 28 | 0.09 | 0.11 | 0.13 | 0.05 | 0.75 | 0.10 | 0.06 | 0.09 | 0.17 | 0.07 | 0.04 | 0.11 | 0.25 | 0.12 | 0.07 | 0.04 | 0.07 | 0.11 |
| 42090 | 1 | pce | Egg/Challah Bread, avg | 40 | 0.14 | 0.15 | 0.21 | 0.08 | 1.14 | 0.13 | 0.08 | 0.15 | 0.28 | 0.12 | 0.08 | 0.19 | 0.38 | 0.20 | 0.12 | 0.04 | 0.12 | 0.18 |
| | | | English Muffins | | | | | | | | | | | | | | | | | | | |
| 42149 | 1 | ea | Mixed grain, avg | 66 | 0.23 | 0.29 | 0.36 | 0.13 | 1.76 | 0.24 | 0.13 | 0.24 | 0.43 | 0.19 | 0.10 | 0.30 | 0.56 | 0.29 | 0.18 | 0.08 | 0.18 | 0.28 |
| 42289 | 1 | ea | Plain, enriched, avg | 57 | 0.16 | 0.17 | 0.23 | 0.09 | 1.37 | 0.16 | 0.10 | 0.13 | 0.31 | 0.14 | 0.08 | 0.22 | 0.46 | 0.21 | 0.14 | 0.05 | 0.13 | 0.20 |
| 42290 | 1 | ea | Plain, unenriched, avg | 57 | 0.16 | 0.17 | 0.23 | 0.09 | 1.37 | 0.16 | 0.10 | 0.13 | 0.31 | 0.14 | 0.08 | 0.22 | 0.46 | 0.21 | 0.14 | 0.05 | 0.13 | 0.20 |
| 42151 | 1 | ea | Raisin cinnamon, avg | 57 | 0.16 | 0.17 | 0.24 | 0.09 | 1.32 | 0.16 | 0.10 | 0.17 | 0.30 | 0.13 | 0.08 | 0.21 | 0.43 | 0.21 | 0.13 | 0.05 | 0.13 | 0.19 |
| 42060 | 1 | ea | Sourdough, avg | 57 | 0.16 | 0.17 | 0.23 | 0.09 | 1.37 | 0.16 | 0.10 | 0.13 | 0.31 | 0.14 | 0.08 | 0.22 | 0.46 | 0.21 | 0.14 | 0.05 | 0.13 | 0.20 |
| 42082 | 1 | ea | Whole wheat, avg | 66 | 0.23 | 0.28 | 0.34 | 0.13 | 1.69 | 0.24 | 0.14 | 0.23 | 0.40 | 0.20 | 0.09 | 0.28 | 0.56 | 0.27 | 0.19 | 0.09 | 0.18 | 0.27 |
| 42043 | 1 | pce | French Bread, avg | 25 | 0.07 | 0.08 | 0.10 | 0.05 | 0.74 | 0.08 | 0.05 | 0.08 | 0.15 | 0.05 | 0.04 | 0.11 | 0.25 | 0.11 | 0.06 | 0.03 | 0.06 | 0.09 |
| 42020 | 1 | ea | Hamburger/Hotdog Rolls, avg | 43 | 0.12 | 0.13 | 0.17 | 0.08 | 1.21 | 0.13 | 0.08 | 0.14 | 0.26 | 0.09 | 0.07 | 0.18 | 0.41 | 0.18 | 0.11 | 0.04 | 0.11 | 0.16 |
| 42162 | 1 | ea | Hamburger/Hotdog Rolls, multigrain, avg | 43 | 0.15 | 0.17 | 0.21 | 0.09 | 1.30 | 0.16 | 0.09 | 0.15 | 0.28 | 0.11 | 0.07 | 0.20 | 0.44 | 0.20 | 0.12 | 0.05 | 0.11 | 0.18 |
| 42132 | 1 | pce | High Calcium Bread, dark Hollywood, avg | 18 | 0.06 | 0.08 | 0.09 | 0.03 | 0.47 | 0.06 | 0.04 | 0.05 | 0.11 | 0.05 | 0.03 | 0.08 | 0.16 | 0.08 | 0.05 | 0.02 | 0.05 | 0.07 |
| 42134 | 1 | pce | High Calcium Bread, light Hollywood, avg | 18 | 0.05 | 0.07 | 0.08 | 0.03 | 0.46 | 0.06 | 0.03 | 0.05 | 0.11 | 0.04 | 0.03 | 0.07 | 0.15 | 0.07 | 0.05 | 0.02 | 0.05 | 0.07 |
| 42118 | 1 | pce | Indian/Navajo Fry Bread | 90 | 0.20 | 0.26 | 0.27 | 0.14 | 2.14 | 0.23 | 0.14 | 0.22 | 0.44 | 0.14 | 0.11 | 0.32 | 0.74 | 0.32 | 0.17 | 0.08 | 0.19 | 0.26 |
| 42119 | 1 | pce | Irish Soda Bread, prep f/recipe, avg | 60 | 0.14 | 0.17 | 0.23 | 0.07 | 1.10 | 0.11 | 0.10 | 0.14 | 0.26 | 0.13 | 0.08 | 0.18 | 0.36 | 0.18 | 0.12 | 0.04 | 0.12 | 0.17 |
| 42046 | 1 | pce | Italian Bread, avg | 30 | 0.09 | 0.09 | 0.11 | 0.06 | 0.90 | 0.09 | 0.06 | 0.10 | 0.18 | 0.06 | 0.05 | 0.13 | 0.30 | 0.13 | 0.07 | 0.03 | 0.07 | 0.11 |
| 42047 | 1 | pce | Multi-grain Bread, mixed, avg | 26 | 0.10 | 0.12 | 0.15 | 0.06 | 0.77 | 0.10 | 0.06 | 0.10 | 0.18 | 0.08 | 0.04 | 0.13 | 0.26 | 0.13 | 0.08 | 0.03 | 0.07 | 0.12 |
| 42069 | 1 | pce | Oat Bran Bread, avg | 30 | 0.11 | 0.13 | 0.16 | 0.07 | 0.95 | 0.12 | 0.07 | 0.12 | 0.22 | 0.09 | 0.05 | 0.16 | 0.32 | 0.15 | 0.09 | 0.04 | 0.10 | 0.14 |
| 42076 | 1 | pce | Oat Bran Bread, low cal, avg | 23 | 0.07 | 0.09 | 0.12 | 0.03 | 0.51 | 0.07 | 0.04 | 0.07 | 0.13 | 0.07 | 0.03 | 0.04 | 0.16 | 0.09 | 0.06 | 0.02 | 0.09 | 0.08 |
| 42049 | 1 | pce | Oatmeal Bread, avg | 27 | 0.09 | 0.11 | 0.14 | 0.06 | 0.65 | 0.09 | 0.05 | 0.09 | 0.16 | 0.07 | 0.04 | 0.11 | 0.21 | 0.11 | 0.07 | 0.03 | 0.07 | 0.11 |
| 42125 | 1 | pce | Oatmeal Bread, low calorie, avg | 23 | 0.06 | 0.08 | 0.10 | 0.04 | 0.51 | 0.06 | 0.04 | 0.07 | 0.13 | 0.06 | 0.03 | 0.09 | 0.18 | 0.09 | 0.05 | 0.02 | 0.06 | 0.08 |
| 42007 | 1 | ea | Pita Bread, white, avg | 60 | 0.18 | 0.20 | 0.24 | 0.12 | 1.82 | 0.19 | 0.12 | 0.21 | 0.38 | 0.13 | 0.10 | 0.27 | 0.61 | 0.26 | 0.15 | 0.06 | 0.15 | 0.24 |
| 42080 | 1 | ea | Pita Bread, whole wheat, avg | 64 | 0.22 | 0.29 | 0.31 | 0.14 | 2.00 | 0.25 | 0.14 | 0.23 | 0.43 | 0.17 | 0.10 | 0.30 | 0.66 | 0.30 | 0.18 | 0.09 | 0.19 | 0.28 |
| 42122 | 1 | pce | Protein Bread, avg | 19 | 0.08 | 0.10 | 0.14 | 0.05 | 0.70 | 0.08 | 0.05 | 0.09 | 0.16 | 0.07 | 0.04 | 0.11 | 0.23 | 0.11 | 0.07 | 0.03 | 0.07 | 0.10 |
| 42006 | 1 | pce | Pumpernickel Bread, avg | 26 | 0.08 | 0.09 | 0.12 | 0.05 | 0.71 | 0.09 | 0.05 | 0.09 | 0.16 | 0.06 | 0.04 | 0.11 | 0.25 | 0.11 | 0.07 | 0.03 | 0.06 | 0.10 |
| 42051 | 1 | pce | Raisin Bread, avg | 26 | 0.07 | 0.09 | 0.09 | 0.04 | 0.61 | 0.07 | 0.04 | 0.07 | 0.13 | 0.05 | 0.03 | 0.09 | 0.22 | 0.09 | 0.06 | 0.02 | 0.05 | 0.09 |
| 42129 | 1 | pce | Rice Bran Bread | 27 | 0.09 | 0.10 | 0.13 | 0.05 | 0.73 | 0.09 | 0.05 | 0.09 | 0.17 | 0.07 | 0.04 | 0.12 | 0.25 | 0.12 | 0.07 | 0.03 | 0.07 | 0.11 |
| 42005 | 1 | pce | Rye Bread, avg | 32 | 0.10 | 0.10 | 0.14 | 0.06 | 0.83 | 0.10 | 0.06 | 0.10 | 0.19 | 0.07 | 0.04 | 0.13 | 0.29 | 0.13 | 0.08 | 0.03 | 0.07 | 0.12 |
| 42127 | 1 | pce | Rye Bread, low calorie, avg | 23 | 0.07 | 0.11 | 0.13 | 0.04 | 0.60 | 0.07 | 0.05 | 0.08 | 0.15 | 0.07 | 0.04 | 0.11 | 0.20 | 0.10 | 0.07 | 0.03 | 0.07 | 0.10 |
| 42045 | 1 | pce | Sourdough Bread, avg | 25 | 0.07 | 0.08 | 0.10 | 0.05 | 0.74 | 0.08 | 0.05 | 0.08 | 0.15 | 0.05 | 0.04 | 0.11 | 0.25 | 0.11 | 0.06 | 0.03 | 0.06 | 0.09 |
| 42044 | 1 | pce | Vienna Bread, avg | 25 | 0.07 | 0.08 | 0.10 | 0.05 | 0.74 | 0.08 | 0.05 | 0.08 | 0.15 | 0.05 | 0.04 | 0.11 | 0.25 | 0.11 | 0.06 | 0.03 | 0.06 | 0.09 |
| | | | Wheat Bread | | | | | | | | | | | | | | | | | | | |
| 42136 | 1 | pce | Bran, avg | 36 | 0.11 | 0.13 | 0.16 | 0.07 | 0.99 | 0.12 | 0.07 | 0.12 | 0.22 | 0.08 | 0.05 | 0.15 | 0.33 | 0.15 | 0.09 | 0.04 | 0.09 | 0.14 |
| 42599 | 1 | pce | Germ, avg | 28 | 0.10 | 0.11 | 0.15 | 0.05 | 0.80 | 0.10 | 0.06 | 0.11 | 0.19 | 0.09 | 0.05 | 0.13 | 0.27 | 0.13 | 0.08 | 0.03 | 0.08 | 0.12 |
| 42095 | 1 | pce | Low calorie, avg | 23 | 0.07 | 0.08 | 0.10 | 0.04 | 0.66 | 0.07 | 0.05 | 0.08 | 0.15 | 0.06 | 0.04 | 0.10 | 0.23 | 0.10 | 0.06 | 0.02 | 0.06 | 0.09 |
| 356 | 1 | ea | Part whole wheat, loaf, avg | 454 | 1.38 | 1.54 | 1.97 | 0.85 | 12.98 | 1.43 | 0.89 | 1.62 | 2.90 | 1.18 | 0.72 | 2.01 | 4.46 | 1.99 | 1.24 | 0.49 | 1.25 | 1.81 |
| | | | White Bread | | | | | | | | | | | | | | | | | | | |
| 42216 | 1 | pce | Average | 30 | 0.08 | 0.09 | 0.12 | 0.05 | 0.80 | 0.09 | 0.05 | 0.10 | 0.17 | 0.07 | 0.04 | 0.12 | 0.26 | 0.12 | 0.07 | 0.03 | 0.07 | 0.11 |
| 42084 | 1 | pce | Low calorie, avg | 23 | 0.07 | 0.08 | 0.12 | 0.03 | 0.56 | 0.06 | 0.05 | 0.09 | 0.15 | 0.08 | 0.04 | 0.10 | 0.20 | 0.10 | 0.07 | 0.02 | 0.07 | 0.10 |
| 42606 | 1 | pce | Prepared f/recipe, w/whole milk, avg | 38 | 0.10 | 0.12 | 0.15 | 0.06 | 0.90 | 0.10 | 0.07 | 0.12 | 0.22 | 0.10 | 0.05 | 0.15 | 0.32 | 0.15 | 0.09 | 0.04 | 0.10 | 0.13 |

TABLE A **Amino Acid Content for Selected Foods *(continued)***

| Code | Amount | | Description | Weight (g) | Alanine (g) | Arginine (g) | Aspartic acid (g) | Cystine (g) | Glutamic acid (g) | Glycine (g) | Histidine (g) | Isoleucine (g) | Leucine (g) | Lysine (g) | Methionine (g) | Phenylalanine (g) | Proline (g) | Serine (g) | Threonine (g) | Tryptophan (g) | Tyrosine (g) | Valine (g) |
|---|---|---|---|---|---|---|---|---|---|---|---|---|---|---|---|---|---|---|---|---|---|---|
| 42073 | 1 | pce | Very low sodium, avg | 25 | 0.07 | 0.08 | 0.10 | 0.04 | 0.66 | 0.07 | 0.04 | 0.08 | 0.14 | 0.06 | 0.04 | 0.10 | 0.22 | 0.10 | 0.06 | 0.02 | 0.06 | 0.09 |
| 42014 | 1 | pce | Whole Wheat Bread, avg | 28 | 0.10 | 0.13 | 0.15 | 0.06 | 0.83 | 0.11 | 0.06 | 0.11 | 0.19 | 0.08 | 0.04 | 0.13 | 0.27 | 0.13 | 0.08 | 0.04 | 0.08 | 0.12 |
| | | | **GRAIN PRODUCTS—CRACKERS** | | | | | | | | | | | | | | | | | | | |
| 1034 | 4 | ea | Armenian cracker bread, avg | 28 | 0.23 | 0.24 | 0.40 | 0.07 | 1.46 | 0.13 | 0.27 | 0.39 | 0.76 | 0.66 | 0.20 | 0.42 | 0.94 | 0.42 | 0.27 | 0.10 | 0.43 | 0.55 |
| 43543 | 9 | ea | Butter flavored, snack type, avg | 27 | 0.06 | 0.08 | 0.08 | 0.04 | 0.67 | 0.07 | 0.04 | 0.07 | 0.14 | 0.04 | 0.04 | 0.10 | 0.23 | 0.10 | 0.05 | 0.02 | 0.06 | 0.08 |
| | | | Cheese Crackers | | | | | | | | | | | | | | | | | | | |
| 43500 | 30 | ea | Average | 30 | 0.09 | 0.12 | 0.14 | 0.05 | 0.91 | 0.09 | 0.07 | 0.13 | 0.22 | 0.13 | 0.06 | 0.15 | 0.33 | 0.16 | 0.09 | 0.04 | 0.10 | 0.14 |
| 43663 | 30 | ea | Low sodium, avg | 30 | 0.09 | 0.12 | 0.14 | 0.05 | 0.91 | 0.09 | 0.07 | 0.13 | 0.22 | 0.13 | 0.06 | 0.15 | 0.33 | 0.16 | 0.09 | 0.04 | 0.10 | 0.14 |
| 43501 | 4 | ea | Peanut butter filling, avg | 28 | 0.13 | 0.27 | 0.28 | 0.06 | 0.94 | 0.16 | 0.08 | 0.13 | 0.24 | 0.12 | 0.05 | 0.18 | 0.28 | 0.18 | 0.11 | 0.04 | 0.12 | 0.15 |
| 43527 | 2 | ea | Graham, chocolate coated, avg | 28 | 0.05 | 0.06 | 0.10 | 0.02 | 0.45 | 0.05 | 0.03 | 0.07 | 0.13 | 0.06 | 0.03 | 0.08 | 0.16 | 0.08 | 0.06 | 0.02 | 0.06 | 0.08 |
| 43502 | 4 | ea | Graham, plain/honey, avg | 28 | 0.06 | 0.08 | 0.09 | 0.04 | 0.64 | 0.07 | 0.04 | 0.07 | 0.13 | 0.05 | 0.03 | 0.10 | 0.22 | 0.10 | 0.05 | 0.03 | 0.06 | 0.08 |
| | | | Matzoh | | | | | | | | | | | | | | | | | | | |
| 43535 | 1 | ea | Egg, avg | 28 | 0.13 | 0.15 | 0.18 | 0.07 | 1.03 | 0.12 | 0.08 | 0.13 | 0.25 | 0.11 | 0.07 | 0.17 | 0.35 | 0.19 | 0.11 | 0.04 | 0.11 | 0.15 |
| 43536 | 1 | ea | Egg & onion, avg | 28 | 0.10 | 0.12 | 0.14 | 0.06 | 0.87 | 0.10 | 0.06 | 0.10 | 0.20 | 0.08 | 0.05 | 0.14 | 0.30 | 0.15 | 0.08 | 0.03 | 0.09 | 0.12 |
| 43534 | 1 | ea | Plain, avg | 28 | 0.09 | 0.10 | 0.11 | 0.06 | 0.98 | 0.10 | 0.06 | 0.10 | 0.19 | 0.05 | 0.05 | 0.14 | 0.33 | 0.14 | 0.07 | 0.03 | 0.08 | 0.12 |
| 43510 | 1 | ea | Whole wheat, avg | 28 | 0.13 | 0.18 | 0.19 | 0.09 | 1.14 | 0.15 | 0.09 | 0.14 | 0.25 | 0.10 | 0.06 | 0.17 | 0.38 | 0.17 | 0.11 | 0.06 | 0.11 | 0.17 |
| | | | Melba Toast | | | | | | | | | | | | | | | | | | | |
| 43509 | 6 | ea | Plain, avg | 30 | 0.12 | 0.13 | 0.16 | 0.08 | 1.23 | 0.13 | 0.08 | 0.14 | 0.25 | 0.08 | 0.06 | 0.18 | 0.41 | 0.18 | 0.10 | 0.04 | 0.10 | 0.16 |
| 43566 | 6 | ea | Plain, w/o salt, avg | 30 | 0.12 | 0.13 | 0.16 | 0.08 | 1.23 | 0.13 | 0.08 | 0.14 | 0.25 | 0.08 | 0.06 | 0.18 | 0.41 | 0.18 | 0.10 | 0.04 | 0.10 | 0.16 |
| 43537 | 6 | ea | Rye, avg | 30 | 0.13 | 0.14 | 0.19 | 0.07 | 1.06 | 0.13 | 0.08 | 0.13 | 0.24 | 0.10 | 0.06 | 0.17 | 0.37 | 0.17 | 0.11 | 0.04 | 0.09 | 0.16 |
| 43538 | 6 | ea | Wheat, avg | 30 | 0.13 | 0.16 | 0.19 | 0.09 | 1.24 | 0.15 | 0.09 | 0.15 | 0.27 | 0.10 | 0.06 | 0.18 | 0.41 | 0.18 | 0.11 | 0.05 | 0.11 | 0.17 |
| 43539 | 3 | ea | Milk cracker, avg | 33 | 0.08 | 0.10 | 0.11 | 0.05 | 0.81 | 0.09 | 0.05 | 0.09 | 0.18 | 0.08 | 0.04 | 0.12 | 0.28 | 0.13 | 0.07 | 0.03 | 0.08 | 0.11 |
| 43507 | 30 | ea | Oyster cracker, avg | 30 | 0.09 | 0.11 | 0.12 | 0.06 | 0.92 | 0.10 | 0.06 | 0.10 | 0.19 | 0.08 | 0.05 | 0.14 | 0.31 | 0.14 | 0.08 | 0.04 | 0.08 | 0.12 |
| 43540 | 3 | ea | Rusk Toast, avg | 30 | 0.18 | 0.19 | 0.28 | 0.08 | 0.96 | 0.15 | 0.09 | 0.18 | 0.30 | 0.21 | 0.09 | 0.20 | 0.31 | 0.23 | 0.15 | 0.05 | 0.14 | 0.21 |
| | | | Rye Crackers | | | | | | | | | | | | | | | | | | | |
| 43504 | 3 | ea | Average | 33 | 0.13 | 0.14 | 0.22 | 0.06 | 0.88 | 0.12 | 0.07 | 0.12 | 0.22 | 0.11 | 0.05 | 0.16 | 0.34 | 0.17 | 0.11 | 0.04 | 0.06 | 0.16 |
| 43541 | 4 | ea | Cheese filled, avg | 28 | 0.09 | 0.11 | 0.14 | 0.05 | 0.76 | 0.09 | 0.06 | 0.10 | 0.18 | 0.09 | 0.05 | 0.12 | 0.27 | 0.13 | 0.08 | 0.03 | 0.08 | 0.12 |
| 43532 | 3 | ea | Crispbread, avg | 30 | 0.10 | 0.11 | 0.17 | 0.05 | 0.64 | 0.09 | 0.05 | 0.09 | 0.17 | 0.09 | 0.04 | 0.12 | 0.24 | 0.13 | 0.08 | 0.03 | 0.05 | 0.12 |
| 43531 | 4 | ea | Crispbread, low sodium, avg | 28 | 0.16 | 0.17 | 0.26 | 0.07 | 0.98 | 0.14 | 0.08 | 0.14 | 0.25 | 0.14 | 0.05 | 0.18 | 0.37 | 0.20 | 0.13 | 0.04 | 0.08 | 0.18 |
| 43542 | 1 | ea | Seasoned, avg | 22 | 0.08 | 0.09 | 0.14 | 0.04 | 0.55 | 0.08 | 0.04 | 0.08 | 0.14 | 0.07 | 0.03 | 0.10 | 0.21 | 0.11 | 0.07 | 0.02 | 0.04 | 0.03 |
| | | | Saltine Crackers | | | | | | | | | | | | | | | | | | | |
| 43506 | 10 | ea | Average | 30 | 0.09 | 0.11 | 0.12 | 0.06 | 0.92 | 0.10 | 0.06 | 0.10 | 0.19 | 0.08 | 0.05 | 0.14 | 0.31 | 0.14 | 0.08 | 0.04 | 0.08 | 0.12 |
| 43553 | 10 | ea | Low sodium, avg | 30 | 0.09 | 0.11 | 0.12 | 0.06 | 0.92 | 0.10 | 0.06 | 0.10 | 0.19 | 0.08 | 0.05 | 0.14 | 0.31 | 0.14 | 0.08 | 0.04 | 0.08 | 0.12 |
| 43664 | 6 | ea | Low sodium, fat-free, avg | 30 | 0.10 | 0.12 | 0.13 | 0.07 | 1.05 | 0.11 | 0.07 | 0.11 | 0.21 | 0.09 | 0.05 | 0.15 | 0.36 | 0.16 | 0.09 | 0.04 | 0.09 | 0.13 |
| 43567 | 10 | ea | Unsalted top, avg | 30 | 0.09 | 0.11 | 0.12 | 0.06 | 0.92 | 0.10 | 0.06 | 0.10 | 0.19 | 0.08 | 0.05 | 0.14 | 0.31 | 0.14 | 0.08 | 0.04 | 0.08 | 0.12 |
| | | | Wheat Crackers | | | | | | | | | | | | | | | | | | | |
| 43548 | 4 | ea | Cheese filled, avg | 28 | 0.09 | 0.11 | 0.14 | 0.05 | 0.84 | 0.09 | 0.06 | 0.11 | 0.20 | 0.10 | 0.05 | 0.13 | 0.29 | 0.14 | 0.08 | 0.04 | 0.08 | 0.12 |
| 43569 | 10 | ea | Low salt, avg | 30 | 0.09 | 0.11 | 0.12 | 0.06 | 0.83 | 0.10 | 0.06 | 0.09 | 0.17 | 0.07 | 0.04 | 0.12 | 0.28 | 0.13 | 0.07 | 0.04 | 0.08 | 0.11 |
| 43549 | 4 | ea | Peanut Butter filled, avg | 28 | 0.14 | 0.29 | 0.30 | 0.07 | 1.02 | 0.18 | 0.09 | 0.14 | 0.25 | 0.12 | 0.06 | 0.19 | 0.30 | 0.19 | 0.12 | 0.05 | 0.13 | 0.16 |
| 43570 | 7 | ea | Whole Wheat, low salt | 28 | 0.09 | 0.12 | 0.13 | 0.06 | 0.78 | 0.10 | 0.06 | 0.09 | 0.17 | 0.07 | 0.04 | 0.12 | 0.26 | 0.12 | 0.07 | 0.04 | 0.07 | 0.11 |
| 43508 | 7 | ea | Whole Wheat, Triscuits | 28 | 0.09 | 0.12 | 0.13 | 0.06 | 0.78 | 0.10 | 0.06 | 0.09 | 0.17 | 0.07 | 0.04 | 0.12 | 0.26 | 0.12 | 0.07 | 0.04 | 0.07 | 0.11 |
| | | | **GRAIN PRODUCTS—FRENCH TOAST** | | | | | | | | | | | | | | | | | | | |
| 42155 | 1 | pce | Frozen, ready to heat, avg | 59 | 0.18 | 0.20 | 0.30 | 0.08 | 1.05 | 0.14 | 0.10 | 0.20 | 0.35 | 0.22 | 0.10 | 0.22 | 0.37 | 0.25 | 0.17 | 0.06 | 0.16 | 0.22 |
| 42156 | 1 | pce | Prepared f/recipe w/2% milk, avg | 65 | 0.22 | 0.24 | 0.37 | 0.10 | 1.11 | 0.16 | 0.12 | 0.24 | 0.40 | 0.27 | 0.12 | 0.25 | 0.38 | 0.30 | 0.20 | 0.06 | 0.18 | 0.27 |
| 42040 | 1 | pce | Prepared f/recipe w/whole milk, avg | 65 | 0.22 | 0.24 | 0.38 | 0.10 | 1.12 | 0.16 | 0.12 | 0.24 | 0.40 | 0.27 | 0.12 | 0.25 | 0.38 | 0.30 | 0.20 | 0.06 | 0.18 | 0.27 |
| | | | **GRAIN PRODUCTS—MUFFINS** | | | | | | | | | | | | | | | | | | | |
| | | | Blueberry Muffins | | | | | | | | | | | | | | | | | | | |
| 44516 | 1 | ea | Average | 57 | 0.12 | 0.14 | 0.18 | 0.06 | 0.87 | 0.11 | 0.07 | 0.13 | 0.24 | 0.11 | 0.07 | 0.16 | 0.30 | 0.17 | 0.10 | 0.04 | 0.10 | 0.15 |
| 44517 | 1 | oz | Dry mix, avg | 28 | 0.04 | 0.05 | 0.06 | 0.03 | 0.45 | 0.05 | 0.03 | 0.05 | 0.09 | 0.05 | 0.02 | 0.06 | 0.15 | 0.07 | 0.04 | 0.02 | 0.04 | 0.06 |
| 44505 | 1 | ea | Prepared f/dry mix, avg | 50 | 0.09 | 0.11 | 0.15 | 0.06 | 0.70 | 0.09 | 0.05 | 0.11 | 0.19 | 0.11 | 0.05 | 0.12 | 0.23 | 0.15 | 0.08 | 0.04 | 0.08 | 0.12 |

TABLE A **Amino Acid Content for Selected Foods *(continued)***

| Code | Amount | Description | Weight (g) | Alanine (g) | Arginine (g) | Aspartic acid (g) | Cystine (g) | Glutamic acid (g) | Glycine (g) | Histidine (g) | Isoleucine (g) | Leucine (g) | Lysine (g) | Methionine (g) | Phenylalanine (g) | Proline (g) | Serine (g) | Threonine (g) | Tryptophan (g) | Tyrosine (g) | Valine (g) |
|---|---|---|---|---|---|---|---|---|---|---|---|---|---|---|---|---|---|---|---|---|---|
| 44520 | 1 ea | Prepared f/recipe w/2% milk, avg | 57 | 0.13 | 0.16 | 0.21 | 0.07 | 1.02 | 0.12 | 0.09 | 0.16 | 0.28 | 0.15 | 0.08 | 0.18 | 0.37 | 0.20 | 0.12 | 0.05 | 0.13 | 0.18 |
| 44501 | 1 ea | Prepared f/recipe w/whole milk, avg | 57 | 0.13 | 0.16 | 0.21 | 0.07 | 1.03 | 0.12 | 0.09 | 0.16 | 0.28 | 0.15 | 0.08 | 0.18 | 0.37 | 0.20 | 0.12 | 0.05 | 0.13 | 0.18 |
| 44518 | 1 ea | Toaster, avg | 33 | 0.06 | 0.10 | 0.16 | 0.02 | 0.32 | 0.06 | 0.04 | 0.07 | 0.12 | 0.09 | 0.02 | 0.07 | 0.10 | 0.08 | 0.06 | 0.02 | 0.05 | 0.07 |
| | | Corn Meal Muffins | | | | | | | | | | | | | | | | | | | |
| 44521 | 1 ea | Average | 57 | 0.16 | 0.18 | 0.27 | 0.06 | 0.75 | 0.13 | 0.09 | 0.14 | 0.29 | 0.16 | 0.07 | 0.17 | 0.27 | 0.18 | 0.13 | 0.04 | 0.12 | 0.17 |
| 44504 | 1 ea | Prepared f/dry mix, avg | 50 | 0.18 | 0.17 | 0.25 | 0.07 | 0.83 | 0.13 | 0.09 | 0.16 | 0.33 | 0.16 | 0.08 | 0.18 | 0.32 | 0.20 | 0.14 | 0.04 | 0.14 | 0.19 |
| 44524 | 1 ea | Prepared f/recipe w/2% milk, avg | 57 | 0.20 | 0.18 | 0.27 | 0.07 | 0.93 | 0.14 | 0.10 | 0.17 | 0.37 | 0.17 | 0.09 | 0.20 | 0.36 | 0.22 | 0.15 | 0.04 | 0.15 | 0.21 |
| 44503 | 1 ea | Prepared f/recipe w/whole milk, avg | 57 | 0.20 | 0.18 | 0.27 | 0.07 | 0.93 | 0.14 | 0.10 | 0.17 | 0.37 | 0.17 | 0.09 | 0.20 | 0.36 | 0.21 | 0.15 | 0.04 | 0.15 | 0.21 |
| 44522 | 1 ea | Toaster, avg | 33 | 0.08 | 0.08 | 0.11 | 0.04 | 0.44 | 0.06 | 0.04 | 0.07 | 0.14 | 0.06 | 0.04 | 0.09 | 0.16 | 0.10 | 0.06 | 0.02 | 0.06 | 0.08 |
| 44514 | 1 ea | Oat Bran, avg | 57 | 0.19 | 0.27 | 0.33 | 0.10 | 0.82 | 0.19 | 0.09 | 0.15 | 0.29 | 0.16 | 0.07 | 0.20 | 0.21 | 0.18 | 0.12 | 0.06 | 0.13 | 0.21 |
| 44515 | 1 ea | Plain, prepared f/recipe w/2% milk, avg | 57 | 0.14 | 0.17 | 0.22 | 0.07 | 1.08 | 0.13 | 0.09 | 0.17 | 0.30 | 0.16 | 0.08 | 0.19 | 0.39 | 0.21 | 0.13 | 0.05 | 0.14 | 0.19 |
| 44500 | 1 ea | Plain, prepared f/recipe w/whole milk, avg | 57 | 0.14 | 0.16 | 0.22 | 0.07 | 1.08 | 0.13 | 0.09 | 0.16 | 0.30 | 0.16 | 0.08 | 0.19 | 0.39 | 0.21 | 0.13 | 0.05 | 0.14 | 0.19 |
| | | Wheat Bran Muffins | | | | | | | | | | | | | | | | | | | |
| 44525 | 1 oz | Dry mix, avg | 28 | 0.08 | 0.11 | 0.11 | 0.05 | 0.51 | 0.09 | 0.05 | 0.07 | 0.13 | 0.07 | 0.03 | 0.08 | 0.17 | 0.10 | 0.06 | 0.03 | 0.06 | 0.09 |
| 44506 | 1 ea | Prepared f/dry mix, avg | 50 | 0.15 | 0.18 | 0.23 | 0.08 | 0.71 | 0.14 | 0.08 | 0.13 | 0.23 | 0.15 | 0.07 | 0.15 | 0.23 | 0.18 | 0.12 | 0.05 | 0.10 | 0.16 |
| 44528 | 1 ea | Prepared f/recipe w/2% milk, avg | 57 | 0.17 | 0.21 | 0.27 | 0.08 | 0.93 | 0.16 | 0.10 | 0.16 | 0.29 | 0.18 | 0.08 | 0.18 | 0.33 | 0.21 | 0.14 | 0.06 | 0.14 | 0.20 |
| 44502 | 1 ea | Prepared f/recipe w/whole milk, avg | 57 | 0.17 | 0.21 | 0.27 | 0.08 | 0.93 | 0.16 | 0.10 | 0.16 | 0.29 | 0.18 | 0.08 | 0.18 | 0.33 | 0.21 | 0.14 | 0.06 | 0.14 | 0.20 |
| 44526 | 1 ea | Toaster, w/raisins, avg | 36 | 0.08 | 0.11 | 0.16 | 0.04 | 0.43 | 0.08 | 0.05 | 0.07 | 0.13 | 0.08 | 0.03 | 0.09 | 0.14 | 0.10 | 0.07 | 0.03 | 0.06 | 0.08 |
| | | **GRAIN PRODUCTS—PANCAKES** | | | | | | | | | | | | | | | | | | | |
| 45023 | 1 ea | Blueberry, Prepared f/recipe, 4", avg | 38 | 0.09 | 0.10 | 0.15 | 0.04 | 0.56 | 0.07 | 0.05 | 0.11 | 0.19 | 0.12 | 0.05 | 0.12 | 0.21 | 0.13 | 0.09 | 0.03 | 0.09 | 0.12 |
| 45024 | 1/4 cup | Buckwheat, incomplete dry mix, avg | 30 | 0.14 | 0.18 | 0.21 | 0.07 | 0.84 | 0.17 | 0.08 | 0.12 | 0.23 | 0.11 | 0.05 | 0.15 | 0.27 | 0.16 | 0.11 | 0.05 | 0.09 | 0.15 |
| 45000 | 1 ea | Buckwheat, prep f/incomplete mix, avg | 30 | 0.10 | 0.12 | 0.17 | 0.04 | 0.50 | 0.09 | 0.06 | 0.11 | 0.19 | 0.13 | 0.05 | 0.11 | 0.18 | 0.13 | 0.09 | 0.03 | 0.08 | 0.13 |
| 45025 | 1 ea | Buttermilk, prepared f/recipe, 4", avg | 38 | 0.10 | 0.11 | 0.17 | 0.05 | 0.62 | 0.08 | 0.06 | 0.12 | 0.21 | 0.13 | 0.06 | 0.13 | 0.23 | 0.14 | 0.10 | 0.03 | 0.09 | 0.14 |
| | | Plain Pancakes | | | | | | | | | | | | | | | | | | | |
| 45019 | 1/4 cup | Dry mix, complete, avg | 32 | 0.14 | 0.14 | 0.20 | 0.06 | 0.82 | 0.11 | 0.08 | 0.13 | 0.28 | 0.13 | 0.07 | 0.16 | 0.31 | 0.17 | 0.12 | 0.04 | 0.11 | 0.16 |
| 45026 | 1 oz | Dry mix, low sodium, w/fructose, avg | 28 | 0.11 | 0.12 | 0.16 | 0.05 | 0.68 | 0.09 | 0.06 | 0.09 | 0.22 | 0.07 | 0.04 | 0.13 | 0.25 | 0.12 | 0.08 | 0.03 | 0.08 | 0.11 |
| 45066 | 1 ea | Frozen, RTE, 4", avg | 36 | 0.07 | 0.08 | 0.11 | 0.04 | 0.49 | 0.06 | 0.04 | 0.08 | 0.15 | 0.08 | 0.04 | 0.09 | 0.18 | 0.10 | 0.07 | 0.02 | 0.06 | 0.09 |
| 45002 | 1 ea | Prepared f/complete dry mix, 4", avg | 38 | 0.08 | 0.08 | 0.12 | 0.04 | 0.51 | 0.06 | 0.05 | 0.08 | 0.17 | 0.08 | 0.04 | 0.10 | 0.19 | 0.10 | 0.07 | 0.02 | 0.07 | 0.10 |
| 45001 | 1 ea | Prepared f/recipe, 4", avg | 38 | 0.09 | 0.11 | 0.16 | 0.04 | 0.60 | 0.08 | 0.06 | 0.11 | 0.19 | 0.12 | 0.06 | 0.12 | 0.22 | 0.14 | 0.09 | 0.03 | 0.09 | 0.13 |
| 45028 | 1/4 cup | Whole Wheat, dry mix, incomplete, avg | 35 | 0.19 | 0.25 | 0.28 | 0.11 | 1.26 | 0.19 | 0.10 | 0.17 | 0.32 | 0.15 | 0.08 | 0.22 | 0.39 | 0.21 | 0.14 | 0.07 | 0.14 | 0.22 |
| 45008 | 1 ea | Whole Wheat, prep f/dry mix, 4", avg | 44 | 0.16 | 0.19 | 0.27 | 0.07 | 0.87 | 0.13 | 0.09 | 0.17 | 0.30 | 0.19 | 0.08 | 0.18 | 0.30 | 0.20 | 0.14 | 0.05 | 0.14 | 0.21 |
| | | **GRAIN PRODUCTS—PASTA** | | | | | | | | | | | | | | | | | | | |
| 38151 | 1 cup | Corn, cooked, avg | 140 | 0.28 | 0.18 | 0.26 | 0.07 | 0.69 | 0.15 | 0.11 | 0.13 | 0.45 | 0.10 | 0.08 | 0.18 | 0.32 | 0.17 | 0.14 | 0.03 | 0.15 | 0.19 |
| 38290 | 1/2 cup | Corn, dry, avg | 52 | 0.29 | 0.19 | 0.27 | 0.07 | 0.73 | 0.16 | 0.12 | 0.14 | 0.48 | 0.11 | 0.08 | 0.19 | 0.34 | 0.18 | 0.15 | 0.03 | 0.16 | 0.20 |
| 38076 | 1 cup | Couscous, cooked, avg | 157 | 0.17 | 0.22 | 0.24 | 0.17 | 2.14 | 0.19 | 0.12 | 0.23 | 0.40 | 0.11 | 0.09 | 0.29 | 0.65 | 0.28 | 0.16 | 0.08 | 0.16 | 0.25 |
| 38281 | 1/2 cup | Couscous, dry, avg | 86 | 0.32 | 0.40 | 0.45 | 0.31 | 3.96 | 0.35 | 0.22 | 0.42 | 0.75 | 0.21 | 0.17 | 0.53 | 1.20 | 0.52 | 0.29 | 0.14 | 0.29 | 0.47 |
| | | Fresh Pasta | | | | | | | | | | | | | | | | | | | |
| 38293 | 2 oz | Plain, avg | 57 | 0.19 | 0.23 | 0.26 | 0.18 | 2.29 | 0.20 | 0.13 | 0.25 | 0.43 | 0.12 | 0.10 | 0.31 | 0.70 | 0.30 | 0.17 | 0.08 | 0.17 | 0.27 |
| 38159 | 2 oz | Prepared f/recipe w/egg, avg | 57 | 0.11 | 0.13 | 0.16 | 0.08 | 0.93 | 0.10 | 0.06 | 0.13 | 0.22 | 0.09 | 0.06 | 0.15 | 0.28 | 0.16 | 0.09 | 0.04 | 0.09 | 0.14 |
| 38093 | 1 cup | Prepared f/recipe w/o egg, avg | 76 | 0.10 | 0.12 | 0.14 | 0.09 | 1.20 | 0.10 | 0.07 | 0.13 | 0.23 | 0.06 | 0.05 | 0.16 | 0.36 | 0.16 | 0.09 | 0.04 | 0.09 | 0.14 |
| 38069 | 2 oz | Spinach, cooked, avg | 57 | 0.10 | 0.12 | 0.15 | 0.08 | 0.88 | 0.09 | 0.06 | 0.12 | 0.21 | 0.09 | 0.05 | 0.14 | 0.27 | 0.15 | 0.09 | 0.04 | 0.08 | 0.14 |
| 38303 | 2 oz | Spinach, dry, avg | 57 | 0.23 | 0.27 | 0.34 | 0.17 | 1.97 | 0.21 | 0.14 | 0.28 | 0.46 | 0.19 | 0.12 | 0.32 | 0.60 | 0.33 | 0.20 | 0.09 | 0.19 | 0.31 |
| | | Noodles | | | | | | | | | | | | | | | | | | | |
| 38048 | 1/2 cup | Chow Mein, dry, avg | 22 | 0.05 | 0.07 | 0.08 | 0.05 | 0.66 | 0.06 | 0.04 | 0.07 | 0.13 | 0.04 | 0.03 | 0.09 | 0.20 | 0.09 | 0.05 | 0.02 | 0.05 | 0.08 |
| 38251 | 1 cup | Egg, enriched, cooked w/salt, avg | 160 | 0.26 | 0.31 | 0.38 | 0.21 | 2.42 | 0.24 | 0.16 | 0.32 | 0.54 | 0.21 | 0.14 | 0.38 | 0.74 | 0.39 | 0.23 | 0.10 | 0.22 | 0.36 |

TABLE A **Amino Acid Content for Selected Foods *(continued)***

| Code | Amount | Description | Weight (g) | Alanine (g) | Arginine (g) | Aspartic acid (g) | Cystine (g) | Glutamic acid (g) | Glycine (g) | Histidine (g) | Isoleucine (g) | Leucine (g) | Lysine (g) | Methionine (g) | Phenylalanine (g) | Proline (g) | Serine (g) | Threonine (g) | Tryptophan (g) | Tyrosine (g) | Valine (g) |
|---|---|---|---|---|---|---|---|---|---|---|---|---|---|---|---|---|---|---|---|---|---|
| 38273 | 1 cup | Egg, unenenriched, cooked w/salt, avg | 160 | 0.26 | 0.31 | 0.38 | 0.21 | 2.42 | 0.24 | 0.16 | 0.32 | 0.54 | 0.21 | 0.14 | 0.38 | 0.74 | 0.39 | 0.23 | 0.10 | 0.22 | 0.36 |
| 38259 | 1/2 cup | Egg, unenriched, dry, avg | 19 | 0.09 | 0.11 | 0.13 | 0.07 | 0.85 | 0.08 | 0.06 | 0.11 | 0.19 | 0.07 | 0.05 | 0.13 | 0.26 | 0.14 | 0.08 | 0.04 | 0.08 | 0.13 |
| 38160 | 1 cup | Egg/Spinach, cooked, avg | 160 | 0.28 | 0.34 | 0.43 | 0.21 | 2.46 | 0.26 | 0.17 | 0.35 | 0.58 | 0.24 | 0.15 | 0.40 | 0.76 | 0.41 | 0.25 | 0.11 | 0.24 | 0.39 |
| 38302 | 1/2 cup | Egg/Spinach, dry, avg | 19 | 0.10 | 0.12 | 0.15 | 0.07 | 0.85 | 0.09 | 0.06 | 0.12 | 0.20 | 0.08 | 0.05 | 0.14 | 0.26 | 0.14 | 0.09 | 0.04 | 0.08 | 0.13 |
| | | Macaroni | | | | | | | | | | | | | | | | | | | |
| 38102 | 1 cup | Enriched, cooked, avg | 140 | 0.20 | 0.25 | 0.27 | 0.19 | 2.40 | 0.21 | 0.14 | 0.26 | 0.46 | 0.13 | 0.10 | 0.32 | 0.73 | 0.31 | 0.18 | 0.09 | 0.17 | 0.28 |
| 38182 | 1 cup | Enriched, protein fortified, cooked, avg | 115 | 0.30 | 0.36 | 0.42 | 0.25 | 3.20 | 0.31 | 0.19 | 0.37 | 0.64 | 0.22 | 0.15 | 0.45 | 0.98 | 0.44 | 0.26 | 0.12 | 0.25 | 0.41 |
| 38258 | 1 cup | Unenriched, cooked, avg | 140 | 0.20 | 0.25 | 0.27 | 0.19 | 2.40 | 0.21 | 0.14 | 0.26 | 0.46 | 0.13 | 0.10 | 0.32 | 0.73 | 0.31 | 0.18 | 0.09 | 0.17 | 0.28 |
| 38272 | 1/2 cup | Unenriched, dry, avg | 52 | 0.19 | 0.24 | 0.27 | 0.19 | 2.39 | 0.21 | 0.13 | 0.26 | 0.45 | 0.13 | 0.10 | 0.32 | 0.73 | 0.31 | 0.18 | 0.09 | 0.17 | 0.28 |
| 38117 | 1 cup | Vegetable, enriched, cooked, avg | 134 | 0.18 | 0.23 | 0.26 | 0.17 | 2.14 | 0.19 | 0.12 | 0.23 | 0.41 | 0.12 | 0.09 | 0.29 | 0.65 | 0.29 | 0.16 | 0.08 | 0.16 | 0.26 |
| 38110 | 1 cup | Whole wheat, cooked, avg | 140 | 0.23 | 0.26 | 0.34 | 0.16 | 2.59 | 0.27 | 0.17 | 0.29 | 0.51 | 0.17 | 0.12 | 0.37 | 0.80 | 0.36 | 0.20 | 0.10 | 0.19 | 0.32 |
| 38295 | 1/2 cup | Whole wheat, dry, avg | 28 | 0.13 | 0.14 | 0.18 | 0.09 | 1.42 | 0.15 | 0.10 | 0.16 | 0.28 | 0.09 | 0.07 | 0.20 | 0.44 | 0.20 | 0.11 | 0.05 | 0.11 | 0.18 |
| 38209 | 1/2 cup | Rice Noodles, dried, avg | 70 | 0.23 | 0.26 | 0.33 | 0.06 | 0.68 | 0.11 | 0.07 | 0.15 | 0.30 | 0.11 | 0.13 | 0.17 | 0.18 | 0.15 | 0.10 | 0.12 | 0.08 | 0.20 |
| 38094 | 1 cup | Soba, Japanese, cooked, avg | 114 | 0.28 | 0.36 | 0.42 | 0.11 | 1.25 | 0.38 | 0.14 | 0.22 | 0.38 | 0.24 | 0.08 | 0.25 | 0.35 | 0.30 | 0.20 | 0.08 | 0.12 | 0.28 |
| 38246 | 2 oz | Soba, Japanese, dry, avg | 57 | 0.40 | 0.51 | 0.60 | 0.15 | 1.77 | 0.54 | 0.19 | 0.32 | 0.53 | 0.35 | 0.12 | 0.35 | 0.49 | 0.42 | 0.29 | 0.12 | 0.17 | 0.40 |
| 38095 | 1 cup | Somen, Japanese, cooked, avg | 176 | 0.21 | 0.26 | 0.29 | 0.20 | 2.53 | 0.22 | 0.14 | 0.27 | 0.48 | 0.14 | 0.11 | 0.34 | 0.77 | 0.33 | 0.19 | 0.09 | 0.18 | 0.30 |
| 38247 | 2 oz | Somen, Japanese, dry, avg | 57 | 0.19 | 0.24 | 0.26 | 0.18 | 2.33 | 0.20 | 0.13 | 0.25 | 0.44 | 0.12 | 0.10 | 0.31 | 0.71 | 0.30 | 0.17 | 0.08 | 0.17 | 0.28 |
| | | Spaghetti noodles | | | | | | | | | | | | | | | | | | | |
| 38121 | 1 cup | Enriched, cooked, avg | 140 | 0.20 | 0.25 | 0.27 | 0.19 | 2.40 | 0.21 | 0.14 | 0.26 | 0.46 | 0.13 | 0.10 | 0.32 | 0.73 | 0.31 | 0.18 | 0.09 | 0.17 | 0.28 |
| 38403 | 1 cup | Enriched, protein fortified, cooked, avg | 140 | 0.36 | 0.44 | 0.51 | 0.31 | 3.88 | 0.38 | 0.24 | 0.45 | 0.78 | 0.27 | 0.18 | 0.55 | 1.18 | 0.53 | 0.32 | 0.14 | 0.31 | 0.49 |
| 38066 | 1 cup | Spinach, cooked, avg | 140 | 0.19 | 0.24 | 0.28 | 0.18 | 2.27 | 0.20 | 0.13 | 0.25 | 0.44 | 0.13 | 0.10 | 0.31 | 0.68 | 0.31 | 0.17 | 0.08 | 0.17 | 0.27 |
| 38062 | 2 oz | Spinach, dry, avg | 57 | 0.23 | 0.28 | 0.33 | 0.21 | 2.70 | 0.24 | 0.15 | 0.29 | 0.52 | 0.16 | 0.12 | 0.37 | 0.81 | 0.36 | 0.21 | 0.10 | 0.20 | 0.33 |
| 38274 | 1 cup | Unenriched, cooked w/salt, avg | 140 | 0.20 | 0.25 | 0.27 | 0.19 | 2.40 | 0.21 | 0.14 | 0.26 | 0.46 | 0.13 | 0.10 | 0.32 | 0.73 | 0.31 | 0.18 | 0.09 | 0.17 | 0.28 |
| 38261 | 2 oz | Unenriched, dry, avg | 57 | 0.21 | 0.27 | 0.30 | 0.21 | 2.62 | 0.23 | 0.15 | 0.28 | 0.50 | 0.14 | 0.11 | 0.35 | 0.80 | 0.34 | 0.19 | 0.09 | 0.19 | 0.31 |
| 38060 | 1 cup | Whole wheat, cooked, avg | 140 | 0.23 | 0.26 | 0.34 | 0.16 | 2.59 | 0.27 | 0.17 | 0.29 | 0.51 | 0.17 | 0.12 | 0.37 | 0.80 | 0.36 | 0.20 | 0.10 | 0.19 | 0.32 |
| 38248 | 2 oz | Whole wheat, dry, avg | 57 | 0.26 | 0.29 | 0.38 | 0.17 | 2.89 | 0.30 | 0.20 | 0.32 | 0.57 | 0.18 | 0.13 | 0.41 | 0.89 | 0.41 | 0.22 | 0.11 | 0.22 | 0.36 |
| | | **GRAIN PRODUCTS—RICE** | | | | | | | | | | | | | | | | | | | |
| 38082 | 1/2 cup | Brown, medium grain, cooked, avg | 98 | 0.13 | 0.17 | 0.21 | 0.03 | 0.46 | 0.11 | 0.06 | 0.10 | 0.19 | 0.09 | 0.05 | 0.12 | 0.11 | 0.12 | 0.08 | 0.03 | 0.09 | 0.13 |
| 38081 | 1/4 cup | Brown, medium grain, dry, avg | 48 | 0.21 | 0.27 | 0.34 | 0.04 | 0.73 | 0.18 | 0.09 | 0.15 | 0.30 | 0.14 | 0.08 | 0.19 | 0.17 | 0.19 | 0.13 | 0.05 | 0.13 | 0.21 |
| | | White Rice | | | | | | | | | | | | | | | | | | | |
| 38157 | 1/2 cup | Enriched, cooked, avg | 93 | 0.13 | 0.18 | 0.21 | 0.04 | 0.43 | 0.10 | 0.05 | 0.09 | 0.18 | 0.08 | 0.05 | 0.12 | 0.10 | 0.12 | 0.08 | 0.03 | 0.07 | 0.13 |
| 38083 | 1/2 cup | Glutinous, cooked, avg | 87 | 0.10 | 0.15 | 0.17 | 0.04 | 0.34 | 0.08 | 0.04 | 0.08 | 0.15 | 0.06 | 0.04 | 0.09 | 0.08 | 0.09 | 0.06 | 0.02 | 0.06 | 0.11 |
| 38285 | 1/4 cup | Glutinous, dry, avg | 46 | 0.18 | 0.26 | 0.29 | 0.06 | 0.61 | 0.14 | 0.07 | 0.14 | 0.26 | 0.11 | 0.07 | 0.17 | 0.15 | 0.16 | 0.11 | 0.04 | 0.10 | 0.19 |
| 38016 | 1/2 cup | Long grain, enriched, cooked, avg | 88 | 0.12 | 0.17 | 0.19 | 0.04 | 0.39 | 0.09 | 0.05 | 0.09 | 0.17 | 0.07 | 0.05 | 0.11 | 0.09 | 0.11 | 0.07 | 0.02 | 0.07 | 0.12 |
| 38019 | 1/2 cup | Long grain, instant, cooked, avg | 82 | 0.10 | 0.14 | 0.16 | 0.03 | 0.33 | 0.08 | 0.04 | 0.07 | 0.14 | 0.06 | 0.04 | 0.09 | 0.08 | 0.09 | 0.06 | 0.02 | 0.06 | 0.10 |
| 38289 | 1/4 cup | Wild, dry, avg | 40 | 0.33 | 0.46 | 0.57 | 0.07 | 1.03 | 0.27 | 0.15 | 0.25 | 0.41 | 0.25 | 0.18 | 0.29 | 0.21 | 0.31 | 0.19 | 0.07 | 0.25 | 0.34 |
| 38021 | 1/2 cup | Wild, cooked, avg | 82 | 0.18 | 0.25 | 0.31 | 0.04 | 0.57 | 0.15 | 0.09 | 0.14 | 0.23 | 0.14 | 0.10 | 0.16 | 0.11 | 0.17 | 0.10 | 0.04 | 0.14 | 0.19 |
| | | **GRAIN PRODUCTS—STUFFING & MIXES** | | | | | | | | | | | | | | | | | | | |
| | | Bread Stuffing | | | | | | | | | | | | | | | | | | | |
| 42145 | 1 ea | Plain, dry mix, avg, 6 oz pkg | 170 | 0.66 | 0.80 | 0.94 | 0.38 | 5.91 | 0.69 | 0.43 | 0.68 | 1.31 | 0.54 | 0.33 | 0.94 | 2.02 | 0.93 | 0.56 | 0.24 | 0.58 | 0.79 |
| 42037 | 1/2 cup | Plain, prep f/dry mix, avg | 100 | 0.11 | 0.14 | 0.16 | 0.06 | 1.00 | 0.12 | 0.07 | 0.12 | 0.23 | 0.10 | 0.06 | 0.16 | 0.34 | 0.16 | 0.10 | 0.04 | 0.10 | 0.14 |
| 42038 | 1/2 cup | Plain, prep f/recipe, avg | 116 | 0.15 | 0.17 | 0.24 | 0.09 | 1.33 | 0.15 | 0.09 | 0.17 | 0.30 | 0.12 | 0.07 | 0.21 | 0.44 | 0.20 | 0.13 | 0.05 | 0.12 | 0.19 |
| 42146 | 1 ea | Cornbread Stuffing, dry mix, avg, 6 oz pkg | 170 | 0.82 | 0.75 | 0.93 | 0.33 | 4.66 | 0.65 | 0.43 | 0.62 | 1.48 | 0.47 | 0.32 | 0.85 | 1.73 | 0.83 | 0.54 | 0.18 | 0.58 | 0.76 |
| 42147 | 1/2 cup | Cornbread Stuffing, prepared f/dry mix, avg | 100 | 0.14 | 0.13 | 0.16 | 0.06 | 0.79 | 0.11 | 0.07 | 0.11 | 0.26 | 0.08 | 0.05 | 0.14 | 0.30 | 0.14 | 0.09 | 0.03 | 0.10 | 0.13 |
| | | **GRAIN PRODUCTS—TORTILLAS** | | | | | | | | | | | | | | | | | | | |
| | | Corn Tortilla | | | | | | | | | | | | | | | | | | | |
| 42023 | 1 ea | 6″, avg | 26 | 0.11 | 0.07 | 0.10 | 0.03 | 0.28 | 0.06 | 0.05 | 0.05 | 0.18 | 0.04 | 0.03 | 0.07 | 0.13 | 0.07 | 0.06 | 0.01 | 0.06 | 0.08 |
| 42297 | 1 ea | 6″, unsalted, avg | 26 | 0.11 | 0.07 | 0.10 | 0.03 | 0.28 | 0.06 | 0.05 | 0.05 | 0.18 | 0.04 | 0.03 | 0.07 | 0.13 | 0.07 | 0.06 | 0.01 | 0.06 | 0.08 |
| 42168 | 1 ea | Taco shell, baked, 5″, avg | 13 | 0.07 | 0.05 | 0.07 | 0.02 | 0.18 | 0.04 | 0.03 | 0.03 | 0.12 | 0.03 | 0.02 | 0.05 | 0.08 | 0.04 | 0.04 | 0.01 | 0.04 | 0.05 |
| 42296 | 1 ea | Taco shell, baked, unsalted, 5″, avg | 13 | 0.07 | 0.05 | 0.07 | 0.02 | 0.18 | 0.04 | 0.03 | 0.03 | 0.12 | 0.03 | 0.02 | 0.05 | 0.08 | 0.04 | 0.04 | 0.01 | 0.04 | 0.05 |

TABLE A **Amino Acid Content for Selected Foods *(continued)***

| Code | Amount | Description | Weight (g) | Alanine (g) | Arginine (g) | Aspartic acid (g) | Cystine (g) | Glutamic acid (g) | Glycine (g) | Histidine (g) | Isoleucine (g) | Leucine (g) | Lysine (g) | Methionine (g) | Phenylalanine (g) | Proline (g) | Serine (g) | Threonine (g) | Tryptophan (g) | Tyrosine (g) | Valine (g) |
|---|---|---|---|---|---|---|---|---|---|---|---|---|---|---|---|---|---|---|---|---|---|
| | | **GRAIN PRODUCTS—WAFFLES** | | | | | | | | | | | | | | | | | | | |
| 45030 | 1 ea | Buttermilk, prepared f/recipe, 7", avg | 75 | 0.23 | 0.27 | 0.40 | 0.11 | 1.53 | 0.19 | 0.15 | 0.29 | 0.50 | 0.31 | 0.14 | 0.31 | 0.57 | 0.35 | 0.23 | 0.08 | 0.23 | 0.33 |
| | | Plain Waffles | | | | | | | | | | | | | | | | | | | |
| 45029 | 1 ea | Frozen, ready to heat, 4", avg | 35 | 0.07 | 0.09 | 0.11 | 0.04 | 0.62 | 0.07 | 0.05 | 0.08 | 0.15 | 0.06 | 0.04 | 0.10 | 0.21 | 0.11 | 0.06 | 0.03 | 0.07 | 0.09 |
| 45004 | 1 ea | Prepared f/complete dry mix, 7", avg | 75 | 0.21 | 0.21 | 0.31 | 0.09 | 1.06 | 0.15 | 0.11 | 0.20 | 0.39 | 0.21 | 0.10 | 0.23 | 0.40 | 0.26 | 0.18 | 0.05 | 0.17 | 0.24 |
| 45003 | 1 ea | Prepared f/recipe, 7", avg | 75 | 0.22 | 0.26 | 0.38 | 0.11 | 1.49 | 0.13 | 0.14 | 0.27 | 0.47 | 0.29 | 0.13 | 0.29 | 0.54 | 0.33 | 0.22 | 0.07 | 0.22 | 0.31 |
| | | **GRANOLA BARS** | | | | | | | | | | | | | | | | | | | |
| 23100 | 1 ea | Almond, hard, avg | 24 | 0.09 | 0.14 | 0.17 | 0.06 | 0.40 | 0.10 | 0.04 | 0.07 | 0.14 | 0.07 | 0.03 | 0.09 | 0.10 | 0.09 | 0.05 | 0.03 | 0.07 | 0.10 |
| 23106 | 1 ea | Chocolate Chip, Graham & Marshmallow, soft, avg | 28 | 0.09 | 0.13 | 0.15 | 0.04 | 0.37 | 0.08 | 0.04 | 0.07 | 0.13 | 0.07 | 0.03 | 0.09 | 0.09 | 0.08 | 0.06 | 0.02 | 0.06 | 0.09 |
| 23101 | 1 ea | Chocolate Chip, hard, avg | 24 | 0.09 | 0.12 | 0.16 | 0.05 | 0.36 | 0.09 | 0.04 | 0.07 | 0.13 | 0.07 | 0.03 | 0.09 | 0.09 | 0.09 | 0.05 | 0.03 | 0.07 | 0.10 |
| 23096 | 1 ea | Chocolate Chip, w/choc coating, soft, avg | 35 | 0.08 | 0.08 | 0.17 | 0.02 | 0.39 | 0.05 | 0.04 | 0.09 | 0.17 | 0.10 | 0.04 | 0.10 | 0.14 | 0.09 | 0.08 | 0.02 | 0.09 | 0.12 |
| 23105 | 1 ea | Chocolate, soft, avg | 42 | 0.14 | 0.20 | 0.25 | 0.06 | 0.59 | 0.14 | 0.07 | 0.11 | 0.21 | 0.12 | 0.05 | 0.15 | 0.15 | 0.13 | 0.10 | 0.04 | 0.10 | 0.16 |
| 23107 | 1 ea | Nut & Raisin, uncoated, soft, avg | 28 | 0.10 | 0.18 | 0.20 | 0.05 | 0.46 | 0.11 | 0.05 | 0.08 | 0.15 | 0.08 | 0.04 | 0.11 | 0.11 | 0.10 | 0.07 | 0.03 | 0.07 | 0.11 |
| 23102 | 1 ea | Peanut, hard, avg | 24 | 0.12 | 0.23 | 0.26 | 0.07 | 0.55 | 0.15 | 0.06 | 0.10 | 0.19 | 0.11 | 0.04 | 0.14 | 0.14 | 0.13 | 0.08 | 0.04 | 0.10 | 0.13 |
| 23109 | 1 ea | Peanut Butter w/Chocolate, uncoated, soft, avg | 28 | 0.11 | 0.29 | 0.31 | 0.04 | 0.55 | 0.15 | 0.07 | 0.10 | 0.18 | 0.10 | 0.04 | 0.14 | 0.12 | 0.13 | 0.09 | 0.03 | 0.11 | 0.12 |
| 23103 | 1 ea | Peanut Butter, Hard, avg | 24 | 0.10 | 0.23 | 0.25 | 0.05 | 0.49 | 0.13 | 0.06 | 0.08 | 0.16 | 0.09 | 0.03 | 0.12 | 0.12 | 0.12 | 0.07 | 0.03 | 0.09 | 0.11 |
| 23108 | 1 ea | Peanut Butter, soft, uncoated, avg | 24 | 0.11 | 0.27 | 0.28 | 0.04 | 0.51 | 0.14 | 0.06 | 0.09 | 0.17 | 0.09 | 0.04 | 0.13 | 0.11 | 0.12 | 0.08 | 0.03 | 0.10 | 0.11 |
| 23095 | 1 ea | Peanut Butter, soft, w/choc coating, avg | 37 | 0.14 | 0.26 | 0.36 | 0.04 | 0.76 | 0.15 | 0.08 | 0.17 | 0.30 | 0.19 | 0.05 | 0.19 | 0.25 | 0.18 | 0.14 | 0.05 | 0.16 | 0.21 |
| 23059 | 1 ea | Plain, hard, avg | 24 | 0.11 | 0.16 | 0.20 | 0.07 | 0.48 | 0.12 | 0.05 | 0.08 | 0.17 | 0.10 | 0.04 | 0.11 | 0.12 | 0.11 | 0.06 | 0.04 | 0.08 | 0.12 |
| 23104 | 1 ea | Plain, uncoated, soft, avg | 28 | 0.10 | 0.14 | 0.18 | 0.05 | 0.42 | 0.10 | 0.05 | 0.08 | 0.15 | 0.08 | 0.04 | 0.11 | 0.17 | 0.09 | 0.07 | 0.03 | 0.07 | 0.11 |
| 23097 | 1 ea | Raisin, soft, avg | 42 | 0.16 | 0.25 | 0.27 | 0.07 | 0.69 | 0.16 | 0.08 | 0.13 | 0.24 | 0.13 | 0.05 | 0.17 | 0.17 | 0.14 | 0.11 | 0.05 | 0.11 | 0.17 |
| | | **INFANT CEREAL** | | | | | | | | | | | | | | | | | | | |
| 60483 | 1 Tbs | Barley Cereal, dry, avg | 2 | 0.01 | 0.01 | 0.01 | 0.01 | 0.06 | 0.01 | 0.00 | 0.01 | 0.02 | 0.01 | 0.00 | 0.01 | 0.03 | 0.01 | 0.01 | 0.00 | 0.01 | 0.01 |
| 60868 | 1 Tbs | Barley Cereal, prepared, avg | 15 | 0.02 | 0.03 | 0.05 | 0.01 | 0.16 | 0.02 | 0.02 | 0.03 | 0.06 | 0.04 | 0.01 | 0.03 | 0.07 | 0.03 | 0.03 | 0.01 | 0.03 | 0.04 |
| 60532 | 1 Tbs | Grits Cereal, w/egg yolk, strained, avg | 14 | 0.01 | 0.01 | 0.02 | 0.00 | 0.05 | 0.01 | 0.01 | 0.01 | 0.03 | 0.02 | 0.01 | 0.01 | 0.02 | 0.01 | 0.01 | 0.00 | 0.01 | 0.01 |
| | | Mixed Cereal | | | | | | | | | | | | | | | | | | | |
| 60571 | 1 Tbs | Applesauce Banana, junior, RTE, avg | 15 | 0.01 | 0.01 | 0.01 | 0.00 | 0.05 | 0.01 | 0.00 | 0.01 | 0.01 | 0.01 | 0.00 | 0.01 | 0.01 | 0.01 | 0.01 | 0.00 | 0.01 | 0.01 |
| 60572 | 1 Tbs | Applesauce Banana, strained, RTE, avg | 15 | 0.01 | 0.01 | 0.01 | 0.00 | 0.05 | 0.01 | 0.00 | 0.01 | 0.01 | 0.01 | 0.00 | 0.01 | 0.01 | 0.01 | 0.01 | 0.00 | 0.01 | 0.01 |
| 60564 | 1 Tbs | Banana, dry, 2nd Foods, Gerber | 2 | 0.01 | 0.01 | 0.02 | 0.00 | 0.05 | 0.01 | 0.01 | 0.01 | 0.02 | 0.01 | 0.00 | 0.01 | 0.02 | 0.01 | 0.01 | 0.00 | 0.01 | 0.01 |
| 60565 | 1 Tbs | Banana, prep w/whole milk, avg | 15 | 0.02 | 0.03 | 0.05 | 0.01 | 0.14 | 0.02 | 0.02 | 0.03 | 0.06 | 0.04 | 0.02 | 0.03 | 0.06 | 0.03 | 0.03 | 0.01 | 0.03 | 0.04 |
| 60566 | 1 Tbs | Plain, dry, avg | 2 | 0.01 | 0.01 | 0.01 | 0.01 | 0.06 | 0.01 | 0.01 | 0.01 | 0.02 | 0.01 | 0.00 | 0.01 | 0.02 | 0.01 | 0.01 | 0.00 | 0.01 | 0.01 |
| 60563 | 1 Tbs | Plain, prep w/water, Earths Best | 15 | 0.03 | 0.03 | 0.05 | 0.01 | 0.16 | 0.02 | 0.02 | 0.04 | 0.06 | 0.04 | 0.02 | 0.04 | 0.06 | 0.04 | 0.03 | 0.01 | 0.03 | 0.04 |
| 60539 | 1 Tbs | Plain, prep w/whole milk, avg | 2 | 0.03 | 0.05 | 0.08 | 0.01 | 0.14 | 0.03 | 0.02 | 0.03 | 0.05 | 0.04 | 0.01 | 0.04 | 0.04 | 0.04 | 0.03 | 0.01 | 0.03 | 0.03 |
| 60540 | 1 Tbs | Plain, prep w/whole milk, high protein, avg | 15 | 0.05 | 0.08 | 0.13 | 0.02 | 0.25 | 0.05 | 0.03 | 0.06 | 0.11 | 0.09 | 0.02 | 0.06 | 0.09 | 0.07 | 0.05 | 0.02 | 0.05 | 0.07 |
| 60505 | 1 Tbs | With egg yolk, junior, avg | 16 | 0.01 | 0.02 | 0.02 | 0.00 | 0.06 | 0.01 | 0.01 | 0.02 | 0.03 | 0.02 | 0.01 | 0.01 | 0.02 | 0.02 | 0.01 | 0.00 | 0.01 | 0.02 |
| 60504 | 1 Tbs | With egg yolk, strained, avg | 16 | 0.01 | 0.02 | 0.02 | 0.00 | 0.06 | 0.01 | 0.01 | 0.02 | 0.03 | 0.02 | 0.01 | 0.01 | 0.02 | 0.02 | 0.01 | 0.00 | 0.01 | 0.02 |
| | | Oatmeal Cereal | | | | | | | | | | | | | | | | | | | |
| 60575 | 1 Tbs | Applesauce Banana, junior, avg | 15 | 0.01 | 0.01 | 0.02 | 0.00 | 0.04 | 0.01 | 0.01 | 0.01 | 0.01 | 0.01 | 0.00 | 0.01 | 0.01 | 0.01 | 0.01 | 0.00 | 0.01 | 0.01 |
| 60576 | 1 Tbs | Applesauce Banana, strained, avg | 15 | 0.01 | 0.01 | 0.02 | 0.00 | 0.04 | 0.01 | 0.01 | 0.01 | 0.01 | 0.01 | 0.00 | 0.01 | 0.01 | 0.01 | 0.01 | 0.00 | 0.01 | 0.01 |
| 60579 | 1 Tbs | Banana, dry, avg | 2 | 0.01 | 0.01 | 0.02 | 0.01 | 0.05 | 0.01 | 0.01 | 0.01 | 0.02 | 0.01 | 0.01 | 0.01 | 0.02 | 0.01 | 0.01 | 0.00 | 0.01 | 0.01 |
| 60580 | 1 Tbs | Banana, prep w/whole milk, avg | 15 | 0.03 | 0.03 | 0.05 | 0.01 | 0.15 | 0.02 | 0.02 | 0.04 | 0.06 | 0.04 | 0.02 | 0.03 | 0.06 | 0.04 | 0.03 | 0.01 | 0.03 | 0.04 |
| 60577 | 1 Tbs | Plain, dry, avg | 2 | 0.01 | 0.02 | 0.02 | 0.01 | 0.06 | 0.01 | 0.00 | 0.01 | 0.02 | 0.01 | 0.01 | 0.01 | 0.01 | 0.01 | 0.01 | 0.00 | 0.01 | 0.02 |
| 60578 | 1 Tbs | Plain, prep f/dry, w/milk, avg | 15 | 0.03 | 0.04 | 0.06 | 0.02 | 0.16 | 0.03 | 0.02 | 0.04 | 0.06 | 0.05 | 0.02 | 0.03 | 0.06 | 0.04 | 0.03 | 0.01 | 0.03 | 0.05 |
| | | Rice Cereal | | | | | | | | | | | | | | | | | | | |
| 60617 | 1 Tbs | Applesauce Banana, strained, RTE, avg | 16 | 0.01 | 0.01 | 0.01 | 0.00 | 0.04 | 0.00 | 0.01 | 0.01 | 0.02 | 0.01 | 0.00 | 0.01 | 0.02 | 0.01 | 0.01 | 0.00 | 0.01 | 0.01 |

## TABLE A **Amino Acid Content for Selected Foods *(continued)***

| Code | Amount | Description | Weight (g) | Alanine (g) | Arginine (g) | Aspartic acid (g) | Cystine (g) | Glutamic acid (g) | Glycine (g) | Histidine (g) | Isoleucine (g) | Leucine (g) | Lysine (g) | Methionine (g) | Phenylalanine (g) | Proline (g) | Serine (g) | Threonine (g) | Tryptophan (g) | Tyrosine (g) | Valine (g) |
|---|---|---|---|---|---|---|---|---|---|---|---|---|---|---|---|---|---|---|---|---|---|
| 60618 | 1 Tbs | Banana, dry, avg | 2 | 0.01 | 0.01 | 0.02 | 0.00 | 0.03 | 0.01 | 0.01 | 0.01 | 0.02 | 0.01 | 0.00 | 0.01 | 0.01 | 0.01 | 0.01 | 0.00 | 0.01 | 0.01 |
| 60615 | 1 Tbs | Banana, prep w/whole milk, avg | 15 | 0.03 | 0.03 | 0.05 | 0.01 | 0.12 | 0.02 | 0.02 | 0.03 | 0.06 | 0.04 | 0.02 | 0.03 | 0.05 | 0.03 | 0.03 | 0.01 | 0.03 | 0.04 |
| 60619 | 1 Tbs | Plain, dry, avg | 2 | 0.01 | 0.01 | 0.01 | 0.00 | 0.02 | 0.01 | 0.00 | 0.01 | 0.01 | 0.01 | 0.00 | 0.01 | 0.01 | 0.01 | 0.01 | 0.00 | 0.01 | 0.01 |
| 60622 | 1 Tbs | Plain, prep w/whole milk, avg | 15 | 0.02 | 0.03 | 0.05 | 0.01 | 0.11 | 0.02 | 0.02 | 0.03 | 0.05 | 0.04 | 0.01 | 0.03 | 0.05 | 0.03 | 0.03 | 0.01 | 0.03 | 0.04 |
| | | **INFANT DESSERTS** | | | | | | | | | | | | | | | | | | | |
| 60525 | 1 Tbs | Cottage Cheese w/pineapple, strained, avg | 14 | 0.01 | 0.01 | 0.02 | 0.00 | 0.06 | 0.01 | 0.01 | 0.01 | 0.03 | 0.02 | 0.00 | 0.01 | 0.03 | 0.01 | 0.01 | 0.00 | 0.01 | 0.02 |
| 60524 | 1 Tbs | Cottage Cheese w/pineapple, junior, avg | 14 | 0.01 | 0.01 | 0.02 | 0.00 | 0.06 | 0.01 | 0.01 | 0.01 | 0.03 | 0.02 | 0.00 | 0.01 | 0.03 | 0.01 | 0.01 | 0.00 | 0.01 | 0.02 |
| | | Puddings | | | | | | | | | | | | | | | | | | | |
| 60518 | 1 Tbs | Chocolate Custard, junior, avg | 14 | 0.01 | 0.01 | 0.02 | 0.00 | 0.05 | 0.01 | 0.01 | 0.01 | 0.03 | 0.02 | 0.01 | 0.01 | 0.02 | 0.01 | 0.01 | 0.00 | 0.01 | 0.02 |
| 60517 | 1 Tbs | Chocolate Custard, strained, avg | 14 | 0.01 | 0.01 | 0.02 | 0.00 | 0.05 | 0.01 | 0.01 | 0.01 | 0.03 | 0.02 | 0.01 | 0.01 | 0.02 | 0.01 | 0.01 | 0.00 | 0.01 | 0.02 |
| 60586 | 1 Tbs | Orange, strained, avg | 16 | 0.01 | 0.01 | 0.02 | 0.00 | 0.03 | 0.00 | 0.00 | 0.01 | 0.02 | 0.01 | 0.00 | 0.01 | 0.02 | 0.01 | 0.01 | 0.00 | 0.01 | 0.01 |
| 60640 | 1 Tbs | Vanilla Custard, junior, avg | 14 | 0.01 | 0.01 | 0.02 | 0.00 | 0.04 | 0.00 | 0.01 | 0.01 | 0.01 | 0.02 | 0.01 | 0.01 | 0.01 | 0.01 | 0.01 | 0.00 | 0.01 | 0.01 |
| 60641 | 1 Tbs | Vanilla Custard, strained, avg | 14 | 0.01 | 0.01 | 0.02 | 0.00 | 0.04 | 0.00 | 0.01 | 0.01 | 0.01 | 0.02 | 0.01 | 0.01 | 0.01 | 0.01 | 0.01 | 0.00 | 0.01 | 0.01 |
| | | **INFANT DINNERS** | | | | | | | | | | | | | | | | | | | |
| 60489 | 1 Tbs | Beef & Noodles, junior, avg | 16 | 0.02 | 0.02 | 0.03 | 0.00 | 0.08 | 0.02 | 0.01 | 0.02 | 0.03 | 0.03 | 0.01 | 0.02 | 0.03 | 0.01 | 0.02 | 0.00 | 0.01 | 0.02 |
| 60492 | 1 Tbs | Beef & Noodles, strained, avg | 16 | 0.02 | 0.02 | 0.03 | 0.00 | 0.07 | 0.02 | 0.01 | 0.02 | 0.03 | 0.03 | 0.01 | 0.02 | 0.03 | 0.01 | 0.01 | 0.00 | 0.01 | 0.02 |
| 60493 | 1 Tbs | Beef & Rice, toddler, avg | 16 | 0.05 | 0.05 | 0.07 | 0.01 | 0.14 | 0.06 | 0.02 | 0.04 | 0.06 | 0.06 | 0.02 | 0.03 | 0.05 | 0.03 | 0.03 | 0.01 | 0.03 | 0.04 |
| | | Beef & Vegetables | | | | | | | | | | | | | | | | | | | |
| 60541 | 1 Tbs | High meat, junior, avg | 14 | 0.06 | 0.05 | 0.08 | 0.01 | 0.13 | 0.07 | 0.03 | 0.04 | 0.07 | 0.06 | 0.02 | 0.03 | 0.05 | 0.03 | 0.03 | 0.01 | 0.03 | 0.04 |
| 60542 | 1 Tbs | High meat, strained, avg | 14 | 0.05 | 0.05 | 0.07 | 0.01 | 0.12 | 0.07 | 0.02 | 0.03 | 0.06 | 0.06 | 0.02 | 0.03 | 0.05 | 0.03 | 0.03 | 0.01 | 0.02 | 0.04 |
| 60660 | 1 Tbs | Junior, avg | 16 | 0.03 | 0.02 | 0.04 | 0.00 | 0.07 | 0.03 | 0.01 | 0.02 | 0.03 | 0.03 | 0.01 | 0.01 | 0.02 | 0.01 | 0.01 | 0.00 | 0.01 | 0.02 |
| 60651 | 1 Tbs | Strained, avg | 16 | 0.02 | 0.02 | 0.03 | 0.00 | 0.06 | 0.02 | 0.01 | 0.01 | 0.02 | 0.02 | 0.01 | 0.01 | 0.02 | 0.01 | 0.01 | 0.00 | 0.01 | 0.02 |
| 60491 | 1 Tbs | Beef Stew, toddler, avg | 16 | 0.05 | 0.06 | 0.08 | 0.01 | 0.13 | 0.06 | 0.02 | 0.04 | 0.06 | 0.06 | 0.02 | 0.03 | 0.05 | 0.03 | 0.03 | 0.01 | 0.03 | 0.04 |
| 60511 | 1 Tbs | Chicken & Noodles, junior, avg | 16 | 0.02 | 0.02 | 0.03 | 0.00 | 0.06 | 0.02 | 0.01 | 0.02 | 0.03 | 0.02 | 0.01 | 0.01 | 0.02 | 0.01 | 0.01 | 0.00 | 0.01 | 0.02 |
| 60515 | 1 Tbs | Chicken & Noodles, strained, avg | 16 | 0.02 | 0.02 | 0.03 | 0.00 | 0.07 | 0.02 | 0.01 | 0.02 | 0.03 | 0.02 | 0.01 | 0.02 | 0.02 | 0.01 | 0.01 | 0.00 | 0.01 | 0.02 |
| | | Chicken & Vegetables | | | | | | | | | | | | | | | | | | | |
| 60537 | 1 Tbs | High meat, junior, avg | 14 | 0.06 | 0.06 | 0.09 | 0.01 | 0.15 | 0.07 | 0.03 | 0.05 | 0.08 | 0.08 | 0.03 | 0.04 | 0.05 | 0.04 | 0.04 | 0.01 | 0.03 | 0.05 |
| 60543 | 1 Tbs | High meat, strained, avg | 14 | 0.05 | 0.06 | 0.08 | 0.01 | 0.14 | 0.06 | 0.03 | 0.04 | 0.07 | 0.07 | 0.02 | 0.03 | 0.05 | 0.03 | 0.04 | 0.01 | 0.03 | 0.04 |
| 60652 | 1 Tbs | Strained, avg | 16 | 0.02 | 0.02 | 0.02 | 0.00 | 0.06 | 0.02 | 0.01 | 0.01 | 0.02 | 0.02 | 0.01 | 0.01 | 0.02 | 0.01 | 0.01 | 0.00 | 0.01 | 0.02 |
| 60523 | 1 Tbs | Chicken Soup, creamed, strained, avg | 14 | 0.02 | 0.02 | 0.03 | 0.00 | 0.06 | 0.02 | 0.01 | 0.02 | 0.03 | 0.03 | 0.01 | 0.01 | 0.02 | 0.01 | 0.01 | 0.00 | 0.01 | 0.02 |
| 60513 | 1 Tbs | Chicken Stew, toddler, avg | 16 | 0.05 | 0.05 | 0.08 | 0.01 | 0.14 | 0.05 | 0.02 | 0.04 | 0.06 | 0.07 | 0.02 | 0.03 | 0.06 | 0.03 | 0.04 | 0.01 | 0.03 | 0.05 |
| | | Ham & Vegetables | | | | | | | | | | | | | | | | | | | |
| 60538 | 1 Tbs | High meat, junior, avg | 14 | 0.05 | 0.05 | 0.08 | 0.01 | 0.13 | 0.05 | 0.03 | 0.04 | 0.07 | 0.07 | 0.02 | 0.03 | 0.05 | 0.03 | 0.03 | 0.01 | 0.02 | 0.04 |
| 60544 | 1 Tbs | High meat, strained, avg | 14 | 0.05 | 0.05 | 0.08 | 0.01 | 0.13 | 0.05 | 0.03 | 0.04 | 0.07 | 0.07 | 0.02 | 0.03 | 0.04 | 0.03 | 0.03 | 0.01 | 0.02 | 0.04 |
| 60661 | 1 Tbs | Junior, avg | 16 | 0.02 | 0.02 | 0.03 | 0.00 | 0.07 | 0.02 | 0.01 | 0.01 | 0.02 | 0.02 | 0.01 | 0.01 | 0.02 | 0.01 | 0.01 | 0.00 | 0.01 | 0.02 |
| 60653 | 1 Tbs | Strained, avg | 16 | 0.02 | 0.02 | 0.03 | 0.00 | 0.06 | 0.01 | 0.01 | 0.01 | 0.02 | 0.02 | 0.01 | 0.01 | 0.01 | 0.01 | 0.01 | 0.00 | 0.01 | 0.01 |
| 60654 | 1 Tbs | Toddler, avg | 14 | 0.03 | 0.04 | 0.07 | 0.01 | 0.10 | 0.03 | 0.02 | 0.03 | 0.05 | 0.04 | 0.01 | 0.03 | 0.03 | 0.02 | 0.02 | 0.01 | 0.02 | 0.03 |
| 60662 | 1 Tbs | Lamb & Vegetables, junior, avg | 16 | 0.02 | 0.02 | 0.03 | 0.00 | 0.07 | 0.02 | 0.01 | 0.02 | 0.02 | 0.02 | 0.00 | 0.01 | 0.02 | 0.01 | 0.01 | 0.00 | 0.01 | 0.02 |
| 60655 | 1 Tbs | Lamb & Vegetables, strained, avg | 15 | 0.02 | 0.02 | 0.03 | 0.00 | 0.06 | 0.02 | 0.01 | 0.01 | 0.02 | 0.02 | 0.00 | 0.01 | 0.02 | 0.01 | 0.01 | 0.00 | 0.01 | 0.01 |
| 60490 | 1 Tbs | Lasagna, beef, toddler, avg | 15 | 0.04 | 0.04 | 0.05 | 0.01 | 0.13 | 0.04 | 0.01 | 0.03 | 0.05 | 0.04 | 0.01 | 0.03 | 0.05 | 0.02 | 0.02 | 0.01 | 0.02 | 0.03 |
| 60663 | 1 Tbs | Liver & Vegetables, junior, avg | 14 | 0.02 | 0.02 | 0.03 | 0.00 | 0.04 | 0.01 | 0.01 | 0.01 | 0.02 | 0.02 | 0.01 | 0.01 | 0.01 | 0.01 | 0.01 | 0.00 | 0.01 | 0.02 |
| 60656 | 1 Tbs | Liver & Vegetables, strained, avg | 14 | 0.02 | 0.02 | 0.03 | 0.00 | 0.05 | 0.02 | 0.01 | 0.01 | 0.03 | 0.02 | 0.01 | 0.01 | 0.02 | 0.01 | 0.01 | 0.00 | 0.01 | 0.02 |
| 60555 | 1 Tbs | Macaroni & Beef, w/tomato, junior, avg | 16 | 0.02 | 0.02 | 0.03 | 0.01 | 0.10 | 0.02 | 0.01 | 0.02 | 0.03 | 0.02 | 0.01 | 0.02 | 0.03 | 0.02 | 0.01 | 0.00 | 0.01 | 0.02 |
| 60556 | 1 Tbs | Macaroni & Beef, w/tomato, strained, avg | 16 | 0.02 | 0.02 | 0.03 | 0.00 | 0.09 | 0.02 | 0.01 | 0.02 | 0.03 | 0.02 | 0.01 | 0.02 | 0.03 | 0.02 | 0.01 | 0.00 | 0.01 | 0.02 |
| 60557 | 1 Tbs | Macaroni & Cheese, junior, avg | 16 | 0.01 | 0.02 | 0.03 | 0.00 | 0.10 | 0.01 | 0.01 | 0.02 | 0.04 | 0.02 | 0.01 | 0.02 | 0.05 | 0.02 | 0.01 | 0.00 | 0.02 | 0.02 |

# TABLE A **Amino Acid Content for Selected Foods *(continued)***

| Code | Amount | | Description | Weight (g) | Alanine (g) | Arginine (g) | Aspartic acid (g) | Cystine (g) | Glutamic acid (g) | Glycine (g) | Histidine (g) | Isoleucine (g) | Leucine (g) | Lysine (g) | Methionine (g) | Phenylalanine (g) | Proline (g) | Serine (g) | Threonine (g) | Tryptophan (g) | Tyrosine (g) | Valine (g) |
|---|---|---|---|---|---|---|---|---|---|---|---|---|---|---|---|---|---|---|---|---|---|---|
| 60559 | 1 | Tbs | Macaroni & Cheese, strained, avg | 16 | 0.01 | 0.02 | 0.03 | 0.01 | 0.11 | 0.01 | 0.01 | 0.02 | 0.04 | 0.02 | 0.01 | 0.02 | 0.05 | 0.02 | 0.01 | 0.01 | 0.02 | 0.02 |
| 60623 | 1 | Tbs | Spaghetti w/meat & tomato sauce, toddler, avg | 16 | 0.04 | 0.04 | 0.07 | 0.01 | 0.20 | 0.04 | 0.02 | 0.04 | 0.06 | 0.05 | 0.02 | 0.04 | 0.07 | 0.03 | 0.03 | 0.01 | 0.03 | 0.04 |
| 60636 | 1 | Tbs | Turkey & Rice, junior, avg | 16 | 0.02 | 0.02 | 0.03 | 0.00 | 0.05 | 0.02 | 0.01 | 0.01 | 0.02 | 0.02 | 0.01 | 0.01 | 0.02 | 0.01 | 0.01 | 0.00 | 0.01 | 0.02 |
| 60637 | 1 | Tbs | Turkey & Rice, strained, avg | 16 | 0.02 | 0.02 | 0.03 | 0.00 | 0.05 | 0.02 | 0.01 | 0.02 | 0.02 | 0.02 | 0.01 | 0.01 | 0.02 | 0.01 | 0.01 | 0.00 | 0.01 | 0.02 |
| | | | Turkey & Vegetables | | | | | | | | | | | | | | | | | | | |
| 60546 | 1 | Tbs | High meat, junior, avg | 14 | 0.05 | 0.05 | 0.08 | 0.01 | 0.13 | 0.05 | 0.03 | 0.04 | 0.07 | 0.07 | 0.02 | 0.03 | 0.05 | 0.03 | 0.04 | 0.01 | 0.03 | 0.04 |
| 60664 | 1 | Tbs | Junior, avg | 16 | 0.02 | 0.02 | 0.03 | 0.00 | 0.04 | 0.02 | 0.01 | 0.01 | 0.02 | 0.02 | 0.01 | 0.01 | 0.01 | 0.01 | 0.01 | 0.00 | 0.01 | 0.02 |
| 60658 | 1 | Tbs | Strained, avg | 16 | 0.02 | 0.02 | 0.03 | 0.00 | 0.04 | 0.02 | 0.01 | 0.01 | 0.02 | 0.02 | 0.01 | 0.01 | 0.01 | 0.01 | 0.01 | 0.00 | 0.01 | 0.02 |
| 60657 | 1 | Tbs | Toddler, avg | 16 | 0.04 | 0.05 | 0.08 | 0.01 | 0.15 | 0.03 | 0.02 | 0.04 | 0.06 | 0.05 | 0.01 | 0.03 | 0.05 | 0.03 | 0.03 | 0.01 | 0.03 | 0.04 |
| 60547 | 1 | Tbs | Veal & Vegetables, high meat, junior, avg | 14 | 0.05 | 0.06 | 0.08 | 0.01 | 0.14 | 0.06 | 0.03 | 0.04 | 0.07 | 0.07 | 0.02 | 0.03 | 0.05 | 0.03 | 0.03 | 0.01 | 0.02 | 0.04 |
| 60548 | 1 | Tbs | Veal & Vegetables, high meat, strained, avg | 14 | 0.05 | 0.06 | 0.08 | 0.01 | 0.14 | 0.06 | 0.03 | 0.04 | 0.07 | 0.07 | 0.02 | 0.03 | 0.05 | 0.03 | 0.03 | 0.01 | 0.02 | 0.04 |
| 60659 | 1 | Tbs | Vegetables & Bacon, junior, avg | 16 | 0.01 | 0.02 | 0.03 | 0.00 | 0.06 | 0.01 | 0.01 | 0.01 | 0.02 | 0.02 | 0.01 | 0.01 | 0.01 | 0.01 | 0.01 | 0.00 | 0.01 | 0.02 |
| 60650 | 1 | Tbs | Vegetables & Bacon, strained, avg | 16 | 0.01 | 0.02 | 0.03 | 0.00 | 0.05 | 0.01 | 0.01 | 0.01 | 0.02 | 0.01 | 0.01 | 0.01 | 0.01 | 0.01 | 0.01 | 0.00 | 0.01 | 0.01 |
| | | | **INFANT MEATS** | | | | | | | | | | | | | | | | | | | |
| | | | Beef | | | | | | | | | | | | | | | | | | | |
| 60494 | 1 | Tbs | Junior, avg | 15 | 0.14 | 0.15 | 0.19 | 0.03 | 0.33 | 0.14 | 0.07 | 0.10 | 0.17 | 0.18 | 0.07 | 0.08 | 0.11 | 0.08 | 0.10 | 0.02 | 0.07 | 0.11 |
| 60495 | 1 | Tbs | Strained, avg | 15 | 0.13 | 0.14 | 0.18 | 0.02 | 0.31 | 0.13 | 0.07 | 0.09 | 0.16 | 0.17 | 0.06 | 0.08 | 0.10 | 0.07 | 0.09 | 0.02 | 0.07 | 0.10 |
| 60496 | 1 | Tbs | With Beef Heart, strained, avg | 14 | 0.12 | 0.12 | 0.16 | 0.02 | 0.28 | 0.12 | 0.05 | 0.09 | 0.14 | 0.15 | 0.05 | 0.07 | 0.09 | 0.06 | 0.07 | 0.02 | 0.05 | 0.10 |
| | | | Chicken | | | | | | | | | | | | | | | | | | | |
| 60516 | 1 | Tbs | Junior, avg | 15 | 0.14 | 0.15 | 0.20 | 0.03 | 0.32 | 0.15 | 0.07 | 0.10 | 0.17 | 0.18 | 0.06 | 0.09 | 0.11 | 0.08 | 0.10 | 0.03 | 0.07 | 0.11 |
| 60514 | 1 | ea | Sticks, junior, avg | 10 | 0.08 | 0.10 | 0.13 | 0.01 | 0.22 | 0.08 | 0.05 | 0.07 | 0.11 | 0.12 | 0.03 | 0.07 | 0.09 | 0.05 | 0.06 | 0.01 | 0.05 | 0.08 |
| 60849 | 1 | Tbs | Strained, avg | 15 | 0.13 | 0.14 | 0.19 | 0.03 | 0.30 | 0.14 | 0.06 | 0.10 | 0.16 | 0.17 | 0.06 | 0.08 | 0.11 | 0.07 | 0.09 | 0.02 | 0.07 | 0.10 |
| 60528 | 1 | Tbs | Egg Yolks, strained, avg | 14 | 0.07 | 0.10 | 0.13 | 0.02 | 0.17 | 0.04 | 0.03 | 0.08 | 0.12 | 0.11 | 0.04 | 0.06 | 0.06 | 0.09 | 0.06 | 0.01 | 0.06 | 0.09 |
| 60535 | 1 | Tbs | Ham, junior, avg | 15 | 0.14 | 0.15 | 0.22 | 0.03 | 0.34 | 0.13 | 0.08 | 0.11 | 0.18 | 0.19 | 0.06 | 0.09 | 0.11 | 0.08 | 0.10 | 0.02 | 0.08 | 0.12 |
| 60536 | 1 | Tbs | Ham, strained, avg | 15 | 0.13 | 0.14 | 0.20 | 0.03 | 0.31 | 0.12 | 0.07 | 0.10 | 0.17 | 0.18 | 0.05 | 0.08 | 0.10 | 0.08 | 0.09 | 0.02 | 0.07 | 0.11 |
| 60552 | 1 | Tbs | Lamb, junior, avg | 15 | 0.14 | 0.15 | 0.21 | 0.03 | 0.35 | 0.13 | 0.06 | 0.11 | 0.18 | 0.20 | 0.07 | 0.09 | 0.13 | 0.09 | 0.10 | 0.02 | 0.08 | 0.12 |
| 60553 | 1 | Tbs | Lamb, strained, avg | 15 | 0.13 | 0.14 | 0.20 | 0.03 | 0.32 | 0.12 | 0.05 | 0.10 | 0.17 | 0.19 | 0.07 | 0.08 | 0.12 | 0.08 | 0.10 | 0.02 | 0.07 | 0.11 |
| 60554 | 1 | Tbs | Liver, strained, avg | 14 | 0.12 | 0.12 | 0.19 | 0.03 | 0.26 | 0.11 | 0.05 | 0.10 | 0.18 | 0.13 | 0.05 | 0.10 | 0.11 | 0.09 | 0.10 | 0.03 | 0.08 | 0.13 |
| 60561 | 1 | ea | Meat Sticks, junior, avg | 10 | 0.08 | 0.09 | 0.11 | 0.01 | 0.20 | 0.07 | 0.05 | 0.07 | 0.10 | 0.10 | 0.03 | 0.06 | 0.08 | 0.05 | 0.06 | 0.01 | 0.05 | 0.07 |
| 60610 | 1 | Tbs | Pork, strained, avg | 15 | 0.13 | 0.14 | 0.20 | 0.02 | 0.32 | 0.11 | 0.07 | 0.10 | 0.17 | 0.17 | 0.06 | 0.09 | 0.11 | 0.08 | 0.09 | 0.02 | 0.08 | 0.11 |
| | | | Turkey | | | | | | | | | | | | | | | | | | | |
| 60639 | 1 | Tbs | Junior, avg | 15 | 0.15 | 0.15 | 0.23 | 0.03 | 0.37 | 0.15 | 0.06 | 0.12 | 0.18 | 0.19 | 0.07 | 0.09 | 0.11 | 0.09 | 0.10 | 0.02 | 0.08 | 0.12 |
| 60638 | 1 | ea | Sticks, junior, avg | 10 | 0.07 | 0.09 | 0.13 | 0.01 | 0.22 | 0.07 | 0.04 | 0.06 | 0.11 | 0.12 | 0.03 | 0.06 | 0.07 | 0.05 | 0.05 | 0.01 | 0.05 | 0.07 |
| 60850 | 1 | Tbs | Strained, avg | 15 | 0.14 | 0.14 | 0.21 | 0.03 | 0.34 | 0.14 | 0.05 | 0.11 | 0.17 | 0.18 | 0.07 | 0.09 | 0.11 | 0.08 | 0.09 | 0.02 | 0.08 | 0.11 |
| 60642 | 1 | Tbs | Veal, junior, avg | 15 | 0.14 | 0.15 | 0.20 | 0.03 | 0.33 | 0.16 | 0.07 | 0.10 | 0.18 | 0.18 | 0.05 | 0.09 | 0.13 | 0.08 | 0.10 | 0.03 | 0.07 | 0.11 |
| 60643 | 1 | Tbs | Veal, strained, avg | 15 | 0.13 | 0.13 | 0.18 | 0.03 | 0.29 | 0.14 | 0.06 | 0.09 | 0.16 | 0.16 | 0.04 | 0.08 | 0.11 | 0.07 | 0.08 | 0.02 | 0.06 | 0.10 |
| | | | **INFANT VEGETABLES** | | | | | | | | | | | | | | | | | | | |
| 60497 | 1 | Tbs | Beets, strained, avg | 14 | 0.01 | 0.00 | 0.01 | 0.00 | 0.04 | 0.00 | 0.00 | 0.01 | 0.01 | 0.00 | 0.00 | 0.00 | 0.00 | 0.01 | 0.00 | 0.00 | 0.00 | 0.01 |
| | | | Carrots | | | | | | | | | | | | | | | | | | | |
| 60501 | 1 | Tbs | Buttered, junior, avg | 14 | 0.01 | 0.01 | 0.02 | 0.00 | 0.03 | 0.00 | 0.00 | 0.00 | 0.00 | 0.00 | 0.00 | 0.00 | 0.00 | 0.00 | 0.00 | 0.00 | 0.00 | 0.00 |
| 60503 | 1 | Tbs | Buttered, strained, avg | 14 | 0.01 | 0.01 | 0.02 | 0.00 | 0.03 | 0.00 | 0.00 | 0.00 | 0.00 | 0.00 | 0.00 | 0.00 | 0.00 | 0.00 | 0.00 | 0.00 | 0.00 | 0.00 |
| 60500 | 1 | Tbs | Junior, avg | 14 | 0.01 | 0.01 | 0.02 | 0.00 | 0.03 | 0.00 | 0.00 | 0.00 | 0.00 | 0.00 | 0.00 | 0.00 | 0.00 | 0.00 | 0.00 | 0.00 | 0.00 | 0.00 |
| 60502 | 1 | Tbs | Strained, avg | 14 | 0.01 | 0.01 | 0.02 | 0.00 | 0.03 | 0.00 | 0.00 | 0.00 | 0.00 | 0.00 | 0.00 | 0.00 | 0.00 | 0.00 | 0.00 | 0.00 | 0.00 | 0.00 |
| 60521 | 1 | Tbs | Corn, creamed, junior, avg | 15 | 0.01 | 0.01 | 0.01 | 0.00 | 0.04 | 0.01 | 0.0 | 0.01 | 0.02 | 0.01 | 0.01 | 0.01 | 0.02 | 0.01 | 0.01 | 0.00 | 0.01 | 0.01 |
| 60522 | 1 | Tbs | Corn, creamed, strained, avg | 15 | 0.01 | 0.01 | 0.01 | 0.00 | 0.04 | 0.01 | 0.0 | 0.01 | 0.02 | 0.01 | 0.01 | 0.01 | 0.02 | 0.01 | 0.01 | 0.00 | 0.01 | 0.01 |
| 60531 | 1 | Tbs | Garden Vegetables, strained, avg | 15 | 0.02 | 0.03 | 0.03 | 0.00 | 0.04 | 0.01 | 0.0 | 0.01 | 0.02 | 0.02 | 0.01 | 0.01 | 0.02 | 0.01 | 0.01 | 0.00 | 0.01 | 0.01 |
| | | | Green Beans | | | | | | | | | | | | | | | | | | | |
| 60485 | 1 | Tbs | Buttered, junior, avg | 14 | 0.01 | 0.01 | 0.04 | 0.00 | 0.02 | 0.01 | 0.0 | 0.01 | 0.01 | 0.01 | 0.00 | 0.01 | 0.01 | 0.01 | 0.01 | 0.00 | 0.01 | 0.01 |
| 60486 | 1 | Tbs | Buttered, strained, avg | 14 | 0.01 | 0.01 | 0.03 | 0.00 | 0.02 | 0.01 | 0.00 | 0.01 | 0.01 | 0.01 | 0.00 | 0.01 | 0.01 | 0.01 | 0.01 | 0.00 | 0.01 | 0.01 |
| 60484 | 1 | Tbs | Creamed, junior, avg | 15 | 0.01 | 0.01 | 0.01 | 0.00 | 0.03 | 0.00 | 0.00 | 0.01 | 0.01 | 0.01 | 0.00 | 0.01 | 0.01 | 0.01 | 0.01 | 0.00 | 0.01 | 0.01 |

## TABLE A Amino Acid Content for Selected Foods *(continued)*

| Code | Amount | Description | Weight (g) | Alanine (g) | Arginine (g) | Aspartic acid (g) | Cystine (g) | Glutamic acid (g) | Glycine (g) | Histidine (g) | Isoleucine (g) | Leucine (g) | Lysine (g) | Methionine (g) | Phenylalanine (g) | Proline (g) | Serine (g) | Threonine (g) | Tryptophan (g) | Tyrosine (g) | Valine (g) |
|---|---|---|---|---|---|---|---|---|---|---|---|---|---|---|---|---|---|---|---|---|---|
| 60487 | 1 Tbs | Junior, avg | 15 | 0.01 | 0.01 | 0.04 | 0.00 | 0.02 | 0.01 | 0.00 | 0.01 | 0.01 | 0.01 | 0.00 | 0.01 | 0.01 | 0.01 | 0.01 | 0.00 | 0.01 | 0.01 |
| 60488 | 1 Tbs | Strained, avg | 15 | 0.01 | 0.01 | 0.04 | 0.00 | 0.03 | 0.01 | 0.01 | 0.01 | 0.01 | 0.01 | 0.00 | 0.01 | 0.01 | 0.01 | 0.01 | 0.00 | 0.01 | 0.01 |
| 60569 | 1 Tbs | Mixed Vegetables, junior, avg | 15 | 0.01 | 0.01 | 0.02 | 0.00 | 0.05 | 0.01 | 0.00 | 0.01 | 0.01 | 0.01 | 0.00 | 0.01 | 0.02 | 0.01 | 0.01 | 0.00 | 0.01 | 0.01 |
| 60568 | 1 Tbs | Mixed Vegetables, strained, avg | 15 | 0.01 | 0.01 | 0.02 | 0.00 | 0.05 | 0.01 | 0.00 | 0.01 | 0.01 | 0.01 | 0.00 | 0.01 | 0.01 | 0.01 | 0.01 | 0.00 | 0.01 | 0.01 |
| | | Peas | | | | | | | | | | | | | | | | | | | |
| 60601 | 1 Tbs | Buttered, junior, avg | 14 | 0.03 | 0.06 | 0.04 | 0.00 | 0.07 | 0.02 | 0.01 | 0.02 | 0.03 | 0.03 | 0.01 | 0.02 | 0.02 | 0.02 | 0.02 | 0.00 | 0.02 | 0.02 |
| 60604 | 1 Tbs | Buttered, strained, avg | 14 | 0.03 | 0.06 | 0.05 | 0.00 | 0.07 | 0.02 | 0.01 | 0.02 | 0.03 | 0.03 | 0.01 | 0.02 | 0.02 | 0.02 | 0.02 | 0.01 | 0.02 | 0.02 |
| 60603 | 1 Tbs | Strained, avg | 15 | 0.03 | 0.06 | 0.05 | 0.00 | 0.08 | 0.02 | 0.01 | 0.02 | 0.04 | 0.04 | 0.01 | 0.02 | 0.02 | 0.02 | 0.02 | 0.01 | 0.02 | 0.03 |
| 60625 | 1 Tbs | Spinach, creamed, strained, avg | 15 | 0.02 | 0.02 | 0.03 | 0.00 | 0.06 | 0.01 | 0.01 | 0.02 | 0.03 | 0.02 | 0.01 | 0.01 | 0.03 | 0.02 | 0.02 | 0.01 | 0.02 | 0.02 |
| | | Squash | | | | | | | | | | | | | | | | | | | |
| 60628 | 1 Tbs | Buttered, junior, avg | 14 | 0.00 | 0.01 | 0.01 | 0.00 | 0.02 | 0.00 | 0.00 | 0.00 | 0.01 | 0.00 | 0.00 | 0.00 | 0.00 | 0.00 | 0.00 | 0.00 | 0.00 | 0.00 |
| 60629 | 1 Tbs | Buttered, strained, avg | 14 | 0.00 | 0.00 | 0.01 | 0.00 | 0.02 | 0.00 | 0.00 | 0.00 | 0.01 | 0.00 | 0.00 | 0.00 | 0.00 | 0.00 | 0.00 | 0.00 | 0.00 | 0.00 |
| 60627 | 1 Tbs | Strained, avg | 14 | 0.00 | 0.01 | 0.01 | 0.00 | 0.02 | 0.00 | 0.00 | 0.00 | 0.01 | 0.00 | 0.00 | 0.00 | 0.00 | 0.00 | 0.00 | 0.00 | 0.00 | 0.01 |
| | | Sweet Potatoes | | | | | | | | | | | | | | | | | | | |
| 60631 | 1 Tbs | Buttered, junior, avg | 14 | 0.01 | 0.01 | 0.02 | 0.00 | 0.01 | 0.01 | 0.00 | 0.01 | 0.01 | 0.00 | 0.00 | 0.01 | 0.01 | 0.01 | 0.01 | 0.00 | 0.00 | 0.01 |
| 60630 | 1 Tbs | Buttered, strained, avg | 14 | 0.01 | 0.01 | 0.02 | 0.00 | 0.01 | 0.01 | 0.00 | 0.01 | 0.01 | 0.01 | 0.00 | 0.01 | 0.01 | 0.01 | 0.01 | 0.00 | 0.00 | 0.01 |
| 60632 | 1 Tbs | Junior, avg | 14 | 0.01 | 0.01 | 0.03 | 0.00 | 0.02 | 0.01 | 0.00 | 0.01 | 0.01 | 0.01 | 0.00 | 0.01 | 0.01 | 0.01 | 0.01 | 0.00 | 0.01 | 0.01 |
| 60633 | 1 Tbs | Strained, avg | 14 | 0.01 | 0.01 | 0.03 | 0.00 | 0.02 | 0.01 | 0.00 | 0.01 | 0.01 | 0.01 | 0.00 | 0.01 | 0.01 | 0.01 | 0.01 | 0.00 | 0.01 | 0.01 |
| | | **MEALS, ENTRÉES AND DISHES** | | | | | | | | | | | | | | | | | | | |
| 56087 | 1 cup | Beef Macaroni, w/tomato sauce, homemade | 226 | 0.85 | 0.91 | 1.38 | 0.23 | 3.40 | 0.77 | 0.49 | 0.68 | 1.18 | 1.09 | 0.36 | 0.64 | 0.88 | 0.63 | 0.63 | 0.18 | 0.50 | 0.73 |
| 11023 | 1 cup | Beef, Pepper Steak, frzn, avg | 217 | 1.73 | 1.81 | 2.60 | 0.32 | 4.30 | 1.56 | 0.98 | 1.29 | 2.26 | 2.39 | 0.73 | 1.12 | 1.26 | 1.10 | 1.25 | 0.32 | 0.96 | 1.39 |
| 11022 | 1 ea | Beef, Swiss Steak, frzn, avg | 170 | 1.19 | 1.25 | 1.80 | 0.22 | 2.98 | 1.08 | 0.68 | 0.89 | 1.56 | 1.64 | 0.51 | 0.77 | 0.87 | 0.76 | 0.86 | 0.22 | 0.66 | 0.96 |
| 15925 | 1 cup | Chicken w/Cheese Sauce, avg | 241 | 0.15 | 1.21 | 0.22 | 0.02 | 0.66 | 0.16 | 0.06 | 0.10 | 0.17 | 0.16 | 0.07 | 0.10 | 0.15 | 0.09 | 0.08 | 0.02 | 0.07 | 0.12 |
| 56001 | 1 cup | Chili w/beans, cnd, avg | 256 | 0.68 | 0.92 | 1.69 | 0.16 | 2.25 | 0.67 | 0.42 | 0.64 | 1.17 | 1.05 | 0.24 | 0.75 | 0.64 | 0.75 | 0.61 | 0.18 | 0.42 | 0.75 |
| 56637 | 1 ea | Chimichanga, w/beef, cheese & red chili peppers, homema | 180 | 0.71 | 0.79 | 1.11 | 0.18 | 3.31 | 0.76 | 0.41 | 0.60 | 1.09 | 0.90 | 0.30 | 0.62 | 1.07 | 0.63 | 0.52 | 0.17 | 0.46 | 0.67 |
| 56293 | 1 ea | Crepes, meat filled, homemade | 119 | 1.21 | 1.28 | 1.86 | 0.27 | 3.41 | 1.07 | 0.68 | 0.96 | 1.68 | 1.66 | 0.54 | 0.87 | 1.05 | 0.89 | 0.91 | 0.24 | 0.73 | 1.05 |
| 38145 | 1/2 cup | Fried Rice, w/bean sprouts & scallions, avg | 83 | 0.13 | 0.19 | 0.22 | 0.05 | 0.45 | 0.11 | 0.05 | 0.10 | 0.19 | 0.08 | 0.05 | 0.12 | 0.11 | 0.12 | 0.08 | 0.03 | 0.08 | 0.14 |
| 56080 | 1 cup | Moussaka, w/lamb, homemade | 250 | 0.92 | 0.94 | 1.53 | 0.20 | 2.55 | 0.72 | 0.48 | 0.79 | 1.27 | 1.32 | 0.40 | 0.69 | 0.75 | 0.69 | 0.69 | 0.19 | 0.56 | 0.89 |
| 66001 | 1 pce | Pizza, Cheese, 1/8 of 12", avg | 63 | 0.23 | 0.30 | 0.47 | 0.08 | 1.92 | 0.18 | 0.23 | 0.32 | 0.63 | 0.55 | 0.17 | 0.37 | 0.76 | 0.39 | 0.25 | 0.09 | 0.35 | 0.40 |
| 56618 | 1 pce | Pizza, Combination, 12", avg | 79 | 0.48 | 0.59 | 0.88 | 0.13 | 3.01 | 0.44 | 0.40 | 0.54 | 1.06 | 0.96 | 0.30 | 0.60 | 1.15 | 0.64 | 0.45 | 0.16 | 0.55 | 0.67 |
| 56619 | 1 pce | Pizza, Pepperoni, 1/8 of 12", avg | 71 | 0.33 | 0.42 | 0.64 | 0.10 | 2.46 | 0.27 | 0.31 | 0.42 | 0.82 | 0.72 | 0.23 | 0.48 | 0.97 | 0.51 | 0.34 | 0.12 | 0.45 | 0.52 |
| 38163 | 1 cup | Rice A Roni, w/pasta, cooked | 202 | 0.24 | 0.33 | 0.38 | 0.11 | 1.32 | 0.21 | 0.11 | 0.21 | 0.39 | 0.15 | 0.10 | 0.26 | 0.36 | 0.26 | 0.16 | 0.06 | 0.18 | 0.28 |
| 38286 | 1/2 cup | Rice A Roni, w/pasta, dry | 82 | 0.36 | 0.50 | 0.56 | 0.16 | 1.98 | 0.31 | 0.17 | 0.32 | 0.59 | 0.23 | 0.16 | 0.39 | 0.55 | 0.39 | 0.24 | 0.09 | 0.27 | 0.41 |
| 56075 | 1 cup | Souffle, Cheese, homemade | 112 | 0.48 | 0.53 | 0.91 | 0.17 | 2.06 | 0.29 | 0.32 | 0.62 | 1.02 | 0.87 | 0.31 | 0.59 | 0.86 | 0.73 | 0.48 | 0.14 | 0.52 | 0.71 |
| 56089 | 1 cup | Tuna Noodle Casserole, homemade | 202 | 0.89 | 0.91 | 1.47 | 0.24 | 3.24 | 0.72 | 0.45 | 0.76 | 1.31 | 1.24 | 0.44 | 0.70 | 0.89 | 0.74 | 0.68 | 0.20 | 0.55 | 0.85 |
| | | **MEALS, ENTRÉES AND DISHES—BREAKFASTS** | | | | | | | | | | | | | | | | | | | |
| | | Biscuits | | | | | | | | | | | | | | | | | | | |
| 56600 | 1 ea | With Egg, avg | 136 | 0.51 | 0.58 | 0.85 | 0.23 | 2.22 | 0.36 | 0.26 | 0.58 | 0.90 | 0.59 | 0.29 | 0.58 | 0.77 | 0.71 | 0.45 | 0.16 | 0.42 | 0.66 |
| 56601 | 1 ea | With Egg & Bacon, avg | 150 | 0.84 | 0.94 | 1.34 | 0.29 | 3.06 | 0.77 | 0.43 | 0.82 | 1.31 | 1.02 | 0.42 | 0.81 | 1.09 | 0.94 | 0.68 | 0.22 | 0.59 | 0.95 |
| 56602 | 1 ea | With Egg & Ham, avg | 192 | 1.06 | 1.19 | 1.73 | 0.37 | 3.77 | 0.84 | 0.59 | 1.00 | 1.65 | 1.38 | 0.54 | 0.99 | 1.19 | 1.10 | 0.87 | 0.27 | 0.73 | 1.08 |
| 66028 | 1 ea | With Egg & Sausage, avg | 180 | 0.97 | 1.07 | 1.54 | 0.33 | 3.53 | 0.83 | 0.50 | 0.92 | 1.50 | 1.20 | 0.49 | 0.90 | 1.21 | 1.07 | 0.79 | 0.25 | 0.68 | 1.05 |
| 56603 | 1 ea | With Egg & Steak, avg | 148 | 0.93 | 1.01 | 1.48 | 0.30 | 3.18 | 0.74 | 0.50 | 0.87 | 1.43 | 1.18 | 0.46 | 0.83 | 1.04 | 0.94 | 0.75 | 0.23 | 0.64 | 0.98 |
| 66029 | 1 ea | With Egg, Cheese & Bacon, avg | 144 | 0.71 | 0.84 | 1.21 | 0.24 | 3.01 | 0.63 | 0.46 | 0.77 | 1.29 | 1.11 | 0.40 | 0.78 | 1.17 | 0.86 | 0.62 | 0.21 | 0.64 | 0.92 |
| 56604 | 1 ea | With Ham, avg | 113 | 0.68 | 0.77 | 1.08 | 0.22 | 2.89 | 0.62 | 0.43 | 0.58 | 1.06 | 0.92 | 0.33 | 0.62 | 0.90 | 0.60 | 0.54 | 0.17 | 0.45 | 0.60 |
| 66030 | 1 ea | With Sausage, avg | 124 | 0.53 | 0.60 | 0.79 | 0.19 | 2.98 | 0.57 | 0.32 | 0.48 | 0.90 | 0.65 | 0.26 | 0.53 | 1.05 | 0.56 | 0.43 | 0.14 | 0.39 | 0.55 |
| 56605 | 1 ea | With Steak, avg | 141 | 0.62 | 0.68 | 0.94 | 0.19 | 2.92 | 0.58 | 0.38 | 0.56 | 1.01 | 0.79 | 0.30 | 0.57 | 0.98 | 0.57 | 0.49 | 0.16 | 0.44 | 0.62 |
| | | Croissants | | | | | | | | | | | | | | | | | | | |
| 56606 | 1 ea | With Egg & Cheese, avg | 127 | 0.47 | 0.60 | 0.89 | 0.19 | 2.60 | 0.33 | 0.39 | 0.63 | 1.06 | 0.92 | 0.33 | 0.66 | 1.06 | 0.72 | 0.47 | 0.18 | 0.57 | 0.76 |
| 56607 | 1 ea | With Egg, Cheese & Bacon, avg | 129 | 0.64 | 0.80 | 1.16 | 0.23 | 3.21 | 0.50 | 0.50 | 0.79 | 1.34 | 1.18 | 0.42 | 0.81 | 1.30 | 0.89 | 0.61 | 0.22 | 0.70 | 0.95 |
| 56608 | 1 ea | With Egg, Cheese & Ham, avg | 152 | 0.90 | 1.04 | 1.52 | 0.31 | 3.57 | 0.70 | 0.59 | 0.90 | 1.54 | 1.37 | 0.49 | 0.92 | 1.23 | 0.99 | 0.77 | 0.26 | 0.73 | 1.01 |

TABLE A **Amino Acid Content for Selected Foods *(continued)***

| Code | Amount | | Description | Weight (g) | Alanine (g) | Arginine (g) | Aspartic acid (g) | Cystine (g) | Glutamic acid (g) | Glycine (g) | Histidine (g) | Isoleucine (g) | Leucine (g) | Lysine (g) | Methionine (g) | Phenylalanine (g) | Proline (g) | Serine (g) | Threonine (g) | Tryptophan (g) | Tyrosine (g) | Valine (g) |
|---|---|---|---|---|---|---|---|---|---|---|---|---|---|---|---|---|---|---|---|---|---|---|
| 56609 | 1 | ea | With Egg, Cheese & Sausage, avg | 160 | 0.93 | 1.08 | 1.54 | 0.30 | 3.78 | 0.30 | 0.58 | 0.95 | 1.60 | 1.41 | 0.51 | 0.95 | 1.40 | 1.07 | 0.79 | 0.26 | 0.78 | 1.11 |
| 42354 | 1 | pce | French Toast, sticks, avg | 28 | 0.07 | 0.07 | 0.10 | 0.03 | 0.46 | 0.06 | 0.04 | 0.07 | 0.12 | 0.06 | 0.03 | 0.08 | 0.15 | 0.08 | 0.06 | 0.02 | 0.06 | 0.08 |
| 42353 | 1 | pce | French Toast w/butter, avg | 68 | 0.23 | 0.26 | 0.39 | 0.10 | 1.13 | 0.18 | 0.12 | 0.27 | 0.41 | 0.25 | 0.12 | 0.27 | 0.39 | 0.32 | 0.20 | 0.07 | 0.17 | 0.31 |
| | | | **MEATS—BEEF** | | | | | | | | | | | | | | | | | | | |
| | | | Dried Beef | | | | | | | | | | | | | | | | | | | |
| 10051 | 1 | ea | Beef Jerky, large pce | 20 | 0.42 | 0.44 | 0.64 | 0.08 | 1.05 | 0.38 | 0.24 | 0.31 | 0.55 | 0.57 | 0.17 | 0.27 | 0.31 | 0.27 | 0.30 | 0.08 | 0.23 | 0.34 |
| 10009 | 5 | pce | Cured | 21 | 0.40 | 0.41 | 0.54 | 0.07 | 0.88 | 0.45 | 0.18 | 0.25 | 0.46 | 0.50 | 0.15 | 0.23 | 0.33 | 0.25 | 0.26 | 0.05 | 0.18 | 0.28 |
| 10052 | 1 | ea | Meat Sticks, smkd | 20 | 0.29 | 0.30 | 0.40 | 0.06 | 0.61 | 0.43 | 0.11 | 0.16 | 0.29 | 0.30 | 0.09 | 0.16 | 0.29 | 0.18 | 0.17 | 0.04 | 0.12 | 0.19 |
| 10106 | 1 | oz | Fat, cooked | 28 | 0.18 | 0.19 | 0.27 | 0.03 | 0.45 | 0.16 | 0.10 | 0.13 | 0.24 | 0.25 | 0.08 | 0.12 | 0.13 | 0.11 | 0.13 | 0.03 | 0.10 | 0.15 |
| | | | Ground Beef | | | | | | | | | | | | | | | | | | | |
| 10454 | 3 | oz | 16% Fat, bkd | 85 | 1.26 | 1.32 | 1.90 | 0.23 | 3.13 | 1.14 | 0.71 | 0.94 | 1.64 | 1.73 | 0.53 | 0.81 | 0.92 | 0.80 | 0.91 | 0.23 | 0.70 | 1.01 |
| 10456 | 3 | oz | 16% Fat, brld | 85 | 1.30 | 1.37 | 1.97 | 0.24 | 3.25 | 1.18 | 0.74 | 0.97 | 1.71 | 1.79 | 0.55 | 0.84 | 0.95 | 0.83 | 0.94 | 0.24 | 0.73 | 1.05 |
| 10261 | 3 | oz | 16% Fat, pan fried | 85 | 1.28 | 1.34 | 1.94 | 0.24 | 3.19 | 1.16 | 0.73 | 0.95 | 1.67 | 1.77 | 0.54 | 0.83 | 0.94 | 0.81 | 0.93 | 0.24 | 0.71 | 1.03 |
| 10453 | 4 | oz | 17% Fat, raw | 113 | 1.38 | 1.42 | 1.93 | 0.20 | 3.32 | 1.57 | 0.67 | 0.91 | 1.69 | 1.76 | 0.49 | 0.80 | 1.07 | 0.82 | 0.89 | 0.26 | 0.66 | 1.02 |
| 10459 | 3 | oz | 18% Fat, bkd | 85 | 1.22 | 1.28 | 1.86 | 0.23 | 3.06 | 1.11 | 0.70 | 0.92 | 1.61 | 1.69 | 0.52 | 0.79 | 0.90 | 0.78 | 0.89 | 0.23 | 0.68 | 0.99 |
| 10673 | 3 | oz | 19% Fat, brld | 85 | 1.27 | 1.33 | 1.92 | 0.24 | 3.15 | 1.15 | 0.72 | 0.94 | 1.66 | 1.75 | 0.54 | 0.82 | 0.93 | 0.80 | 0.92 | 0.24 | 0.71 | 1.02 |
| 8208 | 3 | oz | 19% Fat, fried | 85 | 1.24 | 1.30 | 1.88 | 0.23 | 3.09 | 1.12 | 0.71 | 0.93 | 1.63 | 1.72 | 0.53 | 0.80 | 0.91 | 0.79 | 0.90 | 0.23 | 0.69 | 1.00 |
| 10725 | 3 | oz | 21% Fat, bkd | 85 | 1.16 | 1.22 | 1.77 | 0.22 | 2.91 | 1.05 | 0.66 | 0.87 | 1.53 | 1.61 | 0.49 | 0.75 | 0.85 | 0.74 | 0.84 | 0.22 | 0.65 | 0.94 |
| 10700 | 3 | oz | 21% Fat, brld | 85 | 1.23 | 1.29 | 1.87 | 0.23 | 3.08 | 1.11 | 0.70 | 0.92 | 1.62 | 1.70 | 0.52 | 0.80 | 0.90 | 0.78 | 0.89 | 0.23 | 0.69 | 0.99 |
| 10458 | 4 | oz | 21% Fat, raw | 113 | 1.31 | 1.34 | 1.83 | 0.19 | 3.14 | 1.48 | 0.64 | 0.86 | 1.60 | 1.67 | 0.47 | 0.76 | 1.01 | 0.77 | 0.84 | 0.25 | 0.62 | 0.97 |
| 10464 | 3 | oz | 23% Fat, fried | 85 | 1.22 | 1.28 | 1.86 | 0.23 | 3.05 | 1.11 | 0.70 | 0.92 | 1.61 | 1.69 | 0.52 | 0.79 | 0.90 | 0.78 | 0.89 | 0.23 | 0.68 | 0.99 |
| 10462 | 4 | oz | 27% Fat, raw | 113 | 1.23 | 1.27 | 1.72 | 0.18 | 2.95 | 1.39 | 0.60 | 0.81 | 1.50 | 1.57 | 0.44 | 0.71 | 0.95 | 0.73 | 0.79 | 0.23 | 0.59 | 0.91 |
| | | | Retail Cuts, all grades, lean & fat, 1/8" trim | | | | | | | | | | | | | | | | | | | |
| 10820 | 3 | oz | Average, ckd | 85 | 1.35 | 1.42 | 2.05 | 0.25 | 3.37 | 1.22 | 0.77 | 1.01 | 1.78 | 1.87 | 0.57 | 0.88 | 0.99 | 0.86 | 0.98 | 0.25 | 0.75 | 1.10 |
| 10819 | 4 | oz | Average, raw | 113 | 1.28 | 1.33 | 1.93 | 0.24 | 3.18 | 1.15 | 0.72 | 0.95 | 1.67 | 1.76 | 0.54 | 0.82 | 0.93 | 0.81 | 0.92 | 0.24 | 0.71 | 1.03 |
| 10008 | 1 | cup | Brisket, corned, cnd, ckd | 140 | 2.70 | 2.31 | 3.67 | 0.48 | 6.11 | 3.13 | 1.20 | 1.52 | 2.76 | 2.88 | 0.87 | 1.35 | 2.70 | 1.51 | 1.41 | 0.34 | 1.23 | 1.65 |
| 10787 | 3 | oz | Brisket, corned, ckd | 85 | 1.10 | 0.94 | 1.50 | 0.20 | 2.49 | 1.28 | 0.49 | 0.56 | 1.12 | 1.17 | 0.35 | 0.55 | 1.10 | 0.62 | 0.58 | 0.14 | 0.50 | 0.67 |
| 10485 | 4 | oz | Brisket, corned, raw | 113 | 1.19 | 1.01 | 1.61 | 0.21 | 2.67 | 1.38 | 0.52 | 0.71 | 1.21 | 1.26 | 0.38 | 0.59 | 1.19 | 0.66 | 0.62 | 0.15 | 0.54 | 0.72 |
| 10828 | 3 | oz | Brisket, whole, brsd | 85 | 1.33 | 1.39 | 2.01 | 0.25 | 3.30 | 1.20 | 0.75 | 0.39 | 1.73 | 1.83 | 0.56 | 0.86 | 0.97 | 0.84 | 0.96 | 0.25 | 0.74 | 1.07 |
| 10827 | 4 | oz | Brisket, whole, raw | 113 | 1.25 | 1.31 | 1.90 | 0.23 | 3.13 | 1.14 | 0.71 | 0.94 | 1.65 | 1.73 | 0.53 | 0.81 | 0.92 | 0.80 | 0.91 | 0.23 | 0.70 | 1.01 |
| 10834 | 3 | oz | Chuck, arm pot roast, brsd | 85 | 1.46 | 1.53 | 2.22 | 0.27 | 3.65 | 1.33 | 0.83 | 1.09 | 1.92 | 2.02 | 0.62 | 0.94 | 1.07 | 0.93 | 1.06 | 0.27 | 0.82 | 1.18 |
| 10833 | 4 | oz | Chuck, arm pot roast, raw | 113 | 1.28 | 1.34 | 1.94 | 0.24 | 3.19 | 1.16 | 0.73 | 0.95 | 1.68 | 1.76 | 0.54 | 0.83 | 0.94 | 0.81 | 0.93 | 0.24 | 0.71 | 1.03 |
| 10840 | 3 | oz | Chuck, blade pot roast, brsd | 85 | 1.38 | 1.44 | 2.08 | 0.26 | 3.42 | 1.24 | 0.78 | 1.02 | 1.80 | 1.90 | 0.58 | 0.89 | 1.00 | 0.87 | 0.99 | 0.26 | 0.76 | 1.11 |
| 10839 | 4 | oz | Chuck, blade pot roast, raw | 113 | 1.18 | 1.23 | 1.77 | 0.22 | 2.92 | 1.06 | 0.66 | 0.87 | 1.54 | 1.62 | 0.50 | 0.76 | 0.86 | 0.74 | 0.85 | 0.22 | 0.65 | 0.94 |
| 11487 | 3 | oz | Porterhouse Steak, ckd | 85 | 1.21 | 1.27 | 1.83 | 0.22 | 3.00 | 1.09 | 0.68 | 0.90 | 1.58 | 1.67 | 0.51 | 0.78 | 0.88 | 0.76 | 0.88 | 0.22 | 0.67 | 0.97 |
| 11486 | 4 | oz | Porterhouse Steak, raw | 113 | 1.28 | 1.34 | 1.94 | 0.24 | 3.19 | 1.16 | 0.73 | 0.95 | 1.68 | 1.76 | 0.54 | 0.83 | 0.94 | 0.81 | 0.93 | 0.24 | 0.71 | 1.03 |
| 10859 | 3 | oz | Ribs, large end 6-9, ckd | 85 | 1.11 | 1.16 | 1.67 | 0.20 | 2.75 | 1.00 | 0.63 | 0.82 | 1.45 | 1.52 | 0.47 | 0.71 | 0.81 | 0.70 | 0.80 | 0.20 | 0.62 | 0.89 |
| 10950 | 4 | oz | Ribs, large end 6-9, raw | 113 | 1.11 | 1.16 | 1.68 | 0.21 | 2.76 | 1.00 | 0.63 | 0.83 | 1.46 | 1.53 | 0.47 | 0.72 | 0.81 | 0.70 | 0.80 | 0.21 | 0.62 | 0.89 |
| 10871 | 3 | oz | Ribs, small end 10-12, ckd | 85 | 1.22 | 1.28 | 1.86 | 0.23 | 3.05 | 1.11 | 0.70 | 0.92 | 1.61 | 1.69 | 0.52 | 0.79 | 0.90 | 0.78 | 0.89 | 0.23 | 0.68 | 0.99 |
| 10870 | 4 | oz | Ribs, small end 10-12, raw | 113 | 1.15 | 1.21 | 1.75 | 0.21 | 2.88 | 1.05 | 0.66 | 0.86 | 1.51 | 1.59 | 0.49 | 0.75 | 0.85 | 0.73 | 0.84 | 0.21 | 0.64 | 0.93 |
| 10846 | 3 | oz | Ribs, whole 6-12, ckd | 85 | 1.15 | 1.21 | 1.74 | 0.21 | 2.86 | 1.04 | 0.65 | 0.86 | 1.50 | 1.59 | 0.49 | 0.74 | 0.84 | 0.73 | 0.83 | 0.21 | 0.64 | 0.93 |
| 10845 | 4 | oz | Ribs, whole 6-12, raw | 85 | 0.85 | 0.89 | 1.28 | 0.16 | 2.11 | 0.77 | 0.48 | 0.63 | 1.11 | 1.17 | 0.36 | 0.55 | 0.62 | 0.54 | 0.61 | 0.16 | 0.47 | 0.68 |
| 11410 | 3 | oz | Round, bottom, ckd | 85 | 1.51 | 1.58 | 2.30 | 0.28 | 3.77 | 1.37 | 0.86 | 1.13 | 1.98 | 2.08 | 0.64 | 0.98 | 1.11 | 0.96 | 1.10 | 0.28 | 0.84 | 1.22 |
| 10886 | 4 | oz | Round, bottom, raw | 113 | 1.41 | 1.48 | 2.14 | 0.26 | 3.50 | 1.28 | 0.80 | 1.05 | 1.84 | 1.94 | 0.60 | 0.91 | 1.03 | 0.89 | 1.02 | 0.26 | 0.78 | 1.13 |
| 11425 | 3 | oz | Round, tip, ckd | 85 | 1.41 | 1.48 | 2.13 | 0.26 | 3.50 | 1.28 | 0.80 | 1.05 | 1.84 | 1.94 | 0.60 | 0.91 | 1.03 | 0.89 | 1.02 | 0.26 | 0.78 | 1.14 |
| 11424 | 4 | oz | Round, tip , raw | 113 | 1.33 | 1.40 | 2.02 | 0.25 | 3.32 | 1.21 | 0.76 | 1.00 | 1.75 | 1.84 | 0.57 | 0.86 | 0.98 | 0.85 | 0.97 | 0.25 | 0.74 | 1.08 |
| 11463 | 3 | oz | Sirloin, top, ckd | 85 | 1.45 | 1.51 | 2.19 | 0.27 | 3.60 | 1.31 | 0.82 | 1.08 | 1.90 | 2.00 | 0.61 | 0.94 | 1.06 | 0.92 | 1.05 | 0.27 | 0.81 | 1.16 |
| 10943 | 4 | oz | Sirloin, top, raw | 113 | 1.33 | 1.39 | 2.01 | 0.25 | 3.31 | 1.20 | 0.75 | 0.99 | 1.74 | 1.83 | 0.56 | 0.86 | 0.97 | 0.84 | 0.96 | 0.25 | 0.74 | 1.07 |
| 11491 | 3 | oz | T-bone Steak, ckd | 85 | 1.25 | 1.31 | 1.89 | 0.23 | 3.11 | 1.13 | 0.71 | 0.93 | 1.63 | 1.72 | 0.53 | 0.81 | 0.91 | 0.79 | 0.90 | 0.23 | 0.69 | 1.00 |
| 11490 | 4 | oz | T-bone Steak, raw | 113 | 1.31 | 1.37 | 1.98 | 0.24 | 3.25 | 1.19 | 0.74 | 0.98 | 1.72 | 1.81 | 0.55 | 0.85 | 0.96 | 0.83 | 0.95 | 0.24 | 0.73 | 1.06 |

## TABLE A **Amino Acid Content for Selected Foods *(continued)***

| Code | Amount | Description | Weight (g) | Alanine (g) | Arginine (g) | Aspartic acid (g) | Cystine (g) | Glutamic acid (g) | Glycine (g) | Histidine (g) | Isoleucine (g) | Leucine (g) | Lysine (g) | Methionine (g) | Phenylalanine (g) | Proline (g) | Serine (g) | Threonine (g) | Tryptophan (g) | Tyrosine (g) | Valine (g) |
|---|---|---|---|---|---|---|---|---|---|---|---|---|---|---|---|---|---|---|---|---|---|
| 11451 | 3 oz | Tenderloin, ckd | 85 | 1.32 | 1.38 | 1.99 | 0.24 | 3.27 | 1.19 | 0.75 | 0.98 | 1.72 | 1.81 | 0.56 | 0.85 | 0.96 | 0.83 | 0.95 | 0.24 | 0.73 | 1.06 |
| 10931 | 4 oz | Tenderloin, raw | 113 | 1.23 | 1.29 | 1.86 | 0.23 | 3.06 | 1.11 | 0.70 | 0.92 | 1.62 | 1.69 | 0.52 | 0.80 | 0.90 | 0.78 | 0.89 | 0.23 | 0.68 | 0.99 |
| 11432 | 3 oz | Top Round, ckd | 85 | 1.56 | 1.64 | 2.37 | 0.29 | 3.90 | 1.42 | 0.89 | 1.16 | 2.05 | 2.16 | 0.66 | 1.01 | 1.15 | 0.99 | 1.13 | 0.29 | 0.88 | 1.27 |
| 10907 | 4 oz | Top Round, raw | 113 | 1.49 | 1.56 | 2.25 | 0.28 | 3.71 | 1.34 | 0.84 | 1.11 | 1.95 | 2.06 | 0.63 | 0.96 | 1.09 | 0.94 | 1.08 | 0.28 | 0.83 | 1.20 |
| | | Steaks, Prepared | | | | | | | | | | | | | | | | | | | |
| 10083 | 1 ea | Battered, fried | 243 | 3.45 | 3.62 | 5.22 | 0.64 | 8.60 | 3.13 | 1.96 | 2.58 | 4.54 | 4.79 | 1.47 | 2.25 | 2.53 | 2.19 | 2.50 | 0.64 | 1.93 | 2.79 |
| 10084 | 1 ea | Battered, fried, lean | 165 | 2.61 | 2.74 | 3.94 | 0.48 | 6.50 | 2.36 | 1.48 | 1.93 | 3.42 | 3.60 | 1.11 | 1.70 | 1.91 | 1.65 | 1.90 | 0.48 | 1.45 | 2.11 |
| 10080 | 1 ea | Breaded, brld | 243 | 3.55 | 3.72 | 5.37 | 0.66 | 8.85 | 3.23 | 2.02 | 2.64 | 4.67 | 4.91 | 1.51 | 2.31 | 2.60 | 2.25 | 2.58 | 0.66 | 1.98 | 2.87 |
| 10072 | 1 ea | Fried | 153 | 2.85 | 2.98 | 4.30 | 0.53 | 7.08 | 2.57 | 1.61 | 2.11 | 3.72 | 3.93 | 1.21 | 1.84 | 2.08 | 1.81 | 2.07 | 0.53 | 1.58 | 2.30 |
| 10079 | 1 ea | Fried, lean | 117 | 2.38 | 2.49 | 3.59 | 0.44 | 5.92 | 2.15 | 1.35 | 1.77 | 3.11 | 3.29 | 1.01 | 1.54 | 1.74 | 1.51 | 1.73 | 0.44 | 1.32 | 1.92 |
| | | **MEATS—GAME** | | | | | | | | | | | | | | | | | | | |
| 14052 | 4 oz | Antelope, raw | 113 | 1.47 | 1.66 | 2.40 | 0.22 | 3.81 | 1.14 | 1.21 | 0.97 | 2.14 | 2.11 | 0.72 | 1.00 | 1.16 | 1.07 | 1.18 | 0.00 | 0.88 | 1.12 |
| 14053 | 3 oz | Antelope, rstd | 85 | 1.46 | 1.65 | 2.37 | 0.22 | 3.77 | 1.12 | 1.19 | 0.96 | 2.12 | 2.09 | 0.71 | 0.99 | 1.15 | 1.05 | 1.16 | 0.00 | 0.87 | 1.11 |
| 14067 | 4 oz | Beefalo, raw | 113 | 1.49 | 1.56 | 2.29 | 0.27 | 3.84 | 1.27 | 1.67 | 1.11 | 2.05 | 2.06 | 0.62 | 0.99 | 1.05 | 1.00 | 1.08 | 0.27 | 0.85 | 1.19 |
| 14008 | 3 oz | Beefalo, rstd | 85 | 1.49 | 1.55 | 2.27 | 0.27 | 3.82 | 1.26 | 0.69 | 1.11 | 2.03 | 2.04 | 0.62 | 0.98 | 1.05 | 0.99 | 1.07 | 0.26 | 0.84 | 0.96 |
| 14056 | 4 oz | Bison, raw | 113 | 1.39 | 1.45 | 2.12 | 0.25 | 3.56 | 1.18 | 0.65 | 1.03 | 1.90 | 1.91 | 0.58 | 0.91 | 0.98 | 0.93 | 1.01 | 0.25 | 0.79 | 1.11 |
| 14009 | 3 oz | Bison, rstd | 85 | 1.38 | 1.44 | 2.10 | 0.25 | 3.53 | 1.16 | 0.64 | 1.02 | 1.88 | 1.89 | 0.57 | 0.91 | 0.97 | 0.92 | 0.99 | 0.25 | 0.78 | 1.10 |
| 14057 | 4 oz | Boar, raw | 113 | 1.42 | 1.67 | 2.24 | 0.31 | 3.74 | 1.10 | 1.22 | 1.17 | 1.96 | 2.38 | 0.59 | 0.96 | 0.91 | 0.99 | 1.13 | 0.32 | 0.86 | 1.29 |
| 14010 | 3 oz | Boar, rstd | 85 | 1.42 | 1.66 | 2.22 | 0.31 | 3.71 | 1.09 | 1.21 | 1.16 | 1.94 | 2.35 | 0.59 | 0.95 | 0.90 | 0.98 | 1.12 | 0.32 | 0.85 | 1.28 |
| 14059 | 4 oz | Caribou, raw | 113 | 1.37 | 1.53 | 2.26 | 0.18 | 4.01 | 1.07 | 1.01 | 1.15 | 2.11 | 2.32 | 0.57 | 1.14 | 0.79 | 0.90 | 1.09 | 0.39 | 0.84 | 1.20 |
| 14012 | 3 oz | Caribou, rstd | 85 | 1.35 | 1.50 | 2.24 | 0.18 | 3.97 | 1.06 | 1.00 | 1.15 | 2.09 | 2.30 | 0.57 | 1.12 | 0.79 | 0.89 | 1.08 | 0.39 | 0.83 | 1.19 |
| 14061 | 4 oz | Elk, raw | 113 | 1.63 | 1.79 | 2.54 | 0.00 | 4.12 | 1.10 | 0.83 | 0.84 | 2.19 | 2.41 | 0.62 | 1.03 | 1.12 | 1.13 | 1.13 | 0.47 | 0.93 | 0.92 |
| 14014 | 3 oz | Elk, rstd | 85 | 1.62 | 1.76 | 2.52 | 0.00 | 4.08 | 1.09 | 0.82 | 0.83 | 2.17 | 2.38 | 0.62 | 1.02 | 1.11 | 1.12 | 1.12 | 0.46 | 0.92 | 0.91 |
| 14026 | 4 oz | Horse, raw | 113 | 1.39 | 1.58 | 2.37 | 0.34 | 3.53 | 1.16 | 0.93 | 1.14 | 1.92 | 2.06 | 0.53 | 0.99 | 1.12 | 0.92 | 1.08 | 0.30 | 0.76 | 1.25 |
| 14018 | 3 oz | Horse, rstd | 85 | 1.38 | 1.56 | 2.35 | 0.33 | 3.49 | 1.16 | 0.92 | 1.13 | 1.90 | 2.04 | 0.53 | 0.99 | 1.11 | 0.91 | 1.07 | 0.30 | 0.75 | 1.24 |
| 14062 | 4 oz | Moose, raw | 113 | 1.45 | 1.63 | 2.36 | 0.00 | 4.07 | 1.10 | 0.84 | 1.21 | 2.21 | 2.28 | 0.64 | 1.09 | 1.02 | 0.90 | 1.15 | 0.00 | 0.93 | 1.37 |
| 14019 | 3 oz | Moose, rstd | 85 | 1.44 | 1.61 | 2.34 | 0.00 | 4.03 | 1.09 | 0.84 | 1.20 | 2.19 | 2.26 | 0.64 | 1.07 | 1.01 | 0.89 | 1.14 | 0.00 | 0.92 | 1.35 |
| 14063 | 4 oz | Muskrat, raw | 113 | 1.24 | 1.13 | 2.02 | 0.00 | 2.98 | 1.14 | 0.70 | 0.89 | 1.85 | 1.84 | 0.39 | 0.97 | 0.94 | 0.84 | 0.97 | 0.00 | 0.64 | 1.04 |
| 14020 | 3 oz | Muskrat, rstd | 85 | 1.35 | 1.22 | 2.21 | 0.00 | 3.26 | 1.25 | 0.76 | 0.98 | 2.01 | 2.01 | 0.43 | 1.05 | 1.02 | 0.92 | 1.05 | 0.00 | 0.70 | 1.14 |
| | | Rabbit | | | | | | | | | | | | | | | | | | | |
| 14048 | 4 oz | Raw | 113 | 1.37 | 1.40 | 2.21 | 0.28 | 3.64 | 1.23 | 0.64 | 1.07 | 1.76 | 1.99 | 0.57 | 0.93 | 1.11 | 1.00 | 1.01 | 0.30 | 0.81 | 1.15 |
| 14004 | 3 oz | Roasted | 85 | 1.49 | 1.53 | 2.41 | 0.31 | 3.96 | 1.34 | 0.69 | 1.17 | 1.92 | 2.16 | 0.62 | 1.01 | 1.21 | 1.10 | 1.11 | 0.33 | 0.88 | 1.26 |
| 14049 | 3 oz | Stewed | 85 | 1.56 | 1.60 | 2.52 | 0.32 | 4.14 | 1.40 | 0.72 | 1.22 | 2.01 | 2.26 | 0.65 | 1.06 | 1.27 | 1.15 | 1.16 | 0.34 | 0.92 | 1.31 |
| 14051 | 4 oz | Squirrel, raw | 113 | 1.14 | 1.25 | 1.91 | 0.00 | 3.24 | 1.04 | 0.63 | 0.91 | 1.73 | 1.74 | 0.53 | 0.93 | 0.89 | 0.79 | 0.91 | 0.00 | 0.72 | 0.95 |
| 14024 | 3 oz | Squirrel, rstd | 85 | 1.24 | 1.37 | 2.08 | 0.00 | 3.54 | 1.13 | 0.68 | 0.99 | 1.88 | 1.90 | 0.57 | 1.01 | 0.98 | 0.86 | 0.99 | 0.00 | 0.78 | 1.04 |
| 14060 | 4 oz | Venison, raw | 113 | 1.62 | 1.86 | 2.41 | 0.29 | 3.77 | 1.33 | 1.29 | 1.03 | 2.20 | 2.27 | 0.64 | 1.06 | 1.33 | 1.10 | 1.22 | 0.00 | 0.92 | 1.21 |
| 14013 | 3 oz | Venison, rstd | 85 | 1.61 | 1.85 | 2.38 | 0.29 | 3.73 | 1.32 | 1.27 | 1.01 | 2.18 | 2.24 | 0.63 | 1.05 | 1.33 | 1.09 | 1.21 | 0.00 | 0.91 | 1.20 |
| 14058 | 4 oz | Water Buffalo, raw | 113 | 0.00 | 1.45 | 2.29 | 0.37 | 3.34 | 0.90 | 0.76 | 1.15 | 1.99 | 1.82 | 0.58 | 0.92 | 0.88 | 0.99 | 1.10 | 0.28 | 0.92 | 1.22 |
| 14011 | 3 oz | Water Buffalo, rstd | 85 | 0.00 | 1.43 | 2.28 | 0.36 | 3.31 | 0.89 | 0.75 | 1.15 | 1.96 | 1.80 | 0.57 | 0.92 | 0.88 | 0.98 | 1.09 | 0.28 | 0.92 | 1.22 |
| | | **MEATS—GOAT** | | | | | | | | | | | | | | | | | | | |
| 13528 | 4 oz | Raw | 113 | 0.00 | 1.71 | 0.00 | 0.28 | 0.00 | 0.00 | 0.48 | 1.18 | 1.94 | 1.73 | 0.62 | 0.81 | 0.00 | 0.00 | 1.11 | 0.35 | 0.72 | 1.24 |
| 13623 | 3 oz | Roasted | 85 | 0.00 | 1.69 | 0.00 | 0.27 | 0.00 | 0.00 | 0.48 | 1.16 | 1.92 | 1.72 | 0.62 | 0.80 | 0.00 | 0.00 | 1.10 | 0.34 | 0.71 | 1.23 |
| 14016 | 2 ea | Roasted, ribs | 92 | 0.00 | 1.83 | 0.00 | 0.30 | 0.00 | 0.00 | 0.52 | 1.26 | 2.08 | 1.86 | 0.67 | 0.87 | 0.00 | 0.00 | 1.19 | 0.37 | 0.77 | 1.33 |
| | | **MEATS—LAMB** | | | | | | | | | | | | | | | | | | | |
| 13584 | 1 oz | Fat, ckd | 28 | 0.16 | 0.16 | 0.24 | 0.03 | 0.39 | 0.13 | 0.09 | 0.13 | 0.21 | 0.24 | 0.07 | 0.11 | 0.11 | 0.10 | 0.12 | 0.03 | 0.09 | 0.15 |
| 13583 | 1 oz | Fat, raw | 28 | 0.12 | 0.12 | 0.17 | 0.02 | 0.28 | 0.09 | 0.06 | 0.09 | 0.15 | 0.17 | 0.05 | 0.08 | 0.08 | 0.07 | 0.08 | 0.02 | 0.07 | 0.10 |
| 13524 | 3 oz | Ground, 20% fat, brld | 85 | 1.27 | 1.25 | 1.85 | 0.25 | 3.05 | 1.03 | 0.67 | 1.01 | 1.64 | 1.86 | 0.54 | 0.86 | 0.88 | 0.78 | 0.90 | 0.25 | 0.71 | 1.14 |
| 13578 | 4 oz | Ground, 23% fat, raw | 113 | 1.13 | 1.11 | 1.65 | 0.22 | 2.71 | 0.91 | 0.59 | 0.90 | 1.46 | 1.65 | 0.48 | 0.76 | 0.78 | 0.69 | 0.80 | 0.22 | 0.63 | 1.01 |
| | | Retail Cuts, choice, lean & fat, 1/8" trim | | | | | | | | | | | | | | | | | | | |
| 13628 | 3 oz | Average, ckd | 85 | 1.30 | 1.29 | 1.91 | 0.26 | 3.15 | 1.06 | 0.69 | 1.05 | 1.68 | 1.91 | 0.56 | 0.88 | 0.91 | 0.81 | 0.93 | 0.25 | 0.73 | 1.17 |

TABLE A **Amino Acid Content for Selected Foods *(continued)***

| Code | Amount | | Description | Weight (g) | Alanine (g) | Arginine (g) | Aspartic acid (g) | Cystine (g) | Glutamic acid (g) | Glycine (g) | Histidine (g) | Isoleucine (g) | Leucine (g) | Lysine (g) | Methionine (g) | Phenylalanine (g) | Proline (g) | Serine (g) | Threonine (g) | Tryptophan (g) | Tyrosine (g) | Valine (g) |
|---|---|---|---|---|---|---|---|---|---|---|---|---|---|---|---|---|---|---|---|---|---|---|
| 13627 | 4 | oz | Average, raw | 113 | 1.20 | 1.18 | 1.74 | 0.24 | 2.88 | 0.97 | 0.63 | 0.96 | 1.55 | 1.75 | 0.51 | 0.81 | 0.83 | 0.74 | 0.85 | 0.23 | 0.67 | 1.07 |
| 13630 | 3 | oz | Foreshank, brsd | 85 | 1.45 | 1.44 | 2.13 | 0.29 | 3.50 | 1.18 | 0.75 | 1.16 | 1.88 | 2.13 | 0.52 | 0.99 | 1.01 | 0.90 | 1.03 | 0.28 | 0.81 | 1.30 |
| 13629 | 4 | oz | Foreshank, raw | 113 | 1.29 | 1.27 | 1.89 | 0.26 | 3.11 | 1.04 | 0.68 | 1.03 | 1.66 | 1.89 | 0.55 | 0.87 | 0.90 | 0.79 | 0.92 | 0.25 | 0.72 | 1.15 |
| 13633 | 4 | oz | Leg, shank, raw | 113 | 1.29 | 1.28 | 1.89 | 0.26 | 3.12 | 1.05 | 0.68 | 1.04 | 1.67 | 1.90 | 0.55 | 0.87 | 0.90 | 0.80 | 0.92 | 0.25 | 0.72 | 1.16 |
| 13634 | 3 | oz | Leg, shank, rstd | 85 | 1.37 | 1.35 | 2.00 | 0.27 | 3.30 | 1.11 | 0.72 | 1.10 | 1.77 | 2.01 | 0.58 | 0.93 | 0.95 | 0.84 | 0.97 | 0.27 | 0.76 | 1.22 |
| 13635 | 4 | oz | Leg, sirloin, raw | 113 | 1.18 | 1.15 | 1.72 | 0.23 | 2.83 | 0.95 | 0.62 | 0.94 | 1.51 | 1.72 | 0.50 | 0.79 | 0.82 | 0.72 | 0.83 | 0.23 | 0.65 | 1.05 |
| 13636 | 3 | oz | Leg, sirloin, rstd | 85 | 1.28 | 1.26 | 1.87 | 0.25 | 3.08 | 1.04 | 0.67 | 1.02 | 1.65 | 1.87 | 0.54 | 0.87 | 0.89 | 0.79 | 0.91 | 0.25 | 0.71 | 1.15 |
| 13631 | 4 | oz | Leg, whole, raw | 113 | 1.25 | 1.24 | 1.84 | 0.25 | 3.03 | 1.02 | 0.66 | 1.01 | 1.63 | 1.84 | 0.54 | 0.85 | 0.88 | 0.78 | 0.89 | 0.24 | 0.70 | 1.13 |
| 13632 | 3 | oz | Leg, whole, rstd | 85 | 1.34 | 1.33 | 1.96 | 0.27 | 3.23 | 1.09 | 0.71 | 1.07 | 1.73 | 1.96 | 0.57 | 0.91 | 0.94 | 0.83 | 0.95 | 0.26 | 0.75 | 1.20 |
| 13638 | 1 | ea | Loin, steak, brld | 53 | 0.83 | 0.82 | 1.21 | 0.16 | 2.00 | 0.67 | 0.44 | 0.57 | 1.08 | 1.22 | 0.35 | 0.56 | 0.58 | 0.51 | 0.59 | 0.16 | 0.46 | 0.75 |
| 13637 | 1 | ea | Loin, steak, raw | 79 | 0.81 | 0.81 | 1.19 | 0.16 | 1.97 | 0.66 | 0.43 | 0.55 | 1.06 | 1.20 | 0.35 | 0.55 | 0.57 | 0.50 | 0.58 | 0.16 | 0.46 | 0.73 |
| 13641 | 3 | oz | Rib, brld | 85 | 1.18 | 1.16 | 1.73 | 0.23 | 2.85 | 0.96 | 0.62 | 0.94 | 1.52 | 1.73 | 0.50 | 0.80 | 0.82 | 0.73 | 0.84 | 0.23 | 0.66 | 1.05 |
| 13640 | 4 | oz | Rib, raw | 113 | 1.04 | 1.03 | 1.53 | 0.21 | 2.51 | 0.85 | 0.55 | 0.84 | 1.34 | 1.53 | 0.44 | 0.71 | 0.73 | 0.64 | 0.74 | 0.20 | 0.58 | 0.93 |
| 13642 | 3 | oz | Rib, rstd | 85 | 1.11 | 1.11 | 1.63 | 0.22 | 2.69 | 0.91 | 0.59 | 0.89 | 1.45 | 1.64 | 0.48 | 0.75 | 0.78 | 0.69 | 0.79 | 0.22 | 0.62 | 1.00 |
| 13648 | 3 | oz | Shoulder, arm, steak, brsd | 85 | 1.59 | 1.57 | 2.33 | 0.32 | 3.83 | 1.29 | 0.84 | 1.28 | 2.06 | 2.34 | 0.68 | 1.08 | 1.11 | 0.99 | 1.13 | 0.31 | 0.89 | 1.43 |
| 13649 | 3 | oz | Shoulder, arm, steak, brld | 85 | 1.28 | 1.26 | 1.86 | 0.25 | 3.08 | 1.04 | 0.67 | 1.02 | 1.65 | 1.87 | 0.54 | 0.86 | 0.89 | 0.79 | 0.91 | 0.25 | 0.71 | 1.14 |
| 13647 | 1 | ea | Shoulder, arm, steak, raw | 84 | 0.87 | 0.86 | 1.27 | 0.17 | 2.09 | 0.71 | 0.46 | 0.70 | 1.13 | 1.28 | 0.37 | 0.59 | 0.61 | 0.54 | 0.62 | 0.17 | 0.49 | 0.78 |
| 13652 | 3 | oz | Shoulder, blade, brsd | 85 | 1.48 | 1.46 | 2.17 | 0.29 | 3.57 | 1.20 | 0.78 | 1.19 | 1.91 | 2.17 | 0.63 | 1.00 | 1.03 | 0.92 | 1.05 | 0.29 | 0.83 | 1.33 |
| 13653 | 3 | oz | Shoulder, blade, brld | 85 | 1.20 | 1.19 | 1.76 | 0.24 | 2.90 | 0.98 | 0.63 | 0.96 | 1.56 | 1.76 | 0.51 | 0.81 | 0.84 | 0.74 | 0.86 | 0.23 | 0.67 | 1.08 |
| 13651 | 4 | oz | Shoulder, blade, raw | 113 | 1.15 | 1.14 | 1.69 | 0.23 | 2.79 | 0.94 | 0.61 | 0.93 | 1.49 | 1.69 | 0.49 | 0.78 | 0.81 | 0.71 | 0.82 | 0.22 | 0.65 | 1.04 |
| 13654 | 3 | oz | Shoulder, blade, rstd | 85 | 1.16 | 1.14 | 1.69 | 0.23 | 2.79 | 0.94 | 0.61 | 0.93 | 1.50 | 1.70 | 0.49 | 0.78 | 0.81 | 0.71 | 0.82 | 0.22 | 0.65 | 1.04 |
| 13644 | 3 | oz | Shoulder, whole, brsd | 85 | 1.50 | 1.49 | 2.20 | 0.30 | 3.64 | 1.22 | 0.79 | 1.21 | 1.95 | 2.21 | 0.64 | 1.02 | 1.05 | 0.94 | 1.07 | 0.29 | 0.84 | 1.35 |
| 13645 | 3 | oz | Shoulder, whole, brld | 85 | 1.22 | 1.21 | 1.78 | 0.24 | 2.94 | 0.99 | 0.64 | 0.98 | 1.57 | 1.79 | 0.52 | 0.82 | 0.85 | 0.75 | 0.87 | 0.24 | 0.68 | 1.10 |
| 13643 | 4 | oz | Shoulder, whole, raw | 113 | 1.16 | 1.14 | 1.69 | 0.23 | 2.80 | 0.94 | 0.61 | 0.93 | 1.50 | 1.71 | 0.49 | 0.79 | 0.81 | 0.72 | 0.82 | 0.22 | 0.65 | 1.04 |
| 13646 | 3 | oz | Shoulder, whole, rstd | 85 | 1.16 | 1.15 | 1.70 | 0.23 | 2.80 | 0.94 | 0.61 | 0.94 | 1.50 | 1.70 | 0.49 | 0.79 | 0.81 | 0.72 | 0.83 | 0.23 | 0.65 | 1.05 |
| | | | **MEATS—LUNCHMEATS AND SAUSAGES** | | | | | | | | | | | | | | | | | | | |
| | | | Beef Lunchmeat | | | | | | | | | | | | | | | | | | | |
| 13002 | 1 | pce | Bologna, avg | 23 | 0.20 | 0.17 | 0.27 | 0.04 | 0.45 | 0.23 | 0.09 | 0.12 | 0.20 | 0.21 | 0.06 | 0.10 | 0.20 | 0.11 | 0.10 | 0.03 | 0.09 | 0.12 |
| 13069 | 1 | pce | Bologna, lebanon, avg | 23 | 0.29 | 0.30 | 0.40 | 0.05 | 0.64 | 0.33 | 0.13 | 0.18 | 0.33 | 0.36 | 0.11 | 0.17 | 0.24 | 0.18 | 0.19 | 0.04 | 0.13 | 0.20 |
| 13100 | 1 | oz | Jellied, cured, avg | 28 | 0.37 | 0.37 | 0.45 | 0.06 | 0.74 | 0.50 | 0.14 | 0.20 | 0.37 | 0.41 | 0.12 | 0.19 | 0.35 | 0.21 | 0.21 | 0.04 | 0.14 | 0.23 |
| 13039 | 1 | pce | Loaf, corned beef, jellied, avg | 28 | 0.44 | 0.45 | 0.55 | 0.07 | 0.89 | 0.61 | 0.17 | 0.24 | 0.44 | 0.49 | 0.14 | 0.23 | 0.42 | 0.26 | 0.25 | 0.05 | 0.17 | 0.28 |
| 13038 | 1 | pce | Loaf, pork barbecue, avg | 23 | 0.20 | 0.22 | 0.32 | 0.05 | 0.58 | 0.19 | 0.12 | 0.17 | 0.29 | 0.30 | 0.09 | 0.15 | 0.21 | 0.16 | 0.16 | 0.04 | 0.12 | 0.18 |
| 13067 | 1 | pce | Loaf, slice, avg | 28 | 0.28 | 0.28 | 0.34 | 0.04 | 0.56 | 0.38 | 0.11 | 0.15 | 0.28 | 0.31 | 0.09 | 0.14 | 0.26 | 0.16 | 0.16 | 0.03 | 0.11 | 0.17 |
| 13101 | 1 | oz | Pastrami, avg | 28 | 0.34 | 0.30 | 0.47 | 0.06 | 0.78 | 0.40 | 0.15 | 0.21 | 0.35 | 0.36 | 0.11 | 0.17 | 0.34 | 0.19 | 0.18 | 0.04 | 0.16 | 0.21 |
| 13035 | 1 | pce | Salami, beerwurst, avg | 23 | 0.20 | 0.17 | 0.28 | 0.04 | 0.46 | 0.23 | 0.09 | 0.12 | 0.21 | 0.22 | 0.07 | 0.10 | 0.20 | 0.11 | 0.11 | 0.03 | 0.09 | 0.12 |
| 13023 | 1 | pce | Salami, ckd, avg | 23 | 0.25 | 0.21 | 0.33 | 0.04 | 0.56 | 0.29 | 0.11 | 0.15 | 0.25 | 0.26 | 0.08 | 0.12 | 0.25 | 0.14 | 0.13 | 0.03 | 0.11 | 0.15 |
| 13103 | 1 | oz | Smoked, chopped, cured, avg | 28 | 0.37 | 0.38 | 0.50 | 0.07 | 0.8[illegible] | 0.42 | 0.16 | 0.23 | 0.42 | 0.46 | 0.14 | 0.21 | 0.31 | 0.23 | 0.24 | 0.05 | 0.17 | 0.26 |
| 13000 | 6 | pce | Thin Sliced, avg | 25 | 0.47 | 0.47 | 0.63 | 0.08 | 1.0[illegible] | 0.52 | 0.20 | 0.29 | 0.52 | 0.57 | 0.17 | 0.26 | 0.38 | 0.29 | 0.29 | 0.06 | 0.21 | 0.32 |
| | | | Beef & Pork Lunchmeat | | | | | | | | | | | | | | | | | | | |
| 13032 | 1 | pce | Bologna, avg | 23 | 0.23 | 0.23 | 0.32 | 0.04 | 0.53 | 0.25 | 0.11 | 0.15 | 0.27 | 0.28 | 0.09 | 0.13 | 0.18 | 0.15 | 0.15 | 0.03 | 0.11 | 0.17 |
| 13048 | 1 | pce | Mortadella, avg | 15 | 0.17 | 0.15 | 0.24 | 0.03 | 0.39 | 0.20 | 0.08 | 0.11 | 0.18 | 0.19 | 0.06 | 0.09 | 0.16 | 0.10 | 0.09 | 0.02 | 0.08 | 0.11 |
| 13086 | 1 | pce | Mother's Loaf, avg | 21 | 0.14 | 0.17 | 0.24 | 0.04 | 0.43 | 0.12 | 0.10 | 0.12 | 0.21 | 0.22 | 0.07 | 0.11 | 0.13 | 0.11 | 0.11 | 0.03 | 0.08 | 0.12 |
| 13087 | 1 | pce | Picnic Loaf, avg | 28 | 0.25 | 0.25 | 0.37 | 0.05 | 0.63 | 0.27 | 0.12 | 0.16 | 0.32 | 0.33 | 0.11 | 0.15 | 0.24 | 0.18 | 0.18 | 0.04 | 0.13 | 0.18 |
| 13024 | 1 | pce | Salami, ckd, avg | 28 | 0.25 | 0.24 | 0.36 | 0.05 | 0.54 | 0.33 | 0.10 | 0.19 | 0.26 | 0.31 | 0.08 | 0.13 | 0.23 | 0.15 | 0.15 | 0.03 | 0.15 | 0.19 |
| 13026 | 3 | pce | Salami, dry, avg | 30 | 0.44 | 0.46 | 0.62 | 0.08 | 1.01 | 0.49 | 0.21 | 0.29 | 0.52 | 0.55 | 0.18 | 0.26 | 0.36 | 0.28 | 0.29 | 0.06 | 0.21 | 0.32 |
| 13046 | 1 | pce | Sausage, avg | 23 | 0.22 | 0.25 | 0.35 | 0.06 | 0.47 | 0.26 | 0.11 | 0.17 | 0.28 | 0.32 | 0.08 | 0.14 | 0.19 | 0.14 | 0.15 | 0.04 | 0.13 | 0.19 |
| 13094 | 1 | pce | Chicken roll, light meat, avg | 28 | 0.31 | 0.34 | 0.49 | 0.07 | 0.81 | 0.32 | 0.16 | 0.28 | 0.40 | 0.45 | 0.15 | 0.21 | 0.25 | 0.19 | 0.23 | 0.06 | 0.18 | 0.27 |
| | | | Frankfurters | | | | | | | | | | | | | | | | | | | |
| 13008 | 1 | ea | Beef, avg | 57 | 0.49 | 0.42 | 0.67 | 0.09 | 1.10 | 0.56 | 0.22 | 0.29 | 0.50 | 0.52 | 0.16 | 0.24 | 0.49 | 0.27 | 0.25 | 0.06 | 0.22 | 0.30 |
| 13009 | 1 | ea | Beef & Pork, avg | 57 | 0.44 | 0.48 | 0.64 | 0.07 | 1.05 | 0.47 | 0.20 | 0.28 | 0.47 | 0.52 | 0.13 | 0.20 | 0.31 | 0.26 | 0.23 | 0.05 | 0.18 | 0.27 |

TABLE A **Amino Acid Content for Selected Foods *(continued)***

| Code | Amount | Description | Weight (g) | Alanine (g) | Arginine (g) | Aspartic acid (g) | Cystine (g) | Glutamic acid (g) | Glycine (g) | Histidine (g) | Isoleucine (g) | Leucine (g) | Lysine (g) | Methionine (g) | Phenylalanine (g) | Proline (g) | Serine (g) | Threonine (g) | Tryptophan (g) | Tyrosine (g) | Valine (g) |
|---|---|---|---|---|---|---|---|---|---|---|---|---|---|---|---|---|---|---|---|---|---|
| 13260 | 1 ea | Chicken, avg | 45 | 0.40 | 0.40 | 0.59 | 0.06 | 0.92 | 0.45 | 0.16 | 0.20 | 0.45 | 0.49 | 0.15 | 0.23 | 0.31 | 0.27 | 0.26 | 0.05 | 0.17 | 0.24 |
| 13012 | 1 ea | Turkey, avg | 45 | 0.42 | 0.42 | 0.65 | 0.05 | 1.07 | 0.37 | 0.24 | 0.24 | 0.52 | 0.55 | 0.18 | 0.26 | 0.31 | 0.30 | 0.31 | 0.05 | 0.23 | 0.26 |
| | | Ham/Pork Lunchmeat | | | | | | | | | | | | | | | | | | | |
| 13042 | 1 pce | Cheese Loaf, avg | 28 | 0.26 | 0.31 | 0.43 | 0.07 | 0.74 | 0.21 | 0.19 | 0.21 | 0.38 | 0.42 | 0.12 | 0.19 | 0.22 | 0.19 | 0.20 | 0.06 | 0.16 | 0.22 |
| 13057 | 1 pce | Chopped, sliced, avg | 21 | 0.21 | 0.25 | 0.35 | 0.05 | 0.54 | 0.17 | 0.15 | 0.16 | 0.29 | 0.32 | 0.09 | 0.14 | 0.15 | 0.14 | 0.16 | 0.04 | 0.11 | 0.17 |
| 13033 | 1 ea | Cured, patty, grilled, avg | 60 | 0.47 | 0.51 | 0.75 | 0.11 | 1.28 | 0.41 | 0.29 | 0.35 | 0.63 | 0.68 | 0.21 | 0.34 | 0.34 | 0.32 | 0.36 | 0.09 | 0.26 | 0.35 |
| 13261 | 1 pce | Extra Lean, 5% fat, sliced, avg | 28 | 0.32 | 0.35 | 0.51 | 0.08 | 0.88 | 0.28 | 0.19 | 0.24 | 0.43 | 0.46 | 0.14 | 0.23 | 0.23 | 0.22 | 0.24 | 0.06 | 0.18 | 0.23 |
| 13013 | 1 pce | Minced, avg | 21 | 0.20 | 0.21 | 0.31 | 0.04 | 0.49 | 0.19 | 0.13 | 0.15 | 0.26 | 0.29 | 0.10 | 0.13 | 0.15 | 0.14 | 0.15 | 0.03 | 0.11 | 0.16 |
| 13049 | 1 pce | Olive Loaf, avg | 28 | 0.17 | 0.16 | 0.27 | 0.04 | 0.54 | 0.19 | 0.08 | 0.12 | 0.24 | 0.23 | 0.08 | 0.12 | 0.23 | 0.14 | 0.13 | 0.03 | 0.11 | 0.14 |
| 13263 | 1 pce | Regular, 11% fat, avg | 28 | 0.29 | 0.32 | 0.46 | 0.07 | 0.80 | 0.26 | 0.18 | 0.22 | 0.39 | 0.42 | 0.13 | 0.21 | 0.21 | 0.20 | 0.22 | 0.06 | 0.16 | 0.21 |
| 13031 | 1 pce | Salami, beerwurst, avg | 23 | 0.18 | 0.19 | 0.28 | 0.02 | 0.49 | 0.18 | 0.10 | 0.11 | 0.22 | 0.24 | 0.08 | 0.10 | 0.15 | 0.13 | 0.13 | 0.03 | 0.09 | 0.12 |
| 13090 | 3 pce | Salami, dry, avg | 30 | 0.40 | 0.41 | 0.63 | 0.09 | 1.15 | 0.47 | 0.18 | 0.32 | 0.49 | 0.56 | 0.14 | 0.28 | 0.40 | 0.27 | 0.30 | 0.08 | 0.21 | 0.34 |
| 13083 | 1 pce | Liver Cheese Lunchmeat, avg | 38 | 0.35 | 0.31 | 0.51 | 0.12 | 0.70 | 0.36 | 0.15 | 0.24 | 0.51 | 0.45 | 0.13 | 0.27 | 0.27 | 0.26 | 0.25 | 0.08 | 0.18 | 0.31 |
| 13019 | 1 pce | Liverwurst Lunchmeat, avg | 18 | 0.15 | 0.15 | 0.21 | 0.03 | 0.39 | 0.20 | 0.08 | 0.12 | 0.20 | 0.21 | 0.05 | 0.11 | 0.15 | 0.12 | 0.12 | 0.03 | 0.06 | 0.15 |
| 13021 | 5 pce | Pepperoni, avg | 28 | 0.39 | 0.38 | 0.55 | 0.07 | 0.91 | 0.44 | 0.19 | 0.25 | 0.44 | 0.46 | 0.15 | 0.22 | 0.34 | 0.24 | 0.24 | 0.06 | 0.19 | 0.27 |
| 13096 | 1 Tbs | Pate, Chicken Liver, avg | 13 | 0.10 | 0.11 | 0.16 | 0.03 | 0.25 | 0.09 | 0.05 | 0.10 | 0.16 | 0.12 | 0.04 | 0.09 | 0.09 | 0.09 | 0.08 | 0.03 | 0.06 | 0.11 |
| 13265 | 1 Tbs | Pate, Goose Liver, smkd, avg | 13 | 0.09 | 0.09 | 0.14 | 0.02 | 0.19 | 0.09 | 0.04 | 0.08 | 0.13 | 0.11 | 0.04 | 0.07 | 0.07 | 0.06 | 0.07 | 0.02 | 0.05 | 0.09 |
| 13050 | 1 pce | Peppered Loaf Lunchmeat, avg | 28 | 0.28 | 0.33 | 0.46 | 0.07 | 0.74 | 0.25 | 0.18 | 0.22 | 0.39 | 0.42 | 0.13 | 0.19 | 0.23 | 0.20 | 0.21 | 0.06 | 0.15 | 0.23 |
| 13051 | 1 pce | Pickle/Pimiento Loaf Lunchmeat, w/pork, avg | 28 | 0.19 | 0.19 | 0.29 | 0.03 | 0.54 | 0.21 | 0.10 | 0.14 | 0.27 | 0.25 | 0.07 | 0.12 | 0.23 | 0.16 | 0.15 | 0.03 | 0.11 | 0.16 |
| | | Sausages | | | | | | | | | | | | | | | | | | | |
| 13102 | 1 ea | Beef, link, smoked, avg | 43 | 0.43 | 0.37 | 0.59 | 0.08 | 0.98 | 0.50 | 0.19 | 0.26 | 0.44 | 0.46 | 0.14 | 0.22 | 0.43 | 0.24 | 0.23 | 0.05 | 0.20 | 0.26 |
| 13028 | 1 ea | Beef & Pork, link, smkd, avg | 16 | 0.12 | 0.12 | 0.18 | 0.02 | 0.32 | 0.14 | 0.06 | 0.08 | 0.13 | 0.14 | 0.06 | 0.06 | 0.11 | 0.08 | 0.07 | 0.02 | 0.06 | 0.07 |
| 13089 | 1 ea | Beef & Pork, patty, ckd, avg | 27 | 0.22 | 0.23 | 0.32 | 0.04 | 0.54 | 0.24 | 0.11 | 0.14 | 0.26 | 0.29 | 0.09 | 0.13 | 0.18 | 0.14 | 0.15 | 0.04 | 0.11 | 0.16 |
| 13001 | 1 pce | Berliner, avg | 23 | 0.22 | 0.24 | 0.34 | 0.05 | 0.54 | 0.20 | 0.14 | 0.16 | 0.28 | 0.30 | 0.09 | 0.14 | 0.17 | 0.14 | 0.15 | 0.04 | 0.11 | 0.16 |
| 13077 | 1 pce | Blood, avg | 25 | 0.26 | 0.17 | 0.34 | 0.05 | 0.53 | 0.23 | 0.18 | 0.08 | 0.35 | 0.26 | 0.05 | 0.21 | 0.25 | 0.17 | 0.14 | 0.05 | 0.09 | 0.26 |
| 13078 | 1 ea | Bockwurst, link, avg | 65 | 0.49 | 0.53 | 0.77 | 0.10 | 1.26 | 0.47 | 0.26 | 0.38 | 0.61 | 0.68 | 0.21 | 0.32 | 0.39 | 0.36 | 0.36 | 0.09 | 0.28 | 0.40 |
| 13079 | 1 ea | Bratwurst, link, ckd, avg | 85 | 0.67 | 0.71 | 0.99 | 0.12 | 1.66 | 0.73 | 0.35 | 0.44 | 0.80 | 0.91 | 0.29 | 0.40 | 0.56 | 0.46 | 0.47 | 0.10 | 0.35 | 0.48 |
| 13066 | 1 pce | Braunschweiger, avg | 28 | 0.21 | 0.21 | 0.32 | 0.07 | 0.46 | 0.25 | 0.09 | 0.14 | 0.29 | 0.25 | 0.09 | 0.15 | 0.21 | 0.16 | 0.15 | 0.04 | 0.12 | 0.17 |
| 13036 | 1 ea | Brotwurst, link, avg | 70 | 0.65 | 0.66 | 0.90 | 0.11 | 1.48 | 0.72 | 0.31 | 0.42 | 0.76 | 0.80 | 0.26 | 0.38 | 0.52 | 0.41 | 0.42 | 0.09 | 0.31 | 0.47 |
| 13070 | 1 ea | Chorizo, link, avg | 60 | 0.89 | 0.96 | 1.25 | 0.16 | 2.04 | 0.99 | 0.41 | 1.26 | 0.98 | 1.38 | 0.27 | 0.66 | 0.71 | 0.57 | 0.84 | 0.16 | 0.43 | 0.52 |
| 13015 | 1 ea | Italian, link, ckd, avg | 67 | 0.75 | 0.79 | 1.12 | 0.13 | 1.86 | 0.81 | 0.39 | 0.49 | 0.90 | 1.02 | 0.33 | 0.45 | 0.62 | 0.52 | 0.53 | 0.11 | 0.39 | 0.54 |
| 13082 | 1 ea | Italian, link, raw, avg | 102 | 0.81 | 0.86 | 1.21 | 0.15 | 2.01 | 0.88 | 0.42 | 0.53 | 0.98 | 1.10 | 0.35 | 0.49 | 0.68 | 0.56 | 0.57 | 0.12 | 0.42 | 0.58 |
| 13043 | 1 pce | Kielbasa, avg | 26 | 0.22 | 0.24 | 0.32 | 0.06 | 0.42 | 0.27 | 0.08 | 0.17 | 0.23 | 0.26 | 0.07 | 0.13 | 0.18 | 0.14 | 0.11 | 0.04 | 0.13 | 0.17 |
| 13044 | 1 ea | Knockwurst, link, avg | 68 | 0.46 | 0.48 | 0.69 | 0.10 | 1.10 | 0.48 | 0.25 | 0.32 | 0.56 | 0.63 | 0.20 | 0.28 | 0.37 | 0.32 | 0.33 | 0.07 | 0.25 | 0.35 |
| 13016 | 1 ea | Pork, link, ckd | 13 | 0.14 | 0.15 | 0.21 | 0.03 | 0.35 | 0.15 | 0.07 | 0.09 | 0.17 | 0.19 | 0.06 | 0.09 | 0.12 | 0.10 | 0.10 | 0.02 | 0.07 | 0.10 |
| 13266 | 1 ea | Pork, patty, ckd, avg | 27 | 0.30 | 0.31 | 0.44 | 0.05 | 0.73 | 0.32 | 0.15 | 0.19 | 0.36 | 0.40 | 0.13 | 0.18 | 0.25 | 0.21 | 0.21 | 0.04 | 0.15 | 0.21 |
| 13068 | 1 ea | Pork, patty, raw, avg | 57 | 0.37 | 0.39 | 0.55 | 0.07 | 0.92 | 0.40 | 0.19 | 0.24 | 0.45 | 0.51 | 0.16 | 0.22 | 0.31 | 0.26 | 0.26 | 0.05 | 0.19 | 0.27 |
| 13022 | 1 ea | Pork, polish, avg | 227 | 2.05 | 2.10 | 2.93 | 0.36 | 4.81 | 2.25 | 1.01 | 1.39 | 2.45 | 2.52 | 0.86 | 1.22 | 1.62 | 1.33 | 1.34 | 0.31 | 1.01 | 1.54 |
| 13027 | 1 ea | Pork, smoked, link, avg | 68 | 0.97 | 0.99 | 1.38 | 0.17 | 2.26 | 1.06 | 0.48 | 0.65 | 1.15 | 1.19 | 0.41 | 0.58 | 0.76 | 0.62 | 0.63 | 0.15 | 0.48 | 0.73 |
| 13030 | 1 pce | Thuringer Summer, beef & pork, avg | 23 | 0.26 | 0.22 | 0.35 | 0.05 | 0.58 | 0.30 | 0.11 | 0.16 | 0.26 | 0.28 | 0.08 | 0.13 | 0.26 | 0.14 | 0.14 | 0.03 | 0.12 | 0.16 |
| 13054 | 1 ea | Vienna, beef & pork, cnd, avg | 16 | 0.10 | 0.11 | 0.16 | 0.03 | 0.21 | 0.16 | 0.04 | 0.09 | 0.13 | 0.13 | 0.04 | 0.07 | 0.10 | 0.07 | 0.06 | 0.02 | 0.05 | 0.09 |
| | | Spreads | | | | | | | | | | | | | | | | | | | |
| 13095 | 1 Tbs | Chicken, cnd, avg | 13 | 0.11 | 0.12 | 0.18 | 0.03 | 0.30 | 0.10 | 0.06 | 0.10 | 0.15 | 0.17 | 0.06 | 0.08 | 0.09 | 0.07 | 0.08 | 0.02 | 0.07 | 0.10 |
| 13034 | 1 Tbs | Ham Salad, avg | 15 | 0.08 | 0.09 | 0.13 | 0.01 | 0.20 | 0.07 | 0.05 | 0.06 | 0.11 | 0.12 | 0.03 | 0.05 | 0.06 | 0.06 | 0.06 | 0.01 | 0.04 | 0.07 |
| 13045 | 1 pce | Luncheon Meat, cnd, avg | 21 | 0.18 | 0.18 | 0.24 | 0.04 | 0.39 | 0.23 | 0.08 | 0.12 | 0.20 | 0.20 | 0.07 | 0.10 | 0.14 | 0.10 | 0.10 | 0.03 | 0.08 | 0.14 |

TABLE A **Amino Acid Content for Selected Foods *(continued)***

| Code | Amount | | Description | Weight (g) | Alanine (g) | Arginine (g) | Aspartic acid (g) | Cystine (g) | Glutamic acid (g) | Glycine (g) | Histidine (g) | Isoleucine (g) | Leucine (g) | Lysine (g) | Methionine (g) | Phenylalanine (g) | Proline (g) | Serine (g) | Threonine (g) | Tryptophan (g) | Tyrosine (g) | Valine (g) |
|---|---|---|---|---|---|---|---|---|---|---|---|---|---|---|---|---|---|---|---|---|---|---|
| 13056 | 1 | Tbs | Pork & Beef, avg | 15 | 0.07 | 0.08 | 0.11 | 0.02 | 0.17 | 0.07 | 0.04 | 0.05 | 0.09 | 0.10 | 0.03 | 0.05 | 0.05 | 0.05 | 0.05 | 0.01 | 0.04 | 0.05 |
| 13268 | 1 | Tbs | Poultry Salad, avg | 13 | 0.09 | 0.10 | 0.14 | 0.02 | 0.23 | 0.09 | 0.05 | 0.08 | 0.11 | 0.13 | 0.04 | 0.06 | 0.07 | 0.06 | 0.06 | 0.02 | 0.05 | 0.08 |
| | | | Turkey Lunchmeat | | | | | | | | | | | | | | | | | | | |
| 13007 | 1 | pce | Bologna, avg | 28 | 0.25 | 0.25 | 0.39 | 0.03 | 0.64 | 0.22 | 0.14 | 0.14 | 0.31 | 0.33 | 0.11 | 0.16 | 0.19 | 0.18 | 0.18 | 0.03 | 0.14 | 0.16 |
| 13020 | 1 | pce | Pastrami, avg | 28 | 0.33 | 0.36 | 0.49 | 0.06 | 0.81 | 0.31 | 0.15 | 0.26 | 0.40 | 0.46 | 0.14 | 0.20 | 0.24 | 0.22 | 0.22 | 0.06 | 0.19 | 0.26 |
| 13025 | 1 | pce | Salami, ckd, avg | 28 | 0.29 | 0.32 | 0.44 | 0.05 | 0.72 | 0.27 | 0.14 | 0.23 | 0.35 | 0.41 | 0.13 | 0.18 | 0.21 | 0.20 | 0.20 | 0.05 | 0.17 | 0.24 |
| | | | **MEATS—PORK AND HAM** | | | | | | | | | | | | | | | | | | | |
| | | | Bacon | | | | | | | | | | | | | | | | | | | |
| 12002 | 1 | pce | Canadian, grilled | 23 | 0.28 | 0.30 | 0.46 | 0.07 | 0.77 | 0.24 | 0.20 | 0.21 | 0.39 | 0.44 | 0.15 | 0.18 | 0.21 | 0.21 | 0.22 | 0.06 | 0.17 | 0.22 |
| 12008 | 1 | pce | Canadian, unheated | 28 | 0.29 | 0.32 | 0.48 | 0.07 | 0.80 | 0.25 | 0.21 | 0.22 | 0.41 | 0.46 | 0.16 | 0.19 | 0.22 | 0.22 | 0.23 | 0.06 | 0.17 | 0.23 |
| 12000 | 4 | pce | Cooked | 32 | 0.55 | 0.60 | 0.80 | 0.10 | 1.34 | 0.70 | 0.28 | 0.40 | 0.68 | 0.72 | 0.22 | 0.37 | 0.52 | 0.37 | 0.37 | 0.09 | 0.28 | 0.47 |
| 12165 | 2 | pce | Raw | 57 | 0.28 | 0.30 | 0.41 | 0.05 | 0.68 | 0.35 | 0.14 | 0.20 | 0.34 | 0.37 | 0.11 | 0.19 | 0.26 | 0.19 | 0.19 | 0.05 | 0.14 | 0.24 |
| | | | Fat | | | | | | | | | | | | | | | | | | | |
| 12100 | 1 | Tbs | Cooked | 9 | 0.08 | 0.10 | 0.08 | 0.01 | 0.10 | 0.18 | 0.01 | 0.03 | 0.07 | 0.09 | 0.02 | 0.04 | 0.12 | 0.05 | 0.03 | 0.00 | 0.02 | 0.05 |
| 12153 | 1 | oz | Raw | 28 | 0.03 | 0.05 | 0.05 | 0.00 | 0.08 | 0.02 | 0.01 | 0.01 | 0.03 | 0.04 | 0.01 | 0.02 | 0.02 | 0.02 | 0.02 | 0.00 | 0.01 | 0.02 |
| 12171 | 1 | oz | Salt Pork, raw | 28 | 0.08 | 0.15 | 0.12 | 0.01 | 0.19 | 0.10 | 0.02 | 0.04 | 0.10 | 0.12 | 0.02 | 0.05 | 0.08 | 0.05 | 0.05 | 0.00 | 0.02 | 0.07 |
| | | | Ham, Cured | | | | | | | | | | | | | | | | | | | |
| 12212 | 3 | oz | Boneless, 5% fat, rstd | 85 | 1.05 | 1.16 | 1.68 | 0.27 | 2.90 | 0.93 | 0.64 | 0.78 | 1.41 | 1.51 | 0.47 | 0.77 | 0.76 | 0.73 | 0.79 | 0.21 | 0.58 | 0.77 |
| 12307 | 3 | oz | Boneless, 8% fat, rstd | 85 | 1.02 | 1.12 | 1.63 | 0.26 | 2.81 | 0.89 | 0.62 | 0.75 | 1.37 | 1.46 | 0.45 | 0.74 | 0.74 | 0.71 | 0.77 | 0.21 | 0.56 | 0.75 |
| 12211 | 3 | oz | Boneless, 11% fat, rstd | 85 | 0.99 | 1.10 | 1.60 | 0.25 | 2.75 | 0.88 | 0.60 | 0.74 | 1.33 | 1.43 | 0.45 | 0.73 | 0.72 | 0.69 | 0.75 | 0.20 | 0.55 | 0.73 |
| 12209 | 3 | oz | Canned, 4% fat, rstd | 85 | 1.03 | 1.11 | 1.66 | 0.21 | 2.65 | 0.88 | 0.71 | 0.77 | 1.40 | 1.55 | 0.47 | 0.69 | 0.76 | 0.70 | 0.80 | 0.20 | 0.59 | 0.81 |
| 12226 | 3 | oz | Canned, 7% fat, rstd | 85 | 1.02 | 1.11 | 1.64 | 0.21 | 2.63 | 0.88 | 0.70 | 0.77 | 1.39 | 1.53 | 0.46 | 0.69 | 0.76 | 0.69 | 0.79 | 0.20 | 0.58 | 0.80 |
| 12168 | 3 | oz | Canned, 13% fat, rstd | 85 | 0.99 | 1.08 | 1.62 | 0.21 | 2.58 | 0.86 | 0.69 | 0.75 | 1.36 | 1.50 | 0.45 | 0.67 | 0.74 | 0.68 | 0.78 | 0.20 | 0.57 | 0.78 |
| 12169 | 1 | ea | Patty, 28% fat, unheated | 65 | 0.49 | 0.54 | 0.79 | 0.11 | 1.33 | 0.43 | 0.30 | 0.36 | 0.66 | 0.71 | 0.22 | 0.35 | 0.35 | 0.34 | 0.37 | 0.10 | 0.27 | 0.36 |
| 12175 | 3 | oz | Shoulder arm picnic, 7% fat, rstd | 85 | 1.25 | 1.38 | 2.01 | 0.32 | 3.46 | 1.11 | 0.75 | 0.93 | 1.68 | 1.80 | 0.56 | 0.92 | 0.91 | 0.87 | 0.94 | 0.25 | 0.70 | 0.92 |
| 12174 | 3 | oz | Shoulder arm picnic, 21% fat, rstd | 85 | 0.93 | 1.19 | 1.49 | 0.25 | 2.56 | 0.81 | 0.58 | 0.73 | 1.36 | 1.47 | 0.44 | 0.74 | 0.67 | 0.64 | 0.75 | 0.19 | 0.54 | 0.76 |
| 12177 | 3 | oz | Shoulder blade roll, 24% fat, rstd | 85 | 0.87 | 0.95 | 1.39 | 0.22 | 2.40 | 0.76 | 0.53 | 0.64 | 1.16 | 1.25 | 0.39 | 0.63 | 0.63 | 0.60 | 0.65 | 0.18 | 0.48 | 0.64 |
| 12006 | 3 | oz | Whole, 6% fat, rstd | 85 | 1.26 | 1.39 | 2.01 | 0.32 | 3.47 | 1.11 | 0.76 | 0.94 | 1.69 | 1.80 | 0.56 | 0.92 | 0.91 | 0.88 | 0.94 | 0.26 | 0.70 | 0.93 |
| 12005 | 3 | oz | Whole, 17% fat, rstd | 85 | 1.00 | 1.24 | 1.62 | 0.27 | 2.78 | 0.88 | 0.62 | 0.78 | 1.45 | 1.56 | 0.47 | 0.78 | 0.73 | 0.70 | 0.80 | 0.21 | 0.58 | 0.80 |
| | | | Pork | | | | | | | | | | | | | | | | | | | |
| 12259 | 4 | oz | Back Ribs, raw | 113 | 1.06 | 1.13 | 1.69 | 0.23 | 2.85 | 0.86 | 0.73 | 0.85 | 1.46 | 1.64 | 0.48 | 0.73 | 0.73 | 0.75 | 0.83 | 0.23 | 0.64 | 0.99 |
| 12097 | 3 | oz | Back Ribs, rstd | 85 | 1.20 | 1.28 | 1.91 | 0.26 | 3.23 | 0.98 | 0.82 | 0.97 | 1.66 | 1.85 | 0.55 | 0.82 | 0.83 | 0.85 | 0.94 | 0.26 | 0.72 | 1.12 |
| 12046 | 1 | ea | Chop, center rib, raw | 98 | 1.17 | 1.25 | 1.81 | 0.25 | 3.05 | 1.03 | 0.77 | 0.91 | 1.58 | 1.76 | 0.51 | 0.79 | 0.84 | 0.82 | 0.89 | 0.24 | 0.68 | 1.07 |
| 12050 | 3 | oz | Chop, center rib, rstd | 85 | 1.37 | 1.47 | 2.14 | 0.29 | 3.60 | 1.21 | 0.91 | 1.08 | 1.86 | 2.09 | 0.61 | 0.93 | 0.99 | 0.96 | 1.05 | 0.29 | 0.80 | 1.26 |
| 12309 | 3 | oz | Composite Cuts, ckd | 85 | 1.37 | 1.47 | 2.17 | 0.30 | 3.65 | 1.16 | 0.93 | 1.09 | 1.88 | 2.11 | 0.62 | 0.94 | 0.96 | 0.97 | 1.06 | 0.29 | 0.81 | 1.27 |
| 12118 | 3 | oz | Composite Cuts, lean, ckd | 85 | 1.45 | 1.55 | 2.31 | 0.32 | 3.89 | 1.18 | 0.99 | 1.16 | 2.00 | 2.24 | 0.66 | 0.99 | 1.00 | 1.03 | 1.14 | 0.32 | 0.87 | 1.35 |
| 12137 | 4 | oz | Composite Cuts, lean, raw | 113 | 1.39 | 1.48 | 2.20 | 0.30 | 3.73 | 1.13 | 0.95 | 1.12 | 1.91 | 2.15 | 0.63 | 0.95 | 0.96 | 0.98 | 1.09 | 0.30 | 0.83 | 1.29 |
| 12308 | 4 | oz | Composite Cuts, raw | 113 | 1.25 | 1.36 | 1.97 | 0.27 | 3.30 | 1.11 | 0.83 | 0.99 | 1.71 | 1.92 | 0.56 | 0.85 | 0.91 | 0.88 | 0.97 | 0.26 | 0.73 | 1.15 |
| 12099 | 3 | oz | Ground, ckd | 85 | 1.28 | 1.36 | 2.02 | 0.28 | 3.42 | 1.04 | 0.88 | 1.02 | 1.75 | 1.96 | 0.58 | 0.88 | 0.88 | 0.90 | 0.99 | 0.28 | 0.76 | 1.18 |
| 12281 | 4 | oz | Ground, raw | 113 | 1.11 | 1.19 | 1.77 | 0.24 | 2.98 | 0.91 | 0.76 | 0.89 | 1.53 | 1.72 | 0.51 | 0.76 | 0.77 | 0.79 | 0.87 | 0.24 | 0.66 | 1.04 |
| 12215 | 4 | oz | Leg, ham, raw | 113 | 1.16 | 1.27 | 1.79 | 0.24 | 2.98 | 1.12 | 0.74 | 0.89 | 1.56 | 1.75 | 0.50 | 0.78 | 0.89 | 0.81 | 0.88 | 0.24 | 0.66 | 1.05 |
| 12016 | 3 | oz | Leg, ham, rstd | 85 | 1.35 | 1.46 | 2.08 | 0.28 | 3.47 | 1.27 | 0.87 | 1.04 | 1.80 | 2.03 | 0.58 | 0.90 | 1.02 | 0.94 | 1.02 | 0.28 | 0.77 | 1.22 |
| 12182 | 1 | ea | Loin Chop, raw | 110 | 1.04 | 1.13 | 1.57 | 0.21 | 2.60 | 1.05 | 0.64 | 0.78 | 1.36 | 1.54 | 0.44 | 0.69 | 0.82 | 0.72 | 0.77 | 0.20 | 0.57 | 0.93 |
| 12022 | 3 | oz | Loin Chop, rstd | 85 | 1.20 | 1.31 | 1.82 | 0.25 | 3.02 | 1.21 | 0.75 | 0.90 | 1.58 | 1.78 | 0.51 | 0.80 | 0.94 | 0.83 | 0.89 | 0.24 | 0.67 | 1.07 |
| 12269 | 4 | oz | Ribs, country style, raw | 113 | 1.13 | 1.23 | 1.75 | 0.24 | 2.93 | 1.06 | 0.73 | 0.87 | 1.53 | 1.72 | 0.49 | 0.76 | 0.85 | 0.79 | 0.86 | 0.23 | 0.65 | 1.03 |
| 12235 | 3 | oz | Ribs, country style, rstd | 85 | 1.16 | 1.24 | 1.84 | 0.25 | 3.11 | 0.94 | 0.79 | 0.94 | 1.60 | 1.78 | 0.53 | 0.79 | 0.80 | 0.82 | 0.91 | 0.25 | 0.69 | 1.08 |
| 12042 | 1 | ea | Roast, center loin, raw | 112 | 1.32 | 1.42 | 2.07 | 0.28 | 3.47 | 1.18 | 0.88 | 1.04 | 1.79 | 2.02 | 0.59 | 0.90 | 0.96 | 0.93 | 1.02 | 0.28 | 0.77 | 1.21 |
| 12045 | 3 | oz | Roast, center loin, rstd | 85 | 1.32 | 1.41 | 2.06 | 0.28 | 3.44 | 1.16 | 0.87 | 1.03 | 1.78 | 2.00 | 0.58 | 0.89 | 0.95 | 0.93 | 1.01 | 0.28 | 0.76 | 1.21 |
| 12141 | 1 | ea | Roast, sirloin, raw | 107 | 1.21 | 1.31 | 1.88 | 0.26 | 3.16 | 1.08 | 0.80 | 0.94 | 1.64 | 1.84 | 0.53 | 0.82 | 0.88 | 0.85 | 0.93 | 0.25 | 0.70 | 1.10 |
| 12106 | 3 | oz | Roast, sirloin, rstd | 85 | 1.35 | 1.44 | 2.15 | 0.29 | 3.62 | 1.10 | 0.93 | 1.09 | 1.86 | 2.08 | 0.61 | 0.93 | 0.93 | 0.96 | 1.05 | 0.29 | 0.81 | 1.26 |

TABLE A **Amino Acid Content for Selected Foods *(continued)***

| Code | Amount | | Description | Weight (g) | Alanine (g) | Arginine (g) | Aspartic acid (g) | Cystine (g) | Glutamic acid (g) | Glycine (g) | Histidine (g) | Isoleucine (g) | Leucine (g) | Lysine (g) | Methionine (g) | Phenylalanine (g) | Proline (g) | Serine (g) | Threonine (g) | Tryptophan (g) | Tyrosine (g) | Valine (g) |
|---|---|---|---|---|---|---|---|---|---|---|---|---|---|---|---|---|---|---|---|---|---|---|
| 12285 | 4 | oz | Roast, top loin, raw | 113 | 1.34 | 1.45 | 2.10 | 0.29 | 3.54 | 1.18 | 0.89 | 1.06 | 1.82 | 2.05 | 0.60 | 0.91 | 0.97 | 0.94 | 1.03 | 0.28 | 0.78 | 1.23 |
| 12060 | 3 | oz | Roast, top loin, rstd | 85 | 1.43 | 1.52 | 2.27 | 0.31 | 3.83 | 1.16 | 0.98 | 1.15 | 1.96 | 2.20 | 0.65 | 0.98 | 0.99 | 1.01 | 1.12 | 0.31 | 0.85 | 1.33 |
| 12258 | 4 | oz | Spareribs, raw | 113 | 1.13 | 1.20 | 1.80 | 0.25 | 3.03 | 0.92 | 0.77 | 0.90 | 1.55 | 1.74 | 0.51 | 0.77 | 0.78 | 0.80 | 0.88 | 0.25 | 0.67 | 1.05 |
| 12010 | 3 | oz | Spareribs, brsd | 85 | 1.44 | 1.54 | 2.30 | 0.32 | 3.87 | 1.17 | 0.99 | 1.16 | 1.98 | 2.22 | 0.65 | 0.99 | 0.99 | 1.02 | 1.13 | 0.31 | 0.86 | 1.34 |
| 12289 | 1 | ea | Steak, boston blade, raw | 228 | 2.37 | 2.55 | 3.69 | 0.50 | 6.18 | 2.14 | 1.56 | 1.85 | 3.19 | 3.60 | 1.04 | 1.60 | 1.74 | 1.66 | 1.81 | 0.49 | 1.37 | 2.17 |
| 12115 | 3 | oz | Steak, boston blade, rstd | 85 | 1.16 | 1.25 | 1.80 | 0.25 | 3.01 | 1.05 | 0.76 | 0.90 | 1.56 | 1.75 | 0.51 | 0.78 | 0.85 | 0.81 | 0.88 | 0.24 | 0.67 | 1.05 |
| 12238 | 3 | oz | Tenderloin, rstd | 85 | 1.38 | 1.48 | 2.18 | 0.30 | 3.69 | 1.15 | 0.94 | 1.11 | 1.90 | 2.13 | 0.62 | 0.94 | 0.96 | 0.98 | 1.08 | 0.30 | 0.82 | 1.28 |
| 12221 | 4 | oz | Whole Shoulder, raw | 113 | 1.15 | 1.24 | 1.77 | 0.24 | 2.95 | 1.08 | 0.74 | 0.88 | 1.54 | 1.73 | 0.50 | 0.77 | 0.86 | 0.80 | 0.87 | 0.24 | 0.65 | 1.04 |
| 12109 | 3 | oz | Whole Shoulder, rstd | 85 | 1.17 | 1.28 | 1.79 | 0.24 | 2.99 | 1.13 | 0.75 | 0.89 | 1.56 | 1.76 | 0.50 | 0.78 | 0.90 | 0.82 | 0.88 | 0.24 | 0.66 | 1.05 |
| | | | MEATS—VEAL | | | | | | | | | | | | | | | | | | | |
| 11553 | 1 | oz | Fat, cooked | 28 | 0.16 | 0.16 | 0.23 | 0.03 | 0.42 | 0.14 | 0.10 | 0.13 | 0.21 | 0.22 | 0.06 | 0.11 | 0.11 | 0.10 | 0.12 | 0.03 | 0.08 | 0.15 |
| 11534 | 1 | oz | Fat, raw | 28 | 0.10 | 0.10 | 0.15 | 0.02 | 0.27 | 0.09 | 0.06 | 0.08 | 0.13 | 0.14 | 0.04 | 0.07 | 0.07 | 0.06 | 0.07 | 0.02 | 0.05 | 0.09 |
| 11581 | 4 | oz | Ground, 7% fat, raw | 113 | 1.30 | 1.29 | 1.89 | 0.25 | 3.46 | 1.12 | 0.79 | 1.08 | 1.74 | 1.80 | 0.51 | 0.88 | 0.91 | 0.82 | 0.95 | 0.22 | 0.70 | 1.21 |
| 11530 | 3 | oz | Ground, 8% fat, brld | 85 | 1.23 | 1.22 | 1.78 | 0.23 | 3.28 | 1.06 | 0.75 | 1.02 | 1.65 | 1.71 | 0.48 | 0.84 | 0.87 | 0.78 | 0.91 | 0.21 | 0.66 | 1.15 |
| | | | Retail Cuts | | | | | | | | | | | | | | | | | | | |
| 11531 | 3 | oz | Average, ckd | 85 | 1.52 | 1.50 | 2.21 | 0.29 | 4.05 | 1.32 | 0.93 | 1.26 | 2.04 | 2.11 | 0.60 | 1.04 | 1.07 | 0.96 | 1.12 | 0.26 | 0.82 | 1.41 |
| 11552 | 3 | oz | Average, lean, ckd | 85 | 1.62 | 1.60 | 2.34 | 0.31 | 4.29 | 1.39 | 0.99 | 1.33 | 2.16 | 2.24 | 0.63 | 1.10 | 1.13 | 1.02 | 1.18 | 0.27 | 0.87 | 1.50 |
| 11533 | 4 | oz | Average, lean, raw | 113 | 1.36 | 1.34 | 1.97 | 0.26 | 3.62 | 1.18 | 0.83 | 1.12 | 1.82 | 1.88 | 0.53 | 0.92 | 0.95 | 0.86 | 1.00 | 0.23 | 0.73 | 1.27 |
| 11551 | 4 | oz | Average, raw | 113 | 1.30 | 1.29 | 1.89 | 0.25 | 3.46 | 1.12 | 0.79 | 1.08 | 1.74 | 1.80 | 0.51 | 0.88 | 0.91 | 0.82 | 0.95 | 0.22 | 0.70 | 1.21 |
| 11687 | 3 | oz | Breast, brsd | 85 | 1.37 | 1.35 | 1.98 | 0.26 | 3.63 | 1.18 | 0.83 | 1.13 | 1.83 | 1.89 | 0.54 | 0.93 | 0.96 | 0.86 | 1.00 | 0.23 | 0.73 | 1.27 |
| 11690 | 3 | oz | Breast, lean, brsd | 85 | 1.54 | 1.52 | 2.23 | 0.29 | 4.08 | 1.33 | 0.94 | 1.27 | 2.05 | 2.13 | 0.60 | 1.04 | 1.08 | 0.97 | 1.12 | 0.26 | 0.82 | 1.42 |
| 11686 | 4 | oz | Breast, raw | 113 | 1.18 | 1.16 | 1.71 | 0.22 | 3.12 | 1.01 | 0.72 | 0.97 | 1.57 | 1.63 | 0.46 | 0.80 | 0.82 | 0.74 | 0.86 | 0.20 | 0.63 | 1.09 |
| 11516 | 3 | oz | Leg, lean, rstd | 85 | 1.42 | 1.40 | 2.06 | 0.27 | 3.77 | 1.22 | 0.87 | 1.17 | 1.90 | 1.96 | 0.56 | 0.96 | 0.99 | 0.89 | 1.05 | 0.24 | 0.76 | 1.32 |
| 11555 | 3 | oz | Leg, top round, brsd | 85 | 1.83 | 1.81 | 2.65 | 0.35 | 4.86 | 1.58 | 1.11 | 1.51 | 2.45 | 2.53 | 0.72 | 1.24 | 1.28 | 1.16 | 1.34 | 0.31 | 0.98 | 1.70 |
| 11557 | 3 | oz | Leg, top round, lean, brsd | 85 | 1.85 | 1.84 | 2.69 | 0.35 | 4.94 | 1.61 | 1.13 | 1.54 | 2.48 | 2.58 | 0.73 | 1.26 | 1.30 | 1.17 | 1.36 | 0.32 | 0.99 | 1.73 |
| 11556 | 4 | oz | Leg, top round, lean, raw | 113 | 1.44 | 1.41 | 2.08 | 0.27 | 3.81 | 1.23 | 0.87 | 1.19 | 1.91 | 1.98 | 0.56 | 0.97 | 1.00 | 0.90 | 1.05 | 0.24 | 0.77 | 1.33 |
| 11554 | 4 | oz | Leg, top round, raw | 113 | 1.41 | 1.39 | 2.05 | 0.27 | 3.75 | 1.22 | 0.86 | 1.16 | 1.89 | 1.95 | 0.55 | 0.96 | 0.99 | 0.89 | 1.04 | 0.24 | 0.76 | 1.31 |
| 11509 | 3 | oz | Leg, top round, rstd | 85 | 1.40 | 1.39 | 2.03 | 0.27 | 3.72 | 1.21 | 0.86 | 1.16 | 1.88 | 1.94 | 0.55 | 0.95 | 0.99 | 0.88 | 1.03 | 0.24 | 0.75 | 1.30 |
| 11529 | 3 | oz | Leg/Shoulder, lean, cubed, brsd | 85 | 1.77 | 1.75 | 2.57 | 0.33 | 4.70 | 1.53 | 1.08 | 1.46 | 2.36 | 2.45 | 0.69 | 1.20 | 1.24 | 1.11 | 1.30 | 0.30 | 0.94 | 1.64 |
| 11580 | 4 | oz | Leg/Shoulder, lean, cubed, raw | 113 | 1.37 | 1.34 | 1.98 | 0.26 | 3.63 | 1.18 | 0.83 | 1.13 | 1.82 | 1.89 | 0.53 | 0.92 | 0.96 | 0.86 | 1.00 | 0.23 | 0.73 | 1.27 |
| 11517 | 1 | ea | Loin Chop, brsd | 80 | 1.44 | 1.42 | 2.08 | 0.27 | 3.82 | 1.24 | 0.88 | 1.19 | 1.92 | 1.99 | 0.56 | 0.98 | 1.01 | 0.90 | 1.06 | 0.24 | 0.77 | 1.34 |
| 11504 | 1 | ea | Loin Chop, breaded, fried | 127 | 2.01 | 2.01 | 2.93 | 0.42 | 5.78 | 1.74 | 1.21 | 1.70 | 2.74 | 2.72 | 0.80 | 1.44 | 1.59 | 1.37 | 1.49 | 0.36 | 1.10 | 1.92 |
| 11507 | 1 | ea | Loin Chop, fried | 105 | 1.98 | 1.96 | 2.88 | 0.38 | 5.27 | 1.71 | 1.21 | 1.64 | 2.66 | 2.75 | 0.78 | 1.34 | 1.40 | 1.25 | 1.46 | 0.34 | 1.06 | 1.85 |
| 11518 | 1 | ea | Loin Chop, lean, brsd | 69 | 1.38 | 1.36 | 2.00 | 0.26 | 3.66 | 1.19 | 0.84 | 1.14 | 1.84 | 1.91 | 0.54 | 0.94 | 0.97 | 0.87 | 1.01 | 0.23 | 0.74 | 1.28 |
| 11511 | 1 | ea | Loin Chop, lean, breaded, fried | 101 | 1.67 | 1.66 | 2.42 | 0.34 | 4.77 | 1.44 | 1.01 | 1.40 | 2.27 | 2.26 | 0.66 | 1.18 | 1.30 | 1.13 | 1.23 | 0.30 | 0.91 | 1.59 |
| 11514 | 1 | ea | Loin Chop, lean, fried | 85 | 1.67 | 1.66 | 2.43 | 0.32 | 4.46 | 1.45 | 1.02 | 1.39 | 2.24 | 2.32 | 0.66 | 1.14 | 1.18 | 1.05 | 1.23 | 0.29 | 0.90 | 1.56 |
| 11559 | 1 | ea | Loin Chop, lean, raw | 113 | 1.36 | 1.34 | 1.97 | 0.26 | 3.60 | 1.18 | 0.83 | 1.12 | 1.82 | 1.88 | 0.53 | 0.92 | 0.95 | 0.85 | 1.00 | 0.23 | 0.73 | 1.27 |
| 11560 | 3 | oz | Loin Chop, lean, rstd | 85 | 1.33 | 1.32 | 1.93 | 0.25 | 3.54 | 1.15 | 0.81 | 1.11 | 1.78 | 1.84 | 0.52 | 0.90 | 0.94 | 0.84 | 0.98 | 0.23 | 0.71 | 1.24 |
| 11558 | 4 | oz | Loin Chop, raw | 113 | 1.27 | 1.25 | 1.84 | 0.24 | 3.38 | 1.10 | 0.78 | 1.05 | 1.69 | 1.76 | 0.50 | 0.86 | 0.89 | 0.80 | 0.93 | 0.22 | 0.68 | 1.18 |
| 11595 | 1 | ea | Loin Chop, rstd | 229 | 3.39 | 3.34 | 4.90 | 0.64 | 8.98 | 2.93 | 2.06 | 2.79 | 4.51 | 4.67 | 1.33 | 2.29 | 2.38 | 2.13 | 2.47 | 0.57 | 1.81 | 3.14 |
| 11561 | 3 | oz | Ribs, brsd | 85 | 1.64 | 1.62 | 2.38 | 0.31 | 4.36 | 1.42 | 1.00 | 1.36 | 2.19 | 2.27 | 0.64 | 1.11 | 1.15 | 1.04 | 1.21 | 0.28 | 0.88 | 1.52 |
| 11563 | 3 | oz | Ribs, lean, brsd | 85 | 1.74 | 1.73 | 2.52 | 0.33 | 4.63 | 1.50 | 1.06 | 1.45 | 2.33 | 2.41 | 0.68 | 1.18 | 1.22 | 1.10 | 1.28 | 0.30 | 0.94 | 1.62 |
| 11562 | 4 | oz | Ribs, lean, raw | 113 | 1.34 | 1.33 | 1.94 | 0.25 | 3.57 | 1.16 | 0.82 | 1.11 | 1.80 | 1.86 | 0.53 | 0.91 | 0.94 | 0.85 | 0.99 | 0.23 | 0.72 | 1.24 |
| 11520 | 3 | oz | Ribs, lean, rstd | 85 | 1.30 | 1.29 | 1.89 | 0.25 | 3.46 | 1.12 | 0.79 | 1.08 | 1.74 | 1.80 | 0.51 | 0.88 | 0.92 | 0.82 | 0.96 | 0.22 | 0.70 | 1.21 |
| 11597 | 4 | oz | Ribs, raw | 113 | 1.27 | 1.25 | 1.84 | 0.24 | 3.37 | 1.09 | 0.77 | 1.05 | 1.69 | 1.75 | 0.50 | 0.86 | 0.89 | 0.80 | 0.93 | 0.22 | 0.68 | 1.18 |
| 11519 | 3 | oz | Ribs, rstd | 85 | 1.22 | 1.20 | 1.76 | 0.23 | 3.22 | 1.05 | 0.74 | 1.00 | 1.62 | 1.67 | 0.48 | 0.82 | 0.85 | 0.76 | 0.89 | 0.21 | 0.65 | 1.12 |
| 11521 | 3 | oz | Shoulder, arm/blade, brsd | 85 | 1.62 | 1.61 | 2.35 | 0.31 | 4.31 | 1.40 | 0.99 | 1.34 | 2.17 | 2.24 | 0.64 | 1.10 | 1.14 | 1.02 | 1.19 | 0.28 | 0.87 | 1.50 |
| 11522 | 3 | oz | Shoulder, arm/blade, lean, brsd | 85 | 1.70 | 1.68 | 2.47 | 0.32 | 4.53 | 1.47 | 1.04 | 1.41 | 2.28 | 2.36 | 0.67 | 1.16 | 1.20 | 1.07 | 1.25 | 0.29 | 0.91 | 1.58 |
| 11566 | 4 | oz | Shoulder, arm/blade, lean, raw | 113 | 1.33 | 1.31 | 1.93 | 0.25 | 3.54 | 1.15 | 0.81 | 1.10 | 1.79 | 1.84 | 0.52 | 0.90 | 0.93 | 0.84 | 0.98 | 0.23 | 0.71 | 1.23 |
| 11567 | 3 | oz | Shoulder, arm/blade, lean, rstd | 85 | 1.31 | 1.29 | 1.90 | 0.25 | 3.47 | 1.13 | 0.80 | 1.08 | 1.75 | 1.81 | 0.51 | 0.88 | 0.92 | 0.82 | 0.96 | 0.22 | 0.70 | 1.22 |

TABLE A **Amino Acid Content for Selected Foods *(continued)***

| Code | Amount | Description | Weight (g) | Alanine (g) | Arginine (g) | Aspartic acid (g) | Cystine (g) | Glutamic acid (g) | Glycine (g) | Histidine (g) | Isoleucine (g) | Leucine (g) | Lysine (g) | Methionine (g) | Phenylalanine (g) | Proline (g) | Serine (g) | Threonine (g) | Tryptophan (g) | Tyrosine (g) | Valine (g) |
|---|---|---|---|---|---|---|---|---|---|---|---|---|---|---|---|---|---|---|---|---|---|
| 11564 | 4 oz | Shoulder, arm/blade, raw | 113 | 1.30 | 1.28 | 1.88 | 0.25 | 3.45 | 1.12 | 0.73 | 1.07 | 1.73 | 1.80 | 0.51 | 0.88 | 0.91 | 0.82 | 0.95 | 0.22 | 0.69 | 1.21 |
| 11565 | 3 oz | Shoulder, arm/blade, rstd | 85 | 1.28 | 1.27 | 1.85 | 0.24 | 3.41 | 1.11 | 0.73 | 1.06 | 1.72 | 1.78 | 0.50 | 0.87 | 0.90 | 0.81 | 0.94 | 0.22 | 0.69 | 1.19 |
| 11692 | 3 oz | Shank, brsd | 85 | 1.60 | 1.58 | 2.31 | 0.22 | 4.24 | 1.38 | 0.93 | 1.32 | 2.13 | 2.21 | 0.63 | 1.08 | 1.12 | 1.00 | 1.17 | 0.27 | 0.85 | 1.48 |
| 11694 | 3 oz | Shank, lean, brsd | 85 | 1.63 | 1.62 | 2.36 | 0.31 | 4.34 | 1.41 | 0.93 | 1.35 | 2.18 | 2.26 | 0.64 | 1.11 | 1.15 | 1.03 | 1.20 | 0.28 | 0.88 | 1.51 |
| 11693 | 4 oz | Shank, lean, raw | 113 | 1.30 | 1.29 | 1.88 | 0.25 | 3.45 | 1.12 | 0.73 | 1.07 | 1.73 | 1.80 | 0.51 | 0.88 | 0.91 | 0.82 | 0.95 | 0.22 | 0.69 | 1.20 |
| 11691 | 4 oz | Shank, raw | 113 | 1.29 | 1.28 | 1.86 | 0.25 | 3.42 | 1.11 | 0.73 | 1.07 | 1.72 | 1.79 | 0.51 | 0.87 | 0.90 | 0.81 | 0.94 | 0.22 | 0.69 | 1.20 |
| 11577 | 3 oz | Sirloin, brsd | 85 | 1.58 | 1.56 | 2.30 | 0.30 | 4.20 | 1.37 | 0.97 | 1.31 | 2.12 | 2.19 | 0.62 | 1.07 | 1.11 | 0.99 | 1.16 | 0.27 | 0.85 | 1.47 |
| 11576 | 4 oz | Sirloin, raw | 113 | 1.28 | 1.27 | 1.86 | 0.24 | 3.41 | 1.11 | 0.73 | 1.06 | 1.72 | 1.77 | 0.50 | 0.87 | 0.90 | 0.81 | 0.94 | 0.22 | 0.69 | 1.19 |
| 11527 | 3 oz | Sirloin, rstd | 85 | 1.28 | 1.26 | 1.84 | 0.24 | 3.38 | 1.10 | 0.73 | 1.05 | 1.70 | 1.76 | 0.50 | 0.87 | 0.89 | 0.80 | 0.94 | 0.22 | 0.63 | 1.18 |
| 11579 | 3 oz | Sirloin, lean, brsd | 85 | 1.72 | 1.70 | 2.49 | 0.33 | 4.56 | 1.49 | 1.05 | 1.42 | 2.30 | 2.38 | 0.67 | 1.16 | 1.21 | 1.08 | 1.26 | 0.29 | 0.92 | 1.60 |
| 11528 | 3 oz | Sirloin, lean, rstd | 85 | 1.33 | 1.32 | 1.93 | 0.25 | 3.54 | 1.15 | 0.81 | 1.11 | 1.78 | 1.84 | 0.52 | 0.90 | 0.94 | 0.84 | 0.98 | 0.23 | 0.71 | 1.24 |
| 11578 | 4 oz | Sirloin, lean, raw | 113 | 1.36 | 1.34 | 1.97 | 0.26 | 3.62 | 1.18 | 0.83 | 1.12 | 1.82 | 1.89 | 0.53 | 0.92 | 0.95 | 0.86 | 1.00 | 0.23 | 0.73 | 1.27 |
| | | **MEATS—ORGAN MEATS** | | | | | | | | | | | | | | | | | | | |
| | | Beef | | | | | | | | | | | | | | | | | | | |
| 10468 | 3 oz | Brains, ckd | 85 | 0.52 | 0.51 | 0.84 | 0.17 | 1.15 | 0.44 | 0.24 | 0.36 | 0.71 | 0.56 | 0.20 | 0.48 | 0.39 | 0.54 | 0.45 | 0.08 | 0.33 | 0.46 |
| 10467 | 4 oz | Brains, raw | 85 | 0.46 | 0.45 | 0.75 | 0.15 | 1.02 | 0.39 | 0.21 | 0.32 | 0.62 | 0.50 | 0.17 | 0.42 | 0.35 | 0.48 | 0.40 | 0.07 | 0.30 | 0.41 |
| 10785 | 3 oz | Heart, ckd | 85 | 1.51 | 1.64 | 2.25 | 0.32 | 3.87 | 1.28 | 0.67 | 1.07 | 2.17 | 2.01 | 0.63 | 1.11 | 1.15 | 1.13 | 1.16 | 0.27 | 0.89 | 1.28 |
| 10469 | 4 oz | Heart, raw | 113 | 1.19 | 1.29 | 1.77 | 0.25 | 3.05 | 1.01 | 0.53 | 0.85 | 1.71 | 1.59 | 0.49 | 0.87 | 0.91 | 0.89 | 0.91 | 0.22 | 0.70 | 1.01 |
| 10034 | 3 oz | Kidney, ckd | 85 | 1.22 | 1.28 | 1.91 | 0.07 | 2.52 | 1.32 | 0.57 | 0.88 | 1.73 | 1.45 | 0.45 | 1.04 | 1.24 | 1.06 | 1.05 | 0.29 | 0.81 | 1.35 |
| 10470 | 4 oz | Kidney, raw | 113 | 1.05 | 1.10 | 1.66 | 0.06 | 2.18 | 1.14 | 0.49 | 0.77 | 1.50 | 1.24 | 0.39 | 0.90 | 1.07 | 0.92 | 0.91 | 0.26 | 0.71 | 1.18 |
| 10472 | 3 oz | Liver, brsd | 85 | 1.24 | 1.30 | 1.98 | 0.32 | 2.79 | 1.19 | 0.55 | 0.95 | 1.94 | 1.43 | 0.52 | 1.10 | 1.09 | 0.99 | 0.95 | 0.30 | 0.82 | 1.28 |
| 10471 | 4 oz | Liver, raw | 113 | 1.34 | 1.42 | 2.16 | 0.35 | 3.05 | 1.29 | 0.61 | 1.03 | 2.11 | 1.56 | 0.57 | 1.20 | 1.19 | 1.08 | 1.03 | 0.32 | 0.89 | 1.39 |
| 10474 | 3 oz | Lungs, brsd | 85 | 1.07 | 1.05 | 1.05 | 0.27 | 1.84 | 0.79 | 0.53 | 0.83 | 1.28 | 1.23 | 0.35 | 0.70 | 1.78 | 0.88 | 0.65 | 0.16 | 0.39 | 0.86 |
| 10473 | 4 oz | Lungs, raw | 113 | 1.13 | 1.11 | 1.10 | 0.28 | 1.95 | 0.83 | 0.55 | 0.87 | 1.34 | 1.30 | 0.37 | 0.74 | 1.88 | 0.92 | 0.68 | 0.17 | 0.41 | 0.90 |
| 10477 | 3 oz | Pancreas, brsd | 85 | 1.18 | 1.32 | 2.21 | 0.29 | 1.93 | 1.40 | 0.45 | 1.16 | 1.80 | 1.70 | 0.42 | 0.96 | 1.18 | 0.92 | 1.07 | 0.30 | 1.00 | 1.23 |
| 10476 | 4 oz | Pancreas, raw | 113 | 0.91 | 1.01 | 1.71 | 0.23 | 1.49 | 1.08 | 0.35 | 0.90 | 1.39 | 1.31 | 0.32 | 0.74 | 0.91 | 0.71 | 0.82 | 0.23 | 0.78 | 0.95 |
| 10479 | 3 oz | Spleen, brsd | 85 | 1.65 | 1.23 | 1.50 | 0.62 | 1.95 | 1.29 | 0.75 | 0.82 | 1.89 | 1.55 | 0.39 | 0.86 | 1.29 | 0.74 | 0.84 | 0.22 | 0.61 | 1.28 |
| 10478 | 4 oz | Spleen, raw | 113 | 1.60 | 1.20 | 1.46 | 0.60 | 1.89 | 1.25 | 0.74 | 0.80 | 1.83 | 1.49 | 0.38 | 0.83 | 1.25 | 0.71 | 0.81 | 0.21 | 0.59 | 1.24 |
| 10482 | 3 oz | Thymus, brsd | 85 | 0.95 | 1.22 | 1.78 | 0.24 | 1.56 | 1.13 | 0.38 | 0.63 | 1.24 | 1.55 | 0.26 | 0.53 | 0.95 | 0.74 | 0.67 | 0.14 | 0.39 | 0.80 |
| 10481 | 4 oz | Thymus, raw | 113 | 0.71 | 0.91 | 1.32 | 0.18 | 1.15 | 0.84 | 0.24 | 0.47 | 0.92 | 1.14 | 0.19 | 0.39 | 0.71 | 0.55 | 0.50 | 0.11 | 0.60 | 0.60 |
| 10011 | 3 oz | Tongue, ckd | 85 | 1.08 | 1.20 | 1.72 | 0.25 | 2.59 | 1.13 | 0.49 | 0.81 | 1.40 | 1.45 | 0.40 | 0.78 | 0.88 | 0.76 | 0.82 | 0.14 | 0.61 | 0.90 |
| 10483 | 4 oz | Tongue, raw | 113 | 0.97 | 1.07 | 1.54 | 0.22 | 2.32 | 1.01 | 0.44 | 0.72 | 1.25 | 1.30 | 0.36 | 0.69 | 0.79 | 0.68 | 0.73 | 0.13 | 0.54 | 0.81 |
| 10019 | 3 oz | Tripe, pickled | 85 | 0.64 | 0.69 | 0.78 | 0.12 | 1.34 | 0.82 | 0.25 | 0.41 | 0.66 | 0.72 | 0.22 | 0.33 | 0.80 | 0.46 | 0.35 | 0.08 | 0.27 | 0.42 |
| 10018 | 4 oz | Tripe, raw | 113 | 1.05 | 1.12 | 1.28 | 0.13 | 2.20 | 1.34 | 0.41 | 0.67 | 1.07 | 1.18 | 0.36 | 0.53 | 1.31 | 0.76 | 0.57 | 0.13 | 0.45 | 0.69 |
| | | Chicken | | | | | | | | | | | | | | | | | | | |
| 15106 | 3 oz | Giblets, ckd | 85 | 1.08 | 1.47 | 2.06 | 0.23 | 3.33 | 1.21 | 0.51 | 1.11 | 1.76 | 1.61 | 0.55 | 0.99 | 1.12 | 0.96 | 0.99 | 0.25 | 0.72 | 1.17 |
| 15104 | 4 oz | Giblets, raw | 113 | 0.99 | 1.34 | 1.90 | 0.27 | 3.06 | 1.11 | 0.47 | 1.01 | 1.62 | 1.48 | 0.51 | 0.92 | 1.03 | 0.88 | 0.92 | 0.23 | 0.66 | 1.08 |
| 15025 | 3 oz | Gizzards, ckd | 85 | 0.91 | 1.66 | 2.13 | 0.33 | 3.94 | 1.22 | 0.46 | 1.09 | 1.62 | 1.60 | 0.61 | 0.96 | 1.20 | 1.04 | 1.06 | 0.21 | 0.70 | 1.04 |
| 15107 | 4 oz | Gizzards, raw | 113 | 0.81 | 1.48 | 1.89 | 0.27 | 3.51 | 1.08 | 0.41 | 0.97 | 1.45 | 1.42 | 0.54 | 0.86 | 1.07 | 0.92 | 0.95 | 0.18 | 0.62 | 0.92 |
| 15024 | 3 oz | Heart, ckd | 85 | 1.41 | 1.43 | 2.17 | 0.33 | 3.32 | 1.24 | 0.59 | 1.20 | 1.95 | 1.87 | 0.54 | 1.00 | 1.14 | 0.91 | 1.01 | 0.29 | 0.80 | 1.27 |
| 15108 | 4 oz | Heart, raw | 113 | 1.11 | 1.13 | 1.71 | 0.24 | 2.61 | 0.97 | 0.46 | 0.94 | 1.54 | 1.47 | 0.42 | 0.79 | 0.90 | 0.71 | 0.80 | 0.22 | 0.63 | 0.99 |
| 15215 | 3 oz | Liver, ckd | 85 | 1.21 | 1.27 | 1.97 | 0.23 | 2.69 | 1.21 | 0.55 | 1.10 | 1.87 | 1.56 | 0.49 | 1.03 | 1.03 | 0.89 | 0.92 | 0.29 | 0.73 | 1.31 |
| 15109 | 4 oz | Liver, raw | 113 | 1.18 | 1.24 | 1.93 | 0.27 | 2.63 | 1.18 | 0.54 | 1.08 | 1.83 | 1.54 | 0.48 | 1.01 | 1.01 | 0.87 | 0.90 | 0.29 | 0.71 | 1.28 |
| | | Lamb | | | | | | | | | | | | | | | | | | | |
| 13506 | 3 oz | Brains, brsd | 85 | 0.60 | 0.72 | 0.89 | 0.11 | 1.27 | 0.50 | 0.28 | 0.42 | 0.83 | 0.68 | 0.21 | 0.51 | 0.46 | 0.56 | 0.48 | 0.11 | 0.39 | 0.51 |
| 13537 | 4 oz | Brains, raw | 113 | 0.67 | 0.79 | 0.98 | 0.12 | 1.39 | 0.56 | 0.31 | 0.47 | 0.92 | 0.75 | 0.23 | 0.57 | 0.51 | 0.61 | 0.53 | 0.12 | 0.43 | 0.56 |
| 13504 | 3 oz | Heart, brsd | 85 | 1.29 | 1.39 | 1.83 | 0.18 | 2.71 | 1.03 | 0.49 | 0.92 | 1.80 | 1.60 | 0.46 | 0.92 | 0.96 | 0.82 | 1.00 | 0.23 | 0.66 | 1.05 |
| 13539 | 4 oz | Heart, raw | 113 | 1.13 | 1.22 | 1.60 | 0.16 | 2.37 | 0.90 | 0.43 | 0.81 | 1.58 | 1.40 | 0.41 | 0.80 | 0.84 | 0.72 | 0.88 | 0.20 | 0.58 | 0.93 |
| 13541 | 3 oz | Kidneys, brsd | 85 | 1.09 | 1.16 | 1.73 | 0.23 | 2.18 | 1.17 | 0.51 | 0.80 | 1.51 | 1.30 | 0.41 | 0.94 | 1.03 | 0.94 | 0.94 | 0.27 | 0.71 | 1.18 |
| 13540 | 4 oz | Kidneys, raw | 113 | 0.96 | 1.03 | 1.54 | 0.20 | 1.93 | 1.03 | 0.45 | 0.71 | 1.33 | 1.15 | 0.36 | 0.82 | 0.91 | 0.83 | 0.84 | 0.24 | 0.63 | 1.04 |

TABLE A **Amino Acid Content for Selected Foods *(continued)***

| Code | Amount | Description | Weight (g) | Alanine (g) | Arginine (g) | Aspartic acid (g) | Cystine (g) | Glutamic acid (g) | Glycine (g) | Histidine (g) | Isoleucine (g) | Leucine (g) | Lysine (g) | Methionine (g) | Phenylalanine (g) | Proline (g) | Serine (g) | Threonine (g) | Tryptophan (g) | Tyrosine (g) | Valine (g) |
|---|---|---|---|---|---|---|---|---|---|---|---|---|---|---|---|---|---|---|---|---|---|
| 13505 | 3 oz | Liver, brsd | 85 | 1.30 | 1.45 | 2.24 | 0.27 | 2.81 | 1.26 | 0.61 | 1.12 | 2.13 | 1.40 | 0.56 | 1.16 | 1.24 | 1.12 | 1.12 | 0.30 | 0.93 | 1.43 |
| 13542 | 4 oz | Liver, raw | 113 | 1.15 | 1.29 | 1.99 | 0.24 | 2.49 | 1.11 | 0.54 | 0.99 | 1.89 | 1.24 | 0.50 | 1.03 | 1.10 | 0.99 | 1.00 | 0.27 | 0.82 | 1.27 |
| 13545 | 3 oz | Lungs, brsd | 85 | 1.06 | 1.02 | 1.33 | 0.27 | 1.82 | 1.43 | 0.43 | 0.53 | 1.35 | 1.10 | 0.31 | 0.70 | 1.08 | 0.67 | 0.62 | 0.17 | 0.48 | 0.94 |
| 13544 | 4 oz | Lungs, raw | 113 | 1.19 | 1.14 | 1.49 | 0.30 | 2.03 | 1.59 | 0.47 | 0.60 | 1.51 | 1.22 | 0.34 | 0.78 | 1.21 | 0.75 | 0.69 | 0.19 | 0.53 | 1.04 |
| 13507 | 3 oz | Pancreas, brsd | 85 | 0.99 | 1.15 | 1.33 | 0.25 | 2.70 | 1.21 | 0.56 | 0.68 | 1.24 | 1.67 | 0.28 | 0.65 | 0.99 | 0.78 | 0.71 | 0.25 | 0.47 | 0.84 |
| 13547 | 4 oz | Pancreas, raw | 113 | 0.86 | 0.99 | 1.15 | 0.21 | 2.34 | 1.05 | 0.48 | 0.59 | 1.07 | 1.45 | 0.24 | 0.56 | 0.86 | 0.67 | 0.62 | 0.21 | 0.40 | 0.72 |
| 13550 | 3 oz | Spleen, brsd | 85 | 1.45 | 1.42 | 1.96 | 0.29 | 2.62 | 1.46 | 0.75 | 1.43 | 2.00 | 1.74 | 0.43 | 1.02 | 1.25 | 0.99 | 0.92 | 0.25 | 0.66 | 1.47 |
| 13549 | 4 oz | Spleen, raw | 113 | 1.25 | 1.23 | 1.68 | 0.25 | 2.26 | 1.27 | 0.65 | 1.23 | 1.73 | 1.50 | 0.37 | 0.88 | 1.08 | 0.85 | 0.79 | 0.21 | 0.57 | 1.27 |
| 13527 | 3 oz | Tongue, brsd | 85 | 1.05 | 1.21 | 1.64 | 0.20 | 2.36 | 1.19 | 0.41 | 0.72 | 1.31 | 1.30 | 0.39 | 0.68 | 0.97 | 0.72 | 0.83 | 0.19 | 0.54 | 0.88 |
| 13551 | 4 oz | Tongue, raw | 113 | 1.02 | 1.16 | 1.58 | 0.19 | 2.29 | 1.15 | 0.39 | 0.69 | 1.27 | 1.25 | 0.38 | 0.66 | 0.93 | 0.70 | 0.80 | 0.18 | 0.53 | 0.85 |
| | | Pork | | | | | | | | | | | | | | | | | | | |
| 12143 | 3 oz | Brains, brsd | 85 | 0.56 | 0.54 | 1.03 | 0.18 | 1.21 | 0.50 | 0.28 | 0.48 | 0.90 | 0.81 | 0.20 | 0.53 | 0.56 | 0.54 | 0.48 | 0.13 | 0.43 | 0.59 |
| 12142 | 4 oz | Brains, raw | 113 | 0.64 | 0.61 | 1.16 | 0.21 | 1.36 | 0.56 | 0.31 | 0.54 | 1.01 | 0.91 | 0.23 | 0.59 | 0.64 | 0.62 | 0.54 | 0.15 | 0.49 | 0.66 |
| 12145 | 3 oz | Chitlings, small intestines, ckd | 85 | 0.62 | 0.71 | 0.81 | 0.08 | 1.12 | 0.93 | 0.18 | 0.36 | 0.68 | 0.56 | 0.16 | 0.35 | 0.61 | 0.42 | 0.38 | 0.05 | 0.32 | 0.42 |
| 12144 | 4 oz | Chitlings, small intestines, raw | 113 | 0.83 | 0.90 | 1.06 | 0.10 | 1.51 | 1.33 | 0.23 | 0.44 | 0.86 | 0.72 | 0.19 | 0.42 | 0.84 | 0.53 | 0.47 | 0.10 | 0.36 | 0.53 |
| 12147 | 1 ea | Ears, ckd | 111 | 1.68 | 1.41 | 1.30 | 0.16 | 2.21 | 3.45 | 0.21 | 0.40 | 0.96 | 0.81 | 0.14 | 0.56 | 2.10 | 0.75 | 0.52 | 0.03 | 0.35 | 0.70 |
| 12146 | 1 ea | Ears, raw | 113 | 2.49 | 2.08 | 1.86 | 0.22 | 3.15 | 4.93 | 0.30 | 0.55 | 1.31 | 1.18 | 0.15 | 0.81 | 3.20 | 1.06 | 0.71 | 0.05 | 0.45 | 0.93 |
| 12178 | 3 oz | Feet, ckd | 85 | 1.33 | 1.22 | 1.17 | 0.14 | 1.79 | 2.86 | 0.18 | 0.28 | 0.72 | 0.70 | 0.18 | 0.47 | 1.72 | 0.65 | 0.44 | 0.03 | 0.26 | 0.41 |
| 12208 | 3 oz | Feet, pickled | 85 | 0.94 | 0.86 | 0.83 | 0.10 | 1.27 | 2.01 | 0.13 | 0.20 | 0.51 | 0.49 | 0.13 | 0.33 | 1.21 | 0.46 | 0.31 | 0.02 | 0.18 | 0.29 |
| 12148 | 1 ea | Feet, raw | 190 | 3.52 | 3.19 | 2.94 | 0.37 | 4.58 | 6.95 | 0.50 | 0.67 | 1.76 | 1.80 | 0.42 | 1.13 | 4.62 | 1.68 | 1.09 | 0.08 | 0.63 | 0.97 |
| 12303 | 1 ea | Heart, brsd | 129 | 1.93 | 2.04 | 2.74 | 0.54 | 4.85 | 1.64 | 0.77 | 1.46 | 2.73 | 2.50 | 0.77 | 1.33 | 1.40 | 1.42 | 1.33 | 0.35 | 1.03 | 1.60 |
| 12149 | 1 ea | Heart, raw | 226 | 2.50 | 2.61 | 3.51 | 0.70 | 6.23 | 2.11 | 0.99 | 1.87 | 3.51 | 3.22 | 0.99 | 1.71 | 1.79 | 1.83 | 1.70 | 0.45 | 1.33 | 2.06 |
| 12150 | 4 oz | Jowl, raw | 113 | 0.43 | 0.74 | 0.67 | 0.06 | 1.12 | 0.33 | 0.08 | 0.19 | 0.50 | 0.60 | 0.11 | 0.27 | 0.27 | 0.30 | 0.24 | 0.02 | 0.12 | 0.34 |
| 12152 | 3 oz | Kidneys, brsd | 85 | 1.36 | 1.33 | 2.03 | 0.47 | 2.58 | 1.37 | 0.52 | 1.16 | 1.94 | 1.56 | 0.46 | 1.02 | 1.33 | 1.15 | 0.89 | 0.28 | 0.78 | 1.24 |
| 12151 | 1 ea | Kidneys, raw | 233 | 2.42 | 2.35 | 3.61 | 0.84 | 4.57 | 2.42 | 0.92 | 2.05 | 3.45 | 2.77 | 0.82 | 1.81 | 2.38 | 2.03 | 1.59 | 0.50 | 1.38 | 2.21 |
| 12013 | 3 pce | Liver, brsd | 54 | 0.84 | 0.86 | 1.27 | 0.27 | 1.83 | 0.82 | 0.38 | 0.71 | 1.25 | 1.09 | 0.35 | 0.69 | 0.76 | 0.76 | 0.60 | 0.20 | 0.48 | 0.87 |
| 12154 | 4 oz | Liver, raw | 113 | 1.45 | 1.49 | 2.19 | 0.46 | 3.14 | 1.40 | 0.66 | 1.23 | 2.16 | 1.86 | 0.60 | 1.19 | 1.30 | 1.31 | 1.03 | 0.34 | 0.82 | 1.49 |
| 12156 | 3 oz | Lungs, brsd | 85 | 0.89 | 0.73 | 1.27 | 0.22 | 1.47 | 1.03 | 0.36 | 0.56 | 1.10 | 1.03 | 0.23 | 0.59 | 0.90 | 0.62 | 0.50 | 0.12 | 0.40 | 0.84 |
| 12155 | 4 oz | Lungs, raw | 113 | 1.01 | 0.83 | 1.44 | 0.25 | 1.65 | 1.16 | 0.40 | 0.64 | 1.23 | 1.16 | 0.26 | 0.66 | 1.02 | 0.70 | 0.56 | 0.14 | 0.45 | 0.95 |
| 12159 | 3 oz | Pancreas, brsd | 85 | 1.24 | 1.39 | 2.33 | 0.31 | 2.00 | 1.48 | 0.47 | 1.28 | 1.81 | 1.67 | 0.40 | 1.04 | 1.24 | 0.97 | 1.09 | 0.53 | 1.02 | 1.31 |
| 12158 | 4 oz | Pancreas, raw | 113 | 1.07 | 1.21 | 2.01 | 0.27 | 1.73 | 1.28 | 0.41 | 1.10 | 1.57 | 1.45 | 0.35 | 0.90 | 1.07 | 0.84 | 0.94 | 0.46 | 0.88 | 1.13 |
| 12161 | 3 oz | Spleen, brsd | 85 | 1.55 | 1.31 | 2.11 | 0.31 | 2.75 | 1.54 | 0.57 | 1.07 | 1.96 | 1.79 | 0.44 | 1.03 | 1.33 | 1.05 | 0.96 | 0.25 | 0.67 | 1.30 |
| 12160 | 4 oz | Spleen, raw | 113 | 1.30 | 1.10 | 1.77 | 0.26 | 2.32 | 1.29 | 0.48 | 0.90 | 1.65 | 1.50 | 0.37 | 0.86 | 1.12 | 0.88 | 0.81 | 0.21 | 0.56 | 1.10 |
| 12163 | 4 oz | Tongue, raw | 113 | 0.97 | 1.14 | 1.72 | 0.27 | 2.32 | 1.37 | 0.46 | 0.84 | 1.48 | 1.50 | 0.41 | 0.76 | 0.97 | 0.77 | 0.78 | 0.21 | 0.56 | 0.96 |
| 12180 | 3 oz | Tail, ckd | 85 | 1.07 | 0.99 | 1.22 | 0.19 | 1.86 | 1.92 | 0.26 | 0.33 | 0.81 | 0.87 | 0.26 | 0.43 | 1.22 | 0.62 | 0.51 | 0.09 | 0.29 | 0.43 |
| 12179 | 4 oz | Tail, raw | 113 | 1.45 | 1.34 | 1.56 | 0.26 | 2.41 | 2.67 | 0.34 | 0.46 | 1.02 | 1.14 | 0.36 | 0.54 | 1.71 | 0.78 | 0.62 | 0.10 | 0.36 | 0.58 |
| | | Turkey | | | | | | | | | | | | | | | | | | | |
| 16073 | 3 oz | Giblets, ckd | 85 | 1.12 | 1.50 | 2.12 | 0.30 | 3.41 | 1.25 | 0.53 | 1.14 | 1.82 | 1.66 | 0.56 | 1.03 | 1.15 | 0.99 | 1.02 | 0.26 | 0.75 | 1.22 |
| 16072 | 4 oz | Giblets, raw | 113 | 1.10 | 1.46 | 2.06 | 0.29 | 3.29 | 1.21 | 0.52 | 1.10 | 1.76 | 1.62 | 0.54 | 1.00 | 1.11 | 0.95 | 0.99 | 0.25 | 0.72 | 1.19 |
| 16004 | 1 ea | Gizzard, ckd | 67 | 0.78 | 1.41 | 1.82 | 0.26 | 3.37 | 1.04 | 0.40 | 0.93 | 1.39 | 1.36 | 0.52 | 0.82 | 1.03 | 0.88 | 0.91 | 0.18 | 0.60 | 0.88 |
| 16074 | 1 ea | Gizzard, raw | 113 | 0.85 | 1.55 | 1.99 | 0.28 | 3.68 | 1.13 | 0.44 | 1.02 | 1.51 | 1.49 | 0.57 | 0.90 | 1.12 | 0.97 | 0.99 | 0.19 | 0.66 | 0.97 |
| 16005 | 3 ea | Hearts, ckd | 87 | 1.47 | 1.49 | 2.26 | 0.32 | 3.44 | 1.29 | 0.61 | 1.25 | 2.02 | 1.94 | 0.56 | 1.04 | 1.19 | 0.94 | 1.05 | 0.30 | 0.83 | 1.32 |
| 16075 | 4 ea | Heart, raw | 116 | 1.32 | 1.34 | 2.04 | 0.28 | 3.11 | 1.16 | 0.55 | 1.12 | 1.82 | 1.75 | 0.51 | 0.94 | 1.07 | 0.84 | 0.95 | 0.27 | 0.75 | 1.18 |
| 16007 | 1 ea | Liver, ckd | 75 | 1.04 | 1.10 | 1.71 | 0.24 | 2.33 | 1.04 | 0.48 | 0.95 | 1.62 | 1.36 | 0.43 | 0.89 | 0.89 | 0.77 | 0.80 | 0.25 | 0.63 | 1.13 |
| 16076 | 1 ea | Liver, raw | 102 | 1.18 | 1.25 | 1.94 | 0.27 | 2.64 | 1.18 | 0.54 | 1.08 | 1.85 | 1.55 | 0.48 | 1.02 | 1.01 | 0.88 | 0.91 | 0.29 | 0.72 | 1.29 |
| | | Veal | | | | | | | | | | | | | | | | | | | |
| 11598 | 3 oz | Brain, pan fried | 85 | 0.63 | 0.67 | 1.05 | 0.13 | 1.47 | 0.54 | 0.31 | 0.50 | 0.95 | 0.76 | 0.27 | 0.65 | 0.51 | 0.63 | 0.61 | 0.12 | 0.48 | 0.59 |
| 11535 | 4 oz | Brain, raw | 113 | 0.60 | 0.64 | 0.99 | 0.12 | 1.39 | 0.51 | 0.29 | 0.47 | 0.90 | 0.72 | 0.26 | 0.61 | 0.48 | 0.60 | 0.58 | 0.12 | 0.45 | 0.55 |
| 11501 | 3 oz | Heart, brsd | 85 | 1.54 | 1.54 | 2.30 | 0.27 | 3.57 | 1.35 | 0.67 | 1.19 | 1.95 | 2.13 | 0.56 | 1.07 | 1.15 | 1.15 | 1.10 | 0.26 | 0.81 | 1.29 |
| 11536 | 4 oz | Heart, raw | 113 | 1.21 | 1.21 | 1.81 | 0.21 | 2.80 | 1.06 | 0.52 | 0.93 | 1.53 | 1.67 | 0.44 | 0.84 | 0.90 | 0.90 | 0.86 | 0.21 | 0.64 | 1.01 |

## TABLE A Amino Acid Content for Selected Foods *(continued)*

| Code | Amount | Description | Weight (g) | Alanine (g) | Arginine (g) | Aspartic acid (g) | Cystine (g) | Glutamic acid (g) | Glycine (g) | Histidine (g) | Isoleucine (g) | Leucine (g) | Lysine (g) | Methionine (g) | Phenylalanine (g) | Proline (g) | Serine (g) | Threonine (g) | Tryptophan (g) | Tyrosine (g) | Valine (g) |
|---|---|---|---|---|---|---|---|---|---|---|---|---|---|---|---|---|---|---|---|---|---|
| 11538 | 3 oz | Kidneys, brsd | 85 | 1.18 | 1.38 | 1.94 | 0.25 | 2.08 | 1.32 | 0.54 | 0.95 | 1.81 | 1.49 | 0.47 | 1.06 | 1.10 | 0.98 | 1.02 | 0.29 | 0.86 | 1.18 |
| 11537 | 4 oz | Kidneys, raw | 113 | 0.94 | 1.10 | 1.54 | 0.20 | 1.66 | 1.05 | 0.43 | 0.76 | 1.45 | 1.19 | 0.37 | 0.85 | 0.87 | 0.78 | 0.81 | 0.23 | 0.68 | 0.94 |
| 11500 | 3 oz | Liver, brsd | 85 | 0.99 | 0.88 | 1.70 | 0.20 | 2.19 | 0.94 | 0.40 | 0.81 | 1.50 | 0.83 | 0.23 | 0.89 | 0.80 | 0.78 | 0.78 | 0.19 | 0.66 | 1.03 |
| 11539 | 4 oz | Liver, raw | 113 | 1.09 | 0.97 | 1.86 | 0.22 | 2.41 | 1.02 | 0.44 | 0.89 | 1.64 | 0.91 | 0.32 | 0.98 | 0.88 | 0.85 | 0.86 | 0.21 | 0.73 | 1.13 |
| 11550 | 3 oz | Tongue, brsd | 85 | 1.22 | 1.28 | 1.87 | 0.22 | 2.98 | 1.29 | 0.50 | 0.94 | 1.58 | 1.62 | 0.45 | 0.87 | 1.04 | 0.82 | 0.88 | 0.24 | 0.66 | 1.01 |
| 11549 | 4 oz | Tongue, raw | 113 | 1.08 | 1.14 | 1.65 | 0.19 | 2.63 | 1.14 | 0.44 | 0.83 | 1.40 | 1.42 | 0.40 | 0.77 | 0.92 | 0.72 | 0.78 | 0.21 | 0.58 | 0.89 |
| | | **MEAT SUBSTITUTES, TOFU AND OTHER SOY FOODS** | | | | | | | | | | | | | | | | | | | |
| 7511 | 1 ea | Sausage Substitute, pattie, avg | 25 | 0.19 | 0.34 | 0.52 | 0.07 | 0.94 | 0.18 | 0.12 | 0.22 | 0.36 | 0.28 | 0.05 | 0.24 | 0.25 | 0.24 | 0.18 | 0.06 | 0.16 | 0.23 |
| | | Soybeans | | | | | | | | | | | | | | | | | | | |
| 90028 | 1/2 cup | Cooked, w/salt, avg | 86 | 0.64 | 1.05 | 1.70 | 0.22 | 2.61 | 0.62 | 0.36 | 0.65 | 1.10 | 0.90 | 0.13 | 0.70 | 0.79 | 0.78 | 0.59 | 0.20 | 0.51 | 0.67 |
| 7063 | 1/2 cup | Roasted, dry, avg | 86 | 1.52 | 2.50 | 4.05 | 0.52 | 6.24 | 1.49 | 0.87 | 1.56 | 2.62 | 2.14 | 0.43 | 1.68 | 1.89 | 1.86 | 1.40 | 0.47 | 1.22 | 1.61 |
| 7719 | 1/2 cup | Roasted, mature seeds, unsalted, avg | 86 | 1.35 | 2.22 | 3.60 | 0.46 | 5.54 | 1.32 | 0.77 | 1.39 | 2.33 | 1.90 | 0.39 | 1.50 | 1.67 | 1.66 | 1.24 | 0.42 | 1.08 | 1.43 |
| | | Tofu | | | | | | | | | | | | | | | | | | | |
| 7540 | 1/2 cup | Silken Extra Firm, Morinaga Nutritional Foods | 126 | 0.35 | 0.67 | 1.03 | 0.16 | 1.61 | 0.35 | 0.23 | 0.43 | 0.81 | 0.62 | 0.12 | 0.54 | 0.46 | 0.44 | 0.39 | 0.15 | 0.40 | 0.50 |
| 7542 | 1/2 cup | Silken Firm, Morinaga Nutritional Foods | 126 | 0.34 | 0.65 | 0.97 | 0.13 | 1.48 | 0.34 | 0.21 | 0.44 | 0.74 | 0.58 | 0.13 | 0.50 | 0.44 | 0.42 | 0.36 | 0.11 | 0.38 | 0.49 |
| 7541 | 1/2 cup | Silken Soft, Morinaga Nutritional Foods | 124 | 0.24 | 0.47 | 0.68 | 0.09 | 0.99 | 0.24 | 0.15 | 0.29 | 0.35 | 0.42 | 0.09 | 0.38 | 0.31 | 0.30 | 0.27 | 0.08 | 0.24 | 0.37 |
| | | **NUTS, SEEDS AND PRODUCTS** | | | | | | | | | | | | | | | | | | | |
| | | Acorns | | | | | | | | | | | | | | | | | | | |
| 4639 | 1 oz | Dried, avg | 28 | 0.13 | 0.17 | 0.23 | 0.04 | 0.36 | 0.11 | 0.06 | 0.11 | 0.18 | 0.14 | 0.04 | 0.10 | 0.09 | 0.10 | 0.09 | 0.03 | 0.07 | 0.13 |
| 4679 | 1 oz | Flour, full fat, avg | 28 | 0.12 | 0.16 | 0.22 | 0.04 | 0.34 | 0.10 | 0.06 | 0.10 | 0.17 | 0.13 | 0.04 | 0.09 | 0.08 | 0.09 | 0.08 | 0.03 | 0.06 | 0.12 |
| 4704 | 1 oz | Raw, avg | 28 | 0.10 | 0.13 | 0.18 | 0.03 | 0.28 | 0.08 | 0.05 | 0.08 | 0.14 | 0.11 | 0.03 | 0.08 | 0.07 | 0.07 | 0.07 | 0.02 | 0.05 | 0.10 |
| | | Almonds | | | | | | | | | | | | | | | | | | | |
| 4547 | 1 oz | Blanched, whole, avg | 28 | 0.23 | 0.61 | 0.58 | 0.09 | 1.45 | 0.30 | 0.14 | 0.21 | 0.38 | 0.16 | 0.05 | 0.27 | 0.31 | 0.22 | 0.18 | 0.09 | 0.17 | 0.25 |
| 4721 | 1 oz | Blanched, slivered, Blue Diamond | 28 | 0.27 | 0.68 | 0.63 | 0.11 | 1.43 | 0.39 | 0.14 | 0.20 | 0.37 | 0.19 | 0.03 | 0.31 | 0.25 | 0.25 | 0.17 | 0.04 | 0.16 | 0.24 |
| 4572 | 2 Tbs | Butter, plain, salted, avg | 32 | 0.20 | 0.52 | 0.49 | 0.07 | 1.23 | 0.26 | 0.12 | 0.18 | 0.32 | 0.14 | 0.05 | 0.23 | 0.26 | 0.19 | 0.15 | 0.07 | 0.15 | 0.21 |
| 4534 | 2 Tbs | Butter, plain, unsalted, avg | 32 | 0.20 | 0.52 | 0.49 | 0.07 | 1.23 | 0.26 | 0.12 | 0.18 | 0.32 | 0.14 | 0.05 | 0.23 | 0.26 | 0.19 | 0.15 | 0.07 | 0.15 | 0.21 |
| 4691 | 2 Tbs | Butter, w/honey & cinnamon, salted, avg | 32 | 0.20 | 0.54 | 0.51 | 0.08 | 1.29 | 0.27 | 0.12 | 0.19 | 0.34 | 0.14 | 0.05 | 0.24 | 0.27 | 0.20 | 0.16 | 0.08 | 0.15 | 0.22 |
| 4567 | 2 Tbs | Butter, w/honey & cinnamon, unsalted, avg | 32 | 0.20 | 0.54 | 0.51 | 0.08 | 1.29 | 0.27 | 0.12 | 0.19 | 0.34 | 0.14 | 0.05 | 0.24 | 0.27 | 0.20 | 0.16 | 0.08 | 0.15 | 0.22 |
| 4500 | 1 oz | Dried, avg | 28 | 0.23 | 0.60 | 0.57 | 0.09 | 1.43 | 0.30 | 0.13 | 0.21 | 0.37 | 0.16 | 0.05 | 0.27 | 0.30 | 0.22 | 0.18 | 0.09 | 0.17 | 0.25 |
| 4571 | 1 oz | Dry Roasted, salted, avg | 28 | 0.18 | 0.49 | 0.46 | 0.07 | 1.16 | 0.24 | 0.11 | 0.17 | 0.30 | 0.13 | 0.04 | 0.22 | 0.25 | 0.18 | 0.14 | 0.07 | 0.14 | 0.20 |
| 4549 | 1 oz | Dry Roasted, unsalted, avg | 28 | 0.18 | 0.49 | 0.46 | 0.07 | 1.16 | 0.24 | 0.11 | 0.17 | 0.30 | 0.13 | 0.04 | 0.22 | 0.25 | 0.18 | 0.14 | 0.07 | 0.14 | 0.20 |
| 4687 | 1 oz | Honey Roasted, avg | 28 | 0.21 | 0.55 | 0.51 | 0.08 | 1.30 | 0.27 | 0.12 | 0.19 | 0.34 | 0.15 | 0.05 | 0.24 | 0.27 | 0.20 | 0.16 | 0.08 | 0.15 | 0.22 |
| 4692 | 1 oz | Meal, salted, avg | 28 | 0.45 | 1.18 | 1.11 | 0.17 | 2.83 | 0.59 | 0.27 | 0.41 | 0.74 | 0.32 | 0.11 | 0.53 | 0.60 | 0.43 | 0.35 | 0.17 | 0.34 | 0.49 |
| 4657 | 1 oz | Nut Meal, avg | 28 | 0.45 | 1.18 | 1.11 | 0.17 | 2.83 | 0.59 | 0.27 | 0.41 | 0.74 | 0.32 | 0.11 | 0.53 | 0.60 | 0.43 | 0.35 | 0.17 | 0.34 | 0.49 |
| 4620 | 1 oz | Oil Roasted, salted, avg | 28 | 0.23 | 0.61 | 0.58 | 0.09 | 1.46 | 0.30 | 0.14 | 0.21 | 0.38 | 0.16 | 0.05 | 0.27 | 0.31 | 0.22 | 0.18 | 0.09 | 0.17 | 0.25 |
| 4505 | 1 oz | Oil Roasted, unsalted, avg | 28 | 0.23 | 0.61 | 0.58 | 0.09 | 1.46 | 0.30 | 0.14 | 0.21 | 0.38 | 0.16 | 0.05 | 0.27 | 0.31 | 0.22 | 0.18 | 0.09 | 0.17 | 0.25 |
| 4553 | 2 Tbs | Paste, packed, avg | 29 | 0.11 | 0.28 | 0.26 | 0.04 | 0.67 | 0.14 | 0.06 | 0.10 | 0.17 | 0.07 | 0.03 | 0.12 | 0.14 | 0.10 | 0.08 | 0.04 | 0.08 | 0.12 |
| 4566 | 1 oz | Toasted, whole, avg | 28 | 0.23 | 0.61 | 0.58 | 0.09 | 1.45 | 0.30 | 0.14 | 0.21 | 0.38 | 0.16 | 0.05 | 0.27 | 0.31 | 0.22 | 0.18 | 0.09 | 0.17 | 0.25 |
| 4725 | 1 oz | Whole Natural, Blue Diamond | 28 | 0.26 | 0.66 | 0.63 | 0.11 | 1.42 | 0.39 | 0.13 | 0.21 | 0.38 | 0.18 | 0.03 | 0.30 | 0.25 | 0.24 | 0.17 | 0.04 | 0.15 | 0.25 |
| 4642 | 1 oz | Beechnuts, dried, avg | 28 | 0.12 | 0.12 | 0.30 | 0.05 | 0.22 | 0.09 | 0.05 | 0.07 | 0.10 | 0.10 | 0.04 | 0.07 | 0.09 | 0.09 | 0.06 | 0.02 | 0.05 | 0.10 |
| 4643 | 1 oz | Butternuts, dried, avg | 28 | 0.31 | 1.09 | 0.69 | 0.11 | 1.36 | 0.34 | 0.18 | 0.26 | 0.49 | 0.17 | 0.14 | 0.32 | 0.28 | 0.37 | 0.21 | 0.08 | 0.22 | 0.34 |
| 4535 | 1 oz | Brazil Nuts, dried, avg | 28 | 0.14 | 0.58 | 0.33 | 0.08 | 0.76 | 0.16 | 0.10 | 0.15 | 0.29 | 0.13 | 0.24 | 0.18 | 0.18 | 0.18 | 0.11 | 0.06 | 0.11 | 0.22 |
| | | Breadfruit Seeds | | | | | | | | | | | | | | | | | | | |
| 4606 | 1 oz | Boiled, avg | 28 | 0.06 | 0.09 | 0.14 | 0.02 | 0.18 | 0.08 | 0.04 | 0.03 | 0.10 | 0.10 | 0.02 | 0.14 | 0.07 | 0.09 | 0.07 | 0.02 | 0.10 | 0.09 |
| 4605 | 1 oz | Raw, avg | 28 | 0.08 | 0.12 | 0.20 | 0.03 | 0.26 | 0.11 | 0.05 | 0.11 | 0.14 | 0.14 | 0.02 | 0.20 | 0.09 | 0.12 | 0.10 | 0.03 | 0.13 | 0.13 |
| 4607 | 1 oz | Roasted, avg | 28 | 0.07 | 0.10 | 0.17 | 0.02 | 0.21 | 0.10 | 0.04 | 0.09 | 0.12 | 0.12 | 0.02 | 0.16 | 0.08 | 0.10 | 0.08 | 0.03 | 0.11 | 0.11 |
| | | Cashews | | | | | | | | | | | | | | | | | | | |
| 4662 | 2 Tbs | Butter, salted | 32 | 0.23 | 0.58 | 0.50 | 0.09 | 1.21 | 0.27 | 0.13 | 0.24 | 0.43 | 0.27 | 0.09 | 0.26 | 0.23 | 0.28 | 0.20 | 0.08 | 0.16 | 0.35 |
| 4537 | 2 Tbs | Butter, unsalted, avg | 32 | 0.23 | 0.58 | 0.50 | 0.09 | 1.21 | 0.27 | 0.13 | 0.24 | 0.43 | 0.27 | 0.09 | 0.26 | 0.23 | 0.28 | 0.20 | 0.08 | 0.16 | 0.35 |
| 4519 | 1 oz | Dry Roasted, salted, avg | 28 | 0.18 | 0.44 | 0.38 | 0.07 | 0.92 | 0.20 | 0.10 | 0.19 | 0.33 | 0.21 | 0.07 | 0.20 | 0.18 | 0.22 | 0.15 | 0.06 | 0.12 | 0.26 |

TABLE A **Amino Acid Content for Selected Foods *(continued)***

| Code | Amount | | Description | Weight (g) | Alanine (g) | Arginine (g) | Aspartic acid (g) | Cystine (g) | Glutamic acid (g) | Glycine (g) | Histidine (g) | Isoleucine (g) | Leucine (g) | Lysine (g) | Methionine (g) | Phenylalanine (g) | Proline (g) | Serine (g) | Threonine (g) | Tryptophan (g) | Tyrosine (g) | Valine (g) |
|---|---|---|---|---|---|---|---|---|---|---|---|---|---|---|---|---|---|---|---|---|---|---|
| 4621 | 1 | oz | Dry Roasted, unsalted, avg | 28 | 0.18 | 0.44 | 0.38 | 0.07 | 0.92 | 0.20 | 0.10 | 0.19 | 0.33 | 0.21 | 0.07 | 0.20 | 0.18 | 0.22 | 0.15 | 0.06 | 0.12 | 0.26 |
| 4596 | 1 | oz | Oil Roasted, salted, avg | 28 | 0.19 | 0.47 | 0.41 | 0.08 | 0.97 | 0.22 | 0.11 | 0.20 | 0.35 | 0.22 | 0.07 | 0.21 | 0.19 | 0.23 | 0.16 | 0.06 | 0.13 | 0.28 |
| 4622 | 1 | oz | Oil Roasted, unsalted, avg | 28 | 0.19 | 0.47 | 0.41 | 0.08 | 0.97 | 0.22 | 0.11 | 0.20 | 0.35 | 0.22 | 0.07 | 0.21 | 0.19 | 0.23 | 0.16 | 0.06 | 0.13 | 0.28 |
| | | | Chestnuts | | | | | | | | | | | | | | | | | | | |
| 4648 | 1 | oz | Cooked, European, avg | 28 | 0.04 | 0.04 | 0.10 | 0.02 | 0.07 | 0.03 | 0.02 | 0.02 | 0.03 | 0.03 | 0.01 | 0.02 | 0.03 | 0.03 | 0.02 | 0.01 | 0.02 | 0.03 |
| 4531 | 1 | oz | Dried, peeled, avg | 28 | 0.09 | 0.10 | 0.24 | 0.04 | 0.18 | 0.07 | 0.04 | 0.05 | 0.08 | 0.08 | 0.03 | 0.06 | 0.07 | 0.07 | 0.05 | 0.02 | 0.04 | 0.08 |
| 4570 | 1 | oz | Dried, unpeeled, avg | 28 | 0.12 | 0.13 | 0.31 | 0.06 | 0.23 | 0.09 | 0.05 | 0.07 | 0.11 | 0.11 | 0.04 | 0.08 | 0.09 | 0.09 | 0.06 | 0.02 | 0.05 | 0.10 |
| 4658 | 1 | oz | Raw, Japanese, avg | 28 | 0.05 | 0.04 | 0.11 | 0.02 | 0.10 | 0.03 | 0.01 | 0.03 | 0.03 | 0.04 | 0.01 | 0.02 | 0.03 | 0.03 | 0.02 | 0.01 | 0.02 | 0.03 |
| 4530 | 1 | oz | Raw, peeled, avg | 28 | 0.03 | 0.03 | 0.08 | 0.01 | 0.06 | 0.02 | 0.01 | 0.02 | 0.03 | 0.03 | 0.01 | 0.02 | 0.02 | 0.02 | 0.02 | 0.01 | 0.01 | 0.03 |
| 4568 | 1 | oz | Raw, unpeeled, avg | 28 | 0.04 | 0.05 | 0.12 | 0.02 | 0.09 | 0.03 | 0.02 | 0.03 | 0.04 | 0.04 | 0.02 | 0.03 | 0.04 | 0.03 | 0.02 | 0.01 | 0.02 | 0.04 |
| 4538 | 1 | oz | Roasted, avg | 28 | 0.06 | 0.06 | 0.15 | 0.03 | 0.11 | 0.05 | 0.02 | 0.03 | 0.05 | 0.05 | 0.02 | 0.04 | 0.05 | 0.04 | 0.03 | 0.01 | 0.02 | 0.05 |
| | | | Coconut | | | | | | | | | | | | | | | | | | | |
| 4511 | 2 | Tbs | Dried, sweetened, shredded, avg | 23 | 0.03 | 0.10 | 0.06 | 0.01 | 0.14 | 0.03 | 0.01 | 0.02 | 0.05 | 0.03 | 0.01 | 0.03 | 0.03 | 0.03 | 0.02 | 0.01 | 0.02 | 0.04 |
| 4510 | 2 | Tbs | Dried, unsweetened, avg | 20 | 0.06 | 0.21 | 0.12 | 0.02 | 0.29 | 0.06 | 0.03 | 0.05 | 0.09 | 0.06 | 0.02 | 0.06 | 0.05 | 0.07 | 0.05 | 0.01 | 0.04 | 0.08 |
| 4573 | 2 | Tbs | Flaked, sweetened, cnd, avg | 19 | 0.03 | 0.10 | 0.06 | 0.01 | 0.13 | 0.03 | 0.01 | 0.02 | 0.04 | 0.03 | 0.01 | 0.03 | 0.02 | 0.03 | 0.02 | 0.01 | 0.02 | 0.04 |
| 4507 | 2 | Tbs | Fresh, shredded, avg | 20 | 0.03 | 0.10 | 0.06 | 0.01 | 0.14 | 0.03 | 0.01 | 0.02 | 0.05 | 0.03 | 0.01 | 0.03 | 0.03 | 0.03 | 0.02 | 0.01 | 0.02 | 0.04 |
| 4559 | 1/2 | cup | Milk, cnd, avg | 113 | 0.11 | 0.34 | 0.20 | 0.04 | 0.48 | 0.10 | 0.05 | 0.08 | 0.16 | 0.09 | 0.04 | 0.11 | 0.09 | 0.11 | 0.08 | 0.02 | 0.06 | 0.13 |
| 4560 | 1/2 | cup | Milk, f/fzn, avg | 120 | 0.09 | 0.29 | 0.17 | 0.04 | 0.40 | 0.08 | 0.04 | 0.07 | 0.13 | 0.08 | 0.03 | 0.09 | 0.07 | 0.09 | 0.06 | 0.02 | 0.05 | 0.11 |
| 4528 | 1/2 | cup | Milk, raw, avg | 120 | 0.13 | 0.41 | 0.25 | 0.05 | 0.58 | 0.12 | 0.06 | 0.10 | 0.19 | 0.11 | 0.05 | 0.13 | 0.10 | 0.13 | 0.09 | 0.03 | 0.08 | 0.15 |
| 4575 | 1 | oz | Toasted, dry, avg | 28 | 0.07 | 0.22 | 0.13 | 0.03 | 0.31 | 0.06 | 0.03 | 0.05 | 0.10 | 0.06 | 0.03 | 0.07 | 0.06 | 0.07 | 0.05 | 0.02 | 0.04 | 0.08 |
| 4527 | 1/2 | cup | Water, raw, avg | 120 | 0.04 | 0.13 | 0.08 | 0.02 | 0.18 | 0.04 | 0.02 | 0.03 | 0.06 | 0.04 | 0.01 | 0.04 | 0.03 | 0.04 | 0.03 | 0.01 | 0.02 | 0.05 |
| | | | Filberts/Hazelnuts | | | | | | | | | | | | | | | | | | | |
| 4513 | 1 | oz | Dried, avg | 28 | 0.17 | 0.52 | 0.38 | 0.06 | 0.85 | 0.17 | 0.08 | 0.14 | 0.26 | 0.10 | 0.04 | 0.16 | 0.12 | 0.16 | 0.11 | 0.05 | 0.11 | 0.16 |
| 4650 | 1 | oz | Dried, blanched, avg | 28 | 0.17 | 0.51 | 0.38 | 0.05 | 0.83 | 0.17 | 0.08 | 0.13 | 0.26 | 0.09 | 0.04 | 0.16 | 0.12 | 0.16 | 0.11 | 0.05 | 0.11 | 0.16 |
| 4663 | 1 | oz | Dry Roasted, salted, avg | 28 | 0.13 | 0.40 | 0.30 | 0.04 | 0.66 | 0.13 | 0.06 | 0.11 | 0.20 | 0.07 | 0.03 | 0.13 | 0.09 | 0.12 | 0.08 | 0.04 | 0.08 | 0.12 |
| 4651 | 1 | oz | Dry Roasted, unsalted, avg | 28 | 0.13 | 0.40 | 0.30 | 0.04 | 0.66 | 0.13 | 0.06 | 0.11 | 0.20 | 0.07 | 0.03 | 0.13 | 0.09 | 0.12 | 0.08 | 0.04 | 0.08 | 0.12 |
| 4664 | 1 | oz | Oil Roasted, salted | 28 | 0.19 | 0.57 | 0.42 | 0.06 | 0.94 | 0.19 | 0.09 | 0.15 | 0.29 | 0.11 | 0.04 | 0.18 | 0.13 | 0.18 | 0.12 | 0.06 | 0.12 | 0.17 |
| 4652 | 1 | oz | Oil Roasted, unsalted, avg | 28 | 0.19 | 0.57 | 0.42 | 0.06 | 0.94 | 0.19 | 0.09 | 0.15 | 0.29 | 0.11 | 0.04 | 0.18 | 0.13 | 0.18 | 0.12 | 0.06 | 0.12 | 0.17 |
| 4717 | 1 | oz | Whole Natural, Westnut | 28 | 0.20 | 0.66 | 0.47 | 0.08 | 1.08 | 0.22 | 0.11 | 0.14 | 0.31 | 0.13 | 0.06 | 0.18 | 0.16 | 0.21 | 0.15 | 0.05 | 0.12 | 0.18 |
| | | | Formed Nuts | | | | | | | | | | | | | | | | | | | |
| 4600 | 1 | oz | Macadamia Flavor, unsalted | 28 | 0.17 | 0.22 | 0.28 | 0.05 | 0.58 | 0.16 | 0.09 | 0.13 | 0.23 | 0.21 | 0.06 | 0.14 | 0.21 | 0.16 | 0.13 | 0.04 | 0.12 | 0.17 |
| 4601 | 1 | oz | Other Flavors, unsalted | 28 | 0.21 | 0.27 | 0.33 | 0.06 | 0.67 | 0.19 | 0.10 | 0.15 | 0.27 | 0.24 | 0.08 | 0.16 | 0.23 | 0.18 | 0.15 | 0.05 | 0.13 | 0.20 |
| 4599 | 1 | oz | Unflavored, f/wheat & salt, avg | 28 | 0.23 | 0.30 | 0.35 | 0.07 | 0.69 | 0.21 | 0.11 | 0.15 | 0.28 | 0.25 | 0.08 | 0.17 | 0.24 | 0.19 | 0.16 | 0.05 | 0.13 | 0.20 |
| | | | Macadamia Nuts | | | | | | | | | | | | | | | | | | | |
| 4516 | 1 | oz | Dried, avg | 28 | 0.09 | 0.25 | 0.23 | 0.03 | 0.50 | 0.10 | 0.05 | 0.07 | 0.13 | 0.09 | 0.03 | 0.07 | 0.11 | 0.10 | 0.07 | 0.06 | 0.09 | 0.09 |
| 4587 | 1 | oz | Oil Roasted, salted, avg | 28 | 0.08 | 0.22 | 0.20 | 0.02 | 0.44 | 0.09 | 0.04 | 0.06 | 0.11 | 0.08 | 0.02 | 0.06 | 0.10 | 0.09 | 0.06 | 0.05 | 0.08 | 0.08 |
| 4588 | 1 | oz | Oil Roasted, unsalted, avg | 28 | 0.08 | 0.22 | 0.20 | 0.02 | 0.44 | 0.09 | 0.04 | 0.06 | 0.11 | 0.08 | 0.02 | 0.06 | 0.10 | 0.09 | 0.06 | 0.05 | 0.08 | 0.08 |
| | | | Mixed Nuts | | | | | | | | | | | | | | | | | | | |
| 4592 | 1 | oz | Dry Roasted, salted, avg | 28 | 0.20 | 0.55 | 0.51 | 0.07 | 1.09 | 0.26 | 0.12 | 0.18 | 0.34 | 0.18 | 0.06 | 0.24 | 0.22 | 0.23 | 0.15 | 0.07 | 0.17 | 0.23 |
| 4591 | 1 | oz | Dry Roasted, unsalted, avg | 28 | 0.20 | 0.55 | 0.51 | 0.07 | 1.09 | 0.26 | 0.12 | 0.18 | 0.34 | 0.18 | 0.06 | 0.24 | 0.22 | 0.23 | 0.15 | 0.07 | 0.17 | 0.23 |
| 4593 | 1 | oz | Oil Roasted, salted | 28 | 0.19 | 0.51 | 0.49 | 0.07 | 1.03 | 0.25 | 0.12 | 0.18 | 0.34 | 0.16 | 0.08 | 0.23 | 0.21 | 0.23 | 0.14 | 0.06 | 0.16 | 0.23 |
| 4533 | 1 | oz | Oil Roasted, unsalted | 28 | 0.19 | 0.51 | 0.49 | 0.07 | 1.03 | 0.25 | 0.12 | 0.18 | 0.34 | 0.16 | 0.08 | 0.23 | 0.21 | 0.23 | 0.14 | 0.06 | 0.16 | 0.23 |
| | | | Peanut Butter | | | | | | | | | | | | | | | | | | | |
| 4626 | 2 | Tbs | Chunky, salted, avg | 32 | 0.30 | 0.92 | 0.93 | 0.10 | 1.60 | 0.46 | 0.19 | 0.27 | 0.50 | 0.27 | 0.09 | 0.40 | 0.34 | 0.38 | 0.26 | 0.07 | 0.31 | 0.32 |
| 4576 | 2 | Tbs | Chunky, unsalted, avg | 32 | 0.30 | 0.92 | 0.93 | 0.10 | 1.60 | 0.46 | 0.19 | 0.27 | 0.50 | 0.27 | 0.09 | 0.40 | 0.34 | 0.38 | 0.26 | 0.07 | 0.31 | 0.32 |

TABLE A **Amino Acid Content for Selected Foods *(continued)***

| Code | Amount | | Description | Weight (g) | Alanine (g) | Arginine (g) | Aspartic acid (g) | Cystine (g) | Glutamic acid (g) | Glycine (g) | Histidine (g) | Isoleucine (g) | Leucine (g) | Lysine (g) | Methionine (g) | Phenylalanine (g) | Proline (g) | Serine (g) | Threonine (g) | Tryptophan (g) | Tyrosine (g) | Valine (g) |
|---|---|---|---|---|---|---|---|---|---|---|---|---|---|---|---|---|---|---|---|---|---|---|
| 4637 | 2 | Tbs | Natural, salted, avg | 32 | 0.30 | 0.09 | 0.92 | 0.10 | 1.53 | 0.46 | 0.19 | 0.27 | 0.49 | 0.27 | 0.09 | 0.39 | 0.34 | 0.37 | 0.26 | 0.07 | 0.31 | 0.32 |
| 4668 | 2 | Tbs | Natural, unsalted, avg | 32 | 0.30 | 0.91 | 0.92 | 0.10 | 1.53 | 0.46 | 0.19 | 0.27 | 0.49 | 0.27 | 0.09 | 0.39 | 0.34 | 0.37 | 0.26 | 0.07 | 0.31 | 0.32 |
| 4627 | 2 | Tbs | Smooth, salted, avg | 32 | 0.32 | 0.96 | 0.98 | 0.10 | 1.67 | 0.48 | 0.20 | 0.28 | 0.52 | 0.29 | 0.10 | 0.42 | 0.35 | 0.39 | 0.27 | 0.08 | 0.33 | 0.34 |
| 4636 | 2 | Tbs | Smooth, unsalted, avg | 32 | 0.32 | 0.96 | 0.98 | 0.10 | 1.67 | 0.48 | 0.20 | 0.28 | 0.52 | 0.29 | 0.10 | 0.42 | 0.35 | 0.39 | 0.27 | 0.08 | 0.33 | 0.34 |
| | | | Peanuts | | | | | | | | | | | | | | | | | | | |
| 4753 | 1 | oz | Boiled, avg | 28 | 0.15 | 0.45 | 0.46 | 0.05 | 0.73 | 0.23 | 0.09 | 0.13 | 0.24 | 0.13 | 0.05 | 0.19 | 0.17 | 0.18 | 0.13 | 0.04 | 0.15 | 0.16 |
| 4590 | 1 | oz | Dry Roasted, all types, salted | 28 | 0.26 | 0.79 | 0.80 | 0.08 | 1.37 | 0.40 | 0.17 | 0.23 | 0.43 | 0.24 | 0.08 | 0.34 | 0.29 | 0.32 | 0.23 | 0.06 | 0.27 | 0.28 |
| 4756 | 1 | oz | Dry Roasted, all types, unsalted | 28 | 0.26 | 0.79 | 0.80 | 0.08 | 1.37 | 0.40 | 0.17 | 0.23 | 0.43 | 0.24 | 0.08 | 0.34 | 0.29 | 0.32 | 0.23 | 0.06 | 0.27 | 0.28 |
| 4762 | 1 | oz | Oil Roasted, salted, avg | 28 | 0.29 | 0.88 | 0.89 | 0.09 | 1.53 | 0.44 | 0.19 | 0.26 | 0.48 | 0.26 | 0.09 | 0.38 | 0.32 | 0.36 | 0.25 | 0.07 | 0.30 | 0.31 |
| 4542 | 1 | oz | Oil Roasted, unsalted, avg | 28 | 0.29 | 0.88 | 0.89 | 0.09 | 1.53 | 0.44 | 0.19 | 0.26 | 0.48 | 0.26 | 0.09 | 0.38 | 0.32 | 0.36 | 0.25 | 0.07 | 0.30 | 0.31 |
| 4696 | 1 | oz | Raw, avg | 28 | 0.29 | 0.86 | 0.87 | 0.09 | 1.50 | 0.43 | 0.18 | 0.25 | 0.46 | 0.26 | 0.09 | 0.37 | 0.32 | 0.35 | 0.25 | 0.07 | 0.29 | 0.30 |
| | | | Peanuts, Spanish | | | | | | | | | | | | | | | | | | | |
| 4699 | 1 | oz | Oil Roasted, salted, avg | 28 | 0.31 | 0.93 | 0.95 | 0.10 | 1.62 | 0.47 | 0.20 | 0.27 | 0.50 | 0.28 | 0.10 | 0.40 | 0.34 | 0.38 | 0.27 | 0.08 | 0.32 | 0.33 |
| 4665 | 1 | oz | Oil Roasted, unsalted, avg | 28 | 0.31 | 0.93 | 0.95 | 0.10 | 1.62 | 0.47 | 0.20 | 0.27 | 0.50 | 0.28 | 0.10 | 0.40 | 0.34 | 0.38 | 0.27 | 0.08 | 0.32 | 0.33 |
| 4517 | 1 | oz | Raw, avg | 28 | 0.29 | 0.87 | 0.89 | 0.09 | 1.52 | 0.44 | 0.18 | 0.26 | 0.47 | 0.26 | 0.09 | 0.38 | 0.32 | 0.36 | 0.25 | 0.07 | 0.29 | 0.31 |
| | | | Peanuts, Valencia | | | | | | | | | | | | | | | | | | | |
| 4623 | 1 | oz | Dry Roasted, unsalted, avg | 28 | 0.27 | 0.80 | 0.82 | 0.09 | 1.41 | 0.41 | 0.17 | 0.24 | 0.43 | 0.24 | 0.08 | 0.35 | 0.32 | 0.33 | 0.23 | 0.07 | 0.27 | 0.28 |
| 4701 | 1 | oz | Oil Roasted, salted, avg | 28 | 0.30 | 0.90 | 0.92 | 0.10 | 1.57 | 0.45 | 0.19 | 0.26 | 0.49 | 0.27 | 0.09 | 0.39 | 0.33 | 0.37 | 0.26 | 0.07 | 0.30 | 0.31 |
| 4666 | 1 | oz | Oil Roasted, unsalted, avg | 28 | 0.30 | 0.90 | 0.92 | 0.10 | 1.57 | 0.45 | 0.19 | 0.26 | 0.49 | 0.27 | 0.09 | 0.39 | 0.33 | 0.37 | 0.26 | 0.07 | 0.30 | 0.31 |
| 4700 | 1 | oz | Raw, avg | 28 | 0.28 | 0.83 | 0.85 | 0.09 | 1.45 | 0.42 | 0.18 | 0.24 | 0.45 | 0.25 | 0.09 | 0.36 | 0.31 | 0.34 | 0.24 | 0.07 | 0.28 | 0.29 |
| | | | Peanuts, Virginia | | | | | | | | | | | | | | | | | | | |
| 4703 | 1 | oz | Oil Roasted, salted, avg | 28 | 0.29 | 0.86 | 0.88 | 0.09 | 1.50 | 0.43 | 0.18 | 0.25 | 0.47 | 0.26 | 0.09 | 0.37 | 0.32 | 0.36 | 0.25 | 0.07 | 0.29 | 0.30 |
| 4667 | 1 | oz | Oil Roasted, unsalted, avg | 28 | 0.29 | 0.86 | 0.88 | 0.09 | 1.50 | 0.43 | 0.18 | 0.25 | 0.47 | 0.26 | 0.09 | 0.37 | 0.32 | 0.36 | 0.25 | 0.07 | 0.29 | 0.30 |
| 4702 | 1 | oz | Raw, avg | 28 | 0.28 | 0.84 | 0.85 | 0.09 | 1.46 | 0.42 | 0.18 | 0.25 | 0.45 | 0.25 | 0.09 | 0.36 | 0.31 | 0.34 | 0.24 | 0.07 | 0.28 | 0.29 |
| | | | Pecans | | | | | | | | | | | | | | | | | | | |
| 4578 | 1 | oz | Dried, halves, avg | 28 | 0.09 | 0.30 | 0.19 | 0.06 | 0.41 | 0.10 | 0.06 | 0.09 | 0.14 | 0.08 | 0.05 | 0.11 | 0.10 | 0.10 | 0.07 | 0.05 | 0.08 | 0.10 |
| 4583 | 1 | oz | Dry Roasted, salted, avg | 28 | 0.09 | 0.31 | 0.20 | 0.06 | 0.43 | 0.10 | 0.06 | 0.09 | 0.14 | 0.08 | 0.05 | 0.11 | 0.10 | 0.10 | 0.07 | 0.05 | 0.08 | 0.11 |
| 4582 | 1 | oz | Dry Roasted, unsalted, avg | 28 | 0.09 | 0.31 | 0.20 | 0.06 | 0.43 | 0.10 | 0.06 | 0.09 | 0.14 | 0.08 | 0.05 | 0.11 | 0.10 | 0.10 | 0.07 | 0.05 | 0.08 | 0.11 |
| 4586 | 1 | oz | Oil Roasted, salted, avg | 28 | 0.08 | 0.27 | 0.17 | 0.05 | 0.37 | 0.09 | 0.05 | 0.08 | 0.13 | 0.07 | 0.04 | 0.10 | 0.09 | 0.09 | 0.06 | 0.05 | 0.07 | 0.09 |
| 4584 | 1 | oz | Oil Roasted, unsalted, avg | 28 | 0.08 | 0.27 | 0.17 | 0.05 | 0.37 | 0.09 | 0.05 | 0.08 | 0.13 | 0.07 | 0.04 | 0.10 | 0.09 | 0.09 | 0.06 | 0.05 | 0.07 | 0.09 |
| 4764 | 1 | oz | Pine Nuts, pignolia, dried, avg | 28 | 0.34 | 1.26 | 0.59 | 0.12 | 1.10 | 0.33 | 0.16 | 0.25 | 0.47 | 0.24 | 0.12 | 0.25 | 0.35 | 0.28 | 0.21 | 0.08 | 0.24 | 0.34 |
| 4540 | 1 | oz | Pistachio Nuts, dry roasted, salted, avg | 28 | 0.18 | 0.39 | 0.38 | 0.09 | 0.88 | 0.20 | 0.10 | 0.17 | 0.30 | 0.23 | 0.07 | 0.21 | 0.17 | 0.24 | 0.13 | 0.05 | 0.13 | 0.25 |
| 4654 | 1 | oz | Pistachio Nuts, dry roasted, unsalted, avg | 28 | 0.18 | 0.39 | 0.38 | 0.09 | 0.88 | 0.20 | 0.10 | 0.17 | 0.30 | 0.23 | 0.07 | 0.21 | 0.17 | 0.24 | 0.13 | 0.05 | 0.13 | 0.25 |
| | | | Pumpkin Seeds | | | | | | | | | | | | | | | | | | | |
| 4522 | 1 | oz | Dry, avg | 28 | 0.28 | 0.98 | 0.60 | 0.07 | 1.05 | 0.44 | 0.17 | 0.31 | 0.51 | 0.45 | 0.13 | 0.30 | 0.24 | 0.28 | 0.22 | 0.10 | 0.25 | 0.48 |
| 4564 | 1 | oz | Roasted, salted, avg | 28 | 0.21 | 0.75 | 0.46 | 0.06 | 0.80 | 0.33 | 0.13 | 0.23 | 0.38 | 0.34 | 0.10 | 0.23 | 0.18 | 0.21 | 0.17 | 0.08 | 0.19 | 0.36 |
| 4563 | 1 | oz | Roasted, unsalted, avg | 28 | 0.21 | 0.75 | 0.46 | 0.06 | 0.80 | 0.33 | 0.13 | 0.23 | 0.38 | 0.34 | 0.10 | 0.23 | 0.18 | 0.21 | 0.17 | 0.08 | 0.19 | 0.36 |
| | | | Sesame Seeds | | | | | | | | | | | | | | | | | | | |
| 4683 | 2 | Tbs | Butter Paste, avg | 32 | 0.27 | 0.76 | 0.47 | 0.10 | 1.14 | 0.35 | 0.15 | 0.22 | 0.39 | 0.16 | 0.17 | 0.27 | 0.23 | 0.28 | 0.21 | 0.11 | 0.21 | 0.29 |
| 4523 | 1 | oz | Dried, whole, avg | 28 | 0.23 | 0.65 | 0.41 | 0.09 | 0.98 | 0.30 | 0.13 | 0.19 | 0.33 | 0.14 | 0.14 | 0.23 | 0.20 | 0.24 | 0.18 | 0.10 | 0.18 | 0.24 |
| 4619 | 1 | oz | Meal, part defatted, avg | 28 | 0.22 | 0.62 | 0.39 | 0.08 | 0.94 | 0.29 | 0.12 | 0.18 | 0.32 | 0.13 | 0.14 | 0.22 | 0.19 | 0.23 | 0.17 | 0.09 | 0.18 | 0.23 |
| 4706 | 1 | oz | Toasted, roasted, whole, avg | 28 | 0.22 | 0.62 | 0.39 | 0.08 | 0.94 | 0.29 | 0.12 | 0.18 | 0.32 | 0.13 | 0.14 | 0.22 | 0.19 | 0.23 | 0.17 | 0.09 | 0.18 | 0.23 |
| 4688 | 1 | oz | Toasted, salted, avg | 28 | 0.22 | 0.62 | 0.39 | 0.08 | 0.94 | 0.29 | 0.12 | 0.18 | 0.32 | 0.13 | 0.14 | 0.22 | 0.19 | 0.23 | 0.17 | 0.09 | 0.18 | 0.23 |
| | | | Sunflower Seeds | | | | | | | | | | | | | | | | | | | |
| 4661 | 2 | Tbs | Butter, salted, avg | 32 | 0.28 | 0.60 | 0.62 | 0.11 | 1.41 | 0.37 | 0.16 | 0.29 | 0.42 | 0.24 | 0.12 | 0.29 | 0.30 | 0.27 | 0.23 | 0.09 | 0.17 | 0.33 |
| 4550 | 2 | Tbs | Butter, unsalted, avg | 32 | 0.28 | 0.60 | 0.62 | 0.11 | 1.41 | 0.37 | 0.16 | 0.29 | 0.42 | 0.24 | 0.12 | 0.29 | 0.30 | 0.27 | 0.23 | 0.09 | 0.17 | 0.33 |
| 4551 | 1 | oz | Dry Roasted, unsalted, avg | 28 | 0.24 | 0.52 | 0.53 | 0.10 | 1.21 | 0.32 | 0.14 | 0.25 | 0.36 | 0.20 | 0.11 | 0.25 | 0.25 | 0.23 | 0.20 | 0.08 | 0.14 | 0.29 |
| 4545 | 1 | oz | Kernels, dry, avg | 28 | 0.29 | 0.61 | 0.63 | 0.12 | 1.42 | 0.37 | 0.16 | 0.29 | 0.42 | 0.24 | 0.13 | 0.30 | 0.30 | 0.28 | 0.24 | 0.09 | 0.17 | 0.34 |
| 4597 | 1 | oz | Kernels, dry roasted, salted, avg | 28 | 0.24 | 0.52 | 0.53 | 0.10 | 1.21 | 0.32 | 0.14 | 0.25 | 0.36 | 0.20 | 0.11 | 0.25 | 0.25 | 0.23 | 0.20 | 0.08 | 0.14 | 0.29 |
| 4708 | 1 | oz | Kernels, toasted, salted, avg | 28 | 0.22 | 0.46 | 0.47 | 0.09 | 1.08 | 0.23 | 0.12 | 0.22 | 0.32 | 0.18 | 0.10 | 0.23 | 0.23 | 0.21 | 0.18 | 0.07 | 0.13 | 0.25 |

TABLE A **Amino Acid Content for Selected Foods *(continued)***

| Code | Amount | | Description | Weight (g) | Alanine (g) | Arginine (g) | Aspartic acid (g) | Cystine (g) | Glutamic acid (g) | Glycine (g) | Histidine (g) | Isoleucine (g) | Leucine (g) | Lysine (g) | Methionine (g) | Phenylalanine (g) | Proline (g) | Serine (g) | Threonine (g) | Tryptophan (g) | Tyrosine (g) | Valine (g) |
|---|---|---|---|---|---|---|---|---|---|---|---|---|---|---|---|---|---|---|---|---|---|---|
| 4598 | 1 | oz | Kernels, toasted, unsalted, avg | 28 | 0.22 | 0.46 | 0.47 | 0.09 | 1.08 | 0.28 | 0.12 | 0.22 | 0.32 | 0.18 | 0.10 | 0.23 | 0.23 | 0.21 | 0.18 | 0.07 | 0.13 | 0.25 |
| 4552 | 1 | oz | Oil Roasted, salted, avg | 28 | 0.27 | 0.57 | 0.59 | 0.11 | 1.34 | 0.35 | 0.15 | 0.27 | 0.40 | 0.22 | 0.12 | 0.28 | 0.28 | 0.26 | 0.22 | 0.08 | 0.16 | 0.31 |
| 4546 | 1 | oz | Oil Roasted, unsalted, avg | 28 | 0.27 | 0.57 | 0.59 | 0.11 | 1.34 | 0.35 | 0.15 | 0.27 | 0.40 | 0.22 | 0.12 | 0.28 | 0.28 | 0.26 | 0.22 | 0.08 | 0.16 | 0.31 |
| 4525 | 1 | oz | Walnuts, black, dried, avg | 28 | 0.29 | 1.00 | 0.67 | 0.13 | 1.42 | 0.33 | 0.19 | 0.27 | 0.46 | 0.20 | 0.13 | 0.30 | 0.26 | 0.34 | 0.20 | 0.09 | 0.20 | 0.35 |
| 4557 | 1 | oz | Walnuts, English/Persian, halves, dried, avg | 28 | 0.17 | 0.58 | 0.41 | 0.10 | 0.78 | 0.21 | 0.10 | 0.16 | 0.27 | 0.11 | 0.08 | 0.17 | 0.15 | 0.22 | 0.12 | 0.05 | 0.12 | 0.20 |
| | | | **POULTRY—CHICKEN, BONELESS BROILER/FRYER** | | | | | | | | | | | | | | | | | | | |
| | | | Back | | | | | | | | | | | | | | | | | | | |
| 15116 | 1 | ea | Batter Fried | 240 | 2.98 | 3.22 | 4.54 | 0.73 | 8.50 | 3.26 | 1.52 | 2.62 | 3.86 | 4.10 | 1.38 | 2.11 | 2.81 | 1.96 | 2.15 | 0.60 | 1.71 | 2.57 |
| 15014 | 1 | ea | Flour Fried | 144 | 2.29 | 2.48 | 3.51 | 0.54 | 6.16 | 2.49 | 1.17 | 2.00 | 2.92 | 3.20 | 1.06 | 1.58 | 2.00 | 1.44 | 1.64 | 0.45 | 1.29 | 1.94 |
| 15115 | 1 | ea | Raw | 198 | 1.71 | 1.80 | 2.47 | 0.38 | 3.98 | 2.16 | 0.78 | 1.32 | 1.97 | 2.18 | 0.71 | 1.06 | 1.52 | 1.00 | 1.13 | 0.30 | 0.86 | 1.33 |
| 15118 | 1 | ea | Raw, w/skin | 102 | 1.09 | 1.20 | 1.77 | 0.25 | 2.99 | 0.98 | 0.62 | 1.05 | 1.50 | 1.69 | 0.55 | 0.79 | 0.82 | 0.69 | 0.84 | 0.23 | 0.67 | 0.99 |
| 15015 | 1 | ea | Roasted | 106 | 1.66 | 1.76 | 2.45 | 0.38 | 3.96 | 2.01 | 0.78 | 1.32 | 1.96 | 2.18 | 0.72 | 1.06 | 1.44 | 0.98 | 1.12 | 0.30 | 0.86 | 1.31 |
| 15051 | 1 | ea | Roasted, w/o skin | 80 | 1.23 | 1.36 | 2.01 | 0.29 | 3.38 | 1.11 | 0.70 | 1.19 | 1.70 | 1.92 | 0.62 | 0.90 | 0.93 | 0.78 | 0.95 | 0.26 | 0.76 | 1.12 |
| | | | Breast | | | | | | | | | | | | | | | | | | | |
| 15013 | 1 | ea | Batter Fried | 280 | 3.89 | 4.26 | 6.05 | 0.95 | 11.03 | 4.12 | 2.04 | 3.50 | 5.12 | 5.52 | 1.84 | 2.77 | 3.53 | 2.54 | 2.86 | 0.80 | 2.27 | 3.42 |
| 15003 | 1 | ea | Flour Fried | 196 | 3.51 | 3.82 | 5.55 | 0.82 | 9.33 | 3.55 | 1.88 | 3.19 | 4.61 | 5.15 | 1.69 | 2.45 | 2.84 | 2.18 | 2.61 | 0.71 | 2.06 | 3.06 |
| 15053 | 1 | ea | Raw | 290 | 3.45 | 3.74 | 5.39 | 0.79 | 8.93 | 3.57 | 1.81 | 3.07 | 4.44 | 5.02 | 1.63 | 2.37 | 2.77 | 2.11 | 2.52 | 0.69 | 1.98 | 2.96 |
| 15054 | 1 | ea | Raw, w/o skin | 236 | 2.97 | 3.28 | 4.86 | 0.70 | 8.17 | 2.67 | 1.69 | 2.88 | 4.08 | 4.63 | 1.51 | 2.16 | 2.24 | 1.87 | 2.30 | 0.64 | 1.84 | 2.71 |
| 15001 | 1 | ea | Roasted | 196 | 3.31 | 3.61 | 5.21 | 0.76 | 8.62 | 3.37 | 1.76 | 3.00 | 4.31 | 4.84 | 1.58 | 2.29 | 2.65 | 2.04 | 2.43 | 0.67 | 1.92 | 2.86 |
| 15004 | 1 | ea | Roasted, w/o skin | 172 | 2.91 | 3.22 | 4.75 | 0.68 | 8.00 | 2.61 | 1.66 | 2.82 | 4.01 | 4.54 | 1.48 | 2.12 | 2.20 | 1.84 | 2.25 | 0.62 | 1.81 | 2.65 |
| 15019 | 3 | oz | Canned w/broth | 82 | 1.03 | 1.12 | 1.58 | 0.24 | 2.60 | 1.14 | 0.52 | 0.89 | 1.30 | 1.44 | 0.47 | 0.69 | 0.85 | 0.62 | 0.73 | 0.20 | 0.57 | 0.86 |
| | | | Drumstick | | | | | | | | | | | | | | | | | | | |
| 15030 | 1 | ea | Batter Fried | 72 | 0.89 | 0.96 | 1.38 | 0.22 | 2.52 | 0.93 | 0.47 | 0.80 | 1.17 | 1.25 | 0.42 | 0.63 | 0.80 | 0.58 | 0.65 | 0.18 | 0.52 | 0.78 |
| 15007 | 1 | ea | Flour Fried | 49 | 0.75 | 0.81 | 1.17 | 0.17 | 1.97 | 0.78 | 0.39 | 0.67 | 0.97 | 1.08 | 0.36 | 0.52 | 0.62 | 0.46 | 0.55 | 0.15 | 0.43 | 0.65 |
| 15055 | 1 | ea | Raw | 73 | 0.80 | 0.87 | 1.26 | 0.19 | 2.07 | 0.84 | 0.42 | 0.71 | 1.04 | 1.16 | 0.38 | 0.55 | 0.65 | 0.49 | 0.59 | 0.16 | 0.46 | 0.69 |
| 15056 | 1 | ea | Raw, w/o skin | 62 | 0.69 | 0.77 | 1.14 | 0.16 | 1.91 | 0.63 | 0.40 | 0.68 | 0.96 | 1.09 | 0.35 | 0.51 | 0.53 | 0.44 | 0.54 | 0.15 | 0.43 | 0.63 |
| 15008 | 1 | ea | Roasted | 52 | 0.81 | 0.88 | 1.25 | 0.19 | 2.06 | 0.87 | 0.42 | 0.71 | 1.03 | 1.15 | 0.38 | 0.55 | 0.67 | 0.49 | 0.58 | 0.16 | 0.46 | 0.69 |
| 15035 | 1 | ea | Roasted, w/o skin | 44 | 0.68 | 0.75 | 1.11 | 0.16 | 1.87 | 0.61 | 0.39 | 0.66 | 0.93 | 1.06 | 0.34 | 0.49 | 0.51 | 0.43 | 0.53 | 0.15 | 0.42 | 0.62 |
| | | | Leg | | | | | | | | | | | | | | | | | | | |
| 15151 | 1 | ea | Batter Fried | 158 | 1.93 | 2.10 | 2.99 | 0.47 | 5.50 | 2.04 | 1.01 | 1.74 | 2.53 | 2.72 | 0.91 | 1.37 | 1.75 | 1.26 | 1.41 | 0.40 | 1.12 | 1.69 |
| 15155 | 1 | ea | Flour Fried | 112 | 1.71 | 1.86 | 2.57 | 0.40 | 4.51 | 1.81 | 0.89 | 1.52 | 2.21 | 2.45 | 0.80 | 1.18 | 1.43 | 1.06 | 1.24 | 0.34 | 0.98 | 1.47 |
| 15119 | 1 | ea | Raw | 167 | 1.75 | 1.89 | 2.71 | 0.40 | 4.44 | 1.90 | 0.90 | 1.52 | 2.22 | 2.47 | 0.81 | 1.18 | 1.44 | 1.07 | 1.26 | 0.34 | 0.98 | 1.47 |
| 15121 | 1 | ea | Raw, w/o skin | 130 | 1.43 | 1.57 | 2.33 | 0.34 | 3.93 | 1.29 | 0.81 | 1.38 | 1.96 | 2.22 | 0.72 | 1.04 | 1.08 | 0.90 | 1.11 | 0.31 | 0.88 | 1.30 |
| 15154 | 1 | ea | Roasted | 114 | 1.71 | 1.85 | 2.64 | 0.39 | 4.34 | 1.86 | 0.88 | 1.48 | 2.17 | 2.42 | 0.79 | 1.15 | 1.41 | 1.04 | 1.23 | 0.33 | 0.96 | 1.44 |
| 15156 | 1 | ea | Roasted, w/o skin | 95 | 1.40 | 1.55 | 2.29 | 0.33 | 3.85 | 1.26 | 0.80 | 1.36 | 1.93 | 2.18 | 0.71 | 1.02 | 1.05 | 0.88 | 1.08 | 0.30 | 0.87 | 1.27 |
| | | | Neck | | | | | | | | | | | | | | | | | | | |
| 15124 | 1 | ea | Batter Fried | 52 | 0.62 | 0.66 | 0.39 | 0.15 | 1.61 | 0.81 | 0.28 | 0.48 | 0.73 | 0.76 | 0.26 | 0.40 | 0.62 | 0.39 | 0.41 | 0.11 | 0.32 | 0.49 |
| 15082 | 1 | ea | Flour Fried | 36 | 0.53 | 0.56 | 0.76 | 0.12 | 1.28 | 0.70 | 0.24 | 0.40 | 0.61 | 0.66 | 0.22 | 0.33 | 0.50 | 0.32 | 0.35 | 0.09 | 0.26 | 0.41 |
| 15123 | 1 | ea | Raw | 50 | 0.48 | 0.49 | 0.63 | 0.10 | 0.96 | 0.76 | 0.17 | 0.29 | 0.47 | 0.50 | 0.17 | 0.26 | 0.49 | 0.27 | 0.27 | 0.07 | 0.20 | 0.32 |
| 15125 | 1 | ea | Raw, w/o skin | 20 | 0.19 | 0.21 | 0.31 | 0.04 | 0.53 | 0.17 | 0.11 | 0.19 | 0.26 | 0.30 | 0.10 | 0.14 | 0.14 | 0.12 | 0.15 | 0.04 | 0.12 | 0.17 |
| 15083 | 1 | ea | Simmered | 38 | 0.49 | 0.50 | 0.66 | 0.11 | 1.04 | 0.70 | 0.20 | 0.33 | 0.51 | 0.56 | 0.18 | 0.28 | 0.46 | 0.28 | 0.29 | 0.08 | 0.22 | 0.35 |
| 15085 | 1 | ea | Simmered, w/o skin | 18 | 0.24 | 0.27 | 0.39 | 0.06 | 0.66 | 0.22 | 0.14 | 0.23 | 0.33 | 0.38 | 0.12 | 0.18 | 0.18 | 0.15 | 0.19 | 0.05 | 0.15 | 0.22 |
| | | | Skin | | | | | | | | | | | | | | | | | | | |
| 15100 | 3 | oz | Batter Fried | 85 | 0.54 | 0.54 | 0.63 | 0.15 | 1.72 | 0.95 | 0.17 | 0.31 | 0.56 | 0.42 | 0.17 | 0.34 | 0.85 | 0.40 | 0.30 | 0.09 | 0.23 | 0.38 |
| 15101 | 3 | oz | Flour Fried | 85 | 1.24 | 1.19 | 1.38 | 0.27 | 2.26 | 2.41 | 0.31 | 0.52 | 0.95 | 0.91 | 0.32 | 0.56 | 1.52 | 0.66 | 0.56 | 0.13 | 0.37 | 0.68 |
| 15099 | 4 | oz | Raw | 113 | 1.20 | 1.14 | 1.32 | 0.25 | 1.85 | 2.37 | 0.28 | 0.48 | 0.87 | 0.88 | 0.30 | 0.50 | 1.38 | 0.60 | 0.53 | 0.12 | 0.34 | 0.62 |
| 15102 | 3 | oz | Roasted | 85 | 1.38 | 1.32 | 1.53 | 0.28 | 2.12 | 2.73 | 0.33 | 0.55 | 1.01 | 1.02 | 0.34 | 0.58 | 1.59 | 0.70 | 0.61 | 0.14 | 0.39 | 0.72 |
| | | | Thigh | | | | | | | | | | | | | | | | | | | |
| 15036 | 1 | ea | Batter Fried | 86 | 1.04 | 1.14 | 1.61 | 0.26 | 2.98 | 1.11 | 0.54 | 0.94 | 1.37 | 1.46 | 0.49 | 0.74 | 0.95 | 0.68 | 0.76 | 0.21 | 0.61 | 0.91 |
| 15009 | 1 | ea | Flour Fried | 62 | 0.95 | 1.03 | 1.47 | 0.22 | 2.50 | 1.02 | 0.49 | 0.84 | 1.22 | 1.35 | 0.44 | 0.65 | 0.81 | 0.59 | 0.69 | 0.19 | 0.54 | 0.81 |

# TABLE A Amino Acid Content for Selected Foods *(continued)*

| Code | Amount | | Description | Weight (g) | Alanine (g) | Arginine (g) | Aspartic acid (g) | Cystine (g) | Glutamic acid (g) | Glycine (g) | Histidine (g) | Isoleucine (g) | Leucine (g) | Lysine (g) | Methionine (g) | Phenylalanine (g) | Proline (g) | Serine (g) | Threonine (g) | Tryptophan (g) | Tyrosine (g) | Valine (g) |
|---|---|---|---|---|---|---|---|---|---|---|---|---|---|---|---|---|---|---|---|---|---|---|
| 15060 | 1 | ea | Raw | 94 | 0.95 | 1.02 | 1.45 | 0.22 | 2.37 | 1.07 | 0.47 | 0.81 | 1.17 | 1.32 | 0.43 | 0.63 | 0.80 | 0.57 | 0.67 | 0.18 | 0.52 | 0.79 |
| 15061 | 1 | ea | Raw, w/o skin | 69 | 0.74 | 0.82 | 1.21 | 0.17 | 2.03 | 0.57 | 0.42 | 0.72 | 1.02 | 1.15 | 0.38 | 0.54 | 0.56 | 0.47 | 0.57 | 0.16 | 0.46 | 0.67 |
| 15010 | 1 | ea | Roasted | 62 | 0.90 | 0.97 | 1.38 | 0.21 | 2.28 | 0.39 | 0.46 | 0.73 | 1.13 | 1.27 | 0.41 | 0.60 | 0.74 | 0.55 | 0.64 | 0.17 | 0.50 | 0.76 |
| 15012 | 1 | ea | Roasted, w/o skin | 52 | 0.74 | 0.82 | 1.20 | 0.17 | 2.02 | 0.56 | 0.42 | 0.71 | 1.01 | 1.14 | 0.37 | 0.54 | 0.56 | 0.46 | 0.57 | 0.16 | 0.46 | 0.67 |
| | | | Wing | | | | | | | | | | | | | | | | | | | |
| 15034 | 1 | ea | Batter Fried | 49 | 0.57 | 0.61 | 0.83 | 0.14 | 1.57 | 0.72 | 0.27 | 0.45 | 0.70 | 0.72 | 0.24 | 0.38 | 0.58 | 0.37 | 0.39 | 0.11 | 0.30 | 0.47 |
| 15029 | 1 | ea | Flour Fried | 32 | 0.51 | 0.54 | 0.74 | 0.12 | 1.22 | 0.54 | 0.23 | 0.40 | 0.59 | 0.65 | 0.21 | 0.32 | 0.46 | 0.30 | 0.34 | 0.09 | 0.26 | 0.40 |
| 15062 | 1 | ea | Raw | 49 | 0.56 | 0.58 | 0.80 | 0.12 | 1.28 | 0.73 | 0.25 | 0.42 | 0.63 | 0.70 | 0.23 | 0.34 | 0.50 | 0.32 | 0.36 | 0.10 | 0.27 | 0.43 |
| 15046 | 1 | ea | Raw, w/o skin | 29 | 0.35 | 0.39 | 0.57 | 0.08 | 0.95 | 0.31 | 0.20 | 0.34 | 0.48 | 0.54 | 0.18 | 0.25 | 0.26 | 0.22 | 0.27 | 0.07 | 0.22 | 0.32 |
| 15002 | 1 | ea | Roasted | 34 | 0.56 | 0.59 | 0.82 | 0.13 | 1.31 | 0.72 | 0.25 | 0.43 | 0.65 | 0.71 | 0.23 | 0.35 | 0.50 | 0.33 | 0.37 | 0.10 | 0.28 | 0.44 |
| 15059 | 1 | ea | Roasted, w/o skin | 21 | 0.35 | 0.39 | 0.57 | 0.08 | 0.96 | 0.31 | 0.20 | 0.34 | 0.48 | 0.54 | 0.18 | 0.25 | 0.26 | 0.22 | 0.27 | 0.07 | 0.22 | 0.32 |
| | | | Whole, w/o giblets or neck | | | | | | | | | | | | | | | | | | | |
| 15072 | 3 | oz | Batter Fried | 85 | 1.08 | 1.17 | 1.66 | 0.26 | 3.07 | 1.17 | 0.56 | 0.95 | 1.40 | 1.50 | 0.50 | 0.76 | 1.00 | 0.71 | 0.78 | 0.22 | 0.62 | 0.94 |
| 15113 | 3 | oz | Dark Meat, batter fried | 85 | 1.05 | 1.13 | 1.61 | 0.26 | 2.98 | 1.12 | 0.54 | 0.93 | 1.37 | 1.45 | 0.49 | 0.74 | 0.97 | 0.69 | 0.76 | 0.21 | 0.60 | 0.91 |
| 15112 | 4 | oz | Dark Meat, raw | 113 | 1.11 | 1.19 | 1.68 | 0.25 | 2.75 | 1.28 | 0.55 | 0.93 | 1.37 | 1.53 | 0.50 | 0.73 | 0.94 | 0.67 | 0.78 | 0.21 | 0.60 | 0.91 |
| 15114 | 4 | oz | Dark Meat, raw, w/o skin | 113 | 1.24 | 1.37 | 2.02 | 0.29 | 3.40 | 1.11 | 0.70 | 1.20 | 1.71 | 1.93 | 0.63 | 0.90 | 0.93 | 0.78 | 0.96 | 0.27 | 0.77 | 1.13 |
| 15080 | 3 | oz | Dark Meat, rstd | 85 | 1.29 | 1.39 | 1.97 | 0.30 | 3.22 | 1.46 | 0.65 | 1.10 | 1.60 | 1.79 | 0.58 | 0.86 | 1.09 | 0.78 | 0.91 | 0.25 | 0.71 | 1.07 |
| 15081 | 3 | oz | Dark Meat, stwd | 85 | 1.17 | 1.26 | 1.78 | 0.27 | 2.92 | 1.32 | 0.58 | 0.99 | 1.45 | 1.62 | 0.53 | 0.77 | 0.98 | 0.71 | 0.82 | 0.22 | 0.64 | 0.97 |
| 15219 | 3 | oz | Dark Meat, stwd, w/o skin | 85 | 1.21 | 1.33 | 1.96 | 0.28 | 3.31 | 1.09 | 0.69 | 1.16 | 1.66 | 1.88 | 0.61 | 0.88 | 0.91 | 0.76 | 0.94 | 0.26 | 0.75 | 1.10 |
| 15073 | 6 | oz | Flour Fried | 85 | 1.39 | 1.50 | 2.15 | 0.32 | 3.66 | 1.48 | 0.72 | 1.22 | 1.78 | 1.97 | 0.65 | 0.95 | 1.16 | 0.86 | 1.00 | 0.27 | 0.79 | 1.18 |
| 15214 | 3 | oz | Fried, w/o skin | 85 | 1.41 | 1.56 | 2.30 | 0.33 | 3.94 | 1.28 | 0.80 | 1.37 | 1.95 | 2.19 | 0.72 | 1.04 | 1.09 | 0.90 | 1.10 | 0.30 | 0.88 | 1.29 |
| 15111 | 3 | oz | Light Meat, batter fried | 85 | 1.13 | 1.23 | 1.73 | 0.28 | 3.19 | 1.25 | 0.58 | 0.99 | 1.46 | 1.56 | 0.52 | 0.80 | 1.05 | 0.74 | 0.82 | 0.23 | 0.65 | 0.98 |
| 15076 | 3 | oz | Light Meat, flour fried | 85 | 1.49 | 1.61 | 2.30 | 0.34 | 3.85 | 1.58 | 0.77 | 1.31 | 1.90 | 2.12 | 0.69 | 1.01 | 1.23 | 0.91 | 1.07 | 0.29 | 0.84 | 1.27 |
| 15110 | 4 | oz | Light Meat, raw | 113 | 1.33 | 1.44 | 2.05 | 0.31 | 3.36 | 1.46 | 0.67 | 1.15 | 1.67 | 1.86 | 0.61 | 0.89 | 1.10 | 0.81 | 0.95 | 0.26 | 0.74 | 1.11 |
| 15153 | 4 | oz | Light Meat, raw, w/o skin | 113 | 1.44 | 1.58 | 2.34 | 0.34 | 3.92 | 1.29 | 0.81 | 1.39 | 1.97 | 2.23 | 0.73 | 1.04 | 1.08 | 0.90 | 1.11 | 0.31 | 0.88 | 1.30 |
| 15077 | 3 | oz | Light Meat, rstd | 85 | 1.43 | 1.54 | 2.20 | 0.33 | 3.61 | 1.55 | 0.73 | 1.24 | 1.80 | 2.01 | 0.66 | 0.96 | 1.17 | 0.87 | 1.02 | 0.28 | 0.80 | 1.20 |
| 15216 | 3 | oz | Light Meat, rstd, w/skin | 85 | 1.44 | 1.58 | 2.34 | 0.34 | 3.94 | 1.29 | 0.82 | 1.39 | 1.97 | 2.24 | 0.73 | 1.05 | 1.08 | 0.90 | 1.11 | 0.31 | 0.88 | 1.30 |
| 15078 | 3 | oz | Light Meat, stwd | 85 | 1.28 | 1.39 | 1.98 | 0.29 | 3.26 | 1.39 | 0.66 | 1.12 | 1.62 | 1.82 | 0.59 | 0.87 | 1.05 | 0.78 | 0.92 | 0.25 | 0.72 | 1.08 |
| 15071 | 4 | oz | Raw | 113 | 1.23 | 1.32 | 1.88 | 0.28 | 3.06 | 1.38 | 0.61 | 1.04 | 1.53 | 1.71 | 0.56 | 0.81 | 1.03 | 0.74 | 0.87 | 0.23 | 0.67 | 1.02 |
| 15049 | 4 | oz | Raw, w/o skin | 113 | 1.32 | 1.46 | 2.16 | 0.31 | 3.62 | 1.19 | 0.75 | 1.28 | 1.82 | 2.06 | 0.67 | 0.96 | 0.99 | 0.83 | 1.02 | 0.28 | 0.82 | 1.20 |
| 15074 | 3 | oz | Roasted | 85 | 1.35 | 1.45 | 2.07 | 0.31 | 3.39 | 1.50 | 0.68 | 1.16 | 1.69 | 1.89 | 0.62 | 0.90 | 1.12 | 0.82 | 0.96 | 0.26 | 0.75 | 1.13 |
| 15075 | 3 | oz | Stewed | 85 | 1.22 | 1.32 | 1.87 | 0.28 | 3.07 | 1.34 | 0.62 | 1.05 | 1.53 | 1.71 | 0.56 | 0.82 | 1.01 | 0.74 | 0.87 | 0.23 | 0.68 | 1.02 |
| | | | **POULTRY—TURKEY-ALL TYPES, BONELESS** | | | | | | | | | | | | | | | | | | | |
| 16083 | 4 | oz | Back, raw | 113 | 1.33 | 1.44 | 1.93 | 0.23 | 3.16 | 1.41 | 0.59 | 0.98 | 1.53 | 1.77 | 0.55 | 0.78 | 1.03 | 0.88 | 0.87 | 0.22 | 0.74 | 1.03 |
| 16084 | 3 | oz | Back, rstd | 85 | 1.45 | 1.59 | 2.14 | 0.26 | 3.50 | 1.50 | 0.65 | 1.09 | 1.70 | 1.98 | 0.61 | 0.86 | 1.12 | 0.98 | 0.96 | 0.24 | 0.82 | 1.15 |
| 16085 | 4 | oz | Breast, raw | 113 | 1.55 | 1.72 | 2.36 | 0.27 | 3.91 | 1.45 | 0.74 | 1.23 | 1.90 | 2.23 | 0.69 | 0.96 | 1.13 | 1.08 | 1.07 | 0.27 | 0.93 | 1.27 |
| 16086 | 3 | oz | Breast, rstd | 85 | 1.53 | 1.69 | 2.32 | 0.26 | 3.86 | 1.41 | 0.73 | 1.22 | 1.88 | 2.21 | 0.68 | 0.95 | 1.10 | 1.07 | 1.06 | 0.27 | 0.92 | 1.26 |
| 16050 | 3 | oz | Canned, in broth | 85 | 1.27 | 1.40 | 1.92 | 0.22 | 3.18 | 1.20 | 0.60 | 1.00 | 1.54 | 1.81 | 0.56 | 0.78 | 0.93 | 0.88 | 0.87 | 0.22 | 0.75 | 1.04 |
| 16003 | 3 | oz | Ground, ckd | 85 | 1.42 | 1.61 | 2.24 | 0.24 | 3.75 | 1.14 | 0.72 | 1.20 | 1.83 | 2.17 | 0.67 | 0.91 | 0.96 | 1.02 | 1.02 | 0.26 | 0.91 | 1.22 |
| 16157 | 4 | oz | Ground, raw | 113 | 1.21 | 1.36 | 1.90 | 0.20 | 3.19 | 0.97 | 0.61 | 1.01 | 1.56 | 1.84 | 0.56 | 0.77 | 0.81 | 0.87 | 0.87 | 0.22 | 0.77 | 1.04 |
| 16087 | 4 | oz | Leg, raw | 113 | 1.37 | 1.53 | 2.11 | 0.23 | 3.51 | 1.19 | 0.67 | 1.11 | 1.72 | 2.02 | 0.62 | 0.86 | 0.96 | 0.96 | 0.96 | 0.24 | 0.84 | 1.15 |
| 16159 | 3 | oz | Leg, rstd | 85 | 1.48 | 1.65 | 2.27 | 0.25 | 3.77 | 1.31 | 0.71 | 1.19 | 1.84 | 2.16 | 0.67 | 0.92 | 1.04 | 1.03 | 1.03 | 0.26 | 0.90 | 1.23 |
| 16078 | 3 | oz | Neck, ckd, w/o skin | 85 | 1.39 | 1.57 | 2.19 | 0.23 | 3.67 | 1.12 | 0.70 | 1.17 | 1.79 | 2.12 | 0.65 | 0.90 | 0.94 | 1.00 | 1.00 | 0.26 | 0.89 | 1.20 |
| 16077 | 4 | oz | Neck, raw, w/o skin | 113 | 1.39 | 1.57 | 2.18 | 0.23 | 3.66 | 1.11 | 0.70 | 1.17 | 1.79 | 2.11 | 0.65 | 0.89 | 0.93 | 1.00 | 1.00 | 0.25 | 0.89 | 1.19 |
| | | | Whole, w/o giblets or neck | | | | | | | | | | | | | | | | | | | |
| 16080 | 4 | oz | Dark Meat, raw | 113 | 1.34 | 1.48 | 2.03 | 0.23 | 3.37 | 1.26 | 0.64 | 1.06 | 1.64 | 1.92 | 0.59 | 0.83 | 0.98 | 0.93 | 0.92 | 0.23 | 0.80 | 1.10 |
| 16082 | 4 | oz | Dark Meat, raw, w/o skin | 113 | 1.39 | 1.57 | 2.18 | 0.23 | 3.67 | 1.11 | 0.70 | 1.16 | 1.79 | 2.11 | 0.65 | 0.89 | 0.93 | 1.00 | 1.00 | 0.25 | 0.89 | 1.20 |
| 16028 | 3 | oz | Dark Meat, rstd | 85 | 1.47 | 1.63 | 2.23 | 0.25 | 3.69 | 1.38 | 0.70 | 1.16 | 1.80 | 2.10 | 0.65 | 0.91 | 1.07 | 1.02 | 1.01 | 0.26 | 0.87 | 1.20 |
| 16002 | 3 | oz | Dark Meat, rstd, w/o skin | 85 | 1.49 | 1.67 | 2.34 | 0.25 | 3.92 | 1.19 | 0.75 | 1.25 | 1.92 | 2.26 | 0.70 | 0.95 | 1.00 | 1.07 | 1.07 | 0.27 | 0.95 | 1.28 |
| 16079 | 4 | oz | Light Meat, raw | 113 | 1.54 | 1.70 | 2.33 | 0.26 | 3.84 | 1.46 | 0.72 | 1.20 | 1.87 | 2.19 | 0.68 | 0.94 | 1.12 | 1.06 | 1.05 | 0.27 | 0.91 | 1.26 |

TABLE A **Amino Acid Content for Selected Foods *(continued)***

| Code | Amount | Description | Weight (g) | Alanine (g) | Arginine (g) | Aspartic acid (g) | Cystine (g) | Glutamic acid (g) | Glycine (g) | Histidine (g) | Isoleucine (g) | Leucine (g) | Lysine (g) | Methionine (g) | Phenylalanine (g) | Proline (g) | Serine (g) | Threonine (g) | Tryptophan (g) | Tyrosine (g) | Valine (g) |
|---|---|---|---|---|---|---|---|---|---|---|---|---|---|---|---|---|---|---|---|---|---|
| 16081 | 4 oz | Light Meat, raw, w/o skin | 113 | 1.63 | 1.83 | 2.56 | 0.27 | 4.29 | 1.31 | 0.82 | 1.38 | 2.10 | 2.48 | 0.76 | 1.05 | 1.10 | 1.17 | 1.17 | 0.30 | 1.04 | 1.40 |
| 16027 | 3 oz | Light Meat, rstd | 85 | 1.53 | 1.69 | 2.31 | 0.26 | 3.83 | 1.44 | 0.72 | 1.20 | 1.87 | 2.19 | 0.67 | 0.94 | 1.12 | 1.06 | 1.05 | 0.26 | 0.91 | 1.25 |
| 16158 | 3 oz | Light Meat, rstd, w/o skin | 85 | 1.55 | 1.75 | 2.44 | 0.26 | 4.10 | 1.24 | 0.78 | 1.31 | 2.00 | 2.37 | 0.73 | 1.00 | 1.04 | 1.12 | 1.12 | 0.29 | 0.99 | 1.34 |
| 16068 | 4 oz | Raw | 113 | 1.45 | 1.60 | 2.20 | 0.25 | 3.63 | 1.37 | 0.68 | 1.14 | 1.77 | 2.07 | 0.64 | 0.89 | 1.06 | 1.00 | 0.99 | 0.25 | 0.86 | 1.18 |
| 16069 | 4 oz | Raw, w/o skin | 113 | 1.51 | 1.70 | 2.36 | 0.25 | 3.97 | 1.21 | 0.76 | 1.26 | 1.94 | 2.29 | 0.70 | 0.97 | 1.01 | 1.08 | 1.08 | 0.28 | 0.96 | 1.30 |
| 16026 | 3 oz | Roasted | 85 | 1.50 | 1.66 | 2.28 | 0.26 | 3.76 | 1.41 | 0.71 | 1.18 | 1.83 | 2.15 | 0.66 | 0.92 | 1.09 | 1.04 | 1.03 | 0.26 | 0.90 | 1.23 |
| 16000 | 3 oz | Roasted, w/o skin | 85 | 1.53 | 1.72 | 2.39 | 0.26 | 4.02 | 1.22 | 0.77 | 1.28 | 1.96 | 2.32 | 0.71 | 0.97 | 1.02 | 1.09 | 1.09 | 0.28 | 0.97 | 1.31 |
| 16070 | 4 oz | Skin, raw | 113 | 1.15 | 1.09 | 1.27 | 0.23 | 1.76 | 2.26 | 0.27 | 0.46 | 0.83 | 0.84 | 0.28 | 0.48 | 1.32 | 0.57 | 0.50 | 0.11 | 0.32 | 0.59 |
| 16071 | 3 oz | Skin, rstd | 85 | 1.34 | 1.27 | 1.47 | 0.27 | 2.05 | 2.63 | 0.32 | 0.53 | 0.97 | 0.99 | 0.33 | 0.56 | 1.54 | 0.67 | 0.59 | 0.13 | 0.38 | 0.69 |
| 16088 | 4 oz | Wing, raw | 113 | 1.48 | 1.61 | 2.15 | 0.26 | 3.51 | 1.59 | 0.65 | 1.09 | 1.71 | 1.97 | 0.61 | 0.87 | 1.16 | 0.99 | 0.97 | 0.24 | 0.82 | 1.15 |
| 16089 | 3 oz | Wing, rstd | 85 | 1.50 | 1.64 | 2.20 | 0.26 | 3.59 | 1.59 | 0.67 | 1.12 | 1.75 | 2.02 | 0.63 | 0.89 | 1.17 | 1.01 | 0.99 | 0.25 | 0.84 | 1.18 |
| | | **POULTRY—DUCK, EMU, OSTRICH AND OTHER—BONELESS** | | | | | | | | | | | | | | | | | | | |
| 15241 | 4 oz | Cornish Game Hen, avg | 113 | 1.23 | 1.37 | 2.02 | 0.29 | 3.39 | 1.11 | 0.70 | 1.20 | 1.69 | 1.92 | 0.63 | 0.90 | 0.93 | 0.78 | 0.96 | 0.26 | 0.76 | 1.12 |
| 15242 | 3 oz | Cornish Game Hen, rstd | 85 | 1.08 | 1.20 | 1.77 | 0.25 | 2.97 | 0.97 | 0.61 | 1.05 | 1.49 | 1.68 | 0.55 | 0.79 | 0.81 | 0.68 | 0.84 | 0.23 | 0.67 | 0.99 |
| | | Duck | | | | | | | | | | | | | | | | | | | |
| 16061 | 4 oz | Raw | 113 | 0.87 | 0.86 | 1.23 | 0.20 | 1.92 | 1.04 | 0.32 | 0.60 | 1.01 | 1.02 | 0.33 | 0.51 | 0.77 | 0.55 | 0.53 | 0.16 | 0.44 | 0.64 |
| 16062 | 4 oz | Raw, w/o skin | 113 | 1.30 | 1.31 | 2.01 | 0.32 | 3.21 | 1.14 | 0.54 | 1.05 | 1.73 | 1.75 | 0.55 | 0.86 | 1.01 | 0.88 | 0.88 | 0.28 | 0.78 | 1.07 |
| 14001 | 3 oz | Roasted | 85 | 1.09 | 1.08 | 1.52 | 0.25 | 2.36 | 1.36 | 0.39 | 0.73 | 1.24 | 1.25 | 0.40 | 0.63 | 0.99 | 0.68 | 0.65 | 0.20 | 0.54 | 0.79 |
| 14000 | 3 oz | Roasted, w/o skin | 85 | 1.26 | 1.26 | 1.94 | 0.30 | 3.09 | 1.11 | 0.52 | 1.02 | 1.67 | 1.69 | 0.54 | 0.83 | 0.97 | 0.85 | 0.84 | 0.28 | 0.75 | 1.04 |
| | | Goose | | | | | | | | | | | | | | | | | | | |
| 16064 | 4 oz | Raw | 113 | 1.10 | 1.12 | 1.62 | 0.28 | 2.67 | 1.14 | 0.50 | 0.84 | 1.50 | 1.41 | 0.43 | 0.75 | 0.87 | 0.71 | 0.80 | 0.23 | 0.57 | 0.88 |
| 16065 | 4 oz | Raw, w/o skin | 113 | 1.62 | 1.63 | 2.50 | 0.39 | 4.00 | 1.43 | 0.67 | 1.31 | 2.15 | 2.19 | 0.69 | 1.07 | 1.26 | 1.10 | 1.09 | 0.36 | 0.97 | 1.34 |
| 14003 | 3 oz | Roasted | 85 | 1.32 | 1.33 | 1.92 | 0.33 | 3.18 | 1.35 | 0.60 | 1.00 | 1.79 | 1.69 | 0.52 | 0.90 | 1.04 | 0.85 | 0.95 | 0.28 | 0.68 | 1.05 |
| 14002 | 3 oz | Roasted, w/o skin | 85 | 1.55 | 1.56 | 2.39 | 0.38 | 3.82 | 1.37 | 0.64 | 1.26 | 2.07 | 2.09 | 0.66 | 1.02 | 1.20 | 1.05 | 1.05 | 0.34 | 0.93 | 1.28 |
| 14034 | 4 oz | Guinea Hen, raw | 113 | 1.56 | 1.67 | 2.36 | 0.35 | 3.85 | 1.77 | 0.77 | 1.31 | 1.91 | 2.14 | 0.70 | 1.02 | 1.31 | 0.94 | 1.09 | 0.29 | 0.85 | 1.28 |
| 14035 | 4 oz | Guinea Hen, raw, w/o skin | 113 | 1.28 | 1.41 | 2.08 | 0.30 | 3.49 | 1.14 | 0.72 | 1.23 | 1.75 | 1.98 | 0.65 | 0.93 | 0.96 | 0.80 | 0.99 | 0.27 | 0.79 | 1.15 |
| 16022 | 4 oz | Pheasant, raw | 113 | 1.59 | 1.59 | 2.47 | 0.34 | 3.74 | 1.39 | 0.98 | 1.39 | 2.11 | 2.28 | 0.73 | 0.99 | 1.06 | 1.10 | 1.25 | 0.34 | 0.82 | 1.39 |
| 16023 | 4 oz | Pheasant, raw, w/o skin | 113 | 1.60 | 1.62 | 2.59 | 0.35 | 3.93 | 1.18 | 1.06 | 1.49 | 2.26 | 2.44 | 0.78 | 1.04 | 0.97 | 1.14 | 1.33 | 0.37 | 0.87 | 1.48 |
| 16013 | 4 oz | Quail, raw | 113 | 1.40 | 1.42 | 1.84 | 0.38 | 2.82 | 1.71 | 0.77 | 1.12 | 1.79 | 1.84 | 0.66 | 0.92 | 0.96 | 1.04 | 1.05 | 0.32 | 0.95 | 1.15 |
| 16014 | 4 oz | Quail, raw, w/o skin | 113 | 1.49 | 1.54 | 2.02 | 0.42 | 3.15 | 1.61 | 0.92 | 1.33 | 2.09 | 2.13 | 0.77 | 1.05 | 0.89 | 1.18 | 1.22 | 0.38 | 1.13 | 1.32 |
| 16016 | 4 oz | Squab/Pigeon, raw | 113 | 1.33 | 1.35 | 1.74 | 0.36 | 2.66 | 1.66 | 0.72 | 1.05 | 1.68 | 1.72 | 0.62 | 0.86 | 0.94 | 0.98 | 0.99 | 0.30 | 0.88 | 1.08 |
| 16017 | 4 oz | Squab/Pigeon, raw, w/o skin | 113 | 1.20 | 1.24 | 1.63 | 0.34 | 2.53 | 1.29 | 0.74 | 1.06 | 1.67 | 1.70 | 0.62 | 0.85 | 0.71 | 0.95 | 0.98 | 0.31 | 0.90 | 1.06 |
| | | **SALAD DRESSINGS** | | | | | | | | | | | | | | | | | | | |
| 8013 | 1 Tbs | Blue Cheese/Roquefort, avg | 15 | 0.02 | 0.02 | 0.04 | 0.00 | 0.16 | 0.01 | 0.02 | 0.04 | 0.06 | 0.06 | 0.02 | 0.03 | 0.07 | 0.04 | 0.02 | 0.01 | 0.04 | 0.05 |
| 8066 | 1 Tbs | Caesar, avg | 12 | 0.07 | 0.08 | 0.13 | 0.02 | 0.25 | 0.05 | 0.05 | 0.07 | 0.13 | 0.13 | 0.04 | 0.07 | 0.09 | 0.08 | 0.06 | 0.02 | 0.06 | 0.09 |
| 8046 | 1 Tbs | Mayonnaise, avg | 14 | 0.01 | 0.01 | 0.01 | 0.00 | 0.02 | 0.01 | 0.00 | 0.01 | 0.01 | 0.01 | 0.00 | 0.01 | 0.01 | 0.01 | 0.01 | 0.00 | 0.01 | 0.01 |
| 8148 | 1 Tbs | Mayonnaise, light, low sod, avg | 14 | 0.00 | 0.00 | 0.00 | 0.00 | 0.01 | 0.00 | 0.00 | 0.00 | 0.00 | 0.00 | 0.00 | 0.00 | 0.00 | 0.00 | 0.00 | 0.00 | 0.00 | 0.00 |
| 8022 | 1 Tbs | Russian, avg | 15 | 0.01 | 0.02 | 0.02 | 0.00 | 0.03 | 0.01 | 0.01 | 0.01 | 0.02 | 0.02 | 0.01 | 0.01 | 0.01 | 0.02 | 0.01 | 0.00 | 0.01 | 0.01 |
| 8144 | 1 Tbs | Sesame Seed, avg | 15 | 0.00 | 0.06 | 0.00 | 0.00 | 0.07 | 0.00 | 0.00 | 0.01 | 0.01 | 0.02 | 0.00 | 0.01 | 0.00 | 0.00 | 0.01 | 0.01 | 0.02 | 0.01 |
| 8023 | 1 Tbs | Thousand Island, avg | 15 | 0.01 | 0.01 | 0.01 | 0.00 | 0.01 | 0.00 | 0.00 | 0.01 | 0.01 | 0.01 | 0.00 | 0.01 | 0.00 | 0.01 | 0.01 | 0.00 | 0.01 | 0.01 |
| 8024 | 1 Tbs | Thousand, Island, lo cal, avg | 16 | 0.01 | 0.01 | 0.01 | 0.00 | 0.02 | 0.00 | 0.00 | 0.01 | 0.01 | 0.01 | 0.00 | 0.01 | 0.01 | 0.01 | 0.01 | 0.00 | 0.01 | 0.01 |
| | | **SALADS** | | | | | | | | | | | | | | | | | | | |
| 57510 | 1/2 cup | Three Bean, avg | 104 | 0.16 | 0.22 | 0.45 | 0.04 | 0.53 | 0.14 | 0.10 | 0.16 | 0.28 | 0.24 | 0.06 | 0.19 | 0.15 | 0.20 | 0.16 | 0.04 | 0.10 | 0.19 |
| 56109 | 1/2 cup | Carrot Raisin Salad, avg | 88 | 0.07 | 0.18 | 0.12 | 0.03 | 0.18 | 0.04 | 0.04 | 0.05 | 0.07 | 0.06 | 0.02 | 0.05 | 0.10 | 0.06 | 0.05 | 0.01 | 0.03 | 0.06 |
| 56002 | 1/2 cup | Chicken Salad, w/Celery, avg | 78 | 0.57 | 0.64 | 0.96 | 0.14 | 1.58 | 0.51 | 0.32 | 0.56 | 0.80 | 0.90 | 0.29 | 0.42 | 0.43 | 0.38 | 0.45 | 0.12 | 0.36 | 0.53 |
| | | Green Garden/Tossed Salads | | | | | | | | | | | | | | | | | | | |
| 5677 | 1 cup | Average | 139 | 0.05 | 0.06 | 0.16 | 0.02 | 0.31 | 0.05 | 0.02 | 0.07 | 0.07 | 0.07 | 0.01 | 0.05 | 0.04 | 0.04 | 0.05 | 0.01 | 0.03 | 0.06 |
| 56624 | 1 cup | With Cheese & Egg, avg | 145 | 0.22 | 0.27 | 0.49 | 0.07 | 1.10 | 0.15 | 0.15 | 0.33 | 0.46 | 0.40 | 0.13 | 0.28 | 0.39 | 0.31 | 0.23 | 0.07 | 0.22 | 0.35 |
| 56625 | 1 cup | With Chicken, avg | 145 | 0.62 | 0.69 | 1.06 | 0.15 | 1.75 | 0.56 | 0.35 | 0.61 | 0.85 | 0.96 | 0.31 | 0.46 | 0.47 | 0.40 | 0.49 | 0.13 | 0.38 | 0.57 |
| 56626 | 1 cup | With Pasta & Seafood, avg | 278 | 0.52 | 0.62 | 0.94 | 0.17 | 2.30 | 0.48 | 0.26 | 0.50 | 0.80 | 0.71 | 0.24 | 0.46 | 0.62 | 0.45 | 0.41 | 0.13 | 0.33 | 0.52 |

TABLE A **Amino Acid Content for Selected Foods *(continued)***

| Code | Amount | Description | Weight (g) | Alanine (g) | Arginine (g) | Aspartic acid (g) | Cystine (g) | Glutamic acid (g) | Glycine (g) | Histidine (g) | Isoleucine (g) | Leucine (g) | Lysine (g) | Methionine (g) | Phenylalanine (g) | Proline (g) | Serine (g) | Threonine (g) | Tryptophan (g) | Tyrosine (g) | Valine (g) |
|---|---|---|---|---|---|---|---|---|---|---|---|---|---|---|---|---|---|---|---|---|---|
| 56627 | 1 cup | With Shrimp, avg | 157 | 0.53 | 0.75 | 1.00 | 0.13 | 1.62 | 0.50 | 0.20 | 0.49 | 0.75 | 0.76 | 0.26 | 0.42 | 0.32 | 0.43 | 0.40 | 0.13 | 0.32 | 0.49 |
| 56004 | 1/2 cup | Macaroni, avg | 88 | 0.07 | 0.10 | 0.12 | 0.06 | 0.73 | 0.27 | 0.04 | 0.09 | 0.16 | 0.06 | 0.04 | 0.11 | 0.22 | 0.11 | 0.07 | 0.03 | 0.06 | 0.10 |
| 56005 | 1/2 cup | Potato Salad, avg | 125 | 0.15 | 0.19 | 0.53 | 0.06 | 0.48 | 0.11 | 0.08 | 0.17 | 0.25 | 0.21 | 0.08 | 0.17 | 0.13 | 0.20 | 0.14 | 0.05 | 0.13 | 0.21 |
| 56007 | 1/2 cup | Tuna Salad, avg | 102 | 0.98 | 0.99 | 1.66 | 0.18 | 2.45 | 0.78 | 0.48 | 0.75 | 1.32 | 1.49 | 0.48 | 0.64 | 0.58 | 0.67 | 0.72 | 0.18 | 0.55 | 0.84 |
| 56006 | 1/2 cup | Waldorf Salad, avg | 68 | 0.08 | 0.22 | 0.19 | 0.04 | 0.31 | 0.29 | 0.04 | 0.07 | 0.12 | 0.06 | 0.03 | 0.08 | 0.07 | 0.10 | 0.06 | 0.02 | 0.05 | 0.09 |
| | | **SANDWICHES** | | | | | | | | | | | | | | | | | | | |
| 56023 | 1 ea | Avocado & Cheese, on wheat, avg | 214 | 0.55 | 0.64 | 1.07 | 0.20 | 4.07 | 0.46 | 0.44 | 0.78 | 1.28 | 0.91 | 0.33 | 0.76 | 1.55 | 0.81 | 0.53 | 0.20 | 0.59 | 0.89 |
| 56021 | 1 ea | Avocado & Cheese, on white, avg | 210 | 0.50 | 0.55 | 0.99 | 0.18 | 3.92 | 0.41 | 0.41 | 0.75 | 1.23 | 0.86 | 0.33 | 0.72 | 1.51 | 0.77 | 0.50 | 0.18 | 0.56 | 0.84 |
| 56010 | 1 ea | Bacon, Lettuce & Tomato, on wheat, avg | 137 | 0.55 | 0.63 | 0.85 | 0.20 | 2.77 | 0.54 | 0.30 | 0.49 | 0.83 | 0.62 | 0.22 | 0.52 | 0.92 | 0.52 | 0.41 | 0.15 | 0.36 | 0.57 |
| 56008 | 1 ea | Bacon, Lettuce & Tomato, on white, avg | 133 | 0.50 | 0.56 | 0.77 | 0.17 | 2.63 | 0.50 | 0.28 | 0.46 | 0.78 | 0.57 | 0.22 | 0.50 | 0.88 | 0.49 | 0.39 | 0.12 | 0.32 | 0.52 |
| | | Beef Sandwiches | | | | | | | | | | | | | | | | | | | |
| 56020 | 1 ea | Corned Beef & Swiss, on rye, avg | 156 | 1.49 | 1.51 | 2.28 | 0.34 | 5.31 | 1.52 | 0.89 | 1.19 | 2.10 | 2.07 | 0.63 | 1.14 | 2.27 | 1.20 | 0.97 | 0.30 | 1.04 | 1.31 |
| 56038 | 1 ea | Patty Melt, w/ground beef on rye, avg | 182 | 1.91 | 2.15 | 3.06 | 0.42 | 6.48 | 1.70 | 1.24 | 1.64 | 2.93 | 2.94 | 0.90 | 1.56 | 2.18 | 1.51 | 1.49 | 0.44 | 1.35 | 1.85 |
| 56043 | 1 ea | Roast Beef, on white, avg | 160 | 1.74 | 1.80 | 2.36 | 0.40 | 5.22 | 1.34 | 0.80 | 1.18 | 2.16 | 2.06 | 0.67 | 1.16 | 1.89 | 1.24 | 1.16 | 0.26 | 0.87 | 1.33 |
| 56045 | 1 ea | Roast Beef, on whole wheat, avg | 169 | 1.84 | 1.94 | 2.51 | 0.44 | 5.55 | 2.25 | 0.85 | 1.25 | 2.27 | [illegible] | 0.69 | 1.22 | 1.99 | 1.31 | 1.22 | 0.30 | 0.93 | 1.42 |
| 56669 | 1 ea | Roast Beef, w/cheese, avg | 176 | 1.68 | 1.83 | 2.60 | 0.38 | 5.91 | 1.54 | 1.04 | 1.42 | 2.50 | 2.39 | 0.76 | 1.34 | 1.95 | 1.33 | 1.28 | 0.37 | 1.08 | 1.60 |
| 56670 | 1 ea | Steak, avg | 204 | 1.81 | 1.89 | 2.57 | 0.33 | 5.63 | 2.34 | 0.90 | 1.29 | 2.37 | 2.22 | 0.66 | 1.21 | 1.82 | 1.24 | 1.20 | 0.37 | 0.90 | 1.47 |
| 56014 | 1 ea | Cheese, grilled, on wheat, avg | 132 | 0.57 | 0.84 | 1.15 | 0.23 | 4.70 | 0.48 | 0.67 | 0.84 | 1.58 | 1.46 | 0.43 | 0.97 | 1.96 | 0.93 | 0.62 | 0.28 | 0.89 | 1.07 |
| 56012 | 1 ea | Cheese, grilled, on white, avg | 128 | 0.52 | 0.75 | 1.07 | 0.21 | 4.55 | 0.42 | 0.64 | 0.81 | 1.54 | 1.41 | 0.43 | 0.94 | 1.92 | 0.90 | 0.59 | 0.25 | 0.86 | 1.02 |
| | | Chicken Sandwiches | | | | | | | | | | | | | | | | | | | |
| 56000 | 1 ea | Fillet, avg | 182 | 1.22 | 1.35 | 1.97 | 0.33 | 4.44 | 1.13 | 0.70 | 1.21 | 1.78 | 1.74 | 0.61 | 1.01 | 1.33 | 0.92 | 0.95 | 0.28 | 0.76 | 1.20 |
| 56656 | 1 ea | Fillet, w/cheese, avg | 228 | 1.38 | 1.58 | 2.23 | 0.38 | 5.63 | 1.48 | 0.86 | 1.37 | 2.18 | [illegible] | 0.70 | 1.26 | 2.06 | 1.20 | 1.08 | 0.35 | 1.01 | 1.48 |
| 56018 | 1 ea | Salad, on wheat, avg | 123 | 0.56 | 0.67 | 0.90 | 0.23 | 2.99 | 0.55 | 0.33 | 0.57 | 0.92 | 0.69 | 0.27 | 0.56 | 0.94 | 0.54 | 0.46 | 0.17 | 0.41 | 0.60 |
| 56016 | 1 ea | Salad, on white, avg | 119 | 0.52 | 0.57 | 0.81 | 0.21 | 2.83 | 0.49 | 0.30 | 0.54 | 0.87 | 0.64 | 0.26 | 0.53 | 0.90 | 0.51 | 0.42 | 0.14 | 0.36 | 0.55 |
| 56026 | 1 ea | Egg Salad, on wheat, avg | 130 | 0.27 | 0.33 | 0.40 | 0.16 | 2.18 | 0.28 | 0.17 | 0.28 | 0.50 | 0.23 | 0.11 | 0.34 | 0.71 | 0.34 | 0.22 | 0.10 | 0.22 | 0.33 |
| 56024 | 1 ea | Egg Salad, on white, avg | 126 | 0.22 | 0.24 | 0.31 | 0.14 | 2.01 | 0.23 | 0.14 | 0.25 | 0.45 | [illegible] | 0.11 | 0.31 | 0.67 | 0.31 | 0.19 | 0.07 | 0.19 | 0.28 |
| 66011 | 1 ea | Fish w/Cheese & Tartar Sauce, avg | 183 | 1.01 | 1.08 | 1.72 | 0.25 | 4.14 | 0.55 | 0.59 | 0.92 | 1.63 | 1.55 | 0.53 | 0.90 | 1.31 | 0.93 | 0.80 | 0.25 | 0.70 | 1.08 |
| 66010 | 1 ea | Fish w/Tartar Sauce, avg | 158 | 0.90 | 0.92 | 1.48 | 0.22 | 3.38 | 0.77 | 0.46 | 0.76 | 1.32 | 1.22 | 0.43 | 0.72 | 0.98 | 0.76 | 0.67 | 0.20 | 0.52 | 0.87 |
| | | Hamburgers/Cheeseburgers | | | | | | | | | | | | | | | | | | | |
| 66014 | 1 ea | Cheeseburger, avg | 102 | 0.72 | 0.80 | 1.08 | 0.17 | 3.16 | 0.77 | 0.45 | 0.63 | 1.16 | 1.02 | 0.32 | 0.65 | 1.15 | 0.60 | 0.53 | 0.19 | 0.49 | 0.75 |
| 66016 | 1 ea | Cheeseburger, double, avg | 155 | 1.43 | 1.60 | 2.19 | 0.28 | 5.29 | 1.55 | 0.89 | 1.19 | 2.22 | 2.15 | 0.63 | 1.17 | 1.94 | 1.06 | 1.05 | 0.35 | 0.97 | 1.41 |
| 66013 | 1 ea | Cheeseburger, double, w/condmnts & vegs, avg | 166 | 1.09 | 1.21 | 1.69 | 0.21 | 4.12 | 1.18 | 0.68 | 0.91 | 1.68 | 1.64 | 0.48 | 0.89 | 1.47 | 0.81 | 0.80 | 0.27 | 0.74 | 1.08 |
| 56648 | 1 ea | Cheeseburger, large, avg | 185 | 1.54 | 1.71 | 2.33 | 0.31 | 5.86 | 1.57 | 0.95 | 1.29 | 2.40 | 2.29 | 0.68 | 1.28 | 2.15 | 1.16 | 1.13 | 0.38 | 1.05 | 1.53 |
| 66012 | 1 ea | Cheeseburger, large, double, w/cond&vegs, avg | 258 | 2.10 | 2.27 | 3.12 | 0.39 | 7.12 | 2.32 | 1.18 | 1.62 | 2.99 | 2.92 | 0.85 | 1.55 | 2.45 | 1.39 | 1.47 | 0.47 | 1.24 | 1.89 |
| 56651 | 1 ea | Cheeseburger, large, w/bacon & condmnts, avg | 195 | 1.66 | 1.85 | 2.52 | 0.33 | 5.91 | 1.56 | 0.99 | 1.36 | 2.48 | 2.42 | 0.71 | 1.33 | 2.16 | 1.23 | 1.20 | 0.39 | 1.07 | 1.61 |
| 56649 | 1 ea | Cheeseburger, large, w/condiments & veg, avg | 219 | 1.43 | 1.59 | 2.21 | 0.29 | 5.58 | 1.54 | 0.88 | 1.20 | 2.21 | 2.12 | 0.62 | 1.19 | 1.97 | 1.08 | 1.05 | 0.35 | 0.96 | 1.42 |
| 56650 | 1 ea | Cheeseburger, large, w/ham, cond & vegs, avg | 254 | 2.06 | 2.29 | 3.15 | 0.43 | 7.57 | 2.16 | 1.27 | 1.70 | 3.12 | 3.05 | 0.90 | 1.68 | 2.67 | 1.67 | 1.52 | 0.50 | 1.35 | 1.96 |
| 56652 | 1 ea | Cheeseburger, triple, avg | 304 | 3.28 | 3.50 | 4.74 | 0.57 | 10.00 | 3.55 | 1.76 | 2.40 | 4.47 | 4.41 | 1.27 | 2.26 | 3.44 | 2.29 | 2.23 | 0.70 | 1.83 | 2.78 |
| 56647 | 1 ea | Cheeseburger, w/condiments, avg | 113 | 0.77 | 0.86 | 1.18 | 0.18 | 3.42 | 0.53 | 0.48 | 0.68 | 1.24 | 1.10 | 0.34 | 0.70 | 1.24 | 0.65 | 0.58 | 0.20 | 0.53 | 0.81 |
| 66015 | 1 ea | Cheeseburger, w/condiments & vegs, avg | 154 | 0.86 | 0.96 | 1.33 | 0.20 | 3.85 | 0.93 | 0.54 | 0.76 | 1.39 | 1.22 | 0.38 | 0.78 | 1.37 | 0.73 | 0.65 | 0.22 | 0.59 | 0.91 |
| 66007 | 1 ea | Hamburger, avg | 90 | 0.67 | 0.71 | 0.95 | 0.16 | 2.68 | 0.76 | 0.35 | 0.52 | 0.94 | 0.77 | 0.25 | 0.52 | 0.90 | 0.49 | 0.46 | 0.15 | 0.35 | 0.61 |
| 66009 | 1 ea | Hamburger, double, avg | 176 | 1.78 | 1.85 | 2.50 | 0.33 | 5.56 | 2.01 | 0.89 | 1.26 | 2.32 | 2.16 | 0.65 | 1.19 | 1.83 | 1.22 | 1.17 | 0.36 | 0.88 | 1.45 |
| 66006 | 1 ea | Hamburger, double, w/condiments, avg | 215 | 1.88 | 1.97 | 2.64 | 0.35 | 5.93 | 2.12 | 0.94 | 1.34 | 2.45 | 2.28 | 0.69 | 1.27 | 1.94 | 1.29 | 1.25 | 0.38 | 0.94 | 1.54 |
| 56660 | 1 ea | Hamburger, large, avg | 137 | 1.31 | 1.37 | 1.85 | 0.25 | 4.32 | 1.48 | 0.66 | 0.95 | 1.74 | 1.58 | 0.48 | 0.91 | 1.42 | 0.93 | 0.88 | 0.27 | 0.66 | 1.09 |
| 56662 | 1 ea | Hamburger, large, dbl, w/condmnts & vegs, avg | 226 | 2.04 | 2.13 | 2.92 | 0.37 | 6.33 | 2.31 | 1.02 | 1.44 | 2.64 | 2.51 | 0.75 | 1.35 | 2.03 | 1.38 | 1.35 | 0.41 | 1.01 | 1.65 |

TABLE A **Amino Acid Content for Selected Foods *(continued)***

| Code | Amount | Description | Weight (g) | Alanine (g) | Arginine (g) | Aspartic acid (g) | Cystine (g) | Glutamic acid (g) | Glycine (g) | Histidine (g) | Isoleucine (g) | Leucine (g) | Lysine (g) | Methionine (g) | Phenylalanine (g) | Proline (g) | Serine (g) | Threonine (g) | Tryptophan (g) | Tyrosine (g) | Valine (g) |
|---|---|---|---|---|---|---|---|---|---|---|---|---|---|---|---|---|---|---|---|---|---|
| 56661 | 1 ea | Hamburger, large, w/condiments & vegs, avg | 218 | 1.47 | 1.55 | 2.14 | 0.29 | 5.06 | 1.66 | 0.74 | 1.07 | 1.95 | 1.77 | 0.54 | 1.03 | 1.60 | 1.05 | 0.99 | 0.31 | 0.74 | 1.23 |
| 56663 | 1 ea | Hamburger, triple, w/condiments, avg | 259 | 3.08 | 3.21 | 4.33 | 0.52 | 8.75 | 3.50 | 1.52 | 2.13 | 3.94 | 3.83 | 1.12 | 1.96 | 2.87 | 2.01 | 2.02 | 0.61 | 1.52 | 2.43 |
| 56658 | 1 ea | Hamburger, w/condiments, avg | 107 | 0.67 | 0.72 | 0.96 | 0.16 | 2.73 | 0.76 | 0.35 | 0.53 | 0.95 | 0.77 | 0.26 | 0.53 | 0.90 | 0.54 | 0.47 | 0.15 | 0.35 | 0.61 |
| 56659 | 1 ea | Hamburger, w/condiments & vegetables, avg | 110 | 0.70 | 0.74 | 1.01 | 0.16 | 2.84 | 0.78 | 0.36 | 0.54 | 0.98 | 0.80 | 0.26 | 0.55 | 0.93 | 0.56 | 0.48 | 0.16 | 0.37 | 0.63 |
| | | Ham Sandwiches | | | | | | | | | | | | | | | | | | | |
| 56032 | 1 ea | On rye, avg | 150 | 1.15 | 1.34 | 1.88 | 0.34 | 4.02 | 1.04 | 0.71 | 0.92 | 1.66 | 1.60 | 0.53 | 0.96 | 1.13 | 0.91 | 0.90 | 0.26 | 0.70 | 0.94 |
| 56030 | 1 ea | On wheat, avg | 169 | 1.23 | 1.39 | 1.94 | 0.40 | 4.75 | 1.13 | 0.75 | 0.99 | 1.79 | 1.61 | 0.55 | 1.04 | 1.38 | 1.01 | 0.94 | 0.30 | 0.75 | 1.03 |
| 56028 | 1 ea | On white, avg | 170 | 1.21 | 1.35 | 1.91 | 0.39 | 4.74 | 1.10 | 0.74 | 0.99 | 1.79 | 1.60 | 0.55 | 1.04 | 1.39 | 1.00 | 0.94 | 0.28 | 0.73 | 1.01 |
| 56065 | 1 ea | Salad, on wheat, avg | 144 | 0.60 | 0.70 | 0.93 | 0.19 | 3.00 | 0.58 | 0.38 | 0.53 | 0.94 | 0.70 | 0.26 | 0.56 | 0.95 | 0.58 | 0.48 | 0.16 | 0.38 | 0.61 |
| 56063 | 1 ea | Salad, on white, avg | 140 | 0.55 | 0.61 | 0.85 | 0.17 | 2.84 | 0.53 | 0.35 | 0.50 | 0.89 | 0.65 | 0.25 | 0.53 | 0.91 | 0.54 | 0.45 | 0.12 | 0.35 | 0.56 |
| 56036 | 1 ea | With Cheese, on wheat, avg | 170 | 1.06 | 1.30 | 1.82 | 0.36 | 5.20 | 0.95 | 0.81 | 1.04 | 1.92 | 1.78 | 0.56 | 1.12 | 1.80 | 1.08 | 0.90 | 0.32 | 0.91 | 1.17 |
| 56034 | 1 ea | With Cheese, on white, avg | 166 | 1.01 | 1.21 | 1.74 | 0.33 | 5.04 | 0.89 | 0.78 | 1.01 | 1.87 | 1.73 | 0.56 | 1.09 | 1.76 | 1.05 | 0.87 | 0.29 | 0.88 | 1.12 |
| 56033 | 1 ea | With Swiss, on rye, avg | 150 | 0.99 | 1.24 | 1.73 | 0.30 | 4.43 | 0.86 | 0.76 | 0.97 | 1.78 | 1.75 | 0.54 | 1.03 | 1.55 | 0.99 | 0.85 | 0.28 | 0.87 | 1.07 |
| 66004 | 1 ea | Hotdog, avg | 98 | 0.59 | 0.65 | 0.85 | 0.14 | 2.34 | 0.63 | 0.29 | 0.44 | 0.75 | 0.63 | 0.20 | 0.41 | 0.75 | 0.47 | 0.35 | 0.10 | 0.28 | 0.47 |
| 56667 | 1 ea | Hotdog, w/chili, avg | 114 | 0.75 | 0.84 | 1.13 | 0.18 | 2.90 | 0.81 | 0.37 | 0.57 | 0.97 | 0.83 | 0.25 | 0.53 | 0.91 | 0.60 | 0.47 | 0.13 | 0.36 | 0.61 |
| 56041 | 1 ea | Peanut Butter & Jam, on wheat, avg | 114 | 0.49 | 1.03 | 1.12 | 0.23 | 3.32 | 0.63 | 0.31 | 0.47 | 0.86 | 0.43 | 0.18 | 0.63 | 0.94 | 0.62 | 0.41 | 0.16 | 0.45 | 0.56 |
| 56039 | 1 ea | Peanut Butter & Jam, on white, avg | 110 | 0.44 | 0.94 | 1.04 | 0.20 | 3.17 | 0.57 | 0.28 | 0.44 | 0.81 | 0.38 | 0.18 | 0.60 | 0.90 | 0.58 | 0.38 | 0.13 | 0.42 | 0.51 |
| 69072 | 1 ea | Reuben, avg | 239 | 1.47 | 1.48 | 2.23 | 0.33 | 5.21 | 1.60 | 0.87 | 1.16 | 2.05 | 2.02 | 0.61 | 1.12 | 2.22 | 1.17 | 0.95 | 0.29 | 1.02 | 1.30 |
| | | Submarine Sandwiches | | | | | | | | | | | | | | | | | | | |
| 56671 | 1 ea | Cold Cuts, avg | 228 | 0.86 | 1.01 | 1.46 | 0.29 | 5.31 | 0.88 | 0.62 | 0.90 | 1.59 | 1.29 | 0.44 | 0.99 | 1.91 | 1.04 | 0.74 | 0.25 | 0.75 | 1.10 |
| 56672 | 1 ea | Roast Beef, avg | 216 | 1.55 | 1.64 | 2.35 | 0.36 | 5.40 | 1.44 | 0.88 | 1.25 | 2.18 | 1.98 | 0.66 | 1.18 | 1.67 | 1.18 | 1.15 | 0.32 | 0.89 | 1.39 |
| 56673 | 1 ea | Tuna Salad, avg | 256 | 1.58 | 1.62 | 2.61 | 0.38 | 5.94 | 1.36 | 0.80 | 1.33 | 2.32 | 2.16 | 0.76 | 1.27 | 1.71 | 1.31 | 1.18 | 0.34 | 0.92 | 1.53 |
| 56047 | 1 ea | Tuna Salad, on white, avg | 131 | 0.73 | 0.76 | 1.18 | 0.23 | 3.27 | 0.63 | 0.38 | 0.64 | 1.13 | 0.95 | 0.36 | 0.64 | 0.96 | 0.65 | 0.56 | 0.17 | 0.47 | 0.71 |
| 56049 | 1 ea | Tuna Salad, on whole wheat, avg | 135 | 0.78 | 0.85 | 1.26 | 0.25 | 3.44 | 0.69 | 0.41 | 0.67 | 1.18 | 1.00 | 0.36 | 0.67 | 1.00 | 0.69 | 0.59 | 0.20 | 0.50 | 0.77 |
| | | Turkey Sandwiches | | | | | | | | | | | | | | | | | | | |
| 56055 | 1 ea | Ham & Cheese, on rye, avg | 150 | 1.00 | 1.28 | 1.74 | 0.25 | 4.41 | 0.81 | 0.71 | 1.05 | 1.76 | 1.85 | 0.57 | 0.99 | 1.53 | 1.02 | 0.85 | 0.28 | 0.93 | 1.19 |
| 56058 | 1 ea | Ham & Cheese, on wheat, avg | 170 | 1.08 | 1.33 | 1.82 | 0.30 | 5.16 | 0.91 | 0.75 | 1.12 | 1.90 | 1.86 | 0.58 | 1.08 | 1.78 | 1.11 | 0.89 | 0.31 | 0.97 | 1.27 |
| 56056 | 1 ea | Ham & Cheese, on white, avg | 166 | 1.03 | 1.25 | 1.74 | 0.28 | 5.01 | 0.85 | 0.72 | 1.09 | 1.85 | 1.81 | 0.58 | 1.04 | 1.74 | 1.08 | 0.86 | 0.28 | 0.94 | 1.22 |
| 56103 | 1 ea | Ham, on rye, avg | 150 | 1.19 | 1.39 | 1.89 | 0.26 | 3.97 | 0.98 | 0.62 | 1.04 | 1.64 | 1.72 | 0.56 | 0.88 | 1.10 | 0.95 | 0.88 | 0.25 | 0.79 | 1.09 |
| 56105 | 1 ea | Ham, on wheat, avg | 169 | 1.25 | 1.44 | 1.95 | 0.32 | 4.70 | 1.07 | 0.66 | 1.11 | 1.76 | 1.73 | 0.58 | 0.97 | 1.35 | 1.05 | 0.93 | 0.28 | 0.84 | 1.18 |
| 56107 | 1 ea | Ham, on white, avg | 166 | 1.20 | 1.37 | 1.88 | 0.30 | 4.58 | 1.01 | 0.63 | 1.08 | 1.72 | 1.69 | 0.57 | 0.94 | 1.31 | 1.01 | 0.90 | 0.25 | 0.81 | 1.13 |
| 56053 | 1 ea | On wheat, avg | 169 | 1.43 | 1.65 | 2.23 | 0.35 | 5.17 | 1.22 | 0.75 | 1.26 | 1.98 | 2.00 | 0.66 | 1.08 | 1.47 | 1.18 | 1.06 | 0.32 | 0.95 | 1.33 |
| 56051 | 1 ea | On white, avg | 165 | 1.46 | 1.65 | 2.27 | 0.35 | 5.30 | 1.23 | 0.77 | 1.29 | 2.05 | 2.07 | 0.69 | 1.10 | 1.51 | 1.20 | 1.08 | 0.30 | 0.98 | 1.35 |
| | | **SAUCES** | | | | | | | | | | | | | | | | | | | |
| 53021 | 1/2 cup | Bearnaise Sauce | 73 | 0.12 | 0.16 | 0.22 | 0.04 | 0.33 | 0.07 | 0.06 | 0.12 | 0.21 | 0.19 | 0.06 | 0.10 | 0.12 | 0.19 | 0.12 | 0.03 | 0.11 | 0.14 |
| 53018 | 1/2 cup | Bechamel Sauce, avg | 145 | 0.03 | 0.04 | 0.05 | 0.02 | 0.30 | 0.03 | 0.02 | 0.04 | 0.07 | 0.03 | 0.02 | 0.05 | 0.11 | 0.05 | 0.03 | 0.01 | 0.03 | 0.04 |
| 53019 | 1/2 cup | Bordelaise Sauce, avg | 233 | 0.04 | 0.07 | 0.06 | 0.02 | 0.35 | 0.04 | 0.03 | 0.05 | 0.08 | 0.04 | 0.02 | 0.06 | 0.12 | 0.06 | 0.04 | 0.02 | 0.04 | 0.05 |
| | | Curry Sauce | | | | | | | | | | | | | | | | | | | |
| 53016 | 1/2 cup | Average | 115 | 0.01 | 0.01 | 0.02 | 0.01 | 0.13 | 0.01 | 0.01 | 0.01 | 0.03 | 0.01 | 0.01 | 0.02 | 0.05 | 0.02 | 0.01 | 0.01 | 0.01 | 0.02 |
| 53031 | 1 ea | Dry Mix, pkt, avg | 35 | 0.02 | 0.02 | 0.02 | 0.01 | 0.16 | 0.02 | 0.01 | 0.02 | 0.04 | 0.02 | 0.01 | 0.03 | 0.06 | 0.03 | 0.02 | 0.01 | 0.02 | 0.02 |
| 53108 | 1/2 cup | Dry Mix, prep w/milk, avg | 136 | 0.03 | 0.03 | 0.04 | 0.02 | 0.26 | 0.03 | 0.02 | 0.03 | 0.06 | 0.02 | 0.01 | 0.04 | 0.09 | 0.04 | 0.02 | 0.11 | 0.03 | 0.04 |
| 53017 | 1/2 cup | Mornay Sauce, avg | 172 | 0.37 | 0.47 | 0.77 | 0.11 | 2.37 | 0.24 | 0.35 | 0.59 | 1.02 | 0.89 | 0.28 | 0.55 | 1.09 | 0.65 | 0.45 | 0.15 | 0.55 | 0.70 |
| | | White Sauce | | | | | | | | | | | | | | | | | | | |
| 53468 | 1/4 cup | Medium, prep f/recipe, avg | 62 | 0.07 | 0.07 | 0.14 | 0.02 | 0.40 | 0.04 | 0.05 | 0.12 | 0.19 | 0.15 | 0.05 | 0.09 | 0.18 | 0.10 | 0.09 | 0.03 | 0.09 | 0.13 |
| 53469 | 1/4 cup | Thick, prep f/recipe, avg | 62 | 0.06 | 0.06 | 0.13 | 0.02 | 0.37 | 0.04 | 0.05 | 0.11 | 0.17 | 0.14 | 0.04 | 0.09 | 0.17 | 0.10 | 0.08 | 0.02 | 0.09 | 0.12 |
| 53467 | 1/4 cup | Thin, prep f/recipe, avg | 62 | 0.07 | 0.07 | 0.15 | 0.02 | 0.42 | 0.04 | 0.06 | 0.12 | 0.20 | 0.16 | 0.05 | 0.10 | 0.20 | 0.11 | 0.09 | 0.03 | 0.10 | 0.14 |
| | | **SNACK FOODS—CHIPS, PRETZELS, POPCORN** | | | | | | | | | | | | | | | | | | | |
| 44029 | 1 oz | Bugles, avg | 28 | 0.12 | 0.08 | 0.11 | 0.03 | 0.30 | 0.07 | 0.05 | 0.06 | 0.20 | 0.05 | 0.03 | 0.08 | 0.14 | 0.08 | 0.06 | 0.01 | 0.07 | 0.08 |
| 44030 | 1 oz | Bugles, nacho, avg | 28 | 0.12 | 0.08 | 0.13 | 0.03 | 0.35 | 0.07 | 0.06 | 0.07 | 0.21 | 0.07 | 0.04 | 0.09 | 0.16 | 0.09 | 0.07 | 0.02 | 0.08 | 0.10 |
| 44001 | 1 cup | Cheese Puffs, avg | 20 | 0.08 | 0.06 | 0.13 | 0.03 | 0.28 | 0.04 | 0.04 | 0.07 | 0.16 | 0.09 | 0.03 | 0.06 | 0.11 | 0.07 | 0.08 | 0.02 | 0.05 | 0.08 |

TABLE A **Amino Acid Content for Selected Foods *(continued)***

| Code | Amount | | Description | Weight (g) | Alanine (g) | Arginine (g) | Aspartic acid (g) | Cystine (g) | Glutamic acid (g) | Glycine (g) | Histidine (g) | Isoleucine (g) | Leucine (g) | Lysine (g) | Methionine (g) | Phenylalanine (g) | Proline (g) | Serine (g) | Threonine (g) | Tryptophan (g) | Tyrosine (g) | Valine (g) |
|---|---|---|---|---|---|---|---|---|---|---|---|---|---|---|---|---|---|---|---|---|---|---|
| 44026 | 16 | pce | Corn Chips, barbecue, avg | 29 | 0.14 | 0.11 | 0.17 | 0.03 | 0.36 | 0.08 | 0.06 | 0.03 | 0.22 | 0.08 | 0.04 | 0.10 | 0.15 | 0.10 | 0.08 | 0.02 | 0.08 | 0.10 |
| 44002 | 1 | cup | Corn Chips, plain, avg | 26 | 0.13 | 0.08 | 0.12 | 0.03 | 0.32 | 0.07 | 0.05 | 0.05 | 0.21 | 0.05 | 0.04 | 0.08 | 0.15 | 0.08 | 0.06 | 0.01 | 0.07 | 0.09 |
| | | | Corn Nuts | | | | | | | | | | | | | | | | | | | |
| 44034 | 16 | pce | Barbecue, avg | 29 | 0.19 | 0.13 | 0.18 | 0.05 | 0.49 | 0.11 | 0.08 | 0.09 | 0.32 | 0.07 | 0.05 | 0.13 | 0.23 | 0.12 | 0.10 | 0.02 | 0.11 | 0.13 |
| 44069 | 16 | pce | Nacho, avg | 29 | 0.20 | 0.14 | 0.19 | 0.05 | 0.51 | 0.11 | 0.08 | 0.10 | 0.34 | 0.08 | 0.06 | 0.13 | 0.24 | 0.13 | 0.10 | 0.02 | 0.11 | 0.14 |
| 44031 | 16 | pce | Plain, avg | 29 | 0.18 | 0.12 | 0.17 | 0.04 | 0.46 | 0.10 | 0.08 | 0.09 | 0.30 | 0.07 | 0.05 | 0.12 | 0.22 | 0.12 | 0.09 | 0.02 | 0.10 | 0.12 |
| | | | Fruit Snacks | | | | | | | | | | | | | | | | | | | |
| 44212 | 1 | ea | Leather, bars, avg | 23 | 0.01 | 0.02 | 0.03 | 0.01 | 0.13 | 0.01 | 0.01 | 0.01 | 0.03 | 0.01 | 0.01 | 0.02 | 0.04 | 0.02 | 0.01 | 0.00 | 0.01 | 0.02 |
| 44213 | 1 | ea | Leather, bars, w/cream, avg | 24 | 0.01 | 0.01 | 0.03 | 0.00 | 0.03 | 0.01 | 0.00 | 0.01 | 0.02 | 0.01 | 0.00 | 0.01 | 0.01 | 0.01 | 0.01 | 0.00 | 0.01 | 0.01 |
| 44214 | 1 | ea | Leather, pces, avg | 21 | 0.01 | 0.01 | 0.03 | 0.00 | 0.05 | 0.01 | 0.00 | 0.01 | 0.01 | 0.01 | 0.00 | 0.01 | 0.02 | 0.01 | 0.01 | 0.00 | 0.01 | 0.01 |
| | | | Popcorn | | | | | | | | | | | | | | | | | | | |
| 44014 | 1 | cup | Caramel, avg | 35 | 0.07 | 0.08 | 0.14 | 0.01 | 0.23 | 0.08 | 0.04 | 0.05 | 0.10 | 0.10 | 0.03 | 0.05 | 0.06 | 0.05 | 0.05 | 0.02 | 0.04 | 0.06 |
| 44037 | 1 | cup | Caramel, w/peanuts, avg | 42 | 0.16 | 0.21 | 0.24 | 0.04 | 0.52 | 0.13 | 0.08 | 0.10 | 0.27 | 0.08 | 0.05 | 0.13 | 0.19 | 0.13 | 0.10 | 0.02 | 0.11 | 0.13 |
| 44038 | 1 | cup | Cheese, avg | 11 | 0.06 | 0.04 | 0.08 | 0.02 | 0.19 | 0.03 | 0.03 | 0.04 | 0.11 | 0.05 | 0.02 | 0.04 | 0.08 | 0.05 | 0.05 | 0.01 | 0.04 | 0.05 |
| 44072 | 1 | cup | Plain, air popped, avg | 8 | 0.07 | 0.05 | 0.07 | 0.02 | 0.18 | 0.04 | 0.03 | 0.03 | 0.12 | 0.03 | 0.02 | 0.05 | 0.08 | 0.05 | 0.04 | 0.01 | 0.04 | 0.05 |
| 44013 | 1 | cup | Plain, popped in oil, salted, avg | 11 | 0.07 | 0.05 | 0.07 | 0.02 | 0.19 | 0.04 | 0.03 | 0.04 | 0.12 | 0.03 | 0.02 | 0.05 | 0.09 | 0.05 | 0.04 | 0.01 | 0.04 | 0.05 |
| 44022 | 1 | ea | Popcorn Cakes | 10 | 0.07 | 0.06 | 0.08 | 0.02 | 0.19 | 0.04 | 0.03 | 0.04 | 0.10 | 0.03 | 0.02 | 0.05 | 0.07 | 0.05 | 0.04 | 0.01 | 0.04 | 0.05 |
| 44070 | 1 | ea | Popcorn Cakes, Low Sodium, avg | 9 | 0.05 | 0.05 | 0.06 | 0.01 | 0.14 | 0.03 | 0.02 | 0.03 | 0.08 | 0.02 | 0.02 | 0.04 | 0.05 | 0.04 | 0.03 | 0.01 | 0.03 | 0.04 |
| 44039 | 1 | cup | Pork Skins, barbecue | 32 | 1.74 | 1.45 | 1.37 | 0.16 | 2.33 | 3.50 | 0.23 | 0.44 | 1.03 | 0.86 | 0.15 | 0.60 | 2.16 | 0.79 | 0.56 | 0.04 | 0.38 | 0.74 |
| | | | Potato Chips | | | | | | | | | | | | | | | | | | | |
| 44046 | 20 | pce | Barbecue, avg | 26 | 0.07 | 0.09 | 0.26 | 0.02 | 0.31 | 0.06 | 0.04 | 0.09 | 0.14 | 0.12 | 0.03 | 0.08 | 0.10 | 0.08 | 0.08 | 0.02 | 0.07 | 0.11 |
| 44042 | 1 | cup | Cheese, avg | 20 | 0.06 | 0.08 | 0.30 | 0.02 | 0.29 | 0.05 | 0.04 | 0.08 | 0.12 | 0.11 | 0.02 | 0.08 | 0.08 | 0.07 | 0.07 | 0.01 | 0.07 | 0.10 |
| 44045 | 1 | oz | Cheese, Pringles | 28 | 0.07 | 0.09 | 0.30 | 0.02 | 0.35 | 0.06 | 0.05 | 0.09 | 0.14 | 0.13 | 0.03 | 0.09 | 0.11 | 0.09 | 0.08 | 0.02 | 0.08 | 0.12 |
| 44006 | 15 | ea | Plain, avg | 30 | 0.06 | 0.10 | 0.51 | 0.03 | 0.35 | 0.06 | 0.05 | 0.08 | 0.13 | 0.13 | 0.03 | 0.09 | 0.08 | 0.09 | 0.08 | 0.03 | 0.08 | 0.12 |
| 44043 | 20 | pce | Plain, light, avg | 40 | 0.09 | 0.13 | 0.69 | 0.04 | 0.48 | 0.08 | 0.06 | 0.12 | 0.17 | 0.17 | 0.04 | 0.13 | 0.10 | 0.12 | 0.10 | 0.04 | 0.11 | 0.16 |
| 44024 | 1 | oz | Plain, light, Pringles | 28 | 0.06 | 0.08 | 0.32 | 0.02 | 0.26 | 0.05 | 0.04 | 0.07 | 0.10 | 0.10 | 0.02 | 0.07 | 0.06 | 0.06 | 0.07 | 0.01 | 0.06 | 0.09 |
| 44044 | 1 | oz | Plain, Pringles | 28 | 0.06 | 0.08 | 0.34 | 0.02 | 0.28 | 0.06 | 0.04 | 0.07 | 0.11 | 0.10 | 0.02 | 0.08 | 0.06 | 0.07 | 0.07 | 0.01 | 0.07 | 0.10 |
| 44076 | 1 | oz | Plain, unsalted, avg | 28 | 0.06 | 0.09 | 0.48 | 0.02 | 0.33 | 0.06 | 0.04 | 0.08 | 0.12 | 0.12 | 0.03 | 0.09 | 0.07 | 0.08 | 0.07 | 0.03 | 0.07 | 0.11 |
| 5437 | 1 | oz | Sour Cream & Onion, avg | 28 | 0.09 | 0.07 | 0.25 | 0.04 | 0.37 | 0.05 | 0.04 | 0.11 | 0.18 | 0.16 | 0.04 | 0.08 | 0.13 | 0.10 | 0.12 | 0.03 | 0.07 | 0.12 |
| 44046 | 1 | oz | Sour Cream & Onion, Pringles | 28 | 0.07 | 0.08 | 0.24 | 0.02 | 0.29 | 0.05 | 0.04 | 0.08 | 0.13 | 0.11 | 0.03 | 0.08 | 0.10 | 0.08 | 0.07 | 0.02 | 0.07 | 0.10 |
| 44047 | 1 | cup | Potato Sticks | 36 | 0.07 | 0.11 | 0.59 | 0.03 | 0.40 | 0.07 | 0.05 | 0.10 | 0.15 | 0.15 | 0.04 | 0.11 | 0.09 | 0.10 | 0.09 | 0.04 | 0.09 | 0.14 |
| | | | Pretzels | | | | | | | | | | | | | | | | | | | |
| 44015 | 5 | pce | Hard, avg | 30 | 0.09 | 0.10 | 0.12 | 0.06 | 0.91 | 0.10 | 0.06 | 0.10 | 0.19 | 0.07 | 0.05 | 0.14 | 0.30 | 0.13 | 0.08 | 0.03 | 0.08 | 0.12 |
| 44215 | 3 | ea | Hard, chocolate coated, avg | 33 | 0.09 | 0.10 | 0.14 | 0.05 | 0.72 | 0.09 | 0.05 | 0.09 | 0.18 | 0.08 | 0.04 | 0.12 | 0.25 | 0.12 | 0.08 | 0.03 | 0.08 | 0.11 |
| 44079 | 5 | ea | Hard, unsalted, avg | 30 | 0.09 | 0.10 | 0.12 | 0.06 | 0.91 | 0.10 | 0.06 | 0.10 | 0.19 | 0.07 | 0.05 | 0.14 | 0.30 | 0.13 | 0.08 | 0.03 | 0.08 | 0.12 |
| 44048 | 1 | oz | Whole Wheat, avg | 28 | 0.11 | 0.16 | 0.17 | 0.07 | 0.95 | 0.13 | 0.07 | 0.12 | 0.21 | 0.09 | 0.05 | 0.15 | 0.32 | 0.15 | 0.09 | 0.05 | 0.09 | 0.14 |
| | | | Rice Cakes | | | | | | | | | | | | | | | | | | | |
| 44080 | 1 | ea | Brown, avg | 9 | 0.04 | 0.06 | 0.07 | 0.01 | 0.15 | 0.04 | 0.02 | 0.03 | 0.06 | 0.03 | 0.02 | 0.04 | 0.03 | 0.04 | 0.03 | 0.01 | 0.03 | 0.04 |
| 44021 | 1 | ea | Brown, salted, avg | 9 | 0.04 | 0.06 | 0.07 | 0.01 | 0.15 | 0.04 | 0.02 | 0.03 | 0.06 | 0.03 | 0.02 | 0.04 | 0.03 | 0.04 | 0.03 | 0.01 | 0.03 | 0.04 |
| 44049 | 1 | ea | Brown/Buckwheat, avg | 9 | 0.05 | 0.06 | 0.07 | 0.01 | 0.14 | 0.05 | 0.02 | 0.03 | 0.06 | 0.04 | 0.01 | 0.04 | 0.03 | 0.04 | 0.03 | 0.01 | 0.02 | 0.04 |
| 44050 | 1 | ea | Brown/Corn, avg | 9 | 0.05 | 0.05 | 0.06 | 0.01 | 0.15 | 0.04 | 0.02 | 0.03 | 0.07 | 0.03 | 0.02 | 0.04 | 0.04 | 0.04 | 0.03 | 0.01 | 0.03 | 0.04 |
| 44051 | 1 | ea | Brown/Multi-Grain, avg | 9 | 0.04 | 0.06 | 0.07 | 0.01 | 0.15 | 0.04 | 0.02 | 0.03 | 0.06 | 0.03 | 0.02 | 0.04 | 0.04 | 0.04 | 0.03 | 0.01 | 0.03 | 0.04 |
| 44052 | 1 | ea | Brown/Rye, avg | 9 | 0.04 | 0.05 | 0.06 | 0.01 | 0.16 | 0.04 | 0.02 | 0.03 | 0.06 | 0.03 | 0.01 | 0.04 | 0.05 | 0.04 | 0.03 | 0.01 | 0.02 | 0.04 |
| 44053 | 1 | ea | Brown/Sesame Seed, avg | 9 | 0.04 | 0.05 | 0.06 | 0.01 | 0.14 | 0.03 | 0.02 | 0.03 | 0.06 | 0.03 | 0.02 | 0.04 | 0.03 | 0.04 | 0.03 | 0.01 | 0.03 | 0.04 |
| | | | Snack Sticks | | | | | | | | | | | | | | | | | | | |
| 44217 | 1 | oz | Sesame, avg | 28 | 0.11 | 0.18 | 0.20 | 0.06 | 0.87 | 0.12 | 0.07 | 0.12 | 0.21 | 0.10 | 0.05 | 0.15 | 0.28 | 0.15 | 0.09 | 0.04 | 0.10 | 0.13 |
| 44084 | 1 | oz | Sesame, unsalted, avg | 28 | 0.11 | 0.18 | 0.20 | 0.06 | 0.87 | 0.12 | 0.07 | 0.12 | 0.21 | 0.10 | 0.05 | 0.15 | 0.28 | 0.15 | 0.09 | 0.04 | 0.10 | 0.13 |
| 44020 | 10 | ea | Taro Chips, avg | 23 | 0.03 | 0.04 | 0.07 | 0.01 | 0.06 | 0.03 | 0.01 | 0.02 | 0.04 | 0.02 | 0.01 | 0.03 | 0.02 | 0.03 | 0.02 | 0.01 | 0.02 | 0.03 |
| | | | Tortilla Chips | | | | | | | | | | | | | | | | | | | |
| 44054 | 20 | ea | Nacho, light, avg | 32 | 0.18 | 0.14 | 0.19 | 0.04 | 0.53 | 0.10 | 0.08 | 0.11 | 0.32 | 0.10 | 0.06 | 0.13 | 0.24 | 0.13 | 0.10 | 0.02 | 0.11 | 0.14 |

## TABLE A Amino Acid Content for Selected Foods *(continued)*

| Code | Amount | Description | Weight (g) | Alanine (g) | Arginine (g) | Aspartic acid (g) | Cystine (g) | Glutamic acid (g) | Glycine (g) | Histidine (g) | Isoleucine (g) | Leucine (g) | Lysine (g) | Methionine (g) | Phenylalanine (g) | Proline (g) | Serine (g) | Threonine (g) | Tryptophan (g) | Tyrosine (g) | Valine (g) |
|---|---|---|---|---|---|---|---|---|---|---|---|---|---|---|---|---|---|---|---|---|---|
| 44004 | 1 cup | Nacho, Doritos | 26 | 0.13 | 0.10 | 0.14 | 0.03 | 0.39 | 0.07 | 0.06 | 0.08 | 0.23 | 0.08 | 0.04 | 0.10 | 0.18 | 0.10 | 0.07 | 0.02 | 0.08 | 0.10 |
| 44018 | 16 pce | Plain, avg | 29 | 0.15 | 0.10 | 0.14 | 0.04 | 0.38 | 0.08 | 0.06 | 0.07 | 0.25 | 0.06 | 0.04 | 0.10 | 0.18 | 0.10 | 0.08 | 0.01 | 0.08 | 0.10 |
| 44055 | 16 pce | Ranch, avg | 28 | 0.15 | 0.11 | 0.15 | 0.04 | 0.41 | 0.08 | 0.06 | 0.08 | 0.24 | 0.07 | 0.04 | 0.10 | 0.18 | 0.10 | 0.08 | 0.02 | 0.08 | 0.11 |
| 44057 | 16 pce | Taco, avg | 28 | 0.14 | 0.11 | 0.16 | 0.04 | 0.43 | 0.08 | 0.07 | 0.09 | 0.25 | 0.08 | 0.05 | 0.11 | 0.19 | 0.11 | 0.08 | 0.02 | 0.09 | 0.12 |
| | | Trail Mix | | | | | | | | | | | | | | | | | | | |
| 44058 | 1/2 cup | Average | 75 | 0.44 | 1.14 | 1.14 | 0.16 | 2.26 | 0.58 | 0.27 | 0.39 | 0.67 | 0.39 | 0.15 | 0.49 | 0.47 | 0.49 | 0.36 | 0.12 | 0.34 | 0.49 |
| 44060 | 1/2 cup | Tropical, avg | 70 | 0.20 | 0.41 | 0.49 | 0.08 | 0.98 | 0.19 | 0.15 | 0.16 | 0.25 | 0.16 | 0.10 | 0.18 | 0.16 | 0.15 | 0.16 | 0.05 | 0.11 | 0.21 |
| 44085 | 1/2 cup | Unsalted, avg | 75 | 0.44 | 1.14 | 1.14 | 0.16 | 2.26 | 0.58 | 0.27 | 0.39 | 0.67 | 0.39 | 0.15 | 0.49 | 0.47 | 0.49 | 0.36 | 0.12 | 0.34 | 0.49 |
| 44059 | 1/2 cup | With Chocolate Chips, avg | 73 | 0.42 | 1.10 | 1.12 | 0.14 | 2.20 | 0.56 | 0.26 | 0.41 | 0.70 | 0.43 | 0.16 | 0.50 | 0.50 | 0.48 | 0.37 | 0.12 | 0.37 | 0.51 |
| 44086 | 1/2 cup | With Chocolate Chips, unsalted, avg | 73 | 0.42 | 1.10 | 1.12 | 0.14 | 2.20 | 0.56 | 0.26 | 0.41 | 0.70 | 0.43 | 0.16 | 0.50 | 0.50 | 0.48 | 0.37 | 0.12 | 0.37 | 0.51 |
| | | **SOUPS AND STEWS—CANNED** | | | | | | | | | | | | | | | | | | | |
| | | Asparagus Cream Soup | | | | | | | | | | | | | | | | | | | |
| 50056 | 1/2 cup | Condensed, avg | 152 | 0.11 | 0.10 | 0.21 | 0.04 | 0.71 | 0.08 | 0.06 | 0.12 | 0.20 | 0.14 | 0.05 | 0.12 | 0.25 | 0.13 | 0.09 | 0.03 | 0.09 | 0.14 |
| 50057 | 1 cup | Prep, w/milk, avg | 248 | 0.23 | 0.23 | 0.47 | 0.07 | 1.40 | 0.15 | 0.16 | 0.33 | 0.55 | 0.42 | 0.14 | 0.29 | 0.59 | 0.32 | 0.26 | 0.08 | 0.27 | 0.38 |
| 50058 | 1 cup | Prep, w/water, avg | 244 | 0.09 | 0.09 | 0.17 | 0.03 | 0.59 | 0.07 | 0.05 | 0.10 | 0.16 | 0.11 | 0.04 | 0.10 | 0.20 | 0.10 | 0.08 | 0.03 | 0.08 | 0.11 |
| | | Bean Soup | | | | | | | | | | | | | | | | | | | |
| 50648 | 1/2 cup | Bean & Frank, cond, avg | 132 | 0.50 | 0.53 | 1.12 | 0.11 | 1.85 | 0.48 | 0.26 | 0.49 | 0.83 | 0.68 | 0.13 | 0.56 | 0.45 | 0.50 | 0.41 | 0.11 | 0.30 | 0.55 |
| 50063 | 1 cup | Bean & Frank, prep w/water, avg | 250 | 0.50 | 0.52 | 1.12 | 0.11 | 1.84 | 0.48 | 0.26 | 0.49 | 0.82 | 0.68 | 0.13 | 0.56 | 0.45 | 0.50 | 0.41 | 0.10 | 0.30 | 0.55 |
| 50647 | 1/2 cup | Bean w/Bacon, cond, avg | 134 | 0.39 | 0.41 | 0.88 | 0.09 | 1.45 | 0.38 | 0.21 | 0.38 | 0.65 | 0.54 | 0.10 | 0.44 | 0.36 | 0.39 | 0.33 | 0.08 | 0.24 | 0.43 |
| 50000 | 1 cup | Bean w/Bacon, prep w/water, avg | 253 | 0.39 | 0.41 | 0.88 | 0.09 | 1.45 | 0.38 | 0.20 | 0.38 | 0.65 | 0.54 | 0.10 | 0.44 | 0.36 | 0.39 | 0.33 | 0.08 | 0.24 | 0.44 |
| 50064 | 1 cup | Bean w/Ham, chunky, RTS, avg | 243 | 0.63 | 0.66 | 1.41 | 0.14 | 2.32 | 0.61 | 0.33 | 0.62 | 1.04 | 0.86 | 0.16 | 0.70 | 0.57 | 0.62 | 0.52 | 0.13 | 0.38 | 0.69 |
| 50646 | 1/2 cup | Black Bean, cond, avg | 128 | 0.25 | 0.36 | 0.72 | 0.06 | 1.24 | 0.24 | 0.18 | 0.31 | 0.46 | 0.45 | 0.07 | 0.34 | 0.24 | 0.34 | 0.27 | 0.07 | 0.19 | 0.31 |
| 50060 | 1 cup | Black Bean, prep w/water, avg | 247 | 0.23 | 0.33 | 0.65 | 0.06 | 1.13 | 0.22 | 0.16 | 0.29 | 0.42 | 0.41 | 0.06 | 0.31 | 0.22 | 0.31 | 0.25 | 0.06 | 0.05 | 0.28 |
| | | Beef Soup | | | | | | | | | | | | | | | | | | | |
| 50066 | 1 cup | Chunky, RTS, avg | 240 | 0.72 | 0.61 | 1.15 | 0.12 | 2.10 | 0.68 | 0.28 | 0.59 | 0.90 | 0.93 | 0.25 | 0.48 | 0.54 | 0.41 | 0.47 | 0.11 | 0.35 | 0.64 |
| 50649 | 1/2 cup | Noodle, cond, avg | 126 | 0.22 | 0.20 | 0.36 | 0.06 | 1.34 | 0.23 | 0.11 | 0.19 | 0.32 | 0.26 | 0.09 | 0.20 | 0.31 | 0.17 | 0.15 | 0.05 | 0.13 | 0.21 |
| 50003 | 1 cup | Noodle, prep w/water, avg | 244 | 0.22 | 0.20 | 0.35 | 0.06 | 1.33 | 0.23 | 0.11 | 0.19 | 0.31 | 0.26 | 0.09 | 0.20 | 0.31 | 0.17 | 0.15 | 0.05 | 0.12 | 0.21 |
| 50683 | 1/2 cup | Vegetable Beef, cond, avg | 126 | 0.32 | 0.26 | 0.47 | 0.04 | 1.41 | 0.35 | 0.12 | 0.21 | 0.36 | 0.35 | 0.09 | 0.21 | 0.32 | 0.19 | 0.18 | 0.05 | 0.15 | 0.25 |
| 50014 | 1 cup | Vegetable Beef, prep w/water, avg | 244 | 0.32 | 0.26 | 0.47 | 0.04 | 1.41 | 0.35 | 0.12 | 0.21 | 0.36 | 0.34 | 0.10 | 0.20 | 0.32 | 0.19 | 0.17 | 0.05 | 0.15 | 0.25 |
| 50048 | 1 cup | Brunswick Stew, avg | 250 | 0.80 | 0.83 | 1.36 | 0.18 | 2.30 | 0.66 | 0.43 | 0.73 | 1.09 | 1.11 | 0.36 | 0.58 | 0.62 | 0.54 | 0.59 | 0.16 | 0.48 | 0.72 |
| | | Celery Soup | | | | | | | | | | | | | | | | | | | |
| 50650 | 1/2 cup | Cream of Celery, cond, avg | 126 | 0.06 | 0.06 | 0.12 | 0.02 | 0.39 | 0.05 | 0.04 | 0.08 | 0.12 | 0.07 | 0.03 | 0.08 | 0.14 | 0.08 | 0.06 | 0.02 | 0.05 | 0.09 |
| 50015 | 1 cup | Cream of Celery, prep w/milk, avg | 248 | 0.19 | 0.20 | 0.41 | 0.05 | 1.21 | 0.13 | 0.15 | 0.32 | 0.51 | 0.39 | 0.13 | 0.27 | 0.52 | 0.29 | 0.24 | 0.07 | 0.24 | 0.35 |
| 50016 | 1 cup | Cream of Celery, prep w/water, avg | 244 | 0.06 | 0.06 | 0.11 | 0.02 | 0.38 | 0.05 | 0.04 | 0.08 | 0.12 | 0.07 | 0.03 | 0.08 | 0.14 | 0.08 | 0.06 | 0.02 | 0.05 | 0.09 |
| | | Cheese Soup | | | | | | | | | | | | | | | | | | | |
| 50651 | 1/2 cup | Condensed, avg | 128 | 0.16 | 0.15 | 0.34 | 0.04 | 1.50 | 0.10 | 0.13 | 0.29 | 0.46 | 0.34 | 0.10 | 0.25 | 0.51 | 0.22 | 0.17 | 0.06 | 0.22 | 0.34 |
| 50071 | 1 cup | Prepared, w/milk, avg | 251 | 0.29 | 0.28 | 0.63 | 0.08 | 2.32 | 0.19 | 0.24 | 0.52 | 0.84 | 0.65 | 0.20 | 0.44 | 0.89 | 0.43 | 0.34 | 0.12 | 0.41 | 0.60 |
| 50072 | 1 cup | Prepared, w/water, avg | 247 | 0.16 | 0.15 | 0.34 | 0.04 | 1.50 | 0.10 | 0.13 | 0.29 | 0.46 | 0.34 | 0.10 | 0.25 | 0.51 | 0.22 | 0.17 | 0.06 | 0.22 | 0.34 |
| | | Chicken Soup | | | | | | | | | | | | | | | | | | | |
| 50654 | 1/2 cup | Cream of Chicken, cond, avg | 126 | 0.15 | 0.17 | 0.24 | 0.05 | 0.78 | 0.14 | 0.09 | 0.17 | 0.26 | 0.22 | 0.08 | 0.15 | 0.26 | 0.15 | 0.13 | 0.04 | 0.12 | 0.17 |
| 50006 | 1 cup | Cream of Chicken, prep w/milk, avg | 248 | 0.28 | 0.31 | 0.54 | 0.09 | 1.60 | 0.22 | 0.20 | 0.41 | 0.65 | 0.52 | 0.18 | 0.34 | 0.64 | 0.36 | 0.31 | 0.10 | 0.31 | 0.44 |
| 50018 | 1 cup | Cream of Chicken, prep w/water, avg | 244 | 0.15 | 0.17 | 0.24 | 0.05 | 0.78 | 0.14 | 0.09 | 0.17 | 0.26 | 0.21 | 0.08 | 0.15 | 0.26 | 0.15 | 0.13 | 0.04 | 0.12 | 0.17 |
| 50652 | 1/2 cup | Dumpling, cond, avg | 123 | 0.33 | 0.28 | 0.46 | 0.07 | 1.46 | 0.40 | 0.13 | 0.24 | 0.39 | 0.36 | 0.10 | 0.22 | 0.36 | 0.18 | 0.19 | 0.05 | 0.14 | 0.27 |
| 50074 | 1 cup | Dumpling, prep, avg | 241 | 0.33 | 0.28 | 0.46 | 0.07 | 1.46 | 0.40 | 0.13 | 0.23 | 0.39 | 0.36 | 0.10 | 0.22 | 0.35 | 0.18 | 0.19 | 0.05 | 0.14 | 0.27 |
| 50076 | 1/2 cup | Gumbo, cond, avg | 126 | 0.15 | 0.12 | 0.22 | 0.02 | 0.67 | 0.17 | 0.06 | 0.10 | 0.17 | 0.16 | 0.05 | 0.10 | 0.15 | 0.09 | 0.08 | 0.02 | 0.07 | 0.12 |
| 50077 | 1 cup | Gumbo, prep, avg | 244 | 0.15 | 0.12 | 0.22 | 0.02 | 0.66 | 0.17 | 0.06 | 0.10 | 0.17 | 0.16 | 0.05 | 0.10 | 0.15 | 0.09 | 0.08 | 0.02 | 0.07 | 0.12 |
| 50656 | 1/2 cup | Noodle, cond, avg | 123 | 0.18 | 0.16 | 0.29 | 0.05 | 1.09 | 0.19 | 0.09 | 0.15 | 0.26 | 0.22 | 0.07 | 0.16 | 0.26 | 0.14 | 0.13 | 0.04 | 0.10 | 0.17 |
| 50005 | 1 cup | Noodle, prep w/water, avg | 241 | 0.19 | 0.17 | 0.30 | 0.05 | 1.12 | 0.19 | 0.09 | 0.16 | 0.27 | 0.22 | 0.08 | 0.16 | 0.26 | 0.14 | 0.13 | 0.04 | 0.11 | 0.18 |
| 50081 | 1 cup | Noodle, RTS, chunky, avg | 240 | 0.75 | 0.64 | 1.05 | 0.16 | 3.31 | 0.90 | 0.30 | 0.53 | 0.89 | 0.82 | 0.23 | 0.48 | 0.80 | 0.41 | 0.42 | 0.12 | 0.31 | 0.60 |
| 50048 | 1 cup | Noodle & Meatball, RTS, avg | 248 | 0.80 | 0.83 | 1.36 | 0.18 | 2.30 | 0.66 | 0.43 | 0.73 | 1.09 | 1.11 | 0.36 | 0.58 | 0.62 | 0.54 | 0.59 | 0.16 | 0.48 | 0.72 |

TABLE A **Amino Acid Content for Selected Foods *(continued)***

| Code | Amount | Description | Weight (g) | Alanine (g) | Arginine (g) | Aspartic acid (g) | Cystine (g) | Glutamic acid (g) | Glycine (g) | Histidine (g) | Isoleucine (g) | Leucine (g) | Lysine (g) | Methionine (g) | Phenylalanine (g) | Proline (g) | Serine (g) | Threonine (g) | Tryptophan (g) | Tyrosine (g) | Valine (g) |
|---|---|---|---|---|---|---|---|---|---|---|---|---|---|---|---|---|---|---|---|---|---|
| 50658 | 1/2 cup | Rice, cond, avg | 123 | 0.19 | 0.23 | 0.32 | 0.05 | 0.56 | 0.17 | 0.10 | 0.18 | 0.27 | 0.25 | 0.09 | 0.15 | 0.15 | 0.14 | 0.14 | 0.04 | 0.12 | 0.19 |
| 50020 | 1 cup | Rice, prep w/water, avg | 241 | 0.19 | 0.23 | 0.32 | 0.05 | 0.56 | 0.17 | 0.10 | 0.18 | 0.27 | 0.25 | 0.09 | 0.15 | 0.15 | 0.14 | 0.14 | 0.04 | 0.12 | 0.19 |
| 50085 | 1 cup | Rice, RTS, chunky, avg | 240 | 0.67 | 0.81 | 1.10 | 0.18 | 1.94 | 0.60 | 0.35 | 0.62 | 0.94 | 0.87 | 0.32 | 0.52 | 0.52 | 0.48 | 0.49 | 0.14 | 0.43 | 0.66 |
| 50088 | 1 cup | Vegetable, chunky, RTS, avg | 240 | 0.70 | 0.58 | 1.04 | 0.08 | 3.10 | 0.78 | 0.27 | 0.47 | 0.79 | 0.76 | 0.21 | 0.45 | 0.71 | 0.42 | 0.39 | 0.11 | 0.32 | 0.54 |
| 50659 | 1/2 cup | Vegetable, cond, avg | 123 | 0.21 | 0.17 | 0.31 | 0.02 | 0.91 | 0.23 | 0.08 | 0.14 | 0.23 | 0.22 | 0.06 | 0.13 | 0.21 | 0.12 | 0.11 | 0.03 | 0.09 | 0.16 |
| 50219 | 1 cup | Vegetable, low sod, prep, avg | 241 | 0.70 | 0.58 | 1.04 | 0.08 | 3.11 | 0.77 | 0.27 | 0.47 | 0.79 | 0.76 | 0.21 | 0.45 | 0.71 | 0.42 | 0.39 | 0.10 | 0.32 | 0.54 |
| 50091 | 1 cup | Vegetable, prep, avg | 241 | 0.20 | 0.17 | 0.30 | 0.02 | 0.91 | 0.23 | 0.08 | 0.13 | 0.23 | 0.22 | 0.06 | 0.13 | 0.21 | 0.12 | 0.11 | 0.03 | 0.09 | 0.16 |
| 50660 | 1/2 cup | Chili Soup, beef, cond, avg | 132 | 0.34 | 0.35 | 0.75 | 0.07 | 1.24 | 0.32 | 0.18 | 0.33 | 0.55 | 0.46 | 0.08 | 0.37 | 0.30 | 0.33 | 0.28 | 0.07 | 0.20 | 0.37 |
| 50007 | 1 cup | Chili Soup, beef, prep w/water, avg | 250 | 0.33 | 0.35 | 0.75 | 0.07 | 1.23 | 0.32 | 0.17 | 0.33 | 0.55 | 0.45 | 0.09 | 0.37 | 0.30 | 0.33 | 0.28 | 0.07 | 0.20 | 0.37 |
| | | Clam Chowder | | | | | | | | | | | | | | | | | | | |
| 50662 | 1/2 cup | New England, cond, avg | 126 | 0.29 | 0.26 | 0.51 | 0.06 | 1.59 | 0.26 | 0.16 | 0.21 | 0.33 | 0.29 | 0.10 | 0.18 | 0.21 | 0.16 | 0.17 | 0.06 | 0.14 | 0.22 |
| 50008 | 1 cup | New England, prep w/milk, avg | 248 | 0.42 | 0.41 | 0.81 | 0.10 | 2.42 | 0.34 | 0.27 | 0.45 | 0.72 | 0.61 | 0.20 | 0.37 | 0.60 | 0.37 | 0.35 | 0.12 | 0.34 | 0.49 |
| 50195 | 1 cup | New England, prep w/water, avg | 244 | 0.25 | 0.23 | 0.45 | 0.06 | 1.40 | 0.23 | 0.14 | 0.13 | 0.29 | 0.25 | 0.09 | 0.16 | 0.18 | 0.14 | 0.15 | 0.05 | 0.13 | 0.20 |
| | | Minestrone Soup | | | | | | | | | | | | | | | | | | | |
| 50107 | 1 cup | Chunky, RTS, avg | 240 | 0.30 | 0.24 | 0.44 | 0.04 | 1.46 | 0.47 | 0.08 | 0.15 | 0.28 | 0.22 | 0.05 | 0.18 | 0.39 | 0.17 | 0.12 | 0.04 | 0.10 | 0.21 |
| 50664 | 1/2 cup | Condensed, avg | 123 | 0.25 | 0.20 | 0.37 | 0.03 | 1.23 | 0.39 | 0.07 | 0.13 | 0.24 | 0.18 | 0.04 | 0.15 | 0.33 | 0.15 | 0.10 | 0.03 | 0.08 | 0.18 |
| 50009 | 1 cup | Prepared, w/water, avg | 241 | 0.25 | 0.20 | 0.37 | 0.03 | 1.22 | 0.39 | 0.07 | 0.13 | 0.24 | 0.18 | 0.04 | 0.15 | 0.33 | 0.14 | 0.10 | 0.03 | 0.08 | 0.18 |
| | | Mushroom Soup | | | | | | | | | | | | | | | | | | | |
| 50666 | 1/2 cup | Cream of Mushroom, cond, avg | 126 | 0.08 | 0.08 | 0.14 | 0.03 | 0.46 | 0.07 | 0.05 | 0.10 | 0.16 | 0.11 | 0.04 | 0.09 | 0.17 | 0.10 | 0.08 | 0.03 | 0.08 | 0.11 |
| 50011 | 1 cup | Cream of Mushroom, prep w/milk, avg | 248 | 0.21 | 0.23 | 0.44 | 0.06 | 1.28 | 0.15 | 0.15 | 0.33 | 0.54 | 0.42 | 0.14 | 0.28 | 0.55 | 0.31 | 0.25 | 0.08 | 0.26 | 0.37 |
| 50049 | 1 cup | Cream of Mushroom, prep w/water, avg | 244 | 0.09 | 0.10 | 0.16 | 0.03 | 0.53 | 0.08 | 0.05 | 0.11 | 0.18 | 0.13 | 0.04 | 0.11 | 0.20 | 0.12 | 0.09 | 0.03 | 0.09 | 0.12 |
| | | Pea Soup | | | | | | | | | | | | | | | | | | | |
| 50671 | 1/2 cup | Green, cond, avg | 132 | 0.37 | 0.71 | 0.88 | 0.08 | 1.62 | 0.34 | 0.17 | 0.30 | 0.62 | 0.51 | 0.10 | 0.38 | 0.44 | 0.35 | 0.30 | 0.07 | 0.25 | 0.44 |
| 50185 | 1 cup | Green, low sod, prep w/water, avg | 250 | 0.37 | 0.71 | 0.88 | 0.08 | 1.62 | 0.34 | 0.17 | 0.30 | 0.62 | 0.51 | 0.10 | 0.38 | 0.44 | 0.35 | 0.30 | 0.07 | 0.25 | 0.44 |
| 50117 | 1 cup | Green, prep w/milk, avg | 254 | 0.51 | 0.85 | 1.19 | 0.12 | 2.46 | 0.43 | 0.28 | 0.54 | 1.02 | 0.83 | 0.21 | 0.57 | 0.83 | 0.57 | 0.49 | 0.13 | 0.45 | 0.71 |
| 50050 | 1 cup | Green, prep w/water, avg | 250 | 0.37 | 0.71 | 0.88 | 0.08 | 1.62 | 0.34 | 0.17 | 0.30 | 0.62 | 0.51 | 0.10 | 0.38 | 0.44 | 0.35 | 0.30 | 0.07 | 0.25 | 0.44 |
| 50122 | 1 cup | Pepper Pot Soup, avg | 241 | 0.46 | 0.49 | 0.55 | 0.06 | 1.11 | 0.33 | 0.09 | 0.23 | 0.40 | 0.31 | 0.09 | 0.23 | 0.59 | 0.23 | 0.19 | 0.04 | 0.15 | 0.30 |
| 50673 | 1/2 cup | Pepper Pot Soup, cond, avg | 123 | 0.46 | 0.49 | 0.55 | 0.06 | 1.12 | 0.34 | 0.09 | 0.23 | 0.40 | 0.31 | 0.09 | 0.23 | 0.59 | 0.23 | 0.19 | 0.04 | 0.15 | 0.30 |
| | | Potato Soup | | | | | | | | | | | | | | | | | | | |
| 50674 | 1/2 cup | Cream of Potato, cond, avg | 126 | 0.05 | 0.07 | 0.25 | 0.03 | 0.41 | 0.05 | 0.04 | 0.03 | 0.12 | 0.08 | 0.03 | 0.08 | 0.13 | 0.08 | 0.06 | 0.02 | 0.06 | 0.09 |
| 50197 | 1 cup | Cream of Potato, prep w/water, avg | 244 | 0.05 | 0.08 | 0.25 | 0.03 | 0.41 | 0.05 | 0.04 | 0.03 | 0.12 | 0.08 | 0.03 | 0.08 | 0.13 | 0.08 | 0.06 | 0.02 | 0.06 | 0.09 |
| 50027 | 1 cup | Vichyssoise, avg | 248 | 0.19 | 0.21 | 0.54 | 0.06 | 1.21 | 0.13 | 0.14 | 0.31 | 0.49 | 0.39 | 0.13 | 0.27 | 0.50 | 0.29 | 0.23 | 0.08 | 0.25 | 0.35 |
| 50675 | 1/2 cup | Scotch Broth, condensed, avg | 123 | 0.28 | 0.23 | 0.42 | 0.03 | 1.25 | 0.31 | 0.11 | 0.13 | 0.32 | 0.31 | 0.08 | 0.18 | 0.28 | 0.17 | 0.15 | 0.04 | 0.13 | 0.22 |
| 50124 | 1 cup | Scotch Broth, prepared, w/water, avg | 241 | 0.28 | 0.23 | 0.41 | 0.03 | 1.24 | 0.31 | 0.11 | 0.13 | 0.32 | 0.30 | 0.08 | 0.18 | 0.28 | 0.17 | 0.15 | 0.04 | 0.13 | 0.22 |
| | | Split Pea Soup | | | | | | | | | | | | | | | | | | | |
| 50672 | 1/2 cup | With Ham, cond, avg | 134 | 0.48 | 0.70 | 1.05 | 0.13 | 1.74 | 0.50 | 0.22 | 0.43 | 0.71 | 0.69 | 0.14 | 0.45 | 0.47 | 0.44 | 0.36 | 0.10 | 0.32 | 0.49 |
| 50025 | 1 cup | With Ham, prep w/water, avg | 253 | 0.48 | 0.70 | 1.05 | 0.13 | 1.75 | 0.50 | 0.22 | 0.44 | 0.71 | 0.70 | 0.14 | 0.46 | 0.47 | 0.44 | 0.36 | 0.10 | 0.32 | 0.49 |
| 50118 | 1 cup | With Ham, RTS, chunky, avg | 240 | 0.52 | 0.76 | 1.13 | 0.14 | 1.88 | 0.54 | 0.23 | 0.47 | 0.77 | 0.75 | 0.15 | 0.49 | 0.50 | 0.48 | 0.39 | 0.11 | 0.34 | 0.53 |
| 50677 | 1/2 cup | Stock Pot Soup, cond, avg | 128 | 0.28 | 0.23 | 0.41 | 0.03 | 1.22 | 0.30 | 0.11 | 0.13 | 0.31 | 0.30 | 0.08 | 0.18 | 0.28 | 0.17 | 0.15 | 0.04 | 0.13 | 0.21 |
| 50130 | 1 cup | Stock Pot Soup, prep w/water, avg | 248 | 0.28 | 0.23 | 0.41 | 0.03 | 1.23 | 0.31 | 0.11 | 0.13 | 0.31 | 0.30 | 0.08 | 0.18 | 0.28 | 0.17 | 0.15 | 0.04 | 0.13 | 0.22 |
| | | Tomato Soup | | | | | | | | | | | | | | | | | | | |
| 50678 | 1/2 cup | Beef Noodle, cond, avg | 126 | 0.21 | 0.18 | 0.33 | 0.05 | 1.23 | 0.21 | 0.10 | 0.17 | 0.29 | 0.24 | 0.08 | 0.18 | 0.29 | 0.16 | 0.14 | 0.04 | 0.12 | 0.19 |
| 50132 | 1 cup | Beef Noodle, prep w/water, avg | 244 | 0.20 | 0.18 | 0.33 | 0.05 | 1.23 | 0.21 | 0.10 | 0.17 | 0.29 | 0.24 | 0.08 | 0.18 | 0.29 | 0.16 | 0.14 | 0.04 | 0.11 | 0.19 |
| 50687 | 1/2 cup | Bisque, cond, avg | 128 | 0.06 | 0.07 | 0.20 | 0.02 | 0.77 | 0.05 | 0.04 | 0.03 | 0.13 | 0.09 | 0.03 | 0.08 | 0.14 | 0.09 | 0.07 | 0.02 | 0.06 | 0.09 |
| 50134 | 1 cup | Bisque, prep w/milk, avg | 251 | 0.20 | 0.21 | 0.50 | 0.06 | 1.62 | 0.14 | 0.15 | 0.32 | 0.52 | 0.41 | 0.13 | 0.27 | 0.53 | 0.31 | 0.25 | 0.08 | 0.25 | 0.36 |

TABLE A **Amino Acid Content for Selected Foods *(continued)***

| Code | Amount | Description | Weight (g) | Alanine (g) | Arginine (g) | Aspartic acid (g) | Cystine (g) | Glutamic acid (g) | Glycine (g) | Histidine (g) | Isoleucine (g) | Leucine (g) | Lysine (g) | Methionine (g) | Phenylalanine (g) | Proline (g) | Serine (g) | Threonine (g) | Tryptophan (g) | Tyrosine (g) | Valine (g) |
|---|---|---|---|---|---|---|---|---|---|---|---|---|---|---|---|---|---|---|---|---|---|
| 50135 | 1 cup | Bisque, prep w/water, avg | 247 | 0.06 | 0.07 | 0.20 | 0.02 | 0.78 | 0.05 | 0.04 | 0.08 | 0.13 | 0.09 | 0.03 | 0.08 | 0.14 | 0.09 | 0.07 | 0.02 | 0.06 | 0.09 |
| 50688 | 1/2 cup | Condensed, avg | 126 | 0.06 | 0.06 | 0.16 | 0.03 | 0.78 | 0.05 | 0.04 | 0.06 | 0.10 | 0.05 | 0.02 | 0.07 | 0.13 | 0.08 | 0.05 | 0.02 | 0.04 | 0.07 |
| 50012 | 1 cup | Prepared, w/milk, avg | 248 | 0.19 | 0.21 | 0.47 | 0.06 | 1.62 | 0.14 | 0.15 | 0.30 | 0.49 | 0.37 | 0.12 | 0.27 | 0.53 | 0.30 | 0.23 | 0.08 | 0.24 | 0.33 |
| 50028 | 1 cup | Prepared, w/water, avg | 244 | 0.06 | 0.06 | 0.16 | 0.03 | 0.77 | 0.05 | 0.04 | 0.06 | 0.10 | 0.05 | 0.02 | 0.07 | 0.13 | 0.08 | 0.05 | 0.02 | 0.04 | 0.07 |
| | | Turkey Soup | | | | | | | | | | | | | | | | | | | |
| 50138 | 1 cup | Chunky, RTS, avg | 236 | 0.63 | 0.53 | 1.00 | 0.11 | 1.83 | 0.59 | 0.24 | 0.51 | 0.78 | 0.81 | 0.21 | 0.42 | 0.47 | 0.36 | 0.40 | 0.10 | 0.31 | 0.55 |
| 50680 | 1/2 cup | Noodle, cond, avg | 126 | 0.18 | 0.16 | 0.29 | 0.05 | 1.08 | 0.18 | 0.09 | 0.15 | 0.26 | 0.21 | 0.07 | 0.16 | 0.25 | 0.14 | 0.13 | 0.04 | 0.10 | 0.17 |
| 50141 | 1 cup | Noodle, prep w/water, avg | 244 | 0.18 | 0.16 | 0.29 | 0.05 | 1.08 | 0.18 | 0.09 | 0.15 | 0.25 | 0.21 | 0.07 | 0.16 | 0.25 | 0.14 | 0.12 | 0.04 | 0.10 | 0.17 |
| 50681 | 1/2 cup | Vegetable, cond, avg | 123 | 0.18 | 0.15 | 0.26 | 0.02 | 0.78 | 0.19 | 0.07 | 0.12 | 0.20 | 0.19 | 0.05 | 0.11 | 0.18 | 0.11 | 0.10 | 0.03 | 0.08 | 0.14 |
| 50143 | 1 cup | Vegetable, prep w/water, avg | 241 | 0.18 | 0.14 | 0.26 | 0.02 | 0.78 | 0.19 | 0.07 | 0.12 | 0.20 | 0.19 | 0.05 | 0.11 | 0.18 | 0.11 | 0.10 | 0.03 | 0.08 | 0.13 |
| | | Vegetable Soup | | | | | | | | | | | | | | | | | | | |
| 50144 | 1 cup | Chunky, RTS, avg | 240 | 0.19 | 0.19 | 0.46 | 0.03 | 0.74 | 0.13 | 0.08 | 0.16 | 0.27 | 0.19 | 0.03 | 0.16 | 0.13 | 0.13 | 0.11 | 0.03 | 0.08 | 0.19 |
| 50186 | 1 cup | Low Sodium, avg | 241 | 0.11 | 0.11 | 0.23 | 0.04 | 0.52 | 0.09 | 0.06 | 0.11 | 0.17 | 0.11 | 0.03 | 0.11 | 0.17 | 0.09 | 0.09 | 0.02 | 0.06 | 0.11 |
| 50682 | 1/2 cup | Vegetarian, cond, avg | 123 | 0.10 | 0.10 | 0.20 | 0.02 | 0.45 | 0.08 | 0.05 | 0.10 | 0.15 | 0.10 | 0.02 | 0.10 | 0.15 | 0.08 | 0.08 | 0.01 | 0.05 | 0.10 |
| 50013 | 1 cup | Vegetarian, prep w/water, avg | 241 | 0.10 | 0.10 | 0.20 | 0.02 | 0.45 | 0.07 | 0.05 | 0.10 | 0.15 | 0.10 | 0.02 | 0.10 | 0.15 | 0.07 | 0.07 | 0.01 | 0.05 | 0.10 |
| 50684 | 1/2 cup | With Beef Broth, cond, avg | 123 | 0.17 | 0.14 | 0.25 | 0.02 | 0.85 | 0.27 | 0.05 | 0.09 | 0.16 | 0.13 | 0.03 | 0.11 | 0.23 | 0.10 | 0.07 | 0.02 | 0.06 | 0.13 |
| 50147 | 1 cup | With Beef Broth, prep w/water, avg | 241 | 0.17 | 0.14 | 0.25 | 0.02 | 0.85 | 0.27 | 0.05 | 0.09 | 0.16 | 0.13 | 0.03 | 0.11 | 0.23 | 0.10 | 0.07 | 0.02 | 0.06 | 0.13 |
| | | **SOUPS AND STEWS—DRY AND PREPARED** | | | | | | | | | | | | | | | | | | | |
| 50148 | 1 ea | Asparagus Soup, cream of, dry mix, svg, avg | 14 | 0.08 | 0.07 | 0.14 | 0.03 | 0.49 | 0.06 | 0.04 | 0.08 | 0.14 | 0.09 | 0.03 | 0.08 | 0.17 | 0.09 | 0.07 | 0.02 | 0.06 | 0.10 |
| 50149 | 1 cup | Asparagus Soup, cream of, prep f/dry mix, avg | 251 | 0.09 | 0.08 | 0.17 | 0.03 | 0.56 | 0.07 | 0.05 | 0.09 | 0.16 | 0.11 | 0.04 | 0.09 | 0.20 | 0.10 | 0.08 | 0.03 | 0.07 | 0.11 |
| 50150 | 1 oz | Bean w/Bacon, dry mix, avg | 28 | 0.27 | 0.29 | 0.61 | 0.06 | 1.00 | 0.26 | 0.14 | 0.27 | 0.45 | 0.37 | 0.07 | 0.30 | 0.25 | 0.27 | 0.22 | 0.06 | 0.16 | 0.30 |
| 50151 | 1 cup | Bean w/Bacon, prep f/dry mix, avg | 265 | 0.27 | 0.29 | 0.61 | 0.06 | 1.01 | 0.27 | 0.14 | 0.27 | 0.45 | 0.37 | 0.07 | 0.31 | 0.25 | 0.27 | 0.23 | 0.06 | 0.16 | 0.30 |
| | | Beef Soup | | | | | | | | | | | | | | | | | | | |
| 50152 | 1 ea | Noodle, dry mix, svg, avg | 9 | 0.07 | 0.07 | 0.12 | 0.02 | 0.45 | 0.08 | 0.04 | 0.06 | 0.11 | 0.09 | 0.03 | 0.07 | 0.10 | 0.06 | 0.05 | 0.02 | 0.04 | 0.07 |
| 50153 | 1 cup | Noodle, prep f/mix, avg | 251 | 0.10 | 0.09 | 0.16 | 0.03 | 0.61 | 0.10 | 0.05 | 0.09 | 0.14 | 0.12 | 0.04 | 0.09 | 0.14 | 0.08 | 0.07 | 0.02 | 0.06 | 0.10 |
| 50178 | 1 ea | Vegetable, dry, svg, avg | 16 | 0.17 | 0.14 | 0.25 | 0.02 | 0.76 | 0.19 | 0.07 | 0.11 | 0.19 | 0.19 | 0.05 | 0.11 | 0.17 | 0.10 | 0.09 | 0.03 | 0.08 | 0.13 |
| 50044 | 1 cup | Vegetable, prep f/dry mix, avg | 253 | 0.17 | 0.14 | 0.25 | 0.02 | 0.74 | 0.18 | 0.06 | 0.11 | 0.19 | 0.18 | 0.05 | 0.11 | 0.17 | 0.10 | 0.09 | 0.03 | 0.08 | 0.13 |
| 50156 | 1 ea | Celery Cream Soup, dry, svg, avg | 17 | 0.09 | 0.09 | 0.18 | 0.03 | 0.59 | 0.08 | 0.06 | 0.12 | 0.19 | 0.11 | 0.05 | 0.13 | 0.21 | 0.12 | 0.09 | 0.03 | 0.08 | 0.14 |
| 50157 | 1 cup | Celery Cream Soup, prep f/dry, avg | 254 | 0.07 | 0.07 | 0.13 | 0.02 | 0.45 | 0.06 | 0.04 | 0.91 | 0.14 | 0.09 | 0.04 | 0.09 | 0.16 | 0.09 | 0.07 | 0.02 | 0.06 | 0.10 |
| | | Chicken Soup | | | | | | | | | | | | | | | | | | | |
| 50159 | 1 ea | Noodle, dry mix, svg, avg | 11 | 0.10 | 0.09 | 0.15 | 0.02 | 0.58 | 0.10 | 0.05 | 0.08 | 0.14 | 0.11 | 0.04 | 0.09 | 0.14 | 0.08 | 0.07 | 0.02 | 0.05 | 0.09 |
| 50037 | 1 cup | Noodle, prep f/dry mix, avg | 252 | 0.14 | 0.12 | 0.21 | 0.04 | 0.81 | 0.14 | 0.07 | 0.11 | 0.19 | 0.16 | 0.06 | 0.12 | 0.19 | 0.11 | 0.09 | 0.03 | 0.08 | 0.13 |
| 50160 | 1 ea | Rice, dry mix, svg, avg | 16 | 0.13 | 0.16 | 0.22 | 0.03 | 0.38 | 0.12 | 0.07 | 0.12 | 0.19 | 0.17 | 0.06 | 0.10 | 0.10 | 0.09 | 0.10 | 0.03 | 0.08 | 0.13 |
| 50161 | 1 cup | Rice, prep f/dry mix, avg | 253 | 0.10 | 0.12 | 0.17 | 0.03 | 0.29 | 0.09 | 0.05 | 0.09 | 0.14 | 0.13 | 0.05 | 0.08 | 0.78 | 0.07 | 0.07 | 0.02 | 0.07 | 0.10 |
| 50038 | 1 cup | Vegetable, prep f/dry mix, avg | 251 | 0.15 | 0.13 | 0.23 | 0.02 | 0.68 | 0.17 | 0.06 | 0.10 | 0.17 | 0.17 | 0.05 | 0.10 | 0.16 | 0.09 | 0.08 | 0.02 | 0.07 | 0.12 |
| 50158 | 1 ea | Cream of Chicken, dry pkt, avg | 18 | 0.05 | 0.05 | 0.09 | 0.01 | 0.28 | 0.04 | 0.03 | 0.07 | 0.11 | 0.09 | 0.03 | 0.06 | 0.11 | 0.06 | 0.05 | 0.02 | 0.05 | 0.08 |
| 50036 | 1 cup | Cream of Chicken, prep f/dry pkt, avg | 261 | 0.07 | 0.07 | 0.13 | 0.02 | 0.04 | 0.05 | 0.05 | 0.10 | 0.16 | 0.13 | 0.04 | 0.08 | 0.15 | 0.09 | 0.07 | 0.02 | 0.07 | 0.10 |
| 50164 | 1 ea | Clam Chowder, new england, dry mix, svg, avg | 13 | 0.08 | 0.08 | 0.15 | 0.02 | 0.46 | 0.08 | 0.05 | 0.06 | 0.10 | 0.08 | 0.03 | 0.05 | 0.06 | 0.05 | 0.05 | 0.02 | 0.04 | 0.06 |
| 50169 | 1 ea | Minestrone Soup, dry, svg, avg | 17 | 0.17 | 0.14 | 0.25 | 0.02 | 0.84 | 0.27 | 0.05 | 0.09 | 0.16 | 0.13 | 0.03 | 0.11 | 0.22 | 0.10 | 0.07 | 0.02 | 0.59 | 0.12 |
| 50170 | 1 cup | Minestrone Soup, prep f/dry mix, avg | 254 | 0.20 | 0.16 | 0.30 | 0.03 | 0.99 | 0.32 | 0.06 | 0.11 | 0.19 | 0.15 | 0.04 | 0.12 | 0.26 | 1.19 | 0.09 | 0.03 | 0.07 | 0.15 |
| 50171 | 1 ea | Mushroom Soup, dry mix, svg, avg | 17 | 0.10 | 0.08 | 0.15 | 0.01 | 0.05 | 0.16 | 0.03 | 0.05 | 0.10 | 0.07 | 0.02 | 0.06 | 0.13 | 0.06 | 0.04 | 0.01 | 0.03 | 0.07 |
| 50039 | 1 cup | Mushroom Soup, prep f/dry mix, avg | 253 | 0.13 | 0.10 | 0.19 | 0.02 | 0.64 | 0.20 | 0.04 | 0.07 | 0.12 | 0.10 | 0.02 | 0.08 | 0.17 | 0.08 | 0.05 | 0.02 | 0.04 | 0.09 |
| 50174 | 1 ea | Pea Soup, split, dry mix, svg, avg | 28 | 0.25 | 0.47 | 0.59 | 0.05 | 0.11 | 0.23 | 0.11 | 0.20 | 0.41 | 0.34 | 0.07 | 0.25 | 0.30 | 0.23 | 0.20 | 0.05 | 0.17 | 0.29 |
| 50041 | 1 cup | Pea Soup, split, prep f/dry, avg | 255 | 0.31 | 0.59 | 0.74 | 0.07 | 1.36 | 0.29 | 0.14 | 0.25 | 0.52 | 0.43 | 0.09 | 0.32 | 0.37 | 0.29 | 0.25 | 0.06 | 0.21 | 0.37 |
| 50175 | 1 ea | Tomato Soup, dry, svg, avg | 21 | 0.05 | 0.05 | 0.14 | 0.02 | 0.68 | 0.05 | 0.03 | 0.05 | 0.09 | 0.04 | 0.02 | 0.06 | 0.12 | 0.07 | 0.05 | 0.02 | 0.04 | 0.06 |
| 50042 | 1 cup | Tomato Soup, prep f/dry mix, avg | 265 | 0.07 | 0.07 | 0.19 | 0.03 | 0.92 | 0.06 | 0.04 | 0.07 | 0.12 | 0.06 | 0.03 | 0.08 | 0.16 | 0.10 | 0.06 | 0.02 | 0.05 | 0.08 |
| 50187 | 1 cup | Vegetable Soup, low sodium, prep f/dry mix, avg | 253 | 0.10 | 0.10 | 0.21 | 0.03 | 0.47 | 0.08 | 0.05 | 0.10 | 0.15 | 0.10 | 0.03 | 0.10 | 0.15 | 0.08 | 0.08 | 0.02 | 0.05 | 0.10 |
| | | **SPICES, FLAVORS AND SEASONINGS** | | | | | | | | | | | | | | | | | | | |
| 26001 | 1 tsp | Basil, ground, avg | 2 | 0.01 | 0.01 | 0.03 | 0.00 | 0.03 | 0.01 | 0.01 | 0.01 | 0.02 | 0.01 | 0.00 | 0.01 | 0.01 | 0.01 | 0.01 | 0.00 | 0.01 | 0.01 |
| 26045 | 1 Tbs | Basil, leaves, fresh, chpd, avg | 3 | 0.00 | 0.00 | 0.01 | 0.00 | 0.01 | 0.00 | 0.00 | 0.00 | 0.01 | 0.00 | 0.00 | 0.00 | 0.00 | 0.00 | 0.00 | 0.00 | 0.00 | 0.00 |

TABLE A **Amino Acid Content for Selected Foods *(continued)***

| Code | Amount | Description | Weight (g) | Alanine (g) | Arginine (g) | Aspartic acid (g) | Cystine (g) | Glutamic acid (g) | Glycine (g) | Histidine (g) | Isoleucine (g) | Leucine (g) | Lysine (g) | Methionine (g) | Phenylalanine (g) | Proline (g) | Serine (g) | Threonine (g) | Tryptophan (g) | Tyrosine (g) | Valine (g) |
|---|---|---|---|---|---|---|---|---|---|---|---|---|---|---|---|---|---|---|---|---|---|
| 26018 | 1 tsp | Caraway Seed, avg | 2 | 0.02 | 0.02 | 0.04 | 0.01 | 0.06 | 0.03 | 0.01 | 0.02 | 0.02 | 0.02 | 0.01 | 0.02 | 0.02 | 0.02 | 0.02 | 0.00 | 0.01 | 0.02 |
| 26021 | 1 tsp | Dill Weed, dried, avg | 1 | 0.01 | 0.07 | 0.02 | 0.00 | 0.01 | 0.01 | 0.00 | 0.01 | 0.01 | 0.01 | 0.00 | 0.00 | 0.01 | 0.01 | 0.00 | 0.00 | 0.00 | 0.01 |
| 26047 | 1 Tbs | Dill Weed, fresh, avg | 1 | 0.00 | 0.00 | 0.00 | 0.00 | 0.00 | 0.00 | 0.00 | 0.00 | 0.00 | 0.00 | 0.00 | 0.00 | 0.00 | 0.00 | 0.00 | 0.00 | 0.00 | 0.00 |
| 26105 | 1 tsp | Fennel Seed, avg | 2 | 0.02 | 0.01 | 0.04 | 0.00 | 0.06 | 0.02 | 0.01 | 0.01 | 0.02 | 0.02 | 0.01 | 0.01 | 0.02 | 0.02 | 0.01 | 0.01 | 0.01 | 0.02 |
| 26022 | 1 tsp | Fenugreek Seed, avg | 4 | 0.04 | 0.09 | 0.10 | 0.01 | 0.15 | 0.05 | 0.03 | 0.05 | 0.07 | 0.06 | 0.01 | 0.04 | 0.05 | 0.05 | 0.03 | 0.01 | 0.03 | 0.04 |
| 26023 | 1 tsp | Ginger, ground, avg | 2 | 0.00 | 0.00 | 0.02 | 0.00 | 0.02 | 0.00 | 0.00 | 0.01 | 0.01 | 0.01 | 0.00 | 0.00 | 0.00 | 0.00 | 0.00 | 0.00 | 0.00 | 0.01 |
| 26044 | 1 Tbs | Ginger Root, fresh, avg | 6 | 0.00 | 0.00 | 0.01 | 0.00 | 0.01 | 0.00 | 0.00 | 0.00 | 0.00 | 0.00 | 0.00 | 0.00 | 0.00 | 0.00 | 0.00 | 0.00 | 0.00 | 0.00 |
| 26110 | 1 tsp | Mustard Seed, yellow, avg | 4 | 0.05 | 0.07 | 0.08 | 0.02 | 0.20 | 0.05 | 0.03 | 0.04 | 0.07 | 0.06 | 0.02 | 0.04 | 0.08 | 0.04 | 0.04 | 0.02 | 0.03 | 0.05 |
| 26008 | 1 tsp | Onion Powder, avg | 2 | 0.00 | 0.03 | 0.01 | 0.00 | 0.04 | 0.01 | 0.00 | 0.01 | 0.01 | 0.01 | 0.00 | 0.00 | 0.01 | 0.00 | 0.00 | 0.00 | 0.00 | 0.00 |
| 26628 | 1 Tbs | Peppermint, fresh, avg | 16 | 0.03 | 0.03 | 0.07 | 0.01 | 0.07 | 0.03 | 0.01 | 0.02 | 0.04 | 0.03 | 0.01 | 0.03 | 0.02 | 0.02 | 0.02 | 0.01 | 0.02 | 0.03 |
| 26015 | 1 tsp | Poppyseed, avg | 3 | 0.03 | 0.05 | 0.05 | 0.01 | 0.11 | 0.03 | 0.01 | 0.02 | 0.04 | 0.03 | 0.01 | 0.02 | 0.03 | 0.02 | 0.02 | 0.01 | 0.02 | 0.03 |
| 26631 | 1 tsp | Spearmint, dried, avg | 0 | 0.00 | 0.00 | 0.00 | 0.00 | 0.00 | 0.00 | 0.00 | 0.00 | 0.00 | 0.00 | 0.00 | 0.00 | 0.00 | 0.00 | 0.00 | 0.00 | 0.00 | 0.00 |
| 26630 | 1 Tbs | Spearmint, fresh, avg | 6 | 0.01 | 0.01 | 0.02 | 0.00 | 0.02 | 0.01 | 0.00 | 0.01 | 0.01 | 0.01 | 0.00 | 0.01 | 0.01 | 0.01 | 0.01 | 0.00 | 0.01 | 0.01 |
| 26033 | 1 tsp | Thyme, ground, avg | 1 | 0.00 | 0.00 | 0.00 | 0.00 | 0.00 | 0.00 | 0.00 | 0.00 | 0.00 | 0.00 | 0.00 | 0.00 | 0.00 | 0.00 | 0.00 | 0.00 | 0.00 | 0.01 |
| | | **SWEETS AND SUGARS** | | | | | | | | | | | | | | | | | | | |
| 23054 | 1 Tbs | Jam, avg | 20 | 0.01 | 0.01 | 0.03 | 0.00 | 0.02 | 0.01 | 0.00 | 0.00 | 0.01 | 0.01 | 0.00 | 0.00 | 0.00 | 0.01 | 0.00 | 0.00 | 0.01 | 0.00 |
| 25001 | 1 Tbs | Honey, avg | 21 | 0.00 | 0.00 | 0.01 | 0.00 | 0.00 | 0.00 | 0.00 | 0.00 | 0.00 | 0.00 | 0.00 | 0.00 | 0.02 | 0.00 | 0.00 | 0.00 | 0.00 | 0.00 |
| 25204 | 1 Tbs | Malt Syrup, avg | 24 | 0.07 | 0.07 | 0.13 | 0.02 | 0.24 | 0.06 | 0.03 | 0.05 | 0.09 | 0.06 | 0.03 | 0.06 | 0.11 | 0.06 | 0.05 | 0.02 | 0.04 | 0.07 |
| | | **VEGETABLES AND LEGUMES** | | | | | | | | | | | | | | | | | | | |
| | | Amaranth | | | | | | | | | | | | | | | | | | | |
| 5837 | 1/2 cup | Boiled, salted, avg | 66 | 0.08 | 0.07 | 0.13 | 0.02 | 0.17 | 0.07 | 0.03 | 0.07 | 0.11 | 0.07 | 0.02 | 0.08 | 0.07 | 0.06 | 0.06 | 0.02 | 0.04 | 0.08 |
| 5377 | 1/2 cup | Leaf, boiled, drained, avg | 66 | 0.08 | 0.07 | 0.13 | 0.02 | 0.17 | 0.07 | 0.03 | 0.07 | 0.11 | 0.07 | 0.02 | 0.08 | 0.07 | 0.06 | 0.06 | 0.02 | 0.04 | 0.08 |
| 5375 | 1/2 cup | Raw, chpd, avg | 14 | 0.02 | 0.02 | 0.03 | 0.03 | 0.04 | 0.02 | 0.01 | 0.02 | 0.03 | 0.02 | 0.01 | 0.02 | 0.02 | 0.02 | 0.01 | 0.00 | 0.01 | 0.02 |
| | | Asparagus | | | | | | | | | | | | | | | | | | | |
| 5003 | 1/2 cup | Boiled, avg | 90 | 0.11 | 0.11 | 0.27 | 0.03 | 0.38 | 0.08 | 0.04 | 0.09 | 0.10 | 0.11 | 0.02 | 0.05 | 0.12 | 0.09 | 0.06 | 0.02 | 0.04 | 0.09 |
| 5842 | 1/2 cup | Canned, unsalted, avg | 122 | 0.10 | 0.10 | 0.25 | 0.03 | 0.36 | 0.07 | 0.03 | 0.08 | 0.10 | 0.10 | 0.02 | 0.05 | 0.12 | 0.08 | 0.06 | 0.02 | 0.04 | 0.08 |
| 5245 | 1/2 cup | Canned, w/liquid, avg | 122 | 0.10 | 0.10 | 0.25 | 0.03 | 0.36 | 0.07 | 0.03 | 0.08 | 0.10 | 0.10 | 0.02 | 0.05 | 0.12 | 0.08 | 0.06 | 0.02 | 0.04 | 0.08 |
| 5005 | 1/2 cup | Frozen, boiled, avg | 90 | 0.13 | 0.12 | 0.31 | 0.03 | 0.43 | 0.09 | 0.04 | 0.10 | 0.12 | 0.13 | 0.03 | 0.06 | 0.14 | 0.10 | 0.07 | 0.03 | 0.04 | 0.10 |
| 5001 | 1/2 cup | Raw, avg | 67 | 0.07 | 0.07 | 0.18 | 0.02 | 0.25 | 0.05 | 0.02 | 0.06 | 0.07 | 0.07 | 0.01 | 0.04 | 0.08 | 0.06 | 0.04 | 0.01 | 0.02 | 0.06 |
| | | Bamboo Shoots | | | | | | | | | | | | | | | | | | | |
| 5249 | 1/2 cup | Boiled, avg | 60 | 0.04 | 0.03 | 0.15 | 0.01 | 0.09 | 0.03 | 0.02 | 0.03 | 0.05 | 0.05 | 0.01 | 0.03 | 0.08 | 0.05 | 0.03 | 0.01 | 0.00 | 0.04 |
| 5401 | 1/2 cup | Canned, sliced, avg | 66 | 0.05 | 0.04 | 0.19 | 0.01 | 0.11 | 0.04 | 0.02 | 0.04 | 0.06 | 0.06 | 0.01 | 0.04 | 0.10 | 0.06 | 0.04 | 0.01 | 0.00 | 0.05 |
| 5230 | 1/2 cup | Sliced, raw, avg | 76 | 0.09 | 0.07 | 0.32 | 0.02 | 0.19 | 0.07 | 0.03 | 0.07 | 0.11 | 0.10 | 0.02 | 0.07 | 0.17 | 0.10 | 0.07 | 0.02 | 0.00 | 0.08 |
| | | Beans | | | | | | | | | | | | | | | | | | | |
| 6089 | 1/2 cup | Broadbeans/Fava, boiled, avg | 100 | 0.19 | 0.40 | 0.54 | 0.07 | 0.73 | 0.20 | 0.12 | 0.22 | 0.37 | 0.31 | 0.04 | 0.19 | 0.22 | 0.21 | 0.18 | 0.05 | 0.17 | 0.23 |
| 7026 | 1/2 cup | Broadbeans/Fava, raw, avg | 75 | 0.80 | 1.81 | 2.19 | 0.23 | 3.33 | 0.83 | 0.50 | 0.79 | 1.47 | 1.25 | 0.16 | 0.83 | 0.83 | 0.90 | 0.70 | 0.19 | 0.62 | 0.87 |
| 7001 | 1/2 cup | Garbanzo/Chickpeas, boiled, avg | 82 | 0.31 | 0.68 | 0.85 | 0.10 | 1.27 | 0.30 | 0.20 | 0.31 | 0.52 | 0.49 | 0.10 | 0.39 | 0.30 | 0.37 | 0.27 | 0.07 | 0.18 | 0.31 |
| 7000 | 1/2 cup | Garbanzo/Chickpeas, raw, avg | 100 | 0.83 | 1.82 | 2.27 | 0.26 | 3.38 | 0.80 | 0.53 | 0.83 | 1.37 | 1.29 | 0.25 | 1.03 | 0.80 | 0.97 | 0.72 | 0.19 | 0.48 | 0.81 |
| 7021 | 1/2 cup | Great Northern, boiled, avg | 88 | 0.31 | 0.45 | 0.89 | 0.08 | 1.12 | 0.29 | 0.20 | 0.32 | 0.59 | 0.50 | 0.11 | 0.40 | 0.31 | 0.40 | 0.31 | 0.09 | 0.21 | 0.38 |
| 7008 | 1/2 cup | Kidney, all types, boiled, avg | 88 | 0.32 | 0.47 | 0.92 | 0.08 | 1.16 | 0.30 | 0.21 | 0.34 | 0.61 | 0.52 | 0.11 | 0.41 | 0.32 | 0.42 | 0.32 | 0.09 | 0.21 | 0.40 |
| 5319 | 1/2 cup | Lima, baby, boiled, avg | 85 | 0.22 | 0.39 | 0.62 | 0.07 | 0.75 | 0.23 | 0.20 | 0.37 | 0.45 | 0.38 | 0.06 | 0.29 | 0.09 | 0.36 | 0.25 | 0.08 | 0.19 | 0.36 |
| 5527 | 1/2 cup | Lima, baby, cnd, low sod, avg | 87 | 0.13 | 0.24 | 0.38 | 0.04 | 0.46 | 0.14 | 0.12 | 0.23 | 0.28 | 0.23 | 0.03 | 0.17 | 0.06 | 0.22 | 0.15 | 0.05 | 0.11 | 0.22 |
| 7009 | 1/2 cup | Lima, baby, dry, avg | 101 | 1.05 | 1.26 | 2.67 | 0.23 | 2.93 | 0.87 | 0.63 | 1.09 | 1.79 | 1.38 | 0.26 | 1.19 | 0.94 | 1.37 | 0.89 | 0.24 | 0.73 | 1.24 |
| 5019 | 1/2 cup | Lima, baby, fzn, ckd | 90 | 0.23 | 0.40 | 0.64 | 0.07 | 0.77 | 0.24 | 0.20 | 0.39 | 0.47 | 0.40 | 0.06 | 0.30 | 0.09 | 0.37 | 0.25 | 0.08 | 0.19 | 0.37 |
| 7010 | 1/2 cup | Lima, large, boiled, avg | 94 | 0.37 | 0.45 | 0.94 | 0.08 | 1.03 | 0.31 | 0.22 | 0.38 | 0.63 | 0.49 | 0.09 | 0.42 | 0.33 | 0.49 | 0.32 | 0.09 | 0.26 | 0.44 |
| 7011 | 1/2 cup | Lima, large, cnd, avg | 120 | 0.30 | 0.36 | 0.76 | 0.06 | 0.33 | 0.25 | 0.18 | 0.31 | 0.51 | 0.39 | 0.07 | 0.34 | 0.27 | 0.39 | 0.25 | 0.07 | 0.21 | 0.35 |
| 5247 | 1/2 cup | Lima, large, fzn, ckd, avg | 85 | 0.20 | 0.35 | 0.55 | 0.06 | 0.56 | 0.21 | 0.18 | 0.33 | 0.41 | 0.34 | 0.05 | 0.25 | 0.08 | 0.32 | 0.22 | 0.07 | 0.17 | 0.32 |
| 5680 | 1/2 cup | Lima, large, raw, avg | 78 | 0.20 | 0.36 | 0.57 | 0.06 | 0.59 | 0.21 | 0.18 | 0.34 | 0.42 | 0.35 | 0.05 | 0.26 | 0.08 | 0.33 | 0.23 | 0.07 | 0.17 | 0.33 |
| 7022 | 1/2 cup | Navy, ckd, avg | 91 | 0.33 | 0.49 | 0.96 | 0.09 | 1.21 | 0.31 | 0.22 | 0.35 | 0.63 | 0.54 | 0.12 | 0.43 | 0.34 | 0.43 | 0.33 | 0.09 | 0.22 | 0.41 |
| 7013 | 1/2 cup | Pinto, boiled, avg | 86 | 0.30 | 0.44 | 0.85 | 0.08 | 1.08 | 0.28 | 0.20 | 0.31 | 0.56 | 0.49 | 0.11 | 0.38 | 0.30 | 0.38 | 0.30 | 0.08 | 0.20 | 0.37 |

# TABLE A Amino Acid Content for Selected Foods *(continued)*

| Code | Amount | Description | Weight (g) | Alanine (g) | Arginine (g) | Aspartic acid (g) | Cystine (g) | Glutamic acid (g) | Glycine (g) | Histidine (g) | Isoleucine (g) | Leucine (g) | Lysine (g) | Methionine (g) | Phenylalanine (g) | Proline (g) | Serine (g) | Threonine (g) | Tryptophan (g) | Tyrosine (g) | Valine (g) |
|---|---|---|---|---|---|---|---|---|---|---|---|---|---|---|---|---|---|---|---|---|---|
| 5731 | 3 oz | Pinto, fzn, ckd | 85 | 0.02 | 0.03 | 0.05 | 0.00 | 0.06 | 0.02 | 0.01 | 0.02 | 0.03 | 0.03 | 0.01 | 0.02 | 0.02 | 0.02 | 0.02 | 0.00 | 0.01 | 0.02 |
| 7023 | 1/2 cup | Pork & Beans, w/sweet sauce, cnd, avg | 126 | 0.28 | 0.41 | 0.81 | 0.07 | 1.02 | 0.26 | 0.19 | 0.29 | 0.53 | 0.46 | 0.10 | 0.36 | 0.28 | 0.36 | 0.28 | 0.08 | 0.19 | 0.35 |
| 7004 | 1/2 cup | Pork & Beans, w/tomato sauce, cnd, avg | 126 | 0.27 | 0.40 | 0.79 | 0.07 | 0.99 | 0.25 | 0.18 | 0.29 | 0.52 | 0.45 | 0.10 | 0.35 | 0.28 | 0.35 | 0.27 | 0.08 | 0.18 | 0.34 |
| 7024 | 1/2 cup | Refried, cnd, avg | 126 | 0.29 | 0.43 | 0.84 | 0.08 | 1.05 | 0.27 | 0.19 | 0.30 | 0.55 | 0.48 | 0.10 | 0.37 | 0.29 | 0.38 | 0.29 | 0.08 | 0.20 | 0.36 |
| 7063 | 1/2 cup | Soybeans, dry roasted, avg | 86 | 1.52 | 2.50 | 4.05 | 0.52 | 6.24 | 1.49 | 0.87 | 1.56 | 2.62 | 2.14 | 0.43 | 1.68 | 1.89 | 1.86 | 1.40 | 0.47 | 1.22 | 1.61 |
| 7003 | 1/2 cup | White, boiled, avg | 90 | 0.34 | 0.50 | 0.98 | 0.09 | 1.23 | 0.31 | 0.22 | 0.36 | 0.64 | 0.55 | 0.12 | 0.44 | 0.34 | 0.44 | 0.34 | 0.10 | 0.23 | 0.42 |
| 7002 | 1/2 cup | White, raw, avg | 108 | 0.96 | 1.41 | 2.75 | 0.25 | 3.48 | 0.89 | 0.64 | 1.01 | 1.83 | 1.57 | 0.34 | 1.23 | 0.97 | 1.24 | 0.96 | 0.27 | 0.64 | 1.19 |
| 7031 | 1/2 cup | Winged/Goabean, dry, boiled, avg | 86 | 0.27 | 0.50 | 0.84 | 0.14 | 1.05 | 0.30 | 0.21 | 0.39 | 0.66 | 0.56 | 0.09 | 0.37 | 0.51 | 0.32 | 0.31 | 0.20 | 0.38 | 0.40 |
| 7030 | 1/2 cup | Winged/Goabean, mature, dry, avg | 91 | 0.95 | 1.72 | 2.90 | 0.50 | 3.65 | 1.04 | 0.72 | 1.34 | 2.28 | 1.95 | 0.32 | 1.30 | 1.75 | 1.13 | 1.07 | 0.69 | 1.33 | 1.39 |
| 7033 | 1/2 cup | Yard Long, boiled, avg | 86 | 0.33 | 0.49 | 0.86 | 0.08 | 1.35 | 0.00 | 0.22 | 0.29 | 0.55 | 0.48 | 0.10 | 0.42 | 0.32 | 0.36 | 0.27 | 0.09 | 0.23 | 0.34 |
| 7032 | 1/2 cup | Yard Long, mature, raw, avg | 84 | 0.93 | 1.42 | 2.47 | 0.23 | 3.87 | 0.84 | 0.63 | 0.83 | 1.56 | 1.39 | 0.29 | 1.19 | 0.92 | 1.02 | 0.78 | 0.25 | 0.66 | 0.97 |
| | | Beets | | | | | | | | | | | | | | | | | | | |
| 5022 | 1/2 cup | Boiled, diced, avg | 85 | 0.05 | 0.04 | 0.10 | 0.02 | 0.38 | 0.03 | 0.02 | 0.04 | 0.06 | 0.05 | 0.02 | 0.04 | 0.04 | 0.05 | 0.04 | 0.02 | 0.03 | 0.05 |
| 5309 | 1/2 cup | Canned, w/liquid, avg | 123 | 0.04 | 0.03 | 0.07 | 0.01 | 0.26 | 0.02 | 0.01 | 0.03 | 0.04 | 0.04 | 0.01 | 0.03 | 0.02 | 0.04 | 0.03 | 0.01 | 0.02 | 0.03 |
| 5357 | 1/2 cup | Canned, w/liquid, low sod, avg | 123 | 0.04 | 0.03 | 0.07 | 0.01 | 0.26 | 0.02 | 0.01 | 0.03 | 0.04 | 0.04 | 0.01 | 0.03 | 0.02 | 0.04 | 0.03 | 0.01 | 0.02 | 0.03 |
| 5025 | 1/2 cup | Greens, boiled, avg | 72 | 0.07 | 0.05 | 0.11 | 0.02 | 0.22 | 0.07 | 0.03 | 0.04 | 0.08 | 0.05 | 0.02 | 0.05 | 0.04 | 0.06 | 0.05 | 0.03 | 0.04 | 0.05 |
| 5312 | 1/2 cup | Greens, raw, avg | 38 | 0.03 | 0.02 | 0.04 | 0.01 | 0.08 | 0.03 | 0.01 | 0.01 | 0.03 | 0.02 | 0.01 | 0.02 | 0.02 | 0.02 | 0.02 | 0.01 | 0.02 | 0.02 |
| 5310 | 1/2 cup | Pickled, w/liquid, slices, avg | 114 | 0.03 | 0.02 | 0.06 | 0.01 | 0.24 | 0.02 | 0.01 | 0.03 | 0.04 | 0.03 | 0.01 | 0.03 | 0.02 | 0.03 | 0.03 | 0.01 | 0.02 | 0.03 |
| | | Broccoli | | | | | | | | | | | | | | | | | | | |
| 5030 | 1/2 cup | Frozen, boiled, avg | 92 | 0.12 | 0.15 | 0.22 | 0.02 | 0.38 | 0.10 | 0.05 | 0.11 | 0.13 | 0.14 | 0.03 | 0.09 | 0.12 | 0.10 | 0.09 | 0.03 | 0.06 | 0.13 |
| 5867 | 1/2 cup | Leaves, raw, avg | 44 | 0.05 | 0.06 | 0.09 | 0.01 | 0.16 | 0.04 | 0.02 | 0.05 | 0.06 | 0.06 | 0.01 | 0.04 | 0.05 | 0.04 | 0.04 | 0.01 | 0.03 | 0.06 |
| 5026 | 1/2 cup | Raw, chpd, avg | 44 | 0.05 | 0.06 | 0.09 | 0.01 | 0.16 | 0.04 | 0.02 | 0.05 | 0.06 | 0.06 | 0.01 | 0.04 | 0.05 | 0.04 | 0.04 | 0.01 | 0.03 | 0.06 |
| 5653 | 1/2 cup | Steamed, avg | 78 | 0.09 | 0.11 | 0.17 | 0.02 | 0.29 | 0.07 | 0.04 | 0.09 | 0.10 | 0.11 | 0.03 | 0.07 | 0.09 | 0.08 | 0.07 | 0.02 | 0.05 | 0.10 |
| | | Brussel Sprouts | | | | | | | | | | | | | | | | | | | |
| 5033 | 1/2 cup | Boiled, avg | 78 | 0.00 | 0.12 | 0.00 | 0.01 | 0.00 | 0.00 | 0.04 | 0.08 | 0.09 | 0.09 | 0.02 | 0.06 | 0.00 | 0.00 | 0.07 | 0.02 | 0.00 | 0.09 |
| 5035 | 1/2 cup | Frozen, boiled, avg | 78 | 0.00 | 0.17 | 0.00 | 0.02 | 0.00 | 0.00 | 0.06 | 0.11 | 0.13 | 0.13 | 0.03 | 0.08 | 0.00 | 0.00 | 0.10 | 0.03 | 0.00 | 0.13 |
| 5031 | 1/2 cup | Raw, avg | 44 | 0.00 | 0.09 | 0.00 | 0.01 | 0.00 | 0.00 | 0.03 | 0.06 | 0.07 | 0.07 | 0.01 | 0.04 | 0.00 | 0.00 | 0.05 | 0.02 | 0.00 | 0.07 |
| 6760 | 1/2 cup | Burdock Root, boiled, 1" pces, avg | 62 | 0.02 | 0.09 | 0.15 | 0.00 | 0.13 | 0.03 | 0.03 | 0.03 | 0.03 | 0.06 | 0.01 | 0.03 | 0.04 | 0.02 | 0.02 | 0.00 | 0.01 | 0.03 |
| 6759 | 1/2 cup | Burdock Root, raw, 1" pces, avg | 59 | 0.01 | 0.06 | 0.10 | 0.00 | 0.09 | 0.02 | 0.02 | 0.02 | 0.02 | 0.04 | 0.01 | 0.02 | 0.03 | 0.01 | 0.02 | 0.00 | 0.01 | 0.02 |
| | | Cabbage | | | | | | | | | | | | | | | | | | | |
| 5038 | 1/2 cup | Common, boiled, shred, avg | 75 | 0.03 | 0.04 | 0.07 | 0.01 | 0.17 | 0.02 | 0.01 | 0.04 | 0.04 | 0.04 | 0.01 | 0.02 | 0.15 | 0.04 | 0.03 | 0.01 | 0.01 | 0.03 |
| 5036 | 1 cup | Common, raw, shred, avg | 70 | 0.03 | 0.06 | 0.10 | 0.01 | 0.22 | 0.02 | 0.02 | 0.05 | 0.05 | 0.05 | 0.01 | 0.03 | 0.20 | 0.06 | 0.03 | 0.01 | 0.02 | 0.04 |
| 5041 | 1 cup | Pak Choi/Bok Choy, raw, shred, avg | 70 | 0.06 | 0.06 | 0.08 | 0.01 | 0.25 | 0.03 | 0.02 | 0.06 | 0.06 | 0.06 | 0.01 | 0.03 | 0.02 | 0.03 | 0.03 | 0.01 | 0.02 | 0.05 |
| 5671 | 1/2 cup | Pak Choi/Bok Choy, stmd, avg | 85 | 0.07 | 0.07 | 0.09 | 0.01 | 0.31 | 0.04 | 0.02 | 0.07 | 0.07 | 0.08 | 0.01 | 0.04 | 0.03 | 0.04 | 0.04 | 0.01 | 0.02 | 0.06 |
| 5235 | 1/2 cup | Pe Tsai, boiled, shred | 60 | 0.05 | 0.05 | 0.06 | 0.01 | 0.22 | 0.03 | 0.02 | 0.05 | 0.05 | 0.05 | 0.01 | 0.03 | 0.02 | 0.03 | 0.03 | 0.01 | 0.02 | 0.04 |
| 5040 | 1 cup | Pe Tsai, raw, avg | 76 | 0.05 | 0.05 | 0.07 | 0.01 | 0.22 | 0.03 | 0.02 | 0.05 | 0.05 | 0.05 | 0.01 | 0.03 | 0.02 | 0.03 | 0.03 | 0.01 | 0.02 | 0.04 |
| 5238 | 1/2 cup | Red, boiled, avg | 75 | 0.03 | 0.04 | 0.08 | 0.01 | 0.17 | 0.02 | 0.02 | 0.04 | 0.04 | 0.04 | 0.01 | 0.03 | 0.15 | 0.05 | 0.03 | 0.01 | 0.01 | 0.03 |
| 5533 | 1/2 cup | Red, pickled, avg | 75 | 0.01 | 0.02 | 0.04 | 0.00 | 0.09 | 0.01 | 0.01 | 0.02 | 0.02 | 0.02 | 0.00 | 0.01 | 0.08 | 0.02 | 0.01 | 0.00 | 0.01 | 0.02 |
| 5042 | 1 cup | Red, raw, shred | 70 | 0.03 | 0.05 | 0.09 | 0.01 | 0.21 | 0.02 | 0.02 | 0.05 | 0.05 | 0.04 | 0.01 | 0.03 | 0.19 | 0.06 | 0.03 | 0.01 | 0.02 | 0.04 |
| 5044 | 1/2 cup | Savoy, boiled, avg | 72 | 0.04 | 0.07 | 0.13 | 0.01 | 0.28 | 0.03 | 0.03 | 0.06 | 0.07 | 0.06 | 0.01 | 0.04 | 0.25 | 0.07 | 0.04 | 0.01 | 0.02 | 0.05 |
| 5043 | 1 cup | Savoy, raw, avg | 70 | 0.05 | 0.08 | 0.14 | 0.01 | 0.31 | 0.03 | 0.03 | 0.07 | 0.07 | 0.06 | 0.01 | 0.04 | 0.27 | 0.08 | 0.05 | 0.01 | 0.02 | 0.06 |
| 7263 | 1/2 cup | Cactus/Nopales, ckd, unsalted, avg | 74 | 0.04 | 0.04 | 0.07 | 0.01 | 0.11 | 0.04 | 0.02 | 0.04 | 0.06 | 0.05 | 0.01 | 0.04 | 0.03 | 0.03 | 0.03 | 0.01 | 0.02 | 0.05 |
| 7262 | 1/2 cup | Cactus/Nopales, raw, avg | 43 | 0.02 | 0.02 | 0.04 | 0.00 | 0.06 | 0.02 | 0.01 | 0.02 | 0.03 | 0.03 | 0.01 | 0.02 | 0.02 | 0.02 | 0.02 | 0.01 | 0.01 | 0.03 |
| | | Carrots | | | | | | | | | | | | | | | | | | | |
| 5439 | 1 ea | Baby, raw, avg | 10 | 0.00 | 0.00 | 0.01 | 0.00 | 0.02 | 0.00 | 0.00 | 0.00 | 0.00 | 0.00 | 0.00 | 0.00 | 0.00 | 0.00 | 0.00 | 0.00 | 0.00 | 0.00 |
| 5198 | 1/2 cup | Canned, w/liquid, avg | 123 | 0.04 | 0.03 | 0.09 | 0.01 | 0.14 | 0.02 | 0.01 | 0.03 | 0.03 | 0.03 | 0.00 | 0.02 | 0.02 | 0.02 | 0.03 | 0.01 | 0.01 | 0.03 |
| 5888 | 1/2 cup | Canned, w/liquid, unsalted, avg | 123 | 0.04 | 0.03 | 0.09 | 0.01 | 0.14 | 0.02 | 0.01 | 0.03 | 0.03 | 0.03 | 0.00 | 0.02 | 0.02 | 0.02 | 0.03 | 0.01 | 0.01 | 0.03 |
| 5517 | 1/4 cup | Chips, dried, avg | 18 | 0.09 | 0.07 | 0.21 | 0.01 | 0.31 | 0.05 | 0.02 | 0.06 | 0.07 | 0.06 | 0.01 | 0.05 | 0.05 | 0.05 | 0.06 | 0.02 | 0.03 | 0.07 |
| 5633 | 1/2 cup | Cooked, glzd, avg | 80 | 0.34 | 0.02 | 0.08 | 0.00 | 0.12 | 0.02 | 0.01 | 0.02 | 0.02 | 0.02 | 0.00 | 0.02 | 0.02 | 0.02 | 0.02 | 0.01 | 0.01 | 0.03 |
| 5358 | 1/2 cup | Frozen, boiled, drained, avg | 73 | 0.05 | 0.04 | 0.11 | 0.01 | 0.17 | 0.02 | 0.01 | 0.03 | 0.04 | 0.03 | 0.01 | 0.03 | 0.02 | 0.03 | 0.03 | 0.01 | 0.02 | 0.04 |

| Code | Amount | Description | Weight (g) | Alanine (g) | Arginine (g) | Aspartic acid (g) | Cystine (g) | Glutamic acid (g) | Glycine (g) | Histidine (g) | Isoleucine (g) | Leucine (g) | Lysine (g) | Methionine (g) | Phenylalanine (g) | Proline (g) | Serine (g) | Threonine (g) | Tryptophan (g) | Tyrosine (g) | Valine (g) |
|---|---|---|---|---|---|---|---|---|---|---|---|---|---|---|---|---|---|---|---|---|---|
| 5226 | 1/2 cup | Juice, cnd, avg | 118 | 0.06 | 0.05 | 0.15 | 0.01 | 0.22 | 0.03 | 0.02 | 0.04 | 0.05 | 0.04 | 0.01 | 0.03 | 0.03 | 0.04 | 0.04 | 0.01 | 0.02 | 0.05 |
| 5045 | 1 ea | Raw, 7 1/2", avg | 72 | 0.04 | 0.03 | 0.10 | 0.01 | 0.15 | 0.02 | 0.01 | 0.03 | 0.03 | 0.03 | 0.01 | 0.02 | 0.02 | 0.03 | 0.03 | 0.01 | 0.01 | 0.03 |
| 6772 | 1/2 cup | Raw, chpd, avg | 64 | 0.04 | 0.03 | 0.09 | 0.01 | 0.13 | 0.02 | 0.01 | 0.03 | 0.03 | 0.03 | 0.00 | 0.02 | 0.02 | 0.02 | 0.02 | 0.01 | 0.01 | 0.03 |
| 5655 | 1/2 cup | Steamed, avg | 78 | 0.05 | 0.03 | 0.11 | 0.01 | 0.16 | 0.02 | 0.01 | 0.03 | 0.03 | 0.03 | 0.01 | 0.02 | 0.02 | 0.03 | 0.03 | 0.01 | 0.02 | 0.03 |
| 5625 | 1/2 cup | Cassava, ckd, avg | 68 | 0.05 | 0.20 | 0.11 | 0.04 | 0.29 | 0.04 | 0.28 | 0.04 | 0.06 | 0.06 | 0.02 | 0.04 | 0.05 | 0.05 | 0.04 | 0.03 | 0.03 | 0.05 |
| 5356 | 1/2 cup | Cassava, raw, avg | 103 | 0.04 | 0.14 | 0.08 | 0.03 | 0.21 | 0.03 | 0.02 | 0.03 | 0.04 | 0.05 | 0.01 | 0.03 | 0.03 | 0.03 | 0.03 | 0.02 | 0.02 | 0.04 |
| | | Cauliflower | | | | | | | | | | | | | | | | | | | |
| 5051 | 1/2 cup | Boiled, avg | 62 | 0.06 | 0.06 | 0.13 | 0.01 | 0.15 | 0.04 | 0.02 | 0.04 | 0.07 | 0.06 | 0.02 | 0.04 | 0.05 | 0.06 | 0.04 | 0.01 | 0.02 | 0.06 |
| 5053 | 1/2 cup | Frozen, boiled, avg | 90 | 0.08 | 0.07 | 0.17 | 0.02 | 0.19 | 0.05 | 0.03 | 0.05 | 0.08 | 0.08 | 0.02 | 0.05 | 0.06 | 0.08 | 0.05 | 0.02 | 0.03 | 0.07 |
| 7266 | 1/2 cup | Green, ckd, unsalted, avg | 62 | 0.10 | 0.09 | 0.22 | 0.02 | 0.25 | 0.06 | 0.04 | 0.07 | 0.11 | 0.10 | 0.03 | 0.07 | 0.08 | 0.10 | 0.07 | 0.02 | 0.04 | 0.09 |
| 7265 | 1/2 cup | Green, raw, avg | 32 | 0.05 | 0.05 | 0.11 | 0.01 | 0.13 | 0.03 | 0.02 | 0.04 | 0.06 | 0.05 | 0.01 | 0.03 | 0.04 | 0.05 | 0.03 | 0.01 | 0.02 | 0.05 |
| 5607 | 1/2 ea | Pickled, avg | 14 | 0.01 | 0.01 | 0.03 | 0.00 | 0.03 | 0.01 | 0.00 | 0.01 | 0.01 | 0.01 | 0.00 | 0.01 | 0.01 | 0.01 | 0.01 | 0.00 | 0.00 | 0.01 |
| 5049 | 1/2 cup | Raw, avg | 50 | 0.05 | 0.05 | 0.12 | 0.01 | 0.13 | 0.03 | 0.02 | 0.04 | 0.06 | 0.05 | 0.01 | 0.04 | 0.04 | 0.05 | 0.04 | 0.01 | 0.02 | 0.05 |
| | | Celery | | | | | | | | | | | | | | | | | | | |
| 5606 | 1/2 cup | Pickled, avg | 75 | 0.01 | 0.01 | 0.07 | 0.00 | 0.05 | 0.01 | 0.00 | 0.01 | 0.02 | 0.02 | 0.00 | 0.01 | 0.01 | 0.01 | 0.01 | 0.01 | 0.01 | 0.02 |
| 5054 | 1/2 cup | Raw, avg | 60 | 0.02 | 0.01 | 0.08 | 0.00 | 0.06 | 0.01 | 0.01 | 0.01 | 0.02 | 0.02 | 0.00 | 0.01 | 0.01 | 0.01 | 0.01 | 0.01 | 0.01 | 0.02 |
| 5200 | 1/2 cup | Root/Celeriac, ckd, avg | 78 | 0.04 | 0.02 | 0.08 | 0.00 | 0.06 | 0.02 | 0.01 | 0.02 | 0.04 | 0.04 | 0.01 | 0.02 | 0.02 | 0.02 | 0.02 | 0.01 | 0.01 | 0.04 |
| 5742 | 1/2 cup | Root/Celeriac, raw, avg | 78 | 0.06 | 0.03 | 0.12 | 0.00 | 0.09 | 0.04 | 0.02 | 0.04 | 0.06 | 0.06 | 0.01 | 0.04 | 0.03 | 0.04 | 0.03 | 0.01 | 0.02 | 0.05 |
| 5659 | 1/2 cup | Steamed, avg | 75 | 0.02 | 0.02 | 0.10 | 0.00 | 0.07 | 0.02 | 0.01 | 0.02 | 0.03 | 0.02 | 0.00 | 0.02 | 0.01 | 0.02 | 0.02 | 0.01 | 0.01 | 0.02 |
| 5414 | 1/2 cup | Chayote, boiled, chpd, avg | 80 | 0.03 | 0.02 | 0.06 | 0.00 | 0.08 | 0.02 | 0.01 | 0.03 | 0.05 | 0.02 | 0.00 | 0.03 | 0.03 | 0.03 | 0.02 | 0.01 | 0.02 | 0.04 |
| 6781 | 1/2 cup | Chayote, raw, avg | 66 | 0.03 | 0.02 | 0.06 | 0.00 | 0.08 | 0.03 | 0.01 | 0.03 | 0.05 | 0.03 | 0.00 | 0.03 | 0.03 | 0.03 | 0.03 | 0.01 | 0.02 | 0.04 |
| | | Collards | | | | | | | | | | | | | | | | | | | |
| 5061 | 1/2 cup | Boiled, unsalted, avg | 95 | 0.09 | 0.10 | 0.15 | 0.02 | 0.17 | 0.08 | 0.04 | 0.08 | 0.12 | 0.10 | 0.03 | 0.07 | 0.09 | 0.06 | 0.07 | 0.03 | 0.05 | 0.10 |
| 5062 | 1/2 cup | Frozen, boiled, avg | 85 | 0.11 | 0.13 | 0.19 | 0.03 | 0.21 | 0.10 | 0.05 | 0.10 | 0.16 | 0.12 | 0.03 | 0.09 | 0.11 | 0.08 | 0.09 | 0.03 | 0.07 | 0.12 |
| 5898 | 1/2 cup | Frozen, boiled, salted, avg | 85 | 0.11 | 0.13 | 0.19 | 0.03 | 0.21 | 0.10 | 0.05 | 0.10 | 0.16 | 0.12 | 0.03 | 0.09 | 0.11 | 0.08 | 0.09 | 0.03 | 0.07 | 0.12 |
| 5060 | 1/2 cup | Raw, avg | 18 | 0.02 | 0.02 | 0.03 | 0.00 | 0.04 | 0.02 | 0.01 | 0.02 | 0.03 | 0.02 | 0.01 | 0.02 | 0.02 | 0.01 | 0.02 | 0.01 | 0.01 | 0.02 |
| | | Corn | | | | | | | | | | | | | | | | | | | |
| 5252 | 1/2 cup | White, cnd, avg | 105 | 0.23 | 0.10 | 0.19 | 0.02 | 0.49 | 0.10 | 0.07 | 0.10 | 0.27 | 0.11 | 0.05 | 0.12 | 0.22 | 0.12 | 0.10 | 0.02 | 0.09 | 0.14 |
| 5564 | 1/2 cup | White, cnd, creamed, avg | 128 | 0.20 | 0.09 | 0.17 | 0.02 | 0.43 | 0.09 | 0.06 | 0.09 | 0.24 | 0.09 | 0.05 | 0.10 | 0.20 | 0.10 | 0.09 | 0.02 | 0.08 | 0.13 |
| 7207 | 1/2 cup | White, cnd, creamed, low sod, avg | 128 | 0.20 | 0.09 | 0.17 | 0.02 | 0.43 | 0.09 | 0.06 | 0.09 | 0.24 | 0.09 | 0.05 | 0.10 | 0.20 | 0.10 | 0.09 | 0.02 | 0.08 | 0.13 |
| 6017 | 1/2 cup | White, cnd, unsalted, avg | 105 | 0.23 | 0.10 | 0.19 | 0.02 | 0.49 | 0.10 | 0.07 | 0.10 | 0.27 | 0.11 | 0.05 | 0.12 | 0.22 | 0.12 | 0.10 | 0.02 | 0.09 | 0.14 |
| 7203 | 1/2 cup | White, fresh, boiled, avg | 82 | 0.24 | 0.11 | 0.20 | 0.02 | 0.53 | 0.11 | 0.07 | 0.11 | 0.29 | 0.11 | 0.06 | 0.12 | 0.24 | 0.13 | 0.11 | 0.02 | 0.10 | 0.15 |
| 5393 | 1/2 cup | White, fzn, boiled, avg | 82 | 0.15 | 0.11 | 0.19 | 0.03 | 0.37 | 0.07 | 0.05 | 0.12 | 0.21 | 0.13 | 0.06 | 0.11 | 0.15 | 0.13 | 0.10 | 0.03 | 0.09 | 0.14 |
| 5567 | 1 ea | White, on the cob, fzn, boiled, unsalted, avg | 63 | 0.18 | 0.08 | 0.15 | 0.02 | 0.38 | 0.08 | 0.05 | 0.08 | 0.21 | 0.08 | 0.04 | 0.09 | 0.17 | 0.09 | 0.08 | 0.01 | 0.07 | 0.11 |
| 6015 | 1/2 cup | White, raw, avg | 77 | 0.22 | 0.10 | 0.18 | 0.02 | 0.48 | 0.10 | 0.07 | 0.10 | 0.26 | 0.10 | 0.05 | 0.11 | 0.22 | 0.12 | 0.10 | 0.02 | 0.09 | 0.14 |
| 5067 | 1/2 cup | Yellow, cnd, avg | 105 | 0.23 | 0.10 | 0.19 | 0.02 | 0.49 | 0.10 | 0.07 | 0.10 | 0.27 | 0.11 | 0.05 | 0.12 | 0.22 | 0.12 | 0.10 | 0.02 | 0.09 | 0.14 |
| 5068 | 1/2 cup | Yellow, cnd, creamed, avg | 128 | 0.20 | 0.09 | 0.17 | 0.02 | 0.43 | 0.09 | 0.06 | 0.09 | 0.24 | 0.09 | 0.05 | 0.10 | 0.20 | 0.10 | 0.09 | 0.02 | 0.08 | 0.13 |
| 5243 | 1/2 cup | Yellow, cnd, unsalted, avg | 105 | 0.23 | 0.10 | 0.19 | 0.02 | 0.49 | 0.10 | 0.07 | 0.10 | 0.27 | 0.11 | 0.05 | 0.12 | 0.22 | 0.12 | 0.10 | 0.02 | 0.09 | 0.14 |
| 5379 | 1/2 cup | Yellow, fresh, boiled, avg | 82 | 0.24 | 0.11 | 0.20 | 0.02 | 0.53 | 0.11 | 0.07 | 0.11 | 0.29 | 0.11 | 0.06 | 0.12 | 0.24 | 0.13 | 0.11 | 0.02 | 0.10 | 0.15 |
| 5378 | 1/2 cup | Yellow, fresh, raw, avg | 77 | 0.22 | 0.10 | 0.18 | 0.02 | 0.48 | 0.10 | 0.07 | 0.10 | 0.26 | 0.10 | 0.05 | 0.11 | 0.22 | 0.12 | 0.10 | 0.02 | 0.09 | 0.14 |
| 5065 | 1/2 cup | Yellow, fzn, boiled, avg | 82 | 0.15 | 0.11 | 0.19 | 0.03 | 0.37 | 0.07 | 0.05 | 0.12 | 0.21 | 0.13 | 0.06 | 0.11 | 0.15 | 0.13 | 0.10 | 0.03 | 0.09 | 0.14 |
| 5364 | 1 ea | Yellow, on the cob, fzn, boiled, avg | 63 | 0.18 | 0.08 | 0.15 | 0.02 | 0.38 | 0.08 | 0.05 | 0.08 | 0.21 | 0.08 | 0.04 | 0.09 | 0.17 | 0.09 | 0.08 | 0.01 | 0.07 | 0.11 |
| 5470 | 1/2 cup | Yellow Hominy, cnd, avg | 80 | 0.08 | 0.05 | 0.09 | 0.03 | 0.23 | 0.04 | 0.04 | 0.05 | 0.16 | 0.03 | 0.02 | 0.06 | 0.11 | 0.05 | 0.04 | 0.01 | 0.04 | 0.06 |
| | | Cowpeas/Blackeyed Peas | | | | | | | | | | | | | | | | | | | |
| 7018 | 1/2 cup | Boiled, avg | 86 | 0.30 | 0.46 | 0.80 | 0.07 | 1.26 | 0.27 | 0.21 | 0.27 | 0.51 | 0.45 | 0.09 | 0.39 | 0.30 | 0.33 | 0.25 | 0.08 | 0.22 | 0.32 |
| 7016 | 1/2 cup | Canned, avg | 120 | 0.26 | 0.39 | 0.69 | 0.06 | 1.08 | 0.24 | 0.18 | 0.23 | 0.44 | 0.39 | 0.08 | 0.33 | 0.26 | 0.28 | 0.22 | 0.07 | 0.18 | 0.27 |
| 7017 | 1/2 cup | Raw, avg | 84 | 0.90 | 1.37 | 2.39 | 0.22 | 3.74 | 0.82 | 0.61 | 0.80 | 1.51 | 1.34 | 0.28 | 1.15 | 0.89 | 0.99 | 0.75 | 0.24 | 0.64 | 0.94 |
| 5639 | 1/2 cup | Cucumber, ckd, avg | 90 | 0.02 | 0.04 | 0.04 | 0.00 | 0.17 | 0.02 | 0.01 | 0.02 | 0.03 | 0.03 | 0.01 | 0.02 | 0.01 | 0.02 | 0.02 | 0.00 | 0.01 | 0.02 |
| 5071 | 1/2 cup | Cucumber, w/peel, raw, avg | 52 | 0.01 | 0.02 | 0.02 | 0.00 | 0.10 | 0.01 | 0.01 | 0.01 | 0.02 | 0.02 | 0.00 | 0.01 | 0.01 | 0.01 | 0.01 | 0.00 | 0.01 | 0.01 |
| 6910 | 1/2 cup | Dock/Sorrel, geens, raw, avg | 66 | 0.09 | 0.07 | 0.12 | 0.00 | 0.14 | 0.08 | 0.04 | 0.07 | 0.11 | 0.08 | 0.02 | 0.08 | 0.08 | 0.05 | 0.06 | 0.00 | 0.05 | 0.09 |

## TABLE A Amino Acid Content for Selected Foods *(continued)*

| Code | Amount | Description | Weight (g) | Alanine (g) | Arginine (g) | Aspartic acid (g) | Cystine (g) | Glutamic acid (g) | Glycine (g) | Histidine (g) | Isoleucine (g) | Leucine (g) | Lysine (g) | Methionine (g) | Phenylalanine (g) | Proline (g) | Serine (g) | Threonine (g) | Tryptophan (g) | Tyrosine (g) | Valine (g) |
|---|---|---|---|---|---|---|---|---|---|---|---|---|---|---|---|---|---|---|---|---|---|
| 5418 | 1/2 cup | Dock/Sorrel, greens, ckd, avg | 50 | 0.06 | 0.05 | 0.08 | 0.00 | 0.10 | 0.05 | 0.02 | 0.05 | 0.08 | 0.05 | 0.02 | 0.05 | 0.05 | 0.04 | 0.04 | 0.00 | 0.04 | 0.06 |
| | | Eggplant | | | | | | | | | | | | | | | | | | | |
| 5072 | 1/2 cup | Boiled, avg | 50 | 0.02 | 0.02 | 0.07 | 0.00 | 0.08 | 0.02 | 0.01 | 0.02 | 0.03 | 0.02 | 0.00 | 0.02 | 0.02 | 0.02 | 0.01 | 0.00 | 0.01 | 0.02 |
| 5611 | 1/2 cup | Pickled, avg | 68 | 0.03 | 0.04 | 0.11 | 0.00 | 0.12 | 0.03 | 0.01 | 0.03 | 0.04 | 0.03 | 0.01 | 0.03 | 0.03 | 0.03 | 0.02 | 0.01 | 0.02 | 0.03 |
| 5371 | 1/2 cup | Raw, cubes, avg | 41 | 0.02 | 0.02 | 0.07 | 0.00 | 0.08 | 0.02 | 0.01 | 0.02 | 0.03 | 0.02 | 0.00 | 0.02 | 0.02 | 0.02 | 0.02 | 0.00 | 0.01 | 0.02 |
| | | Green Beans | | | | | | | | | | | | | | | | | | | |
| 5011 | 1/2 cup | Snap/String, boiled, avg | 62 | 0.05 | 0.05 | 0.16 | 0.01 | 0.12 | 0.04 | 0.02 | 0.04 | 0.07 | 0.06 | 0.01 | 0.04 | 0.04 | 0.06 | 0.05 | 0.01 | 0.03 | 0.06 |
| 5017 | 1/2 cup | Snap/String, cnd w/liquid, avg | 120 | 0.04 | 0.04 | 0.13 | 0.01 | 0.10 | 0.03 | 0.02 | 0.03 | 0.06 | 0.05 | 0.01 | 0.03 | 0.03 | 0.05 | 0.04 | 0.01 | 0.02 | 0.05 |
| 5013 | 1/2 cup | Snap/String, fzn, boiled, avg | 68 | 0.05 | 0.04 | 0.14 | 0.01 | 0.10 | 0.04 | 0.02 | 0.04 | 0.06 | 0.05 | 0.01 | 0.04 | 0.04 | 0.06 | 0.04 | 0.01 | 0.02 | 0.05 |
| 5009 | 1/2 cup | Snap/String, raw, avg | 55 | 0.05 | 0.04 | 0.14 | 0.01 | 0.10 | 0.04 | 0.02 | 0.04 | 0.06 | 0.05 | 0.01 | 0.04 | 0.04 | 0.05 | 0.04 | 0.01 | 0.02 | 0.05 |
| 5231 | 1/2 cup | String, cnd w/liquid, low sod, avg | 120 | 0.04 | 0.04 | 0.13 | 0.01 | 0.10 | 0.03 | 0.02 | 0.03 | 0.06 | 0.05 | 0.01 | 0.03 | 0.03 | 0.05 | 0.04 | 0.01 | 0.02 | 0.05 |
| 5420 | 1/2 cup | Jute/Potherb, boiled, avg | 44 | 0.09 | 0.09 | 0.20 | 0.01 | 0.17 | 0.07 | 0.04 | 0.08 | 0.13 | 0.08 | 0.02 | 0.07 | 0.09 | 0.06 | 0.06 | 0.01 | 0.05 | 0.09 |
| 5419 | 1/2 cup | Jute/Potherb, raw, avg | 14 | 0.04 | 0.03 | 0.08 | 0.01 | 0.07 | 0.03 | 0.02 | 0.03 | 0.05 | 0.03 | 0.01 | 0.03 | 0.03 | 0.03 | 0.02 | 0.00 | 0.02 | 0.03 |
| | | Kale | | | | | | | | | | | | | | | | | | | |
| 5075 | 1/2 cup | Boiled, drained, unsalted, avg | 65 | 0.06 | 0.07 | 0.11 | 0.02 | 0.14 | 0.06 | 0.03 | 0.07 | 0.09 | 0.07 | 0.01 | 0.06 | 0.07 | 0.05 | 0.06 | 0.01 | 0.04 | 0.07 |
| 5076 | 1/2 cup | Frozen, boiled, avg | 65 | 0.09 | 0.10 | 0.17 | 0.02 | 0.21 | 0.09 | 0.04 | 0.11 | 0.13 | 0.11 | 0.02 | 0.09 | 0.11 | 0.08 | 0.08 | 0.02 | 0.07 | 0.10 |
| 5208 | 1 cup | Raw, chpd, avg | 67 | 0.11 | 0.12 | 0.20 | 0.03 | 0.25 | 0.11 | 0.05 | 0.13 | 0.15 | 0.13 | 0.02 | 0.11 | 0.13 | 0.09 | 0.10 | 0.03 | 0.08 | 0.12 |
| 5079 | 1/2 cup | Kohlrabi, boiled, drained, unsalted, avg | 82 | 0.00 | 0.09 | 0.00 | 0.01 | 0.00 | 0.00 | 0.02 | 0.07 | 0.06 | 0.05 | 0.01 | 0.03 | 0.00 | 0.00 | 0.04 | 0.01 | 0.00 | 0.04 |
| 5078 | 1/2 cup | Kohlrabi, raw, avg | 68 | 0.00 | 0.07 | 0.00 | 0.00 | 0.00 | 0.00 | 0.01 | 0.05 | 0.05 | 0.04 | 0.01 | 0.03 | 0.00 | 0.00 | 0.03 | 0.01 | 0.00 | 0.03 |
| 5203 | 1/2 cup | Leeks, boiled, drained, unsalted, avg | 52 | 0.02 | 0.02 | 0.04 | 0.01 | 0.06 | 0.02 | 0.01 | 0.01 | 0.03 | 0.02 | 0.01 | 0.02 | 0.02 | 0.03 | 0.02 | 0.00 | 0.01 | 0.02 |
| 5205 | 1/2 cup | Leeks, raw, chpd, avg | 44 | 0.03 | 0.03 | 0.06 | 0.01 | 0.10 | 0.03 | 0.01 | 0.02 | 0.04 | 0.03 | 0.01 | 0.02 | 0.03 | 0.04 | 0.03 | 0.01 | 0.02 | 0.02 |
| 7006 | 1/2 cup | Lentils, boiled, avg | 99 | 0.37 | 0.69 | 0.99 | 0.12 | 1.39 | 0.36 | 0.25 | 0.39 | 0.65 | 0.62 | 0.08 | 0.44 | 0.37 | 0.41 | 0.32 | 0.08 | 0.24 | 0.44 |
| 7005 | 1/2 cup | Lentils, raw, avg | 96 | 1.12 | 2.08 | 2.98 | 0.35 | 4.18 | 1.09 | 0.76 | 1.16 | 1.95 | 1.88 | 0.23 | 1.32 | 1.12 | 1.24 | 0.97 | 0.24 | 0.72 | 1.33 |
| | | Lettuce | | | | | | | | | | | | | | | | | | | |
| 5080 | 1 cup | Butterhead, avg | 56 | 0.03 | 0.04 | 0.08 | 0.01 | 0.10 | 0.03 | 0.01 | 0.05 | 0.04 | 0.05 | 0.01 | 0.03 | 0.03 | 0.02 | 0.03 | 0.01 | 0.02 | 0.04 |
| 5083 | 1 cup | Iceberg, avg | 55 | 0.03 | 0.03 | 0.07 | 0.01 | 0.09 | 0.03 | 0.01 | 0.04 | 0.04 | 0.04 | 0.01 | 0.03 | 0.02 | 0.02 | 0.03 | 0.00 | 0.02 | 0.03 |
| 5086 | 1 cup | Looseleaf, avg | 56 | 0.03 | 0.04 | 0.08 | 0.01 | 0.10 | 0.03 | 0.01 | 0.05 | 0.04 | 0.05 | 0.01 | 0.03 | 0.03 | 0.02 | 0.03 | 0.01 | 0.02 | 0.04 |
| 5637 | 1 cup | Mixed Salad Greens, raw, avg | 55 | 0.04 | 0.05 | 0.10 | 0.01 | 0.13 | 0.04 | 0.02 | 0.06 | 0.06 | 0.06 | 0.01 | 0.04 | 0.03 | 0.03 | 0.04 | 0.01 | 0.02 | 0.05 |
| 5088 | 1 cup | Romaine, avg | 56 | 0.04 | 0.05 | 0.10 | 0.01 | 0.13 | 0.04 | 0.02 | 0.06 | 0.05 | 0.06 | 0.01 | 0.04 | 0.03 | 0.03 | 0.04 | 0.01 | 0.02 | 0.05 |
| 5392 | 1/2 cup | Lotus Root, boiled, drained, sliced, avg | 60 | 0.02 | 0.03 | 0.13 | 0.01 | 0.05 | 0.06 | 0.01 | 0.02 | 0.03 | 0.03 | 0.01 | 0.02 | 0.05 | 0.02 | 0.02 | 0.01 | 0.01 | 0.02 |
| 5391 | 10 ea | Lotus Root, raw, slices, avg | 81 | 0.04 | 0.07 | 0.30 | 0.02 | 0.11 | 0.13 | 0.03 | 0.04 | 0.06 | 0.08 | 0.02 | 0.04 | 0.11 | 0.05 | 0.04 | 0.02 | 0.02 | 0.04 |
| | | Mixed Vegetables | | | | | | | | | | | | | | | | | | | |
| 5548 | 1/2 cup | Canned, avg | 122 | 0.07 | 0.12 | 0.18 | 0.02 | 0.24 | 0.06 | 0.04 | 0.08 | 0.12 | 0.10 | 0.02 | 0.07 | 0.04 | 0.08 | 0.07 | 0.02 | 0.05 | 0.09 |
| 5516 | 1/2 cup | Canned, low sod, avg | 91 | 0.05 | 0.09 | 0.13 | 0.01 | 0.17 | 0.05 | 0.03 | 0.01 | 0.08 | 0.08 | 0.02 | 0.05 | 0.03 | 0.06 | 0.05 | 0.01 | 0.03 | 0.07 |
| 5515 | 1/2 cup | Corn w/Red & Green Peppers, cnd w/liquid, avg | 114 | 0.23 | 0.11 | 0.21 | 0.02 | 0.51 | 0.10 | 0.07 | 0.11 | 0.28 | 0.11 | 0.05 | 0.12 | 0.23 | 0.12 | 0.11 | 0.02 | 0.10 | 0.15 |
| 5549 | 3 oz | Frozen, avg | 85 | 0.12 | 0.19 | 0.30 | 0.03 | 0.39 | 0.10 | 0.07 | 0.14 | 0.19 | 0.17 | 0.03 | 0.12 | 0.07 | 0.13 | 0.11 | 0.03 | 0.07 | 0.15 |
| 5187 | 1/2 cup | Frozen, boiled, avg | 91 | 0.11 | 0.18 | 0.28 | 0.02 | 0.35 | 0.09 | 0.07 | 0.13 | 0.17 | 0.15 | 0.03 | 0.11 | 0.06 | 0.12 | 0.10 | 0.03 | 0.07 | 0.14 |
| 5281 | 1/2 cup | Peas & Carrots, cnd, avg | 128 | 0.13 | 0.21 | 0.26 | 0.02 | 0.39 | 0.09 | 0.05 | 0.10 | 0.16 | 0.16 | 0.04 | 0.10 | 0.09 | 0.09 | 0.10 | 0.02 | 0.06 | 0.12 |
| 5123 | 1/2 cup | Peas & Carrots, fzn, ckd, avg | 80 | 0.11 | 0.19 | 0.24 | 0.02 | 0.35 | 0.08 | 0.05 | 0.09 | 0.14 | 0.14 | 0.04 | 0.09 | 0.08 | 0.08 | 0.09 | 0.02 | 0.05 | 0.11 |
| 5577 | 1/2 cup | Peas & Onions, cnd, avg | 60 | 0.09 | 0.16 | 0.18 | 0.01 | 0.27 | 0.07 | 0.04 | 0.07 | 0.11 | 0.11 | 0.03 | 0.07 | 0.06 | 0.07 | 0.07 | 0.01 | 0.04 | 0.08 |
| 6090 | 1/2 cup | Peas & Onions, fzn, ckd, avg | 90 | 0.10 | 0.19 | 0.20 | 0.02 | 0.32 | 0.08 | 0.04 | 0.08 | 0.13 | 0.13 | 0.03 | 0.08 | 0.07 | 0.08 | 0.08 | 0.02 | 0.05 | 0.10 |
| 5251 | 1/2 cup | Succotash, boiled, avg | 96 | 0.27 | 0.28 | 0.47 | 0.05 | 0.73 | 0.19 | 0.15 | 0.27 | 0.43 | 0.29 | 0.07 | 0.24 | 0.19 | 0.28 | 0.20 | 0.05 | 0.17 | 0.30 |
| 5601 | 1/2 cup | Succotash, cnd, avg | 128 | 0.18 | 0.19 | 0.32 | 0.04 | 0.50 | 0.13 | 0.11 | 0.19 | 0.29 | 0.19 | 0.04 | 0.16 | 0.13 | 0.19 | 0.14 | 0.04 | 0.11 | 0.20 |
| 5154 | 1/2 cup | Succotash, fzn, ckd, avg | 85 | 0.20 | 0.21 | 0.36 | 0.04 | 0.55 | 0.15 | 0.12 | 0.21 | 0.32 | 0.21 | 0.05 | 0.18 | 0.14 | 0.21 | 0.15 | 0.04 | 0.12 | 0.22 |
| 5805 | 3 oz | Succotash, raw, avg | 85 | 0.24 | 0.25 | 0.42 | 0.05 | 0.64 | 0.17 | 0.14 | 0.24 | 0.38 | 0.25 | 0.06 | 0.21 | 0.17 | 0.25 | 0.18 | 0.05 | 0.15 | 0.26 |
| 5600 | 1/2 cup | Succotash, w/creamed corn, cnd, avg | 133 | 0.19 | 0.20 | 0.34 | 0.04 | 0.53 | 0.14 | 0.11 | 0.20 | 0.31 | 0.20 | 0.05 | 0.17 | 0.14 | 0.20 | 0.15 | 0.04 | 0.12 | 0.21 |
| | | Mung Bean Sprouts | | | | | | | | | | | | | | | | | | | |
| 5197 | 1/2 cup | Canned, drained, avg | 62 | 0.03 | 0.06 | 0.15 | 0.01 | 0.05 | 0.02 | 0.02 | 0.04 | 0.06 | 0.05 | 0.01 | 0.04 | 0.00 | 0.01 | 0.02 | 0.01 | 0.02 | 0.04 |
| 5020 | 1/2 cup | Raw, avg | 52 | 0.05 | 0.10 | 0.25 | 0.01 | 0.08 | 0.03 | 0.04 | 0.07 | 0.09 | 0.09 | 0.02 | 0.06 | 0.00 | 0.02 | 0.04 | 0.02 | 0.03 | 0.07 |
| 5246 | 1/2 cup | Stir Fried, avg | 62 | 0.10 | 0.19 | 0.47 | 0.02 | 0.16 | 0.06 | 0.07 | 0.13 | 0.17 | 0.16 | 0.03 | 0.11 | 0.00 | 0.03 | 0.08 | 0.04 | 0.05 | 0.13 |

TABLE A **Amino Acid Content for Selected Foods *(continued)***

| Code | Amount | Description | Weight (g) | Alanine (g) | Arginine (g) | Aspartic acid (g) | Cystine (g) | Glutamic acid (g) | Glycine (g) | Histidine (g) | Isoleucine (g) | Leucine (g) | Lysine (g) | Methionine (g) | Phenylalanine (g) | Proline (g) | Serine (g) | Threonine (g) | Tryptophan (g) | Tyrosine (g) | Valine (g) |
|---|---|---|---|---|---|---|---|---|---|---|---|---|---|---|---|---|---|---|---|---|---|
| 6828 | 1/2 cup | Mountain Yam, ckd, avg | 72 | 0.05 | 0.10 | 0.13 | 0.02 | 0.15 | 0.04 | 0.03 | 0.04 | 0.08 | 0.05 | 0.02 | 0.06 | 0.04 | 0.07 | 0.04 | 0.01 | 0.03 | 0.05 |
| 6827 | 1/2 cup | Mountain Yam, raw, avg | 68 | 0.04 | 0.08 | 0.09 | 0.01 | 0.11 | 0.03 | 0.02 | 0.03 | 0.06 | 0.04 | 0.01 | 0.04 | 0.03 | 0.05 | 0.03 | 0.01 | 0.02 | 0.04 |
| | | Mushrooms | | | | | | | | | | | | | | | | | | | |
| 5094 | 1/2 cup | Canned, drained, avg | 78 | 0.11 | 0.07 | 0.14 | 0.00 | 0.26 | 0.07 | 0.04 | 0.06 | 0.09 | 0.15 | 0.03 | 0.06 | 0.11 | 0.07 | 0.07 | 0.03 | 0.03 | 0.07 |
| 5614 | 1/2 cup | Pickled, avg | 78 | 0.64 | 0.04 | 0.08 | 0.00 | 0.15 | 0.04 | 0.02 | 0.03 | 0.05 | 0.09 | 0.02 | 0.03 | 0.06 | 0.04 | 0.04 | 0.02 | 0.02 | 0.04 |
| 5090 | 1/2 cup | Raw, sliced, avg | 35 | 0.05 | 0.04 | 0.07 | 0.00 | 0.12 | 0.03 | 0.02 | 0.03 | 0.04 | 0.07 | 0.01 | 0.03 | 0.05 | 0.03 | 0.03 | 0.02 | 0.02 | 0.03 |
| 5385 | 1/2 cup | Shiitake, ckd, pces, avg | 72 | 0.06 | 0.06 | 0.07 | 0.02 | 0.25 | 0.04 | 0.02 | 0.04 | 0.07 | 0.03 | 0.02 | 0.05 | 0.04 | 0.05 | 0.05 | 0.00 | 0.03 | 0.05 |
| 5383 | 4 ea | Shiitake, dried, avg | 15 | 0.08 | 0.10 | 0.11 | 0.03 | 0.38 | 0.06 | 0.02 | 0.06 | 0.10 | 0.05 | 0.03 | 0.07 | 0.06 | 0.08 | 0.07 | 0.00 | 0.05 | 0.07 |
| 5657 | 1/2 cup | Steamed, sliced, avg | 78 | 0.12 | 0.08 | 0.15 | 0.00 | 0.28 | 0.07 | 0.04 | 0.06 | 0.10 | 0.17 | 0.03 | 0.06 | 0.12 | 0.07 | 0.07 | 0.04 | 0.04 | 0.07 |
| 5096 | 1/2 cup | Mustard Greens, boiled, avg | 70 | 0.00 | 0.12 | 0.00 | 0.02 | 0.00 | 0.00 | 0.03 | 0.06 | 0.05 | 0.07 | 0.01 | 0.04 | 0.00 | 0.00 | 0.04 | 0.02 | 0.03 | 0.06 |
| | | Okra | | | | | | | | | | | | | | | | | | | |
| 5100 | 1/2 cup | Frozen, boiled, avg | 92 | 0.07 | 0.08 | 0.14 | 0.02 | 0.26 | 0.04 | 0.03 | 0.07 | 0.10 | 0.08 | 0.02 | 0.06 | 0.04 | 0.04 | 0.06 | 0.02 | 0.03 | 0.09 |
| 5775 | 1/2 cup | Raw, avg | 50 | 0.04 | 0.04 | 0.07 | 0.01 | 0.14 | 0.02 | 0.02 | 0.03 | 0.05 | 0.04 | 0.01 | 0.03 | 0.02 | 0.02 | 0.03 | 0.01 | 0.04 | 0.05 |
| 5099 | 1/2 cup | Raw, boiled, avg | 80 | 0.05 | 0.06 | 0.11 | 0.01 | 0.20 | 0.03 | 0.02 | 0.05 | 0.08 | 0.06 | 0.02 | 0.05 | 0.03 | 0.03 | 0.05 | 0.01 | 0.05 | 0.07 |
| | | Onions | | | | | | | | | | | | | | | | | | | |
| 5108 | 1/2 cup | Boiled, avg | 105 | 0.04 | 0.19 | 0.08 | 0.03 | 0.23 | 0.06 | 0.02 | 0.05 | 0.05 | 0.07 | 0.01 | 0.04 | 0.04 | 0.04 | 0.03 | 0.02 | 0.04 | 0.03 |
| 5574 | 1/2 cup | Canned, avg | 112 | 0.03 | 0.12 | 0.05 | 0.02 | 0.15 | 0.04 | 0.01 | 0.03 | 0.03 | 0.04 | 0.01 | 0.02 | 0.03 | 0.03 | 0.02 | 0.01 | 0.02 | 0.02 |
| 5113 | 1 Tbs | Flakes, dehydrated, avg | 4 | 0.01 | 0.05 | 0.02 | 0.01 | 0.06 | 0.01 | 0.01 | 0.01 | 0.01 | 0.02 | 0.00 | 0.01 | 0.01 | 0.01 | 0.01 | 0.01 | 0.01 | 0.01 |
| 5300 | 1/2 cup | Frozen, chpd, boiled, avg | 105 | 0.02 | 0.11 | 0.04 | 0.01 | 0.13 | 0.03 | 0.01 | 0.03 | 0.03 | 0.04 | 0.01 | 0.02 | 0.03 | 0.02 | 0.02 | 0.01 | 0.02 | 0.02 |
| 5530 | 1/2 cup | Pearl, pickled, avg | 92 | 0.02 | 0.11 | 0.05 | 0.01 | 0.13 | 0.03 | 0.01 | 0.03 | 0.03 | 0.04 | 0.01 | 0.02 | 0.03 | 0.02 | 0.02 | 0.01 | 0.02 | 0.02 |
| 5101 | 1/2 cup | Raw, chpd, avg | 80 | 0.03 | 0.12 | 0.05 | 0.02 | 0.15 | 0.04 | 0.02 | 0.03 | 0.03 | 0.04 | 0.01 | 0.02 | 0.03 | 0.03 | 0.02 | 0.01 | 0.02 | 0.02 |
| 5190 | 2 ea | Rings, fzn, ckd, avg | 20 | 0.03 | 0.06 | 0.05 | 0.02 | 0.33 | 0.04 | 0.02 | 0.04 | 0.07 | 0.03 | 0.02 | 0.05 | 0.10 | 0.05 | 0.03 | 0.01 | 0.03 | 0.04 |
| 5114 | 1/2 cup | Spring/Green, avg | 50 | 0.04 | 0.07 | 0.08 | 0.01 | 0.19 | 0.05 | 0.02 | 0.04 | 0.05 | 0.05 | 0.01 | 0.03 | 0.06 | 0.04 | 0.04 | 0.01 | 0.03 | 0.04 |
| 5649 | 1/2 cup | Steamed, avg | 105 | 0.03 | 0.17 | 0.07 | 0.02 | 0.20 | 0.05 | 0.02 | 0.04 | 0.04 | 0.06 | 0.01 | 0.03 | 0.04 | 0.04 | 0.03 | 0.02 | 0.03 | 0.03 |
| 5650 | 1/2 cup | Stir Fried, avg | 105 | 0.03 | 0.17 | 0.07 | 0.02 | 0.20 | 0.05 | 0.02 | 0.04 | 0.04 | 0.06 | 0.01 | 0.03 | 0.04 | 0.04 | 0.03 | 0.02 | 0.03 | 0.03 |
| 7270 | 1/2 cup | Palm Hearts, cnd, avg | 73 | 0.08 | 0.13 | 0.12 | 0.01 | 0.22 | 0.08 | 0.04 | 0.07 | 0.12 | 0.07 | 0.03 | 0.07 | 0.06 | 0.06 | 0.07 | 0.02 | 0.04 | 0.08 |
| 5212 | 1/2 cup | Parsnips, raw, boiled, avg | 78 | 0.05 | 0.11 | 0.10 | 0.00 | 0.10 | 0.03 | 0.02 | 0.04 | 0.05 | 0.06 | 0.01 | 0.04 | 0.03 | 0.04 | 0.04 | 0.01 | 0.02 | 0.05 |
| 5211 | 1/2 cup | Parsnips, raw, sliced, avg | 66 | 0.04 | 0.08 | 0.08 | 0.00 | 0.07 | 0.03 | 0.01 | 0.03 | 0.04 | 0.05 | 0.01 | 0.03 | 0.03 | 0.03 | 0.03 | 0.01 | 0.02 | 0.04 |
| | | Peas | | | | | | | | | | | | | | | | | | | |
| 5117 | 1/2 cup | Green, boiled, avg | 80 | 0.19 | 0.34 | 0.39 | 0.03 | 0.59 | 0.15 | 0.08 | 0.15 | 0.26 | 0.25 | 0.06 | 0.16 | 0.14 | 0.14 | 0.16 | 0.03 | 0.09 | 0.19 |
| 5214 | 1/2 cup | Green, cnd w/liquid, avg | 124 | 0.17 | 0.31 | 0.36 | 0.02 | 0.54 | 0.13 | 0.08 | 0.14 | 0.24 | 0.23 | 0.06 | 0.15 | 0.13 | 0.13 | 0.15 | 0.03 | 0.08 | 0.17 |
| 5267 | 1/2 cup | Green, cnd w/liquid, unsalted, avg | 124 | 0.17 | 0.31 | 0.36 | 0.02 | 0.54 | 0.13 | 0.08 | 0.14 | 0.24 | 0.23 | 0.06 | 0.15 | 0.13 | 0.13 | 0.15 | 0.03 | 0.08 | 0.17 |
| 5118 | 1/2 cup | Green, fzn, boiled, avg | 80 | 0.18 | 0.33 | 0.38 | 0.02 | 0.56 | 0.14 | 0.08 | 0.15 | 0.25 | 0.24 | 0.06 | 0.15 | 0.13 | 0.14 | 0.15 | 0.03 | 0.09 | 0.18 |
| 5116 | 1/2 cup | Green, raw, avg | 72 | 0.17 | 0.31 | 0.36 | 0.02 | 0.53 | 0.13 | 0.08 | 0.14 | 0.23 | 0.23 | 0.06 | 0.14 | 0.12 | 0.13 | 0.15 | 0.03 | 0.08 | 0.17 |
| 5783 | 1/2 cup | Pigeon, boiled, avg | 76 | 0.20 | 0.27 | 0.45 | 0.05 | 1.05 | 0.17 | 0.16 | 0.16 | 0.32 | 0.32 | 0.05 | 0.39 | 0.20 | 0.21 | 0.16 | 0.04 | 0.11 | 0.20 |
| 5781 | 1/2 cup | Pigeon, raw, avg | 77 | 0.25 | 0.33 | 0.55 | 0.06 | 1.29 | 0.20 | 0.20 | 0.20 | 0.40 | 0.39 | 0.06 | 0.48 | 0.24 | 0.26 | 0.20 | 0.05 | 0.14 | 0.24 |
| 7020 | 1/2 cup | Split, boiled, avg | 98 | 0.36 | 0.73 | 0.96 | 0.12 | 1.40 | 0.36 | 0.20 | 0.34 | 0.59 | 0.59 | 0.08 | 0.38 | 0.34 | 0.36 | 0.29 | 0.09 | 0.24 | 0.39 |
| 7019 | 1/2 cup | Split, raw, avg | 98 | 1.06 | 2.15 | 2.84 | 0.37 | 4.12 | 1.07 | 0.59 | 0.99 | 1.72 | 1.73 | 0.25 | 1.11 | 0.99 | 1.06 | 0.85 | 0.27 | 0.70 | 1.14 |
| | | Peas, Edible Pods | | | | | | | | | | | | | | | | | | | |
| 5296 | 1/2 cup | Frozen, boiled, avg | 80 | 0.06 | 0.13 | 0.23 | 0.03 | 0.45 | 0.07 | 0.02 | 0.16 | 0.23 | 0.20 | 0.01 | 0.09 | 0.06 | 0.13 | 0.10 | 0.03 | 0.10 | 0.27 |
| 5122 | 1/2 cup | Snow, boiled, avg | 80 | 0.05 | 0.13 | 0.21 | 0.03 | 0.42 | 0.07 | 0.02 | 0.15 | 0.21 | 0.19 | 0.01 | 0.08 | 0.06 | 0.12 | 0.09 | 0.03 | 0.09 | 0.26 |
| 6836 | 1/2 cup | Snow, raw, chpd, avg | 49 | 0.03 | 0.07 | 0.11 | 0.02 | 0.22 | 0.04 | 0.01 | 0.08 | 0.11 | 0.10 | 0.01 | 0.04 | 0.03 | 0.06 | 0.05 | 0.01 | 0.05 | 0.13 |
| 5665 | 1/2 cup | Steamed, avg | 82 | 0.05 | 0.11 | 0.19 | 0.03 | 0.37 | 0.06 | 0.01 | 0.13 | 0.19 | 0.17 | 0.01 | 0.07 | 0.05 | 0.10 | 0.08 | 0.02 | 0.08 | 0.22 |
| | | Peppers, Hot | | | | | | | | | | | | | | | | | | | |
| 7260 | 1 Tbs | Chile, sun dried, avg | 2 | 0.01 | 0.01 | 0.03 | 0.00 | 0.03 | 0.01 | 0.00 | 0.01 | 0.01 | 0.01 | 0.00 | 0.01 | 0.01 | 0.01 | 0.01 | 0.00 | 0.00 | 0.01 |
| 5399 | 1/4 cup | Green Chili, raw, chpd, avg | 38 | 0.03 | 0.04 | 0.11 | 0.01 | 0.10 | 0.03 | 0.02 | 0.02 | 0.04 | 0.03 | 0.01 | 0.02 | 0.03 | 0.03 | 0.03 | 0.01 | 0.02 | 0.03 |
| 5063 | 1/4 cup | Green Chili, cnd, chpd, avg | 34 | 0.01 | 0.01 | 0.04 | 0.01 | 0.04 | 0.01 | 0.01 | 0.01 | 0.02 | 0.01 | 0.00 | 0.01 | 0.01 | 0.01 | 0.01 | 0.00 | 0.01 | 0.01 |
| 5293 | 1/4 cup | Jalapenos, cnd, avg | 34 | 0.01 | 0.01 | 0.04 | 0.01 | 0.04 | 0.01 | 0.01 | 0.01 | 0.02 | 0.01 | 0.00 | 0.01 | 0.01 | 0.01 | 0.01 | 0.00 | 0.01 | 0.01 |
| 5291 | 1/4 cup | Red Chili, cnd, avg | 34 | 0.01 | 0.01 | 0.04 | 0.01 | 0.04 | 0.01 | 0.01 | 0.01 | 0.02 | 0.01 | 0.00 | 0.01 | 0.01 | 0.01 | 0.01 | 0.00 | 0.01 | 0.01 |
| 5288 | 1/4 cup | Red Chili, raw, avg | 38 | 0.03 | 0.04 | 0.11 | 0.01 | 0.10 | 0.03 | 0.02 | 0.02 | 0.04 | 0.03 | 0.01 | 0.02 | 0.03 | 0.03 | 0.03 | 0.01 | 0.02 | 0.03 |

TABLE A **Amino Acid Content for Selected Foods *(continued)***

| Code | Amount | Description | Weight (g) | Alanine (g) | Arginine (g) | Aspartic acid (g) | Cystine (g) | Glutamic acid (g) | Glycine (g) | Histidine (g) | Isoleucine (g) | Leucine (g) | Lysine (g) | Methionine (g) | Phenylalanine (g) | Proline (g) | Serine (g) | Threonine (g) | Tryptophan (g) | Tyrosine (g) | Valine (g) |
|---|---|---|---|---|---|---|---|---|---|---|---|---|---|---|---|---|---|---|---|---|---|
| | | Peppers, Sweet | | | | | | | | | | | | | | | | | | | |
| 5126 | 1/2 cup | Green, boiled, chpd, avg | 68 | 0.03 | 0.03 | 0.09 | 0.01 | 0.08 | 0.02 | 0.01 | 0.02 | 0.03 | 0.03 | 0.01 | 0.02 | 0.03 | 0.03 | 0.02 | 0.01 | 0.01 | 0.03 |
| 5578 | 1/2 cup | Green, cnd, avg | 70 | 0.02 | 0.03 | 0.08 | 0.01 | 0.07 | 0.02 | 0.01 | 0.02 | 0.03 | 0.03 | 0.01 | 0.02 | 0.02 | 0.02 | 0.02 | 0.01 | 0.01 | 0.02 |
| 5284 | 1/2 cup | Green, fzn, boiled, avg | 68 | 0.03 | 0.03 | 0.09 | 0.01 | 0.09 | 0.02 | 0.01 | 0.02 | 0.03 | 0.03 | 0.01 | 0.02 | 0.03 | 0.03 | 0.02 | 0.01 | 0.01 | 0.03 |
| 5214 | 1/2 cup | Green, raw, chpd, avg | 74 | 0.10 | 0.19 | 0.22 | 0.01 | 0.32 | 0.08 | 0.05 | 0.08 | 0.14 | 0.14 | 0.04 | 0.09 | 0.08 | 0.08 | 0.09 | 0.02 | 0.05 | 0.10 |
| 5661 | 1/2 cup | Green, stmd, avg | 68 | 0.02 | 0.03 | 0.09 | 0.01 | 0.08 | 0.02 | 0.01 | 0.02 | 0.03 | 0.03 | 0.01 | 0.02 | 0.03 | 0.02 | 0.02 | 0.01 | 0.01 | 0.03 |
| 5568 | 1/2 cup | Red, cnd, avg | 70 | 0.02 | 0.03 | 0.08 | 0.01 | 0.07 | 0.02 | 0.01 | 0.02 | 0.03 | 0.03 | 0.01 | 0.02 | 0.02 | 0.02 | 0.02 | 0.01 | 0.01 | 0.02 |
| 5278 | 1/2 cup | Red, ckd, avg | 68 | 0.03 | 0.03 | 0.09 | 0.01 | 0.08 | 0.02 | 0.01 | 0.02 | 0.03 | 0.03 | 0.01 | 0.02 | 0.03 | 0.03 | 0.02 | 0.01 | 0.01 | 0.03 |
| 5286 | 1/2 cup | Red, fzn, boiled, avg | 68 | 0.03 | 0.03 | 0.09 | 0.01 | 0.09 | 0.02 | 0.01 | 0.02 | 0.03 | 0.03 | 0.01 | 0.02 | 0.03 | 0.03 | 0.02 | 0.01 | 0.01 | 0.03 |
| 5218 | 1/2 cup | Red, raw, avg | 74 | 0.03 | 0.03 | 0.10 | 0.01 | 0.09 | 0.03 | 0.01 | 0.02 | 0.04 | 0.03 | 0.01 | 0.02 | 0.03 | 0.03 | 0.03 | 0.01 | 0.01 | 0.03 |
| 5663 | 1/2 cup | Red, stmd, avg | 68 | 0.02 | 0.03 | 0.09 | 0.01 | 0.08 | 0.02 | 0.01 | 0.02 | 0.03 | 0.03 | 0.01 | 0.02 | 0.03 | 0.02 | 0.02 | 0.01 | 0.01 | 0.03 |
| 5441 | 1 ea | Yellow, raw, large, avg | 180 | 0.07 | 0.09 | 0.26 | 0.03 | 0.24 | 0.07 | 0.04 | 0.06 | 0.09 | 0.08 | 0.02 | 0.06 | 0.08 | 0.07 | 0.07 | 0.02 | 0.04 | 0.08 |
| | | Potatoes, Plain | | | | | | | | | | | | | | | | | | | |
| 5334 | 1 ea | Baked, long, avg | 202 | 0.14 | 0.21 | 1.14 | 0.06 | 0.78 | 0.14 | 0.10 | 0.19 | 0.28 | 0.28 | 0.07 | 0.21 | 0.17 | 0.20 | 0.17 | 0.07 | 0.17 | 0.26 |
| 5328 | 1 ea | Boiled, f/fzn, avg | 70 | 0.04 | 0.06 | 0.34 | 0.02 | 0.23 | 0.04 | 0.03 | 0.06 | 0.08 | 0.08 | 0.02 | 0.06 | 0.05 | 0.06 | 0.05 | 0.02 | 0.05 | 0.08 |
| 5586 | 1/2 cup | Canned, w/liquid, avg | 150 | 0.59 | 0.76 | 2.97 | 0.20 | 2.87 | 0.53 | 0.38 | 0.77 | 1.17 | 1.08 | 0.23 | 0.76 | 0.77 | 0.71 | 0.72 | 0.15 | 0.67 | 0.99 |
| 5129 | 1 ea | Flesh, baked, avg | 156 | 0.09 | 0.14 | 0.75 | 0.04 | 0.51 | 0.09 | 0.07 | 0.12 | 0.18 | 0.19 | 0.05 | 0.14 | 0.11 | 0.13 | 0.11 | 0.05 | 0.11 | 0.17 |
| 5136 | 1/2 cup | Flesh, boiled, avg | 78 | 0.04 | 0.06 | 0.33 | 0.02 | 0.22 | 0.04 | 0.03 | 0.05 | 0.08 | 0.08 | 0.02 | 0.06 | 0.05 | 0.06 | 0.05 | 0.02 | 0.05 | 0.07 |
| 5345 | 1 ea | Flesh, microwaved, avg | 156 | 0.10 | 0.15 | 0.80 | 0.04 | 0.55 | 0.10 | 0.07 | 0.13 | 0.20 | 0.20 | 0.05 | 0.15 | 0.12 | 0.14 | 0.12 | 0.05 | 0.12 | 0.18 |
| 5582 | 1/2 cup | Flesh, raw, diced, avg | 75 | 0.05 | 0.07 | 0.38 | 0.02 | 0.26 | 0.05 | 0.03 | 0.06 | 0.09 | 0.09 | 0.02 | 0.07 | 0.06 | 0.07 | 0.06 | 0.02 | 0.06 | 0.09 |
| 5340 | 1 ea | Microwaved, avg | 202 | 0.15 | 0.23 | 1.20 | 0.06 | 0.83 | 0.15 | 0.11 | 0.20 | 0.30 | 0.30 | 0.08 | 0.22 | 0.18 | 0.21 | 0.18 | 0.08 | 0.18 | 0.28 |
| 5339 | 1 ea | Skin, baked, avg | 58 | 0.08 | 0.12 | 0.61 | 0.03 | 0.42 | 0.07 | 0.05 | 0.09 | 0.14 | 0.15 | 0.04 | 0.11 | 0.09 | 0.11 | 0.09 | 0.04 | 0.09 | 0.14 |
| 5368 | 1 ea | Skin, boiled, avg | 34 | 0.03 | 0.05 | 0.24 | 0.01 | 0.16 | 0.03 | 0.02 | 0.04 | 0.06 | 0.06 | 0.01 | 0.04 | 0.04 | 0.04 | 0.04 | 0.02 | 0.03 | 0.06 |
| 5350 | 1 ea | Skin, microwaved, avg | 58 | 0.08 | 0.12 | 0.62 | 0.03 | 0.43 | 0.07 | 0.05 | 0.10 | 0.15 | 0.16 | 0.04 | 0.11 | 0.10 | 0.11 | 0.10 | 0.04 | 0.09 | 0.15 |
| 5784 | 1 ea | Skin, raw, avg | 38 | 0.03 | 0.05 | 0.24 | 0.01 | 0.16 | 0.03 | 0.02 | 0.04 | 0.01 | 0.06 | 0.01 | 0.04 | 0.04 | 0.04 | 0.04 | 0.02 | 0.03 | 0.06 |
| | | Potato Dishes | | | | | | | | | | | | | | | | | | | |
| 5786 | 1/2 cup | Au Gratin, prep f/recipe, w/butter, avg | 122 | 0.18 | 0.23 | 0.65 | 0.05 | 1.30 | 0.13 | 0.17 | 0.32 | 0.51 | 0.43 | 0.13 | 0.29 | 0.53 | 0.31 | 0.22 | 0.08 | 0.26 | 0.37 |
| 6177 | 1 ea | Baked, w/cheese sauce, avg | 296 | 0.40 | 0.56 | 1.71 | 0.10 | 3.02 | 0.30 | 0.42 | 0.76 | 1.16 | 1.04 | 0.31 | 0.69 | 1.20 | 0.74 | 0.49 | 0.19 | 0.62 | 0.87 |
| 6178 | 1 ea | Baked, w/cheese sauce & bacon, avg | 299 | 0.59 | 0.78 | 2.10 | 0.14 | 3.68 | 0.52 | 0.54 | 0.94 | 1.45 | 1.35 | 0.40 | 0.86 | 1.46 | 0.91 | 0.65 | 0.23 | 0.75 | 1.09 |
| 6179 | 1 ea | Baked, w/cheese sauce & broccoli, avg | 339 | 0.40 | 0.54 | 1.55 | 0.10 | 2.72 | 0.29 | 0.38 | 0.69 | 1.03 | 0.95 | 0.28 | 0.62 | 1.06 | 0.67 | 0.46 | 0.17 | 0.55 | 0.80 |
| 6180 | 1 ea | Baked, w/cheese sauce & chili, avg | 395 | 0.76 | 1.00 | 2.62 | 0.18 | 4.66 | 0.64 | 0.67 | 1.15 | 1.82 | 1.67 | 0.49 | 1.06 | 1.75 | 1.13 | 0.81 | 0.29 | 0.91 | 1.33 |
| 5790 | 10 ea | French Fries, fzn, avg | 65 | 0.05 | 0.07 | 0.35 | 0.01 | 0.26 | 0.05 | 0.03 | 0.07 | 0.09 | 0.08 | 0.02 | 0.07 | 0.05 | 0.05 | 0.07 | 0.02 | 0.04 | 0.08 |
| 5332 | 10 ea | French Fries, fzn, cottage, oven htd, avg | 50 | 0.06 | 0.08 | 0.40 | 0.01 | 0.27 | 0.06 | 0.03 | 0.07 | 0.10 | 0.09 | 0.02 | 0.07 | 0.06 | 0.06 | 0.08 | 0.02 | 0.04 | 0.09 |
| 5961 | 10 ea | French Fries, fzn, prep, salted, avg | 50 | 0.05 | 0.07 | 0.34 | 0.01 | 0.25 | 0.05 | 0.03 | 0.07 | 0.09 | 0.08 | 0.02 | 0.07 | 0.05 | 0.05 | 0.06 | 0.02 | 0.04 | 0.08 |
| 5330 | 1 cup | French Fries, fzn, prep in veg oil, avg | 57 | 0.08 | 0.11 | 0.53 | 0.01 | 0.36 | 0.08 | 0.04 | 0.10 | 0.14 | 0.12 | 0.03 | 0.10 | 0.07 | 0.08 | 0.10 | 0.03 | 0.06 | 0.12 |
| 5589 | 1/2 cup | Hash Browns, fzn, avg | 105 | 0.07 | 0.10 | 0.50 | 0.01 | 0.34 | 0.08 | 0.04 | 0.09 | 0.13 | 0.12 | 0.02 | 0.09 | 0.07 | 0.08 | 0.10 | 0.03 | 0.05 | 0.11 |
| 5140 | 1/2 cup | Hash Browns, prep f/fzn, avg | 78 | 0.09 | 0.12 | 0.57 | 0.02 | 0.38 | 0.09 | 0.04 | 0.11 | 0.15 | 0.13 | 0.03 | 0.11 | 0.08 | 0.09 | 0.11 | 0.03 | 0.06 | 0.13 |
| 5273 | 1 cup | Hash Browns, prep f/recipe, avg | 156 | 0.13 | 0.18 | 0.87 | 0.02 | 0.59 | 0.14 | 0.06 | 0.16 | 0.23 | 0.20 | 0.04 | 0.16 | 0.12 | 0.14 | 0.17 | 0.05 | 0.10 | 0.19 |
| 5590 | 1 ea | Hash Browns, w/butter sauce, fzn, avg | 170 | 0.11 | 0.15 | 0.74 | 0.02 | 0.50 | 0.12 | 0.05 | 0.14 | 0.19 | 0.17 | 0.04 | 0.14 | 0.10 | 0.11 | 0.14 | 0.04 | 0.08 | 0.16 |
| 5591 | 1/2 cup | Hash Browns, w/butter sauce, prep f/fzn, avg | 72 | 0.06 | 0.08 | 0.41 | 0.01 | 0.28 | 0.06 | 0.03 | 0.08 | 0.11 | 0.09 | 0.02 | 0.08 | 0.06 | 0.06 | 0.08 | 0.02 | 0.04 | 0.09 |
| 5464 | 1/2 cup | Mashed, prep f/flakes, w/whole milk & butter, | 105 | 0.07 | 0.09 | 0.30 | 0.02 | 0.36 | 0.06 | 0.05 | 0.10 | 0.15 | 0.14 | 0.03 | 0.09 | 0.12 | 0.09 | 0.09 | 0.02 | 0.08 | 0.12 |
| 5138 | 1/2 cup | Mashed, prep f/flakes, w/whole milk & marg, avg | 105 | 0.07 | 0.09 | 0.30 | 0.02 | 0.36 | 0.06 | 0.05 | 0.10 | 0.15 | 0.14 | 0.03 | 0.09 | 0.12 | 0.09 | 0.09 | 0.02 | 0.08 | 0.12 |
| 5585 | 1/2 cup | Mashed, prep f/granules, w/milk & butter, avg | 105 | 0.07 | 0.09 | 0.26 | 0.02 | 0.41 | 0.06 | 0.05 | 0.11 | 0.18 | 0.15 | 0.04 | 0.10 | 0.15 | 0.10 | 0.09 | 0.02 | 0.09 | 0.13 |
| 5469 | 1/2 cup | Mashed, prep f/granules, w/milk & marg, avg | 105 | 0.07 | 0.09 | 0.26 | 0.02 | 0.41 | 0.06 | 0.05 | 0.11 | 0.18 | 0.15 | 0.04 | 0.10 | 0.15 | 0.10 | 0.09 | 0.02 | 0.09 | 0.13 |
| 5137 | 1/2 cup | Mashed, w/whole milk, avg | 105 | 0.06 | 0.09 | 0.41 | 0.02 | 0.36 | 0.06 | 0.05 | 0.09 | 0.14 | 0.13 | 0.04 | 0.09 | 0.10 | 0.09 | 0.08 | 0.03 | 0.08 | 0.12 |
| 5569 | 1/2 cup | Mashed, w/whole milk & butter, avg | 105 | 0.06 | 0.08 | 0.39 | 0.02 | 0.35 | 0.05 | 0.05 | 0.09 | 0.14 | 0.13 | 0.04 | 0.09 | 0.10 | 0.09 | 0.08 | 0.03 | 0.08 | 0.12 |
| 5787 | 1/2 cup | O'Brien, fzn, avg | 97 | 0.06 | 0.09 | 0.41 | 0.02 | 0.29 | 0.05 | 0.04 | 0.07 | 0.10 | 0.10 | 0.03 | 0.08 | 0.06 | 0.08 | 0.06 | 0.03 | 0.06 | 0.10 |
| 5269 | 1/2 cup | O'Brien, prep f/fzn, avg | 97 | 0.07 | 0.11 | 0.50 | 0.03 | 0.36 | 0.07 | 0.05 | 0.09 | 0.13 | 0.13 | 0.03 | 0.09 | 0.08 | 0.09 | 0.08 | 0.03 | 0.08 | 0.12 |
| 5268 | 1/2 cup | O'Brien, prep f/recipe, avg | 97 | 0.07 | 0.11 | 0.36 | 0.03 | 0.45 | 0.06 | 0.05 | 0.11 | 0.16 | 0.14 | 0.04 | 0.10 | 0.14 | 0.11 | 0.09 | 0.03 | 0.09 | 0.13 |
| 5263 | 1 ea | Pancakes, prep f/recipe, avg | 76 | 0.20 | 0.25 | 0.75 | 0.09 | 0.76 | 0.15 | 0.11 | 0.22 | 0.33 | 0.29 | 0.11 | 0.23 | 0.20 | 0.27 | 0.19 | 0.06 | 0.18 | 0.27 |

TABLE A **Amino Acid Content for Selected Foods *(continued)***

| Code | Amount | Description | Weight (g) | Alanine (g) | Arginine (g) | Aspartic acid (g) | Cystine (g) | Glutamic acid (g) | Glycine (g) | Histidine (g) | Isoleucine (g) | Leucine (g) | Lysine (g) | Methionine (g) | Phenylalanine (g) | Proline (g) | Serine (g) | Threonine (g) | Tryptophan (g) | Tyrosine (g) | Valine (g) |
|---|---|---|---|---|---|---|---|---|---|---|---|---|---|---|---|---|---|---|---|---|---|
| 5788 | 1/2 cup | Puffs, fzn, avg | 64 | 0.06 | 0.08 | 0.40 | 0.01 | 0.27 | 0.06 | 0.03 | 0.07 | 0.10 | 0.09 | 0.02 | 0.07 | 0.05 | 0.06 | 0.08 | 0.02 | 0.04 | 0.09 |
| 5785 | 1/2 cup | Scalloped, prep f/recipe, w/butter, avg | 122 | 0.11 | 0.14 | 0.52 | 0.04 | 0.68 | 0.09 | 0.08 | 0.17 | 0.27 | 0.23 | 0.07 | 0.16 | 0.24 | 0.17 | 0.14 | 0.05 | 0.14 | 0.21 |
| 5270 | 1/2 cup | Scalloped, prep f/recipe, w/marg, avg | 122 | 0.11 | 0.14 | 0.52 | 0.04 | 0.68 | 0.09 | 0.08 | 0.17 | 0.27 | 0.23 | 0.07 | 0.16 | 0.24 | 0.17 | 0.14 | 0.05 | 0.14 | 0.21 |
| | | Pumpkin | | | | | | | | | | | | | | | | | | | |
| 5396 | 1/2 cup | Boiled, avg | 122 | 0.02 | 0.05 | 0.09 | 0.00 | 0.16 | 0.02 | 0.01 | 0.03 | 0.04 | 0.05 | 0.01 | 0.03 | 0.02 | 0.04 | 0.03 | 0.01 | 0.04 | 0.03 |
| 5142 | 1/2 cup | Canned, avg | 122 | 0.04 | 0.07 | 0.14 | 0.00 | 0.25 | 0.04 | 0.02 | 0.04 | 0.06 | 0.07 | 0.01 | 0.04 | 0.04 | 0.06 | 0.04 | 0.02 | 0.05 | 0.05 |
| 5793 | 1/2 cup | Raw, avg | 58 | 0.02 | 0.03 | 0.06 | 0.00 | 0.11 | 0.02 | 0.01 | 0.02 | 0.03 | 0.03 | 0.01 | 0.02 | 0.02 | 0.03 | 0.02 | 0.01 | 0.02 | 0.02 |
| 5426 | 1/2 cup | Purslane, boiled, avg | 58 | 0.03 | 0.03 | 0.04 | 0.01 | 0.13 | 0.03 | 0.01 | 0.03 | 0.05 | 0.04 | 0.01 | 0.03 | 0.04 | 0.03 | 0.03 | 0.01 | 0.01 | 0.04 |
| 5425 | 1/2 cup | Purslane, raw, avg | 22 | 0.01 | 0.01 | 0.01 | 0.00 | 0.04 | 0.01 | 0.00 | 0.01 | 0.02 | 0.01 | 0.00 | 0.01 | 0.01 | 0.01 | 0.01 | 0.00 | 0.00 | 0.01 |
| | | Radishes | | | | | | | | | | | | | | | | | | | |
| 5593 | 1/2 cup | Oriental, boiled, avg | 74 | 0.02 | 0.03 | 0.03 | 0.00 | 0.09 | 0.02 | 0.01 | 0.02 | 0.03 | 0.02 | 0.00 | 0.02 | 0.01 | 0.01 | 0.02 | 0.00 | 0.01 | 0.02 |
| 5594 | 1/2 cup | Oriental, dried, avg | 58 | 0.14 | 0.26 | 0.31 | 0.04 | 0.86 | 0.14 | 0.03 | 0.20 | 0.24 | 0.23 | 0.04 | 0.15 | 0.12 | 0.14 | 0.19 | 0.02 | 0.09 | 0.21 |
| 5144 | 1/2 cup | Red, slices, avg | 58 | 0.01 | 0.02 | 0.03 | 0.00 | 0.08 | 0.01 | 0.01 | 0.02 | 0.02 | 0.02 | 0.00 | 0.01 | 0.01 | 0.01 | 0.02 | 0.00 | 0.01 | 0.02 |
| 5550 | 1/2 cup | White Icicle, raw, avg | 50 | 0.02 | 0.03 | 0.04 | 0.00 | 0.10 | 0.02 | 0.01 | 0.02 | 0.03 | 0.03 | 0.00 | 0.02 | 0.01 | 0.02 | 0.02 | 0.00 | 0.01 | 0.03 |
| 7225 | 1/2 cup | Rutabaga, boiled, cubes, avg | 85 | 0.03 | 0.14 | 0.08 | 0.01 | 0.13 | 0.03 | 0.03 | 0.05 | 0.03 | 0.04 | 0.01 | 0.03 | 0.00 | 0.03 | 0.04 | 0.01 | 0.02 | 0.04 |
| 7214 | 1/2 cup | Rutabaga, raw, avg | 70 | 0.02 | 0.10 | 0.06 | 0.01 | 0.10 | 0.02 | 0.02 | 0.04 | 0.03 | 0.03 | 0.01 | 0.02 | 0.00 | 0.02 | 0.03 | 0.01 | 0.02 | 0.03 |
| | | Seaweed | | | | | | | | | | | | | | | | | | | |
| 5256 | 1/2 cup | Kelp, raw, avg | 40 | 0.05 | 0.03 | 0.05 | 0.04 | 0.11 | 0.04 | 0.01 | 0.03 | 0.03 | 0.03 | 0.01 | 0.02 | 0.03 | 0.04 | 0.02 | 0.02 | 0.01 | 0.03 |
| 5257 | 1/2 cup | Laver, raw, avg | 40 | 0.26 | 0.11 | 0.23 | 0.04 | 0.22 | 0.15 | 0.05 | 0.10 | 0.20 | 0.09 | 0.06 | 0.11 | 0.10 | 0.12 | 0.09 | 0.02 | 0.10 | 0.16 |
| 5260 | 1/4 cup | Spirulina, dried, avg | 4 | 0.18 | 0.16 | 0.23 | 0.03 | 0.33 | 0.12 | 0.04 | 0.13 | 0.20 | 0.12 | 0.05 | 0.11 | 0.09 | 0.12 | 0.12 | 0.04 | 0.10 | 0.14 |
| 5836 | 3 oz | Spirulina, raw, avg | 85 | 0.39 | 0.36 | 0.50 | 0.06 | 0.73 | 0.27 | 0.09 | 0.28 | 0.43 | 0.26 | 0.10 | 0.24 | 0.21 | 0.26 | 0.26 | 0.08 | 0.22 | 0.30 |
| 5261 | 1/2 cup | Wakame, raw, avg | 40 | 0.05 | 0.04 | 0.07 | 0.01 | 0.08 | 0.04 | 0.01 | 0.03 | 0.10 | 0.04 | 0.03 | 0.04 | 0.04 | 0.03 | 0.07 | 0.01 | 0.02 | 0.08 |
| 5428 | 1 Tbs | Shallots, freeze dried, chpd, avg | 1 | 0.01 | 0.01 | 0.01 | 0.00 | 0.03 | 0.01 | 0.00 | 0.01 | 0.01 | 0.01 | 0.00 | 0.00 | 0.01 | 0.01 | 0.00 | 0.00 | 0.00 | 0.01 |
| 5427 | 1 Tbs | Shallots, raw, chpd, avg | 10 | 0.01 | 0.02 | 0.02 | 0.00 | 0.05 | 0.01 | 0.00 | 0.01 | 0.01 | 0.01 | 0.00 | 0.01 | 0.02 | 0.01 | 0.01 | 0.00 | 0.01 | 0.01 |
| 5259 | 1/2 cup | Soybeans, green, boiled, avg | 90 | 0.50 | 0.89 | 1.30 | 0.10 | 2.09 | 0.46 | 0.30 | 0.49 | 0.79 | 0.67 | 0.14 | 0.50 | 0.52 | 0.62 | 0.44 | 0.14 | 0.40 | 0.49 |
| 5258 | 1/2 cup | Soybeans, green, raw, avg | 128 | 0.74 | 1.33 | 1.93 | 0.15 | 3.11 | 0.59 | 0.45 | 0.73 | 1.19 | 0.99 | 0.20 | 0.75 | 0.78 | 0.92 | 0.66 | 0.20 | 0.59 | 0.74 |
| | | Spinach | | | | | | | | | | | | | | | | | | | |
| 5147 | 1/2 cup | Boiled, avg | 90 | 0.13 | 0.15 | 0.22 | 0.03 | 0.32 | 0.13 | 0.05 | 0.14 | 0.21 | 0.16 | 0.05 | 0.12 | 0.10 | 0.10 | 0.11 | 0.04 | 0.10 | 0.15 |
| 5595 | 1/2 cup | Canned, w/liquid, avg | 117 | 0.12 | 0.14 | 0.21 | 0.03 | 0.30 | 0.12 | 0.05 | 0.13 | 0.19 | 0.15 | 0.05 | 0.11 | 0.10 | 0.09 | 0.11 | 0.03 | 0.09 | 0.14 |
| 5973 | 1/2 cup | Canned, w/liquid, unsalted, avg | 117 | 0.12 | 0.14 | 0.21 | 0.03 | 0.30 | 0.12 | 0.05 | 0.13 | 0.19 | 0.15 | 0.05 | 0.11 | 0.10 | 0.09 | 0.11 | 0.03 | 0.09 | 0.14 |
| 5148 | 1/2 cup | Frozen, boiled, drained, unsalted, avg | 95 | 0.15 | 0.17 | 0.25 | 0.04 | 0.36 | 0.14 | 0.07 | 0.15 | 0.23 | 0.18 | 0.06 | 0.13 | 0.12 | 0.11 | 0.13 | 0.04 | 0.11 | 0.17 |
| 5146 | 1 cup | Raw, chpd, avg | 30 | 0.04 | 0.05 | 0.07 | 0.01 | 0.10 | 0.04 | 0.02 | 0.04 | 0.07 | 0.05 | 0.02 | 0.04 | 0.03 | 0.03 | 0.04 | 0.01 | 0.03 | 0.05 |
| 5670 | 1/2 cup | Steamed, avg | 95 | 0.13 | 0.15 | 0.23 | 0.03 | 0.33 | 0.13 | 0.06 | 0.04 | 0.21 | 0.17 | 0.05 | 0.12 | 0.11 | 0.10 | 0.12 | 0.04 | 0.10 | 0.15 |
| 5669 | 1/2 cup | Stir Fried, avg | 90 | 0.13 | 0.15 | 0.22 | 0.03 | 0.31 | 0.12 | 0.06 | 0.13 | 0.20 | 0.16 | 0.05 | 0.12 | 0.10 | 0.09 | 0.11 | 0.04 | 0.10 | 0.14 |
| | | Sprouts | | | | | | | | | | | | | | | | | | | |
| 5725 | 1/2 cup | Kidney Bean, boiled, avg | 64 | 0.13 | 0.17 | 0.40 | 0.04 | 0.38 | 0.11 | 0.09 | 0.14 | 0.22 | 0.18 | 0.03 | 0.16 | 0.12 | 0.17 | 0.13 | 0.03 | 0.11 | 0.16 |
| 5724 | 1/2 cup | Kidney Bean, raw, avg | 92 | 0.16 | 0.21 | 0.50 | 0.04 | 0.47 | 0.13 | 0.11 | 0.17 | 0.28 | 0.22 | 0.04 | 0.20 | 0.16 | 0.21 | 0.16 | 0.04 | 0.13 | 0.20 |
| 5458 | 1/2 cup | Soybeans, raw, avg | 35 | 0.19 | 0.32 | 0.62 | 0.05 | 0.69 | 0.18 | 0.12 | 0.20 | 0.33 | 0.26 | 0.05 | 0.22 | 0.24 | 0.23 | 0.18 | 0.06 | 0.17 | 0.22 |
| 5459 | 1/2 cup | Steamed, avg | 47 | 0.17 | 0.27 | 0.54 | 0.05 | 0.60 | 0.15 | 0.11 | 0.18 | 0.29 | 0.23 | 0.04 | 0.20 | 0.20 | 0.20 | 0.15 | 0.05 | 0.15 | 0.19 |
| 5795 | 1/2 cup | Stir Fried, avg | 62 | 0.34 | 0.56 | 1.10 | 0.10 | 1.22 | 0.31 | 0.22 | 0.36 | 0.58 | 0.47 | 0.09 | 0.40 | 0.42 | 0.40 | 0.31 | 0.10 | 0.30 | 0.38 |
| | | Squash | | | | | | | | | | | | | | | | | | | |
| 5314 | 1/2 cup | Acorn, baked, avg | 102 | 0.05 | 0.06 | 0.12 | 0.01 | 0.20 | 0.04 | 0.02 | 0.04 | 0.07 | 0.04 | 0.01 | 0.04 | 0.04 | 0.04 | 0.03 | 0.02 | 0.04 | 0.05 |
| 5800 | 1/2 cup | Acorn, raw, cubes, avg | 70 | 0.02 | 0.03 | 0.06 | 0.00 | 0.10 | 0.02 | 0.01 | 0.02 | 0.03 | 0.02 | 0.01 | 0.02 | 0.02 | 0.02 | 0.02 | 0.01 | 0.02 | 0.02 |
| 5318 | 1/2 cup | Butternut, bkd, mshd, avg | 122 | 0.05 | 0.06 | 0.12 | 0.01 | 0.19 | 0.04 | 0.02 | 0.04 | 0.06 | 0.04 | 0.01 | 0.04 | 0.04 | 0.04 | 0.03 | 0.02 | 0.04 | 0.05 |
| 5274 | 1/2 cup | Butternut, ckd f/fzn, avg | 120 | 0.06 | 0.08 | 0.16 | 0.01 | 0.26 | 0.05 | 0.03 | 0.06 | 0.08 | 0.05 | 0.02 | 0.06 | 0.05 | 0.06 | 0.04 | 0.02 | 0.05 | 0.06 |
| 5801 | 1/2 cup | Butternut, raw, avg | 70 | 0.03 | 0.04 | 0.07 | 0.01 | 0.12 | 0.03 | 0.01 | 0.03 | 0.04 | 0.03 | 0.01 | 0.03 | 0.03 | 0.03 | 0.02 | 0.01 | 0.02 | 0.03 |
| 5322 | 1/2 cup | Crookneck, ckd, avg | 90 | 0.04 | 0.03 | 0.10 | 0.01 | 0.09 | 0.03 | 0.02 | 0.03 | 0.05 | 0.04 | 0.01 | 0.03 | 0.03 | 0.03 | 0.02 | 0.01 | 0.02 | 0.04 |
| 5321 | 1/2 cup | Crookneck, raw, avg | 65 | 0.03 | 0.03 | 0.07 | 0.01 | 0.07 | 0.02 | 0.01 | 0.02 | 0.04 | 0.03 | 0.01 | 0.02 | 0.02 | 0.02 | 0.01 | 0.01 | 0.02 | 0.03 |
| 5453 | 1/2 cup | Hubbard, bkd, avg | 120 | 0.07 | 0.10 | 0.19 | 0.02 | 0.31 | 0.07 | 0.03 | 0.07 | 0.10 | 0.07 | 0.02 | 0.07 | 0.06 | 0.07 | 0.05 | 0.03 | 0.06 | 0.08 |
| 5803 | 1/2 cup | Hubbard, raw, avg | 58 | 0.05 | 0.06 | 0.12 | 0.01 | 0.20 | 0.04 | 0.02 | 0.05 | 0.07 | 0.04 | 0.01 | 0.05 | 0.04 | 0.05 | 0.03 | 0.02 | 0.04 | 0.05 |

TABLE A **Amino Acid Content for Selected Foods *(continued)***

| Code | Amount | Description | Weight (g) | Alanine (g) | Arginine (g) | Aspartic acid (g) | Cystine (g) | Glutamic acid (g) | Glycine (g) | Histidine (g) | Isoleucine (g) | Leucine (g) | Lysine (g) | Methionine (g) | Phenylalanine (g) | Proline (g) | Serine (g) | Threonine (g) | Tryptophan (g) | Tyrosine (g) | Valine (g) |
|---|---|---|---|---|---|---|---|---|---|---|---|---|---|---|---|---|---|---|---|---|---|
| 5325 | 1/2 cup | Scallop, boiled, mshd, unsalted, avg | 120 | 0.06 | 0.05 | 0.15 | 0.01 | 0.13 | 0.05 | 0.03 | 0.04 | 0.07 | 0.07 | 0.02 | 0.04 | 0.04 | 0.05 | 0.03 | 0.01 | 0.03 | 0.06 |
| 5323 | 1/2 cup | Scallop, raw, avg | 65 | 0.04 | 0.03 | 0.10 | 0.01 | 0.08 | 0.03 | 0.02 | 0.03 | 0.05 | 0.04 | 0.01 | 0.03 | 0.02 | 0.03 | 0.02 | 0.01 | 0.02 | 0.04 |
| 5455 | 1/2 cup | Spaghetti, boiled, avg | 78 | 0.02 | 0.03 | 0.05 | 0.00 | 0.08 | 0.02 | 0.01 | 0.02 | 0.03 | 0.02 | 0.01 | 0.02 | 0.02 | 0.02 | 0.01 | 0.01 | 0.02 | 0.02 |
| 5804 | 1/2 cup | Spaghetti, raw, avg | 50 | 0.01 | 0.02 | 0.03 | 0.00 | 0.05 | 0.01 | 0.01 | 0.01 | 0.02 | 0.01 | 0.00 | 0.01 | 0.01 | 0.01 | 0.01 | 0.00 | 0.01 | 0.01 |
| 5152 | 1/2 cup | Summer, boiled, unsalted, avg | 90 | 0.04 | 0.03 | 0.10 | 0.01 | 0.09 | 0.03 | 0.02 | 0.03 | 0.05 | 0.04 | 0.01 | 0.03 | 0.03 | 0.03 | 0.02 | 0.01 | 0.02 | 0.04 |
| 5597 | 1/2 cup | Summer, cnd, drained, unsalted, avg | 108 | 0.03 | 0.03 | 0.08 | 0.01 | 0.07 | 0.02 | 0.01 | 0.02 | 0.04 | 0.04 | 0.01 | 0.02 | 0.02 | 0.03 | 0.02 | 0.01 | 0.02 | 0.03 |
| 5797 | 1/2 cup | Summer, ckd f/fzn, avg | 96 | 0.06 | 0.05 | 0.15 | 0.01 | 0.13 | 0.05 | 0.03 | 0.04 | 0.07 | 0.07 | 0.02 | 0.04 | 0.04 | 0.05 | 0.03 | 0.01 | 0.03 | 0.06 |
| 5151 | 1/2 cup | Summer, raw, avg | 56 | 0.03 | 0.03 | 0.08 | 0.01 | 0.07 | 0.02 | 0.01 | 0.02 | 0.04 | 0.04 | 0.01 | 0.02 | 0.02 | 0.03 | 0.02 | 0.01 | 0.02 | 0.03 |
| 5599 | 1/2 cup | Zucchini, cnd, italian style, avg | 114 | 0.06 | 0.05 | 0.14 | 0.01 | 0.13 | 0.04 | 0.03 | 0.04 | 0.07 | 0.06 | 0.02 | 0.04 | 0.04 | 0.05 | 0.03 | 0.01 | 0.03 | 0.05 |
| 5598 | 1/2 cup | Zucchini, ckd f/fzn, avg | 112 | 0.07 | 0.05 | 0.16 | 0.01 | 0.14 | 0.05 | 0.03 | 0.05 | 0.08 | 0.07 | 0.02 | 0.04 | 0.04 | 0.05 | 0.03 | 0.01 | 0.03 | 0.06 |
| 5624 | 1/2 cup | Zucchini, pickled, avg | 85 | 0.04 | 0.03 | 0.09 | 0.01 | 0.08 | 0.03 | 0.02 | 0.27 | 0.04 | 0.04 | 0.11 | 0.03 | 0.02 | 0.03 | 0.02 | 0.01 | 0.02 | 0.03 |
| 5667 | 1/2 cup | Zucchini, stmd, avg | 90 | 0.05 | 0.04 | 0.13 | 0.01 | 0.11 | 0.04 | 0.02 | 0.04 | 0.06 | 0.06 | 0.02 | 0.04 | 0.03 | 0.04 | 0.03 | 0.01 | 0.03 | 0.05 |
| 5668 | 1/2 cup | Zucchini, stir fried, avg | 90 | 0.05 | 0.04 | 0.13 | 0.01 | 0.11 | 0.04 | 0.02 | 0.04 | 0.06 | 0.06 | 0.02 | 0.04 | 0.03 | 0.04 | 0.03 | 0.01 | 0.03 | 0.05 |
| 5326 | 1/2 cup | Zucchini, raw, avg | 65 | 0.04 | 0.03 | 0.09 | 0.01 | 0.08 | 0.03 | 0.02 | 0.03 | 0.04 | 0.04 | 0.01 | 0.03 | 0.02 | 0.03 | 0.02 | 0.01 | 0.02 | 0.03 |
| 5304 | 1/2 cup | Winter, bkd, mshd, avg | 122 | 0.05 | 0.06 | 0.12 | 0.01 | 0.19 | 0.04 | 0.02 | 0.04 | 0.06 | 0.04 | 0.01 | 0.04 | 0.04 | 0.04 | 0.03 | 0.02 | 0.04 | 0.05 |
| 5833 | 1/2 cup | Winter, raw, avg | 58 | 0.04 | 0.05 | 0.09 | 0.01 | 0.15 | 0.03 | 0.02 | 0.03 | 0.05 | 0.03 | 0.01 | 0.03 | 0.03 | 0.03 | 0.02 | 0.01 | 0.03 | 0.04 |
| | | Sweet Potatoes/Yams | | | | | | | | | | | | | | | | | | | |
| 5158 | 1/2 cup | Baked, avg | 100 | 0.09 | 0.08 | 0.29 | 0.01 | 0.17 | 0.08 | 0.03 | 0.09 | 0.13 | 0.09 | 0.04 | 0.10 | 0.08 | 0.09 | 0.09 | 0.02 | 0.07 | 0.11 |
| 5161 | 1/2 cup | Boiled, avg | 164 | 0.15 | 0.13 | 0.46 | 0.02 | 0.26 | 0.12 | 0.05 | 0.13 | 0.20 | 0.13 | 0.07 | 0.16 | 0.12 | 0.14 | 0.13 | 0.03 | 0.11 | 0.18 |
| 5162 | 1/2 cup | Canned, mshd, avg | 128 | 0.14 | 0.12 | 0.43 | 0.02 | 0.25 | 0.11 | 0.05 | 0.13 | 0.19 | 0.12 | 0.06 | 0.15 | 0.11 | 0.13 | 0.13 | 0.03 | 0.10 | 0.17 |
| 5552 | 1/2 cup | Canned, w/syrup, avg | 114 | 0.06 | 0.05 | 0.19 | 0.01 | 0.11 | 0.05 | 0.02 | 0.06 | 0.08 | 0.05 | 0.03 | 0.07 | 0.05 | 0.06 | 0.06 | 0.01 | 0.05 | 0.07 |
| 5542 | 1/2 cup | Frozen, bkd, avg | 88 | 0.08 | 0.07 | 0.26 | 0.01 | 0.15 | 0.07 | 0.03 | 0.08 | 0.11 | 0.07 | 0.04 | 0.09 | 0.07 | 0.08 | 0.07 | 0.02 | 0.06 | 0.10 |
| 6880 | 1/2 cup | Raw, avg | 66 | 0.06 | 0.05 | 0.19 | 0.01 | 0.11 | 0.05 | 0.02 | 0.05 | 0.08 | 0.05 | 0.03 | 0.07 | 0.05 | 0.06 | 0.05 | 0.01 | 0.04 | 0.07 |
| 5059 | 1/2 cup | Swiss Chard, boiled, avg | 88 | 0.00 | 0.11 | 0.00 | 0.00 | 0.00 | 0.00 | 0.03 | 0.14 | 0.12 | 0.09 | 0.02 | 0.10 | 0.00 | 0.00 | 0.08 | 0.02 | 0.00 | 0.10 |
| 5057 | 1/2 cup | Swiss Chard, raw, avg | 18 | 0.00 | 0.02 | 0.00 | 0.00 | 0.00 | 0.00 | 0.01 | 0.03 | 0.02 | 0.02 | 0.00 | 0.02 | 0.00 | 0.00 | 0.01 | 0.00 | 0.00 | 0.02 |
| 5369 | 1/2 cup | Taro, raw, slices, avg | 52 | 0.04 | 0.05 | 0.10 | 0.02 | 0.09 | 0.04 | 0.02 | 0.03 | 0.06 | 0.03 | 0.01 | 0.04 | 0.03 | 0.05 | 0.04 | 0.01 | 0.03 | 0.04 |
| | | Tomatoes | | | | | | | | | | | | | | | | | | | |
| 6927 | 1/2 cup | Canned, crushed, avg | 55 | 0.02 | 0.02 | 0.12 | 0.01 | 0.31 | 0.02 | 0.01 | 0.02 | 0.03 | 0.03 | 0.01 | 0.02 | 0.02 | 0.02 | 0.02 | 0.01 | 0.01 | 0.02 |
| 5474 | 1/2 cup | Canned, stewed, avg | 128 | 0.03 | 0.03 | 0.17 | 0.02 | 0.45 | 0.03 | 0.02 | 0.03 | 0.04 | 0.04 | 0.01 | 0.03 | 0.02 | 0.03 | 0.03 | 0.01 | 0.02 | 0.03 |
| 5179 | 1/2 cup | Canned, unsalted, avg | 120 | 0.03 | 0.03 | 0.15 | 0.01 | 0.41 | 0.03 | 0.02 | 0.03 | 0.04 | 0.04 | 0.01 | 0.03 | 0.02 | 0.03 | 0.03 | 0.01 | 0.02 | 0.03 |
| 5545 | 1/2 cup | Canned, wedges in tomato juice, avg | 130 | 0.03 | 0.02 | 0.14 | 0.01 | 0.38 | 0.03 | 0.02 | 0.02 | 0.04 | 0.04 | 0.01 | 0.03 | 0.02 | 0.03 | 0.03 | 0.01 | 0.02 | 0.03 |
| 5471 | 1/2 cup | Canned, whole, unsalted, avg | 120 | 0.03 | 0.03 | 0.15 | 0.01 | 0.41 | 0.03 | 0.02 | 0.03 | 0.04 | 0.04 | 0.01 | 0.03 | 0.02 | 0.03 | 0.03 | 0.01 | 0.02 | 0.03 |
| 5546 | 1/2 cup | Canned, w/green chilies, avg | 120 | 0.02 | 0.02 | 0.12 | 0.01 | 0.31 | 0.02 | 0.01 | 0.02 | 0.03 | 0.03 | 0.01 | 0.02 | 0.02 | 0.02 | 0.02 | 0.01 | 0.01 | 0.02 |
| 5519 | 1/2 cup | Green, raw, chpd, avg | 90 | 0.03 | 0.03 | 0.15 | 0.01 | 0.40 | 0.03 | 0.02 | 0.03 | 0.04 | 0.04 | 0.01 | 0.03 | 0.02 | 0.03 | 0.03 | 0.01 | 0.02 | 0.03 |
| 5473 | 1/2 cup | Paste, avg | 131 | 0.15 | 0.10 | 0.60 | 0.03 | 1.93 | 0.08 | 0.08 | 0.09 | 0.13 | 0.14 | 0.02 | 0.10 | 0.11 | 0.11 | 0.11 | 0.03 | 0.07 | 0.10 |
| 5181 | 1/2 cup | Paste, unsalted, avg | 131 | 0.15 | 0.10 | 0.60 | 0.03 | 1.93 | 0.08 | 0.08 | 0.09 | 0.13 | 0.14 | 0.02 | 0.10 | 0.11 | 0.11 | 0.11 | 0.03 | 0.07 | 0.10 |
| 5476 | 1/2 cup | Puree, avg | 125 | 0.07 | 0.04 | 0.26 | 0.01 | 0.85 | 0.04 | 0.03 | 0.04 | 0.06 | 0.06 | 0.01 | 0.04 | 0.05 | 0.05 | 0.05 | 0.01 | 0.03 | 0.04 |
| 5225 | 1/2 cup | Puree, unsalted, avg | 125 | 0.07 | 0.04 | 0.26 | 0.01 | 0.85 | 0.04 | 0.03 | 0.04 | 0.06 | 0.06 | 0.01 | 0.04 | 0.05 | 0.05 | 0.05 | 0.01 | 0.03 | 0.04 |
| 5178 | 1/2 cup | Raw, boiled, unsalted, avg | 120 | 0.04 | 0.03 | 0.18 | 0.02 | 0.47 | 0.03 | 0.02 | 0.03 | 0.05 | 0.05 | 0.01 | 0.03 | 0.02 | 0.03 | 0.03 | 0.01 | 0.02 | 0.03 |
| 5627 | 1 ea | Raw, brld, avg | 123 | 0.04 | 0.03 | 0.19 | 0.02 | 0.50 | 0.03 | 0.02 | 0.03 | 0.05 | 0.05 | 0.01 | 0.04 | 0.03 | 0.04 | 0.03 | 0.01 | 0.02 | 0.04 |
| 5170 | 1/2 cup | Raw, chpd, avg | 90 | 0.02 | 0.02 | 0.11 | 0.01 | 0.28 | 0.02 | 0.01 | 0.02 | 0.03 | 0.03 | 0.01 | 0.02 | 0.01 | 0.02 | 0.02 | 0.01 | 0.01 | 0.02 |
| 5628 | 1 ea | Raw, fried, avg | 101 | 0.07 | 0.06 | 0.36 | 0.03 | 0.97 | 0.06 | 0.04 | 0.06 | 0.10 | 0.10 | 0.02 | 0.07 | 0.05 | 0.07 | 0.06 | 0.02 | 0.05 | 0.07 |
| 5468 | 1/2 cup | Raw, stewed, avg | 50 | 0.03 | 0.03 | 0.09 | 0.01 | 0.32 | 0.03 | 0.02 | 0.03 | 0.05 | 0.03 | 0.01 | 0.04 | 0.06 | 0.04 | 0.03 | 0.01 | 0.02 | 0.04 |
| 5180 | 1/2 cup | Sauce, cnd, avg | 122 | 0.05 | 0.03 | 0.20 | 0.01 | 0.65 | 0.03 | 0.03 | 0.03 | 0.05 | 0.05 | 0.01 | 0.03 | 0.04 | 0.04 | 0.04 | 0.01 | 0.02 | 0.03 |
| 5446 | 1/2 cup | Sun Dried, avg | 27 | 0.11 | 0.09 | 0.53 | 0.05 | 1.40 | 0.09 | 0.06 | 0.09 | 0.14 | 0.14 | 0.03 | 0.10 | 0.07 | 0.10 | 0.10 | 0.03 | 0.07 | 0.10 |
| 7482 | 1/2 cup | Sun Dried, packed in oil, drained, avg | 55 | 0.08 | 0.07 | 0.39 | 0.04 | 1.03 | 0.07 | 0.04 | 0.07 | 0.10 | 0.10 | 0.02 | 0.07 | 0.05 | 0.07 | 0.07 | 0.02 | 0.05 | 0.07 |
| | | Turnips | | | | | | | | | | | | | | | | | | | |
| 5184 | 1/2 cup | Boiled, mshd, unsalted, avg | 58 | 0.02 | 0.01 | 0.03 | 0.00 | 0.06 | 0.01 | 0.01 | 0.02 | 0.02 | 0.02 | 0.01 | 0.01 | 0.01 | 0.01 | 0.01 | 0.00 | 0.01 | 0.01 |
| 5819 | 1/2 cup | Frozen, boiled, avg | 78 | 0.05 | 0.03 | 0.08 | 0.01 | 0.17 | 0.03 | 0.02 | 0.05 | 0.04 | 0.05 | 0.01 | 0.02 | 0.04 | 0.04 | 0.03 | 0.01 | 0.02 | 0.04 |
| 5820 | 1/2 cup | Greens, cnd, w/liquid, avg | 117 | 0.11 | 0.10 | 0.16 | 0.02 | 0.21 | 0.09 | 0.04 | 0.08 | 0.14 | 0.10 | 0.04 | 0.09 | 0.07 | 0.06 | 0.08 | 0.03 | 0.06 | 0.11 |

TABLE A **Amino Acid Content for Selected Foods *(continued)***

| Code | Amount | Description | Weight (g) | Alaninine (g) | Arginine (g) | Aspartic acid (g) | Cystine (g) | Glutamic acid (g) | Glycine (g) | Histidine (g) | Isoleucine (g) | Leucine (g) | Lysine (g) | Methionine (g) | Phenylalanine (g) | Proline (g) | Serine (g) | Threonine (g) | Tryptophan (g) | Tyrosine (g) | Valine (g) |
|---|---|---|---|---|---|---|---|---|---|---|---|---|---|---|---|---|---|---|---|---|---|
| 5186 | 1/2 cup | Greens, fzn, boiled, avg | 82 | 0.18 | 0.17 | 0.28 | 0.03 | 0.36 | 0.16 | 0.06 | 0.14 | 0.24 | 0.17 | 0.05 | 0.16 | 0.13 | 0.11 | 0.15 | 0.05 | 0.10 | 0.18 |
| 5185 | 1/2 cup | Greens, raw, boiled, avg | 72 | 0.05 | 0.05 | 0.08 | 0.01 | 0.11 | 0.05 | 0.02 | 0.04 | 0.07 | 0.05 | 0.02 | 0.05 | 0.04 | 0.03 | 0.04 | 0.01 | 0.03 | 0.05 |
| 5547 | 1/2 cup | Greens, raw, chpd, avg | 27 | 0.03 | 0.02 | 0.04 | 0.00 | 0.05 | 0.02 | 0.01 | 0.02 | 0.04 | 0.03 | 0.01 | 0.02 | 0.02 | 0.02 | 0.02 | 0.01 | 0.02 | 0.03 |
| 5623 | 10 ea | Pickled, avg | 70 | 0.02 | 0.02 | 0.04 | 0.00 | 0.09 | 0.02 | 0.01 | 0.02 | 0.02 | 0.02 | 0.01 | 0.01 | 0.02 | 0.02 | 0.02 | 0.01 | 0.01 | 0.02 |
| 5182 | 1/2 cup | Raw, avg | 65 | 0.02 | 0.02 | 0.04 | 0.00 | 0.08 | 0.02 | 0.01 | 0.02 | 0.02 | 0.02 | 0.01 | 0.01 | 0.02 | 0.02 | 0.02 | 0.01 | 0.01 | 0.02 |
| 5823 | 1/2 cup | With Greens, fzn, boiled, avg | 86 | 0.11 | 0.09 | 0.17 | 0.02 | 0.25 | 0.09 | 0.04 | 0.09 | 0.13 | 0.10 | 0.04 | 0.09 | 0.07 | 0.07 | 0.08 | 0.03 | 0.06 | 0.10 |
| 5222 | 1/2 cup | Watercress, fresh, avg | 17 | 0.02 | 0.03 | 0.03 | 0.00 | 0.03 | 0.02 | 0.01 | 0.02 | 0.03 | 0.02 | 0.00 | 0.02 | 0.02 | 0.01 | 0.02 | 0.01 | 0.01 | 0.02 |
| 5436 | 1/2 cup | Yambean/Jicama, boiled, avg | 50 | 0.01 | 0.02 | 0.10 | 0.00 | 0.02 | 0.01 | 0.01 | 0.01 | 0.01 | 0.01 | 0.00 | 0.01 | 0.01 | 0.01 | 0.01 | 0.00 | 0.01 | 0.01 |
| 5224 | 1/2 cup | Yambean/Jicama, raw, avg | 60 | 0.02 | 0.04 | 0.23 | 0.01 | 0.05 | 0.02 | 0.02 | 0.02 | 0.03 | 0.03 | 0.00 | 0.02 | 0.03 | 0.03 | 0.02 | 0.00 | 0.01 | 0.03 |
| | | Yellow Wax Beans | | | | | | | | | | | | | | | | | | | |
| 5194 | 1/2 cup | Boiled, avg | 62 | 0.05 | 0.05 | 0.16 | 0.01 | 0.12 | 0.04 | 0.02 | 0.04 | 0.07 | 0.06 | 0.01 | 0.04 | 0.04 | 0.06 | 0.05 | 0.01 | 0.03 | 0.06 |
| 5195 | 1/2 cup | Frozen, boiled, avg | 68 | 0.05 | 0.04 | 0.14 | 0.01 | 0.10 | 0.04 | 0.02 | 0.04 | 0.06 | 0.05 | 0.01 | 0.04 | 0.04 | 0.06 | 0.04 | 0.01 | 0.02 | 0.05 |
| 6095 | 1/2 cup | Snap, cnd, avg | 120 | 0.04 | 0.04 | 0.13 | 0.01 | 0.10 | 0.03 | 0.02 | 0.03 | 0.06 | 0.05 | 0.01 | 0.03 | 0.03 | 0.05 | 0.04 | 0.01 | 0.02 | 0.05 |
| 6094 | 1/2 cup | Snap, cnd, low sod, avg | 120 | 0.04 | 0.04 | 0.13 | 0.01 | 0.10 | 0.03 | 0.02 | 0.03 | 0.06 | 0.05 | 0.01 | 0.03 | 0.03 | 0.05 | 0.04 | 0.01 | 0.02 | 0.05 |
| 5320 | 1/2 cup | Snap, raw, avg | 55 | 0.05 | 0.04 | 0.14 | 0.01 | 0.10 | 0.04 | 0.02 | 0.04 | 0.06 | 0.05 | 0.01 | 0.04 | 0.04 | 0.05 | 0.04 | 0.01 | 0.02 | 0.05 |
| | | **MISCELLANEOUS** | | | | | | | | | | | | | | | | | | | |
| 27000 | 1 Tbs | Catsup, avg | 15 | 0.01 | 0.00 | 0.03 | 0.00 | 0.09 | 0.00 | 0.00 | 0.00 | 0.01 | 0.01 | 0.00 | 0.00 | 0.00 | 0.01 | 0.01 | 0.00 | 0.00 | 0.00 |
| 27032 | 1 Tbs | Catsup, low salt, avg | 15 | 0.01 | 0.00 | 0.03 | 0.00 | 0.09 | 0.00 | 0.00 | 0.00 | 0.01 | 0.01 | 0.00 | 0.00 | 0.00 | 0.01 | 0.01 | 0.00 | 0.00 | 0.00 |
| 53015 | 1 Tbs | Cheese Sauce, avg | 13 | 0.04 | 0.05 | 0.08 | 0.01 | 0.30 | 0.02 | 0.04 | 0.07 | 0.11 | 0.09 | 0.03 | 0.06 | 0.13 | 0.07 | 0.05 | 0.02 | 0.06 | 0.08 |
| 53097 | 1 Tbs | Cheese Sauce, lowfat, avg | 15 | 0.04 | 0.06 | 0.09 | 0.01 | 0.29 | 0.03 | 0.05 | 0.07 | 0.12 | 0.13 | 0.04 | 0.07 | 0.14 | 0.07 | 0.05 | 0.02 | 0.07 | 0.08 |
| 30000 | 1 Tbs | Cornstarch, avg | 8 | 0.00 | 0.00 | 0.00 | 0.00 | 0.00 | 0.00 | 0.00 | 0.00 | 0.00 | 0.00 | 0.00 | 0.00 | 0.00 | 0.00 | 0.00 | 0.00 | 0.00 | 0.00 |
| 27019 | 1 Tbs | Cranberry Orange Relish, avg | 17 | 0.00 | 0.00 | 0.00 | 0.00 | 0.00 | 0.00 | 0.00 | 0.00 | 0.00 | 0.00 | 0.00 | 0.00 | 0.00 | 0.00 | 0.00 | 0.00 | 0.00 | 0.00 |
| 27053 | 1 Tbs | Pickle Relish, hamburger, avg | 15 | 0.00 | 0.01 | 0.01 | 0.00 | 0.02 | 0.00 | 0.00 | 0.00 | 0.00 | 0.00 | 0.00 | 0.00 | 0.00 | 0.00 | 0.00 | 0.00 | 0.00 | 0.00 |
| 27051 | 1 Tbs | Pickle Relish, hot dog, avg | 15 | 0.01 | 0.01 | 0.01 | 0.00 | 0.05 | 0.01 | 0.00 | 0.01 | 0.01 | 0.01 | 0.00 | 0.01 | 0.01 | 0.01 | 0.01 | 0.00 | 0.00 | 0.01 |
| | | Pickles | | | | | | | | | | | | | | | | | | | |
| 27012 | 1 ea | Dill, avg | 65 | 0.01 | 0.03 | 0.02 | 0.00 | 0.12 | 0.01 | 0.01 | 0.01 | 0.02 | 0.02 | 0.00 | 0.01 | 0.01 | 0.01 | 0.01 | 0.00 | 0.01 | 0.01 |
| 27039 | 1 ea | Dill, low salt, avg | 65 | 0.01 | 0.03 | 0.02 | 0.00 | 0.11 | 0.01 | 0.01 | 0.01 | 0.02 | 0.02 | 0.00 | 0.01 | 0.01 | 0.01 | 0.01 | 0.00 | 0.01 | 0.01 |
| 27023 | 1 ea | Sour, medium, avg | 35 | 0.00 | 0.01 | 0.01 | 0.00 | 0.03 | 0.00 | 0.00 | 0.00 | 0.00 | 0.00 | 0.00 | 0.00 | 0.00 | 0.00 | 0.00 | 0.00 | 0.00 | 0.00 |
| 27026 | 1 ea | Sour, medium, low salt, avg | 35 | 0.00 | 0.01 | 0.01 | 0.00 | 0.03 | 0.00 | 0.00 | 0.00 | 0.00 | 0.00 | 0.00 | 0.00 | 0.00 | 0.00 | 0.00 | 0.00 | 0.00 | 0.00 |
| 27016 | 1 ea | Sweet, medium, avg | 35 | 0.00 | 0.01 | 0.01 | 0.00 | 0.04 | 0.00 | 0.00 | 0.00 | 0.01 | 0.01 | 0.00 | 0.00 | 0.00 | 0.00 | 0.00 | 0.00 | 0.00 | 0.00 |
| 27030 | 1 ea | Sweet, medium, low salt, avg | 35 | 0.00 | 0.01 | 0.01 | 0.00 | 0.04 | 0.00 | 0.00 | 0.00 | 0.01 | 0.01 | 0.00 | 0.00 | 0.00 | 0.00 | 0.00 | 0.00 | 0.00 | 0.00 |
| 90035 | 1 Tbs | Soy Sauce, low sodium, avg | 18 | 0.04 | 0.06 | 0.09 | 0.02 | 0.21 | 0.04 | 0.02 | 0.04 | 0.07 | 0.05 | 0.01 | 0.05 | 0.06 | 0.05 | 0.04 | 0.01 | 0.03 | 0.04 |
| | | Yeast | | | | | | | | | | | | | | | | | | | |
| 28007 | 1 ea | Bakers, compressed cake, avg | 17 | 0.09 | 0.08 | 0.14 | 0.02 | 0.21 | 0.07 | 0.04 | 0.03 | 0.11 | 0.12 | 0.03 | 0.07 | 0.06 | 0.07 | 0.07 | 0.02 | 0.06 | 0.09 |
| 28001 | 1 ea | Bakers, dry active, pkt, avg | 7 | 0.18 | 0.15 | 0.27 | 0.04 | 0.39 | 0.13 | 0.07 | 0.15 | 0.21 | 0.22 | 0.05 | 0.13 | 0.11 | 0.13 | 0.14 | 0.03 | 0.11 | 0.16 |
| 40072 | 1/2 oz | Torula, avg | 7 | 0.01 | 0.01 | 0.01 | 0.03 | 0.03 | 0.01 | 0.00 | 0.01 | 0.01 | 0.01 | 0.00 | 0.01 | 0.01 | 0.01 | 0.00 | 0.00 | 0.01 | 0.01 |

TABLE B **Alcoholic Content of Selected Foods**

| ESHA | Amount | | Description | Wgt (g) | Alcohol (g) |
|---|---|---|---|---|---|
| | | | **ALCOHOLIC BEVERAGES** | | |
| | | | Beer, 12 fl oz | | |
| 22824 | 1 | ea | Bud Dry | 356 | 13.90 |
| 22822 | 1 | ea | Bud Light | 356 | 15.30 |
| 22737 | 1 | ea | Budweiser | 357 | 13.90 |
| 22739 | 1 | ea | Coors Premium | 360 | 14.76 |
| 22632 | 1 | ea | Icehouse | 355 | 17.75 |
| 22610 | 1 | ea | Lowenbrau Dark | 355 | 17.40 |
| 22743 | 1 | ea | Lowenbrau Malt Liquor | 356 | 21.00 |
| 22744 | 1 | ea | Lowenbrau Special | 356 | 17.44 |
| 22745 | 1 | ea | Magnum | 356 | 21.00 |
| 22747 | 1 | ea | Meister Brau | 356 | 16.02 |
| 22748 | 1 | ea | Meister Brau, light | 356 | 16.02 |
| 22749 | 1 | ea | Miller Genuine Draft | 356 | 17.83 |
| 22750 | 1 | ea | Miller Genuine Draft, light | 356 | 16.02 |
| 22751 | 1 | ea | Miller High Life | 356 | 17.83 |
| 22753 | 1 | ea | Miller High Life, light | 356 | 16.02 |
| 22752 | 1 | ea | Miller High Life Ice | 356 | 20.03 |
| 22754 | 1 | ea | Miller Lite | 356 | 16.02 |
| 22755 | 1 | ea | Miller Lite Ice 5.0 | 356 | 17.83 |
| 22758 | 1 | ea | Miller Reserve Lager | 356 | 17.83 |
| 22759 | 1 | ea | Miller Reserve Velvet Stout | 356 | 18.13 |
| 22760 | 1 | ea | Milwaukee's Best | 356 | 16.42 |
| 22761 | 1 | ea | Milwaukee's Best Ice | 356 | 20.03 |
| 22762 | 1 | ea | Milwaukee's Best, light | 356 | 16.02 |
| 22691 | 1 | ea | Near Beer, nonalcoholic | 356 | 1.07 |
| 22826 | 1 | ea | O'Doul's, nonalcoholic | 361 | 1.10 |
| 22764 | 1 | ea | Red Dog | 356 | 17.83 |
| | | | Distilled Spirits, 80 Proof, avg, 1.5 fl oz | | |
| 22696 | 1 | ea | Bourbon | 42 | 14.03 |
| 22692 | 1 | ea | Brandy | 42 | 14.03 |
| 22693 | 1 | ea | Gin | 42 | 14.03 |
| 22729 | 1 | ea | Rum | 42 | 14.03 |
| 22731 | 1 | ea | Vodka | 42 | 14.03 |
| 22694 | 1 | ea | Tequila | 42 | 14.03 |
| 22695 | 1 | ea | Whiskey | 42 | 14.03 |
| | | | Liqueur or Cordial, avg, 1.5 fl oz | | |
| 22547 | 1 | ea | Amaretto | 30 | 7.73 |
| 22548 | 1 | ea | Anisette | 30 | 7.73 |
| 22597 | 1 | ea | Cherry Brandy | 48 | 9.12 |
| 22734 | 1 | ea | Coffee Liqueur | 52 | 11.28 |
| 22736 | 1 | ea | Coffee Liqueur, w/cream | 47 | 6.49 |
| 22732 | 1 | ea | Crème De Menthe | 50 | 14.90 |
| 22549 | 1 | ea | Drambuie | 30 | 7.73 |
| 22550 | 1 | ea | Grenadine | 30 | 7.73 |
| 22551 | 1 | ea | Kahlua | 30 | 7.73 |
| 22552 | 1 | ea | Sloe Gin | 30 | 7.73 |
| 22553 | 1 | ea | Tia Maria | 30 | 7.73 |
| 22554 | 1 | ea | Triple Sec | 30 | 7.73 |
| | | | Mixed Drinks, avg | | |
| 22555 | 1 | ea | Bacardi Cocktail | 63 | 13.77 |
| 22563 | 1 | ea | Black Russian | 90 | 26.11 |
| 22795 | 1 | ea | Bloody Mary | 238 | 22.37 |
| 22796 | 1 | ea | Bourbon & Soda | 232 | 30.16 |
| 22802 | 1 | ea | Coffee Royale | 211 | 13.21 |
| 22797 | 1 | ea | Coquito, P.R., coconut & rum | 263 | 27.22 |
| 22682 | 1 | ea | Gibson | 213 | 68.20 |

TABLE B *(continued)*

| ESHA | Amount | | Description | Wgt (g) | Alcohol (g) |
|---|---|---|---|---|---|
| 125 | 1 | ea | Gin Fizz | 225 | 17.12 |
| 22800 | 1 | ea | Gin & Tonic | 240 | 17.04 |
| 22559 | 1 | ea | Harvey Wallbanger | 213 | 15.15 |
| 22556 | 1 | ea | High Ball | 160 | 15.08 |
| 22808 | 1 | ea | Hot Buttered Rum | 211 | 23.55 |
| 22801 | 1 | ea | Irish Coffee | 211 | 13.21 |
| 22566 | 1 | ea | Mai Tai | 126 | 27.49 |
| 22804 | 1 | ea | Manhattan | 228 | 69.77 |
| 22557 | 1 | ea | Margarita | 77 | 18.38 |
| 22805 | 1 | ea | Martini | 226 | 80.32 |
| 22805 | 1 | ea | Martini | 226 | 72.32 |
| 22803 | 1 | ea | Mexican Eggnog, rompope | 243 | 14.82 |
| 22558 | 1 | ea | Mint Julep | 65 | 20.29 |
| 22568 | 1 | ea | Long Island Iced Tea | 125 | 12.25 |
| 22805 | 1 | ea | Pina Colada | 251 | 80.32 |
| 22805 | 1 | ea | Pina Colada | 251 | 72.32 |
| 22809 | 1 | ea | Screwdriver | 243 | 16.04 |
| 22565 | 1 | ea | Singapore Sling | 225 | 26.21 |
| 22560 | 1 | ea | Slo-Screw | 213 | 15.15 |
| 22562 | 1 | ea | Sloe Gin Fizz | 222 | 15.93 |
| 22810 | 1 | ea | Tequila Sunrise | 250 | 27.25 |
| 22812 | 1 | ea | Tom Collins | 237 | 17.06 |
| 22564 | 1 | ea | White Russian | 100 | 26.10 |
| 22813 | 1 | ea | Whiskey Sour | 243 | 34.26 |
| | | | Wine, Table, 6 fl oz | | |
| 22769 | 1 | ea | All table types | 177 | 16.46 |
| 22780 | 1 | ea | Chinese wine | 177 | 16.46 |
| 22778 | 1 | ea | Japanese Mirin wine | 178 | 24.03 |
| 22779 | 1 | ea | Japanese Plum wine | 178 | 21.36 |
| 22782 | 1 | ea | Japanese Rice wine | 177 | 28.50 |
| 22794 | 1 | ea | Japanese Sake/Saki wine | 178 | 28.66 |
| 22790 | 1 | ea | Red wine | 177 | 16.46 |
| 22792 | 1 | ea | Red Burgundy wine | 176 | 16.37 |
| 22793 | 1 | ea | Red Claret wine | 176 | 16.37 |
| 22771 | 1 | ea | Red Rose' wine | 177 | 16.46 |
| 22791 | 1 | ea | Red Sherry wine, dry | 176 | 16.37 |
| 22770 | 1 | ea | Sangria wine | 177 | 9.65 |
| 22768 | 1 | ea | White wine, medium | 177 | 16.46 |
| 22765 | 1 | ea | Wine Cooler, 12 fl oz | 340 | 31.62 |
| 22766 | 1 | ea | Wine Spritzer, 12 fl oz | 340 | 18.84 |
| | | | Wine, Cooking | | |
| 22603 | 2 | Tbs | Burgundy | 30 | 3.60 |
| 22605 | 2 | Tbs | Chablis | 30 | 3.60 |
| 22608 | 2 | Tbs | Red, Fleischmann's | 30 | 3.60 |
| 27074 | 2 | Tbs | Sauterne, Regina | 30 | 0.35 |
| 22607 | 2 | Tbs | Sherry, Fleischmann's | 30 | 5.10 |
| | | | Wine, Dessert, 6 fl oz | | |
| 22785 | 1 | ea | Dry dessert wine | 177 | 27.08 |
| 22789 | 1 | ea | Madeira dessert wine | 177 | 27.08 |
| 22787 | 1 | ea | Marsala dessert wine | 177 | 27.08 |
| 22788 | 1 | ea | Port dessert wine | 177 | 27.08 |
| 22786 | 1 | ea | Sweet dessert wine | 177 | 27.08 |
| 22784 | 1 | ea | Sweet vermouth dessert wine | 180 | 27.54 |
| | | | **OTHER FOODS** | | |
| 1440 | 1 | Tbs | American Cheese Fondue, avg | 14 | 0.04 |
| 26624 | 1 | tsp | Vanilla Extract, avg | 4 | 1.38 |
| 26625 | 1 | tsp | Vanilla Extract, imitation, avg | 4 | 1.32 |

TABLE C **Caffeine Content of Selected Foods**

| Code | Amount | Description | Wgt (g) | Caffeine (g) |
|---|---|---|---|---|
| | | **BEVERAGES** | | |
| 22734 | 1 ea | Alcoholic, coffee liqueur, 1.5 fl oz | 52 | 13.52 |
| 22736 | 1 ea | Alcoholic, coffee liqueur, w/cream, 1.5 fl oz | 47 | 7.05 |
| | | Carbonated, 1 1/2 cups, 12 fl oz | | |
| 20171 | 1 1/2 cup | Cherry Cola, Shasta | 360 | 0.04 |
| 20481 | 1 1/2 cup | Cherry Cola, diet, Shasta | 360 | 0.04 |
| 20148 | 1 1/2 cup | Coca Cola, Classic | 373 | 46.46 |
| 20149 | 1 1/2 cup | Coca Cola, Cherry | 375 | 46.48 |
| 20515 | 1 1/2 cup | Coca Cola, Cherry, diet | 359 | 46.47 |
| 20271 | 1 1/2 cup | Mountain Dew | 360 | 55.00 |
| 20272 | 1 1/2 cup | Mountain Dew, Diet | 360 | 55.00 |
| 20166 | 1 1/2 cup | Pepsi Cola | 360 | 37.00 |
| 20167 | 1 1/2 cup | Pepsi Cola, Diet | 360 | 36.00 |
| 20270 | 1 1/2 cup | Pepsi Cola, Wild Cherry | 360 | 38.00 |
| 20518 | 1 1/2 cup | Root Beer, Barqs | 376 | 22.51 |
| 20165 | 1 1/2 cup | Tab | 359 | 46.47 |
| | | Coffee | | |
| 20012 | 1 cup | Brewed Coffee, avg | 237 | 137.46 |
| 20065 | 1 cup | Brewed Coffee, decaf, avg | 240 | 2.40 |
| 20044 | 1 cup | Cappuccino w/sugar, avg | 256 | 99.84 |
| 20439 | 1 cup | Espresso, brewed, avg | 237 | 502.44 |
| 20064 | 1 cup | Espresso, brewed, decaf, avg | 240 | 4.80 |
| 20108 | 1 cup | Instant, French, w/sugar, prep f/pwd, avg | 252 | 68.04 |
| 20109 | 1 cup | Instant, Mocha, w/sugar, prep f/pwd, avg | 250 | 45.00 |
| 20089 | 1 cup | Instant, pre-lightened, prep, avg | 180 | 100.80 |
| 20023 | 1 cup | Instant, prep f/pwd, avg | 238 | 76.16 |
| 20091 | 1 cup | Instant, prep f/pwd, decaf, avg | 179 | 1.79 |
| 20087 | 1 cup | Instant, pre-swtnd w/sugar, prep, avg | 180 | 100.80 |
| 20088 | 1 cup | Instant, pre-swtnd w/sugar & pre-lightnd, prep, avg | 180 | 95.40 |
| 20043 | 1 cup | Instant, Swiss mocha, prep, avg | 188 | 40.98 |
| 20093 | 1 cup | Instant, w/chicory, prep f/pwd, avg | 179 | 37.59 |
| | | Chocolate | | |
| 39 | 1 cup | Chocolate Drink, Prep w/milk, avg | 266 | 7.98 |
| 151 | 1 cup | Chocolate Drink, Prep w/water, sugar free, avg | 272 | 5.44 |
| 38 | 1 cup | Chocolate Malt, prep f/mix, avg | 265 | 5.30 |
| 19 | 1 cup | Chocolate Milk, Lowfat, 1%, avg | 250 | 5.00 |
| 18 | 1 cup | Chocolate Milk, Lowfat, 2%, avg | 250 | 5.00 |
| 59 | 1 cup | Chocolate Milk, Nonfat, avg | 250 | 7.50 |
| 70 | 1 cup | Chocolate Milk, Prep w/whole milk & syrup, avg | 263 | 2.63 |
| 197 | 1 cup | Chocolate Milk Shake, avg | 227 | 4.54 |
| 20 | 1 cup | Chocolate Milk, Whole, avg | 250 | 5.00 |
| | | Cocoa | | |
| 48 | 1 cup | Hot, prep w/water, avg | 275 | 5.50 |
| 77 | 1 cup | Hot, prep w/water, low cal, avg | 256 | 20.48 |
| 21 | 1 cup | Hot, prep w/whole milk, avg | 250 | 5.00 |
| 73 | 1 cup | Prep w/water, avg | 279 | 8.37 |
| | | Tea | | |
| 20014 | 1 cup | Brewed Tea, black, avg | 237 | 47.40 |
| 20040 | 1 cup | Instant Iced Tea, Lemon, diet, prep, avg | 237 | 35.55 |
| 20541 | 1 cup | RTS, Earl Grey, Nestea | 246 | 33.03 |

TABLE C *(continued)*

| Code | Amount | | Description | Wgt (g) | Caffeine (g) |
|---|---|---|---|---|---|
| 20543 | 1 | cup | RTS, Extra Sweet w/Lemon, Nestea | 249 | 17.01 |
| 20540 | 1 | cup | RTS, Lemon, diet, Nestea | 240 | 11.02 |
| 20542 | 1 | cup | RTS, Lemon, swtnd, Nestea | 247 | 10.99 |
| | | | **CANDIES AND CONFECTIONS** | | |
| | | | Baking Chocolate and Coating | | |
| 23208 | 1 | oz | Bittersweet Coating, Blue Ribbon | 28 | 17.36 |
| 23044 | 1 | ea | Bittersweet Square, avg | 28 | 29.68 |
| 23418 | 1 | ea | Mexican Squares, avg | 20 | 7.00 |
| 23209 | 1 | oz | Milk Chocolate Coating, avg | 28 | 7.00 |
| 23200 | 1/2 | cup | Semi-Sweet Chocolate, w/butter, avg | 85 | 52.70 |
| 23178 | 1 | oz | Unsweetened, ChocoBake, pre-mltd | 28 | 29.40 |
| 23010 | 1 | ea | Unsweetened Square, avg | 28 | 57.12 |
| 23011 | 1/2 | cup | Unsweetened Square, grated, avg | 66 | 134.64 |
| 23179 | 1 | oz | Unsweetened Bar, Nestle | 28 | 22.96 |
| | | | Baking Chips & Morsels | | |
| 23207 | 1/2 | cup | Chocolate Bittersweet Chips, Ambrosia | 86 | 53.32 |
| 23378 | 2 | Tbs | Crunch Pieces, choc&crspd rice, Nestle | 24 | 5.76 |
| 23423 | 1 | Tbs | Milk Chocolate, M&M's mini bits | 14 | 2.48 |
| 23181 | 1/2 | cup | Milk Chocolate Morsel Chips, Toll House | 86 | 29.24 |
| 23012 | 1/2 | cup | Semi-Sweet Chocolate Chips, avg | 84 | 52.08 |
| 23421 | 1 | Tbs | Semi-Sweet Chocolate Mini Bits, M&M's | 14 | 9.10 |
| 23182 | 1/2 | cup | Semi-Sweet Chocolate Morsels, Toll House | 86 | 46.44 |
| | | | Candy & Candy Bars | | |
| 23049 | 1 | ea | Almond Joy, 1.73 oz bar | 49 | 4.90 |
| 23405 | 1 | ea | Almond Joy, fun size, .7 oz bar | 20 | 2.00 |
| 23077 | 1 | ea | Alpine, white chocolate & almonds, 1.23 oz bar | 35 | 1.75 |
| 23110 | 1 | ea | Baby Ruth , 2.12 oz bar | 60 | 2.40 |
| 23269 | 1 | ea | Baby Ruth, fun size, .5 oz bar | 14 | 0.56 |
| 23111 | 1 | ea | Bar None, 1.52 oz bar | 43 | 11.18 |
| 23116 | 1 | ea | Caramello, 1.6 oz bar | 45 | 1.80 |
| 23117 | 5 | ea | Caramels, chocolate flvd roll, avg | 25 | 0.50 |
| 23020 | 1/2 | cup | Chocolate Coated Almonds, avg | 82 | 3.67 |
| 23113 | 1 | ea | Chocolate Covered Banana, w/nuts, avg | 145 | 17.40 |
| 23023 | 5 | ea | Chocolate Covered Fondant/Mints, avg | 55 | 3.30 |
| 23122 | 1 | ea | Chunky, 1.4 oz. bar | 40 | 11.60 |
| 23099 | 1 | ea | Crisped Rice Chocolate Chip bar, 1 oz, avg | 28 | 1.40 |
| 23133 | 1 | ea | Crunch, milk chocolate bar, 1.4 oz | 40 | 9.60 |
| 23134 | 1 | ea | Crunch, milk chocolate mini bar, .35 oz | 10 | 2.40 |
| 23079 | 5 | ea | Dietetic Chocolate Cvrd Candy, avg | 80 | 8.80 |
| 23125 | 1 | ea | 5TH Avenue, 2 oz bar | 57 | 3.99 |
| 23078 | 1 | pce | Candy Corn, chocolate cvrd, avg | 14 | 0.56 |
| 23025 | 1 | pce | Fudge, chocolate, recipe, avg | 17 | 2.38 |
| 23026 | 1 | pce | Fudge, chocolate w/nuts, recipe, avg | 19 | 2.66 |
| 23126 | 1 | pce | Fudge chocolate marshmallow, recipe, avg | 20 | 2.80 |
| 23127 | 1 | pce | Fudge chocolate marsh w/nuts recipe, avg | 22 | 3.52 |
| 23129 | 1 | ea | Golden Almond Chocolate, 3 oz bar | 85 | 15.30 |
| 23130 | 1 | ea | Golden Almond Solitaires, 2.75 oz pkg | 78 | 12.48 |
| 23131 | 1 | ea | Golden III Chocolate, 3.2 oz bar | 91 | 14.56 |
| 23257 | 1/2 | cup | Goobers, milk chocolate cvrd peanuts | 82 | 18.04 |
| 23060 | 1 | ea | Kit Kat, 1.48 oz bar | 42 | 5.04 |

TABLE C *(continued)*

| Code | Amount | | Description | Wgt (g) | Caffeine (g) |
|---|---|---|---|---|---|
| 23016 | 1 | ea | Kisses, milk chocolate, 1.6oz pkg, Hershey's | 44 | 11.44 |
| 23063 | 6 | pce | Kisses, milk chocolate, 1 oz, Hershey's | 28 | 6.89 |
| 23061 | 1 | ea | Krackel, chocolate & crisped rice bar, 1.45 oz | 41 | 7.38 |
| 23479 | 1 | ea | M&M's, peanut, 25 pces, 1.74 oz pkg | 49 | 5.39 |
| 23480 | 1 | ea | M&M's, plain, 69 pces, 1.69 oz pkg | 48 | 8.64 |
| 23037 | 1 | ea | Mars Almond bar, 1.76 oz | 50 | 2.00 |
| 23192 | 1 | ea | Milk Chocolate candy bar, 1.45 oz, Nestle | 41 | 12.71 |
| 23058 | 1 | ea | Milk Chocolate candy bar w/crsp rice, 1.4 oz, avg | 40 | 9.20 |
| 23019 | 1 | ea | Milk Chocolate candy bar w/peanuts, 1 oz, avg | 28 | 3.15 |
| 23022 | 1/2 | cup | Milk Chocolate Cvrd Raisins, avg | 95 | 23.75 |
| 23419 | 5 | pce | Milk Chocolate Coated Peanuts, 5 pces | 20 | 4.40 |
| 23193 | 1 | pce | Milk Chocolate After 8 Mint, Nestle | 8 | 1.60 |
| 23018 | 1 | ea | Milk chocolate w/almonds, 1.45 oz bar, avg | 41 | 9.02 |
| 23038 | 1 | ea | Milky Way bar, 2.12 oz | 60 | 4.80 |
| 23039 | 1 | ea | Milky Way bar, fun size, .63 oz | 18 | 1.44 |
| 23035 | 1 | ea | Mounds, 1.87 oz bar | 53 | 9.01 |
| 23062 | 1 | ea | Mr. Goodbar, 1.73 oz bar | 49 | 9.80 |
| 23194 | 5 | pce | Nips Chocolate Parfait candy | 36 | 3.46 |
| 23191 | 5 | pce | Nips Coffee candy | 25 | 10.25 |
| 23189 | 1 | oz | Nips Licorice candy | 28 | 0.28 |
| 23135 | 1 | ea | Oh Henry, 2 oz bar | 57 | 5.70 |
| 23214 | 1 | ea | Raisinets, milk choc cvrd raisins, 1.59 oz pkg | 45 | 11.25 |
| 23424 | 5 | ea | Reese's Peanut Butter Cups, mini, 1.2 oz | 35 | 3.50 |
| 23043 | 1 | ea | Reese's Peanut Butter Cups, 1.76 oz pkg | 50 | 5.00 |
| 23436 | 1 | ea | Reese's Pieces candy, 1.6 oz pkg | 46 | 5.52 |
| 23426 | 1 | ea | Rolo Caramels, milk chocolate, 1.87 oz pkg | 53 | 7.95 |
| 23485 | 1 | ea | Skittles, bite size candy, 2.17 oz pkg | 62 | 15.50 |
| 23036 | 1 | ea | Skor English Toffee, 1.38 oz bar | 39 | 3.66 |
| 23040 | 1 | ea | Snickers, 2 oz. bar | 57 | 3.99 |
| 23041 | 1 | ea | Snickers, fun size, .5 oz. bar | 15 | 1.05 |
| 23057 | 1 | ea | Special Dark Chocolate, 1.45 oz bar, Hershey's | 41 | 29.93 |
| 23145 | 1 | ea | Sweet Chocolate bar, 1.45 oz, avg | 41 | 27.06 |
| 23146 | 1 | ea | Symphony Milk Chocolate bar, 1.4 oz | 40 | 26.40 |
| 23136 | 1 | ea | 1000 Grand bar, 1.5 oz | 43 | 11.18 |
| 23375 | 1 | ea | 1000 Grand mini bar, .74 oz | 21 | 5.46 |
| 23075 | 1 | ea | 3 Musketeers bar, 2.12 oz | 60 | 6.60 |
| 23076 | 1 | ea | 3 Musketeers, fun size bar, .58 oz | 16 | 1.76 |
| 23148 | 1 | pce | Truffles candy, homemade, avg | 12 | 1.20 |
| 23123 | 1 | pce | Turtles, choc, caramel & pecans candy, Nestle | 17 | 0.68 |
| 23149 | 1 | ea | Twix Caramel Cookie bar, 2 oz pkg | 57 | 1.71 |
| 23150 | 1 | ea | Twix Peanut Butter Cookie bar, 1.9 oz pkg | 54 | 4.86 |
| 23151 | 1 | ea | Whatchamacallit, 1.69 oz bar | 48 | 2.88 |
| 23084 | 10 | ea | Whoppers, malted milk balls | 29 | 6.67 |
| 23152 | 1 | ea | York Peppermint Patty, 1.48 oz pkg | 42 | 4.20 |
| | | | **CEREALS, BREAKFAST** | | |
| 40102 | 1 | cup | Cocoa Krispies, Kellogg's | 41 | 1.64 |
| 40425 | 1 | cup | Cocoa Puffs, General Mills | 30 | 0.60 |
| 40324 | 1 | cup | Cookie Crisp, Ralston Purina | 30 | 0.60 |
| 40402 | 1 | cup | Count Chocula, General Mills | 30 | 0.90 |
| 40014 | 1 | cup | Malt-o-Meal, ckd, avg | 240 | 2.40 |

TABLE C *(continued)*

| Code | Amount | | Description | Wgt (g) | Caffeine (g) |
|---|---|---|---|---|---|
| 40188 | 1 | cup | Malt-o-Meal, Chocolate, ckd w/salt, avg | 240 | 2.40 |
| | | | **DESSERTS** | | |
| | | | Brownies | | |
| 47030 | 1 | ea | Low Calorie, low sodium, avg | 22 | 2.42 |
| 47683 | 1 | oz | Low Calorie, low sodium, dry mix, avg | 28 | 3.08 |
| 47000 | 1 | ea | With Nuts, avg | 61 | 13.42 |
| 47028 | 1 | ea | Without Nuts, avg | 33 | 3.15 |
| 47027 | 1 | oz | Without Nuts, dry mix, avg | 28 | 2.67 |
| | | | Cakes | | |
| 46002 | 1 | pce | Boston Cream Pie, coml prep, avg | 92 | 4.83 |
| 46052 | 1 | pce | Boston Cream Pie, prep f/rec, avg | 93 | 5.58 |
| 46013 | 1 | pce | Chocolate, commercial prep, w/frosting, avg | 64 | 7.42 |
| 46066 | 1 | pce | Chocolate, German, w/icing, avg | 11 | 0.52 |
| 46061 | 1 | pce | Chocolate, low sod, w/fructose, avg | 38 | 2.65 |
| 46059 | 1 | pce | Chocolate, prep f/mix, avg | 65 | 4.53 |
| 46117 | 1 | pce | Chocolate, w/cream cheese icing, avg | 103 | 6.97 |
| 46120 | 1 | pce | Chocolate, w/fluffy white icing, avg | 91 | 4.74 |
| 46118 | 1 | pce | Chocolate, w/vanilla icing, avg | 103 | 4.53 |
| 46096 | 1 | pce | Coffee, crème filled, w/chocolate frosting, avg | 90 | 5.40 |
| 46119 | 1 | pce | Marble, prep w/chocolate icing, avg | 111 | 6.05 |
| 46069 | 1 | pce | Marble, pudding type, prep f/mix, avg | 73 | 1.73 |
| 46011 | 1 | ea | Snack, chocolate creme filled, w/icing, avg | 50 | 1.50 |
| 46426 | 1 | ea | Snack, chocolate w/frosting, low fat, avg | 43 | 0.86 |
| 46115 | 1 | pce | Sponge, chocolate, w/o icing, avg | 66 | 4.60 |
| 46012 | 1 | pce | Yellow w/chocolate frosting, avg | 64 | 5.47 |
| 49017 | 1 | pce | Cheesecake, chocolate, avg | 128 | 3.84 |
| | | | Cookies | | |
| 47036 | 1 | ea | Chocolate Chip, baked f/refrig dough, avg | 12 | 1.42 |
| 47022 | 1 | ea | Chocolate Chip, diet, avg | 5 | 0.45 |
| 47032 | 1 | ea | Chocolate Chip, low fat, avg | 10 | 0.70 |
| 47033 | 1 | ea | Chocolate Chip, no sodium, w/fructose, avg | 7 | 0.56 |
| 47035 | 1 | ea | Chocolate Chip, prep f/mix, avg | 16 | 1.89 |
| 47037 | 1 | ea | Chocolate Chip, prep f/recipe, avg | 16 | 1.89 |
| 47013 | 1 | ea | Chocolate Chip, refrig dough, avg | 16 | 1.44 |
| 47001 | 1 | ea | Chocolate Chip, soft, avg | 15 | 1.05 |
| 47044 | 1 | ea | Chocolate Fudge cookie, avg | 21 | 1.99 |
| 47039 | 1 | ea | Chocolate Sandwich, low sod, w/fructose, avg | 10 | 0.30 |
| 47038 | 1 | ea | Chocolate Sandwich w/chocolate icing, avg | 17 | 2.01 |
| 47040 | 1 | ea | Chocolate Sandwich w/extra crème, avg | 13 | 1.30 |
| 47041 | 1 | ea | Chocolate Wafer, avg | 6 | 0.54 |
| 47046 | 1 | ea | Marshmallow w/choc coating, avg | 13 | 1.17 |
| 45524 | 1 | ea | Doughnut, chocolate cake, iced, avg | 43 | 0.86 |
| 45508 | 1 | ea | Doughnut, chocolate eclair, avg | 112 | 8.92 |
| | | | Ice Cream | | |
| 2050 | 1/2 | cup | Chocolate, avg | 66 | 1.98 |
| 2051 | 1/2 | cup | Chocolate, soft serve, avg | 86 | 2.58 |
| 2483 | 1/2 | cup | Chocolate, Breyers | 70 | 2.10 |
| | | | Ice Cream Bars | | |
| 2055 | 1 | ea | Chocolate, avg | 101 | 10.10 |
| 2085 | 1 | ea | Chocolate, caramel covered, avg | 54 | 1.62 |

TABLE C *(continued)*

| Code | Amount | Description | Wgt (g) | Caffeine (g) |
|---|---|---|---|---|
| 2084 | 1 ea | Chocolate, choc cvrd, avg | 68 | 5.44 |
| 2026 | 1 ea | Chocolate, pudding pop, avg | 47 | 2.47 |
| 2029 | 1 ea | Drumstick, avg | 60 | 3.60 |
| 2030 | 1 ea | Fudgesicle, avg | 73 | 2.90 |
| | | Ice Cream Cones | | |
| 2113 | 1 ea | Chocolate, avg | 78 | 2.34 |
| 2092 | 1 ea | Chocolate Dipped, avg | 78 | 2.34 |
| 2090 | 1 ea | Chocolate Dipped, w/nuts, avg | 78 | 2.34 |
| 2057 | 1/2 cup | Ice Milk, chocolate, avg | 66 | 1.98 |
| 2667 | 1/2 cup | Mousse, chocolate, avg | 202 | 10.10 |
| 48071 | 1 pce | Pie, chocolate cream, prep f/rec, 1/8 of 9", avg | 142 | 6.25 |
| | | Pudding | | |
| 2634 | 1/2 cup | Chocolate, prep f/mix w/2% milk, avg | 147 | 2.94 |
| 2605 | 1/2 cup | Chocolate, prep f/mix, w/whl milk, avg | 147 | 2.94 |
| 2637 | 1/2 cup | Chocolate, prep f/rec, w/2% milk, avg | 157 | 4.71 |
| 2601 | 1/2 cup | Chocolate, prep f/rec, w/whl milk, avg | 157 | 4.71 |
| 2610 | 1 ea | Chocolate, RTE, cnd, avg | 142 | 7.10 |
| 2618 | 1 ea | Chocolate, RTE, low cal, cnd, avg | 142 | 7.10 |
| 2659 | 1/2 cup | Chocolate, rennin, prep f/mix, w/2%milk, avg | 136 | 1.36 |
| 2660 | 1/2 cup | Chocolate, rennin, prep f/mix, w/whl milk, avg | 136 | 1.36 |
| 2069 | 1 ea | Sundae, chocolate w/whippd cream, small, avg | 165 | 6.93 |
| 2563 | 1 ea | Yogurt, chocolate, whole milk, 8 oz, avg | 245 | 7.35 |
| 2039 | 1/2 cup | Yogurt, frozen, chocolate, fat free, avg | 96 | 2.88 |
| 2071 | 1/2 cup | Yogurt, frozen, chocolate, lowfat, avg | 96 | 2.88 |
| | | **DESSERT TOPPINGS** | | |
| | | Frosting | | |
| 46034 | 2 Tbs | Chocolate, prep f/mix, w/butter, avg | 34 | 1.36 |
| 46035 | 2 Tbs | Chocolate, prep f/mix, w/marg, avg | 34 | 1.36 |
| 46032 | 2 Tbs | Chocolate, prep f/recipe, avg | 34 | 3.91 |
| 46037 | 2 Tbs | Chocolate, RTE, avg | 29 | 0.58 |
| | | Sprinkles | | |
| 23268 | 2 Tbs | Buncha Crunch, topping, Nestle | 20 | 4.40 |
| 23267 | 1 Tbs | Butterfinger, candy topping, Nestle | 25 | 1.00 |
| 23186 | 1 oz | Sno Caps, sweet choc topping, Nestle | 28 | 9.72 |
| 23056 | 2 Tbs | Syrup, chocolate, avg | 38 | 5.32 |
| 23014 | 2 Tbs | Syrup, chocolate fudge, avg | 42 | 2.52 |
| | | **SNACKS AND BARS** | | |
| | | Granola Bars | | |
| 23106 | 1 ea | Chocolate Chip, Graham & Marshmallow, soft, av | 28 | 1.12 |
| 23101 | 1 ea | Chocolate Chip, hard, avg | 24 | 0.96 |
| 23096 | 1 ea | Chocolate Chip, w/choc coating, soft, avg | 35 | 2.80 |
| 23105 | 1 ea | Chocolate, soft, avg | 42 | 1.68 |
| 23109 | 1 ea | Peanut Butter w/Chocolate, uncoated, soft, avg | 28 | 1.40 |
| 23095 | 1 ea | Peanut Butter, soft, w/choc coating, avg | 37 | 2.22 |
| 62278 | 1 ea | Power Bar, chocolate | 65 | 15.00 |
| 62280 | 1 ea | Power Bar, mocha | 65 | 20.00 |
| 44059 | 1/2 cup | Trail Mix w/chocolate chips, avg | 73 | 4.38 |

TABLE D **Phytosterol Content of Selected Foods**

| ESHA | Amount | | Description | Wgt (g) | Phytos (mg) |
|---|---|---|---|---|---|
| | | | **CANDY** | | |
| | | | Fudge | | |
| 23026 | 1 | pce | Chocolate w/nuts, recipe, avg | 19 | 2.66 |
| 23127 | 1 | pce | Chocolate marsh w/nuts recipe, avg | 22 | 1.54 |
| 23128 | 1 | pce | Peanut butter, recipe, avg | 16 | 1.76 |
| 23124 | 1 | pce | Penuche w/brn sugar & nuts, avg | 14 | 2.10 |
| 23028 | 1 | pce | Vanilla w/nuts, recipe, avg | 15 | 2.25 |
| 23081 | 1/2 | cup | Peanut Brittle, recipe, avg | 74 | 47.36 |
| 23138 | 1 | pce | Praline Candy, recipe, avg | 39 | 15.21 |
| 23148 | 1 | pce | Truffles candy, homemade, avg | 12 | 0.24 |
| | | | **DAIRY SUBSTITUTES** | | |
| 534 | 1 | Tbs | Creamer, coffee whitener, avg | 15 | 1.95 |
| 506 | 1 | Tbs | Creamer, powder, avg | 6 | 1.92 |
| 513 | 2 | Tbs | Dessert Topping, dry mix, avg | 3 | 1.08 |
| 514 | 2 | Tbs | Dessert Topping, pressurized, avg | 9 | 1.80 |
| 505 | 2 | Tbs | Sour Cream, imitation, avg | 29 | 5.22 |
| | | | **DESSERTS** | | |
| 49005 | 1/2 | cup | Brown Betty, apple, avg | 103 | 0.07 |
| 46013 | 1 | pce | Cake, chocolate, coml prep, w/frosting, avg | 64 | 13.18 |
| 47011 | 1 | ea | Cookie, Snickerdoodle, avg | 20 | 0.10 |
| 49003 | 1 | pce | Cobbler, apple, avg | 104 | 30.05 |
| 49009 | 1 | pce | Crisp, peach, avg | 139 | 26.77 |
| 49006 | 1 | ea | Dumpling, apple, avg | 151 | 48.64 |
| 23156 | 1/2 | cup | Gelatin, prep, w/added fruit, avg | 106 | 3.18 |
| | | | Pies | | |
| 48082 | 1 | pce | Lemon Meringue, rts, 1/6 of 8" pie, avg | 113 | 8.23 |
| 48083 | 1 | pce | Mince, prep f/rec, 1/8 of 9", avg | 165 | 0.54 |
| 48087 | 1 | pce | Peach, prep f/Recipe, 1/8 of 9 " pie, avg | 139 | 6.65 |
| | | | Puddings | | |
| 2617 | 1/2 | cup | Bread w/Raisins, avg | 126 | 7.56 |
| 2637 | 1/2 | cup | Chocolate, prep f/rec, w/2% milk, avg | 157 | 3.14 |
| 2601 | 1/2 | cup | Chocolate, prep f/rec, w/whl milk, avg | 157 | 3.14 |
| | | | **EGGS, SUBSTITUTES, EGG DISHES** | | |
| | | | Eggs | | |
| 19509 | 1 | ea | Fried, avg | 46 | 6.44 |
| 19534 | 1 | ea | Omelet, plain, w/milk & butter, avg | 61 | 6.10 |
| 19516 | 1 | ea | Scrambled, avg | 61 | 6.10 |
| 19524 | 1/4 | cup | Egg Substitute, frozen, avg | 60 | 57.00 |
| 19525 | 1/4 | cup | Egg Substitute, liquid, avg | 63 | 2.52 |
| | | | **FATS** | | |
| | | | Margarines | | |
| 8052 | 1 | tsp | Corn Oil, hard, avg | 5 | 28.50 |
| 8061 | 1 | tsp | Corn Oil, soft, avg | 5 | 24.15 |
| 8053 | 1 | tsp | Corn Oil, w/soybean/cottonseed oils, hard, avg | 5 | 21.25 |
| 8344 | 1 | tsp | Corn Oil, w/soybean/cottonseed oils, w/o salt, hard, avg | 5 | 13.25 |
| 8263 | 1 | tsp | Coconut/safflower/palm Oils, hard, avg | 5 | 13.25 |
| 8241 | 1 | tsp | Lard, hard, avg | 5 | 2.15 |
| 8155 | 1 | tsp | Light, tub, Fleishmann's | 5 | 13.50 |
| 8249 | 1 | tsp | Palm Oil, hard, imitation, avg | 5 | 6.50 |
| 8058 | 1 | tsp | Safflower Oil, soft, avg | 5 | 10.00 |

TABLE D *(continued)*

| ESHA | Amount | | Description | Wgt (g) | Phytos (mg) |
|---|---|---|---|---|---|
| 8179 | 1 | tsp | Soybean Oil, hard, avg | 5 | 10.95 |
| 8247 | 1 | tsp | Soybean Oil, soft, avg | 5 | 10.30 |
| 8234 | 1 | tsp | Soybean Oil, w/cottonseed oil, hard, avg | 5 | 13.25 |
| 8250 | 1 | tsp | Soybean Oil, w/cottonseed oil, hard, imitation, avg | 5 | 5.30 |
| 8243 | 1 | tsp | Soybean Oil, w/cottonseed oil, soft, avg | 5 | 9.45 |
| 8239 | 1 | tsp | Soybean Oil, w/palm oil, hard, avg | 5 | 6.80 |
| 8345 | 1 | tsp | Soybean Oil, w/palm oil, soft, avg | 5 | 7.95 |
| 8265 | 1 | tsp | Soybean Oil, w/safflower oil, soft, avg | 5 | 10.00 |
| 8242 | 1 | tsp | Soybean Oil, w/o salt, soft, avg | 5 | 7.20 |
| 8262 | 1 | tsp | Sunflower oil, hard, avg | 5 | 21.25 |
| 8059 | 1 | tsp | Sunflower/cottonseed/peanut oils, soft, avg | 5 | 10.00 |
| 8042 | 1 | tsp | Unspecified Oils, hard, avg | 5 | 13.25 |
| 8041 | 1 | tsp | Unspecified Oils, hard, imitation, avg | 5 | 7.50 |
| 8244 | 1 | tsp | Unspecified Oils, soft, avg | 5 | 8.50 |
| | | | Oils, Vegetable | | |
| 8078 | 1 | Tbs | Almond, avg | 14 | 37.24 |
| 8079 | 1 | Tbs | Apricot kernel, avg | 14 | 37.24 |
| 8080 | 1 | Tbs | Cocoa butter, avg | 14 | 28.14 |
| 8037 | 1 | Tbs | Coconut, avg | 14 | 12.04 |
| 8009 | 1 | Tbs | Corn, avg | 14 | 135.52 |
| 8081 | 1 | Tbs | Cottonseed, avg | 14 | 45.36 |
| 8047 | 1 | Tbs | Grapeseed, avg | 14 | 25.20 |
| 8048 | 1 | Tbs | Hazelnut, avg | 14 | 16.80 |
| 8008 | 1 | Tbs | Olive, avg | 14 | 30.94 |
| 8083 | 1 | Tbs | Palm kernel, avg | 14 | 13.30 |
| 8026 | 1 | Tbs | Peanut, avg | 14 | 28.98 |
| 8049 | 1 | Tbs | Poppyseed, avg | 14 | 38.64 |
| 8050 | 1 | Tbs | Rice bran, avg | 14 | 166.60 |
| 8010 | 1 | Tbs | Safflower, avg | 14 | 62.16 |
| 8027 | 1 | Tbs | Sesame, avg | 14 | 121.10 |
| 8108 | 1 | Tbs | Soybean | 14 | 35.00 |
| 8011 | 1 | Tbs | Sunflower, avg | 14 | 14.00 |
| 8351 | 1 | Tbs | Tomato seed, avg | 14 | 14.00 |
| 8085 | 1 | Tbs | Walnut, avg | 14 | 24.64 |
| 8038 | 1 | Tbs | Wheat germ, avg | 14 | 77.42 |
| 8007 | 1 | Tbs | Shortening, multipurpose, soybean/cottonseed, oils, avg | 13 | 26.00 |
| | | | **FRUITS** | | |
| 3000 | 1 | ea | Apple, raw, w/peel, avg | 138 | 16.56 |
| 3657 | 1/2 | cup | Apricot, raw, pitted, fresh, sliced, avg | 82 | 14.76 |
| 3021 | 1/2 | cup | Banana, raw, slices, avg | 75 | 12.00 |
| 3075 | 1/2 | cup | Cantaloupe, cubes, avg | 80 | 8.00 |
| | | | Cherries, Sour | | |
| 3402 | 1/2 | cup | Canned in light syrup, avg | 126 | 5.92 |
| 3035 | 1/2 | cup | Canned in water, avg | 122 | 5.86 |
| 3159 | 1/2 | cup | Frozen, unsweetened, avg | 78 | 5.90 |
| | | | Cherries, Sweet | | |
| 3336 | 1/2 | cup | Canned in juice, avg | 125 | 6.45 |
| 3405 | 1/2 | cup | Canned in light syrup, avg | 126 | 5.29 |
| 3404 | 1/2 | cup | Canned in water, avg | 124 | 6.20 |
| 3158 | 1/2 | cup | Frozen, sweetened, avg | 130 | 9.24 |

TABLE D *(continued)*

| ESHA | Amount | Description | Wgt (g) | Phytos (mg) |
|---|---|---|---|---|
| 3037 | 1/2 cup | Raw, w/o pits, avg | 72 | 8.64 |
| 3160 | 1 ea | Fig, raw, medium, avg | 50 | 15.50 |
| 3058 | 1/2 cup | Grapes, European type/adherent skin, avg | 80 | 3.20 |
| 3686 | 1/2 cup | Grapefruit, white, avg | 115 | 19.55 |
| 3418 | 1 ea | Lemon, fresh, w/peel, avg | 108 | 12.96 |
| 3639 | 1 ea | Loquats, raw, medium, avg | 16 | 0.32 |
| 3715 | 1/2 cup | Orange, California navel, avg | 82 | 19.68 |
| 3096 | 1 ea | Peach, fresh, whole, medium, avg | 98 | 9.80 |
| 3104 | 1/2 cup | Pear, fresh, avg | 82 | 6.56 |
| 3111 | 1/2 cup | Pineapple, fresh, chunks, avg | 78 | 4.68 |
| 3123 | 1/2 cup | Plum, fresh, slices, avg | 82 | 5.74 |
| 3197 | 1 ea | Pomegranate, fresh, avg | 154 | 26.18 |
| 3135 | 1/2 cup | Strawberries, fresh, slices, avg | 83 | 9.96 |
| 3142 | 1/2 cup | Watermelon, fresh, diced, avg | 76 | 1.52 |
| | | **GRAIN PRODUCTS, PREPARED AND BAKED GOODS** | | |
| | | Breads | | |
| 42039 | 1 pce | Banana Bread, prep f/recipe, w/marg, avg | 60 | 20.40 |
| 42116 | 1 pce | Cornbread, prepared f/recipe w/2% milk, avg | 65 | 7.80 |
| 42090 | 1 pce | Egg/Challah Bread, avg | 40 | 2.80 |
| 42118 | 1 pce | Indian/Navajo Fry Bread | 90 | 13.50 |
| 42119 | 1 pce | Irish Soda Bread, prep f/recipe, avg | 60 | 7.80 |
| 42124 | 1 pce | Pumpernickel Bread, prepared f/recipe, avg | 60 | 17.40 |
| 42040 | 1 pce | French Toast, prepared f/recipe w/whole milk, avg | 65 | 2.65 |
| 44503 | 1 ea | Muffin, corn meal, prepared f/recipe w/whole milk, avg | 57 | 14.25 |
| 45008 | 1 ea | Pancakes, whole wheat, prep f/dry mix, 4", avg | 44 | 2.75 |
| 38159 | 2 oz | Pasta, fresh, prepared f/recipe w/egg, avg | 57 | 0.57 |
| 38093 | 1 cup | Pasta, fresh, prepared f/recipe w/o egg, avg | 76 | 1.52 |
| | | **NUTS, SEEDS AND PRODUCTS** | | |
| 4500 | 1 oz | Almonds, dried, avg | 28 | 40.04 |
| 4621 | 1 oz | Cashews, dry roasted, unsalted, avg | 28 | 44.24 |
| 4568 | 1 oz | Chestnuts, raw, unpeeled, avg | 28 | 6.16 |
| 4507 | 2 Tbs | Coconut, fresh, shredded, avg | 20 | 9.40 |
| 4528 | 1/2 cup | Coconut Milk, raw, avg | 120 | 1.20 |
| | | Peanut Butter | | |
| 4626 | 2 Tbs | Chunky, salted, avg | 32 | 32.64 |
| 4576 | 2 Tbs | Chunky, unsalted, avg | 32 | 32.64 |
| 4627 | 2 Tbs | Smooth, salted, avg | 32 | 32.64 |
| 4636 | 2 Tbs | Smooth, unsalted, avg | 32 | 32.64 |
| 4696 | 1 oz | Peanuts, raw, avg | 28 | 61.60 |
| 4578 | 1 oz | Pecans, dried, halves, avg | 28 | 30.24 |
| 4764 | 1 oz | Pine Nuts, pignolia, dried, avg | 28 | 39.48 |
| 4523 | 1 oz | Sesame Seeds, dried, whole, avg | 28 | 199.92 |
| 4545 | 1 oz | Sunflower Seeds, kernels, dry, avg | 28 | 149.52 |
| 4557 | 1 oz | Walnuts, English/Persian, halves, dried, avg | 28 | 30.24 |
| | | **SALAD DRESSINGS AND MAYONNAISE** | | |
| 8046 | 1 Tbs | Mayonnaise, avg | 14 | 31.22 |
| 8231 | 1 Tbs | Mayonnaise, imitation, no choles, avg | 14 | 30.24 |
| | | Salad Dressings | | |
| 8013 | 1 Tbs | Blue Cheese/Roquefort, avg | 15 | 19.50 |
| 8014 | 1 Tbs | French, low calorie, avg | 16 | 2.40 |

TABLE D *(continued)*

| ESHA | Amount | Description | Wgt (g) | Phytos (mg) |
|---|---|---|---|---|
| 8016 | 1 Tbs | Italian, low calorie, avg | 15 | 3.75 |
| 8144 | 1 Tbs | Sesame Seed, avg | 15 | 16.95 |
| 8024 | 1 Tbs | Thousand Island, avg | 16 | 15.52 |
| 8023 | 1 Tbs | Thousand Island, low calorie, avg | 15 | 4.05 |
| | | **SALADS** | | |
| 56109 | 1/2 cup | Carrot Raisin Salad, avg | 88 | 44.44 |
| 56002 | 1/2 cup | Carrot Raisin Salad, w/celery, avg | 78 | 62.73 |
| 5677 | 1 cup | Green Garden/Tossed Salads, avg | 139 | 12.72 |
| 56004 | 1/2 cup | Macaroni Salad, avg | 88 | 53.90 |
| 56006 | 1/2 cup | Waldorf Salad, avg | 68 | 52.65 |
| | | **SANDWICHES** | | |
| 56023 | 1 ea | Avocado & Cheese, on wheat, avg | 214 | 32.48 |
| 56010 | 1 ea | Bacon, Lettuce & Tomato, on wheat, avg | 137 | 33.26 |
| | | Beef | | |
| 56020 | 1 ea | Corned Beef & Swiss, on rye, avg | 156 | 30.76 |
| 56038 | 1 ea | Patty Melt, w/ground beef on rye, avg | 182 | 50.87 |
| 56043 | 1 ea | Roast Beef, on white, avg | 160 | 20.46 |
| 56014 | 1 ea | Cheese, grilled, on wheat, avg | 132 | 20.11 |
| 56018 | 1 ea | Chicken Salad, on wheat, avg | 123 | 62.28 |
| 56026 | 1 ea | Egg Salad, on wheat, avg | 130 | 30.88 |
| | | Ham | | |
| 56032 | 1 ea | On rye, avg | 150 | 20.58 |
| 56030 | 1 ea | On wheat, avg | 169 | 20.46 |
| 56028 | 1 ea | On white, avg | 170 | 30.74 |
| 56065 | 1 ea | Salad, on wheat, avg | 144 | 30.82 |
| 56036 | 1 ea | With Cheese, on wheat, avg | 170 | 20.57 |
| 56041 | 1 ea | Peanut Butter & Jam, on wheat, avg | 114 | 24.63 |
| 69072 | 1 ea | Reuben, avg | 239 | 60.66 |
| 56049 | 1 ea | Tuna Salad, on whole wheat, avg | 135 | 30.76 |
| | | Turkey | | |
| 56055 | 1 ea | Ham & Cheese, on rye, avg | 150 | 20.58 |
| 56058 | 1 ea | Ham & Cheese, on wheat, avg | 170 | 20.57 |
| 56103 | 1 ea | Ham, on rye, avg | 150 | 20.58 |
| 56105 | 1 ea | Ham, on wheat, avg | 169 | 20.46 |
| 56107 | 1 ea | Ham, on white, avg | 166 | 20.57 |
| 56051 | 1 ea | On white, avg | 165 | 30.78 |
| | | **SPICES, FLAVORS AND SEASONINGS** | | |
| 26000 | 1 tsp | Allspice, ground, avg | 2 | 1.22 |
| 26001 | 1 tsp | Basil, ground, avg | 2 | 2.12 |
| 26018 | 1 tsp | Caraway Seed, avg | 2 | 1.52 |
| 26039 | 1 tsp | Cardamom, ground, avg | 2 | 0.92 |
| 26027 | 1 tsp | Cayenne/Red Pepper, dried, avg | 2 | 1.66 |
| 26040 | 1 tsp | Celery Seed, avg | 2 | 1.20 |
| 26002 | 1 tsp | Chili powder, avg | 2 | 1.66 |
| 26003 | 1 tsp | Cinnamon, avg | 2 | 0.52 |
| 26019 | 1 tsp | Cloves, ground, avg | 2 | 5.12 |
| 26041 | 1 tsp | Coriander/Cilantro seed, avg | 2 | 0.92 |
| 26036 | 1 tsp | Cumin Seed, avg | 2 | 1.36 |
| 26004 | 1 tsp | Curry Powder, avg | 2 | 1.44 |
| 26109 | 1 tsp | Dill Seed, avg | 2 | 2.48 |

TABLE D *(continued)*

| ESHA | Amount | Description | Wgt (g) | Phytos (mg) |
|---|---|---|---|---|
| 26105 | 1 tsp | Fennel Seed, avg | 2 | 1.32 |
| 26022 | 1 tsp | Fenugreek Seed, avg | 4 | 5.60 |
| 26023 | 1 tsp | Ginger, ground, avg | 2 | 1.66 |
| 26044 | 1 Tbs | Ginger, root, fresh, avg | 6 | 0.90 |
| 26024 | 1 tsp | Mace, ground, avg | 2 | 1.46 |
| 26025 | 1 tsp | Marjoram, dried, avg | 1 | 0.60 |
| 26110 | 1 tsp | Mustard Seed, yellow, avg | 4 | 4.72 |
| 26026 | 1 tsp | Nutmeg, ground, avg | 2 | 1.24 |
| 26008 | 1 tsp | Onion Powder, avg | 2 | 1.74 |
| 26009 | 1 tsp | Oregano, ground, avg | 2 | 4.06 |
| 26010 | 1 tsp | Paprika, avg | 2 | 3.50 |
| 26016 | 1 tsp | Pepper, black, avg | 2 | 1.84 |
| 26037 | 1 tsp | Pepper, white, avg | 2 | 1.10 |
| 26628 | 1 Tbs | Peppermint, fresh, avg | 16 | 2.08 |
| 26015 | 1 tsp | Poppyseed, avg | 3 | 2.67 |
| 26029 | 1 tsp | Pumpkin Pie, avg | 2 | 1.42 |
| 26031 | 1 tsp | Sage, ground, avg | 1 | 2.44 |
| 26112 | 1 tsp | Savory, ground, avg | 2 | 0.62 |
| 26631 | 1 tsp | Spearmint, dried, avg | 0 | 0.00 |
| 26630 | 1 Tbs | Spearmint, fresh, avg | 6 | 0.60 |
| 26032 | 1 tsp | Tarragon, ground, avg | 2 | 1.62 |
| 26033 | 1 tsp | Thyme, ground, avg | 1 | 1.63 |
| 26034 | 1 tsp | Turmeric, ground, avg | 2 | 1.64 |
| | | **VEGETABLES AND LEGUMES** | | |
| 5003 | 1/2 cup | Asparagus, boiled, avg | 90 | 21.60 |
| 5001 | 1/2 cup | Asparagus, raw, avg | 67 | 16.08 |
| 5230 | 1/2 cup | Bamboo Shoots, sliced, raw, avg | 76 | 14.44 |
| 5312 | 1/2 cup | Beet greens, raw, avg | 38 | 7.98 |
| 7026 | 1/2 cup | Broadbeans/Fava, raw, avg | 75 | 93.00 |
| 5031 | 1/2 cup | Brussels Sprouts raw, avg | 44 | 10.56 |
| 5036 | 1 cup | Cabbage, common, raw, shred, avg | 70 | 7.70 |
| | | Carrots | | |
| 5045 | 1 ea | Raw, 7 1/2", avg | 72 | 8.64 |
| 6772 | 1/2 cup | Raw, chpd, avg | 64 | 7.68 |
| 5655 | 1/2 cup | Steamed, avg | 78 | 9.36 |
| 5049 | 1/2 cup | Cauliflower, raw, avg | 50 | 9.00 |
| 5054 | 1/2 cup | Celery, raw, avg | 60 | 3.60 |
| 5659 | 1/2 cup | Celery, steamed, avg | 75 | 4.51 |
| 5071 | 1/2 cup | Cucumber, w/peel, raw, avg | 52 | 7.28 |
| 5371 | 1/2 cup | Eggplant, raw, cubes, avg | 41 | 2.87 |
| 7000 | 1/2 cup | Garbanzo/Chickpeas, raw, avg | 100 | 35.00 |
| 5083 | 1 cup | Lettuce, iceberg, avg | 55 | 5.50 |
| 5086 | 1 cup | Lettuce, looseleaf, avg | 56 | 21.28 |
| 5020 | 1/2 cup | Mung Bean Sprouts, raw, avg | 52 | 7.80 |
| 5775 | 1/2 cup | Okra, raw, avg | 50 | 12.00 |
| | | Onions | | |
| 5108 | 1/2 cup | Boiled, avg | 105 | 18.90 |
| 5101 | 1/2 cup | Raw, chpd, avg | 80 | 12.00 |
| 5649 | 1/2 cup | Steamed, avg | 105 | 15.96 |
| 5650 | 1/2 cup | Stir Fried, avg | 105 | 15.96 |

TABLE D *(continued)*

| ESHA | Amount | Description | Wgt (g) | Phytos (mg) |
|---|---|---|---|---|
| 7019 | 1/2 cup | Peas, split, raw, avg | 98 | 132.30 |
| | | Peppers, Sweet | | |
| 5126 | 1/2 cup | Green, boiled, chpd, avg | 68 | 6.12 |
| 5661 | 1/2 cup | Green, stmd, avg | 68 | 6.13 |
| 5278 | 1/2 cup | Red, ckd, avg | 68 | 6.12 |
| 5663 | 1/2 cup | Red, stmd, avg | 68 | 6.13 |
| 5263 | 1 ea | Potato Pancakes, prep f/recipe, avg | 76 | 21.28 |
| 5582 | 1/2 cup | Potatoes, flesh, raw, diced, avg | 75 | 3.75 |
| 5469 | 1/2 cup | Potatoes, mashed, prep f/granules, w/milk & marg, avg | 105 | 14.70 |
| 5793 | 1/2 cup | Pumpkin, raw, avg | 58 | 6.96 |
| 5144 | 1/2 cup | Radishes, red, slices, avg | 58 | 4.06 |
| 5427 | 1 Tbs | Shallots, raw, chpd, avg | 10 | 0.50 |
| 5259 | 1/2 cup | Soybeans, green, boiled, avg | 90 | 45.00 |
| 5258 | 1/2 cup | Soybeans, green, raw, avg | 128 | 64.00 |
| 5146 | 1 cup | Spinach, raw, chpd, avg | 30 | 2.70 |
| 5670 | 1/2 cup | Spinach, steamed, avg | 95 | 8.57 |
| 6880 | 1/2 cup | Sweet Potatoes/Yams, raw, avg | 66 | 7.92 |
| 5369 | 1/2 cup | Taro, raw, slices, avg | 52 | 9.88 |
| | | Tomatoes | | |
| 5178 | 1/2 cup | Raw, boiled, unsalted, avg | 120 | 10.80 |
| 5170 | 1/2 cup | Raw, chpd, avg | 90 | 6.30 |
| 5468 | 1/2 cup | Raw, stewed, avg | 50 | 7.00 |
| 5547 | 1/2 cup | Turnips, greens, raw, chpd, avg | 27 | 3.24 |
| 5182 | 1/2 cup | Turnips, raw, avg | 65 | 4.55 |
| | | **MISCELLANEOUS, CONDIMENTS** | | |
| 27000 | 1 Tbs | Catsup, avg | 15 | 1.05 |
| 27032 | 1 Tbs | Catsup, low salt, avg | 15 | 1.05 |
| 53015 | 1 Tbs | Cheese Sauce, avg | 13 | 3.85 |
| 27004 | 1 Tbs | Horseradish, avg | 15 | 1.35 |
| | | Pickles | | |
| 27012 | 1 ea | Dill, avg | 65 | 9.10 |
| 27023 | 1 ea | Sour, medium, avg | 35 | 4.90 |
| 27026 | 1 ea | Sour, medium, low salt, avg | 35 | 4.90 |
| 27016 | 1 ea | Sweet, medium, avg | 35 | 4.90 |
| 27030 | 1 ea | Sweet, medium, low salt, avg | 35 | 4.90 |

TABLE E **Pectin Content of Selected Foods**

| Code | Amount | Description | Wgt (g) | Pectin (g) |
|---|---|---|---|---|
| | | **BEVERAGES** | | |
| | | Alcoholic Beverages | | |
| 22738 | 1 1/2 cup | Beer, 12 fl oz | 356 | 0.71 |
| 22813 | 1 ea | Whisky Sour | 106 | 0.11 |
| 20109 | 1 cup | Coffee, mocha flavor, prep f/pow, sugar sweetened | 240 | 0.28 |
| 20000 | 1 cup | Lemonade, prep f/frozen conc | 240 | 0.25 |
| | | **FRUIT** | | |
| | | Apple | | |
| 3000 | 1 ea | Raw, w/skin | 138 | 1.48 |
| 3003 | 1 ea | Raw, w/o skin | 128 | 0.49 |
| 3388 | 1/2 cup | Boiled, w/o skin | 86 | 0.23 |
| 3148 | 1/2 cup | Canned, sliced, sweetened | 102 | 0.44 |
| 3392 | 1/2 cup | Frozen, unsweetened | 86 | 0.40 |
| 3331 | 1/2 cup | Applesauce, cnd, sweetened | 128 | 0.38 |
| 3858 | 1 ea | Kiwifruit | 76 | 0.32 |
| | | **NUTS** | | |
| 4500 | 1 oz | Almonds, dried (24 nuts) | 28 | 0.38 |
| 4538 | 1 oz | Chestnuts, roasted (3-1/2 nuts) | 28 | 0.34 |
| | | **VEGETABLES** | | |
| 5030 | 1/2 cup | Broccoli, frzn, chpd, boiled | 92 | 0.92 |
| 5035 | 1/2 cup | Brussels Sprouts, frzn, boiled | 78 | 1.09 |
| 5045 | 1 ea | Carrot, raw | 72 | 0.72 |
| 5393 | 1/2 cup | Corn, sweet, frzn, boiled | 82 | 0.33 |
| 5013 | 1/2 cup | Green Beans, frzn, boiled | 68 | 0.61 |
| 5118 | 1/2 cup | Green Peas, frzn, boiled | 80 | 0.48 |
| | | Spinach | | |
| 5146 | 1/2 cup | Raw | 28 | 0.22 |
| 5147 | 1/2 cup | Boiled | 90 | 0.72 |
| 5148 | 1/2 cup | Frozen, boiled | 95 | 1.05 |
| | | Summer Squash | | |
| 5151 | 1/2 cup | All varieties, raw | 65 | 0.39 |
| 5152 | 1/2 cup | All varieties, boiled | 90 | 0.45 |
| 5321 | 1/2 cup | Crookneck, raw | 65 | 0.39 |
| 5322 | 1/2 cup | Crookneck, boiled | 90 | 0.45 |
| 5158 | 1 ea | Sweet Potato, baked w/skin | 114 | 0.91 |
| 5542 | 1/2 cup | Sweet Potato, frzn, baked | 88 | 0.70 |

TABLE F **Theobromine Content of Selected Foods**

| ESHA | Amount | | Description | Wgt (g) | Theobromine (mg) |
|---|---|---|---|---|---|
| | | | **COFFEE** | | |
| 20094 | 2 | tsp | Mocha, instant w/sugar, dry pwd, avg | 12 | 23.28 |
| 20109 | 1 | cup | Mocha, instant w/sugar, prep f/pwd, avg | 250 | 30.00 |
| | | | **DAIRY MIXED DRINKS AND MIXES** | | |
| | | | Chocolate Drinks and Mixes | | |
| 14 | 1 | Tbs | Mix, avg | 26 | 315.12 |
| 74 | 1 | ea | Mix, sugar free, avg, dry env | 21 | 165.90 |
| 39 | 1 | cup | Prep w/milk, avg | 266 | 263.34 |
| 151 | 1 | cup | Prep w/water, sugar free, avg | 272 | 225.76 |
| 37 | 1 | Tbs | Chocolate Malt, dry mix, avg | 5 | 17.25 |
| 38 | 1 | cup | Chocolate Malt, prep f/mix, avg | 265 | 71.55 |
| | | | Chocolate Milk | | |
| 19 | 1 | cup | Lowfat, 1%, avg | 250 | 57.50 |
| 18 | 1 | cup | Lowfat, 2%, avg | 250 | 57.50 |
| 70 | 1 | cup | Prep w/whole milk & syrup, avg | 263 | 165.69 |
| 20 | 1 | cup | Whole, avg | 250 | 57.50 |
| | | | Cocoa | | |
| 48 | 1 | cup | Hot, prep w/water, avg | 275 | 231.00 |
| 77 | 1 | cup | Hot, prep w/water, low cal, avg | 256 | 1546.24 |
| 21 | 1 | cup | Hot, prep w/whole milk, avg | 250 | 57.50 |
| 61 | 1 | ea | Hot Mix, dry pkt, avg | 31 | 187.86 |
| 75 | 1 | ea | Hot Mix, low cal, dry pkt, avg | 19 | 220.21 |
| 73 | 1 | cup | Prep w/water, avg | 279 | 234.36 |
| 197 | 1 | cup | Milk Shakes, chocolate, avg | 227 | 52.21 |
| | | | **CANDIES AND CONFECTIONS** | | |
| | | | Baking Chocolate and Coating | | |
| 23418 | 1 | ea | Mexican Squares, avg | 20 | 42.00 |
| 23200 | 1/2 | cup | Semi-Sweet Chocolate, w/butter, avg | 85 | 413.10 |
| 23010 | 1 | ea | Unsweetened Square, avg | 28 | 346.36 |
| 23011 | 1/2 | cup | Unsweetened Square, grated, avg | 66 | 816.42 |
| | | | Baking Chips & Morsels | | |
| 23378 | 2 | Tbs | Crunch Pieces, choc&crspd rice, Nestle | 24 | 37.44 |
| 23012 | 1/2 | cup | Semi-Sweet Chocolate Chips, avg | 84 | 408.24 |
| | | | Candy & Candy Bars | | |
| 23110 | 1 | ea | Baby Ruth , 2.12 oz bar | 60 | 26.40 |
| 23269 | 1 | ea | Baby Ruth, fun size, .5 oz bar | 14 | 6.16 |
| 23117 | 5 | ea | Caramels, chocolate flvd roll, avg | 25 | 13.25 |
| 23023 | 5 | ea | Chocolate Covered Fondant/Mints, avg | 55 | 73.15 |
| 23122 | 1 | ea | Chunky, 1.4 oz. bar | 40 | 62.80 |
| 23133 | 1 | ea | Crunch, milk chocolate bar, 1.4 oz | 40 | 62.40 |
| 23134 | 1 | ea | Crunch, milk chocolate mini bar, .35 oz | 10 | 15.60 |
| 23125 | 1 | ea | 5TH Avenue, 2 oz bar | 57 | 27.93 |
| 23025 | 1 | pce | Fudge, chocolate, recipe, avg | 17 | 14.79 |
| 23026 | 1 | pce | Fudge, chocolate w/nuts, recipe, avg | 19 | 16.53 |
| 23127 | 1 | pce | Fudge chocolate marsh w/nuts recipe, avg | 22 | 28.38 |
| 23257 | 1/2 | cup | Goobers, milk chocolate cvrd peanuts | 82 | 89.38 |
| 23060 | 1 | ea | Kit Kat, 1.48 oz bar | 42 | 30.24 |
| 23016 | 1 | ea | Kisses, milk chocolate, 1.6 oz pkg, Hershey's | 44 | 74.36 |
| 23479 | 1 | ea | M&M's, peanut, 25 pces, 1.74 oz pkg | 49 | 37.24 |
| 23480 | 1 | ea | M&M's, plain, 69 pces, 1.69 oz pkg | 48 | 55.68 |

TABLE F *(continued)*

| ESHA | Amount | | Description | Wgt (g) | Theobromine (mg) |
|---|---|---|---|---|---|
| 23037 | 1 | ea | Mars Almond bar, 1.76 oz | 50 | 14.50 |
| 23058 | 1 | ea | Milk Chocolate candy bar w/crsp rice, 1.4 oz, avg | 40 | 62.00 |
| 23022 | 1/2 | cup | Milk Chocolate Cvrd Raisins, avg | 95 | 120.65 |
| 23419 | 5 | pce | Milk Chocolate Coated Peanuts, 5 pces | 20 | 21.80 |
| 23193 | 1 | pce | Milk Chocolate After 8 Mint, Nestle | 8 | 11.36 |
| 23018 | 1 | ea | Milk chocolate w/almonds, 1.45 oz bar, avg | 41 | 64.78 |
| 23038 | 1 | ea | Milky Way bar, 2.12 oz | 60 | 55.20 |
| 23039 | 1 | ea | Milky Way bar, fun size, .63 oz | 18 | 16.56 |
| 23035 | 1 | ea | Mounds, 1.87 oz bar | 53 | 69.96 |
| 23062 | 1 | ea | Mr. Goodbar, 1.73 oz bar | 49 | 63.70 |
| 23135 | 1 | ea | Oh Henry, 2 oz bar | 57 | 38.19 |
| 23214 | 1 | ea | Raisinets, milk choc cvrd raisins, 1.59 oz pkg | 45 | 57.15 |
| 23424 | 5 | ea | Reese's Peanut Butter Cups, mini, 1.2 oz | 35 | 23.10 |
| 23043 | 1 | ea | Reese's Peanut Butter Cups, 1.76 oz pkg | 50 | 33.00 |
| 23426 | 1 | ea | Rolo Caramels, milk chocolate, 1.87 oz pkg | 53 | 54.06 |
| 23040 | 1 | ea | Snickers, 2 oz. bar | 57 | 27.36 |
| 23041 | 1 | ea | Snickers, fun size, .5 oz. bar | 15 | 7.20 |
| 23057 | 1 | ea | Special Dark Chocolate, 1.45 oz bar, Hershey's | 41 | 181.63 |
| 23145 | 1 | ea | Sweet Chocolate bar, 1.45 oz, avg | 41 | 174.66 |
| 23136 | 1 | ea | 100 Grand bar, 1.5 oz | 43 | 31.82 |
| 23375 | 1 | ea | 100 Grand mini bar, .74 oz | 21 | 15.54 |
| 23075 | 1 | ea | 3 Musketeers bar, 2.12 oz | 60 | 52.20 |
| 23076 | 1 | ea | 3 Musketeers, fun size bar, .58 oz | 16 | 13.92 |
| 23123 | 1 | pce | Turtles, choc, caramel & pecans candy, Nestle | 17 | 8.16 |
| 23149 | 1 | ea | Twix Caramel Cookie bar, 2 oz pkg | 57 | 51.30 |
| 23150 | 1 | ea | Twix Peanut Butter Cookie bar, 1.9 oz pkg | 54 | 30.78 |
| 23151 | 1 | ea | Whatchamacallit, 1.69 oz bar | 48 | 18.72 |
| | | | **CEREALS, BREAKFAST TYPE** | | |
| 40102 | 1 | cup | Cocoa Krispies, Kellogg's | 41 | 49.20 |
| 40425 | 1 | cup | Cocoa Puffs, General Mills | 30 | 6.60 |
| 40324 | 1 | cup | Cookie Crisp, Ralston Purina | 30 | 6.60 |
| 40402 | 1 | cup | Count Chocula, General Mills | 30 | 28.50 |
| | | | Malt-o-Meal | | |
| 40188 | 1 | cup | Chocolate, ckd w/salt, avg | 240 | 16.80 |
| 40187 | 1/4 | cup | Chocolate, dry, avg | 41 | 39.77 |
| 40014 | 1 | cup | Plain, ckd, avg | 240 | 16.80 |
| | | | **DESSERTS** | | |
| 46011 | 1 | ea | Cake, chocolate creme filled, w/icing, avg | 50 | 56.00 |
| 46426 | 1 | ea | Cake, chocolate w/frosting, low fat, avg | 43 | 35.69 |
| | | | Cookie, Chocolate Chip | | |
| 47672 | 1 | oz | Dry Mix, avg | 28 | 25.48 |
| 47032 | 1 | ea | Low Fat, avg | 10 | 5.50 |
| 47033 | 1 | ea | No Sodium, w/fructose, avg | 7 | 4.27 |
| 47013 | 1 | ea | Refrig Dough, avg | 16 | 11.52 |
| 47001 | 1 | ea | Soft, avg | 15 | 8.70 |
| 47039 | 1 | ea | Cookie, Chocolate Sand, low sod, w/fructose, avg | 10 | 2.00 |
| 43527 | 2 | ea | Cracker, chocolate coated graham, avg | 28 | 101.64 |
| 45524 | 1 | ea | Doughnut, chocolate, iced, avg | 43 | 29.24 |
| 23095 | 1 | ea | Granola Bar, peanut butter, soft, w/choc coating, avg | 37 | 15.54 |
| 2050 | 1/2 | cup | Ice Cream, chocolate, avg | 66 | 40.92 |

TABLE F *(continued)*

| ESHA | Amount | | Description | Wgt (g) | Theobromine (mg) |
|---|---|---|---|---|---|
| 48096 | 1 | pce | Pie, chocolate cream, RTS, 1/8 of 8" pie, avg | 113 | 14.69 |
| | | | Pudding | | |
| 2635 | 1 | oz | Chocolate, mix, avg | 28 | 101.36 |
| 2634 | 1/2 | cup | Chocolate, prep f/mix w/2% milk, avg | 147 | 91.14 |
| 2605 | 1/2 | cup | Chocolate, prep f/mix, w/whl milk, avg | 147 | 91.14 |
| 2610 | 1 | ea | Chocolate, RTE, cnd, avg | 142 | 88.04 |
| 2658 | 1 | oz | Chocolate, rennin, dry mix, avg | 28 | 118.72 |
| 2659 | 1/2 | cup | Chocolate, rennin, prep f/mix, w/2%milk, avg | 136 | 57.12 |
| 2660 | 1/2 | cup | Chocolate, rennin, prep f/mix, w/whl milk, avg | 136 | 57.12 |
| | | | **DESSERT TOPPINGS** | | |
| 23267 | 1 | Tbs | Butterfinger, candy topping, Nestle | 25 | 8.50 |
| | | | Chocolate Frosting | | |
| 46033 | 1 | oz | Creamy, dry mix, avg | 28 | 52.64 |
| 46034 | 2 | Tbs | Prep f/Mix, w/butter, avg | 34 | 49.30 |
| 46035 | 2 | Tbs | Prep f/Mix, w/marg, avg | 34 | 49.30 |
| 46037 | 2 | Tbs | RTE, avg | 29 | 22.91 |
| 23056 | 2 | Tbs | Chocolate Syrup, avg | 38 | 178.98 |
| 23014 | 2 | Tbs | Chocolate Fudge Syrup, avg | 42 | 83.16 |

TABLE G **The Glycemic Index of Selected Foods (using the Glycemic Index of white bread equal to 100)**

| Food | Glycemic Index |
|---|---|
| Breads | |
| Rye (crispbread) | 95 |
| Rye (wholemeal) | 89 |
| Pumpernickel | 68 |
| Wheat (white) | 100 |
| Wheat (wholemeal) | 100 |
| Pasta | |
| Macaroni (white) | 64 |
| Spaghetti (brown) | 61 |
| Spaghetti (white) | 67 |
| Star Pasta (white) | 54 |
| Cereal Grains | |
| Barley (pearled) | 36 |
| Buckwheat | 78 |
| Bulgur | 65 |
| Millet | 103 |
| Rice (brown) | 81 |
| Rice (instant, boiled 1 min) | 65 |
| Rice (polished, boiled 5 min) | 58 |
| Rice (polished, boiled 10-25 min) | 81 |
| Rice (parboiled, boiled 5 min) | 54 |
| Rice (parboiled, boiled 15 min) | 68 |
| Rye kernels | 47 |
| Sweet corn | 80 |
| Wheat kernels | 63 |
| Breakfast Cereals | |
| "All Bran" | 74 |
| Cornflakes | 121 |
| Muesli | 96 |
| Porridge oats | 89 |
| Puffed rice | 132 |
| Puffed wheat | 110 |
| Shredded wheat | 97 |
| "Weetabix" | 109 |
| Cookies | |
| Digestive | 82 |
| Oatmeal | 78 |
| "Rich tea" | 80 |
| Plain crackers (water biscuits) | 100 |
| Shortbread cookies | 88 |
| Root Vegetables | |
| Potato (instant) | 120 |
| Potato (mashed) | 98 |
| Potato (new/white boiled) | 80 |
| Potato (Russett, baked) | 116 |
| Potato (sweet) | 70 |
| Yam | 74 |
| Legumes | |
| Baked beans (canned) | 70 |
| Bengal gram dal | 12 |
| Butter Beans | 46 |
| Chick peas (dried) | 47 |
| Chick peas (canned) | 60 |
| Green peas (canned) | 50 |
| Green peas (dried) | 65 |

TABLE G *(continued)*

| Food | Glycemic Index |
|---|---|
| Haricot beans (white, dried) | 54 |
| Kidney beans (dried) | 43 |
| Kidney beans (canned) | 74 |
| Lentils (green, dried) | 36 |
| Lentils (green, canned) | 74 |
| Lentils (red, dried) | 38 |
| Pinto beans (dried) | 60 |
| Pinto beans (canned) | 64 |
| Peanuts | 15 |
| Soya beans (dried) | 20 |
| Soya beans (canned) | 22 |
| Fruit | |
| Apple | 52 |
| Apple Juice | 45 |
| Banana | 84 |
| Orange | 59 |
| Orange juice | 71 |
| Raisins | 93 |
| Sugars | |
| Fructose | 26 |
| Glucose | 138 |
| Honey | 126 |
| Lactose | 57 |
| Maltose | 152 |
| Sucrose | 83 |
| Dairy Products | |
| Custard | 59 |
| Ice Cream | 69 |
| Skim milk | 46 |
| Whole milk | 44 |
| Yogurt | 52 |
| Snack Foods | |
| Corn chips | 99 |
| Potato chips | 77 |

Source: Wolever, T.M.S.: World Rev Nutr Diet, 62:120–185, 1990.

# INDEX

Page numbers followed by t denote tables.

# C

## D

## E



## F

G